DIAGNOSTIC IMAGING
GYNECOLOGY

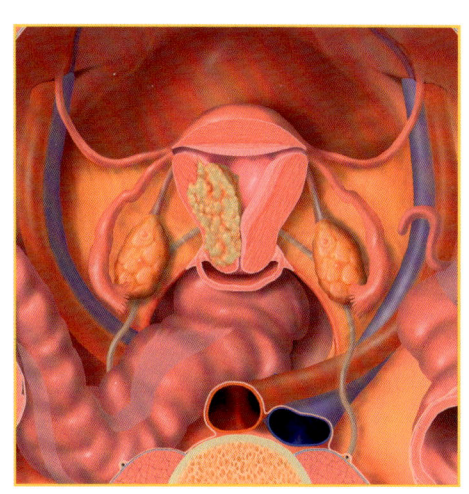

DIAGNOSTIC IMAGING
GYNECOLOGY

Hedvig Hricak, MD, PhD, Dr hc
Chairman, Department of Radiology
Carroll and Milton Petrie Chair
Memorial Sloan-Kettering Cancer Center

Professor of Radiology
Weill Medical College of Cornell University
New York, NY

Oguz Akin, MD
Assistant Attending Radiologist
Department of Radiology
Memorial Sloan-Kettering Cancer Center

Assistant Professor of Radiology
Weill Medical College of Cornell University
New York, NY

Evis Sala, MD, PhD, FRCR
University Lecturer
Department of Radiology
University of Cambridge
United Kingdom

Susan M. Ascher, MD
Professor of Radiology
Georgetown University Medical College

Director, Division of Abdominal Imaging
Georgetown University Hospital
Washington, DC

Deborah Levine, MD
Associate Radiologist-in-Chief of Academic Affairs
Co-chief of Ultrasound
Director of Ob/Gyn Ultrasound
Beth Israel Deaconess Medical Center
Boston, MA

Caroline Reinhold, MD, MSc
Professor of Radiology
Director, MR Imaging
Adjunct Professor of Obstetrics and Gynecology
MGill University Health Center
Montreal, Québec, Canada

Medical Director, Oncology
Synarc Inc.
San Francisco, CA

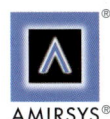

AMIRSYS®
Names you know, content you trust®

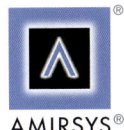

Names you know, content you trust®

First Edition

Text and Radiologic Images - Copyright © 2007 Oguz Akin, MD, Sandra J. Allison, MD, Susan M. Ascher, MD, Mostafa Atri, MD, FRCPC, Dip, Epid, Ilse Castro-Aragon, MD, BSc, Devish Dixit, MD, John Feeney, MD, Nyree Griffin, MD, Winnie Y. Hahn, MD, Olga Hatsiopoulou, MD, Hedvig Hricak, MD, PhD, Drhc, Marcia C. Javitt, MD, FACR, Shephard S. Kosut, MD, Deborah Levine, MD, Svetlana Mironov, MD, Patricia Noël, MD, Maria L. O'Donovan MB, MD, MRCPath, Khashayar Rafat Zand, MD, Caroline Reinhold, MD, MSc, Evis Sala, MD, PhD, FRCR, Tamar Sella, MD, Robert N. Troiano, MD

Drawings - Copyright © 2007 Amirsys Inc.

Compilation - Copyright © 2007 Amirsys Inc.

All rights reserved. No part of this publication may be reproduced, stored in a retrieval system, or transmitted, in any form or media or by any means, electronic, mechanical, photocopying, recording, or otherwise, without prior written permission from Amirsys Inc.

Composition by Amirsys Inc, Salt Lake City, Utah

Printed in Canada by Friesens, Altona, Manitoba, Canada

ISBN-13: 978-1-4160-3338-7
ISBN-10: 1-4160-3338-6
ISBN-13: 978-0-8089-2381-7 (International English Edition)
ISBN-10: 0-8089-2381-1 (International English Edition)

Notice and Disclaimer

The information in this product ("Product") is provided as a reference for use by licensed medical professionals and no others. It does not and should not be construed as any form of medical diagnosis or professional medical advice on any matter. Receipt or use of this Product, in whole or in part, does not constitute or create a doctor-patient, therapist-patient, or other healthcare professional relationship between Amirsys Inc. ("Amirsys") and any recipient. This Product may not reflect the most current medical developments, and Amirsys makes no claims, promises, or guarantees about accuracy, completeness, or adequacy of the information contained in or linked to the Product. The Product is not a substitute for or replacement of professional medical judgment. Amirsys and its affiliates, authors, contributors, partners, and sponsors disclaim all liability or responsibility for any injury and/or damage to persons or property in respect to actions taken or not taken based on any and all Product information.

In the cases where drugs or other chemicals are prescribed, readers are advised to check the Product information currently provided by the manufacturer of each drug to be administered to verify the recommended dose, the method and duration of administration, and contraindications. It is the responsibility of the treating physician relying on experience and knowledge of the patient to determine dosages and the best treatment for the patient.

To the maximum extent permitted by applicable law, Amirsys provides the Product AS IS AND WITH ALL FAULTS, AND HEREBY DISCLAIMS ALL WARRANTIES AND CONDITIONS, WHETHER EXPRESS, IMPLIED OR STATUTORY, INCLUDING BUT NOT LIMITED TO, ANY (IF ANY) IMPLIED WARRANTIES OR CONDITIONS OF MERCHANTABILITY, OF FITNESS FOR A PARTICULAR PURPOSE, OF LACK OF VIRUSES, OR ACCURACY OR COMPLETENESS OF RESPONSES, OR RESULTS, AND OF LACK OF NEGLIGENCE OR LACK OF WORKMANLIKE EFFORT. ALSO, THERE IS NO WARRANTY OR CONDITION OF TITLE, QUIET ENJOYMENT, QUIET POSSESSION, CORRESPONDENCE TO DESCRIPTION OR NON-INFRINGEMENT, WITH REGARD TO THE PRODUCT. THE ENTIRE RISK AS TO THE QUALITY OF OR ARISING OUT OF USE OR PERFORMANCE OF THE PRODUCT REMAINS WITH THE READER.

Amirsys disclaims all warranties of any kind if the Product was customized, repackaged or altered in any way by any third party.

The views expressed in these chapters are those of the author and do not reflect the official policy of the Department of Army, Department of Defense, or U.S. Government

Library of Congress Cataloging-in-Publication Data

Diagnostic imaging. Gynecology / [edited by] Hedvig Hricak. -- 1st ed.
   p. ; cm.
 Includes bibliographical references and index.
 ISBN-13: 978-1-4160-3338-7
 ISBN-10: 1-4160-3338-6
 ISBN-13: 978-0-8089-2381-7 (international English ed.)
 ISBN-10: 0-8089-2381-1 (international English ed.)
 1. Generative organs, Female--Imaging--Handbooks, manuals, etc. I. Hricak, Hedvig. II. Title: Gynecology.
 [DNLM: 1. Genital Diseases, Female--diagnosis--Handbooks. 2. Diagnostic Imaging--Handbooks. 3. Genitalia, Female--pathology--Handbooks. WP 39 D5365 2007]
 RG107.5.I4D53 2007
 618.1'075--dc22
                            2007035169

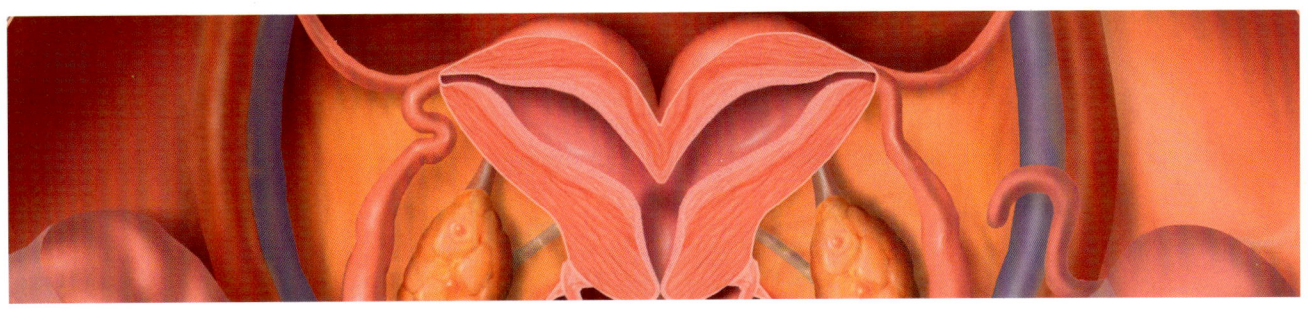

CONTRIBUTORS

Consultant

Maria L. O'Donovan MB, MD, MRCPath
Consultant Histopathologist
Addenbrooke's Hospital, Cambridge University Hospitals NHS Trust
Cambridge, UK

Contributing Authors

Sandra J. Allison, MD
Assistant Professor of Radiology
Georgetown University Medical College
Director, Ultrasound
Division of Abdominal Imaging
Georgetown University Hospital
Washington, DC

Mostafa Atri, MD, FRCPC, Dip, Epid
Professor of Radiology
Head, Abdominal Division & Director of CME
Department of Medical Imaging
University of Toronto
Head, Ultrasound Section
University Health Network/Mount Sinai Hospital/Women's College Hospital
Toronto, Canada

Ilse Castro-Aragon, MD, BSc
Instructor of Radiology
Boston University School of Medicine
Boston, Massachusetts

Devish Dixit, MD
Body Imaging Fellow,
Department of Radiology
Memorial Sloan-Kettering Cancer Center
New York, NY

John Feeney, MD
Body Imaging Fellow,
Department of Radiology
Memorial Sloan-Kettering Cancer Center
New York, NY

Nyree Griffin, MD
Fellow in Cross Sectional Radiology
Addenbrooke's Hospital, Cambridge University Hospitals NHS Trust
Cambridge, UK

Winnie Y. Hahn, MD
Assistant Professor of Radiology
Georgetown University Medical College
Division of Abdominal Imaging
Georgetown University Hospital
Washington, DC

Olga Hatsiopoulou, MD
Specialist Registar, Diagnostic Radiology
Addenbrooke's Hospital, Cambridge University Hospitals NHS Trust
Cambridge, UK
Royal Liverpool and Broadgreen University Hospitals NHS Trust, Liverpool, UK

Marcia C. Javitt, MD, FACR
Adjunct Professor of Radiology
Uniformed Services University of the Health Sciences
Section Head of Body MR
Section Head of Genitourinary Radiology
Walter Reed Army Medical Center
Washington, DC

Shephard S. Kosut, MD
Department of Radiology
Walter Reed Army Medical Center
Washington, DC

Svetlana Mironov, MD
Assistant Attending Radiologist
Department of Radiology
Memorial Sloan-Kettering Cancer Center
Assistant Professor of Radiology
Weill Medical College of Cornell University
New York, NY

Patricia Noël, MD
Staff Radiologist
CHUQ, Hôtel-Dieu de Québec
Clinical Professor of Radiology
Université Laval
Québec City, Québec, Canada

Khashayar Rafat Zand, MD
Radiology Resident
MGill University Health Center
Montreal, Québec, Canada

Tamar Sella, MD
University Lecturer
Abdominal and Women's imaging sections
Hadassah-Hebrew University Hospital
Jerusalem, Israel

Robert N. Troiano, MD
Associate Professor of Radiology and Obstetrics & Gynecology
Weill Medical College of Cornell University
New York, NY

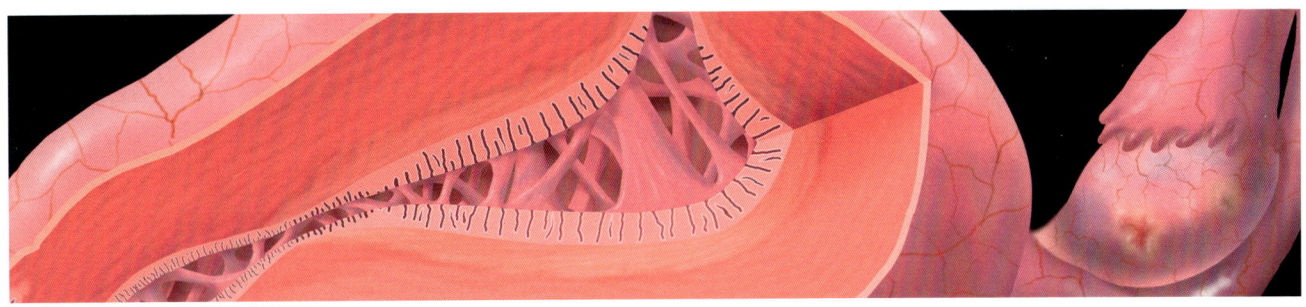

DIAGNOSTIC IMAGING: GYNECOLOGY

We at Amirsys and Elsevier are proud to present Diagnostic Imaging: Gynecology, the fourteenth volume in our acclaimed Diagnostic Imaging (DI) series. We began this precedent-setting, image- and graphic-rich series with David Stoller's DI: Orthopaedics. The next volumes, DI: Brain, DI: Head and Neck, DI: Abdomen, DI: Spine, DI: Pediatrics, DI: Obstetrics, DI: Chest, DI: Breast, DI: Ultrasound, DI: Pediatric Neuroradiology, DI: Emergency, and DI: Nuclear Medicine are now joined by Hedvig Hricak's fabulous new textbook, DI: Gynecology.

Women's health has become a real subspecialty with ever-increasing demand for both clinical and imaging services. DI: Gynecology shows you—whether gynecologist or radiologist--just what to look for and includes both common and less common presentations of many diseases that can be quickly and accurately diagnosed with a variety of imaging techniques. Case examples using a spectrum of modalities including multi-detector row CT, high-resolution MR, and ultrasound are beautifully illustrated.

Again, the unique bulleted format of the DI series allows our authors to present approximately twice the information and four times the images per diagnosis compared to the old-fashioned traditional prose textbook. All the DI books follow the same format, which means that our many readers find the same information in the same place—every time! And in every body part! The innovative visual differential diagnosis "thumbnail" provides you with an at-a-glance look at entities that can mimic the diagnosis in question and has been highly popular (and much copied). "Key Facts" boxes provide a succinct summary for quick, easy review.

In summary, Diagnostic Imaging: Gynecology is a product designed with you, the reader, in mind. Modern women's health providers demand efficiency in both image performance and interpretation. Many generalists increasingly find themselves faced with cases that require subspecialty expertise. Having Diagnostic Imaging: Gynecology on your shelf is like having a group of subspecialty experts at your fingertips. We think you'll find this new volume a highly efficient and wonderfully rich resource that will significantly enhance your practice—and find a welcome place on your bookshelf. Enjoy!

Anne G. Osborn, MD
Executive Vice President & Editor-in-Chief, Amirsys, Inc.

H. Ric Harnsberger, MD
CEO & Chairman, Amirsys, Inc.

Paula J. Woodward, MD
Senior Vice President & Medical Director, Amirsys, Inc.

B.J. Manaster, MD
Vice President & Associate Medical Director, Amirsys, Inc.

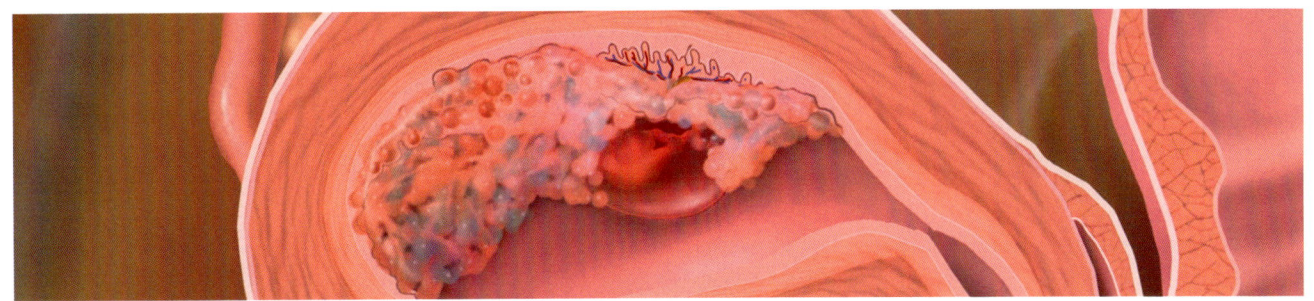

FOREWORD

Imaging has always been important in the diagnosis and management of diseases of the female genital tract. The role of imaging for better diagnosis and treatment in gynecology has expanded greatly due to significant advances in imaging equipment and the increasing knowledge of experts in the field of imaging. As a gynecologist who has spent most of his career treating women with gynecologic cancer, I have learned to depend on the radiologist as an essential member of the multidisciplinary team managing the patient suspected of, or diagnosed with, female genital cancer.

I worked with Dr. Hedvig Hricak in national and international organizations for several years before she was recruited to Memorial Sloan-Kettering Cancer Center as Chairperson of the Department of Radiology. After her arrival, I had the great fortune to work directly with her in the care of patients. Dr. Hricak immediately became an essential member of our gynecologic cancer disease team. Her extensive knowledge of imaging and gynecology allowed her to improve patient care, and her extraordinary ability to teach, improved the educational program for both radiology residents and gynecologic oncology fellows. It is clear that she has directed the same extraordinary abilities and educational commitment in the writing of this book on imaging in gynecology.

Dr. Hricak has brought together an international team of experts in order to produce this outstanding volume of Diagnostic Imaging in Gynecology. The format of all of the books in this series allows for the comprehensive coverage of each topic, using bullet points to avoid verboseness and maximizing the use of illustrations and images. The illustrations and images have been chosen with care to clearly demonstrate each and every abnormality. The standardized format of terminology, imaging findings, differential diagnosis, pathology, and clinical issues is followed by a diagnostic checklist and pertinent references. The authors have covered each topic comprehensively and succinctly. The images are pertinent and clear.

Having spent several years observing Dr. Hricak teaching both radiologists and gynecologists in multidisciplinary patient care conferences, it is easy to see that this book is designed to be an invaluable text for both radiologists and gynecologists. This concise but comprehensive book should be on the shelf of every radiologist who reads pelvic images and every gynecologist who uses imaging to diagnose and treat women. Just as Dr. Hricak has championed multidisciplinary care in her practice and teaching, she has now produced the ideal multidisciplinary text of diagnostic imaging in gynecology.

William J. Hoskins, MD
Executive Director of Surgical Activities,
Attending Surgeon, Gynecology Service
Department of Surgery
Memorial Sloan-Kettering Cancer Center
New York, NY

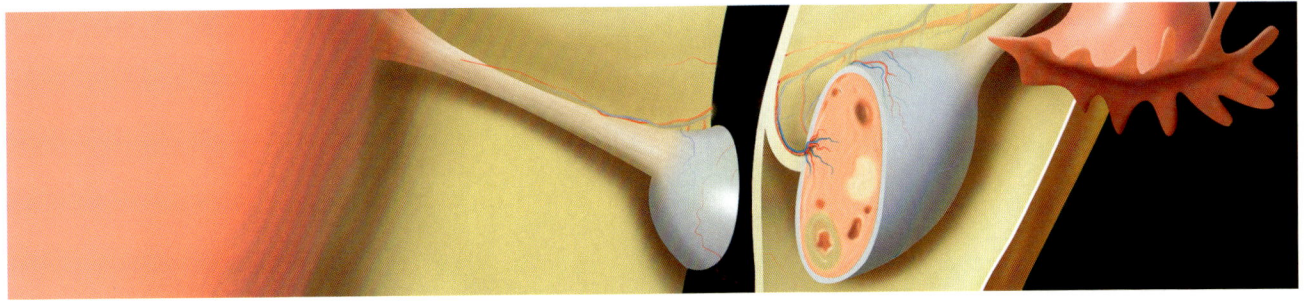

PREFACE

Diagnostic Imaging: Gynecology is intended as a guide for radiologists in training, general radiologists, specialists in women's imaging, and all physicians interested in gynecologic imaging. The breadth and depth of the book's contents, as well as its design, make it suitable as a basic textbook as well as a reference work for clinical practice. It provides details about current imaging techniques and describes the imaging characteristics of normal anatomy and gynecologic pathologies. Each diagnosis is presented in a separate chapter that includes information about differential diagnoses, pathologic features, and key clinical issues, and each chapter is enhanced by a rich image gallery. We have incorporated not only the usual list of topics covered in textbooks, but also a variety of topics not commonly discussed, including many rare diagnoses. The resulting volume is comprehensive, detailed, and concise all at once.

This book was made possible by the unselfish collaboration and dedication of the editors. Each of them came to the task with a slightly different expertise, from benign disease to cancer, from ultrasound to magnetic resonance imaging. They carefully reviewed and commented on each others' work and suggested additions where appropriate. As a result, the diagnostic approaches described are extraordinarily balanced between all the imaging modalities. The team of contributing authors was spectacular, further enhancing the educational value of the book. The radiological expertise of the editors and contributing authors was supplemented by that of a consultant histopathologist, who ensured that all image-pathologic correlation was current and correct. Moreover, due to the generosity of the editors, contributing authors, and case contributors from all over the world, the book contains an unprecedented number of high-quality images of both common and rare diagnoses.

Working on this book was not only highly educational, but personally rewarding. During the process, the team members became increasingly close and respectful of each other—and ever more invested in the book. I would like to thank all the editors and contributing authors from the bottom of my heart for their dedication and mutual support. I am extremely proud of the final product, and I hope readers will appreciate the unique combination of comprehensiveness and accessibility that the editors, contributing authors, and the publisher worked so hard to provide.

Hedvig Hricak, MD, PhD, Drhc
Chairman, Department of Radiology
Carroll and Milton Petrie Chair
Memorial Sloan-Kettering Cancer Center

Professor of Radiology
Weill Medical College of Cornell University
New York, NY

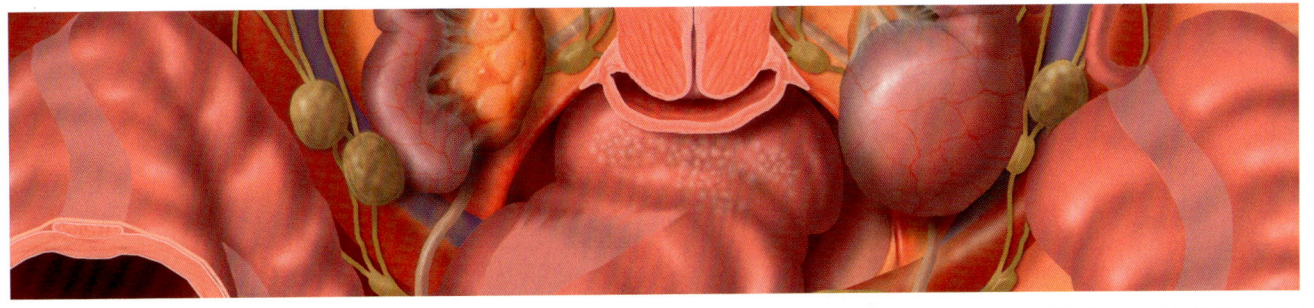

ACKNOWLEDGMENTS

Illustrations
Richard Coombs, MS
Lane R. Bennion, MS
R. Annie Gough, CMI

Image/Text Editing
Douglas Grant Jackson
Amanda Hurtado

Case Management
Christopher B. Odekirk
Roth LaFleur

Case Contributors
Carlo Martinoli, MD – Genoa, Italy
Douglas Levine, MD – New York, NY, USA
Donald Mitchell, MD – Philadelphia, PA, USA
Eric Outwater, MD – Tucson, AZ, USA
Jo Hugil, MD – Cambridge, United Kingdom
Kaori Togashi, MD – Kyoto, Japan
Kay Park, MD – New York, NY, USA
Oksana H. Baltarowich, MD – Philadelphia, PA, USA
Paula J. Woodward, MD – Salt Lake City, UT, USA
Rosemarie Forstner, MD – Salzburg, Austria
Teresa Cunha, MD – Lisbon, Portugal
Seung Hyup Kim, MD – Seoul, Korea

Associate Editor
Kaerli Main

Production Lead
Melissa A. Hoopes

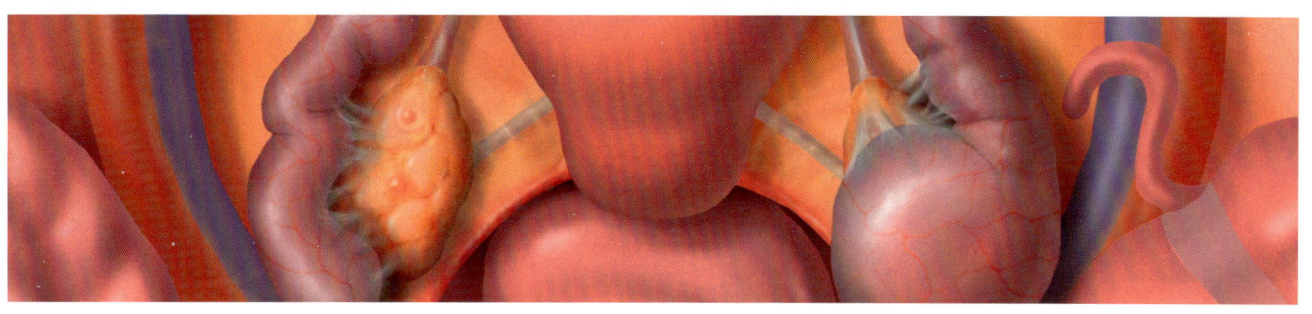

SECTIONS

Pelvis 1

Uterus 2

Uterus-Cervix 3

Vagina 4

Vulva 5

Urethra 6

Ovary 7

Fallopian Tubes 8

Peritoneum 9

Ectopic Pregnancy 10

Placenta 11

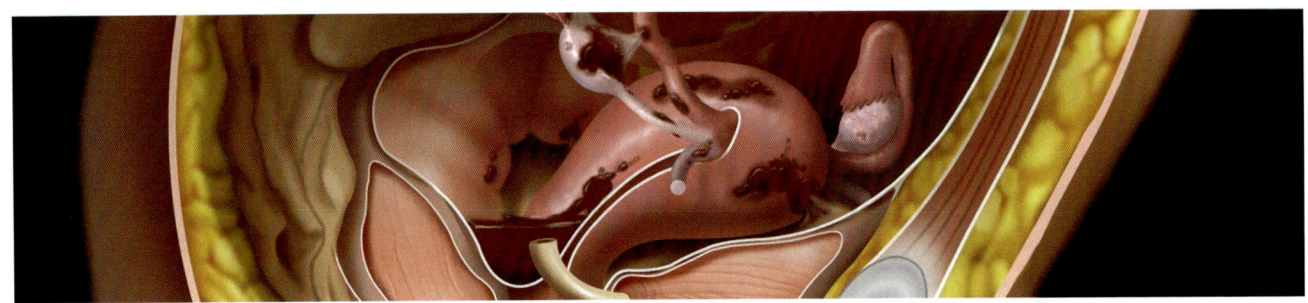

TABLE OF CONTENTS

SECTION 1
Pelvis

Techniques

Ultrasound Technique & Anatomy *Deborah Levine, MD*	1-2
Hysterosalpingography *Evis Sala, MD, PhD & Jo Hugill, MD*	1-6
CT Technique & Anatomy *Olga Hatsiopoulou, MD & Evis Sala, MD, PhD*	1-10
MR Technique & Anatomy *Olga Hatsiopoulou, MD & Evis Sala, MD, PhD*	1-16
PET/CT Technique & Imaging Issues *Evis Sala, MD, PhD*	1-22

Neoplasm

Sacral Teratoma *Devesh Dixit, MD & Oguz Akin, MD*	1-28
Extraperitoneal Sarcoma *Devesh Dixit, MD & Oguz Akin, MD*	1-32
Hemangioma, Pelvis *Oguz Akin, MD*	1-36

Miscellaneous

Ovarian Vein Thrombosis *Winnie Y. Hahn, MD*	1-40
Spinal Meningeal Cysts *Patricia Noël, MD & Caroline Reinhold, MD*	1-44
Bladder Flap Hematoma *Marcia Javitt, MD & Shephard S. Kosut, MD*	1-48
Pelvic Congestion Syndrome *Susan M. Ascher, MD*	1-52
Pelvic Floor Descent *Mostafa Atri, MD & Caroline Reinhold, MD*	1-56
Vaginocele/Cystocele *Mostafa Atri, MD & Caroline Reinhold, MD*	1-60
Enterocele/Rectocele *Mostafa Atri, MD & Caroline Reinhold, MD*	1-64
Pelvic Lipomatosis *Evis Sala, MD, PhD*	1-68
Post-Radiation Pelvis *Evis Sala, MD, PhD*	1-70
Post-Operative Pelvis *Evis Sala, MD, PhD*	1-74

SECTION 2
Uterus

Introduction and Overview

Uterine Anatomy & Imaging Issues *Deborah Levine, MD*	2-2

Techniques

Sonohysterography *Deborah Levine, MD*	2-8

Normal Variants

Age-Related Physiologic Alterations *Patricia Noël, MD & Caroline Reinhold, MD*	2-12
Endometrial Atrophy *Sandra J. Allison, MD*	2-18
Uterine Peristalsis *Susan M. Ascher, MD*	2-22
Normal Post C-Section Change *Marcia Javitt, MD* *Susan M. Ascher, MD & Shephard S. Kosut, MD*	2-26

Congenital

Uterine Hypoplasia/Agenesis *Nyree Griffin, MD* *Caroline Reinhold, MD & Evis Sala, MD, PhD*	2-30
Unicornuate *Nyree Griffin, MD* *Caroline Reinhold, MD & Evis Sala, MD, PhD*	2-34
Didelphys *Nyree Griffin, MD* *Caroline Reinhold, MD & Deborah Levine, MD*	2-40
Bicornuate *Caroline Reinhold, MD & Khashayar Rafat Zand, MD*	2-46
Septate *Susan M. Ascher, MD*	2-52

Arcuate 2-58
Nyree Griffin, MD
Evis Sala, MD, PhD & Caroline Reinhold, MD

DES-Exposed 2-60
Nyree Griffin, MD
Evis Sala, MD, PhD & Caroline Reinhold, MD

Complex Anomalies 2-64
Nyree Griffin, MD
Caroline Reinhold, MD & Evis Sala, MD, PhD

Inflammation/Infection

Asherman Syndrome 2-68
Ilse Castro-Aragon, MD, BSc

Endometrial Synechiae 2-74
Sandra J. Allison, MD

Endometritis 2-78
Ilse Castro-Aragon, MD, BSc

Pyomyoma 2-82
Susan M. Ascher, MD

Neoplasm

Intravenous Leiomyomatosis 2-86
Ilse Castro-Aragon, MD, BSc

Disseminated Peritoneal Leiomyomatosis 2-90
Ilse Castro-Aragon, MD, BSc & Deborah Levine, MD

Neoplasm, Benign

Leiomyoma, Submucosal 2-92
Mostafa Atri, MD & Susan M. Ascher, MD

Leiomyoma, Intramural 2-98
Sandra J. Allison, MD

Leiomyoma, Subserosal 2-104
Sandra J. Allison, MD

Leiomyoma, Degeneration 2-110
Sandra J. Allison, MD

Leiomyoma, Parasitic 2-114
Marcia Javitt, MD & Shephard S. Kosut, MD

Benign Metastasizing Leiomyoma 2-118
Winnie Y. Hahn, MD

Diffuse Leiomyomatosis, Uterus 2-122
Oguz Akin, MD

Lipomatous Uterine Tumors 2-124
Patricia Noël, MD & Caroline Reinhold, MD

Endometrial Polyps 2-128
Mostafa Atri, MD & Caroline Reinhold, MD

Endometrial Hyperplasia 2-134
Mostafa Atri, MD & Caroline Reinhold, MD

Neoplasm, Malignant

Endometrial Cancer, Characterization 2-140
Oguz Akin, MD

Endometrial Cancer, Early Stage 2-144
Caroline Reinhold, MD & Khashayar Rafat Zand, MD

Endometrial Cancer, Late Stage 2-150
Caroline Reinhold, MD & Khashayar Rafat Zand, MD

Endometrial Cancer, Recurrence 2-156
Patricia Noël, MD & Caroline Reinhold, MD

Endometrial Stromal Sarcoma 2-162
Caroline Reinhold, MD & Khashayar Rafat Zand, MD

Adenosarcoma 2-166
Evis Sala, MD, PhD

Malignant Mixed Mesodermal Tumor 2-172
Oguz Akin, MD

Leiomyosarcoma, Uterus 2-176
Oguz Akin, MD

Lymphoma, Uterus 2-180
Svetlana Mironov, MD & Evis Sala, MD, PhD

Choriocarcinoma, Uterus 2-184
Deborah Levine, MD

Metastases, Uterus 2-188
Evis Sala, MD, PhD

Miscellaneous

Adenomyosis 2-192
Caroline Reinhold, MD & Khashayar Rafat Zand, MD

Adenomyoma 2-198
Caroline Reinhold, MD & Khashayar Rafat Zand, MD

Cystic Adenomyosis 2-202
Caroline Reinhold, MD & Khashayar Rafat Zand, MD

Uterine AVM 2-206
Caroline Reinhold, MD & Khashayar Rafat Zand, MD

Uterine Artery Embolization Imaging 2-212
Susan M. Ascher, MD

Failed Uterine Artery Embolization 2-218
Winnie Y. Hahn, MD

Complications, Uterine Artery Embolization 2-222
Susan M. Ascher, MD

Uterine Rupture 2-228
Winnie Y. Hahn, MD

Retained Products of Conception 2-232
Deborah Levine, MD

Tamoxifen-Induced Changes 2-238
Susan M. Ascher, MD

Intrauterine Device Evaluation 2-242
Deborah Levine, MD

SECTION 3
Uterus-Cervix

Inflammation/Infection

Cervical Stenosis 3-2
Sandra J. Allison, MD

Neoplasm, Benign

Endocervical Polyp 3-6
Sandra J. Allison, MD

Leiomyoma, Cervix 3-10
Sandra J. Allison, MD

Neoplasm, Malignant

Cervical Cancer, Characterization 3-14
Oguz Akin, MD

Cervical Cancer, Stage IB-IIA *Oguz Akin, MD*	3-20
Cervical Cancer, Stage IIB-IVB *Oguz Akin, MD*	3-22
Cervical Adenocarcinoma *Patricia Noël, MD & Caroline Reinhold, MD*	3-26
Small Cell Carcinoma, Cervix *Nyree Griffin, MD & Evis Sala, MD, PhD*	3-30
Cervical Cancer, Recurrence *Oguz Akin, MD*	3-34
Adenoma Malignum *Oguz Akin, MD*	3-38
Lymphoma, Cervix *Oguz Akin, MD*	3-40
Sarcoma, Cervix *Nyree Griffin, MD & Evis Sala, MD, PhD*	3-44
Endometrioid Cervical Adenocarcinoma *Nyree Griffin, MD & Evis Sala, MD, PhD*	3-48
Melanoma, Cervix *Nyree Griffin, MD & Evis Sala, MD, PhD*	3-52
Metastasis, Cervix *Nyree Griffin, MD & Evis Sala, MD, PhD*	3-56

Miscellaneous

Nabothian Cysts *Susan M. Ascher, MD*	3-60
Cervical Glandular Hyperplasia *Patricia Noël, MD & Caroline Reinhold, MD*	3-64
Cervical Incompetence *Sandra J. Allison, MD*	3-68
Post Trachelectomy Appearances *Nyree Griffin, MD & Evis Sala, MD, PhD*	3-72
Post-Radiation Cervix *Oguz Akin, MD*	3-76

SECTION 4
Vagina

Introduction and Overview

Vaginal Anatomy & Imaging Issues *John Feeney, MD & Oguz Akin, MD*	4-2

Congenital

MRKH Syndrome *Nyree Griffin, MD & Evis Sala, MD, PhD*	4-4
Vaginal Atresia *Robert Troiano, MD & Caroline Reinhold, MD*	4-8
Imperforate Hymen *Robert Troiano, MD & Caroline Reinhold, MD*	4-10
Vaginal Septae *Robert Troiano, MD & Caroline Reinhold, MD*	4-12
Androgen Insensitivity Syndrome *Caroline Reinhold, MD & Khashayar Rafat Zand, MD*	4-14
Ambiguous Genitalia *Tamar Sella, MD*	4-18
Gonadal Dysgenesis *Caroline Reinhold, MD & Khashayar Rafat Zand, MD*	4-22
Gartner Duct Cysts *Winnie Y. Hahn, MD*	4-26

Inflammation/Infection

Bartholinitis *Olga Hatsiopoulou, MD & Evis Sala, MD, PhD*	4-30
Vaginal Fistula *Olga Hatsiopoulou, MD & Evis Sala, MD, PhD*	4-32

Neoplasm, Benign

Leiomyoma, Vagina *Olga Hatsiopoulou, MD & Evis Sala, MD, PhD*	4-38

Neoplasm, Malignant

Vaginal Carcinoma *Oguz Akin, MD*	4-40
Lymphoma, Vagina *Oguz Akin, MD*	4-46
Leiomyosarcoma, Vagina *Olga Hatsiopoulou, MD & Evis Sala, MD, PhD*	4-48
Embryonal Rhabdomyosarcoma, Vagina *Olga Hatsiopoulou, MD & Evis Sala, MD, PhD*	4-50
Yolk Sac Tumor, Vagina *Olga Hatsiopoulou, MD & Evis Sala, MD, PhD*	4-52
Bartholin Gland Cancer *Olga Hatsiopoulou, MD & Evis Sala, MD, PhD*	4-54
Metastasis, Vagina *Oguz Akin, MD*	4-56

Miscellaneous

Bartholin Cysts *Winnie Y. Hahn, MD*	4-58
Foreign Bodies, Vagina *Olga Hatsiopoulou, MD & Evis Sala, MD, PhD*	4-62

SECTION 5
Vulva

Introduction and Overview

Vulvar Anatomy & Imaging Issues *John Feeney, MD & Oguz Akin, MD*	5-2

Neoplasm, Malignant

Carcinoma, Vulva *Svetlana Mironov, MD & Evis Sala, MD, PhD*	5-4
Leiomyosarcoma, Vulva *Nyree Griffin, MD & Evis Sala, MD, PhD*	5-10
Melanoma, Vulva *Svetlana Mironov, MD & Evis Sala, MD, PhD*	5-12
Aggressive Angiomyxoma, Vulva *Evis Sala, MD, PhD & Jo Hugill, MD*	5-16
Lymphoma, Vulva *Evis Sala, MD, PhD & Jo Hugill, MD*	5-20
Merkel Cell Tumor, Vulva *Svetlana Mironov, MD & Oguz Akin, MD*	5-22

Miscellaneous

Hemangioma, Vulva — 5-24
Oguz Akin, MD

SECTION 6
Urethra

Introduction and Overview

Urethral Anatomy & Imaging Issues — 6-2
Oguz Akin, MD

Neoplasm, Benign

Leiomyoma, Urethra — 6-6
Oguz Akin, MD

Schwannoma, Urethra — 6-8
John Feeney, MD & Oguz Akin, MD

Neoplasm, Malignant

Carcinoma, Urethra — 6-10
Oguz Akin, MD

Metastasis, Urethra — 6-14
Patricia Noël, MD & Caroline Reinhold, MD

Miscellaneous

Diverticulum, Urethra — 6-18
Oguz Akin, MD

Prolapse, Urethra — 6-22
Winnie Y. Hahn, MD

SECTION 7
Ovary

Introduction and Overview

Ovarian Anatomy & Imaging Issues — 7-2
Deborah Levine, MD

Normal Variants

Follicular Cyst — 7-8
Mostafa Atri, MD

Corpus Luteal Cyst — 7-12
Mostafa Atri, MD

Theca Lutein Cysts — 7-16
Patricia Noël, MD & Caroline Reinhold, MD

Luteoma of Pregnancy — 7-20
Deborah Levine, MD

Neoplasm, Benign

Dermoid (Mature Teratoma) — 7-22
Sandra J. Allison, MD & Deborah Levine, MD

Fibrothecoma, Ovary — 7-28
Mostafa Atri, MD & Susan M. Ascher, MD

Adenofibroma — 7-32
Ilse Castro-Aragon, MD, BSc

Granulosa Cell Tumor — 7-34
Ilse Castro-Aragon, MD, BSc

Sclerosing Stromal Tumor — 7-40
Evis Sala, MD, PhD

Cystadenofibroma — 7-44
Sandra J. Allison, MD

Serous Cystadenoma — 7-48
Marcia Javitt, MD
Shephard S. Kosut MD & Deborah Levine, MD

Mucinous Cystadenoma — 7-54
Winnie Y. Hahn, MD & Deborah Levine, MD

Brenner Tumor — 7-60
Evis Sala, MD, PhD

Neoplasm, Malignant

Mucinous Cystadenocarcinoma — 7-64
Oguz Akin, MD & Deborah Levine, MD

Serous Cystadenocarcinoma — 7-70
Oguz Akin, MD

Endometrioid Carcinoma, Ovary — 7-74
Patricia Noël, MD
Caroline Reinhold, MD & Deborah Levine, MD

Sertoli-Leydig Cell Tumor — 7-80
Oguz Akin, MD

Dysgerminoma — 7-84
Oguz Akin, MD

Yolk Sac Tumor, Ovary — 7-88
Evis Sala, MD, PhD

Lymphoma, Ovary — 7-92
Oguz Akin, MD

Clear Cell Carcinoma, Ovary — 7-96
Oguz Akin, MD

Immature Teratoma, Ovary — 7-100
Svetlana Mironov, MD & Evis Sala, MD, PhD

Metastases, Ovary — 7-106
Oguz Akin, MD

Ovarian Cancer, Characterization & Staging — 7-112
Oguz Akin, MD

Ovarian Cancer, Recurrent; Resectable — 7-118
Oguz Akin, MD

Ovarian Cancer, Recurrent; Unresectable — 7-122
Oguz Akin, MD

Choriocarcinoma, Ovary — 7-126
Evis Sala, MD, PhD

Struma Ovarii — 7-130
Svetlana Mironov, MD & Evis Sala, MD, PhD

Carcinoid, Ovary — 7-134
Evis Sala, MD, PhD

Undifferentiated Carcinoma, Ovary — 7-138
Sandra J. Allison, MD

Embryonal Carcinoma, Ovary — 7-142
Evis Sala, MD, PhD

Mixed Mullerian Tumor, Ovary — 7-146
Evis Sala, MD, PhD

Krukenberg Tumor — 7-150
Ilse Castro-Aragon, MD, BSc

Miscellaneous

Inclusion Cyst, Ovary *Patricia Noël, MD & Caroline Reinhold, MD*	7-154
Ovarian Hyperstimulation Syndrome *Olga Hatsiopoulou, MD & Evis Sala, MD, PhD*	7-158
Paraovarian Cyst *Ilse Castro-Aragon, MD, BSc*	7-162
Endometrioma *Mostafa Atri, MD & Caroline Reinhold, MD*	7-166
Endometriosis *Mostafa Atri, MD* *Caroline Reinhold, MD & Deborah Levine, MD*	7-170
Adnexal Torsion *Mostafa Atri, MD & Caroline Reinhold, MD*	7-176
Massive Ovarian Edema *Deborah Levine, MD*	7-182
Polycystic Ovary Syndrome *Patricia Noël, MD & Caroline Reinhold, MD*	7-186
Fibromatosis, Ovary *Winnie Y. Hahn, MD*	7-190
Hemorrhagic Cysts, Ovary *Ilse Castro-Aragon, MD, BSc*	7-192
Meigs Syndrome *Oguz Akin, MD*	7-198

SECTION 8
Fallopian Tubes

Congenital

Paratubal Cysts *Marcia Javitt, MD & Shephard S. Kosut MD*	8-2

Inflammation/Infection

Hydrosalpinx *Sandra J. Allison, MD*	8-6
Salpingitis *Mostafa Atri, MD & Caroline Reinhold, MD*	8-10
Genital Tuberculosis *Caroline Reinhold, MD & Khashayar Rafat Zand, MD*	8-14
Actinomycosis *Caroline Reinhold, MD & Khashayar Rafat Zand, MD*	8-18
Salpingitis Isthmica Nodosa *Ilse Castro-Aragon, MD, BSc & Deborah Levine, MD*	8-22
Tubo-Ovarian Abscess *Nyree Griffin, MD* *Evis Sala, MD, PhD & Deborah Levine, MD*	8-26

Neoplasm, Benign

Leiomyoma, Fallopian Tube *Patricia Noël, MD & Caroline Reinhold, MD*	8-32

Neoplasm, Malignant

Tubal Carcinoma, Characterization *Oguz Akin, MD*	8-36
Tubal Carcinoma, Staging/Prognosis *Sandra J. Allison, MD*	8-42
Metastases, Tubal *Winnie Y. Hahn, MD*	8-48

Miscellaneous

Hematosalpinx *Mostafa Atri, MD & Susan M. Ascher, MD*	8-50

SECTION 9
Peritoneum

Pseudolesions

Peritoneal Inclusion Cysts *Oguz Akin, MD*	9-2

Neoplasm, Malignant

Pseudomyxoma Peritonei *Oguz Akin, MD*	9-6
Peritoneal Mesothelioma *Susan M. Ascher, MD*	9-8
Peritoneal Metastases *Svetlana Mironov, MD & Evis Sala, MD, PhD*	9-12

SECTION 10
Ectopic Pregnancy

Ectopic Pregnancy, Endometrium *Deborah Levine, MD*	10-2
Ectopic Pregnancy, Tubal *Deborah Levine, MD*	10-4
Ectopic Pregnancy, Interstitial *Deborah Levine, MD*	10-10
Ectopic Pregnancy, Cervical *Deborah Levine, MD*	10-16
Ectopic Pregnancy, Ovarian *Deborah Levine, MD*	10-20
Ectopic Pregnancy, Heterotopic *Deborah Levine, MD*	10-22
Ectopic Pregnancy, Abdominal *Deborah Levine, MD*	10-26
Ectopic Pregnancy, Rupture *Deborah Levine, MD*	10-28

SECTION 11
Placenta

Neoplasm, Benign

Teratoma, Placenta *Tamar Sella, MD*	11-2
Hydatiform Mole, Complete Mole *Sandra J. Allison, MD & Deborah Levine, MD*	11-4
Hydatiform Mole, Partial Mole *Ilse Castro-Aragon, MD, BSc & Deborah Levine, MD*	11-10

Neoplasm, Malignant

Invasive Mole 11-16
Winnie Y. Hahn, MD

Placental Site Trophoblastic Tumor 11-20
Winnie Y. Hahn, MD

Miscellaneous

Hematoma, Placenta 11-24
Ilse Castro-Aragon, MD, BSc & Deborah Levine, MD

Chorioangioma, Placenta 11-30
Tamar Sella, MD

DIAGNOSTIC IMAGING
GYNECOLOGY

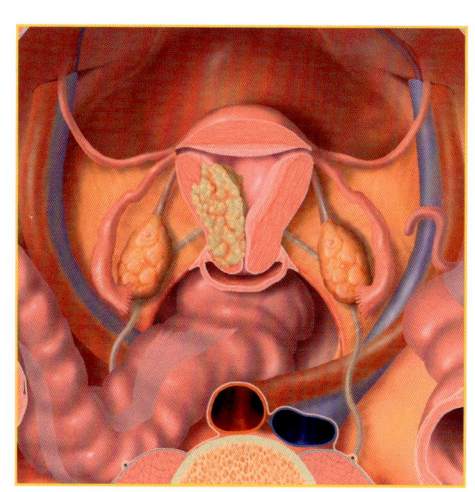

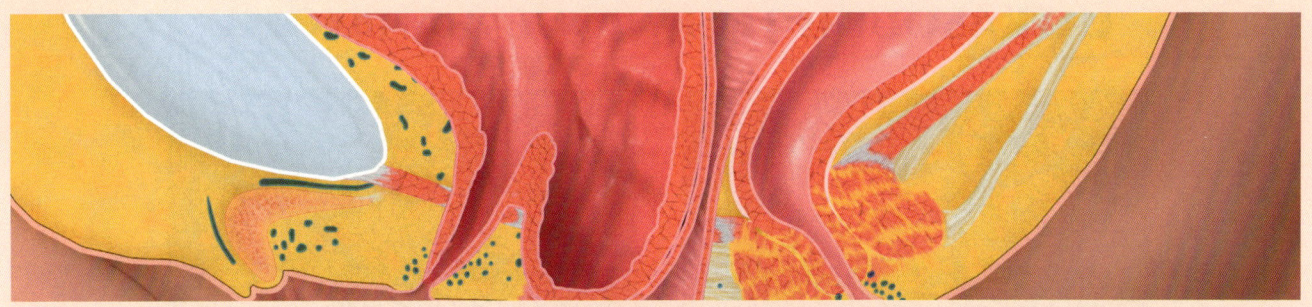

SECTION 1: Pelvis

Techniques

Ultrasound Technique & Anatomy	1-2
Hysterosalpingography	1-6
CT Technique & Anatomy	1-10
MR Technique & Anatomy	1-16
PET/CT Technique & Imaging Issues	1-22

Neoplasm

Sacral Teratoma	1-28
Extraperitoneal Sarcoma	1-32
Hemangioma, Pelvis	1-36

Miscellaneous

Ovarian Vein Thrombosis	1-40
Spinal Meningeal Cysts	1-44
Bladder Flap Hematoma	1-48
Pelvic Congestion Syndrome	1-52
Pelvic Floor Descent	1-56
Vaginocele/Cystocele	1-60
Enterocele/Rectocele	1-64
Pelvic Lipomatosis	1-68
Post-Radiation Pelvis	1-70
Post-Operative Pelvis	1-74

ULTRASOUND TECHNIQUE & ANATOMY

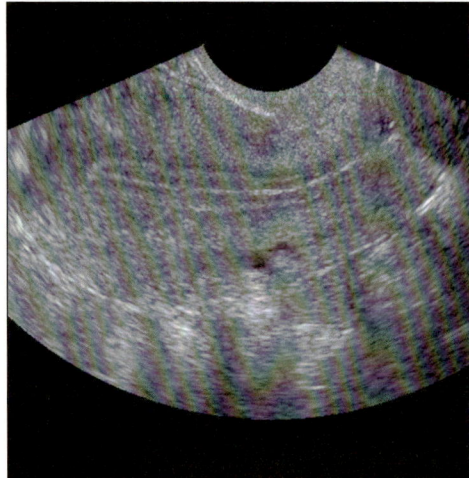

Sagittal transvaginal ultrasound shows the normal appearance of the midcycle endometrium.

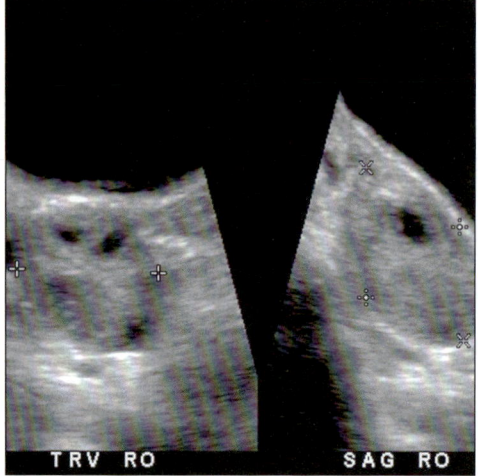

Transabdominal ultrasound in transverse and axial planes shows the normal appearance of an ovary (calipers) with developing follicles.

TERMINOLOGY

Abbreviations
- Transabdominal sonography (TAS)
- Transvaginal sonography (TVS)
- Sonohysterography (SHG)
- Peak systolic velocity (PSV)
- End diastolic velocity (EDV)

Definitions
- Ultrasound machine is an imaging device that uses sound waves to generate images
  - TAS gives wide field of view
    - Due to lower frequency and distance of organ to probe often gives lower resolution
    - Use for large masses
    - Use for superficial lesions and lesions out of range of vaginal probe
  - TVS gives higher resolution images of uterus, cervix, and adnexa
    - Limited field of view
    - Use in cases with abnormal bleeding
    - Use in early pregnancy
- Doppler ultrasound uses frequency shifts to detect flowing blood
  - Use Doppler for assessment of focal endometrial lesions and complex adnexal masses
  - Focal endometrial lesions may have a single vessel, polyp, or complex vascularity suggesting other etiology
  - Doppler helpful in assessing if mass in adnexal is cystic or solid
  - Resistive index: (PSV-EDV)/PSV
    - Low resistive index (< 0.4) is associated with malignancy, but also can be seen in corpus luteum, metabolically active mass, inflammatory mass
    - High resistive index (> 0.7) associated with benign lesions
    - Carefully scan all of mass, as velocities can differ in varied solid components

PRE-PROCEDURE

Indications
- Pelvic pain, pelvic mass, abnormal bleeding, staging for cancer

Contraindications
- TAS can be uncomfortable due to full bladder
- TVS should be avoided in patients with an intact hymen
  - Transperineal sonography can be performed when needed
  - Patients may decline study due to being uncomfortable with the procedure

Getting Started
- Things to Check
  - Full bladder for TAS
  - Empty bladder for TVS
    - Describe to patient use of transvaginal probe
    - Only a portion of the probe is inserted
    - Exam should be relatively painless
- Equipment List
  - Ultrasound machine
  - Appropriate transducers
    - 2-7 MHz for transabdominal scans
    - 5-12 MHz for transvaginal scans
    - Condom to cover transvaginal probe
  - Safety issues
    - 100 mW/cm² is the intensity below which no significant biologic effects in mammalian tissues in vivo

ULTRASOUND TECHNIQUE & ANATOMY

Key Facts

Terminology
- Resistive index: (PSV-EDV)/PSV
- Low resistive index (< 0.4) is associated with malignancy, but also can be seen in corpus luteum, metabolically active mass, inflammatory mass

Pre-procedure
- Full bladder for TAS
- Empty bladder for TVS

Procedure
- TVS gives highest definition images of myometrium, endometrium, and ovaries
- Patients with abnormal bleeding and/or pelvic masses should have TVS, unless contraindicated
- Probes cleansed according to manufacturers and local institutional guidelines
- Rinse probes prior to use to avoid chemical irritation from disinfectants
- Measure endometrium perpendicular to long axis
- Exclude hypoechoic subendometrial zone in endometrial measurement
- If ovaries are difficult to find, obtain a coronal view of uterine fundus and angle laterally to region of broad ligament
- Gentle pressure on anterior abdominal wall can move bowel gas out of the way to improve ovarian visualization

Post-procedure
- No harmful effects from pelvic sonography
- If scanning is performed for infertility, water or saline may be used as a lubricant to avoid adverse effect on sperm motility

- Thermal index < 2 and mechanical index < 0.3 are safe levels for routine use
  - Use probe cover for TVS
    - If latex allergy: Do not use latex probe covers

PROCEDURE

Patient Position/Location
- Best procedure approach
  - TVS gives highest definition images of myometrium, endometrium, and ovaries
  - Patients with abnormal bleeding and/or pelvic masses should have TVS, unless contraindicated
  - Patient in lithotomy position if bed with stirrups
  - Pillow under buttocks can be utilized if needed
- TVS-first approach, only perform transabdominal scan if TVS insufficient
- TAS-first approach, in cases with large masses
  - Some centers begin with TAS, but do not make patient fill bladder
    - Limited TAS to assess uterine size, large masses
    - Proceed to TVS
    - Repeat TAS with full bladder only in cases when TVS insufficient
- Transperineal scan
  - Utilized for visualization of labial and vaginal anomalies
  - Utilized for assessment of primary amenorrhea in patients with an intact hymen
  - Sector transducer covered with condom

Equipment Preparation
- Probes cleansed according to manufacturers and local institutional guidelines
- Rinse probes prior to use to avoid chemical irritation from disinfectants

Procedure Steps
- Primary imaging mode (TAS or TVS) should include
  - Uterine imaging
    - Sagittal midline in long axis of uterus to include all of cervix to uterine fundus for uterine length
    - Perpendicular to sagittal long axis for anteroposterior measurement
    - Transverse in image showing greatest dimension, likely near fundus
    - Measure 2 largest leiomyomas/masses in 3 planes
    - Measure exophytic masses in 3 planes
    - Multiple parasagittal and transverse images to include all of uterus and cervix
  - High resolution image of endometrium
    - Measure endometrium perpendicular to long axis
    - Include both layers of endometrium
    - Exclude any fluid
    - Exclude hypoechoic subendometrial zone in endometrial measurement
    - If focal endometrial lesion, color and pulsed Doppler may be helpful
  - Ovarian imaging
    - If ovaries are difficult to find, obtain a coronal view of uterine fundus and angle laterally to region of broad ligament
    - Gentle pressure on anterior abdominal wall can move bowel gas out of the way to improve ovarian visualization
    - Ovaries measured in parasagittal oblique plane to include long axis and in transverse plane
    - Measure largest cyst or any atypical appearing adnexal lesion in 3 planes
    - Determine if cyst/mass arises from ovary or is separate from ovary
    - Doppler can be helpful to distinguish between a vessel and an adnexal cyst
    - Doppler can be helpful to determine if cyst contents are solid (increasing likelihood of malignancy) or clot
    - Bladder filling and/or emptying can help determine the etiology and location of a pelvic cyst in cases where a large cyst is mistaken for the urinary bladder
  - Scan between uterus and ovaries to assess for other adnexal masses, in particular in first trimester at risk for ectopic pregnancy
  - Check cul-de-sac for fluid

ULTRASOUND TECHNIQUE & ANATOMY

- TAS also includes screening image of kidneys for hydronephrosis (if part of laboratory protocol, and in cases of pelvic masses)
- TVS scanning should include gentle insertion of the vaginal probe
  - Watch the image as the probe is being inserted to assess for vaginal masses
  - Scan generally performed through the anterior vaginal wall
  - If uterus is retroverted or retroflexed scan may be performed through posterior vaginal wall
  - Angle probe gently to avoid pain
  - Some patients have pain when cervix is manipulated, so avoid pressure on cervix
  - In patients with bowel gas obscuring visualization of ovary, gentle abdominal pressure can bring ovary into focus
- Transperineal scan
  - Sagittal midline view of vagina, cervix, and lower uterus
  - Parasagittal views as indicated
- Transrectal scan is occasionally helpful
- In patients with focal tenderness or pain, specifically assess region of pain with probe

Findings and Reporting
- Uterine size
- Myometrial echotexture
- Leiomyoma location and largest size
- Endometrial thickness
- Endometrial masses, fluid, or abnormal thickening
- Ovary appearance
- Cysts out of the physiologic range
- Free fluid
- Other masses

Alternative Procedures/Therapies
- Radiologic
  - MR
    - Overview of pelvic anatomy
    - Better for soft tissue characterization
  - CT
    - Not indicated for screening
    - Used for staging pelvic malignancies
  - Hysterosalpingography
    - Tubal patency assessment
- Surgical
  - Blind endometrial biopsy for abnormal bleeding
  - Hysteroscopic biopsy for focal endometrial lesions

POST-PROCEDURE

Expected Outcome
- No harmful effects from pelvic sonography

Things To Do
- Cleanse probes according to manufacturers and institutional guidelines
- Must have gel both inside the probe cover and outside the probe cover
- If scanning is performed for infertility, water or saline may be used as a lubricant to avoid adverse effect on sperm motility

Things To Avoid
- Male sonographers/sonologist should always have female chaperone in cases of transvaginal scans

PROBLEMS & COMPLICATIONS

Problems
- Post-menopausal women with atrophic vaginitis may be uncomfortable with TVS
  - Use small probe
  - Use extra lubricating gel
  - Allow patient (if she desires) to insert probe herself

SELECTED REFERENCES

1. Jermy K et al: The characterization of common ovarian cysts in premenopausal women. Ultrasound Obstet Gynecol. 17(2):140-4, 2001
2. Brown DL et al: Benign and malignant ovarian masses: selection of the most discriminating gray-scale and Doppler sonographic features. Radiology. 208(1):103-10, 1998
3. Lee W: How to interpret the ultrasound output display standard for higher acoustic output diagnostic ultrasound devices. J Ultrasound Med. 17(8):535-8, 1998
4. Langer RD et al: Transvaginal ultrasonography compared with endometrial biopsy for the detection of endometrial disease. Postmenopausal Estrogen/Progestin Interventions Trial. N Engl J Med. 337(25):1792-8, 1997
5. Lev-Toaff AS: Sonohysterography: evaluation of endometrial and myometrial abnormalities. Semin Roentgenol. 31(4):288-98, 1996
6. Levine D et al: Sonography of ovarian masses: poor sensitivity of resistive index for identifying malignant lesions. AJR Am J Roentgenol. 162(6):1355-9, 1994
7. Freimanis MG et al: Transvaginal ultrasonography. Radiol Clin North Am. 30(5):955-76, 1992
8. Levine D et al: Simple adnexal cysts: the natural history in postmenopausal women. Radiology. 184(3):653-9, 1992
9. Lyons EA et al: Transvaginal sonography of normal pelvic anatomy. Radiol Clin North Am. 30(4):663-75, 1992
10. Platt JF et al: Ultrasound of the normal nongravid uterus: correlation with gross and histopathology. J Clin Ultrasound. 18(1):15-9, 1990
11. Forrest TS et al: Cyclic endometrial changes: US assessment with histologic correlation. Radiology. 167(1):233-7, 1988
12. Fleischer AC et al: Sonographic depiction of normal and abnormal endometrium with histopathologic correlation. J Ultrasound Med. 5(8):445-52, 1986
13. Schwimer SR et al: The effect of ultrasound coupling gels on sperm motility in vitro. Fertil Steril. 42(6):946-7, 1984

ULTRASOUND TECHNIQUE & ANATOMY

IMAGE GALLERY

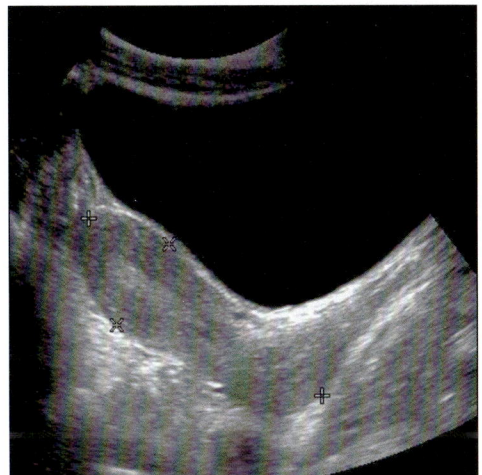
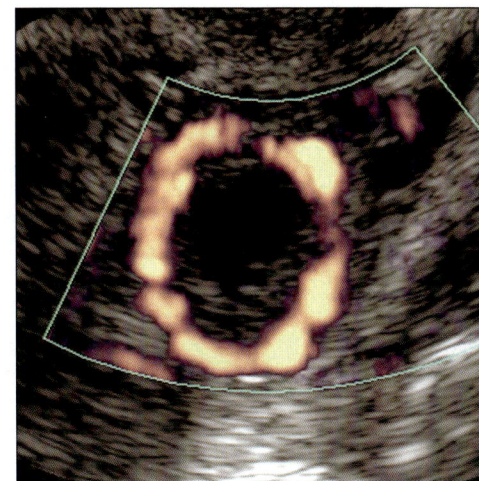

(Left) Sagittal transabdominal ultrasound shows the normal appearance of the uterus (calipers). *(Right)* Transverse power Doppler ultrasound shows a hemorrhagic corpus luteum cyst with a thick hyperemic wall.

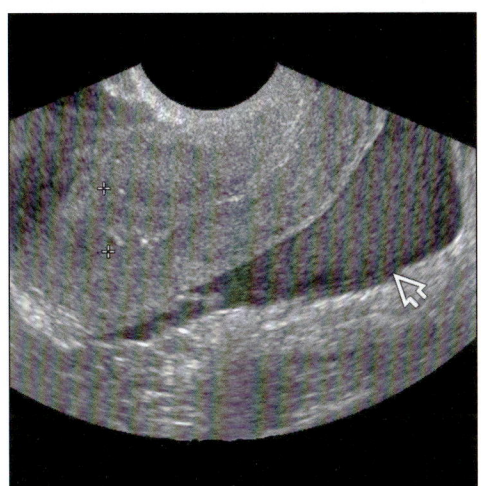
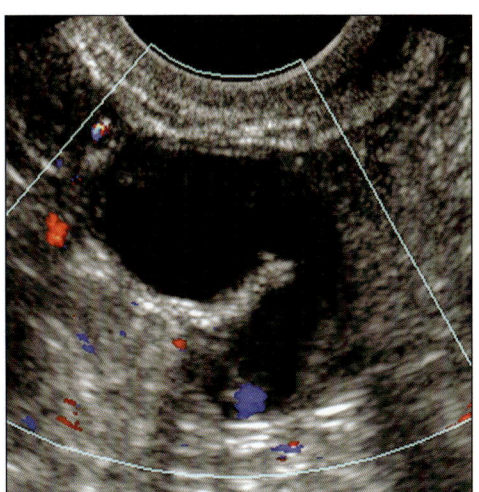

(Left) Sagittal transvaginal ultrasound in a pregnant patient shows fluid with debris ➤ in cul-de-sac in a patient with an ectopic pregnancy. Calipers denote the endometrium. *(Right)* Lateral color Doppler ultrasound shows an anechoic tubular structure folded on itself, without flow, consistent with hydrosalpinx.

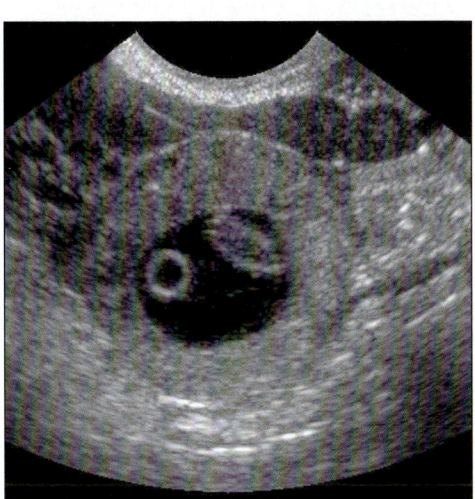
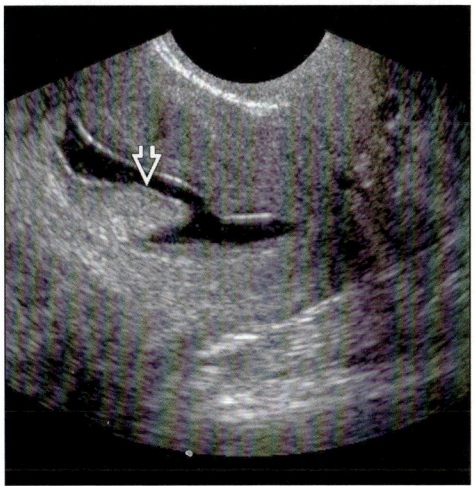

(Left) Transverse transvaginal ultrasound shows an ectopic pregnancy. *(Right)* Sagittal transvaginal ultrasound during sonohysterogram shows a focal endometrial lesion ➤. This is the classic appearance of an endometrial polyp, although histology is needed to exclude malignancy in patients with bleeding.

HYSTEROSALPINGOGRAPHY

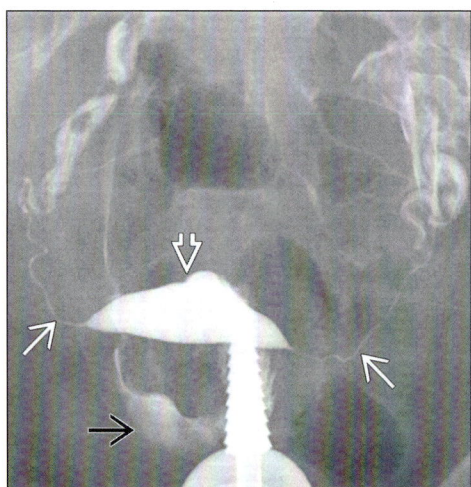

Frontal projection of HSG shows normal appearances of the endometrial cavity ➡ and fallopian tubes ➡, with free bilateral intraperitoneal spill of contrast medium ➡.

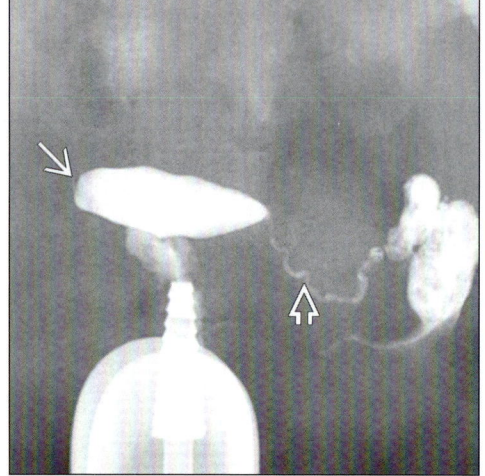

Frontal projection of HSG shows complete blockage of the right fallopian tube ➡. Left fallopian tube is patent ➡ but there is loculated peritoneal spillage indicating adhesions.

TERMINOLOGY

Abbreviations
- Hysterosalpingography (HSG)

Definitions
- Radiographic evaluation of the uterus and fallopian tubes

Advantages
- Best method to assess fallopian tubes
- Relatively easy to perform
- No use of anesthetic but anxiolytic if required

Disadvantages
- Invasive procedure
- Uses ionizing radiation
- Maybe painful

PRE-PROCEDURE

Indications
- Main indication: Infertility
  - First line investigation
  - Routine work-up in most centers
- Indication: Recurrent spontaneous abortions
  - Can assess for mechanical causes
  - Anatomical variants or acquired abnormalities of uterus or fallopian tubes
- Indication: Uterine abnormalities
  - Müllerian duct fusion anomalies
  - Polyps
  - Leiomyomas
  - Adhesions: Post surgical, Asherman syndrome or post infection/inflammatory
  - Adenomyosis
  - Endometrial hyperplasia
- Indication: Tubal abnormalities
  - Tubal occlusion
    - Proximal or distal occlusion: Different therapy available
    - Most common cause remains pelvic inflammatory disease
  - Tubal disease
    - Hydrosalpinx
    - Peritubal adhesions
    - Salpingitis isthmica nodosa
    - Cornual polyps
- Indication: Following tubal surgery
  - To assess patency following tubal ligation or reversal of tubal ligation

Contraindications
- Contraindication: Pregnancy
  - Risks related to ionizing radiation
  - Displacement of embryo leading to potential for miscarriage
- Contraindication: Pelvic inflammatory disease (PID)
  - PID or history of PID in preceding 6 months
    - Can cause progression of infection to septicemia
- Contraindication: Severe iodine allergy
  - Extremely rare with use of currently available low-osmolar non-ionic contrast agents
- Relative contraindication: Active menstrual bleeding
  - Due to risk of intravasation
    - However, lymphatic or vascular intravasation is clinically insignificant and not dangerous
  - Can cause difficulty in interpretation

Getting Started
- Things to Check
  - Date of last menstrual cycle
    - Examination scheduled during days 7-12 of the menstrual cycle as endometrium is thin which facilitates image interpretation

HYSTEROSALPINGOGRAPHY

Key Facts

Terminology
- Radiographic evaluation of the uterus and fallopian tubes

Pre-procedure
- Main indication: Infertility
- Indication: Recurrent spontaneous abortions
- Indication: Following tubal surgery
- Contraindication: Pregnancy
- Contraindication: Pelvic inflammatory disease (PID)

Procedure
- Obtain a scout radiograph of pelvis with catheter in place before contrast medium is instilled
- **Obtain 4 spot radiographs**
- 1. Early filling of the uterus: Evaluate any filling defects or contour abnormalities
- 2. Uterus fully distended: Evaluate shape of the uterus
- 3. Demonstrate and evaluate fallopian tubes
- 4. Image free intraperitoneal spillage of contrast material
- If cornual spasm then glucagon or Buscopan may be administered and further views obtained

Problems & Complications
- Failure to cannulate the cervical os
- Inadequate uterine filling either due to pain or inadequate seal
- Tubal spasm may lead to false negative result
- Irradiation of an early unsuspected pregnancy: Appropriate timing of the procedure and negative pregnancy test should minimize the risk
- Pain
- Infection

- ○ Abstinence from sexual intercourse from time menstrual bleeding ends until the day of the study
  - ▪ Reduce potential for early pregnancy
- ○ If irregular menstrual cycle, or pregnancy is a possibility then serum B-human chorionic gonadotropin level should be evaluated
- ○ Active PID
  - ▪ Erythrocyte sedimentation rate (ESR) to check for active PID
  - ▪ Negative gonorrhea and chlamydia cultures are acceptable in patients with coexistent inflammatory conditions (i.e., arthritis, sarcoidosis, collagen vascular disease)
  - ▪ No routine prophylactic antibiotic treatment in patients with a history of PID
- ○ History of severe iodine allergy
- Medications
  - ○ Glucagon or Buscopan can be used to prevent tubal spasm
  - ○ Contra-indication to glucagon
    - ▪ Phaeochromocytoma
    - ▪ Insulinoma
  - ○ Anxiolytic if required
- Equipment List
  - ○ Private fluoroscopic screening room with adequate lighting
  - ○ Sterile equipment
    - ▪ Vaginal speculum
    - ▪ 5-F HSG balloon catheter
  - ○ Water soluble, non-ionic contrast medium
  - ○ Oil-based agents have been thought to increase fertility rates post-procedure
    - ▪ Larger studies dispute this claim with no statistical difference between oil and water-soluble contrast
    - ▪ More complications (oil emboli and granuloma formation) with oil-based agents

PROCEDURE

Patient Position/Location
- Best procedure approach: Supine, in lithotomy or modified lithotomy position

Equipment Preparation
- Sterile pack

Procedure Steps
- Careful explanation and patient reassurance vital
- Perineum is prepared with cleansing solution and draped with sterile towels
- Insert speculum into vagina and obtain clear view of cervical os
- Cannulate cervical os with a 5-F HSG catheter
- Fully inflate the balloon
- Obtain a scout radiograph of pelvis with catheter in place before contrast medium is instilled
- Under fluoroscopic control slowly instill water-soluble contrast medium
  - ○ Avoid air bubbles as they can hinder interpretation
- **Obtain 4 spot radiographs**
  - ○ 1. Early filling of the uterus: Evaluate any filling defects or contour abnormalities
  - ○ 2. Uterus fully distended: Evaluate shape of the uterus
  - ○ 3. Demonstrate and evaluate fallopian tubes
  - ○ 4. Image free intraperitoneal spillage of contrast material
- Additional spot radiographs to document any abnormality seen
- Oblique views of fallopian tubes if needed to "elongate" the tube or displace superimposed structures
- If no free intraperitoneal spill of contrast visualized repeat contrast medium injection ± prone view
- If cornual spasm then glucagon or Buscopan may be administered and further views obtained

Findings and Reporting
- Normal findings

HYSTEROSALPINGOGRAPHY

- Normal outlined uterine cavity, narrow patent fallopian tubes and free bilateral peritoneal spillage of contrast medium
- Other findings
  - Uterine abnormalities: Congenital or acquired
    - Congenital abnormalities of the uterine shape
    - Abnormalities of uterine contour
    - Luminal filling defects
  - Tubal occlusion (infertility of after ligation procedure)
  - Tubal patency (normal finding or after reversal of ligation procedure)
  - Other tubal abnormalities: Hydrosalpinx, tubal adhesions, loculated spillage (indicative of local adhesions)

Alternative Procedures/Therapies
- Radiologic
  - Sonohysterography
    - Similar technique
    - No ionizing radiation
    - Real time imaging
    - Best for evaluation of endometrium (abnormal uterine bleeding, polyps) and ovaries
    - Less accurate for tubal patency
  - MR
    - No ionizing radiation
    - Assessment of the entire female pelvis during the same examination
    - Multiplanar imaging capability and superb tissue contrast
    - Best used for evaluation of uterine congenital anomalies, myometrium and ovaries
- Surgical
  - Laparoscopic and dye test
    - Requires general anesthetic
    - Uterine cannulation is performed under direct visualization
    - Methylene blue contrast is injected into uterine cavity
    - Spill of methylene blue is visualized via laparoscope into the peritoneal cavity
    - Visualize ovaries and uterine cavity
  - This is deemed gold standard technique for infertility although imperfect
- Other
  - Hormone profile as part of infertility work-up
  - Chlamydia serology for PID
  - Sperm count

POST-PROCEDURE

Expected Outcome
- No complications
- Minor pain
  - Secondary to uterotubal distension or peritoneal spill
    - Reduced by slow injection of contrast medium
    - Responds to simple analgesics
- Minor bleeding: Light spotting after the procedure, usually lasting less than 24 hours

Things To Do
- Instruct patients to watch for sign of possible infection
  - Development of fever or foul-smelling vaginal discharge for 2-4 days following HSG

PROBLEMS & COMPLICATIONS

Problems
- Failure to cannulate the cervical os
- Inadequate uterine filling either due to pain or inadequate seal
  - Inject contrast medium slower if pain occurs
  - Use of different cannula if problems with seal
- Tubal spasm may lead to false negative result
  - Repeat injection or give antispasmodic (glucagon)

Complications
- Most feared complication(s): Irradiation of an early unsuspected pregnancy: Appropriate timing of the procedure and negative pregnancy test should minimize the risk
- Other complications
  - Pain
    - Cramping pain is generally minor and well-tolerated by majority of patients
  - Infection
    - More common in the context of PID
    - If hydrosalpinx identified then a routine course of antibiotics is required
  - Vasovagal reaction
    - Secondary to cervical manipulation or inflation of occlusive balloon
  - Uterine or tubal perforation (extremely rare)

SELECTED REFERENCES

1. Perquin DA et al: Routine use of hysterosalpingography prior to laparoscopy in the fertility workup: a multicentre randomized controlled trial. Hum Reprod. 2006
2. Simpson WL Jr et al: Hysterosalpingography: a reemerging study. Radiographics. 26(2):419-31, 2006
3. Spring DB et al: Enhanced fertility after diagnostic hysterosalpingography may be a myth. AJR Am J Roentgenol. 183(6):1728, 2004
4. Unterweger M et al: Three-dimensional dynamic MR-hysterosalpingography; a new, low invasive, radiation-free and less painful radiological approach to female infertility. Hum Reprod. 17(12):3138-41, 2002
5. Mol BW et al: Comparison of hysterosalpingography and laparoscopy in predicting fertility outcome. Hum Reprod. 14(5):1237-42, 1999
6. Strandell A et al: The assessment of endometrial pathology and tubal patency: a comparison between the use of ultrasonography and X-ray hysterosalpingography for the investigation of infertility patients. Ultrasound Obstet Gynecol. 14(3):200-4, 1999
7. Cundiff G et al: Infertile couples with a normal hysterosalpingogram. Reproductive outcome and its relationship to clinical and laparoscopic findings. J Reprod Med. 40(1):19-24, 1995
8. Swart P et al: The accuracy of hysterosalpingography in the diagnosis of tubal pathology: a meta-analysis. Fertil Steril. 64(3):486-91, 1995

HYSTEROSALPINGOGRAPHY

IMAGE GALLERY

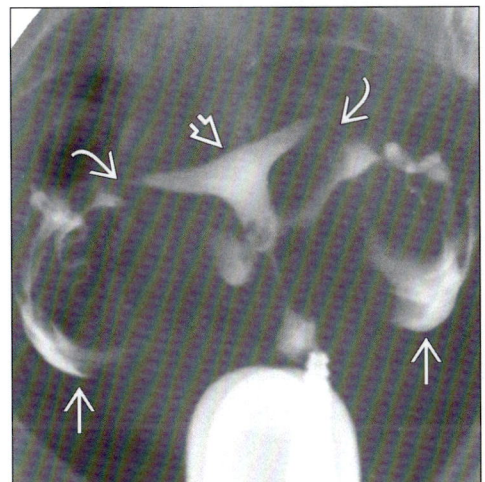
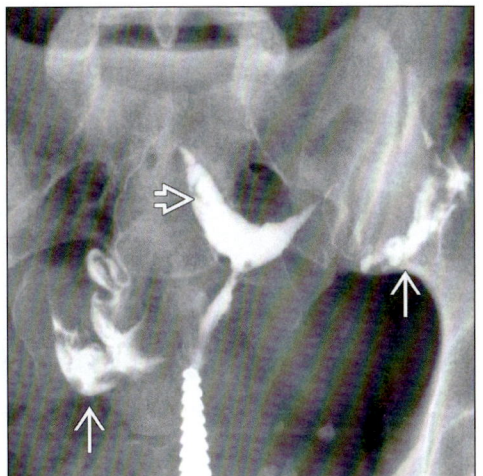

(Left) Frontal projection of HSG shows normal appearances to the uterus ⇨ and fallopian tubes ⇨ with free bilateral intraperitoneal spill of contrast medium ⇨. (Right) Frontal projection shows intrauterine distortion ⇨ in keeping with Asherman syndrome. Note that both fallopian tubes are patent and intraperitoneal spill of contrast medium is demonstrated ⇨.

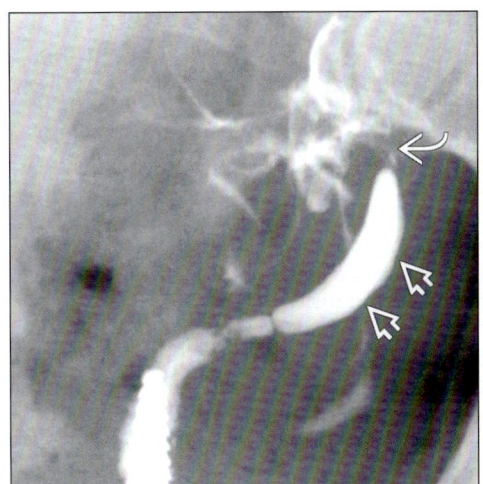
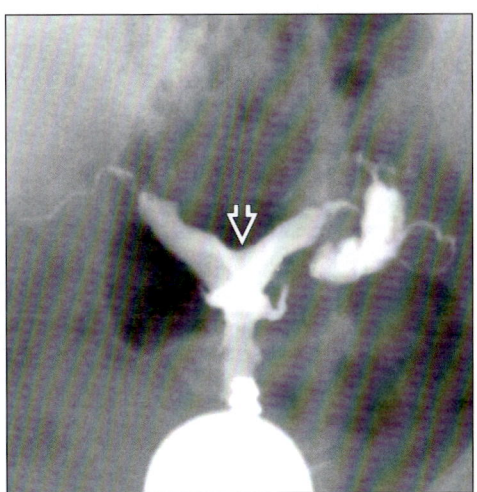

(Left) Magnified frontal projection of HSG a single lateral-flexed uterine horn ⇨ with a single fallopian tube ⇨. (Right) Frontal projection of HSG shows indentation ⇨ in the uterine fundal contour and wide separation of uterine horns suggesting bicornate uterus.

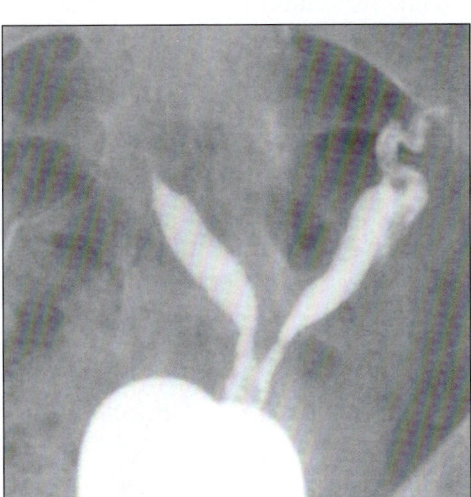
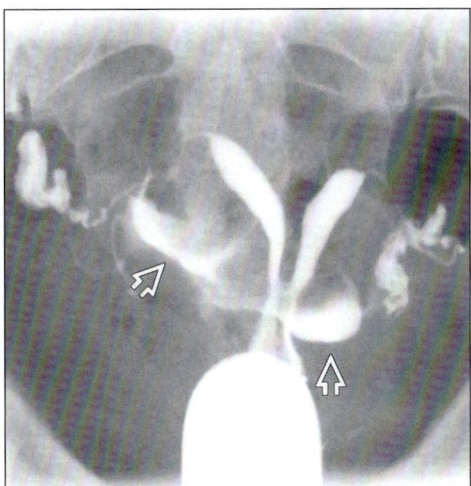

(Left) Frontal projection of HSG shows presence of a didelphys uterus. Note this is early filling phase and therefore no definite spill of contrast medium into the peritoneal cavity is demonstrated. (Right) Frontal projection of HSG delayed filling phase image of the same patient as previous image, demonstrates clear intraperitoneal spill ⇨.

CT TECHNIQUE & ANATOMY

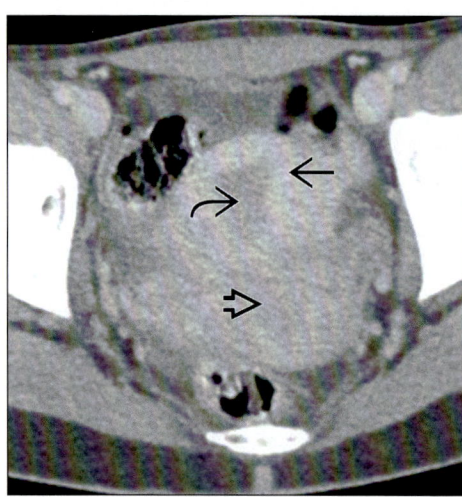

Axial CECT shows a normal low-attenuation, fluid-filled uterine cavity ⇨ & lower degree of enhancement of cervix ⇨ compared to myometrium ⇨, not to be confused with cervical pathology.

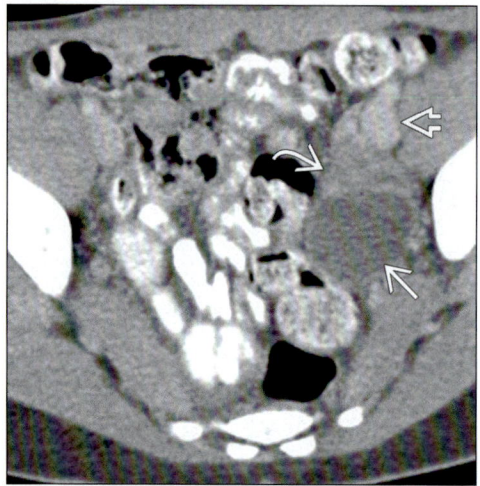

Axial CECT shows a normal left ovary ⇨ located posterior to the external iliac vessels ⇨. Note the low-attenuation dominant follicle ⇨.

TERMINOLOGY

Abbreviations
- Computed tomography (CT)

PROCEDURE

Indications
- **CT used in:**
- Staging of ovarian cancer
  - Evaluate extent of disease
  - Triage patients to surgery or neoadjuvant chemotherapy
- Staging of advanced pelvic malignancies (MR modality of choice)
  - Uterine carcinoma
  - Cervical carcinoma
- Treatment follow-up of gynecologic malignancy
- Assessing tumor recurrence
- Assessing post-operative complications
  - Abscess
  - Fistula
  - Lymphocele
- CT-guided biopsy
  - Providing histological diagnosis
  - Differentiating tumor recurrence vs. post surgical/radiation fibrosis
- CT-guided drainage of pelvic collection

Relative Contraindications (CI)
- CT is not contraindicated in pregnancy but should be used judiciously
  - Ultrasound and MR should be considered first
  - Avoid intravenous contrast

Advantages
- Oral and rectal contrast opacification of the gastrointestinal tract
  - Allows differentiation of bowel from pelvic viscera
- Intravenous contrast-enhancement of blood vessels and viscera
  - Helps differentiation
    - Pelvic blood vessels vs. lymph nodes vs. parametrial tumor extension
  - Enhancement pattern differentiates tumor from myometrium
  - Allows opacification of bladder and ureters
- Multidetector CT provides very fast data acquisition
  - Rapid coverage of the whole body
  - High spatial resolution with improved Z-axis resolution
    - Better multiplanar reconstruction
  - Rapid predictable acquisition
    - Allows different circulatory phases to be acquired

Disadvantages
- Ionizing radiation
- Degradation of image quality by
  - Body habitus
  - Metallic hip prosthesis
- Use of iodinated contrast agents associated with morbidity and mortality
- Limited application in early-stage cancer

CT Technique
- Patient position
  - Supine
  - Prone may be of use in CT-guided biopsy or drainage
- Oral contrast medium
  - 750-1000 mL diluted oral contrast 2 hour prior to examination

CT TECHNIQUE & ANATOMY

Key Facts

Procedure
- CT used in:
- Staging of ovarian cancer
- Staging of advanced pelvic malignancies (MR modality of choice)
- Treatment follow-up of gynecologic malignancy
- Assessing tumor recurrence
- Assessing post-operative complications
- CT-guided biopsy
- Providing histological diagnosis
- Differentiating tumor recurrence vs. post surgical/radiation fibrosis
- CT-guided drainage of pelvic collection
- CECT: Myometrium enhances, helps to delineate the endometrium
- CECT: Early phase: Endometrium low attenuation in the central part of uterus
- CECT: Delayed phase: Endometrium further enhances to CT attenuation similar or higher than myometrium
- Pitfall: Overestimation of endometrial thickness on axial and coronal plane, hence accurate measurements on sagittal reformats only
- CECT: Cervix of similar CT attenuation as myometrium
- Pitfall: Cervix lower attenuation at early CECT, should not be confused with cervical pathology
- Parametrial vessels enhance to similar or higher degree than cervix

---

- o Prolonged oral contrast medium (48 hours) may be of use if slow transit time
- IV contrast medium
  - o 100-150 mL iodinated contrast medium
  - o Injection rate 2-3 mL/sec
  - o Images 70-120 seconds post IV
  - o Delayed
    - 3-5 minutes for pelvic vein imaging (thrombus)
    - 5-10 minutes for bladder visualization
  - o CT angiogram of pelvic vessels
    - Faster injection rate (4-5 mL/sec) and earlier scan time (bolus tracking technique recommended to detect peak enhancement)
- 5 mm collimation (thinner for 3D or small lesion characterization)

CT Anatomy
- Uterus
  - o Appearances depend on
    - Age
    - Position of uterus
    - Presence of leiomyoma, adenomyosis
  - o Triangular or ovoid soft-tissue structure
  - o Posterior to urinary bladder
  - o Secretions within endometrial canal demonstrate centrally located decreased attenuation
  - o CECT: Myometrium enhances, helps to delineate the endometrium
  - o CECT: Early phase: Endometrium low attenuation in the central part of uterus
  - o CECT: Delayed phase: Endometrium further enhances to CT attenuation similar or higher than myometrium
  - o Pitfall: Overestimation of endometrial thickness on axial and coronal plane, hence accurate measurements on sagittal reformats only
- Cervix
  - o More rounded than corpus
  - o At inferior aspect of uterus
  - o CECT: Cervix of similar CT attenuation as myometrium
    - Pitfall: Cervix lower attenuation at early CECT, should not be confused with cervical pathology
  - o Parametrial vessels enhance to similar or higher degree than cervix
- Ovaries
  - o Routinely seen in premenopausal women
  - o Small, not always seen postmenopausally
  - o Uniform soft-tissue density
    - Small low density cystic regions represent follicles
  - o Position variable
    - Usually posterolateral to uterine corpus
    - Anterior and medial to ureter
    - Posterior to round ligament
    - Medial or posteromedial to external iliac vessels
    - Ovarian mass displaces ureter laterally and posteriorly vs. nodal mass lying lateral to ureter
- Pelvic ligaments
  - o Broad ligament
    - Two layers of peritoneum
    - Extend laterally from uterus to pelvic sidewall
    - Not usually seen unless ascites is present
  - o Round ligament
    - Thin soft tissue attenuation band
    - Extends laterally from a broad base at fundus
    - Tapers distally
    - Frequently seen
  - o Uterosacral ligament
    - Extends posteriorly from lateral vagina and cervix
    - Tapers towards anterior body of S2 or S3
    - May be seen as soft tissue arc-like structure from cervix to sacrum
  - o Cardinal ligament
    - Extends laterally from cervix and upper vagina
    - Merges with pelvic sidewall
    - May be seen as triangular soft tissue structure
  - o Ovarian ligament
    - Extends medially from ovary to uterus
    - Inferior and posterior to fallopian tubes
    - Position varies with that of ovaries
    - Not usually identified

Pelvic Pathology
- Leiomyoma
  - o Usually incidental finding
  - o CT not recommended for detection or evaluation

CT TECHNIQUE & ANATOMY

- Uterine enlargement, distortion most common
- Heterogeneous mass, variable appearances
- Soft-tissue density similar to myometrium
- Areas of low-attenuation
- Coarse calcification
- Benign ovarian lesions (US primary imaging modality)
  - Functional cysts
    - Physiologic cysts
    - Common in premenopausal women
    - Greater than 2.5 cm
    - Typically resolve over time
    - Usually unilocular, simple, low-attenuation
  - Theca-lutein cysts
    - Associated with gestational trophoblastic disease
    - Associated with ovarian hyperstimulation syndrome
    - Multiple, bilateral
    - Massive ovarian enlargement common
  - Endometriomas (MR better for lesion characterization)
    - Single or multiple
    - Fluid or higher than fluid attenuation depending on amount and timing of hemorrhage
  - Mature cystic teratoma (dermoid)
    - Cystic tumor
    - Composed of at least two types of tissue (ectoderm, mesoderm, endoderm)
    - Most common benign tumor in younger women
    - Well-defined adnexal mass, usually unilocular
    - Fat attenuation within a cyst ± calcification (e.g., teeth) diagnostic
    - Dermoid plug (nodule of hair and tissue)
- Ovarian carcinoma
  - Unilateral or bilateral
  - Complex adnexal masses
  - Mixed solid/cystic attenuation
  - Enhancing nodules
  - Thick irregular septations
  - Ascites
  - Omental cake
  - Nodular peritoneal deposits
    - Occasionally calcification of peritoneal implants
    - Scalloping of liver
  - Enlarged lymph nodes
  - Distant metastases
- Endometrial carcinoma
  - Heterogeneous mass
  - May fill or expand uterine cavity
  - Central low-attenuation
    - Necrosis
    - Fluid or blood (hydrometra or hematometra) secondary to cervical obstruction
  - Myometrial or extrauterine extension better assessed on MR
  - CT useful in assessment of
    - Advanced disease
    - Lymphadenopathy
    - Bladder, bowel invasion
    - Distant metastasis
    - Disease recurrence
- Cervical carcinoma
  - Heterogeneous mass
  - CECT: Tumor necrosis/ulceration seen as low-attenuation
  - Tumor mass may
    - Expand cervix
    - Obstruct endocervical canal causing hydro/hematometra
  - CT useful in assessment of
    - Ureteric obstruction
    - Bladder or bowel involvement
    - Distant metastases
    - Lymphadenopathy
- Metastases to the ovary
  - Common
    - Gastrointestinal tract (stomach, colorectal, pancreas, biliary tract)
    - Breast
    - Pelvic malignancy
  - Krukenberg tumor
    - Mucinous metastases usually from carcinoma of gastric antrum
    - Massive solid bilateral ovarian enlargement
    - Cystic degeneration
    - Ascites not usually present
- Miscellaneous
  - Tubo-ovarian abscess
  - Ovarian torsion

SELECTED REFERENCES

1. Choi HJ et al: Computed tomography findings of ovarian metastases from colon cancer: comparison with primary malignant ovarian tumors. J Comput Assist Tomogr. 29(1):69-73, 2005
2. Funt SA et al: Role of CT in the management of recurrent ovarian cancer. AJR Am J Roentgenol. 182(2):393-8, 2004
3. Saksouk FA et al: Recognition of the ovaries and ovarian origin of pelvic masses with CT. Radiographics. 24 Suppl 1:S133-46, 2004
4. Fielding JR: MR imaging of the female pelvis. Radiol Clin North Am. 41(1):179-92, 2003
5. Follen M et al: Imaging in cervical cancer. Cancer. 98(9 Suppl):2028-38, 2003
6. Jeong YY et al: Uterine cervical carcinoma after therapy: CT and MR imaging findings. Radiographics. 23(4):969-81; discussion 981, 2003
7. Kido A et al: Diffusely enlarged uterus: evaluation with MR imaging. Radiographics. 23(6):1423-39, 2003
8. Pannu HK et al: Multidetector CT of peritoneal carcinomatosis from ovarian cancer. Radiographics. 23(3):687-701, 2003
9. Togashi K: Ovarian cancer: the clinical role of US, CT, and MRI. Eur Radiol. 13 Suppl 4:L87-104, 2003
10. Outwater EK et al: Ovarian teratomas: tumor types and imaging characteristics. Radiographics. 21(2):475-90, 2001
11. Pannu HK et al: CT evaluation of cervical cancer: spectrum of disease. Radiographics. 21(5):1155-68, 2001
12. Hopper KD et al: Body CT and oncologic imaging. Radiology. 215(1):27-40, 2000
13. Hricak H et al: Complex adnexal masses: detection and characterization with MR imaging--multivariate analysis. Radiology. 214(1):39-46, 2000
14. Jeong YY et al: Imaging evaluation of ovarian masses. Radiographics. 20(5):1445-70, 2000
15. Kawamoto S et al: CT of epithelial ovarian tumors. Radiographics. 19 Spec No:S85-102; quiz S263-4, 1999
16. Kubik-Huch RA: Female pelvis. Eur Radiol. 9(9):1715-21, 1999

CT TECHNIQUE & ANATOMY

IMAGE GALLERY

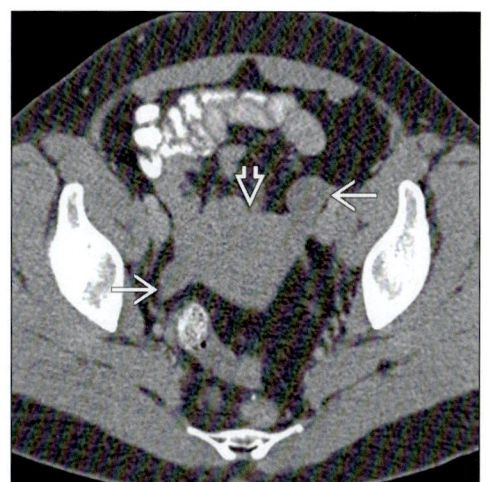
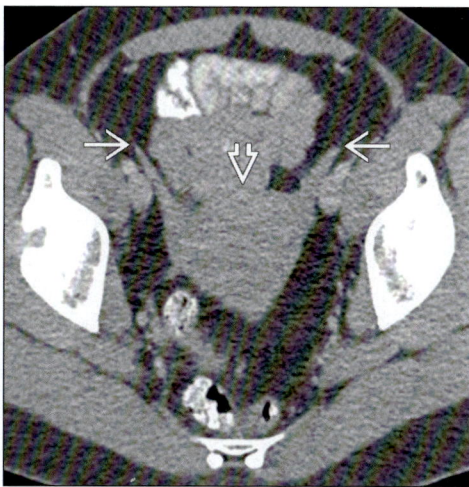

(Left) Axial CECT shows normal appearances of the uterus ⇨ (at the level of the fundus) and both ovaries → in a premenopausal patient. *(Right)* Axial CECT shows the triangular-shaped uterine corpus ⇨ in the same patient. Both round ligaments are well-delineated → as they taper distally.

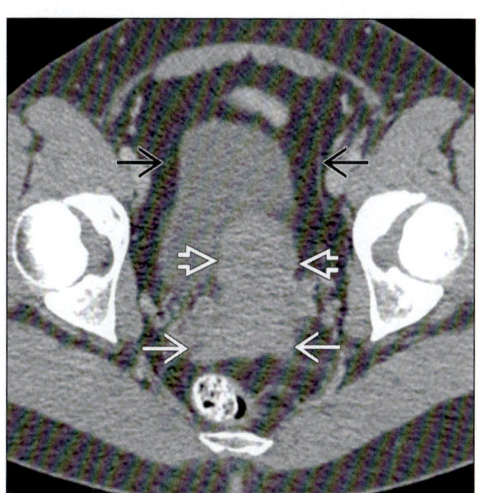
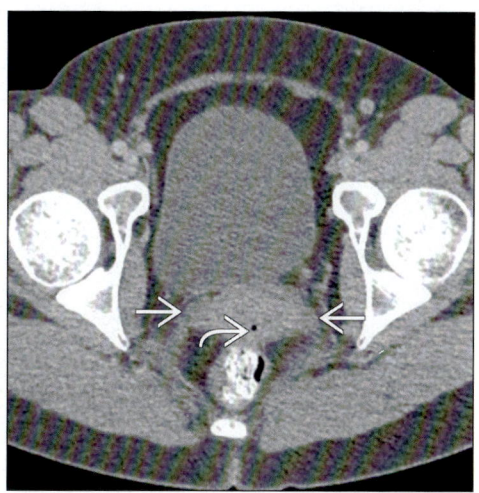

(Left) Axial CECT shows normal appearances of the uterine cervix ⇨. Normal vagina → is also visualized just posterior to the cervix in the same patient as previous image. Note the presence of round ligaments bilaterally →. *(Right)* Axial CECT shows normal appearances of the vaginal vault → in the same premenopausal patient. A fleck of air is also seen within the vagina →.

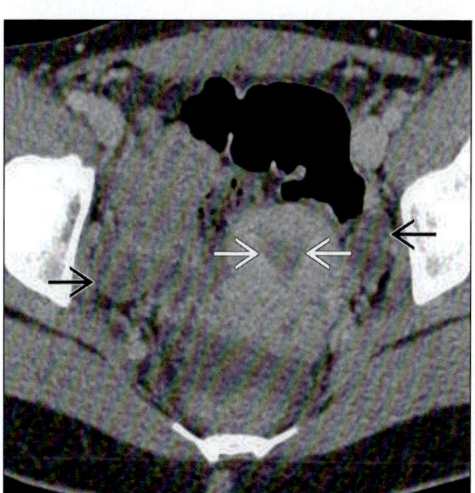
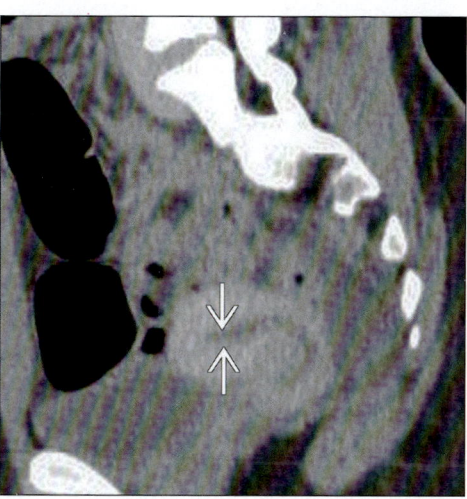

(Left) Axial CECT shows normal enhancement of the myometrium delineating the endometrial canal →. Normal premenopausal ovaries containing multiple follicles are also seen bilaterally →. *(Right)* Sagittal CECT shows normal enhancement of the myometrium delineating the endometrial canal →. The endometrial thickness should always be measured in the sagittal plane to avoid overestimation.

CT TECHNIQUE & ANATOMY

IMAGE GALLERY

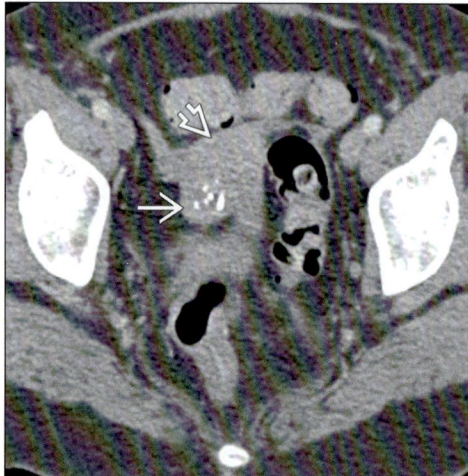
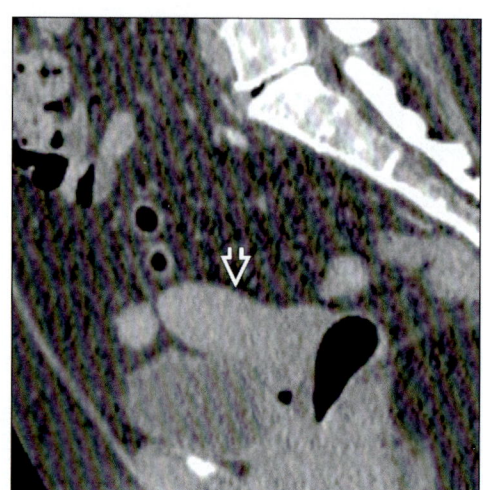

(Left) Axial CECT shows normal appearances of the uterus ➡ in a postmenopausal patient. Note the presence of a calcified subserosal leiomyoma ➡. (Right) Sagittal CECT shows normal appearances of the uterus ➡ in the same patient. The endometrial canal cannot be visualized in this postmenopausal patient.

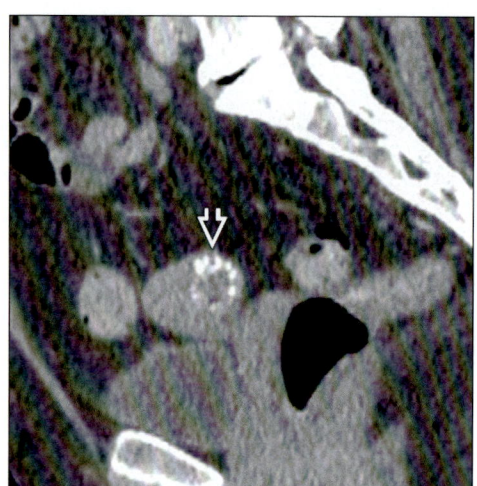
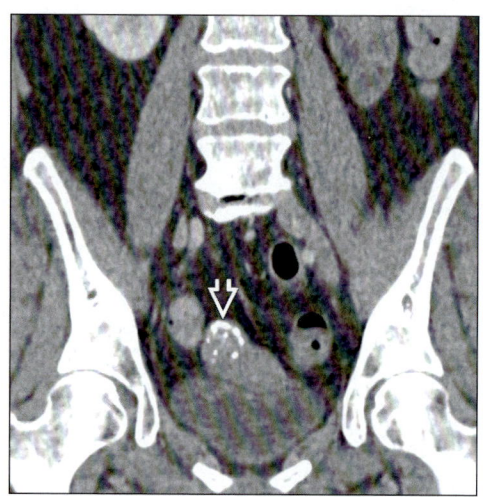

(Left) Sagittal CECT shows the calcified subserosal leiomyoma ➡ in the same postmenopausal patient as in previous images. (Right) Coronal CECT shows normal appearances of the uterus containing a subserosal leiomyoma ➡ in the same postmenopausal patient.

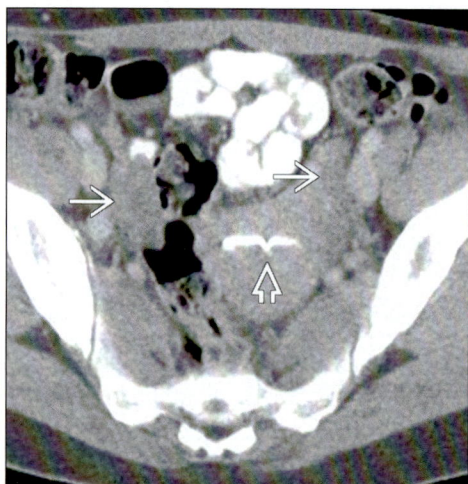
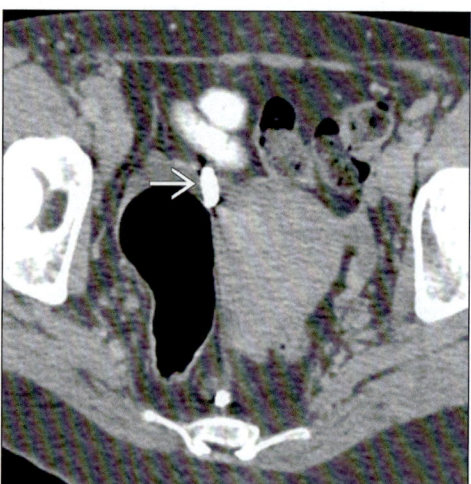

(Left) Axial CECT shows an intrauterine contraceptive device ➡ in a premenopausal patient. Normal ovaries ➡ are also visualized bilaterally medial to the external iliac vessels. (Right) Axial CECT shows a right tubal ligation clip in situ ➡ in a premenopausal patient.

CT TECHNIQUE & ANATOMY

IMAGE GALLERY

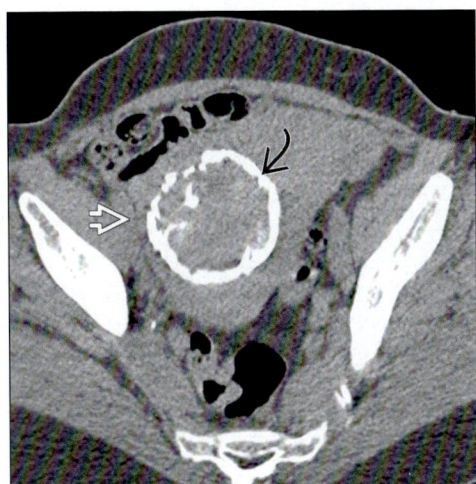
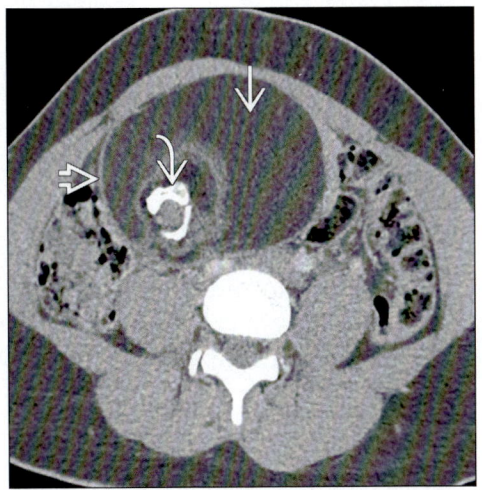

(Left) Axial NECT shows a large uterine leiomyoma ➡. Note the coarse rim-calcification ➡, characteristic of a uterine leiomyoma. *(Right)* Axial CECT shows a mature ovarian teratoma (dermoid) ➡. Note the presence of macroscopic fat ➡ containing areas of soft tissue and a tooth ➡, characteristic of mature ovarian teratoma.

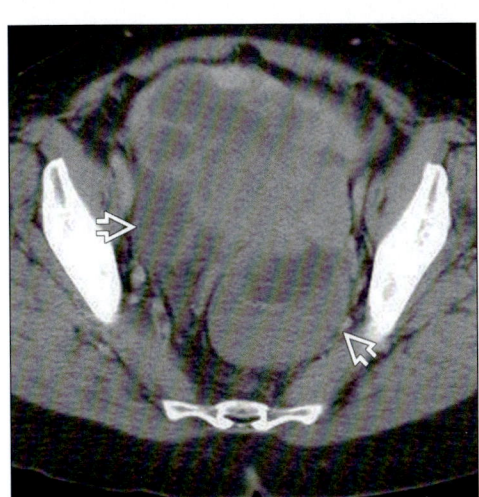
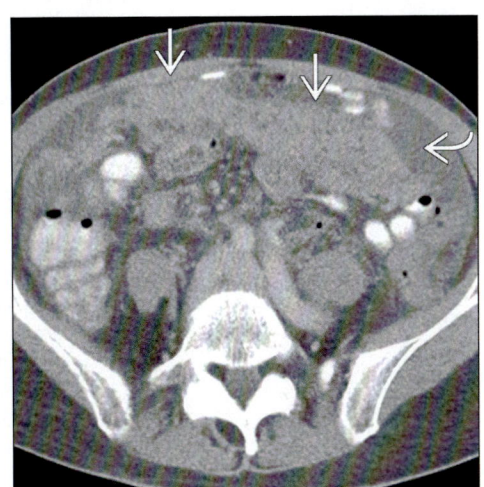

(Left) Axial CECT shows large bilateral adnexal masses of mixed cystic and solid attenuation consistent with bilateral ovarian carcinoma ➡. *(Right)* Axial CECT of the same patient as previous image with advanced ovarian cancer, shows presence of omental cake ➡ overlying the bowel and the presence of ascites ➡.

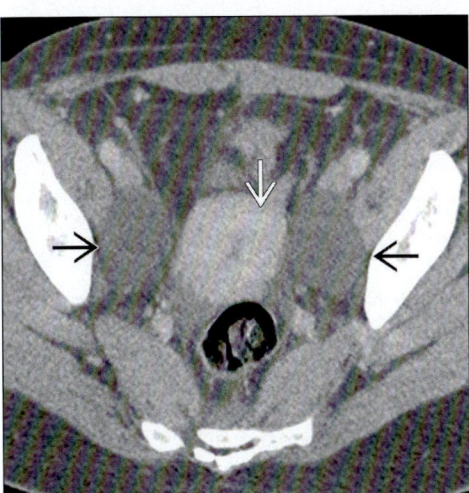
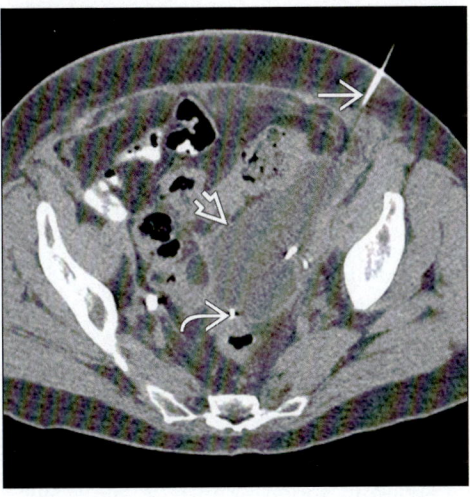

(Left) Axial CECT shows bilateral, low-attenuation lymphoceles ➡. Also note the low-attenuation, fluid-filled uterine cavity and the higher degree of enhancement of the myometrium ➡. *(Right)* Axial NECT shows a CT-guided ➡ drainage of a pelvic collection ➡ in a patient who underwent hysterectomy and bilateral oophorectomy for endometrial carcinoma. Note a drain in situ ➡.

MR TECHNIQUE & ANATOMY

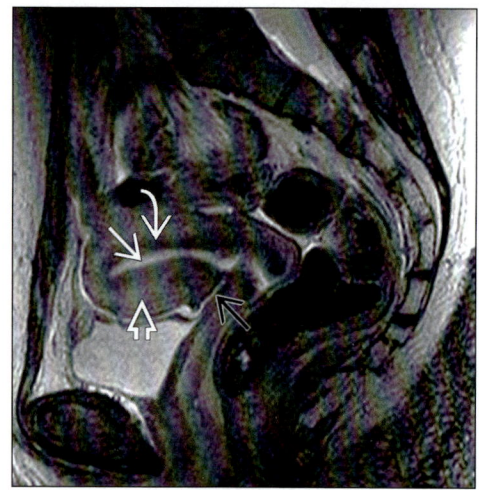

Sagittal T2WI MR shows zonal anatomy at 3T: Intermediate SI outer myometrium ➡, low SI junctional zone ➡ & high SI endometrium ➡ in premenopausal patient. Note anterior scar ➡ related to C-section.

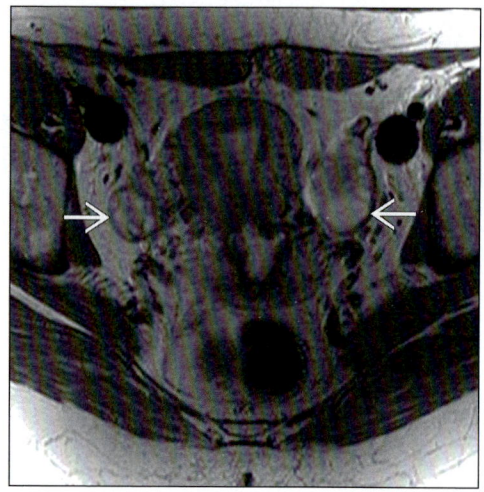

Axial T2WI FS MR shows uterus with normal zonal anatomy. Also note high SI foci within both ovaries ➡ representing normal ovarian follicles.

TERMINOLOGY

Abbreviations
- Magnetic resonance (MR) imaging

PROCEDURE

Indications
- Evaluation of congenital anomalies
- Characterization of adnexal masses
- Staging of pelvic malignancies
- Evaluation of lymphadenopathy
- Treatment follow-up
- Pelvic floor assessment
- Pelvimetry
- Pregnant patients (not 1st trimester)

Contraindications
- Particular caution is advised in patients with
  - Cochlear implants and pacemakers (may be severely impaired by the static magnetic field)
  - Implanted surgical clips or suspected ferromagnetic material (e.g., intraocular foreign body)
  - Tattoos including permanent eye liner
  - Compromised thermoregulatory systems
  - Prosthetic heart valves
  - Pregnancy (1st trimester only)
  - Breastfeeding (if gadolinium is required)
  - Patients who suffer with claustrophobia

Advantages
- No ionizing radiation
- Multiplanar capability
- Excellent spatial and tissue contrast resolution which is improved with higher field magnets (e.g., 3 Tesla)
- Fast imaging (breath-hold and breathing independent)
- Allows definitive noninvasive diagnosis of certain malignant tumors and benign conditions

Patient Preparation
- Patient
  - To limit artifacts due to small bowel peristalsis
    - Fasting for 4-6 hours before MR examination
    - Use of antiperistaltic agents (hyoscine butyl bromide or glucagon) is optional
  - Empty bladder
- Coil selection
  - Image supine using pelvic surface array multichannel coil
  - Body coil shown to provide similar staging accuracy to pelvis surface coil
  - Phase-array coil increases resolution and decreases imaging time
  - Endoluminal coils (endorectal and endovaginal coils)
    - Advantage: High-resolution images especially in the context of small tumors of cervix or those with limited parametrial invasion
    - Disadvantage: Limited field of view that proves inadequate in assessing large tumors and extrauterine tumor extent

MR Technique
- Imaging planes: Axial, sagittal and coronal
  - Axial plane
    - Anatomy seen best (uterus, ovaries, presence of lymph nodes)
    - Evaluation of parametrium (parametrial tumor extension)
  - Sagittal plane
    - Evaluation of uterine zonal anatomy
    - Evaluation of tumor extension to the bladder, cervix and vagina
  - Coronal plane

MR TECHNIQUE & ANATOMY

Key Facts

Procedure
- Evaluation of congenital anomalies
- Characterization of adnexal masses
- Staging of pelvic malignancies
- Evaluation of lymphadenopathy
- Treatment follow-up
- Pelvic floor assessment
- Pelvimetry
- Pregnant patients (not 1st trimester)
- Image supine using pelvic surface array multichannel coil
- Imaging planes: Axial, sagittal and coronal
- Sequences utilized (depends on the clinical problem)
- T1WI: Excellent pelvic outline and valuation of lymph nodes and bone marrow
- T2WI: Superb tissue contrast resolution demonstrating uterine and vaginal zonal anatomy as well as ovaries
- **T1WI FS**
- Differentiates between fat and hemorrhage
- **T1 C+**
- Characterization of adnexal lesions
- Ovarian cancer staging (when CT can not be used)
- **Dynamic Contrast Enhanced 3D GRE T1WI**
- Useful in endometrial cancer staging (myometrial and cervical invasion)
- Can be helpful in detection of small cervical tumors as well as distinguish radiotherapy changes vs. recurrence
- **MR Lymphography**
- Able to detect metastases in normal size lymph nodes with a very high sensitivity and specificity

---

- Complementary information in assessment of uterus, cervix, parametrium, vagina and ovaries
- Evaluation of lymphadenopathy and adnexal masses
  - Oblique planes (axial and/or coronal)
    - Crucial for accurate evaluation of parametria in patients with cervical cancer
- Sequences utilized (depends on the clinical problem)
  - T1WI: Excellent pelvic outline and valuation of lymph nodes and bone marrow
  - T2WI: Superb tissue contrast resolution demonstrating uterine and vaginal zonal anatomy as well as ovaries
  - T1WI FS
    - Differentiates between fat and hemorrhage
    - Improves detection and conspicuity of hyperintense lesions surrounded by fat
- T1 C+
  - Characterization of adnexal lesions
  - Ovarian cancer staging (when CT can not be used)
  - Cervical cancer staging: Evaluation of bladder and rectal invasion as well as presence of fistulae
- **Dynamic Contrast Enhanced 3D GRE T1WI**
  - Shorter sequence with less motion artifact
  - Useful in endometrial cancer staging (myometrial and cervical invasion)
  - Can be helpful in detection of small cervical tumors as well as distinguish radiotherapy changes vs. recurrence
  - Subendometrial enhancement line (early phases) if present helps differentiating stage IA from IB endometrial cancer
  - Maximum inner/outer myometrium contrast at 1 minute
  - Maximum tumor/myometrium contrast in the equilibrium phase (2-3 minutes)
  - Endocervical mucosa enhancement in the late phase (4-5 minutes)
  - Compact fibrous stroma of the cervix remains of low SI (poor enhancement) compared to endocervical mucosa and outer smooth muscle of cervix
  - Parametrial tissues and vaginal walls also enhance
- Perfusion MR
  - Displays information about tissue perfusion and permeability
  - Lesion detection and characterization, improving accuracy of tumor staging, predicting and monitoring response to treatment
- BOLD (Blood Oxygenation Level Dependent) MR
  - Uses intrinsic-susceptibility contrast of tissues
  - Interrogates both the functionality of tumor vasculature and tumor blood volume
  - Provides clinical indices of tumor pathophysiology such as grade and response to radiotherapy
- DWI-MR
  - Displays information about water mobility, tissue cellularity and integrity of cellular membranes
  - Diagnosis and grading of tumors, predicting and assessing response to anti-cancer treatment and therapy planning
- **MR Lymphography**
  - Able to detect metastases in normal size lymph nodes with a very high sensitivity and specificity
  - Requires intravenous injection of ultra small particles iron oxide (USPIO)
  - USPIO is taken up by normal lymph nodes, whereas metastatic lymph nodes show no uptake

MR Anatomy

- Uterine and cervical zonal anatomy
  - Uterus: Average length and width
    - Reproductive age: 8 x 5 cm
    - Postmenopausal: 5 x 2 cm
  - T1WI: Uterus of intermediate to low signal intensity
  - T2WI: Three distinct layers differentiated: Endometrium, junctional zone and myometrium
    - Endometrium: High SI, occupies central portion of uterus, thickness varies with menstrual cycle
    - Endometrial thickness: Width (both leaflets) sagittally at its thinnest after menstruation and at beginning of proliferative phase (1-3 mm), and thickest at mid secretory phase (up to 7 mm)
    - Junctional zone: Innermost myometrium layer of low SI that separates endometrium from outer myometrial layer

MR TECHNIQUE & ANATOMY

- Myometrium: Intermediate SI, higher than striated muscle, increases in SI in mid secretory phase
  - Parametrium: Intermediate SI on T1WI and variable SI on T2WI
  - Cervical zonal anatomy demonstrated with T2WI
  - Inner central zone of normal cervix
    - High SI on T2WI due to high percentage of mucus & endocervical glands
  - Surrounding cervical stroma
    - Low SI on T2WI due to high concentration of elastic fibrous tissue
  - Periphery of cervix
    - Intermediate SI similar to that of myometrium on all sequences
    - Occasionally, intermediate SI cervical mucosal folds (plicae palmatae) demonstrated between low SI cervical stroma and high SI endocervical canal
- Physiological variation
  - Pre-pubertal females
    - Endometrial layer: Either absent or minimal on T2WI
    - Myometrium: Lower SI than in women of reproductive age
  - At menstruation
    - Zonal anatomy ill defined and irregularly thick
    - Menstrual blood as low SI band in middle of endometrium
  - Postmenopausal
    - If not receiving exogenous hormones, uterine zonal anatomy often indistinct, endometrium less than 3 mm
    - If receiving exogenous hormones, appearance of uterus similar to women of reproductive age
  - Post-partum uterus: Vaginal delivery
    - Shortly after delivery zonal appearance different from non pregnant uterus
    - Endometrium: SI variable (fluid, blood), changes resolve after 1 week
    - Junctional zone: Usually not identifiable for approximately 6 weeks
    - Myometrium: Heterogeneous with engorged vessels of variable SI
    - Cervical stroma: High SI up to 30 hours after delivery, subsequently intermediate SI
  - Post-partum uterus: Cesarean section
    - Low SI scar visible anteriorly
    - Delay in involutionary changes: Uterine enlargement persists longer compared to vaginal delivery
    - Zonal anatomy: Identifiable from 6 months post cesarean section
- Exogenous therapy
  - Oral contraceptive pill causes increase in SI of myometrium on T1WI and T2WI (more pronounced with higher concentrations of hormone)
    - Myometrium may appear swollen and globular
    - Endometrium may become atrophic due to smooth muscle hypertrophy, sinusoidal dilatation, edema
  - Gonadotrophin releasing hormones result in involutional changes
    - Uterus similar SI as in postmenopausal state
  - Tamoxifen
    - Endometrium: Can appear thickened and heterogeneous ranging from hyperplasia to endometrial cancer
    - Junctional zone: Can appear thickened

Tissue Characterization (SI Compared to the SI of Outer Myometrium)

- Fat
  - High T1WI SI, intermediate T2WI SI, no enhancement
  - Examples: Normal pelvic fat, mature cystic teratoma
- Simple, uncomplicated fluid
  - Low T1WI SI, high T2WI SI, no enhancement
  - Examples: Urine, simple ascites, ovarian follicles
- Blood
  - Intracellular methemoglobin: High T1WI SI, low T2WI SI, no enhancement
  - Extracellular methemoglobin: High T1WI SI, high T2WI SI, no enhancement
  - Examples of methemoglobin: Subacute hematomas, endometriomas
  - Ferritin/hemosiderin: Low T1WI SI and T2WI SI, no enhancement
  - Example of ferritin/hemosiderin: In rim of endometriomas
- Smooth muscle and fibrous tissue
  - Isointense T1WI SI, low T2WI SI, variable enhancement
  - Examples: Adenomyosis, solid endometriosis, scar tissue
- Solid malignant tissue
  - Isointense T1WI SI, and T2WI SI, variable enhancement
  - Example: Endometrial carcinoma
- Mucin
  - Variable T1WI SI depending on amount of hydration of mucinous tissue, high T2WI SI, peripheral enhancement
  - Example: Mucinous ovarian carcinoma

SELECTED REFERENCES

1. Morakkabati-Spitz N et al: 3.0-T high-field magnetic resonance imaging of the female pelvis: preliminary experiences. Eur Radiol. 15(4):639-44, 2005
2. Padhani AR et al: Perfusion MR imaging of extracranial tumor angiogenesis. Top Magn Reson Imaging. 15(1):41-57, 2004
3. Kido A et al: Diffusely enlarged uterus: evaluation with MR imaging. Radiographics. 23(6):1423-39, 2003
4. Hamm B et al: MR imaging and CT of the female pelvis: radiologic-pathologic correlation. Eur Radiol. 9(1):3-15, 1999
5. Kubik-Huch RA: Female pelvis. Eur Radiol. 9(9):1715-21, 1999
6. Shiraiwa M et al: Cervical carcinoma: efficacy of thin-section oblique axial T2-weighted images for evaluating parametrial invasion. Abdom Imaging. 24(5):514-9, 1999
7. Siegelman ES et al: Tissue characterization in the female pelvis by means of MR imaging. Radiology. 212(1):5-18, 1999
8. Hricak K et al: MRI of the Pelvis: A Text Atlas. 1st ed. Norwalk, Appleton & Lange. 95-7, 1991

MR TECHNIQUE & ANATOMY

IMAGE GALLERY

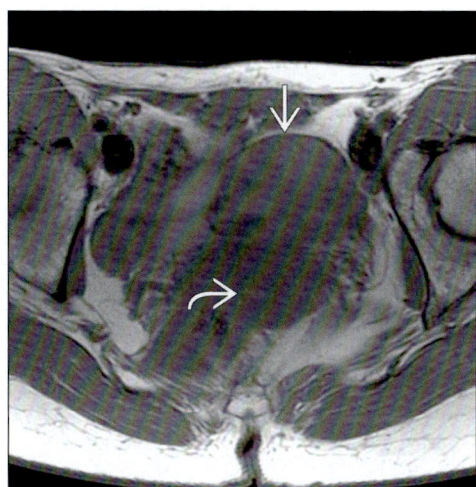
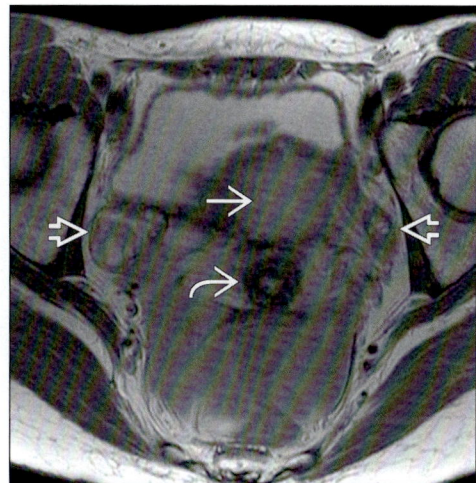

(Left) Axial T1WI MR shows uterine corpus ➡ and cervix ➡. Note that the uterine zonal anatomy is indistinct on T1W images. (Right) Axial T2WI MR shows an intermediate signal intensity myometrium ➡ at the level of the fundus and low signal intensity cervix ➡ containing high signal intensity secretions. Note normal appearances of both ovaries ➡ containing multiple follicles in this premenopausal woman.

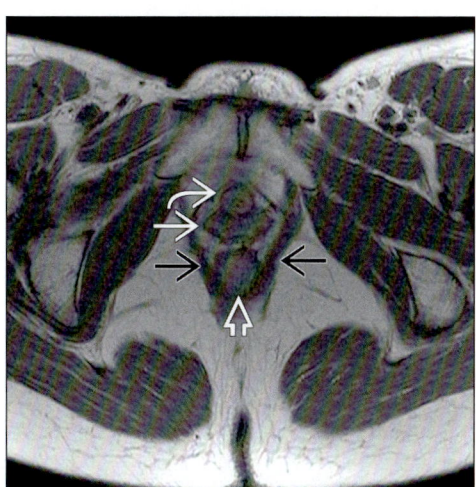
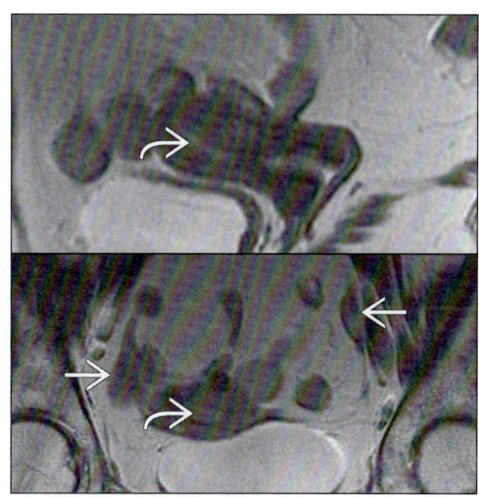

(Left) Axial T2WI MR at the level of lower vagina shows normal appearances of lower vagina ➡ situated posterior to the urethra ➡ and anterior to the rectum ➡. The levator sling ➡ is also elegantly demonstrated. (Right) Sagittal and coronal T2WI MR show typical appearances of the uterus in a postmenopausal woman. Note the indistinct zonal anatomy. The endometrium ➡ is thin. Both ovaries ➡ are small and do not contain any follicles.

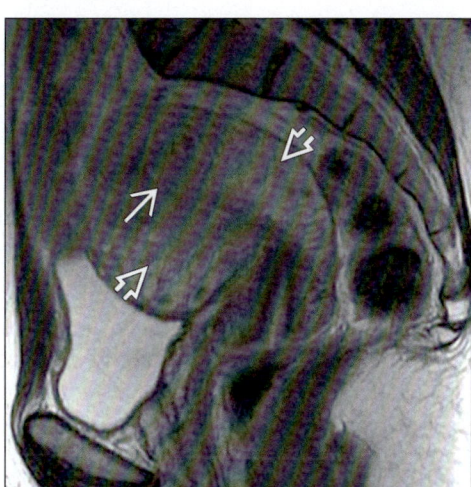
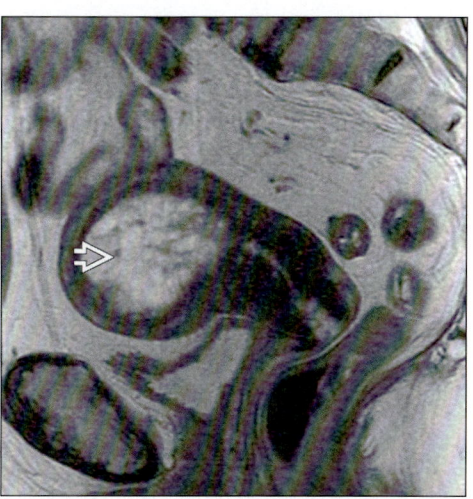

(Left) Sagittal T2WI MR shows the uterus in a woman on oral contraceptives. The myometrium ➡ is of high signal intensity and appears globular. The endometrium ➡ appears atrophic. (Right) Sagittal T2WI MR shows the uterus in a patient receiving tamoxifen for breast cancer treatment. The endometrium ➡ is thickened and heterogeneous. Pathology showed endometrial hyperplasia.

MR TECHNIQUE & ANATOMY

IMAGE GALLERY

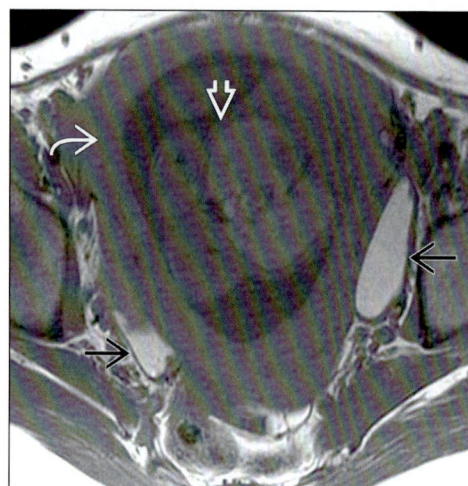 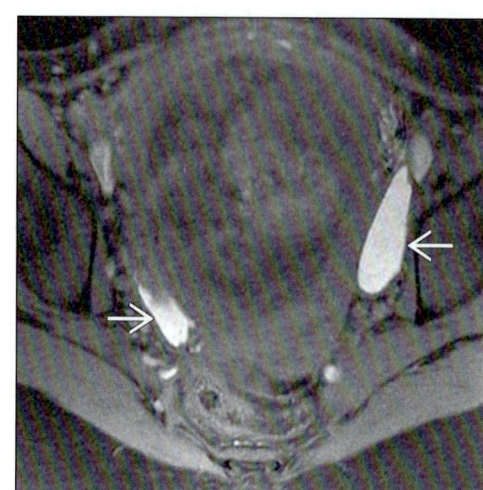

(Left) Axial T1WI MR shows bilateral high signal intensity adnexal lesions ➔ in a pregnant patient. Note the gravid uterus ➔ containing fetal parts ➔. (Right) Axial T1WI FS MR in the same patient as previous image shows bilateral adnexal lesions ➔ which remain of high signal intensity after fat suppression. The appearances are those of bilateral endometriomas.

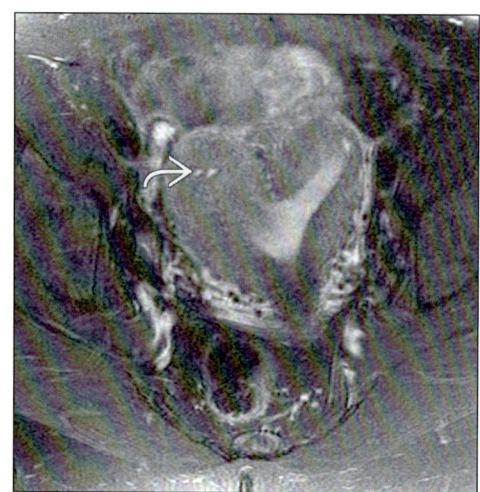 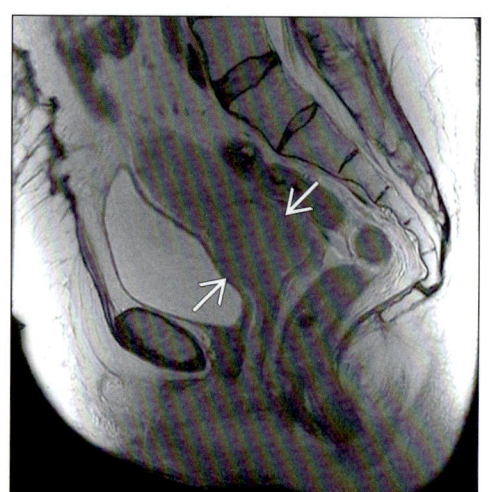

(Left) Axial T2WI FS MR shows a bicornuate uterus. Also note presence of adenomyosis as thickened junctional zone which contains foci of endometrial rests of high signal intensity ➔. (Right) Sagittal T2WI MR shows a large mass ➔ expanding the cervix and involving both anterior and posterior lips.

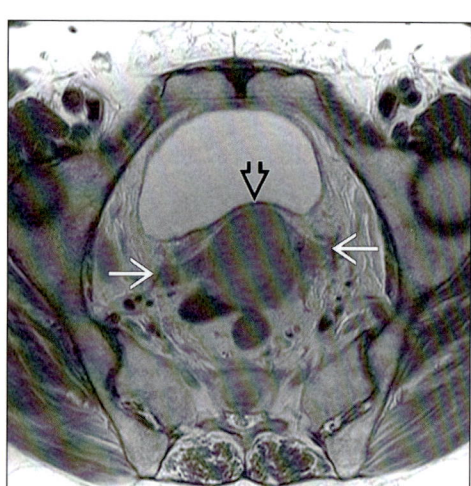 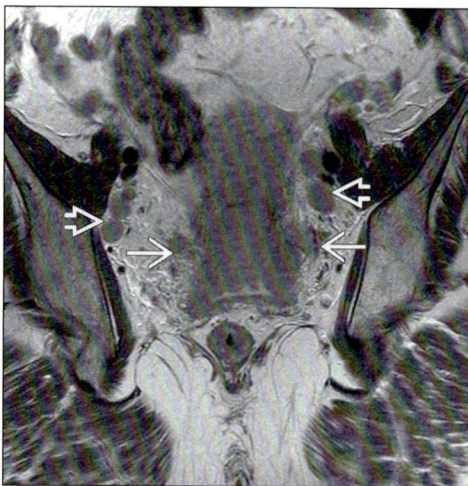

(Left) Axial oblique T2WI MR in the same patient as above right shows a large cervical mass ➔ extending to both parametria ➔. (Right) Coronal oblique T2WI MR in the same patient shows bilateral parametrial extension ➔ of the cervical tumor. Also note the presence of enlarged external iliac lymph nodes ➔ bilaterally. The oblique planes are crucial for accurate evaluation of parametrial invasion.

MR TECHNIQUE & ANATOMY

IMAGE GALLERY

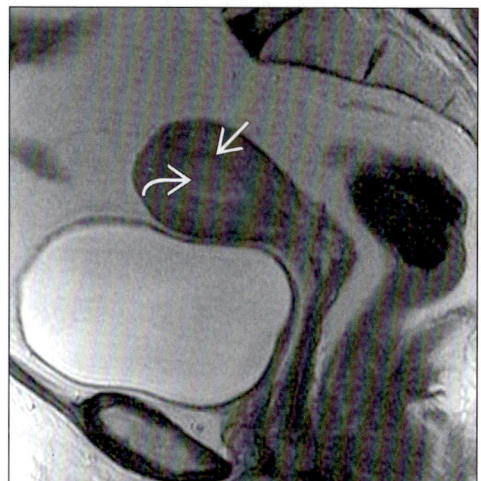
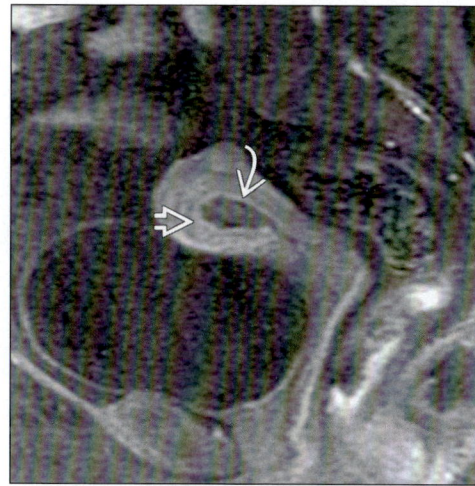

(Left) Sagittal T2WI MR shows thickening of the endometrium ➡ in a postmenopausal patient. Note the intact junctional zone ➡. *(Right)* Sagittal DCE T1WI FS MR (early phase) confirms the presence of thickened endometrium which enhances less than the adjacent myometrium ➡. Note the intact band of subendometrial enhancement ➡ indicating a stage IA endometrial cancer.

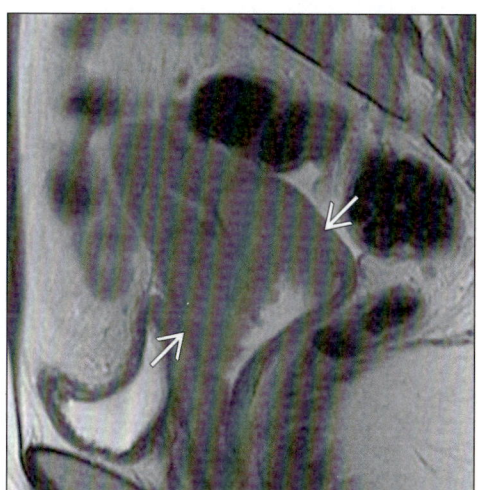
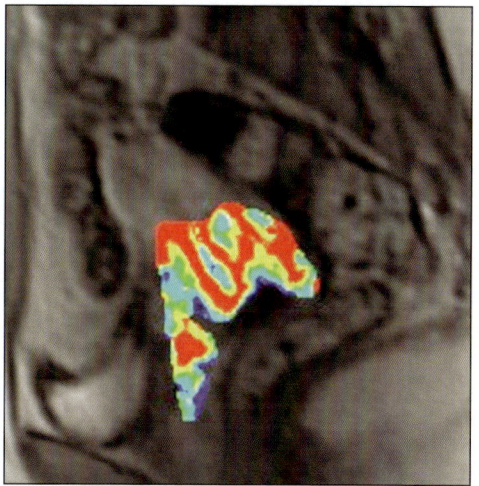

(Left) Sagittal T2WI MR shows a large cervical mass ➡ involving both anterior and posterior lips of the cervix. *(Right)* Color parametric data superimposed on 3D GRE T1WI (in the same patient as previous image) prior to start of radiochemotherapy shows a very heterogeneous tumor. Red represents areas of high perfusion and blue those of low perfusion.

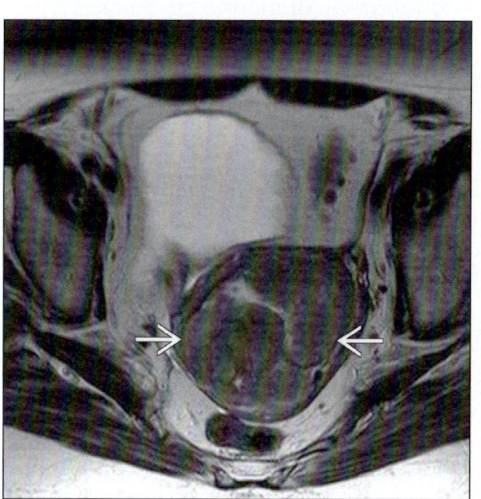
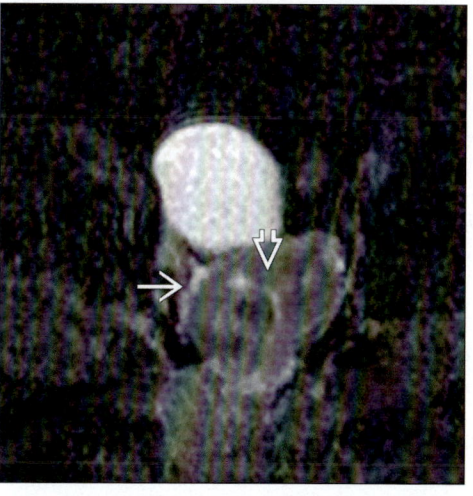

(Left) Axial T2WI MR shows a heterogeneous endometrial mass ➡ in a postmenopausal patient. *(Right)* Apparent diffusion coefficient (ADC) map calculated from different b-value images (0-1000) shows low ADC values in endometrial carcinoma ➡. Note high ADC values in the remaining intact myometrium ➡. (Courtesy A. Padhani, MD).

PET/CT TECHNIQUE & IMAGING ISSUES

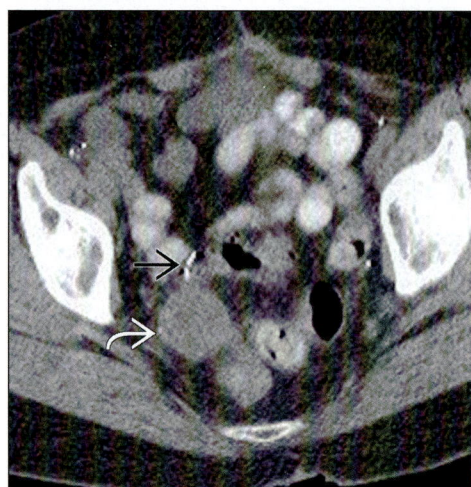 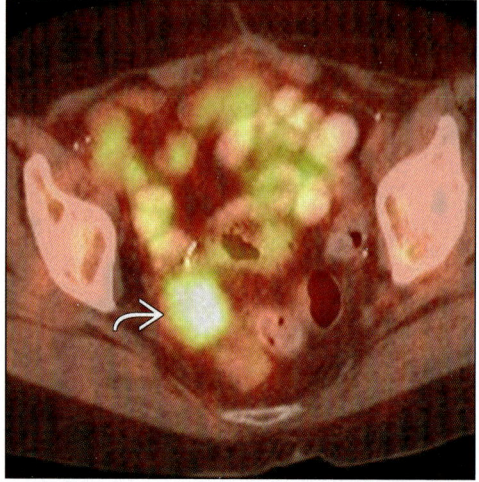

Axial NECT shows a cystic mass in the right adnexa in a patient with previous ovarian cancer. Note presence of surgical clips related to previous surgery for ovarian carcinoma.

Axial fused PET/CT (same patient as previous image) shows high FDG uptake within the right adnexal lesion in keeping with tumor recurrence.

TERMINOLOGY

Synonyms
- 18Fluorodeoxyglucose (18-FDG) PET/CT
  - 18-FDG is the most widely used tracer in the clinical practice, however other tracers are available

Definitions
- Combined metabolic (PET) and morphologic (CT) information

PRE-PROCEDURE

Indications
- Primary staging of pelvic malignancies, only in cases of equivocal CT and/or MR findings
- Restaging of pelvic malignancies, particularly if follow-up surgery is being considered
- Radiation therapy planning
  - Planning radiotherapy target volume
  - Curative versus palliative radiation therapy
- Site-specific indications
  - **Endometrial carcinoma**
    - Evaluation of treatment response
    - Detection of recurrent disease
    - Detection of lymph node metastases
    - Limited sensitivity in detecting metastatic lymph nodes < 1 cm
  - **Cervical carcinoma**
    - Detection of metastatic lymph nodes with better sensitivity and specificity than MR
    - Can be helpful in differentiating tumor recurrence from radiation changes
    - Has added value in patients with recurrent cervical cancer who undergo salvage therapy, as it can provide precise re-staging information
  - Vagina & vulva carcinoma
    - Evaluation of the extent of lymph node metastases
  - **Ovarian carcinoma**
    - Differentiation between residual and recurrent disease
    - To confirm the presence of solitary local recurrence prior to pelvic exenteration
    - Useful for an accurate selection of patients with late recurrent disease who may benefit from secondary cytoreductive surgery
    - Valuable when conventional studies are inconclusive or negative and tumor markers are rising
    - It is particularly useful for detecting tumor deposits in mesentery and bowel serosa
    - Sensitivity in detecting small tumor implants is limited
  - Other rare pelvic malignancies
    - Staging and follow-up of uterine sarcomas
    - Staging and follow-up of uterine lymphoma

Contraindications
- Pregnancy
- Breastfeeding

Advantages
- Precise localization of lesions on FDG PET scans within the anatomic reference frame provided by CT leading to increased specificity of the examination
- On PET/CT scanners the emission data can be corrected for photon attenuation using the CT scan to generate an attenuation map
  - Less statistical noise from CT compared with germanium 68 transmission data on stand-alone PET scanners
  - Due to fast CT data acquisition PET/CT examination time is 15-20 minutes shorter than PET with radioactive source transmission correction

PET/CT TECHNIQUE & IMAGING ISSUES

Key Facts

Pre-procedure
- **Endometrial carcinoma**
- Detection of lymph node metastases
- **Cervical carcinoma**
- Detection of metastatic lymph nodes with better sensitivity and specificity than MR
- Can be helpful in differentiating tumor recurrence from radiation changes
- Has added value in patients with recurrent cervical cancer who undergo salvage therapy, as it can provide precise re-staging information
- **Ovarian carcinoma**
- To confirm the presence of solitary local recurrence prior to pelvic exenteration
- Valuable when conventional studies are inconclusive or negative and tumor markers are rising
- Sensitivity in detecting small tumor implants is limited

Post-procedure
- Premenopausal endometrial FDG uptake changes cyclically, increasing during ovulatory and menstrual phases
- Postmenopausal endometrial FDG uptake is abnormal (unless patient is on HRT)
- Premenopausal ovarian FDG uptake may be functional as corpus luteum cysts can transiently increase ovarian uptake
- Postmenopausal ovarian FDG uptake is associated with malignancy
- Wait at least 6 weeks for PET/CT if tumor recurrence is suspected in the surgical or irradiated bed

---

  - More efficient use of fast-decaying PET pharmaceuticals
  - Need for PET transmission hardware and the cost of replacing germanium source rods is eliminated
- CECT acquired at the end of PET/CT examination offers a "one-stop shopping" imaging protocol in PET/CT
- Images can be transferred to a radiation therapy planning system

Disadvantages
- Increase in radiation dose compared to PET or CT when performed alone
- Artifacts due to use of CT data for attenuation correction
  - Use of concentrated CT contrast agents
  - Beam hardening artifacts due to metallic implants
  - Physiologic motion

New Developments
- 64-slice PET/CT scanners
- PET/MR scanners particularly useful in uterine malignancies
- New tumor-specific radiotracers

Patient Preparation
- Patients with insulin-dependent diabetes mellitus (IDDM) should be instructed to
  - Drink plenty of water (at least 1 litre) in the 6 hours leading up to the procedure
  - Not to fast in order to prevent disruption of blood glucose levels
- Patients without insulin-dependent diabetes mellitus (IDDM) should be instructed to
  - Drink plenty of water prior to the procedure
  - Abstain from food at least 4-6 hours prior to the procedure
- Patient should be comfortably warm prior to procedure as this aids relaxation and reduces unwanted muscle and physiological brown fat uptake
- 5 mg of oral diazepam may be administered one hour prior to imaging in order to reduce physiological brown fat uptake
  - This is not particularly important for pelvic malignancies but can be very helpful in head and neck lymph node imaging

Recommended Imaging Protocol
- Measurement of blood glucose level and injection of rapid-acting insulin if glucose level is above 8 mmol/L
- Administration of 1 L dilute oral contrast agent 1 hour before examination
- Administration of 10 mCi FDG 45-90 minutes before examination
- Bladder voiding just before examination to eliminate renally excreted FDG
- Comfortable head fixation with arms raised above the head
- Low-dose CT (20-60 mAs, according to body habitus) with no IV contrast agent
- PET starting at pelvic floor and moving cephalad to minimize pelvic image misregistration due to bladder filling
- Both PET and CT performed during free breathing
- Subsequent CECT tailored to the diagnostic problem

PROCEDURE

Procedure Steps
- Patient interview
  - Menstrual status
  - Phase of menstrual cycle if premenopausal
- Radiotracer injection
  - DOSE injected via the antecubital vein
  - Note if extravasation occurs in order to avoid confusion with pathological causes of subcutaneous tracer uptake
- Patient positioning
  - Patients are routinely imaged with their arms raised above their head in order to prevent beam hardening artifact on the CT component of the study

PET/CT TECHNIQUE & IMAGING ISSUES

Findings and Reporting
- Dedicated PET/CT workstation is mandatory for optimal viewing of the combined scans
  - Review CT data with appropriate window settings
  - Examine displays of both attenuation-corrected and non-attenuation-corrected PET data
  - Review fused PET/CT data set for accurate and reproducible correlation of a hypermetabolic focus seen on PET with correct anatomic equivalent on CT
  - Special fusion software can be employed to fuse PET/CT images with MR images
- Gynecological malignancies, peritoneal implants and metastatic lymph nodes are FDG-avid
  - Necrosis within a tumor and/or lymph node can appear as a photopenic area
- Standardized uptake values (SUV) should be routinely measured and reported
  - It is generally accepted that SUV > 2-3 indicates malignancy, while SUV < 2 is associated with benign lesions
  - Multiple SUV comparisons are mandatory for evaluation of tumor response to treatment provided same model PET/CT scanner and, tracer dose and post-injection imaging time are used

POST-PROCEDURE

Things To Avoid
- Contact with young children for 10 hours following injection of the radiotracer

Specific Interpretation Issues
- Attenuation correction
  - Overestimation of true FDG activity with CT-based attenuation correction due to overcorrection of photopenic areas corresponding to high-attenuation structures on CT
    - Concentrated CT contrast agents
    - CT beam hardening artifact due to metallic implants such as hip replacements, IUCD or surgical clips
  - Artifacts representing intense focal accumulation of positive oral contrast material can be resolved by
    - Viewing CT and non-attenuation-corrected PET images, which are not affected by high-density material
    - Use of diluted or negative-attenuation oral contrast material
    - Recently shown that coregistration with CECT data does not result in significant artifacts following CT attenuation correction
- Misregistration
  - False positive or negative PET/CT findings results from superimposition of FDG activity on inappropriate anatomic structures seen at CT due to
    - Breathing, patient motion, bowel motility, distention of urinary bladder
  - Normal "free" breathing (expiratory phase) is more suitable than maximum inspiratory or expiratory phases for acquisition of CT scans for coregistration
    - However, use of breath-hold imaging has distinct advantages in terms of CT image quality
  - Minimizing time delay between PET and CT is important in reducing patient motion between scans

Pearls and Pitfalls
- Physiological uptake
  - Uterus
    - Premenopausal endometrial FDG uptake changes cyclically, increasing during ovulatory and menstrual phases
    - Postmenopausal endometrial FDG uptake is abnormal (unless patient is on HRT)
  - Ovary
    - Premenopausal ovarian FDG uptake may be functional as corpus luteum cysts can transiently increase ovarian uptake
    - Corpus luteum cysts characteristically appear as small, rim-enhancing cyst at CECT
    - Increased FDG uptake in solid part of ovary which does not correspond to a corpus luteum cyst on CT should be regarded as suspicious for malignancy
    - Postmenopausal ovarian FDG uptake is associated with malignancy
- Nonneoplastic hypermetabolic lesions
  - Granulomatous disease, abscess, surgical changes, radiation changes, foreign body reaction
    - CT component can readily reveal clinically pertinent nonneoplastic conditions
    - Use of CECT can augment CT performance and avoid false-positive interpretation
    - Wait at least 6 weeks for PET/CT if tumor recurrence is suspected in the surgical or irradiated bed
    - Interpreting physicians should be aware of any pertinent clinical symptoms which may point to underlying inflammatory disease
- Benign tumors
  - Leiomyoma, benign endometrial abnormalities, benign ovarian tumors
- High background or neighboring FDG activity
  - CT often provides complimentary diagnostic information when there is high background FDG activity adjacent or surrounding a malignancy

SELECTED REFERENCES

1. Suzuki R et al: Validity of positron emission tomography using fluoro-2-deoxyglucose for the preoperative evaluation of endometrial cancer. Int J Gynecol Cancer, 2007
2. Unger JB et al: The prognostic value of pretreatment 2-[F]-fluoro-2-deoxy-d-glucose positron emission tomography scan in women with cervical cancer. Int J Gynecol Cancer, 2007
3. Blake MA et al: Pearls and pitfalls in interpretation of abdominal and pelvic PET-CT. Radiographics. 26(5):1335-53, 2006
4. von Schulthess GK et al: Integrated PET/CT: current applications and future directions. Radiology. 238(2):405-22, 2006
5. Lerman H et al: Normal and abnormal 18F-FDG endometrial and ovarian uptake in pre- and postmenopausal patients: assessment by PET/CT. J Nucl Med. 45(2):266-71, 2004

PET/CT TECHNIQUE & IMAGING ISSUES

IMAGE GALLERY

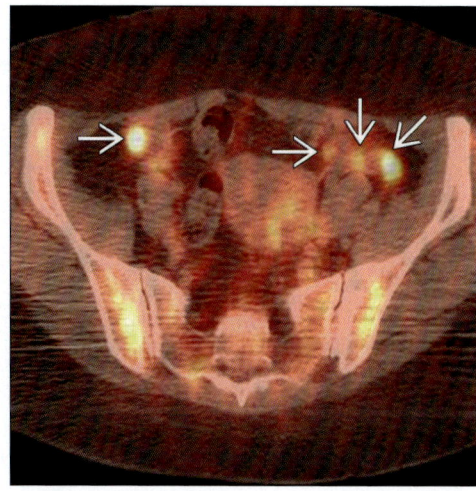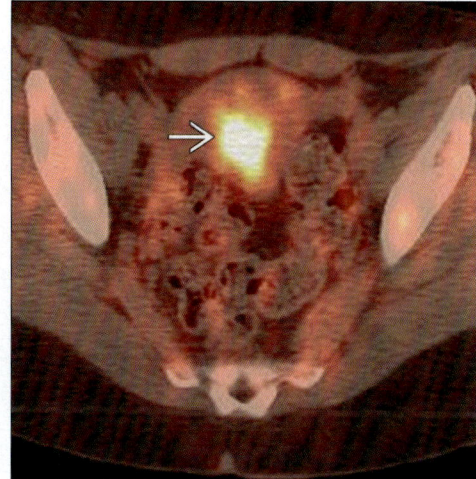

(Left) Axial fused PET/CT shows increased FDG uptake within multiple ovarian follicles ➡ in both ovaries. This is a normal finding in premenopausal women and should not be confused with malignancy. *(Right)* Axial fused PET/CT shows increased FDG uptake within the endometrial canal ➡ in a patient which is actively menstruating. This is a normal finding in premenopausal women and should not be confused with malignancy.

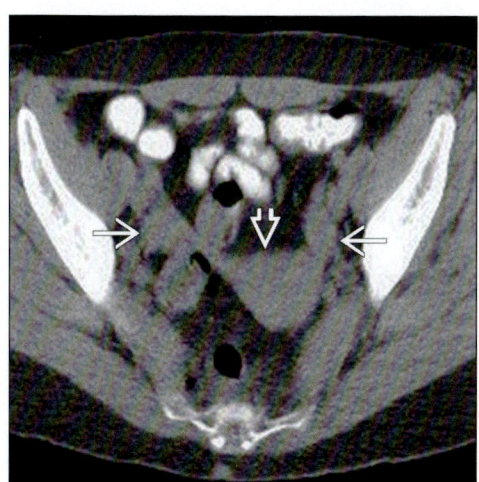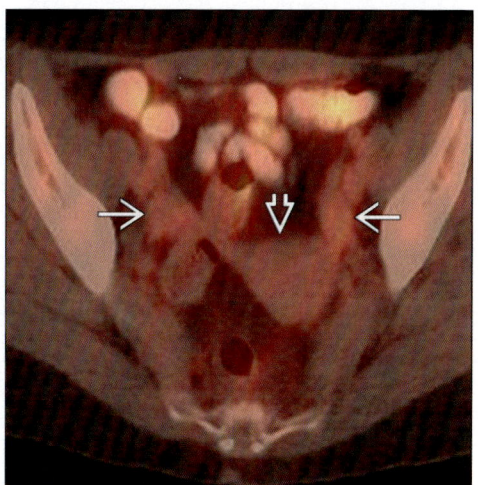

(Left) Axial NECT shows normal appearances to the uterus ➡ and both ovaries ➡ in a postmenopausal patient. Note the lack of follicles in both ovaries. *(Right)* Axial fused PET/CT shows no FDG uptake in uterus ➡ and both ovaries ➡ in the same patient as previous image. These are normal appearances in a postmenopausal patient.

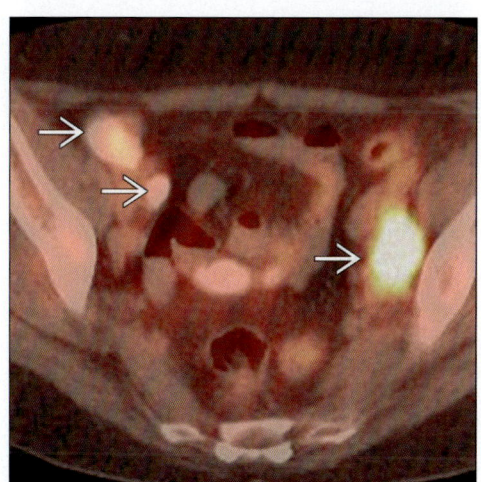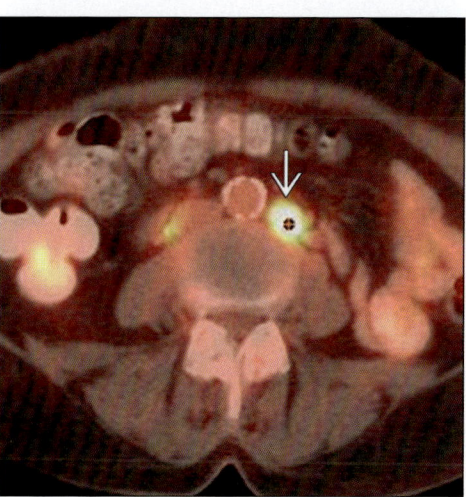

(Left) Axial fused PET/CT shows increased FDG uptake ➡ within enlarged bilateral external iliac lymph nodes in a patient with recurrent cervical cancer. *(Right)* Axial fused PET/CT shows increased FDG uptake ➡ within an enlarged left paraaortic lymph node (in same patient as previous image) with recurrent cervical cancer.

PET/CT TECHNIQUE & IMAGING ISSUES

IMAGE GALLERY

(Left) Axial NECT shows a nodal mass ➡ in the right inguinal region in a patient with recurrent cervical cancer. Note the thickening of the right pectineus muscle ➡. (Right) Axial fused PET/CT in the same patient as previous image shows increased FDG uptake ➡ within the right inguinal lymph node mass. Also note increased FDG uptake extending to the right pectineus muscle ➡ suggesting muscle involvement by tumor.

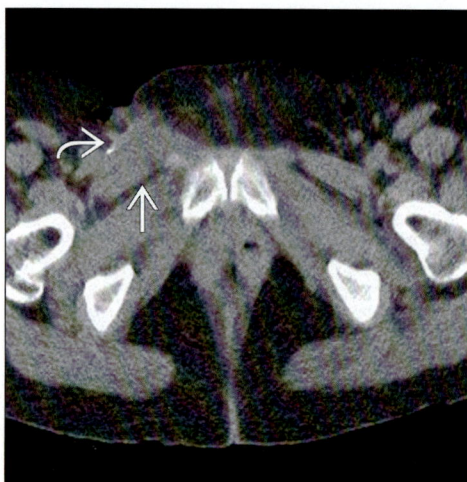
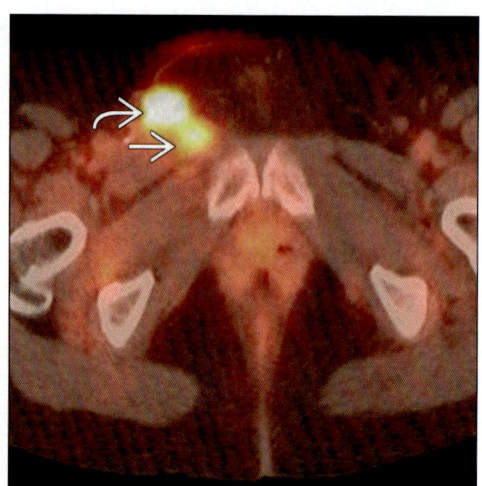

(Left) Axial NECT shows a soft tissue mass ➡ in the cervix in a patient with previous stage 2B cervical cancer treated with radiochemotherapy. (Right) Axial fused PET/CT in the same patient as previous image shows increased FDG ➡ uptake within the cervical soft tissue mass suggestive of tumor recurrence. Pathology: Recurrent adenocarcinoma of the cervix. Note physiological FDG uptake within the bladder ➡.

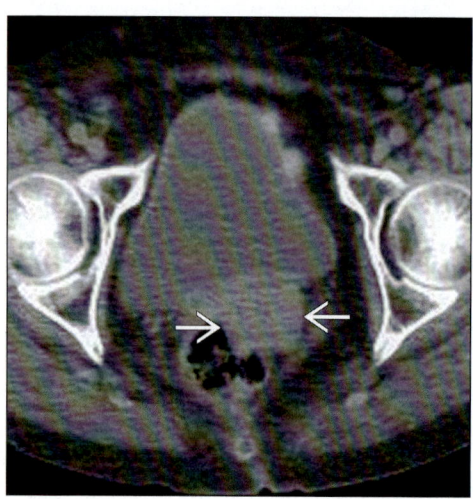
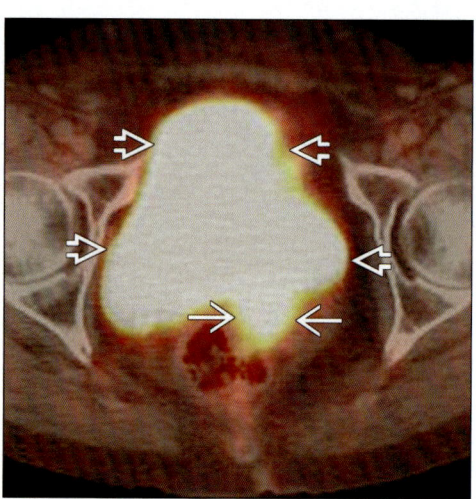

(Left) Axial NECT shows a vulva mass ➡ in a patient with vulva carcinoma. Also note the presence of a soft tissue mass ➡ in the right inguinal region. (Right) Axial fused PET/CT in the same patient as previous image shows avid FDG uptake in the vulva mass ➡. Also note the increased FDG uptake within the right inguinal lymph node mass ➡.

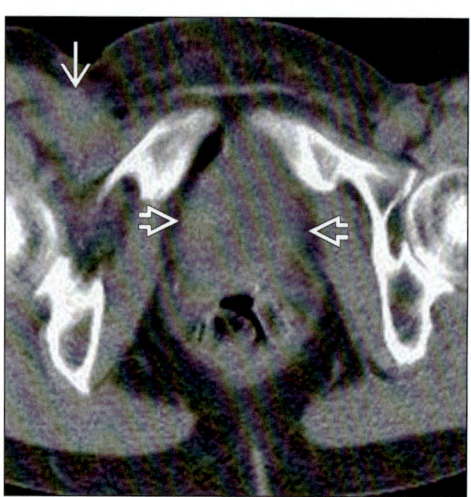
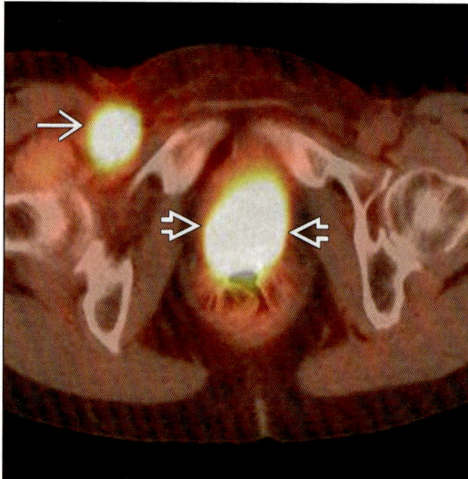

PET/CT TECHNIQUE & IMAGING ISSUES

IMAGE GALLERY

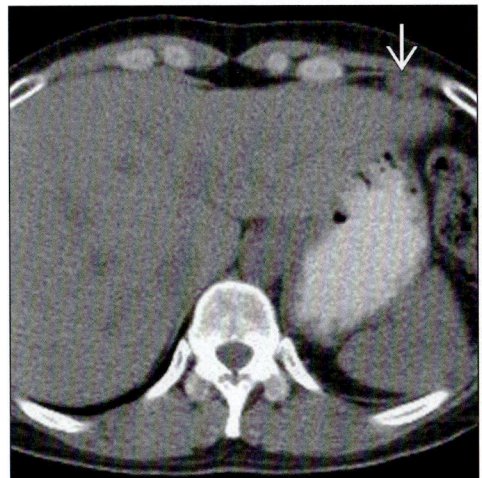
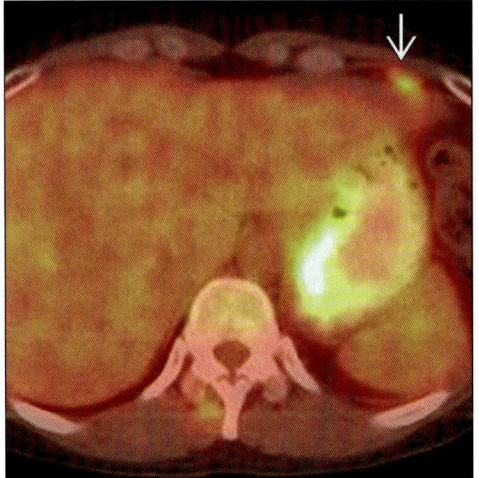

(Left) Axial NECT in a patient with stage 3 ovarian cancer shows a small peritoneal deposit ➡ indenting the liver surface on the left lobe. *(Right)* Axial fused PET/CT in the same patient as previous image shows increased FDG uptake within the peritoneal deposit ➡ along the liver capsule on the left in keeping with a tumor implant.

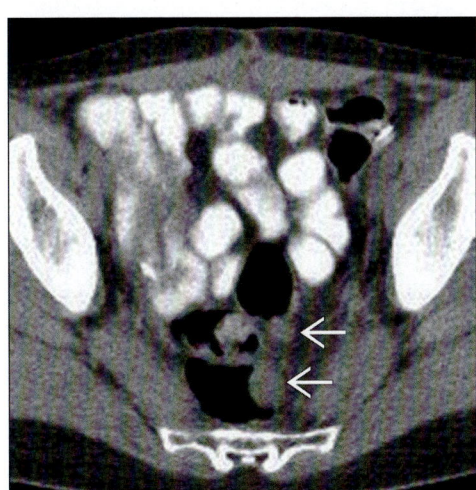
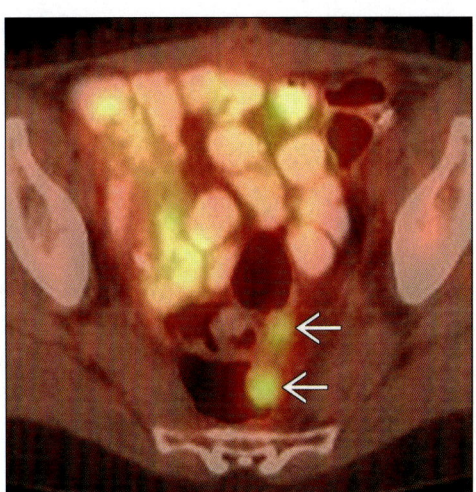

(Left) Axial NECT in the same patient as previous image shows small serosal implants ➡ along the sigmoid colon. *(Right)* Axial fused PET/CT in the same patient as previous image shows increased FDG uptake within the small serosal implants ➡ along the sigmoid colon, confirming presence of tumor implants.

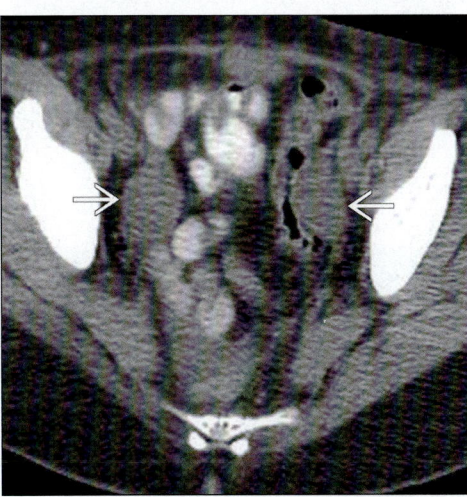
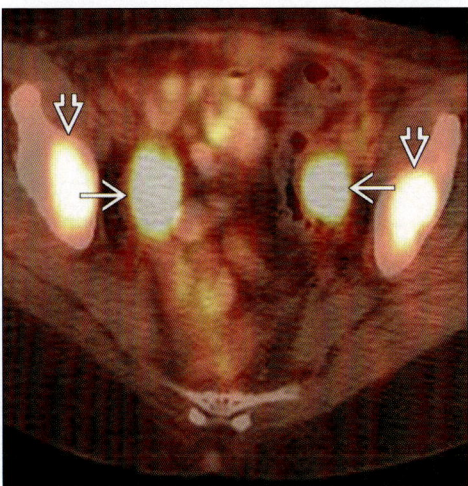

(Left) Axial NECT in a young patient with metastatic breast cancer shows solid appearances to both ovaries ➡ which are otherwise of normal size. *(Right)* Axial fused PET/CT in the same patient as previous image shows avid FDG uptake in both ovaries ➡ in keeping with bilateral ovarian metastases. Patient was on chemotherapy-induced menopause for 3 years. Also note the presence of FDG-avid bone metastases ➡ bilaterally.

SACRAL TERATOMA

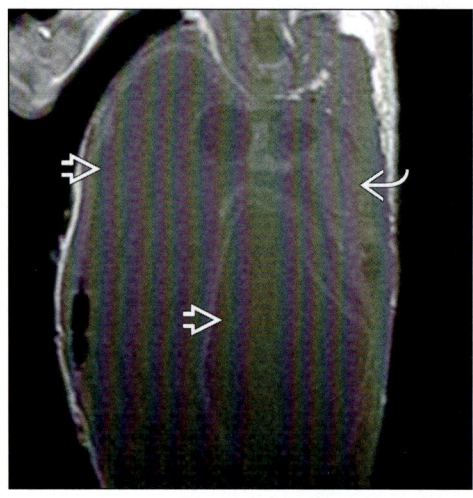

Sagittal T1WI MR shows a large heterogeneous mass with cystic ⇨ and solid ⇨ components in the sacrococcygeal region.

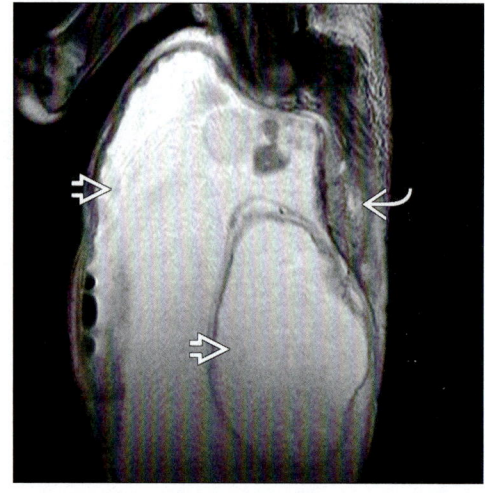

Sagittal T2WI MR shows a large sacrococcygeal mass with high signal intensity cystic ⇨ and intermediate signal intensity solid ⇨ components.

TERMINOLOGY

Abbreviations and Synonyms
- Sacrococcygeal teratoma

Definitions
- Derived from the Greek word "teratos" meaning "monster"
- Neoplasm composed of all three germ cell layers (ectoderm, mesoderm, and endoderm)
- Occurs in the midline and gonads, most commonly in the sacrococcygeal region

IMAGING FINDINGS

General Features
- Best diagnostic clue: Complex cystic and solid sacral region mass in the fetus or newborn
- Location
  - Often arise from tissues around tip of coccyx, rarely invading coccyx unless malignant
  - May extend posteriorly into buttocks and pelvis, or anteriorly displacing and compressing organs (rectum, vagina, urinary tract) without involving them
  - Occasional extension into spinal canal
- Size
  - Usually 5-15 cm, can be up to 30 cm
  - Immature forms tend to be larger than mature
  - Size does not predict biologic behavior
- Morphology: Usually cystic and solid, often with fat, calcifications and septations; purely cystic in 15%

Ultrasonographic Findings
- Cystic component is anechoic or hypoechoic; may have septations
- Echogenicity may represent solid component, diffusely microcystic component or hemorrhage
- Doppler US to evaluate tumor vascularity
- Polyhydramnios often present; placentomegaly, cardiomegaly, or non-immune hydrops fetalis are poor prognostic indicators
- Need to assess for other fetal anomalies

DDx: Sacral Masses

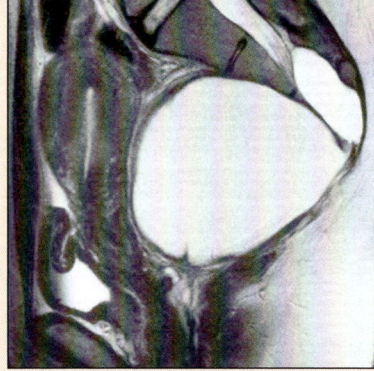
Anterior Meningocele

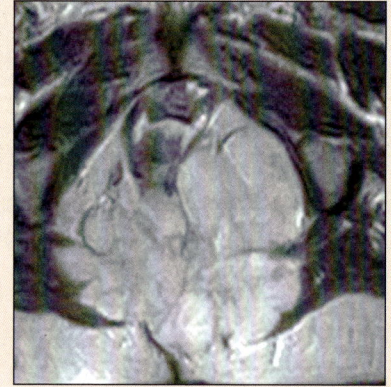
Sacrococcygeal Chordoma

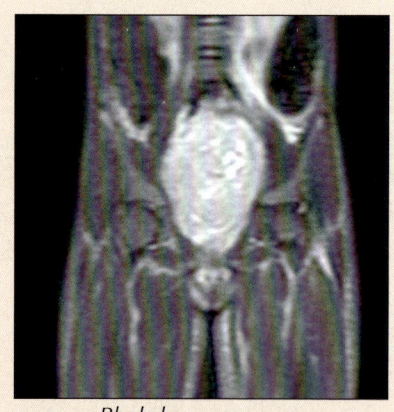
Rhabdomyosarcoma

SACRAL TERATOMA

Key Facts

Imaging Findings
- Usually 5-15 cm, can be up to 30 cm
- Size does not predict biologic behavior
- Morphology: Usually cystic and solid, often with fat, calcifications and septations; purely cystic in 15%
- MR allows multiplanar evaluation of tumor extent, tumor content, presence of hemorrhage: Factors known to influence prognosis
- Assess intrapelvic and intraabdominal extent, relationship to pelvic viscera, presence of urologic complications (common) and extension into spinal canal
- Polyhydramnios often present; placentomegaly, cardiomegaly, or non-immune hydrops fetalis are poor prognostic indicators
- Best imaging tool: MR

Top Differential Diagnoses
- Myelomeningocele, Especially Anterior Sacral Meningocele

Pathology
- Epidemiology: Most common congenital neoplasm, affecting 1 in 40,000 infants
- Mature or immature types, composed of all three germ cell lines

Clinical Issues
- Most present in newborn as a large exophytic sacral mass, usually immature form and benign
- Gender: Female preponderance 4:1
- Malignant transformation occurs in 5-10% of tumors found before age 2 months, 50-90% in tumors discovered at age 2-4 months

CT Findings
- Complex mass with low attenuation fat, fluid-attenuation cystic and dense calcific components
- CT better depicts the boney and cartilaginous elements of mature teratomas than MR

MR Findings
- MR allows multiplanar evaluation of tumor extent, tumor content, presence of hemorrhage: Factors known to influence prognosis
- Fat (high T1 and T2, suppresses with fat-saturation) differentiated from hemorrhage (usually high T1, variable T2)
- Assess intrapelvic and intraabdominal extent, relationship to pelvic viscera, presence of urologic complications (common) and extension into spinal canal
- Useful for deciding mode of delivery and planning postpartum surgery

Imaging Recommendations
- Best imaging tool: MR
- Protocol advice: T1 weighted with and without fat-saturation, T2 weighted, and fat-saturated post-contrast sequences

DIFFERENTIAL DIAGNOSIS

Myelomeningocele, Especially Anterior Sacral Meningocele
- Neural tube defect and sacral anomaly are present
- Meningeal outpouching communicating with spinal subarachnoid space through a defect in the sacrum

Developmental Cyst (Tail-Gut Cyst, Dermoid Cyst, Epidermoid Cyst)
- Uni- or multilocular complex cystic mass derived from a single germ cell layer

Duplication Cyst
- Cystic mass with well-formed dual layers of smooth muscle and neural plexuses

Sacrococcygeal Chordoma
- Midline, expansile and destructive bone tumor

Pelvic Sarcomas
- Rhabdomyosarcoma is the most common pelvic sarcoma in this age group

Extrarenal Wilms Tumor
- Rare tumor developing primarily outside the kidneys, and not as a metastatic renal Wilms tumor
- Heterogeneous solid mass with necrosis and/or hemorrhage, and absence of teratomatous elements
- Located in the pelvis, inguinal region, retroperitoneum and thorax

PATHOLOGY

General Features
- Genetics
  - No known chromosomal aberration
  - Rarely presents as part of the autosomal dominant Currarino anomaly consisting of triad of presacral mass (more commonly anterior meningocele), partial sacral agenesis, and anorectal defects
- Etiology: Thought to arise in early gestation from pluripotent germ cells originating in the primitive streak and developing in Hensen node, a remnant at the tip or anterior surface of the coccyx
- Epidemiology: Most common congenital neoplasm, affecting 1 in 40,000 infants
- Associated abnormalities: Genitourinary (hydronephrosis, renal dysplasia, urethral atresia, duplication of uterus or vagina, undescended testes), gastrointestinal (rectal atresia or stenosis), vertebral (spina bifida, sacral agenesis, meningocele), limb (hip dislocation)

SACRAL TERATOMA

Gross Pathologic & Surgical Features
- Midline, encapsulated mass with gray-tan nodules consisting of varying portions of solid tissue, myxoid, hemorrhagic, and cystic areas
- Mature forms may contain fat, bone, cartilage, hair, occasionally a partly or fully developed body part
- Cysts may be filled with serous, mucoid, sebaceous or cerebrospinal fluid and lined by true epithelium

Microscopic Features
- Mature or immature types, composed of all three germ cell lines
- Predominance of ectodermal (especially neural) and mesodermal elements
- Immature elements consist mainly of primitive neuroglial tissue and neuroepithelial rosettes
- Histological grading based on proportion of immature tissue and presence of malignant elements (yolk sac, embryonal, choriocarcinoma); histologic grade does not correlate directly with prognosis

Staging, Grading or Classification Criteria
- Classified according to a system developed by Altman and associates of the Surgical Section of the American Academy of Pediatrics
- 4 types based on the amount of mass present externally versus internally
  - Type I: Mass developing only outside the fetus
  - Type II: Extrafetal and intrapelvic presacral extent
  - Type III: Extrafetal and abdominopelvic extent
  - Type IV: Mass developing completely in the fetal pelvis

CLINICAL ISSUES

Presentation
- Most common signs/symptoms
  - May present prenatally as uterus size greater than dates due to tumor and/or polyhydramnios
  - Most can be detected between the 22nd and the 34th week of gestation
- Other signs/symptoms: Tumor markers (alpha-fetoprotein, Beta-HCG) may be elevated, especially in malignant teratomas

Demographics
- Age
  - Most present in newborn as a large exophytic sacral mass, usually immature form and benign
  - Mixed malignant sacral teratomas more commonly found in older infants and children
  - Completely presacral tumors (type 4) may remain undetected until after age 4, occasionally presenting in adulthood
- Gender: Female preponderance 4:1

Natural History & Prognosis
- Prenatal maternal complications (up to 80%) include polyhydramnios, oligohydramnios, preterm labor, preeclampsia, hemolysis, elevated liver enzymes, low platelets (HELLP) syndrome
- Mortality rate 15-35%; 5% for diagnosis at birth, 50% when discovered prenatally
- Poor prognostic indicators: Hydrops and cardiac failure from vascular steal by tumor, solid composition (vs. cystic), high vascularity, tumor hemorrhage or rupture, intrapelvic extension, early gestational age
- Malignant transformation occurs in 5-10% of tumors found before age 2 months, 50-90% in tumors discovered at age 2-4 months
- Resectable tumors, regardless of tumor type, have excellent prognosis, with > 90% event-free survival
- Prognosis worse if surgical margins are positive due to high recurrence rate, but recurrences can be successfully treated with surgery and/or chemotherapy

Treatment
- Treatment options include open fetal surgery and radio frequency ablation, as well as complete tumor resection and chemotherapy following delivery

DIAGNOSTIC CHECKLIST

Consider
- Large heterogeneous cystic and solid presacral mass in a fetus or neonate

Image Interpretation Pearls
- Often discovered on antenatal obstetric ultrasound, presenting as a complex pelvic mass
- May be associated with other congenital anomalies, but absence of sacral dysraphism excludes meningocele or myelomeningocele
- CT and MR show a complex mass with varying amounts of fat, calcification, bone, cartilage and other mesenchymal elements, depending on level of maturity
- MR is useful for assessing local extent and planning delivery and surgery

SELECTED REFERENCES

1. Woodward PJ et al: From the archives of the AFIP: a comprehensive review of fetal tumors with pathologic correlation. Radiographics. 25(1):215-42, 2005
2. Hedrick HL et al: Sacrococcygeal teratoma: prenatal assessment, fetal intervention, and outcome. J Pediatr Surg. 39(3):430-8; discussion 430-8, 2004
3. Avni FE et al: MR imaging of fetal sacrococcygeal teratoma: diagnosis and assessment. AJR Am J Roentgenol. 178(1):179-83, 2002
4. Perrelli L et al: Sacrococcygeal teratoma. Outcome and management. An analysis of 17 cases. J Perinat Med. 30(2):179-84, 2002
5. Westerburg B et al: Sonographic prognostic factors in fetuses with sacrococcygeal teratoma. J Pediatr Surg. 35(2):322-5; discussion 325-6, 2000
6. Chisholm CA et al: Prenatal diagnosis and perinatal management of fetal sacrococcygeal teratoma. Am J Perinatol. 16(1):47-50, 1999
7. Rescorla FJ et al: Long-term outcome for infants and children with sacrococcygeal teratoma: a report from the Childrens Cancer Group. J Pediatr Surg. 33(2):171-6, 1998
8. Keslar PJ et al: Germ cell tumors of the sacrococcygeal region: radiologic-pathologic correlation. Radiographics. 14(3):607-20; quiz 621-2, 1994

SACRAL TERATOMA

IMAGE GALLERY

Typical

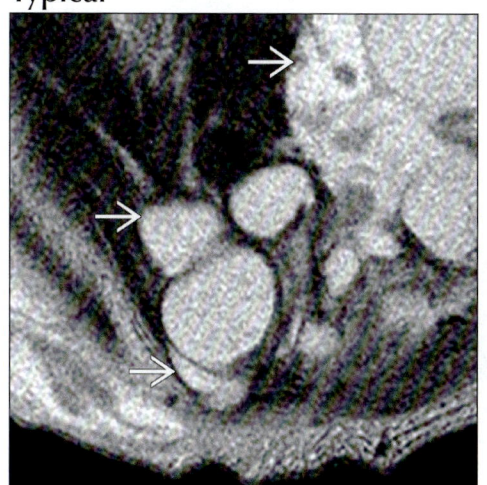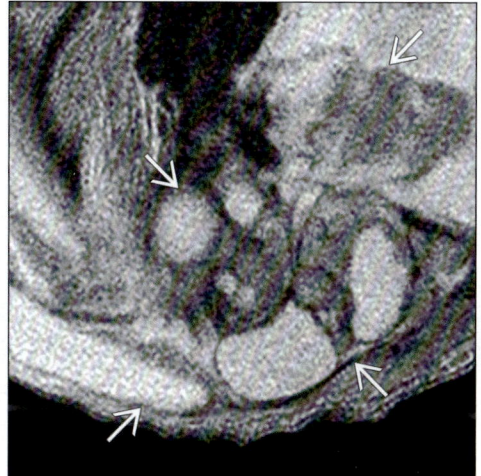

(Left) Axial T2WI MR shows that the tumor ➡ involves the sacrum and extends into the pelvis anteriorly on the left side. *(Right)* Axial T2WI MR shows that the coccyx is also replaced by heterogeneous cystic and solid mass ➡.

Typical

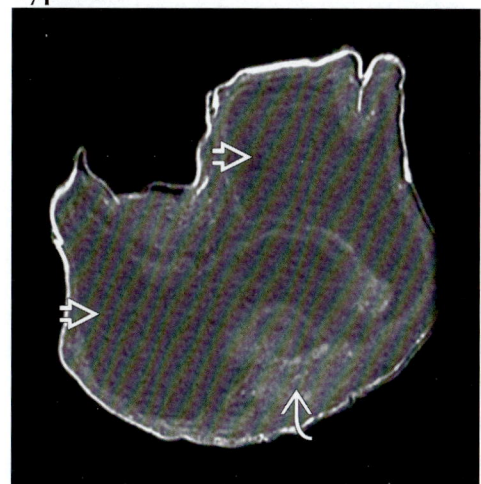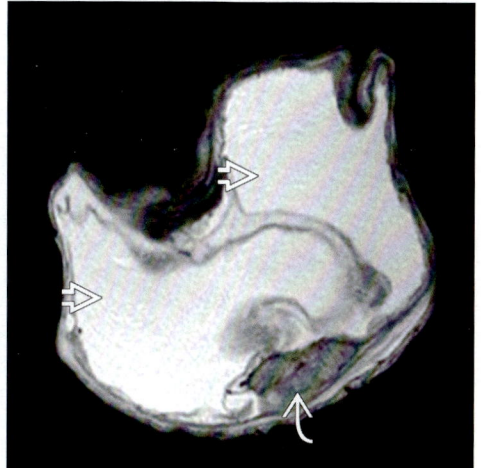

(Left) Axial T1WI MR shows the midsection of the tumor with encapsulated cystic ➡ and solid ➡ components. *(Right)* Axial T2WI MR shows high signal intensity cystic ➡ and intermediate signal intensity solid ➡ components of the mass.

Typical

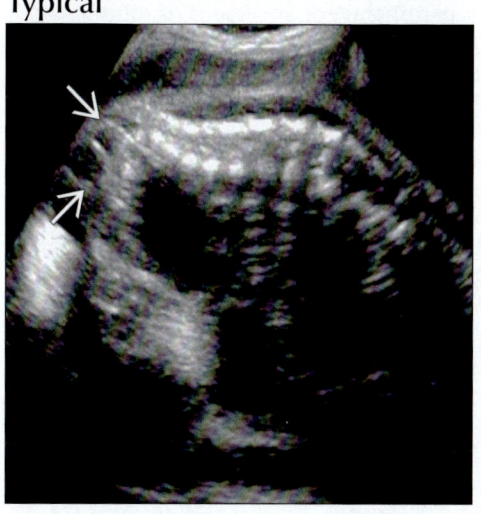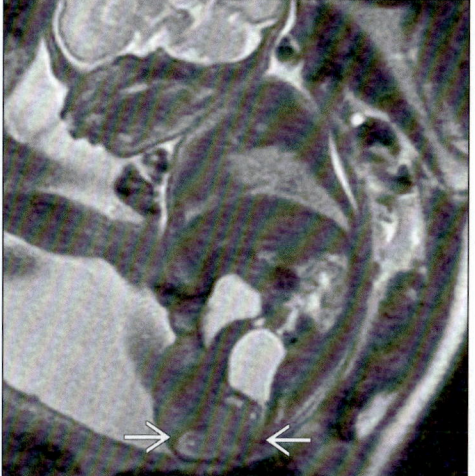

(Left) Sagittal transabdominal ultrasound shows a cystic sacral teratoma ➡ detected antenatally. *(Right)* Sagittal T2WI MR shows a sacrococcygeal teratoma ➡ seen on fetal MR.

EXTRAPERITONEAL SARCOMA

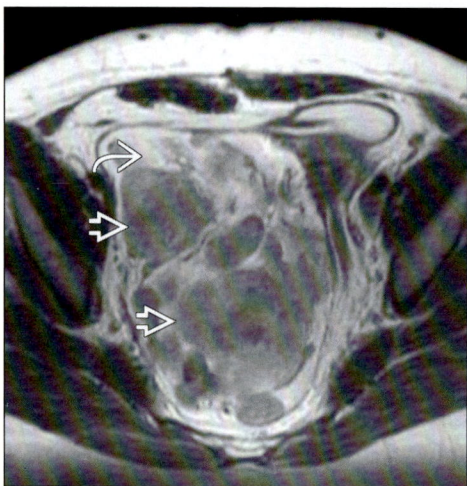

Axial T2WI MR shows a large right pelvic liposarcoma with multiple soft tissue intensity nodular ⇨ and fatty ➥ components.

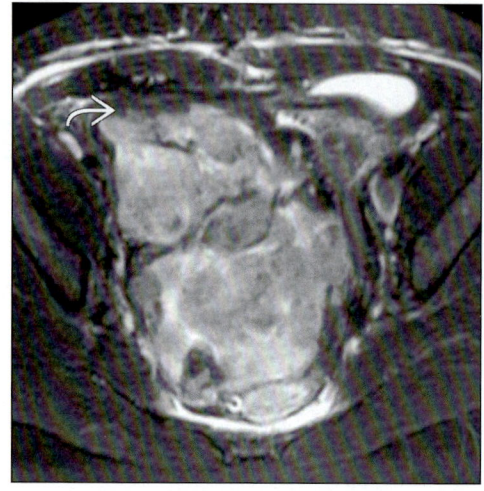

Axial T2WI FS MR shows that the fatty ➥ components of the mass lose signal.

TERMINOLOGY

Definitions
- Tumors of mesenchymal origin including muscle, endothelium, peripheral nerves, cartilage and connective tissue

IMAGING FINDINGS

General Features
- Best diagnostic clue
  - Lobulated heterogeneous masses with variable solid, necrotic, and hemorrhagic components
  - May contain fat (liposarcoma) or calcifications
- Location
  - Those originating in true pelvis arise between pelvic inlet (bounded by symphysis pubis, iliopectineal line and sacral promontory) and pelvic outlet (anterior pubic arch, ischial tuberosities and coccyx)
  - May extend to retroperitoneum and/or to thigh
  - May invade or displace adjacent pelvic viscera, sidewall, muscle, neurovascular structures, abdominal wall, bone, joint
- Size: Large at presentation, mean 5-15 cm
- Morphology
  - Depends on subtype and grade
  - Liposarcoma may be predominantly fatty if well-differentiated
  - Higher grade tumors may contain necrosis and hemorrhage

CT Findings
- NECT
  - Well-differentiated liposarcoma is predominantly of fatty density with thick septa and/or nodular soft tissue masses
  - Other sarcomas are usually of soft tissue density, and heterogeneous with central areas of low attenuation, corresponding to myxoid regions, hemorrhage or necrosis
  - Useful for assessing involvement of adjacent bone
- CECT
  - Nodular or peripheral enhancement of solid components of the mass
  - Well-differentiated liposarcoma may show subtle nodular or septal enhancement

DDx: Pelvic Masses

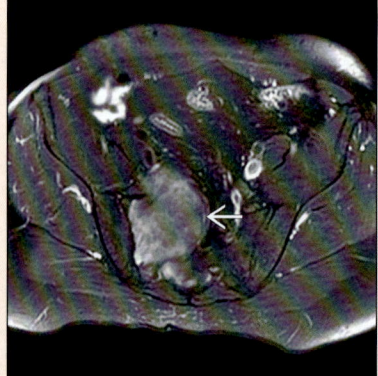
Schwannoma

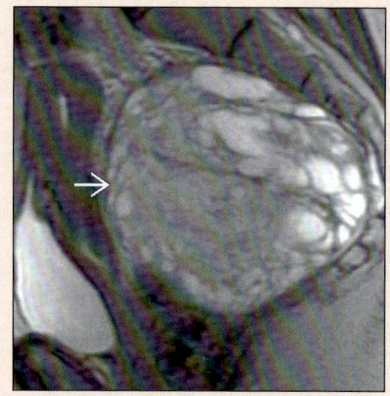
Hemangiopericytoma

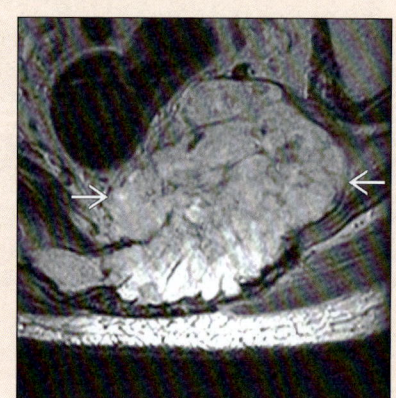
Sacral Chordoma

EXTRAPERITONEAL SARCOMA

Key Facts

Terminology
- Tumors of mesenchymal origin including muscle, endothelium, peripheral nerves, cartilage and connective tissue

Imaging Findings
- T1WI: Usually low to intermediate; may have hyperintense hemorrhagic component
- T2WI: Usually intermediate to hyperintense; low signal foci may represent fibrous or calcific elements
- Nodular or peripheral enhancement of solid components
- Best imaging tool: MR provides excellent soft tissue definition, and multiplanar capability shows relationship of tumor to surrounding structures

Pathology
- As degree of histologic differentiation declines, determination of cellular origin becomes increasingly difficult

Clinical Issues
- Most common signs/symptoms: Present late with vague abdominal pain, constipation, urinary or neurological symptoms related to large tumor size and adjacent organ invasion
- Prognosis related to tumor size, histologic grade, resectability with negative margins and presence of metastases are negative prognostic features
- Lymph node involvement is rare
- Large size at presentation and adjacent organ invasion make surgical resection with negative margins difficult

---

  ○ Staging evaluation of lungs and liver usually performed with CT

MR Findings
- T1WI: Usually low to intermediate; may have hyperintense hemorrhagic component
- T2WI: Usually intermediate to hyperintense; low signal foci may represent fibrous or calcific elements
- T2WI FS: Well-differentiated liposarcoma is hyperintense on T1WI and T2WI and loses signal with fat-saturation
- T1 C+
  ○ Nodular or peripheral enhancement of solid components
  ○ Well-differentiated liposarcoma may show subtle nodular or internal lace-like enhancement

Nuclear Medicine Findings
- PET
  ○ Useful in detection of local and systemic recurrences
  ○ Intensity of uptake by tumor correlates with grade of malignancy

Imaging Recommendations
- Best imaging tool: MR provides excellent soft tissue definition, and multiplanar capability shows relationship of tumor to surrounding structures
- Protocol advice: T1WI, T2WI FS, T1 C+ FS

DIFFERENTIAL DIAGNOSIS

Different Types of Sarcomas
- Malignant fibrous histiocytoma, liposarcoma, leiomyosarcoma, rhabdomyosarcoma (pediatric group), malignant peripheral nerve sheath tumor, undifferentiated sarcoma, hemangiopericytoma, etc.
- Histopathologic examination required to distinguish various types of sarcomas
- Imaging can provide clues in some cases

Tumors Originating from other Pelvic Organs such as Bone, Uterus, Ovary or Rectum
- Imaging evaluation help identify site of origin and extent of disease

Neurogenic Tumor, such as Neurofibroma, Schwannoma
- Occur in presacral region and may expand sacral neural foramina
- "Ancient schwannoma" contains extensive degenerative changes and may mimic a sarcoma on imaging

Myxoma
- Benign soft tissue tumor containing gelatinous material

Lymphoma
- May present as pelvic mass, usually with other involved lymph nodes (unusual with sarcoma)

PATHOLOGY

General Features
- General path comments
  ○ Classified according to cellular differentiation
  ○ As degree of histologic differentiation declines, determination of cellular origin becomes increasingly difficult
- Etiology
  ○ Prior exposure to radiation, rarely chemical agents
  ○ Increased frequency in hereditary cancer syndromes, such as neurofibromatosis type 1, Li-Fraumeni syndrome (p53 mutation), Gardner syndrome

Gross Pathologic & Surgical Features
- Gray-white to yellow in appearance
  ○ Mucoid nodules present in myxoid variants of malignant fibrous histiocytoma and liposarcoma

EXTRAPERITONEAL SARCOMA

- ○ Well-differentiated liposarcomas contain variable proportions of relatively mature fat and fibrocollagenous tissues
- Solid multilobulated mass with well-circumscribed or ill-defined infiltrative borders
  - ○ May be enclosed by pseudocapsule consisting of compressed tumor cells and a fibrovascular zone of reactive tissue with variable inflammatory component
  - ○ High grade sarcomas have a poorly-defined reactive zone that may be locally invaded by tumor
- High grade sarcomas vary from pink-tan to brown and may have extensive hemorrhage and necrosis

Microscopic Features

- Wide range of histologies depending on particular mesenchymal tissue present; a few are given
  - ○ Malignant fibrous histiocytoma: Pleomorphic spindle cells form fascicular or typical storiform patterns, and fibroblasts, histiocyte-like cells and inflammatory cells also present
  - ○ Liposarcoma: Lipoblasts present and subtypes may have mature fat (well-differentiated type), myxoid ground substance and delicate vascular network (myxoid type), poorly-differentiated round cells (round cell type), or bizarre lipoblasts and atypical stromal cells (pleomorphic type)
  - ○ Leiomyosarcoma: Interlacing bundles of smooth muscle cells with variable uniformity, anaplasia with atypical nuclei and multinucleated cells, and mitoses according to histologic grade

Staging, Grading or Classification Criteria

- Classified according to cell of origin
  - ○ Immunostaining, electron microscopy, cytogenetic analysis, and molecular markers for gene rearrangements may all be used in determining diagnosis depending on degree of differentiation of specific tumor
- Staged according to American Joint Committee on Cancer criteria based on tumor histologic grade, size, location, nodal status and presence of metastases
  - ○ Histopathological features (cellularity, growth pattern, matrix production, cell size and shape, atypia and anaplasia, mitoses, necrosis) determine tumor grade (low, intermediate, high)
  - ○ Higher grade lesions have higher propensity to recur locally and metastasize

CLINICAL ISSUES

Presentation

- Most common signs/symptoms: Present late with vague abdominal pain, constipation, urinary or neurological symptoms related to large tumor size and adjacent organ invasion

Demographics

- Age
  - ○ Malignant fibrous histiocytoma, liposarcoma and most other sarcomas usually develop in adults
  - ○ Rhabdomyosarcoma is usually seen in children under age of 15

Natural History & Prognosis

- Prognosis related to tumor size, histologic grade, resectability with negative margins and presence of metastases are negative prognostic features
- Overall poor prognosis, with 5 year survival 20-60%
- Lymph node involvement is rare
- Local recurrence is common
- Metastases present in up to 25% at presentation, usually from high grade tumors

Treatment

- Wide surgical excision
  - ○ Large size at presentation and adjacent organ invasion make surgical resection with negative margins difficult
  - ○ High rate of morbidity and complications after pelvic surgery
  - ○ Resection of local recurrence may be possible and can improve survival, especially in low grade tumors
- Adjuvant radiation therapy
  - ○ Pre-operative radiation uses a smaller field, shrinks the primary tumor and may allow more extensive resection while preserving adjacent structures
  - ○ Post-operative radiation covers the entire surgical field, with lower rate of wound complications
  - ○ Brachytherapy sometimes delivers short-duration high dose localized radiation to tumor bed
- Adjuvant chemotherapy
  - ○ May be used pre-operatively or in patients with metastatic disease and may improve time to local and distant recurrence

DIAGNOSTIC CHECKLIST

Consider

- Major role of imaging is to define local extent of sarcomas

Image Interpretation Pearls

- Large non-visceral pelvic mass
- Multilobulated heterogeneous mass locally infiltrating adjacent tissues
- High grade tumors may have areas of necrosis and metastases at presentation
- Variable composition of tumor produces wide spectrum of appearances on imaging
- If intervening fat plane is not visible, report as "contact"; diagnose invasion only if gross interdigitation is evident

SELECTED REFERENCES

1. Keyzer-Dekker CMG et al: Adult pelvic sarcomas: a heterogeneous collection of sarcomas? Sarcoma. 8(1):19-24, 2004
2. Lewis SJ et al: Soft tissue sarcomas involving the pelvis. J Surg Oncol. 77(1):8-14; discussion 15, 2001
3. Nishimura H et al: MR imaging of soft-tissue masses of the extraperitoneal spaces. Radiographics. 21(5):1141-54, 2001
4. Pui MH et al: Imaging diagnosis of abdominal and pelvic sarcomas. Australas Radiol. 43(2):134-41, 1999
5. Foshager MC et al: Masses simulating gynecologic diseases at CT and MR imaging. Radiographics. 16(5):1085-99, 1996

EXTRAPERITONEAL SARCOMA

IMAGE GALLERY

Typical

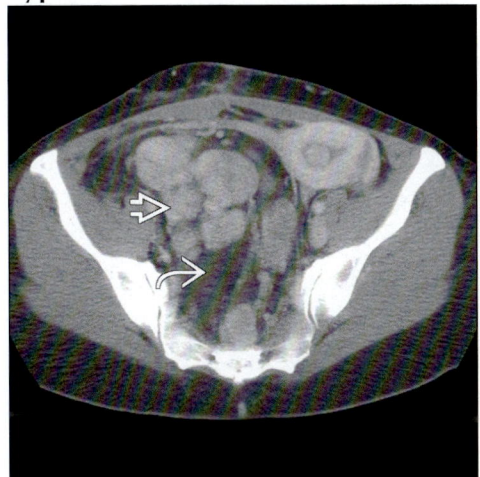
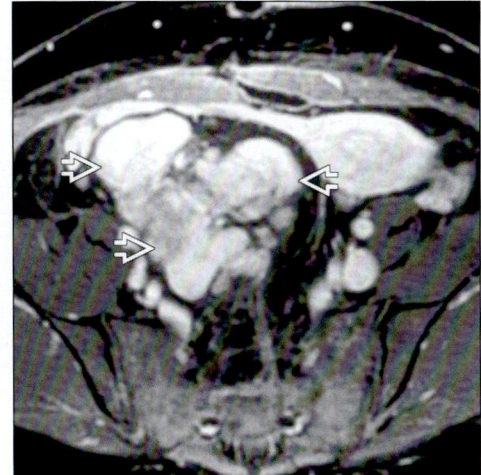

(Left) Axial CECT shows right pelvic mass with soft tissue density nodular ⮕ and low density fatty ⮕ components. *(Right)* Axial T1 C+ FS MR shows that nodular components ⮕ of the mass markedly enhance.

Typical

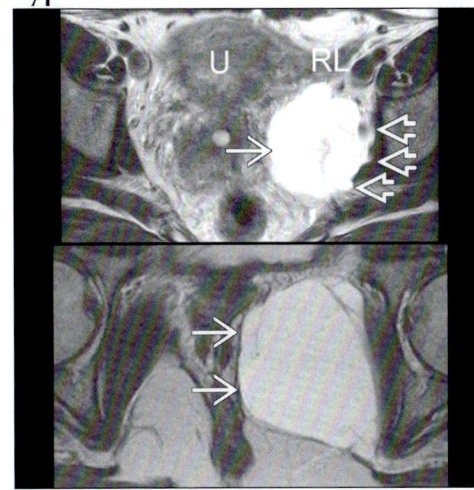
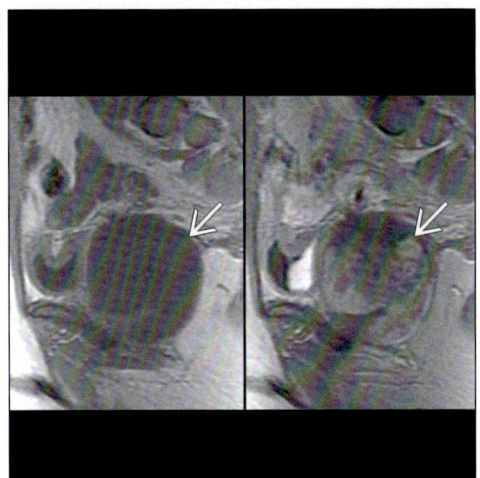

(Left) Axial T2WI MR shows high signal intensity myxoid liposarcoma ⮕. Note scalloped margin of mass with internal obturator muscle ⮕. Uterus (U) and round ligament (RL) are also seen. *(Right)* Sagittal T1 C+ MR (left) before and (right) after administration of contrast shows heterogeneous enhancement throughout the mass ⮕.

Typical

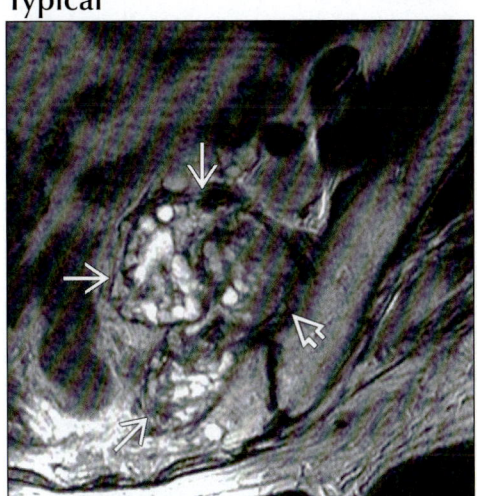
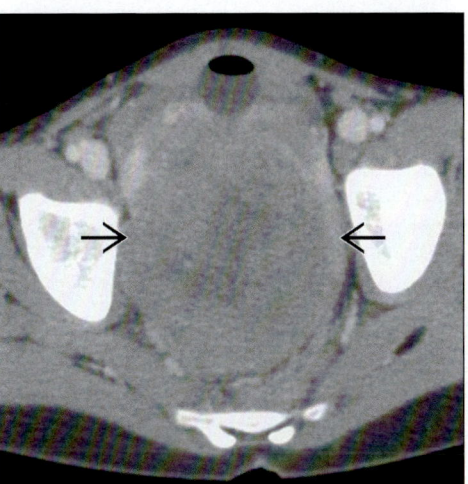

(Left) Axial T2WI MR shows malignant fibrous histiocytoma ⮕ which demonstrates heterogeneous signal intensity. Note that the mass contacts the adjacent bone ⮕. *(Right)* Axial CECT shows a large, heterogeneously enhancing rhabdomyosarcoma ⮕ in the pelvis.

HEMANGIOMA, PELVIS

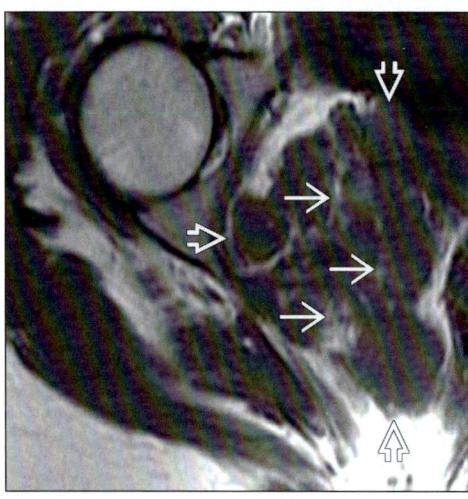

Axial T1WI MR shows lobulated soft tissue mass in lower right pelvis. Key finding indicating hemangioma is linear fatty deposits within mass.

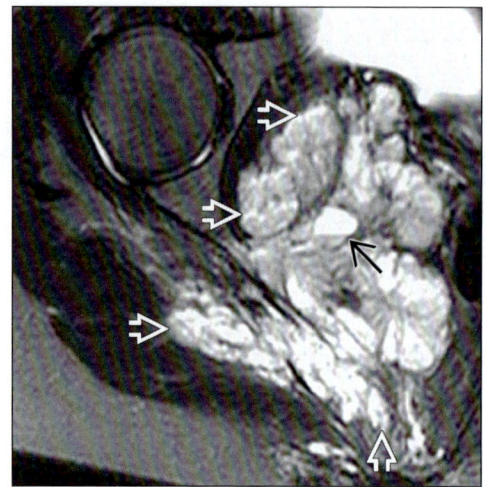

Axial T2WI MR shows well-defined, gyriform architecture of a high signal intensity hemangioma with fluid-fluid level.

TERMINOLOGY

Definitions
- Hemangioma is a benign vascular neoplasm that closely resembles normal vessels

IMAGING FINDINGS

General Features
- Best diagnostic clue: Lobulated, enhancing mass containing linear fatty deposits and phlebolith(s)
- Location
  - Hemangiomas can be found in all organs of the human body
  - Soft tissue hemangiomas are usually located superficially but may involve deep structures
- Size: Varies
- Morphology
  - Hemangiomas are often rounded, lobulated masses
  - They may exhibit "gyriform" architecture
  - They can invade adjacent bone, with serpentine lytic pattern
  - They usually have sharply-defined margins, despite infiltrative growth pattern

Radiographic Findings
- Plain radiographs show calcified thrombi (phleboliths) within hemangioma in up to 50% of cases
- Bony overgrowth of affected extremity may occur

Ultrasonographic Findings
- Grayscale Ultrasound
  - Hemangiomas are seen as complex masses
  - Phleboliths may cause acoustic shadowing
- Color Doppler: Doppler evaluation may show low-resistance arterial flow with forward flow during both systole and diastole

CT Findings
- NECT
  - May show fatty streaks or septa within lobulated mass
  - Calcified thrombi (which may have lucent centers) are well-demonstrated
- CECT: Hemangiomas show intense enhancement, similar to that of other vessels

DDx: Pelvic Masses

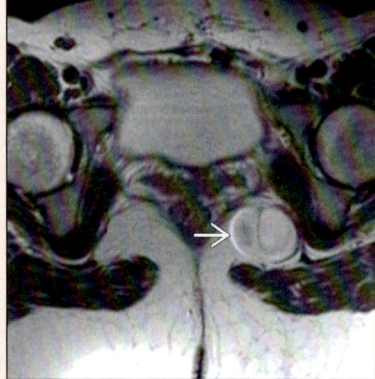

Neurofibroma

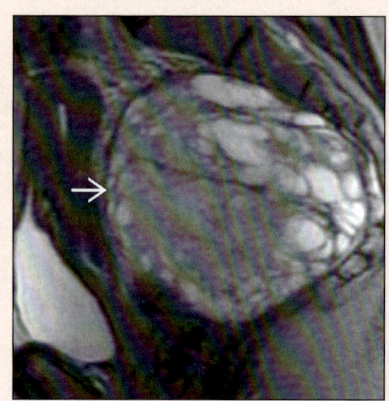

Hemangiopericytoma

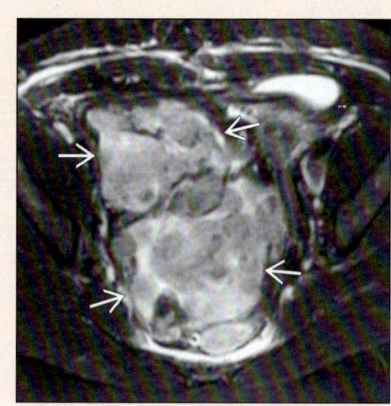

Liposarcoma

HEMANGIOMA, PELVIS

Key Facts

Terminology
- Hemangioma is a benign vascular neoplasm that closely resembles normal vessels

Imaging Findings
- Best diagnostic clue: Lobulated, enhancing mass containing linear fatty deposits and phlebolith(s)
- Hemangiomas can be found in all organs of the human body
- Hemangiomas are often rounded, lobulated masses
- They may exhibit "gyriform" architecture
- They usually have sharply-defined margins, despite infiltrative growth pattern
- MR is most useful to characterize and determine anatomic extent due to superior contrast resolution
- Plain radiographs or CT are better than MR for demonstrating phleboliths

Pathology
- Benign tumor resembling normal vessels
- Linear fatty components represent reactive overgrowth of fat
- Hemangiomas are the most frequently encountered vascular soft tissue tumors

Clinical Issues
- Hemangiomas generally have a good prognosis, although post-treatment recurrences do occur

Diagnostic Checklist
- Imaging is often diagnostic for soft tissue hemangiomas, thus, biopsy can usually be avoided

MR Findings
- T1WI
  - Hemangiomas usually demonstrate intermediate signal intensity between that of muscle and fat
  - Fatty septa between lobules of mass may be seen
- T2WI
  - Hemangiomas have extensive areas of heterogeneous multiple high signal intensity lobules
    - This appearance is due to cavernous or cystic vascular spaces containing stagnant blood
  - Central low signal areas in mass may be due to thrombi or flow
- T1 C+: Hemangiomas demonstrate extensive enhancement after contrast administration

Angiographic Findings
- Puddling of contrast within mass is seen
- Enlarged feeding vessels are common

Nuclear Medicine Findings
- Tc-99m Labeled Red Cell Scintigraphy: Hemangiomas demonstrate increased focal radiotracer activity that progresses over time

Imaging Recommendations
- Best imaging tool
  - MR is most useful to characterize and determine anatomic extent due to superior contrast resolution
  - Plain radiographs or CT are better than MR for demonstrating phleboliths

DIFFERENTIAL DIAGNOSIS

Angiomatosis
- Diffuse infiltration of soft tissue by hemangioma or lymphangioma

Angiolipoma
- Benign subcutaneous lesions
- Often in trunk or upper extremity
- Contains fat

Plexiform Neurofibroma
- Occurs in neurofibromatosis I
- May demonstrate "target sign" on T2WI, with central low signal as in hemangioma
- Central low signal enhances with gadolinium, unlike in hemangioma

Hemangiopericytomas
- Uncommon tumors that arise from the cells of Zimmerman that are located around vessels
- Have both benign and malignant forms; presence of intratumoral necrosis indicates malignancy
- On MR, they appear as a well-circumscribed masses with intermediate signal intensity on T1WI and mildly high signal intensity on T2WI

Hemangioendothelioma
- Intermediately aggressive vascular neoplasms of the endothelial cells
- MR imaging findings are not specific and may be identical to that of a hemangioma

Soft Tissue Sarcoma
- Fat deposits in well-differentiated liposarcoma typically more mass-like than in hemangioma
- Sarcomas are typically more heterogeneous in appearance, with areas of necrosis

PATHOLOGY

General Features
- General path comments
  - Benign tumor resembling normal vessels
  - Linear fatty components represent reactive overgrowth of fat
- Epidemiology
  - Hemangiomas are the most frequently encountered vascular soft tissue tumors
  - They comprise 7% of all benign soft tissue tumors
- Associated abnormalities
  - Maffucci syndrome

HEMANGIOMA, PELVIS

- Consists of multiple enchondromas and soft tissue cavernous hemangiomas
- Malignant transformation occurs in both enchondromas and soft tissue hemangiomas
○ Kasabach-Merritt syndrome
- Consists of large hemangiomas, thrombocytopenia and purpura
- This syndrome is due to intravascular coagulation, clotting, and fibrinolysis within the hemangioma
○ Klippel-Trenaunay-Weber syndrome
- Consists of the triad of cutaneous hemangioma, bone and soft tissue hypertrophy, and varicose veins

Gross Pathologic & Surgical Features
- Hemangiomas are seen as red-blue spongy masses

Microscopic Features
- Hemangiomas are nonencapsulated
- Dilated, blood-filled cystic spaces lined by flattened endothelium
- May contain fat, fibrous tissue, thrombus, hemosiderin

CLINICAL ISSUES

Presentation
- Most common signs/symptoms
  ○ Large hemangiomas may manifest as a smooth, palpable soft tissue mass
  ○ Most patients experience chronic pain or intermittent swelling
  ○ A characteristic bluish discoloration of the overlying skin may be seen
  ○ Physical exertion can result in retrograde flow in the arterial segment distal to the hemangioma and results in ischemia of the surrounding tissues
  ○ Occasionally, a bruit may be heard in the region
- Other signs/symptoms
  ○ Hemangiomas may enlarge during pregnancy
  ○ A soft tissue hemangioma may cause osseous overgrowth secondary to chronic hyperemia

Demographics
- Age
  ○ Hemangiomas are the most frequently diagnosed soft tissue neoplasms in children
  ○ Often noted at birth or during first few decades
- Gender: More common in women

Natural History & Prognosis
- Hemangiomas generally have a good prognosis, although post-treatment recurrences do occur

Treatment
- None required if asymptomatic
- Laser therapy, embolotherapy, sclerotherapy, or surgical resection may relieve symptoms

DIAGNOSTIC CHECKLIST

Image Interpretation Pearls
- Imaging is often diagnostic for soft tissue hemangiomas, thus, biopsy can usually be avoided
  ○ Biopsy attempts in cavernous hemangiomas usually do not provide sufficient solid tissue for histologic analysis
  ○ Additionally, biopsy of soft tissue hemangiomas may lead to bleeding complications

SELECTED REFERENCES

1. Olsen KI et al: Soft-tissue cavernous hemangioma. Radiographics. 24(3):849-54, 2004
2. Vilanova JC et al: Hemangioma from head to toe: MR imaging with pathologic correlation. Radiographics. 24(2):367-85, 2004
3. Tang P et al: Surgical treatment of hemangiomas of soft tissue. Clin Orthop Relat Res. (399):205-10, 2002
4. Goto T et al: Soft-tissue haemangioma and periosteal new bone formation on the neighbouring bone. Arch Orthop Trauma Surg. 121(10):549-53, 2001
5. Donnelly LF et al: Vascular malformations and hemangiomas: a practical approach in a multidisciplinary clinic. AJR Am J Roentgenol. 174(3):597-608, 2000
6. Kern S et al: Differentiation of vascular birthmarks by MR imaging. An investigation of hemangiomas, venous and lymphatic malformations. Acta Radiol. 41(5):453-7, 2000
7. Paltiel HJ et al: Soft-tissue vascular anomalies: utility of US for diagnosis. Radiology. 214(3):747-54, 2000
8. Munk PL et al: Deep soft tissue hemangiomas. Skeletal Radiol. 28(1):57-8, 1999
9. Dubois J et al: Soft-tissue hemangiomas in infants and children: diagnosis using Doppler sonography. AJR Am J Roentgenol. 171(1):247-52, 1998
10. Sung MS et al: Regional bone changes in deep soft tissue hemangiomas: radiographic and MR features. Skeletal Radiol. 27(4):205-10, 1998
11. Meyer JS et al: Biological classification of soft-tissue vascular anomalies: MR correlation. AJR Am J Roentgenol. 157(3):559-64, 1991

HEMANGIOMA, PELVIS

IMAGE GALLERY

Typical

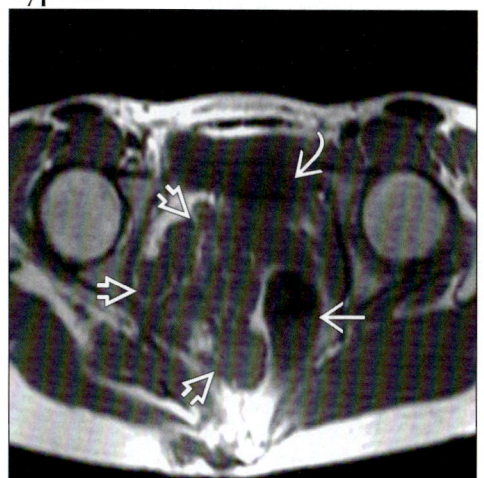
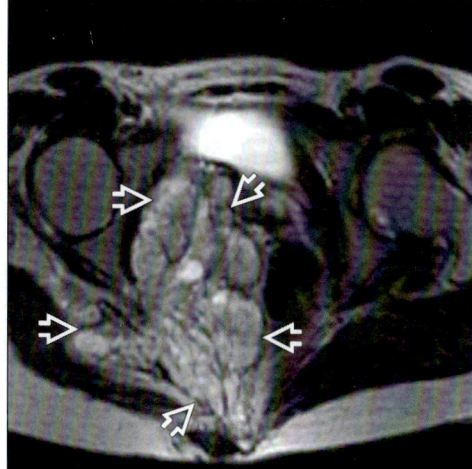

(Left) Axial T1WI MR shows a large right pelvic hemangioma ➡ displacing rectosigmoid ➡ and bladder ➡. (Right) Axial T2WI MR shows well-defined, lobulated high signal intensity hemangioma ➡ in the right pelvis extending to right gluteal region.

Typical

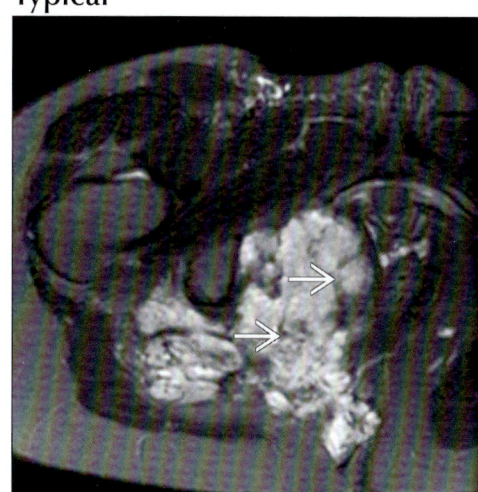
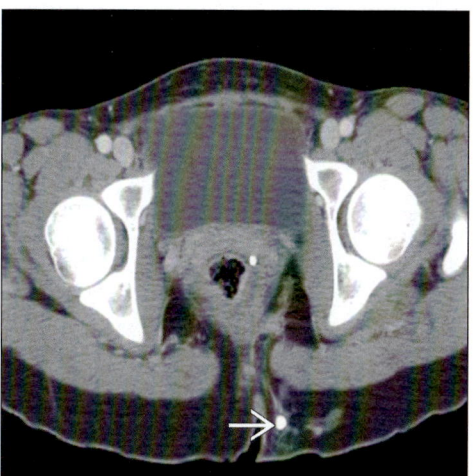

(Left) Axial T2WI FS MR shows that only the linear fatty deposits ➡ within the hemangioma loose signal. (Right) Axial CECT shows a phlebolith ➡ in the superior aspect of a left gluteal hemangioma.

Typical

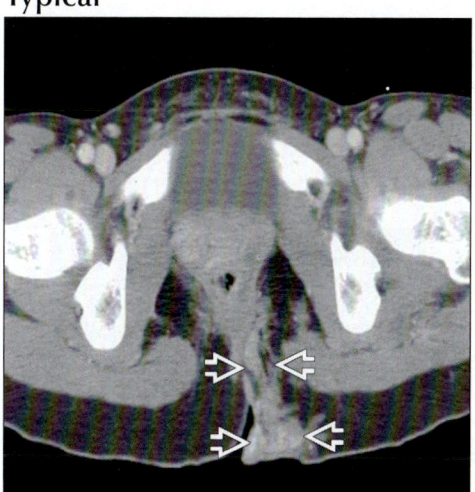
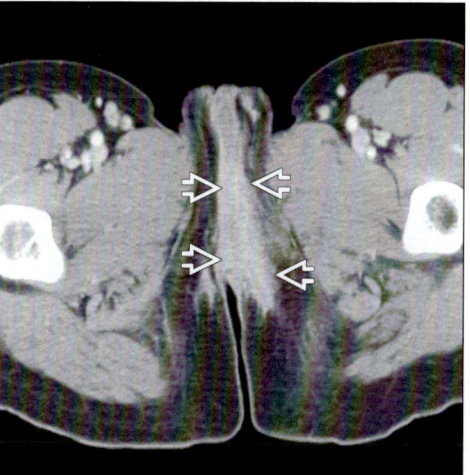

(Left) Axial CECT shows an markedly enhancing hemangioma ➡ extending from the left gluteal region to left ischiorectal fossa. (Right) Axial CECT shows that the mass ➡ extends to left perineum and vulva.

OVARIAN VEIN THROMBOSIS

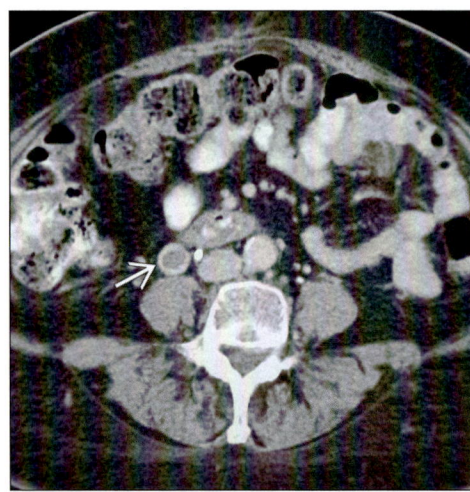

Axial CECT shows an enlarged right ovarian vein with a low-attenuation lumen thrombus ➡. Note the bright wall enhancement. (Courtesy C. Cooper, MD).

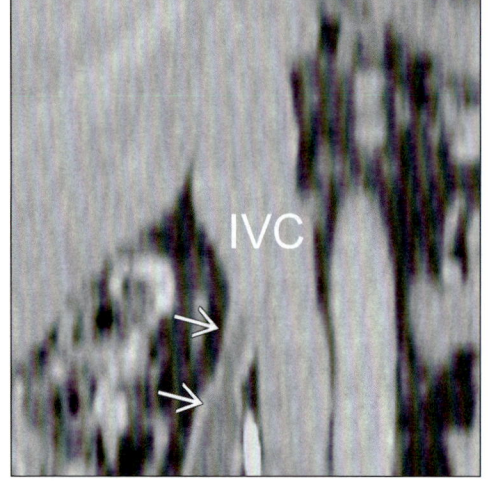

Coronal CECT multiplanar reconstruction shows extensive thrombus along the course of the right ovarian vein ➡ as it joins the inferior vena cava (IVC). (Courtesy C. Cooper, MD).

TERMINOLOGY

Abbreviations and Synonyms
- Ovarian vein thrombosis (OVT)
- Gonadal vein thrombosis

Definitions
- Rare: Usually associated with ascending postpartum ovarian vein thrombophlebitis or can be seen after pelvic surgery

IMAGING FINDINGS

General Features
- Best diagnostic clue
  - Enlarged, well-defined, tubular retroperitoneal structure extending from pelvis to infrarenal inferior vena cava (IVC) along expected course of ovarian vein without demonstrable flow
    - Enhancement of venous wall
    - Perivascular inflammation
- Location
  - Usually involves the right ovarian vein in postpartum patients
    - 80% patients on the right
    - 14% patients on both sides
    - 6% patients on the left
- Size: Range from small partially occlusive thrombus to complete occlusion
- Morphology: Round, tubular

Ultrasonographic Findings
- Grayscale Ultrasound
  - Tubular structure in adnexa representing thrombosed ovarian vein
  - Variable echogenicity of thrombus
  - Tubular mass lateral to aorta or IVC
- Color Doppler: Partial or absent flow within vein

CT Findings
- NECT: Hyperintense to isointense thrombus relative to venous wall
- CECT
  - Enlarged ovarian vein
  - Low-attenuation central lumen (filling defect)
  - Sharply-defined enhancing wall
  - Perivascular fat stranding suggest thrombophlebitis

DDx: Ovarian Vein Thrombosis

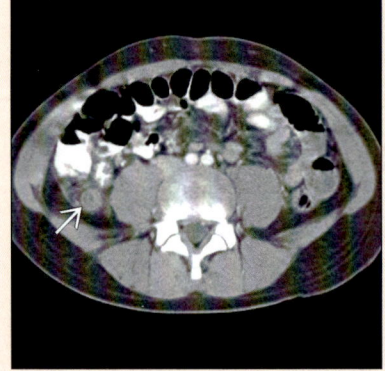

Appendicitis

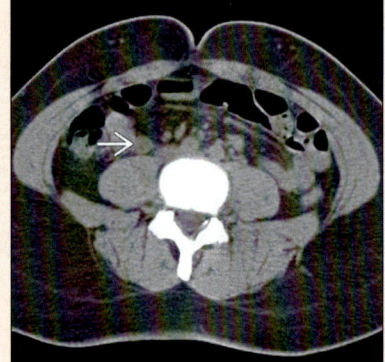

Dilated Right Ureter

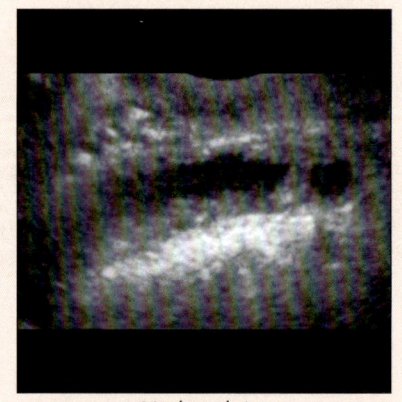

Hydrosalpinx

OVARIAN VEIN THROMBOSIS

Key Facts

Terminology
- Gonadal vein thrombosis
- Rare: Usually associated with ascending postpartum ovarian vein thrombophlebitis or can be seen after pelvic surgery

Imaging Findings
- Enlarged, well-defined, tubular retroperitoneal structure extending from pelvis to infrarenal inferior vena cava (IVC) along expected course of ovarian vein without demonstrable flow
- Enhancement of venous wall
- Perivascular inflammation
- Usually involves the right ovarian vein in postpartum patients
- CT less expensive and more available than MR
- Protocol advice: Delayed imaging often necessary to make diagnosis

Top Differential Diagnoses
- Appendicitis
- Hydrosalpinx/Pyosalpinx
- Dilated Ureter
- Thrombosis of Duplicated IVC
- Adnexal Torsion

Pathology
- 1:600 deliveries
- 1-2% following cesarian section complicated by endometritis

---

- Can extend into IVC, renal vein
- Imaging pitfall: Right ovarian vein pseudothrombosis
  - Asymmetric ovarian vein opacification: Left > right
  - Etiology: Early reflux of contrast medium down left ovarian vein
- Follow ovarian vein to the IVC or left renal vein in order to distinguish it from the ureter

MR Findings
- T1WI: Intermediate to high signal intensity intraluminal clot
- T2WI: High signal intensity intraluminal clot
- T1 C+
  - Filling defect within vein
  - Enhancement of vessel wall
- Time-of-flight
  - May demonstrate thrombus but artifacts are common
- True FISP
  - May demonstrate thrombus but artifacts are common

Imaging Recommendations
- Best imaging tool
  - CT less expensive and more available than MR
  - MR useful in patients with iodinated contrast allergy
- Protocol advice: Delayed imaging often necessary to make diagnosis

DIFFERENTIAL DIAGNOSIS

Appendicitis
- Symptoms may mimic OVT, but initial pain is periumbilical that moves to right lower quadrant
- Short tubular abnormality connects to cecum; patent right ovarian vein

Hydrosalpinx/Pyosalpinx
- Tubular structure with thickened longitudinal folds and echogenic luminal contents

Dilated Ureter
- Follow ureter from the collecting system to the urinary bladder to distinguish from ovarian vein

Thrombosis of Duplicated IVC
- Duplicated IVC originates from left common iliac vein

Adnexal Torsion
- Torsion: Enlarged avascular ovary with heterogeneity (hemorrhage), free intraperitoneal fluid

Broad Ligament Hematoma or Phlegmon
- Heterogeneous mass-like area in region of broad ligament

Necrotic Lymphadenopathy
- Necrotic retroperitoneal lymphadenopathy may be confused with thrombosed ovarian vein
- Lymphadenopathy is not tubular and scrolling through images helps in correct diagnosis

PATHOLOGY

General Features
- Etiology
  - Pregnancy and puerperium
    - Hypercoagulability (pregnancy & puerperium associated with increased levels of factors I, II, VII, IX & X)
    - Alterations in vein wall (secondary to high estrogen levels, surgical insult and/or endometritis)
    - Stasis of blood flow (venous blood flow decreases during pregnancy and postpartum venous velocity drops sharply)
    - Compression of veins by gravid uterus, particularly in third trimester; minimal adventitial sheaths of the ovarian veins make them vulnerable to compression
  - Other predisposing conditions
    - Pelvic inflammatory disease
    - Gynecologic surgery

OVARIAN VEIN THROMBOSIS

- Malignancy
- Chemotherapy
- Lupus anticoagulant
- Protein S deficiency
- Factor V Leiden mutation
- Epidemiology
  - 1:600 deliveries
  - 1-2% following cesarian section complicated by endometritis
  - < 0.2% following vaginal delivery

Gross Pathologic & Surgical Features

- Thrombosed, distended ovarian vein

CLINICAL ISSUES

Presentation

- Most common signs/symptoms
  - Common triad
    - Right lower abdominal or flank pain
    - Fever
    - Rope-like palpable abdominal mass
- Clinical Profile
  - Early in puerperium; most within 10 days of delivery
  - May be asymptomatic
  - Elevated white blood cell count
  - Elevated C-reactive protein

Demographics

- Age: Usually of child-bearing age
- Gender: Females

Natural History & Prognosis

- Overall: Good
- Spontaneous resolution may be seen in some patients (e.g., malignancy)
- Complications: May result in infection and pulmonary emboli
- Death rate: 18/1,000,000 pregnancies
- Can cause ipsilateral ureteral obstruction

Treatment

- Anticoagulation with heparin and warfarin
- Intravenous broad spectrum antibiotics
- Surgical intervention (vein interruption/ligation) for patients who fail medical therapy
- If incidental finding in asymptomatic patients, no need for therapy

DIAGNOSTIC CHECKLIST

Consider

- OVT in postpartum patients with fever unresponsive to antibiotics

Image Interpretation Pearls

- Enlarged, well-defined, tubular structure with central low attenuation along expected course of ovarian vein

SELECTED REFERENCES

1. Persaud T et al: Puerperal ovarian vein thrombosis (2006: 1b). Eur Radiol. :1-4 [Epub ahead of print] No abstract available, 2006
2. Leyendecker JR et al: MR imaging of maternal diseases of the abdomen and pelvis during pregnancy and the immediate postpartum period. Radiographics. 24(5):1301-16, 2004
3. Morales-Rosello J et al: Postpartum ovarian vein thrombosis with positive lupus anticoagulant. Int J Gynaecol Obstet. 87(2):163-4, 2004
4. Prieto-Nieto MI et al: Acute appendicitis-like symptoms as initial presentation of ovarian vein thrombosis. Ann Vasc Surg. 18(4):481-3, 2004
5. Benfayed WH et al: Detection of pulmonary emboli resulting from ovarian vein thrombosis. AJR Am J Roentgenol. 181(5):1430-1, 2003
6. Kubik-Huch RA et al: Role of duplex color Doppler ultrasound, computed tomography, and MR angiography in the diagnosis of septic puerperal ovarian vein thrombosis. Abdom Imaging. 24(1):85-91, 1999
7. Salomon O et al: Risk factors associated with postpartum ovarian vein thrombosis. Thromb Haemost. 82(3):1015-9, 1999
8. Twickler DM et al: Imaging of puerperal septic thrombophlebitis: prospective comparison of MR imaging, CT, and sonography. AJR Am J Roentgenol. 169(4):1039-43, 1997
9. Zuckerman J et al: Imaging of pelvic postpartum complications. AJR Am J Roentgenol. 168(3):663-8, 1997
10. Zuckerman J et al: Imaging of postpartum complications. Am J Roentgenol. 170:1395-6, 1997
11. Rooholamini SA et al: Imaging of pregnancy-related complications. Radiographics. 13(4):753-70, 1993
12. Toland KC et al: Postpartum ovarian vein thrombosis presenting as ureteral obstruction: a case report and review of the literature. J Urol. 149(6):1538-40, 1993
13. Leclerc JR et al: Venous thromboembolic disorders. Burrow GN et al eds. Medical Complications During Pregnancy. Philadelphia, Saunders. 204-23, 1988
14. Angel JL et al: Computed tomography in diagnosis of puerperal ovarian vein thrombosis. Obstet Gynecol. 63(1):61-4, 1984
15. Munsick RA et al: A review of the syndrome of puerperal ovarian vein thrombophlebitis. Obstet Gynecol Surv. 36(2):57-66, 1981
16. Brown TK et al: Puerperal ovarian vein thrombophlebitis: a syndrome. Am J Obstet Gynecol. 109(2):263-73, 1971
17. Ikard RW et al: Lower limb venous dynamics in pregnant women. Surg Gynecol Obstet. 132(3):483-8, 1971
18. Goodrich SM et al: Peripheral venous distensibility and velocity of venous blood flow during pregnancy or during oral contraceptive therapy. Am J Obstet Gynecol. 90:740-4, 1964
19. Kerr MG et al: Studies of the inferior vena cava in late pregnancy. Br Med J. 1(5382):532-3, 1964

OVARIAN VEIN THROMBOSIS

IMAGE GALLERY

Typical

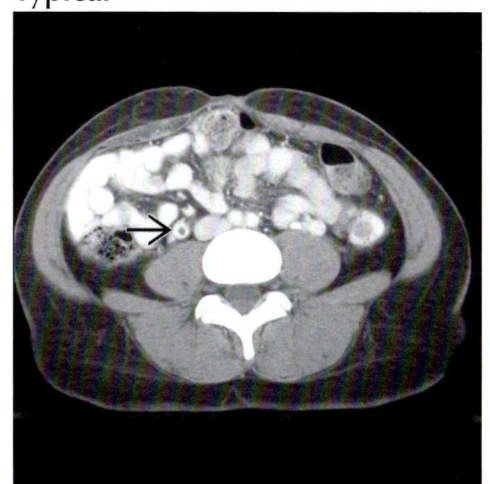
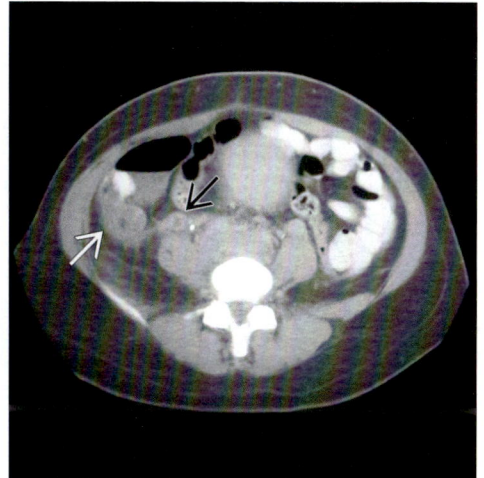

(Left) Axial CECT shows partial occlusive thrombus within the right ovarian vein ➡. *(Courtesy C. Cooper, MD).* *(Right)* Axial CECT shows right sided OVT ➡ associated with stranding of the surrounding fat ➡, consistent with thrombophlebitis. Note that these inflammatory changes can abut the nearby cecum, thereby mimicking appendicitis.

Typical

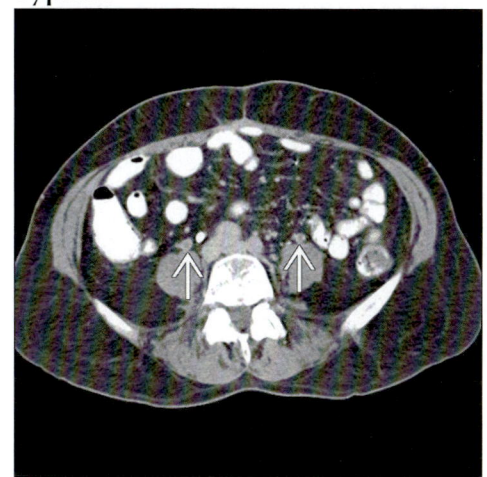
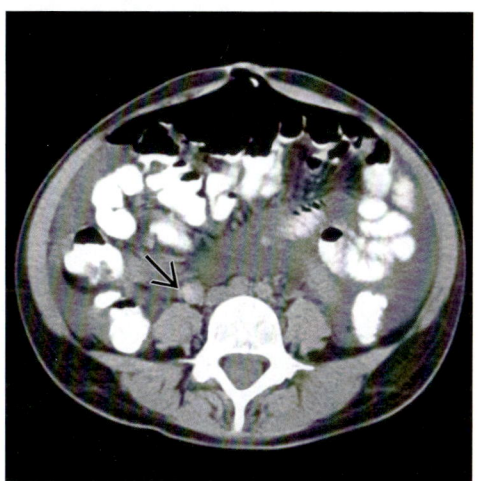

(Left) Axial CECT shows bilateral ovarian vein thromboses ➡. *(Right)* Axial NECT shows hyperdense thrombus ➡ within the right ovarian vein.

Typical

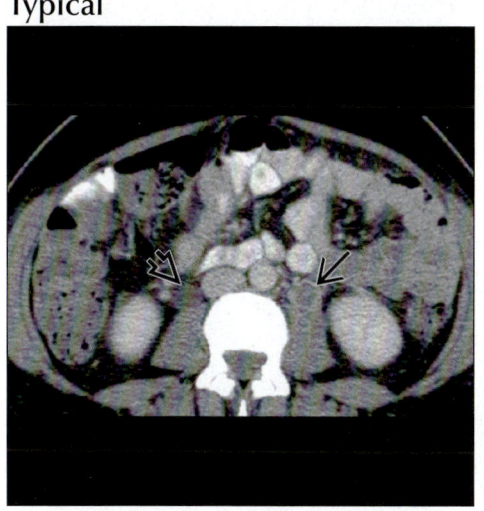
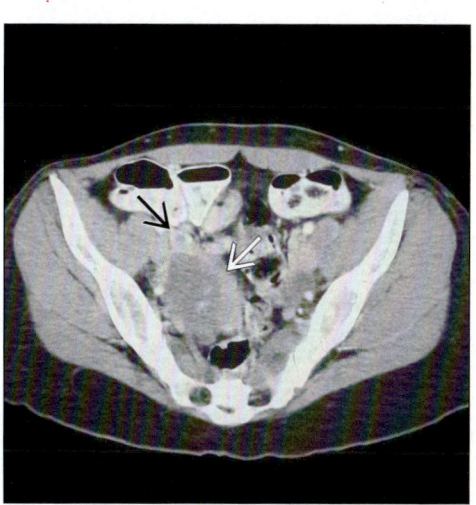

(Left) Axial CECT shows filling defect within the left ovarian vein ➡ consistent with thrombosis. On the right, there is a dilated ureter ➡ which should not be confused for OVT. *(Right)* Axial CECT shows right sided ovarian thrombosis ➡ adjacent to an enlarged, postpartum uterus ➡.

SPINAL MENINGEAL CYSTS

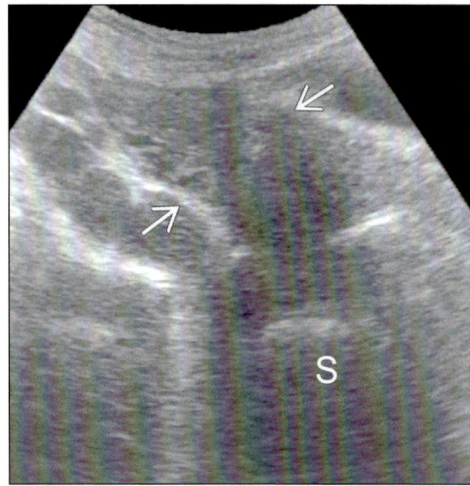

Axial ultrasound shows a hypoechoic mass ➡ located in the right adnexa with low level echoes and thin septations. Enhanced through transmission confirms cystic nature. Ovaries were not identified. Sacrum (S).

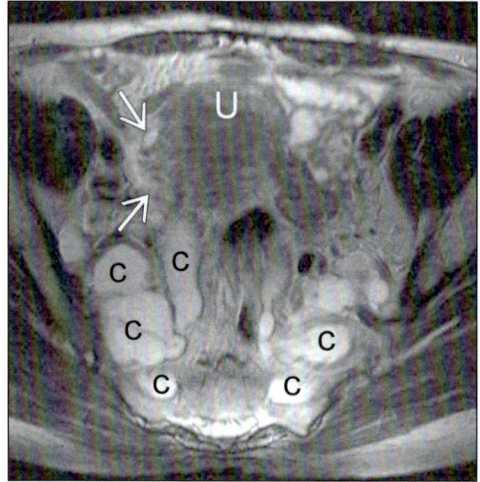

Axial T2WI MR shows perineural cysts (C) (type 2) herniating through sacral foramina and connecting with thecal sac. The right ovary ➡ is identified separately adjacent to the uterus (U).

TERMINOLOGY

Abbreviations and Synonyms
- Arachnoid cysts, Tarlov cysts, perineural cysts, cysts of sacral nerve root sheath, anterior sacral meningoceles

Definitions
- Diverticula of the spinal meningeal sac, nerve root sheath, or arachnoid
- Several entities intermixed under general label of spinal meningeal cysts
- Nabors classification: 3 types of spinal meningeal cysts
  - Type 1: Extradural meningeal cyst without spinal nerve root fibers
    - Type 1A: Extradural arachnoid cyst
    - Type 1B: Sacral meningocele
  - Type 2: Extradural meningeal cyst with spinal nerve root fibers (perineural cyst or Tarlov cyst)
  - Type 3: Intradural meningeal cyst

IMAGING FINDINGS

General Features
- Best diagnostic clue
  - Posteriorly located extraovarian adnexal cystic mass
  - Cystic structures accompanying sacrococcygeal nerve roots with widening of sacral foramina ± erosion of adjacent sacrum
- Location: Extraperitoneal pre-sacral cyst
- Size: Variable
- Morphology: Unilocular or multilocular
- Unilateral or bilateral
- Imaging appearance ranges from simple unilocular cyst to complex cystic mass
- Ovaries identified as separate structures
- Mass located posterior to ovaries and anterior to sacrum
- Extraperitoneal
- Uncommon presentation at transvaginal sonography (TVS)
- Subgroup that presents as an adnexal mass on TVS more commonly shows imaging findings of a complex cystic mass
  - Frequently multilocular

DDx: Multilocular Adnexal Cyst

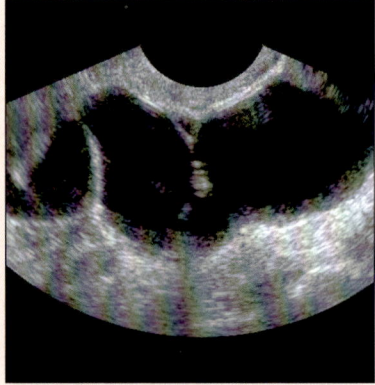
Hydrosalpinx

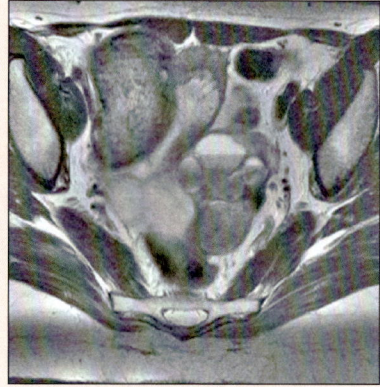
Endometrioma

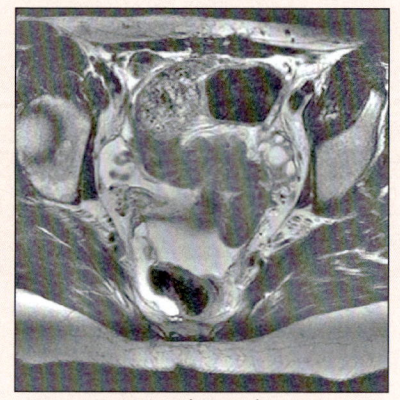
Peritoneal Pseudocyst

SPINAL MENINGEAL CYSTS

Key Facts

Terminology
- Arachnoid cysts, Tarlov cysts, perineural cysts, cysts of sacral nerve root sheath, anterior sacral meningoceles
- Diverticula of the spinal meningeal sac, nerve root sheath, or arachnoid
- Several entities intermixed under general label of spinal meningeal cysts

Imaging Findings
- Posteriorly located extraovarian adnexal cystic mass
- Cystic structures accompanying sacrococcygeal nerve roots with widening of sacral foramina ± erosion of adjacent sacrum
- Location: Extraperitoneal pre-sacral cyst
- Uncommon presentation at transvaginal sonography (TVS)
- Subgroup that presents as an adnexal mass on TVS more commonly shows imaging findings of a complex cystic mass
- MR findings diagnostic by showing ventral herniation through sacral foramina and connection with thecal sac

Top Differential Diagnoses
- Hydrosalpinx
- Paraovarian/Paratubal Cyst
- Cystic Ovarian Neoplasm/Endometrioma
- Peritoneal Inclusion Cyst or Peritoneal Pseudocyst

Diagnostic Checklist
- Pelvic extension of a sacral process in the case of a complex cystic extraovarian mass discovered on US

- Internal septa with debris
- No thickening of wall or septa (≤ 2 mm in thickness)
- No mural or septal nodularity
- No vascularity of wall or septa

Radiographic Findings
- Radiography
  - Widened sacral foramina
  - Thinned pedicles
  - Posterior vertebral scalloping

Ultrasonographic Findings
- Grayscale Ultrasound
  - Unilateral or bilateral complex cystic "adnexal" mass
    - Common: Thin-walled, multiloculated cyst with internal debris
    - Uncommon: Unilocular simple cyst
  - Fixed to pelvic side wall (lack of movement with respiration)
  - Ventral extension through anterior sacral foramina
- Color Doppler: No flow

CT Findings
- Uniform masses with water density (< 10 HU) anterior to the sacrum
- Multilocular cystic masses
- No enhancement
- Widened sacral foramina ± erosion of adjacent sacrum
  - CT myelography
    - Intrathecal contrast filling of cyst, initially or on delayed imaging

MR Findings
- T1WI
  - Low signal intensity [follows signal of cerebrospinal fluid (CSF)]
  - May be higher than CSF if increased protein content
- T2WI
  - High signal intensity (follows signal of CSF)
  - Signal may be higher than CSF due to absence of flow related T2 shortening
  - Signal intensity may be heterogeneous if internal debris
- PD/Intermediate: CSF intensity
- T1 C+: No enhancement
- Multiplanar acquisition shows ventral herniation through sacral foramina
- Connection with thecal sac

Imaging Recommendations
- Best imaging tool: MR and CT are essential to confirm continuity with thecal sac or nerve roots
- MR findings diagnostic by showing ventral herniation through sacral foramina and connection with thecal sac

DIFFERENTIAL DIAGNOSIS

Hydrosalpinx
- Intraperitoneal, usually mobile but may be fixed due to adhesions
- More elongated and tubular than perineural cysts as seen on TVS
- Incomplete septae due to folding or kinking in dilated tube

Paraovarian/Paratubal Cyst
- Typically unilocular, simple cyst
- Mobile, intraperitoneal

Cystic Ovarian Neoplasm/Endometrioma
- Intraperitoneal
- No normal ovary identified separately
- Extra-ovarian endometriosis rarely cystic
- Absence of connection to thecal sac
- MR: T2 shading of endometrioma

Peritoneal Inclusion Cyst or Peritoneal Pseudocyst
- Intraperitoneal
- Loculated ascites contained by fibrous bands/adhesions
- Separate from ovaries

SPINAL MENINGEAL CYSTS

- Absence of connection to thecal sac

PATHOLOGY

General Features
- General path comments
  - Depends on type of meningeal cyst
  - Nabors classification of spinal meningeal cysts
  - Type 1A: Extradural meningeal cyst without spinal nerve root fibers - extradural arachnoid cyst
    - Herniation of arachnoid through congenital or acquired dural defect
    - Begins as diverticulum & subsequently enlarge
    - Valve-like mechanism
    - At histology, either no epithelial lining or attenuated lining of arachnoid-like cells
  - Type 1B: Extradural meningeal cyst without spinal nerve root fibers - sacral meningocele
    - Herniation of dura through sacral defect
    - Diverticulum of the meningeal sac
    - Pedicle connecting to dural sac
    - Association with other spinal anomalies, congenital
  - Type 2: Extradural meningeal cyst with spinal nerve root fibers (perineural cyst or Tarlov cyst)
    - Dilatation of the nerve root sleeve
    - No pedicle
    - Part of lining of perineural cysts contains nerve fibers ± ganglion cells
    - Cyst cavity occupies space between perineurium (arachnoid covering the root) and endoneurium (outer layer of pia)
    - Arise in sacrococcygeal nerve roots: Most commonly second and third sacral nerve root levels
    - Communicate with subarachnoid space
    - Relatively common: 5% of lumbosacral MR examinations
    - Often multiple
  - Type 3: Intradural meningeal cyst
    - Loculation of arachnoid
    - Typically at level of thoracic spine
    - Posterior to cord and may be multiple
    - Most communicate with subarachnoid space through narrow neck
    - May cause symptomatic compressive myelopathy
- Etiology
  - Type 1
    - Most are congenital
  - Type 2: Etiology uncertain
    - Traumatic: Hemorrhage post-trauma impedes venous drainage leading to rupture and subsequent cyst formation
    - Congenital: Caused by arachnoidal proliferations within root sleeve leading to obstruction of normal CSF pathways
    - Mechanism of cyst formation: Stenosis of nerve root sheath ostium, leading to ball-valve phenomenon of CSF entering cyst
  - Type 3
    - Congenital: Weakness of arachnoid, bulging with variations in CSF pressure
    - Acquired: Arachnoiditis caused by trauma, hemorrhage, inflammation

CLINICAL ISSUES

Presentation
- Most common signs/symptoms
  - Sacral type 1
    - Bowel or bladder dysfunction
  - Type 2
    - Most asymptomatic (99%)
    - Radicular pain, urinary dysfunction rare
  - Type 3
    - May cause symptomatic compressive myelopathy

Treatment
- Type 1: Closing of ostium between cyst and subarachnoid space
- Type 2: Most require no treatment
  - Percutaneous guided needle aspiration (high recurrence rate)
    - Allows documentation of pain relief
  - Sacral laminectomy, partial resection and oversewing of cyst wall, or total excision of cyst with nerve root
  - Microsurgical cyst fenestration, and cyst imbrication
- Type 3: Total excision

DIAGNOSTIC CHECKLIST

Consider
- Pelvic extension of a sacral process in the case of a complex cystic extraovarian mass discovered on US

Image Interpretation Pearls
- MR diagnostic by showing extension from the spinal canal through sacral foramina
- Spinal meningeal cysts include several pathologic entities which share herniation through sacral foramina and possible confusion with an adnexal mass

SELECTED REFERENCES
1. Khosla A et al: CT myelography and MR imaging of extramedullary cysts of the spinal canal in adult and pediatric patients. AJR Am J Roentgenol. 178(1):201-7, 2002
2. Diel J et al: The sacrum: pathologic spectrum, multimodality imaging, and subspecialty approach. Radiographics. 21(1):83-104, 2001
3. McClure MJ et al: Perineural cysts presenting as complex adnexal cystic masses on transvaginal sonography. AJR Am J Roentgenol. 177(6):1313-8, 2001
4. Paulsen RD et al: Prevalence and percutaneous drainage of cysts of the sacral nerve root sheath (Tarlov cysts). AJNR Am J Neuroradiol. 15(2):293-7; discussion 298-9, 1994
5. Davis SW et al: Sacral meningeal cysts: evaluation with MR imaging. Radiology. 187(2):445-8, 1993
6. Nabors MW et al: Updated assessment and current classification of spinal meningeal cysts. J Neurosurg. 68(3):366-77, 1988

SPINAL MENINGEAL CYSTS

IMAGE GALLERY

Typical

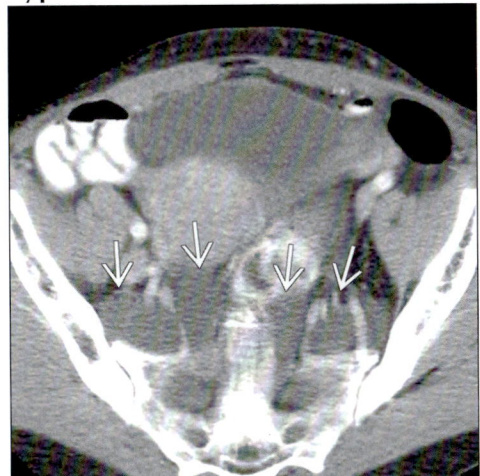 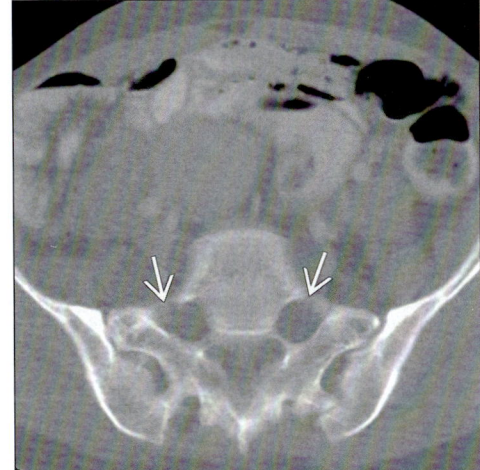

(Left) Axial CECT shows perineural cysts herniating ➔ through enlarged sacral foramina. *(Right)* Axial CECT with bone windows shows enlarged sacral foramina ➔ secondary to perineural cysts.

Typical

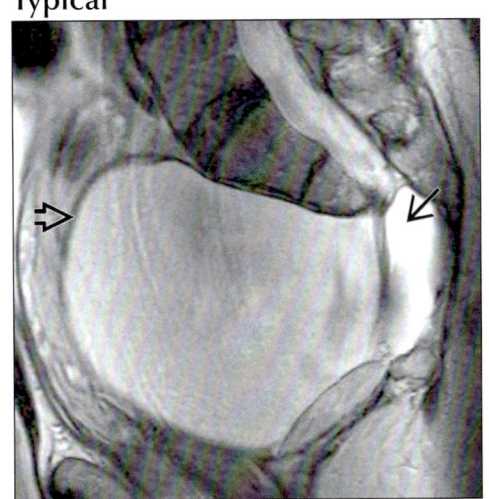 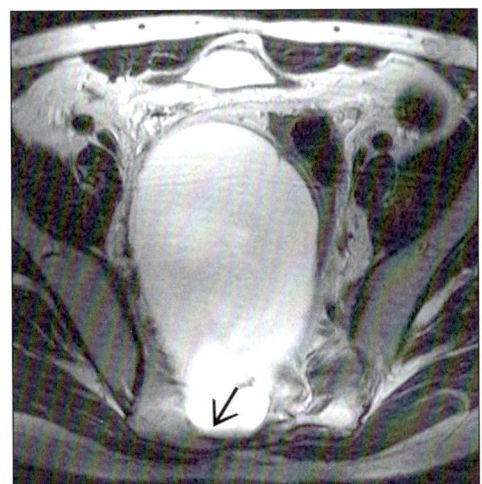

(Left) Sagittal T2WI MR shows a cystic mass ➔ projecting in the pre-sacral space, arising from the spinal canal and herniating through a sacral defect ➔ corresponding to an anterior meningocele. *(Right)* Axial T2WI MR shows the cystic pre-sacral mass herniating through a hypoplastic right sacrum ➔. Type 1B (sacral meningocele).

Typical

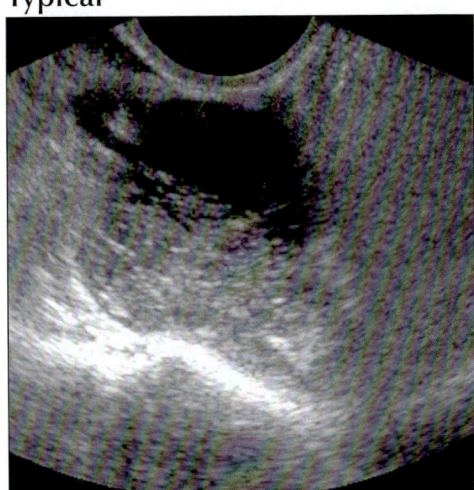 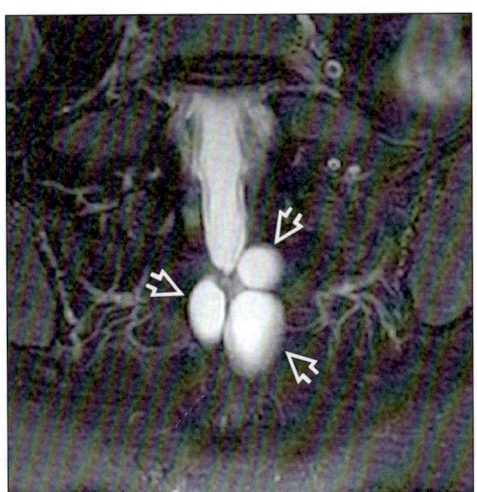

(Left) Oblique transvaginal ultrasound shows a complex cystic pelvic mass containing internal debris. The ovaries were not identified separately. *(Right)* Coronal T2WI FS MR shows the multiloculated presacral cystic lesion ➔ in the same patient as previous image connecting with the thecal sac confirming sacral perineural cysts (type 2). (Courtesy M. Haider, MD).

BLADDER FLAP HEMATOMA

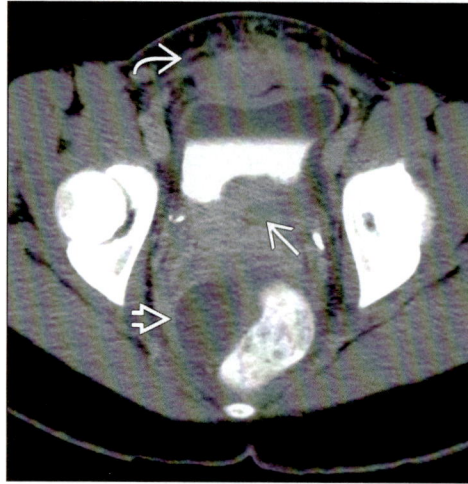

Axial CECT shows bladder flap hematoma ➔, and right cul-de-sac post-operative collection ➔. Note post-operative changes in anterior abdominal wall fat and right rectus muscle ➔.

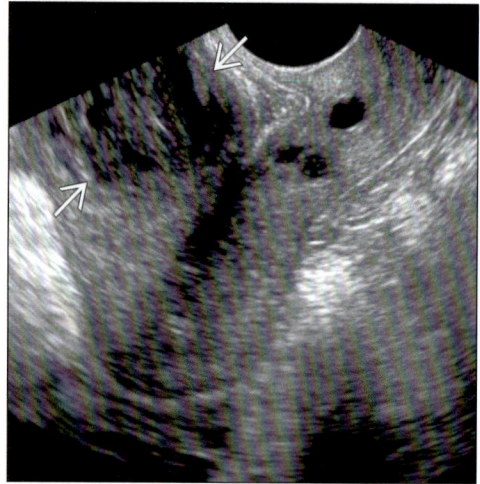

Sagittal transabdominal ultrasound shows complex hypoechoic fluid collection ➔ of a bladder flap hematoma abutting the anterior lower uterine segment.

TERMINOLOGY

Definitions
- Extraperitoneal blood collection at site of cesarian section incision, between lower uterine segment and posterior bladder

IMAGING FINDINGS

General Features
- Best diagnostic clue: Complex fluid collection between bladder and lower uterine segment in post-cesarian section patient
- Location
  - Bladder flap is adjacent to low transverse uterine incision formed by reflected peritoneum
    - Hematoma covered by fold of peritoneum that was incised, reflected, and reapproximated during surgery
  - Hematoma may remain contained or extend into surrounding structures
    - Laterally via broad ligaments into retroperitoneum
    - Into uterine subserosa
- Size
  - Can range in size from 1-2 cm to greater than 10 cm
  - Less than 2 cm are often normal post-operative findings
    - Generally asymptomatic
  - Greater than 2 cm have been associated with significant symptoms
  - Greater than 5 cm should prompt evaluation for possible uterine dehiscence
- Morphology: Variable depending on size and age of blood products

Ultrasonographic Findings
- Transabdominal and transvaginal US
  - Heterogeneous collection between lower uterine segment & bladder adjacent to the incision
  - Three criteria
    - Mass ≥ 2 cm in diameter
    - Posterior to bladder
    - Anterior to lower uterine segment
  - Borders of hematoma are ill-defined
- **Blood can dissect**:
  - Subserosally along uterus

DDx: Bladder Flap Hematoma

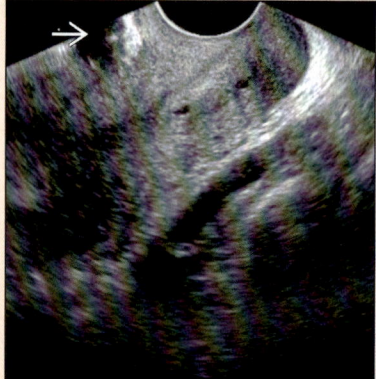
Non-Distended Bladder

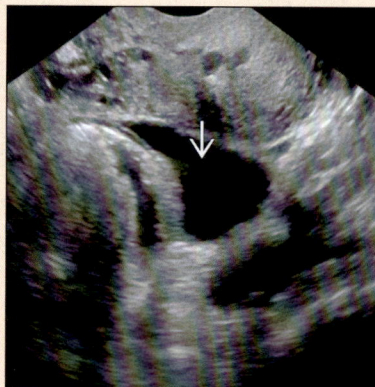
Cul-de-Sac Fluid

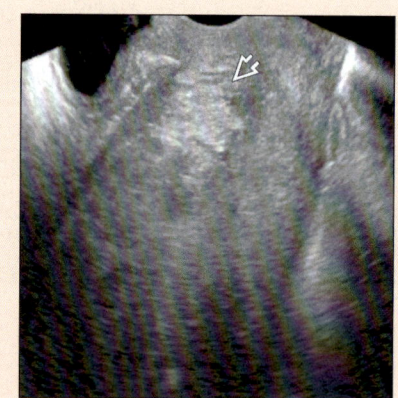
Blood in C-Section Incision

BLADDER FLAP HEMATOMA

Key Facts

Terminology
- Extraperitoneal blood collection at site of cesarian section incision, between lower uterine segment and posterior bladder

Imaging Findings
- Bladder flap is adjacent to low transverse uterine incision formed by reflected peritoneum
- Can range in size from 1-2 cm to greater than 10 cm
- Less than 2 cm are often normal post-operative findings
- **Transabdominal and transvaginal US**
- Heterogeneous collection between lower uterine segment & bladder adjacent to the incision
- **Blood can dissect**:
- Subserosally along uterus
- Laterally along broad ligaments and into retroperitoneum

Top Differential Diagnoses
- Normal Post-Cesarian Section Change
- Abscess
- Free Pelvic Fluid
- Non-Distended Bladder
- Subfascial Hematoma
- Dehiscence

Clinical Issues
- Most common signs/symptoms: Dropping hematocrit in post-partum, cesarian section patient
- Conservative treatment often results in spontaneous resolution

○ Laterally along broad ligaments and into retroperitoneum
- Transperineal US
  ○ Complementary to transabdominal and transvaginal US
    ▪ Limited field of view does not allow evaluation of endometrium nor uterine body and fundus in enlarged post-partum uterus
  ○ More comfortable than scanning over skin incision
  ○ Empty bladder or markedly overdistended bladder interfere with transperineal imaging

CT Findings
- Heterogeneous increased density on both NECT & CECT interposed between bladder and lower uterine segment consistent with subacute blood
- Underlying serosal and myometrial layers should be intact
  ○ Important finding to excluded dehiscence
- Presence of gas raises possibility of abscess
  ○ Clinical history is important in making diagnosis
    ▪ Post-cesarian section patients can normally have gas in the endometrial canal extending into the bladder flap hematoma

MR Findings
- T1WI
  ○ Mixed signal intensity
    ▪ Increased signal intensity (SI) representing subacute hemorrhage with areas of low SI edema
- T2WI
  ○ Usually high SI representing hemorrhage and edema
  ○ Underlying serosal and myometrial layers should be intact, excluding dehiscence

Imaging Recommendations
- Best imaging tool: Ultrasound

DIFFERENTIAL DIAGNOSIS

Normal Post-Cesarian Section Change
- Hypoechoic area less than 2 cm immediately posterior to bladder
- Symmetrically localized to region of the uterine incision
- May be hyperechoic if blood within incision

Abscess
- Gas within collection aids diagnosis
- Clinical history aids diagnosis

Free Pelvic Fluid
- Cul-de-sac fluid is remote from bladder & posterior to uterus

Non-Distended Bladder
- Posterior bladder wall may be mistaken for bladder flap hematoma

Subfascial Hematoma
- Occur at level of skin incision
- Results from extraperitoneal hemorrhage from epigastric vessels within the prevesical space
  ○ Posterior to rectus muscle and transversalis fascia
  ○ Anterior to peritoneum and umbilicovesical fascia
- Often occur in conjunction with bladder flap hematoma
- Subfascial hematoma may extend inferiorly into the space of Retzius (prevesicular space in the retropubic region)
  ○ May be difficult to detect with transabdominal US
- Potential for significant blood loss
  ○ Can accommodate up to 2500 mL before evidence of abdominal wall mass

Dehiscence
- Discontinuity of serosal or myometrial layers of uterus
- Need to carefully evaluate for fluid or blood tracking through incision site

BLADDER FLAP HEMATOMA

PATHOLOGY

General Features
- Etiology
  - Hematoma forms in potential space between bladder and lower uterine segment adjacent to the incision
  - Potential space is created during cesarian section when
    - Peritoneum covering uterus is reflected, and
    - Blunt dissection is performed between bladder & lower uterine segment
- Epidemiology
  - Up to 9% of women will have a bladder flap hematoma
  - Presence of bladder flap hematoma
    - Not predictive of post-operative fever
    - Not synonymous with post-partum complication
- Associated abnormalities: Subfascial hematomas are often present in patients with bladder flap hematomas

Gross Pathologic & Surgical Features
- Clot interposed between posterior bladder and lower uterine segment at level of cesarian section incision

Microscopic Features
- Blood products

CLINICAL ISSUES

Presentation
- Most common signs/symptoms: Dropping hematocrit in post-partum, cesarian section patient
- Other signs/symptoms: Post-operative fever

Demographics
- Age: No age predilection
- Gender: Post-cesarian section women

Natural History & Prognosis
- May spread along subserosally along uterus and along broad ligaments into retroperitoneum
- Most resolve without therapy

Treatment
- Conservative treatment often results in spontaneous resolution
- Laparotomy and surgical drainage if bleeding persists
- Surgical drainage requires incision of peritoneum

DIAGNOSTIC CHECKLIST

Consider
- Bladder flap hematoma in a patient post-cesarian section patient with a drop in hematocrit and/or fever
- CT for possible extension of hematoma into the retroperitoneum

Image Interpretation Pearls
- Always evaluate uterine wall to rule out dehiscence

SELECTED REFERENCES

1. Rivlin ME et al: Diagnostic imaging in uterine incisional necrosis/dehiscence complicating cesarean section. J Reprod Med. 50(12):928-32, 2005
2. Nagayama M et al: Fast MR imaging in obstetrics. Radiographics. 22(3):563-80; discussion 580-2, 2002
3. Gemer O et al: Sonographically diagnosed pelvic hematomas and postcesarean febrile morbidity. Int J Gynaecol Obstet. 65(1):7-9, 1999
4. Maldjian C et al: MR appearance of uterine dehiscence in the post-cesarean section patient. J Comput Assist Tomogr. 22(5):738-41, 1998
5. Hertzberg BS et al: Complications of cesarean section: role of transperineal US. Radiology. 188(2):533-6, 1993
6. Woo GM et al: The pelvis after cesarean section and vaginal delivery: normal MR findings. AJR Am J Roentgenol. 161(6):1249-52, 1993
7. Baker ME et al: Sonography of the low transverse incision, cesarean section: a prospective study. J Ultrasound Med. 7(7):389-93, 1988
8. Wiener MD et al: Sonography of subfascial hematoma after cesarean delivery. AJR Am J Roentgenol. 148(5):907-10, 1987
9. Winsett MZ et al: Sonographic demonstration of bladder-flap hematoma. J Ultrasound Med. 5(9):483-7, 1986
10. Baker ME et al: Sonography of post-cesarean-section bladder-flap hematoma. AJR Am J Roentgenol. 144(4):757-9, 1985
11. Faustin D et al: Relationship of ultrasound findings after cesarean section to operative morbidity. Obstet Gynecol. 66(2):195-8, 1985

BLADDER FLAP HEMATOMA

IMAGE GALLERY

Typical

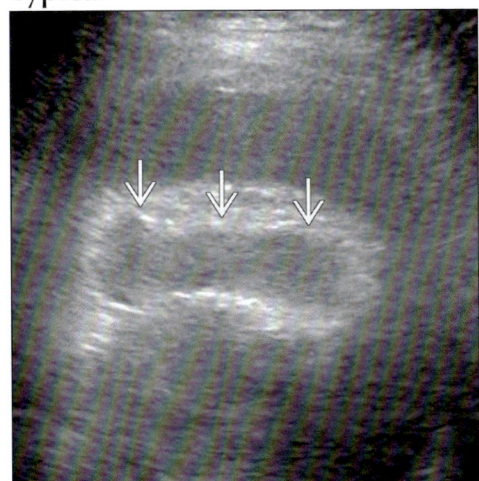
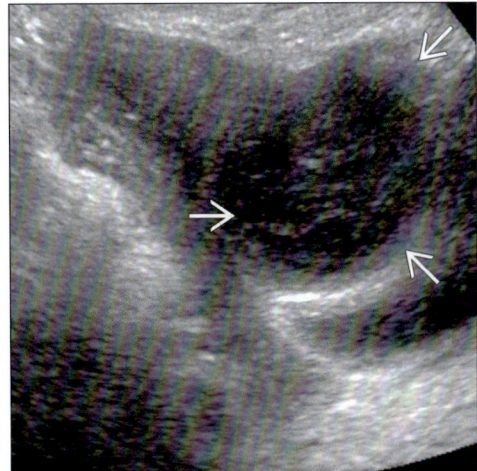

(Left) Axial transabdominal ultrasound shows hypoechoic hematoma with internal echoes ➡ at the typical location between bladder and anterior lower uterus. (Right) Sagittal transabdominal ultrasound shows large hypoechoic collection of blood ➡ from bladder flap hematoma.

Variant

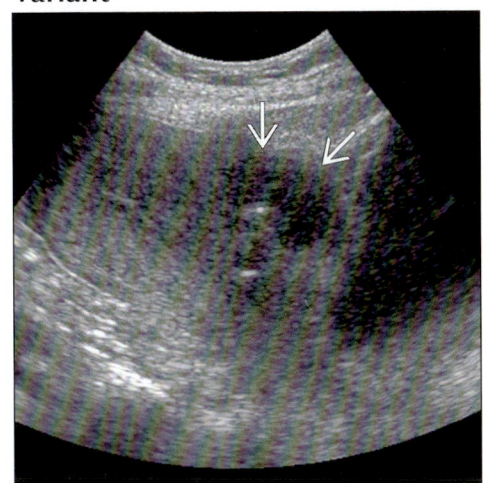
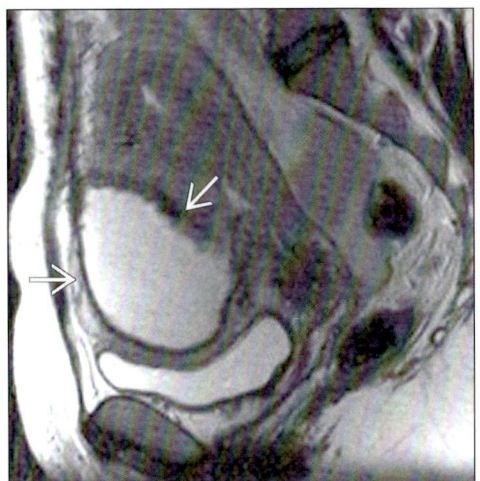

(Left) Sagittal transvaginal ultrasound shows a heterogeneous collection ➡ between the bladder and lower uterine segment in a febrile patient at the level of the cesarian section incision. (Right) Sagittal T2WI MR in the same patient as previous image, shows high signal intensity fluid collection ➡ of an infected bladder flap hematoma.

Variant

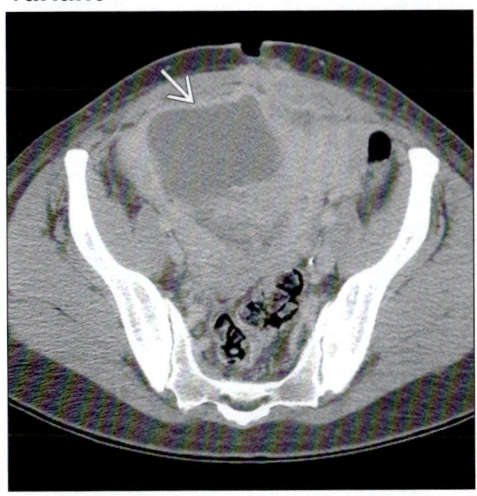
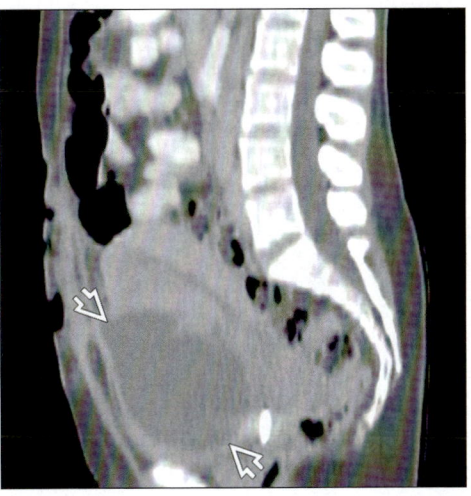

(Left) Axial NECT in the same patient as previous image, shows the collection ➡ anterior to the uterus. (Right) Sagittal NECT multiplanar reconstruction in the same patient as previous image, shows the large infected bladder flap hematoma ➡.

PELVIC CONGESTION SYNDROME

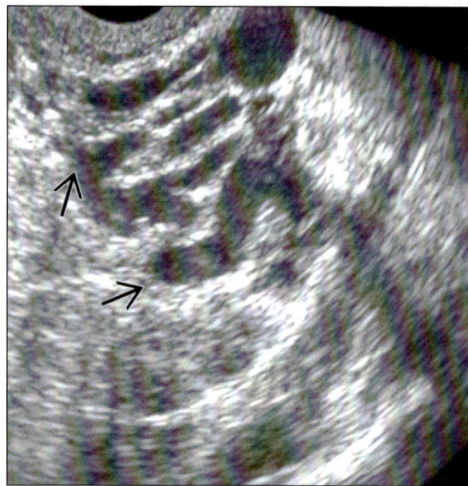

Sagittal transvaginal ultrasound shows serpentine hypoechoic tubular structures ➔ in a parauterine location. Doppler (not shown) confirmed venous waveforms.

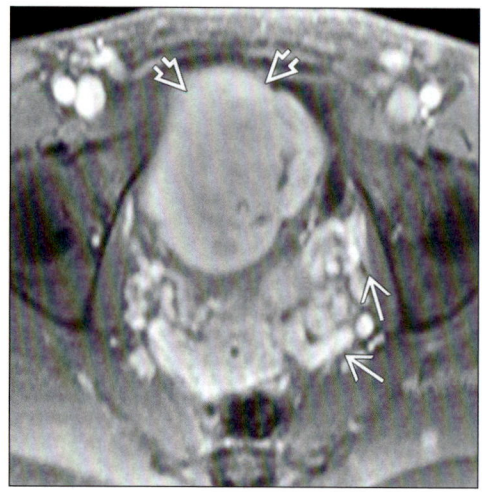

Axial T1 C+ FS MR shows markedly dilated left parauterine veins ➔ in a woman with chronic pelvic pain. The patient's pain may also be related to a leiomyoma ➔.

TERMINOLOGY

Abbreviations and Synonyms
- PCS, pelvic varices, pelvic venous incompetence, pelvic vein syndrome

Definitions
- Non-cyclical chronic pelvic pain caused by dilated veins in broad ligament & ovarian plexus
  - Sidewall, paravaginal and internal iliac varicosities may be present
  - Occasionally pelvic varices communicate with vulval & lower extremity varicosities
- First described by Richet in 1857
  - Chronic dull pelvic pain, pressure and heaviness: A result of dilated tortuous & congested veins caused by retrograde flow through incompetent ovarian vein valves
- Underdiagnosed treatable cause of chronic pelvic pain
  - Pelvic varicoceles are found in approximately 1/2 of women with chronic pelvic pain

IMAGING FINDINGS

General Features
- Best diagnostic clue
  - Dilated and tortuous parauterine tubular structures on contrast venography, ultrasound, CT, and/or MR
    - 50% of patients with associated cystic ovaries
- Varices may extend laterally in broad ligament and/or inferiorly to communicate with paravaginal venous plexus
- Most cross-sectional studies are not performed erect; therefore, subjective assessment by the radiologist is important for final diagnosis

Ultrasonographic Findings
- Grayscale Ultrasound
  - **Transvaginal ultrasound (TVS): 3 criteria:**
    - Tortuous pelvic vein with a diameter > 4 mm (some investigators use > 5 mm)
    - Slow blood flow (about 3 cm/sec)
    - Dilated arcuate vein in the myometrium that communicates between bilateral pelvic varicose veins
  - Single institution study

DDx: Pelvic Congestion Syndrome

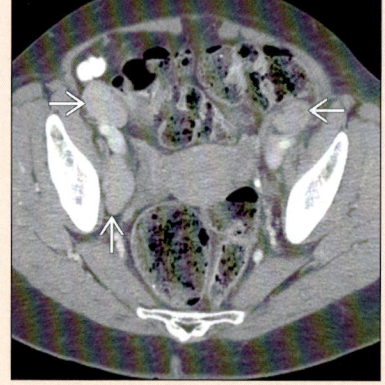

Lymphadenopathy

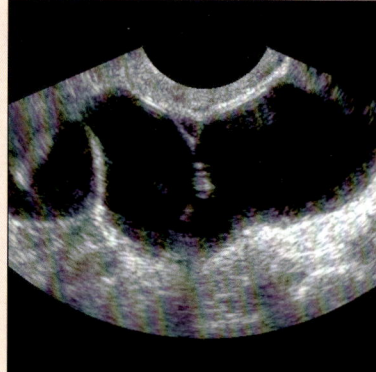

Hydrosalpinx

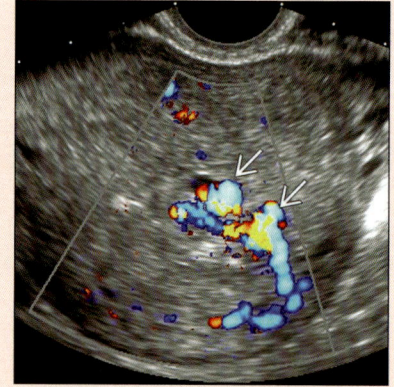

Arteriovenous Malformation

PELVIC CONGESTION SYNDROME

Key Facts

Terminology
- PCS, pelvic varices, pelvic venous incompetence, pelvic vein syndrome
- Non-cyclical chronic pelvic pain caused by dilated veins in broad ligament & ovarian plexus

Imaging Findings
- Dilated and tortuous parauterine tubular structures on contrast venography, ultrasound, CT, and/or MR
- **Transvaginal ultrasound (TVS): 3 criteria:**
- Tortuous pelvic vein with a diameter > 4 mm (some investigators use > 5 mm)
- Slow blood flow (about 3 cm/sec)
- Dilated arcuate vein in the myometrium that communicates between bilateral pelvic varicose veins

Top Differential Diagnoses
- Pelvic Lymphadenopathy
- Hydrosalpinx
- Arteriovenous Malformation

Pathology
- Primary valvular deficiency
- Hormonal vasodilation
- "Nutcracker" phenomenon: Left renal vein entrapment between aorta & superior mesenteric artery
- Other obstructing anatomic anomalies: Left ovarian vein obstruction by retroaortic left renal vein or right common iliac artery

Clinical Issues
- Treat with transcatheter embolization

- PCS: Mean diameter of left & right pelvic veins: .68 and .64 cm, respectively
- Controls: Mean diameter of left & right pelvic veins: .42 and .35 cm, respectively
- Transabdominal US showed enlarged (.79 cm) left ovarian vein draining into left renal vein in PCS patients
- Color Doppler
  - Large venous structures engorging uterus & ovaries
  - If vulval varices, loud "reflux" with Valsalva maneuver
  - For "Nutcracker" syndrome: Color flow in gonadal & retroperitoneal collaterals
  - Valsalva maneuver: Variable color Doppler waveform

CT Findings
- CECT
  - At least 4 ipsilateral tortuous parauterine veins of varying caliber, at least one of which is > 4 mm in maximum diameter, or an ovarian vein diameter > 8 mm
  - Varices are isodense with other pelvic veins

MR Findings
- T1WI: Serpentine flow void
- T2WI
  - Serpentine flow void
  - May have high or heterogeneous signal intensity because of relative slow flow in dilated veins
  - Same diagnostic criteria as CECT
    - At least 4 ipsilateral tortuous parauterine veins of varying caliber, at least one of which is > 4 mm in maximum diameter, or an ovarian vein diameter > 8 mm
- T1 C+
  - Delayed enhancement of dilated & tortuous involved veins
    - Around the uterus and ovary and may extend into broad ligament, pelvic sidewall and paravaginal venous plexus
- MRV: High-signal-intensity ovarian and/or parauterine veins

Angiographic Findings
- Retrograde ovarian venography (patient in semi-erect position with Valsalva maneuver performed as needed)
  - Ovarian vein > 8-10 mm
  - Uterine venous engorgement
  - Congestion of the ovarian plexus
  - Filling of pelvic veins across midline and/or filling of vulvovaginal & thigh varicosities

Imaging Recommendations
- Best imaging tool: Color and Doppler TVS
- Protocol advice
  - IF TVS is equivocal or non-diagnostic
    - Noninvasive: MR or CECT
    - Invasive: Retrograde ovarian vein venography

DIFFERENTIAL DIAGNOSIS

Pelvic Lymphadenopathy
- Soft tissue masses that are not tubular, nor enhance in a similar fashion to pelvic venous structures

Hydrosalpinx
- Dilated anechoic fallopian tube without flow
- Pyosalpinx may have low level echogenic debris

Arteriovenous Malformation
- Congenital or acquired condition in the uterus or parauterine tissues, not purely venous
- CECT or CEMR: Briskly enhancing soft tissue masses versus delayed enhancement of pelvic varices in pelvic congestion

PATHOLOGY

General Features
- General path comments
  - Incompetent ovarian and/or internal iliac veins are usually present but not causative
  - Pelvic/ovarian varices can be seen in asymptomatic women

PELVIC CONGESTION SYNDROME

- Prevalence in general population approaches 10%
- Passive reflux into left gonadal vein is common
- Genetics: Hereditary risk factors have been suggested
- Etiology
  - Not well understood but related to the physiologic increase in blood flow in pelvic veins during puberty & pregnancy
  - Multifactorial: Possible factors
    - Primary valvular deficiency
    - Hormonal vasodilation
    - "Nutcracker" phenomenon: Left renal vein entrapment between aorta & superior mesenteric artery
    - Other obstructing anatomic anomalies: Left ovarian vein obstruction by retroaortic left renal vein or right common iliac artery
    - Psychomotor venodilation
  - Risk factors: Heredity, pelvic surgery, retroverted uterus, history of varicose veins
  - Secondary PCS is associated with portal hypertension & acquired inferior vena cava syndrome
- Epidemiology: Multiparous women of reproductive age
- Classification system of parauterine venous plexus
  - Normal: Veins are small, straight, similar in caliber & easily recognized
  - Moderate congestion: Veins are tortuous, variable in caliber & difficult to resolve separately
  - Severe congestion: Veins are wide, markedly tortuous & vary greatly in caliber

Gross Pathologic & Surgical Features

- Primary pelvic varices are positively associated with absent or incompetent valves and parity
  - Pelvic varices and PCS can occur independently

CLINICAL ISSUES

Presentation

- Most common signs/symptoms
  - Chronic pelvic pain: May be relieved when recumbent
    - Dull/heavy aching pain that is associated with movement, posture and activities that increase abdominal pressure
    - Pain may be unilateral or bilateral and is often asymmetric
  - Dyspareunia (71%), dysmenorrhea (66%), and postcoital ache (65%)
- Other signs/symptoms
  - Pain while walking
  - May have sharp exacerbations of pain and/or rectal discomfort and/or urinary frequency
  - Physical exam may show: Varicose veins (in the vulva, buttocks and legs) & ovarian point tenderness upon palpation
- Clinical Profile: Women in their reproductive years

Demographics

- Age
  - Most often found in multiparous women of reproductive age
  - Pelvic varices occur in approximately 10% of the female population
    - Up to 59% develop PCS
    - 77% may benefit from treatment

Treatment

- Treat with transcatheter embolization
  - Sclerosing agent and/or coils
  - High rate of technical success (96-99%)
  - Coil embolization: Significant decrease in (50-80%) in pain without notable impact on menstrual cycle; 60% report complete resolution of symptoms
- Resection or ligation (open surgical or laparoscopic management)
  - Increased incidence of morbidity compared with embolic therapy
  - Bilateral ligation: Pilot study with complete remission of pain and absence of varicose veins for 1 year
- Hormonal manipulation (pharmacologic ovarian suppression)

DIAGNOSTIC CHECKLIST

Consider

- PCS in women with non-cyclic chronic pelvic pain and dilated pelvic veins

SELECTED REFERENCES

1. Cheong Y et al: Chronic pelvic pain: aetiology and therapy. Best Pract Res Clin Obstet Gynaecol. 20(5):695-711, 2006
2. Kim HS et al: Embolotherapy for pelvic congestion syndrome: long-term results. J Vasc Interv Radiol. 17(2 Pt 1):289-97, 2006
3. Koc Z et al: Association of left renal vein variations and pelvic varices in abdominal MDCT. Eur Radiol. 2006
4. Nicholson T et al: Pelvic congestion syndrome, who should we treat and how? Tech Vasc Interv Radiol. 9(1):19-23, 2006
5. Kuligowska E et al: Pelvic pain: overlooked and underdiagnosed gynecologic conditions. Radiographics. 25(1):3-20, 2005
6. Siddall KA et al: Multidetector CT of the female pelvis. Radiol Clin North Am. 43(6):1097-118, ix, 2005
7. Park SJ et al: Diagnosis of pelvic congestion syndrome using transabdominal and transvaginal sonography. AJR Am J Roentgenol. 182(3):683-8, 2004
8. Belenky A et al: Ovarian varices in healthy female kidney donors: incidence, morbidity, and clinical outcome. AJR Am J Roentgenol. 179(3):625-7, 2002
9. Nascimento AB et al: Ovarian veins: magnetic resonance imaging findings in an asymptomatic population. J Magn Reson Imaging. 15(5):551-6, 2002
10. Venbrux AC et al: Pelvic congestion syndrome (pelvic venous incompetence): impact of ovarian and internal iliac vein embolotherapy on menstrual cycle and chronic pelvic pain. J Vasc Interv Radiol. 13(2 Pt 1):171-8, 2002
11. Rozenblit AM et al: Incompetent and dilated ovarian veins: a common CT finding in asymptomatic parous women. AJR Am J Roentgenol. 176(1):119-22, 2001
12. Coakley FV et al: CT and MRI of pelvic varices in women. J Comput Assist Tomogr. 23(3):429-34, 1999

PELVIC CONGESTION SYNDROME

IMAGE GALLERY

Typical

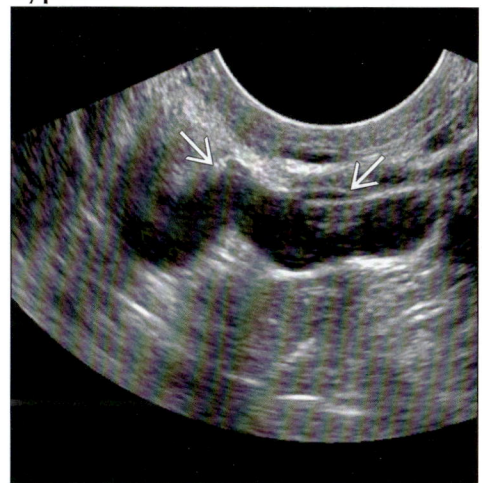
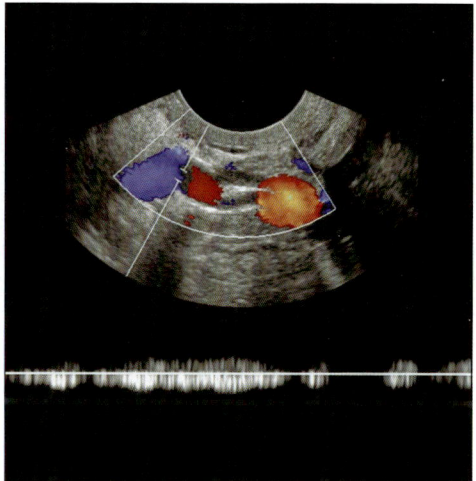

(Left) Sagittal transvaginal ultrasound shows a hypoechoic tubular structure ➡ in the left adnexa with a diameter > 5 mm, consistent with a pelvic varix. *(Right)* Sagittal color Doppler ultrasound in the same patient as previous image, shows venous flow within the vessel.

Typical

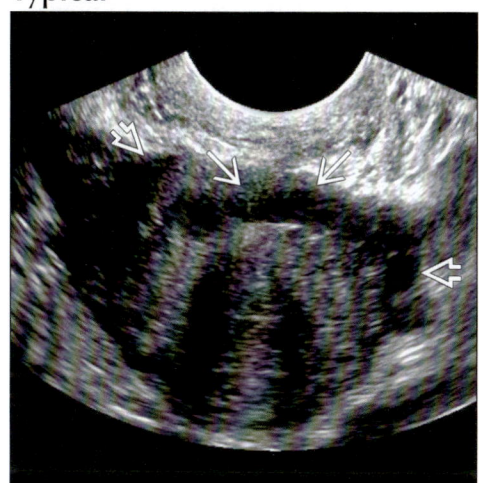
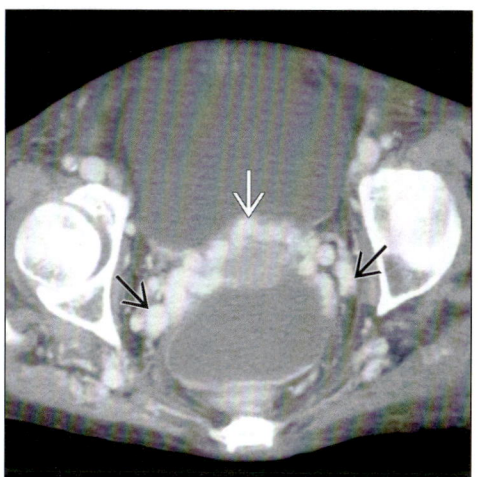

(Left) Axial transvaginal ultrasound shows a dilated arcuate vein ➡ within the myometrium that communicates with bilateral pelvic varices ➡. *(Right)* Axial CECT shows a dilated enhancing myometrial arcuate vein ➡ that communicates with bilateral varicose veins ➡.

Typical

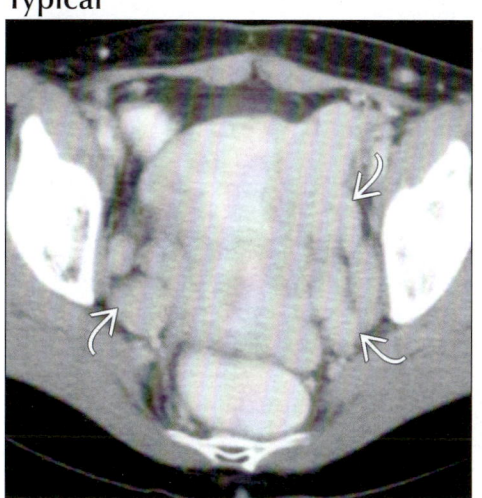
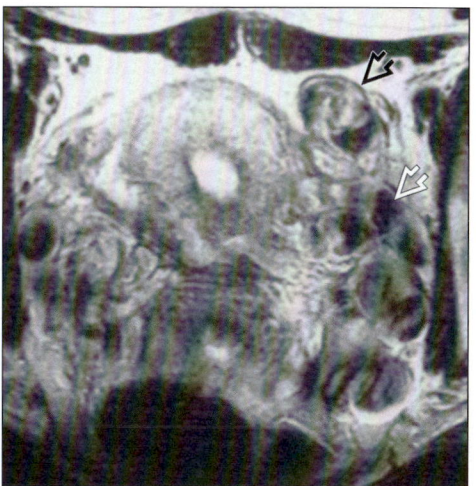

(Left) Axial CECT markedly dilated enhancing veins ➡ in a patient with chronic pelvic pain. *(Right)* Axial T2WI MR in the same patient as previous image, shows the dilated veins may image as primarily signal voids ➡ or have a more heterogeneous appearance ➡ because of slow flow.

PELVIC FLOOR DESCENT

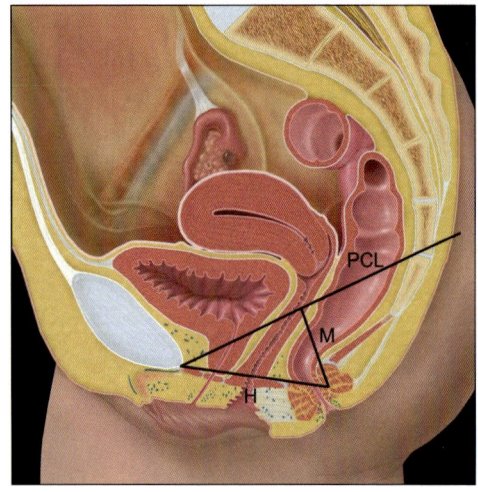

Sagittal graphic shows the pubococcygeal line (PCL), M line and H line.

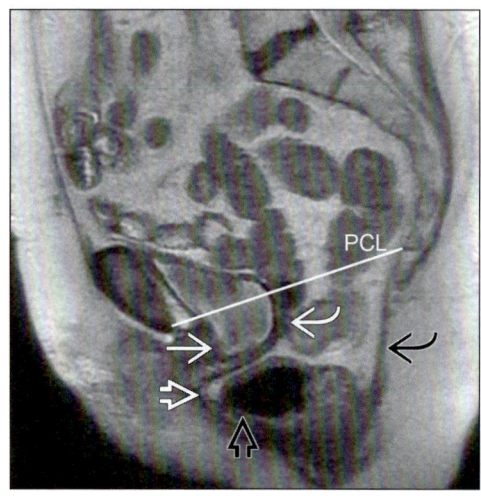

Sagittal T2WI MR with straining shows urethrovesical (UV) junction ➔, and vaginal cuff ➔ below the PCL. Note the peritoneocele ⬧, anterior rectocele ⬧ and vertical orientation of the levator plate ➔.

TERMINOLOGY

Abbreviations and Synonyms
- Pelvic organ prolapse, pelvic floor relaxation

Definitions
- Pelvic floor descent encompasses three different compartments; each needs to be corrected separately
  - Anterior: Bladder and urethra
  - Middle: Vagina, cervix, and uterus
  - Posterior: Enterocele, rectocele

IMAGING FINDINGS

General Features
- Best diagnostic clue: Puborectalis insertion on rectum > 2 cm below pubococcygeal line (PCL)
- Imaging findings must be interpreted in conjunction with physical examination and symptoms
- Mechanism is weakness of pelvic floor fascia, muscles, ligaments
  - Pelvic floor supporting structures
    - Anterior compartment: Puborectalis/pubovaginalis component of levator ani muscle, pubourethral/pubovesical ligaments
    - Middle compartment: Uterosacral and cardinal ligaments, parametrium, paracolpium, and rectovaginal fascia
    - Posterior compartment: Iliococcygeus component of levator ani and levator plate in continuity with external anal sphincter
- Anatomical landmarks
  - PCL: Between lower symphysis pubis and last mobile coccygeal joint (site of insertion of levator plate)
  - H line (levator hiatus): Between lower symphysis pubis and puborectalis insertion on rectum
  - M line: Perpendicular line between H line and PCL, at insertion of H line to rectum
- Normal landmark values/appearance
  - Levator plate parallels PCL
  - H line < 5 cm
  - M line < 2 cm

MR Findings
- T2WI

DDx: Low Midline Pelvic Mass

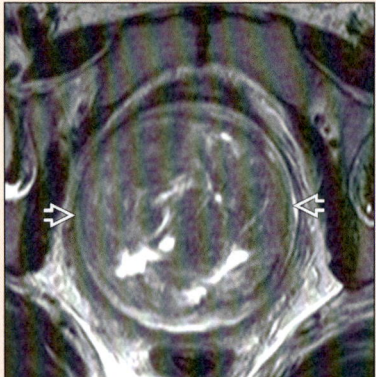

Prolapsing Leiomyoma

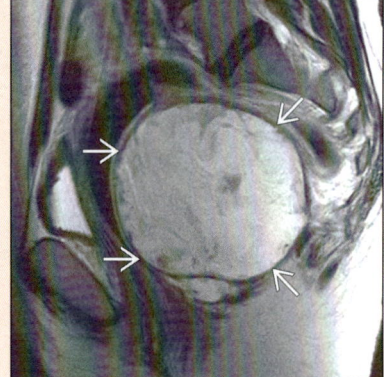

Mucinous Rectal Cancer

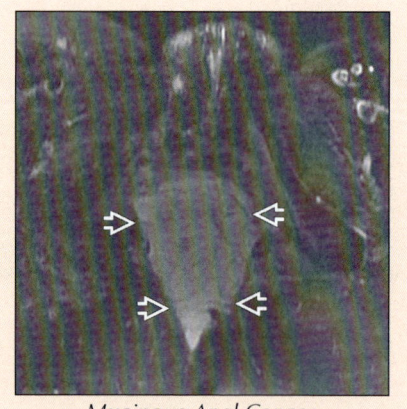

Mucinous Anal Cancer

PELVIC FLOOR DESCENT

Key Facts

Terminology
- Pelvic organ prolapse, pelvic floor relaxation

Imaging Findings
- Best diagnostic clue: Puborectalis insertion on rectum > 2 cm below pubococcygeal line (PCL)
- Imaging findings must be interpreted in conjunction with physical examination and symptoms
- PCL: Between lower symphysis pubis and last mobile coccygeal joint (site of insertion of levator plate)
- H line (levator hiatus): Between lower symphysis pubis and puborectalis insertion on rectum
- M line: Perpendicular line between H line and PCL, at insertion of H line to rectum
- Elongation of H line > 5 cm
- Elongation of M line > 2 cm
- Mild descent: Displacement > 1 cm and ≤ 2 cm of urethrovesical junction, cervix/vaginal cuff, anorectal junction below PCL on straining views
- Marked descent: Displacement > 2 cm below PCL on straining views; requires surgery
- Levator plate does not parallel PCL: Inclination relative to PCL > 10°

Clinical Issues
- Lack of recognition of multi-compartment disease a cause for up to 30% treatment failure
- Each segment must be reported to optimize patient management

Diagnostic Checklist
- Coach the patient to achieve optimal straining
- Acquire dynamic images using Cine MR

- Pelvic relaxation indicated in a symptomatic patient when
  - Elongation of H line > 5 cm
  - Elongation of M line > 2 cm
  - Mild descent: Displacement > 1 cm and ≤ 2 cm of urethrovesical junction, cervix/vaginal cuff, anorectal junction below PCL on straining views
  - Marked descent: Displacement > 2 cm below PCL on straining views; requires surgery
  - Levator plate does not parallel PCL: Inclination relative to PCL > 10°
  - Lateral convexity of levator ani on axial and inferior convexity on coronal images
  - Inferior bulge of perineal body

Fluoroscopic Findings
- Colpocystodefecography (CCD) using findings similar to MR to diagnosis pelvic floor descent

Imaging Recommendations
- Best imaging tool
  - MR is the modality of choice since it optimally depicts the supporting structures of the pelvic floor
    - Maximal sensitivity attained with an open magnet and sitting position to optimize straining
  - MR is indicated under the following circumstances
    - Suboptimal physical examination
    - To establish multi-compartment disease
    - To establish other compartment disease when surgery fails
  - Alternative exam: Fluoroscopic CCD
    - Many surgeons prefer this exam over supine MR due to upright position
- Protocol advice
  - Axial breath-hold fast spin-echo (FSE)
    - To delineate anatomy and exclude underlying pathology
    - Slice thickness ≤ 6 mm
  - Dynamic Cine MR is mainstay of pelvic floor assessment
    - Single shot FSE (SSFSE), Half-Fourier Snapshot Turbo Spin-Echo (HASTE), or true Fast Imaging with Steady-state Precession (true FISP)
    - Sequential images with a 1 to 2 second temporal resolution
    - Continuous evaluation with Cine MR improves evaluation during straining
    - 6-10 mm slice thickness
    - Basic protocol: Midline sagittal, relaxed and straining sequences
    - Optional protocol: Coronal, relaxed and straining sequences

DIFFERENTIAL DIAGNOSIS

Cystitis
- Differential diagnosis for urinary incontinence
- Symptoms of infection
- No clinical evidence of pelvic floor descent

Atrophic Urethritis/Vaginitis
- Cause of incontinence in as many as 80% of elderly women
- Associated symptoms of infection
- No clinical evidence of pelvic descent

Rectal Intussusception
- Secondary to chronic straining
  - Typically present during evacuation
  - Frequent association with rectocele
- Infolding of the rectal wall
- May be intra-rectal, intra-anal or complete rectal prolapse
- No associated cystocele

Low Midline Pelvic Mass
- Pressure on pelvic organs can mimic symptoms of pelvic floor descent
- Mass can bulge out pelvic floor

PATHOLOGY

General Features
- General path comments

PELVIC FLOOR DESCENT

- Abnormal descent in up to 50% of women > 50 years of age
- Rare in men presumably because of strong levator ani
- Genetics: Higher incidence in some families
- Etiology
  - Increasing age and stress related to multiple pregnancies even in absence of vaginal delivery
  - Hysterectomy
  - Obesity
  - Chronic cough associated with smoking
- Epidemiology
  - 50% of women over 50 years of age
  - 10-20% symptomatic
- Associated abnormalities
  - Vesical, vaginal, rectal prolapse
  - Constipation, rectal ulceration, hemorrhoids
  - Ureteral obstruction

CLINICAL ISSUES

Presentation
- Most common signs/symptoms
  - Urinary, stool incontinence
  - 10% to 20% symptomatic
- Other signs/symptoms
  - Back/pelvic pain
  - Difficulty emptying bladder, ureteral obstruction
  - Urinary and fecal stress or total incontinence
  - Constipation and rectal ulceration, hemorrhoids
  - Organ prolapse (bladder, uterus, rectum)
- Clinical Profile: Woman with history of hysterectomy and multiple pregnancies

Demographics
- Age
  - ≥ 45 years of age
  - Increased incidence after menopause
- Ethnicity: Most common amongst Caucasian women, followed by Hispanic, Asian and black women

Natural History & Prognosis
- Lack of recognition of multi-compartment disease a cause for up to 30% treatment failure

Treatment
- Different approaches for
  - Anterior vaginal wall prolapse
  - Posterior vaginal wall prolapse
  - Enterocele and prolapse of vaginal vault
  - Uterine prolapse
- Each segment must be reported to optimize patient management
- > 2 cm descent below PCL requires surgery

DIAGNOSTIC CHECKLIST

Consider
- Coach the patient to achieve optimal straining
- Acquire dynamic images using Cine MR

Image Interpretation Pearls
- Levator plate does not parallel PCL
- Elongation of M line > 2 cm

SELECTED REFERENCES

1. Schofield ML et al: MRI findings following laparoscopic sacrocolpopexy. Clin Radiol. 60(3):333-9, 2005
2. Pannu HK: MRI of pelvic organ prolapse. Eur Radiol. 14(8):1456-64, 2004
3. Grodstein F et al: Association of age, race, and obstetric history with urinary symptoms among women in the Nurses' Health Study. Am J Obstet Gynecol. 189(2):428-34, 2003
4. Fielding JR: Practical MR imaging of female pelvic floor weakness. Radiographics. 22(2):295-304, 2002
5. Barbaric ZL et al: Magnetic resonance imaging of the perineum and pelvic floor. Top Magn Reson Imaging. 12(2):83-92, 2001
6. Goh V et al: Dynamic MR imaging of the pelvic floor in asymptomatic subjects. AJR Am J Roentgenol. 174(3):661-6, 2000
7. Pannu HK et al: Dynamic MR imaging of pelvic organ prolapse: spectrum of abnormalities. Radiographics. 20(6):1567-82, 2000
8. Gufler H et al: Pelvic floor descent: dynamic MR imaging using a half-Fourier RARE sequence. J Magn Reson Imaging. 9(3):378-83, 1999
9. Vanbeckevoort D et al: Pelvic floor descent in females: comparative study of colpocystodefecography and dynamic fast MR imaging. J Magn Reson Imaging. 9(3):373-7, 1999
10. Raz S et al: Vaginal reconstructive surgery for incontinence and prolapse in Campbell's urology. W.B. Saunders company. 1059-94, 1998
11. Steiner RA et al: Patterns of prolapse in women with symptoms of pelvic floor weakness: magnetic resonance imaging and laparoscopic treatment. Curr Opin Obstet Gynecol. 10(4):295-301, 1998
12. Lienemann A et al: Dynamic MR colpocystorectography assessing pelvic-floor descent. Eur Radiol. 7(8):1309-17, 1997
13. Yang A et al: Pelvic floor descent in women: dynamic evaluation with fast MR imaging and cinematic display. Radiology. 179(1):25-33, 1991

PELVIC FLOOR DESCENT

IMAGE GALLERY

Typical

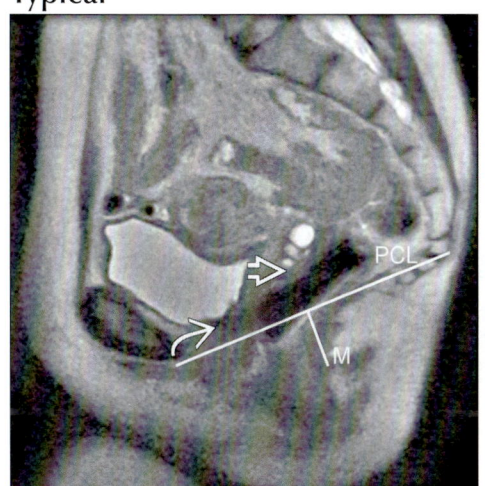
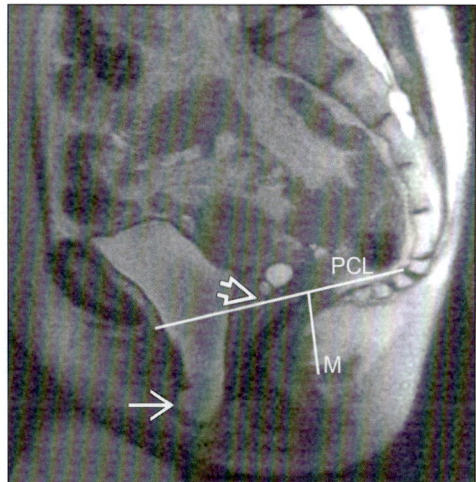

(Left) Sagittal T2WI MR without straining. The UV junction ➔ and exocervix ➔ lie above the PCL. The M line measures less than 2 cm. *(Right)* Sagittal T2WI MR with straining in the same patient as previous image. The UV junction ➔ has descended below the PCL indicating a cystocele, and the exocervix ➔ has descended to the level of the PCL. The M line measures between 2 and 4 cm consistent with a grade 1 descent.

Typical

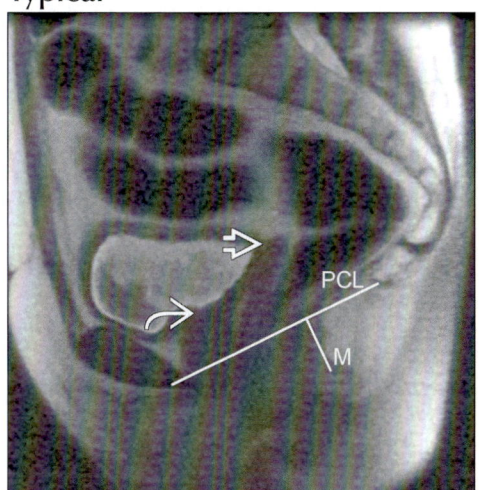
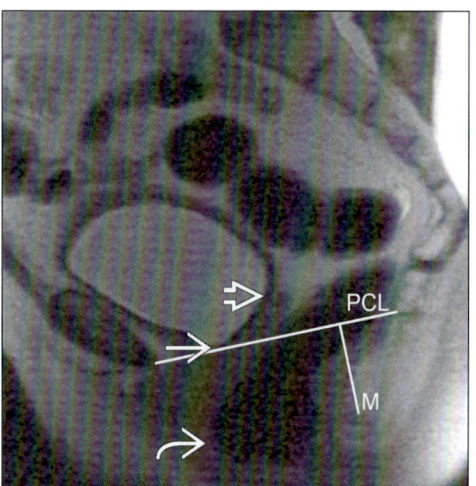

(Left) Sagittal T2WI MR without straining shows the UV junction ➔ and vaginal cuff ➔ to lie above the PCL. The M line measures less than 2 cm. Note position of the rectum. *(Right)* Sagittal T2WI MR with straining in the same patient as previous image. Both the UV junction ➔ and vaginal cuff ➔ have descended close to the PCL. Note the significant descent and anterior bulge of the rectum ➔. The M line measures between 2 and 4 cm consistent with a grade 1 descent.

Typical

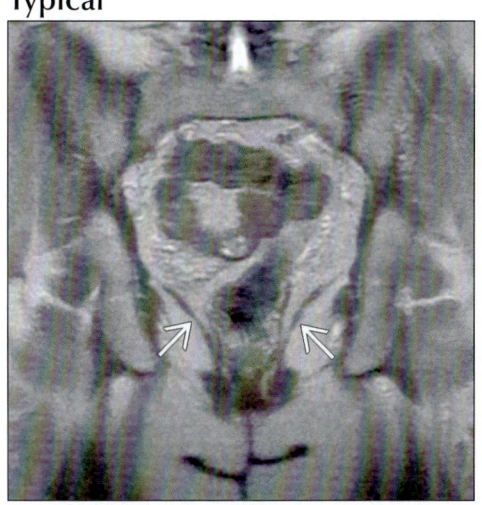
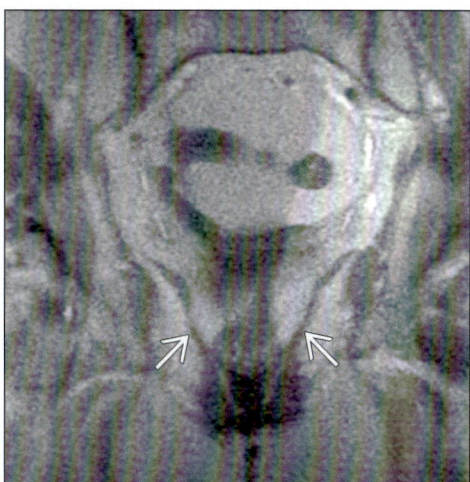

(Left) Coronal T2WI MR without straining shows the normal inferolateral concavity ➔ and symmetric appearance of both levator plates. *(Right)* Coronal T2WI MR with straining in a different patient shows the inferolateral convexity ➔ of the levator plates due to pelvic floor prolapse.

VAGINOCELE/CYSTOCELE

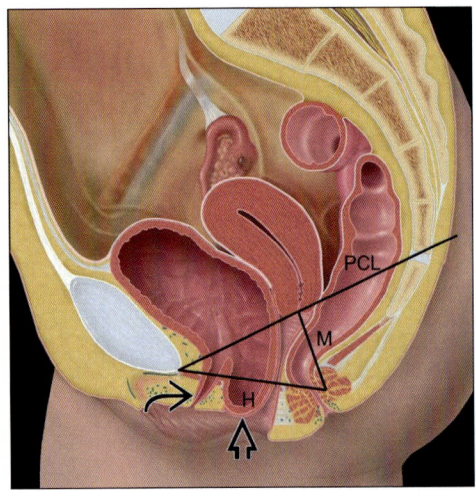

Sagittal graphic shows the pubococcygeal line (PCL), M line and H line. There is a urethrovesical (UV) junction ➔ and bladder ➔ prolapse.

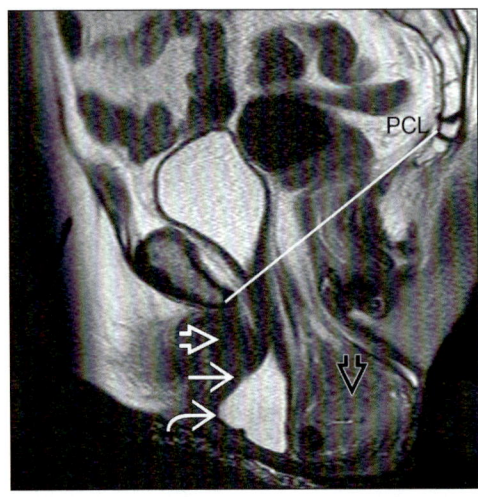

Sagittal T2WI MR on straining shows a large cystocele ➔. The UV junction ➔ is significantly below the PCL and the urethral axis ➔ is reversed. Note the prolapsed uterus ➔ protruding through the vagina.

TERMINOLOGY

Abbreviations and Synonyms
- Anterior vaginal wall prolapse, urethral hypermobility

Definitions
- Lateral cystocele (70-80%): Weakness or disruption of lateral attachment of vesicopelvic fascia
- Central cystocele (5-15%): Attenuated central vesicopelvic fascia

IMAGING FINDINGS

General Features
- Best diagnostic clue
  - Descent of UV junction on resting or strain > 1 cm below pubococcygeal line (PCL)
  - Descent of vaginal cuff below PCL
- Pelvic floor descent encompasses three different compartments; each needs to be corrected separately
  - Anterior: Bladder, urethra
  - Middle: Vagina, cervix, urethra
  - Posterior: Rectum, rectovaginal septum
- Imaging findings must be interpreted in conjunction with physical examination and symptoms
- Pelvic floor supporting structures
  - Anterior compartment: Puborectalis/pubovaginalis component of levator ani muscle, pubourethral/pubovesical ligaments
  - Middle compartment: Uterosacral and cardinal ligaments, parametrium, paracolpium, and rectovaginal fascia
- Anatomical landmarks
  - PCL: Between lower symphysis pubis and last mobile coccygeal joint (insertion of levator plate)
  - H line (levator hiatus): Between lower symphysis pubis and puborectalis insertion on rectum
  - M line: Perpendicular line between H line and PCL, at insertion of H line to rectum
  - VUA (vesicourethral angle): Angle between base of bladder and urethral plane
  - UI (urethral inclination): Angle between urethra and the vertical plane
- Normal landmark values/appearance
  - H-shaped vagina on axial T2WI
  - Symmetric thickness of levator ani on axial

DDx: Periurethral Masses

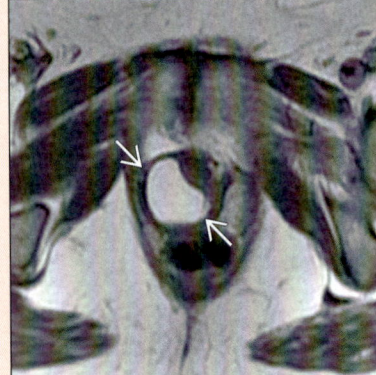

Urethral Diverticulum

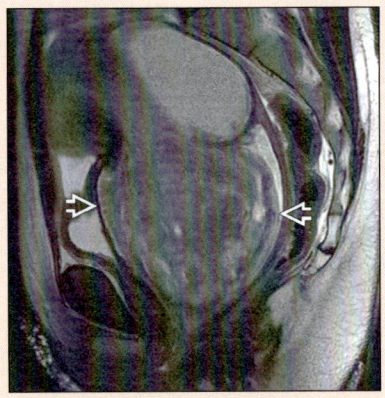

Prolapsed Submucosal Leiomyoma

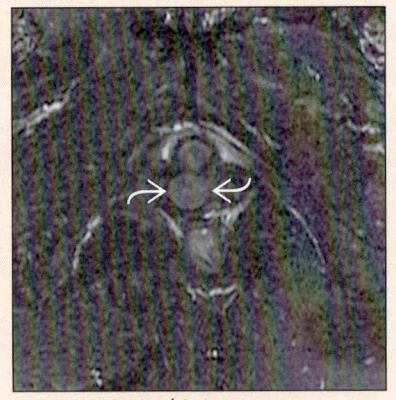

Vaginal Leiomyoma

VAGINOCELE/CYSTOCELE

Key Facts

Terminology
- Anterior vaginal wall prolapse, urethral hypermobility

Imaging Findings
- Descent of UV junction on resting or strain > 1 cm below pubococcygeal line (PCL)
- Descent of vaginal cuff below PCL
- PCL: Between lower symphysis pubis and last mobile coccygeal joint (insertion of levator plate)
- H line (levator hiatus): Between lower symphysis pubis and puborectalis insertion on rectum
- M line: Perpendicular line between H line and PCL, at insertion of H line to rectum
- Indentation of anterior vaginal wall by bladder base
- Horizontal orientation of urethra
- VUA > 115 degrees
- Elongation of H line > 5 cm
- Elongation of M line > 2 cm
- Convexity of levator ani muscle on axial and coronal planes

Pathology
- General path comments: Abnormal descent in up to 50% of women > 50 years old

Clinical Issues
- Lack of recognition of multi-compartment disease a cause for up to 30% treatment failure

Diagnostic Checklist
- Coach the patient to achieve optimal straining
- Apparent thinning of right levator ani due to chemical shift artifact

---

- At times apparent thinning of right side due to chemical shift artifact when phase encoding is in the AP direction
- Straight or concave levator ani on axial
- Vertical orientation of urethra
- H line < 5 cm, M line < 2 cm, VUA < 115°

Ultrasonographic Findings
- Grayscale Ultrasound
  - Transvesical US used to measure pre-void bladder volume, post-void residue and bladder wall thickness
  - Bladder base descent and VUA can be assessed by transvaginal, transrectal or transperineal sonography

MR Findings
- T2WI
  - Descent of UV junction on strain > 1 cm below PCL
  - Descent of vaginal cuff/cervix on strain below PCL
  - Indentation of anterior vaginal wall by bladder base
  - Horizontal orientation of urethra
    - UI > 30 degrees from the vertical
    - VUA > 115 degrees
  - Elongation of H line > 5 cm
  - Elongation of M line > 2 cm
  - Thinning of levator muscle on axial
  - Convexity of levator ani muscle on axial and coronal planes
  - Convex iliococcygeal muscle on coronal
- Related pathology i.e., urethral diverticulum, ureteral dilatation, vesicovaginal fistula detected by MR

Non-Vascular Interventions
- US is used to guide injection of periurethral collagen
- US/MR used for monitoring injected material

Fluoroscopic Findings
- Voiding cystourethrography with bead chain
  - Stress incontinence: Correlates with increasing urethral hypermobility
  - Cystocele: Descent of bladder base below inferior aspect of symphysis pubis, > 1 cm urethral descent
  - Literature contradictory with some studies showing positive and others no correlation with stress incontinence of the above findings

Imaging Recommendations
- Best imaging tool
  - MR is the modality of choice to assess pelvic floor
  - Good correlation between physical examination and dynamic Cine MR
  - MR is indicated under the following circumstances
    - Suboptimal physical examination
    - To establish multi-compartment disease
    - To establish other compartment disease when surgery fails
- Protocol advice
  - Axial breath-hold fast spin-echo (FSE)
    - To delineate anatomy and exclude underlying pathology; slice thickness ≤ 6 mm
  - Dynamic Cine MR is mainstay of pelvic floor assessment
    - Single shot FSE (SSFSE), Half-Fourier Snapshot Turbo Spin-Echo (HASTE), or true Fast Imaging with Steady-state Precession (true FISP)
    - Sequential images, 1-2 second temporal resolution, 6-10 mm slice thickness
    - Basic protocol: Midline sagittal, relaxed and straining sequences
    - Optional protocol: Coronal, relaxed and straining sequences
    - Too much bladder fullness prevents vaginal prolapse

DIFFERENTIAL DIAGNOSIS

Cystitis
- Transient, symptoms of infection
- No clinical evidence of cystovaginocele

Atrophic Urethritis/Vaginitis
- Cause of incontinence in as many as 80% of elderly women
- Associated symptoms of infection

VAGINOCELE/CYSTOCELE

- No clinical evidence of cystovaginocele

Periurethral Mass
- No clinical evidence of cystovaginocele

PATHOLOGY

General Features
- General path comments: Abnormal descent in up to 50% of women > 50 years old
- Genetics: Higher incidence in some families
- Etiology
  - Urethrocystocele
    - Anatomic weakness due to weak anterior vaginal wall (urethral hypermobility)
    - Anatomic weakness due to damaged pubovaginal fascia (bladder prolapse)
    - Intrinsic urethral abnormality
    - Increasing age and stress related to multiple pregnancies even in absence of vaginal delivery
    - Hysterectomy, obesity, smoking (chronic cough)
  - Uterovaginal prolapse
    - Damaged uterosacral and cardinal ligaments
    - Damaged pubovaginal ligament
- Epidemiology: Vaginal prolapse reported in 0.2-43% post hysterectomy
- Associated abnormalities
  - Vaginal, rectal prolapse
  - Ureteral obstruction

Staging, Grading or Classification Criteria
- Clinical staging includes
  - Grade 1: Descent of bladder base toward introitus in straining
  - Grade 2: Descent of bladder base to level of introitus in straining
  - Grade 3: Descent of bladder base outside introitus in straining
  - Grade 4: Descent of bladder base outside introitus at rest
- Above grading also used for uterine prolapse with cervix being landmark

CLINICAL ISSUES

Presentation
- Most common signs/symptoms: Grade 1 and 2 asymptomatic unless urethral hypermobility causes urinary incontinence
- Other signs/symptoms: Vaginal mass, recurrent infection, back pain, hydronephrosis
- Clinical Profile: History of hysterectomy and multiple pregnancies

Demographics
- Age: ≥ 45 years of age, more common after menopause
- Ethnicity: Most common amongst Caucasian women, followed by Hispanic, Asian and black women

Natural History & Prognosis
- Lack of recognition of multi-compartment disease a cause for up to 30% treatment failure

Treatment
- Retropubic (Burch) colposuspension for cystocele to suspend urethra anteriorly
- Paravaginal repair
- Fixation of vaginal wall to sidewall
- Vaginal hysterectomy and uterosacral suspension for uterine prolapse
- Periurethral collagen injection for urethral sphincter deficiency

DIAGNOSTIC CHECKLIST

Consider
- Coach the patient to achieve optimal straining
- Assess for other compartment involvement

Image Interpretation Pearls
- Descent of urethrovesical junction on strain to > 1 cm below PCL
- Descent of vaginal cuff/cervix on strain below PCL
- Apparent thinning of right levator ani due to chemical shift artifact

SELECTED REFERENCES

1. Poon CI et al: Three-dimensional ultrasonography to assess long-term durability of periurethral collagen in women with stress urinary incontinence due to intrinsic sphincter deficiency. Urology. 65(1):60-4, 2005
2. Dietz HP: Ultrasound imaging of the pelvic floor. Part I: two-dimensional aspects. Ultrasound Obstet Gynecol. 23(1):80-92, 2004
3. Grodstein F et al: Association of age, race, and obstetric history with urinary symptoms among women in the Nurses' Health Study. Am J Obstet Gynecol. 189(2):428-34, 2003
4. Tunn R et al: Introital and transvaginal ultrasound as the main tool in the assessment of urogenital and pelvic floor dysfunction: an imaging panel and practical approach. Ultrasound Obstet Gynecol. 22(2):205-13, 2003
5. Fielding JR: Practical MR imaging of female pelvic floor weakness. Radiographics. 22(2):295-304, 2002
6. Stoker J et al: Pelvic floor imaging. Radiology. 218(3):621-41, 2001
7. Raz S et al: Vaginal reconstructive surgery for incontinence and prolapse. In Campbell's Urology. W.B. Saunders. 1059-94, 1998
8. Pelsang RE et al: Voiding cystourethrography in female stress incontinence. AJR Am J Roentgenol. 166(3):561-5, 1996
9. Yang A et al: Pelvic floor descent in women: dynamic evaluation with fast MR imaging and cinematic display. Radiology. 179(1):25-33, 1991
10. Greenwald SW et al: Cystourethrography as a diagnostic aid in stress incontinence. An evaluation. Obstet Gynecol. 29(3):324-7, 1967

VAGINOCELE/CYSTOCELE

IMAGE GALLERY

Typical

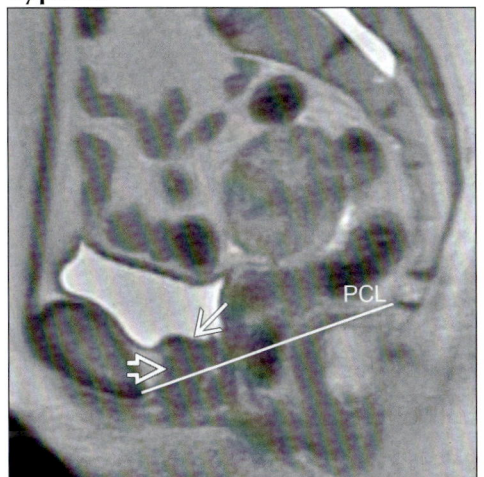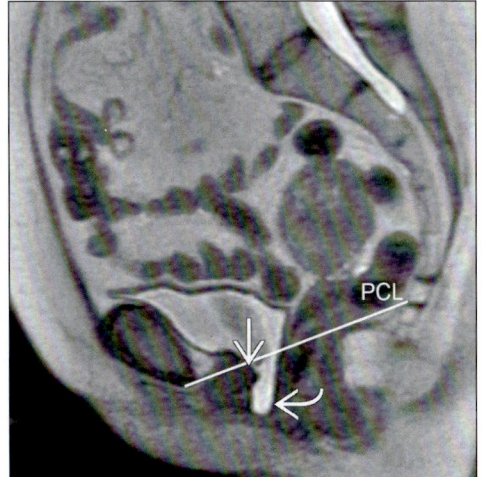

(Left) Sagittal T2WI MR acquired without straining in a supine position shows the UV junction ➜ above the PCL. Note the near vertical orientation of the urethra ➜. *(Right)* Sagittal T2WI MR with straining in the same patient as previous shows a cystocele ➜ below the PCL. Note the slight descent of the UV junction ➜ relative to the PCL as compared to the relaxed view.

Typical

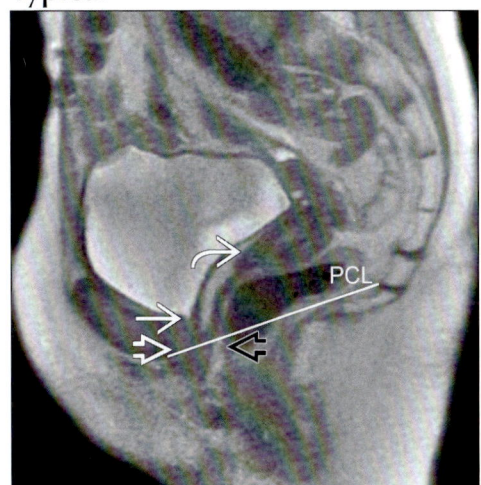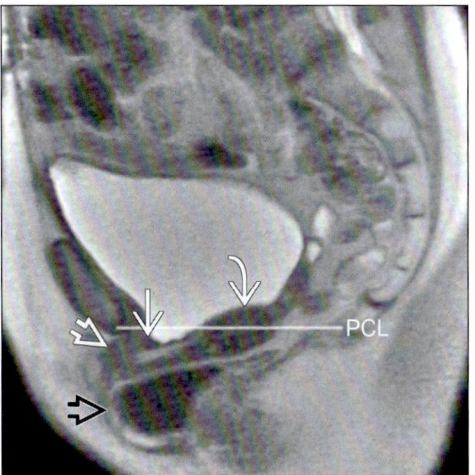

(Left) Sagittal T2WI MR without straining shows the UV junction ➜ and vaginal cuff ➜ to lie above the PCL. Note the position of the anterior wall of the rectum ➜. The urethra ➜ has a vertical orientation. *(Right)* Sagittal T2WI MR with attempted straining in the same patient as previous shows descent of the UV junction ➜ relative to the PCL, a horizontal orientation of the urethra ➜, descent of the uterus ➜ as well as vagina, and an anterior rectocele ➜.

Typical

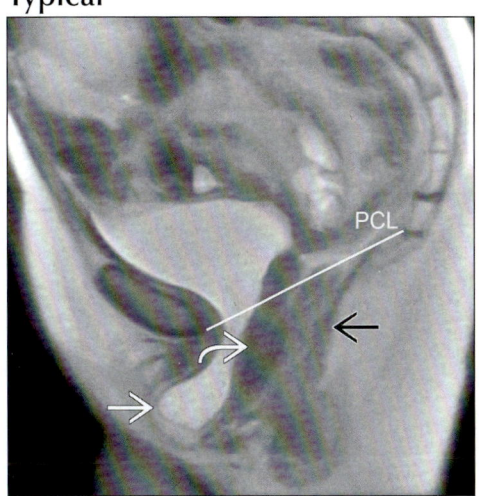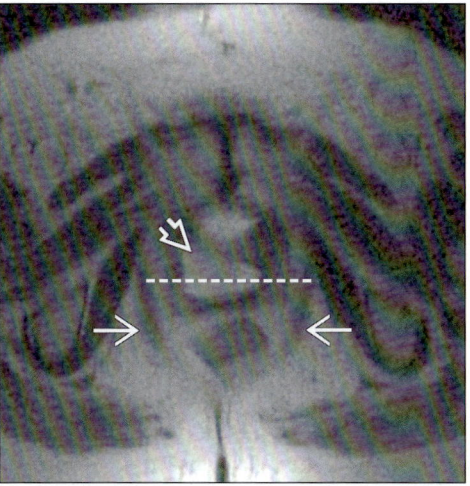

(Left) Sagittal T2WI cine MR, now with improved straining, shows greater descent of the cystocele ➜. The entire uterus ➜ is below the PCL. Note more vertical position of levator plate ➜. These images show the importance of adequate strain & evacuation. Rectocele, if not emptied, may prevent visualization of a cystocele or enterocele. *(Right)* Axial T2WI MR shows widening of the transverse hiatus (dotted line), lateral convexity of the levator muscles ➜ & a cystocele ➜.

ENTEROCELE/RECTOCELE

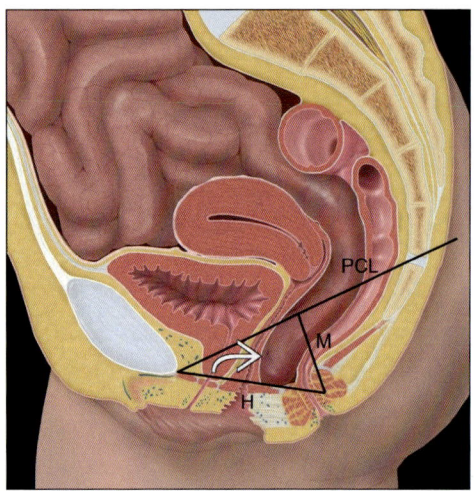

Sagittal graphic shows the pubococcygeal line (PCL), M line and H line. In addition, a peritoneocele ➔ is depicted.

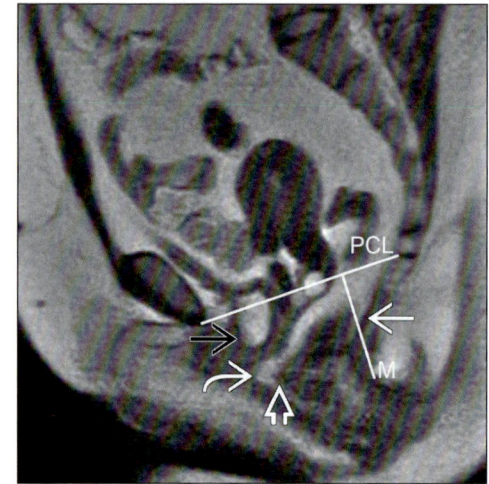

Sagittal T2WI MR with straining shows descent of the peritoneum ➔ below the PCL, and angulation of the anterior rectal wall ➔. The M line ➔ measures > 2 cm and the levator plate is vertical. There is a cystocele ➔.

TERMINOLOGY

Abbreviations and Synonyms
- Posterior vaginal wall prolapse, peritoneocele

Definitions
- Enterocele/peritoneocele: Herniation of peritoneum (peritoneocele) and contents (small bowel - enterocele, sigmoid - sigmoidocele) through rectovaginal septum between vagina and rectum
- Rectocele: Herniation of rectal wall (usually anterior) through posterior vaginal wall

IMAGING FINDINGS

General Features
- Best diagnostic clue
  ○ Enterocele
    ▪ Descent of bowel, peritoneum, or intraperitoneal fluid more than 2 cm below pubococcygeal line (PCL)
    ▪ Descent of bowel, peritoneum, or fluid between rectum and vagina
  ○ Rectocele
    ▪ Anterior rectal wall bulge > 2 cm ventral to a line along anterior wall of anal canal
  ○ Enterocele and rectocele frequently co-exist
- Location
  ○ Enterocele typically located midline in rectovaginal space, occasionally situated laterally or anterior to vagina
  ○ Rectocele usually involves anterior wall of rectum, less commonly lateral or posterior wall
- Size: May extend out through introitus
- Pelvic floor descent consists of three different compartments; each needs to be corrected separately
  ○ Anterior: Bladder and urethra
  ○ Middle: Vagina, cervix, uterus
  ○ Posterior: Rectum, rectovaginal septum
- Anatomical landmarks
  ○ PCL: Between lower symphysis pubis and last mobile coccygeal joint (site of insertion of levator plate)
  ○ H line (levator hiatus): Between lower symphysis pubis and puborectalis insertion on rectum
  ○ M line: Perpendicular line between H line and PCL, at insertion of H line to rectum

DDx: Anorectal Mass

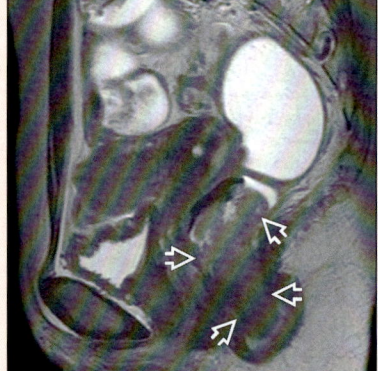
Prolapsing Rectal Cancer

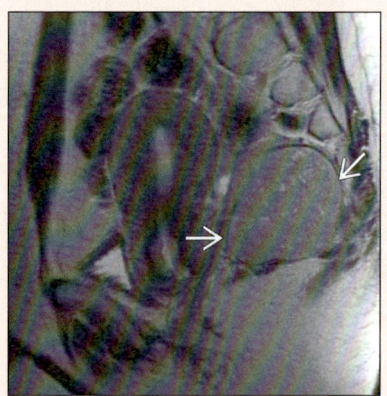
Rectum Duplication Cyst

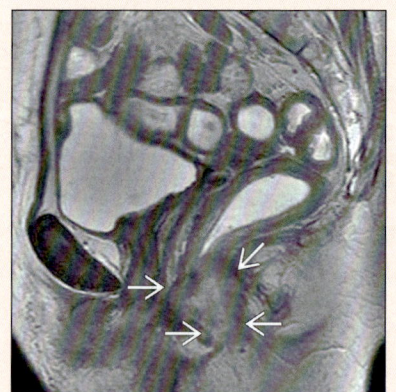
Anal Cancer

ENTEROCELE/RECTOCELE

Key Facts

Terminology
- Enterocele/peritoneocele: Herniation of peritoneum (peritoneocele) and contents (small bowel - enterocele, sigmoid - sigmoidocele) through rectovaginal septum between vagina and rectum
- Rectocele: Herniation of rectal wall (usually anterior) through posterior vaginal wall

Imaging Findings
- Descent of bowel, peritoneum, or intraperitoneal fluid more than 2 cm below pubococcygeal line (PCL)
- Descent of bowel, peritoneum, or fluid between rectum and vagina
- Anterior rectal wall bulge > 2 cm ventral to a line along anterior wall of anal canal
- Enterocele and rectocele frequently co-exist
- Inclination of levator plate relative to PCL > 10°
- Elongation of M line > 2 cm
- MR superior to PE for peritoneocele/enterocele
- MR inferior to PE for rectocele when rectal gel is not used and evacuation sequences are not performed
- Without rectal evacuation, significant defects can be missed during MR in supine position

Pathology
- Abnormal descent in up to 50% of women > 50 years of age
- Asymptomatic rectocele present in up to 80% of patients with multi-compartment disease

Diagnostic Checklist
- Consider routine use of rectal gel and evacuation sequences for accurate evaluation of posterior compartment defects

---

- Normal landmark values/appearance
  - Levator plate parallels PCL
  - H line < 5 cm
  - M line < 2 cm
  - Anterior rectal wall < 2 cm ventral to a line along anterior wall of anal canal

MR Findings
- T2WI
  - Enterocele may contain fat, small bowel, sigmoid colon, or fluid
    - Small bowel more commonly present than colon
    - Descent of peritoneum or bowel between rectum and vagina, more than 2 cm below PCL
  - Rectocele with anterior bulging of rectum
    - Anterior rectal wall more than 2 cm ventral to a line drawn along anterior wall of anal canal
  - Inferior descent of rectum/rectovaginal septum
    - Inclination of levator plate relative to PCL > 10°
    - Inferior bulge of perineal body
    - Elongation of M line > 2 cm
  - Isolated enterocele or anterior rectocele: Levator plate often maintains its normal angulation, M and H lines are normal or only minimally elongated

Fluoroscopic Findings
- Fluoroscopic defecography using findings similar to MR to diagnose rectocele/enterocele

Imaging Recommendations
- Best imaging tool
  - Closed MR system in a supine position most commonly used
    - Sensitivity and specificity for detecting rectocele is 76-100% and 50%, respectively
    - Improved sensitivity with sitting position in open magnet
  - Advantages/limitations of MR
    - MR superior to physical examination (PE) to show multi-compartment involvement
    - MR superior to PE for peritoneocele/enterocele
    - MR inferior to PE for rectocele when rectal gel is not used and evacuation sequences are not performed
- Protocol advice
  - Axial breath-hold fast spin-echo (FSE)
    - To delineate anatomy and exclude underlying pathology
    - Slice thickness ≤ 6 mm
  - Dynamic Cine MR is mainstay of pelvic floor assessment
    - Single shot FSE (SSFSE), Half-Fourier Snapshot Turbo Spin-Echo (HASTE), or true Fast Imaging with Steady-state Precession (true FISP)
    - Sequential images with a 1 to 2 second temporal resolution
    - Continuous evaluation with Cine MR improves evaluation during straining
    - 6-10 mm slice thickness
    - Basic protocol: Midline sagittal, relaxed and straining sequences
    - Optional protocol: Coronal, relaxed and straining sequences
    - T1W gradient echo imaging may be used for dynamic MR with open magnet
  - For posterior compartment defects, rectal gel with complete evacuation must be performed routinely
    - Judgment of adequacy of strain is difficult, especially for technologists
    - Without rectal evacuation, significant defects can be missed during MR in supine position

DIFFERENTIAL DIAGNOSIS

Rectal Intussusception
- Secondary to chronic straining
  - Typically present during evacuation
  - Frequent association with rectocele
- Infolding of rectal wall
- May be intra-rectal, intra-anal or complete rectal prolapse
- No associated cystocele

ENTEROCELE/RECTOCELE

Pelvic Mass
- Pelvic mass compressing rectum on MR

PATHOLOGY

General Features
- Etiology
  - Increasing age and stress related to multiple pregnancies even in absence of vaginal delivery
  - Hysterectomy, obesity
  - Two types of enteroceles
    - Traction: Follows vaginal/uterine prolapse
    - Pulsion: Occurs with chronic pressure on vaginal vault
  - Mechanism
    - Damaged iliococcygeal muscle
    - Damaged vaginorectal fascia
- Epidemiology
  - Abnormal descent in up to 50% of women > 50 years of age
  - Enterocele occurs in up to 27% after retropubic (Burch) colposuspension for cystocele
  - Asymptomatic rectocele present in up to 80% of patients with multi-compartment disease
- Associated abnormalities: Intussusception: Infolding of rectal wall that may cause obstruction

Gross Pathologic & Surgical Features
- Rectocele: Ventral herniation of anterior rectal wall
- Rectal descent: Inferior descent of anorectal junction

Staging, Grading or Classification Criteria
- Grade 1: Separation of fourchette and perineal skin
- Grade 2: Separation of muscles and fascia of perineal body
- Grade 3: Separation of perineal body and anal sphincter
- Grade 4: Separation of anal sphincter and exposure of rectal lumen

CLINICAL ISSUES

Presentation
- Most common signs/symptoms
  - Enterocele: Symptomatic when grade 2 or more
  - Rectocele: Obstructed defecation or incomplete evacuation
    - Patients may feel need to manually place pressure on posterior vaginal wall or perineum to empty rectum
- Other signs/symptoms
  - 75% of enteroceles associated with vault prolapse (complex enterocele)
  - Bulge along supero-posterior wall of vagina on physical examination due to enterocele or anterior rectal prolapse
  - Perineal fullness, dyspareunia, low back pain

Demographics
- Age: > 45 years of age, increased incidence after menopause
- Ethnicity: Most common amongst Caucasian women, followed by Hispanic, Asian and African descent women

Natural History & Prognosis
- Recurrent vault prolapse in 0-25% after treatment

Treatment
- Excision of hernial sac
- Enterocele/peritoneocele: Approximation of rectovaginal and cardinal ligaments
  - Enterocele repair requires reapproximation of the rectovaginal fascia
- Rectocele: Posterior colporrhaphy (posterior fixation of rectum)
  - Rectocele is treated with rectovaginal fascial repair

DIAGNOSTIC CHECKLIST

Consider
- Consider routine use of rectal gel and evacuation sequences for accurate evaluation of posterior compartment defects

Image Interpretation Pearls
- Descent of peritoneum or bowel between rectum and vagina, more than 2 cm below PCL
- Anterior rectal wall more than 2 cm ventral to a line drawn along anterior wall of anal canal

SELECTED REFERENCES

1. Schofield ML et al: MRI findings following laparoscopic sacrocolpopexy. Clin Radiol. 60(3):333-9, 2005
2. Dvorkin LS et al: Open-magnet MR defaecography compared with evacuation proctography in the diagnosis and management of patients with rectal intussusception. Colorectal Dis. 6(1):45-53, 2004
3. Pannu HK: MRI of pelvic organ prolapse. Eur Radiol. 14(8):1456-64, 2004
4. Bertschinger KM et al: Dynamic MR imaging of the pelvic floor performed with patient sitting in an open-magnet unit versus with patient supine in a closed-magnet unit. Radiology. 223(2):501-8, 2002
5. Fielding JR: Practical MR imaging of female pelvic floor weakness. Radiographics. 22(2):295-304, 2002
6. Stoker J et al: Imaging of the posterior pelvic floor. Eur Radiol. 12(4):779-88, 2002
7. Matsuoka H et al: A comparison between dynamic pelvic magnetic resonance imaging and videoproctography in patients with constipation. Dis Colon Rectum. 44(4):571-6, 2001
8. Rentsch M et al: Dynamic magnetic resonance imaging defecography: a diagnostic alternative in the assessment of pelvic floor disorders in proctology. Dis Colon Rectum. 44(7):999-1007, 2001
9. Lamb GM et al: Upright dynamic MR defaecating proctography in an open configuration MR system. Br J Radiol. 73(866):152-5, 2000
10. Vanbeckevoort D et al: Pelvic floor descent in females: comparative study of colpocystodefecography and dynamic fast MR imaging. J Magn Reson Imaging. 9(3):373-7, 1999
11. Yang A et al: Pelvic floor descent in women: dynamic evaluation with fast MR imaging and cinematic display. Radiology. 179(1):25-33, 1991

ENTEROCELE/RECTOCELE

IMAGE GALLERY

Typical

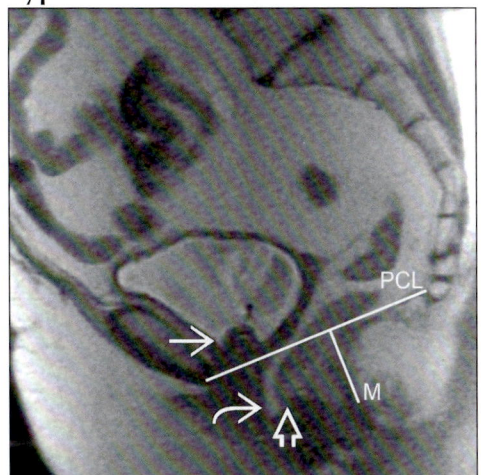
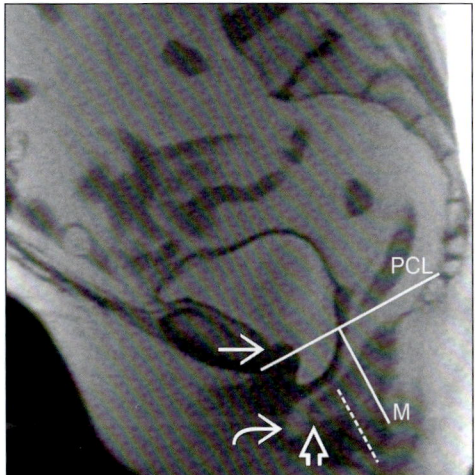

(Left) Sagittal T2WI MR without straining shows the urethrovesical (UV) junction ➡ above the PCL, descent of the peritoneal fat ➡ below, and a slight anterior rectal wall bulge ➡. The M line measures 2 cm. *(Right)* Straining view of the same patient as previous image, shows the UV junction ➡ at the PCL but the bladder base below. Note further descent of the peritoneocele ➡, a more pronounced rectal wall bulge ➡ extending anterior to the anus (dotted line) and lengthening of the M line.

Typical

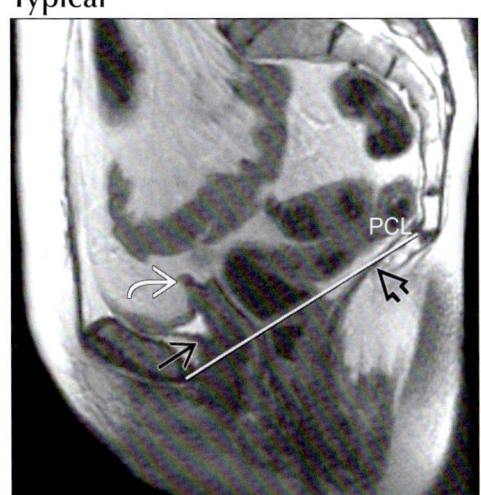
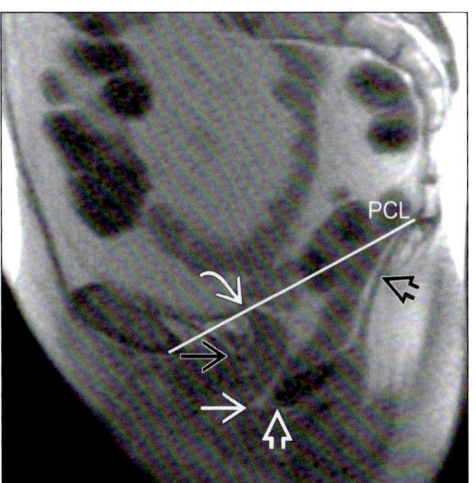

(Left) Sagittal T2WI MR without straining shows UV junction ➡ & vaginal cuff ➡ above PCL. Contour of anterior rectal wall is normal. Note the horizontal orientation of the levator plate ➡. *(Right)* Straining view (same patient as previous image) shows descent of peritoneum ➡ below PCL, anterior rectal wall bulge ➡, descent of UV junction ➡ & vaginal cuff ➡, indicating prolapse of all compartments. Note the more steep orientation of the levator plate ➡.

Typical

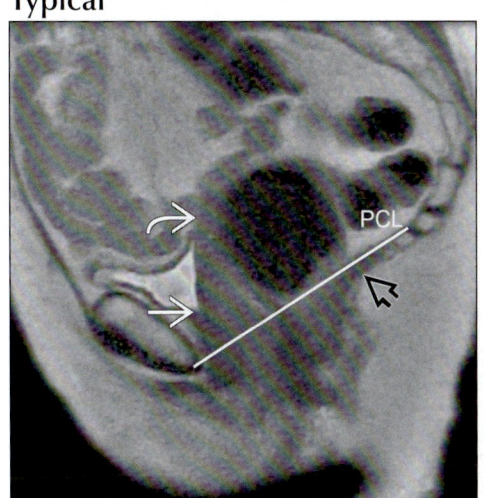
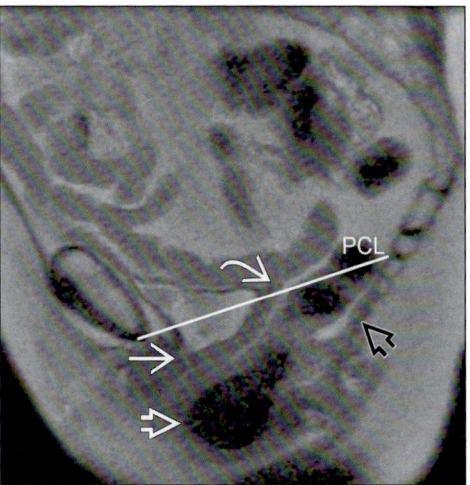

(Left) Sagittal T2WI MR without straining shows UV junction ➡ & vaginal cuff ➡ above the PCL. There is no anterior rectal wall bulge. Note the horizontal orientation of the levator plate ➡ relative to the PCL. *(Right)* Straining view (same patient as previous image) shows a rectal wall bulge ➡ & descent of the UV junction ➡ indicating rectal prolapse with cystocele. Note the steep orientation of the levator plate ➡. Vaginal cuff ➡ remains above the PCL.

PELVIC LIPOMATOSIS

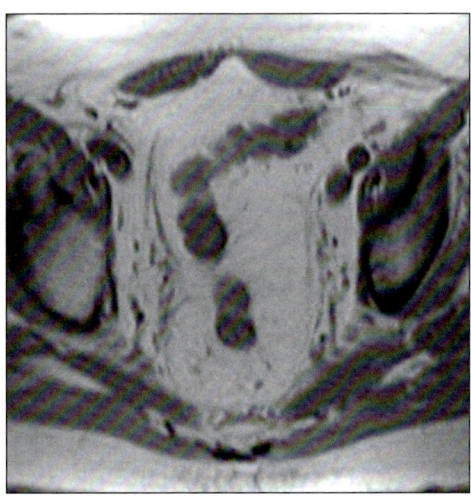

Axial T1WI MR shows excess intrapelvic fat compressing the rectosigmoid colon.

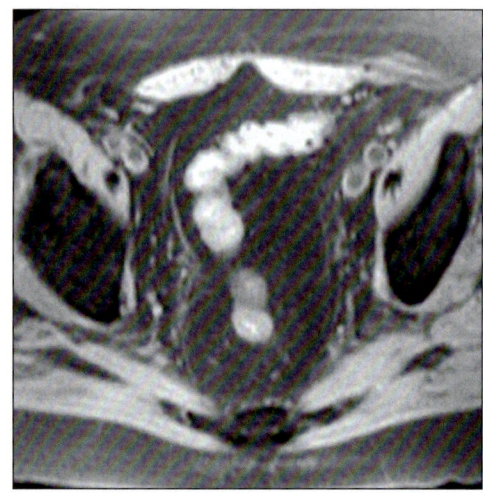

Axial T1WI FS MR shows excess intrapelvic fat of identical signal intensity to subcutaneous fat.

TERMINOLOGY

Abbreviations and Synonyms
- Pelvic lipomatosis (PL), fibrolipomatosis

Definitions
- Nonmalignant overgrowth of adipose tissue compressing soft tissue structures within pelvis

IMAGING FINDINGS

General Features
- Best diagnostic clue: Elongation and elevation of the urinary bladder with symmetric inverted pear shape; elevation of rectosigmoid colon out of pelvis; pelvic radiolucency

Radiographic Findings
- Radiography
  o Increased lucency around urinary bladder
  o Tubular narrowing of rectosigmoid colon
- IVP
  o High positioned, pear shaped or inverted teardrop bladder
  o Dilated tortuous medially displaced ureters

CT Findings
- Excess intrapelvic fat surrounding pelvic organs symmetrically
- May contain strands with higher attenuation than fat (fibrolipomatosis)

MR Findings
- Cranial displacement of bladder base
- Elongation of bladder neck and posterior urethra
- Elevation of prostate gland and medial and superior displacement of seminal vesicles
- Fatty tissue separating prostate gland from the rectum

Fluoroscopic Findings
- Contrast Enema
  o Increase in pre-sacral space > 10 mm (lateral view)
  o Elongation and symmetric extrinsic compression of rectum and cranial displacement of sigmoid

Imaging Recommendations
- Best imaging tool: CT is confirmatory

DDx: Widened Pre-Sacral Space

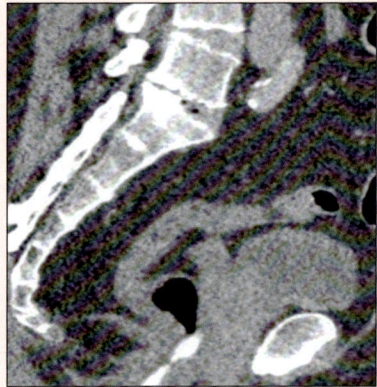
Pelvic Lipomatosis

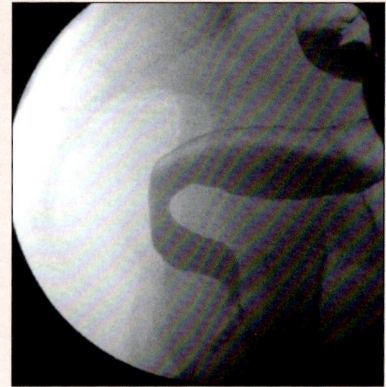
Ulcerative Colitis

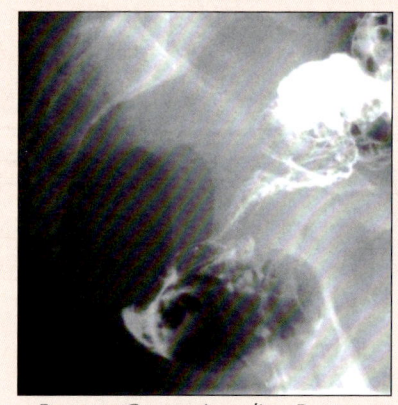
Prostate Cancer Invading Rectum

PELVIC LIPOMATOSIS

Key Facts

Imaging Findings
- Best diagnostic clue: Elongation and elevation of the urinary bladder with symmetric inverted pear shape; elevation of rectosigmoid colon out of pelvis; pelvic radiolucency
- Best imaging tool: CT is confirmatory

Top Differential Diagnoses
- Proctitis
- Ulcerative Colitis
- Normal Variant
- External Compression/Invasion of Rectum

Pathology
- General path comments: Nonmalignant condition

Diagnostic Checklist
- MRI follow-up to monitor ureteric obstruction
- Use CT to differentiate from other pathologies

DIFFERENTIAL DIAGNOSIS

Proctitis
- History of radiation therapy to the pelvis

Ulcerative Colitis
- Multiple ulcerations & loss of haustral pattern
- Lead pipe rectosigmoid colon in chronic phase

Normal Variant
- Large iliopsoas muscles & narrow bony pelvis

External Compression/Invasion of Rectum
- E.g., advanced prostate cancer, retroperitoneal tumor

PATHOLOGY

General Features
- General path comments: Nonmalignant condition
- Associated abnormalities: Cystitis glandularis

CLINICAL ISSUES

Presentation
- Most common signs/symptoms
  - Asymptomatic
  - ↑ Urinary frequency, hematuria, flank pain, fever
  - Constipation, rectal bleeding, tenesmus
  - Edema of lower extremities

Demographics
- Age: 9-80 years old, peak 25-60 years old
- Gender: M:F = 10:1
- Ethnicity: No racial predominance

Natural History & Prognosis
- Ureteric obstruction that may lead to renal failure
- Inferior vena cava obstruction

Treatment
- Urinary diversion to relieve obstruction

DIAGNOSTIC CHECKLIST

Consider
- MRI follow-up to monitor ureteric obstruction

Image Interpretation Pearls
- Use CT to differentiate from other pathologies

SELECTED REFERENCES

1. Heyns CF: Pelvic lipomatosis: a review of its diagnosis and management. J Urol. 146(2):267-73, 1991
2. Demas BE et al: Pelvic lipomatosis: diagnosis and characterization by magnetic resonance imaging. Urol Radiol. 10(4):198-202, 1988
3. Klein FA et al: Pelvic lipomatosis: 35-year experience. J Urol. 139(5):998-1001, 1988

IMAGE GALLERY

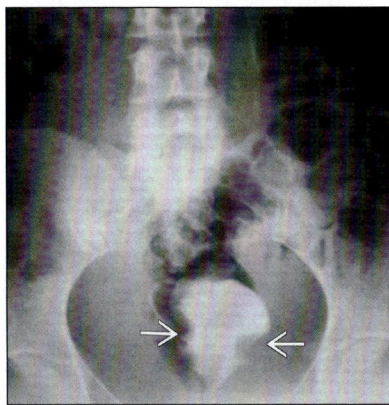 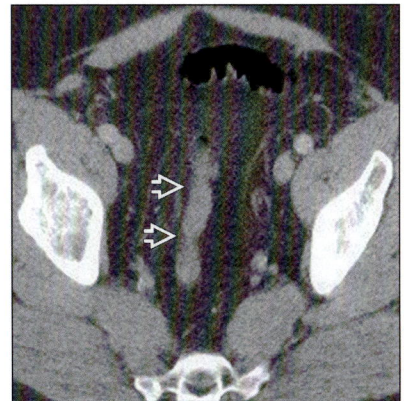 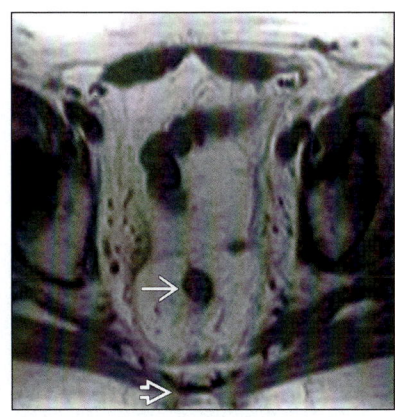

(Left) Frontal IVP shows high positioned inverted pear shape or teardrop bladder ➡. *(Center)* Axial CECT shows tubular narrowing of the sigmoid colon ➡ due to adipose tissue overgrowth in a patient with pelvic lipomatosis. *(Right)* Axial T1WI MR shows excess intrapelvic fat elevating the rectum ➡ from the sacrum ➡.

POST-RADIATION PELVIS

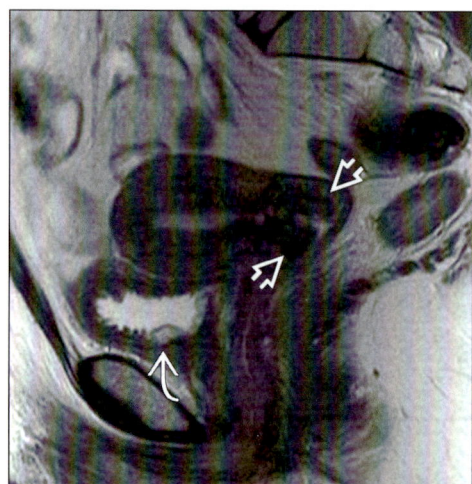

Sagittal T2WI MR shows homogeneous low signal intensity cervical stroma ➤ at completion of radiotherapy for stage 2B cervical cancer. Bullous edema ➤ of the bladder wall is also noted.

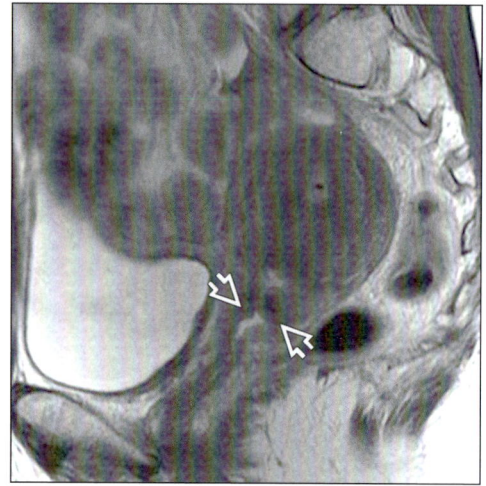

Sagittal T2WI MR shows presence of fluid within a short and irregular cervical canal ➤ in keeping with radiation necrosis following radiotherapy for stage 2B cervical cancer.

TERMINOLOGY

Abbreviations and Synonyms
- Post-radiotherapy (RT) treatment appearances

Definitions
- Radiation-induced changes to the uterus, ovaries, colon, bladder, soft tissues and bone marrow

IMAGING FINDINGS

General Features
- Best diagnostic clue
  - Reconstitution of normal zonal anatomy of the cervix and homogeneous low signal intensity cervical stroma reliable indicators of tumor-free post-radiation cervix
  - High signal intensity sigmoid colon, rectum and bladder wall on T2WI
  - High signal intensity pelvic muscles on T2WI
  - High signal intensity bone marrow on T1WI

Radiographic Findings
- Sigmoid colon & rectum: Fluoroscopic-guided barium enema (double contrast preferred)
  - Acute radiation colitis
    - Disrupted or distorted mucosal pattern
  - Chronic radiation colitis
    - Diffuse or focal narrowing with tapered margins
    - Colonic stricture or fistula
    - Widening of presacral space of more than 1.5 cm at the S4/5 vertebral level on the lateral view
- Bladder: Intravenous urogram
  - Bladder often normal in acute cystitis
  - Acute radiation cystitis
    - Thickened mucosal folds with cobblestone appearances
    - Bullous edema of the bladder mucosa
  - Chronic radiation cystitis
    - Irregular, thick-walled bladder
- Bones
  - Osteopenia (1 year after radiation), periostitis
  - Avascular necrosis, insufficiency fractures

DDx: Cervical Cancer Recurrence after Radiotherapy

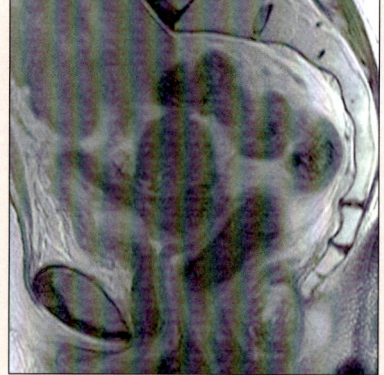

At RT Completion

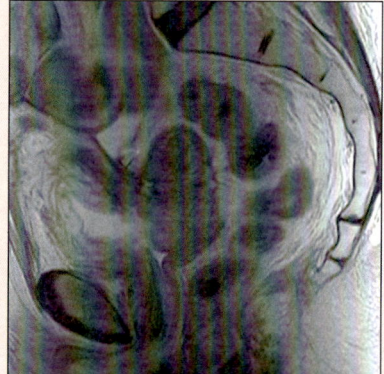

Recurrence (T2WI)

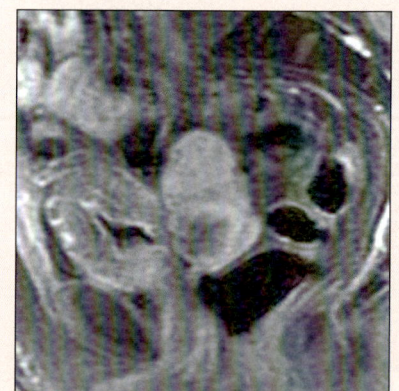

Recurrence (T1 C+)

POST-RADIATION PELVIS

Key Facts

Imaging Findings
- Reconstitution of normal zonal anatomy of the cervix and homogeneous low signal intensity cervical stroma reliable indicators of tumor-free post-radiation cervix
- High signal intensity sigmoid colon, rectum and bladder wall on T2WI
- High signal intensity bone marrow on T1WI
- In postmenopausal women radiation therapy does not significantly change the size & signal intensity of the uterus
- MR best imaging technique for tumor recurrence vs. radiation fibrosis, acute radiation colitis, cystitis and insufficiency fractures
- Protocol advice: DCE-MR and serial follow-up imaging to differentiate tumor recurrence from radiation fibrosis

Top Differential Diagnoses
- Tumor Recurrence
- Diverticulitis
- Bone Metastases

Diagnostic Checklist
- PET/CT to differentiate between radiation fibrosis and recurrent tumor
- Mild, moderate or severe changes can be seen in bladder or rectum on MR at any time during or after radiation

Ultrasonographic Findings
- Radiation cystitis: Hypoechoic, edematous bladder wall

CT Findings
- CECT
  - Uterus & ovaries
    - Ovaries may not be identified
    - Small uterus and ovaries (premenopausal women only)
  - Sigmoid colon & rectum
    - Uniform bowel wall thickening
    - Mild pericolonic inflammation
    - "Target sign" due to submucosal circumferential lucency
    - Proliferation of the perirectal fat > 15 mm
    - Thickening of the perirectal fascia
    - "Halo effect" due to pararectal fibrosis
    - Luminal narrowing or stricture
    - Sinuses and/or fistulae may be present
  - Bladder
    - Bladder wall thickening and/or hypodense bladder wall
- Bone CT
  - Osteopenia, periostitis
  - Fracture line, cortical disruption
  - Endosteal callus
  - No soft tissue mass

MR Findings
- Uterus, vagina & ovaries
  - In postmenopausal women radiation therapy does not significantly change the size & signal intensity of the uterus
  - Acute (< 6 months)
    - T2WI: Decrease in signal intensity of the tumor due to progressive replacement by radiation fibrosis
    - T2WI: Reconstitution of normal zonal anatomy of the cervix and homogeneous low signal intensity cervical stroma
    - T2WI: Low signal intensity myometrium (as early as 1 month after treatment)
    - T2WI: No differentiation between the junctional zone (JZ) and outer myometrium (premenopausal women only)
    - T2WI: Intermediate or high signal intensity endometrium
    - T2WI: Hyperintense vaginal wall
  - Chronic (> 6 months)
    - T2WI: Decrease in size and loss of normal zonal anatomy of uterus (premenopausal women only)
    - T2WI: Low signal intensity thin endometrium (premenopausal women only)
    - T2WI: Cervical os stenosis (3-6 months)
    - T2WI: Hypointense vaginal wall and vaginal atrophy
    - T2WI: Smaller ovaries of decrease signal intensity
  - Vaginal ulceration and fistula formation (severe radiation injury)
- Sigmoid colon & rectum
  - Acute
    - T2WI: High signal intensity submucosa (earliest change)
    - T2WI: Outer muscle layer retains its normal low signal intensity
    - T2WI: High signal intensity outer muscle layer leading to loss of differentiation between mucosa and muscle layers
    - T1 C+: Bowel wall enhancement with no distinction between component layers
    - T2WI FS: Fistulae or sinus track from the rectum (most severe changes)
  - Chronic
    - Thickened rectal wall of > 6 mm when distended
    - Luminal narrowing or stricture
    - Thickening of the perirectal fascia
    - Widening of the presacral space
- Bladder
  - Acute
    - T2WI: High signal intensity bladder wall that starts at the bladder trigone (mild injury)

POST-RADIATION PELVIS

- T2WI: Bladder wall thickening (> 5 mm) of high signal intensity (severe injury)
- T1 C+: Differential enhancement of the bladder mucosa
  - Chronic
    - T2WI: Low signal intensity inner bladder wall due to radiation-induced fibrosis
    - T2WI: High signal intensity outer bladder wall
    - Fistula and sinus track formation (only in severe radiation injury)
- Pelvic fat and striated muscles
  - T1WI + T2WI: Heterogeneous decrease in signal intensity within the pelvic fat
  - T2WI: Symmetric high signal intensity within the pelvic muscles
  - T1 C+: Diffuse enhancement in muscles of the radiation field
- Bone marrow
  - T1WI + T2WI: Diffuse high signal intensity at the end of radiotherapy
  - Bone edema
    - T1WI: Low signal intensity
    - T2WI: Heterogeneous signal intensity
    - STIR: High signal intensity
  - Insufficiency fracture
    - SI joints 61%, S1-S2 28%, S3-S5 4%, pubis 4% and ischium 3%
    - T1WI: Low signal intensity
    - T2WI: Variable signal intensity

Nuclear Medicine Findings
- Bone Scan: Insufficiency fractures: Symmetric area of increased radionuclide uptake in the sacro-iliac region: "Honda sign"

Imaging Recommendations
- Best imaging tool
  - MR best imaging technique for tumor recurrence vs. radiation fibrosis, acute radiation colitis, cystitis and insufficiency fractures
  - CT best imaging technique for chronic radiation colitis
- Protocol advice: DCE-MR and serial follow-up imaging to differentiate tumor recurrence from radiation fibrosis

DIFFERENTIAL DIAGNOSIS

Tumor Recurrence
- Occurs at least 6 months after treated lesion has regressed
- Mass of high signal intensity on T2WI similar to corresponding primary tumor
- Early enhancement (at 45 sec)
- Biopsy is sometimes necessary to establish diagnosis

Diverticulitis
- Less uniform wall thickening, more pericolonic inflammation

Bone Metastases
- Soft tissue mass common
- Occur outside radiation field

PATHOLOGY

General Features
- Epidemiology
  - Incidence of complications increases with a total radiation dose of 50 Gy or greater
  - Incidence of radiation cystitis: 12%
  - Incidence of radiation colitis: 5%
  - Radiation colitis can occur up to 20 years following radiotherapy

Microscopic Features
- No pathognomonic morphologic features, but characteristic enough to be recognized
- Epithelial atrophy, necrosis, metaplasia, atypia, dysplasia and neoplasia
- Stromal fibrosis and necrosis
- Intimal fibrosis, occlusive thrombosis and vasculitis leading to ischemia
- Bone marrow hypoplasia and aplasia

CLINICAL ISSUES

Presentation
- Most common signs/symptoms
  - Tenesmus, diarrhea, bleeding, constipation
  - Dysuria, increased frequency, urgency, hematuria
  - Back pain, hip pain

DIAGNOSTIC CHECKLIST

Consider
- PET/CT to differentiate between radiation fibrosis and recurrent tumor

Image Interpretation Pearls
- Mild, moderate or severe changes can be seen in bladder or rectum on MR at any time during or after radiation

SELECTED REFERENCES
1. Fajardo LF: The pathology of ionizing radiation as defined by morphologic patterns. Acta Oncol. 44(1):13-22, 2005
2. Jeong YY et al: Uterine cervical carcinoma after therapy: CT and MR imaging findings. Radiographics. 23(4):969-81; discussion 981, 2003
3. Iyer RB et al: Imaging findings after radiotherapy to the pelvis. AJR Am J Roentgenol. 177(5):1083-9, 2001
4. Kinkel K et al: Differentiation between recurrent tumor and benign conditions after treatment of gynecologic pelvic carcinoma: value of dynamic contrast-enhanced subtraction MR imaging. Radiology. 204(1):55-63, 1997
5. Blomlie V et al: Incidence of radiation-induced insufficiency fractures of the female pelvis: evaluation with MR imaging. AJR Am J Roentgenol. 167(5):1205-10, 1996
6. Sugimura K et al: Postirradiation changes in the pelvis: assessment with MR imaging. Radiology. 175(3):805-13, 1990
7. Arrive L et al: Radiation-induced uterine changes: MR imaging. Radiology. 170(1 Pt 1):55-8, 1989

POST-RADIATION PELVIS

IMAGE GALLERY

Typical

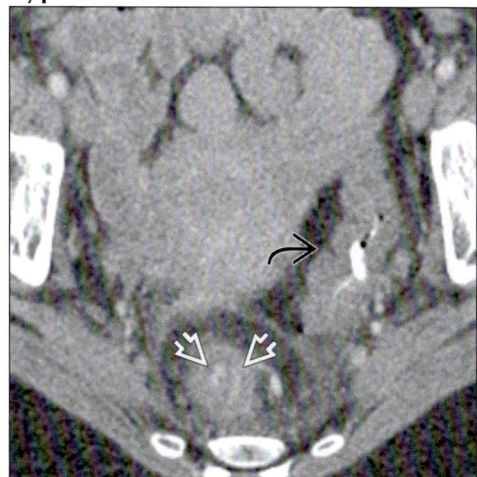
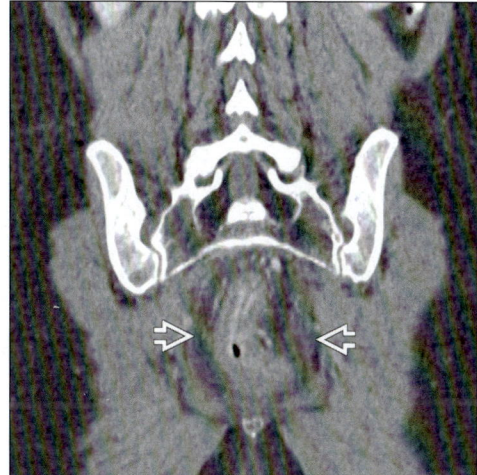

(Left) Axial CECT shows "target sign" ➡ due to rectal submucosal circumferential lucency in a patient with radiation proctitis. Note also thickening of the wall of the sigmoid colon ➚. *(Right)* Coronal CECT shows uniform wall thickening of the rectum with associated mild pericolonic inflammation ➡ following radiotherapy for recurrent ovarian cancer.

Typical

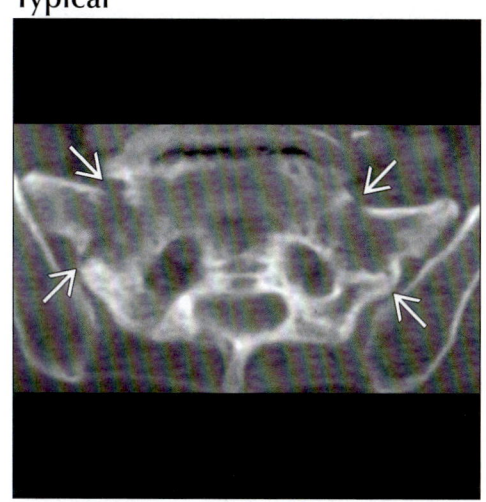
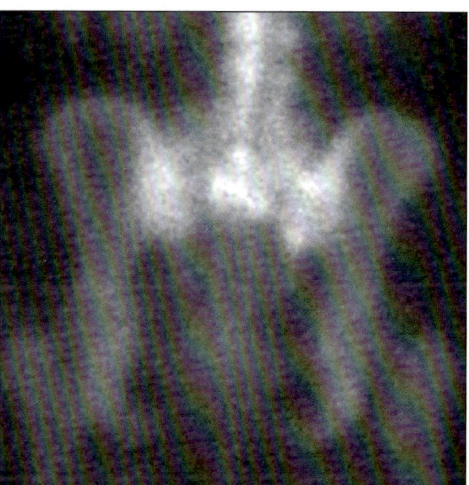

(Left) Axial NECT shows bilateral symmetrical cortical disruption ➡ within the sacral bone in keeping with a sacral insufficiency fractures in following radiotherapy for carcinoma of the cervix. *(Right)* Frontal skeletal scintigraphy confirms the presence of a sacral insufficiency fracture as a symmetric area of increased radionuclide uptake in the sacro-iliac region: "Honda sign".

Variant

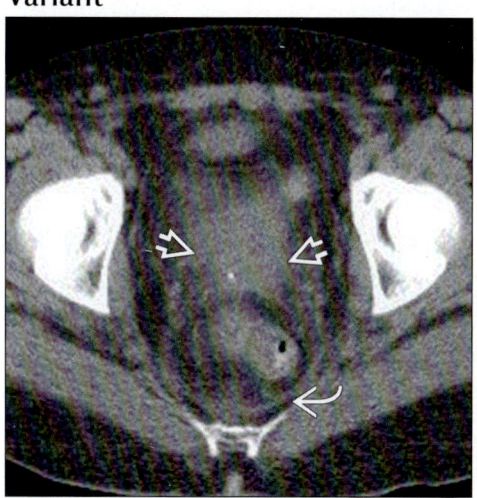
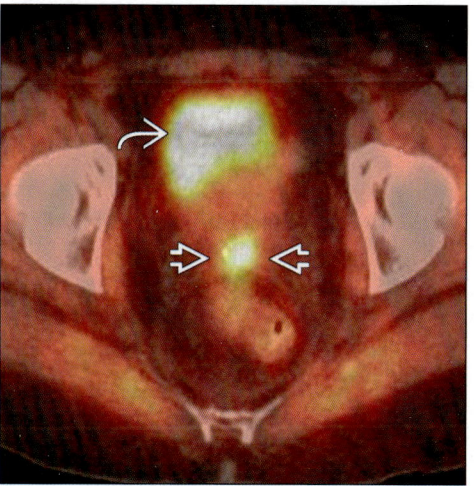

(Left) CT component of a PET CT study shows a soft tissue mass at the level of the cervix ➡ in a patient undergoing radiotherapy for stage 2B cervical carcinoma. Also note radiation-related perirectal inflamation ➚. *(Right)* Axial fused PET/CT shows increased FDG uptake centered in the cervix ➡ in keeping with residual cervical carcinoma. Physiological bladder uptake ➡ is also noted.

POST-OPERATIVE PELVIS

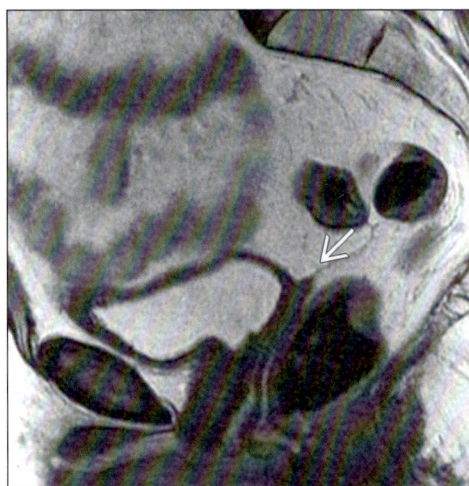

Sagittal T2WI MR shows absence of the uterus and smooth configuration of the vaginal vault ➡.

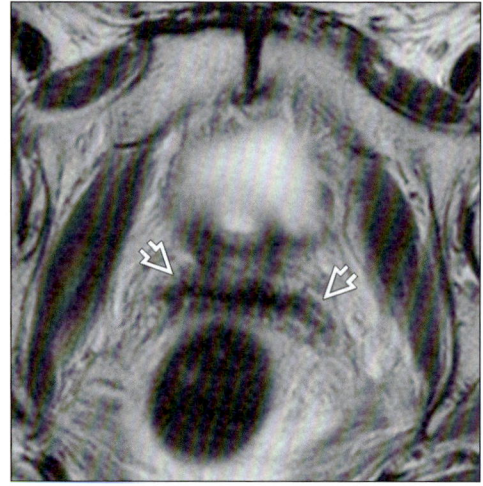

Axial T2WI MR confirms the linear soft tissue configuration of the vaginal fornices ➡ in a patient who underwent TAH & BSO for stage IB1 squamous cell carcinoma of the cervix.

TERMINOLOGY

Abbreviations and Synonyms
- Post-surgical appearances to the pelvis
- Total abdominal hysterectomy (TAH) and bilateral salpingo-oophorectomy (BSO)

Definitions
- Normal appearances to the female pelvis after surgery for benign or malignant gynecological conditions
- Post-operative complications such as hematoma, abscess, lymphocele and fistula or sinus tract

IMAGING FINDINGS

General Features
- Best diagnostic clue
  - Post conization: Extensive shortening of the cervix
  - Post trachelectomy: Absent cervix with uterine corpus anastomosing with the vagina
  - Post supracervical hysterectomy: Absent uterine corpus with preservation of cervix and vagina
  - Post TAH & BSO: Absence of the uterus and ovaries, linear soft tissue configuration of the vaginal fornices +/- metallic clips along pelvic sidewall and/or para-aortic region at the site of lymph node dissection
  - Total pelvic exenteration: Absence of bladder, urethra, uterus, vagina, ovaries, rectum and all the pelvic supportive and connective tissues; colostomy and urinary diversion are seen
  - Anterior pelvic exenteration: Rectum is preserved and sometimes occupies a more anterior position; potential space in the anterior pelvis is filled by bowel
  - Posterior pelvic exenteration: Retention of the urethra and bladder which extends into the posterior pelvis

Ultrasonographic Findings
- TAH & BSO: Absence of the uterus and ovaries, smooth vaginal vault
- Supracervical hysterectomy: Absence of uterine corpus, preserved cervix and vagina
- Hematoma: Varied echogenicity, can appear similar to an abscess

DDx: Post-Operative Pelvis

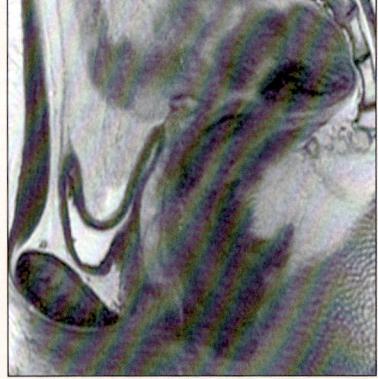

MRKH Syndrome

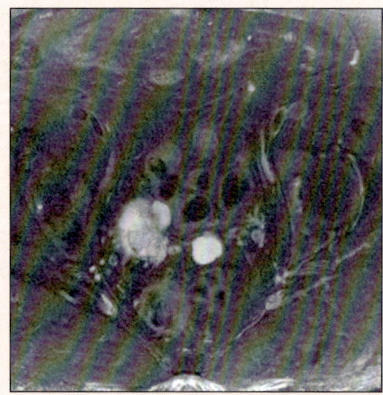

Vaginal Vault Recurrence

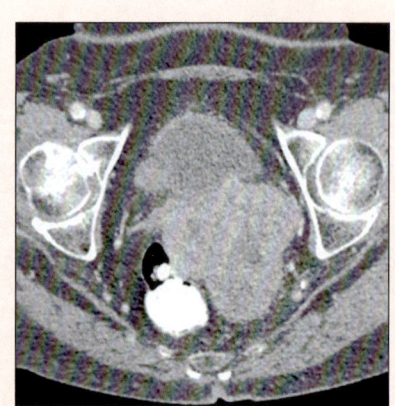

Vaginal Vault Recurrence

POST-OPERATIVE PELVIS

Key Facts

Terminology
- Normal appearances to the female pelvis after surgery for benign or malignant gynecological conditions
- Post-operative complications such as hematoma, abscess, lymphocele and fistula or sinus tract

Imaging Findings
- Post TAH & BSO: Absence of the uterus and ovaries, linear soft tissue configuration of the vaginal fornices +/- metallic clips along pelvic sidewall and/or para-aortic region at the site of lymph node dissection
- Best imaging tool: CT for post-operative complications; MR for detection of tumor recurrence
- Protocol advice: MR: DCE-MR to distinguish tumor recurrence from fibrotic scar; T1 C+ FS to improve fistula detection

Top Differential Diagnoses
- Müllerian Agenesis (Mayer-Rokitansky-Küster-Hauser Syndrome)
- Tumour Recurrence in the Vaginal Vault

Clinical Issues
- Abscess: Image guided percutaneous catheter drainage or surgical intervention
- Lymphocele: Aspiration, percutaneous catheter drainage +/- sclerotherapy if large and symptomatic
- Fistula: Surgical intervention

Diagnostic Checklist
- In most cases, a normal vaginal cuff is confirmed by visualizing a smooth, low signal intensity muscular wall on T2WI MR

- Lymphocele: Anechoic round or oval shape structures along the pelvic sidewall

CT Findings
- Normal post-operative appearances
  - Absence of uterus and/or ovaries, smooth linear configuration of the vaginal vault
  - Metallic clips along pelvic side wall and/or para-aortic region at the site of lymph node dissection
  - Total exenteration: Pelvis is devoid of bladder, urethra, uterus and rectum; urinary diversion and colostomy are present
- Hematoma
  - Attenuation values depend on the age of hemorrhage
  - Acute
    - NECT: Hyperdensity is specific for acute hematoma
    - NECT: Higher attenuation value (+70 to +90 HU) than circulating blood as clot formation and retraction cause greater concentration of red blood cells
    - CECT: May show active arterial extravasation as focal high density area surrounded by a large hematoma or diffuse area of high density
  - Subacute
    - Often shows a lucent halo and a soft tissue density center
    - Can be confused with a retroperitoneal tumor
  - Chronic
    - Low density (+20 to +40 HU) mass with a thick dense rim
    - Peripheral calcifications may be present
    - May have similar appearances to an abscess, lymphocele, cyst or urinoma
- Abscess
  - Appearances depend on the age of abscess
    - Early stage: Mass of near soft tissue attenuation
    - Mature stage: Central region of near water attenuation (necrosis) surrounded by a higher attenuation rim which enhances on CECT
    - 30% contain small bubbles of air or an air fluid level
    - Ancillary findings include displacement of surrounding structures, thickening and obliteration of the adjacent fascial planes
- Fistulae or sinus tract
  - Not easily visualized unless large and associated with a pelvic abscess
  - CT fistulogram (injection of iodinated contrast agent at a concentration of 5-10% through the fistula) may improve fistula visualization and establish the presence of communication with adjacent abscesses or the genitourinary tract
- Lymphocele
  - Well-circumscribed oval structures of low attenuation seen along the pelvic sidewall
  - May contain multiple septa

MR Findings
- Normal post-operative appearances
  - T1WI + T2WI
    - Absence of uterus and/or ovaries, smooth linear configuration of the vaginal vault, metallic clips at the sites of lymph node dissection
    - Total exenteration: Absence of bladder, urethra, uterus and rectum; urinary diversion and colostomy
  - T1WI: Linear, nodular or full vaginal fornices
  - T2WI
    - Smooth vaginal cuff of low signal intensity muscular wall
    - Intermediate signal intensity vaginal cuff if fibrotic scar tissue is present
    - Short residual vagina after radical hysterectomy
- Hematoma
  - Appearances depend on the age of hematoma
  - Acute
    - Nonspecific findings as abscesses and tumors may have similar appearances
    - T1WI: Signal intensity similar to muscle; a fluid-fluid level with higher signal intensity on the dependent layer may be seen in large hematomas

POST-OPERATIVE PELVIS

- T2WI: Marked low signal intensity due to intracellular deoxyhemoglobin
  - Subacute
    - T1WI: 3 distinct layers: Low signal intensity rim corresponding to the hemosiderin-laden fibrous capsule, high signal intensity peripheral zone, intermediate signal intensity central core
    - T2WI: Low signal intensity rim with a central core of a higher signal intensity than the peripheral zone
  - Chronic
    - T1WI + T2WI: Central core (retracted clot) decreases in size leading to a homogeneous high signal intensity mass with a low signal intensity rim
- Abscess
  - T1WI: Mass of intermediate signal intensity
  - T2WI: Mass of high signal intensity
  - Necrosis produces heterogeneous appearances
  - The presence of a long air fluid level as opposed to small discreet bubbles suggests communication with GI tract
- Fistulae or sinus tract
  - T2WI: Fistulae appear as fluid filled tracks surrounded by lower signal intensity tissue representing fibrosis, granulation or tumor
  - Key finding: Focal interruption in the low signal intensity muscle of the bladder rectum or vagina
  - Use of gadolinium improves fistula detection
  - Sinus tracts: Linear or tubular structures that run from the pelvis to the skin surface, usually perineum
- Lymphocele
  - T2WI: High signal intensity due to high protein content

Imaging Recommendations
- Best imaging tool: CT for post-operative complications; MR for detection of tumor recurrence
- Protocol advice: MR: DCE-MR to distinguish tumor recurrence from fibrotic scar; T1 C+ FS to improve fistula detection

DIFFERENTIAL DIAGNOSIS

Müllerian Agenesis (Mayer-Rokitansky-Küster-Hauser Syndrome)
- Young age at presentation, no history of pelvic surgery
- Ovaries are usually present, absent uterus and upper two thirds of the vagina with varying degrees of development of the lower vagina

Tumor Recurrence in the Vaginal Vault
- T2WI: Mass of high signal intensity similar to the primary tumor, which obliterates the muscle layer of the vagina
- T2WI: Predominantly cystic vaginal vault mass (atypical)
- T1C+: Heterogeneous enhancement

PATHOLOGY

General Features
- Epidemiology: Prevalence of post-operative complications is about 4%

CLINICAL ISSUES

Presentation
- Most common signs/symptoms
  - Abscess & fistula: Pain, fever, palpable pelvic mass, vaginal discharge
  - Hematoma & lymphocele: Asymptomatic when small, considerable discomfort when large

Natural History & Prognosis
- Most of hematomas and lymphoceles resolve spontaneously

Treatment
- Abscess: Image guided percutaneous catheter drainage or surgical intervention
- Lymphocele: Aspiration, percutaneous catheter drainage +/- sclerotherapy if large and symptomatic
- Fistula: Surgical intervention

DIAGNOSTIC CHECKLIST

Image Interpretation Pearls
- In most cases, a normal vaginal cuff is confirmed by visualizing a smooth, low signal intensity muscular wall on T2WI MR

SELECTED REFERENCES

1. Sahdev A et al: MR imaging appearances of the female pelvis after trachelectomy. Radiographics. 25(1):41-52, 2005
2. Jeong YY et al: Uterine cervical carcinoma after therapy: CT and MR imaging findings. Radiographics. 23(4):969-81; discussion 981, 2003
3. Sugimura K et al: Postsurgical pelvis: treatment follow-up. Radiol Clin North Am. 40(3):659-80, viii, 2002
4. Fulcher AS et al: Recurrent cervical carcinoma: typical and atypical manifestations. Radiographics. 19 Spec No:S103-16; quiz S264-5, 1999
5. Kim JK et al: Postoperative pelvic lymphocele: treatment with simple percutaneous catheter drainage. Radiology. 212(2):390-4, 1999
6. Yamashita Y et al: Dynamic MR imaging of recurrent postoperative cervical cancer. J Magn Reson Imaging. 6(1):167-71, 1996
7. Kasales CJ et al: Pelvic pathology after hysterectomy. A pictorial essay. Clin Imaging. 19(3):210-7, 1995
8. Outwater E et al: Pelvic fistulas: findings on MR images. AJR Am J Roentgenol. 160(2):327-30, 1993
9. Brown JJ et al: MR appearance of the normal and abnormal vagina after hysterectomy. AJR Am J Roentgenol. 158(1):95-9, 1992
10. Petru E et al: Pelvic and paraaortic lymphocysts after radical surgery because of cervical and ovarian cancer. Am J Obstet Gynecol. 161(4):937-41, 1989

POST-OPERATIVE PELVIS

IMAGE GALLERY

Typical

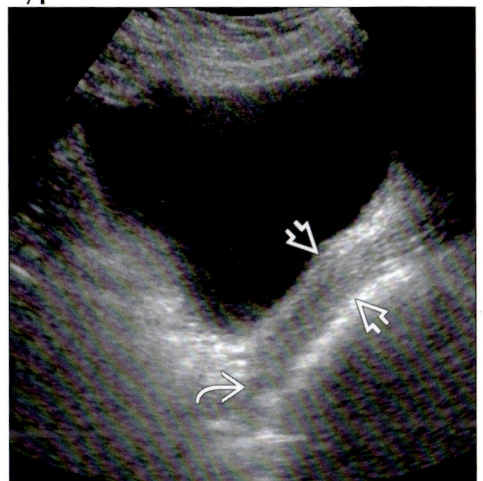 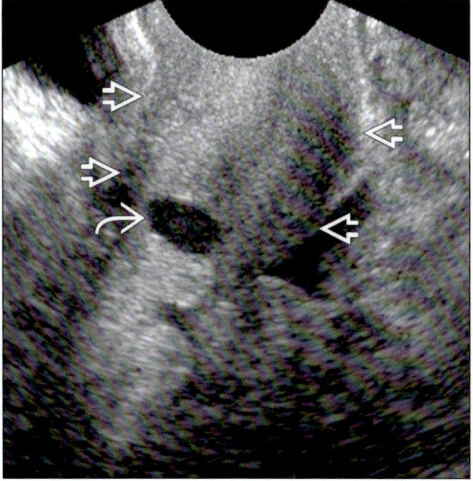

(Left) Sagittal transabdominal ultrasound shows normal appearances to the vagina ➡ following hysterectomy. Note the smooth configuration of the normal vaginal vault ➡. *(Right)* Sagittal transvaginal ultrasound shows normal appearances to the uterine cervix ➡ following supracervical hysterectomy for leiomyomas. Also note presence of a Nabothian cyst ➡.

Typical

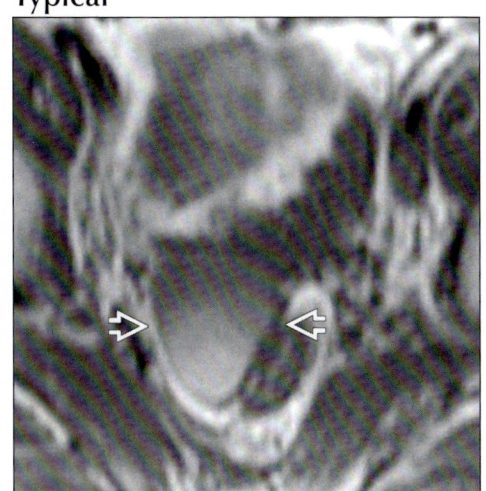 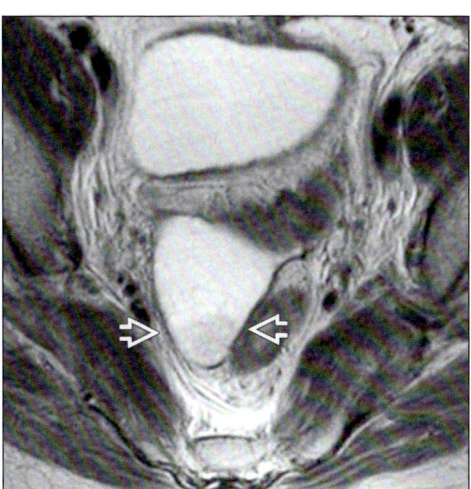

(Left) Axial T1WI MR shows a moderate size pelvic hematoma ➡ of signal intensity similar to muscle. Note the presence of a fluid-fluid level with higher signal intensity on the dependent layer. *(Right)* Axial T2WI MR confirms the presence of blood layering within the pelvic hematoma ➡ following TAH & BSO in a patient with stage IB1 squamous cell carcinoma of the cervix.

Typical

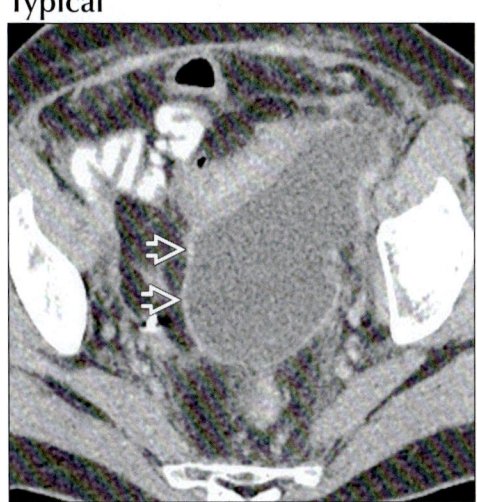 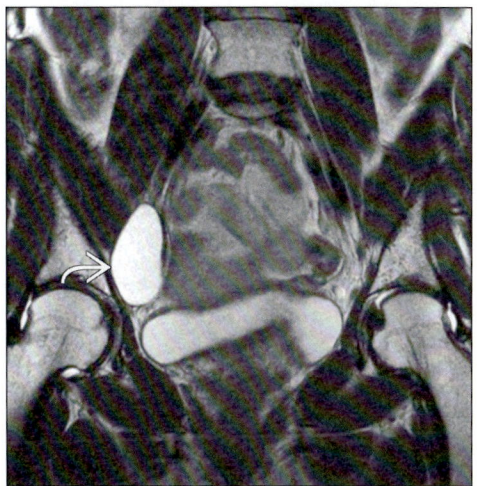

(Left) Axial CECT shows fluid collection within pelvis demonstrating avid rim-enhancement ➡. Findings are consistent with an abscess following TAH & BSO in a patient with stage IIA adenocarcinoma of the cervix. *(Right)* Coronal T2WI MR shows a well-circumscribed high SI oval structure ➡ along the right pelvic sidewall, representing a lymphocele following pelvic node dissection & radiotherapy in a patient with stage 2B squamous cell carcinoma of the cervix.

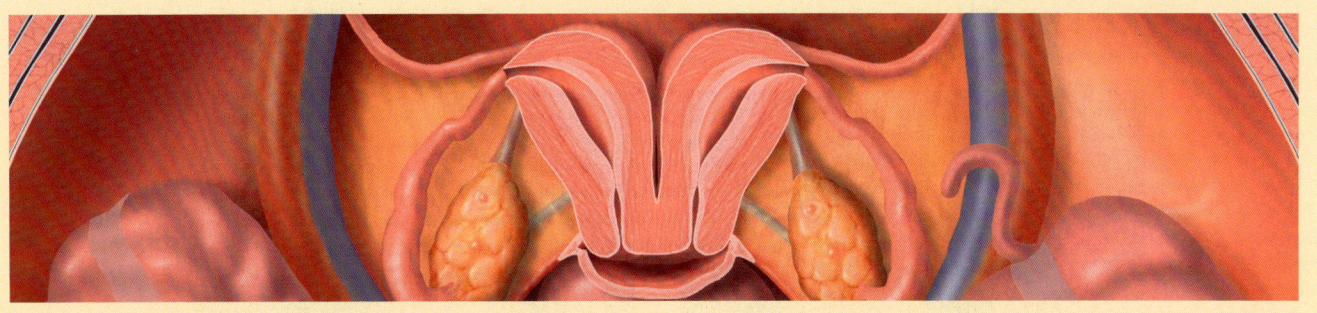

SECTION 2: Uterus

Introduction and Overview
Uterine Anatomy & Imaging Issues 2-2

Techniques
Sonohysterography 2-8

Normal Variants
Age-Related Physiologic Alterations 2-12
Endometrial Atrophy 2-18
Uterine Peristalsis 2-22
Normal Post C-Section Change 2-26

Congenital
Uterine Hypoplasia/Agenesis 2-30
Unicornuate 2-34
Didelphys 2-40
Bicornuate 2-46
Septate 2-52
Arcuate 2-58
DES-Exposed 2-60
Complex Anomalies 2-64

Inflammation/Infection
Asherman Syndrome 2-68
Endometrial Synechiae 2-74
Endometritis 2-78
Pyomyoma 2-82

Neoplasm
Intravenous Leiomyomatosis 2-86
Disseminated Peritoneal Leiomyomatosis 2-90

Neoplasm, Benign
Leiomyoma, Submucosal 2-92
Leiomyoma, Intramural 2-98
Leiomyoma, Subserosal 2-104
Leiomyoma, Degeneration 2-110
Leiomyoma, Parasitic 2-114
Benign Metastasizing Leiomyoma 2-118
Diffuse Leiomyomatosis, Uterus 2-122
Lipomatous Uterine Tumors 2-124
Endometrial Polyps 2-128
Endometrial Hyperplasia 2-134

Neoplasm, Malignant
Endometrial Cancer, Characterization 2-140
Endometrial Cancer, Early Stage 2-144
Endometrial Cancer, Late Stage 2-150
Endometrial Cancer, Recurrence 2-156
Endometrial Stromal Sarcoma 2-162
Adenosarcoma 2-166
Malignant Mixed Mesodermal Tumor 2-172
Leiomyosarcoma, Uterus 2-176
Lymphoma, Uterus 2-180
Choriocarcinoma, Uterus 2-184
Metastases, Uterus 2-188

Miscellaneous
Adenomyosis 2-192
Adenomyoma 2-198
Cystic Adenomyosis 2-202
Uterine AVM 2-206
Uterine Artery Embolization Imaging 2-212
Failed Uterine Artery Embolization 2-218
Complications, Uterine Artery Embolization 2-222
Uterine Rupture 2-228
Retained Products of Conception 2-232
Tamoxifen-Induced Changes 2-238
Intrauterine Device Evaluation 2-242

UTERINE ANATOMY & IMAGING ISSUES

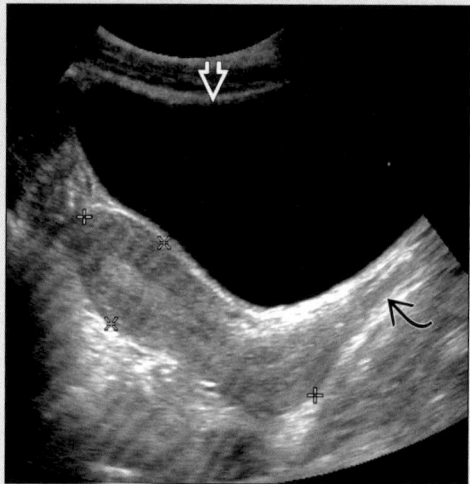

Sagittal transabdominal ultrasound shows uterus (calipers). Note the uterine measurement includes the cervix. The uterus is visualized through the full bladder ➡. The vagina is also visualized ➢.

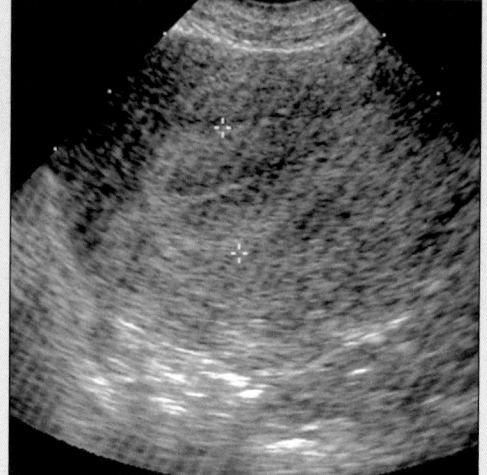

Sagittal transvaginal ultrasound shows mid-cycle three layer endometrium (calipers).

TERMINOLOGY

Abbreviations
- Transvaginal sonography (TVS)
- Transabdominal sonography (TAS)
- Hysterosalpingography (HSG)

Definitions
- Endometrial appearance changes with phase of menstrual cycle
  - Menstrual cycle 28 days (23-35 days in 90% of women)
  - Menstrual phase (days 1-5 typically)
    - Hypoechoic material can be seen centrally in endometrial cavity due to blood and tissue
  - Proliferative phase (days 6-14 typically)
    - Endometrial glands are straight
    - Endometrium is thin initially, increases later in cycle
  - Mid-cycle
    - Endometrium has multilayered appearance
    - Echogenic line centrally
    - Hypoechoic band surrounding interface
    - Echogenic outer rim
  - Secretory phase (days 15-28 typically)
    - Endometrial thickness increases as glands become tortuous and filled with mucin and glycogen
    - Endometrial echogenicity increases with increased through transmission
    - If endometrium homogeneously thick, can re-scan early in next menstrual cycle, after cessation of menses
- Uterine position is described with respect to position at cervix/vagina and at isthmus of uterus
  - Version at angle of cervix to vaginal (anteverted, retroverted)
  - Flexion at angle of body of uterus at isthmus (anteflexed, retroflexed)
  - Normal uterus is anteverted and anteflexed
  - Uterine position can change between transabdominal and transvaginal studies
  - When uterus is retroverted or retroflexed it is difficult to evaluate transabdominally and should be scanned with vaginal probe

IMAGING ANATOMY

General Anatomic Considerations
- Uterus located in midline
- Uterine measurement in sagittal plane includes the cervix
- TVS allows for improved visualization of the endometrium compared to TAS since TVS uses a higher frequency transducer, located closer to endometrium

Anatomic Relationships
- Sagittal midline view shows vagina, cervix, bladder, and mid-uterus
- Ovaries located to either side of uterus

ANATOMY-BASED IMAGING ISSUES

Key Concepts or Questions
- How does the post-menopausal uterus differ from the uterus of a younger woman?
  - Uterus decreases in size after menopause, eventually obtaining infantile configuration with body of uterus smaller than cervix
  - Arcuate artery calcifications may be present along outer 1/3 of myometrium
  - Endometrial thickness should be thin, except in patients taking hormones
    - Continuous combined estrogen/progesterone should have thin endometrium
    - Sequential estrogen/progesterone can have endometrial thickness that varies with phase of hormone cycle, and should be scanned early in cycle to visualize endometrium at thinnest

Imaging Approaches
- Ultrasound screening method of choice

UTERINE ANATOMY & IMAGING ISSUES

Key Facts

Multiple Factors Affect Uterine Size
- Uterine size changes with age, parity, and menopausal status
- An enlarged uterus is most often due to normal variant, adenomyosis, or leiomyomas
- Rarely an enlarged uterus will be due to endometrial carcinoma, cervical carcinoma, or sarcoma

Uterine Duplication Anomalies are Common and are Frequently Asymptomatic
- Septate uterus associated with increased incidence of spontaneous abortion
- Bicornuate uterus associated with incompetent cervix
- Müllerian hypoplasia/agenesis associated with primary amenorrhea
- Arcuate uterus is a normal variant

In Patients with Abnormal Bleeding
- TVS is best mode to assess endometrium, and should be performed unless there is a contraindication
- Sonohysterography is helpful to determine cause of a focal endometrial lesion
  - Focal endometrial lesion is best biopsied under direct hysteroscopic visualization
- A heterogeneous endometrium can be due to submucosal leiomyomas, blood clots, secretory phase, polyps, hyperplasia, or carcinoma
- Thick homogeneous endometrium can be assessed with blind endometrial biopsy
- Blind endometrial biopsy misses 50% of focal endometrial lesions

---

  - TVS for best visualization of endometrium
  - Color and pulsed Doppler to assess focal endometrial lesions
  - Sonohysterography to assess for focal endometrial lesions
  - 3D ultrasound helpful in assessing duplication anomalies
- CT not indicated
- MR
  - Staging endometrial cancer
  - Assessing adenomyosis
  - Assessing patients pre- and post-uterine artery embolization
  - May be needed for complete assess of congenital anomalies
- HSG used to assess tubal patency not for uterine anatomy

Normal Measurements
- Normal size of uterus varies with patient age and parity
  - Neonatal
    - Body of uterus slightly larger than cervix due to stimulation from maternal hormones
  - Early childhood
    - Body of uterus rapidly decreases in size after birth to tubular shape with body being smaller than cervix
  - Pre-menarche
    - Body of uterus smaller than cervix, but enlarges as menarche approaches
    - Uterine volume increases from 1.6-43 ml with uterine growth continuing for several years after menarche
  - Menstrual age
    - Body of uterus larger than cervix, typically twice the size of cervix
    - 8 cm length x 4 cm width x 4 cm anteroposterior
    - Can be larger in multiparous patients, up to 1 cm greater in each dimension
  - Postpartum
    - Enlarged, slowly decreasing in size over 3 months postpartum
  - Post-menopausal
    - Slowly reverts to infantile appearance
- Range of endometrial thickness varies with phase of the menstrual cycle and with menopausal status
  - Proliferative phase up to 8 mm
  - Secretory phase up to 16 mm
  - Post-menopausal not bleeding up to 8 mm
    - Post-menopausal endometrium up to 8 mm may contain asymptomatic polyps
    - Women taking hormones may have endometrial thickness that varies with the phase of the hormone cycle
  - Post-menopausal with bleeding up to 4 mm

PATHOLOGIC ISSUES

General Pathologic Considerations
- Is the uterus enlarged?
  - Enlarged uterus can be due to multiparity, leiomyomas, or adenomyosis
- Is the myometrium homogeneous?
  - Heterogeneous myometrium can be due to leiomyomas or adenomyosis
  - Enlarging focal myometrial lesion is worrisome for leiomyosarcoma
- Is the endometrium abnormally thick?
  - Assess thickness with respect to phase of menstrual cycle
  - Thick endometrium can be due to polyps, hyperplasia, cancer, secretory phase
- Is the endometrium homogeneous?
  - Heterogeneous endometrium can be due to polyps, hyperplasia, polyps, or distortion from leiomyomas
- Is there a mass in the cervix?
  - Most common mass in cervix is nabothian cyst
  - Leiomyomas may be present in cervix
  - Unlikely for initial diagnosis of cervical cancer to be made on ultrasound, since typically found by Pap smear first

UTERINE ANATOMY & IMAGING ISSUES

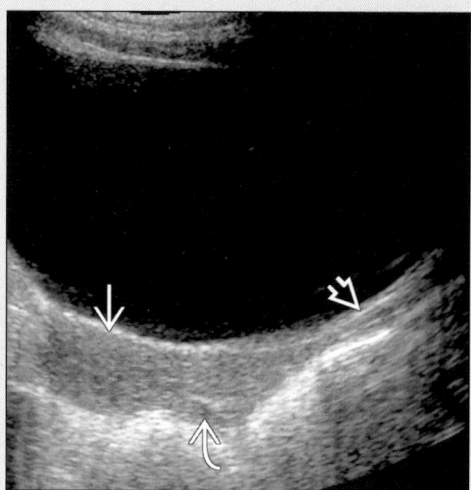

Sagittal transabdominal ultrasound through a full bladder shows body of uterus ➡, cervix ➢, and vagina ➡.

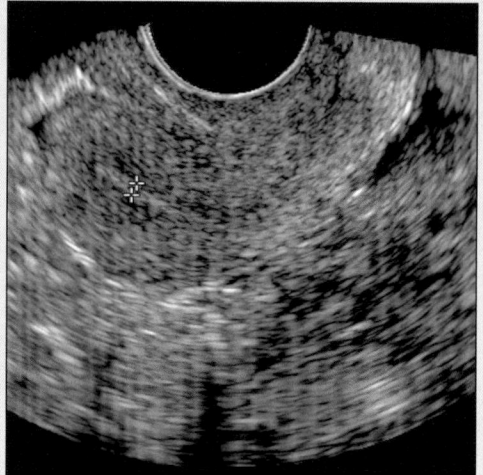

Sagittal transvaginal ultrasound shows thin endometrium (calipers).

PATHOLOGY-BASED IMAGING ISSUES

Key Concepts or Questions

- How should a woman with abnormal bleeding be assessed?
  - Transvaginal sonography to assess for endometrial thickness and/or focal lesion
    - Thick homogeneous endometrium can be assessed with blind endometrial biopsy
    - Blind endometrial biopsy misses 50% of focal endometrial lesions
    - Focal endometrial lesion is best biopsied under direct hysteroscopic visualization
  - If focal lesion present, assess with color Doppler
  - If study is indeterminate, sonohysterography can be helpful

Imaging Pitfalls

- Arcuate vessels in periphery of uterus can be visualized as a segmented hypoechoic band in outer third of myometrium
  - Flow void on Doppler
  - In post-menopausal women with hypertension, diabetes or renal failure, arcuate arteries can calcify
- Leiomyomas with submucosal extent can deviate the endometrium
  - Distorted endometrium can be difficult to assess for focal lesion

EMBRYOLOGY

Embryologic Events

- At 6 weeks Müllerian ducts develop lateral to Wolffian ducts
- Wolffian ducts degenerate in normal females
- Müllerian ducts fuse by 12 weeks to become uterus and upper 2/3 of vagina

Practical Implications

- If fusion fails to occur then a duplication anomaly of uterus will be present
  - Duplication anomalies of uterus occur in 0.5-5% of women
  - Duplication anomalies are usually asymptomatic
    - Septate uterus associated with increased incidence of spontaneous abortion
    - Bicornuate uterus associated with incompetent cervix
    - Müllerian hypoplasia/agenesis associated with primary amenorrhea

CLINICAL IMPLICATIONS

Function-Dysfunction

- Primary amenorrhea defined as lack of menses by age 16
  - Can be hormonal, karyotypic, or anatomic
  - Imaging important to determine pelvic anatomy
  - Identify uterine tissue, determine length of agenetic segment, describe obstructed uterus/vagina

RELATED REFERENCES

1. Reinhold C et al: Primary amenorrhea: evaluation with MR imaging. Radiology. 203:383-90, 1997
2. Holm K et al: Pubertal maturation of the internal genitalia: an ultrasound evaluation of 166 healthy girls. Ultrasound Obstet Gynecol. 6:175-81, 1995
3. Moore K et al: The Developing Human. 5th edition. Philadelphia, WB Saunders, 1993
4. Blask AR et al: Obstructed uterovaginal anomalies: demonstration with sonography. Part I. Neonates and infants. Radiology. 179:79-83, 1991
5. Siegel M: Pediatric gynecologic sonography. Radiology. 179:583-600, 1991
6. Platt JF et al: Ultrasound of the normal nongravid uterus: correlation with gross and histopathology. J Clin Ultrasound. 18:15-9, 1990

UTERINE ANATOMY & IMAGING ISSUES

IMAGE GALLERY

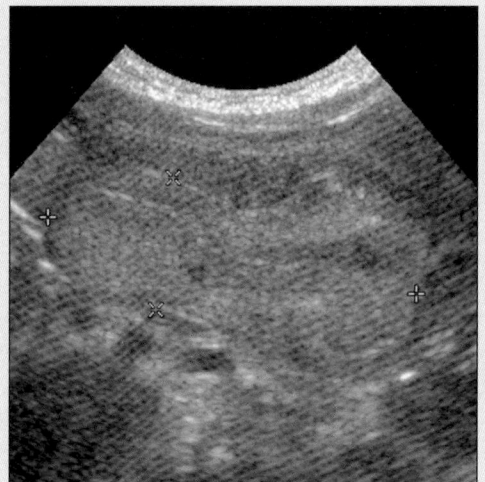
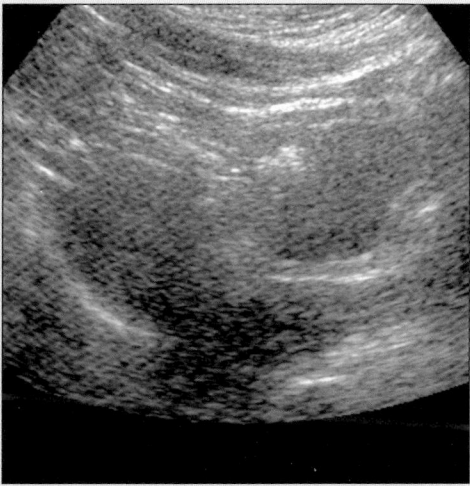

(Left) Sagittal transabdominal ultrasound shows neonatal uterus (calipers). *(Right)* Sagittal transabdominal ultrasound shows appearance of uterus in a large patient with an empty bladder. This emphasizes the importance of a full bladder scan when transvaginal scanning is inadequate.

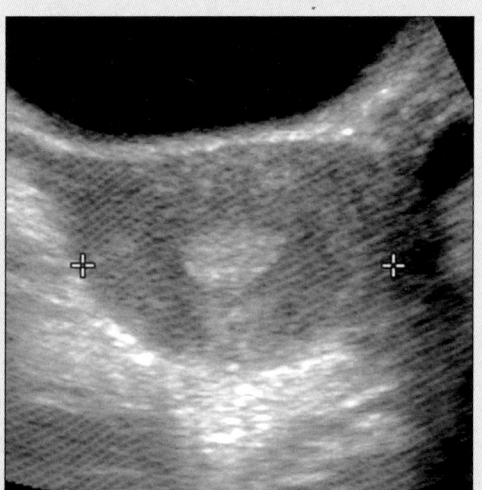
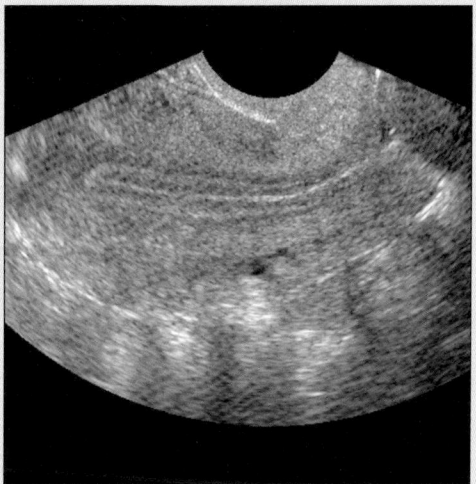

(Left) Transverse transabdominal ultrasound shows normal appearing uterus (calipers). *(Right)* Sagittal transvaginal ultrasound shows midcycle appearance to endometrium with three layers.

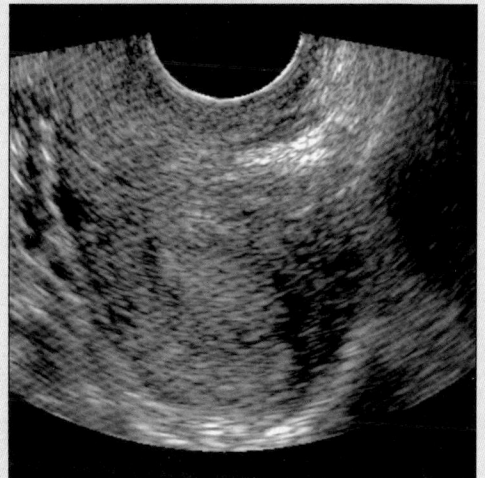
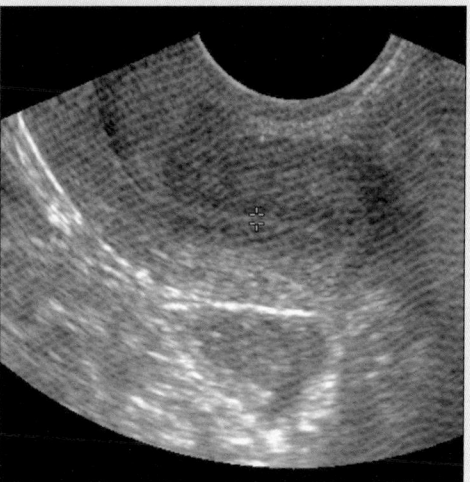

(Left) Sagittal transvaginal ultrasound shows retroflexed uterus. *(Right)* Sagittal transvaginal ultrasound in postmenopausal woman shows retroflexed uterus with thin endometrium (calipers).

UTERINE ANATOMY & IMAGING ISSUES

IMAGE GALLERY

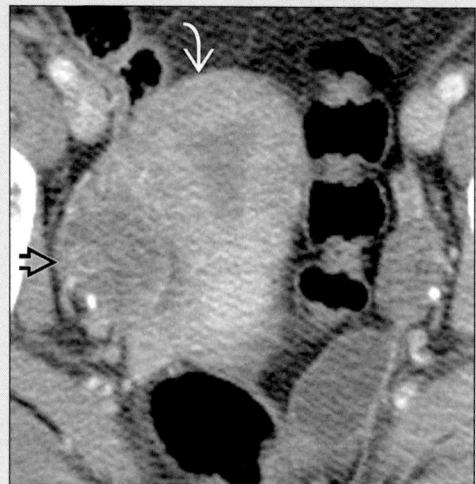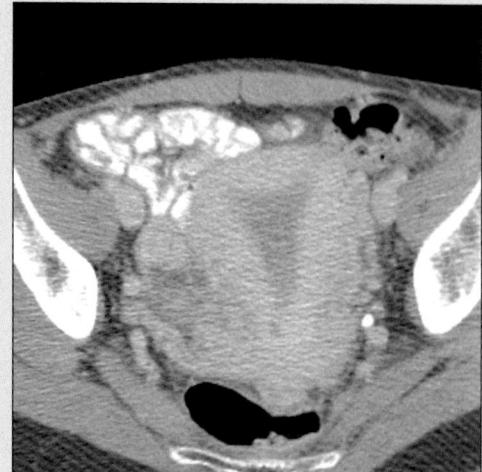

(Left) Axial CECT shows uterus ➡ and right ovary ➡. (Right) Axial CECT shows uterus in coronal plane.

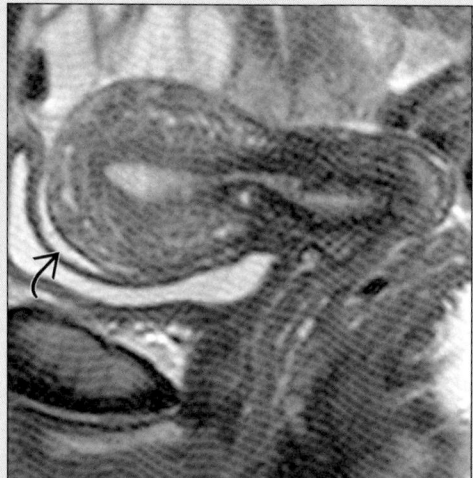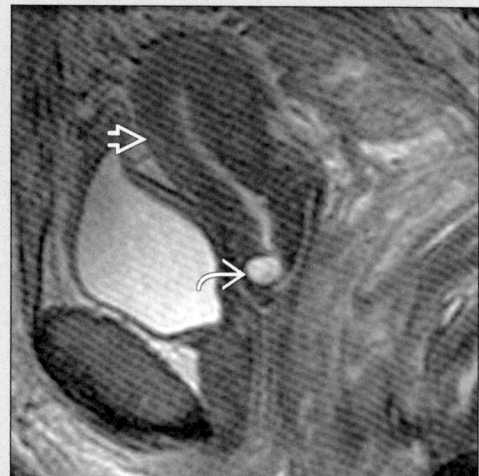

(Left) Sagittal T2WI MR shows normal uterus. Note small amount of surrounding fluid ➡. (Right) Sagittal T2WI MR shows uterus ➡ with nabothian cyst in cervix ➡.

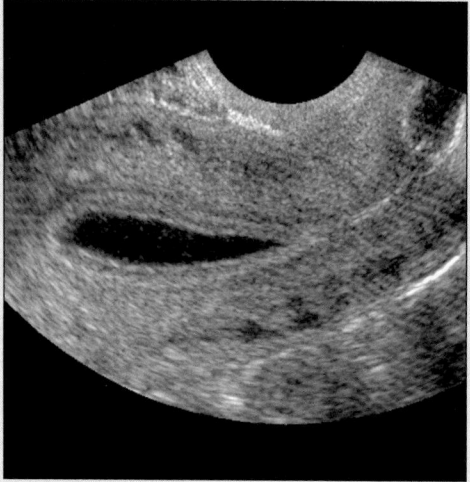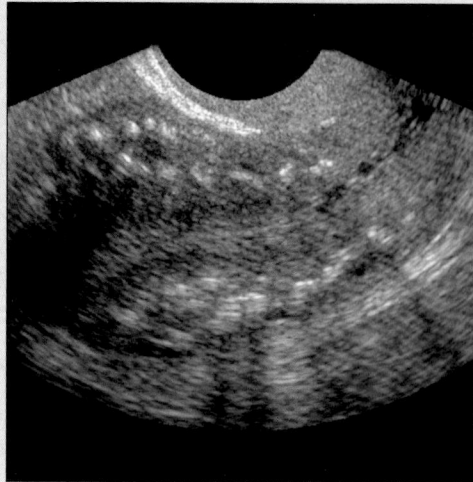

(Left) Sagittal transvaginal ultrasound during sonohysterogram shows normal endometrial cavity. (Right) Sagittal transvaginal ultrasound shows arcuate artery calcifications in the out third of the myometrium.

UTERINE ANATOMY & IMAGING ISSUES

IMAGE GALLERY

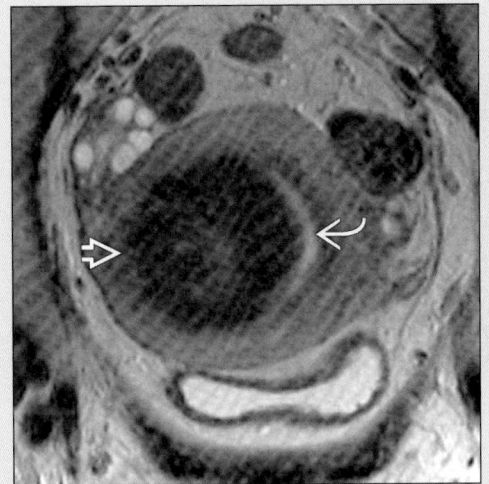
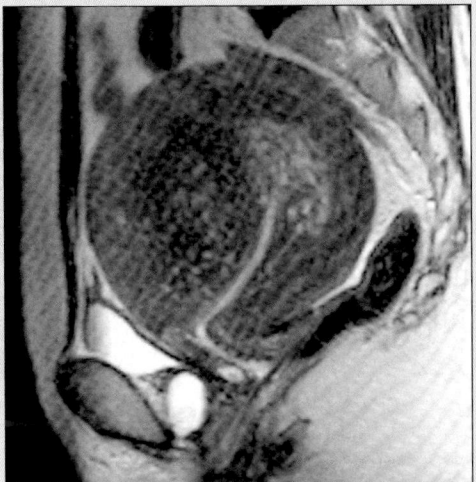

(Left) Coronal T2WI MR shows uterus with intramural fibroid ➡, deviating endometrium ➡ to the left. *(Right)* Sagittal T2WI MR in woman with adenomyosis shows enlarged uterus with multiple small cysts in the myometrium and thickened junctional zone.

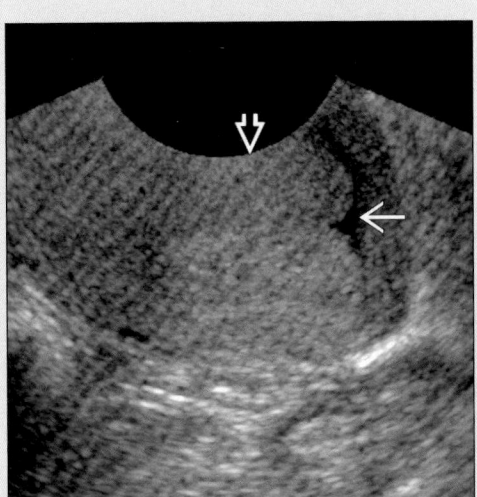
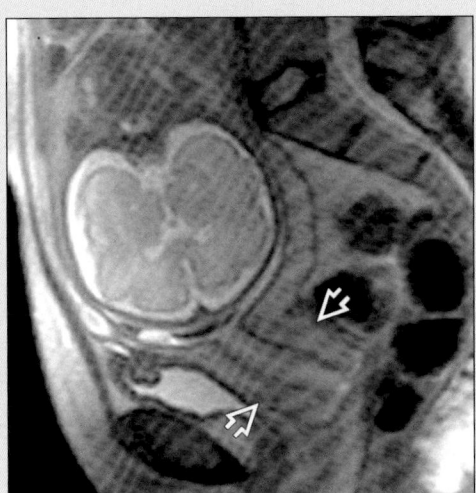

(Left) Sagittal transvaginal ultrasound shows cervix ➡ with a small amount of fluid ➡ outlining the external os. *(Right)* Sagittal T2WI MR in pregnant patient shows fetal head and cervix ➡.

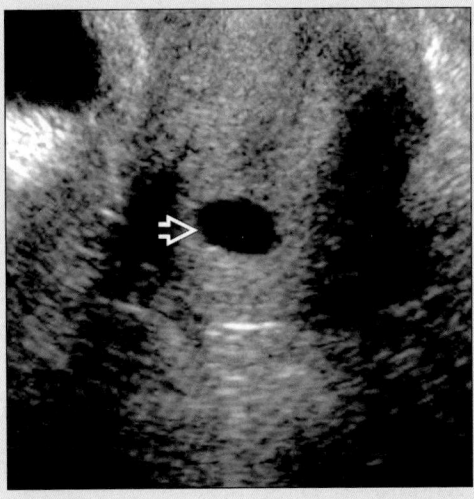
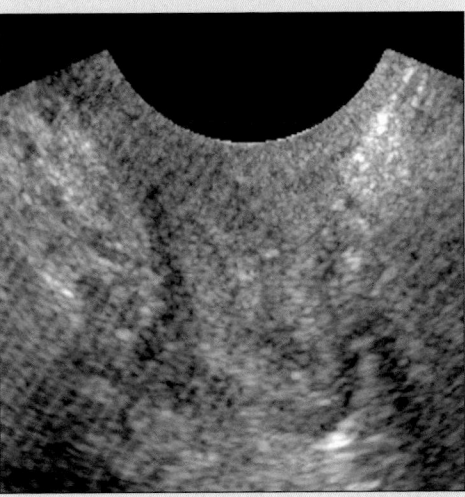

(Left) Sagittal transvaginal ultrasound shows cervix in patient with history of supracervical hysterectomy. Note nabothian cyst ➡. *(Right)* Sagittal transvaginal ultrasound with probe at introitus shows blind-ending vagina in patient after hysterectomy.

SONOHYSTEROGRAPHY

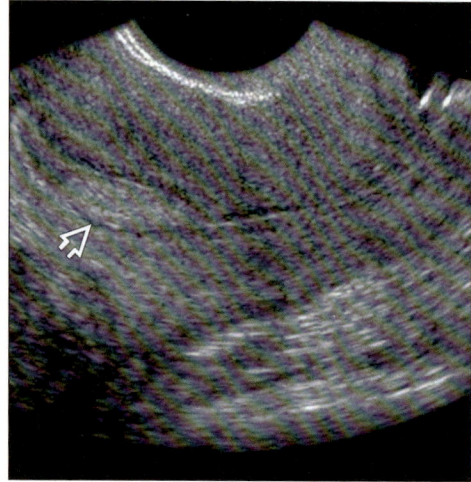

Sagittal transvaginal ultrasound prior to sonohysterogram shows focal echogenic mass ➡ in endometrium suggestive of polyp.

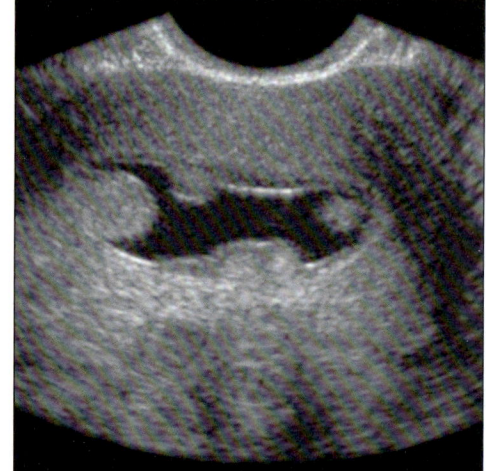

Axial transvaginal ultrasound in same patient as previous image shows multiple endometrial polyps outlined by fluid during sonohysterogram.

TERMINOLOGY

Abbreviations
- Sonohysterogram (SHG)

Synonyms
- Hysterosonography
- Saline infused sonography

Definitions
- SHG describes infusion of sterile saline into endometrial and cervical cavities to outline pathology
- Sonosalpingography describes assessment of the fallopian tubes with saline/gas mixture

PRE-PROCEDURE

Indications
- Abnormal bleeding
  o Most common indication
  o Safe, non-invasive, inexpensive mode for triage of further procedures
    ▪ No further evaluation if thin and normal appearing
    ▪ Blind endometrial sampling for a global endometrial process
    ▪ Visually directed endometrial sampling when pathology is focal
- Focal mass on sonography
- Assessment of endometrium in patients taking tamoxifen
  o SHG improves accuracy of diagnosis of intrauterine mass in asymptomatic postmenopausal tamoxifen-treated patients
  o Size of the intrauterine mass correlates with the severity of the endometrial pathology
- Heterogeneous endometrium on sonography, unclear if mass present
- Location of leiomyomas with respect to endometrial cavity for triage of treatment
  o Leiomyomas with greater than 50% of volume in endometrial cavity are typically amenable to hysteroscopic removal
- Tubal patency in patients with contraindication to hysterosalpingography
- Infertility or recurrent miscarriage
- Suspected synechiae
- Suspected uterine duplication abnormality

Contraindications
- Pelvic inflammatory disease
  o If dilated tubes found pre-procedure and patient has not been treated with prophylactic antibiotics, then procedure should be delayed until treatment can be administered
  o If hydrosalpinx found during procedure then give antibiotics at time of examination
- Pregnancy
- Secretory phase
- Unexplained pelvic pain that could be secondary to chronic pelvic inflammatory disease
- Relative contraindication is acute vaginal bleeding due to theoretic risk of causing endometriosis

Getting Started
- Things to Check
  o Patient should be in first 10 days of menstrual cycle after cessation of menstruation
    ▪ If currently bleeding there is theoretic risk of inducing endometriosis
  o Patient should not be pregnant
  o Confirm no current pelvic inflammatory disease or vaginal infection

SONOHYSTEROGRAPHY

Key Facts

Pre-procedure
- Abnormal bleeding
- Focal mass on sonography
- Assessment of endometrium in patients taking tamoxifen
- Heterogeneous endometrium on sonography, unclear if mass present
- Location of leiomyomas with respect to endometrial cavity for triage of treatment
- Patient should be in first 10 days of menstrual cycle after cessation of menstruation
- If currently bleeding there is theoretic risk of inducing endometriosis
- Patient should not be pregnant
- Confirm no current pelvic inflammatory disease or vaginal infection
- Ibuprofen 1 hour prior to procedure decreases cramping
- Balloon catheter gives better occlusion but is more painful for patient
- Straight catheter easier to use for experienced practitioner, but can slip out of place

Procedure
- 3D sweep of endometrium may obviate need for multiple sagittal and transverse images
- Focal lesions may benefit from use of color and pulsed Doppler

Post-procedure
- Mild cramping
- Mild spotting

- Patients with infection can have spread of disease with the procedure
- Medications
  - Ibuprofen 1 hour prior to procedure decreases cramping
  - If unexpected hydrosalpinx found, patients should be given appropriate antibiotics
- Equipment List
  - Ultrasound machine with transvaginal probe
  - Written informed consent
  - Speculum
  - Swabs to cleanse cervix
  - Betadine to cleanse cervix
  - Sterile saline in 20 cc syringe
  - Catheter
    - Balloon catheter gives better occlusion but is more painful for patient
    - Straight catheter easier to use for experienced practitioner, but can slip out of place
    - If straight catheter needs to be re-introduced, cervical mucus plug may be dislodged and it will no longer be possible to distend the endometrial cavity

PROCEDURE

Patient Position/Location
- Best procedure approach: Lithotomy position

Procedure Steps
- Pre-procedure assessment of endometrium
  - Measure bilayer endometrial thickness in sagittal plane
  - Document focal lesions
- Pre-procedure documentation of fluid in cul-de-sac
- Written informed consent
- Insert speculum to visualize cervix
- If obvious vaginal infection, abort procedure and have patient treated appropriately
- Cleanse cervix with betadine
  - If external os is not clearly visualized, gentle pressure above symphysis pubis may move external os into view
- Insert catheter
  - If using balloon catheter, place balloon in mid cervix
  - If using straight catheter, place tip of catheter in lower uterus
  - Stenotic cervix may need to be dilated pre-procedure
- Remove speculum
- Insert vaginal probe
- Inject saline while observing position of catheter
  - If balloon catheter in mid uterus, deflate balloon and reposition
  - If balloon catheter in lower uterus, perform procedure and at end of procedure, deflate balloon withdraw slightly, and assess lower endometrium
- Assess endometrium while scanning in sagittal plane
- Document endometrium in sagittal and bilateral parasagittal planes
- Assess endometrium while scanning in transverse plane
- Document endometrium at multiple levels in transverse plane
- 3D sweep of endometrium may obviate need for multiple sagittal and transverse images
- Focal lesions may benefit from use of color and pulsed Doppler
- If patient with infertility, agitate saline with small amount of air, and inject, observing flow of contrast through cornua, and into peritoneal cavity, documenting tubal patency
- If uterus is large, transabdominal images may be needed to fully evaluate the endometrium

Findings and Reporting
- Procedure note
- Pre-procedure endometrial thickness
- Pre-procedure endometrial appearance
- Distensibility of endometrial cavity
- Focal endometrial lesions
- If leiomyomas, document what percentage of the leiomyomas project into endometrium

SONOHYSTEROGRAPHY

- If patient with infertility, comment on tubal patency
  - If more fluid present in peritoneal cavity after procedure than before procedure, at least one tube is patent

Alternative Procedures/Therapies
- Radiologic
  - Hysterosalpingography
    - Better for tubal assessment
    - Worse for endometrial lesions
    - Uses ionizing radiation
    - Uses iodinated contrast (with associated risks)
- Surgical
  - Hysteroscopy
    - Requires anesthesia
    - More invasive
    - More expensive
    - Allows for concurrent biopsy of lesions
- Other: SHG may be used to guide focal endometrial lesion biopsy

POST-PROCEDURE

Expected Outcome
- Mild cramping
  - Similar to light day of menstruation
  - Treat with ibuprofen
- Mild spotting
  - Similar to light day of menstruation

PROBLEMS & COMPLICATIONS

Problems
- Performing the procedure in the secretory phase can lead to false positive diagnosis since the endometrium can have a lumpy irregular appearance
- Blood clot in the endometrial cavity can simulate a mass
  - Clot should be mobile
  - Clot should not have blood flow

Complications
- Most feared complication(s)
  - Pelvic inflammatory disease and septicemia
    - Patients with hydrosalpinx at risk
    - Patients with underlying infection at risk
  - Spill of malignant cells into peritoneal cavity in patients with endometrial carcinoma
    - Microscopic spill occurs in up to 25% of patients with malignancy according to an intraoperative study
- Other complications
  - Performance of procedure in pregnant patient
    - History should exclude this possibility
    - Pregnancy test prior to procedure for anyone unsure of pregnancy status
  - Vasovagal reaction
    - Secondary to manipulation of cervix
    - Secondary to inflation of balloon catheter

SELECTED REFERENCES

1. Dessole S et al: Risks and usefulness of sonohysterography in patients with endometrial carcinoma. Am J Obstet Gynecol. 194(2):362-8, 2006
2. Valenzano MM et al: Transvaginal sonohysterographic evaluation of uterine malformations. Eur J Obstet Gynecol Reprod Biol. 124(2):246-9, 2006
3. Wei AY et al: Saline contrast sonohysterography and directed extraction, resection and biopsy of intrauterine pathology using a Uterine Explora Curette. Ultrasound Obstet Gynecol. 27(2):202-5, 2006
4. Ragni G et al: Effectiveness of sonohysterography in infertile patient work-up: a comparison with transvaginal ultrasonography and hysteroscopy. Gynecol Obstet Invest. 59(4):184-8, 2005
5. Salim R et al: A comparative study of three-dimensional saline infusion sonohysterography and diagnostic hysteroscopy for the classification of submucous fibroids. Hum Reprod. 20(1):253-7, 2005
6. ACOG technology assessment. International J Gynecol Obstet. 84:95-8, 2004
7. Goldstein SR: Menorrhagia and abnormal bleeding before the menopause. Best Pract Res Clin Obstet Gynaecol. 18(1):59-69, 2004
8. Markovitch O et al: The value of sonohysterography in the prediction of endometrial pathologies in asymptomatic postmenopausal breast cancer tamoxifen-treated patients. Gynecol Oncol. 94(3):754-9, 2004
9. Laifer-Narin S et al: False-normal appearance of the endometrium on conventional transvaginal sonography: comparison with saline hysterosonography. AJR Am J Roentgenol. 178(1):129-33, 2002
10. Hann LE et al: Sonohysterography for evaluation of the endometrium in women treated with tamoxifen. AJR Am J Roentgenol. 177(2):337-42, 2001
11. Bree RL et al: US evaluation of the uterus in patients with postmenopausal bleeding: A positive effect on diagnostic decision making. Radiology. 216(1):260-4, 2000
12. Laifer-Narin SL et al: Transvaginal saline hysterosonography: characteristics distinguishing malignant and various benign conditions. AJR Am J Roentgenol. 172(6):1513-20, 1999
13. Schwartz LB et al: The use of transvaginal ultrasound and saline infusion sonohysterography for the evaluation of asymptomatic postmenopausal breast cancer patients on tamoxifen. Ultrasound Obstet Gynecol. 11(1):48-53, 1998
14. Lev-Toaff AS et al: Value of sonohysterography in the diagnosis and management of abnormal uterine bleeding. Radiology. 201(1):179-84, 1996
15. Lev-Toaff AS: Sonohysterography: evaluation of endometrial and myometrial abnormalities. Semin Roentgenol. 31(4):288-98, 1996
16. Dubinsky TJ et al: Transvaginal hysterosonography in the evaluation of small endoluminal masses. J Ultrasound Med. 14(1):1-6, 1995
17. Cohen JR et al: Sonohysterography for the diagnosis of endometrial thickening in postmenopausal bleeding-a preliminary report. J AM Assoc Gynecol Laparosc. 1:S7-8, 1994
18. Goldstein SR: Use of ultrasonohysterography for triage of perimenopausal patients with unexplained uterine bleeding. Am J Obstet Gynecol. 170(2):565-70, 1994
19. Parsons AK et al: Sonohysterography for endometrial abnormalities: preliminary results. J Clin Ultrasound. 21(2):87-95, 1993

SONOHYSTEROGRAPHY

IMAGE GALLERY

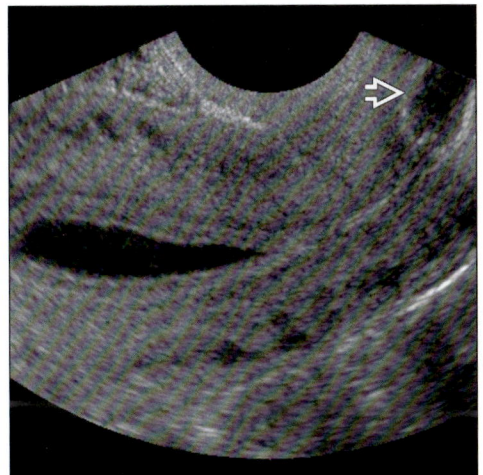
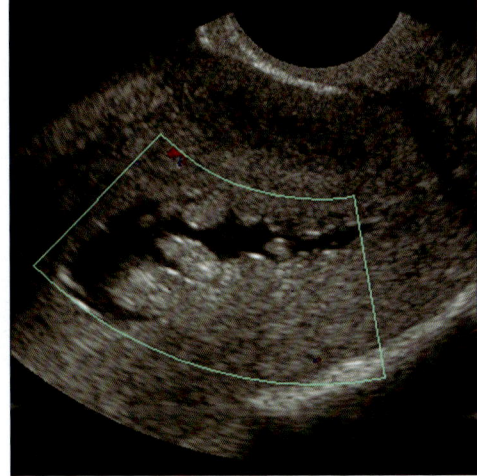

(Left) Sagittal transvaginal ultrasound shows normal appearance to endometrium during sonohysterogram. Note balloon catheter ➔ in cervix. *(Right)* Sagittal transvaginal ultrasound during sonohysterogram shows multiple polypoid lesions projecting into endometrial cavity in patient with complex hyperplasia with atypia.

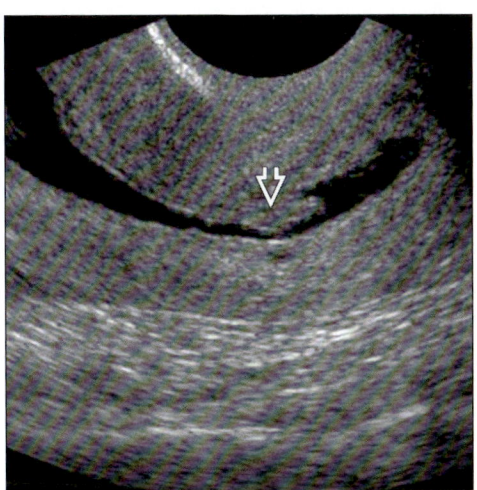
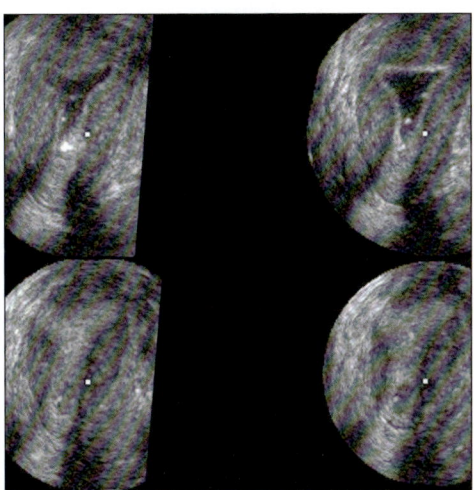

(Left) Sagittal transvaginal ultrasound after removal of sonohysterography catheter shows small polyp ➔ in cervix. *(Right)* Coronal transvaginal ultrasound shows 3D reconstructions during sonohysterogram.

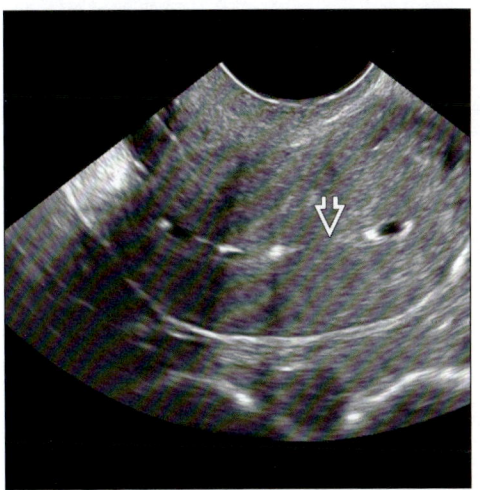
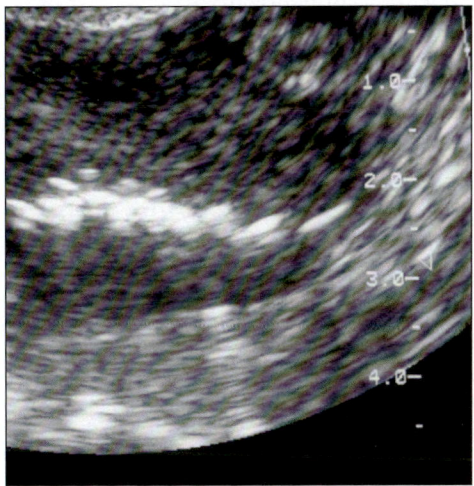

(Left) Sagittal transvaginal ultrasound in retroflexed uterus during SHG shows poorly distensible endometrial cavity with band of tissue extending across endometrial cavity ➔ consistent with scar. *(Right)* Coronal oblique transvaginal ultrasound during SHG for tubal patency shows injection of air/saline mix with bubbles extending out interstitial portion of tube.

AGE-RELATED PHYSIOLOGIC ALTERATIONS

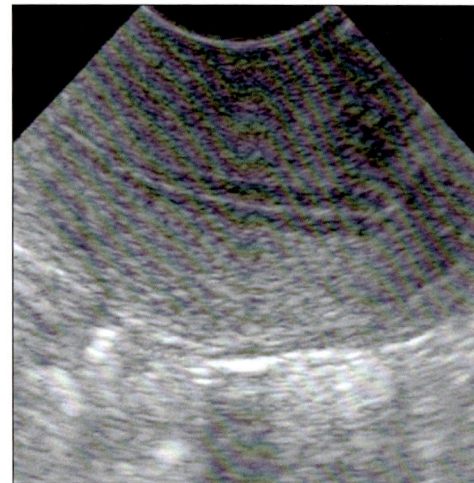

Sagittal transvaginal ultrasound of a normal early proliferative phase uterus shows a trilaminar appearance of the endometrium.

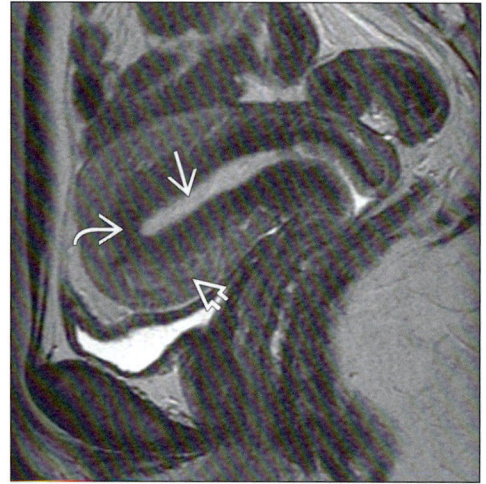

Sagittal T2WI MR shows a normal proliferative phase uterus. The endometrium is hyperintense and thin ➔, the junctional zone hypointense ➔ and the myometrium ➔ of intermediate signal intensity.

TERMINOLOGY

Definitions
- Cyclic variation of uterus and ovaries on imaging in hormonally active female
- Variation of uterine and ovarian appearance with age and hormonal status

IMAGING FINDINGS

General Features
- Best diagnostic clue: Uterus has a changing appearance throughout life and menstrual cycle
- Size
  - Average length and width of uterus during reproductive years (8 x 5 cm)
    - Uterine volume greatest during secretory phase
  - Uterus small in pre-menarchal and postmenopausal women (5 x 2 cm)
    - Corpus and cervix have equal length
  - **Endometrial thickness variation**
    - Proliferative phase: 3-8 mm
    - Secretory phase: 5-16 mm
    - Postmenopausal (no bleeding): ≤ 8 mm, thickness may vary with phase if receiving exogenous hormones
    - Postmenopausal (bleeding): ≤ 5 mm

Ultrasonographic Findings
- Pre-menarche
  - Inverse pear-shaped uterus (cervix anteroposterior diameter greater than fundus)
  - Ovaries small, ovoid-shaped, solid appearing
    - May show millimetric cysts
- Reproductive age
  - Proliferative phase
    - Trilaminar appearance of endometrium
    - Central echogenic line corresponding to endometrial interface
    - Functionalis layer: Hypoechoic superficial layer of endometrium (4-8 mm)
    - Basalis layer: Hyperechoic, deep (juxtamyometrial) layer of endometrium
    - Subendometrial halo (inner myometrium): Hypoechoic
    - Myometrium: Intermediate echogenicity, outer and middle layers separated by arcuate vessels

DDx: Mimics of Age-Related Physiologic Alterations

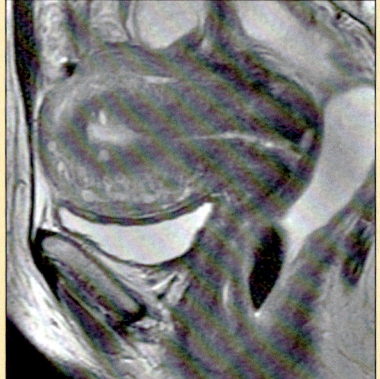
Adenomyosis

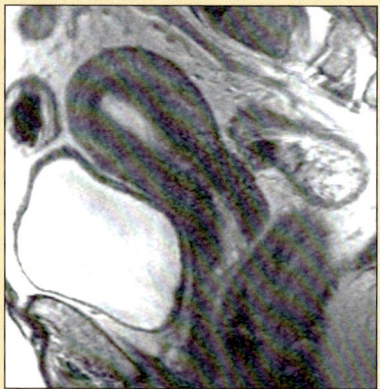
Endometrial Carcinoma

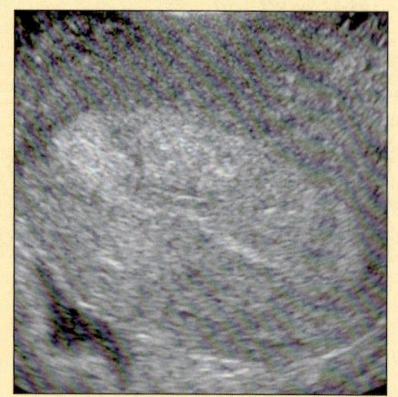
Endometrial Polyp

AGE-RELATED PHYSIOLOGIC ALTERATIONS

Key Facts

Terminology
- Variation of uterine and ovarian appearance with age and hormonal status

Imaging Findings
- Average length and width of uterus during reproductive years (8 x 5 cm)
- Uterine volume greatest during secretory phase
- **Endometrial thickness variation**
- Proliferative phase: 3-8 mm
- Secretory phase: 5-16 mm
- Postmenopausal (no bleeding): ≤ 8 mm, thickness may vary with phase if receiving exogenous hormones
- Postmenopausal (bleeding): ≤ 5 mm
- Best imaging tool: TVS and sagittal T2WI MR offer best depiction of uterine zonal anatomy
- Protocol advice: Real-time TVS or cine MR may be performed during menstrual/periovulatory phases to differentiate pseudothickening of JZ due to uterine peristalsis from pathologic thickening

Top Differential Diagnoses
- Endometrial Carcinoma
- Endometrial Hyperplasia
- Endometrial Polyp
- Adenomyosis

Diagnostic Checklist
- Hormonal status and phase of menstrual cycle must be known when performing TVS or MR examination
- Normal hormonal variations can influence detection of pathology

---

- Ovary: Cortex hypoechoic, medulla slightly hyperechoic
- Anechoic follicular cysts develop, one of them dominant
- Secretory phase
  - Thickening of endometrium which becomes diffusely hyperechoic (with posterior acoustic enhancement)
  - Thin hypoechoic subendometrial halo remains
- Menstrual phase
  - Endometrium: Thin, broken echogenic line
- Post-menopause
  - Calcifications of arcuate arteries (peripheral linear echogenic areas with shadowing)
  - Endometrium: Thin echogenic line
  - Small ovaries, homogeneous, no follicles

CT Findings
- NECT: Postmenopausal uterus: Crescent-shaped calcifications in outer one third of myometrium (calcified arcuate arteries)
- CECT
  - Limited zonal anatomy depiction
  - On early phase acquisition, hypodense endometrium relative to myometrium
  - May see early enhancement of junctional zone (JZ) during menstrual phase

MR Findings
- T1WI
  - Uterus: Homogeneous intermediate signal intensity
    - Isointense to muscle
    - No zonal anatomy depicted
- T2WI
  - Best delineation of zonal anatomy variation
  - Pre-menarche
    - Corpus and cervix equal length
    - Thin endometrium, no cyclic change in endometrial appearance
    - Intermediate signal intensity (SI) myometrium, lower than in women of reproductive age
  - Reproductive age
    - Zonal anatomy of uterine corpus well-depicted
    - Endometrial complex: High SI
    - Outer myometrium: Intermediate SI
    - JZ: Low SI inner myometrium, ≤ 8 mm
    - Appearance varies with menstrual cycle
  - Proliferative phase: Thin endometrium
  - Periovulatory phase: Zonal anatomy well-depicted
  - Secretory phase: Increased thickness of endometrium and myometrium
    - Outer myometrium increased SI
    - Decreased thickness of junctional zone
    - Pre-menstrual (24 hours): Low SI of endometrium
  - Menstrual phase: Uterine corpus of diminished volume
    - JZ ill-defined and irregularly thickened due to uterine peristalsis/contractions
    - Thin endometrium, low SI line in the endometrial cavity (menstrual blood)
  - Oral contraceptive pill (OCP)
    - Marked endometrial atrophy
    - Little temporal variation of endometrial thickness (average 2 mm)
    - JZ often thin or not visible
    - Myometrium hyperintense, may appear swollen (smooth muscle hyperplasia)
  - Cervical zonal anatomy: No significant change with hormonal status
  - Ovarian zonal anatomy
    - Outer cortex: Low SI
    - Central medulla: Intermediate SI
  - Post-menopause
    - Atrophic endometrium without cyclic variation
    - Myometrium decreases in SI, becomes isointense with JZ
    - Zonal anatomy becomes indistinct after menopause
    - With exogenous estrogens, zonal anatomy can be restored
    - Ovary: Low SI cortex and medulla
- T1 C+
  - Depends on hormonal status
  - Proliferative phase
    - Early enhancement of thin subendometrial layer

AGE-RELATED PHYSIOLOGIC ALTERATIONS

- Delayed enhancement of remaining myometrium
- Secretory phase
  - Early enhancement of outer myometrium
  - Endometrial delayed enhancement, isointense or hyperintense to myometrium
- Menstrual phase
  - Early enhancement of JZ
- Cervix: Rapid enhancement of endocervical mucosa, more gradual enhancement of fibrous stroma
- Postmenopausal
  - Same as proliferative phase: Early enhancement of thin subendometrial layer
- Ovary
  - Premenopausal: Enhances less than myometrium
  - Postmenopausal: Enhancement equivalent to myometrium

Imaging Recommendations
- Best imaging tool: TVS and sagittal T2WI MR offer best depiction of uterine zonal anatomy
- Protocol advice: Real-time TVS or cine MR may be performed during menstrual/periovulatory phases to differentiate pseudothickening of JZ due to uterine peristalsis from pathologic thickening

DIFFERENTIAL DIAGNOSIS

Endometrial Carcinoma
- Can overlap with secretory phase endometrium
- Usually more heterogeneous than normal endometrium on TVS
- Typically lower SI than normal endometrium on T2WI
- Hypovascular compared to myometrium on delayed T1 C+

Endometrial Hyperplasia
- Can overlap with secretory phase endometrium
- Iso- to slightly hypointense to endometrium on T2WI
- May show cystic changes: Hyperintense foci on T2WI

Endometrial Polyp
- Separate endometrial lining may be seen
- Stalk flow on color Doppler
- Hypointense central fibrous stalk on T2WI
- On early T1 C+, stand out against hypointense endometrium

Adenomyosis
- Diffuse/segmental thickening of JZ persisting during successive MR sequences or cine MR allows to differentiate from peristalsis/contractions
- Bright SI foci in JZ found in adenomyosis

PATHOLOGY

Microscopic Features
- Endometrium: Superficial functionalis layer and deep basalis layer
- Inner myometrium
  - Compact, linear arrangement of muscle fibers parallel to basal layer of endometrium
  - Higher nuclear-to-cytoplasm ratio, lower water content
- Outer myometrium
  - Smooth muscle less compact
  - Greater extracellular matrix, increased water content
  - Numerous venous structures
- OCP: Smooth muscle hypertrophy, sinusoidal dilatation, edema
- Post-menopause
  - Atrophic endometrium
  - Moderate fibrosis of endometrial stroma
  - Small vessels, irregular distribution
- Ovary
  - Ovarian cortex: Stroma more cellular
  - Ovarian medulla: Stroma made of looser, vascularized connective tissue; higher free water content
  - Post-menopause: Replacement of medulla with corpora albicans, increased stromal cells and absence of small follicles

DIAGNOSTIC CHECKLIST

Consider
- Hormonal status and phase of menstrual cycle must be known when performing TVS or MR examination
- Normal hormonal variations can influence detection of pathology

Image Interpretation Pearls
- Sagittal T2WI offers the best zonal anatomy depiction on a single slice

SELECTED REFERENCES

1. Chaudhry S et al: Benign and malignant diseases of the endometrium. Top Magn Reson Imaging. 14(4):339-57, 2003
2. Kido A et al: Diffusely enlarged uterus: evaluation with MR imaging. Radiographics. 23(6):1423-39, 2003
3. Siegelman ES et al: Tissue characterization in the female pelvis by means of MR imaging. Radiology. 212(1):5-18, 1999
4. Rumack CM et al: Diagnostic Ultrasound. Vol 1. 2nd ed. St-Louis, Mosby. 524-8, 1998
5. Noci I et al: Morphological and functional aspects of the endometrium of asymptomatic post-menopausal women: does the endometrium really age? Hum Reprod. 11(10):2246-50, 1996
6. Brown HK et al: Uterine junctional zone: correlation between histologic findings and MR imaging. Radiology. 179(2):409-13, 1991
7. Mitchell DG et al: Zones of the uterus: discrepancy between US and MR images. Radiology. 174(3 Pt 1):827-31, 1990
8. Demas BE et al: Uterine MR imaging: effects of hormonal stimulation. Radiology. 159(1):123-6, 1986
9. Haynor DR et al: Changing appearance of the normal uterus during the menstrual cycle: MR studies. Radiology. 161(2):459-62, 1986
10. Hricak H: MRI of the female pelvis: a review. AJR Am J Roentgenol. 146(6):1115-22, 1986
11. McCarthy S et al: Female pelvic anatomy: MR assessment of variations during the menstrual cycle and with use of oral contraceptives. Radiology. 160(1):119-23, 1986

AGE-RELATED PHYSIOLOGIC ALTERATIONS

IMAGE GALLERY

Typical

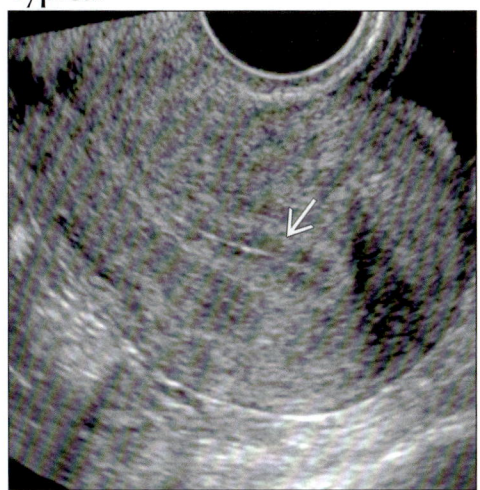
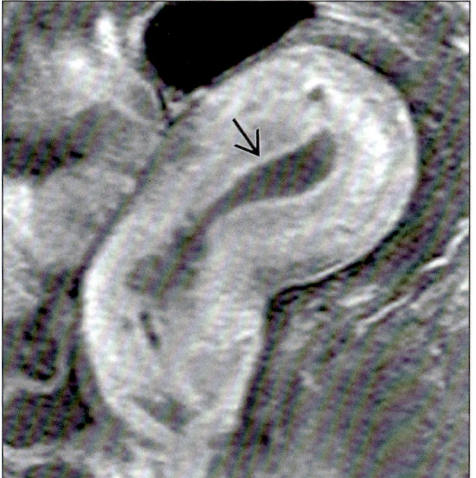

(Left) Sagittal transvaginal ultrasound of a late proliferative phase uterus shows progressive thickening and hyperechogenicity of the functionalis ➡ endometrial layer. *(Right)* Sagittal T1 C+ FS MR shows a proliferative phase uterus with early enhancement of a thin subendometrial layer ➡. This type of enhancement can also be found in postmenopausal patients.

Typical

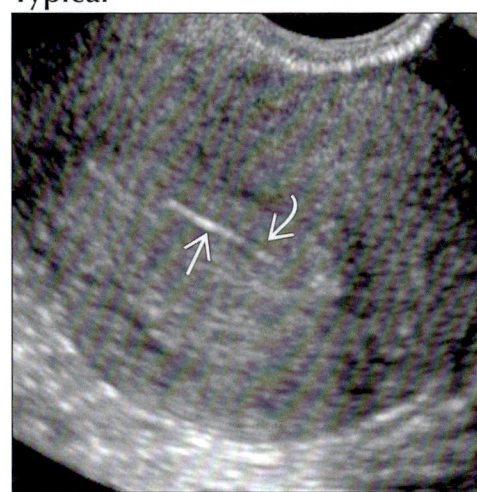
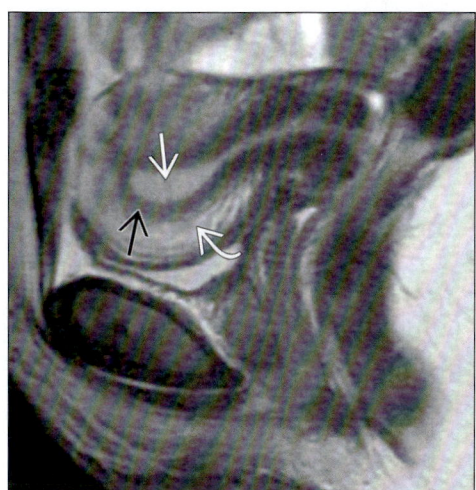

(Left) Sagittal transvaginal ultrasound shows a secretory phase endometrium with a thickened and echogenic functionalis layer ➡. The central endometrial interface is seen as a thin, echogenic line ➡. *(Right)* Sagittal T2WI MR shows a secretory phase uterus with a thickened endometrium ➡. The junctional zone is thin ➡ while the outer myometrium is hyperintense and thickened ➡.

Typical

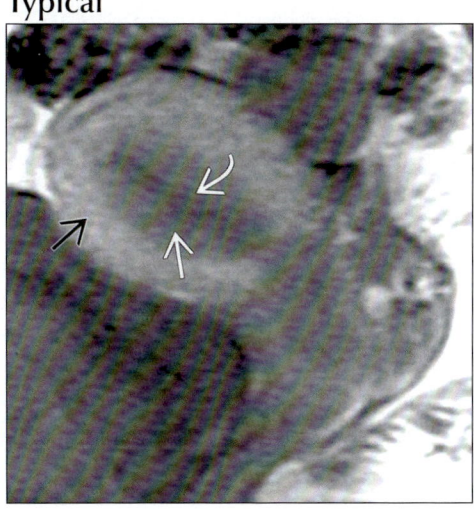
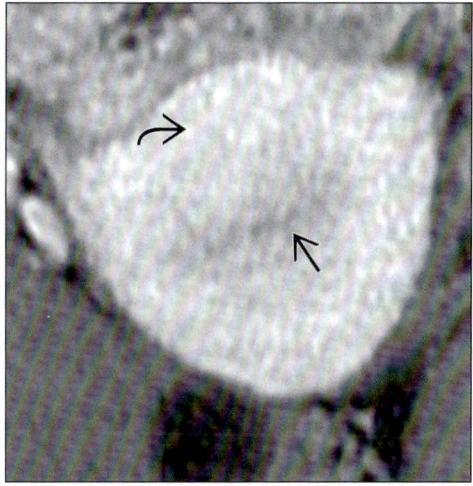

(Left) Sagittal T1 C+ MR shows early enhancement of the outer myometrium ➡ of a secretory phase uterus. The endometrium ➡ and junctional zone ➡ remain relatively hypovascular during the early arterial phase. *(Right)* Axial T1WI FS MR during the secretory phase shows delayed enhancement of the endometrium ➡ becoming isointense or hyperintense to myometrium ➡.

AGE-RELATED PHYSIOLOGIC ALTERATIONS

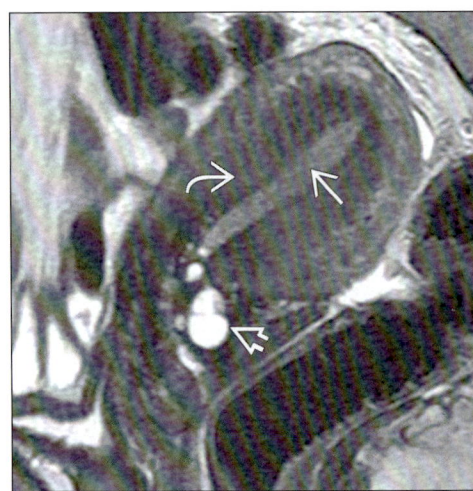

Typical

(Left) Sagittal T2WI MR shows a menstrual phase uterus with a diffusely hypointense endometrium ➔. The junctional zone ➔ appears thickened and ill-defined. Incidental cervical nabothian cyst ➔. *(Right)* Sagittal T2WI MR shows a menstrual phase uterus. There is a thin low signal intensity (SI) line within the endometrial cavity representing blood ➔ and an ill-defined low SI area within the myometrium ➔ in keeping with a myometrial contraction.

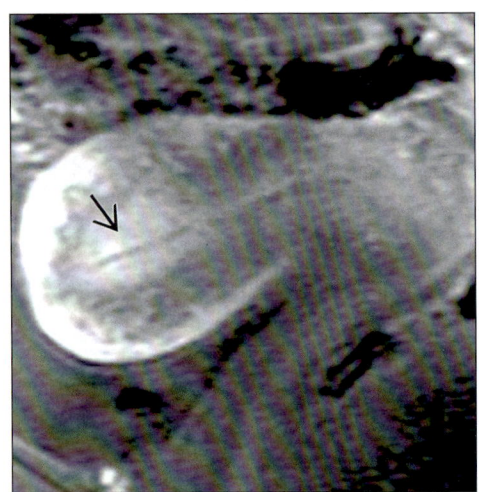 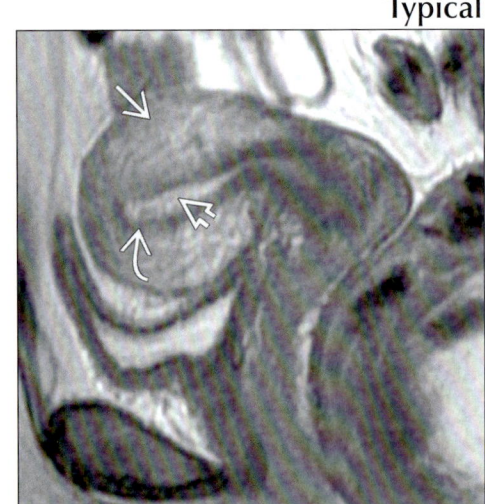

Typical

(Left) Sagittal T1 C+ FS MR shows early enhancement of the junctional zone ➔ and inner myometrium in a menstrual phase uterus. *(Right)* Sagittal T2WI MR shows a uterus in a woman under continuous oral contraceptives with a thin endometrium ➔. The myometrium is bright ➔, the junctional zone ➔ thin and ill-defined.

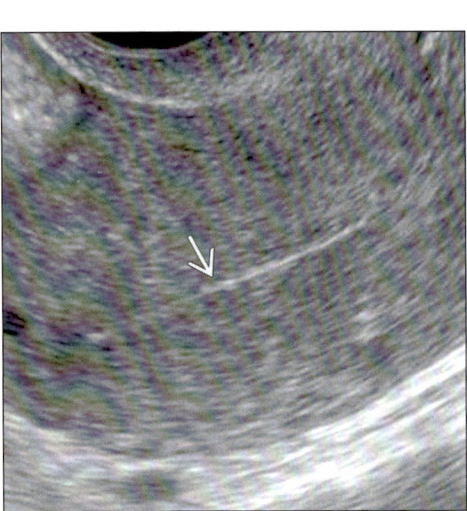 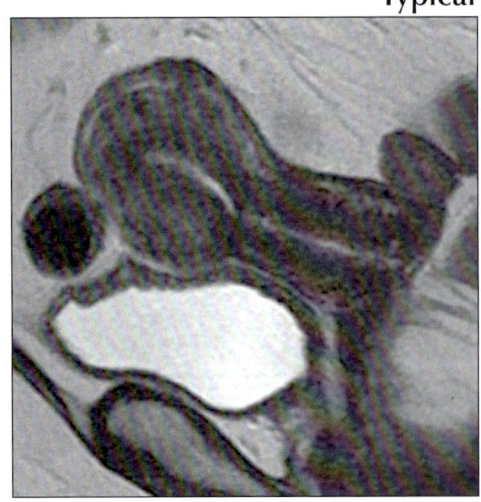

Typical

(Left) Sagittal transvaginal ultrasound shows an atrophic endometrium in a postmenopausal patient, visible as a thin echogenic line ➔. *(Right)* Sagittal T2WI MR shows a small postmenopausal uterus with an atrophic endometrium. There is loss of zonal anatomy with both the myometrium and junctional zone appearing hypointense.

AGE-RELATED PHYSIOLOGIC ALTERATIONS

Typical

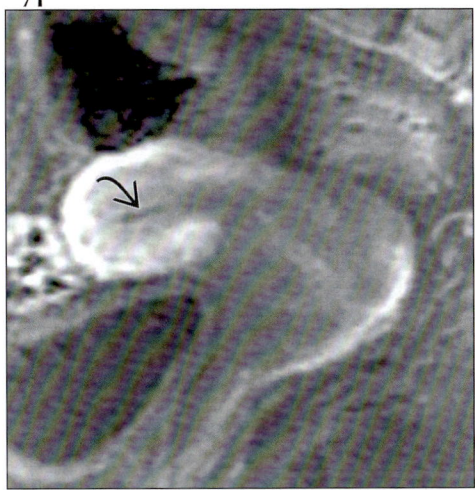 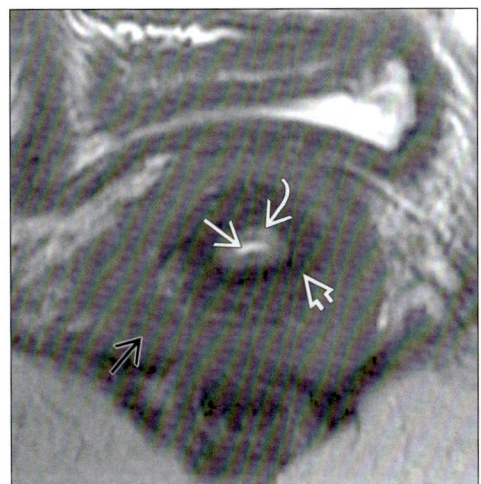

(Left) Sagittal T1 C+ FS MR of a postmenopausal uterus early after contrast administration shows a thin layer ⇨ of subendometrial enhancement. (Right) Axial oblique T2WI MR shows the normal cervical zonal anatomy. From inner layer to outer layer: Fluid ⇨, mucosa ⇨, fibrous stroma ⇨, and outer cervical stroma ⇨.

Typical

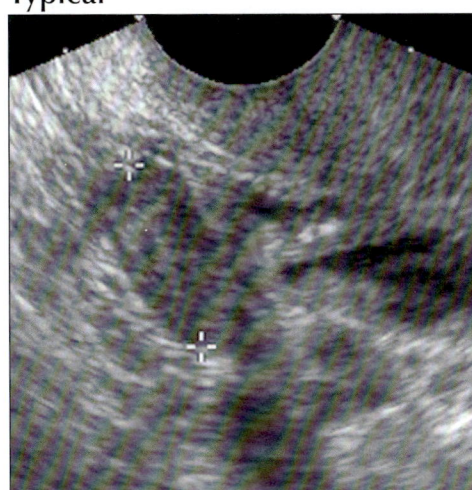 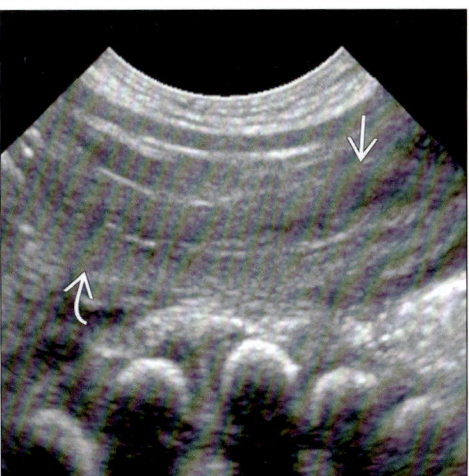

(Left) Sagittal transvaginal ultrasound shows a postmenopausal ovary (calipers). The ovary is small, ovoid in shape, relatively homogeneous and hypoechoic. (Right) Sagittal transabdominal ultrasound of a female newborn uterus shows that the anteroposterior diameter of the cervix ⇨ is greater than that of the uterine corpus ⇨.

Typical

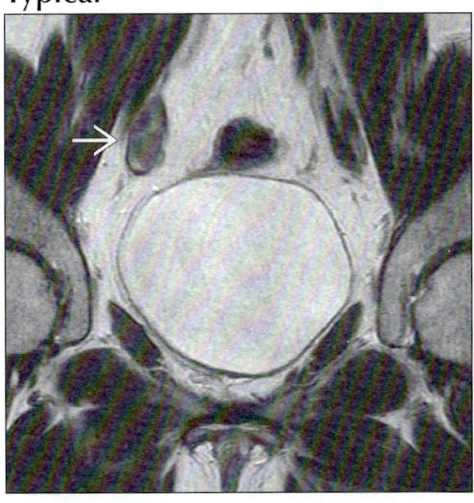 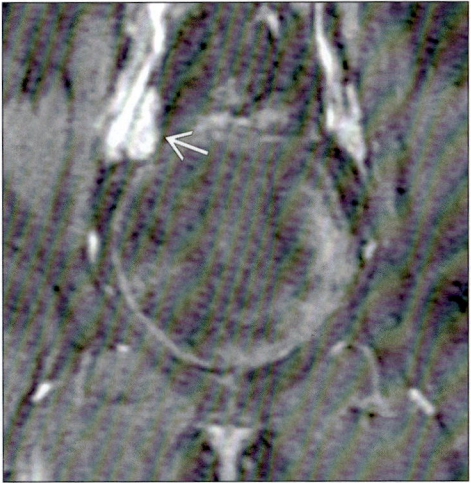

(Left) Coronal T2WI MR shows a normal low signal intensity postmenopausal right ovary ⇨. Note the absence of follicles and isointensity of the cortex and stroma. (Right) Axial T1 C+ FS MR in the same patient as previous image, shows normal homogeneous and intense enhancement of the right ovary ⇨. The enhancement is typically isointense to myometrium.

ENDOMETRIAL ATROPHY

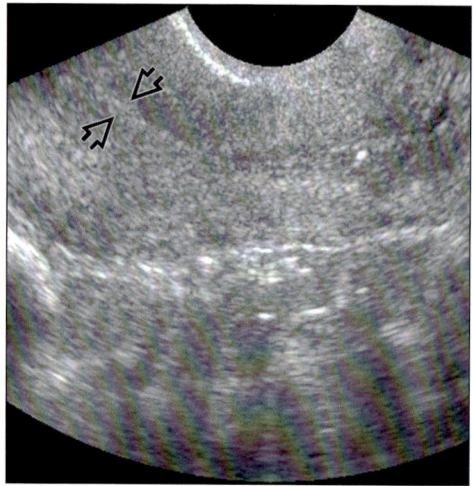

Sagittal transvaginal ultrasound shows a thin endometrial stripe less than 4 mm ➤ in this postmenopausal woman with endometrial atrophy.

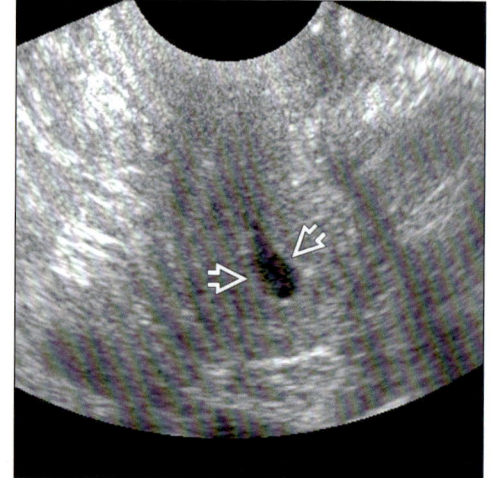

Sagittal transvaginal ultrasound sonohysterography in a woman with postmenopausal bleeding. The endometrial leaflets are thin ➤ without evidence of a focal mass.

TERMINOLOGY

Abbreviations and Synonyms
- Senile atrophy (when present in postmenopausal women)

Definitions
- Common response of endometrium to any condition that results in a hypoestrogenic state

IMAGING FINDINGS

General Features
- Best diagnostic clue: Thin endometrium (< 4 mm)
- Other features: May see cystically dilated endometrial glands in cases of cystic atrophy (e.g., patients on Tamoxifen therapy and/or longstanding hypoestrogenic state)
- Anatomy: Thinned endometrium without masses

Ultrasonographic Findings
- Transvaginal ultrasound (TVS)
  - Thin echogenic endometrium < 4 mm (double-layer thickness)
  - Endometrial thickness is determined by measuring anterior and posterior layers of endometrium in sagittal plane at level of maximum estimated thickness
  - May see "spurious" widening secondary to cystic atrophy with cysts "projecting" into endometrial cavity on TVS
  - Small uterus with corpus:cervix ratio approaching 1:1 (pre-pubescent)
  - When intrauterine fluid is present, measurement of endometrial thickness only includes endometrial leaflets and excludes intervening fluid
  - When endometrium cannot be seen, follow-up with sonohysterography or hysteroscopy is recommended
- Sonohysterography
  - Thinned endometrium
  - No focal endometrial mass
  - Single layer thickness equal to or less then 2 mm
  - May see cystically dilated glands below endometrial surface

DDx: Endometrial Atrophy

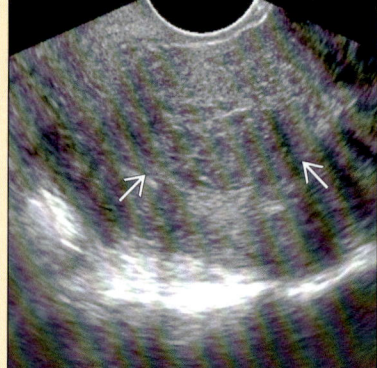

Obscuration by Leiomyoma

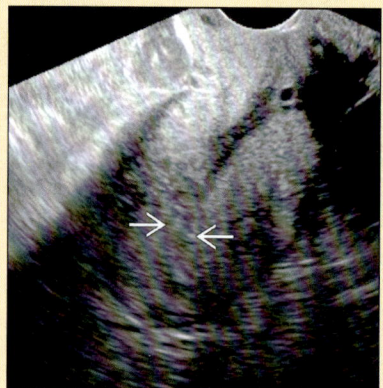

Cystic Polyp

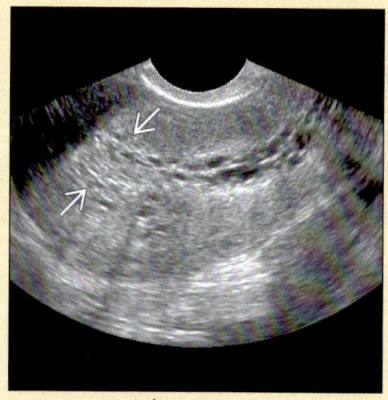

Adenomyosis

ENDOMETRIAL ATROPHY

Key Facts

Terminology
- Senile atrophy (when present in postmenopausal women)
- Common response of endometrium to any condition that results in a hypoestrogenic state

Imaging Findings
- Best diagnostic clue: Thin endometrium (< 4 mm)
- When intrauterine fluid is present, measurement of endometrial thickness only includes endometrial leaflets and excludes intervening fluid
- Transvaginal ultrasound should be initial modality for evaluation of endometrial cavity in symptomatic women
- If sonohysterography is not available or cannot be performed because of cervical stenosis, MR can be performed

Pathology
- Atrophy of endometrium proceeds progressively after menopause; in some cases this may take years
- Atrophy can also be result of any condition that induces a prolonged hypoestrogenic state
- Menopause (most common etiology)

Clinical Issues
- Typically normal finding in postmenopausal women
- Reported in clinical literature to be most common cause of postmenopausal bleeding

---

  - Even if endometrial atrophy is detected, other causes of bleeding may be present and only obvious with sonohysterography

MR Findings
- T1WI: Small uterus with a corpus:cervix ratio approaching 1:1
- T2WI
  - High signal intensity endometrium < 3 mm (not on hormone replacement therapy)
    - May see subendometrial cysts (especially women on tamoxifen)
    - Junctional zone may not be apparent
- MR C+: Variable, may see enhancement of thin endometrium; cystically dilated glands do not enhance

Imaging Recommendations
- Best imaging tool
  - TVS
  - Sonohysterography if inconclusive or non-diagnostic TVS
- Transvaginal ultrasound should be initial modality for evaluation of endometrial cavity in symptomatic women
- If inconclusive or non-diagnostic, sonohysterography should be performed
- If sonohysterography is not available or cannot be performed because of cervical stenosis, MR can be performed
- Biopsies of endometria thinner than 5 mm are nearly always negative or result in tissue insufficient for diagnosis
- Hysteroscopy & endometrial sampling is often performed in symptomatic women regardless of imaging findings, especially if endometrial thickness is > 5 mm

DIFFERENTIAL DIAGNOSIS

Endometrial Polyp (Cystic)
- Cystic mass within endometrial canal (versus cystically dilated glands in cystic atrophy)
- Sonohysterography confirms diagnosis

Obscured Endometrium
- Occurs in premenopausal women with leiomyomas
- Seen in the setting of adenomyosis
- Endometrial disease that causes endometrium to be isoechoic with myometrium

PATHOLOGY

General Features
- General path comments
  - Atrophy of endometrium proceeds progressively after menopause; in some cases this may take years
  - Atrophy can also be result of any condition that induces a prolonged hypoestrogenic state
- Etiology
  - Conditions that produce a prolonged hypoestrogenic state
    - Menopause (most common etiology)
    - Surgical or radiotherapeutic castration
    - Tamoxifen use
    - Prolonged oral contraception
    - Total ovarian functional insufficiency in certain disease states (e.g., Sheehan & Schmidt syndromes)

Gross Pathologic & Surgical Features
- Atrophic mucosa: Pale, thin and smooth
- Measures approximately 4 mm in thickness

Microscopic Features
- Atrophic mucosa: Scant glands of regular contour and small caliber
  - Glands are lined by a single layer of small cylindrical cells
  - Stroma is dense & composed of small round cells

ENDOMETRIAL ATROPHY

- Vascularization is poorly developed; arteriosclerotic lesions are present
- In the absence of estrogen after menopause, the functional layer is inactive and atrophies leaving only the shallow basalis layer
- Collapsed endometrial surfaces contain little or no fluid to prevent intracavitary friction, resulting in micro-erosion of the surface epithelium and subsequent chronic inflammatory reaction
- Cystic atrophy develops in longstanding hypoestrogenic states (usually postmenopausal women > 65 years)
  - Cysts form in response to obstruction of gland necks with subsequent dilation
  - Cystic spaces are lined by an atrophic endometrium with a small amount of fibrous stroma
  - Cystic spaces may be situated within endometrium or extend into endometrial-myometrial junction to form subendometrial cysts
  - Some elongated glands take an orientation parallel to mucosal surface
  - Cystic atrophy can be seen in patients on Tamoxifen therapy
  - Biopsy is insensitive in this population because tissue sample is often inadequate for diagnosis
- In extreme cases, there is endometrial stromal fibrosis & only surface epithelium and rare glands remain lined by low cuboidal cells; this can result in cervical stenosis
- Atrophy of endometrium exposes vessels in underlying myometrium

CLINICAL ISSUES

Presentation
- Most common signs/symptoms: Postmenopausal bleeding
- Most patients are asymptomatic
- Typically normal finding in postmenopausal women
- Reported in clinical literature to be most common cause of postmenopausal bleeding
- Postmenopausal bleeding is any vaginal bleeding in a postmenopausal woman not on hormone replacement therapy or unscheduled bleeding in a woman on hormone replacement therapy
- Endometrial atrophy bleeding is a function of
  - Myometrial arteriosclerosis and/or
  - Venous bleeding accompanying rupture of atrophic endometrial cysts

Natural History & Prognosis
- Atrophy is end result to prolonged hypoestrogenic state
- Good prognosis
- Risk of carcinoma when the endometrium is 4 mm or less in thickness is low
  - As little as 1 in 20 chance of cancer in a postmenopausal woman with bleeding

Treatment
- Endometrial visualization and/or sampling to rule out other potential causes of dysfunctional uterine bleeding
- Endometrial sampling is less successful in women with a thin endometrial stripe on ultrasound than in women with real endometrial pathologic condition
- Symptomatic relief with over-the-counter treatments
- Hormone replacement therapy

DIAGNOSTIC CHECKLIST

Image Interpretation Pearls
- Thin endometrium which may have cystically dilated glands

SELECTED REFERENCES

1. Litta P et al: Role of hysteroscopy with endometrial biopsy to rule out endometrial cancer in postmenopausal women with abnormal uterine bleeding. Maturitas. 50(2):117-23, 2005
2. Dubinsky TJ: Value of sonography in the diagnosis of abnormal vaginal bleeding. J Clin Ultrasound. 32(7):348-53, 2004
3. Smith-Bindman R et al: How thick is too thick? When endometrial thickness should prompt biopsy in postmenopausal women without vaginal bleeding. Ultrasound Obstet Gynecol. 24(5):558-65, 2004
4. Davidson KG et al: Ultrasonographic evaluation of the endometrium in postmenopausal vaginal bleeding. Radiol Clin North Am. 41(4):769-80, 2003
5. Ferenczy A: Pathophysiology of endometrial bleeding. Maturitas. 45(1):1-14, 2003
6. Gupta JK et al: Ultrasonographic endometrial thickness for diagnosing endometrial pathology in women with postmenopausal bleeding: a meta-analysis. Acta Obstet Gynecol Scand. 81(9):799-816, 2002
7. Kubik-Huch RA et al: Uterus and Cervix. In: Abdominal-Pelvic MRI. RC Semelka (ed). New York, Wiley-Liss; 1049-122, 2002
8. Alcazar JL et al: Transvaginal ultrasonographic measurement of endometrial thickness: an intra-observer and interobserver reproducibility study. Radiography. 7:101, 2001
9. Goldstein RB et al: Evaluation of the woman with postmenopausal bleeding: Society of Radiologists in Ultrasound-Sponsored Consensus Conference statement. J Ultrasound Med. 20(10):1025-36, 2001
10. Bree RL et al: US evaluation of the uterus in patients with postmenopausal bleeding: A positive effect on diagnostic decision making. Radiology. 216(1):260-4, 2000
11. Gull B et al: Transvaginal ultrasonography of the endometrium in women with postmenopausal bleeding: is it always necessary to perform an endometrial biopsy? Am J Obstet Gynecol. 182(3):509-15, 2000
12. Dubinsky TJ et al: The role of transvaginal sonography and endometrial biopsy in the evaluation of peri- and postmenopausal bleeding. AJR Am J Roentgenol. 169(1):145-9, 1997
13. Ferrazzi E et al: Sonographic endometrial thickness: a useful test to predict atrophy in patients with postmenopausal bleeding. An Italian multicenter study. Ultrasound Obstet Gynecol. 7(5):315-21, 1996
14. Karlsson B et al: Transvaginal ultrasonography of the endometrium in women with postmenopausal bleeding--a Nordic multicenter study. Am J Obstet Gynecol. 172(5):1488-94, 1995
15. Weigel M et al: Measuring the thickness--is that all we have to do for sonographic assessment of endometrium in postmenopausal women? Ultrasound Obstet Gynecol. 6(2):97-102, 1995

ENDOMETRIAL ATROPHY

IMAGE GALLERY

Typical

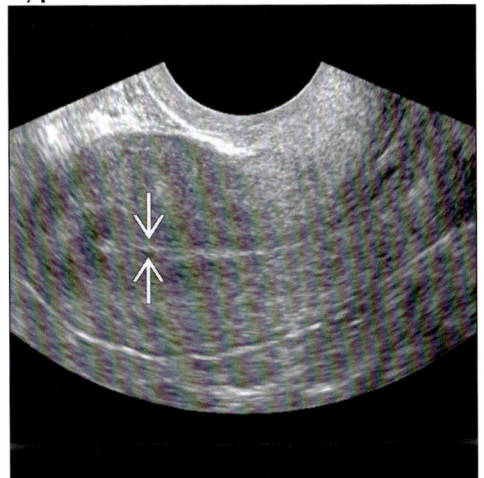
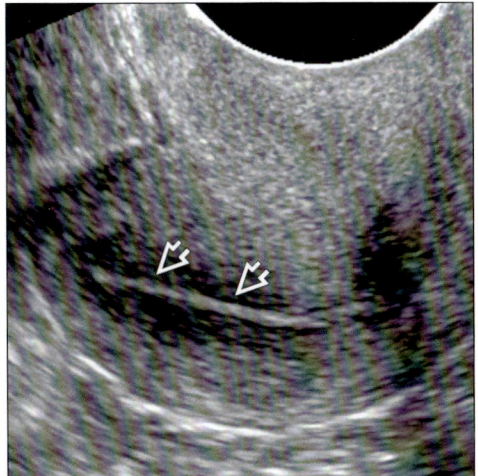

(Left) Sagittal transvaginal ultrasound shows a thin echogenic endometrium ➡ less than 4 mm in this postmenopausal woman. *(Right)* Sagittal transvaginal ultrasound shows a postmenopausal uterus with pencil-thin echogenic atrophic endometrium ➡.

Variant

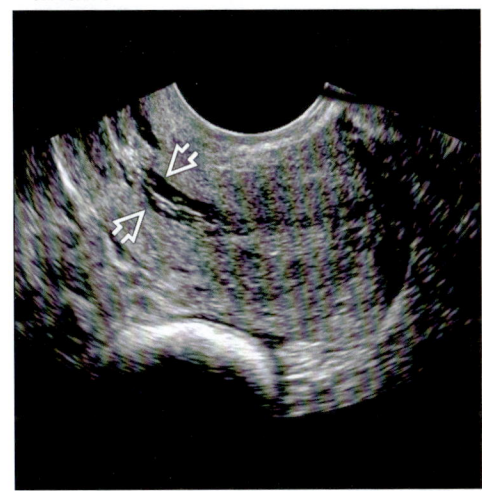
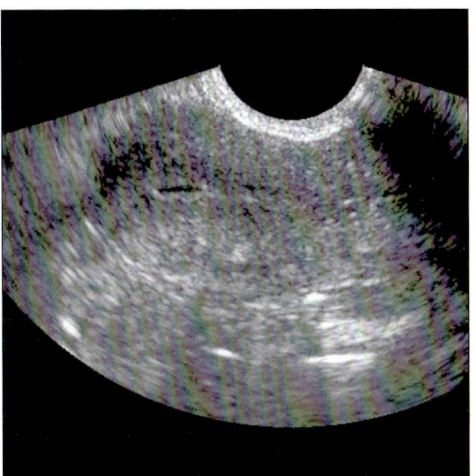

(Left) Sagittal transvaginal ultrasound shows retroverted uterus with thin endometrium and cystic changes in the lower uterine segment ➡. Compatible with cystic atrophy in this patient receiving Tamoxifen therapy. *(Right)* Sagittal transvaginal ultrasound shows endometrial thickness of 1.4 mm compatible with atrophy. Note that the measurement does not include the fluid in the canal.

Typical

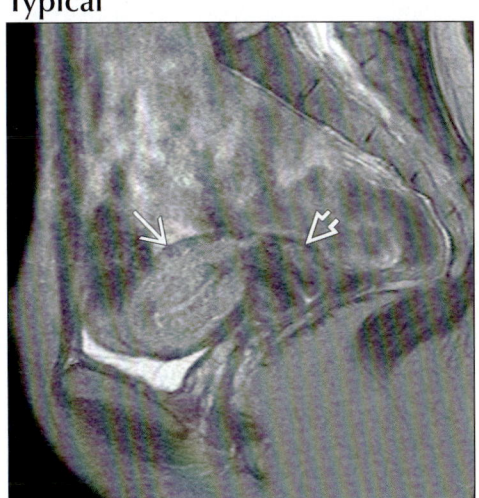
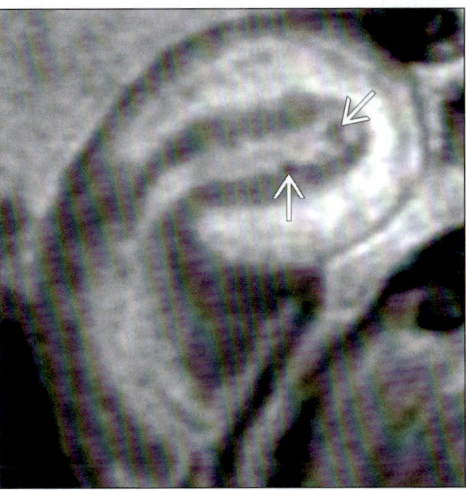

(Left) Sagittal T1WI FS MR shows postmenopausal uterus (corpus ➡ to cervix ➡ ratio approaches 1:1) with a thin endometrium. *(Right)* Sagittal T1 C+ MR shows small signal void foci ➡ in the endometrium in a patient with cystic atrophy on Tamoxifen therapy.

UTERINE PERISTALSIS

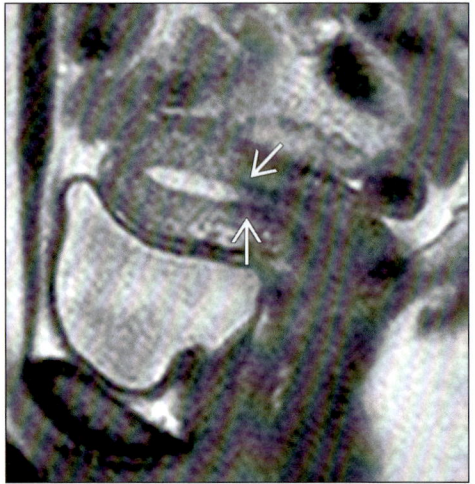

Sagittal T2WI MR SS FSE shows early changes of cervico-fundal uterine peristalsis with thickening of the inner myometrium at the lower uterine segment ➔.

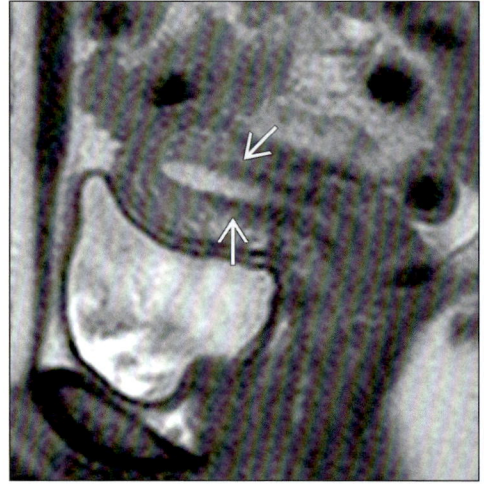

Sagittal T2WI MR SS FSE in the same patient as previous image, shows propagation of cervico-fundal uterine peristalsis approaching the mid fundus ➔.

TERMINOLOGY

Abbreviations and Synonyms
- Uterine kinematics

Definitions
- Spontaneous subtle rhythmic contractions of uterus
  - Frequency of conduction: 2-3 times/minute
  - Pattern changes with phase of menstrual cycle

IMAGING FINDINGS

General Features
- Best diagnostic clue
  - Cine MR to identify conduction of low signal intensity (SI) wave
    - Rhythmic contractions with change in configuration & SI of inner myometrium or low SI endometrial stripping movement
    - May distort the endometrium
    - Cine T2 single shot fast spin echo (SS FSE): Best imaging sequence to identify peristalsis
- Location
  - Inner myometrium (subendometrium) and/or endometrium
  - May distort endometrium
- Size: Variable amplitude and frequency
- Morphology: Variable
- May involve all layers, subendometrial layer of myometrium or endometrium
- At real time: Contractions progress antegrade or retrograde depending on phase of menstrual cycle
- Morphology varies: Focal, diffuse, round, or oval

Ultrasonographic Findings
- Transvaginal ultrasound (TVS) findings: Usually interpreted in conjunction with intracavitary pressure transducer
  - Three distinct phases
  - Luteofollicular (menses)
    - Antegrade from fundus to cervix: Discharge of menstrual blood
    - All layers involved but may not be observed even at real time
    - High amplitude contractions
  - Late follicular (peri-ovulatory)

DDx: Uterine Peristalsis

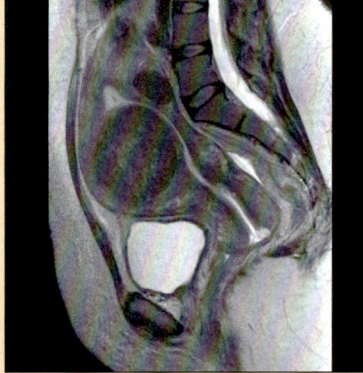
Submucosal/Intramural Leiomyoma

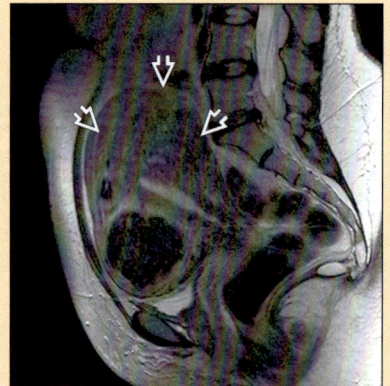
Adenomyosis

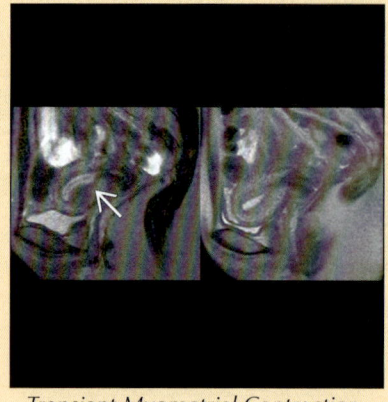
Transient Myometrial Contraction

UTERINE PERISTALSIS

Key Facts

Terminology
- Uterine kinematics
- Spontaneous subtle rhythmic contractions of uterus
- Pattern changes with phase of menstrual cycle

Imaging Findings
- Cine T2 single shot fast spin echo (SS FSE): Best imaging sequence to identify peristalsis
- Cine: Low SI wave-like changes in the inner myometrium and/or endometrial stripping wave
- Pattern changes with menstrual cycle: Three patterns
- **Luteofollicular (menses)**
- Antegrade: Fundus to cervix
- **Late follicular (periovulatory)**
- Retrograde: Cervix to fundus
- **Luteal phase**
- Quiescent
- Transvaginal ultrasound (TVS) findings: Usually interpreted in conjunction with intracavitary pressure transducer
- Best imaging tool: Cine MR

Top Differential Diagnoses
- Submucosal Leiomyoma
- Adenomyosis/Adenomyoma
- Myometrial Contraction

Clinical Issues
- Majority of patients asymptomatic

Diagnostic Checklist
- Must view images in cine mode at real time or greater than real time
- Static image interpretation may lead to pseudolesions

- Retrograde from cervix to fundus: Transport sperm to fallopian tube
- Subendometrial layer
- Highest frequency of contractions in cycle
  ○ Luteal phase
    ■ Quiescent: Promote implantation

MR Findings
- T2WI
  ○ Cine: Low SI wave-like changes in the inner myometrium and/or endometrial stripping wave
    ■ Low SI may relate to regional decrease in vascularity
    ■ Static images may lead to pseudolesion due to summation of contractions
  ○ Pattern changes with menstrual cycle: Three patterns
  ○ Luteofollicular (menses)
    ■ Antegrade: Fundus to cervix
    ■ Discharge of menstrual blood
  ○ Late follicular (periovulatory)
    ■ Retrograde: Cervix to fundus
    ■ Sperm transport
    ■ Peak frequency during this phase
  ○ Luteal phase
    ■ Quiescent
    ■ Promote implantation

Imaging Recommendations
- Best imaging tool: Cine MR
- Protocol advice
  ○ May need to view cine MR faster than real-time (12x) to facilitate movement evaluation
  ○ Must correlate imaging findings with phase of menstrual cycle
  ○ Scan during periovulatory phase to see highest frequency of contractions

DIFFERENTIAL DIAGNOSIS

Submucosal Leiomyoma
- Permanent
- Homogeneous, round and protrude into endometrial canal
- Low SI on T2WI if not degenerated

Adenomyosis/Adenomyoma
- Permanent
- Diffuse or focal widening of junctional zone that usually does not have marked mass effect
- Ill-defined mass in myometrium
- May have ancillary findings (punctate high SI foci on T1WI and/or T2WI)

Myometrial Contraction
- Transient myometrial contraction in non-gravid uterus
- Classic: Distort endometrial complex but do not deform outer uterine contour
- Usually resolves in 45 minutes

PATHOLOGY

General Features
- General path comments
  ○ Inherent uterine contractility
    ■ Identifiable pattern of myometrial/endometrial contractility throughout cycle
    ■ Reproducible patterns from cycle to cycle
- Etiology
  ○ Unknown but may be a function of hormone levels
    ■ Stimulatory effect of estrogen at midcycle
    ■ Inhibitory effect of estrogen plus progesterone at luteal phase

Staging, Grading or Classification Criteria
- No formal MR grading system but several characteristics described
  ○ Frequency of stripping wave
  ○ Direction of stripping wave
  ○ Amplitude of low SI myometrial changes

UTERINE PERISTALSIS

CLINICAL ISSUES

Presentation
- Most common signs/symptoms
  - Majority of patients asymptomatic
  - Symptomatic patients: Dysmenorrhea and/or infertility may be linked to
    - Abnormal or dyskinetic peristalsis
    - Increased transient thickness of inner myometrium
    - Increased endometrial distortion

Natural History & Prognosis
- Reproducibility of patterns from cycle to cycle
- Dyskinesis and/or other abnormalities of uterine contractions may affect fertility and be a factor in dysmenorrhea

DIAGNOSTIC CHECKLIST

Consider
- Uterine peristalsis if transient changes of submucosal leiomyoma and/or adenomyosis/adenomyoma

Image Interpretation Pearls
- Must view images in cine mode at real time or greater than real time
- Static image interpretation may lead to pseudolesions

SELECTED REFERENCES

1. Orisaka M et al: A comparison of uterine peristalsis in women with normal uteri and uterine leiomyoma by cine magnetic resonance imaging. Eur J Obstet Gynecol Reprod Biol. 2007
2. Togashi K: Uterine contractility evaluated on cine Magnetic Resonance Imaging. Ann N Y Acad Sci. 2007
3. Kido A et al: Cine MR imaging of uterine peristalsis in patients with endometriosis. Eur Radiol. 2006
4. Kido A et al: Investigation of uterine peristalsis diurnal variation. Magn Reson Imaging. 24(9):1149-55, 2006
5. Kunz G et al: Control and function of uterine peristalsis during the human luteal phase. Reprod Biomed Online. 13(4):528-40, 2006
6. Mueller A et al: Role of estrogen and progesterone in the regulation of uterine peristalsis: results from perfused non-pregnant swine uteri. Hum Reprod. 21(7):1863-8, 2006
7. Mueller A et al: Uterine contractility in response to different prostaglandins: results from extracorporeally perfused non-pregnant swine uteri. Hum Reprod. 21(8):2000-5, 2006
8. Ogura T et al: Magnetic resonance imaging of morphological and functional changes of the uterus induced by sacral surface electrical stimulation. Tohoku J Exp Med. 208(1):65-73, 2006
9. Kataoka M et al: Dysmenorrhea: evaluation with cine-mode-display MR imaging--initial experience. Radiology. 235(1):124-31, 2005
10. Kido A et al: A semiautomated technique for evaluation of uterine peristalsis. J Magn Reson Imaging. 21(3):249-57, 2005
11. Kido A et al: Oral contraceptives and uterine peristalsis: evaluation with MRI. J Magn Reson Imaging. 22(2):265-70, 2005
12. Nishino M et al: Uterine contractions evaluated on cine MR imaging in patients with uterine leiomyomas. Eur J Radiol. 53(1):142-6, 2005
13. Fujiwara T et al: Kinematics of the uterus: cine mode MR imaging. Radiographics. 24(1):e19, 2004
14. Kissler S et al: Uterine contractility and directed sperm transport assessed by hysterosalpingoscintigraphy (HSSG) and intrauterine pressure (IUP) measurement. Acta Obstet Gynecol Scand. 83(4):369-74, 2004
15. Nakai A et al: Uterine peristalsis: comparison of transvaginal ultrasound and two different sequences of cine MR imaging. J Magn Reson Imaging. 20(3):463-9, 2004
16. Nakai A et al: Uterine peristalsis shown on cine MR imaging using ultrafast sequence. J Magn Reson Imaging. 18(6):726-33, 2003
17. Eytan O et al: Characteristics of uterine peristalsis in spontaneous and induced cycles. Fertil Steril. 76(2):337-41, 2001
18. Kunz G et al: Sonographic evidence for the involvement of the utero-ovarian counter-current system in the ovarian control of directed uterine sperm transport. Hum Reprod Update. 4(5):667-72, 1998
19. Kunz G et al: Uterine peristalsis during the follicular phase of the menstrual cycle: effects of oestrogen, antioestrogen and oxytocin. Hum Reprod Update. 4(5):647-54, 1998
20. Kunz G et al: The uterine peristaltic pump. Normal and impeded sperm transport within the female genital tract. Adv Exp Med Biol. 424:267-77, 1997
21. Kunz G et al: The dynamics of rapid sperm transport through the female genital tract: evidence from vaginal sonography of uterine peristalsis and hysterosalpingoscintigraphy. Hum Reprod. 11(3):627-32, 1996
22. Togashi K et al: Sustained uterine contractions: a cause of hypointense myometrial bulging. Radiology. 187(3):707-10, 1993
23. Togashi K et al: Uterine contractions: possible diagnostic pitfall at MR imaging. J Magn Reson Imaging. 3(6):889-93, 1993
24. Lyons EA et al: Characterization of subendometrial myometrial contractions throughout the menstrual cycle in normal fertile women. Fertil Steril. 55(4):771-4, 1991

UTERINE PERISTALSIS

IMAGE GALLERY

Typical

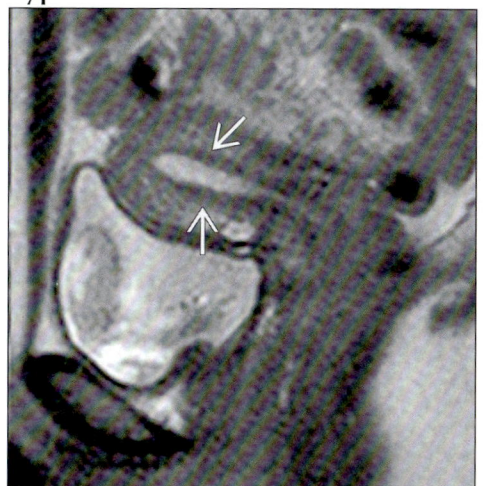 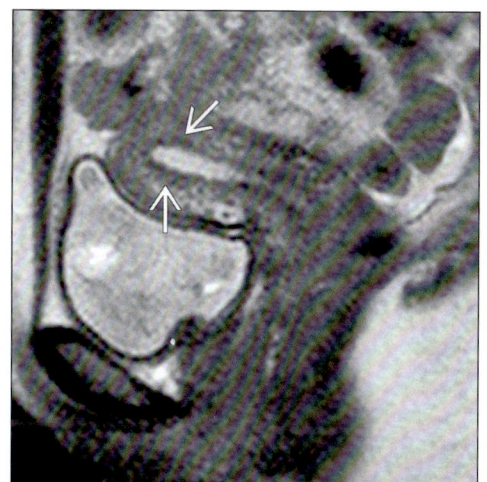

(Left) Sagittal T2WI MR SS FSE in the same patient as previous image, shows propagation of cervico-fundal uterine peristalsis with progressive thickening of the inner myometrium of the mid fundus ➡. *(Right)* Sagittal T2WI MR SS FSE in the same patient as previous image, shows propagation of the cervico-fundal uterine peristalsis with progressive thickening of the inner myometrium approaching the fundus ➡.

Typical

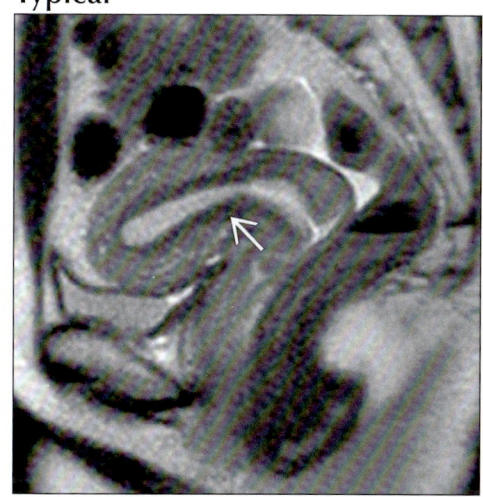 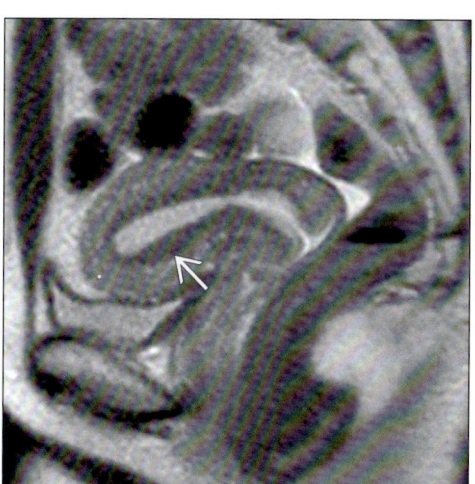

(Left) Sagittal T2WI MR SS FSE shows early change of cervico-fundal uterine peristalsis with thickening of the subendometrial myometrium in the lower uterine segment ➡. *(Right)* Sagittal T2WI MR SS FSE in the same patient as previous image, shows propagation of cervico-fundal uterine peristalsis at the mid fundus ➡.

Typical

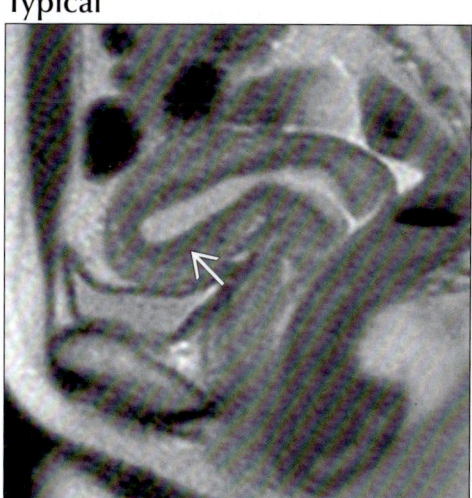 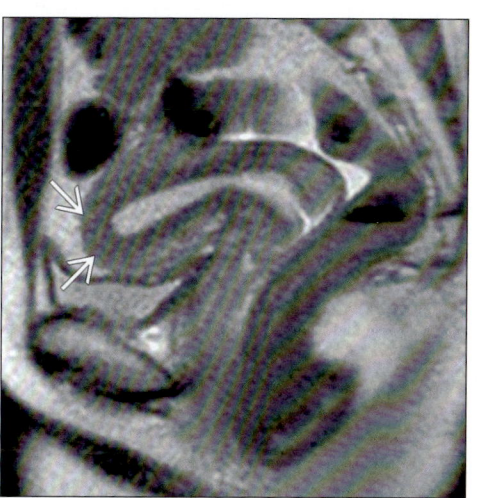

(Left) Sagittal T2WI MR SS FSE in the same patient as previous image, shows propagation of cervico-fundal uterine peristalsis approaching the fundus ➡. *(Right)* Sagittal T2WI MR SS FSE in the same patient as previous image, shows propagation of cervico-fundal uterine peristalsis at the fundus ➡.

NORMAL POST C-SECTION CHANGE

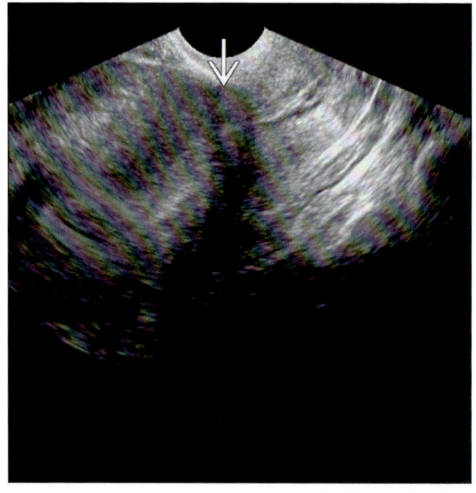

Sagittal ultrasound shows focal thinning of the myometrium in the anterior lower uterine segment above the internal os ➡ from C-section scar.

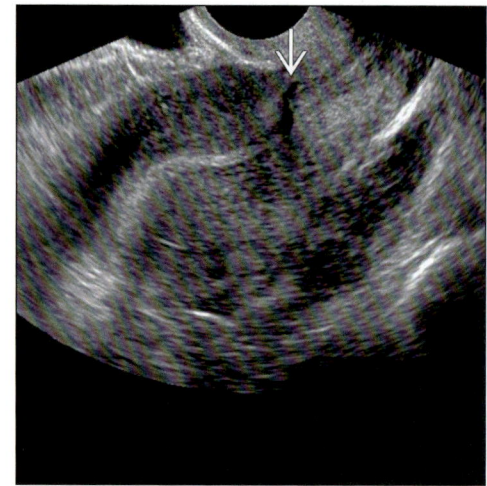

Sagittal ultrasound shows fluid ➡ tracking within the thinned anterior lower uterine segment myometrium above the internal os at site of the C-section scar.

TERMINOLOGY

Abbreviations and Synonyms
- C-section scar, niche, filling defect, pouch, hiatus, diverticula

Definitions
- Focal thinning of the myometrium in the anterior lower uterine segment above the internal os at site of prior cesarian delivery (low-transverse incision)
  - Triangular "defect" underlies scar
  - May have fluid within the triangular "defect"

IMAGING FINDINGS

General Features
- Best diagnostic clue
  - Focal thinning of anterior myometrium in the lower uterine segment above the internal os
    - May or may not have fluid within triangular "defect" resulting from myometrial thinning
- Location: Anterior lower uterine segment above the internal os at site of the previous cesarian section
- Size
  - Mean lower uterine segment myometrial thickness at the level of the scar is: 1.9 ± 1.4 mm
    - Versus nulliparous control: 2.3 ± 1.1 mm and multiparous control: 3.4 ± 2.2 mm
  - Mean depth of triangular "defect": 6.17 ± 3.6 mm
    - Range: 2.5-11.5 mm
- Morphology
  - Focal thinning of the anterior myometrium at lower uterine segment above the internal os
  - Triangular "defect" underlies scar

Ultrasonographic Findings
- Grayscale Ultrasound
  - Focal thinning of the myometrium in the lower uterine segment above the internal os
    - Anechoic fluid may reside within triangular "defect" formed by focal myometrial thinning
  - Sonohysterography: Triangular "defect" fills with saline at level cesarean section scar

CT Findings
- Only on sagittal reformatted images will CT show defect
- CT soft tissue contrast is not as good as MR

DDx: Mimics of Scar

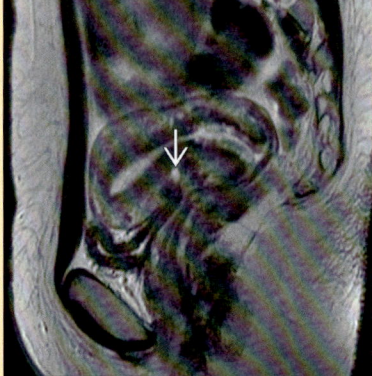

Myometrial Cyst

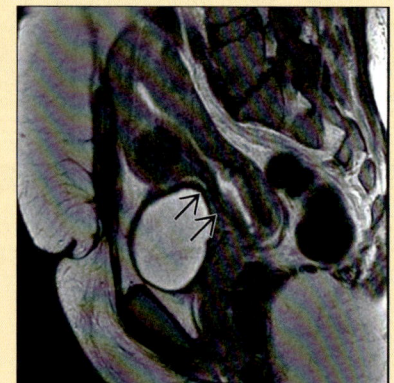

Post Myomectomy

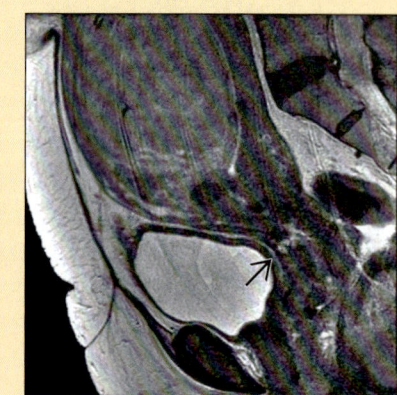

Myomectomy Scar

NORMAL POST C-SECTION CHANGE

Key Facts

Terminology
- C-section scar, niche, filling defect, pouch, hiatus, diverticula
- Focal thinning of the myometrium in the anterior lower uterine segment above the internal os at site of prior cesarian delivery (low-transverse incision)
- Triangular "defect" underlies scar

Imaging Findings
- Mean lower uterine segment myometrial thickness at the level of the scar is: 1.9 ± 1.4 mm
- Mean depth of triangular "defect": 6.17 ± 3.6 mm
- Anechoic fluid may reside within triangular "defect" formed by focal myometrial thinning
- Sonohysterography: Triangular "defect" fills with saline at level cesarean section scar
- TVS & sonohysterography are best imaging tools

Top Differential Diagnoses
- Myomectomy Scar
- Marked Uterine Anteflexion
- Myometrial Cyst

Pathology
- Epidemiology: No correlation between the number of cesarean section deliveries and mean size of the scar or residual thickness of myometrium

Clinical Issues
- More than 3 prior cesarean sections results in much greater risk of uterine rupture during labor
- Other signs/symptoms: Cesarian scar pregnancies may progress to term unlike cervical ectopic pregnancies
- Abnormal implantation in scar

MR Findings
- T1WI: Isointense to myometrium
- T2WI
  - Low signal intensity (SI) focal thinning of myometrium in the anterior lower uterine segment above the internal os
    - Focally disrupts normal uterine zonal anatomy
  - May see triangular high SI "defect" underlying scar
    - Fluid and/or retracted endometrium

Imaging Recommendations
- Best imaging tool
  - TVS & sonohysterography are best imaging tools
    - Safe
    - Inexpensive
    - Widely available
    - Saline infusion sonohysterography: "Defect" will fill with fluid subjcent to focal myometrial scar/thinning
- Protocol advice
  - Search entire lower uterine segment on US or on MR
    - Need to image in both sagittal and axial planes

DIFFERENTIAL DIAGNOSIS

Myomectomy Scar
- History and location of finding aid diagnosis
- Usually less focal
- Typically no associated triangular "defect"

Marked Uterine Anteflexion
- True long axis images aid diagnosis
- Search for the true sagittal plane
- Endocervical and endometrial canal should be visible on a single image
- Assess the myometrial thickness and integrity on the sagittal scan

Myometrial Cyst
- No associated myometrial thinning

PATHOLOGY

General Features
- Etiology: Status post cesarean section with low transverse incision
- Epidemiology: No correlation between the number of cesarean section deliveries and mean size of the scar or residual thickness of myometrium
- Associated abnormalities
  - Uterine dehiscence
  - Abnormal placentation in future pregnancies
    - Acreta
    - Increta
    - Percreta

Gross Pathologic & Surgical Features
- 3 types of cesarean section scars are described in resected uteri
  - 1) Thick muscle layer with shallow groove
  - 2) Lack of muscle layer replaced by connective tissue
  - 3) Lack of muscle layer

Microscopic Features
- Scarring
- Retraction
- Growth of fibrous tissue
- Suture material
- Occasional congested endometrium above scar recess

CLINICAL ISSUES

Presentation
- Most common signs/symptoms
  - Most are asymptomatic but some patients have abnormal uterine bleeding
  - Rates of primary and repeat cesarean deliveries have increased since 1996, having previously declined in 1980s
  - Advantages of cesarean section include lower frequency of the following conditions
    - Postpartum hemorrhage
    - Perineal laceration

NORMAL POST C-SECTION CHANGE

- Urinary incontinence
- Obstetrical trauma
- Neonatal intracranial hemorrhage
- Neonatal asphyxia/encephalopathy
- Brachial plexus birth injury
- Neonatal infections
○ Disadvantage of cesarian section
  - General anesthesia and higher risk of subsequent placental previa
○ Compared with vaginal delivery, cesarian delivery is associated with
  - Greater length of stay
  - More general anesthesia
  - Higher risk of subsequent placenta previa
  - Greater risk of uterine rupture during vaginal birth after cesarean section
  - Respiratory morbidity in newborn infants
○ More than one prior cesarian section with low transverse incision results in slightly increased risk of uterine rupture during labor
○ More than 3 prior cesarian sections results in much greater risk of uterine rupture during labor
- Other signs/symptoms: Cesarian scar pregnancies may progress to term unlike cervical ectopic pregnancies

Demographics
- Age
  ○ Women of child bearing age and older
  ○ In 2004, 1.2 million or 29.1% of live births in United States were by cesarian section

Natural History & Prognosis
- Most patients are asymptomatic
- Complications include
  ○ Uterine rupture or dehiscence
  ○ Adherent placenta (acreta, increta or percreta)
  ○ Abnormal implantation in scar
  ○ Abnormal uterine bleeding

Treatment
- Surgery for patients with intractable bleeding and with possible interference with embryo implantation from blood in defect
  ○ Hysteroscopic guidance to resect fibrotic tissue that overhangs scar to reduce blood pooling and improve menstrual drainage

DIAGNOSTIC CHECKLIST

Image Interpretation Pearls
- Myometrial thinning in the anterior lower uterine segment above the internal os
- Triangular fluid-filled area in the "defect" caused by myometrial thinning

SELECTED REFERENCES

1. NIH State-of-the-Science Conference: Cesarean Delivery on Maternal Request, http://consensus.nih.gov/2006/2006CesareanSOS027html.htm March 27-29, 2006, accessed April 4, 2006
2. Ben Nagi J et al: First-trimester cesarean scar pregnancy evolving into placenta previa/accreta at term. J Ultrasound Med. 24(11):1569-73, 2005
3. Shukunami K et al: Sonographic appearance of previous cesarian scars in pregnant women as 3 macroscopic types. J Ultrasound Med. 24(3):394-5, 2005
4. Cheung VY et al: Sonographic evaluation of the lower uterine segment in patients with previous cesarean delivery. J Ultrasound Med. 23(11):1441-7, 2004
5. Fabres C et al: The cesarean delivery scar pouch: clinical implications and diagnostic correlation between transvaginal sonography and hysteroscopy. J Ultrasound Med. 22(7):695-700; quiz 701-2, 2003
6. Nagayama M et al: Fast MR imaging in obstetrics. Radiographics. 22(3):563-80; discussion 580-2, 2002
7. Lydon-Rochelle M et al: Risk of uterine rupture during labor among women with a prior cesarean delivery. N Engl J Med. 345:3-8, 2001
8. Monteagudo A et al: Saline infusion sonohysterography in nonpregnant women with previous cesarean delivery: the "niche" in the scar. J Ultrasound Med. 20(10):1105-15, 2001
9. Gotoh H et al: Prediction incomplete uterine rupture with vaginal sonography during the late second trimester in women with prior cesarean. Obstet Gynecol. 95:596-600, 2000
10. Suzuki S et al: Preoperative diagnosis of dehiscence of the lower uterine segment in patients with a single previous Cesarean section. Aust NZ J Obstet Gyencol. 40:402-404, 2000
11. Erikson SS et al: Intermenstrual bleeding secondary to cesarean scar diverticuli: Report of three cases. Obstet Gynecol. 93:802-805, 1999
12. Thurmond AS et al: Cesarean section scar as a cause of abnormal vaginal bleeding: Diagnosis by sonohysterography. J Ultrasound Med. 18:13-16, 1999
13. Maldjian C et al: MR appearance of uterine dehiscence in the post-cesarean section patient. J Comput Assist Tomogr. 22(5):738-41, 1998
14. Fernandez E et al: Hysteroscopic correction of cesarean section scars in women with abnormal bleeding. J Am Assoc Gynecol Laparosc. 3(suppl):S13, 1996
15. Rozenberg P et al: Ultrasonographic measurement of lower uterine segment to assess risk of defects of scarred uterus. Lancet. 347:281-284, 1996
16. Lonky NM et al: Prediction of cesarean section scars with ultrasound imaging during pregnancy. J. Ultrasound Med. 8:15-19, 1989
17. Michaels WH et al: Ultrasound diagnosis of defects in the scarred lower uterine segment during pregnancy. Obstet Gynecol. 243: 221-224, 1988

NORMAL POST C-SECTION CHANGE

IMAGE GALLERY

Typical

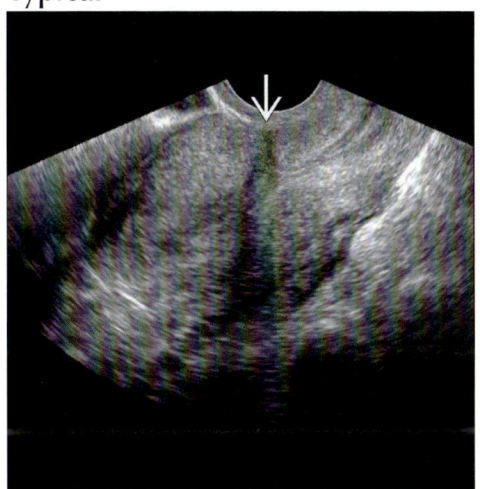
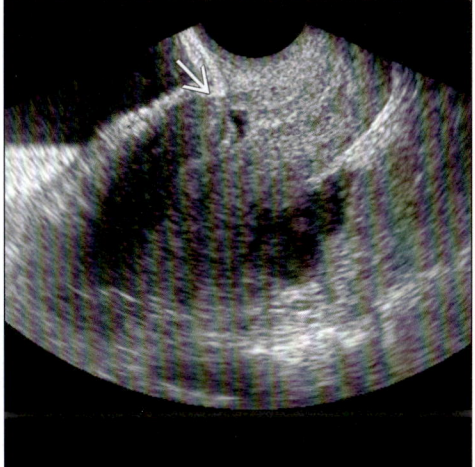

(Left) Sagittal T2WI MR shows an area of myometrial thinning and scarring ➡ at anterior lower uterine segment at the cesarian section site. *(Right)* Sagittal ultrasound shows triangular fluid-filled "defect" ➡ at location of myometrial thinning and scarring from prior C-section.

Typical

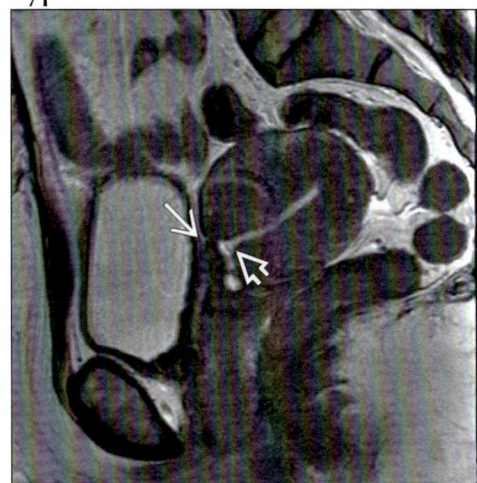
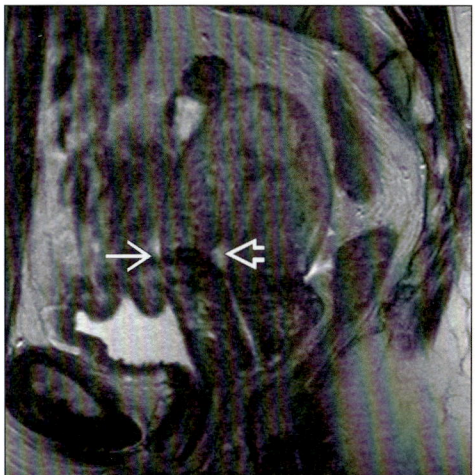

(Left) Sagittal T2WI MR shows marked thinning of myometrium at C-section scar ➡ and associated triangular fluid-filled "defect" and/or retracted endometrium ➡. *(Right)* Sagittal T2WI MR shows typical scar ➡ and retracted endometrium and/or triangular fluid collection ➡ underlying the myometrial thinning.

Typical

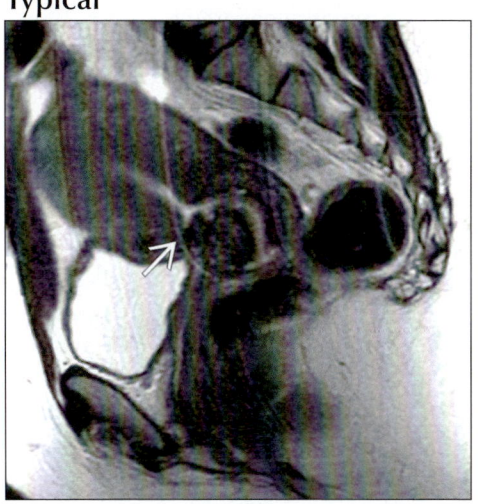
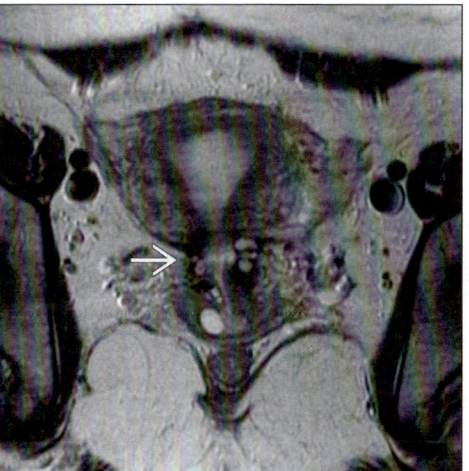

(Left) Sagittal T2WI MR shows typical scar ➡ with fluid and/or retracted endometrium at the site of prior cesarian section. *(Right)* Coronal oblique T2WI MR shows Nabothian cysts and thinning of myometrium ➡ associated with cesarian section.

UTERINE HYPOPLASIA/AGENESIS

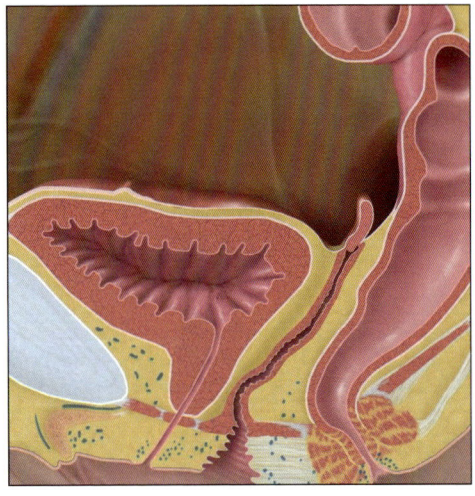

Graphic of uterine hypoplasia shows a small uterine remnant. The upper 2/3 of the vagina is hypoplastic.

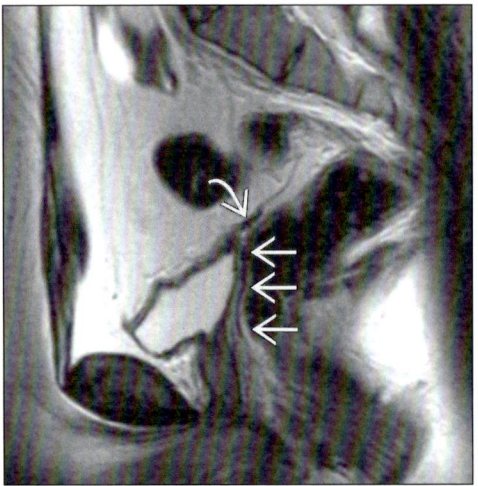

Sagittal T2WI MR shows a small soft tissue uterine remnant ➔ in the expected location of the uterus. The upper 2/3 of the vagina ➔ is hypoplastic and atretic without normal zonal anatomy.

TERMINOLOGY

Definitions
- Class I Müllerian duct anomaly (MDA)
  - Based on Buttram & Gibbons/American Fertility Society (AFS) classification system
- Absence or hypoplasia of uterus ± vagina and fallopian tube due to variable failure of Müllerian ducts to develop prior to fusion

IMAGING FINDINGS

General Features
- Best diagnostic clue
  - Uterine hypoplasia: Small hypoplastic uterine soft tissue remnant
  - Uterine agenesis: Connective tissue (fibrous remnant) and veins in expected location of uterus
  - Upper 2/3 of vagina: Absent or atretic in both uterine hypoplasia and agenesis
  - Normal ovaries in majority of patients
- Morphology
  - Uterine hypoplasia
    - Decreased intercornual distance (normal range: 2-4 cm)
    - May have a bicornuate or unicornuate configuration
    - Rarely a contracted endometrial cavity is present resulting in hematometra at menarche
  - Mayer-Rokitansky-Küster-Hauser (MRKH) syndrome: Most common class I Müllerian anomaly
    - Type 1: Vaginal agenesis with associated uterine agenesis in 90% of cases
      - Fallopian tubes usually normal
    - Type 2: Vaginal agenesis with associated uterine hypoplasia in 10% of cases
      - Typically two separate uterine horns
      - Hypoplastic uterine horns can be symmetric or asymmetric; rarely associated with functioning endometrial tissue
      - ± Hypoplasia or aplasia of one or both fallopian tubes
    - Ovaries normal in majority of patients
      - Often situated more cranially in lower quadrants of abdomen

DDx: Absent Uterus

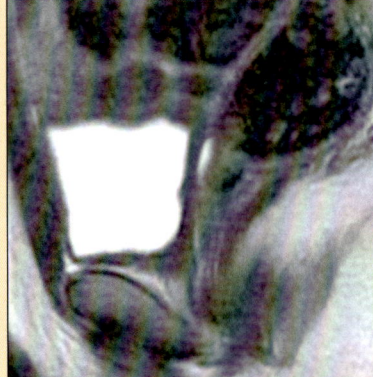

Male Pseudohermaphrodite

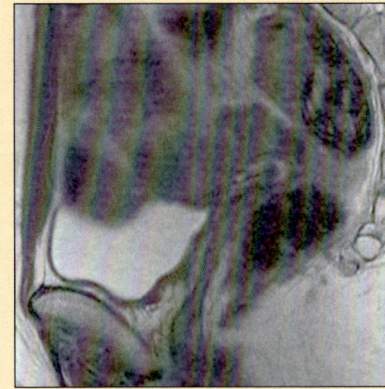

Androgen Insensitivity Syndrome

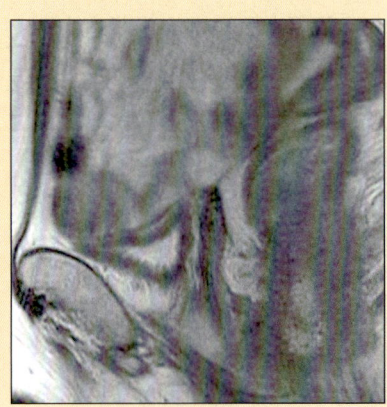

Total Hysterectomy

UTERINE HYPOPLASIA/AGENESIS

Key Facts

Terminology
- Class I Müllerian duct anomaly (MDA)
- Absence or hypoplasia of uterus ± vagina and fallopian tube due to variable failure of Müllerian ducts to develop prior to fusion

Imaging Findings
- Uterine hypoplasia: Small hypoplastic uterine soft tissue remnant
- Uterine agenesis: Connective tissue (fibrous remnant) and veins in expected location of uterus
- Upper 2/3 of vagina: Absent or atretic in both uterine hypoplasia and agenesis
- Normal ovaries in majority of patients

Top Differential Diagnoses
- Gonadal Dysgenesis
- Androgen Insensitivity Syndrome
- Pseudohermaphrodite (Male)
- DES-Exposure

Pathology
- 46 XX female karyotype
- Increased incidence of renal anomalies (40-50%)

Clinical Issues
- Little or no reproductive potential
- In patients with associated vaginal agenesis; vaginal dilatation or reconstruction performed to allow normal sexual functioning

Diagnostic Checklist
- Uterine hypoplasia/agenesis as a cause of primary amenorrhea in a young woman with normal secondary sexual characteristics

Radiographic Findings
- Hysterosalpingography (HSG)
  - No role in the evaluation of uterine hypoplasia or agenesis

Ultrasonographic Findings
- Grayscale Ultrasound
  - Uterine agenesis: No identifiable uterus at anticipated level of vaginal apex
  - Uterine hypoplasia: Small uterus typically without echogenic endometrial complex
    - Endometrial complex rarely present, results in distension of endometrial cavity with low level echoes at menarche
  - Vaginal agenesis: Echogenic connective tissue in the expected location of vagina between urethra and rectum
  - Vaginal hypoplasia/atresia: Thin hypoechoic band in expected location of vagina without normal zonal anatomy

CT Findings
- No role in the evaluation of uterine hypoplasia or agenesis

MR Findings
- T1WI FS: Hematometra presents as high signal intensity (SI) fluid within endometrial cavity
- T2WI
  - Uterine agenesis: No identifiable uterus at anticipated level of vaginal apex
    - Important not to mistake connective tissue/veins around a tiny fibrous remnant as uterus
  - Uterine hypoplasia
    - Abnormal low SI myometrium with poorly delineated zonal anatomy
    - Endometrial cavity (if present) and myometrium reduced in size
    - May have a unicornuate or bicornuate configuration
  - Vaginal agenesis: Only veins and connective tissue demonstrated in expected location of vagina
  - Vaginal hypoplasia/atresia: Low SI band in expected location of vagina without normal zonal anatomy

Imaging Recommendations
- Best imaging tool
  - Ultrasound (US) and MR provide complementary information
  - MR modality of choice for complete mapping of anatomy
- Protocol advice
  - Transabdominal US used to screen for associated renal tract abnormalities and to locate ovaries
    - Provides limited information regarding uterine agenesis/hypoplasia
  - Vaginal agenesis with US best assessed using a transrectal/transperineal approach
  - MR: Phased array body coil
  - Single shot fast spin echo (SS FSE) T2 coronal image through the abdomen and pelvis to assess kidneys
  - High resolution FSE T2WI, ≤ 4 mm slice thickness
    - Hypoplastic uterus best visualized on sagittal imaging with mildly distended urinary bladder
    - Vaginal agenesis best visualized on axial images
  - Axial T1WI ± FS to confirm hematometra

DIFFERENTIAL DIAGNOSIS

Gonadal Dysgenesis
- Hypoplastic uterus with atrophic vagina
- Streak gonads

Androgen Insensitivity Syndrome
- Androgen insensitivity
- Absent uterus, upper 2/3 vagina, ovaries
- Testes (usually undescended)
- Male karyotype (46 XY)

Pseudohermaphrodite (Male)
- Variable development of uterus, upper 2/3 vagina
- Partial masculinization of external genitalia
- Male karyotype (46 XY)

DES-Exposure
- Hypoplastic uterus with T-shaped endometrial cavity
- Myometrial constriction bands
- Vagina present

Total Hysterectomy
- Absent uterus
- Vagina present with normal zonal anatomy

PATHOLOGY

General Features
- Genetics
  - MRKH syndrome
    - Polygenic multifactorial inheritance with a 1-2% recurrence risk
    - In familial cases, syndrome transmitted as autosomal dominant with incomplete penetrance and variable expressivity
    - Associated with HNF-1β gene mutations in conjunction with renal anomalies and diabetes
  - 46 XX female karyotype
- Epidemiology
  - Incidence 1:5,000
  - Approximately 5-10% of MDAs
- Associated abnormalities
  - Increased incidence of renal anomalies (40-50%)
    - e.g., renal agenesis, ectopia, horseshoe kidneys
  - Associated skeletal or spinal anomalies in 10-12% of cases
  - Conductive or sensorineural hearing loss in 10-25% of cases

CLINICAL ISSUES

Presentation
- Most common signs/symptoms
  - Primary amenorrhea
    - MRKH syndrome is the second most common cause of primary amenorrhea after gonadal dysgenesis
- Other signs/symptoms: Rarely cyclic pelvic pain
- Clinical Profile
  - Complete agenesis and uterine hypoplasia without functioning endometrium presents with primary amenorrhea
    - No reproductive potential
  - Uterine hypoplasia with functioning endometrium
    - Primary amenorrhea with severe cyclic pain if associated with vaginal agenesis; results in hematometra
    - Little or no reproductive potential
  - Secondary sexual characteristics present with normal ovarian function
  - Normal external genitalia

Demographics
- Age: Developmental abnormality that remains undiagnosed until puberty or early adulthood
- Ethnicity: No ethnic predilection

Natural History & Prognosis
- Little or no reproductive potential

Treatment
- In patients with associated vaginal agenesis; vaginal dilatation or reconstruction performed to allow normal sexual functioning
  - Vaginal dilatation (Frank's method)
  - Skin graft (McIndoe procedure)
  - Laparoscopic creation of neovagina (modified Vecchietti technique)
  - Construction of neovagina with segment of sigmoid colon (sigmoid colpoplasty)

DIAGNOSTIC CHECKLIST

Consider
- Uterine hypoplasia/agenesis as a cause of primary amenorrhea in a young woman with normal secondary sexual characteristics

Image Interpretation Pearls
- Absent or hypoplastic uterus ± agenesis of upper 2/3 of vagina

SELECTED REFERENCES
1. Morcel K et al: Mayer-Rokitansky-Kuster-Hauser (MRKH) syndrome. Orphanet J Rare Dis. 2:13, 2007
2. Guerrier D et al: The Mayer-Rokitansky-Kuster-Hauser syndrome (congenital absence of uterus and vagina)--phenotypic manifestations and genetic approaches. J Negat Results Biomed. 5:1, 2006
3. Pittock ST et al: Mayer-Rokitansky-Kuster-Hauser anomaly and its associated malformations. Am J Med Genet A. 2005
4. Janssens F et al: Mayer-Rokitansky-Kuster-Hauser syndrome. JBR-BTR. 2004
5. Kula S et al: Mayer-Rokitansky-Kuster-Hauser syndrome associated with pulmonary stenosis. Acta Paediatr. 2004
6. Basile C et al: Renal abnormalities in Mayer-Rokitanski-Kuster-Hauser syndrome. J Nephrol. 2001
7. LeRoy S: Vaginal reconstruction in adolescent females with Mayer-Rokitansky-Kuster-Hauser syndrome. Plast Surg Nurs. 21(1):23-7, 39, 2001
8. Reinhold C et al: Primary amenorrhea: evaluation with MR imaging. Radiology. 203(2):383-90, 1997
9. Chapron C et al: Laparoscopic management of asymmetric Mayer-Rokitansky-Kuster-Hauser syndrome. Hum Reprod. 1995
10. Strubbe EH et al: The Mayer-Rokitansky-Kuster-Hauser (MRKH) syndrome without and with associated features: two separate entities? Clin Dysmorphol. 3(3):192-9, 1994
11. Strubbe EH et al: Mayer-Rokitansky-Kuster-Hauser syndrome: distinction between two forms based on excretory urographic, sonographic, and laparoscopic findings. AJR Am J Roentgenol. 160(2):331-4, 1993
12. Fedele L et al: Magnetic resonance imaging in Mayer-Rokitansky-Kuster-Hauser syndrome. Obstet Gynecol. 76(4):593-6, 1990

UTERINE HYPOPLASIA/AGENESIS

IMAGE GALLERY

Typical

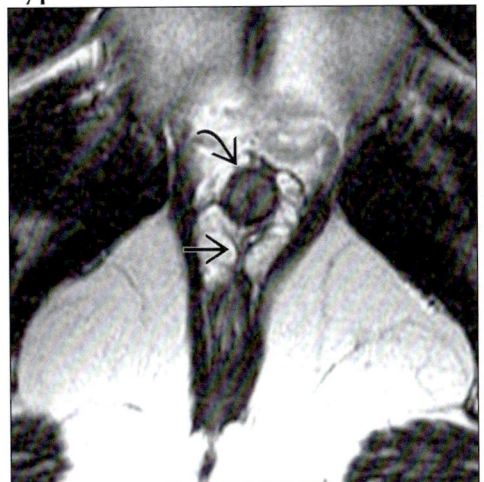
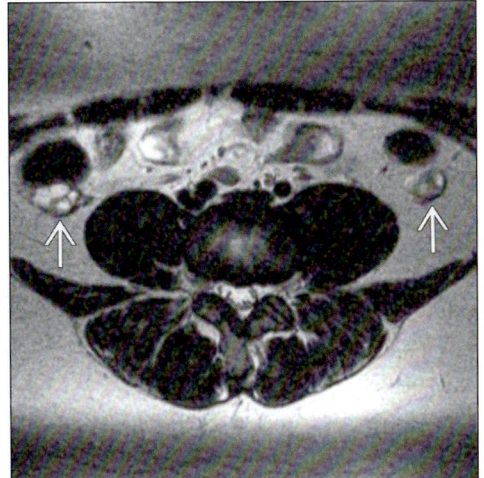

(Left) Axial T2WI MR in a patient with uterine agenesis and MRKH syndrome shows the upper 2/3 of the vagina to be atretic ➡ without normal zonal anatomy. Note the target appearance of the normal urethra ➡ anteriorly. (Right) Axial T2WI MR in the same patient as previous image, shows the ovaries ➡ located more cranially than usual in the right and left lower quadrants.

Typical

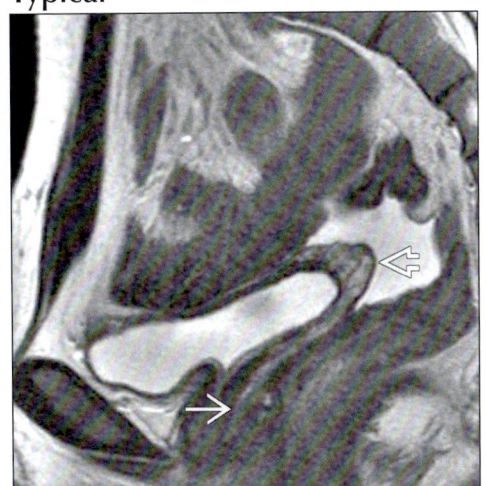
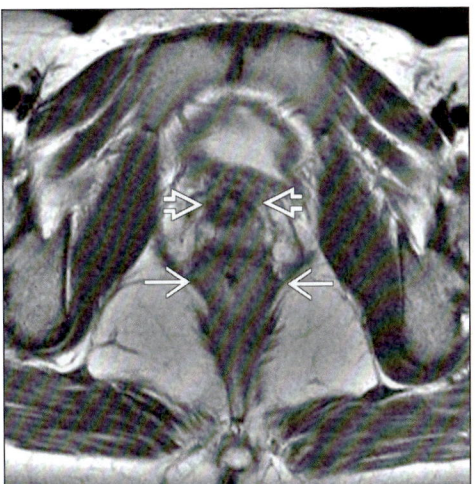

(Left) Sagittal T2WI MR shows Müllerian duct agenesis with connective tissue and veins present in the expected location of the uterus ➡ and upper two-thirds of the vagina. The lower third of the vagina ➡ is present. (Right) Axial T2WI MR in the same patient as previous image, shows vaginal agenesis with only the urethra ➡ and rectum ➡ visible on this image.

Typical

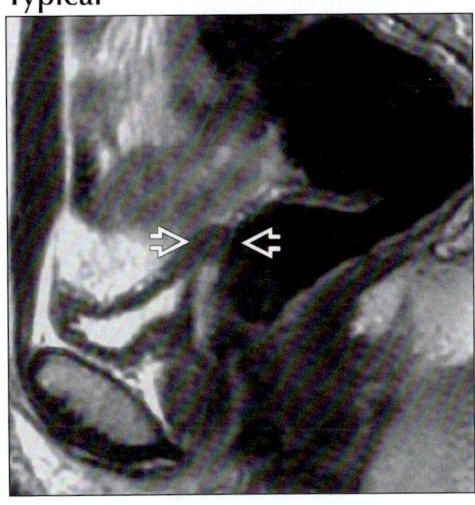
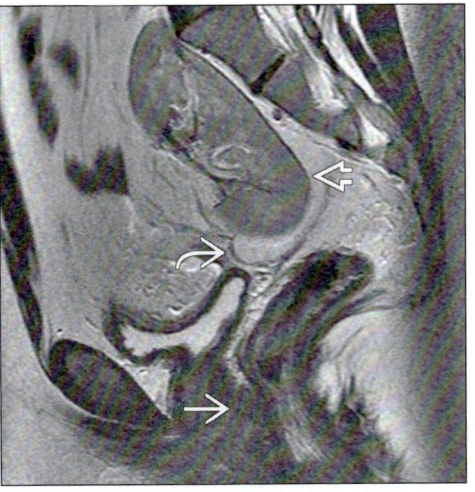

(Left) Axial T2WI MR in another patient with Müllerian duct agenesis shows absence of the uterine corpus, cervix and upper two-thirds of the vagina. A small soft tissue uterine remnant ➡ in the expected location of the uterus is demonstrated. (Right) Sagittal T2WI MR shows agenesis of the uterus ➡ and upper 2/3 of the vagina. The lower vagina ➡ is present. There is an ectopic left pelvic kidney ➡.

UNICORNUATE

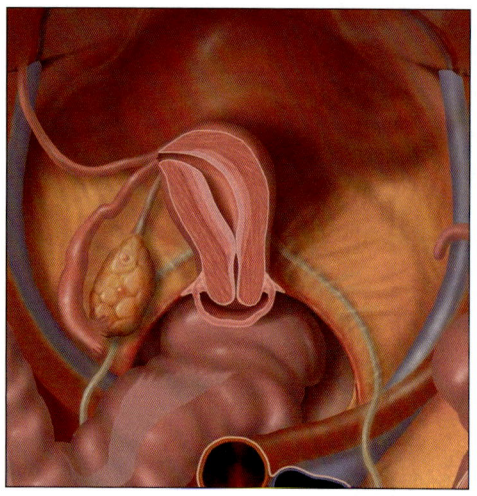

Graphic of a unicornuate uterus shows a small uterus shifted off midline with smooth tapering of fundal myometrium. The endometrial canal communicates with a solitary fallopian tube.

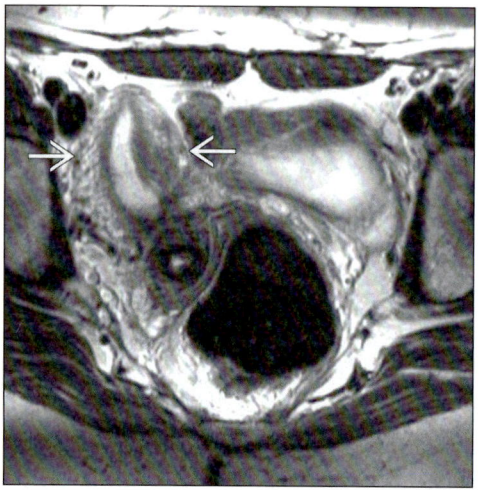

Axial T2WI MR shows a unicornuate uterus ➔ located off midline. Note the curved configuration of the uterus with the elongated tapering fundal segment resulting in a "banana shape."

TERMINOLOGY

Definitions
- Class II Müllerian duct anomaly (MDA)
  - Based on Buttram & Gibbons/American Fertility Society (AFS) classification system
- Failure of one Müllerian duct to elongate causing an asymmetric uterus with or without a small rudimentary horn

IMAGING FINDINGS

General Features
- Best diagnostic clue
  - Small, elliptical uterus, deviated to one side of pelvis with a single cornua
  - "Banana" configuration of uterus
- Size: Corpus uteri generally smaller than the nulliparous uterus
- Small, elliptical uterus, shifted off midline, without or with small residual rudimentary horn
- Solitary uterine horn and cervix: 35%
- Associated rudimentary horn: 65%
  - Non-cavitary (no endometrial segment): 33%
  - Cavitary (endometrial segment present): 32%
    - May or may not communicate with endometrial cavity of dominant uterine horn
    - Non-communicating (22%)
    - Communicating (10%)
- Fallopian tube of nondominant horn
  - Absent in unicornuate uterus without a rudimentary horn and in presence of a small atretic residual horn
  - Both fallopian tubes are present with most other rudimentary horns
- Both ovaries present and normal

Radiographic Findings
- Hysterosalpingography (HSG)
  - Opacified endometrial cavity shifted off midline
  - Fusiform configuration of opacified endometrial cavity, tapers at apex
  - Endometrial cavity drains into one fallopian tube
  - Opacification of a small communicating rudimentary horn may be seen if present
  - Will not demonstrate non communicating rudimentary horn, although presence may be suspected by

DDx: Mimics of Unicornuate Uterus

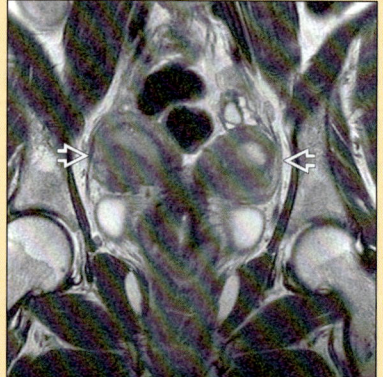

Bicornuate Uterus

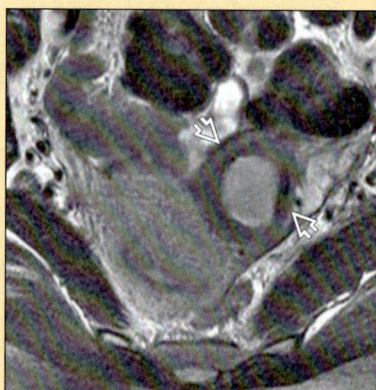

Cystic Adenomyosis

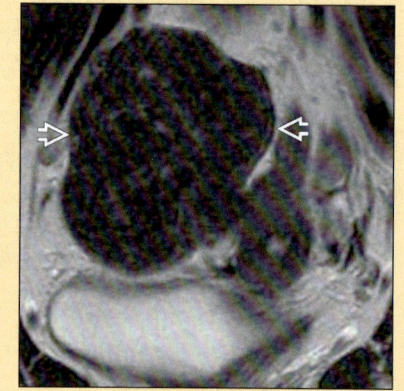

Subserosal Fibroid

UNICORNUATE

Key Facts

Terminology
- Class II Müllerian duct anomaly (MDA)
- Based on Buttram & Gibbons/American Fertility Society (AFS) classification system

Imaging Findings
- Small, elliptical uterus, deviated to one side of pelvis with a single cornua
- "Banana" configuration of uterus
- Associated rudimentary horn: 65%

Top Differential Diagnoses
- Bicornuate Uterus
- Uterus Didelphys
- Pedunculated Leiomyoma
- Hemorrhagic Degeneration of Leiomyoma
- Cystic Adenomyosis

Pathology
- Highest associated incidence of renal anomalies of MDAs (40%)

Clinical Issues
- Risk of ectopic pregnancy in cavitary rudimentary horn
- Increased incidence of endometriosis in patients with obstructed horn, possibly due to retrograde expulsion of menstrual products
- Obstetric complications among highest of MDAs

Diagnostic Checklist
- "Banana" configuration of unicornuate uterus on long-axis T2WI
- Improve detection rate by systematically identifying both cornua in all patients

---

- More medial position of dominant horn (compared to simple unicornuate uterus) due to partial fusion of Müllerian ducts

Ultrasonographic Findings
- Transvaginal ultrasound (TVS)
  - Often difficult to detect, especially if not suspected
  - Small, elliptical uterus
  - Single cornua
  - Small, echogenic rudimentary horn (if present)
    - May mimic prominent cervix
    - May mimic pedunculated leiomyoma
    - Small, echogenic endometrial complex in cavitary rudimentary horn
  - Improve detection rate by systematically identifying both cornua

CT Findings
- CT not indicated in characterizing Müllerian duct anomalies

MR Findings
- T1WI
  - Obstructed segment of high signal intensity
  - Associated complications, hematosalpinx and endometriosis also of high signal intensity
- T2WI
  - Uterus curved, elongated with tapering fundal segment off midline: "Banana" configuration
  - Dominant horn: Uterine volume reduced
    - Single cornua
    - Endometrium uniformly narrowed or "bullet"-shaped tapering at cornua
    - Endometrial/myometrial width and ratio preserved
    - Normal uterine zonal anatomy maintained
  - Rudimentary horn: Variable
    - Absence of endometrium: Adjacent low-signal-intensity soft tissue mass with loss of normal zonal anatomy
    - Presence of endometrium: High-signal-intensity endometrium without or with preserved normal zonal anatomy
- T1 C+ FS: Dominant and rudimentary horns show normal myometrial enhancement

Imaging Recommendations
- Best imaging tool: MR allows accurate classification of unicornuate uterus
- Protocol advice
  - Phased array body coil
  - Single shot fast spin echo (FSE) coronal image through the abdomen and pelvis to assess kidneys
  - High resolution FSE T2WI, ≤ 4 mm slice thickness
    - Axial oblique (long-axis) view to diagnose unicornuate uterus
    - Coronal oblique (short-axis) view to document rudimentary horn and assess endometrial segment
  - Axial T1WI ± FS images through the pelvis
    - To confirm blood products in obstructed segments and demonstrate complications such as hematosalpinx and endometriosis
    - T1 C+ FS may help to demonstrate rudimentary horn if T2WI indeterminate

DIFFERENTIAL DIAGNOSIS

Bicornuate Uterus
- Symmetric duplication of uterine horns with communicating endometrial cavities

Uterus Didelphys
- Complete, symmetric duplication of uterine corpus and cervix

Pedunculated Leiomyoma
- Uterus of normal volume with two cornua
- Leiomyomas are typically round in configuration

Hemorrhagic Degeneration of Leiomyoma
- Mimics an obstructed cavitary rudimentary horn
- Blood products appear bright on T1WI FS

Cystic Adenomyosis
- Mimics an obstructed cavitary rudimentary horn
- Uterus of normal volume with two cornua

UNICORNUATE

- Well-circumscribed, thick-walled, complex cystic mass of myometrial origin
- Contains blood products which appear bright on T1WI FS
- Cyst wall of lower signal on T2WI than normal myometrium

PATHOLOGY

General Features
- General path comments
  - Failure of one Müllerian duct to elongate causing an asymmetric uterus with or without a small rudimentary horn
  - "Banana" configuration of uterus
  - Fallopian tube of nondominant horn
    - Absent in unicornuate uterus without a rudimentary horn and in presence of a small atretic residual horn
    - Both fallopian tubes are present with most other rudimentary horns
  - Ovaries usually normal; occasionally malpositioned or elongated
  - In unicornuate uterus with non communicating cavitary rudimentary horn, retrograde expulsion of menstrual products occurs via ipsilateral fallopian tube during menses
- Genetics: Majority of cases sporadic or multifactorial in nature
- Epidemiology: Accounts for 20% of MDAs
- Associated abnormalities
  - Highest associated incidence of renal anomalies of MDAs (40%)
    - Always ipsilateral to absent or rudimentary horn
    - Include ectopic kidney, renal agenesis, cystic dysplasia and duplicated collecting system

Staging, Grading or Classification Criteria
- Unicornuate uterus, no rudimentary horn: Class IId
- Unicornuate uterus with rudimentary horn
  - Noncavitary: Class IIc
  - Cavitary, noncommunicating: Class IIb
  - Cavitary, communicating: Class IIa

CLINICAL ISSUES

Presentation
- Most common signs/symptoms
  - Unicornuate uterus ± communicating rudimentary horn are usually incidental findings in the adult during investigation for infertility or other pelvic pathology
  - Present at puberty with cyclical pelvic pain in cases of cavitary, non communicating uterine horn with partially obstructed or aplastic fallopian tube
- Risk of ectopic pregnancy in cavitary rudimentary horn
  - Approximately 90% of rudimentary horn pregnancies end in rupture of the horn
- Increased incidence of endometriosis in patients with obstructed horn, possibly due to retrograde expulsion of menstrual products

Natural History & Prognosis
- Obstetric complications among highest of MDAs
  - Spontaneous abortion rate: 50%
  - Pre-term birth rate: 15%
  - Fetal survival rate: 40%

Treatment
- Solitary without a rudimentary horn
  - Expectant
- Solitary with a noncavitary rudimentary horn
  - Expectant
- Cavitary uterine horn
  - Communicating type
    - Laparoscopic salpingectomy to reduce risk of pregnancy in rudimentary horn
  - Non communicating type
    - Excision of rudimentary horn (usually via a laparoscopic approach) for symptomatic relief of hematometra and prevention of endometriosis

DIAGNOSTIC CHECKLIST

Consider
- The possibility of unicornuate uterus
  - In a female patient being investigated for infertility
  - In a post-pubertal patient presenting with cyclical pelvic pain

Image Interpretation Pearls
- "Banana" configuration of unicornuate uterus on long-axis T2WI
- Improve detection rate by systematically identifying both cornua in all patients

SELECTED REFERENCES

1. Troiano RN et al: Mullerian duct anomalies: imaging and clinical issues. Radiology. 2004
2. Chakravarti S et al: Rudimentary uterine horn: management of a diagnostic enigma. Acta Obstet Gynecol Scand. 2003
3. Marten K et al: MRI in the evaluation of mullerian duct anomalies. Clin Imaging. 2003
4. Scarsbrook AF et al: MRI appearances of mullerian duct abnormalities. Clin Radiol. 2003
5. Troiano RN: Magnetic resonance imaging of mullerian duct anomalies of the uterus. Top Magn Reson Imaging. 2003
6. Brody JM et al: Unicornuate uterus: imaging appearance, associated anomalies, and clinical implications. AJR Am J Roentgenol. 171(5):1341-7, 1998

UNICORNUATE

IMAGE GALLERY

Typical

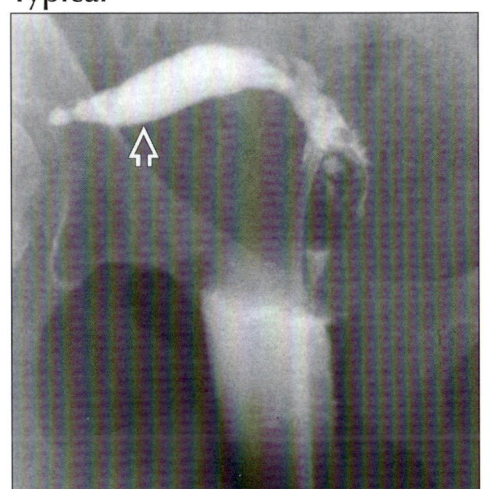
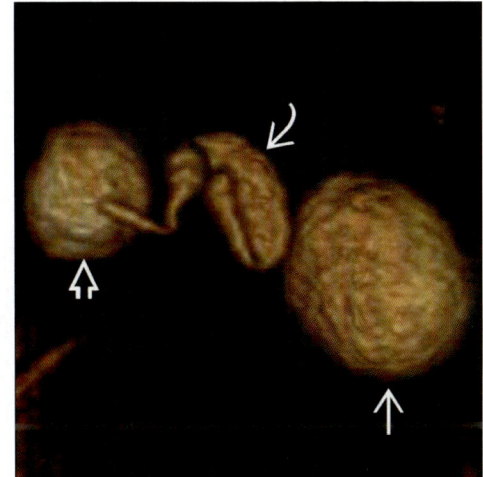

(Left) Anteroposterior hysterosalpingogram shows a typical case of unicornuate uterus ➡. The cervix has been cannulated. *(Right)* Anteroposterior volume rendering MR of an obstructed rudimentary horn ➡, hematosalpinx ➡ and endometrioma ➡ in a patient with a unicornuate uterus.

Typical

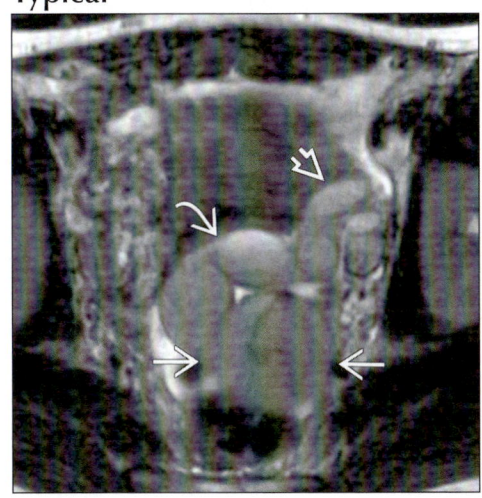
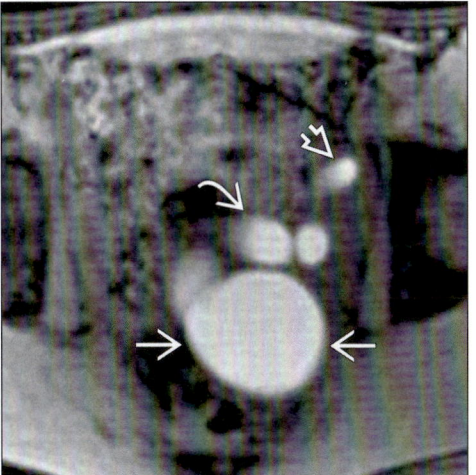

(Left) Axial T2WI MR of the preceding patient shows the obstructed rudimentary horn ➡, hematosalpinx ➡ and endometrioma ➡. Note heterogeneous intermediate signal in keeping with blood products. *(Right)* Axial T1WI FS MR in the same patient as previous image confirms the presence of blood products in the obstructed rudimentary horn ➡, hematosalpinx ➡ and endometrioma ➡.

Typical

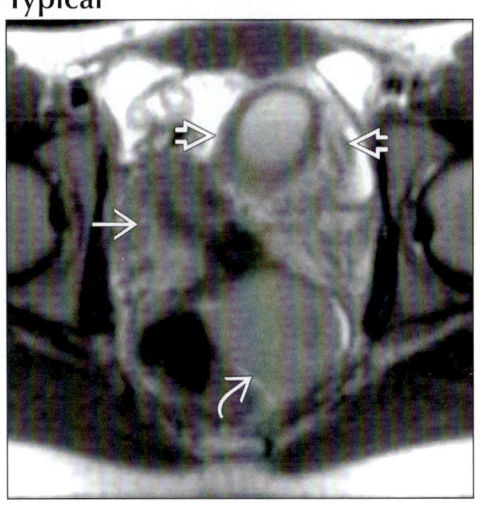
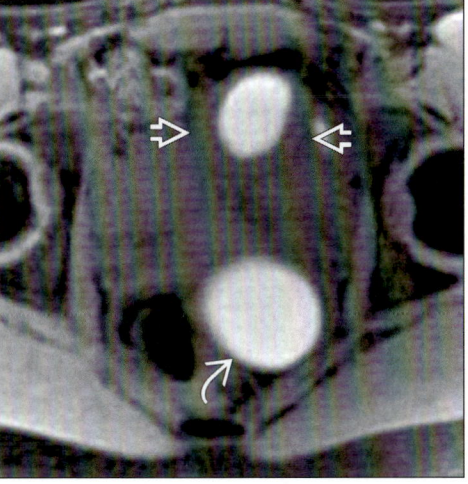

(Left) Axial T2WI MR in the preceding patient at a different slice location shows the unicornuate uterus ➡ with an obstructed rudimentary horn ➡ complicated by an endometrioma ➡. *(Right)* Axial T1WI FS MR in the same patient as previous image, shows high signal intensity within the obstructed rudimentary horn ➡ and endometrioma ➡, denoting blood products.

UNICORNUATE

(Left) Axial transvaginal ultrasound shows a unicornuate uterus ➡ with a non-cavitary rudimentary horn ➡. *(Right)* Axial T2WI MR in the same patient as previous image, shows the typical configuration of a unicornuate uterus with the dominant horn ➡ located to the left of the midline. A noncavitary rudimentary horn is present ➡.

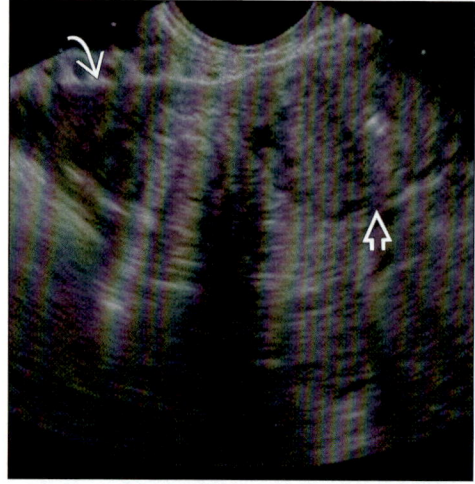
Typical

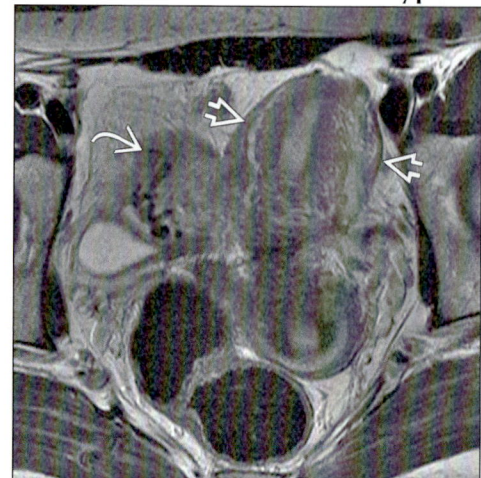
Typical

(Left) Longitudinal transvaginal ultrasound shows a unicornuate uterus with the typical "banana-shaped" configuration ➡. Note the decreased uterine volume. No rudimentary horn was seen. *(Right)* Axial T2WI MR in the same patient as previous image, shows the "banana-shaped" configuration of the dominant horn which is deviated to the right of the midline ➡. Incidental note is made of a small leiomyoma ➡.

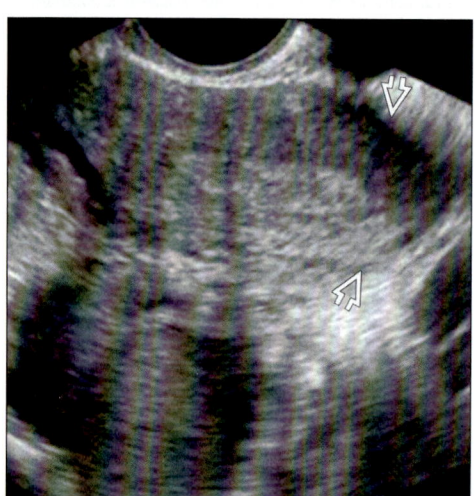

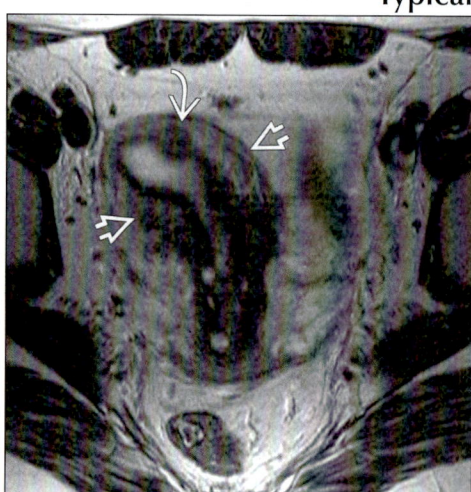
Typical

(Left) Coronal T2WI MR in the same patient as previous image, acquired at a different slice level, shows the unicornuate uterus ➡ with a noncavitary rudimentary horn ➡. *(Right)* Coronal oblique T2WI MR in the same patient as previous image, shows to better advantage the noncavitary rudimentary horn ➡.

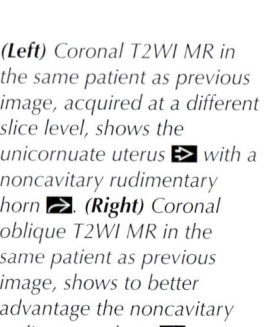

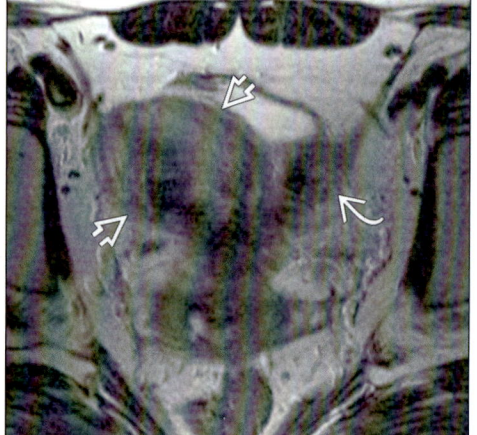

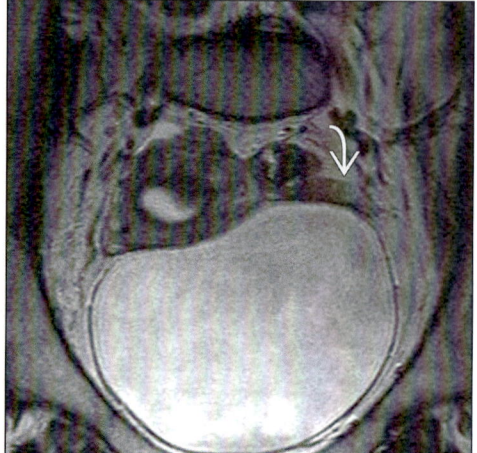
Typical

UNICORNUATE

Typical

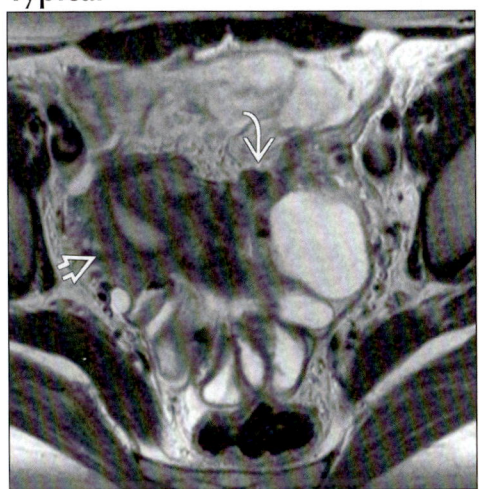
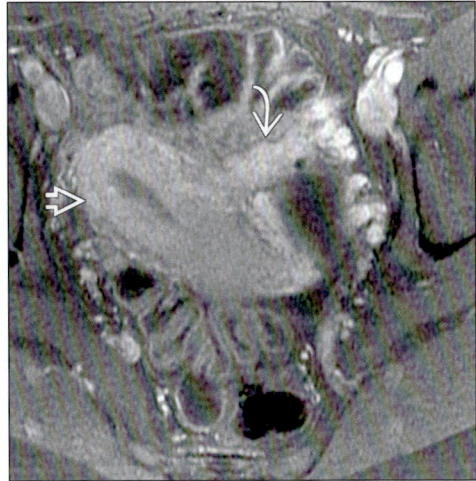

(Left) Axial T2WI MR shows a unicornuate uterus ➡ of diminished volume with a non cavitary rudimentary horn ➡. *(Right)* Axial T1 C+ FS MR in the same patient as previous image, shows the normal myometrial enhancement of both the dominant ➡ and non-cavitary rudimentary horn ➡.

Typical

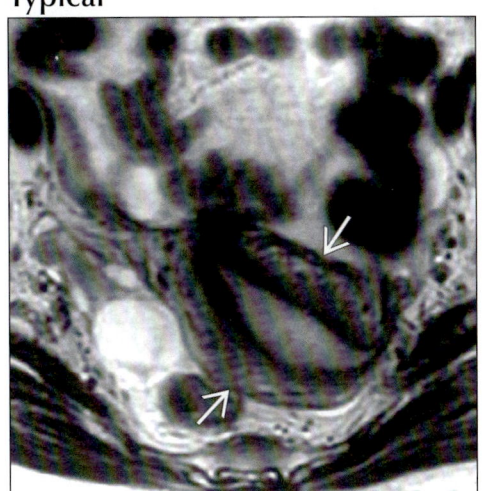
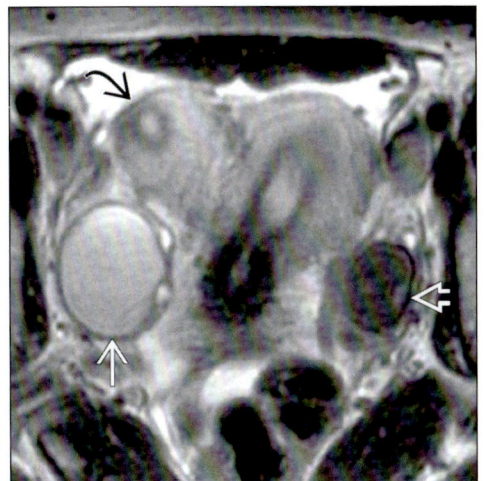

(Left) Axial T2WI MR shows the banana configuration of a left-sided unicornuate uterus ➡ without a rudimentary horn. *(Right)* Axial T2WI MR shows a unicornuate uterus with a cavitary rudimentary horn ➡. The endometrial segment is non-communicating. There is a hemorrhagic right ovarian cyst ➡ and an endometrioma ➡ arising from the left ovary.

Typical

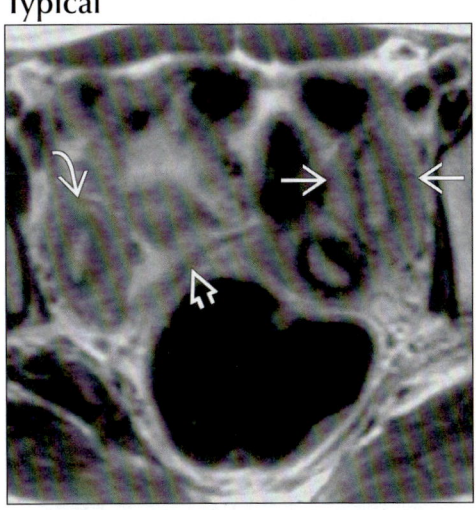
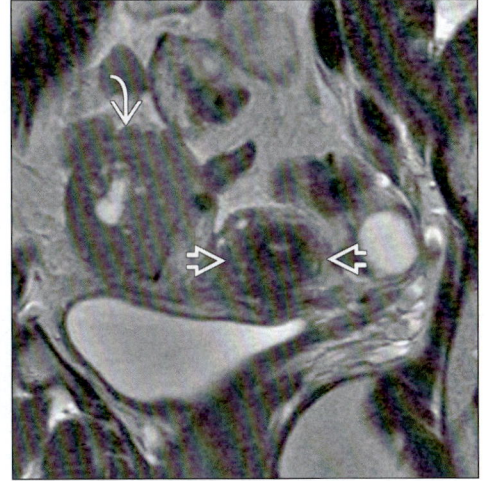

(Left) Axial T2WI MR shows a unicornuate uterus ➡ with a cavitary rudimentary horn ➡. The endometrial segment is non-communicating and is connected to the dominant horn by a thin low signal intensity band ➡. *(Right)* Coronal oblique T2WI MR shows a unicornuate uterus with the cervix of the dominant horn to the left of midline ➡. There is an obstructed rudimentary horn ➡ which is enlarged due the presence of diffuse adenomyosis.

DIDELPHYS

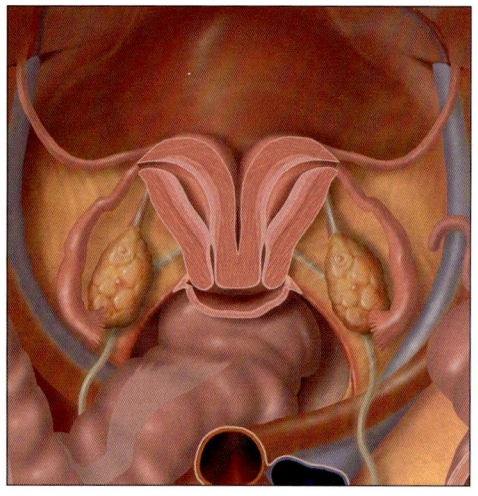

Graphic of uterus didelphys shows complete duplication of uterine horns and cervices with no communication of the endometrial cavities.

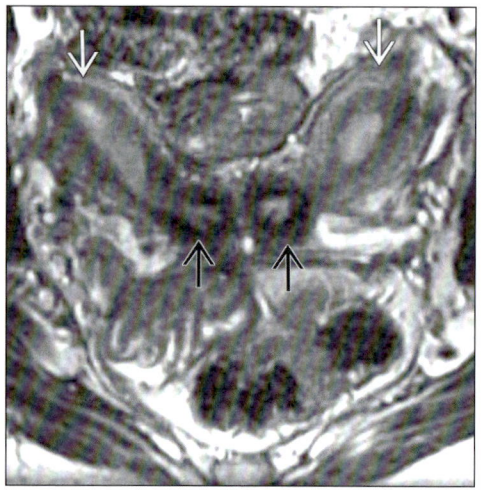

Coronal oblique T2WI MR shows two completely separate corpus uteri ➡ and cervices ➡. The cornual segments of the uterine horns are widely divergent. Note preservation of zonal anatomy.

TERMINOLOGY

Definitions
- **Class III Müllerian duct anomaly (MDA)**
  - Based on Buttram & Gibbons/American Fertility Society (AFS) classification system
- Complete nonfusion of uterovaginal horns

IMAGING FINDINGS

General Features
- Best diagnostic clue
  - Complete duplication of uterine horns and cervices
  - No communication between duplicated endometrial or endocervical cavities
- Size: Uterine volume in each duplicated segment reduced
- Two symmetric uterine horns and cervices with minor degree of fusion at most caudal margin
- Longitudinal vaginal septum present in 75%
  - Occasionally complicated by transverse vaginal septum causing obstruction

Radiographic Findings
- Hysterosalpingography (HSG)
  - Two separate opacified endocervical canals opening into separate, symmetric fusiform endometrial cavities
  - Each cavity ends in a solitary fallopian tube
  - No communication between opacified endocervical and endometrial cavities
  - Pitfall: Only one cervical os may be cannulated; endometrial configuration then mimics unicornuate uterus

Ultrasonographic Findings
- Transabdominal ultrasound (US)
  - Widely divergent uterine horns
  - 3D ultrasound may aid in diagnosis, but typically two separate uterine horns are well-visualized at real-time scanning
- Transvaginal ultrasound (TVS)
  - Divergent, symmetric, endometrial echogenic complexes without communication
  - Two distinct cervices need to be documented

DDx: Mimics of Uterus Didelphys

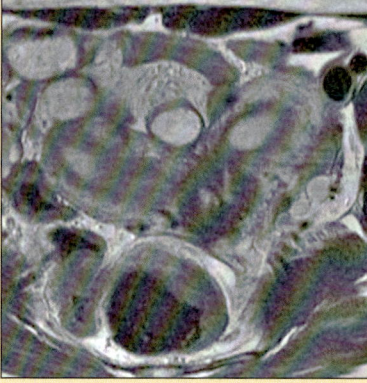

Complex Duplication Anomaly

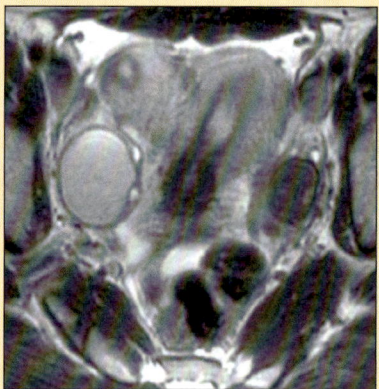

Unicornuate, Rudimentary Horn

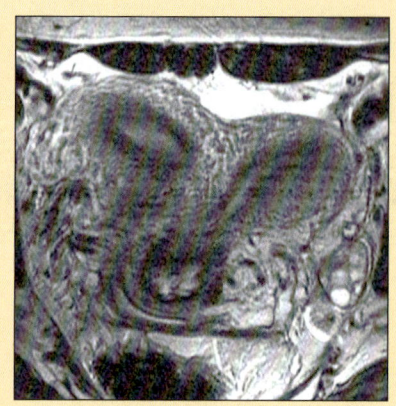

Bicornuate Uterus

DIDELPHYS

Key Facts

Terminology
- **Class III Müllerian duct anomaly (MDA)**
- Based on Buttram & Gibbons/American Fertility Society (AFS) classification system
- Complete nonfusion of uterovaginal horns

Imaging Findings
- Complete duplication of uterine horns and cervices
- No communication between duplicated endometrial or endocervical cavities
- Longitudinal vaginal septum present in 75%
- Occasionally complicated by transverse vaginal septum causing obstruction

Top Differential Diagnoses
- Bicornuate Bicollis Uterus
- Unicornuate Uterus
- Complex Duplication Anomalies

Pathology
- Renal anomalies: Agenesis, duplex or pelvic kidney
- Increased incidence of endometriosis in the obstructed type due to retrograde menstrual flow

Clinical Issues
- Second highest probability of a successful pregnancy after arcuate uterus
- Hysteroscopic resection of vaginal septum in patients with an obstructing vaginal septum

Diagnostic Checklist
- Uterus didelphys with obstruction in a patient presenting at menarche with cyclical dysmenorrhea and pelvic mass

CT Findings
- CT has no role in characterization of uterus didelphys

MR Findings
- T1WI
  - High signal intensity (SI) hematometrocolpos
    - Caused by obstruction of transverse vaginal septum
    - Associated complications: Hematosalpinx, endometriosis
- T2WI
  - Two separate uteri and cervices
  - Uterine volume of each horn reduced
    - Normal uterine/cervical zonal anatomy
  - Cornual segments of horns widely divergent; cervices usually in close approximation
  - Longitudinal vaginal septum: Longitudinal low SI band extending through vagina which may be complete or incomplete
  - Obstructed unilateral transverse vaginal septum
    - Transverse low SI band anywhere along vagina, usually at junction of upper and middle thirds
    - Marked deformity of uterus due to hematometrocolpos with dilatation of vaginal segment and lesser dilatation of endometrial segment
    - Variable SI of hematometrocolpos depending on stage of hemorrhage
    - Hematosalpinx and/or endometriosis may be present

Imaging Recommendations
- Best imaging tool
  - 2D and 3D US can be used as initial imaging modality
  - Pelvic MR modality of choice
    - Optimal depiction of uterine duplication anomaly and evaluation of associated hematometrocolpos and endometriosis
- Protocol advice
  - Phased array body coil
  - Single shot fast spin echo (SS FSE) coronal T2WI through abdomen and pelvis to assess kidneys
  - High resolution FSE T2WI, ≤ 4 mm slice thickness
    - Imaging plane parallel to long axis of uterus to assess degree of divergence of uterine horns and cervical duplication
    - Short-axis view of vagina to delineate vaginal septum
  - T1WI ± FS
    - FS images will confirm the presence of blood products due to persistent high SI

DIFFERENTIAL DIAGNOSIS

Bicornuate Bicollis Uterus
- Nonfusion confined to uterine corpus compared to didelphys where nonfusion of both uterus and cervix occurs
- Central myometrium extends to external cervical os
  - Communication between uterine horns must be present
  - Caudal end of septum may be fibrous: Low SI on T2 and T1WI
- Vaginal obstruction is rare

Unicornuate Uterus
- Asymmetric horns with smaller rudimentary horn
- Solitary cervix

Complex Duplication Anomalies
- Comprise features of more than one class of MDAs
- Most common scenario: Degree of nonfusion less than didelphys, greater than bicornuate uterus
  - Variable fundal duplication of uterine horns with midline, lower uterine septum
  - Solitary or duplicated cervix

PATHOLOGY

General Features
- Genetics

DIDELPHYS

- Majority of cases sporadic or multifactorial in origin
- May be caused by an autosomal dominant or recessive gene in certain cases
- Hepatocyte nuclear factor (HNF-1) β mutations reported in association with renal anomalies and diabetes
- Etiology: Complete nonfusion of uterovaginal horns
- Epidemiology: Accounts for 5% of MDAs
- Associated abnormalities
  - Renal anomalies: Agenesis, duplex or pelvic kidney
  - Uterus didelphys with obstructed hemivagina
    - Renal agenesis: 85-100%, ipsilateral to side of obstruction
    - Contralateral renal anomalies: 50%
  - Nonobstructive uterus didelphys
    - Renal agenesis: 15%
  - Increased incidence of endometriosis in the obstructed type due to retrograde menstrual flow
    - Especially in subset with unilateral obstruction secondary to transverse septum

CLINICAL ISSUES

Presentation
- Most common signs/symptoms
  - Nonobstructive uterus didelphys
    - Usually asymptomatic
    - Diagnosis made during investigation of recurrent spontaneous abortions and premature delivery
  - Uterus didelphys with obstructed hemivagina
    - Frequently symptomatic at menarche with pelvic mass (hematometrocolpos) and dysmenorrhea
    - Hematometrocolpos may cause acute urinary retention or other pressure effects
    - Superinfection presents with fever, peritonitis and vaginal discharge
- Other signs/symptoms: Rarely acute rupture of hematosalpinx, presenting with peritonitis

Demographics
- Age: Developmental abnormality which usually presents at menarche or later
- Ethnicity: No ethnic predilection

Natural History & Prognosis
- Compared to other uterine anomalies
  - Second highest probability of a successful pregnancy after arcuate uterus
  - Reproductive outcomes slightly better than unicornuate uterus
    - Possibly secondary to better uterine perfusion
- Simultaneous pregnancy in both uteri reported
- Breech presentation with pregnancy is common (45%)
- Spontaneous abortion rate: 45% (range 32-52%)
- Premature birth rate: 40% (range 20-45%)
- Fetal survival rate: 55% (range 41-64%)

Treatment
- Expectant
- Metroplasty leaving duplicated cervix intact in selected patients with recurrent spontaneous abortions and premature deliveries
  - Traditionally performed abdominally via a Pfannenstiel approach (e.g., Strassman metroplasty)
  - Currently performed by a combined hysteroscopic and laparoscopic approach
  - Benefits of metroplasty unclear
- Hysteroscopic resection of vaginal septum in patients with an obstructing vaginal septum

DIAGNOSTIC CHECKLIST

Consider
- Uterus didelphys with obstruction in a patient presenting at menarche with cyclical dysmenorrhea and pelvic mass

Image Interpretation Pearls
- Two separate uteri and cervices identified on T2WI

SELECTED REFERENCES

1. Bhattacharya K et al: Uterus didelphys with fibroid uterus and ovarian cyst--rare Muellerian malformation. J Indian Med Assoc. 104(6):336-7, 2006
2. Madureira AJ et al: Case 94: Uterus didelphys with obstructing hemivaginal septum and ipsilateral renal agenesis. Radiology. 239(2):602-6, 2006
3. Prada Arias M et al: Uterus didelphys with obstructed hemivagina and multicystic dysplastic kidney. Eur J Pediatr Surg. 15(6):441-5, 2005
4. Montevecchi L et al: Resectoscopic treatment of complete longitudinal vaginal septum. Int J Gynaecol Obstet. 2004
5. Troiano RN et al: Mullerian duct anomalies: imaging and clinical issues. Radiology. 2004
6. Dalkalitsis N et al: Unicornuate uterus and uterus didelphys indications and techniques for surgical reconstruction: a review. Clin Exp Obstet Gynecol. 30(2-3):137-43, 2003
7. Hinckley MD et al: Management of uterus didelphys, obstructed hemivagina and ipsilateral renal agenesis. A case report. J Reprod Med. 48(8):649-51, 2003
8. Takagi H et al: Magnetic resonance imaging in the evaluating of double uterus and associated urinary tract anomalies: a report of five cases. J Obstet Gynaecol. 23(5):525-7, 2003
9. Troiano RN: Magnetic resonance imaging of mullerian duct anomalies of the uterus. Top Magn Reson Imaging. 2003
10. Woodward PJ et al: MR imaging in the evaluation of female infertility. Radiographics. 1993
11. Pellerito JS et al: Diagnosis of uterine anomalies: relative accuracy of MR imaging, endovaginal sonography, and hysterosalpingography. Radiology. 183(3):795-800, 1992
12. Carrington BM et al: Mullerian duct anomalies: MR imaging evaluation. Radiology. 176(3):715-20, 1990
13. Fedele L et al: Magnetic resonance evaluation of double uteri. Obstet Gynecol. 74(6):844-7, 1989

DIDELPHYS

IMAGE GALLERY

Typical

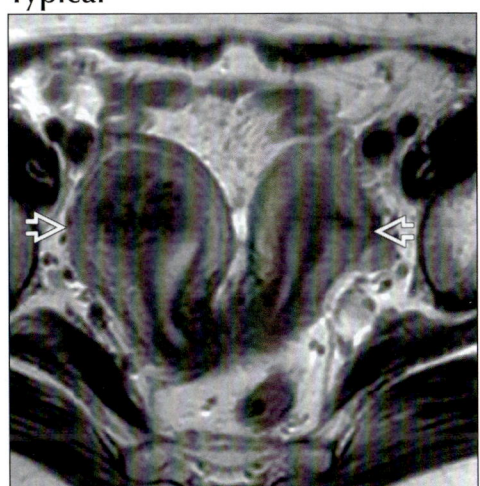 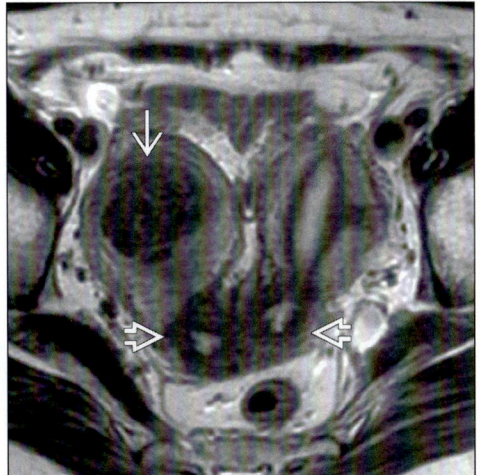

(Left) Coronal oblique T2WI MR shows an example of uterine didelphys with completely separate and divergent uterine horns ➡. (Right) Coronal oblique T2WI MR in the same patient as previous image, shows complete duplication of the cervix ➡ in keeping with uterine didelphys. Incidentally there is an intramural leiomyoma in the right uterine horn ➡.

Typical

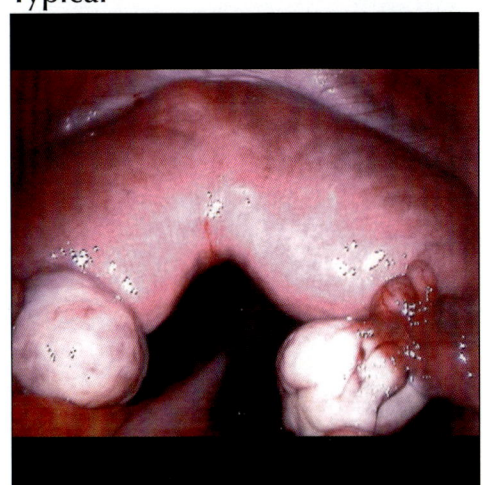 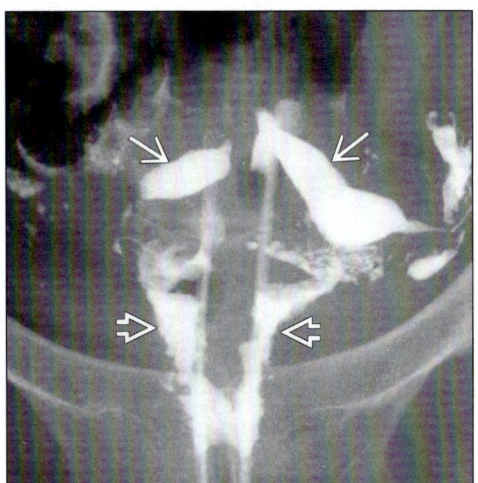

(Left) Anteroposterior intra-operative photograph in a patient with uterus didelphys. Note the widely divergent and separate uterine horns. (Courtesy T. Tulandi, MD). (Right) Anteroposterior hysterosalpingogram shows a case of uterus didelphys. Two completely separate opacified endocervical canals ➡ and uterine cavities ➡ are clearly demonstrated.

Typical

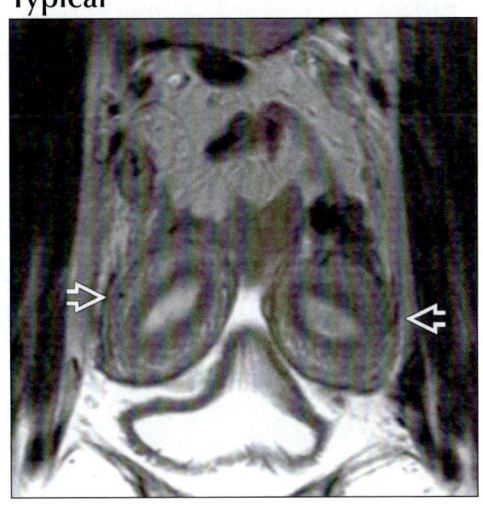 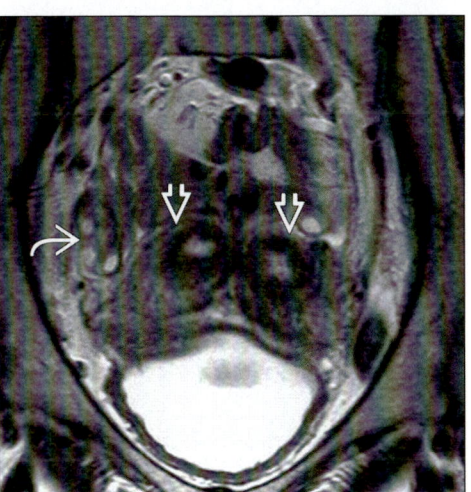

(Left) Coronal T2WI MR shows a patient with uterus didelphys. Note the completely separate and widely divergent uterine horns ➡. The zonal anatomy is preserved. (Right) Coronal T2WI MR in the same patient as previous image, shows the two duplicated but closely approximated cervices ➡. Note presence of a normal right ovary ➡.

DIDELPHYS

(Left) Transverse transabdominal ultrasound through a full bladder shows a gestational sac within the right horn ➡ and an empty left horn ➡ of a uterus didelphys. *(Right)* Sagittal transabdominal ultrasound shows an empty right renal fossa in a patient with uterus didelphys. Since duplication anomalies are associated with renal agenesis, it is important to assess the kidneys.

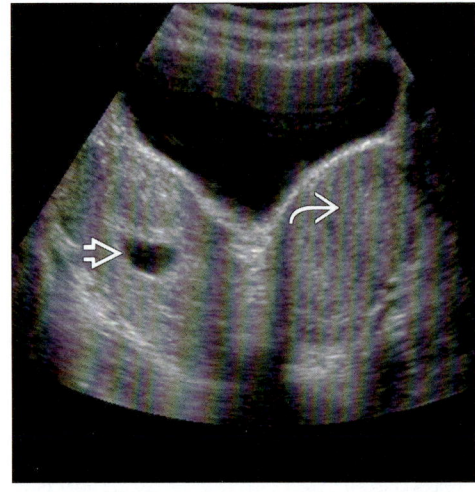
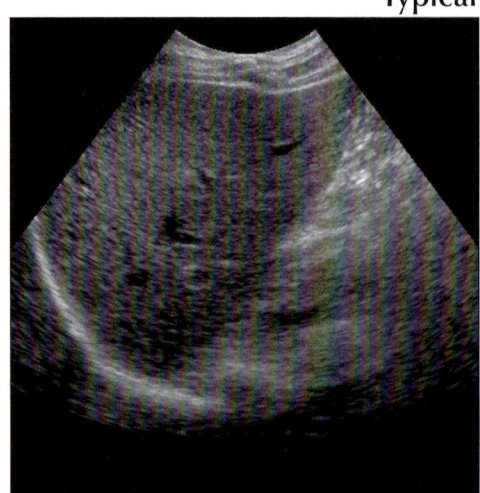

(Left) Transverse transabdominal ultrasound shows two widely divergent uterine horns of a uterus didelphys with a gestational sac ➡ in the right horn. *(Right)* Transverse transvaginal ultrasound in same patient as previous image, shows again the two separate uterine horns with a pregnancy in the right horn. In this image the yolk sac ➡ and embryonic pole ➡ are visible.

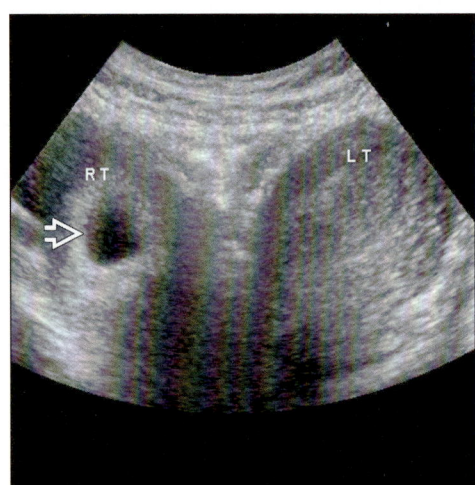
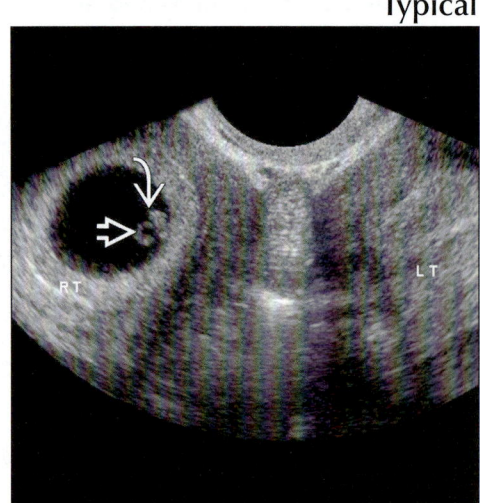

(Left) Transverse transabdominal ultrasound shows two separate and widely divergent uterine horns. *(Right)* Sagittal oblique transvaginal ultrasound in the same patient as previous image, shows two separate cervices ➡. Cervical assessment is best performed using a transvaginal approach.

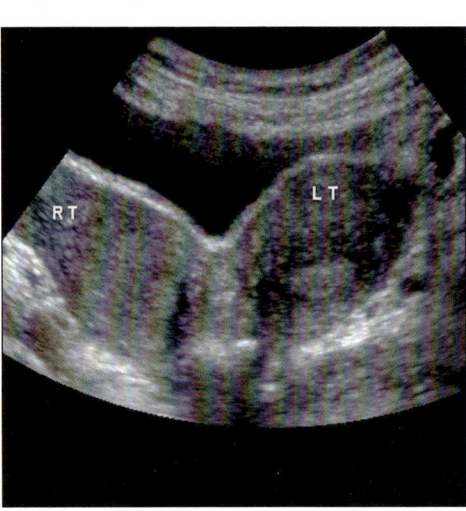
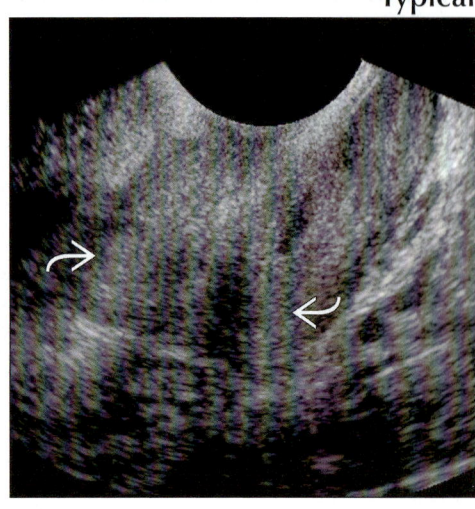

DIDELPHYS

Typical

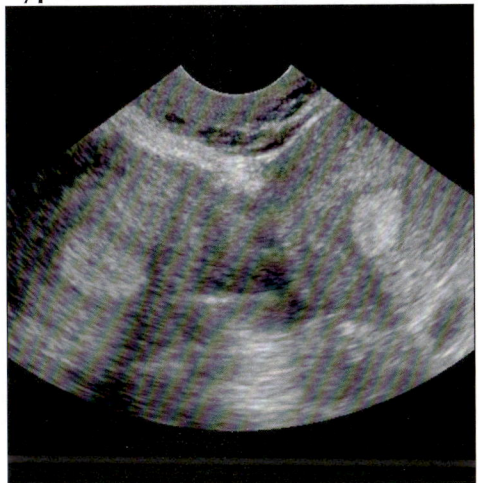
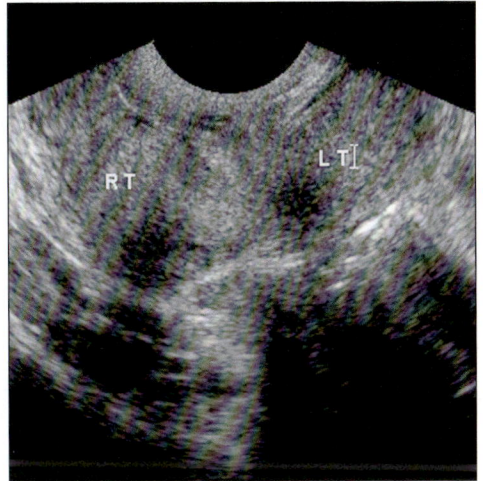

(Left) Transverse transvaginal ultrasound shows two symmetric and divergent uterine horns. *(Right)* Transverse transvaginal ultrasound in the same patient as previous image, shows non-communicating uterine horns at a more caudal level in this patient with uterus didelphys.

Typical

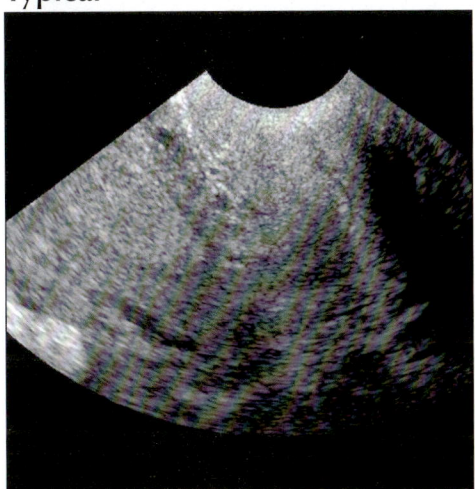
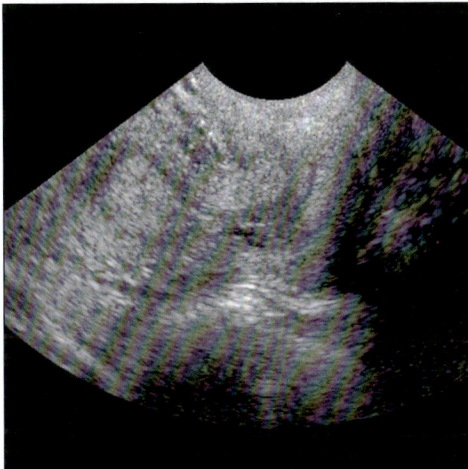

(Left) Sagittal transvaginal ultrasound shows a separate left uterine horn and cervix. *(Right)* Sagittal transvaginal ultrasound in same patient as previous image, shows a separate right uterine horn and cervix. It is important to assess each uterine horn and endometrial cavity separately.

Typical

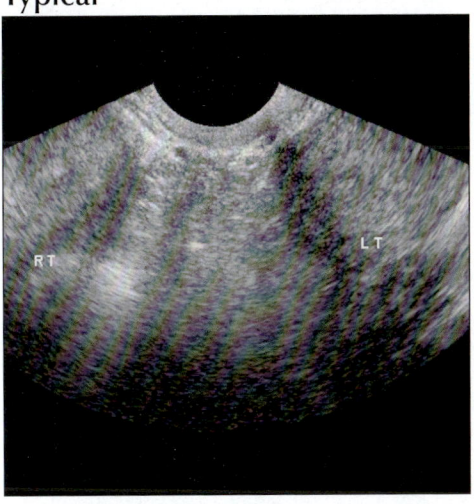
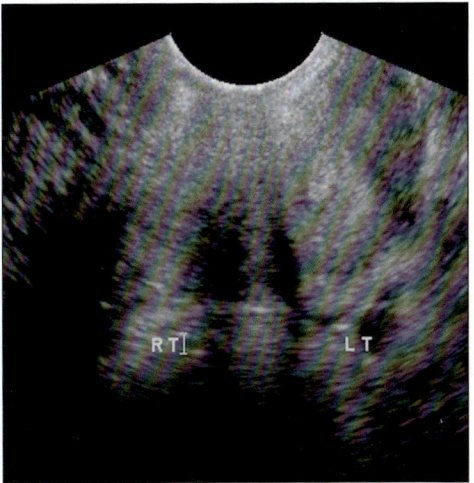

(Left) Transverse transvaginal ultrasound shows two widely divergent uterine horns. *(Right)* Transverse transvaginal ultrasound shows complete duplication of the cervices in a patient with uterus didelphys.

BICORNUATE

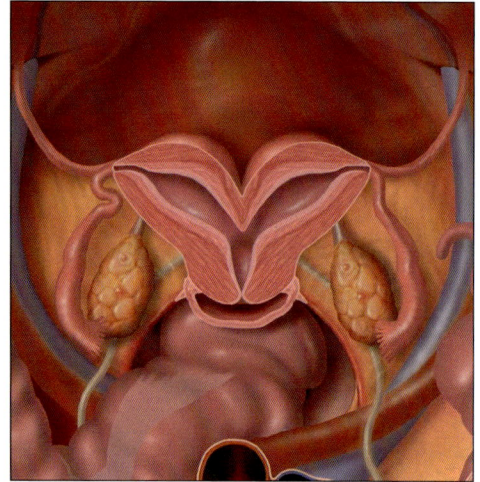

Graphic of a bicornuate uterus shows incomplete fusion of fundal myometrium with cleft separating divergent, symmetric horns. There is communication of the caudal segment of the endometrial cavities.

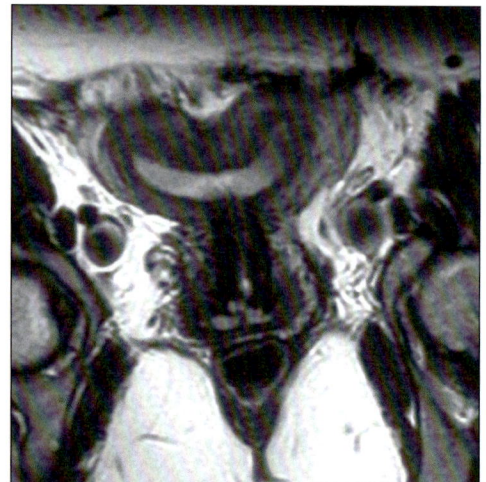

Axial T2WI MR shows a bicornuate unicollis uterus. Note the symmetry and normal zonal anatomy of each horn. There is wide communication of the endometrial cavities.

TERMINOLOGY

Definitions
- Class IV Müllerian duct anomaly (MDA)
  - Based on Buttram & Gibbons/American Fertility Society (AFS) classification system
  - Complete (IVa): Fundal cleft extending to internal cervical os
  - Partial (IVb): Fundal cleft variable in length, ending proximal to internal os
- Incomplete fusion of fundal myometrium with two symmetric, communicating uterine horns

IMAGING FINDINGS

General Features
- Best diagnostic clue
  - Fundal cleft > 1 cm separating divergent, symmetric uterine horns
  - Uterine horns symmetric in size and appearance
  - Communication between uterine horns must be present to make diagnosis
    - Most commonly at proximal isthmus
- Morphology
  - Bicornuate unicollis: Solitary cervix
  - Bicornuate bicollis: Duplicated cervix
    - Communication at endometrial or endocervical level; uncommonly may only be fenestrations

Radiographic Findings
- Radiography
  - Hysterosalpingography (HSG)
    - Fusiform symmetric uterine cavities, tapering at cornua, ending each in one fallopian tube
    - Significant overlap of findings with septate uterus
    - High divergence angle (> 105°) between opacified endometrial cavities suggestive of bicornuate uterus
    - Acute angle (< 75°) between uterine horns suggestive of septate uterus
    - Intercornual distance > 4 cm favoring bicornuate uterus
  - Pitfall: Secondary distortion and widening of divergence angles with septal adenomyosis or insinuated leiomyoma
  - Accuracy of HSG for differentiating septate from bicornuate uterus: 55%

DDx: Mimics of Bicornuate Uterus

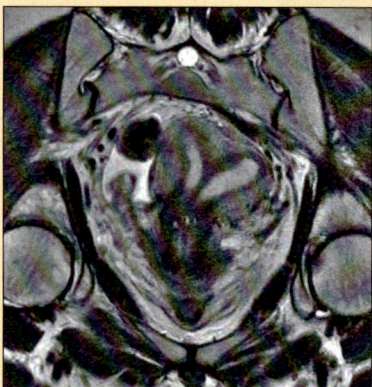

Septate Uterus

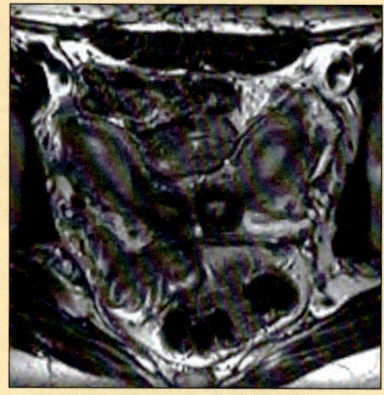

Uterus Didelphys

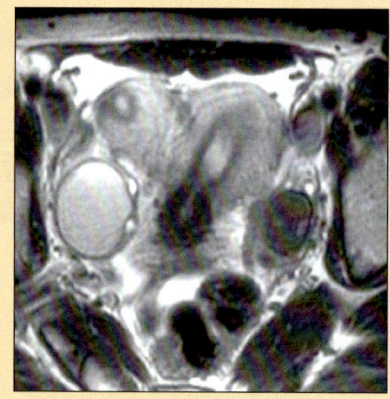

Unicornuate, Rudimentary Horn

BICORNUATE

Key Facts

Terminology
- Class IV Müllerian duct anomaly (MDA)
- Based on Buttram & Gibbons/American Fertility Society (AFS) classification system
- Complete (IVa): Fundal cleft extending to internal cervical os
- Partial (IVb): Fundal cleft variable in length, ending proximal to internal os

Imaging Findings
- Fundal cleft > 1 cm separating divergent, symmetric uterine horns
- Uterine horns symmetric in size and appearance
- Communication between uterine horns must be present to make diagnosis
- Bicornuate unicollis: Solitary cervix
- Bicornuate bicollis: Duplicated cervix

Top Differential Diagnoses
- Septate Uterus
- Uterus Didelphys
- Complex Duplication Anomaly
- Unicornuate with Rudimentary Horn
- Arcuate Uterus

Clinical Issues
- Adverse reproductive outcomes: Increased rates of spontaneous abortions and premature deliveries
- Significant improvement in reproductive capacity and fetal survival rates after metroplasty

Diagnostic Checklist
- Distinction from septate uterus critical due to different surgical treatments

---

- Accuracy improved if contrast spilled from tubes is used to outline fundal contour spilled from tubes
- Accuracy increased to 90% if combined with sonohysterography

Ultrasonographic Findings
- Grayscale Ultrasound
  - True orthogonal view along the long axis essential for diagnosis
    - Large fundal cleft > 1 cm
    - Fundal indentation of external contour below, or ≤ 5 mm above interostial line
  - Widely divergent, symmetric, normal appearing echogenic endometrial complexes
  - Endometrial complexes convergent at caudal extent
  - Echogenicity of tissue separating horns identical to myometrium
  - Pitfall: Extreme anteflexion or retroflexion and co-existing fundal leiomyomas causing convexity of fundal contour
  - Accuracy of transvaginal ultrasound (TVS): 90-92%

MR Findings
- T1WI: Inferior portion of septum low signal intensity (SI) if fibrous
- T2WI
  - Uterine horns separated by intervening cleft in external fundal myometrium > 1.0 cm
    - Measured from apex of fundal cleft to the line connecting serosal contour of uterine horns
  - Symmetric uterine horns, each with normal circumferential zonal anatomy
    - Communication between endometrial or endocervical canal essential for diagnosis
  - SI of the tissue separating the horns identical to myometrium on all sequences
    - Low SI of inferior portion of septum if fibrous
  - Accuracy of MR: 100%

Imaging Recommendations
- Best imaging tool
  - 2D and 3D ultrasound can be used as initial imaging modality
  - MR modality of choice in patients with adverse reproductive outcomes: 100% accuracy for differentiating septate from bicornuate uterus, and bicornuate from complex duplication anomaly
    - Optimal assessment of co-existing uterine pathologies affecting fertility (leiomyomas, adenomyosis, endometriosis)
- Protocol advice
  - Phased array body coil
  - Single shot fast spin echo (SSFSE) coronal T2WI through abdomen and pelvis to assess kidneys
  - High resolution FSE T2WI, ≤ 4 mm slice thickness
    - Imaging plane parallel to long axis of uterus to assess fundal cleft
  - T1WI parallel to the long axis for characterization of external uterine contour, if not well-delineated on T2WI

DIFFERENTIAL DIAGNOSIS

Septate Uterus
- Fused external fundal myometrium
- External uterine contour convex, flat or concave < 1.0 cm

Uterus Didelphys
- Near complete duplication of uterus
- Normal zonal anatomy of corpus and cervix within each hemiuterus
- No communication between endometrial cavities

Complex Duplication Anomaly
- Comprise features of more than one class of MDAs
- Most common scenario: Degree of nonfusion less than didelphys, greater than bicornuate uterus
  - May result in a "bicornuate configuration" of uterine horns without a communicating segment

Unicornuate with Rudimentary Horn
- Asymmetric uterine horns
- Diminutive rudimentary horn with small, contracted endometrial segment

BICORNUATE

Arcuate Uterus
- Fused external fundal myometrium
- Mild indentation of myometrium on endometrial cavity

PATHOLOGY

General Features
- Genetics
  - Majority of cases sporadic or multifactorial in nature
  - Occasional associated syndromes
    - Autosomal dominant syndromes: Apert
    - Autosomal recessive syndromes: Donahue (Leprechaunism), Fraser, Fryns, Meckel, Roberts, Rüdiger
  - 46 XX female karyotype
- Etiology
  - Abnormality of lateral fusion of normally developed Müllerian (paramesonephric) ducts
    - Incomplete fusion of cephalad extent of uterovaginal horns
- Epidemiology: Accounts for 10% of MDAs
- Associated abnormalities
  - Highest association with cervical incompetence (38%) among MDAs
  - Associated anomalies due to defects of vertical fusion, mesonephric induction and uterovaginal septum resorption
    - Renal anomalies, most commonly agenesis
    - Associated longitudinal vaginal septa in 25%
    - Occasional association with transverse vaginal septa

Gross Pathologic & Surgical Features
- Two uterine horns, each with uterine cavity, endometrium, myometrium, and covering serosa

Microscopic Features
- Septum comprised of either myometrium, or myometrium and fibrous tissue combined
  - Septum covered by normal functional endometrium

Staging, Grading or Classification Criteria
- Complete versus partial
- Unicollis versus bicollis

CLINICAL ISSUES

Presentation
- Most common signs/symptoms
  - Adverse reproductive outcomes: Increased rates of spontaneous abortions and premature deliveries
    - Greater with complete than partial configuration
    - Spontaneous abortion rate: 30%
    - Preterm birth rate: 20%
    - Fetal survival rate: 60%

Natural History & Prognosis
- Asymptomatic during childhood or at puberty if unaccompanied by obstruction
- Minimal, if any impact on fertility in absence of extrauterine causes
- Increasing length of subsequent gestations with increasing parity
- Significant improvement in reproductive capacity and fetal survival rates after metroplasty

Treatment
- Prophylactic cervical cerclage in selected patients associated with increased fetal survival rates
- Hysteroscopic partial restoration of uterine cavity in partial bicornuate uterus
- Metroplasty (variation of Strassman) using a hysteroscopic and laparoscopic approach reserved for patients with recurrent second- and third-trimester pregnancy loss
  - Wedge resection of medial aspect of each uterine horn with subsequent unification of cavities
  - No increased risk of complications in subsequent pregnancies

DIAGNOSTIC CHECKLIST

Consider
- Distinction from septate uterus critical due to different surgical treatments

Image Interpretation Pearls
- External uterine contour crucial for differentiating septate from bicornuate uterus
- Mild concavity (≤ 1 cm) of external uterine contour not to be construed as "partial" bicornuate configuration

SELECTED REFERENCES

1. Papp Z et al: Reproductive performance after transabdominal metroplasty: a review of 157 consecutive cases. J Reprod Med. 51(7):544-52, 2006
2. Troiano RN et al: Mullerian duct anomalies: imaging and clinical issues. Radiology. 233(1):19-34, 2004
3. Troiano RN: Magnetic resonance imaging of mullerian duct anomalies of the uterus. Top Magn Reson Imaging. 14(4):269-79, 2003
4. Grimbizis GF et al: Clinical implications of uterine malformations and hysteroscopic treatment results. Hum Reprod Update. 7(2):161-74, 2001
5. Ascher SM: MR imaging of the female pelvis: the time has come. Radiographics. 18(4):931-45, 1998
6. Wu MH et al: Detection of congenital mullerian duct anomalies using three-dimensional ultrasound. J Clin Ultrasound. 25(9):487-92, 1997
7. Pellerito JS et al: Diagnosis of uterine anomalies: relative accuracy of MR imaging, endovaginal sonography, and hysterosalpingography. Radiology. 183(3):795-800, 1992
8. Carrington BM et al: Mullerian duct anomalies: MR imaging evaluation. Radiology. 176(3):715-20, 1990
9. Fedele L et al: Magnetic resonance evaluation of double uteri. Obstet Gynecol. 74(6):844-7, 1989
10. Reuter KL et al: Septate versus bicornuate uteri: errors in imaging diagnosis. Radiology. 172(3):749-52, 1989

BICORNUATE

IMAGE GALLERY

Typical

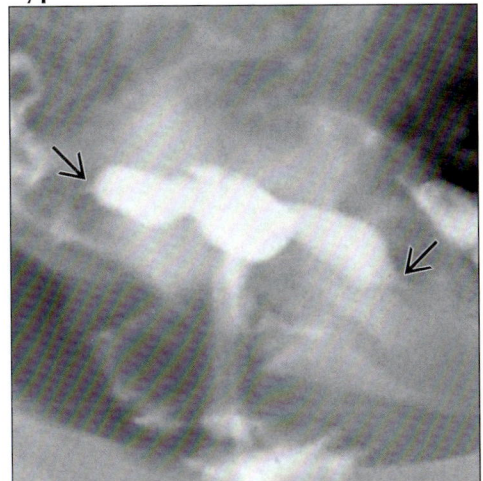
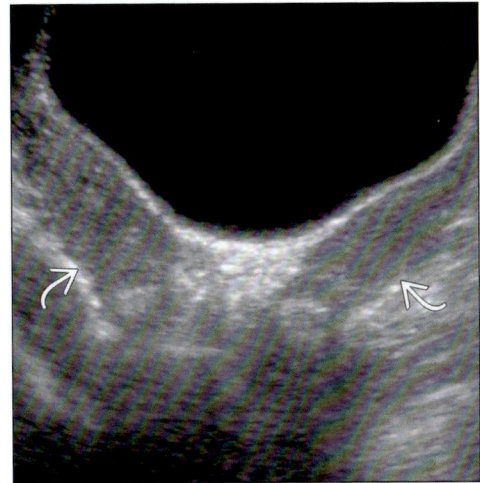

(Left) Coronal hysterosalpingogram shows widely divergent (> 105° and > 4 cm) symmetric uterine horns with connecting endometrial cavities inferiorly. Each cornua communicates with the corresponding right and left fallopian tube ➡. *(Right)* Axial transabdominal ultrasound in the same patient as previous image, shows symmetric uterine horns ➡ widely diverging. The communicating endometrial segments are not shown.

Typical

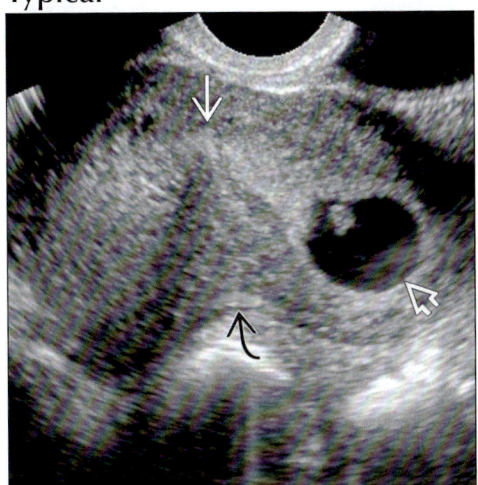
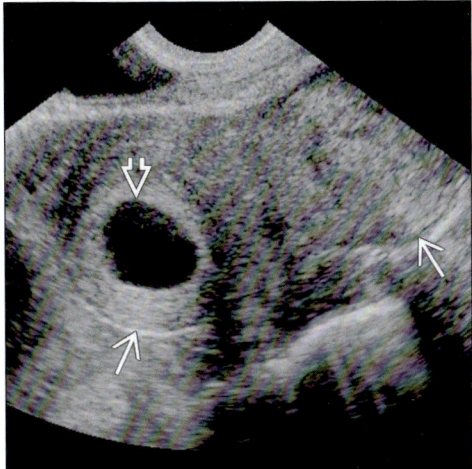

(Left) Axial transvaginal ultrasound shows a large fundal cleft ➡ with communicating ➡ uterine cavities and a gestational sac ➡ within the left uterine horn. *(Right)* Axial transvaginal ultrasound at the level of the mid-corpus shows two symmetric uterine horns ➡, with a gestational sac ➡ within the right uterine horn of a bicornuate uterus.

Typical

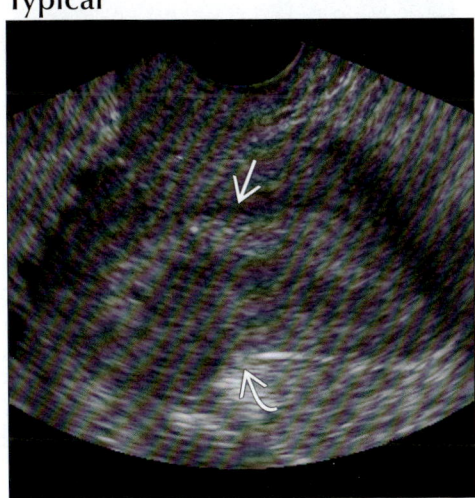
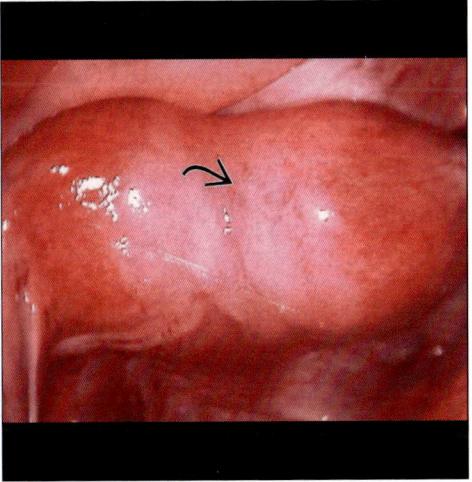

(Left) Axial transvaginal ultrasound shows a large fundal cleft ➡, symmetric uterine horns and connecting endometrial cavities ➡. These findings are characteristic of a bicornuate uterus. *(Right)* Intra-operative laparoscopic photograph shows a deep fundal cleft ➡ and normal-appearing symmetric uterine horns characteristic of a bicornuate uterus. *(Courtesy T. Tulandi, MD).*

BICORNUATE

Typical

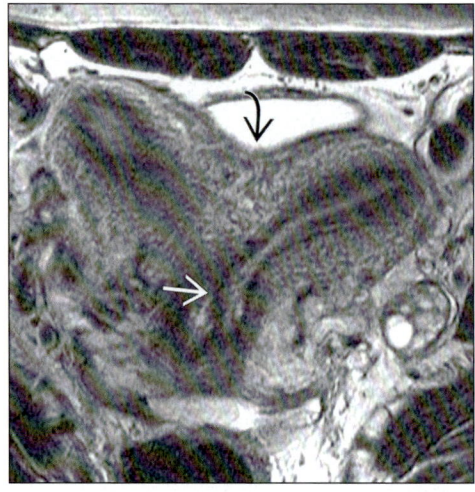 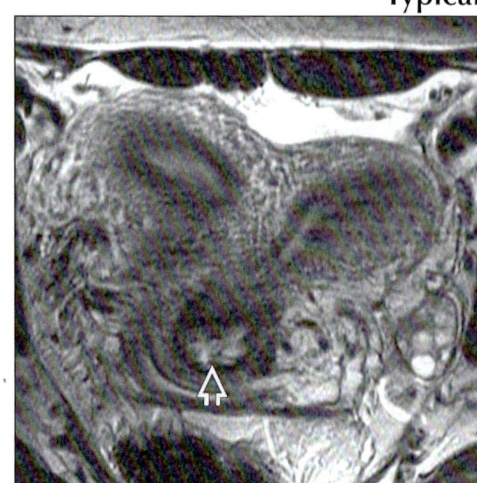

(Left) Axial oblique T2WI MR shows a deep fundal cleft (> 1 cm) ➔ in a patient with symmetric duplication of the uterine horns. The septum extends to the level of the cervix ➔. The degree of fusion is more than expected for a didelphys uterus. (Right) Axial oblique T2WI MR in the same patient as previous image, shows the communication of the two horns more caudally at the level of the endocervical canal ➔ consistent with a bicornuate uterus.

Typical

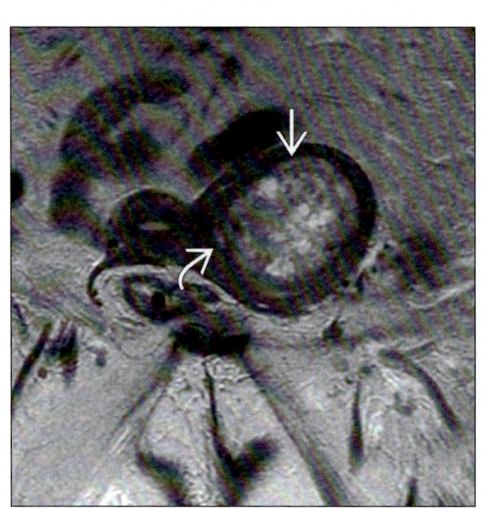 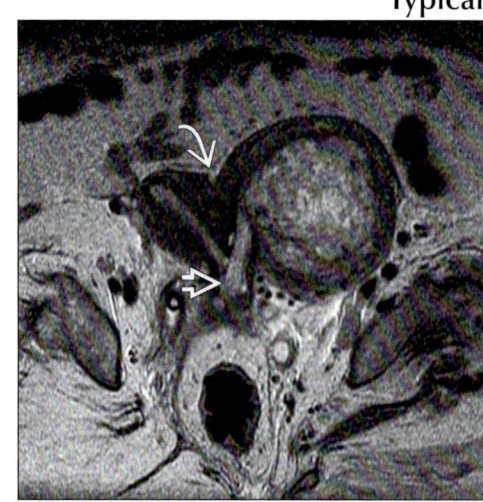

(Left) Coronal oblique T2WI MR shows a bicornuate uterus with a normal right horn. The left horn is enlarged due to a myometrial leiomyoma ➔, which displaces the corresponding endometrial cavity medially ➔. (Right) Axial oblique T2WI MR (long-axis view) in the same patient as previous image, shows the fundal cleft ➔ and interconnecting endometrial cavities ➔ diagnostic of a bicornuate uterus.

Typical

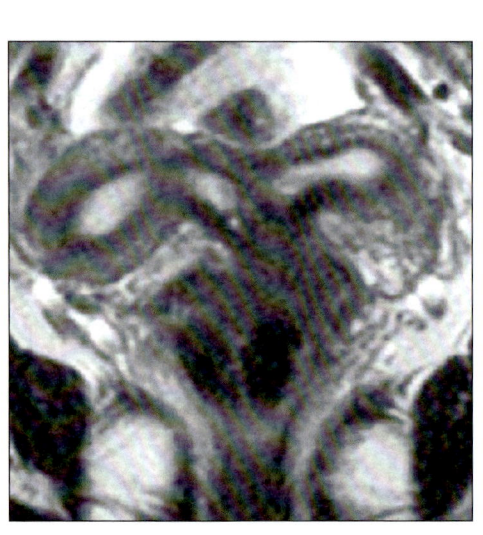 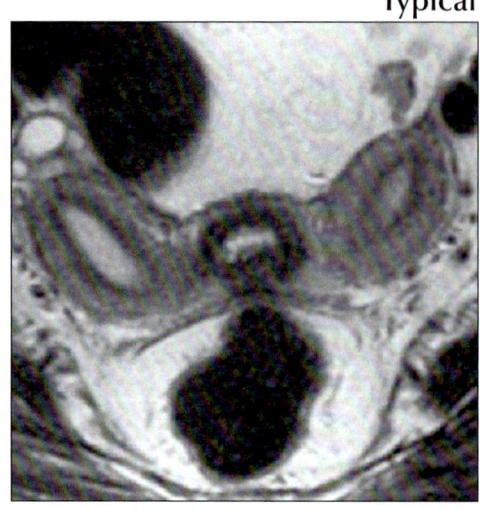

(Left) Coronal T2WI MR shows fundal duplication of the uterine horns with fusion of the caudal uterine body and cervix. There is a wide intervening fundal cleft with significant divergence of the uterine horns. (Right) Coronal T2WI MR acquired more caudally in the same patient as previous image, illustrates communication of the endocervical canals.

BICORNUATE

Typical

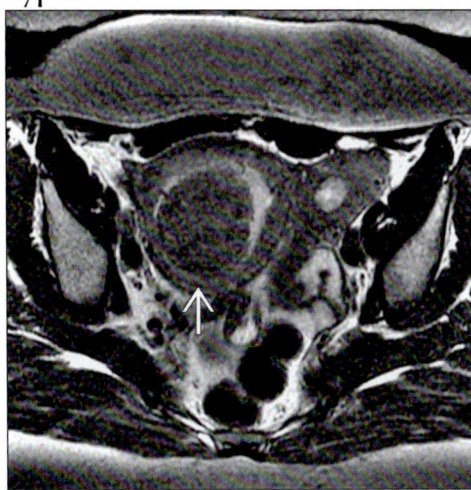
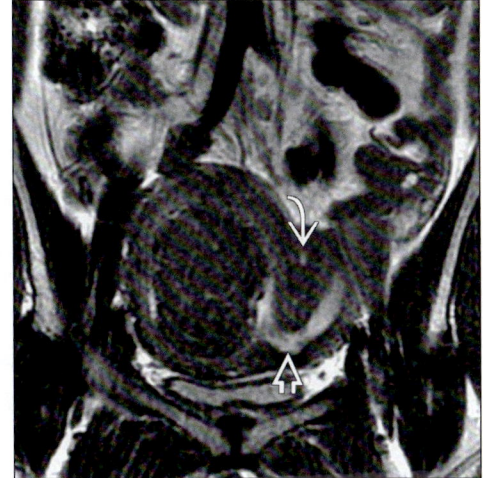

(Left) Axial T2WI MR shows the right endometrial cavity expanded by a submucosal leiomyoma ➡. The left horn has normal zonal anatomy. *(Right)* Coronal oblique T2WI MR (long-axis view) in the same patient as previous image, shows the caudal communication of the endometrial cavities ➡ and partial effacement of the deep fundal cleft ➡ due to the mass effect exerted by the leiomyoma.

Typical

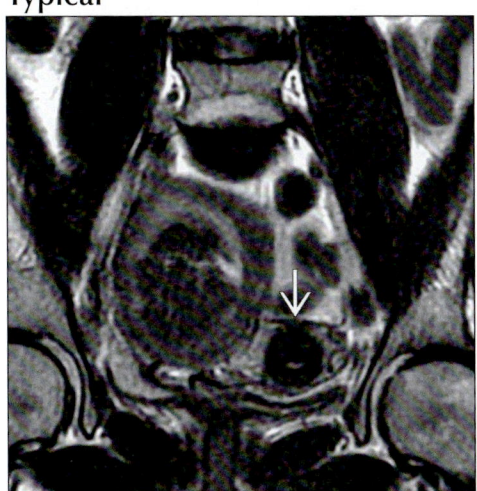
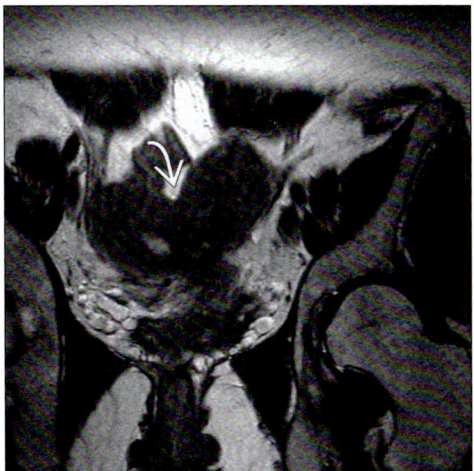

(Left) Coronal T2WI MR in the preceding patient, acquired more posteriorly, shows the expanded right horn and solitary cervix ➡ consistent with a bicornuate unicollis uterus. *(Right)* Coronal oblique T2WI MR shows a deep fundal cleft ➡ and symmetric uterine horns.

Typical

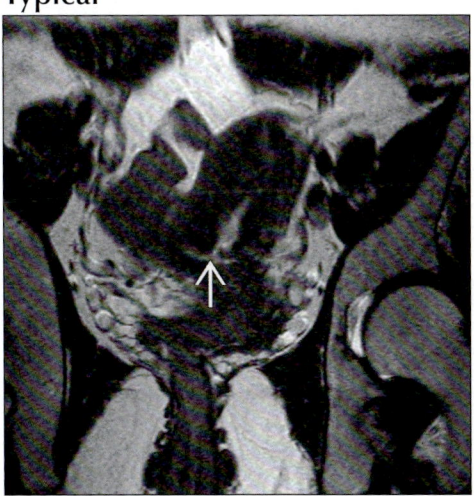
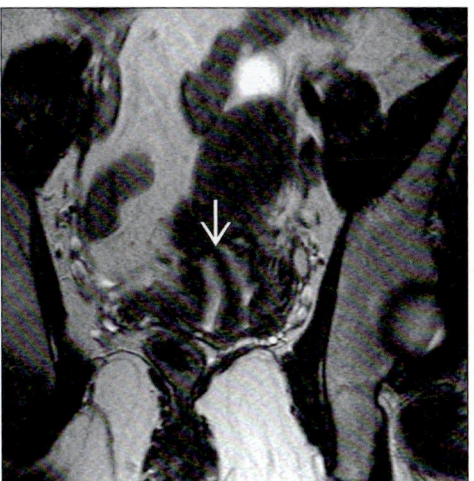

(Left) Coronal oblique T2WI MR in the preceding patient, acquired more posteriorly, shows communication of the endometrial cavities ➡ at the level of the lower uterine segment. *(Right)* Coronal oblique T2WI MR in the same patient as previous image, shows the septum ➡ extending down into the cervix, classifying this as a bicornute bicollis uterus.

SEPTATE

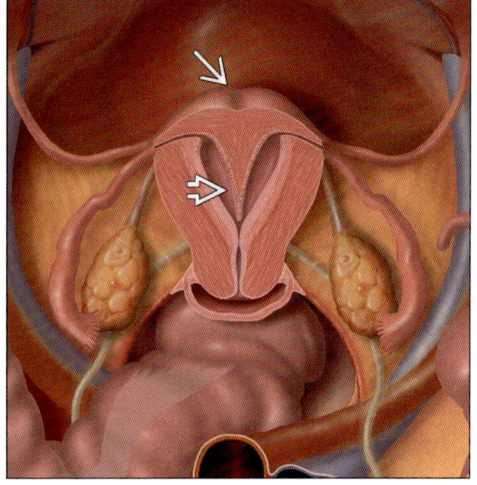

Coronal graphic shows complete fusion of the fundal myometrium with a slight concavity of the external contour ➡. This is a partial septate with the septum ➡ approaching the internal os.

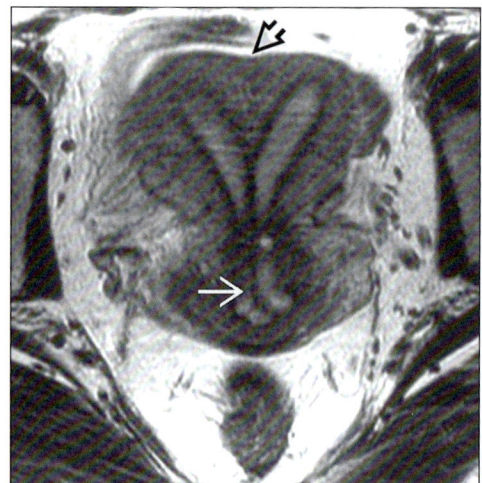

Axial oblique T2WI MR shows a complete septate uterus with a nearly flat fundal contour ➡ and a septum that extends to the external os ➡.

TERMINOLOGY

Definitions
- Class V Müllerian duct anomaly (MDA) based on Buttram & Gibbons & American Fertility Society (AFS) classification systems
- Incomplete resorption of medial uterovaginal septum
  ○ Complete: Septum extends to the external os
  ○ Partial: Variable length septum ending proximal to external cervical os
- Most common MDA

IMAGING FINDINGS

General Features
- Best diagnostic clue
  ○ **Midline septum with fusion of fundal myometrium**
    ▪ Uterine fundal contour is flat, convex or mildly concave ≤ 1 cm
    ▪ Complete: Septum extends to external cervical os
    ▪ Partial: Variable length septum
    ▪ Symmetric small & narrow endometrial cavities
- Size: Normal size uterus, but each endometrial cavity is narrower & smaller than normal
- Morphology
  ○ External uterine fundal contour: Convex, flat or concave ≤ 1 cm
  ○ Septum arises midline in fundus
  ○ Superior segment of septum is myometrial in composition
  ○ Inferior segment of septum is fibrous
    ▪ Complete: All with inferior fibrous septum
    ▪ Partial: Small subset with inferior fibrous septum
  ○ Endometrial cavities are narrower & smaller
  ○ Extension of septum to upper 1/3 vagina in 25%
  ○ Duplication of cervix with complete septa included in classification

Radiographic Findings
- Hysterosalpingography (HSG) findings
  ○ Symmetric endometrial cavities that are narrower & smaller than normal
  ○ Significant degree of overlap of findings with bicornuate uterus
    ▪ Acute angle (< 75°) between opacified endometrial cavities suggestive of septate uterus

DDx: Septate Uterus

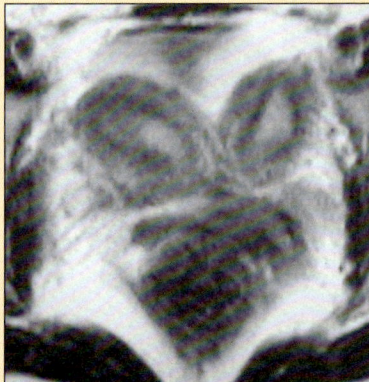

Bicornuate Uterus

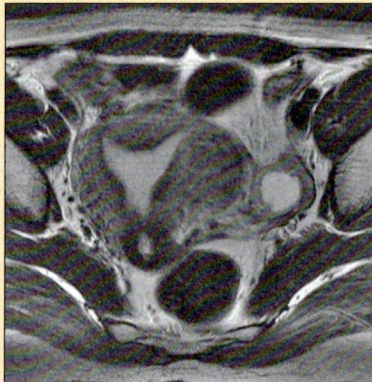

Arcuate Uterus

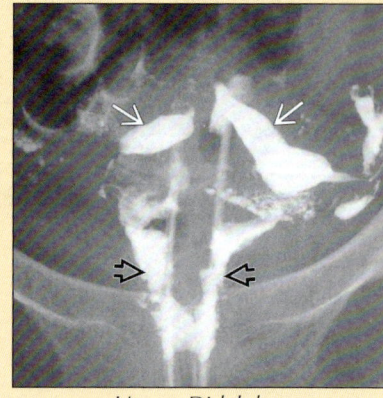

Uterus Didelphys

SEPTATE

Key Facts

Terminology
- Class V Müllerian duct anomaly (MDA) based on Buttram & Gibbons & American Fertility Society (AFS) classification systems
- Incomplete resorption of medial uterovaginal septum

Imaging Findings
- **Midline septum with fusion of fundal myometrium**
- Uterine fundal contour is flat, convex or mildly concave ≤ 1 cm
- Complete: Septum extends to external cervical os
- Partial: Variable length septum
- Symmetric small & narrow endometrial cavities
- **T2 MR is the most accurate imaging modality**
- Oblique imaging parallel to long axis of uterus to obtain true fundal contour
- Coronal large field of view of the body to assess if associated renal anomalies

Top Differential Diagnoses
- Bicornuate Uterus
- Arcuate Uterus
- Didelphys Uterus

Clinical Issues
- Worst obstetric outcome of all MDA's
- **Reproductive outcome after hysteroscopic septal resection is good**
- Spontaneous abortion rate: 6%
- Successful delivery rate: 85%

Diagnostic Checklist
- Distinction from bicornuate uterus critical due to different surgical treatments

---

- Intercornual distance < 4.0 cm favors a septate uterus but is unreliable
  - HSG accuracy for diagnosis of septate uterus: 29%
    - Accuracy of HSG for differentiating septate from bicornuate uterus: 55%

Ultrasonographic Findings
- Transvaginal ultrasound (TVS) findings
  - Echogenic endometrial cavities separated by intermediate echogenicity of fundal myometrium in all partial and fundal segments of complete septa, corresponding to myometrial component
  - Inferior segment hypoechoic in complete septa corresponding to fibrous component
  - Fundal indentation > 5 mm over interostial line (line drawn between apices of endometrial cavities at ostia on true orthogonal view)
  - Accuracy: 92%; sensitivity: 100%; specificity 80%
- 3-D sonohysterography to improve visualization of external & internal uterine features

MR Findings
- T2WI
  - Imaging performed parallel to long axis of uterus to characterize external uterine fundal contour
  - External uterine contour convex, flat, or concavity ≤ 1 cm
  - Superior segment of septum is isointense with myometrium
    - Includes: All partial septae uteri & fundal portion of complete septate uteri
  - Inferior segment of septum is low signal intensity (SI)
    - Includes: All complete septate uteri & small subset of partial septate uteri
  - Symmetric small & narrow endometrial canals
  - Complete duplication of normal cervical zonal anatomy in complete septa with 2 cervices
  - Accuracy: 100%; sensitivity: 100%; specificity: 100%
- T1 C+: May help define uterine fundal contour if difficult to identify on T2 WI because of bowel applied to the uterus

Imaging Recommendations
- Best imaging tool
  - T2 MR is the most accurate imaging modality
  - Role of 3-D sonohysterography emerging
- Protocol advice
  - High resolution FSE T2 WI
  - Phased array body coil
  - Oblique imaging parallel to long axis of uterus to obtain true fundal contour
  - Coronal large field of view of the body to assess if associated renal anomalies

DIFFERENTIAL DIAGNOSIS

Bicornuate Uterus
- Non-fusion fundal myometrium
- Intervening cleft > 1.0 cm

Arcuate Uterus
- Mild indentation of fundal myometrium on endometrial cavity
- Defining depth to differentiate arcuate from broad septum not established
- Variable obstetric outcomes reported

Didelphys Uterus
- Near complete duplication of uterus
- Normal zonal anatomy of corpus & cervix within each hemiuterus
- No communication between endometrial canals

Unicornuate Uterus with Rudimentary Horn
- Asymmetric uterine horns
- Fundal cleft typically > 1 cm

PATHOLOGY

General Features
- General path comments: Length of septum does not correlate with obstetric outcome
- Genetics

SEPTATE

- ○ Majority of MDA's are considered sporadic or multifactorial
- ○ Polygenic & genetic patterns of inheritance have been described in the expression of MDA's
  - ▪ Absence of Bcl-22 gene has been implicated in persistence of uterine septum
- Etiology: Unknown, but likely multifactorial with both extrauterine & intrauterine environmental factors
- Epidemiology: Most common Müllerian duct anomaly: Approximately 55%

Gross Pathologic & Surgical Features
- Fundal contour is flat, convex or mildly concave
- Morphologic narrowing of the endometrial cavity by septum

Microscopic Features
- Deficient septal composition
  - ○ Increased amount of muscular tissue: Perhaps leading to increased contractility
  - ○ Decreased connective tissue: May result in poor decidualization
- Septal endometrium is irregular by electron microscopy

Staging, Grading or Classification Criteria
- Complete
- Partial

CLINICAL ISSUES

Presentation
- Most common signs/symptoms
  - ○ Recurrent pregnancy loss
    - ▪ Spontaneous abortion rate: 32-94% (65% pooled)
    - ▪ Etiology: Increased contractility, poor decidualization and/or reduction in endometrial capacity
- Other signs/symptoms: Increased incidence of renal anomalies

Natural History & Prognosis
- Worst obstetric outcome of all MDA's
- Reproductive outcome before surgery is poor
  - ○ Spontaneous abortion rate: 65%
  - ○ Preterm birth rate: 20%
  - ○ Fetal survival rate: 30%
- **Reproductive outcome after hysteroscopic septal resection is good**
  - ○ Spontaneous abortion rate: 6%
  - ○ Successful delivery rate: 85%

Treatment
- Hysteroscopic resection of septum with history of poor reproductive outcome
- Residual septum < 1 cm following resection considered optimal

DIAGNOSTIC CHECKLIST

Image Interpretation Pearls
- Duplication of endometrial cavity with fusion of fundal myometrium leading to a flat, convex or mildly concave fundal contour is diagnostic
- Distinction from bicornuate uterus critical due to different surgical treatments

SELECTED REFERENCES

1. Takeuchi M et al: Pathologies of the uterine endometrial cavity: usual and unusual manifestations and pitfalls on magnetic resonance imaging. Eur Radiol. 15(11):2244-55, 2005
2. Patton PE et al: The diagnosis and reproductive outcome after surgical treatment of the complete septate uterus, duplicated cervix and vaginal septum. Am J Obstet Gynecol. 190(6):1669-75; discussion 1675-8, 2004
3. Marten K et al: MRI in the evaluation of mullerian duct anomalies. Clin Imaging. 27(5):346-50, 2003
4. Takagi H et al: Magnetic resonance imaging in the evaluating of double uterus and associated urinary tract anomalies: a report of five cases. J Obstet Gynaecol. 23(5):525-7, 2003
5. Byrne J et al: Prevalence of Mullerian duct anomalies detected at ultrasound. Am J Med Genet. 94(1):9-12, 2000
6. Kupesic S et al: Septate uterus: detection and prediction of obstetrical complications by different forms of ultrasonography. J Ultrasound Med. 17(10):631-6, 1998
7. Lee DM et al: Localization of Bcl-2 in the human fetal mullerian tract. Fertil Steril. 70(1):135-40, 1998
8. Zreik TG et al: Myometrial tissue in uterine septa. J Am Assoc Gynecol Laparosc. 5(2):155-60, 1998
9. Letterie GS et al: A comparison of pelvic ultrasound and magnetic resonance imaging as diagnostic studies for mullerian tract abnormalities. Int J Fertil Menopausal Stud. 40(1):34-8, 1995
10. Ozsarlak O et al: Septate uterus: hysterosalpingography and magnetic resonance imaging findings. Eur J Radiol. 21(2):122-5, 1995
11. Woodward PJ et al: Congenital uterine malformations. Curr Probl Diagn Radiol. 24(5):178-97, 1995
12. Woodward PJ et al: MR imaging in the evaluation of female infertility. Radiographics. 13(2):293-310, 1993
13. Doyle MB: Magnetic resonance imaging in mullerian fusion defects. J Reprod Med. 37(1):33-8, 1992
14. Markham SM et al: Structural anomalies of the reproductive tract. Curr Opin Obstet Gynecol. 4(6):867-73, 1992
15. Pellerito JS et al: Diagnosis of uterine anomalies: relative accuracy of MR imaging, endovaginal sonography, and hysterosalpingography. Radiology. 183(3):795-800, 1992
16. Carrington BM et al: Mullerian duct anomalies: MR imaging evaluation. Radiology. 176(3):715-20, 1990
17. Fedele L et al: Magnetic resonance evaluation of double uteri. Obstet Gynecol. 74(6):844-7, 1989
18. Reuter KL et al: Septate versus bicornuate uteri: errors in imaging diagnosis. Radiology. 172(3):749-52, 1989
19. Buttram VC Jr et al: Mullerian anomalies: a proposed classification. (An analysis of 144 cases). Fertil Steril. 32(1):40-6, 1979

SEPTATE

IMAGE GALLERY

Typical

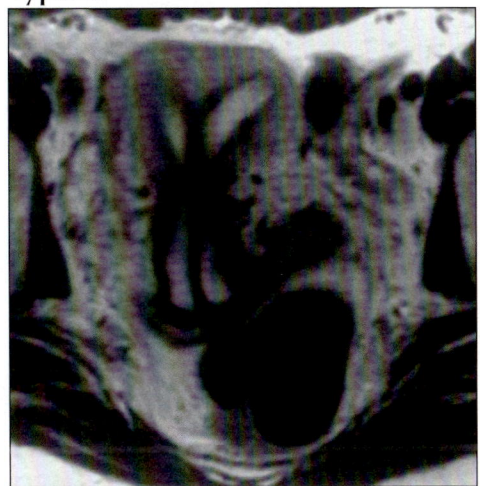
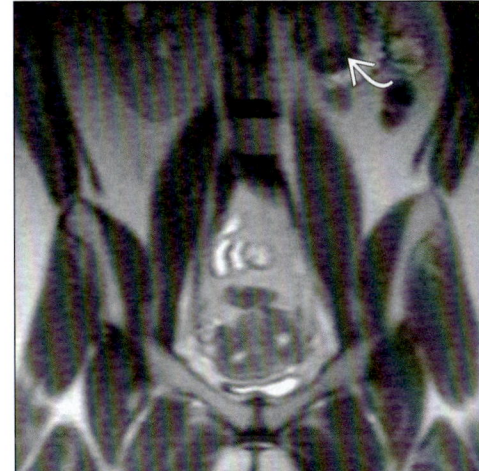

(Left) Axial oblique T2WI MR shows a complete septate uterus with a flat external fundal contour and primarily low signal intensity septum bisecting the endometrial and endocervical canals. *(Right)* Coronal T2WI MR in the same patient shows the two endometrial canals. The large field of view allows diagnosis of left renal agenesis with bowel occupying the renal fossa ➡.

Typical

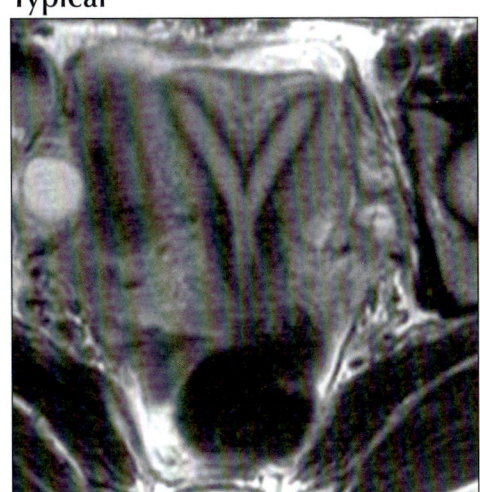
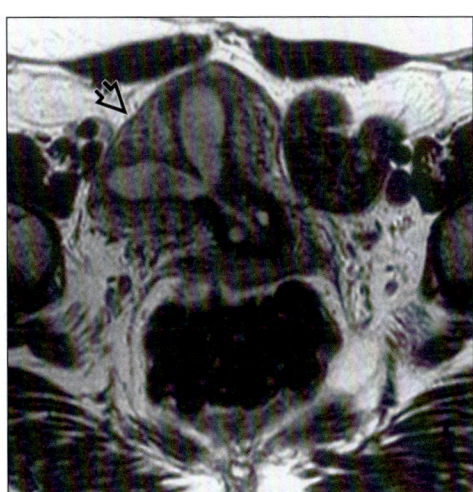

(Left) Axial oblique T2WI MR shows a partial septate uterus. Note that the upper portion of the septum is myometrial in composition. *(Right)* Axial oblique T2WI MR shows a partial septate uterus with a slightly convex fundal contour ➡.

Typical

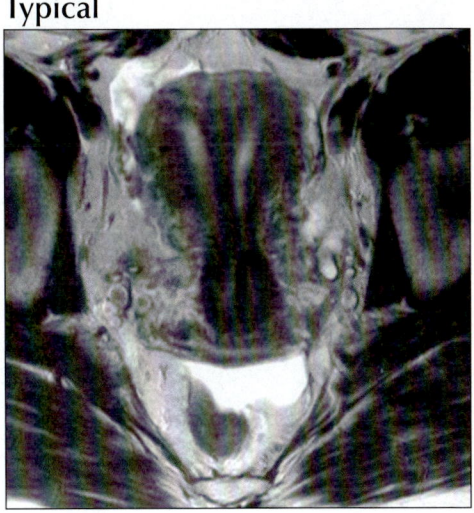
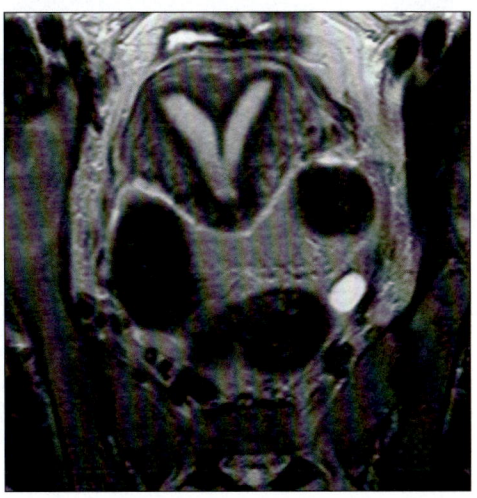

(Left) Axial oblique T2WI MR shows a complete septate uterus. The external fundal contour is flat. *(Right)* Axial oblique T2WI MR shows a patient with a partial septate uterus.

SEPTATE

(Left) Axial oblique T2WI FS MR shows a partial septate uterus. The septum is primarily myometrium. *(Right)* Coronal oblique radiograph HSG in a patient with a septate uterus shows a fundal cleft > 1.5 cm ➡ and an intercornual distance < 4 cm. There is significant overlap in the imaging features of a bicornate uterus.

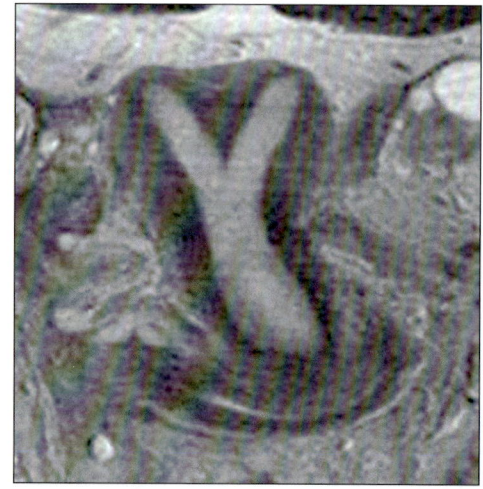
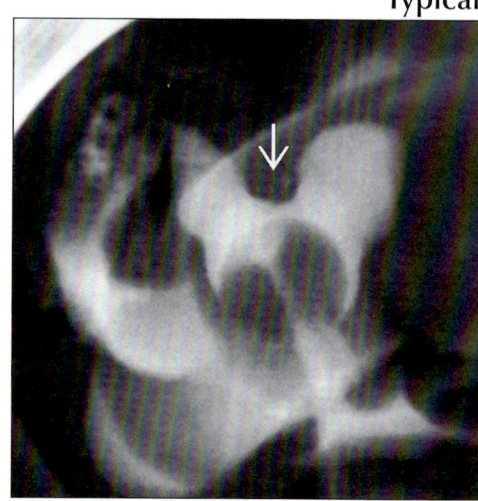

Typical

(Left) Axial oblique transvaginal ultrasound shows two separate endometrial canals in a patient with a septate uterus. A subtle intrauterine pregnancy is visible in the left horn ➡. *(Right)* Axial oblique transabdominal ultrasound shows minimal indentation of the fundal contour and two separate endometrial stripes.

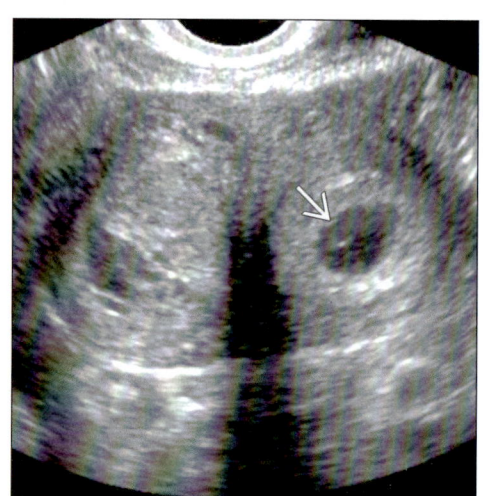
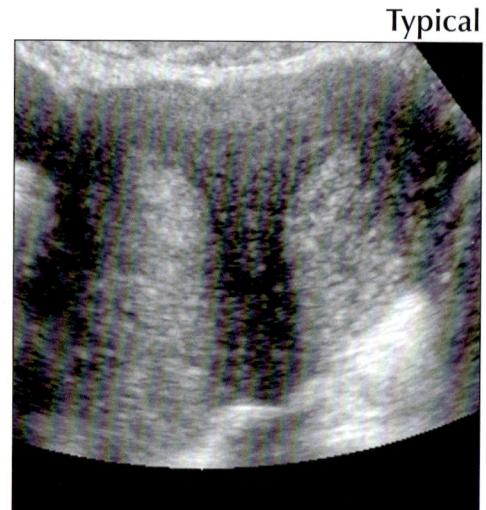

Typical

(Left) Coronal oblique 3D ultrasound performed after hysteroscopic saline infusion shows a slightly convex uterine fundal contour ➡ and distended fluid-filled endometrial canals ➡. *(Right)* Axial oblique 3D ultrasound following sonohysterography in the same patient shows the distended endometrial canals ➡. The fundal contour is not visualized in the plane.

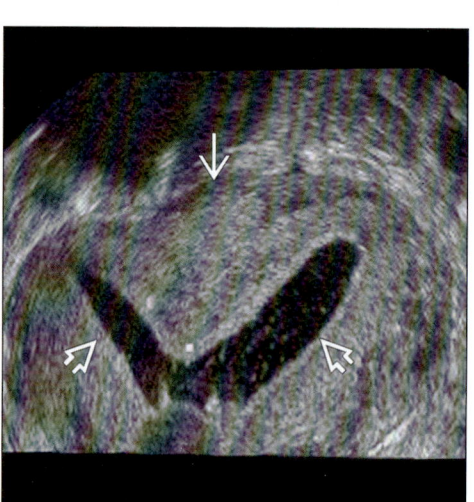
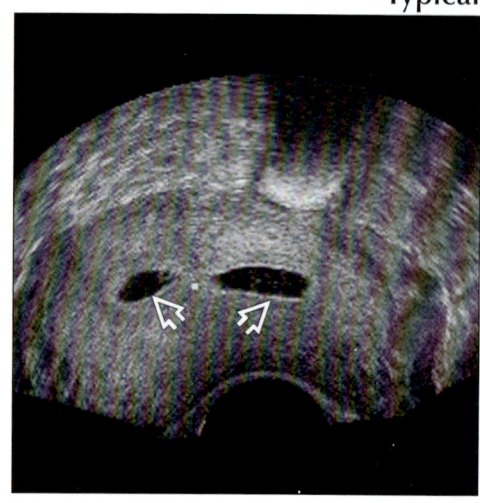

Typical

SEPTATE

Typical

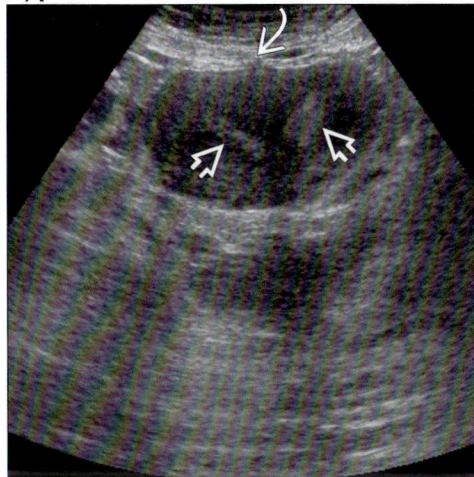
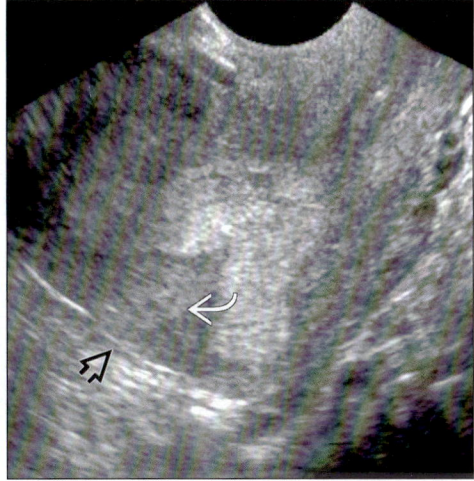

(Left) Coronal oblique transabdominal ultrasound shows two echogenic endometrial canals ⇨ with a straight fundal contour ➔ in a patient with a septate uterus. *(Right)* Coronal oblique transvaginal ultrasound shows a convex external fundal contour ➔ in a patient with a partial septate uterus. The septum ➔ has similar echogenicity as the normal endometrium.

Typical

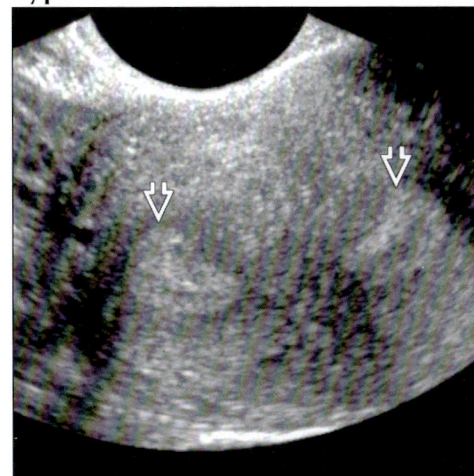
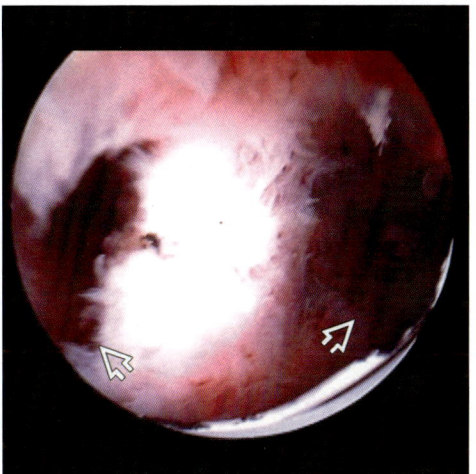

(Left) Axial oblique transvaginal ultrasound shows two echogenic endometrial horns ⇨ with intervening myometrium in a patient with a septate uterus. *(Right)* Axial oblique clinical photograph shows two endometrial cavities ⇨ separated by tissue in a patient with a septate uterus.

Variant

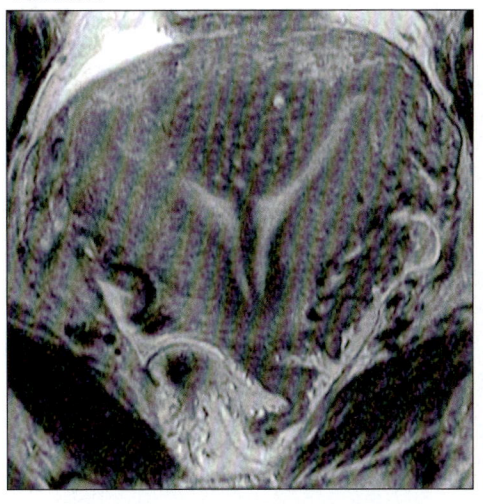
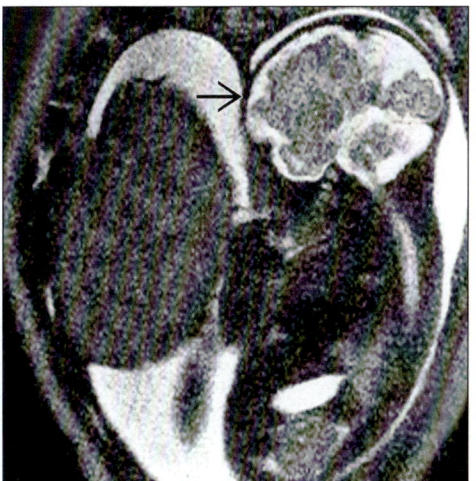

(Left) Coronal oblique T2WI MR shows a septate uterus with concomitant adenomyosis in the uterine fundus. *(Right)* Coronal T2WI MR shows an intrauterine pregnancy following hysteroscopic resection of a uterine septum. A remnant of the septum is visible ➔. The patient went on to deliver a term baby.

ARCUATE

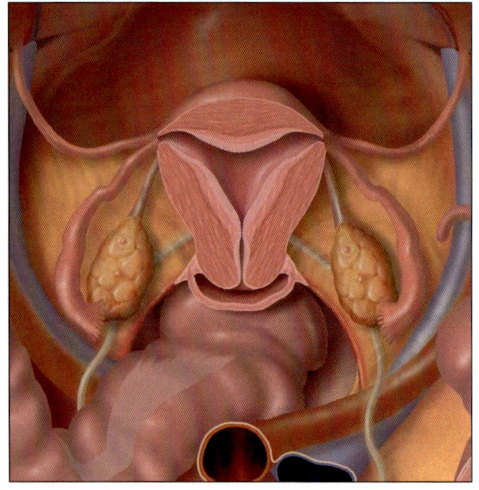

Graphic of an arcuate uterus shows mild thickening of the fundal myometrium causing a broad, smooth indentation on the endometrial cavity.

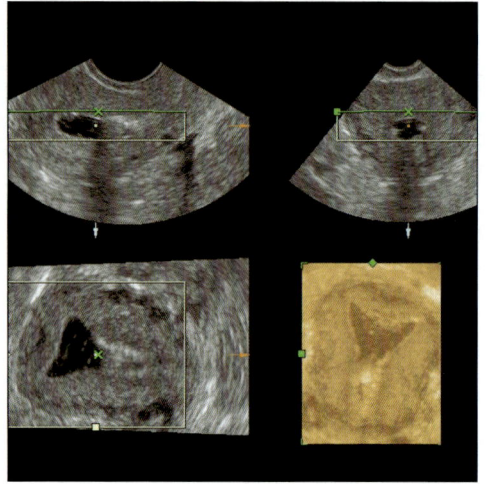

3D reconstruction from hysterosonogram showing arcuate uterus. Note the smooth external contour and only mild indentation of the endometrial cavity.

TERMINOLOGY

Definitions
- Class VI Müllerian duct anomaly (MDA)
  - Based on Buttram & Gibbons/American Fertility Society (AFS) classification system
  - Classification can be difficult: Normal variant versus true anomaly

IMAGING FINDINGS

General Features
- Best diagnostic clue: Mild, focal thickening of fundal myometrium with a fused external uterine contour
- Smooth, broad focal midline thickening of myometrium with minor indentation on endometrial cavity
- External uterine contour fused with fundal cleft ≤ 1.0 cm; outer contour convex or flat

Radiographic Findings
- Hysterosalpingography (HSG)
  - Single opacified endometrial cavity with broad, saddle-shaped indentation at uterine fundus
  - Ratio ≤ 10% between height of fundal indentation and distance between apices at uterine cornua

Ultrasonographic Findings
- Transvaginal ultrasound (TVS)
  - Normal external uterine contour on true orthogonal plane
  - Subtle, focal duplication of echogenic endometrial complexes on transverse plane at level of fundus
  - Smooth, broad fundal indentation, isoechoic to myometrium

MR Findings
- T2WI
  - Smooth, broad fundal indentation of endometrial complex, isointense to myometrium
  - No low signal intensity fibrous component present
  - Fused external uterine contour

Imaging Recommendations
- Best imaging tool: TVS and MR
- Protocol advice
  - High resolution FSE T2WI, ≤ 4 mm slice thickness

DDx: Mimics of Arcuate Uterus

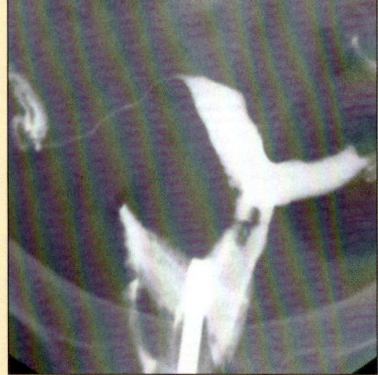

Corrected Septate Uterus

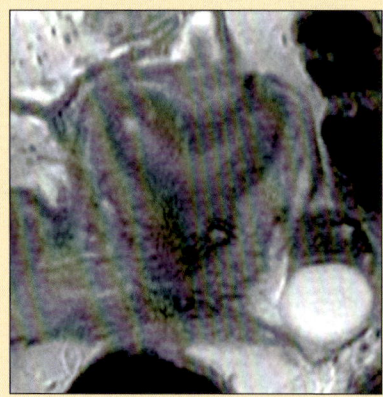

Partial Septate

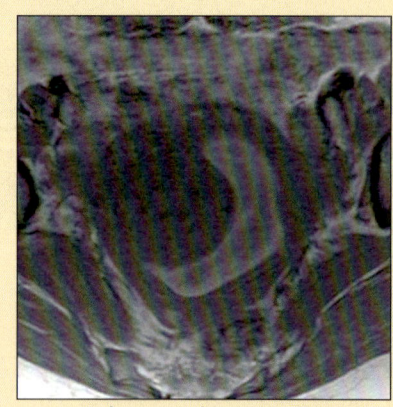

Submucosal Leiomyoma

ARCUATE

Key Facts

Terminology
- Class VI Müllerian duct anomaly (MDA)
- Classification can be difficult: Normal variant versus true anomaly

Imaging Findings
- Best diagnostic clue: Mild, focal thickening of fundal myometrium with a fused external uterine contour
- No low signal intensity fibrous component present

Top Differential Diagnoses
- Partial Septate Uterus
- Partial Bicornuate Uterus
- Submucosal Leiomyoma

Clinical Issues
- Data regarding reproductive outcomes very limited
- Generally compatible with normal term gestations; delivery rate of 85%

- Oblique imaging performed parallel to long axis of uterus

DIFFERENTIAL DIAGNOSIS

Partial Septate Uterus
- Fundal indentation of myometrium more extensive ± small caudal fibrous component

Partial Bicornuate Uterus
- Fundal myometrium divided by intervening cleft > 1.0 cm

Submucosal Leiomyoma
- Distortion/displacement of junctional zone on MR

PATHOLOGY

General Features
- Epidemiology: Accounts for 20% of MDAs

CLINICAL ISSUES

Presentation
- Most common signs/symptoms: Usually asymptomatic

Natural History & Prognosis
- Data regarding reproductive outcomes very limited
- Both good and poor reproductive outcomes reported
  - Generally compatible with normal term gestations; delivery rate of 85%
- Good reproductive outcome if ratio of < 10% between the height of the fundal indentation and distance between the lateral apices of the horns

Treatment
- Expectant management
- Hysteroscopic resection of prominent arcuate configuration in select patients with recurrent pregnancy loss and extrauterine factors for infertility excluded

DIAGNOSTIC CHECKLIST

Image Interpretation Pearls
- Mild focal thickening of fundal myometrium with a fused external uterine contour on T2WI

SELECTED REFERENCES
1. Troiano RN et al: Mullerian duct anomalies: imaging and clinical issues. Radiology. 2004
2. Gell JS: Mullerian anomalies. Semin Reprod Med. 2003
3. Scarsbrook AF et al: MRI appearances of mullerian duct abnormalities. Clin Radiol. 2003
4. Lin PC et al: Female genital anomalies affecting reproduction. Fertil Steril. 2002
5. Tulandi T et al: Arcuate and bicornuate uterine anomalies and infertility. Fertil Steril. 34(4):362-4, 1980

IMAGE GALLERY

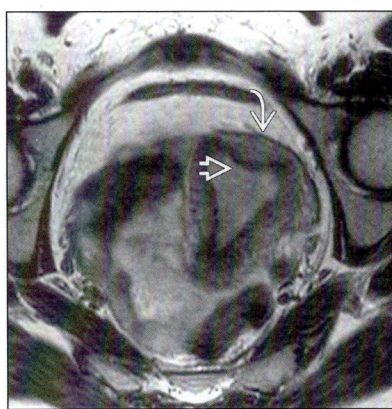 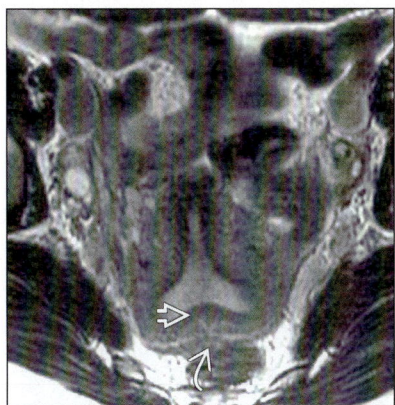 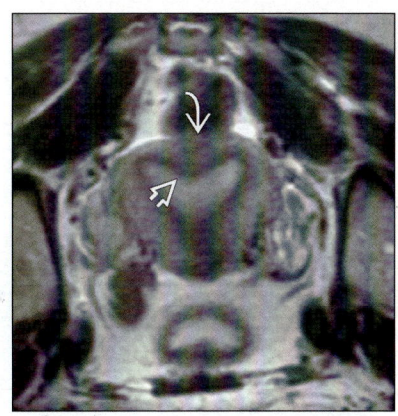

(Left) Axial T2WI MR (long-axis view) shows a patient with an arcuate uterus. Note the mild focal thickening of the fundal myometrium ➡ with a convex uterine contour ➡. *(Center)* Axial T2WI MR in a patient with a retroverted uterus shows an arcuate configuration of the endometrial cavity with focal myometrial thickening ➡ at the fundus. Note a small external fundal cleft ➡. *(Right)* Axial T2WI MR shows a broad midline thickening of the myometrium with only mild indentation of the endometrial cavity ➡. There is a convex outer uterine contour ➡.

DES-EXPOSED

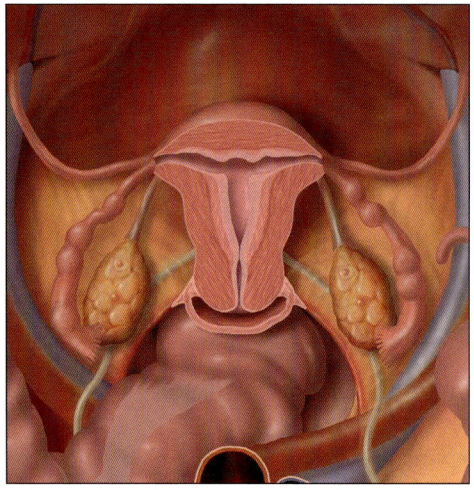

Graphic of DES-exposed uterus shows a small uterus with constriction bands and T-shaped configuration of the endometrial cavity. The fallopian tubes show sacculations and areas of narrowing at the fimbrial ends.

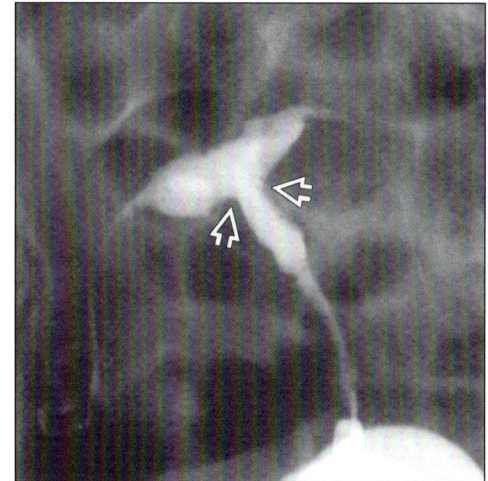

Anteroposterior hysterosalpingogram (HSG) shows the characteristic T-shape of the endometrial cavity with myometrial constriction bands ▸. (Courtesy S. McCarthy, MD).

TERMINOLOGY

Definitions
- Class VII Müllerian duct anomaly (MDA)
  - Based on Buttram & Gibbons/American Fertility Society (AFS) classification system
- Anomaly often associated with in-utero exposure to diethylstilboestrol (DES)

IMAGING FINDINGS

General Features
- Best diagnostic clue
  - Narrowed T-shaped configuration of endometrial cavity
  - Associated myometrial constriction bands
- Uterine corpus
  - T-shaped configuration of endometrial cavity
    - Most common manifestation: 31%
  - Small, hypoplastic uterus
  - Constriction bands
  - Narrowed fundal segment of endometrium
  - Irregular endometrial margins
  - Widened lower uterine segment
- Uterine cervix
  - Hypoplasia, or stenosis (25%)
  - Anterior ridge and "collar"
  - Pseudopolyps
  - Abnormal cervical finding is associated with abnormal corpus uterine changes in 86% of cases
- Fallopian tubes
  - Shortened
  - Sacculations
  - Fimbrial deformities and stenosis

Radiographic Findings
- Hysterosalpingography (HSG)
  - Cannulation of endocervical canal may be difficult due to cervical hypoplasia or stenosis
  - Uterine abnormalities detected in 69%
    - Narrow, irregular, opacified endocervical canal
    - Small endometrial cavity with shortened upper uterine segment with characteristic T-shape
    - Constriction bands, often mid-fundal
    - Bands cause narrowing of the interstitial segments of the fallopian tubes
  - Fallopian tubes are short with irregular contours

DDx: T-Shaped Uterus

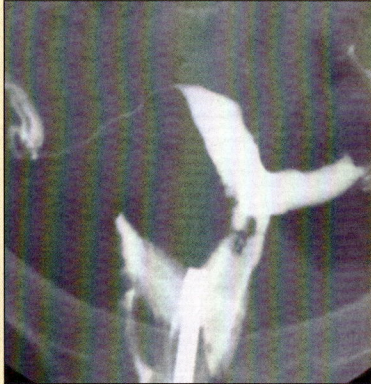

Septate Uterus

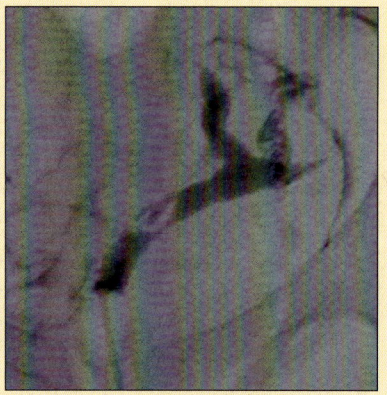

Asherman Syndrome

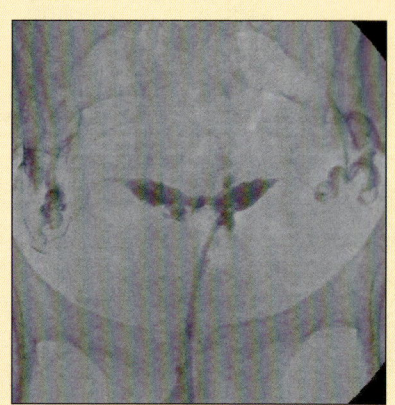

Asherman Syndrome

DES-EXPOSED

Key Facts

Terminology
- Class VII Müllerian duct anomaly (MDA)
- Based on Buttram & Gibbons/American Fertility Society (AFS) classification system
- Anomaly often associated with in-utero exposure to diethylstilboestrol (DES)

Imaging Findings
- T-shaped configuration of endometrial cavity
- Small, hypoplastic uterus
- Constriction bands
- Fallopian tubes are short with irregular contours

Top Differential Diagnoses
- Morphologic Changes
- Asherman Syndrome
- Uterine Hypoplasia
- Arcuate/Partial Septate Uterus

Pathology
- Increased incidence of clear cell carcinoma of vagina

Clinical Issues
- Infertility
- Ectopic pregnancy
- Spontaneous abortion

Diagnostic Checklist
- Consider DES-exposed uterus in a female patient presenting with infertility or spontaneous abortions, with history of in utero exposure to DES
- T-shaped configuration of endometrial cavity on HSG and T2WI

Ultrasonographic Findings
- Grayscale Ultrasound
  - Findings often difficult to characterize
  - Length of uterus does not exceed 6 cm
  - Endometrial cavity length and surface area significantly smaller than normal
  - Endometrial thickness smaller than normal
  - Extreme narrowing of vertical and horizontal limbs of echogenic endometrial cavity resulting in a T-shaped configuration to endometrial cavity
  - Cervical length markedly shorter than normal
- Pulsed Doppler
  - Increased uterine arterial pulsatility index found in DES-exposed women
    - Reflects reduced uterine perfusion

CT Findings
- CT has no role in characterization of uterine anomalies

MR Findings
- T2WI
  - T-shaped configuration: Narrowing of vertical and horizontal limbs of endometrial cavity
  - Constriction bands present
    - Focal thickening of junctional zone causing small indentations on endometrial cavity

Imaging Recommendations
- Best imaging tool
  - HSG is the primary imaging modality and best demonstrates
    - Characteristic T-shaped configuration to endometrial cavity and presence of constriction bands
    - Fallopian tube abnormalities
  - MR useful in imaging this anomaly due to its high soft tissue contrast resolution and multiplanar ability
- Protocol advice
  - MR pelvis with multicoil array
  - High-resolution T2WI, ≤ 4 mm slice thickness
  - Oblique imaging plane parallel to long axis of uterus
  - Axial T2WI images to evaluate vagina, cervix and ovaries

DIFFERENTIAL DIAGNOSIS

Morphologic Changes
- Rare, similar morphologic changes reported in women without DES-exposure

Asherman Syndrome
- Usually late sequelae of uterine curettage after delivery or abortion; can develop after endometrial infections e.g., tuberculosis
- Intrauterine synechiae or adhesions develop
- Nondistensible endometrial cavity on HSG
- HSG shows multiple lacunar-shaped, intracavitary filling defects of variable size
- Low signal intensity fibrous adhesions on T2WI

Uterine Hypoplasia
- Small uterine soft tissue remnant with or without small endometrial cavity
- Normal configuration of endometrial cavity
- Decreased intercornual distance in uterine hypoplasia

Arcuate/Partial Septate Uterus
- Mild focal thickening of fundal myometrium with fused external uterine contour in arcuate uterus
- Fundal indentation of myometrium more extensive ± small caudal fibrous component in septate uterus

PATHOLOGY

General Features
- Etiology
  - DES is a synthetic estrogen; introduced in 1948
  - Prescribed for women with recurrent spontaneous abortions (SABs) and poor reproductive outcomes

DES-EXPOSED

- ○ DES discontinued in 1971 once teratogenic effects in utero realized
- ○ Structural abnormalities not likely to occur
  - ▪ If DES given to pregnant mother early in the first trimester or after 22 weeks gestation
- ○ Structural abnormalities also depend on amount of DES given to pregnant mother
- ○ Similar spectrum of morphologic changes reported without history of DES exposure
  - ▪ Suggests this may represent a rare müllerian anomaly of the uterus that becomes expressed following in utero exposure to DES
- Epidemiology: 1.0-1.5 million offspring exposed in utero
- Associated abnormalities
  - ○ Increased incidence of benign vaginal adenosis: 67%
    - ▪ When present, associated uterine abnormalities are present in 82% of cases
  - ○ Increased incidence of clear cell carcinoma of vagina
    - ▪ 0.14-1.4 per 1,000 women exposed
  - ○ Only congenital uterine abnormality not associated with increased prevalence of renal abnormalities

CLINICAL ISSUES

Presentation
- Most common signs/symptoms
  - ○ Infertility
    - ▪ Uncorrected fertility rate of approximately 65%
    - ▪ If T-shaped uterus with constriction of upper uterine cavity, odds ratio for inability to conceive is 2.6
  - ○ Ectopic pregnancy
    - ▪ Nine-fold increased risk
  - ○ Spontaneous abortion
    - ▪ Two-fold increased risk: Spontaneous abortion occurs in 24% of DES exposed women compared to 12% in the unexposed population
    - ▪ Can occur in 1st or 2nd trimester

Demographics
- Ethnicity: No ethnic predilection

Natural History & Prognosis
- Increased risk of adverse obstetric outcomes
  - ○ Ectopic pregnancy
  - ○ Spontaneous abortion
  - ○ Premature birth rates
    - ▪ Incidence of preterm delivery 3 times as great as in the unexposed population (approximately 16%)
- Increased incidence of clear cell carcinoma of vagina

Treatment
- Expectant management
- Consideration to cervical cerclage given in patients
  - ○ Predisposed to cervical incompetence due to structural abnormality, abnormal smooth muscle to collagen ratio and decreased cervical elastin
  - ○ History of second trimester losses and preterm births
- Hysteroscopic metroplasty can be performed for small uteri in patients with primary infertility who wish to become pregnant
  - ○ Following metroplasty, 17 out of 23 women exposed to DES in utero experienced 26 pregnancies, leading to 13 live born babies

DIAGNOSTIC CHECKLIST

Consider
- Consider DES-exposed uterus in a female patient presenting with infertility or spontaneous abortions, with history of in utero exposure to DES

Image Interpretation Pearls
- T-shaped configuration of endometrial cavity on HSG and T2WI

SELECTED REFERENCES

1. Troiano RN et al: Mullerian duct anomalies: imaging and clinical issues. Radiology. 233(1):19-34, 2004
2. Imaoka I et al: MR imaging of disorders associated with female infertility: use in diagnosis, treatment, and management. Radiographics. 23(6):1401-21, 2003
3. Kruse K et al: Clinical implications of DES. Nurse Pract. 28(7 Pt 1):26-32,35, table of contents; quiz 35-7, 2003
4. Troiano RN: Magnetic resonance imaging of mullerian duct anomalies of the uterus. Top Magn Reson Imaging. 14(4):269-79, 2003
5. Swan SH: Intrauterine exposure to diethylstilbestrol: long-term effects in humans. APMIS. 108(12):793-804, 2000
6. Woodward PJ et al: MR imaging in the evaluation of female infertility. Radiographics. 13(2):293-310, 1993
7. Milhan D: DES exposure: implications for childbearing. Int J Childbirth Educ. 7(4):21-8, 1992
8. Carrington BM et al: Mullerian duct anomalies: MR imaging evaluation. Radiology. 176(3):715-20, 1990
9. Kaufman RH et al: Upper genital tract changes and infertility in diethylstilbestrol-exposed women. Am J Obstet Gynecol. 154(6):1312-8, 1986
10. Glaze GM: Diethylstilbestrol exposure in utero: review of literature. J Am Osteopath Assoc. 83(6):435-8, 1984
11. Nunley WC Jr et al: Upper reproductive tract radiographic findings in DES-exposed female offspring. AJR Am J Roentgenol. 142(2):337-9, 1984
12. Stillman RJ et al: Diethylstilbestrol exposure in utero and endometriosis in infertile females. Fertil Steril. 41(3):369-72, 1984
13. Haney AF et al: Infertility in women exposed to diethylstilbestrol in utero. J Reprod Med. 28(12):851-6, 1983
14. Kaufman RH: Structural changes of the genital tract associated with in utero exposure to diethylstilbestrol. Obstet Gynecol Annu. 11:187-202, 1982
15. Kinch RA: Diethylstilbestrol in pregnancy: an update. Can Med Assoc J. 127(9):812-3, 1982
16. Ben-Baruch G et al: Uterine anomalies in diethylstilbestrol-exposed women with fertility disorders. Acta Obstet Gynecol Scand. 60(4):395-7, 1981
17. Berger MJ et al: Impaired reproductive performance in DES-exposed women. Obstet Gynecol. 55(1):25-7, 1980
18. Kaufman RH: Upper genital tract changes and pregnancy outcome in offspring exposed in utero to diethylstilbestrol. Am J Obstet Gynecol. 137(3):299-308, 1980
19. Rennell CL: T-shaped uterus in diethylstilbestrol (DES) exposure. AJR Am J Roentgenol. 132(6):979-80, 1979
20. Kaufman RH et al: Genital tract anomalies associated with in utero exposure to diethylstilbestrol. Isr J Med Sci. 14(3):353-62, 1978

DES-EXPOSED

IMAGE GALLERY

Typical

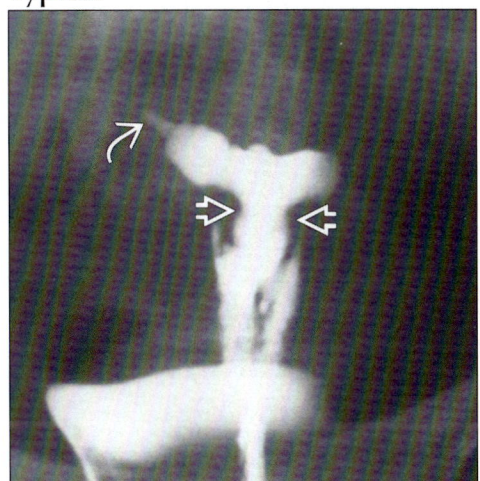
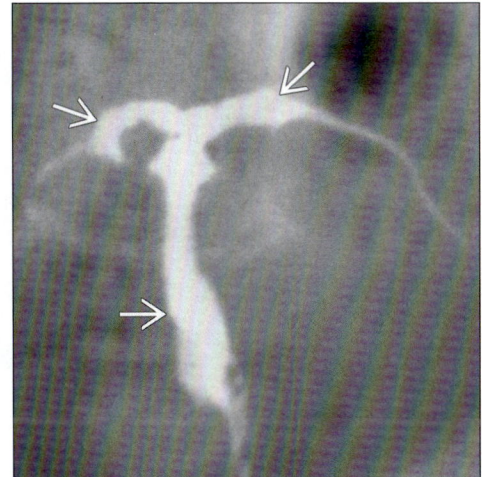

(Left) Anteroposterior hysterosalpingogram shows a T-shaped endometrial cavity with a large constriction band in the lower uterine segment ➡. The right fallopian tube is shortened ➡. *(Right)* Anteroposterior hysterosalpingogram shows a typical narrow, irregular T-shaped endometrial cavity outlined by contrast medium ➡. Note also the elongated lower uterine segment.

Typical

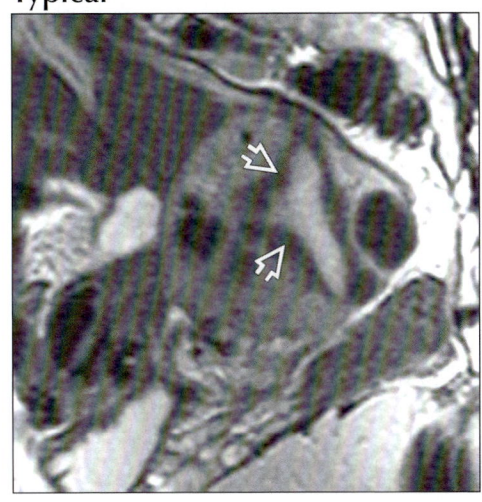
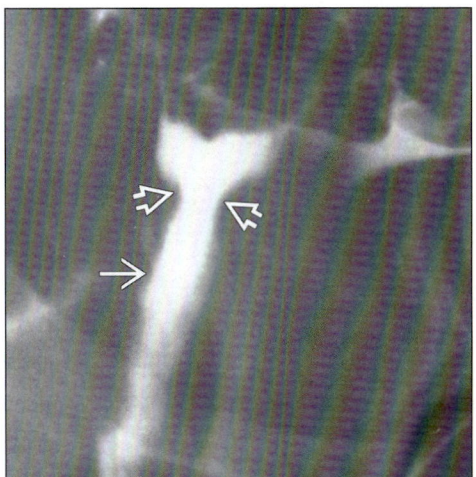

(Left) Sagittal oblique T2WI MR shows characteristic T-shape of endometrial cavity with myometrial constriction bands ➡. Note thickening of junctional zone (JZ) at level of constriction bands. Small leiomyomas are present. *(Right)* Anteroposterior hysterosalpingogram (same patient as previous image) shows a DES-exposed uterus. Note T-shaped endometrial cavity with widened lower uterine segment ➡ & constriction bands ➡.

Typical

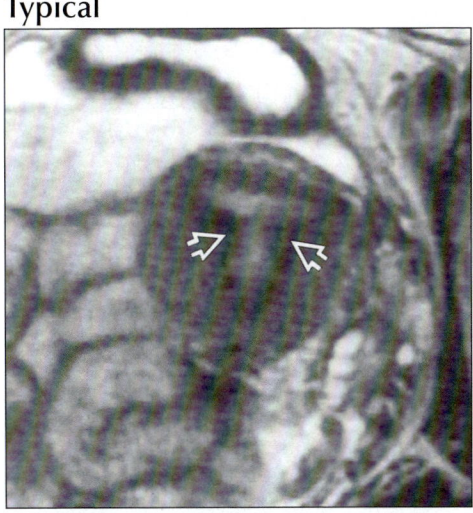
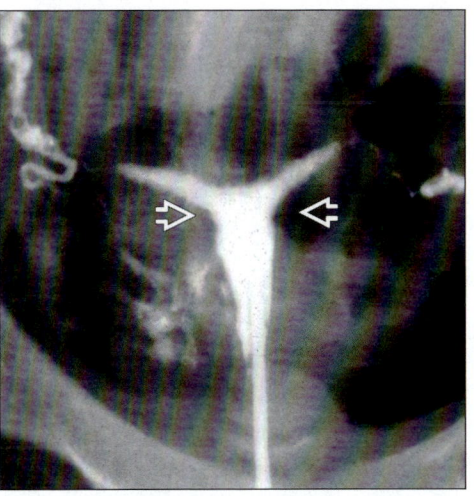

(Left) Axial T2WI MR shows the characteristic T-shape of the endometrial cavity with myometrial constriction bands ➡. Note the thickening of the junctional zone at the level of the constriction bands. (Courtesy S. McCarthy, MD). *(Right)* Anteroposterior hysterosalpingogram shows a DES-exposed uterus with a T-shaped endometrial cavity ➡. The fallopian tubes are unremarkable.

COMPLEX ANOMALIES

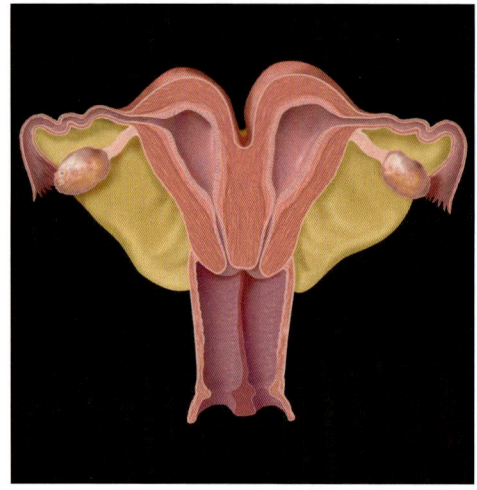

Graphic shows a complex duplication anomaly with fundal duplication of the uterine horns, a solitary cervix with a septum and complete duplication of the vagina.

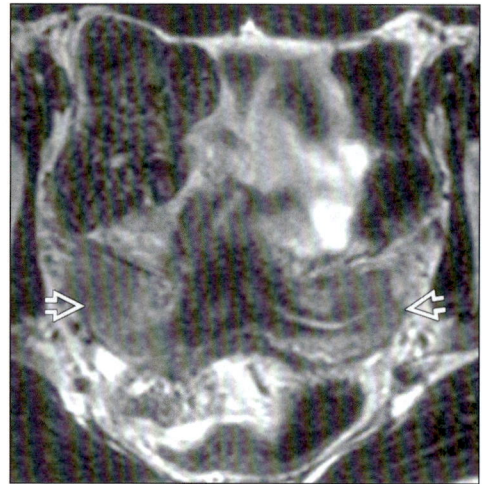

Coronal oblique T2WI MR shows a complex duplication anomaly with fundal duplication of the uterine horns ➡. There is a solitary cervix with a septum and complete duplication of the vagina (ensuing images).

TERMINOLOGY

Abbreviations and Synonyms
- Complex duplication anomalies

Definitions
- Comprise features of more than one class of Müllerian duct anomalies (MDAs)
  - Based on Buttram & Gibbons/American Fertility Society (AFS) classification system
- Includes a combination of dysgenesis, vertical and lateral fusion defects

IMAGING FINDINGS

General Features
- Best diagnostic clue
  - Complex duplication anomaly which cannot be categorized into a single class
  - Classical imaging appearance: Variable, fundal duplication of uterine horns with lower uterine midline septum
  - Degree of nonfusion less than didelphys, greater than bicornuate uterus
    - Frequently misclassified as uterus didelphys
    - May present as "bicornuate" configuration without communicating endometrial segments
- Morphology
  - Variable imaging appearance
  - Uterine horns
    - Two uterine horns connected at caudal margins
    - Midline lower uterine body septum
    - Endometrial cavities noncommunicating
    - Solitary or duplicated cervix
  - Vagina
    - With or without upper vaginal septum
    - Obstruction of cavity with associated transverse vaginal septum
    - May be completely duplicated

Radiographic Findings
- Hysterosalpingography (HSG)
  - Variable degrees of divergence of endometrial cavities
  - Two separate opacified endocervical canals connected to separate fusiform endometrial cavities

DDx: Mimics of Complex Duplication Anomalies

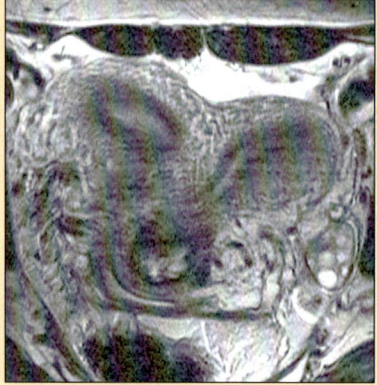

Bicornuate Uterus

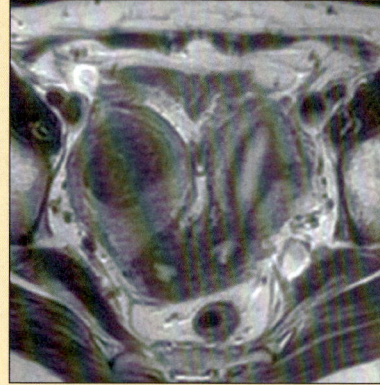

Uterus Didelphys

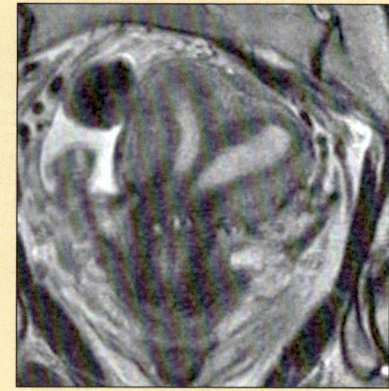

Septate Uterus

COMPLEX ANOMALIES

Key Facts

Terminology
- Comprise features of more than one class of Müllerian duct anomalies (MDAs)

Imaging Findings
- Complex duplication anomaly which cannot be categorized into a single class
- Classical imaging appearance: Variable, fundal duplication of uterine horns with lower uterine midline septum
- Degree of nonfusion less than didelphys, greater than bicornuate uterus
- Frequently misclassified as uterus didelphys
- May present as "bicornuate" configuration without communicating endometrial segments

Top Differential Diagnoses
- Bicornuate Uterus
- Didelphys Uterus
- Septate Uterus

Clinical Issues
- Difficult to assess reproductive outcomes given lack of data, frequency, and misclassification as didelphys
- Unrecognized obstructive MDA results in hematocolpos and hematometra

Diagnostic Checklist
- In patients with complex duplication anomalies reporting of defects should include a separate description of uterine, cervical and vaginal segments

---

  - Each cavity ends in solitary fallopian tube
  - No communication between uterine horns

Ultrasonographic Findings
- Transvaginal ultrasound (TVS)
  - Divergent endometrial echogenic complexes without communication
  - Wide fundal cleft of variable depth
  - Lower uterine septum primarily hypoechoic corresponding to fibrous component
  - Echogenic distention of endometrial cavity and upper vagina with unilateral obstruction (distention greater in vaginal segment)

CT Findings
- CT has no role in evaluation of complex uterine anomalies

MR Findings
- T1WI: Obstructed segments in case of transverse vaginal septum: High signal intensity
- T2WI
  - Uterine horns separated by fundal cleft of variable depth
  - Normal zonal anatomy within each horn
  - Endometrial cavities usually symmetric
  - Lower midline uterine septum
    - Superior segment isointense to myometrium if myometrial component present
    - Inferior or complete segment low signal intensity corresponding to fibrous component
  - Partial or complete duplication of cervical zonal anatomy
  - Obstructed segments in case of transverse vaginal septum
    - Distention of vagina greater than endometrial cavity
    - Low to intermediate signal intensity

Imaging Recommendations
- Best imaging tool
  - 2D and 3D ultrasound can be used as initial imaging modality
  - MR modality of choice in patients with adverse reproductive outcomes and obstructed segments
    - Best at defining uterine anatomy; less accurate at defining cervical and vaginal anatomy when compared to findings at surgery
- Protocol advice
  - Phased array body coil
  - Single shot fast spin echo (SSFSE) coronal image through abdomen and pelvis to assess kidneys
  - High resolution FSE T2WI, ≤ 4 mm slice thickness
    - Imaging plane parallel to long axis of uterus to assess degree of divergence of uterine horns and cervical duplication
    - Short-axis view of vagina to delineate vaginal septum/duplication
  - T1WI ± FS
    - To confirm blood products in obstructed segments

DIFFERENTIAL DIAGNOSIS

Bicornuate Uterus
- Symmetric duplicated uterine horns
- Communication of endometrial cavities at caudal extent
- Degree of nonfusion less than complex anomaly

Didelphys Uterus
- Near complete duplication of uterus
- Each hemiuterine corpus and cervix with preserved zonal anatomy
- Degree of nonfusion greater than complex anomaly

Septate Uterus
- Convex, flat or mildly concave external uterine contour
- Septum has an upper myometrial segment and lower fibrous segment extending to external cervical os

COMPLEX ANOMALIES

PATHOLOGY

General Features
- Genetics
  - Majority of cases sporadic or multifactorial in nature
  - 46 XX female karyotype
- Associated abnormalities
  - Increased incidence of bladder, cloaca and urogenital disorders due to close embryological development
    - e.g., Renal agenesis, ectopic kidney, cystic dysplasia and duplicated collecting system

CLINICAL ISSUES

Presentation
- Most common signs/symptoms
  - Nonobstructive complex duplication anomaly
    - Usually asymptomatic
    - Diagnosis made during investigation of recurrent spontaneous abortions, premature labor
  - Complex duplication anomaly with obstructed segments
    - Development of cyclical pelvic pain at menarche
  - Normal secondary sexual characteristics

Demographics
- Age: Developmental abnormality which usually presents at menarche or later
- Ethnicity: No ethnic predilection

Natural History & Prognosis
- Difficult to assess reproductive outcomes given lack of data, frequency, and misclassification as didelphys
- Unrecognized obstructive MDA results in hematocolpos and hematometra
  - If untreated, tubal damage and endometriosis may occur
    - Fertility is further compromised
    - Incidence of ectopic pregnancy increased

Treatment
- Appropriate description of defects directs treatment and intervention
  - Reporting of defects should include a separate description of uterine, cervical and vaginal segments
- Expectant
- Septae within vagina and uterus can be removed hysteroscopically
  - Resection of uterine septum with recurrent pregnancy loss
  - Resection of transverse vaginal septum with obstruction
- Correction of "bicornuate" configuration requires a combined laparoscopic and hysteroscopic approach if metroplasty is considered
- "Didelphys" configuration without vaginal septae typically requires no surgery

DIAGNOSTIC CHECKLIST

Consider
- In patients with complex duplication anomalies reporting of defects should include a separate description of uterine, cervical and vaginal segments

Image Interpretation Pearls
- Degree of nonfusion less than didelphys, greater than bicornuate uterus

SELECTED REFERENCES

1. Gassner I et al: Ultrasound of female genital anomalies. Eur Radiol. 2004
2. Troiano RN et al: Mullerian duct anomalies: imaging and clinical issues. Radiology. 2004
3. Gell JS: Mullerian anomalies. Semin Reprod Med. 2003
4. Imaoka I et al: MR imaging of disorders associated with female infertility: use in diagnosis, treatment, and management. Radiographics. 23(6):1401-21, 2003
5. Scarsbrook AF et al: MRI appearances of mullerian duct abnormalities. Clin Radiol. 2003
6. Troiano RN: Magnetic resonance imaging of mullerian duct anomalies of the uterus. Top Magn Reson Imaging. 2003
7. Colacurci N et al: The significance of hysteroscopic treatment of congenital uterine malformations. Reprod Biomed Online. 4 Suppl 3:52-4, 2002
8. MacLaughlin DT et al: Mullerian inhibiting substance: an update. Adv Exp Med Biol. 2002
9. Siewart B et al: Problems and pitfalls in MR evaluation of uterine anomalies. Journal of Women's Imaging. 4:100-7, 2002
10. Burgis J: Obstructive Mullerian anomalies: case report, diagnosis, and management. Am J Obstet Gynecol. 2001
11. Folch M et al: Mullerian agenesis: etiology, diagnosis, and management. Obstet Gynecol Surv. 2000
12. Colacurci N et al: Hysteroscopic metroplasty. J Am Assoc Gynecol Laparosc. 5(2):171-4, 1998
13. Muram D: Persistent Mullerian duct syndrome. J Pediatr Adolesc Gynecol. 1998
14. Woodward PJ et al: Congenital uterine malformations. Curr Probl Diagn Radiol. 1995
15. Woodward PJ et al: MR imaging in the evaluation of female infertility. Radiographics. 1993
16. Markham SM et al: Structural anomalies of the reproductive tract. Curr Opin Obstet Gynecol. 1992
17. Pellerito JS et al: Diagnosis of uterine anomalies: relative accuracy of MR imaging, endovaginal sonography, and hysterosalpingography. Radiology. 183(3):795-800, 1992
18. Carrington BM et al: Mullerian duct anomalies: MR imaging evaluation. Radiology. 1990
19. Golan A et al: Congenital anomalies of the mullerian system. Fertil Steril. 1989
20. Reuter KL et al: Septate versus bicornuate uteri: errors in imaging diagnosis. Radiology. 172(3):749-52, 1989

COMPLEX ANOMALIES

IMAGE GALLERY

Typical

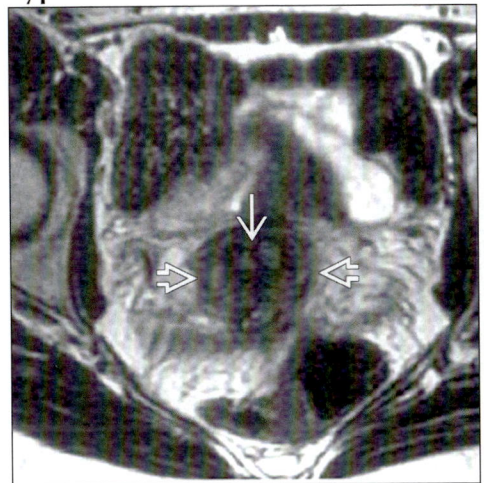
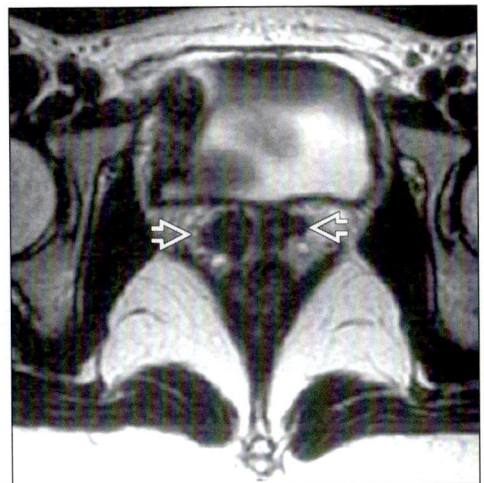

(Left) Axial T2WI MR of the same patient as previous image shows a solitary cervix ➡ with a septum ➡ dividing the endocervical canal. *(Right)* Axial T2WI MR in the same patient as previous image shows complete duplication of the vagina ➡.

Typical

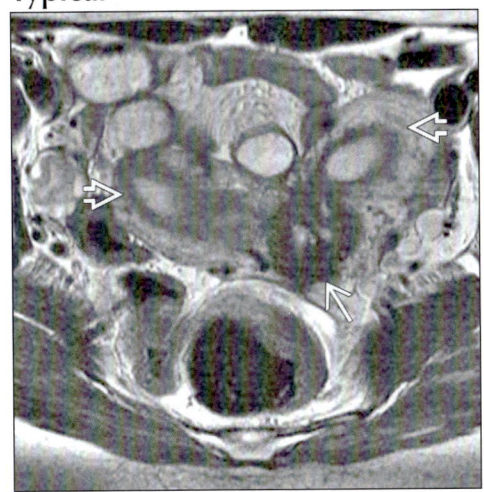
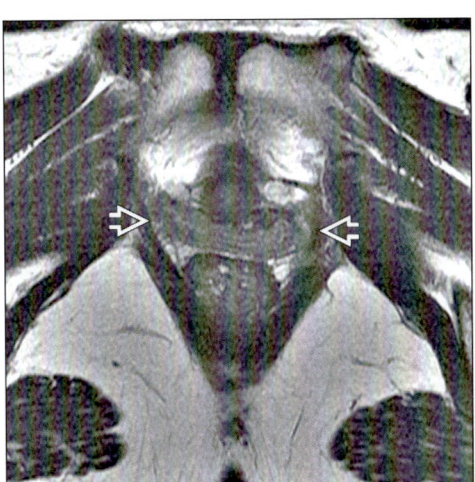

(Left) Axial T2WI MR shows a complex anomaly with divergent non-communicating uterine horns ➡ (didelphys configuration) and incomplete duplication of the cervix ➡. *(Right)* Axial T2WI MR in the same patient as previous image shows the presence of a single vagina ➡.

Typical

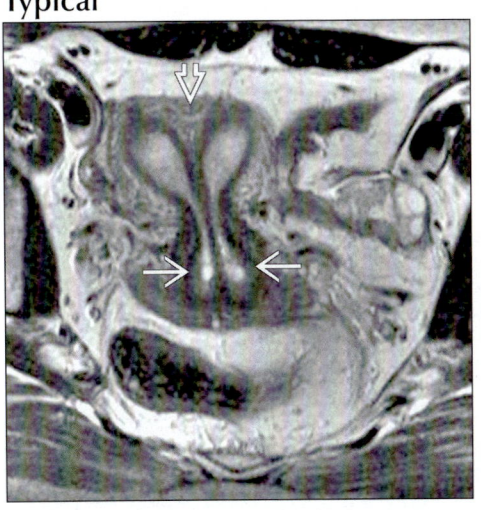
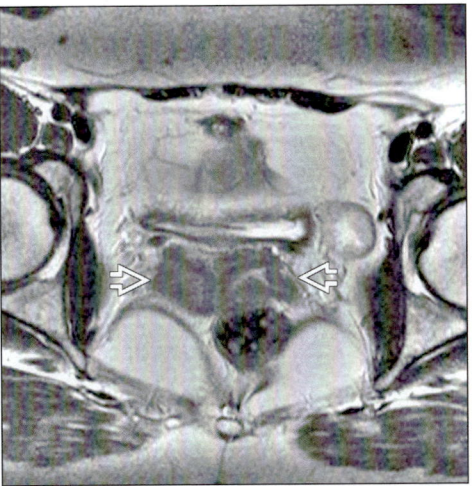

(Left) Axial T2WI MR in a patient with a complex anomaly shows a septate configuration of the uterus ➡ with a partial duplication of the cervix ➡. *(Right)* Axial T2WI MR in the same patient as previous image shows the complete duplication of the vagina ➡.

ASHERMAN SYNDROME

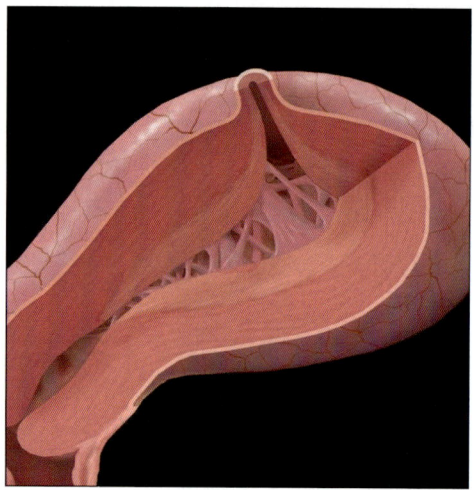

Sagittal graphic shows extensive intrauterine adhesions obliterating the internal os, lower uterine segment, uterine body and sparing the cornua.

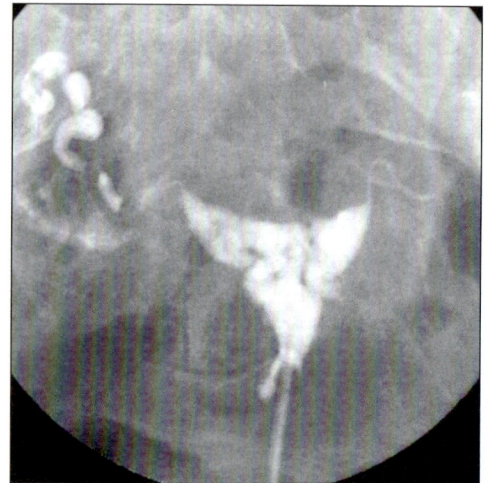

Anteroposterior view from HSG shows multiple, small filling defects, partially obliterating the uterine cavity but sparing the cornual regions and endocervix.

TERMINOLOGY

Abbreviations and Synonyms
- Intrauterine adhesions (IUA)

Definitions
- Permanent adherence of uterine walls in variable sites, partial or complete obliteration of uterine cavity and/or internal cervical os and clinical symptoms including menstrual abnormalities, infertility and recurrent pregnancy loss

IMAGING FINDINGS

General Features
- Best diagnostic clue: Nondistensible endometrial cavity during hysterosalpingogram (HSG)
- Location
  ○ Endometrial cavity
    ▪ Adhesions may be centrally or peripherally located
    ▪ Usually do not involve cornual regions
    ▪ Complete obliteration of endometrial cavity at internal cervix or lower uterine segment in severe cases
    ▪ Endometrial cavity including cornual regions may be lost entirely in tuberculous endometritis
- Morphology: Filling defects are irregular, angulated, have sharp contours

Ultrasonographic Findings
- Grayscale Ultrasound
  ○ IUA appear as eccentric echogenic areas; rarely have calcifications
  ○ Sonohysterogram (SHG): Echogenic bands traversing distended endometrial canal extending side to side of uterine wall

MR Findings
- T2WI
  ○ Low signal intensity fibrous adhesions
  ○ Loss of normal, high-endometrial signal intensity
- T1 C+: Adhesions will enhance, especially in early phase after contrast administration

DDx: Intrauterine Adhesion

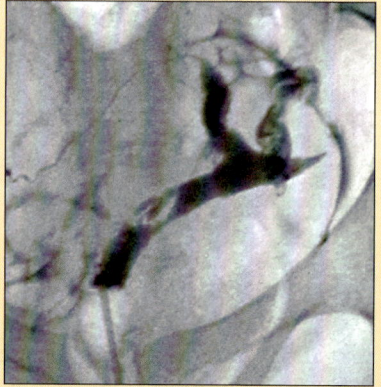

Synechiae

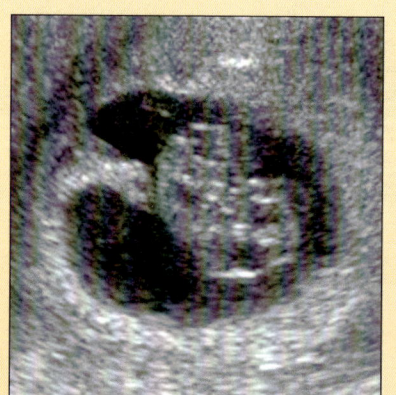

Synechiae/Pregnancy

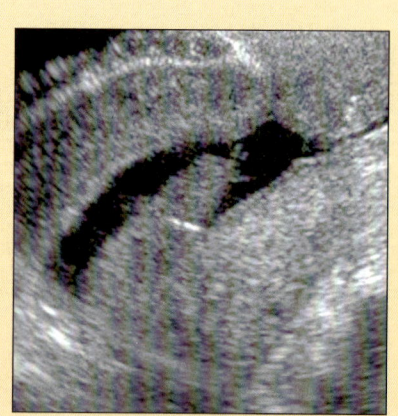

Endometrial Polyp

ASHERMAN SYNDROME

Key Facts

Terminology
- Permanent adherence of uterine walls in variable sites, partial or complete obliteration of uterine cavity and/or internal cervical os and clinical symptoms including menstrual abnormalities, infertility and recurrent pregnancy loss

Imaging Findings
- Best diagnostic clue: Nondistensible endometrial cavity during hysterosalpingogram (HSG)
- HSG shows multiple, lacunar-shaped, intracavitary filling defects of variable sizes
- Patient can have pain during injection of contrast due to poor distensibility of cavity
- Low signal intensity fibrous adhesions
- Loss of normal, high-endometrial signal intensity
- IUA appear as eccentric echogenic areas; rarely have calcifications
- Sonohysterogram (SHG): Echogenic bands traversing distended endometrial canal extending side to side of uterine wall
- Must be present on every film to distinguish synechiae from polyps

Diagnostic Checklist
- Suspect diagnosis in patient with secondary amenorrhea and history of postpartum or postabortion curettage
- US and/or MR to image uterine cavity above adhesions and demonstrate remnants of normal endometrium

Fluoroscopic Findings
- HSG shows multiple, lacunar-shaped, intracavitary filling defects of variable sizes
- Lack of or incomplete communication between cornua and cervical canal due to adhesions
- Patient can have pain during injection of contrast due to poor distensibility of cavity

Imaging Recommendations
- Best imaging tool
  - HSG
    - Correlation between the diagnosis by hysterosalpingogram and hysteroscopy: 72% for synechiae of the cervix, 73% for mild synechiae, 83% for moderate synechiae and 75% for severe synechiae
- Protocol advice
  - Document involvement of cornual areas, upper/lower uterine cavity and cervix
  - Document size and number
  - Must be present on every film to distinguish synechiae from polyps
  - Minimize technical problems during HSG
    - Instill contrast medium slowly under fluoroscopic guidance
    - If contrast is difficult to inject due to poor distensibility, the procedure may need to be terminated prior to visualization of entire endometrial cavity
  - Define position and flexion of uterine cavity to plan treatment

DIFFERENTIAL DIAGNOSIS

Uterine Synechia
- Few bands of tissue that do not limit distensibility of uterine cavity and are usually asymptomatic

Endometrial Polyp
- Polypoid mass protrudes and distends endometrial canal
- Will not extend from one wall of the uterus to another

Endometrial Blood Clot
- Filling defect of variable morphology
- May be mobile during HSG or SHG

Submucosal Leiomyoma
- Round mass protrudes into and distends endometrial canal

PATHOLOGY

General Features
- Etiology
  - Endometrial trauma to basalis layer
    - Most common: Late sequelae of uterine curettage after delivery or abortion
    - Less common: Surgery such as cesarian section, myomectomy, diagnostic curettage, pelvic irradiation, endometrial necrosis from uterine artery embolization, intrauterine contraceptive device, tubercular endometritis, and septic abortion
  - Postpartum uterus predisposed to develop adhesions
    - Related to temporary hypoestrogenic state
    - Increased fragility of the uterine lining and likelihood of damage during curettage
    - Curettage between second and fourth week postpartum is most likely to cause adhesions
    - Higher risk for adhesion formation in women who breast feed because of prolonged estrogen deficiency and delayed endometrial proliferation
- Epidemiology
  - Prevalence of IUA difficult to determine
    - 4-23% in women with postpartum bleeding
    - 5-39% in women with recurrent miscarriages
    - 68% of women with secondary infertility who have history of two or more uterine curettages
- Associated abnormalities: IUA rarely accompanied by deeply invasive adenomyosis

ASHERMAN SYNDROME

Gross Pathologic & Surgical Features
- Formation of fibrous adhesions and endometrial sclerosis involving uterine cavity and sometimes the internal cervical os
- Most commonly patients have multiple adhesions that bridge anterior and posterior uterine walls
- Evolve from thin endometrial strands to thick fibrous bands

Microscopic Features
- Avascular strands of fibrous tissue with varying amounts of white-cell infiltration
- Some patients have no adhesions but only sclerotic, atrophic endometrium

CLINICAL ISSUES

Presentation
- Most common signs/symptoms
  - Menstrual abnormalities (secondary amenorrhea, irregular menses or dysmenorrhea)
  - Infertility, recurrent pregnancy loss, or premature delivery
  - Abdominal pain, dyspareunia
- Other signs/symptoms: May be asymptomatic and pelvic examination does not reveal abnormalities

Natural History & Prognosis
- If untreated natural history of adhesions is unknown
  - Spontaneous resolution and successful pregnancies have been reported
  - Adhesive process may be progressive
- Myometrial adhesions carry poor prognosis
  - Endometrial basalis is necessary for new endometrium to proliferate following adhesiolysis and estrogen treatment
- Patients with atrophic endometrium have extremely poor prognosis
- Endometrial sclerosis following radiation or tuberculous endometritis not amenable to any type of therapy
- If no endometrial proliferation after high dose estrogen therapy, suspect complete obliteration by muscular adhesions or endometrial sclerosis and no further surgery recommended
- After one hysteroscopic treatment, 90% of patients have normal follow-up hysteroscopy or HSG
  - Most others need a second procedure, few women need three to five operations
- After hysteroscopic treatment of severe Asherman syndrome, half of the patients become pregnant and a third have live births
  - High incidence of preterm delivery (up to 50% in large series)
  - High incidence of abnormal placentation such as placenta previa and placenta accreta (8%)

Treatment
- Options, risks, complications
  - Aims are to restore the normal size and shape of the uterine cavity by removing adhesions and preventing the formation of new adhesions
  - Uncover functional endometrium and make pregnancy possible
  - Even when satisfying anatomical result is obtained, normal endometrial function not guaranteed
  - Lysis of adhesions under direct vision with hysteroscopy is safest, least traumatic and most precise method
    - Other methods: Surgical reconstruction of the uterine cavity (vaginal route or abdominal hysterotomy), curettage, adhesiolysis with electrosurgery, laser, or intrauterine balloon
    - Laparoscopy and intra-operative ultrasound used to define pelvic anatomy and monitor treatment
  - Following hysteroscopic treatment
    - Loop IUD frequently placed in uterine cavity and retained for 2 months, reduces chance of adherence
    - High dose sequential estrogen-progestin treatment stimulates the endometrium so scarred surfaces are re-epithelialized
- Post treatment complications
  - Perforation, hemorrhage, residual intrauterine synechia, infertility

DIAGNOSTIC CHECKLIST

Consider
- Suspect diagnosis in patient with secondary amenorrhea and history of postpartum or postabortion curettage

Image Interpretation Pearls
- Multiple filling defects and partial or complete obliteration of the uterine cavity on HSG
- US and/or MR to image uterine cavity above adhesions and demonstrate remnants of normal endometrium

SELECTED REFERENCES
1. Zikopoulos KA et al: Live delivery rates in subfertile women with Asherman's syndrome after hysteroscopic adhesiolysis using the resectoscope or the Versapoint system. Reprod Biomed Online. 8(6):720-5, 2004
2. Capella-Allouc S et al: Hysteroscopic treatment of severe Asherman's syndrome and subsequent fertility. Hum Reprod. 14(5):1230-3, 1999
3. McComb PF et al: Simplified therapy for Asherman's syndrome. Fertil Steril. 68(6):1047-50, 1997
4. Schenker JG: Etiology of and therapeutic approach to synechia uteri. Eur J Obstet Gynecol Reprod Biol. 65(1):109-13, 1996
5. Bacelar AC et al: The value of MRI in the assessment of traumatic intra-uterine adhesions (Asherman's syndrome). Clin Radiol. 50(2):80-3, 1995
6. March CM: Intrauterine adhesions. Obstet Gynecol Clin North Am. 22(3):491-505, 1995
7. Schlaff WD et al: Preoperative sonographic measurement of endometrial pattern predicts outcome of surgical repair in patients with severe Asherman's syndrome. Fertil Steril. 63(2):410-3, 1995

ASHERMAN SYNDROME

IMAGE GALLERY

Typical

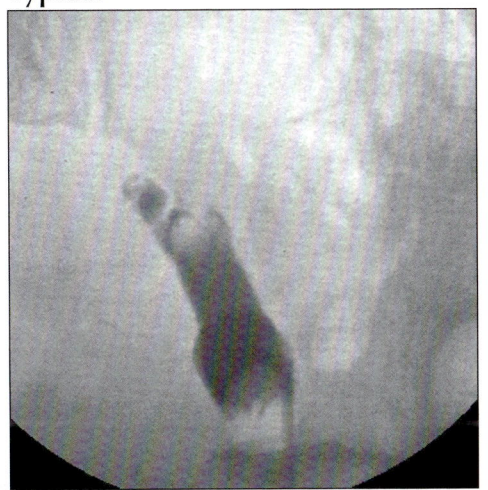
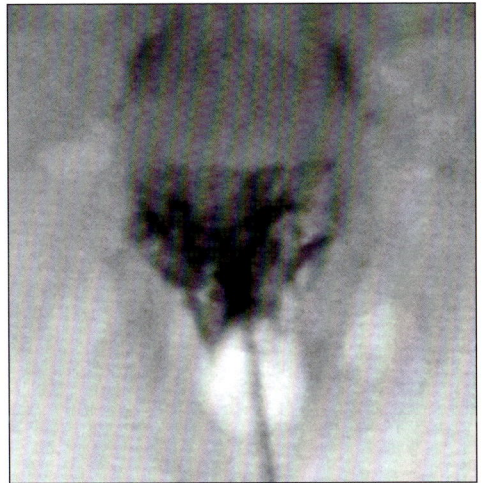

(Left) Anteroposterior view after instillation of contrast material, shows abnormal contour of the lower uterine segment and complete obliteration of the cavity. *(Right)* Anteroposterior view from HSG shows partial distensibility of the uterine cavity and multiple irregular filling defects from multiple adhesions.

Typical

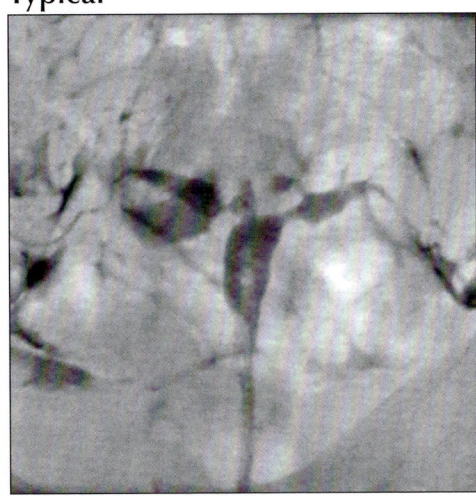
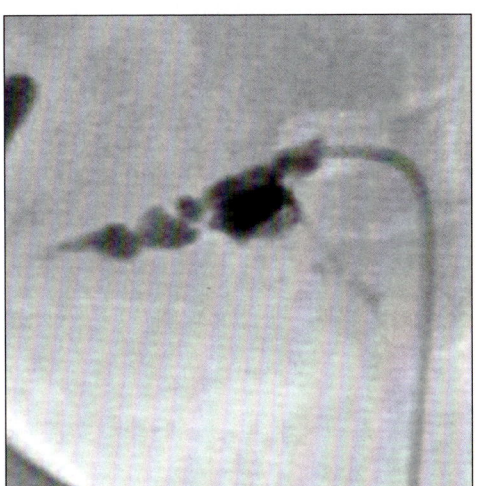

(Left) Anteroposterior radiograph from HSG shows small and distorted uterine cavity with multiple filling defects related to IUA. *(Right)* Anteroposterior view from HSG shows multiple sharply demarcated filling defects in the uterine cavity causing partial obliteration.

Typical

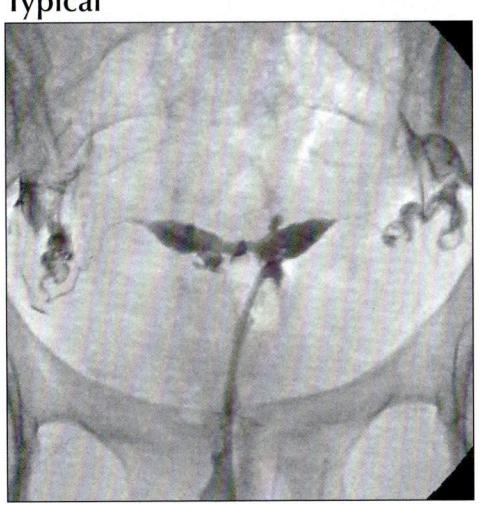
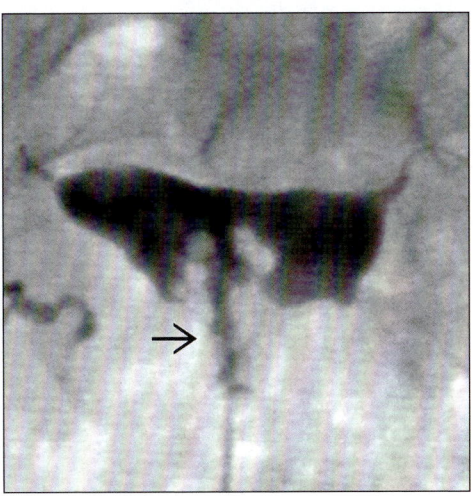

(Left) Anteroposterior view from HSG shows obliteration of the mid- and lower-uterine segments as well as the internal cervical os in a patient with progressive IUA after curettage for mild synechiae. *(Right)* Anteroposterior view from HSG in a patient with prior myomectomy shows poor distensibility of the lower uterine segment and ➔ multiple small filling defects.

ASHERMAN SYNDROME

(Left) Oblique radiograph from HSG shows multiple, irregular filling defects ➔ in the right fundal region from adhesions, which prevent filling of the right fallopian tube. (Right) Anteroposterior view from HSG shows a large, sharply angulated, filling defect ➔ from thick adhesion partially obliterating the right side of the fundus.

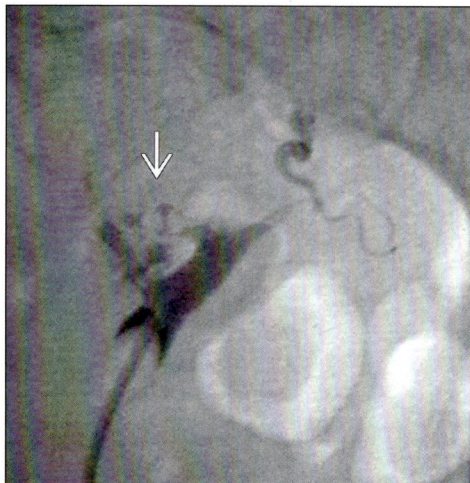
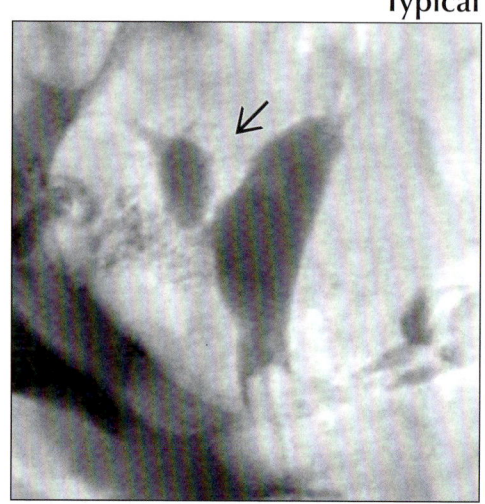

(Left) Anteroposterior view from HSG shows large, centrally located uterine adhesions which spare the cornual regions and endocervical canal. (Right) Anteroposterior view from HSG shows well-demarcated filling defect involving the mid-body, associated with partial distention of the endometrial cavity.

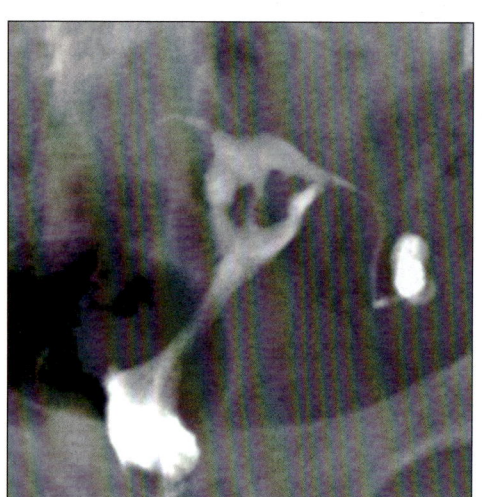
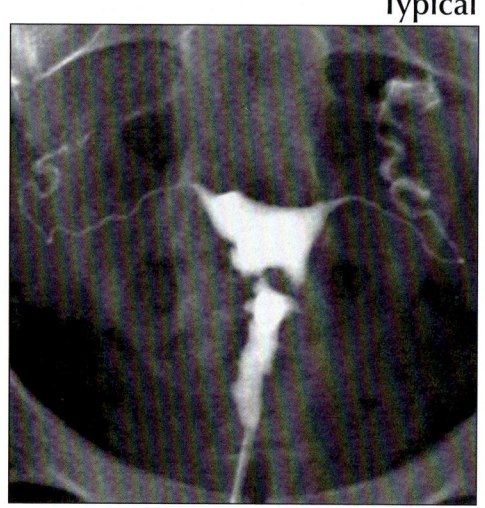

(Left) Sagittal T2WI MR shows distorted and partially distended endometrial cavity which contains bands ➔ of low signal intensity fibrous adhesions that are outlined by fluid. (Right) Coronal T2WI MR ➔ shows a fundal, low signal intensity, linear band of tissue, which is outlined by fluid trapped in the endometrial cavity.

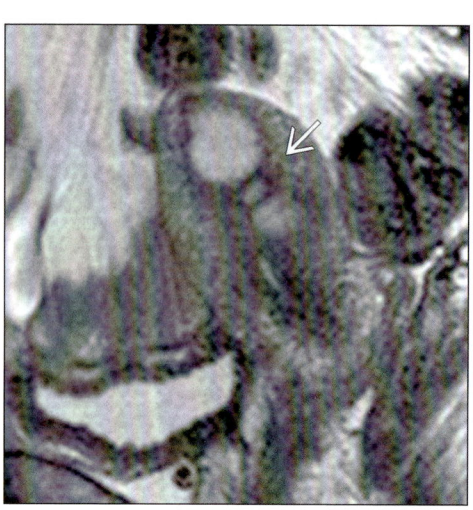
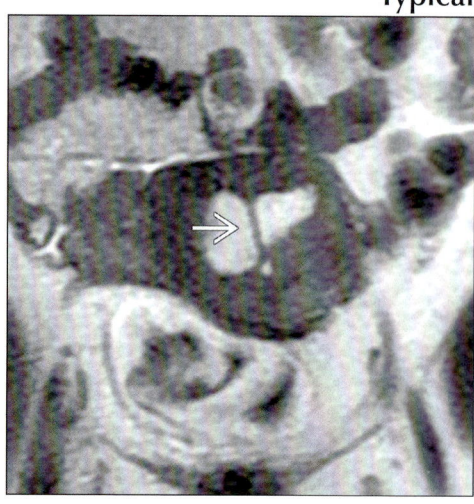

ASHERMAN SYNDROME

Typical

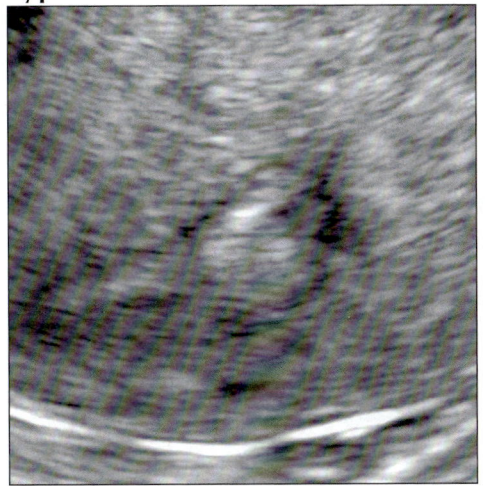 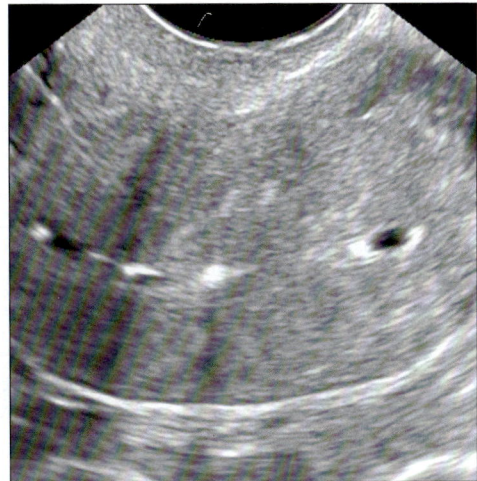

(Left) Sagittal transvaginal ultrasound shows echogenic foci, eccentric to the endometrial stripe which on subsequent imaging proved to be an intrauterine adhesion. *(Right)* Sagittal view from a hysterosalpingogram, shows poor distention of the uterine cavity from intrauterine adhesions.

Typical

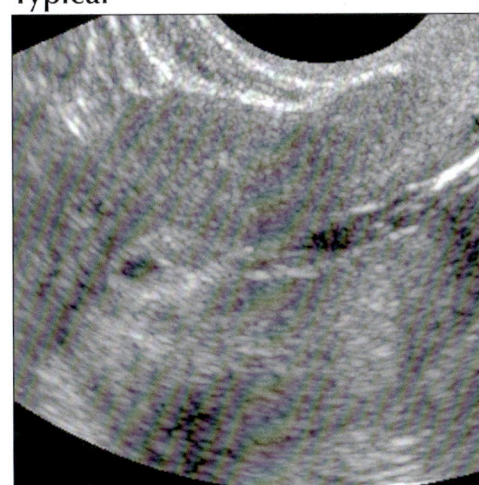 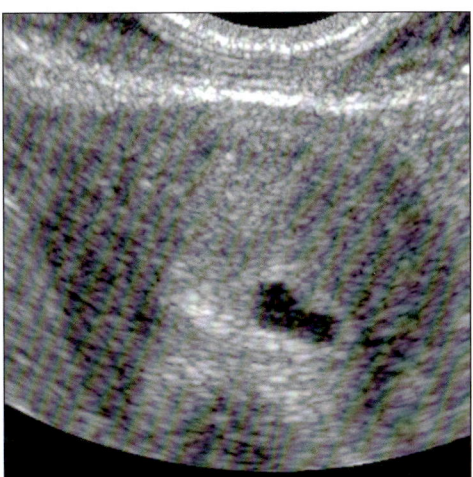

(Left) Sagittal transvaginal ultrasound during SHG demonstrates multiple uterine adhesions and poor distensibility of the uterine cavity. *(Right)* Axial view from SHG demonstrates pocket of fluid in the fundus of the uterus and lack of distention of the right fundal region due to IUA.

Typical

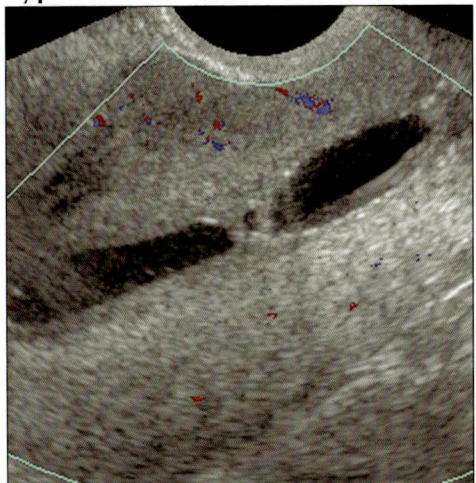 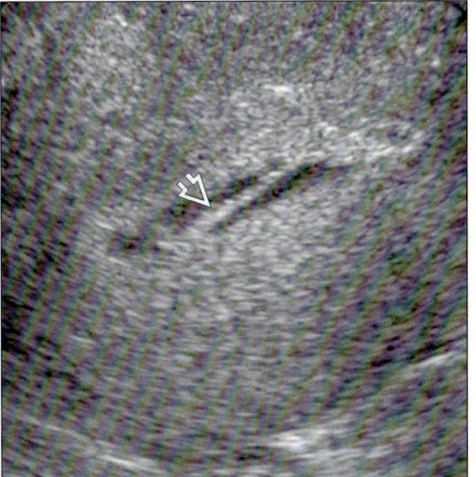

(Left) Sagittal transvaginal ultrasound during SHG shows a band of echogenic tissue within the endometrial cavity which contributes to poor distensibility. *(Right)* Sagittal transvaginal ultrasound during SHG shows thin, echogenic band of tissue ➡ crossing endometrial cavity.

ENDOMETRIAL SYNECHIAE

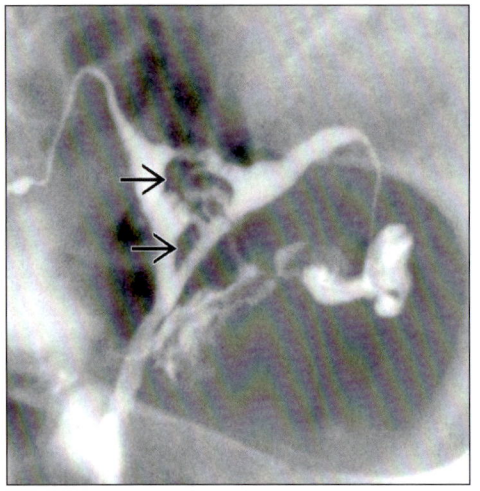

Coronal oblique radiograph from hysterosalpingogram shows filling defects ➡ traversing the endometrial canal.

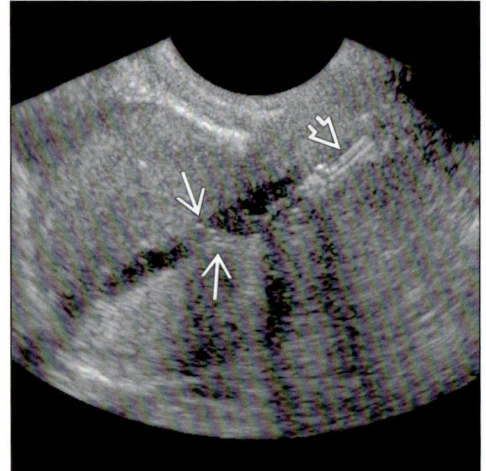

Sagittal transvaginal ultrasound demonstrates thick echogenic adhesion ➡ that spans the endometrial canal. The sonohysterography catheter ➡ is visible in the lower uterine segment.

TERMINOLOGY

Abbreviations and Synonyms
- Intrauterine adhesions, webs, scarring
- Asherman syndrome: In setting of infertility or recurrent pregnancy loss

Definitions
- Permanent adherence of uterine walls, with variable site(s) of these adhesions
- Formed when walls of uterus adhere to each other & cause partial or total obliteration of cavity

IMAGING FINDINGS

General Features
- Best diagnostic clue
  - Irregular, well-demarcated, angular and/or straight tissue bridges spanning endometrial cavity
  - Endometrial cavity may be partially distorted or completely obliterated
  - When completely obliterated, non-filling of the endometrial cavity on hysterosalpingography or sonohysterography
- Location: Cervical, cervicocorporeal & corporeal

Radiographic Findings
- Hysterosalpingography (HSG) findings
  - Highly sensitive but lacks specificity
  - "Lacunar pattern": Multiple or single serpentine, sharply angulated or straight filling defect(s)
  - Complete non-filling of endometrial cavity at cervical or lower uterine segment level
  - Extensive adhesions distort size and shape of uterine cavity
  - Total obliteration of the uterine chamber with severe involvement
  - Incomplete distension of the cavity, folds and contractions can mimic synechiae

Ultrasonographic Findings
- Transvaginal ultrasound (TVS) and sonohysterography findings
  - Endometrium may appear normal

DDx: Endometrial Synechiae

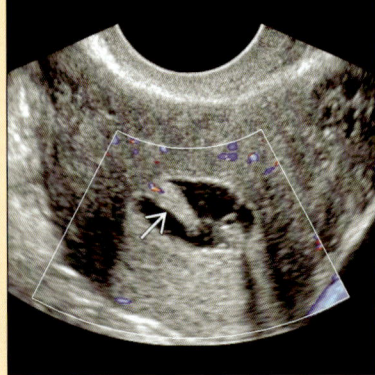

Endometrial Polyp

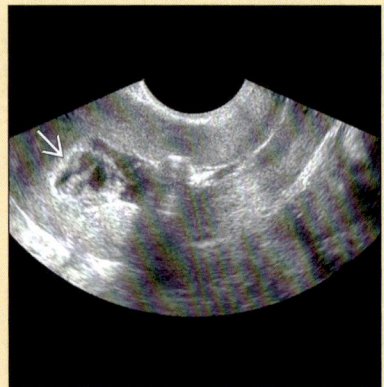

Blood Clot

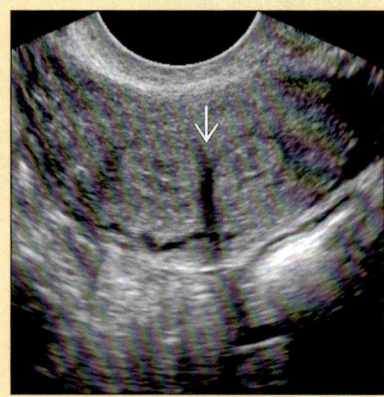

Partial Uterine Septum

ENDOMETRIAL SYNECHIAE

Key Facts

Terminology
- Intrauterine adhesions, webs, scarring
- Asherman syndrome: In setting of infertility or recurrent pregnancy loss
- Permanent adherence of uterine walls, with variable site(s) of these adhesions

Imaging Findings
- Irregular, well-demarcated, angular and/or straight tissue bridges spanning endometrial cavity
- Endometrial cavity may be partially distorted or completely obliterated
- When completely obliterated, non-filling of the endometrial cavity on hysterosalpingography or sonohysterography
- Incomplete distension of the cavity, folds and contractions can mimic synechiae

- Best imaging tool: Sonohysterography is considered to be almost as reliable as hysteroscopy in diagnosis of presence and extent of intrauterine adhesions

Pathology
- Factors causing destruction of endometrium allow for myometrial adhesions from opposing uterine walls
- Predisposing factors include: Gravid uterus, infection, missed abortion

Clinical Issues
- Scant or absent menstrual flow
- Secondary infertility (43%) and repeated spontaneous abortions
- Treat via hysteroscopic resection/lysis of adhesions

- If not distended, may just see endometrial thickening with or without "cysts" (fluid trapped in between synechiae)
- Echogenic bands traverse fluid-filled canal
- Synechiae may appear straight or serpentine
- Fibrous bands may calcify
- Absent endometrial stripe if canal is completely obliterated
- Synechiae may also be thin and filmy and appear to undulate in the fluid
- Difficult to distend the endometrial cavity with saline if adhesions are extensive or thick
- Endometrial cavity may appear distorted
- 3D ultrasound
  - Good supplement to TVS which only obtains images in two planes
  - Can better depict extent and locations of synechiae

MR Findings
- T2WI
  - Low signal intensity adhesions
  - Loss of normal endometrial high signal of lower uterine segment extending to external cervical os
- T1 C+: Adhesions will enhance, especially in early phase after contrast administration

Imaging Recommendations
- Best imaging tool: Sonohysterography is considered to be almost as reliable as hysteroscopy in diagnosis of presence and extent of intrauterine adhesions
- Hysterosalpingography (HSG) can detect filling defects in canal but is not specific
- Sonohysterography allows further characterization of filling defects and aids diagnosis and management
- Hysteroscopy allows for both diagnosis and treatment in a single procedure

DIFFERENTIAL DIAGNOSIS

Endometrial Polyp
- Polypoid mass(es) protrude into/distend endometrial canal

Focal Endometrial Hyperplasia
- Endometrial thickening with or without cysts

Endometrial Cancer
- Variable morphology, but may be polypoid or irregular
- Myometrial invasion is diagnostic of malignant process

Endometrial Blood Clot
- Variable morphology
- Passage of clot or evolution of clot with time

Partial Uterine Septum
- Congenital
- Unique characteristic site

Tuberculous Endometritis
- Filling defects with distortion of the cavity
- Distinguished by the presence of uterine fistulas

Nondistention of Endometrial Cavity
- During sonohysterography or hysterosalpingography: May be related to other causes such as fibroids

PATHOLOGY

General Features
- General path comments
  - Fibromuscular band with/without surrounding superficial epithelial cells
  - No significant inflammation
  - Partial or complete obliteration the endometrial cavity or obstruction of the cervical canal
- Etiology
  - Factors causing destruction of endometrium allow for myometrial adhesions from opposing uterine walls
  - Common denominator in all various etiologies is sustained apposition of injured intrauterine surfaces
  - Predisposing factors include: Gravid uterus, infection, missed abortion

ENDOMETRIAL SYNECHIAE

- Gravid uterus and trauma to the endometrial basal layer and myometrium during post partum period
- Infection
- Missed abortion
- Curettage or endometrial ablation
- Surgery, myomectomy (when involving surface of endometrium)
- Genital tuberculosis, tuberculous endometritis
- Caustic chemicals
- Foreign body reaction (intrauterine packing)
- Epidemiology
  - Universal incidence is steadily increasing
  - Incidence increases with number of D&Cs
    - 16% after first and up to 32% after three procedures

Gross Pathologic & Surgical Features

- Linear tissue spanning and/or obliterating endometrial canal
- Cervico-isthmic area is less commonly affected
- Calcifications are rarely seen
- Failure of re-epithelialization and subsequent development of fibromuscular adhesions
- Synechiae may be delicate, consisting solely of attenuated endometrial stroma but more commonly may consist of hypertrophic fibromuscular tissue extending between walls of uterine cavity
- Degree of distortion and obliteration of cavity is proportional to extent of pathologic change
- May be classified according to location

Microscopic Features

- Islands of granulation tissue from opposing uterine walls join to form bridges of scar tissue
- Bridges of scar tissue may be infiltrated by myometrium & inflammatory cells & on occasion may be covered with endometrium
- Fibrosis, distorted inactive endometrial glands, fibrous stroma with round cell infiltration and scant or absent vasculature on histologic examination
- Endometrium may be normal, atrophic, and ± lymphocyte infiltration
- Adenomyosis often coexists

CLINICAL ISSUES

Presentation

- Most common signs/symptoms
  - Scant or absent menstrual flow
  - Secondary infertility (43%) and repeated spontaneous abortions
- Menstrual disorders in 62%: Amenorrhea (37%), hypomenorrhea, and dysmenorrhea; most associated with cervico-isthmic adhesions
- Pregnancy, if achieved, may be complicated by habitual abortion, premature labor, placenta previa and placenta accreta
- Normal ovulatory hormonal profile

Natural History & Prognosis

- Following successful hysteroscopic treatment of severe synechiae
  - 28.7-57.4% intrauterine pregnancy rate
  - 28.7-32.1% live birth rate
  - Women < 35 years of age have better results (62.5% pregnancy rate)
- Even with satisfying results, normal endometrial function not guaranteed
- Spontaneous recovery has been reported

Treatment

- Goals of treatment: To eradicate adhesions and prevent their reformation
  - Treat via hysteroscopic resection/lysis of adhesions
    - Myometrial scoring is an alternative technique
  - Insertion of an intrauterine device to promote canal patency
  - Sequential hormonal therapy to build a good endometrium
  - Post-operative sonohysterography is important for documenting the adequacy of lysis of adhesions

DIAGNOSTIC CHECKLIST

Image Interpretation Pearls

- Endometrium may appear normal on transvaginal ultrasound
- Sonohysterography ideal for detection of adhesion and differentiation from other filling defects

SELECTED REFERENCES

1. Simpson WL Jr et al: Hysterosalpingography: a reemerging study. Radiographics. 26(2):419-31, 2006
2. Roma Dalfo A et al: Diagnostic value of hysterosalpingography in the detection of intrauterine abnormalities: a comparison with hysteroscopy. AJR Am J Roentgenol. 183(5):1405-9, 2004
3. Imaoka I et al: MR imaging of disorders associated with female infertility: use in diagnosis, treatment, and management. Radiographics. 23(6):1401-21, 2003
4. Davis PC et al: Sonohysterographic findings of endometrial and subendometrial conditions. Radiographics. 22(4):803-16, 2002
5. Kupesic S et al: Screening for uterine abnormalities by three-dimensional ultrasound improves perinatal outcome. J Perinat Med. 30(1):9-17, 2002
6. Nalaboff KM et al: Imaging the endometrium: disease and normal variants. Radiographics. 21(6):1409-24, 2001
7. Richenberg J et al: Ultrasound of the uterus. In: Ultrasonography in Obstetrics & Gynecology. Callen PW (ed.) W.B. Saunders, Philadelphia ; 814-846, 2000
8. Fedele L et al: Intrauterine adhesions: detection with transvaginal US. Radiology. 199(3):757-9, 1996
9. Schenker JG: Etiology of and therapeutic approach to synechia uteri. Eur J Obstet Gynecol Reprod Biol. 65(1):109-13, 1996
10. Bacelar AC et al: The value of MRI in the assessment of traumatic intra-uterine adhesions (Asherman's syndrome). Clin Radiol. 50(2):80-3, 1995
11. Cullinan JA et al: Sonohysterography: a technique for endometrial evaluation. Radiographics. 15(3):501-14; discussion 515-6, 1995
12. Atri M et al: Transvaginal US appearance of endometrial abnormalities. Radiographics. 14(3):483-92, 1994

ENDOMETRIAL SYNECHIAE

IMAGE GALLERY

Typical

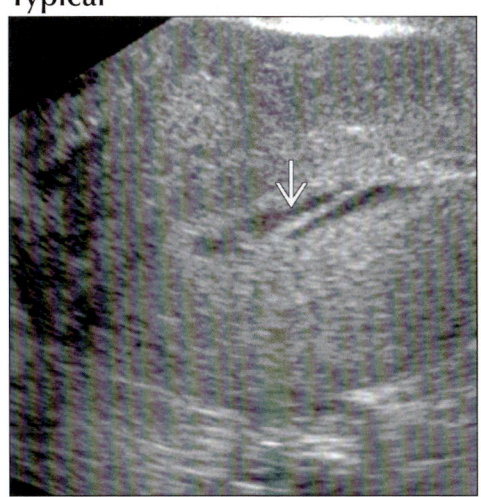
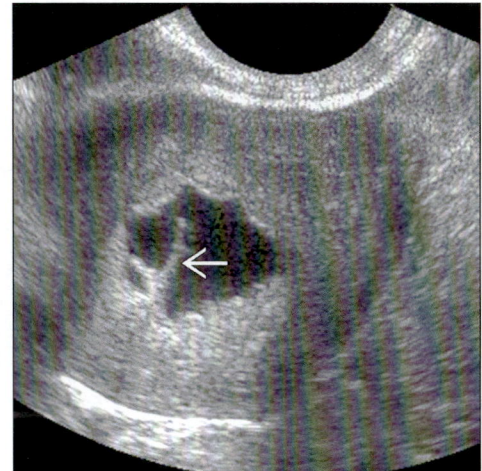

(Left) Sagittal transvaginal ultrasound shows echogenic band ➡ traversing the fluid-filled endometrial canal. *(Right)* Coronal transvaginal ultrasound shows thin, filmy echogenic structure ➡ which appeared to undulate as fluid was instilled during sonohysterogram.

Typical

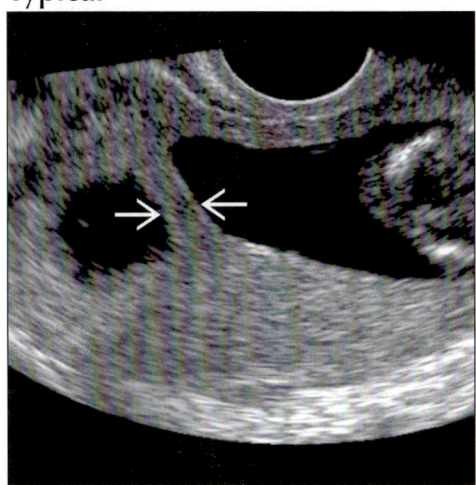
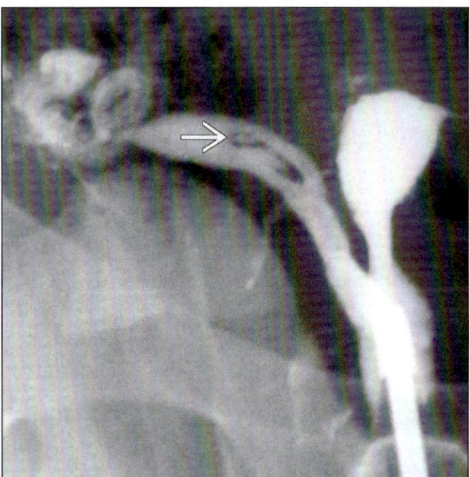

(Left) Coronal ultrasound shows myometrial to myometrial bridging septation ➡. *(Right)* Coronal oblique radiograph hysterosalpingogram shows a linear filling defect ➡ in the right horn of a known septate uterus.

Typical

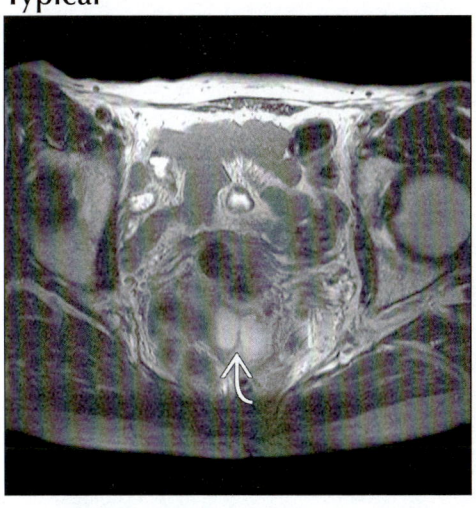
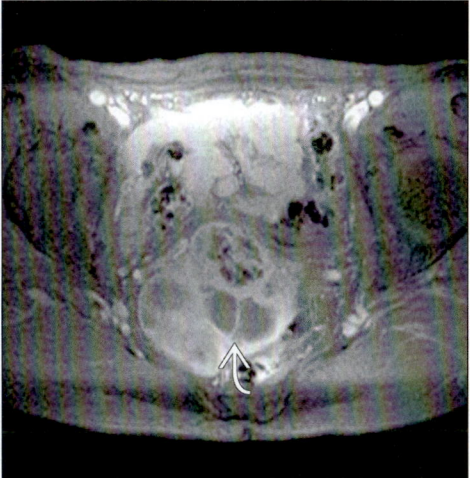

(Left) Axial T2WI MR shows a thin low signal intensity band ➡ coursing through the endometrial cavity. *(Right)* Axial T1 C+ FS MR in the same patient as previous image shows the enhancing synechia ➡.

ENDOMETRITIS

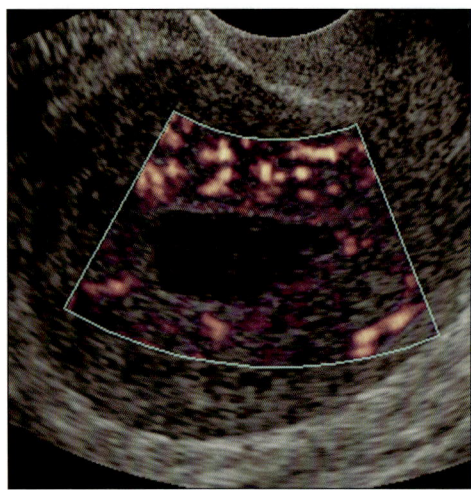

Sagittal power Doppler ultrasound shows fluid in the endometrial cavity in a patient with pelvic pain and fever who presents two weeks after a therapeutic abortion.

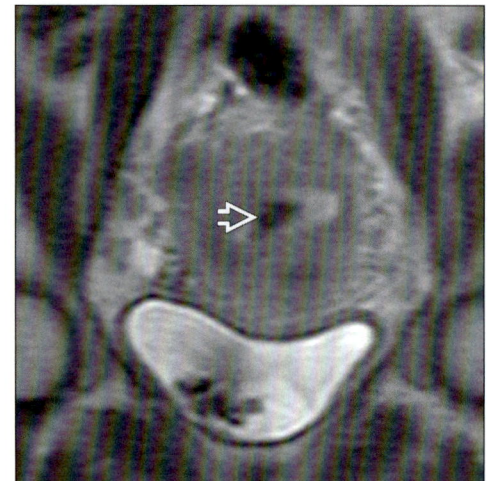

Coronal oblique T2WI MR in a febrile patient with pelvic pain after dilatation and curettage after miscarriage, shows a low signal intensity blood clot ⇨ surrounded by fluid within the endometrial cavity.

TERMINOLOGY

Definitions
- Polymicrobial infection originates from upward spread of infecting organisms through cervix and into uterus

IMAGING FINDINGS

General Features
- Best diagnostic clue: Increasing fluid and gas in endometrial cavity in postpartum patient with fever and pelvic tenderness

Ultrasonographic Findings
- Grayscale Ultrasound
  - Uterus may be enlarged
    - Patient may be tender to palpation, limiting ability to perform ultrasound examination
  - Thickened, heterogeneous endometrium and endometrial fluid with or without internal echoes representing gas
    - Within first 3 weeks postpartum intrauterine gas frequently a normal finding
  - Large volume of echogenic material in uterine cavity is normal immediately postpartum
  - Increase in amount of fluid and/or gas worrisome for endometritis
  - If associated with pelvic inflammatory disease (PID), heterogeneous collection in adnexa
- Color Doppler: Increased flow in inflamed pelvic structures (fallopian tubes or adnexal masses)

CT Findings
- Thickened endometrium, fluid or gas in endometrial cavity
- Parametrial inflammatory changes better seen than with ultrasound

MR Findings
- Thickened endometrial stripe, fluid or gas in endometrial cavity
  - Gas appears as a signal void on both T1WI and T2WI
- Contrast-enhanced MR increases the conspicuity of fluid collections
  - Low signal intensity areas adjacent to enhancing endometrium and myometrium

DDx: Endometritis

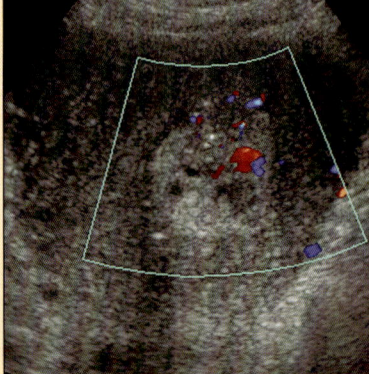
Retained Products of Conception

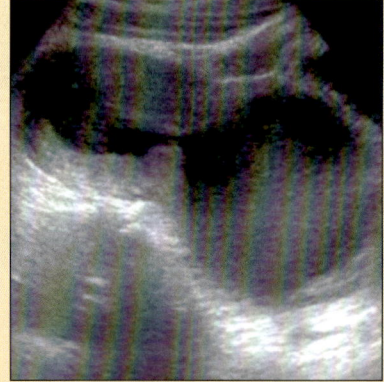
Cervical Stenosis

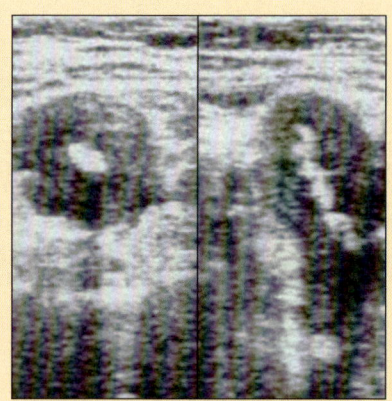
Endometrial Calcifications

ENDOMETRITIS

Key Facts

Terminology
- Polymicrobial infection originates from upward spread of infecting organisms through cervix and into uterus

Imaging Findings
- Best diagnostic clue: Increasing fluid and gas in endometrial cavity in postpartum patient with fever and pelvic tenderness
- Within first 3 weeks postpartum intrauterine gas frequently a normal finding

Pathology
- Most common cause of fever during postpartum period
- Increased risk with chorioamnionitis, premature rupture of the membranes, prolonged labor, retained clots, RPOC
- Endometritis (infectious and noninfectious) reported in 0.5% of UAE

Clinical Issues
- Risk of endometritis after vaginal delivery is 2-3%, after elective cesarian section 7%

Diagnostic Checklist
- Endometritis is a clinical diagnosis
- Imaging is requested for patients with refractory fever or pain to exclude any additional abnormality
- Imaging findings are frequently normal in uncomplicated endometritis

---

- If related to uterine artery embolization (UAE) or postpartum may be associated with uterine enlargement and intracavitary hematoma

Imaging Recommendations
- Best imaging tool: Transvaginal ultrasound
- Protocol advice
  - If an endometrial mass is seen, it could be retained products of conception or blood clot
  - Serial examinations may be needed to distinguish normal postpartum endometrial fluid from endometritis

DIFFERENTIAL DIAGNOSIS

Retained Products of Conception (RPOC)
- Echogenic endometrial mass, usually has high velocity, low resistance flow in color Doppler US
- Lack of increased flow does not eliminate the possibility of RPOC

Intrauterine Clot and Debris
- Fluid or complex fluid collection which changes in appearance over time
- Seen in 24% of cases after delivery

Gas in Endometrial Cavity
- 21% of patients after uncomplicated vaginal delivery have sonographic evidence of gas in endometrial cavity during the first 3 postpartum weeks, with no evidence of endometritis

Endometrial Calcifications
- Usually incidental finding associated with benign endometrial tissue, polyps, marked atrophy, postpartum or trauma from prior instrumentation
- Curvilinear calcifications have been reported in endometrial stromal sarcoma

PATHOLOGY

General Features
- Etiology
  - Etiologic agent often never identified
  - Common causal agents are Chlamydia trachomatis, Neisseria gonorrhoeae, genital tract mycoplasmas, aerobic and anaerobic vaginal flora (including those involved in bacterial vaginosis)
  - Postpartum endometritis is usually polymicrobial and involves anaerobes
  - Risk factors for endometritis: Gonococcal and chlamydial infection, current intrauterine device use, recent douching, proliferative phase of the menstrual cycle, postpartum
- Epidemiology
  - Most common cause of fever during postpartum period
  - Increased risk with chorioamnionitis, premature rupture of the membranes, prolonged labor, retained clots, RPOC
  - Endometritis (infectious and noninfectious) reported in 0.5% of UAE
    - Noninfective endometritis has high incidence with use of gold-colored gelatin microspheres
- Associated abnormalities
  - Tubo-ovarian abscess
  - Salpingitis
  - Pelvic fluid or abnormal fluid collections
  - Ovarian vein thrombosis

Gross Pathologic & Surgical Features
- Laparoscopy may demonstrate edema, erythema and purulent exudate, but cases of proven upper tract infection can be missed
  - Laparoscopy has a sensitivity of 50% and a specificity of 80% for salpingitis; if there is endometritis without salpingitis laparoscopy is frequently normal

Microscopic Features
- Acute endometritis

ENDOMETRITIS

- Histological diagnosis of acute endometritis is difficult during menstruation due to overlap of features
- Moderate - large numbers of neutrophils in non bleeding endometrium
- Aggregates of neutrophils in the stroma (microabscesses)
- Neutrophils filling and disrupting endometrial glands
- Chronic endometritis
  - Diagnosis is based on presence of plasma cells
  - Macrophages, lymphocytes and neutrophils may also be present
- 10-30% of cases of upper tract infection may be missed if diagnosis based on endometrial findings alone
- Plasma cell endometritis has been seen in 9% of asymptomatic, uninfected women

CLINICAL ISSUES

Presentation
- Most common signs/symptoms
  - Postpartum endometritis
    - Enlarged tender uterus on examination
    - Elevated white blood cell count
    - Fever
    - Increasing fluid/gas in endometrial cavity
  - Clinical abnormalities on physical examination of the women with non-postpartum endometritis less pronounced than in salpingitis
    - Lower abdominal pain, dyspareunia, fever, back pain, and vomiting
    - Elevated erythrocyte sedimentation rate, white blood counts and C-reactive protein levels
    - Adnexal tenderness on bimanual examination has sensitivity of 95% for histologic endometritis
    - Spectrum of endometritis alone encompasses asymptomatic women who may outnumber women with symptoms and signs suggestive of acute PID
- Other signs/symptoms
  - Spectrum of disease ranges from subclinical or asymptomatic to severe and life threatening
  - Frequently associated with symptoms of lower genital tract infection such as abnormal vaginal discharge, bleeding, itching, odor
  - Sequelae include chronic pelvic pain, ectopic pregnancy, infertility
  - Psychological distress due to association with sexually transmitted infection and potential for serious sequelae

Demographics
- Age: Any, more common in sexually active women
- Gender: Female

Natural History & Prognosis
- Postpartum
  - Risk of endometritis after vaginal delivery is 2-3%, after elective cesarian section 7%
  - Risk of endometritis for non-elective cesarian section is 19% in those who receive intraoperative antibiotics and 30% in those who don't
    - Incidence as high as 85% in women with cesarian delivery 6 hours or more after membranes have ruptured
- Non-postpartum, PID patients
  - In a study of women with suspected PID 28% had neither endometritis nor salpingitis, 17% had endometritis alone and 55% had salpingitis; 85% of the women with salpingitis had endometritis
- Prognosis of endometritis in the absence of laparoscopic signs of salpingitis remains largely undefined
- Potential for progression to salpingitis and subsequent infertility risks warrant aggressive antimicrobial therapy

Treatment
- Parenteral therapy necessary for patients with tuboovarian abscess, pregnant, severely ill, unable to follow treatment or unable to tolerate oral antibiotics
- Patients are hospitalized if surgical emergency cannot be excluded or if no clinical improvement occurs after three days

DIAGNOSTIC CHECKLIST

Consider
- Endometritis is a clinical diagnosis
  - 80% of women with persistent postpartum fever and endometritis have complicating factors besides resistant organisms that may be identified with imaging studies and change management
- Imaging is requested for patients with refractory fever or pain to exclude any additional abnormality
- Imaging findings are frequently normal in uncomplicated endometritis

Image Interpretation Pearls
- Suspect diagnosis in symptomatic or postpartum patient with increasing air in endometrial cavity or increasing thickness of heterogeneous endometrium

SELECTED REFERENCES

1. Crossman SH: The challenge of pelvic inflammatory disease. Am Fam Physician. 73(5):859-64, 2006
2. Kitamura Y et al: Imaging manifestations of complications associated with uterine artery embolization. Radiographics. 25 Suppl 1:S119-32, 2005
3. Eckert LO et al: Endometritis: the clinical-pathologic syndrome. Am J Obstet Gynecol. 186(4):690-5, 2002
4. Boardman LA et al: Endovaginal sonography for the diagnosis of upper genital tract infection. Obstet Gynecol. 90(1):54-7, 1997
5. Zuckerman J et al: Imaging of pelvic postpartum complications. AJR Am J Roentgenol. 168(3):663-8, 1997
6. Cacciatore B et al: Transvaginal sonographic findings in ambulatory patients with suspected pelvic inflammatory disease. Obstet Gynecol. 80(6):912-6, 1992
7. Wachsberg RH et al: Gas within the endometrial cavity at postpartum US: a normal finding after spontaneous vaginal delivery. Radiology. 183(2):431-3, 1992
8. Lev-Toaff AS et al: Diagnostic imaging in puerperal febrile morbidity. Obstet Gynecol. 78(1):50-5, 1991

ENDOMETRITIS

IMAGE GALLERY

Typical

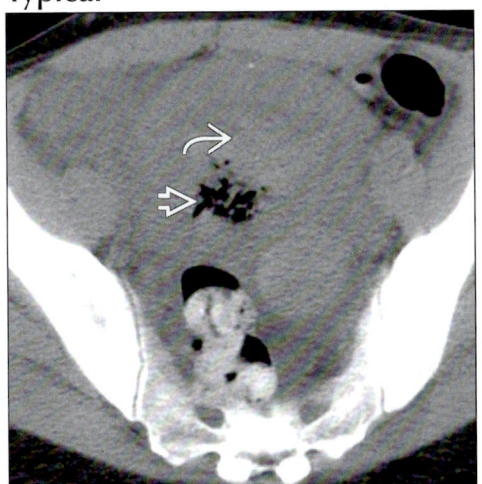
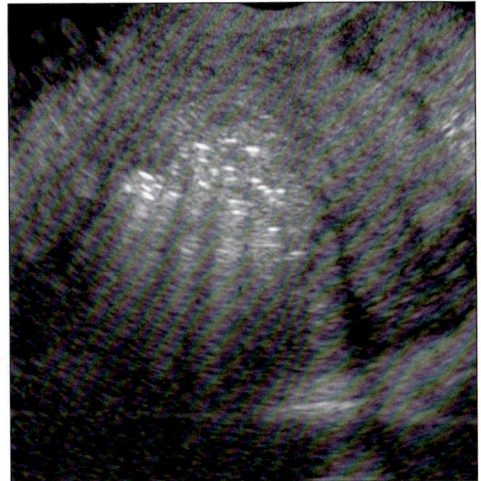

(Left) Axial NECT in patient with history of fever and abdominal pain two months after UAE shows large amount of gas ➡ near endometrial cavity and thickened endometrium ➡. *(Right)* Transverse transvaginal ultrasound shows heterogeneous increased echogenicity in endometrial cavity with "dirty shadowing" due to gas.

Typical

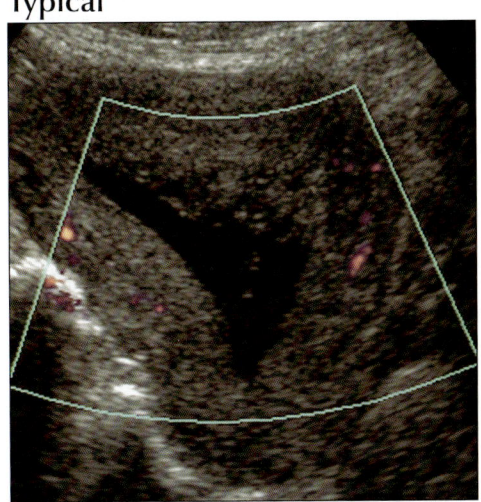
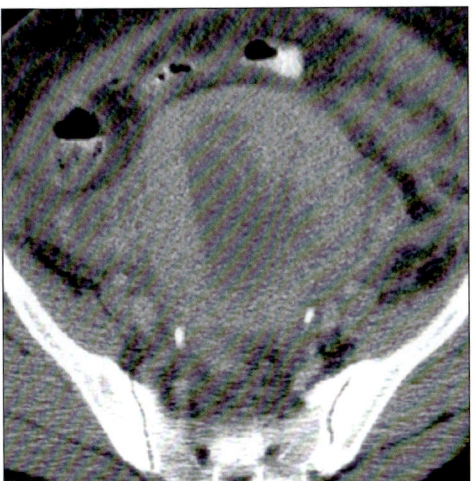

(Left) Sagittal power Doppler ultrasound in a postpartum patient with fever and abdominal pain shows echogenic debris and fluid in the endometrial cavity. *(Right)* Axial CECT in postpartum patient with fever and abdominal pain shows enlarged uterus with heterogeneous low attenuation debris in the endometrial cavity.

Typical

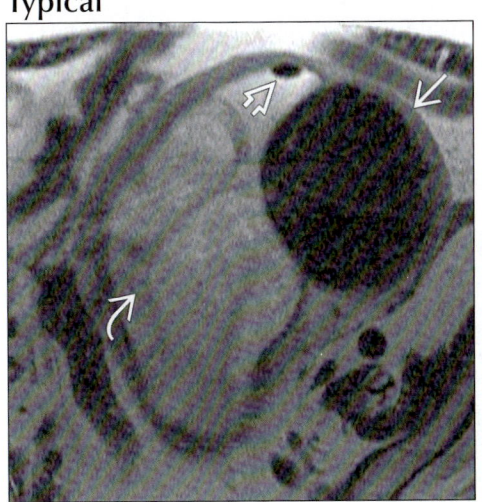
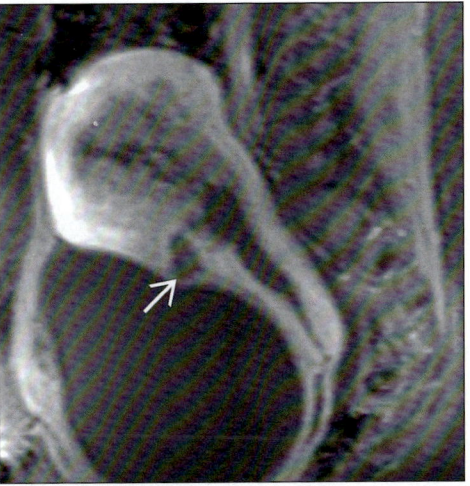

(Left) Axial T2WI MR in patient with purulent discharge shows fibroid uterus with large fibroid ➡, large mass from endometrial cancer ➡, and small amount of gas in endometrial cavity ➡. *(Right)* Sagittal T1 C+ MR shows endometrial cavity with fluid and debris in a postpartum patient with fever. Note cesarian section defect in the anterior wall of the lower uterine segment ➡.

PYOMYOMA

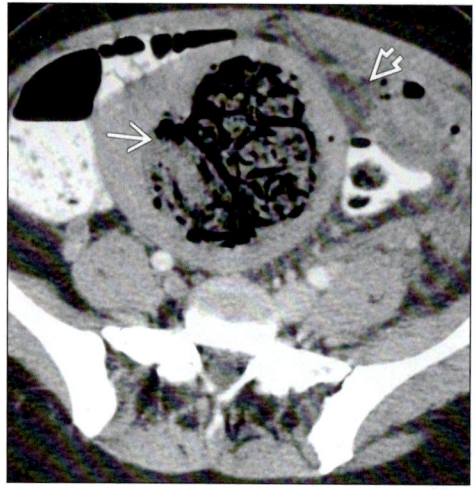

Axial CECT shows enlarged postpartum leiomyomatous uterus in a septic patient. A large gas-filled fundal leiomyoma ➡ is present with associated stranding ➡ of the adjacent pelvic fat.

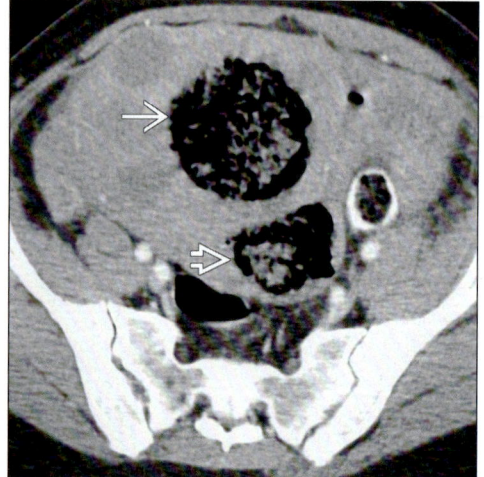

Axial CECT in the same patient as previous image shows two suppurative leiomyomas: The fundal pyomyoma ➡ and a second posterior and inferior pyomyoma ➡.

TERMINOLOGY

Abbreviations and Synonyms
- Suppurative leiomyoma, uterine pyomyoma

Definitions
- Infected leiomyoma

IMAGING FINDINGS

General Features
- Best diagnostic clue: Gas and debris within a leiomyoma in a symptomatic patient
- Location
  - Uterine
    - Intramural
    - Submucosal
    - Subserosal
- Size
  - Variable
  - May be multiple
- Morphology: Round, may rupture

Ultrasonographic Findings
- Grayscale Ultrasound
  - Transvaginal ultrasound (TVS)
    - Enlarging pelvic mass or discrete leiomyoma
    - Heterogeneous pelvic mass or discrete leiomyoma with cystic and solid components
    - Leiomyoma with debris
    - Development of increasing echogenicity with reverberation artifact (gas) within leiomyoma

CT Findings
- NECT: Enlarged uterus with gas within leiomyoma
- CECT
  - Leiomyoma with gas and internal debris
  - Heterogeneous leiomyoma with solid and cystic components
  - Multiplanar reformation may help identify pyomyoma rupture with discontinuity of leiomyoma wall
  - Intraperitoneal fluid and gas if associated uterine rupture

DDx: Pyomyoma

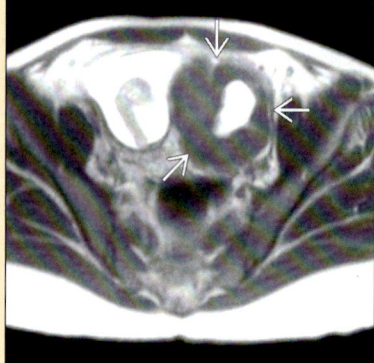

Degenerated Leiomyoma

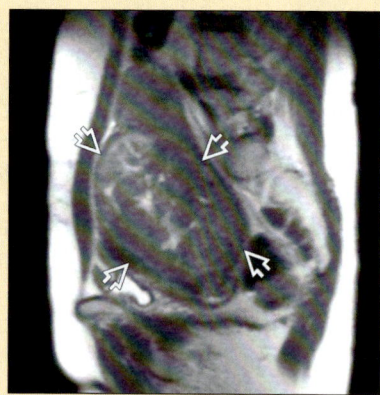

Leiomyosarcoma

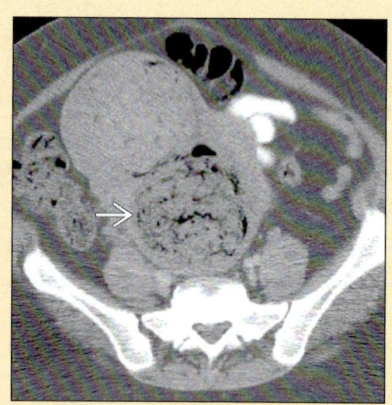

Normal Post-UAE Uterus

PYOMYOMA

Key Facts

Terminology
- Suppurative leiomyoma, uterine pyomyoma
- Infected leiomyoma

Imaging Findings
- Best diagnostic clue: Gas and debris within a leiomyoma in a symptomatic patient
- Heterogeneous leiomyoma with solid and cystic components
- Multiplanar reformation may help identify pyomyoma rupture with discontinuity of leiomyoma wall
- Development of increasing echogenicity with reverberation artifact (gas) within leiomyoma

Top Differential Diagnoses
- Leiomyoma with Hemorrhagic Infarction
- Degenerated Leiomyoma
- Leiomyosarcoma
- Endometritis

Pathology
- Rare
- Decline in cases secondary to the advent of antibiotic therapy

Clinical Issues
- Most common signs/symptoms: Triad: Leiomyoma, bacteremia, and sepsis
- Usually develop slowly over days or weeks, especially after delivery or abortion
- Mortality rates approach 21-30%
- Hysterectomy or myomectomy usually necessary
- Aggressive antibiotic therapy

Imaging Recommendations
- Best imaging tool: Ultrasound or CT showing gas & debris within leiomyoma in symptomatic patient
- Protocol advice: Interpret imaging findings in light of clinical history

DIFFERENTIAL DIAGNOSIS

Leiomyoma with Hemorrhagic Infarction
- Iatrogenic: Following uterine artery embolization (UAE)
- Spontaneous: Outgrow blood supply
- Variable appearance
  - CT: May see gas within infarcted leiomyoma; on NECT may see areas of high attenuation (blood); calcified rim may form post UAE
  - TVS early: Heterogeneous increased echogenicity, may also see echogenic foci with reverberation artifact (gas)
  - TVS late: May be hypoechoic with calcified rim ("fetal head sign")
  - MR: Homogeneous high SI on T1WI and low SI on T2WI
- Presence of gas is not synonymous with infection
- Patients may complain of pain, but are not septic

Degenerated Leiomyoma
- Heterogeneous leiomyoma
  - CECT: Calcified rim if calcific degeneration
  - TVS: May see shadowing echogenic foci if calcific degeneration
  - MR: High and low SI on T2WI
  - Imaging findings not specific for most types of degeneration
- Patients are not symptomatic

Leiomyosarcoma
- Patients are not septic
- Enlarging heterogeneous leiomyoma
  - CECT: Enhancing mass with irregular areas of necrosis; enhancement is less than normal myometrium
  - TVS: Heterogeneous echotexture secondary to solid, necrotic or hemorrhagic regions; color Doppler with increased vascularity
  - MR: Areas of necrosis and hemorrhage; enhancement is less than normal myometrium
- Necrosis and hemorrhage are common, but not specific

Endometritis
- Confined to endometrium
- Most common cause of postpartum fever
- Variable imaging appearance
  - Normal
  - Thickened heterogeneous endometrium
  - Intracavitary fluid
  - Intracavitary air

PATHOLOGY

General Features
- Etiology
  - Associated with several clinical conditions
    - Pregnancy
    - Post-abortion
    - Postpartum: Vaginal or cesarian delivery
    - Ascending uterine infection
    - Cervical stenosis
    - Post-uterine artery embolization
    - Postmenopausal patients secondary to ischemia resulting from hypertension, diabetes or atherosclerosis
  - Mechanisms of spread
    - Contiguous spread from endometrium
    - Direct extension from adjacent bowel or adnexa
    - Hematogenous/lymphatic spread from distant infection
- Epidemiology
  - Rare
    - 1871-1945: 75 reported cases

PYOMYOMA

- 1945-1990: 10 cases
- Decline in cases secondary to the advent of antibiotic therapy

Gross Pathologic & Surgical Features
- Enlarged uterus
- Gray-white friable leiomyoma

Microscopic Features
- Coagulation necrosis
- Purulent inflammation
- Multiple organisms
  - Streptococcus
  - Staphylococcus
  - Proteus
  - Serratia
  - Actinomyces
  - Enterococcus
  - Edwardsiella

CLINICAL ISSUES

Presentation
- Most common signs/symptoms: Triad: Leiomyoma, bacteremia, and sepsis
- Other signs/symptoms
  - Fever
  - Leukocytosis
  - Endocarditis
  - Deep venous thrombosis

Demographics
- Age
  - Variable
    - Reproductive age women
    - Postmenopausal women

Natural History & Prognosis
- Usually develop slowly over days or weeks, especially after delivery or abortion
- If untreated, may rupture or penetrate into
  - Abdominal cavity
  - Adjacent pelvic structure
  - Abdominal wall
  - Endometrial cavity
- Mortality rates approach 21-30%

Treatment
- Hysterectomy or myomectomy usually necessary
- Aggressive antibiotic therapy

DIAGNOSTIC CHECKLIST

Consider
- Pyomyoma in a woman with unexplained sepsis and leiomyoma
- Two patient populations
  - Pregnant, postpartum or postabortal women
  - Postmenopausal women

Image Interpretation Pearls
- Think pyomyoma in a septic patient with gas-containing leiomyoma

SELECTED REFERENCES

1. Kitamura Y et al: Imaging manifestations of complications associated with uterine artery embolization. Radiographics. 25 Suppl 1:S119-32, 2005
2. Mason TC et al: Postpartum pyomyoma. J Natl Med Assoc. 97(6):826-8, 2005
3. Sah SP et al: Pyomyoma in a postmenopausal woman: a case report. Southeast Asian J Trop Med Public Health. 36(4):979-81, 2005
4. Rajan DK et al: Risk of intrauterine infectious complications after uterine artery embolization. J Vasc Interv Radiol. 15(12):1415-21, 2004
5. de Blok S et al: Fatal sepsis after uterine artery embolization with microspheres. J Vasc Interv Radiol. 14(6):779-83, 2003
6. Karcaaltincaba M et al: CT of a ruptured pyomyoma. AJR Am J Roentgenol. 181(5):1375-7, 2003
7. Lin YH et al: Pyomyoma after a cesarean section. Acta Obstet Gynecol Scand. 81(6):571-2, 2002
8. Genta PR et al: Streptococcus agalactiae endocarditis and giant pyomyoma simulating ovarian cancer. South Med J. 94(5):508-11, 2001
9. Grune B et al: Sepsis in second trimester of pregnancy due to an infected myoma. A case report and a review of the literature. Fetal Diagn Ther. 16(4):245-7, 2001
10. Gupta B et al: Pyomyoma: a case report. Aust N Z J Obstet Gynaecol. 39(4):520-1, 1999
11. Vashisht A et al: Fatal septicaemia after fibroid embolisation. Lancet. 354(9175):307-8, 1999
12. Yang CH et al: Edwardsiella tarda bacteraemia--complicated by acute pancreatitis and pyomyoma. J Infect. 38(2):124-6, 1999
13. Prahlow JA et al: Uterine pyomyoma as a complication of pregnancy in an intravenous drug user. South Med J. 89(9):892-5, 1996
14. Tobias DH et al: Pyomyoma after uterine instrumentation. A case report. J Reprod Med. 41(5):375-8, 1996
15. Greenspoon JS et al: Pyomyoma associated with polymicrobial bacteremia and fatal septic shock: case report and review of the literature. Obstet Gynecol Surv. 45(9):563-9, 1990
16. Prichard JG et al: Streptococcus milleri pyomyoma simulating infective endocarditis. Obstet Gynecol. 68(3 Suppl):46S-49S, 1986

PYOMYOMA

IMAGE GALLERY

Typical

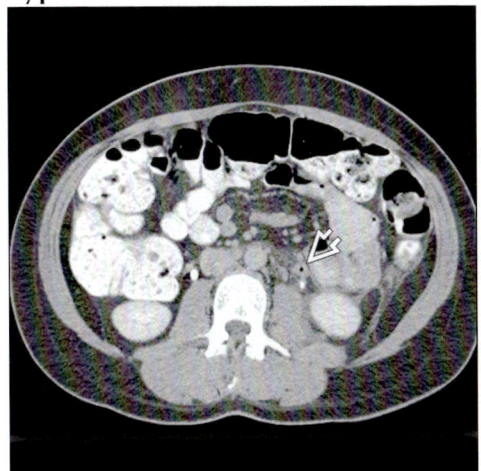
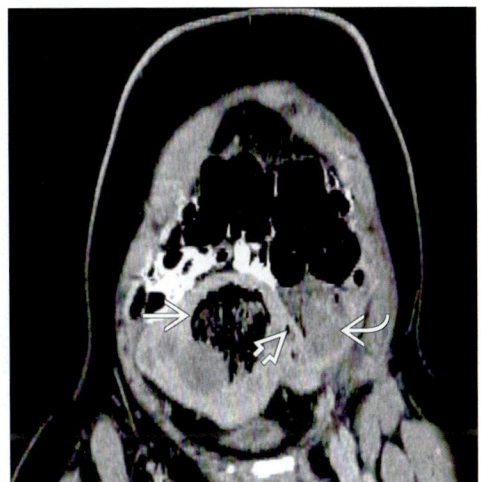

(Left) Axial CECT in the same patient as previous image shows air within an enlarged left ovarian vein ➡ with stranding in the surrounding fat. Septic thrombophlebitis may be seen in association with pyomyoma. *(Right)* Coronal CECT multiplanar reconstruction in the same patient as previous image shows the fundal pyomyoma ➡ and an associated pyosalpinx with punctate foci of gas ➡. A left ovarian abscess is also present ➡.

Typical

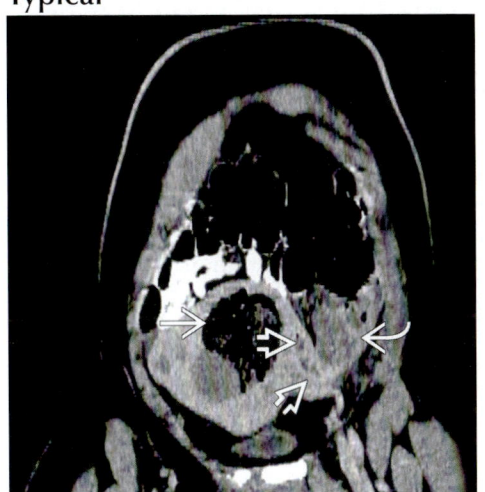
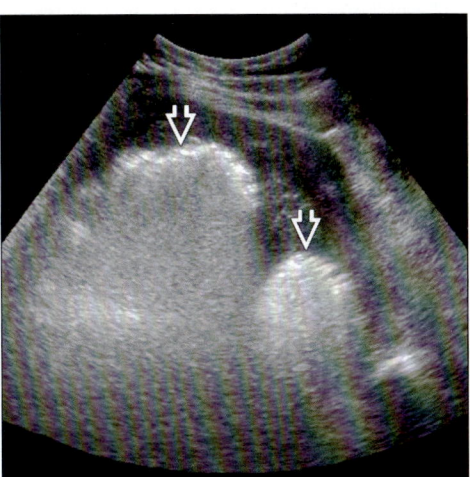

(Left) Coronal CECT multiplanar reconstruction in the same patient as previous image shows the infected leiomyoma ➡ and increased enhancement of the associated tubular pyosalpinx ➡. A left ovarian abscess is also seen ➡. *(Right)* Sagittal transabdominal ultrasound in the same patient as previous image shows two echogenic regions with reverberation artifact within the uterus corresponding to gas within two leiomyomas ➡.

Typical

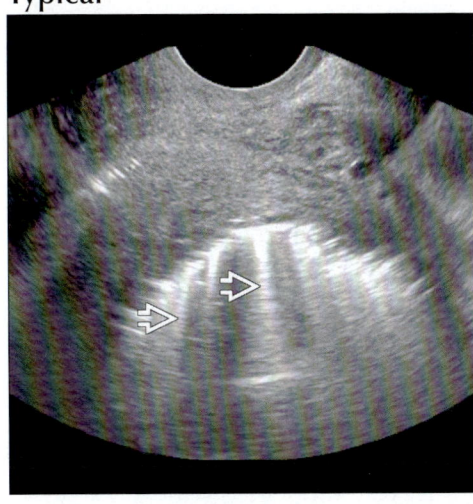
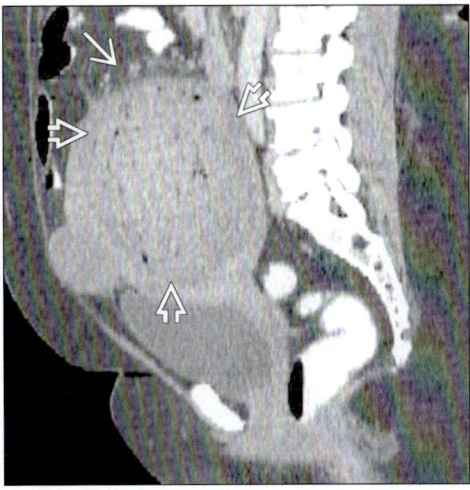

(Left) Axial transvaginal ultrasound in the same patient as previous image. The improved spatial resolution of TVS increases the conspicuity of the ring-down artifact ➡ secondary to gas within the fundal pyomyoma. *(Right)* Sagittal CECT multiplanar reconstruction in a septic patient post uterine artery embolization shows gas within a hemorrhagic leiomyoma ➡ and fat stranding in the surrounding fat ➡ consistent with pyomyoma.

INTRAVENOUS LEIOMYOMATOSIS

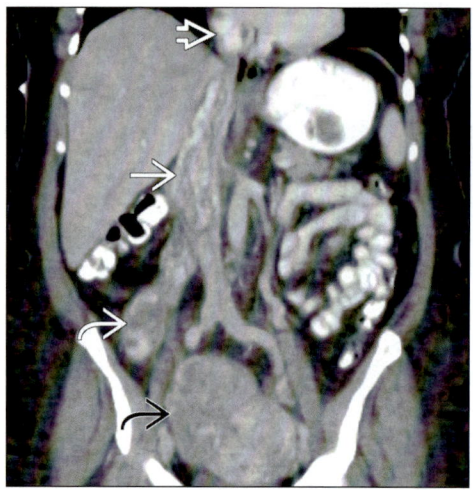

Coronal reformatted CT shows enlarged, irregularly enhancing uterus, large enhancing pelvic veins, enhancing tumor in the right ovarian vein, subphrenic segment of the IVC, and heart.

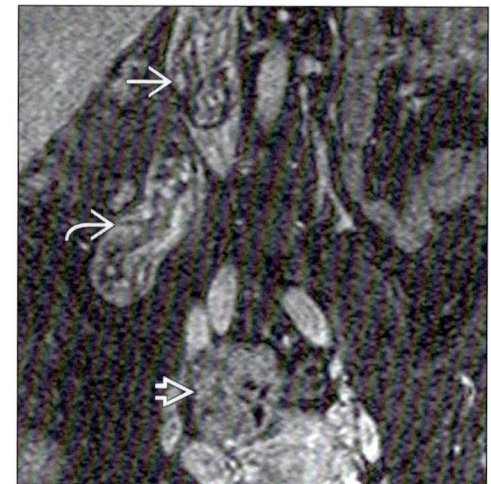

Coronal T1 C+ MR shows heterogeneously enhancing uterus, enlarged pelvic veins, long and irregularly enhancing filling defects in the right ovarian vein and subphrenic segment of the IVC.

TERMINOLOGY

Abbreviations and Synonyms
- Intravenous leiomyomatosis (IVL)

Definitions
- Uncommon uterine tumor characterized by intravascular nodular masses of histologically benign smooth muscle that may extend variable distances

IMAGING FINDINGS

General Features
- Best diagnostic clue: Enlarged uterus with mass in adjacent veins
- Location
  - 80% of tumors extend from uterus to extrauterine pelvic veins
    - Majority of cases involve unilateral venous system, uterine vein more common than ovarian vein
    - 40% extend into inferior vena cava (IVC) and heart
    - Cardiac involvement in up to 10% of cases
    - Tumor may extend to retroperitoneal veins

Ultrasonographic Findings
- Grayscale Ultrasound
  - Enlarged uterus with heterogeneous mass
  - Intravascular extension of tumor has multiple venous attachments within involved vessels
- Color Doppler: Demonstrates flow around tumor and circulation within intravascular tumor

CT Findings
- CTA
  - Defines extravascular, intravascular and intracardiac extension of tumor
    - Involved vessels are enlarged and distended with enhancing tumor
    - Direct extension may involve pulmonary arteries and branches, although tumor embolus is rare
- CECT
  - Enlarged uterus with heterogeneously enhancing mass and variable intravenous growth to veins of uterus and broad ligaments
    - Uterine mass may undergo cystic degeneration
    - Intravascular tumor may calcify

DDx: Intravenous Leiomyomatosis

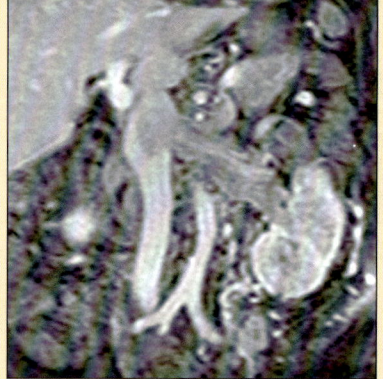
Renal Cell Cancer

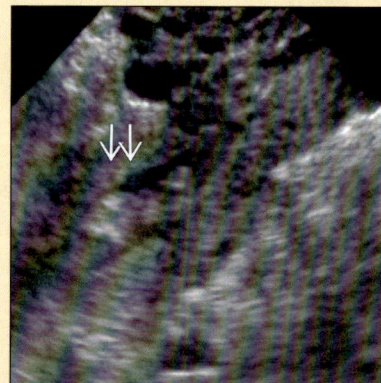
Ovarian Vein Thrombosis

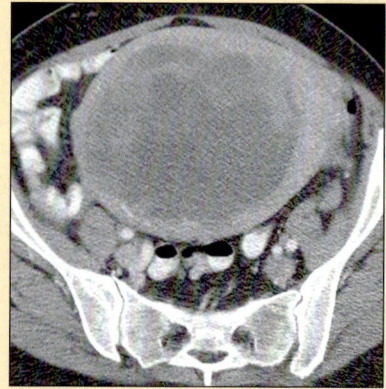
Leiomyosarcoma

INTRAVENOUS LEIOMYOMATOSIS

Key Facts

Imaging Findings
- Enlarged uterus with heterogeneously enhancing mass and variable intravenous growth to veins of uterus and broad ligaments
- Enhancing tumor may extend to iliac, uterine or gonadal veins, IVC, heart and pulmonary arteries
- Low signal intensity uterine mass with worm-like, tubular projections that involve myometrium
- Prominent signal voids in tubular projections
- Intravenous tumor has multiple venous or cardiac attachments

Pathology
- Under-diagnosed since it is easily missed in early stages
- Neoplastic cells have minimal nuclear atypia and low mitotic index

Clinical Issues
- Long term prognosis very good after resection
- 30% of patients may have persistent or continued growth of incompletely excised intravenous tumor
- Avoid exogenous estrogens (especially if resection is incomplete) because tumor is estrogen dependent

Diagnostic Checklist
- Pre-operative imaging delineates extent of tumor but does not differentiate between benign and malignant etiologies
- When tumor is inside small vessels of the myometrium it is not detected on preoperative imaging

---

  - Enhancing tumor may extend to iliac, uterine or gonadal veins, IVC, heart and pulmonary arteries
  - Ureters may be dilated (compression from pelvic tumor)
  - Bladder may be anteriorly displaced but not infiltrated by tumor

MR Findings
- T2WI
  - Low signal intensity uterine mass with worm-like, tubular projections that involve myometrium
  - Prominent signal voids in tubular projections
- T1 C+
  - Heterogeneous, avidly enhancing mass in uterus
  - Intravenous growth to veins of uterus and broad ligaments
  - Can extend into IVC and heart

Angiographic Findings
- Inferior vena cavography
  - Demonstrates IVC occlusion with multiple intravascular filling defects and collateral circulation

Echocardiographic Findings
- Echocardiogram
  - Elongated, mobile masses extending from lower body veins including IVC and azygos vein
  - Intravenous tumor has multiple venous or cardiac attachments
  - Tumor fills veins, right heart chambers and rarely pulmonary arteries
  - Valvular disease such as tricuspid regurgitation
  - Transesophageal echocardiogram helps define extent

Imaging Recommendations
- Best imaging tool: Contrast-enhanced MR or CT
- Protocol advice
  - Coronal plane demonstrates extent of disease
  - Cardiac involvement determines surgical approach
  - Determine adherence of intravascular tumor to venous wall
  - Patency of iliac and femoral veins important for surgical planning

DIFFERENTIAL DIAGNOSIS

Leiomyosarcoma
- No grossly visible vascular involvement

Diffuse Leiomyomatosis
- Replacement of myometrium by multiple, confluent, benign leiomyomatous nodules

Disseminated Leiomyomatosis
- Multiple, benign leiomyomas in peritoneal cavity

Benign Metastasizing Leiomyomatosis
- Benign leiomyomas in solid organs, most common in lung or liver

Renal Cell Carcinoma Invading IVC
- Rarely have endocardial attachments
- Mass-like appearance, not long mobile structures
- Enters IVC from renal veins

Right Sided Heart Thrombus-in-Transit
- Elongated mobile masses without multiple points of attachment in heart chambers
- No flow on color Doppler, no enhancement

Ovarian Vein Thrombosis
- Occurs in febrile, postpartum patient with pain
- No enhancement of thrombus

PATHOLOGY

General Features
- Etiology: Unclear, tumor may arise from uterine leiomyoma, walls of uterine vessel or myometrium
- Epidemiology
  - About 200 cases reported in literature
  - Under-diagnosed since it is easily missed in early stages

INTRAVENOUS LEIOMYOMATOSIS

Gross Pathologic & Surgical Features
- Enlargement of the uterus by solitary or multiple mural or submucosal leiomyomas
  - Most are well-demarcated from surrounding myometrium, but can be poorly circumscribed
  - Masses are typically lobulated or multinodular (grape-like), rubbery and have fluid accumulation
  - Color is tan, gray or reddish-blue
  - Cystic degeneration
  - Tumor frequently extends to the broad ligament or parametrium
- Worm-like plugs of tumor within myometrial or cervical veins are frequently not appreciated on initial examination (40-60%) but almost always visible upon re-examination of the hysterectomy specimen

Microscopic Features
- Endothelium-covered proliferations of benign smooth muscle within lumen of myometrial vessels
  - Most of vessels are veins, some lymphatics
  - Intravascular tumor can be unattached or have delicate to broad-based intimal attachments
  - Tumor has thick-walled blood vessels
- In typical cases, intravascular tumor closely resembles uterine leiomyoma
  - May have zones of hyalinization
  - Contrary to leiomyoma, it is a highly vascular neoplasm with elevated microvessel counts
- Neoplastic cells have minimal nuclear atypia and low mitotic index
  - Histologic variants of IVL differ in cellular composition but resemble typical IVL in clinical behavior
  - Variants should be distinguished from endometrial stromal sarcoma and leiomyosarcoma
  - Variable histologic appearance can lead to difficultly in recognition of smooth muscle nature

CLINICAL ISSUES

Presentation
- Most common signs/symptoms
  - Pelvic or lower abdominal mass from enlarged uterus
  - Abnormal uterine bleeding
  - Pelvic pain
- Other signs/symptoms
  - Uterine prolapse, stress incontinence
  - Right-sided congestive symptoms: Lower limb swelling, dyspnea, congestive heart failure, ascites
  - Syncope (from obstruction at tricuspid valve)
  - Systemic embolism, sudden death
  - Asymptomatic (cases of intermediate extension limited to the IVC)

Demographics
- Age
  - 25-75 years, median age 42 years
  - Usually premenopausal
  - 90% of reported cases have had pregnancies

Natural History & Prognosis
- Long term prognosis very good after resection
- 30% of patients may have persistent or continued growth of incompletely excised intravenous tumor
  - Recurrences reported up to 15 years after resection
- Death from tumor is rare, intraoperative deaths have occurred from massive retroperitoneal hemorrhage

Treatment
- Options, risks, complications
  - Total abdominal hysterectomy, bilateral salpingo-oophorectomy and excision of extrauterine tumor
  - May necessitate sternotomy (using cardiopulmonary bypass or circulatory arrest) as well as laparotomy in a single or two-stage operation
  - Avoid exogenous estrogens (especially if resection is incomplete) because tumor is estrogen dependent
  - Tamoxifen can be used to help control growth of unresectable tumor

DIAGNOSTIC CHECKLIST

Consider
- Pre-operative imaging delineates extent of tumor but does not differentiate between benign and malignant etiologies
- CT and MR are ideal techniques to demonstrate full extent of tumor from pelvis to thorax
- When tumor is inside small vessels of the myometrium it is not detected on preoperative imaging
- There is often a past history of hysterectomy with ovarian preservation

SELECTED REFERENCES
1. Moorjani N et al: Intravenous uterine leiomyosarcomatosis with intracardial extension. J Card Surg. 20(4):382-5, 2005
2. Lam PM et al: Intravenous leiomyomatosis: two cases with different routes of tumor extension. J Vasc Surg. 39(2):465-9, 2004
3. Kullo IJ et al: Intracardiac leiomyomatosis: echocardiographic features. Chest. 115(2):587-91, 1999
4. Bertrand P et al: Intravenous leiomyomatosis with caval involvement: report of a case with radical resection and venous replacement. Arch Surg. 133(4):460-2, 1998
5. Gawne-Cain ML et al: Case report: intravenous leiomyomatosis, an unusual cause of intracardiac filling defect. Clin Radiol. 50(2):123-5, 1995
6. Clement PB et al: Intravenous leiomyomatosis of the uterus. A clinicopathological analysis of 16 cases with unusual histologic features. Am J Surg Pathol. 12(12):932-45, 1988

INTRAVENOUS LEIOMYOMATOSIS

IMAGE GALLERY

Typical

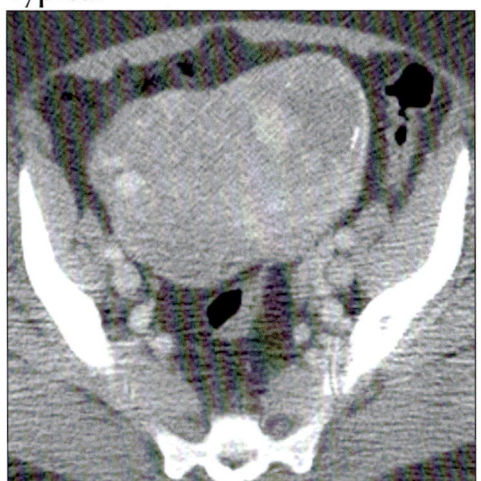
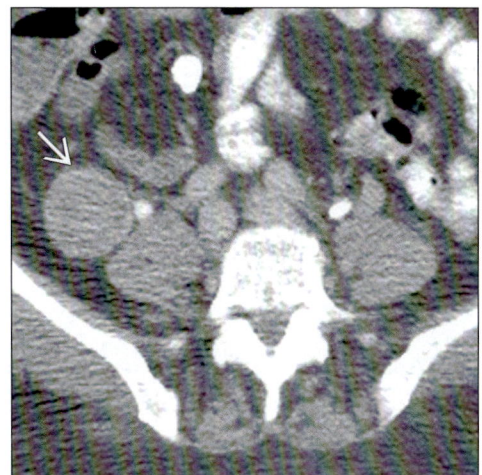

(Left) Axial CECT in the arterial phase shows enlarged, heterogeneously enhancing uterus surrounded by enlarged, enhancing pelvic vessels that contain intravenous tumor. (Right) Axial CECT during late venous phase shows enlargement of right ovarian vein due to enhancing tumor ➡.

Typical

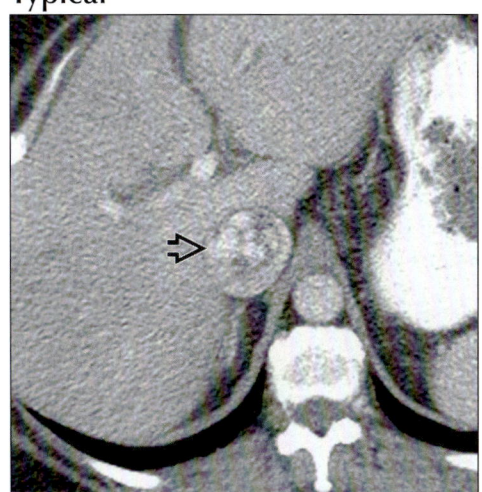
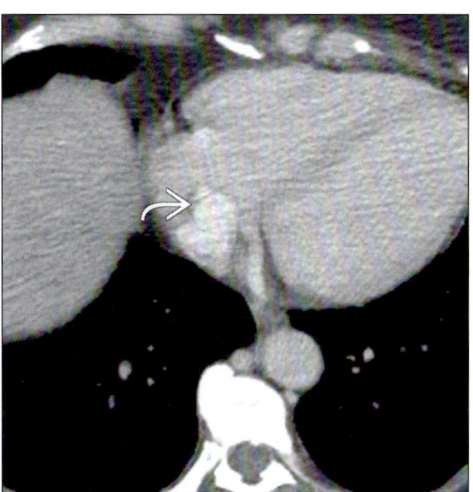

(Left) Axial CECT in the arterial phase shows enlarged retrohepatic IVC with enhancing tumor ➡. (Right) Axial CECT in arterial phase shows enhancing tumor ➡ within the right atrium, which does not extend to the right ventricle.

Typical

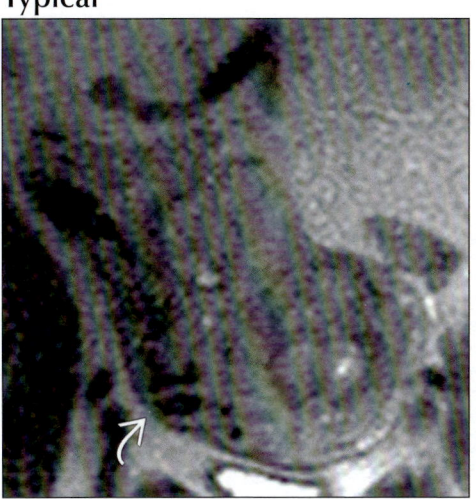
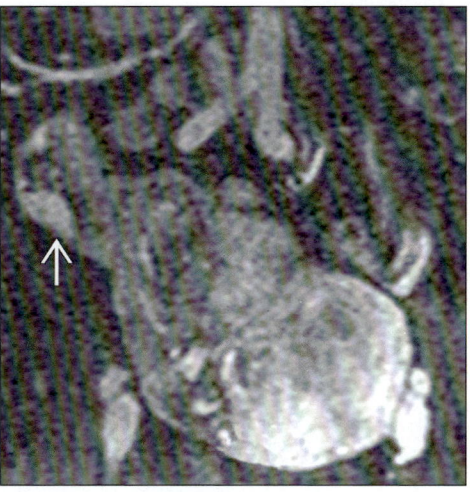

(Left) Coronal T1WI MR shows enlarged uterus with multiple low signal intensity masses and tubular flow voids ➡ in the myometrium, consistent with intravenous extension of high flow tumor. (Right) Coronal T1 C+ MR shows enlarged uterus with multiple heterogeneously enhancing leiomyomas and filling defects in large right ovarian vein ➡.

DISSEMINATED PERITONEAL LEIOMYOMATOSIS

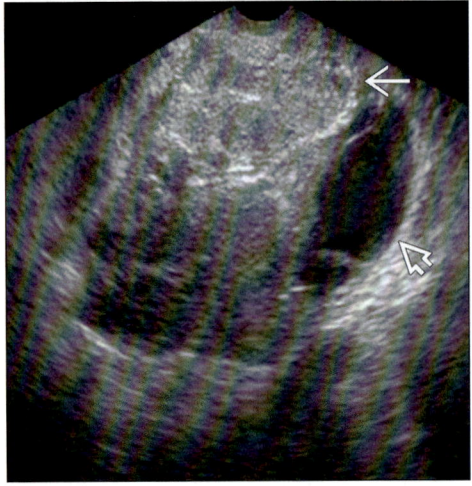

Transvaginal ultrasound shows uterus distorted by leiomyomas ➡. There is a left hydrosalpinx caused by a left retroperitoneal and pelvic mass ➡. Reproduced with permission from AJR.

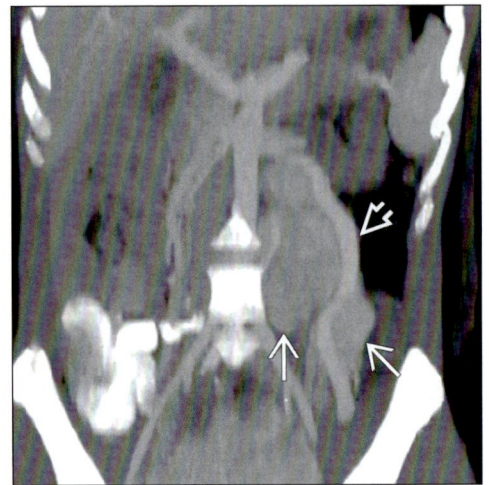

Coronal CECT shows a heterogeneously enhancing left retroperitoneal mass ➡ which encases and displaces the left gonadal vein ➡. Reproduced with permission from AJR.

TERMINOLOGY

Definitions
- Typically benign condition characterized by multiple smooth muscle nodules arising in pelvic and abdominal cavities

IMAGING FINDINGS

General Features
- Size: Few millimeters to several centimeters

Ultrasonographic Findings
- Solid or complex soft tissue peritoneal masses

CT Findings
- CECT
  - Solid and complex soft tissue masses in the peritoneum, uterus, broad ligaments, ovaries, mesentery, intestines, omentum
  - Enhancement similar to uterus or heterogeneous
  - Not associated with infiltration of omentum, ascites or liver metastases

MR Findings
- T1WI: Masses similar in signal intensity to skeletal muscle or uterine parenchyma
- T2WI: Low signal intensity due to smooth muscle
- T1 C+: Variable enhancement

Nuclear Medicine Findings
- PET: Peritoneal nodules do not show increased uptake of F-18 FDG as would be seen in leiomyosarcoma

DIFFERENTIAL DIAGNOSIS

Metastatic Malignant Neoplasm
- Nodules on peritoneal surface

Leiomyosarcoma
- Higher mitotic index, nuclear atypia, tumor necrosis and infiltrative growth into adjacent structures

Multiple Pedunculated Uterine Leiomyomas
- Look for attachment of leiomyomas to uterus

Benign Metastasizing Leiomyomas
- Smooth muscle tumor in liver or lung

DDx: Disseminated Peritoneal Leiomyomatosis

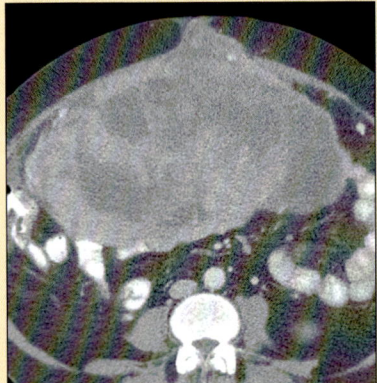
Metastatic Leiomyosarcoma

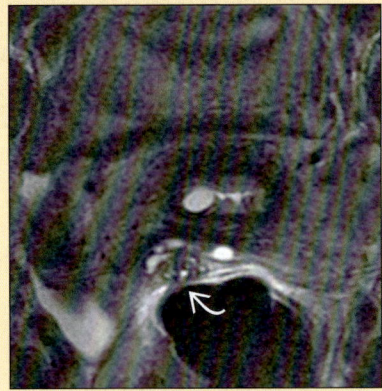
Endometriosis Implants

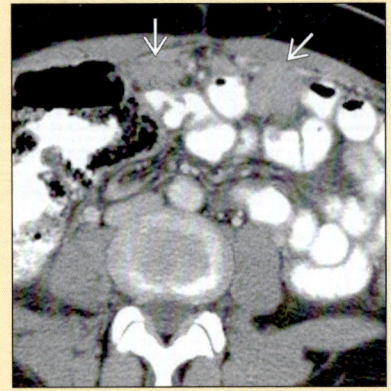
Peritoneal Carcinomatosis

DISSEMINATED PERITONEAL LEIOMYOMATOSIS

Key Facts

Terminology
- Typically benign condition characterized by multiple smooth muscle nodules arising in pelvic and abdominal cavities

Imaging Findings
- Solid and complex soft tissue masses in the peritoneum, uterus, broad ligaments, ovaries, mesentery, intestines, omentum
- Enhancement similar to uterus or heterogeneous
- Not associated with infiltration of omentum, ascites or liver metastases

Pathology
- Grossly malignant but histologically benign

Clinical Issues
- Spontaneous regression when ↓ exposure to estrogen

Diagnostic Checklist
- Mimics peritoneal carcinomatosis

Intravenous Leiomyomatosis
- Extension of uterine leiomyoma into venous channels

PATHOLOGY

General Features
- Etiology
  - Smooth muscle metaplasia of subperitoneal pluripotent mesenchymal stem cells
  - Many cases associated with pregnancy, granulosa cell tumor, or oral contraceptive use
- Epidemiology: Rare, over 100 cases reported
- Associated abnormalities: Endometrial hyperplasia, leiomyomas, endometriosis

Gross Pathologic & Surgical Features
- Grossly malignant but histologically benign
- Well-circumscribed, firm, subperitoneal masses

Microscopic Features
- Subperitoneal smooth muscle proliferation with little mitotic activity, absent cell atypia and tumor necrosis
  - Cells arranged in interdigitating fascicles
- Nodules may contain fibroblasts, myofibroblasts, decidual and endometrial stromal cells
- Six cases have described sarcomatous changes

CLINICAL ISSUES

Presentation
- Most common signs/symptoms: Pelvic pain, uterine bleeding, urinary frequency, peritonitis, asymptomatic

Demographics
- Age: Reproductive age, rare in postmenopausal
- Gender: Female; reported case in a male

Natural History & Prognosis
- Benign course; recurrence has been reported
- Spontaneous regression when ↓ exposure to estrogen

Treatment
- Conservative, GnRH agonists or bilateral salpingooophorectomy ± hysterectomy

DIAGNOSTIC CHECKLIST

Consider
- Mimics peritoneal carcinomatosis

SELECTED REFERENCES
1. Advincula AP et al: Images in reproductive medicine. Disseminated leiomyomatosis peritonei. Fertil Steril. 84(5):1505-7, 2005
2. Bekkers RL et al: Leiomyomatosis peritonealis disseminata: does malignant transformation occur? A literature review. Gynecol Oncol. 75(1):158-63, 1999

IMAGE GALLERY

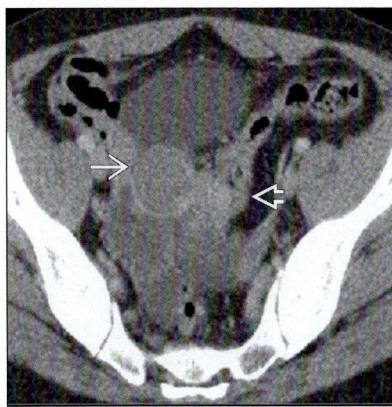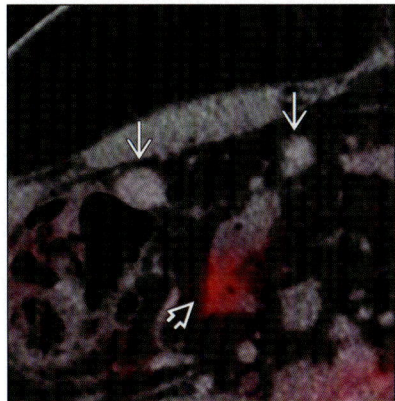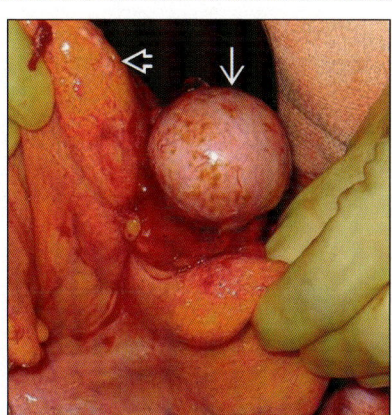

(Left) Axial CECT shows a round, solid, enhancing mass ➡ adjacent to the sigmoid colon ➡ in a 36 year old with abdominal pain. Reproduced with permission from AJR. (Center) Axial fused PET/CT shows nodules ➡ which do not show increased F-18 FDG uptake. Physiologic intestinal uptake is seen in a loop of small bowel ➡. Reproduced with permission from AJR. (Right) Intra-operative photograph confirms the round mass ➡ seen on CT and also demonstrates radiologically occult, 4 mm peritoneal nodules ➡. Reproduced with permission from AJR.

LEIOMYOMA, SUBMUCOSAL

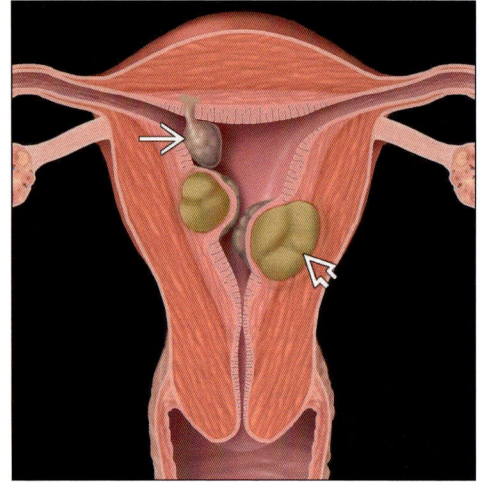

Graphic demonstrates several submucosal leiomyomas protruding into and distorting the endometrial canal. Submucosal leiomyomas may be sessile ➔ or pedunculated ➔.

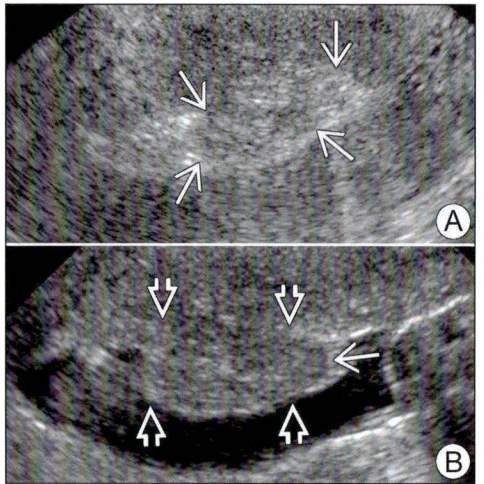

(A) Sagittal TVS shows an endometrial hypoechoic mass ➔ with edge shadows. (B) Sonohysterogram shows mass ➔ stretching the endometrium ➔. The entire mass protrudes into the endometrial cavity.

TERMINOLOGY

Abbreviations and Synonyms
- Submucosal fibroid, myoma, fibroleiomyoma, fibroma

Definitions
- Leiomyomas that originate from myometrium underlying the endometrium

IMAGING FINDINGS

General Features
- Best diagnostic clue
  - Subendometrial solid mass indenting or stretching overlying endometrium
  - Subendometrial solid mass that protrudes into the uterine cavity
- Location
  - Subendometrial myometrium
  - Intracavitary
- Size: Wide range: Can fill the whole female pelvis
- Morphology: Round to elongated
- May extend into uterine cavity & present as polypoid intracavitary mass
- Intracavitary mass can become pedunculated & prolapse through cervix

Ultrasonographic Findings
- Grayscale Ultrasound
  - Transvaginal sonography (TVS) findings
    - Hypoechoic subendometrial mass
    - Stretched but intact overlying echogenic endometrium
    - In continuity with myometrium
    - May attenuate sound or cause edge shadows
- Pulsed Doppler: Variable resistive indices depending on its vascularity
- Color Doppler
  - Wide range of vascularity depending on cellularity or presence of degeneration
    - Highly vascular lesions show central vascularity as well as vessels draped around the mass
    - Broad based: Multiple vascular pedicles (single vascular pedicle uncommon)
- Power Doppler: Wide range of vascularity depending on cellularity or presence of degeneration

DDx: Intrauterine/Subendometrial Mass

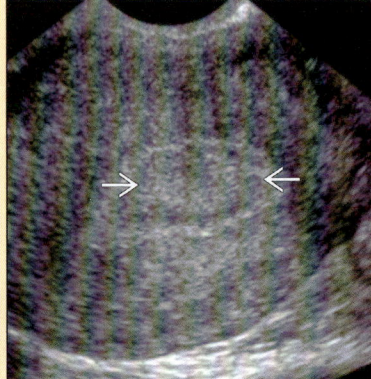
Endometrial Polyp

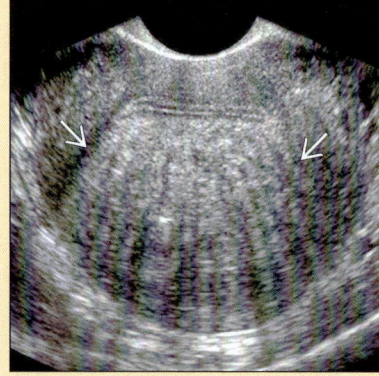
Adenomyoma

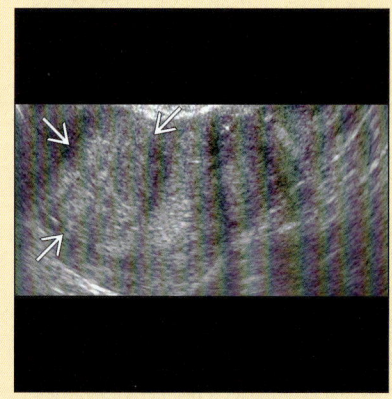
Myometrial Contraction

LEIOMYOMA, SUBMUCOSAL

Key Facts

Imaging Findings
- Subendometrial solid mass indenting or stretching overlying endometrium
- Homogeneous isointense to myometrium on T1
- If hemorrhagic degeneration: Hyperintense on T1
- Homogeneous hypointense to myometrium on T2
- Cannot normally differentiate types of degeneration; heterogeneous appearance with varied cellularity or degeneration
- Hypoechoic subendometrial mass
- Stretched but intact overlying echogenic endometrium
- May attenuate sound or cause edge shadows
- Broad based: Multiple vascular pedicles (single vascular pedicle uncommon)
- Intraluminal thickness should be > 50% of total thickness to be eligible for hysteroscopic removal
- TVS for initial imaging & diagnosis

Top Differential Diagnoses
- Endometrial Polyp
- Adenomyosis
- Endometrial Carcinoma
- Myometrial Contraction

Pathology
- Estrogen dependent

Clinical Issues
- Increase in size during pregnancy & regress with menopause

CT Findings
- NECT: Mass isodense to the uterus
- CECT: Variable degrees of enhancement from no enhancement to significant enhancement

MR Findings
- T1WI
  - Homogeneous isointense to myometrium on T1
  - If hemorrhagic degeneration: Hyperintense on T1
- T2WI
  - Homogeneous hypointense to myometrium on T2
    - May be partially surrounded by high signal intensity distended endometrial canal
- T1 C+ FS: Variable enhancement; mass enhances less than normal myometrium on delayed phase
- Generally well-defined mass originating from myometrium
- Cannot normally differentiate types of degeneration; heterogeneous appearance with varied cellularity or degeneration

Angiographic Findings
- Conventional
  - Variable vascularity with vascular lesions showing central vascularity as well as vessels draped around the mass
  - Blood supply from either uterine or ovarian vessels

Other Modality Findings
- Sonohysterography (SHG)
  - Mass indenting the endometrial cavity
  - Intraluminal mass
  - Intraluminal thickness should be > 50% of total thickness to be eligible for hysteroscopic removal
  - SHG evaluates the thickness of overlying myometrium

Imaging Recommendations
- Best imaging tool
  - TVS for initial imaging & diagnosis
  - Sonohysterography for surgical planning
  - MR before surgical planning when
    - Multiple leiomyomas cause significant uterine distortion
    - In some cases to differentiate leiomyoma from adenomyoma or polyp
- TVS for initial imaging & diagnosis
- Sonohysterography for surgical planning
- MR before surgical planning when
  - Multiple leiomyomas causing significant uterine distortion
  - In some cases to differentiate leiomyoma from adenomyoma or polyp

DIFFERENTIAL DIAGNOSIS

Endometrial Polyp
- TVS: No stretched endometrial lining overlying the mass
  - No continuity with underlying myometrium
  - Single vascular pedicle
- MR: High signal intensity on T2WI
  - Endometrial origin on T2WI or C+ MR

Adenomyosis
- TVS: Ill-defined area of heterogeneous echogenicity which may have associated cystic spaces
  - Disproportionally lower mass effect considering the size of mass
- MR: Focal widening of low signal intensity junctional zone on T2WI
  - More elliptical in shape and oriented along endometrial axis
  - May have punctate foci of high signal intensity on T1WI & T2WI
  - Disproportionately lower mass effect considering the size of mass

Endometrial Carcinoma
- TVS: Usually no endometrial stripe
- MR: Heterogeneous signal intensity on T2WI and C+ MR

LEIOMYOMA, SUBMUCOSAL

Myometrial Contraction
- Transient nature on both US and MR
- May take up to 45 minutes to resolve

PATHOLOGY

General Features
- General path comments
  - Benign neoplasms of smooth muscle origin
  - Comprise 5-10% of all leiomyomas
  - Estrogen dependent
- Genetics: More common in some families
- Etiology: No known etiology
- Epidemiology: Occurs in 20-30% of women > than 30 years of age & more common in black women and women with a positive family history
- Associated abnormalities: Adenomyosis

Gross Pathologic & Surgical Features
- Demarcated from surrounding myometrium by pseudocapsule
- Smooth-muscle cells are arranged whorl-like, with intervening collagen
- Cellular type leiomyomas are variant, composed of densely packed cells
- Larger leiomyomas tend to undergo degeneration and are heterogeneous

Microscopic Features
- Proliferation of disorderly arranged, nodularly circumscribed, spindle-shaped, smooth muscle cells; rare mitotic figures
- Degenerative changes include: Hyaline fibrosis, hemorrhage, edema, cystic or myxoid degeneration, and calcification
- Degeneration more likely during pregnancy & with progestational agents

Staging, Grading or Classification Criteria
- For surgical approach, they are divided into 3 grades
  - Grade 0: No protrusion into uterine cavity
  - Grade I: < 50% of height protruding into cavity
  - Grade II: ≥ 50% of height protruding into cavity

CLINICAL ISSUES

Presentation
- Most common signs/symptoms: Abnormal uterine bleeding in both pre- and postmenopausal women
- Other signs/symptoms
  - Passage of necrotic tissue in pedunculated intra-cavitary type
  - Pregnancy related: Infertility, 2nd trimester abortion, pain from degeneration, bleeding resulting in hemoperitoneum
- Clinical profile
  - Most symptomatic type of leiomyoma

Demographics
- Age: 20-30% of women > 30 years of age
- Gender: Female
- Ethnicity: More common in black women

Natural History & Prognosis
- Increase in size during pregnancy & regress with menopause
- Very small percentage may undergo malignant transformation
- Benign disease in the overwhelming majority of patients
- Very small percentage may undergo malignant transformation
- Intracavitary submucosal leiomyoma may slough off completely, presumably because of torsion
- US for rapid growth that may suggest malignant transformation

Treatment
- Surgical
  - Grade 0 and I: Transabdominal myomectomy
  - Grade II: Hysteroscopic myomectomy
  - Hysterectomy when extensive disease is present
- Uterine artery embolization as alternative to hysterectomy
- GnRH analogue therapy: Cellular type responds better

DIAGNOSTIC CHECKLIST

Consider
- US for rapid growth that may suggest malignant transformation
- Consider malignancy when poorly defined

Image Interpretation Pearls
- Hypoechoic attenuating central uterine mass on TVS
- Multiple vascular pedicles on TVS
- Hypointense mass on T2WI
- Continuity with myometrium

SELECTED REFERENCES

1. Aviram R et al: Uterine sarcomas versus leiomyomas: gray-scale and Doppler sonographic findings. J Clin Ultrasound. 33(1):10-3, 2005
2. Park HR et al: Uterine restoration after repeated sloughing of fibroids or vaginal expulsion following uterine artery embolization. Eur Radiol. 15(9):1850-4, 2005
3. Salim R et al: A comparative study of three-dimensional saline infusion sonohysterography and diagnostic hysteroscopy for the classification of submucous fibroids. Hum Reprod. 20(1):253-7, 2005
4. Dubinsky TJ: Value of sonography in the diagnosis of abnormal vaginal bleeding. J Clin Ultrasound. 32(7):348-53, 2004
5. Ojili V et al: Uterine artery embolization for the treatment of symptomatic fibroids. Int J Gynaecol Obstet. 87(3):249-51, 2004
6. Murase E et al: Uterine leiomyomas: histopathologic features, MR imaging findings, differential diagnosis, and treatment. Radiographics. 19(5):1179-97, 1999
7. Ueda H et al: Unusual appearances of uterine leiomyomas: MR imaging findings and their histopathologic backgrounds. Radiographics. 19 Spec No:S131-45, 1999
8. Mayer DP et al: Ultrasonography and magnetic resonance imaging of uterine fibroids. Obstet Gynecol Clin North Am. 22(4):667-725, 1995
9. Atri M et al: Transvaginal US appearance of endometrial abnormalities. Radiographics. 14(3):483-92, 1994

LEIOMYOMA, SUBMUCOSAL

IMAGE GALLERY

Typical

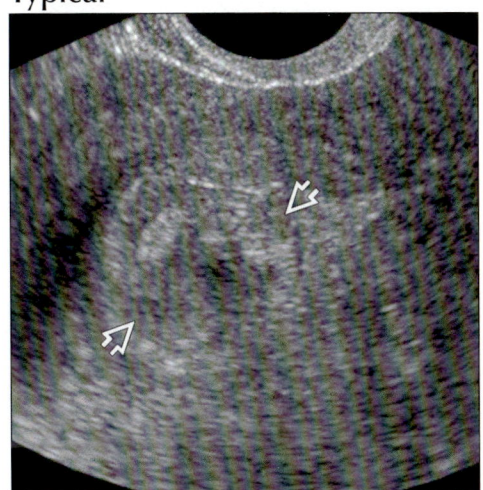 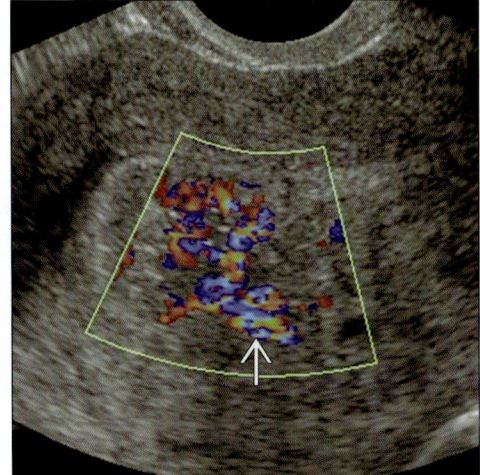

(Left) Sagittal transvaginal ultrasound shows a heterogeneous intrauterine mass ➡ in the uterine cavity. *(Right)* Sagittal color Doppler ultrasound of the same patient as previous image shows broad-based vascular supply ➡.

Typical

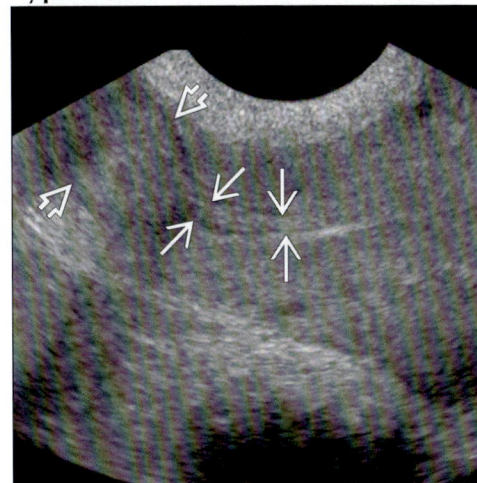 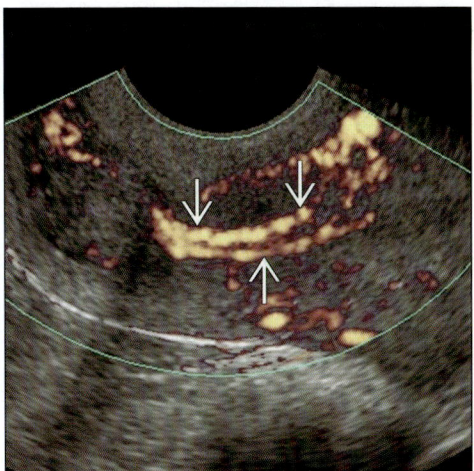

(Left) Sagittal transvaginal ultrasound shows an isoechoic intrauterine mass ➡ attached to the myometrium by a long narrow pedicle ➡. *(Right)* Sagittal power Doppler ultrasound in the same patient as previous image shows significant vascularity running in the long pedicle ➡.

Typical

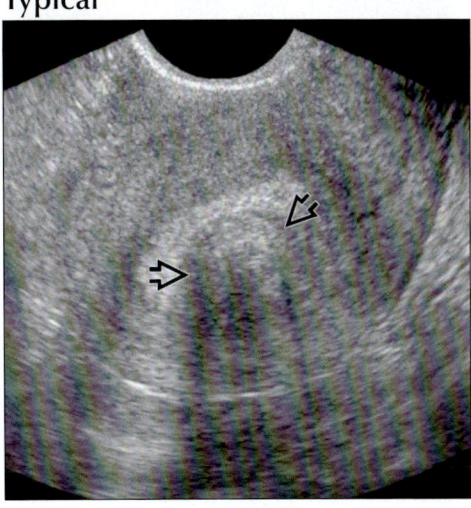 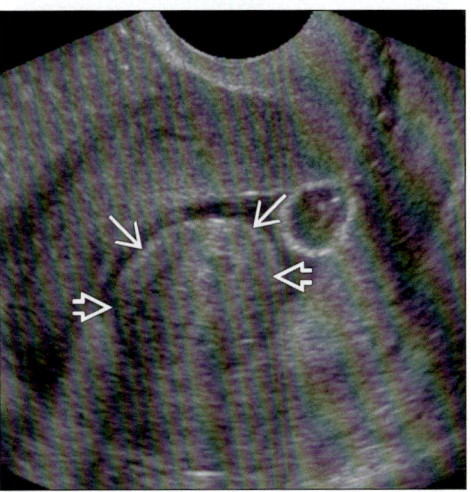

(Left) Axial transvaginal ultrasound shows a hypoechoic attenuating mass ➡ distorting the endometrium consistent with a submucosal leiomyoma. *(Right)* Sagittal transvaginal ultrasound SHG shows an attenuating mass ➡ stretching the endometrium ➡ with more than 50% of the diameter protruding into the uterine cavity.

LEIOMYOMA, SUBMUCOSAL

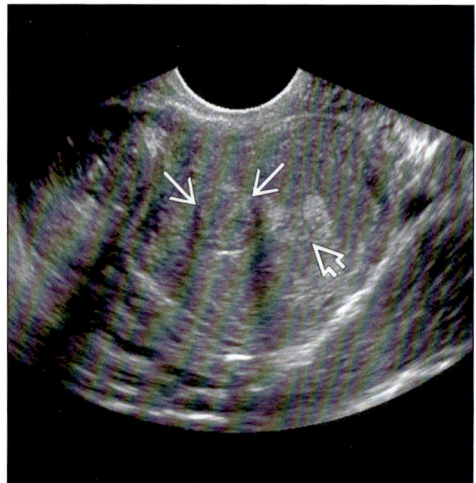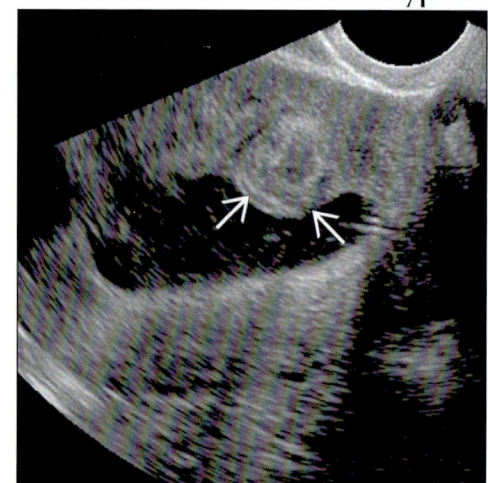

(Left) Axial transvaginal ultrasound shows a mass with attenuating sides ➡ abutting the endometrium ➡. *(Right)* Sagittal transvaginal ultrasound SHG in the same patient as previous image shows the mass to be a submucosal leiomyoma ➡ protruding into the endometrium.

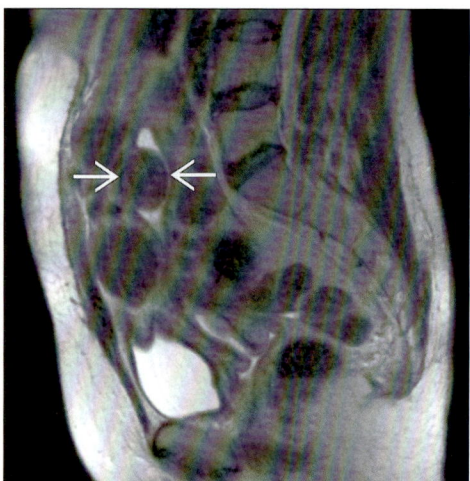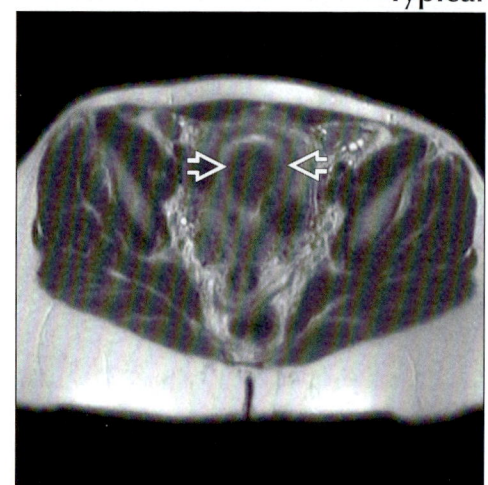

(Left) Sagittal T2WI MR shows multiple leiomyomas with a moderately-sized submucosal leiomyoma ➡ distending the endometrial canal. *(Right)* Axial T2WI MR shows a homogeneous, round, low SI, submucosal leiomyoma ➡ within the endometrial canal.

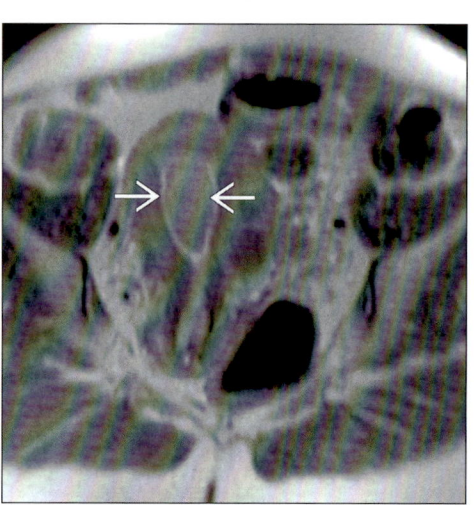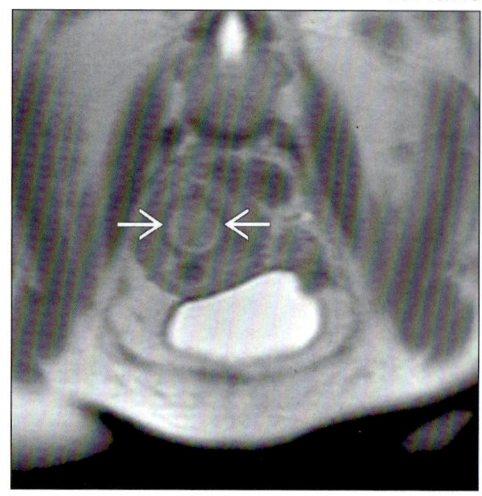

(Left) Axial T2WI MR shows a mass ➡ within the endometrial canal. Its signal intensity is higher than myometrium suggesting a submucosal leiomyoma with cellular histology. *(Right)* Coronal T2WI MR in the same patient as previous image shows the cellular leiomyoma ➡ distending the endometrial canal.

LEIOMYOMA, SUBMUCOSAL

Typical

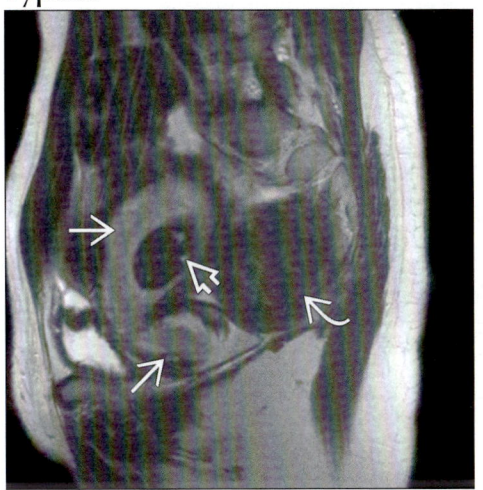
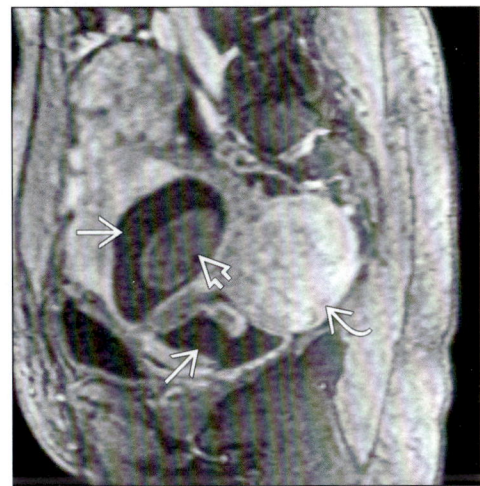

(Left) Sagittal T2WI MR shows a submucosal leiomyoma ➡ projecting into endometrial canal. Heterogeneous SI in endometrial and endocervical canals ➡ is consistent with blood. A subserosal leiomyoma is also present ➡. (Right) Sagittal T1 C+ FS MR in the same patient shows minimal enhancement of the submucosal leiomyoma ➡ and marked enhancement of the subserosal one ➡. The blood clots do not enhance ➡.

Typical

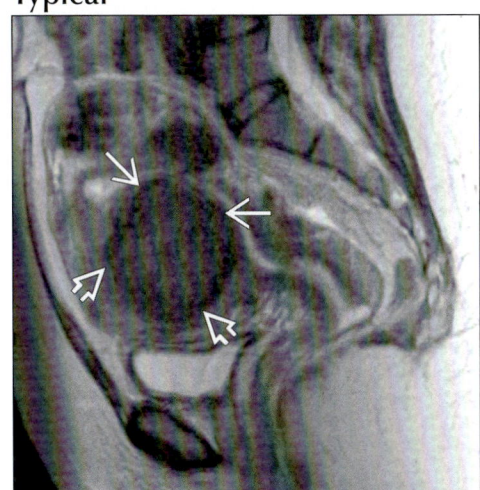
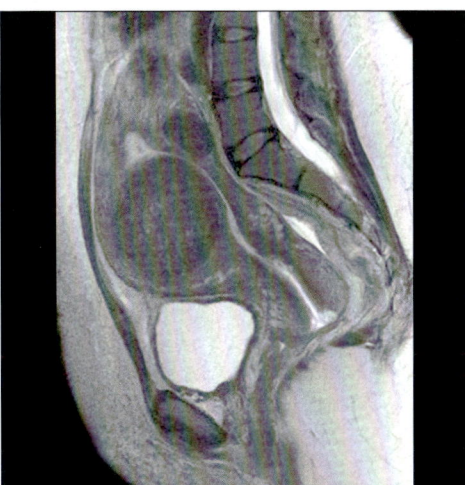

(Left) Sagittal T2WI MR shows a leiomyoma with both submucosal ➡ and intramural ➡ components obtained on a 1.5T system. (Right) Sagittal T2WI MR of the same patient as previous image obtained on a 3.0T system has improved spatial resolution. The image quality of the dominant leiomyoma with submucosal and intramural components is superior.

Typical

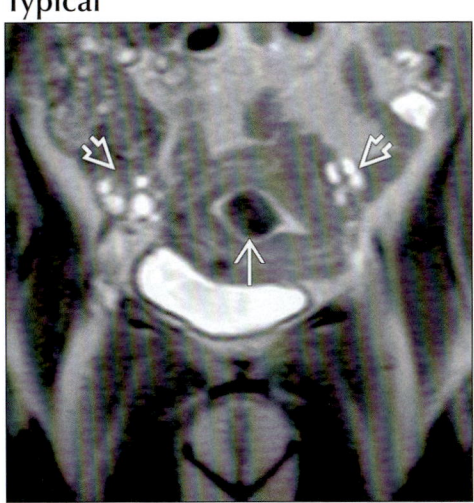
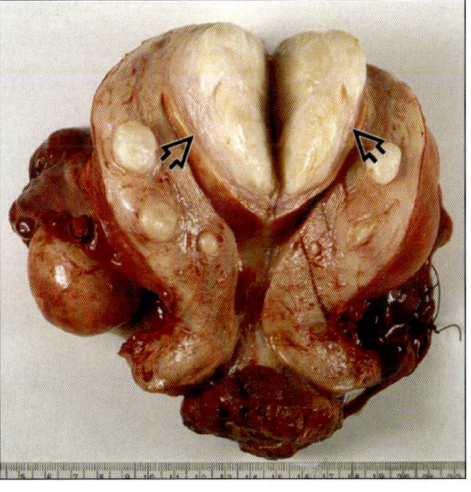

(Left) Coronal T2WI MR shows a submucosal leiomyoma ➡ distending the endometrial canal. The normal ovaries are well seen ➡. (Right) Coronal gross pathology shows a bivalved hysterectomy specimen with a large broad-based submucosal leiomyoma ➡ distending the endometrial canal. (Courtesy B. Hamm, MD).

LEIOMYOMA, INTRAMURAL

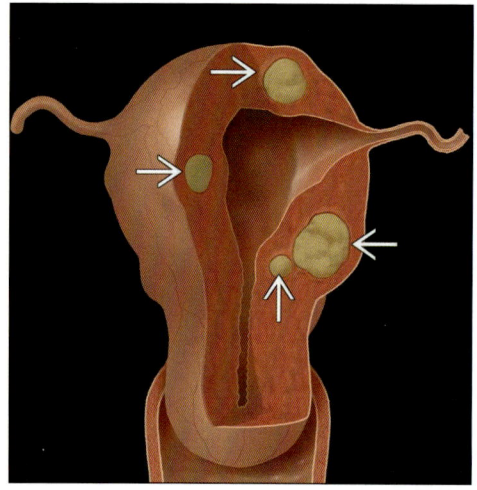

Coronal graphic shows a uterus with multiple intramural leiomyomas ➔.

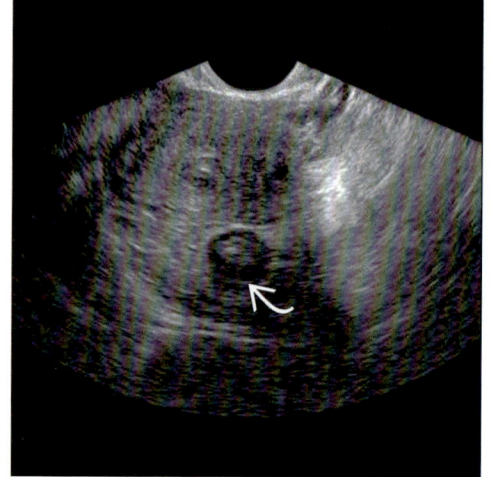

Oblique transvaginal ultrasound shows a well-defined hypoechoic mass ➔ in the posterior uterus surrounded by myometrium.

TERMINOLOGY

Abbreviations and Synonyms
- Intramural fibroid, fibroleiomyoma, myoma

Definitions
- Benign tumor of uterine smooth muscle cells

IMAGING FINDINGS

General Features
- Best diagnostic clue: Homogeneous, round, well-defined myometrial mass
- Location
  ○ Intramural: Most common leiomyoma location
  ○ Anatomy: Normal myometrium circumscribes mass
- Size
  ○ Few millimeters to several centimeters
  ○ Often degenerated if > 8 cm

Radiographic Findings
- Radiography: May see calcifications in leiomyoma or displacement of bowel loops by enlarged uterus
- IVP: Mass effect on bladder & displacement of ureters

Ultrasonographic Findings
- Grayscale Ultrasound
  ○ Enlarged lobulated uterus
    ▪ Areas of sound attenuation, and/or shadowing and/or obscuration of deeper tissues
- Color Doppler: Marked peripheral flow with decreased central flow or an avascular core
- Transvaginal ultrasound (TVS) findings
  ○ Homogeneous hypoechoic mass
    ▪ Poor sound attenuation if not degenerated & primarily composed of smooth muscle
  ○ Heterogeneous, with or without calcification if degenerated
  ○ May be hyperechoic with increased sound through transmission as leiomyoma degenerates
  ○ Calcification: Echogenic foci with shadowing
  ○ Radiations of sharp discrete shadowing: Related to interfaces between fibrous tissue and smooth muscle

CT Findings
- NECT
  ○ Homogeneous attenuation similar to myometrium
    ▪ Uniform solid attenuation

DDx: Intramural Leiomyoma

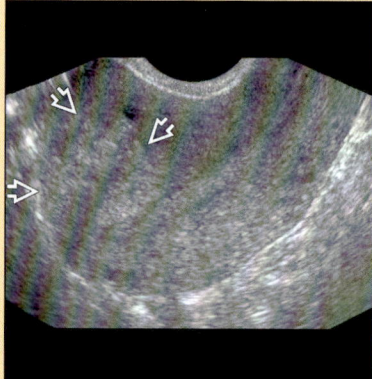

Focal Adenomyosis (Adenomyoma)

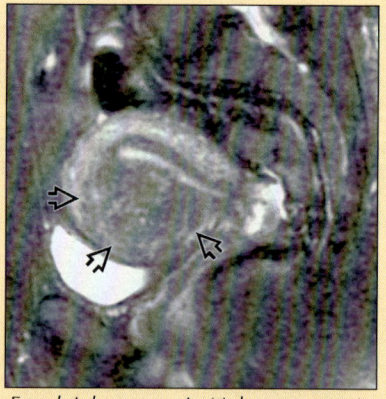

Focal Adenomyosis (Adenomyoma)

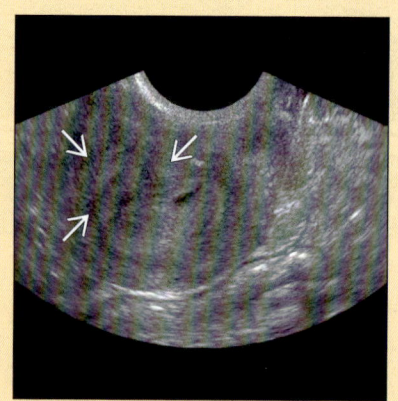

Uterine Sarcoma

LEIOMYOMA, INTRAMURAL

Key Facts

Terminology
- Intramural leiomyoma, fibroleiomyoma, myoma
- Benign tumor of uterine smooth muscle cells

Imaging Findings
- Best diagnostic clue: Homogeneous, round, well-defined myometrial mass
- Intramural: Most common leiomyoma location
- Anatomy: Normal myometrium circumscribes mass
- US is primary modality to evaluate abnormal uterine bleeding, uterine enlargement or pelvic mass but is limited by its field of view
- MR is the most accurate to diagnose leiomyomas (size, number and location)

Top Differential Diagnoses
- Adenomyosis
- Malignant Uterine Neoplasms

Pathology
- Most common uterine neoplasm: 40% of women after age 35

Clinical Issues
- Majority are asymptomatic
- Symptomatic in 25-30% of women
- Abnormal uterine bleeding is most common symptom and main indication for therapy
- Malignant transformation is rare at 0.2-0.3%
- Definitive: Hysterectomy (total or supracervical)
- Myomectomy: 11-15% re-intervention rate
- Uterine artery embolization: At least 5 year durability has been demonstrated

---

  - Enlarged uterus with deformed contour
  - May see calcifications and/or necrosis if degenerated
- CECT
  - Initially enhances less than myometrium
  - Usually homogeneous enhancement but large/degenerated leiomyomas may enhance heterogeneously

MR Findings
- T1WI
  - Intermediate signal intensity (SI)
  - Lobulated appearance to the uterus
  - If not degenerated: Isointense to myometrium
  - If degenerated: High and low SI
- T2WI
  - Most useful sequence for detecting leiomyomas
  - Homogeneous, well-defined and hypointense to myometrium
    - Pseudocapsule of compressed normal myometrium
    - Hyperintense rim: Edema, dilated lymphatics & veins
  - Homogeneous high SI: Cellular histology
  - Heterogeneity is not specific for type of degeneration
    - Myxoid, hyaline and cystic most common
- T2* GRE: If calcified: Foci of SI loss (susceptibility)
- T1 C+
  - Contrast not necessary to make the diagnosis
  - Well marginated with variable enhancement
  - Enhancing halo of dilated lymphatics and veins
  - Nonenhancing regions of hemorrhagic, necrotic or cystic degeneration
- Fat sat T1WI
  - Carneous (hemorrhagic) degeneration: High SI

Other Modality Findings
- HSG: No findings unless mass effect on endometrium

Imaging Recommendations
- US is primary modality to evaluate abnormal uterine bleeding, uterine enlargement or pelvic mass but is limited by its field of view
- Transabdominal scanning is essential for multiple leiomyomas: Get overall uterine size & leiomyoma locations
- Transvaginal scanning improves spatial resolution
  - Caveat: Structures deep to leiomyomas may be obscured by poor sound penetration
- MR is the most accurate to diagnose leiomyomas (size, number and location)
  - Helps select patients for invasive treatment
  - Assists in surgical planning (e.g., road map)
  - Monitors treatment response

DIFFERENTIAL DIAGNOSIS

Adenomyosis
- Poorly marginated, may be diffuse or focal
- When focal, can differentiate from leiomyoma by its elliptical shape and minimal mass effect
- Ultrasound: Poorly defined abnormal myometrial echotexture
  - May see myometrial cysts and/or echogenic striations into myometrium
- T2WI: Widening of junctional zone ≥ 12 mm or ill-defined low SI myometrial mass
  - Ancillary features: High SI punctate foci and/or high SI striations radiating into myometrium

Malignant Uterine Neoplasms
- Irregular morphology; not well demarcated
- Heterogeneous echogenicity or high SI on T2WI
- Leiomyosarcoma: Rare, often misdiagnosed as leiomyomas but on follow-up exhibit rapid growth and metastases

PATHOLOGY

General Features
- General path comments
  - Well-defined, pseudoencapsulated mass within myometrium

LEIOMYOMA, INTRAMURAL

- Most common uterine neoplasm: 40% of women after age 35
  - Account for 1/3-1/2 of hysterectomies in North America
- Genetics: No hereditary factor clearly identified
- Etiology: Unclear; likely multifactorial
- Epidemiology
  - Most common gynecologic tumor in women of the reproductive age group: Up to 30%
  - Increased incidence in Black/African American women

Gross Pathologic & Surgical Features
- Spherical, firm, white and elastic in consistency

Microscopic Features
- Uniform, anastomosed & whorled smooth muscle cells
- Variable amounts of fibrous connective tissue
- Small, infrequent blood vessels
- No significant mitosis, atypia or necrosis

CLINICAL ISSUES

Presentation
- Most common signs/symptoms
  - Majority are asymptomatic
  - Symptomatic in 25-30% of women
  - Abnormal uterine bleeding is most common symptom and main indication for therapy
    - Typical: Menorrhagia or polymenorrhea
    - Metromenorrhagia or intermenstrual bleeding
    - Bleeding related to location, size & number
  - Pressure effects and pain: Proportional to leiomyoma size
    - May present as heaviness, a dull ache or bloating
    - May compress the nerve supply to the pelvis and the legs causing back or leg pain, or suprapubic pain
    - May produce urinary symptoms, constipation or dyspareunia from general pressure effects
    - Acute pain can occur due to degeneration
  - Infertility: Relationship with leiomyoma is controversial
    - Faulty implantation or compression on fallopian tube by leiomyomas located near cornua
    - Associated with spontaneous abortion, preterm labor, placenta previa, malpresentation or dystocia
    - Risk of placental abruption greatest when leiomyoma is subplacental in location
- Clinical Profile
  - Enlarged, bulky or lobular uterus with or without symptoms
  - Size is hormonally responsive
    - Estrogen: Stimulates; increase in pregnancy
    - Progesterone: Inhibits; decrease after menopause

Demographics
- Age: Most common during reproductive years
- Ethnicity
  - Black/African American women
    - 3x increased incidence & more severe disease

Natural History & Prognosis
- Good prognosis, most women are asymptomatic
- If symptomatic, most women benefit from treatment
- Malignant transformation is rare at 0.2-0.3%

Treatment
- Definitive: Hysterectomy (total or supracervical)
  - Leiomyomas are leading indication for surgery in women
- Uterine sparing alternatives
  - Medical therapy: GnRH analog: Regrowth with cessation
  - Myomectomy: 11-15% re-intervention rate
    - Increasing number of leiomyomas associated with worse outcomes
  - Uterine artery embolization: At least 5 year durability has been demonstrated
    - 80-90% successful in improving symptoms
    - Similar success rate to myomectomy with fewer adverse events, shorter recovery time and use of fewer postoperative narcotics
  - Thermoablative techniques: Myolysis, cryomyolysis, laser ablation and focused ultrasound (FUS)
    - Not widespread: Limited by size and location

DIAGNOSTIC CHECKLIST

Image Interpretation Pearls
- Round, well-defined, homogeneous myometrial mass

SELECTED REFERENCES

1. Goodwin SC et al: Uterine artery embolization versus myomectomy: a multicenter comparative study. Fertil Steril. 85(1):14-21, 2006
2. Spies JB et al: Long-term outcome of uterine artery embolization of leiomyomata. Obstet Gynecol. 106(5 Pt 1):933-9, 2005
3. Day Baird D et al: High cumulative incidence of uterine leiomyoma in black and white women: ultrasound evidence. Am J Obstet Gynecol. 188(1):100-7, 2003
4. Kido A et al: Diffusely enlarged uterus: evaluation with MR imaging. Radiographics. 23(6):1423-39, 2003
5. Razavi MK et al: Abdominal myomectomy versus uterine fibroid embolization in the treatment of symptomatic uterine leiomyomas. AJR Am J Roentgenol. 180(6):1571-5, 2003
6. American College of Obstetricians and Gynecologists. Surgical alternatives to hysterectomy in the management of leiomyomas, 2000
7. Murase E et al: Uterine leiomyomas: histopathologic features, MR imaging findings, differential diagnosis, and treatment. Radiographics. 19(5):1179-97, 1999
8. Mayer DP et al: Ultrasonography and magnetic resonance imaging of uterine fibroids. Obstet Gynecol Clin North Am. 22(4):667-725, 1995
9. Karasick S et al: Imaging of uterine leiomyomas. AJR Am J Roentgenol. 158(4):799-805, 1992

LEIOMYOMA, INTRAMURAL

IMAGE GALLERY

Typical

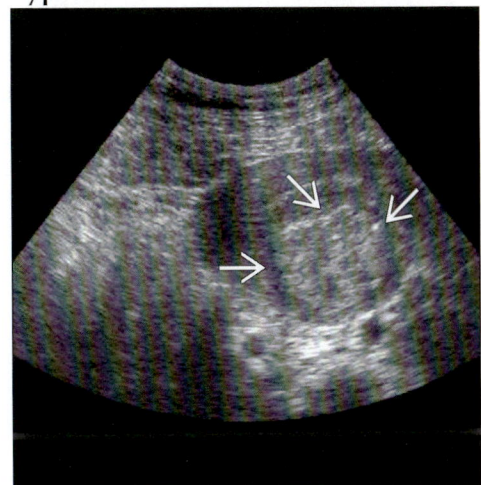
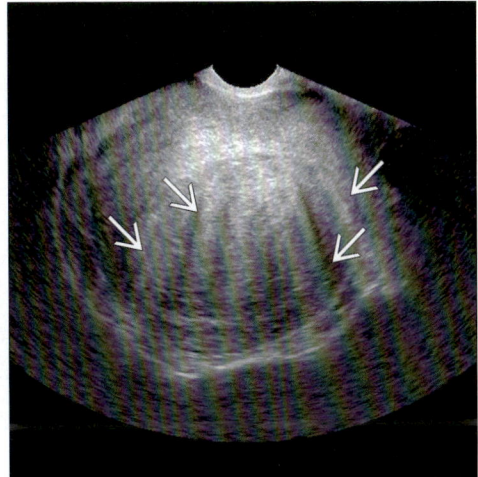

(Left) Sagittal transabdominal ultrasound shows a well-defined, hyperechoic, intramural leiomyoma ➡ which does not attenuate sound. *(Right)* Axial transvaginal ultrasound shows a mixed-echogenicity mass in the posterior myometrium. The sharp radiating shadows ➡ are related to tissue interfaces and not calcification.

Typical

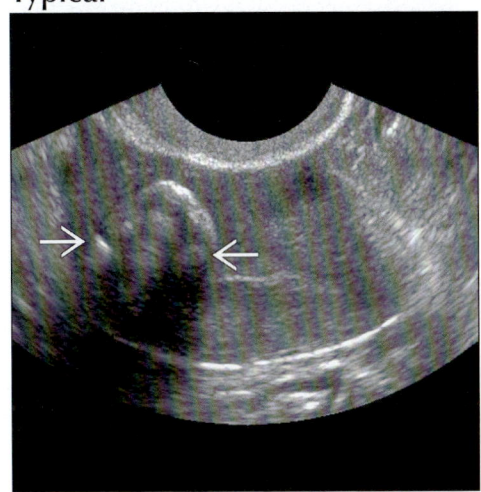
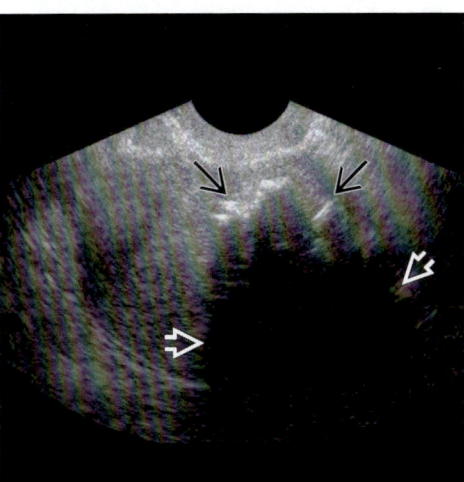

(Left) Axial transvaginal ultrasound shows a well-defined intramural mass with highly echogenic components causing well-defined posterior acoustic shadows ➡, compatible with degenerating leiomyoma. *(Right)* Coronal transvaginal ultrasound shows a degenerating leiomyoma ➡. The posterior shadowing ➡ prevents evaluation of deeper portions of myometrium.

Typical

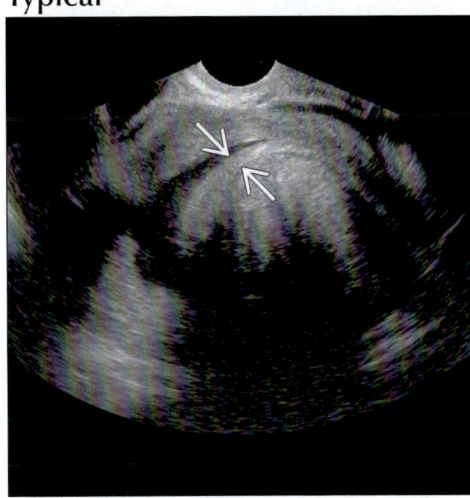
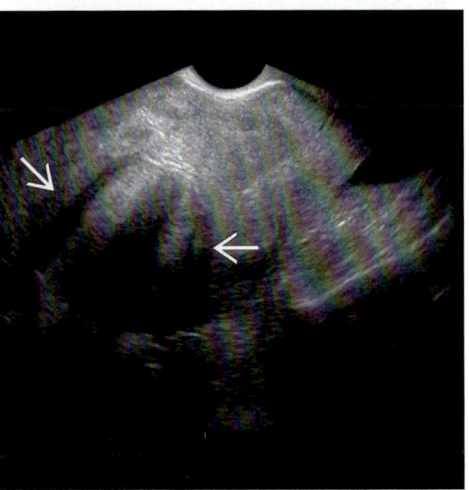

(Left) Sagittal transvaginal ultrasound shows a thin strip of myometrium ➡ between the leiomyoma and endometrium. *(Right)* Sagittal transvaginal ultrasound shows displacement of the endometrium anteriorly by an ill-defined leiomyoma with sharp radiating shadows ➡.

LEIOMYOMA, INTRAMURAL

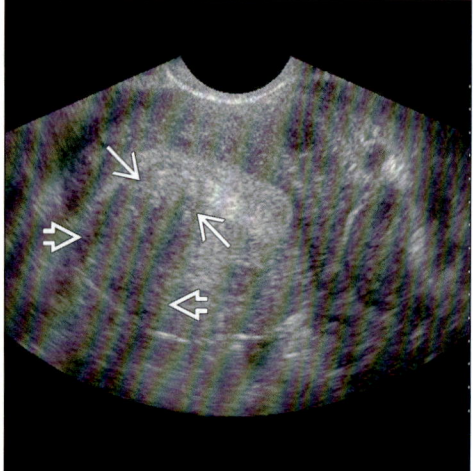 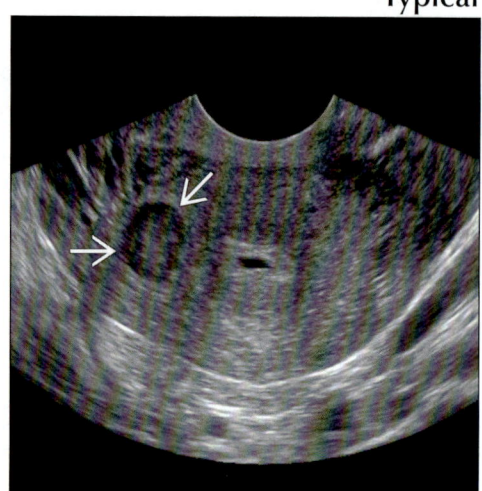

(Left) Sagittal oblique transvaginal ultrasound shows an ill-defined heterogeneous mass. Although adenomyosis may have a similar appearance, the attenuation of sound ➡ and mass effect on the endometrium ➡, favors the diagnosis of leiomyoma. (Right) Coronal transvaginal ultrasound shows a well-defined, hypoechoic, intramural leiomyoma ➡. This type slightly enhances sound instead of attenuating it.

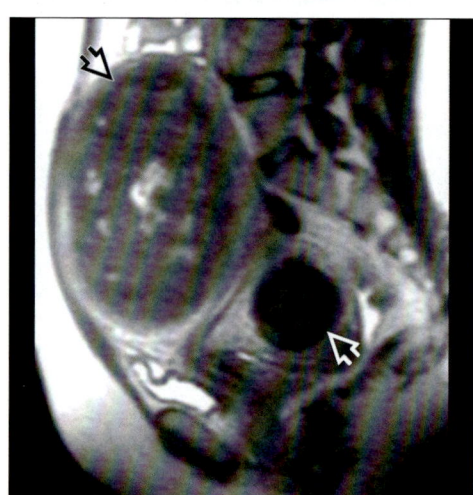 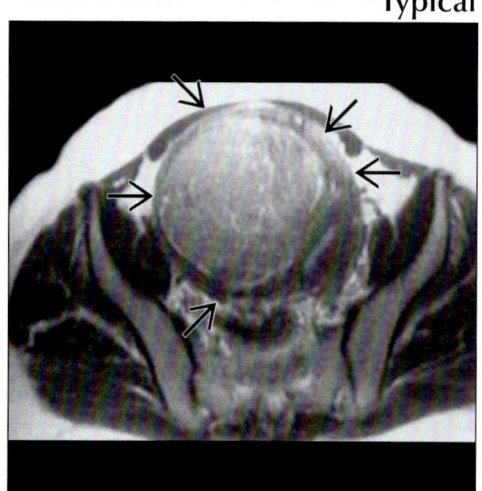

(Left) Sagittal T2WI MR shows two intramural leiomyomas surrounded by myometrium: One anterior ➡, and the other posterior ➡ to the endometrium. (Right) Axial T2WI MR shows an intramural leiomyoma surrounded by myometrium ➡. The leiomyoma has higher SI than myometrium consistent with cellular histology.

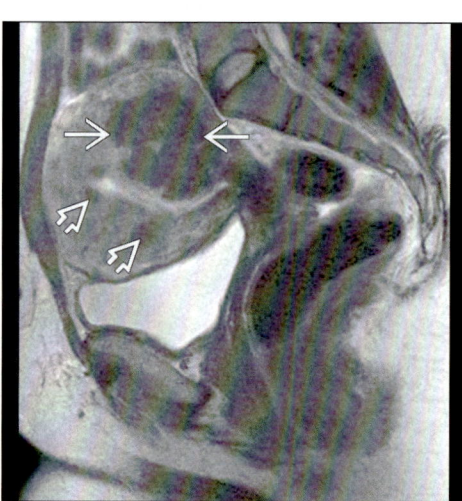 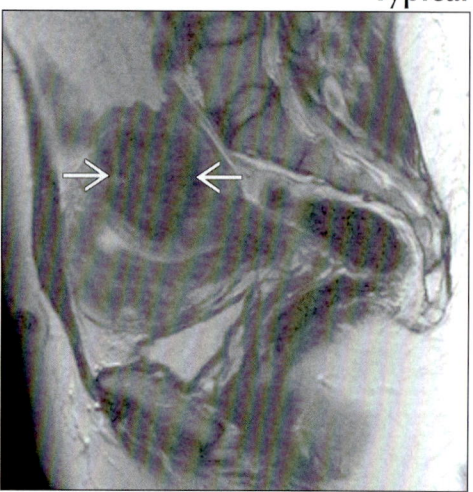

(Left) Sagittal T2WI MR at 3.0T shows the same intramural leiomyoma ➡ as previous image. Note the improved spatial resolution associated with with a 3.0T system improves the conspicuity of smaller leiomyomas ➡. (Right) Sagittal T2WI MR at 1.5T shows a low signal intensity intramural leiomyoma ➡.

LEIOMYOMA, INTRAMURAL

Typical

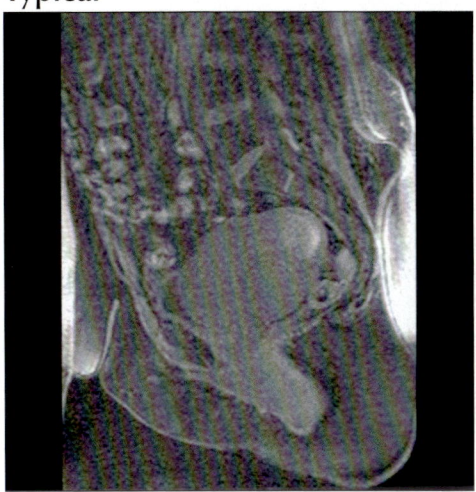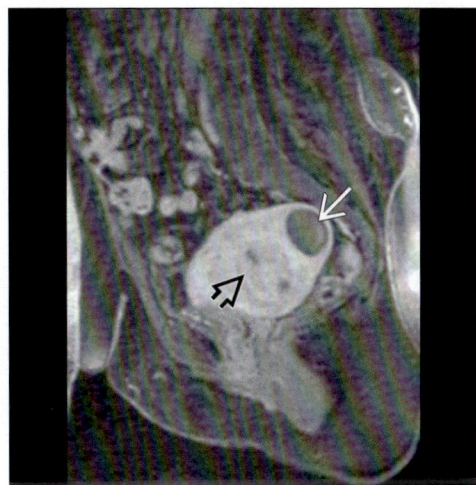

(Left) Sagittal T1WI FS MR shows rounded high SI, blood products, surrounded by myometrium in the posterior corpus in a women with multiple leiomyomas. (Right) Sagittal T1 C+ FS MR in the same patient as previous image shows no enhancement in this intramural leiomyoma ➡ consistent with hemorrhagic (carneous) degeneration. Note the adjacent viable leiomyoma ⬧.

Typical

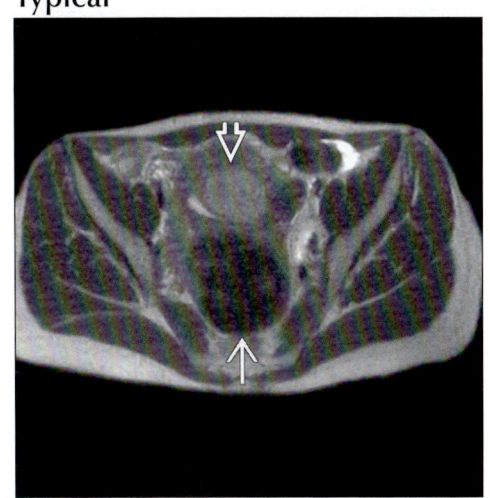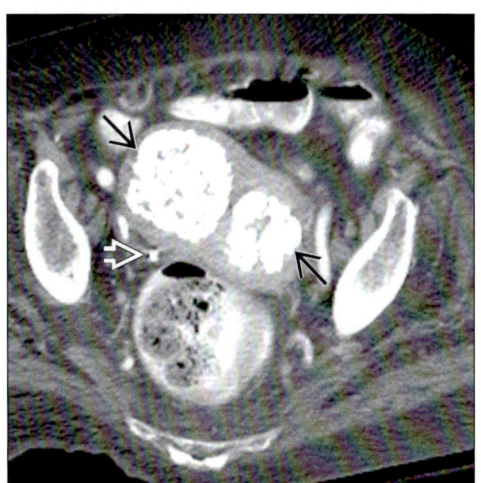

(Left) Axial T2WI MR shows a high SI cellular intramural leiomyoma ⬧ approaching the endometrium. A low SI subserosal leiomyoma is also seen ➡. (Right) Axial CECT shows two calcified leiomyomas ➡ within the myometrium. Incidental note is made of a right ureteral stent ⬧.

Typical

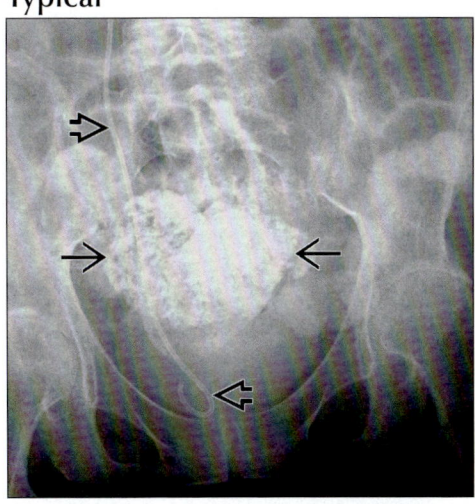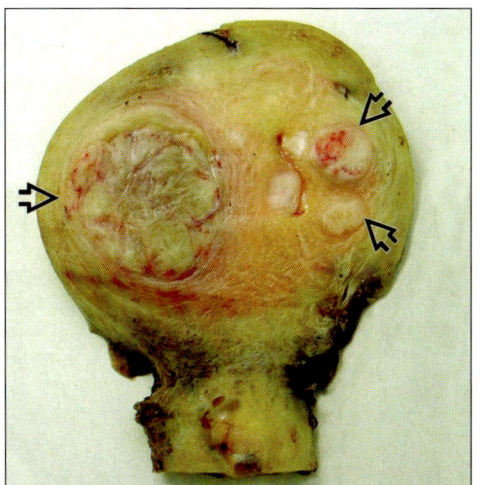

(Left) Anteroposterior radiograph in the same patient as previous image, shows the calcified leiomyomas projecting within the pelvis ➡. Incidental note is made of a right ureteral stent ⬧. (Right) Coronal gross pathology shows a hysterectomy specimen with multiple intramural leiomyomas ⬧. (Courtesy B. Hamm, MD).

LEIOMYOMA, SUBSEROSAL

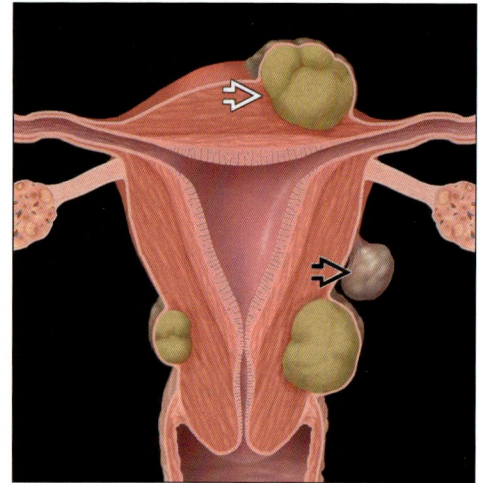

Schematic shows multiple subserosal leiomyomas that originate beneath the uterine serosa and are not surrounded by myometrium. They may be sessile ⇨ or pedunculated ⇨.

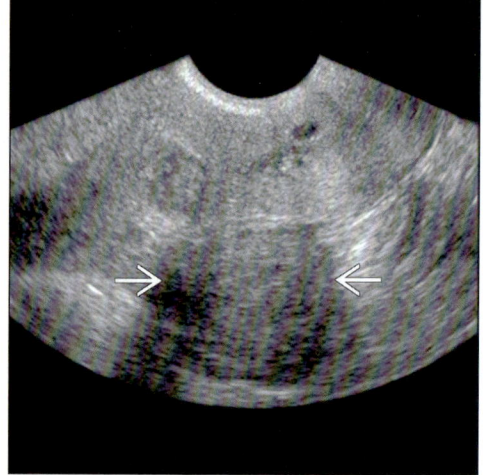

Sagittal transvaginal ultrasound shows well-defined, hypoechoic mass → extending from posterior lower uterine segment, not surrounded by myometrium.

TERMINOLOGY

Abbreviations and Synonyms
- Subserosal fibroid, myoma, fibroleiomyoma

Definitions
- Benign, smooth muscle tumor originating just deep to and abutting serosa

IMAGING FINDINGS

General Features
- Best diagnostic clue: Homogeneous, round, well-defined mass
- Location: Originates just deep to and abuts serosa
- Size: Few millimeters to several centimeters
- Morphology: Sessile or pedunculated
- Anatomy: Normal myometrium does not surround entire mass

Radiographic Findings
- Radiography: Bowel loops displaced by enlarged uterus
- IVP
  - Mass effect on bladder & displacement of ureters
  - Ureteral dilatation if compressed by leiomyomas

Ultrasonographic Findings
- Grayscale Ultrasound
  - Enlarged lobulated uterus
  - May not be detectable by transvaginal (TVS) approach: Transabdominal (TAS) scan may be only way to visualize pedunculated subtype
- Color Doppler
  - Peripheral flow with decreased central flow or avascular core
  - Pedunculated: Vessels in stalk
  - By identifying blood supply, can identify uterine origin
- Transvaginal ultrasound findings
  - Homogeneous, round, well-defined, hypoechoic mass
    - Poor sound transmission if not degenerated & primarily composed of smooth muscle
  - Portion of the mass is not surrounded by myometrium
  - If degenerated: Heterogeneous with or without calcification

DDx: Subserosal Leiomyoma

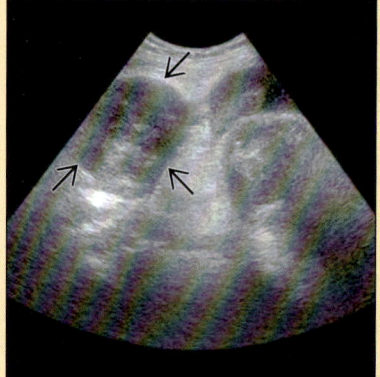

Parasitizing Leiomyoma

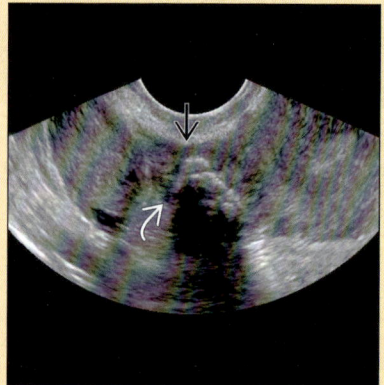

Broad Ligament Leiomyoma

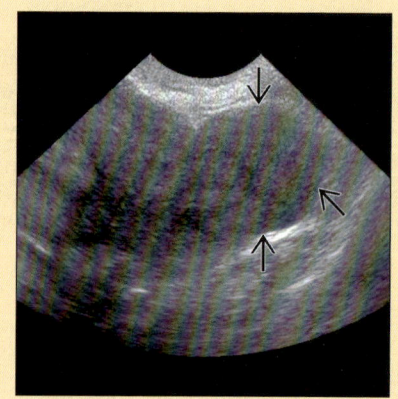

Solid Ovarian Mass

LEIOMYOMA, SUBSEROSAL

Key Facts

Terminology
- Subserosal leiomyoma, myoma, fibroleiomyoma
- Benign, smooth muscle tumor originating just deep to and abutting serosa

Imaging Findings
- Best diagnostic clue: Homogeneous, round, well-defined mass
- Morphology: Sessile or pedunculated
- Anatomy: Normal myometrium does not surround entire mass
- May not be detectable by transvaginal (TVS) approach: Transabdominal (TAS) scan may be only way to visualize pedunculated subtype
- Homogeneous, round, well-defined, hypoechoic mass
- Protocol advice: Need to perform both TAS and TVS
- Pedunculated leiomyomata may be beyond TVS' FOV; need TAS to diagnose
- MR useful to establish uterine origin and determine if pedunculated or broad-based

Top Differential Diagnoses
- Ovarian Neoplasm
- Broad Ligament Leiomyoma
- Parasitic Leiomyoma

Clinical Issues
- Majority are asymptomatic
- Symptomatic in 25-30% of women
- Pressure effects and pain
- Ethnicity: African American women have increased incidence and more severe disease
- Definitive: Hysterectomy

  - Calcification: Echogenic foci with shadowing
  - May be hyperechoic with increased sound through transmission as leiomyoma degenerates
  - Limited field of view (FOV)

CT Findings
- NECT: Protrudes from uterus with similar attenuation to myometrium
- CECT
  - Most enhance less than normal myometrium
  - May see calcifications and/or necrosis if degenerated
  - Claw of myometrium partially surrounding tumor can establish connection to uterus

MR Findings
- T1WI
  - Hypo- to isointense to myometrium
    - No fat plane separating mass from uterine surface
    - May or may not see pedicle
  - High signal intensity (SI) if carneous (hemorrhagic) degeneration present
- T2WI
  - Most useful sequence for detecting leiomyomas
    - Claw of myometrium partially surrounding tumor can establish diagnosis
  - Homogeneous, well-defined low SI mass protruding from uterus
  - Homogeneous high SI: Cellular histology
  - Low SI pedicle if present
  - Heterogeneity is not specific for degeneration type
- T1 C+: Enhance heterogeneously; degenerated areas may not enhance

Imaging Recommendations
- Protocol advice: Need to perform both TAS and TVS
- US is primary modality to diagnose & evaluate
- Pedunculated leiomyomata may be beyond TVS' FOV; need TAS to diagnose
- Can perform limited scan of kidneys to exclude hydronephrosis
- MR for equivocal cases or for patients prior to invasive therapy
- MR useful to establish uterine origin and determine if pedunculated or broad-based
- Correct diagnosis and localization impacts surgical management (hysterectomy vs. uterine sparing treatment)

DIFFERENTIAL DIAGNOSIS

Ovarian Neoplasm
- Originates from and inseparable from ovary

Broad Ligament Leiomyoma
- Originates in broad ligament, no identifiable connection to uterus

Parasitic Leiomyoma
- Arises when leiomyoma adheres to surrounding structures and develops auxiliary blood supply
- Eventually it may lose original attachment to uterus

PATHOLOGY

General Features
- General path comments
  - Well-defined, pseudoencapsulated mass originating beneath serosa
  - Subserosal location is less common than intramural
- Genetics: No hereditary factor clearly identified
- Etiology: Unclear
- Epidemiology
  - 40% of women > 35 years (most common tumor in reproductive years)
  - African Americans, 2-3x greater risk compared with Caucasians and disproportionately affected by more multiple and larger leiomyomas
  - Present in as many as 80% of women by age 50

Gross Pathologic & Surgical Features
- Spherical, firm, white & elastic in consistency
- Ranges in size from several millimeters to many centimeters

LEIOMYOMA, SUBSEROSAL

- Not wholly surrounded by myometrium; one aspect abutting or covered by serosa

Microscopic Features
- Uniform, anastomosed & whorled, smooth muscle cells
- Variable amounts of fibrous connective tissue
- Small, few internal blood vessels
- No significant mitosis, atypia or necrosis

CLINICAL ISSUES

Presentation
- Most common signs/symptoms
  - Majority are asymptomatic
  - Symptomatic in 25-30% of women
  - Pressure effects and pain
    - Directly proportional to size
    - May present as heaviness, a dull ache or bloating
    - May produce urinary symptoms, constipation or dyspareunia from general pressure effects
    - Acute pain can occur from leiomyoma degeneration
    - Carneous degeneration, which occurs during pregnancy, can present with abdominal pain, low grade fever and leukocytosis
    - Pedunculated type may twist on its pedicle, torse, infarct and necrose; may detach and become infected
    - May experience severe dysmenorrhea during a menstrual cycle especially when they coexist with pelvic inflammatory disease, adhesions or endometriosis
  - Infertility
    - Thought to be related to compression on fallopian tube by pedunculated type
- Other signs/symptoms: If large: Pelvic or lower limb thrombosis, respiratory difficulty, polycythemia, sciatic neuropathy & pressure symptoms
- Clinical Profile
  - Palpation of enlarged, bulky or lobular uterus with or without symptoms
  - Hormonally responsive

Demographics
- Age: Reproductive age group
- Gender: Female
- Ethnicity: African American women have increased incidence and more severe disease

Natural History & Prognosis
- Grow during reproductive years under estrogen stimulation
- Regress with menopause or induced hypoestrogenemia
- Rapid unexpected growth may indicate malignant transformation
- Malignant transformation is rare at 0.2-0.3%
- May become parasitic

Treatment
- Definitive: Hysterectomy
- Uterine sparing alternatives
  - Medical therapy: Gonadotropin-releasing hormone analog
  - Myomectomy
    - Principal mode of treatment for those who wish to maintain fertility
    - Up to 15% require re-intervention
    - Increasing number of leiomyomata is associated with worse outcome
  - Uterine artery embolization (UAE)
    - Majority of patients report improvement in symptoms (5 year durability reported)
    - Dominant leiomyoma with thin pedicle: Relative contraindication for UAE because of theoretical risk of pedicle infarction and subsequent detachment of infarcted leiomyoma into peritoneal cavity
  - Thermoablation: Myolysis, cryomyolysis, laser ablation and high frequency focused US

DIAGNOSTIC CHECKLIST

Image Interpretation Pearls
- Round, well-defined, homogeneous mass originating from uterine surface

SELECTED REFERENCES

1. Goodwin SC et al: Uterine artery embolization versus myomectomy: a multicenter comparative study. Fertil Steril. 85(1):14-21, 2006
2. Katsumori T et al: Long-term outcomes of uterine artery embolization using gelatin sponge particles alone for symptomatic fibroids. AJR Am J Roentgenol. 186(3):848-54, 2006
3. Stewart EA et al: Clinical outcomes of focused ultrasound surgery for the treatment of uterine fibroids. Fertil Steril. 85(1):22-9, 2006
4. West S et al: Abdominal myomectomy in women with very large uterine size. Fertil Steril. 85(1):36-9, 2006
5. Spies JB et al: Long-term outcome of uterine artery embolization of leiomyomata. Obstet Gynecol. 106(5 Pt 1):933-9, 2005
6. Day Baird D et al: High cumulative incidence of uterine leiomyoma in black and white women: ultrasound evidence. Am J Obstet Gynecol. 188(1):100-7, 2003
7. Kido A et al: Diffusely enlarged uterus: evaluation with MR imaging. Radiographics. 23(6):1423-39, 2003
8. Razavi MK et al: Abdominal myomectomy versus uterine fibroid embolization in the treatment of symptomatic uterine leiomyomas. AJR Am J Roentgenol. 180(6):1571-5, 2003
9. Murase E et al: Uterine leiomyomas: histopathologic features, MR imaging findings, differential diagnosis, and treatment. Radiographics. 19(5):1179-97, 1999
10. Fried AM et al: Benign pelvic masses: sonographic spectrum. Radiographics. 16(2):321-34, 1996
11. Mayer DP et al: Ultrasonography and magnetic resonance imaging of uterine fibroids. Obstet Gynecol Clin North Am. 22(4):667-725, 1995
12. Karasick S et al: Imaging of uterine leiomyomas. AJR Am J Roentgenol. 158(4):799-805, 1992
13. Casillas J et al: CT appearance of uterine leiomyomas. Radiographics. 10(6):999-1007, 1990

LEIOMYOMA, SUBSEROSAL

IMAGE GALLERY

Typical

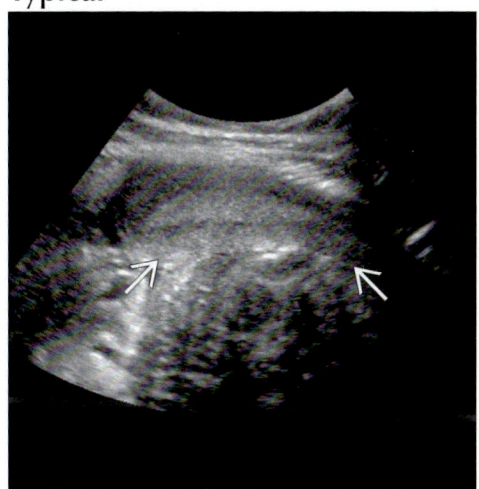
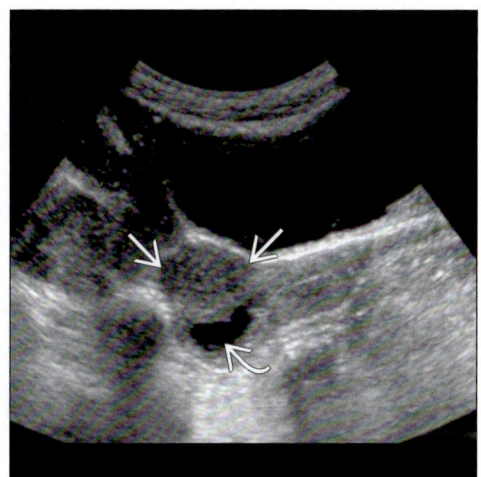

(Left) Sagittal transabdominal ultrasound shows posterior sound attenuating mass displacing uterus anteriorly representing subserosal leiomyoma with broad based attachment ➡. *(Right)* Sagittal transabdominal ultrasound shows hypoechoic, well-defined, subserosal leiomyoma ➡ arising from anterior body. Note fluid in endometrial cavity ➡.

Typical

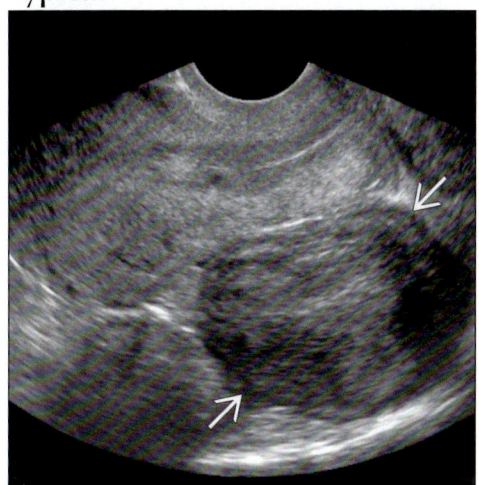
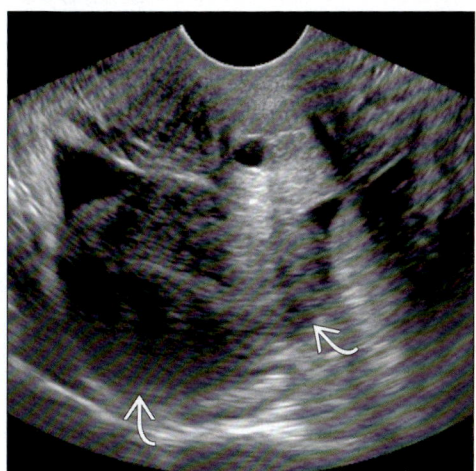

(Left) Sagittal transvaginal ultrasound shows a hypoechoic mass posterior to the cervix ➡. The site of origin or attachment is not obvious. *(Right)* Coronal transvaginal ultrasound in the same patient as previous image shows the well-defined, hypoechoic mass posterior to the cervix ➡.

Typical

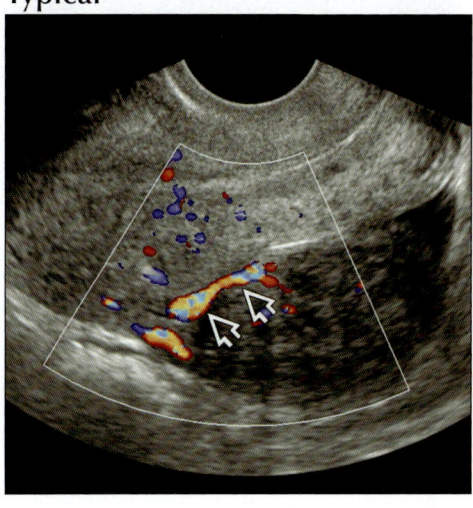
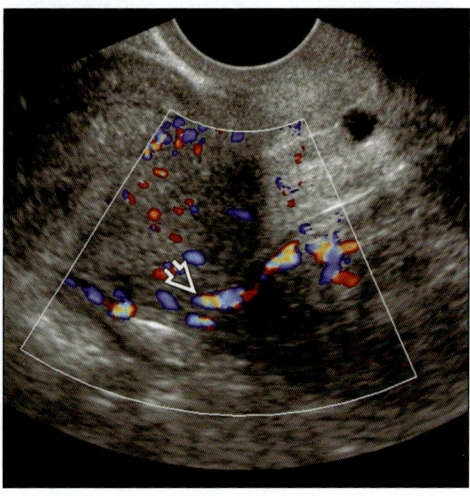

(Left) Sagittal color Doppler ultrasound in the same patient as previous image shows feeding vessels ➡ arising from posterior body and confirms the diagnosis of pedunculated subserosal leiomyoma. *(Right)* Sagittal color Doppler ultrasound in the same patient as previous image shows feeding vessels within pedicle ➡. Note the vessels drape around the leiomyoma, with relatively little internal flow within the lesion.

LEIOMYOMA, SUBSEROSAL

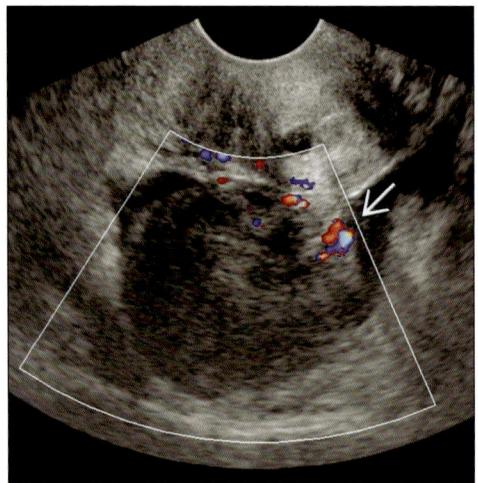 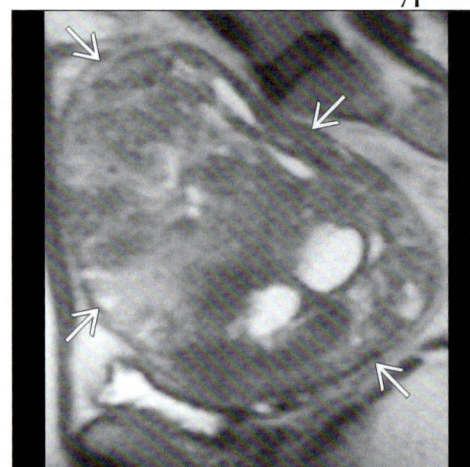

(Left) Coronal color Doppler ultrasound in the same patient as previous image shows lack of internal vascularity typical of leiomyomas. The feeding vessel is seen in the periphery of the lesion ➡. (Right) Sagittal T2WI MR shows a heterogeneous mass in the mid pelvis ➡.

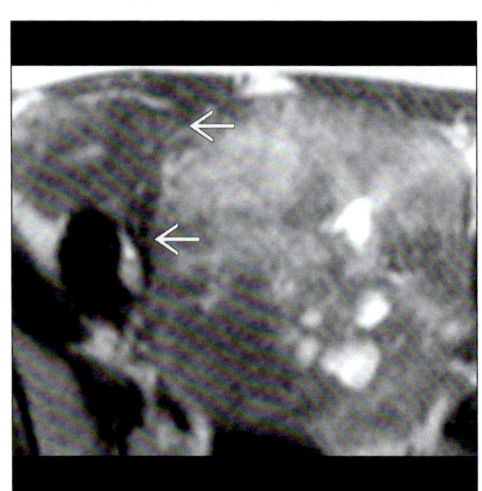 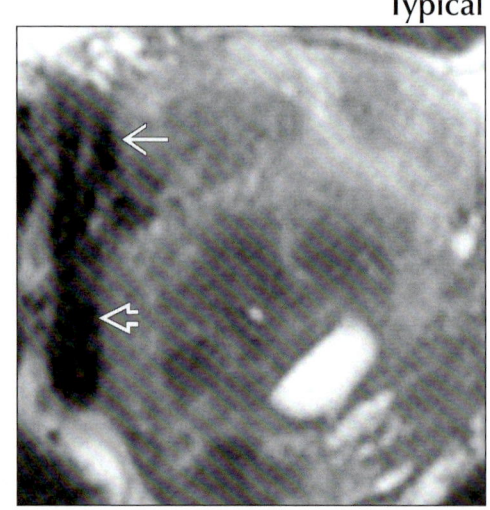

(Left) Axial T2WI MR in the same patient as previous image shows the uterine corpus in the right side of the pelvis with "claws" of myometrium ➡ partially surrounding the large degenerated subserosal leiomyoma. (Right) Axial T2WI MR in the same patient as previous image shows the degenerated subserosal leiomyoma applied to the left side of the uterine corpus ➡ and cervix ➡.

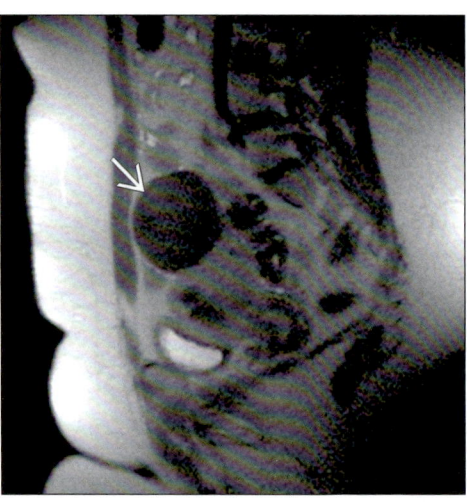 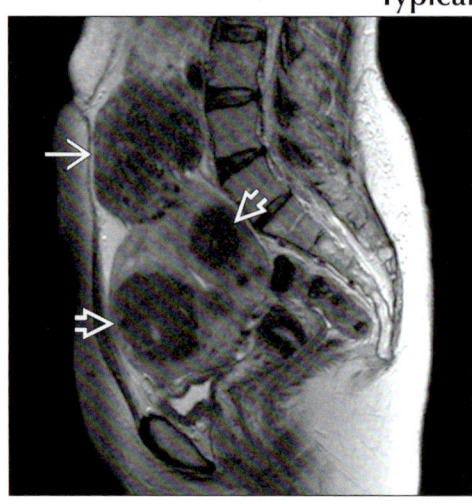

(Left) Sagittal T2WI MR shows exophytic, broad-based, subserosal leiomyoma arising from the fundus ➡. This was not visible on TVS. (Right) Sagittal T2WI MR shows multiple intramural leiomyomas ➡ and one broad-based subserosal leiomyoma ➡ arising from the fundus.

LEIOMYOMA, SUBSEROSAL

Typical

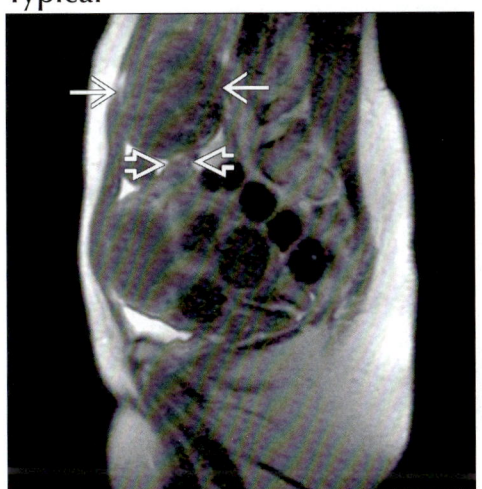
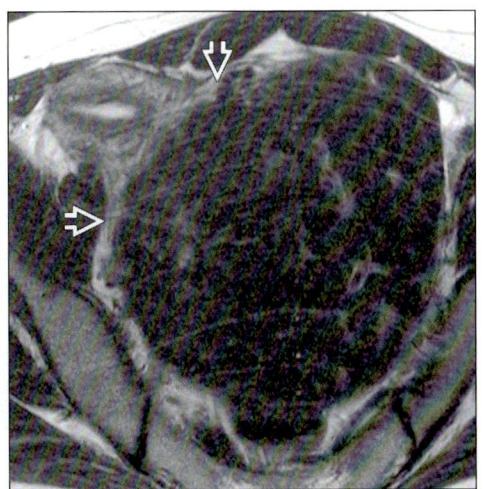

(Left) Sagittal T2WI MR shows multiple intramural leiomyomata and a pedunculated subserosal leiomyoma ➡ arising from the fundus. Note the thin pedicle ➡. (Right) Axial T2WI MR shows large broad-based mass with very low signal intensity arising from left uterine corpus. Note the myometrial "claws" ➡ that only partially surround the leiomyoma.

Typical

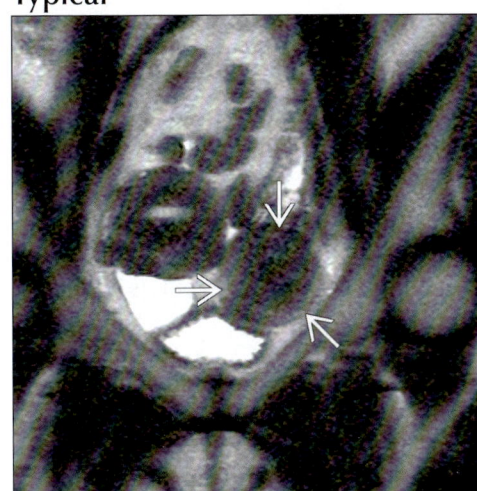
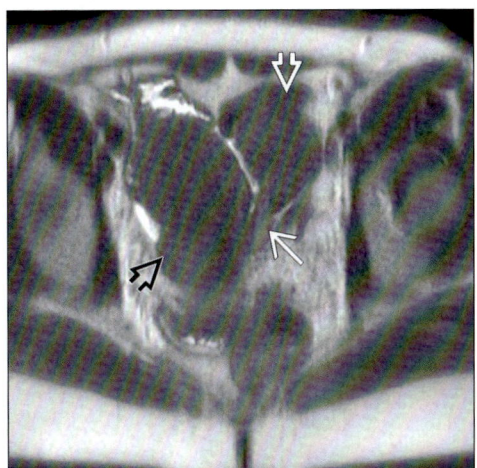

(Left) Coronal T2WI MR shows a round, low signal intensity, subserosal leiomyoma ➡. (Right) Axial T2WI MR shows a myometrial stalk ➡ connecting the leiomyoma ➡ to the uterus. A broad-based, low signal intensity, right-sided, subserosal leiomyoma is also present ➡.

Typical

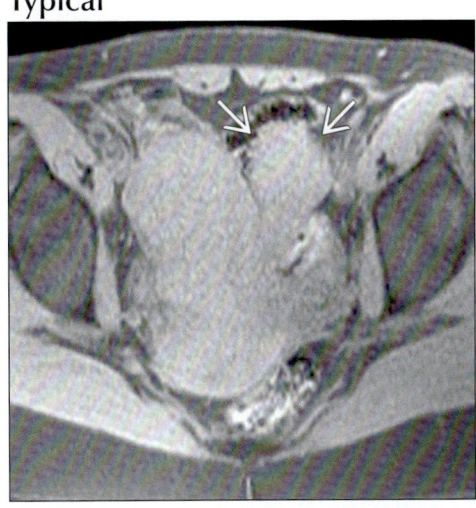
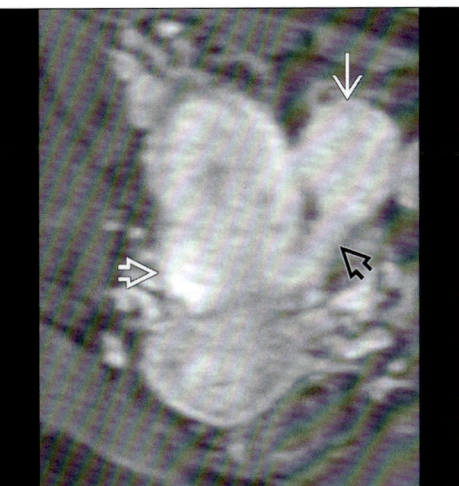

(Left) Axial T1WI FS MR in the same patient as previous image shows the subserosal leiomyoma ➡ is isointense to the rest of the uterus. (Right) Axial oblique T1 C+ FS MR in the same patient as previous image shows enhancement of the pedunculated leiomyoma ➡, including its stalk ➡. The broad-based subserosal leiomyoma ➡ also enhances.

LEIOMYOMA, DEGENERATION

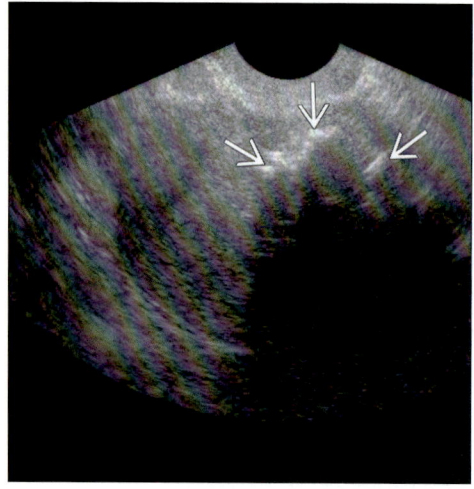

Axial transvaginal ultrasound shows an arc of increased echogenicity ➡ with posterior acoustic shadowing, consistent with a calcified degenerated leiomyoma.

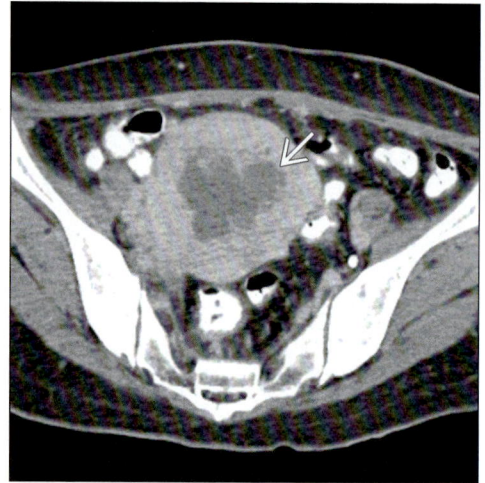

Axial CECT shows uterine mass lacking central enhancement ➡ in the degenerating portion of the leiomyoma.

TERMINOLOGY

Abbreviations and Synonyms
- Degenerated fibroid, fibroleiomyoma or myoma

Definitions
- Degenerated, benign, smooth muscle tumor

IMAGING FINDINGS

General Features
- Best diagnostic clue: Heterogeneous, well-defined uterine mass with either cystic changes or coarse calcifications
- Size: The larger the leiomyoma, the more likely it is that some form of degeneration is present
- Imaging may provide explanation for pain as well as treatment options
- Heterogeneity depends on amount and type of degeneration
- Imaging may not be able to differentiate types of degeneration

Ultrasonographic Findings
- Transvaginal ultrasound (TVS) findings
  - Heterogeneous mass when degenerated (nonspecific)
    - Hemorrhagic or cystic: Anechoic or hypoechoic cystic spaces within leiomyoma
    - Calcific: Clusters of high-level echoes with distal shadowing
  - Relatively avascular on Doppler or color US compared to myometrium

CT Findings
- NECT
  - Heterogeneous attenuation compared to myometrium
    - Calcification and acute hemorrhage: Higher attenuation
    - Cystic: Lower attenuation
    - Hyaline degeneration: Cystic appearance with diminished contrast-enhancement
- CECT: Areas of necrosis will not enhance

MR Findings
- T1WI
  - Hemorrhagic: Diffuse increased signal intensity (SI)

DDx: Leiomyoma (Degenerating)

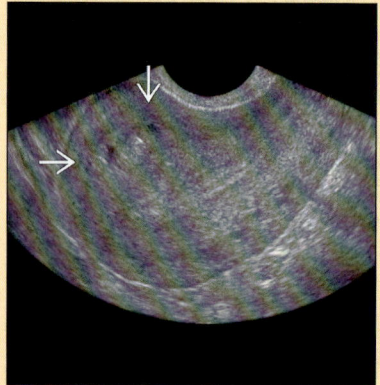

Focal Adenomyosis

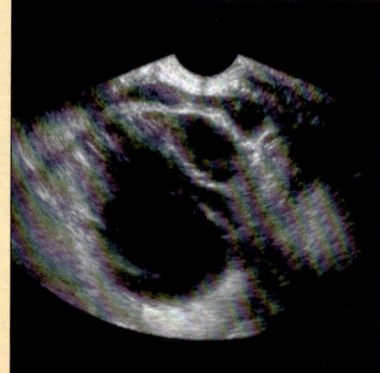

Cystic Adnexal Mass

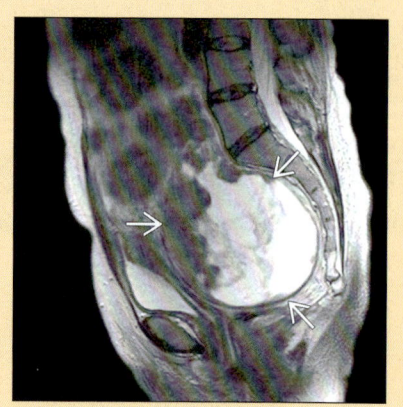

Leiomyosarcoma

LEIOMYOMA, DEGENERATION

Key Facts

Terminology
- Degenerated fibroid, fibroleiomyoma or myoma

Imaging Findings
- Best diagnostic clue: Heterogeneous, well-defined uterine mass with either cystic changes or coarse calcifications
- Size: The larger the leiomyoma, the more likely it is that some form of degeneration is present
- Imaging may provide explanation for pain as well as treatment options
- Heterogeneity depends on amount and type of degeneration
- Imaging may not be able to differentiate types of degeneration
- Relatively avascular on Doppler or color US compared to myometrium

Top Differential Diagnoses
- Focal Adenomyosis/Adenomyoma
- Cystic Adnexal Mass
- Leiomyosarcoma
- Abscess/Tuboovarian Abscess

Pathology
- 2/3 of leiomyomas show some form of degeneration
- Often degenerated if > 5-8 cm
- Commonly occurs when outgrow blood supply associated with rapid growth, pregnancy, trauma, & postmenopausal atrophy

Clinical Issues
- If symptomatic, present with: Acute pelvic pain, localized tenderness, mild leukocytosis, pyrexia and/or nausea and vomiting

---

  - Carneous/red: Diffuse increased SI (early); high SI rim (late) which corresponds to obstructed vein
  - Cystic: Low SI within cystic spaces
  - Hyaline: Variable, may have high SI
  - Calcific: Punctate signal voids within or circumscribing leiomyoma
  - Myxoid: Variable
  - Edema: Diffuse low SI
- T2WI
  - Round, well-defined and often heterogeneous
  - Hemorrhagic: Diffuse low SI
  - Carneous/red: Low SI peripheral rim corresponds to obstructed veins at the periphery, variable SI in center of lesion
  - Cystic: Increased SI within the cystic spaces
  - Hyaline: Decreased SI
  - Calcific: Foci of signal voids
  - Myxoid: Increased SI
  - Edema: Entire lesion with high SI due to the accumulation of fluid
- T1 C+
  - No enhancement if cystic degeneration
  - No enhancement within entire lesion if carneous/red degeneration which indicates complete interruption of blood flow
  - With extensive edema there is marked enhancement which is explained by the retention of contrast material within the abundant interstitial spaces

DIFFERENTIAL DIAGNOSIS

Focal Adenomyosis/Adenomyoma
- Poorly-marginated ectopic endometrial glands and stroma in myometrium
- US: Poorly-defined area of abnormal heterogeneous echotexture in myometrium with cysts simulates cystic degeneration
- T2WI: Focal widening of junctional zone ≥ 12 mm and/or ill-defined low-signal-intensity mass with or without punctate bright foci

Cystic Adnexal Mass
- Uterus is separate from mass

Leiomyosarcoma
- Contains areas of hemorrhage and necrosis
- Overlap in imaging features with degenerated leiomyoma
- T1WI: Variable appearance, may have hemorrhagic high SI components
- T2WI: Heterogeneous, irregular, ill-defined
- Secondary signs of malignancy are present, such as ascites, lymphadenopathy, peritoneal implants and invasion of adjacent structures

Pelvic or Tubo-Ovarian Abscess
- Complex cystic adnexal mass inseparable from ovary

PATHOLOGY

General Features
- General path comments
  - 2/3 of leiomyomas show some form of degeneration
  - Often degenerated if > 5-8 cm
  - Commonly occurs when outgrow blood supply associated with rapid growth, pregnancy, trauma, & postmenopausal atrophy
    - Also seen following uterine artery embolization (UAE)
  - Type of degenerative change seems to depend on the degree & rapidity of the onset of vascular insufficiency
  - Edema is not a phenomenon of degeneration but is a common histopathologic finding & is present in around 50% of leiomyomas
    - May change into various degrees of collagen deposition and cystic degeneration
    - May antedate hyalinization
    - Usually scattered throughout lesion in speckled pattern but frequently prominent at periphery
  - Hyaline degeneration
    - Occurs in more than 60% of leiomyomas

LEIOMYOMA, DEGENERATION

- Accounts for the typical low signal intensity on T2WI relative to myometrium and intermediate signal intensity on T1WI
- When advanced may develop a fatty component
- Secondary calcification occurs in hyalinized tissue in about 4%, seen more often after menopause
- Calcifications usually dense and amorphous
- Ring-like peripheral calcification is a rare pattern which represents thrombosed veins from past red degeneration
  - Cystic degeneration
    - Extreme sequela of edema and is observed in about 4% of leiomyomas
    - Other theories include liquefaction of hyalinized areas due to a decreased blood supply
    - Cystic spaces appear as round, well-demarcated areas with fluid signal intensity
    - Corresponds to areas of necrosis
  - Myxoid degeneration
    - Soft mucoid areas, sometimes with cystic change
    - This type of degeneration may also be seen in leiomyosarcomas and other malignant tumors
  - Carneous/red degeneration
    - Involves massive hemorrhagic infarction
    - Due to obstruction of drainage veins at the periphery of the lesion
    - Degeneration related to extensive coagulation necrosis that involves the entire lesion
    - Occurs during pregnancy & with oral contraceptives
  - Hemorrhage and necrosis (separate from red degeneration)
    - Usually seen after UAE
    - Relates to damaged smooth muscle which will eventually be replaced by firm collagenous tissue
    - More important to recognize as clues in the diagnosis of sarcoma

Gross Pathologic & Surgical Features
- Soft consistency
- Hyaline: Smooth homogeneous translucent zone
- Myxoid: Cystic masses filled with gelatinous material
- Carneous/red: Loss of whorled appearance of cut surface, softer consistency
- Necrotic: Yellow foci
- Hemorrhagic: Red foci

Microscopic Features
- Hyaline: Eosinophilic bands or plaques in the extracellular space, begins in the stromal component that separates the smooth muscle cells and then progresses to extensive replacement of the smooth muscle cells by collagen
- Myxoid: Hyaluronic acid-rich mucopolysaccharides make up the gelatinous component
- Carneous/ed: Peripheral venous thrombosis, ghosts of the muscle cells
- Cystic degeneration: May be large or small cystic spaces, develop in the edematous acellular center
- Edema: Fluid seen in the stroma of the leiomyoma, often in association with collagen

CLINICAL ISSUES

Presentation
- Most common signs/symptoms
  - Most degenerating leiomyomas are asymptomatic
  - If symptomatic, present with: Acute pelvic pain, localized tenderness, mild leukocytosis, pyrexia and/or nausea and vomiting
  - Risk for pain increases with size and is high in lesions that are larger than 5 cm in diameter
  - Pain typically presents in the late first or early second trimester, which corresponds to the period of greatest rate of leiomyoma growth
  - Red degeneration can cause systemic symptoms and has been shown to incite premature labor
- Other signs/symptoms: Massive intraperitoneal hemorrhage due to leiomyomas, which is uncommon

Natural History & Prognosis
- Good, most women are asymptomatic
- If symptomatic, most women benefit from treatment
- Rapid unexpected growth may indicate malignant transformation

Treatment
- If symptomatic: Medical (GnRH analog), surgical (hysterectomy or myomectomy) and/or minimally invasive (UAE) therapy

SELECTED REFERENCES

1. Fogata ML et al: Degenerating cystic uterine fibroid mimics an ovarian cyst in a pregnant patient. J Ultrasound Med. 25(5):671-4, 2006
2. Ouyang DW et al: Obstetric complications of fibroids. Obstet Gynecol Clin North Am. 33(1):153-69, 2006
3. Birchard KR et al: MRI of acute abdominal and pelvic pain in pregnant patients. AJR Am J Roentgenol. 184(2):452-8, 2005
4. Pelage JP et al: Uterine fibroid vascularization and clinical relevance to uterine fibroid embolization. Radiographics. 25 Suppl 1:S99-117, 2005
5. Low SC et al: A case of cystic leiomyoma mimicking an ovarian malignancy. Ann Acad Med Singapore. 33(3):371-4, 2004
6. Bennett GL et al: Gynecologic causes of acute pelvic pain: spectrum of CT findings. Radiographics. 22(4):785-801, 2002
7. Coronado GD et al: Complications in pregnancy, labor, and delivery with uterine leiomyomas: a population-based study. Obstet Gynecol. 95(5):764-9, 2000
8. Murase E et al: Uterine leiomyomas: histopathologic features, MR imaging findings, differential diagnosis, and treatment. Radiographics. 19(5):1179-97, 1999
9. Ueda H et al: Unusual appearances of uterine leiomyomas: MR imaging findings and their histopathologic backgrounds. Radiographics. 19 Spec No:S131-45, 1999
10. Yarwood RL et al: Cystic degeneration of a uterine leiomyoma masquerading as a postmenopausal ovarian cyst. A case report. J Reprod Med. 44(7):649-52, 1999
11. Cohen JR et al: Ultrasonic "honeycomb" appearance of uterine submucous fibroids undergoing cystic degeneration. J Clin Ultrasound. 23(5):293-6, 1995

LEIOMYOMA, DEGENERATION

IMAGE GALLERY

Typical

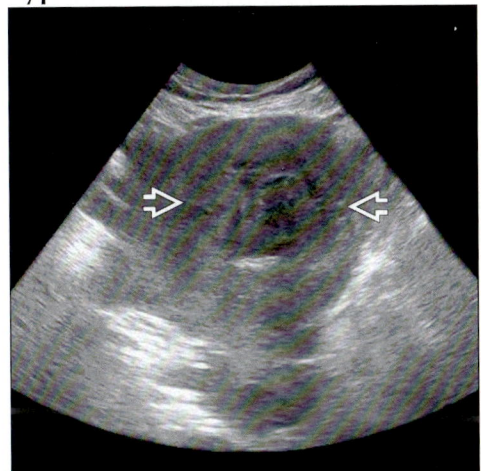
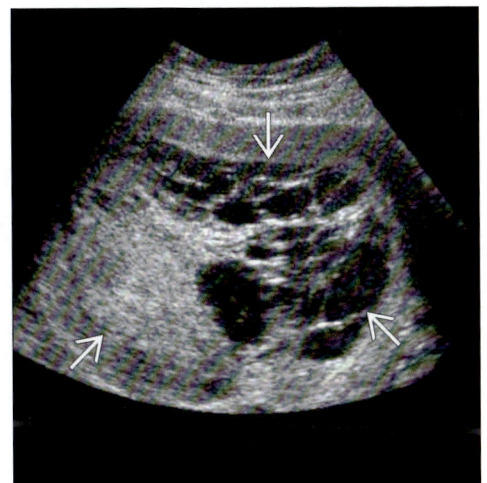

(Left) Axial transabdominal ultrasound in this emergency room patient with pelvic pain shows a cystic uterine mass ➡. *(Right)* Coronal transvaginal ultrasound of the same patient as previous image, better shows the internal cystic change of the mass ➡. The mass was a degenerating leiomyoma on subsequent MR.

Typical

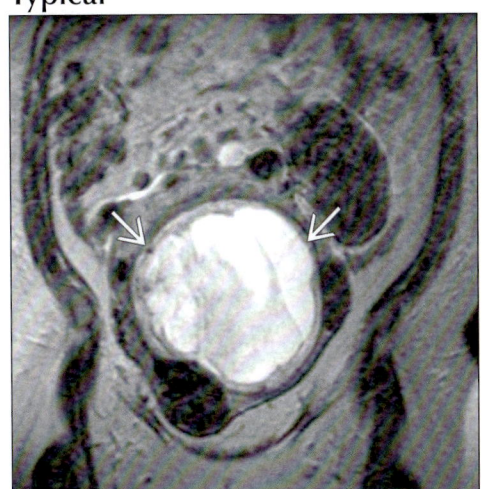
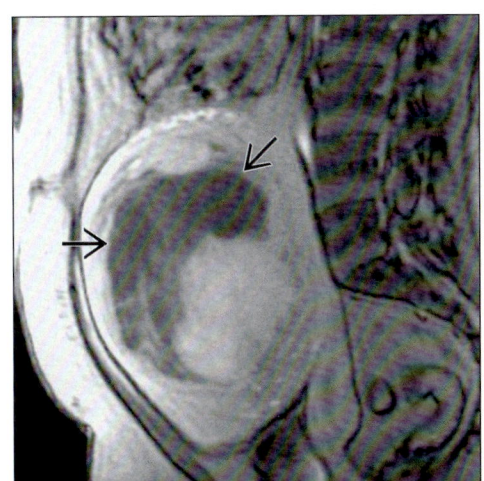

(Left) Coronal T2WI MR shows an intramural leiomyoma with primarily high signal intensity ➡. *(Right)* Sagittal T1 C+ MR in the same patient as previous image, shows the areas of high signal intensity on T2WI are cystic areas of degeneration ➡.

Typical

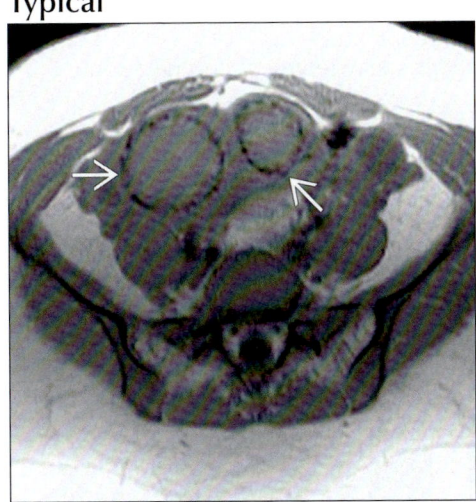
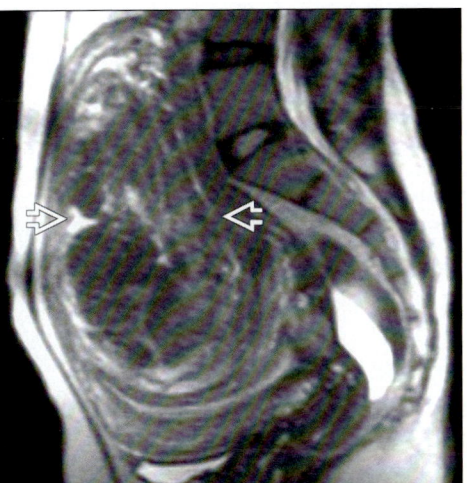

(Left) Axial T1WI MR shows discontinuous signal voids ➡, calcifications, circumscribing two intramural leiomyomas. *(Right)* Sagittal T2WI MR shows a heterogeneous, intramural fundal leiomyoma ➡. The exact type of degeneration cannot be determined because of overlap in SI of the different types of degeneration.

LEIOMYOMA, PARASITIC

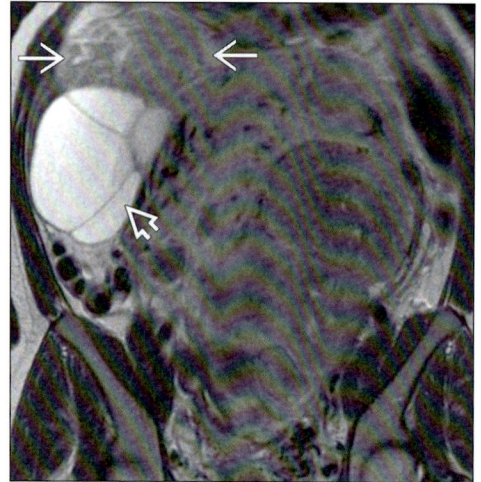

Coronal T2WI MR shows hyperstimulated right ovary ➡ elevated into abdomen by an enlarged leiomyomatous uterus. The parasitic leiomyoma ➡ is contiguous with right ovary and right fundus.

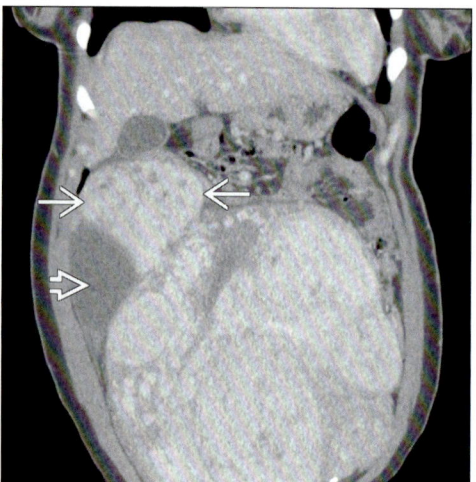

Coronal CECT in the same patient as previous image shows hyperstimulated right ovary ➡ and adjacent parasitic leiomyoma ➡ cephalad to enlarged uterus.

TERMINOLOGY

Abbreviations and Synonyms
- Parasitic fibroid

Definitions
- Uterine leiomyoma (either free in pelvis or still attached to uterus by a stalk) that recruits blood supply from nearby structures

IMAGING FINDINGS

General Features
- Best diagnostic clue
  - Subserosal, pedunculated or freely detached leiomyoma with clearly defined arterial supply from nearby pelvic/abdominal structures
    - May even recruit flow from omentum and intestines
  - Recruits neovascularization from surrounding structures
  - May see large draining veins
  - If torsed from uterine blood supply, lesion can be free in the peritoneum
  - Multiplanar imaging is key to definition of surrounding organ involvement including bladder, ureters, and neovascularity
  - Surgical planning relies on detailed cross-sectional imaging to define extent of lesion and blood supply
- Location
  - Parasitic leiomyomas are almost exclusively subserosal in location and often pedunculated
  - Many are often detached from the uterus and free within pelvis or attached to nearby organs/viscera
  - Common sites of attachment and/or arterial recruitment are fallopian tubes, broad ligament, and omentum
- Size: Variable
- Morphology: Identical in size, shape, morphology, and histology to typical uterine leiomyomas

Ultrasonographic Findings
- Heterogeneous echotexture
- Cystic central areas may represent degeneration

DDx: Mimics of Parasitic Leiomyoma

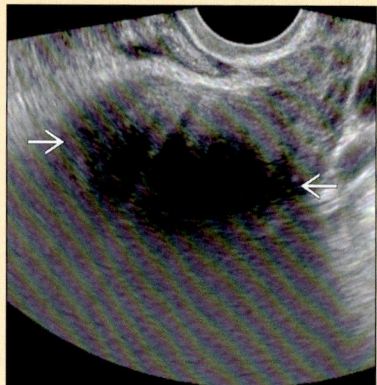

Ovarian Fibroma

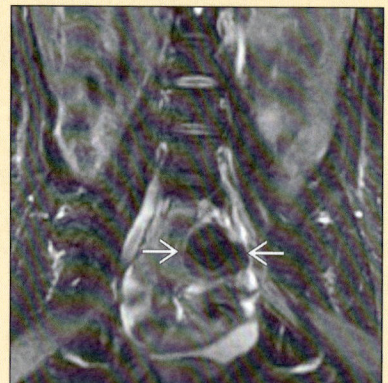

Ovarian Fibroma

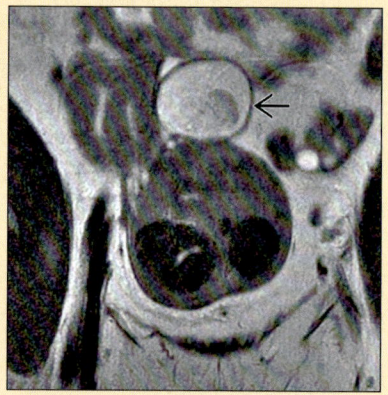

Dermoid

LEIOMYOMA, PARASITIC

Key Facts

Terminology
- Parasitic leiomyoma
- Uterine leiomyoma (either free in pelvis or still attached to uterus by a stalk) that recruits blood supply from nearby structures

Imaging Findings
- Subserosal, pedunculated or freely detached leiomyoma with clearly defined arterial supply from nearby pelvic/abdominal structures
- Multiplanar imaging is key to definition of surrounding organ involvement including bladder, ureters, and neovascularity
- Surgical planning relies on detailed cross-sectional imaging to define extent of lesion and blood supply
- Parasitic leiomyomas are almost exclusively subserosal in location and often pedunculated
- Many are often detached from the uterus and free within pelvis or attached to nearby organs/viscera
- Common sites of attachment and/or arterial recruitment are fallopian tubes, broad ligament, and omentum
- Morphology: Identical in size, shape, morphology, and histology to typical uterine leiomyomas
- Absence of color flow Doppler signal does not necessarily indicate acute torsion because leiomyomas may show absent flow or low flow without torsion
- Presence of color flow Doppler signal does not exclude intermittent torsion of parasitic leiomyoma
- Best imaging tool: Gadolinium enhanced MR of pelvis is most sensitive modality for defining size, location, and arterial supply of a parasitic leiomyoma

---

- Absence of color flow Doppler signal does not necessarily indicate acute torsion because leiomyomas may show absent flow or low flow without torsion
  - Presence of color flow Doppler signal does not exclude intermittent torsion of parasitic leiomyoma

CT Findings
- Usually uniform, solid soft tissue density with Hounsfield units similar to normal uterine myometrium
- Calcifications can be seen in 3-10% of all leiomyomas
- Contrast-enhancement similar to typical leiomyomas
- CTA may show arterial supply and venous drainage of parasitic leiomyoma

MR Findings
- Signal characteristics are similar to typical non-degenerated uterine leiomyomas
  - Subserosal (broad-based or pedunculated) pelvic mass
    - T1WI: Isointense to myometrium
    - T2WI: Hypointense to myometrium
  - Mass may be separate from uterus within pelvis if a pedunculated leiomyoma has torsed "free"
- Degenerative changes are also identical to uterine leiomyomas
  - Cystic and myxoid degeneration
    - Focal areas of low signal intensity on T1WI and increased signal intensity on T2WI
    - Variable enhancement on gadolinium T1WI
  - Hemorrhagic degeneration: High signal intensity areas on T1 with rim of low T2 signal
- MRA and post contrast images
  - Enhancing vasculature that can be traced to "parasitized" end organ: Often distinctly separate from normal uterine artery
  - May see draining veins
- Careful scrutiny of enhanced vessels or flow voids should be made
- Relationships to fallopian tubes, broad ligaments, omentum, and any intervening structures must be noted

Imaging Recommendations
- Best imaging tool: Gadolinium enhanced MR of pelvis is most sensitive modality for defining size, location, and arterial supply of a parasitic leiomyoma
- Protocol advice: Multiplanar pre and post gadolinium images with small field of view centered over pelvis or region of interest

DIFFERENTIAL DIAGNOSIS

Lymphadenopathy
- Often there are other pathologically enlarged lymph nodes throughout pelvis

Ovarian Stromal Tumor
- Continuity with ovary/adnexa
- Inability to demonstrate normal ovaries
- Ovarian fibromas and Brenner tumors may have similar imaging characteristics due to fibrous content

Other Adnexal Neoplasms (Benign and Malignant)
- Cystadenoma, cystadenocarcinoma, Müllerian carcinoma, teratoma, leiomyosarcoma, malignant fibrous histiocytoma

Other Adnexal Lesions
- Endometriosis, ectopic pregnancy

Leiomyosarcoma
- Often a pathologic diagnosis
  - Imaging features are not specific: Irregular margins, necrosis and hemorrhage may suggest diagnosis
  - Rapid increase in size in postmenopausal woman
  - Features of aggressive invasion into surrounding soft tissues

Inflammatory Lesions of Fallopian Tube
- Salpingitis from gonococcus or Chlamydia, fungus, tuberculosis
- Crohn disease, sarcoidosis

LEIOMYOMA, PARASITIC

PATHOLOGY

General Features
- Epidemiology
  - Leiomyomas are the most common gynecologic neoplasm occurring in 20-30% of women
    - Incidence of parasitic leiomyomas has not been reported
    - Leiomyoma: Most common solid broad ligament tumor

Gross Pathologic & Surgical Features
- Identical to typical uterine leiomyomas
- Spherical, firm, white and elastic in consistency

Microscopic Features
- Identical to typical uterine leiomyomas
- Uniform, anastomosed & whorled smooth muscle cells
- Variable amounts of fibrous connective tissue
- Small, infrequent blood vessels
- No significant mitosis, atypia or necrosis

CLINICAL ISSUES

Presentation
- Most common signs/symptoms
  - Pelvic pain
    - Pressure on adjacent organs (i.e., bladder, rectum)
    - Torsion
  - Infertility
  - Small/large bowel obstruction
- Other signs/symptoms: May recur after resection

Demographics
- Age
  - Premenopausal females
    - Usually develops in premenopausal females, but may become clinically evident in pre or postmenopausal patients
  - May be hormone responsive
    - Can shrink with menopause

Natural History & Prognosis
- May be asymptomatic depending on size and menstrual status
  - Hormone responsive and may enlarge to cause mass effect on nearby structures

Treatment
- Often surgical removal for symptomatic relief or for impingement on nearby structures
- Because differential diagnosis includes malignancy, tissue sampling is usually required to confirm benign parasitic leiomyoma
  - Once benign tissue is confirmed, treatment options include
    - Medical management (analgesia, hormone manipulation)
    - Surgical management (myomectomy)

DIAGNOSTIC CHECKLIST

Consider
- Since lesion is separate from uterus, it is easily mistaken for an adnexal mass
- Identification of lesion as separate from both uterus and ovaries is key to excluding adnexal mass
- If uterus, ovaries and lesion are contiguous, primary source of lesion can be difficult to identify
  - Search for vascular supply of lesion - if uterine, likely parasitic leiomyoma on stalk
  - If blood supply is completely neovascular with no stalk, source of lesion remains unknown

Image Interpretation Pearls
- Locate lesion separate from uterus and ovaries
- Pedicle may not be visible especially on sonography

SELECTED REFERENCES

1. Cohen et al: Uterine smooth-muscle tumors with unusual growth patterns. Imaging with pathologic correlation. AJR. 188:246-55, 2007
2. Muffly T et al: Massive leiomyoma of the broad ligament. Obstet Gynecol. 109(2 Pt2):563-5, 2007
3. Pelage et al: Uterine fibroid vascularization and clinical relevance to uterine fibroid embolization. Radiographics. 25:S99-S117, 2005
4. Murase et al: Uterine leiomyomas: histopathologic features, MR imaging findings, differential diagnosis, and treatment. Radiographics. 19:1179-97, 1999
5. Ueda et al: Unusual appearances of uterine leiomyomas: MR imaging findings and their histologic backgrounds. Radiographics. 19:S131-45, 1999
6. Yeh et al: Parasitic and pedunculated leiomyomas: ultrasonographic features. J Ultrasound Med. 18:789-94, 1999

LEIOMYOMA, PARASITIC

IMAGE GALLERY

Typical

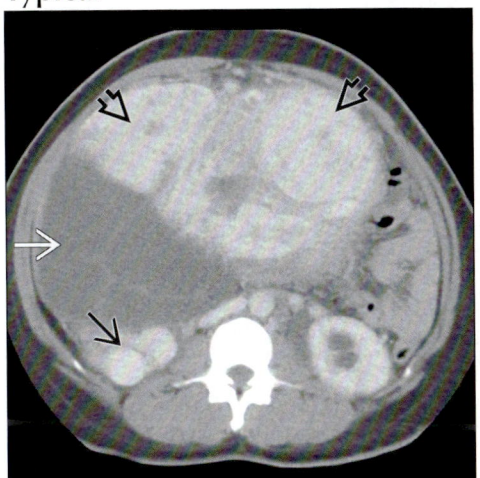
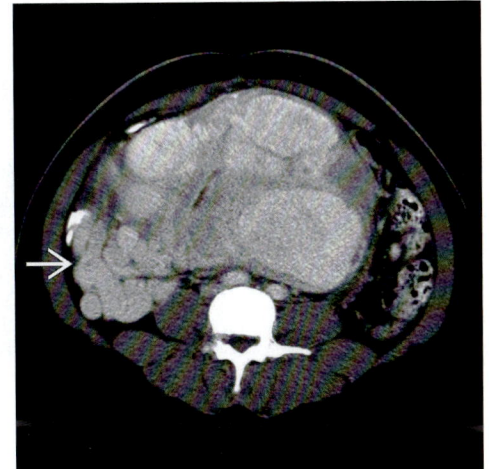

(Left) Axial CECT in the same patient as previous images shows hyperstimulated right ovary ➡ and large collateral draining veins ➡ adjacent to leiomyomatous uterus ➡. *(Right)* Axial CECT shows large enhanced venous collaterals ➡ in a patient with parasitic leiomyomas.

Typical

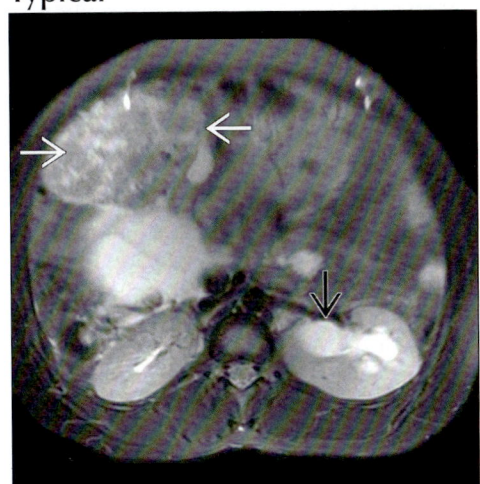
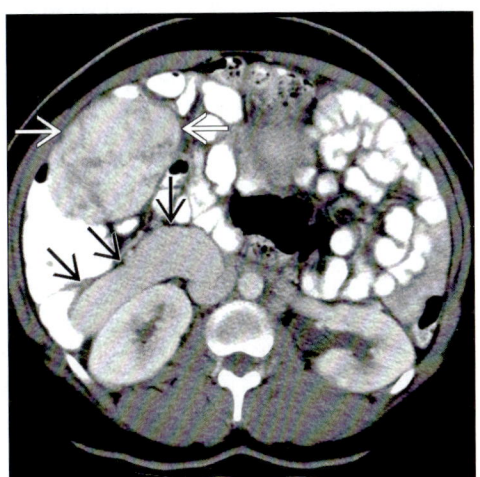

(Left) Axial T2WI FS MR shows a parasitic leiomyoma ➡. Note left hydronephrosis ➡ from compression by enlarged uterus. *(Right)* Axial CECT in the same patient as previous image shows a parasitic leiomyoma ➡ with a huge draining vein ➡ emptying into the inferior vena cava.

Typical

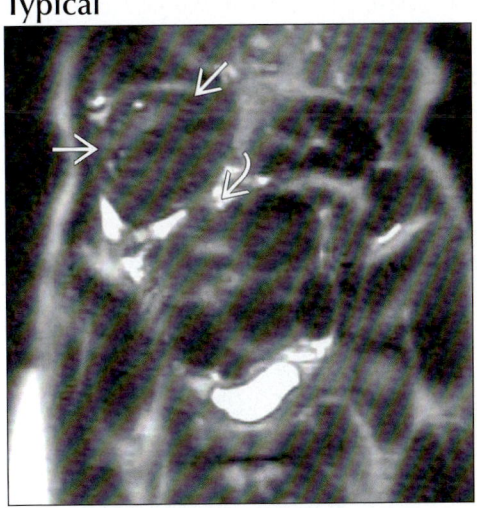
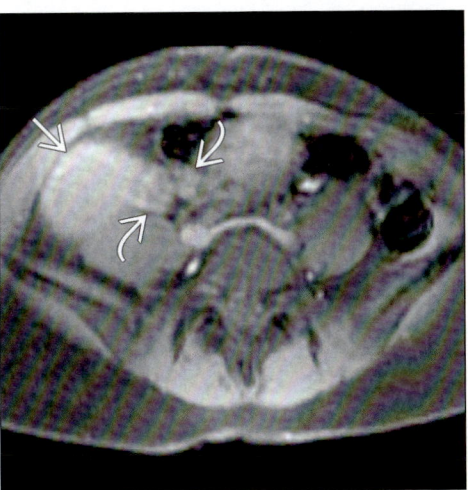

(Left) Coronal T2WI MR shows a patient with a parasitic subserosal pedunculated leiomyoma ➡. Note the stalk ➡ connecting the leiomyoma to the right uterine fundus. *(Right)* Axial T1 C+ FS MR in the same patient as previous image shows enhancing parasitized vessels ➡ supplying the parasitic leiomyoma ➡.

BENIGN METASTASIZING LEIOMYOMA

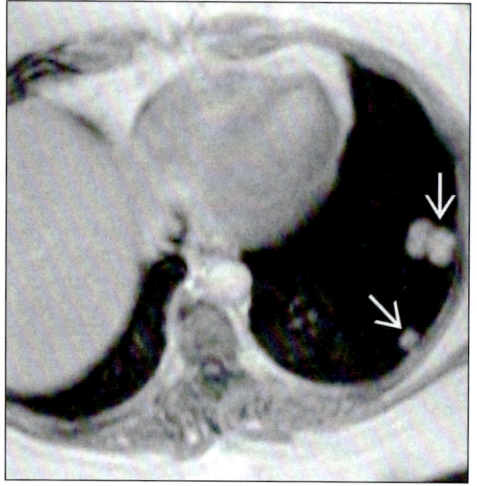

Axial T1 C+ MR shows multiple enhancing nodules ➡ in a patient with BML. Reprinted by permission of John Wiley & Sons, Inc. In: Abdominal-Pelvic MRI, Semelka RC (ed), Copyright 2002 by Wiley-Liss, Inc.

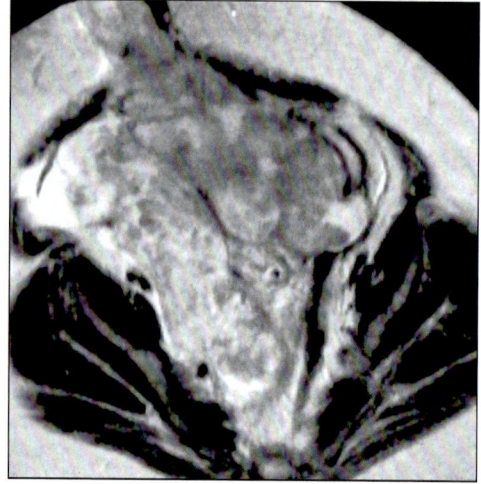

Axial T2WI MR shows a pelvic heterogeneous mass consistent with fibroids. Reprinted by permission of John Wiley & Sons, Inc. In: Abdominal-Pelvic MRI, Semelka RC (ed), Copyright 2002 by Wiley-Liss, Inc.

TERMINOLOGY

Abbreviations and Synonyms
- Metastatic leiomyomas, multiple fibroleiomyomatous hamartomas

Definitions
- Asymptomatic extra-uterine benign leiomyomas
  - Usually affects women after hysterectomy for leiomyomas

IMAGING FINDINGS

General Features
- Best diagnostic clue: Incidental well-circumscribed pulmonary nodules in otherwise healthy woman
- Location
  - Multiple extrauterine sites affected (3 months to 20 years post hysterectomy)
    - Lung is most common site
    - Other sites include: Lymph nodes, peritoneum and retroperitoneum
- Size: Range from few mm to cm in diameter
- Morphology: Most are smooth & well-circumscribed

Radiographic Findings
- Chest radiograph findings
  - Multiple bilateral well-defined pulmonary nodules
  - Less common presentations
    - Miliary pattern
    - Pedunculated pulmonary mass with large cyst
    - Giant cyst with multiple pulmonary nodules
  - No associated calcifications, pleural effusion or mediastinal lymphadenopathy
  - Can be associated with pneumothorax
- Often found on chest radiograph as incidental finding

Ultrasonographic Findings
- Grayscale Ultrasound
  - Usually heterogeneous, well-defined uterine mass
  - May be isoechoic, hyperechoic, or hypoechoic compared to normal myometrium
- Color Doppler: Vascular supply contiguous with myometrium

CT Findings
- Multiple bilateral well-defined pulmonary nodules
- Less common: Cavitary lung nodules

DDx: Benign Metastasizing Leiomyoma

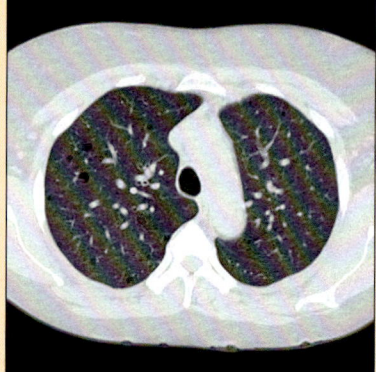

Lymphangioleiomyomatosis

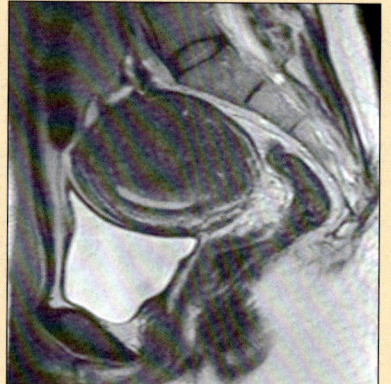

Adenomyosis

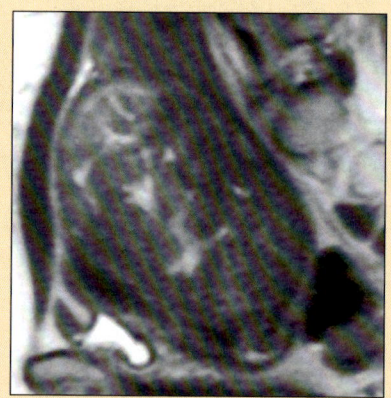

Leiomyosarcoma

BENIGN METASTASIZING LEIOMYOMA

Key Facts

Terminology
- Metastatic leiomyomas, multiple fibroleiomyomatous hamartomas
- Asymptomatic extra-uterine benign leiomyomas
- Usually affects women after hysterectomy for leiomyomas

Imaging Findings
- Best diagnostic clue: Incidental well-circumscribed pulmonary nodules in otherwise healthy woman
- Multiple extrauterine sites affected (3 months to 20 years post hysterectomy)
- Lung is most common site
- Other sites include: Lymph nodes, peritoneum and retroperitoneum
- Morphology: Most are smooth & well-circumscribed
- MR for evaluation of leiomyomas
- CT for evaluation of lung nodules

Top Differential Diagnoses
- Leiomyomatosis Peritonealis Disseminata
- Lymphangioleiomyomatosis (LAM)
- Metastatic Leiomyosarcoma

Pathology
- General path comments: Benign smooth muscle proliferation
- Hematogenous metastases from benign uterine leiomyomas
- Rare; 75 reported cases in literature

Clinical Issues
- Indolent: Majority of affected women die from other causes

- No associated calcifications
- No pleural effusion
- No significant mediastinal lymphadenopathy
- Do not enhance significantly after contrast

MR Findings
- T1WI: Intermediate signal intensity masses in the uterus
- T2WI: Low signal intensity masses in the uterus
- T1 C+: Degree of enhancement of the leiomyomas can vary greatly depending on vascularity

Imaging Recommendations
- Best imaging tool
  - MR for evaluation of leiomyomas
  - CT for evaluation of lung nodules
- Protocol advice
  - Multiplanar T2WI of uterus
  - Axial T1WI with and without fat-saturation
  - Post-gadolinium T1WI with fat-saturation
- CT guided percutaneous biopsy

DIFFERENTIAL DIAGNOSIS

Leiomyomatosis Peritonealis Disseminata
- Proliferation of benign smooth muscle cells on peritoneal surfaces
- Affects women during reproductive years & may present during pregnancy
- Promoted or initiated by hormonal factors; leiomyomas regress after hormonal manipulation is stopped
- No extraperitoneal manifestations

Lymphangioleiomyomatosis (LAM)
- Benign smooth muscle cell proliferation from lymphatic walls in lung and lymph nodes
- Young women present with spontaneous pneumothorax, chylous pleural effusion or progressive dyspnea
- No association with uterine leiomyomas
- Imaging findings: Pulmonary hyperinflation & numerous thin-walled cysts

Metastatic Leiomyosarcoma
- Primary tumor: Uterine leiomyosarcoma
- Metastases with cytologic atypia and increased mitoses mimicking primary tumor

Other Causes of Multiple Pulmonary Nodules
- Metastases from other primary cancers
- Infectious or inflammatory disease
- Collagen-vascular disease

Other Cause of Uterine Mass
- Adenomyosis
  - Ectopic endometrial tissue within the myometrium
  - On MR, thickened junctional zone, T2 hyperintense foci within the myometrium
  - In contrast to leiomyomas, focal adenomas are poorly-defined and demonstrate minimal mass effect on the endometrium

PATHOLOGY

General Features
- General path comments: Benign smooth muscle proliferation
- Etiology
  - Hematogenous metastases from benign uterine leiomyomas
  - Mechanism of spread theory
    - Extension from uterus into pelvic venous channels
    - Tumors gain venous access from surgical trauma during hysterectomy
- Epidemiology
  - Women post hysterectomy (few cases diagnosed with intact uterus)
  - Rare; 75 reported cases in literature

BENIGN METASTASIZING LEIOMYOMA

Gross Pathologic & Surgical Features
- Solid, white-tan homogeneous nodules
- Circumscribed large lesions without encapsulation
- Less well-defined small lesions
- Some can be cystic, multiloculated

Microscopic Features
- Proliferation of smooth muscle cells with varying amounts of intervening collagen
- Well-differentiated, benign-appearing
- No anaplasia or vascular invasion
- Rare mitotic figures
- Some lesions less cellular with moderate amounts of collagen
- Immunohistochemistry: Strong reactivity for desmin & muscle-specific actin
- Estrogen and progesterone receptors
- Lung: Metaplastic, low cuboidal epithelium present on alveolar septa at periphery of lesion with extension and entrapment of similarly lined clefts and tubular spaces in nodule interior
- Nodules have benign glandular component lined by simple cuboidal to columnar epithelium
  - In cystic nodules, there is cystic dilatation of these glands

Staging, Grading or Classification Criteria
- Proposed classification system for multiple lung smooth muscle lesions
  - Benign metastasizing leiomyoma: Uterine source in mature women
  - Metastatic leiomyoma: Extrauterine source in children and men
  - Multiple fibroleiomyomatous hamartoma: No extrapulmonary source
- Low grade leiomyosarcoma if increased mitotic activity (controversial)

CLINICAL ISSUES

Presentation
- Most common signs/symptoms: Usually asymptomatic
- Other signs/symptoms
  - Fever, nonproductive cough, chest pain, dyspnea
  - Little correlation between disease extent and pulmonary symptoms
  - Abdominal pain if peritoneal or retroperitoneal structures affected

Demographics
- Age: Large age range from premenopausal to postmenopausal
- Gender: Female

Natural History & Prognosis
- Indolent: Majority of affected women die from other causes
- Prognosis usually excellent
- Hormonally responsive: Progression with estrogen, regression with progesterone
- Prognosis can depend on patient's estrogen status
  - Indolent in post-menopausal women
  - In premenopausal women, reports of disease progression, even leading to death

Treatment
- No standard treatment
- Therapy is not always indicated: May regress without therapy (e.g., with menopause)
- Detection of estrogen and progesterone receptors in biopsy specimens can help optimize therapy
- Hormonal manipulation: Progesterone or luteinizing hormone-releasing hormone analogues
- Hysterectomy and oophorectomy
- Anecdotal success with chemotherapy

DIAGNOSTIC CHECKLIST

Image Interpretation Pearls
- Pulmonary nodules in an otherwise healthy woman with history of hysterectomy for leiomyomas

SELECTED REFERENCES
1. Abramson S et al: Benign metastasizing leiomyoma: clinical, imaging and pathologic correlation. Am J Roentgen. 176:1409-113, 2001
2. Koh DM et al: Benign metastasizing leiomyoma with intracaval leiomyatosis. The British Journal of Radiology. 73:435-7, 2000
3. Ueda H et al: Unusual appearances of uterine leiomyomas: MR imaging findings and their histopathologic backgrounds. Radiographics. 19:S131-S145, 1999
4. Maredia R et al: Benign metastasizing leiomyoma in the lung. Radiographics. 18:779-82, 1998
5. Abu-Rustum NR et al: Regression of uterine low-grade smooth-muscle tumors metastatic to the lung after oophorectomy. Obstet Gynecol. 89:850-2, 1997
6. Papdatos D et al: CT of leiomyomatosis peritonealis disseminata mimicking peritoneal carcinomatosis. AJR. 167:475-6, 1996
7. Shin MS et al: Unusual computed tomographic manifestations of benign metastasizing leiomyomas as cavitary nodular lesions or interstitial lung disease. Clin Imaging 20:45-9, 1996
8. Mark AS et al: Adenomyosis and leiomyoma: differential diagnosis with MR imaging. Radiology. 163:527-9, 1987
9. Dryer L et al: Leiomatosis peritonealis disseminata: a report of two cases and review of the literature. Br J Obstet Gynaecol. 92:856-61, 1985
10. Horstmann JP et al: Spontaneous regression of pulmonary leiomyomas during pregnancy. Cancer. 39:614-21, 1977
11. Lefebvre R et al: Leiomyoma of the uterus with bilateral pulmonary metastases. Can Med Assoc J. 105:501-3, 1971
12. Harper RS et al: Intravenous leiomyomatosis of uterus. Obstet Gynecol 18:519-29, 1961

BENIGN METASTASIZING LEIOMYOMA

IMAGE GALLERY

Typical

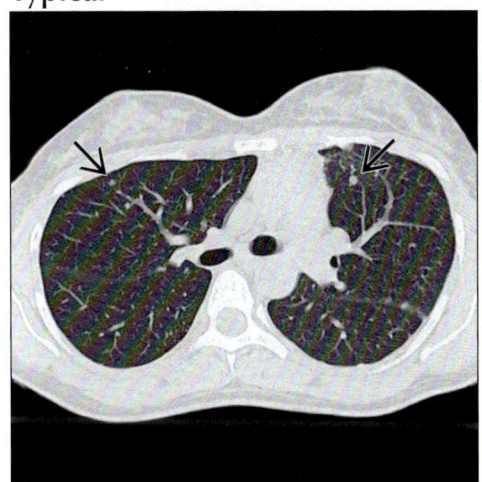
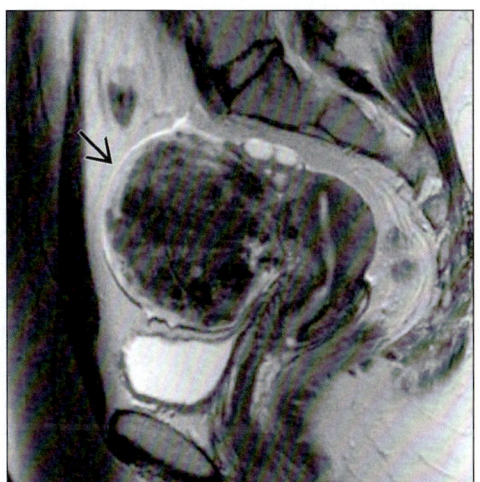

(Left) Axial NECT shows multiple bilateral pulmonary nodules ➡. *(Right)* Sagittal T2WI MR shows fairly well-circumscribed hypointense mass ➡ emanating from the anterior uterine body.

Variant

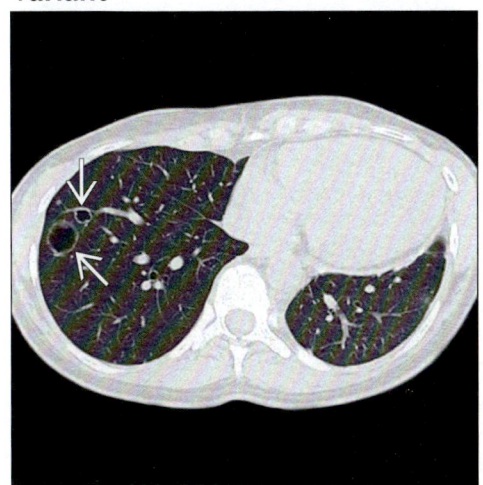
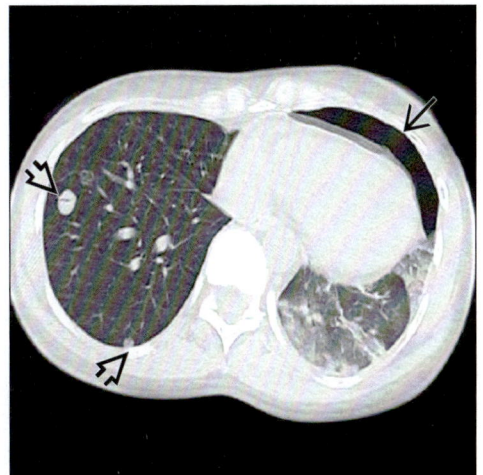

(Left) Axial CECT shows cavitary pulmonary nodules ➡. *(Right)* Axial NECT shows several pulmonary nodules, some of which are cavitary ➡. A left pneumothorax ➡ is also noted.

Typical

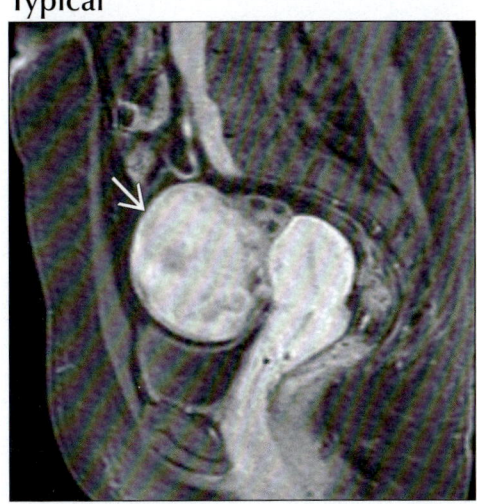
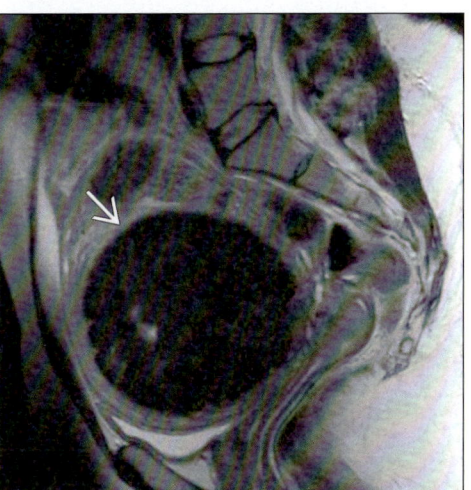

(Left) Sagittal T1 C+ FS MR shows mildly heterogeneous enhancement of the leiomyoma ➡. *(Right)* Sagittal T2WI MR shows a large well-circumscribed, homogeneous T2 hypointense leiomyoma ➡ in the anterior uterus.

DIFFUSE LEIOMYOMATOSIS, UTERUS

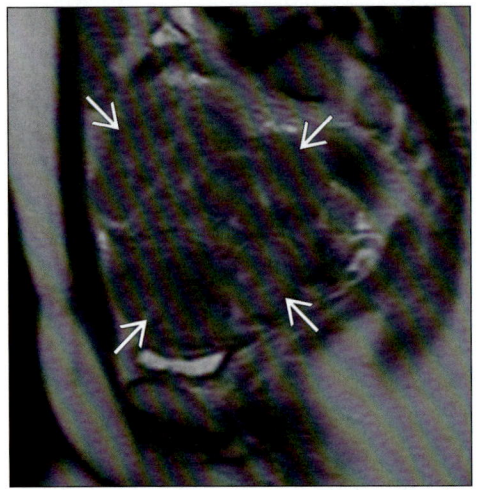

Sagittal T2WI MR shows enlargement of uterus with multiple nodules ➔ in a patient with diffuse leiomyomatosis. (Courtesy T. Kroencke, MD).

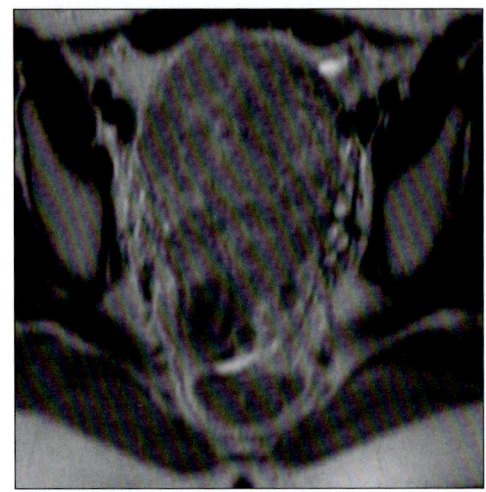

Axial T2WI MR shows ill-defined innumerable nodules with variable sizes in enlarged uterus. (Courtesy T. Kroencke, MD).

TERMINOLOGY

Abbreviations and Synonyms
- Diffuse uterine leiomyomatosis

Definitions
- Rare condition in which smooth muscle proliferation with unusual growth pattern involves uterus

IMAGING FINDINGS

General Features
- Best diagnostic clue: Innumerable ill-defined nodules with symmetric enlargement of uterus
- Location: Myometrium is diffusely involved
- Size: Smooth muscle nodules range from microscopic to 3 cm in size
- Morphology: Uterus is often diffusely enlarged and lobulated

Ultrasonographic Findings
- Grayscale Ultrasound: Multiple nodules and enlarged uterus with heterogeneous echogenicity

CT Findings
- CECT: Multiple enhancing nodules causing diffuse thickening in myometrium

MR Findings
- T1WI: Nodules are isointense to muscle
- T2WI: Nodules are ill-defined and have intermediate signal intensity
- T1 C+: Diffuse and marked enhancement of nodules

Imaging Recommendations
- Best imaging tool: MR is method of choice

DIFFERENTIAL DIAGNOSIS

Multiple Uterine Leiomyomas
- Leiomyomas are well-circumscribed unlike diffuse leiomyomatosis nodules that are ill-defined

Disseminated Peritoneal Leiomyomatosis
- Multiple smooth muscle nodules involving uterus with dissemination in peritoneal cavity

DDx: Uterine Masses

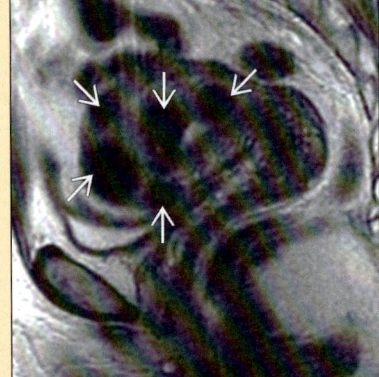

Multiple Leiomyomas

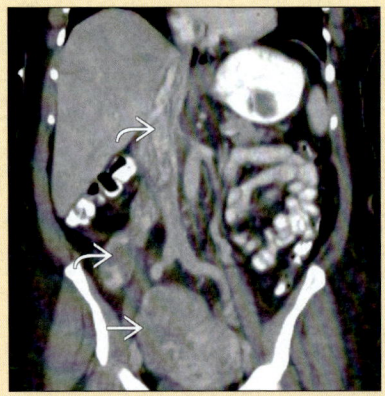

Intravenous Leiomyomatosis

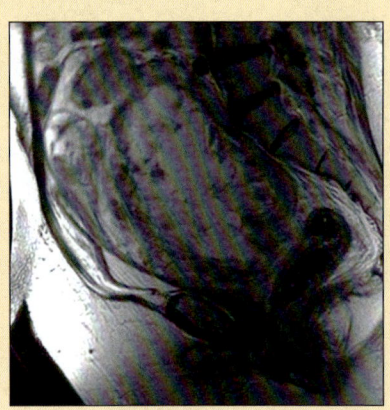

Leiomyosarcoma

DIFFUSE LEIOMYOMATOSIS, UTERUS

Key Facts

Terminology
- Rare condition in which smooth muscle proliferation with unusual growth pattern involves uterus

Imaging Findings
- Best diagnostic clue: Innumerable ill-defined nodules with symmetric enlargement of uterus
- Size: Smooth muscle nodules range from microscopic to 3 cm in size

Top Differential Diagnoses
- Multiple Uterine Leiomyomas
- Disseminated Peritoneal Leiomyomatosis
- Intravenous Leiomyomatosis
- Uterine Sarcoma

Pathology
- Nodules are composed of uniform, spindled smooth muscle cells

Intravenous Leiomyomatosis
- Enlarged uterus with masses extending into extrauterine veins
- IVC and heart may be involved

Uterine Sarcoma
- More aggressive, heterogeneous mass which may have evidence of metastasis at presentation

PATHOLOGY

Gross Pathologic & Surgical Features
- Innumerable nodules that are less circumscribed than leiomyomata

Microscopic Features
- Nodules are composed of uniform, spindled smooth muscle cells

CLINICAL ISSUES

Presentation
- Most common signs/symptoms
  - Menorrhagia and/or dysmenorrhea
  - Abdominal pain and/or pressure
  - Infertility

Demographics
- Age: Usually younger women

Natural History & Prognosis
- This is a benign condition
- Complications such as hemorrhage or uterine rupture are reported

Treatment
- Hysterectomy is treatment of choice because of diffuse nature of disease
- Alternatively uterine artery embolization may be performed to control symptoms and reduce uterine volume
- In young women who prefer to preserve uterine function and fertility, conservative treatment may be offered
  - Extensive myomectomy with sparing sufficient myometrial tissue for uterine reconstruction
  - GnRH analogues may be administered to reduce size of lesions

SELECTED REFERENCES

1. Cohen DT et al: Uterine smooth-muscle tumors with unusual growth patterns: imaging with pathologic correlation. AJR Am J Roentgenol. 188(1):246-55, 2007
2. Thomas EO et al: Diffuse uterine leiomyomatosis with uterine rupture and benign metastatic lesions of the bone. Obstet Gynecol. 109:528-30, 2007
3. Fedele L et al: Conservative treatment of diffuse uterine leiomyomatosis. Fertil Steril. 82(2):450-3, 2004
4. Kido A et al: Uterine arterial embolization for the treatment of diffuse leiomyomatosis. J Vasc Interv Radiol. 14(5):643-7, 2003

IMAGE GALLERY

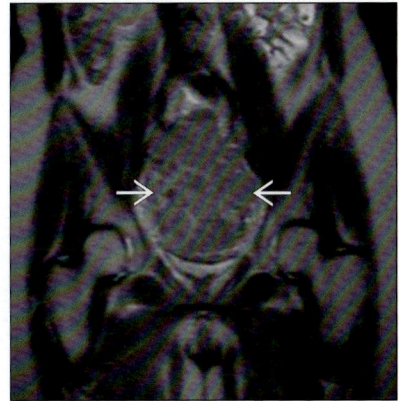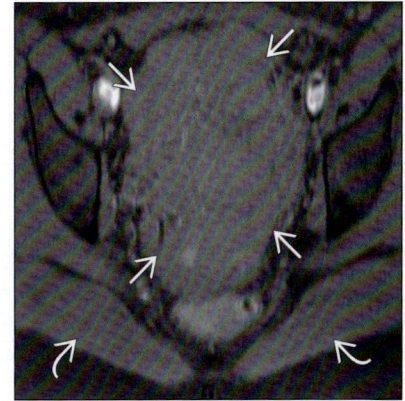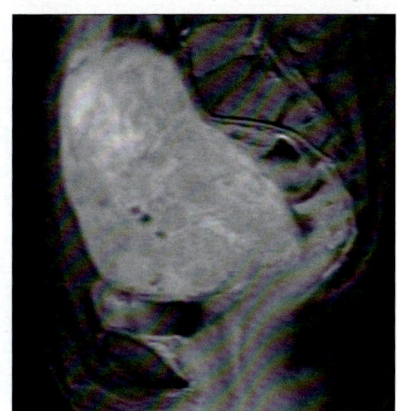

(Left) Coronal T2WI MR shows enlarged uterus with multiple nodular masses ➡. (Center) Axial T1WI FS MR shows lobulated contours of enlarged uterus with multiple nodular masses ➡ that are isointense to muscle ➡. (Right) Sagittal T1 C+ FS MR shows marked enhancement of multiple nodular masses in uterus. (Courtesy T. Kroencke, MD).

LIPOMATOUS UTERINE TUMORS

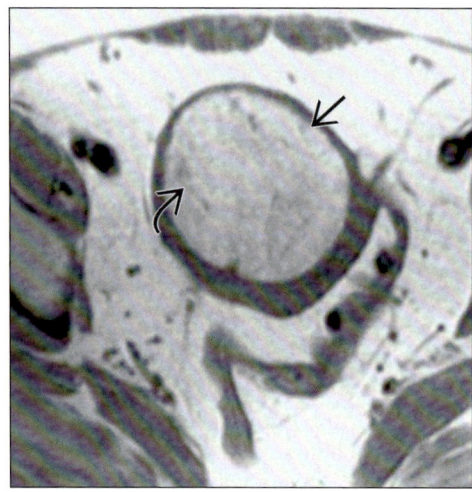

Axial T1WI MR shows an intramural hyperintense uterine mass ➔ with fine hypointense internal septations ➚.

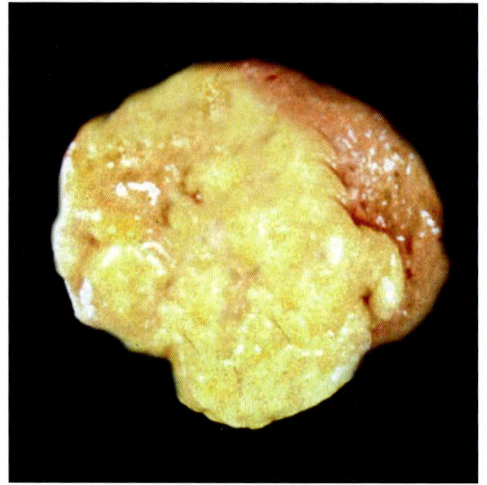

Gross pathology from the hysterectomy specimen shows a soft, well-defined yellow mass which proved to be a predominantly fatty lipoleiomyoma.

TERMINOLOGY

Abbreviations and Synonyms
- Lipomatous uterine tumors (LUT), uterine lipomatous neometaplasia, lipoleiomyoma (LLM), lipoma, fibromyolipoma (FML), angiolipoleiomyoma (ALLM)

Definitions
- Uterine tumors composed entirely, or in part, of adult-type adipose tissue, with or without intermixed smooth muscle and fibrous tissue

IMAGING FINDINGS

General Features
- Best diagnostic clue: Fat containing mass of uterine origin
- Location
  ○ Uterine corpus (90%), less commonly cervix
  ○ Intramural (60%), subserosal (35%), rarely submucosal
- Size: Variable, mean 5-10 cm
- Morphology
  ○ Spherical or ovoid mass
  ○ Well-circumscribed, encapsulated
  ○ Heterogeneous contents
  ○ Uterine origin difficult to establish for pedunculated or exophytic lesions, especially on CT or ultrasound

Radiographic Findings
- Radiography: Radiolucent pelvic mass partially surrounded by radiodense rind

Ultrasonographic Findings
- Hyperechoic well-defined mass
- Hypoechoic internal foci, septations
- Posterior attenuation
- May be partially surrounded by hypoechoic rind

CT Findings
- Fat density (range -120 to -20 HU) with variable areas of soft tissue density
- Can show calcifications

MR Findings
- T1WI
  ○ High signal intensity foci, isointense with subcutaneous fat

DDx: Lipomatous Tumors of Uterus

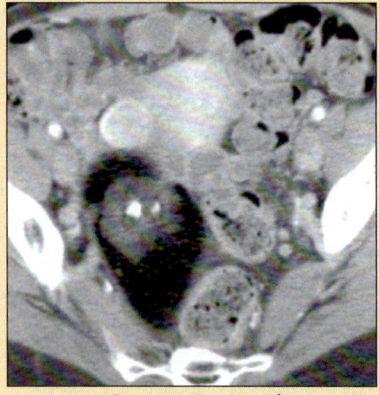

Ovarian Dermoid

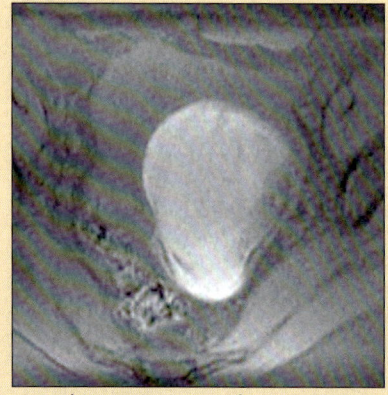

Red Degeneration of Leiomyoma

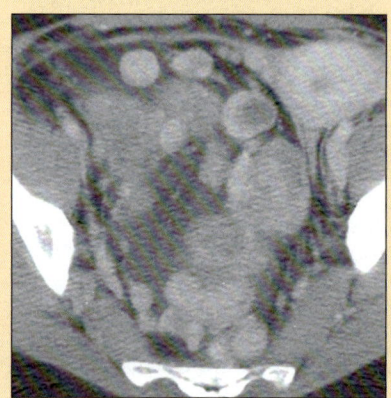

Pelvic Liposarcoma

LIPOMATOUS UTERINE TUMORS

Key Facts

Terminology
- Uterine tumors composed entirely, or in part, of adult-type adipose tissue, with or without intermixed smooth muscle and fibrous tissue

Imaging Findings
- Best diagnostic clue: Fat containing mass of uterine origin
- Uterine corpus (90%), less commonly cervix
- CT often diagnostic, especially for intramural lipomatous tumors
- MR modality of choice for diagnosis
- High sensitivity and specificity for presence of fat
- Most accurate modality to establish uterine origin in exophytic or pedunculated masses
- Protocol advice: T1WI and T1WI FS must be obtained to confirm bright signal represents fat rather than hemorrhagic or high mucin content leiomyoma

Top Differential Diagnoses
- Benign Cystic Ovarian Teratoma
- Benign Degenerated Uterine Leiomyoma
- Malignant Mixed Mesodermal Tumor (MMMT)

Pathology
- Associated abnormalities: High prevalence of concomitant uterine leiomyoma

Diagnostic Checklist
- Establish uterine origin of mass
- Presence of fat within uterus virtually diagnostic of LUT

- Areas of low signal due to presence of smooth muscle
- Chemical shift artifact on in- and opposed-phase imaging (frequency encode direction)
- T1WI FS
  - Lipomatous areas become low signal intensity (follows the signal of subcutaneous fat)
  - Hemorrhagic or mucinous cystic degenerated leiomyoma will maintain high signal intensity
- T2WI
  - Intermediate or high signal intensity, isointense to subcutaneous fat
  - Chemical shift artifact may be first clue as to lipomatous contents of mass
- T1 C+ FS
  - Smooth muscle component enhances slightly
  - Capsule demonstrates moderate vascularity
- Lipomatous component isointense with subcutaneous fat on all sequences
- Uterine origin confirmed by multiplanar capabilities

Imaging Recommendations
- Best imaging tool
  - Typically discovered as an incidental finding on ultrasound
  - CT often diagnostic, especially for intramural lipomatous tumors
  - MR modality of choice for diagnosis
    - High sensitivity and specificity for presence of fat
    - Most accurate modality to establish uterine origin in exophytic or pedunculated masses
- Protocol advice: T1WI and T1WI FS must be obtained to confirm bright signal represents fat rather than hemorrhagic or high mucin content leiomyoma

DIFFERENTIAL DIAGNOSIS

Benign Cystic Ovarian Teratoma
- Most common fat-containing pelvic mass
- Extra-uterine mass of ovarian origin
- Occurs mainly during reproductive years rather than after menopause
- At imaging contains fat, calcium, fluid and soft tissue
- Teeth, fat/fluid level and dermoid plug are diagnostic
- 1-2% malignant degeneration (prominent soft tissue component suspicious)

Benign Degenerated Uterine Leiomyoma
- Red (hemorrhagic) degeneration
  - Hyperintense signal T1WI and T1WI FS
  - Often low signal T2WI
- Increased risk for degeneration during pregnancy
- Mucinous cystic degeneration
  - Hyperintense signal T1WI and T1WI FS
  - Bright signal T2WI

Malignant Mixed Mesodermal Tumor (MMMT)
- Large broad-based uterine mass with aggressive myometrial invasion
- May show foci of signal loss on opposed-phase images due to small quantities of intravoxel fat

Non Teratomatous Lipomatous Ovarian Tumor
- Ovarian rather than uterine origin
- Extremely rare
- Ovarian lipoma or lipoleiomyoma

Sarcomatous Degeneration of Uterine Leiomyoma
- Inhomogeneous mass of myometrial origin
- Cystic degeneration and necrosis, absence of fat
- Hemorrhagic and hyaline degeneration, remain bright on T1WI FS
- No definite imaging criteria allowing differentiation of degenerated benign leiomyoma from leiomyosarcoma

Benign Pelvic Lipoma
- Extraperitoneal
- Well-circumscribed
- Homogeneous fat containing mass
- Distinct from uterus

LIPOMATOUS UTERINE TUMORS

Pelvic Liposarcoma
- Usually extraperitoneal rather than intraperitoneal
- Heterogeneous soft tissue mass
- Variable amounts of fat

PATHOLOGY

General Features
- Etiology
  - Various theories suggested
    - Originates from misplaced embryonal mesodermal rests with potential for lipoblastic differentiation
    - Pericapillary pluripotential mesenchymal cells
    - Lipoblasts migrating along uterine arteries and nerves
    - Metaplasia of stromal or smooth muscle cells in pre-existing leiomyoma
- Epidemiology: 0.03-0.2% of hysterectomy specimen
- Associated abnormalities: High prevalence of concomitant uterine leiomyoma

Gross Pathologic & Surgical Features
- Well-circumscribed, usually encapsulated
- Consistency varies with proportion of different components
  - Soft, pale yellow mass in rare cases of pure lipomas
  - Firm grey-white mass, with soft yellow areas (LLM)
  - Vascular patches, especially at periphery (ALLM)

Microscopic Features
- Lipomatous and smooth muscle cell neoplasia in all tumors (except pure lipoma)
- Usually leiomyomatous component more abundant than adipose tissue
- FML: Hyalinized fibrous stroma
- ALLM: Marked proliferation of abnormal blood vessels

CLINICAL ISSUES

Presentation
- Most common signs/symptoms
  - Usually asymptomatic
  - If symptomatic, symptoms parallel uterine leiomyomas
    - Chronic pelvic discomfort
    - Heaviness
    - Pressure
    - Uterine bleeding

Demographics
- Age
  - Most occur in postmenopausal women
  - 90% older than 40 years old

Natural History & Prognosis
- Almost invariably benign
- Rare case reports of intravascular lipoleiomyomatosis
- One case report of leiomyosarcoma arising from uterine lipoleiomyoma

Treatment
- None if asymptomatic
- Hysterectomy in selected symptomatic patients

DIAGNOSTIC CHECKLIST

Consider
- MR most accurate modality to confirm uterine origin
- MR most sensitive and specific modality to confirm presence of fat

Image Interpretation Pearls
- Establish uterine origin of mass
- Presence of fat within uterus virtually diagnostic of LUT

SELECTED REFERENCES

1. Avritscher R et al: Lipoleiomyoma of the uterus. AJR Am J Roentgenol. 177(4):856, 2001
2. Prieto A et al: Uterine lipoleiomyomas: US and CT findings. Abdom Imaging. 25(6):655-7, 2000
3. Murase E et al: Uterine leiomyomas: histopathologic features, MR imaging findings, differential diagnosis, and treatment. Radiographics. 19(5):1179-97, 1999
4. Ishigami K et al: Uterine lipoleiomyoma: MRI appearances. Abdom Imaging. 23(2):214-6, 1998
5. Semelka et al: MRI of the abdomen and pelvis. 1st ed. New York, Wiley-Liss, Inc., John Wiley & Sons. 613, 1997
6. Tsushima Y et al: Uterine lipoleiomyoma: MRI, CT and ultrasonographic findings. Br J Radiol. 70(838):1068-70, 1997
7. Hashiguchi J et al: Intravascular leiomyomatosis with uterine lipoleiomyoma. Gynecol Oncol. 52(1):94-8, 1994
8. Aizenstein R et al: CT and MRI of uterine lipoleiomyoma. Gynecol Oncol. 40(3):274-6, 1991
9. Dodd GD 3rd et al: Lipomatous tumors of the pelvis in women: spectrum of imaging findings. AJR Am J Roentgenol. 155(2):317-22, 1990
10. Dodd GD 3rd et al: Lipomatous uterine tumors: diagnosis by ultrasound, CT, and MR. J Comput Assist Tomogr. 14(4):629-32, 1990
11. Sieinski W: Lipomatous neometaplasia of the uterus. Report of 11 cases with discussion of histogenesis and pathogenesis. Int J Gynecol Pathol. 8(4):357-63, 1989
12. Jacobs JE et al: CT diagnosis of uterine lipoma. AJR Am J Roentgenol. 150(6):1335-6, 1988
13. Oppenheimer DA et al: Lipoleiomyoma of the uterus. J Comput Assist Tomogr. 6(3):640-2, 1982
14. Pounder DJ: Fatty tumours of the uterus. J Clin Pathol. 35(12):1380-3, 1982
15. Houser LM et al: Lipomatous tumour of the uterus: radiographic and ultrasonic appearance. Br J Radiol. 52(624):992-3, 1979
16. Brandfass RT et al: Lipomatous tumors of the uterus; a review of the world's literature with report of a case of true lipoma. Am J Obstet Gynecol. 70(2):359-67, 1955

LIPOMATOUS UTERINE TUMORS

IMAGE GALLERY

Typical

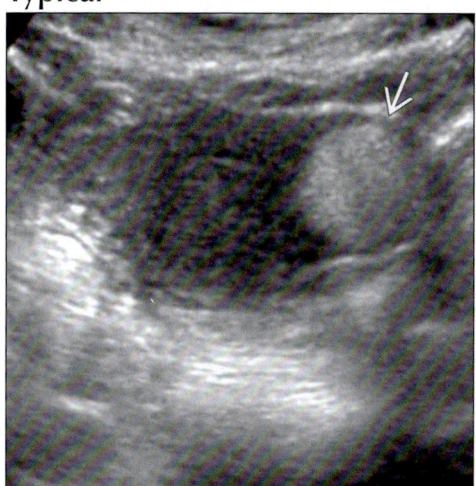
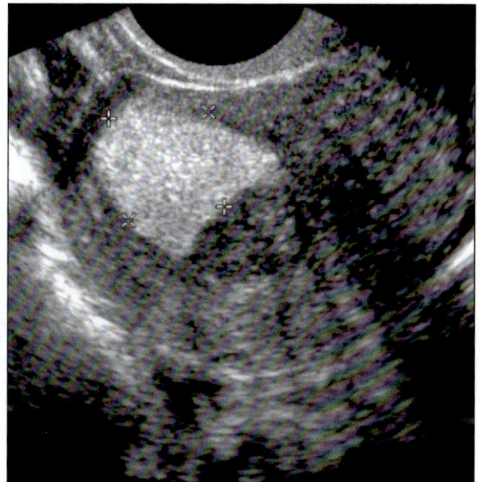

(Left) Axial transabdominal ultrasound shows an echogenic lesion with subtle attenuation in the left uterus ➔ consistent with a lipomatous lesion. *(Right)* Sagittal oblique transvaginal ultrasound in the same patient as previous image shows a well-defined echogenic lesion (calipers) in the myometrium.

Variant

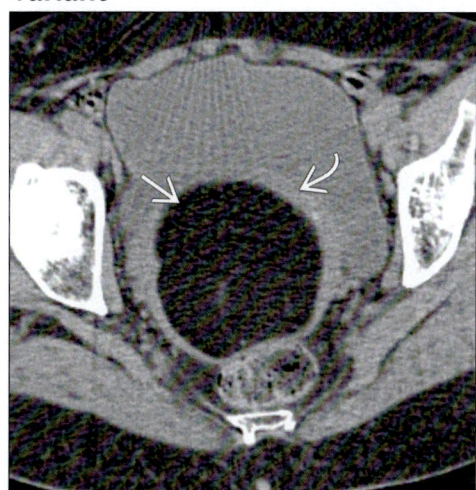
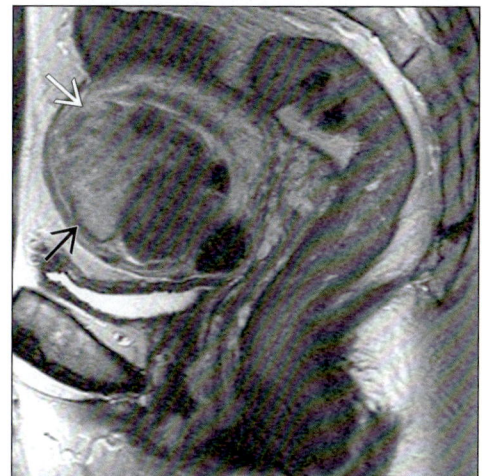

(Left) Axial NECT shows a lipoma ➔ of uterine origin isodense with subcutaneous fat. The uterine origin is confirmed by a surrounding rind of myometrium ➔. *(Right)* Sagittal T2WI MR shows a chemical shift artifact ➔ in the frequency encode direction at the edge of a hyperintense uterine lipoadenofibroma ➔. (Courtesy Ref. 5).

Typical

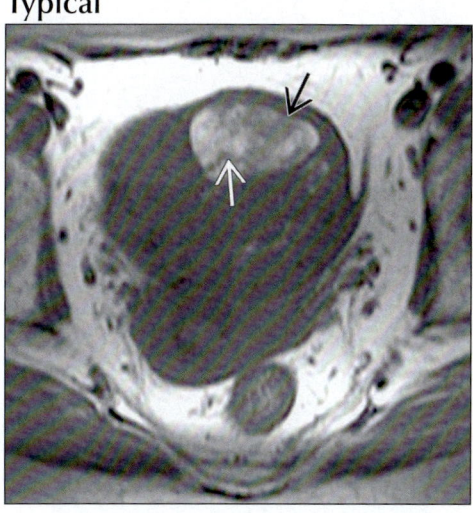
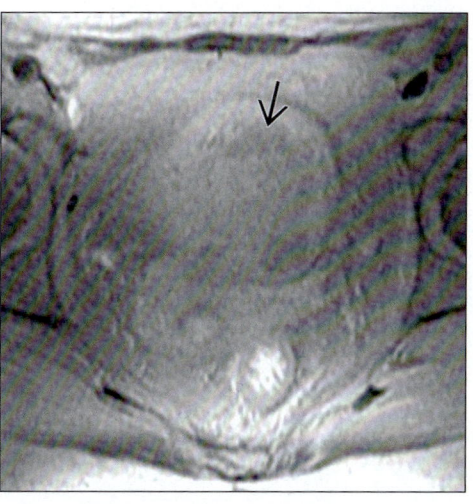

(Left) Axial T1WI MR in the same patient as previous image shows a hyperintense intramural uterine mass ➔ with internal intermediate signal intensity strands ➔. (Courtesy Ref. 5). *(Right)* Axial T1WI FS MR in the same patient as previous image shows signal loss of the uterine mass ➔ confirming its adipose contents. It proved to be a uterine lipoadenofibroma. (Courtesy Ref. 5).

ENDOMETRIAL POLYPS

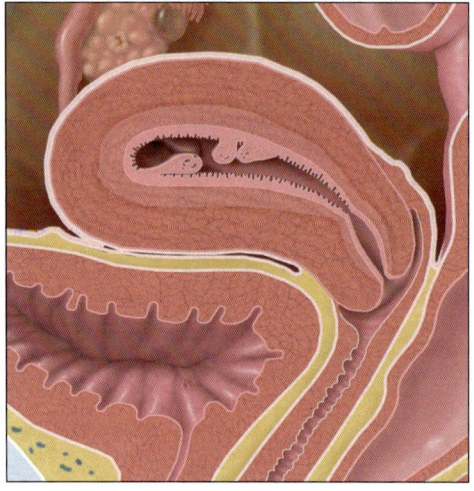

Sagittal graphic shows the presence of three endometrial polyps.

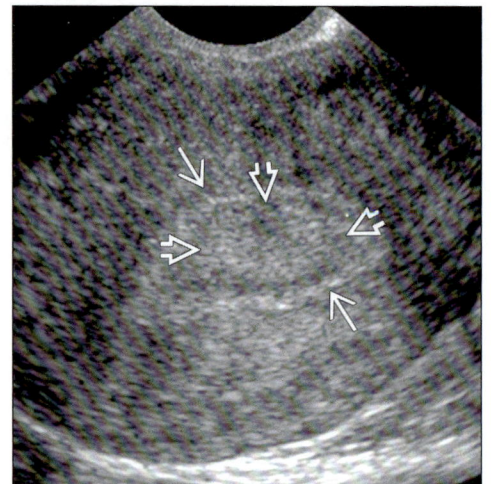

Axial transvaginal ultrasound shows an endometrial polyp ➡ surrounded by a complete endometrial stripe ➡ in a premenopausal woman.

TERMINOLOGY

Definitions
- Polypoid focal endometrial hyperplasia

IMAGING FINDINGS

General Features
- Best diagnostic clue
  - Intraluminal pedunculated endometrial mass on TVS
  - Visualization of a separate, completely intact endometrial stripe on TVS
  - Hypointense fibrous core or stalk on T2WI
  - Hypervascular endometrial mass on early dynamic enhanced scan
- Location: Most common origin cornual and fundus, rarely prolapsing through exo-cervix
- Size: 1 mm to a few cms
- Morphology: Broad-based to pedunculated

Ultrasonographic Findings
- Grayscale Ultrasound
  - Partially or completely intact separate endometrial stripe (82%) specificity on TVS
  - ± Cysts representing dilated glands on TVS
  - Nonspecific focal endometrial thickening/mass on TVS
  - Predominantly echogenic
  - Intact overlying endometrium or hypoechoic subendometrial halo on TVS
- Pulsed Doppler: Low to high resistance
- Color Doppler: Single stalk flow unless there are multiple polyps
- Power Doppler: Single stalk flow unless there are multiple polyps

CT Findings
- NECT: Central uterine mass isodense to the uterus
- CECT: Enhancing central uterine mass in the portal phase CT

MR Findings
- T1WI: Isointense to endometrium, may contain hypointense components
- T2WI

DDx: Focal Endometrial Mass

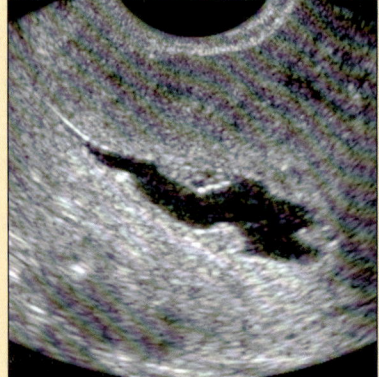

Focal Hyperplasia

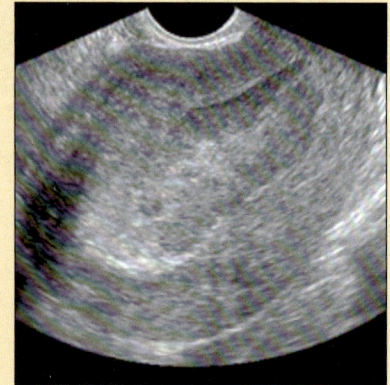

Cancer

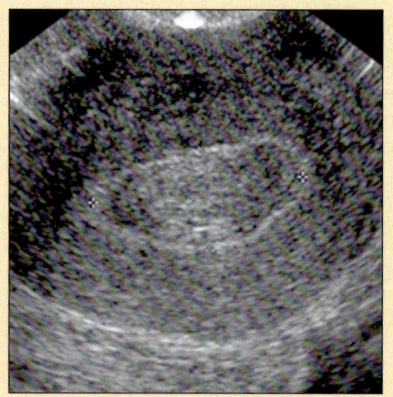

Hematometra

ENDOMETRIAL POLYPS

Key Facts

Terminology
- Polypoid focal endometrial hyperplasia

Imaging Findings
- Intraluminal pedunculated endometrial mass on TVS
- Visualization of a separate, completely intact endometrial stripe on TVS
- Ranges from mildly hypointense to isointense relative to normal endometrium, cystic changes, hypointense central fibrous core
- Homogeneous or heterogeneous enhancement, small polyps stand out best against hypointense endometrium on early arterial phase
- Color Doppler: Single stalk flow unless there are multiple polyps
- Pedicle often originating from one cornual

Top Differential Diagnoses
- Focal Hyperplasia
- Submucosal Leiomyoma
- Endometrial Carcinoma
- Hematometra

Pathology
- Etiology: More common in patients receiving tamoxifen or on hormone replacement

Clinical Issues
- Small polyps may slough with menstruation

Diagnostic Checklist
- SHG if endometrium is suboptimally seen or central endometrial interface not seen in its entirety

---

  - Ranges from mildly hypointense to isointense relative to normal endometrium, cystic changes, hypointense central fibrous core
  - May see hypointense stalk in a pedunculated polyp
- T1 C+ FS
  - Homogeneous or heterogeneous enhancement, small polyps stand out best against hypointense endometrium on early arterial phase
  - Later phase may show focal endometrial thickening
- MR features may be nonspecific

Other Modality Findings
- Sonohysterography (SHG)
  - Sessile or pedunculated endometrial mass and intact overlying endometrium
  - Pedicle often originating from one cornual

Imaging Recommendations
- Best imaging tool
  - TVS: Modality of choice with 56-96% sensitivity and 82% specificity
  - SHG: Consider using when TVS is suboptimal or shows nonspecific thickening of endometrium
  - MR: May increase probability of polyp diagnosis in cases when biopsy not possible
- Protocol advice
  - SHG: Optimal distension of the uterine cavity with normal saline is mandatory
  - MR: T1 C+ FS improves sensitivity

DIFFERENTIAL DIAGNOSIS

Focal Hyperplasia
- Lack of overlying endometrium on biopsy
- Cannot be differentiated from small broad-based polyp on imaging

Submucosal Leiomyoma
- Hypoechoic
- ± Attenuation
- Endometrium stretched overlying the intracavitary mass
- Intact overlying endometrium and continuity with myometrium

Endometrial Carcinoma
- Poor definition of the adjacent endometrium/myometrium
- Multiple vascular supplies
- Early dynamic T1 C+ FS: Hypovascular

Hematometra
- Complete endometrial stripe surrounding the clot
- No vascularity

PATHOLOGY

General Features
- General path comments
  - 20% multiple
  - Focal glandular and stromal hyperplasia covered by endometrium
  - Three types
    - Hyperplastic: Resembles glands in endometrial hyperplasia
    - Atrophic: Occur in postmenopausal women; composed of atrophic cystically dilated glands
    - Functional: Rare, follow cyclic endometrial changes
  - Adenomyomatous polyp: Variant with glandular and muscle elements
- Genetics: No known genetic predisposition
- Etiology: More common in patients receiving tamoxifen or on hormone replacement
- Epidemiology: 10% of autopsies, most asymptomatic
- Associated abnormalities: Endometrial changes such as hyperplasia, atrophy or carcinoma when associated with Tamoxifen use

Gross Pathologic & Surgical Features
- Smooth surfaced sessile or pedunculated with thick or slender stalk

ENDOMETRIAL POLYPS

Microscopic Features
- Focal overgrowth of endometrial glands and stroma with intact overlying endometrium on three sides

CLINICAL ISSUES

Presentation
- Most common signs/symptoms: Postmenopausal bleeding
- Other signs/symptoms
  - Menorrhagia or menometrorrhagia
  - Intermenstrual bleeding
  - Mucous discharge
  - Infertility
- Clinical Profile
  - Often incidental finding on TVS
  - Frequently missed on Pipelle biopsy or D&C
  - Hysteroscopy most accurate diagnostic tool

Demographics
- Age: Both pre and postmenopausal

Natural History & Prognosis
- No indication of transformation to endometrial cancer
- Slow growth
- 0.5% malignant
- 15-35% of patients with endometrial cancer have associated polyp(s)
- Develop more cystic changes and become less vascular postmenopause
- Small polyps may slough with menstruation

Treatment
- Polypectomy, if benign
- Hysterectomy, if atypical hyperplasia or carcinoma in polyp
- Observation in older asymptomatic patients

DIAGNOSTIC CHECKLIST

Consider
- SHG if endometrium is suboptimally seen or central endometrial interface not seen in its entirety

Image Interpretation Pearls
- Focal endometrial thickening with a separate endometrial stripe
- Single vascular pedicle

SELECTED REFERENCES

1. Takeuchi M et al: Pathologies of the uterine endometrial cavity: usual and unusual manifestations and pitfalls on magnetic resonance imaging. Eur Radiol. 15(11):2244-55, 2005
2. Grasel RP et al: Endometrial polyps: MR imaging features and distinction from endometrial carcinoma. Radiology. 214(1):47-52, 2004
3. Chaudhry S et al: Benign and malignant diseases of the endometrium. Top Magn Reson Imaging. 14(4):339-57, 2003
4. Goldstein SR et al: Evaluation of endometrial polyps. Am J Obstet Gynecol. 186(4):669-74, 2002
5. Jorizzo JR et al: Endometrial polyps: sonohysterographic evaluation. AJR Am J Roentgenol. 176(3):617-21, 2001
6. Caspi B et al: The bright edge of the endometrial polyp. Ultrasound Obstet Gynecol. 15:327-30, 2000
7. Dijkhuizen FP et al: Comparison of transvaginal ultrasonography and saline infusion sonography for the detection of intracavitary abnormalities in premenopausal women. Ultrasound Obstet Gynecol. 15(5):372-6, 2000
8. Grasel RP et al: Endometrial polyps: MR imaging features and distinction from endometrial carcinoma. Radiology. 214:47-52, 2000
9. Strauss HG et al: Significance of endovaginal ultrasonography in assessing tamoxifen-associated changes of the endometrium. A prospective study. Acta Obstet Gynecol Scand. 79(8):697-701, 2000
10. Baldwin MT et al: Focal intracavitary masses recognized with the hyperechoic line sign at endovaginal US and characterized with hysterosonography. Radiographics. 19(4):927-35, 1999
11. Farrell T et al: The significance of an 'insufficient' Pipelle sample in the investigation of post-menopausal bleeding. Acta Obstet Gynecol Scand. 78(9):810-2, 1999
12. La Torre R et al: Transvaginal sonographic evaluation of endometrial polyps: a comparison with two dimensional and three dimensional contrast sonography. Clin Exp Obstet Gynecol. 26(3-4):171-3, 1999
13. Laifer-Narin SL et al: Transvaginal saline hysterosonography: characteristics distinguishing malignant and various benign conditions. AJR Am J Roentgenol. 172(6):1513-20, 1999
14. Senoh D et al: Clinical application of intrauterine sonography with high-frequency, real-time miniature transducer in gynecologic disorders. Preliminary report. Gynecol Obstet Invest. 47(2):108-13, 1999
15. Smith-Bindman R et al: Endovaginal ultrasound to exclude endometrial cancer and other endometrial abnormalities. JAMA. 280(17):1510-7, 1998
16. Atri M et al: Transvaginal ultrasound appearance of endometrial abnormalities. Radiographics. 14:483-92, 1994
17. Grasel RP et al: Endometrial polyps: MR imaging features and distinction from endometrial carcinoma. 214(1):47-52, Radiology.

ENDOMETRIAL POLYPS

IMAGE GALLERY

Typical

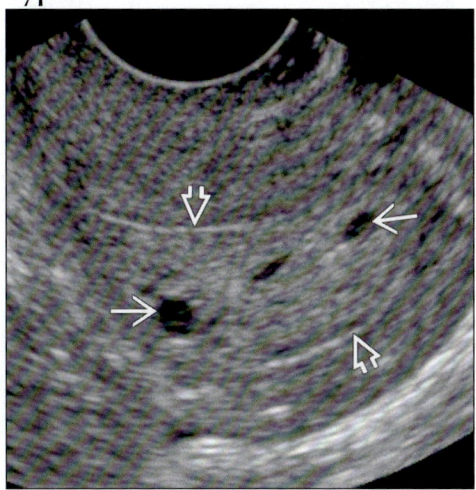 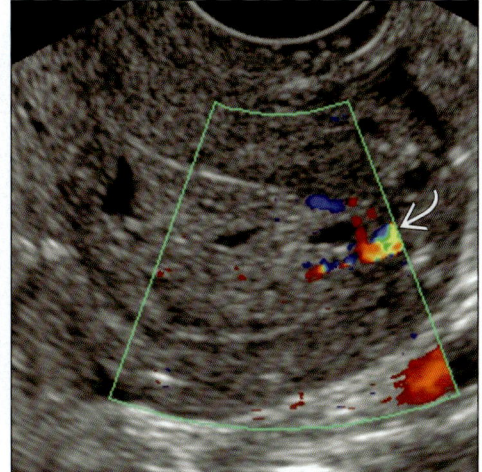

(Left) Sagittal transvaginal ultrasound shows a predominantly solid polyp with cystic spaces ➡ surrounded by an incomplete thin atrophic endometrial stripe ➡ in a postmenopausal woman. *(Right)* Axial color Doppler ultrasound of the image to the left shows a single vascular pedicle ➡ originating from the left cornual.

Typical

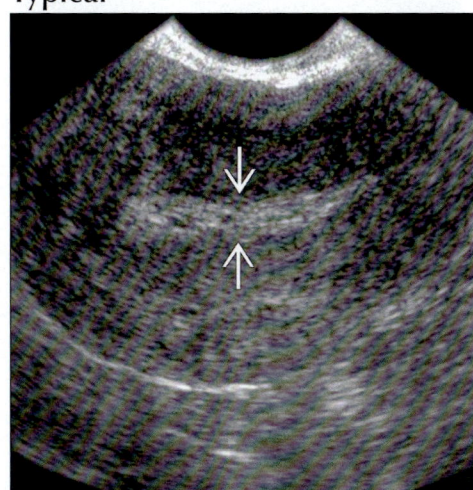 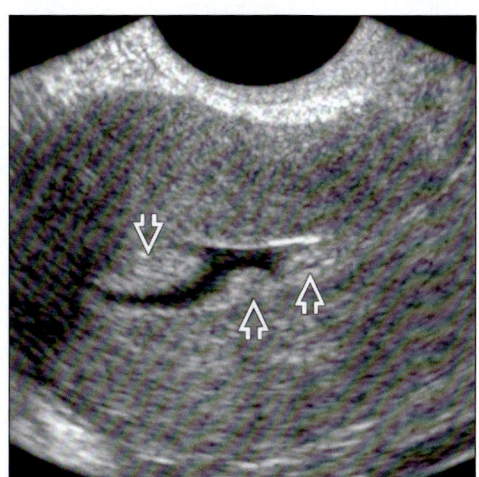

(Left) Sagittal transvaginal ultrasound shows an endometrial thickness of 5 mm ➡ without focal abnormality. *(Right)* Sagittal sonohysterogram in the same patient as previous image demonstrates three endometrial polyps ➡.

Typical

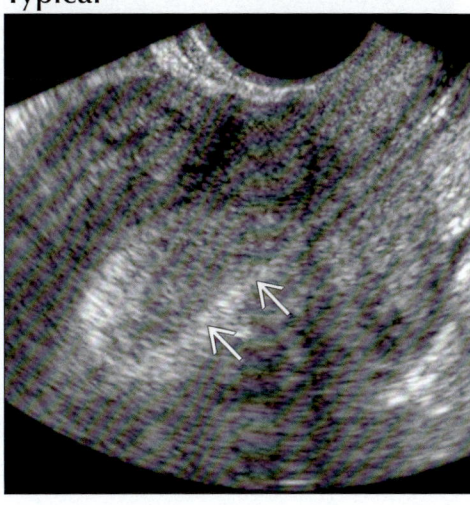 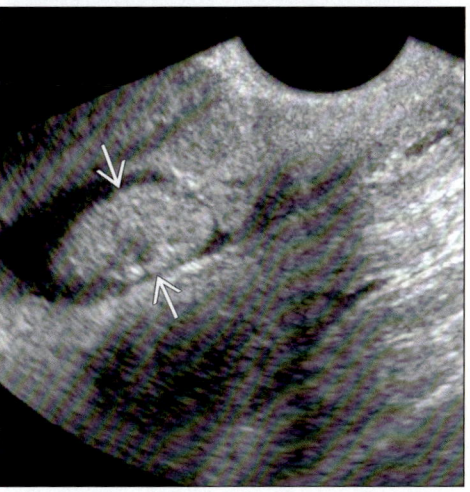

(Left) Sagittal transvaginal ultrasound shows a complete endometrial stripe ➡ surrounding focal endometrial thickening. *(Right)* Sagittal sonohysterogram in the same patient as previous image demonstrates the presence of an endometrial polyp ➡.

ENDOMETRIAL POLYPS

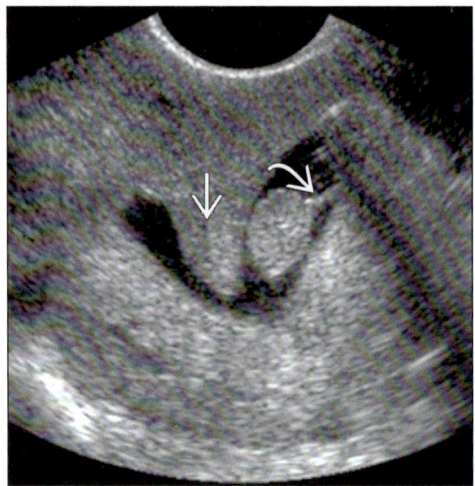
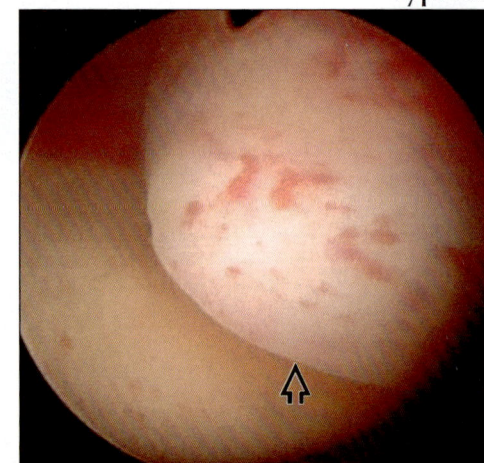

(Left) Axial sonohysterogram shows one pedunculated ➡ and one broad-based ➡ polyp. (Right) Hysteroscopic photograph shows the endometrial polyp ➡ with multiple hemorrhagic foci on the surface.

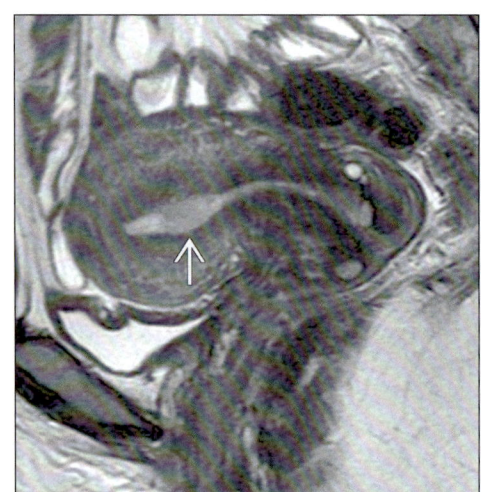
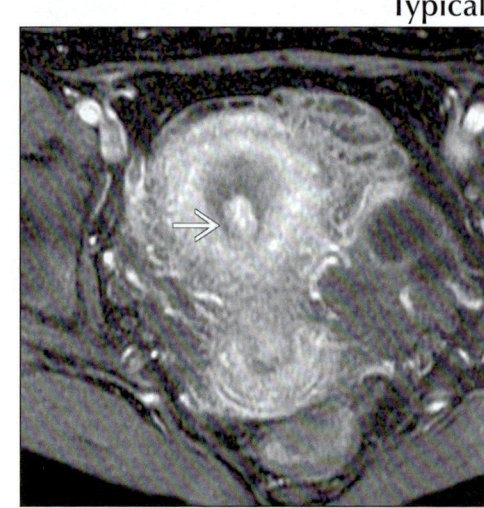

(Left) Sagittal T2WI MR shows focal endometrial thickening ➡ with a slightly decreased signal intensity relative to the normal endometrium. (Right) Axial T1 C+ FS MR in the same patient as previous image shows early enhancement ➡ of the focal mass relative to the surrounding endometrium. These findings are typical of an endometrial polyp.

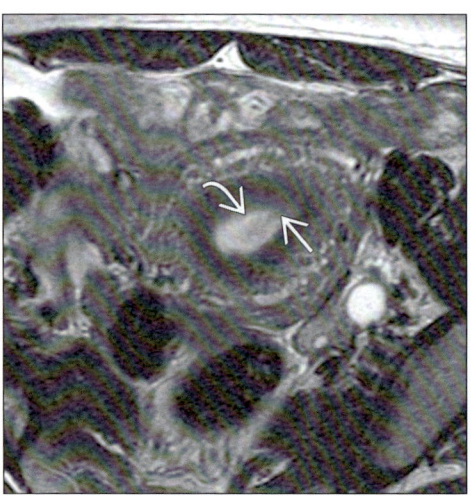
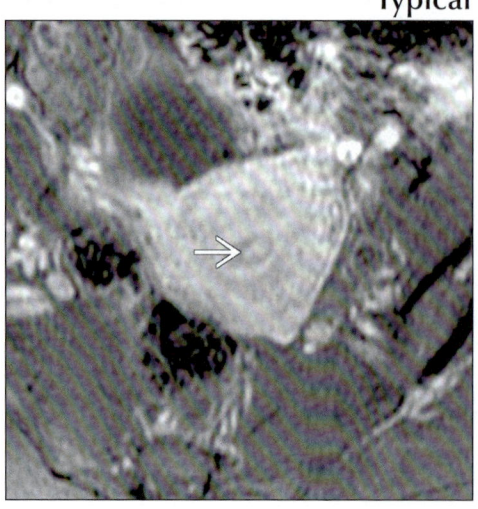

(Left) Axial T2WI MR shows a slightly hypointense mass within the endometrial cavity. Note a faint hyperintense rim ➡. A hypointense stalk ➡ is seen arising from the left cornual. (Right) Axial T1 C+ FS MR in the same patient as previous image shows early enhancement ➡ of the focal mass relative to the surrounding endometrium.

ENDOMETRIAL POLYPS

Typical

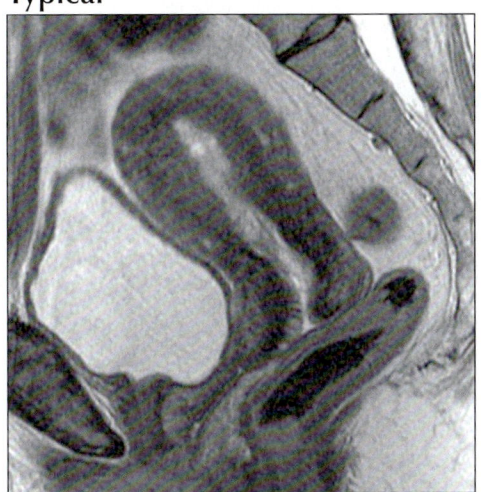
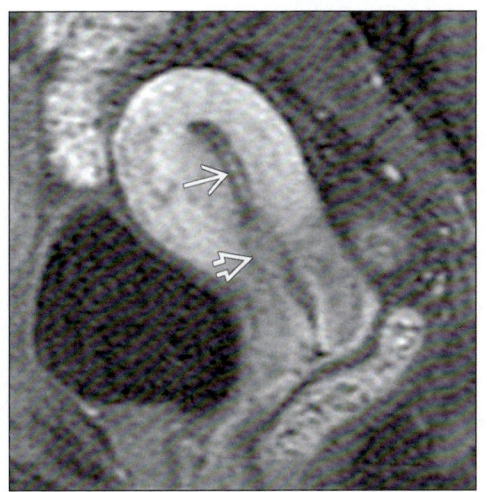

(Left) Sagittal T2WI MR shows nonspecific thickening of the endometrial complex which is of slightly decreased signal intensity and heterogeneous. (Right) Sagittal T1 C+ FS MR shows a pedunculated endometrial polyp ➡ in the lower uterine segment and upper cervix with a long vascular stalk ➡ arising from the fundus.

Typical

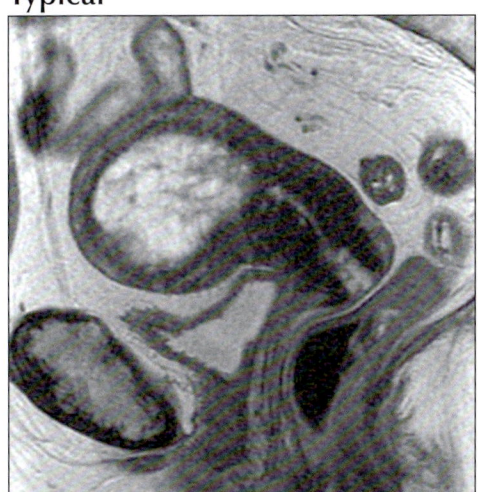
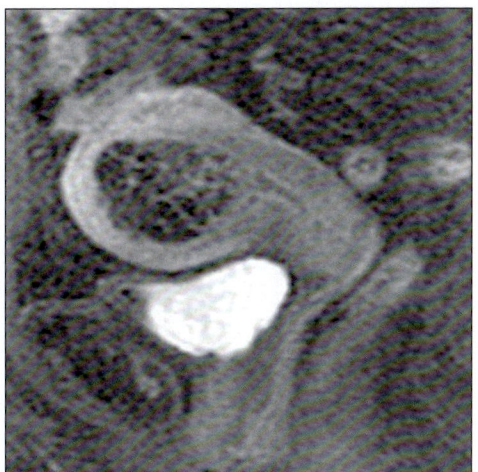

(Left) Sagittal T2WI MR in a patient receiving Tamoxifen shows a large heterogeneous, predominately hyperintense endometrial mass with hypointense linear bands. Proven benign endometrial polyp. (Right) Sagittal T1 C+ FS MR in the same patient as left shows a "lattice-like" pattern of enhancement of the endometrial polyp.

Typical

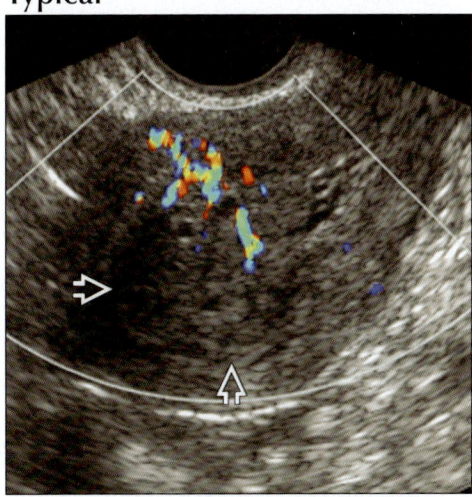
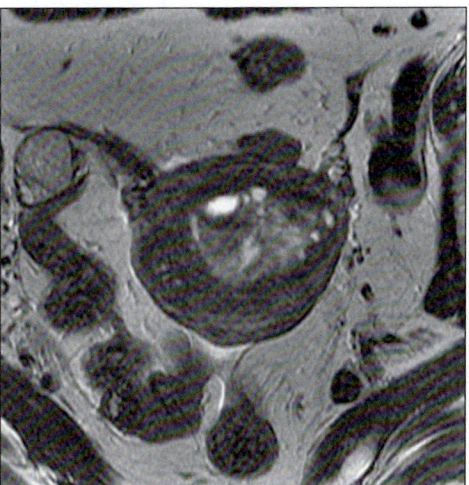

(Left) Sagittal color Doppler ultrasound in a patient receiving tamoxifen shows an iso- to slightly hyperechoic endometrial-based mass ➡ with multiple feeding vessels entering the mass ventrally. (Right) Axial T2WI MR in the same patient as left shows a heterogeneous mass with cystic areas proven to be a benign endometrial polyp.

ENDOMETRIAL HYPERPLASIA

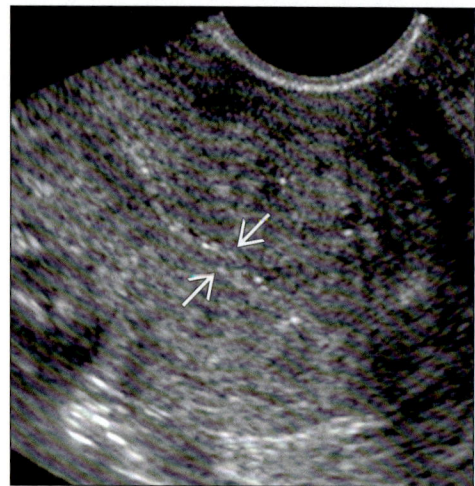

Sagittal transvaginal ultrasound shows a 4 mm thick endometrium ➡ in a postmenopausal woman with vaginal bleeding.

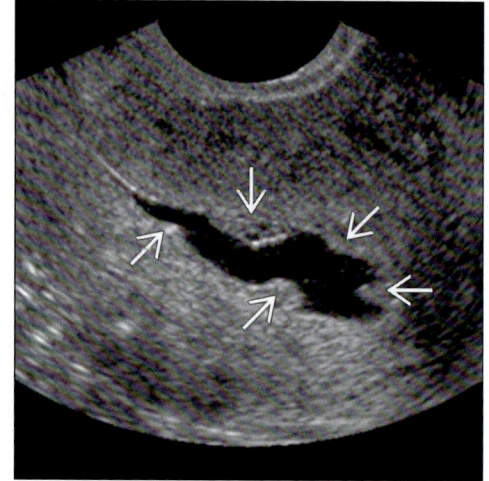

Sagittal sonohysterogram (SHG) in the same patient as previous image shows multiple focal endometrial thickenings ➡ consistent with focal hyperplasia.

TERMINOLOGY

Abbreviations and Synonyms
- Endometrial hyperplasia with or without atypia

Definitions
- Excessive proliferation of endometrial glands with an increased ratio of glands to stroma

IMAGING FINDINGS

General Features
- Best diagnostic clue
  - Postmenopausal women presenting with bleeding ± hormonal replacement therapy (HRT), and endometrial thickness (ET) > 5 mm on transvaginal ultrasound (TVS)
    - Sensitivity/specificity for detecting cancer 96/61%
    - Sensitivity/specificity for detecting pathology 92/81%
  - Postmenopausal women on HRT without bleeding, limited data on TVS
    - Unopposed estrogen: ET > 8 mm is abnormal
    - Sequential estrogen/progesterone: Image just after withdrawal bleeding or in the progesterone phase, ET > 5 mm is abnormal
    - Continuous combined estrogen/progesterone: ET > 5 mm is abnormal
  - Premenopausal women: No reliable threshold value, limited data on TVS in the literature suggests
    - ET > 8 mm during proliferative phase is abnormal
    - ET > 16 mm during secretory phase is abnormal
  - Extrapolate criteria for ET from the TVS literature to MR, paucity of MR data
- Location: Endometrium
- Thickening may be focal or nodular
- Cystic changes may be present
- Endometrial borders remain well-defined

Ultrasonographic Findings
- Grayscale Ultrasound
  - Diffusely thickened, homogeneously echogenic endometrium
  - Focal endometrial thickening
  - Cystic changes present as small anechoic foci
  - Uncommonly hypoechoic/heterogeneous areas may be present with atypical hyperplasia

DDx: Nodular Endometrial Thickening

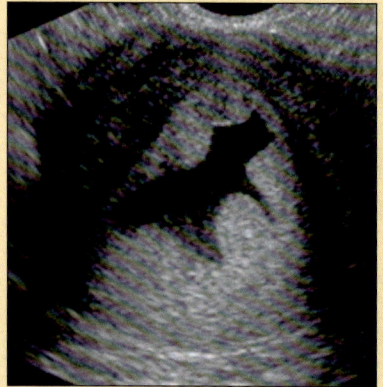

Secretary Phase (SHG)

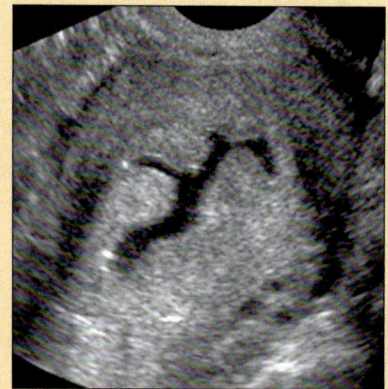

Multiple Polyps (SHG)

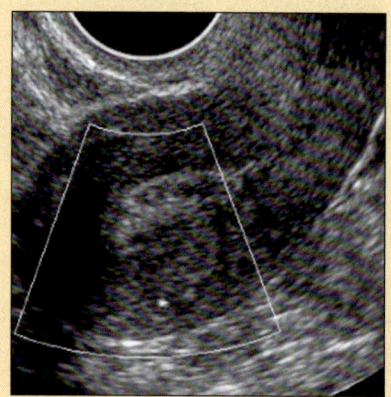

Endometrial Cancer

ENDOMETRIAL HYPERPLASIA

Key Facts

Terminology
- Excessive proliferation of endometrial glands with an increased ratio of glands to stroma

Imaging Findings
- Postmenopausal women presenting with bleeding ± hormonal replacement therapy (HRT), and endometrial thickness (ET) > 5 mm on transvaginal ultrasound (TVS)
- Thickening may be focal or nodular
- Cystic changes may be present
- Isointense or slightly hypointense relative to normal endometrium on T2WI
- Early C+: Hypointense relative to myometrium
- Delayed C+: Iso or hyperintense relative to myometrium
- Diffusely thickened, homogeneously echogenic endometrium
- Multiple feeding vessels, sparse vascularity on color Doppler

Top Differential Diagnoses
- Secretory Endometrium
- Endometrial Carcinoma
- Endometrial Polyp
- Endometritis

Diagnostic Checklist
- SHG if the central interface is not seen in its entirety on TVS, and therefore the two layers of endometrium are not seen distinctly
- Look for focal endometrial thickening on TVS or SHG to triage patient for targeted biopsy

---

- Sonohysterography (SHG)
  - Similar findings to TVS
  - Differentiates diffuse from focal endometrial thickening
  - Helps triage patients to office Pipelle vs. hysteroscopically-guided biopsy
- Pulsed Doppler
  - Wide range of resistive index from high to low
- Color Doppler
  - No definite criteria to reliably differentiate hyperplasia from carcinoma
  - Multiple feeding vessels, sparse vascularity on color Doppler
- Power Doppler
  - No definite criteria to reliably differentiate hyperplasia from carcinoma
  - Multiple feeding vessels, sparse vascularity

MR Findings
- T1WI: Isointense to myometrium on T1WI
- T2WI
  - Isointense or slightly hypointense relative to normal endometrium on T2WI
  - Cystic changes present as small hyperintense foci on T2WI
- T1 C+ FS
  - Early C+: Hypointense relative to myometrium
  - Delayed C+: Iso or hyperintense relative to myometrium
    - Cystic changes present as small hypointense foci on contrast-enhanced images

Imaging Recommendations
- Best imaging tool: TVS along with SHG (if individual layers are not seen on TVS) are best screening tools
- Protocol advice
  - Measure ET where the outer contours of the two layers of endometrium parallel each other
  - Subtract fluid within endometrial cavity for measuring ET
  - Focal fundal endometrial thickening when endometrium is thin in the lower uterine segment may be a normal variant

DIFFERENTIAL DIAGNOSIS

Secretory Endometrium
- Imaging findings completely overlap with findings of hyperplasia

Endometrial Carcinoma
- May coexist with endometrial hyperplasia
- Imaging findings can completely overlap with those of hyperplasia in 30% of cases
- Irregular endometrial thickening ± mass
- Ill-defined borders with myometrium
- TVS: Heterogeneous with areas of decreased echogenicity (60%)
- MR
  - T2WI: Hypointense relative to normal endometrium
  - T1 C+ FS: Hypointense relative to myometrium

Endometrial Polyp
- May coexist with endometrial hyperplasia
- Sessile polyps may mimic appearance of focal endometrial hyperplasia
- Separate endometrial lining (endometrial stripe sign)
- Color Doppler: Single feeding vessel in a pedunculated polyp
- SHG: Highest accuracy for differentiating hyperplasia from a large endometrial polyp filling endometrial cavity
- Fibrous stalk on MR

Endometritis
- Diffuse hypervascular endometrial thickening
- Uterine cavity fluid
- Adnexal changes of pelvic inflammatory disease
- Clinical presentation and endometrial sampling help differentiation

PATHOLOGY

General Features
- General path comments

ENDOMETRIAL HYPERPLASIA

- Accounts for 4-8% of cases of postmenopausal bleeding
- In postmenopausal women most often due to unopposed estrogen stimulation
- Excessive proliferation of endometrial glands and increased ratio of glands to stroma ± cystic dilatation of glands
- Broadly classified into two categories: Endometrial hyperplasia without cellular atypia; endometrial hyperplasia with cellular atypia or atypical hyperplasia
    - Endometrial hyperplasia without cellular atypia: Risk of endometrial carcinoma small < 2%; trial of progesterone therapy with follow-up transvaginal sonography (TVS) ± endometrial biopsy
    - Endometrial hyperplasia with cellular atypia or atypical hyperplasia: 25% harbor co-existing foci of endometrial carcinoma or will develop endometrial carcinoma in future; treated with hysterectomy
- Etiology
    - Estrogen excess despite relative progesterone deficiency
        - Chronic anovulatory states
        - Unopposed exogenous estrogen use
        - Tamoxifen
        - Obesity
        - Estrogen-secreting ovarian tumors
- Epidemiology
    - Risk factors for endometrial hyperplasia are similar to endometrial cancer and include unopposed estrogen and obesity
    - Long-term use of oral contraceptives decreases risk
- Associated abnormalities: Endometrial polyp, endometrial cancer

Gross Pathologic & Surgical Features
- Diffuse endometrial hyperplasia is not distinctive grossly, but focal hyperplasia can simulate a polyp

Microscopic Features
- Increase in the number of glands relative to stroma
    - Simple hyperplasia: Gross or minimally cystically dilated glands
    - Complex hyperplasia: Highly complex, crowded glands with epithelial stratification but little stroma
    - Hyperplasia with atypia: Increase in the number of glands lined by cells displaying cytologic atypia

Staging, Grading or Classification Criteria
- Hyperplasia without atypia: Subdivided into simple hyperplasia and complex hyperplasia
- Hyperplasia with atypia

CLINICAL ISSUES

Presentation
- Most common signs/symptoms: Bleeding, especially in postmenopausal women
- Other signs/symptoms: Menorrhagia, menometrorrhagia

Natural History & Prognosis
- Risk of progression to endometrial cancer is 1-25% depending on the age and type of hyperplasia
- Prognosis is excellent with early detection and appropriate treatment

Treatment
- Simple and complex hyperplasia: Conservative or hormonal therapy
- Hyperplasia with atypia: Curettage or simple hysterectomy depending on the age of patient
- Hyperplasia in patients on HRT: Cessation of HRT and re-biopsy

DIAGNOSTIC CHECKLIST

Consider
- SHG if the central interface is not seen in its entirety on TVS, and therefore the two layers of endometrium are not seen distinctly

Image Interpretation Pearls
- Look for focal endometrial thickening on TVS or SHG to triage patient for targeted biopsy

SELECTED REFERENCES

1. Davidson KG et al: Ultrasonographic evaluation of the endometrium in postmenopausal vaginal bleeding. Radiol Clin North Am. 41(4):769-80, 2003
2. Farquhar C et al: A systematic review of transvaginal ultrasonography, sonohysterography and hysteroscopy for the investigation of abnormal uterine bleeding in premenopausal women. Acta Obstet Gynecol Scand. 82(6):493-504, 2003
3. Davis PC et al: Sonohysterographic findings of endometrial and subendometrial conditions. Radiographics. 22(4):803-16, 2002
4. Gupta JK et al: Ultrasonographic endometrial thickness for diagnosing endometrial pathology in women with postmenopausal bleeding: a meta-analysis. Acta Obstet Gynecol Scand. 81(9):799-816, 2002
5. Reinhold C et al: Postmenopausal bleeding: value of imaging. Radiol Clin North Am. 40(3):527-62, 2002
6. Nalaboff KM et al: Imaging the endometrium: disease and normal variants. Radiographics. 21(6):1409-24, 2001
7. Smith-Bindman R et al: Endovaginal ultrasound to exclude endometrial cancer and other endometrial abnormalities. JAMA. 280(17):1510-7, 1998
8. Lerner JP et al: Use of transvaginal sonography in the evaluation of endometrial hyperplasia and carcinoma. Obstet Gynecol Surv. 51(12):718-25, 1996

ENDOMETRIAL HYPERPLASIA

IMAGE GALLERY

Typical

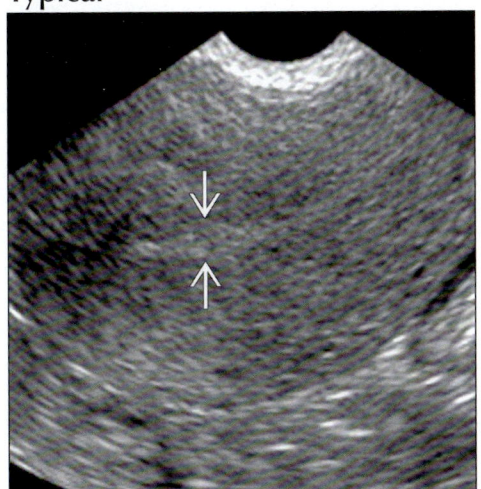
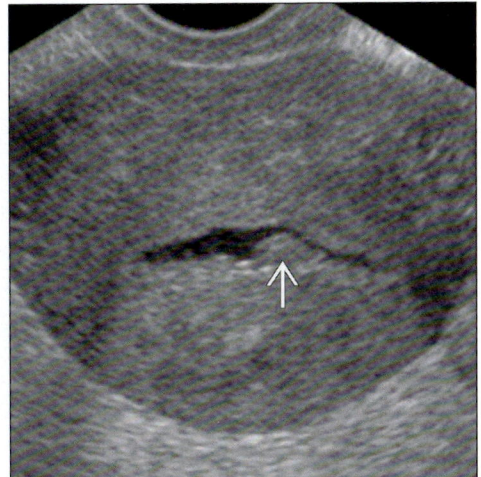

(Left) Sagittal transvaginal ultrasound shows focal endometrial thickening ➡ in a patient with postmenopausal bleeding. *(Right)* Axial SHG in the same patient as previous image shows focal endometrial thickening ➡ of the dorsal endometrial lining.

Typical

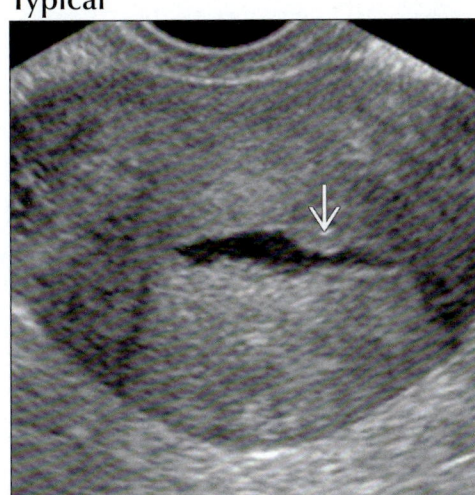
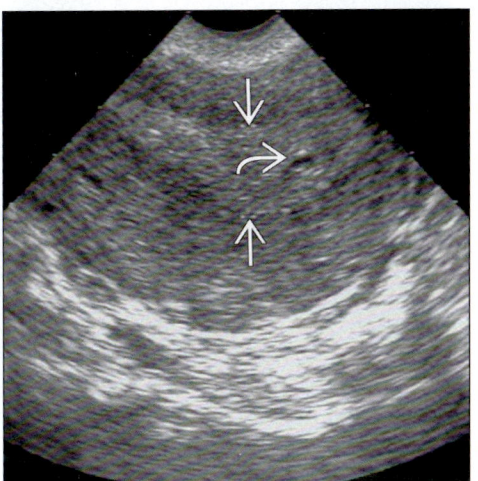

(Left) Axial SHG in the same patient as previous image shows focal endometrial thickening ➡ of the ventral endometrial lining. *(Right)* Sagittal transvaginal ultrasound shows diffuse endometrial thickening ➡ (14 mm) and a small endometrial cyst ➡. No separate endometrial lining is identified.

Typical

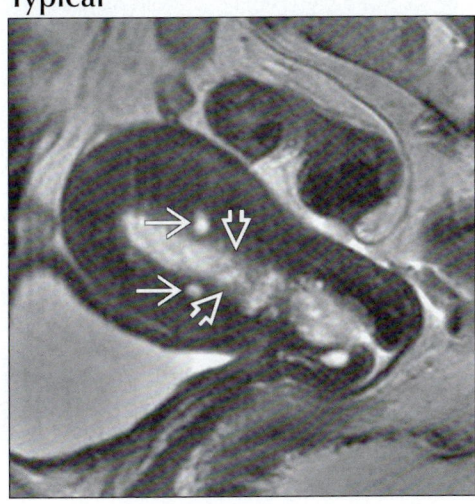
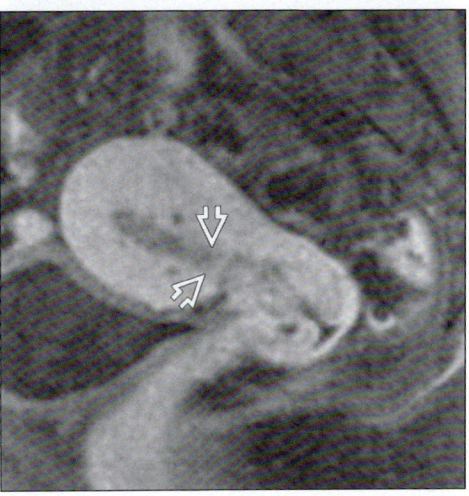

(Left) Sagittal T2WI MR shows heterogeneous endometrial thickening ➡. Cystic changes in the underlying myometrium ➡ are consistent with adenomyosis. *(Right)* Sagittal T1 C+ FS MR in the same patient as previous image shows heterogeneous enhancement of the thickened endometrium ➡. Cystic hyperplasia was present at biopsy.

ENDOMETRIAL HYPERPLASIA

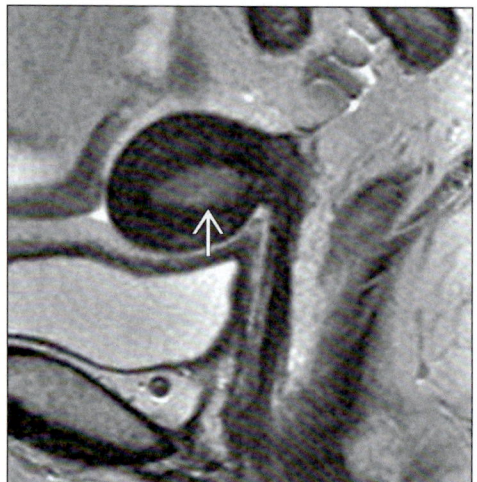 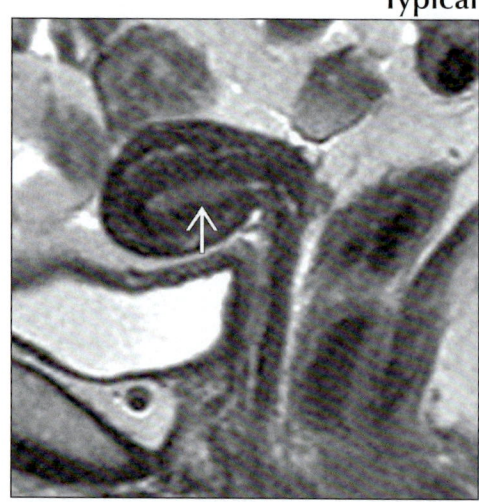

(Left) Sagittal T2WI MR shows the endometrium to be diffusely thickened ➡ and of homogeneous decreased signal intensity. Endometrial curettage revealed hyperplasia with cellular atypia. (Right) Sagittal T2WI MR in the same patient as previous image after progesterone therapy shows decreased endometrial thickening ➡. Repeat biopsy revealed no evidence of malignancy.

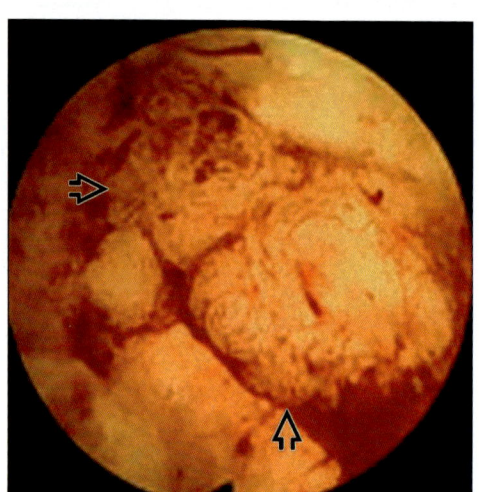 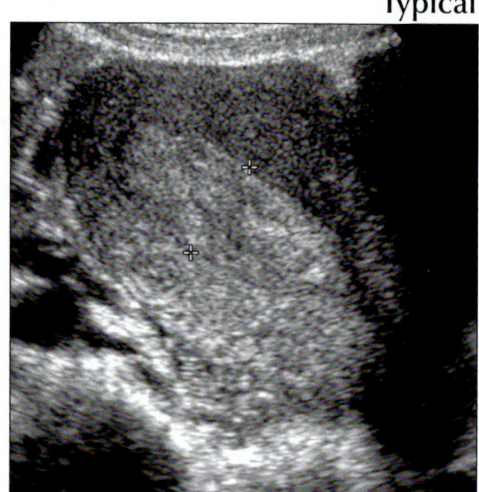

(Left) Hysteroscopic view of the endometrial cavity shows focal hyperplasia ➡. (Right) Sagittal transabdominal ultrasound shows thickened heterogeneous endometrium (calipers) in patient with complex hyperplasia.

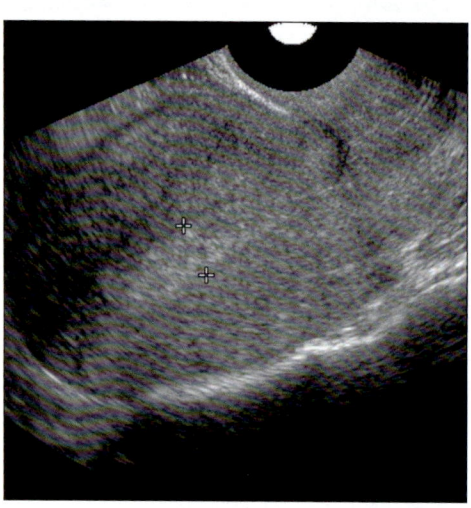 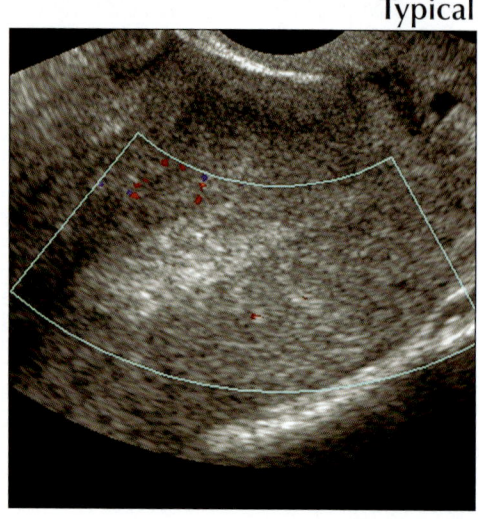

(Left) Sagittal transvaginal ultrasound shows 9 mm slightly heterogeneous endometrium (calipers). (Right) Sagittal color Doppler ultrasound in the same case as previous image shows no flow to the endometrium. Histology was complex hyperplasia.

ENDOMETRIAL HYPERPLASIA

Typical

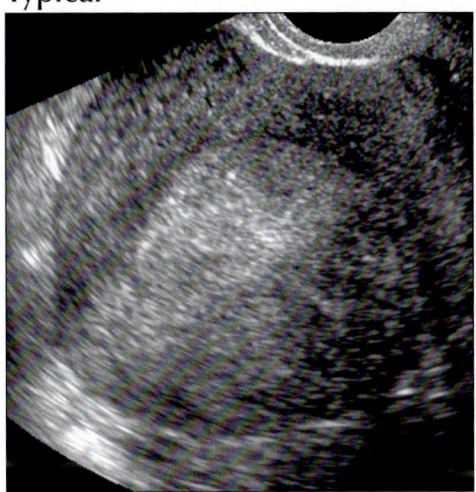 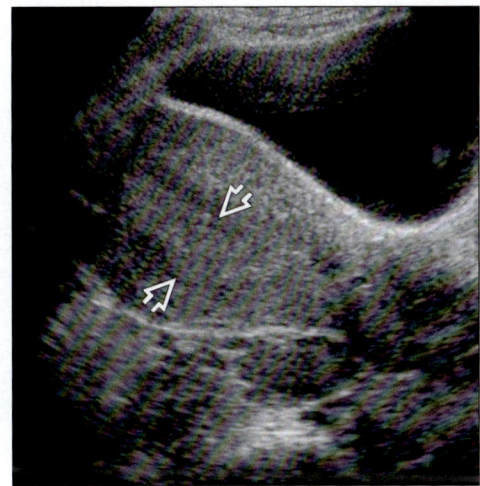

(Left) Sagittal transvaginal ultrasound shows thickened slightly heterogeneous endometrium in patient with endometrial hyperplasia. *(Right)* Sagittal transabdominal ultrasound shows a region of focal endometrial thickening ➡ in a patient with endometrial hyperplasia.

Typical

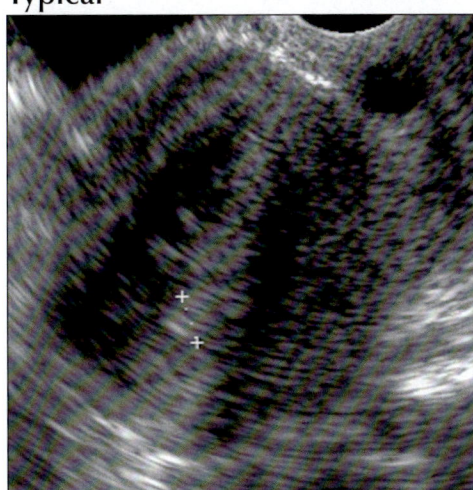 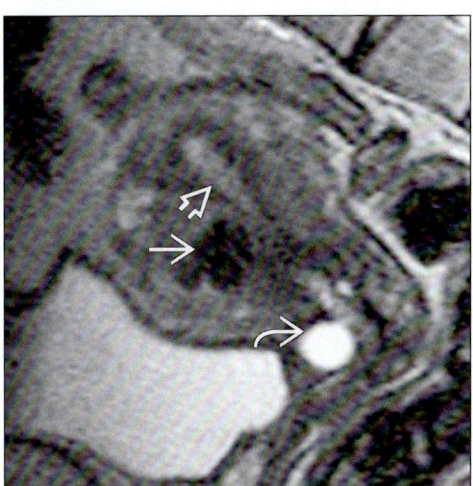

(Left) Sagittal transvaginal ultrasound shows 6 mm endometrial thickness (calipers) in a postmenopausal woman with bleeding. Histology was endometrial hyperplasia. *(Right)* Sagittal T2WI MR shows slightly heterogeneous endometrium ➡ in postmenopausal woman with abnormal bleeding. Note also leiomyoma ➡ and nabothian cyst ➡.

Typical

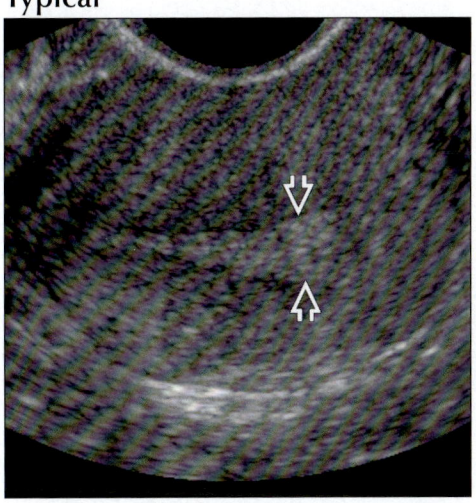 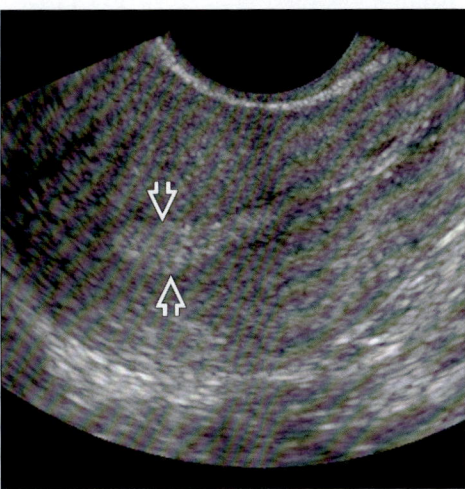

(Left) Transverse transvaginal ultrasound shows an area of focal thickening ➡ of the endometrium in a patient with endometrial hyperplasia. *(Right)* Sagittal transvaginal ultrasound in same patient as previous image shows focal thickening ➡ near the fundus.

ENDOMETRIAL CANCER, CHARACTERIZATION

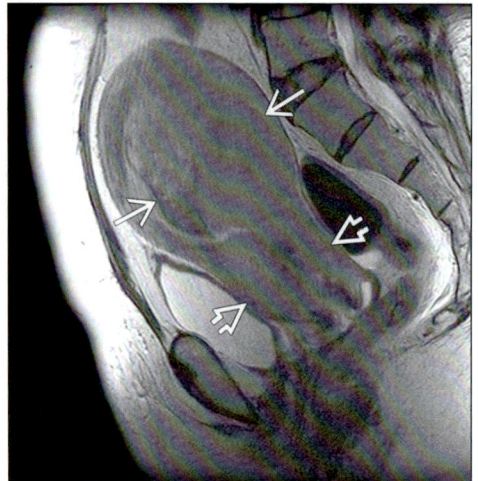

Sagittal T2WI MR shows large mass invading myometrium ➡, extending into the cervix, and invading the cervical stroma ➡. Adenocarcinoma of the endometrium.

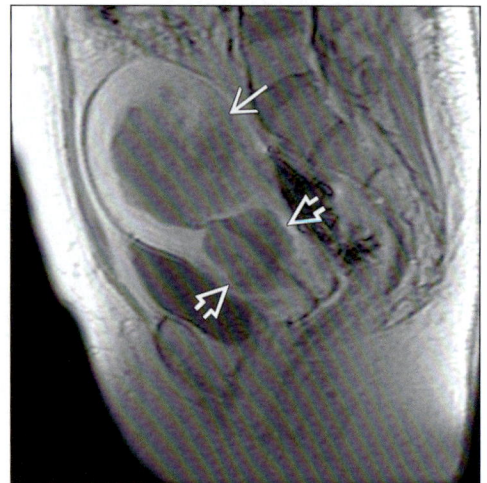

Sagittal T1 C+ MR shows a mass enhancing less avidly than myometrium, making diagnosis of deep myometrial ➡ and cervical stromal ➡ invasion more conspicuous on early contrast-enhanced sagittal T1WI.

TERMINOLOGY

Abbreviations and Synonyms
- Carcinoma of endometrium

Definitions
- Malignant neoplasm of endometrium

IMAGING FINDINGS

General Features
- Best diagnostic clue
  - Mass in endometrial cavity causing expansion in the endometrial cavity
  - Localized tumors: Polypoid masses with superficial attachment to endometrium
  - Diffuse tumors: Extensive invasion of entire endometrium
- Location
  - Endometrial cavity of uterus
  - Some cases may show invasion into myometrium, cervix or adjacent structures
- Size: Varies from small to large lesions
- Morphology: Polypoid masses or diffuse thickening in the endometrial cavity

Ultrasonographic Findings
- 3D: 3D ultrasound provides endometrial cancer volume measurement that may be better than thickness measurement for the detection of endometrial cancer
- Transvaginal ultrasound (TVS) findings
  - Initial study obtained in women with suspected endometrial cancer
  - Endometrial cancer appears as a polypoid mass or diffuse thickening in the endometrial cavity
  - Disruption of subendometrial halo suggests myometrial invasion
  - TVS is limited for the evaluation of cervix, parametrium, and lymph nodes

CT Findings
- NECT: Difficult to differentiate endometrial cancer from the normal uterus
- CECT
  - Diffuse thickening or a discrete mass could be seen in the endometrial cavity

DDx: Uterine Masses

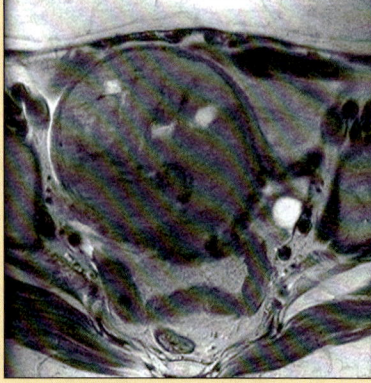

Leiomyosarcoma

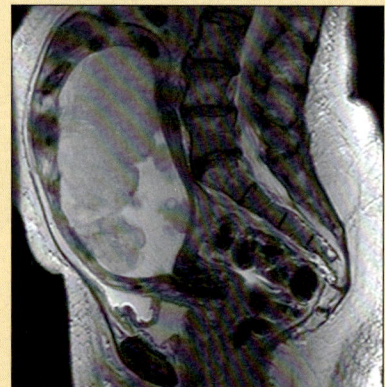

Malignant Mixed Mesodermal Tumor

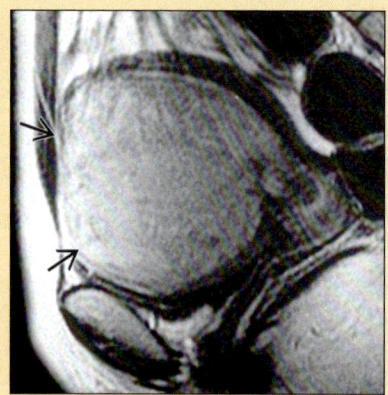

Endometrial Stromal Sarcoma

ENDOMETRIAL CANCER, CHARACTERIZATION

Key Facts

Terminology
- Malignant neoplasm of endometrium

Imaging Findings
- Mass in endometrial cavity causing expansion in the endometrial cavity

Top Differential Diagnoses
- Endometrial Hyperplasia or Polyps
- Imaging methods cannot differentiate stage IA endometrial carcinoma from hyperplasia or polyps
- Invasion to myometrium and/or cervix indicates malignancy
- Uterine Sarcomas
- Difficult to differentiate endometrial cancer from much less common uterine sarcomas
- Uterine sarcomas tend to be larger, heterogeneous and more aggressive

Pathology
- Adenocarcinoma (90%)
- Epidemiology: Most common invasive gynecologic malignancy

Diagnostic Checklist
- TVS as initial imaging test in women with abnormal uterine bleeding
- MR for local staging and treatment planning
- CT for advanced cases with distant metastasis
- Mass causing expansion in the endometrial cavity
- Disruption of junctional zone and an irregular endometrium-myometrium interface suggest myometrial invasion

---

- Endometrial cancer remains relatively low attenuation compared to myometrium
- Irregular tumor-myometrial border indicates myometrial invasion
- Limited in local staging due to inability to accurately demonstrate deep myometrial invasion and cervical involvement
- Commonly used in the assessment of lymphadenopathy and distant metastases

MR Findings
- T1WI: Low to same signal intensity relative to normal endometrium
- T2WI
  - Heterogeneous intermediate signal intensity relative to normal endometrium
    - If junctional zone intact: Deep myometrial invasion excluded
    - If junctional zone not well seen (e.g., postmenopausal women): Irregular endometrium/myometrium interface suggests myometrial invasion
- T1 C+
  - Endometrial cancer enhances less avidly compared to myometrium and cervix
  - Dynamic post-contrast images are very useful in the depiction of myometrial and cervical invasion
  - Post-contrast images are also useful to differentiate endometrial cancer from fluid or blood filling the endometrial cavity

Nuclear Medicine Findings
- PET: F-18 FDG PET is useful in detecting metastases and and surveillance for recurrent disease

Imaging Recommendations
- Best imaging tool
  - TVS may be used for initial evaluation especially in women with abnormal uterine bleeding
  - Role of CT and MR is to determine the stage of disease for treatment planning once the diagnosis is established
  - MR is the most accurate imaging technique for local staging
  - CT and MR are equally good for the assessment of pelvic and paraaortic lymph nodes
- Protocol advice
  - MR imaging protocol should include
    - T1WI: Axial, large field of view including entire pelvis
    - T2WI: Axial, sagittal and coronal small field of view
    - T1 C+: Dynamic; sagittal

DIFFERENTIAL DIAGNOSIS

Endometrial Hyperplasia or Polyps
- Imaging methods cannot differentiate stage IA endometrial carcinoma from hyperplasia or polyps
- Invasion to myometrium and/or cervix indicates malignancy

Submucosal Leiomyoma
- Low signal intensity on T2WI
- Displaces rather than expanding endometrial stripe

Uterine Sarcomas
- Difficult to differentiate endometrial cancer from much less common uterine sarcomas
- Uterine sarcomas tend to be larger, heterogeneous and more aggressive

PATHOLOGY

General Features
- General path comments
  - Adenocarcinoma (90%)
  - Other types: Adenocarcinoma with squamous differentiation, adenosquamous carcinoma, papillary serous carcinoma and clear cell carcinoma
- Etiology
  - Unopposed estrogen stimulation causing hyperplasia-carcinoma cycle

ENDOMETRIAL CANCER, CHARACTERIZATION

- Spontaneous carcinoma arising from atrophic or inert endometrium
- Epidemiology: Most common invasive gynecologic malignancy

Gross Pathologic & Surgical Features
- Polypoid masses or diffuse thickening in endometrial cavity with various levels of myometrial invasion

Staging, Grading or Classification Criteria
- FIGO staging system
  - 0: Carcinoma in situ
  - I: Tumor confined to corpus
    - IA: Limited to endometrium
    - IB: Invasion less than half of myometrium
    - IC: Invasion more than half of myometrium
  - II: Tumor invades cervix
    - IIA: Endocervical glandular involvement
    - IIB: Cervical stromal involvement
  - III: Tumor extends beyond uterus but not outside true pelvis
    - IIIA: Invasion of serosa or adnexa or positive peritoneal cytology
    - IIIB: Vaginal involvement
    - IIIC: Metastases to pelvic or paraaortic lymph nodes
  - IV: Adjacent organ invasion or distant metastases
    - IVA: Invasion of bladder, bowel or both
    - IVB: Distant metastases including intraabdominal and inguinal lymph nodes
  - Grading
    - Well-differentiated (grade I) to anaplastic (grade III)

CLINICAL ISSUES

Presentation
- Most common signs/symptoms: Abnormal uterine bleeding
- Other signs/symptoms: Signs secondary to metastases in advanced cases
- Clinical Profile
  - Most commonly postmenopausal women with abnormal vaginal bleeding
  - Diagnosis made by dilatation and curettage

Demographics
- Age: Commonly in women at 6th and 7th decades of life

Natural History & Prognosis
- Most important prognostic factors
  - Histologic grade of tumor
  - Depth of myometrial invasion
  - Stage of disease
  - Lymph node involvement
- 5 year survival rates: 90% for stage I, 80% for stage II, 15-20% for stage III-IV

Treatment
- Multimodality approach depending on tumor stage
  - Surgery: Total abdominal hysterectomy (TAH) + bilateral salpingo-oophorectomy (BSO)
  - Pre-operative and post-operative radiation treatment
  - Chemotherapy or hormonal treatment

DIAGNOSTIC CHECKLIST

Consider
- TVS as initial imaging test in women with abnormal uterine bleeding
- MR for local staging and treatment planning
- CT for advanced cases with distant metastasis
- Imaging studies should be directed to determine the following prognostic factors
  - Depth of myometrial invasion
  - Stage of disease
  - Lymph node involvement

Image Interpretation Pearls
- Mass causing expansion in the endometrial cavity
- Disruption of junctional zone and an irregular endometrium-myometrium interface suggest myometrial invasion

SELECTED REFERENCES

1. Ioffe OB. Related Articles et al: Recent developments and selected diagnostic problems in carcinomas of the endometrium. Am J Clin Pathol. 124 Suppl:S42-51, 2005
2. Manfredi R et al: Endometrial cancer: magnetic resonance imaging. Abdom Imaging. 30(5):626-36, 2005
3. Pandit-Taskar N. Related Articles et al: Oncologic imaging in gynecologic malignancies. J Nucl Med. 46(11):1842-50, 2005
4. Manfredi R et al: Local-regional staging of endometrial carcinoma: role of MR imaging in surgical planning. Radiology. 231(2):372-8, 2004
5. Utsunomiya D et al: Endometrial carcinoma in adenomyosis: assessment of myometrial invasion on T2-weighted spin-echo and gadolinium-enhanced T1-weighted images. AJR Am J Roentgenol. 182(2):399-404, 2004
6. Ascher SM et al: Imaging of cancer of the endometrium. Radiol Clin North Am. 40(3):563-76, 2002
7. Frei KA et al: Prediction of deep myometrial invasion in patients with endometrial cancer: clinical utility of contrast-enhanced MR imaging-a meta-analysis and Bayesian analysis. Radiology. 216(2):444-9, 2000
8. Hardesty LA et al: Use of preoperative MR imaging in the management of endometrial carcinoma: cost analysis. Radiology. 215(1):45-9, 2000
9. Saez F et al: Endometrial carcinoma: assessment of myometrial invasion with plain and gadolinium-enhanced MR imaging. J Magn Reson Imaging. 12(3):460-6, 2000
10. Seki H et al: Myometrial invasion of endometrial carcinoma: assessment with dynamic MR and contrast-enhanced T1-weighted images. Clin Radiol. 52(1):18-23, 1997
11. Gruboeck K et al: The diagnostic value of endometrial thickness and volume measurements by three-dimensional ultrasound in patients with postmenopausal bleeding. Ultrasound Obstet Gynecol. 8(4):272-6, 1996
12. Yamashita Y et al: Assessment of myometrial invasion by endometrial carcinoma: transvaginal sonography vs contrast-enhanced MR imaging. AJR Am J Roentgenol. 161(3):595-9, 1993

ENDOMETRIAL CANCER, CHARACTERIZATION

IMAGE GALLERY

Typical

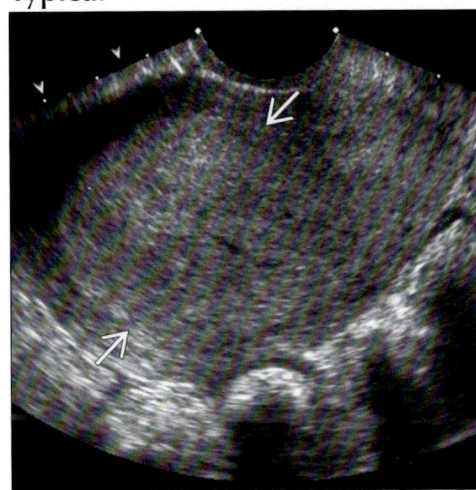
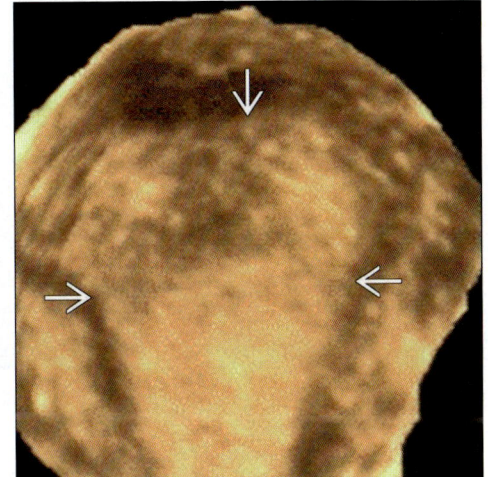

(Left) Sagittal transvaginal ultrasound shows a large mass ➡ which expands the endometrial cavity. *(Right)* Coronal 3D ultrasound shows endometrial mass ➡ with irregular margins in the endometrial cavity. (Courtesy of C. Lulla, MD).

Typical

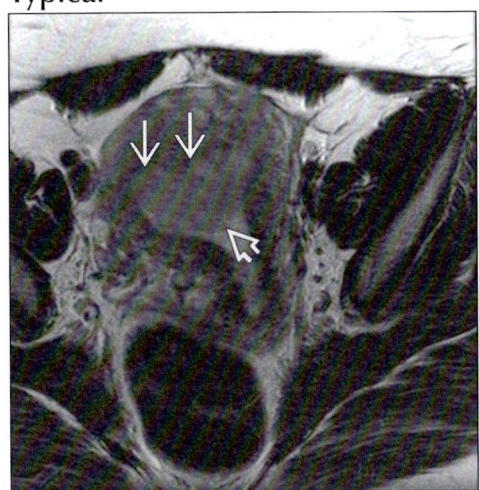
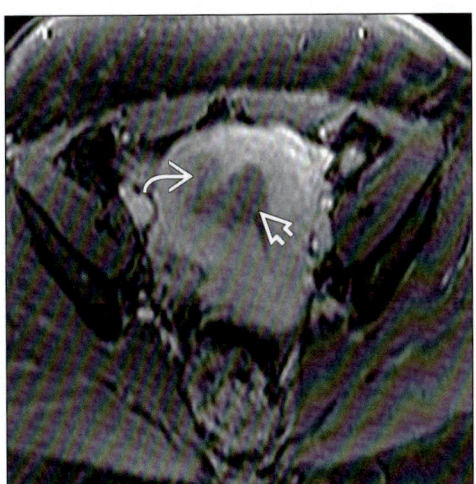

(Left) Axial T2WI MR shows a large polypoid mass ➡ in the endometrial cavity. Note that the junctional zone ➡ is ill-defined and irregular indicating myometrial invasion. *(Right)* Axial T1 C+ FS MR shows that the endometrial mass ➡ remains hypointense relative to myometrium. Irregular low signal intensity area ➡ in the myometrium indicates myometrial invasion.

Typical

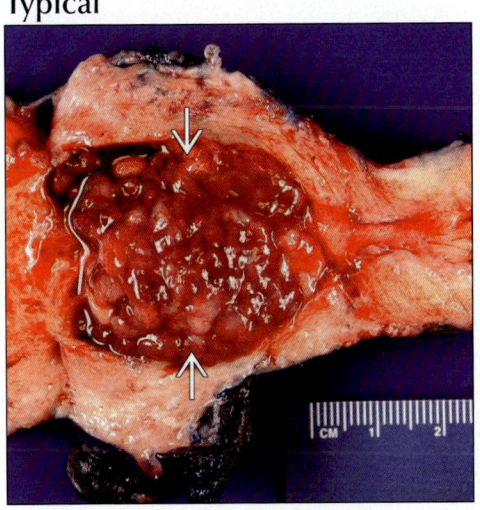
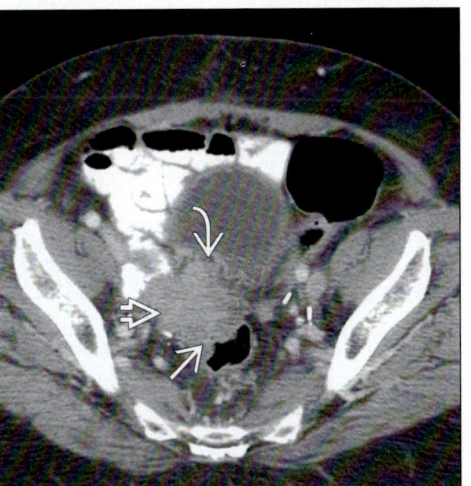

(Left) Gross pathology shows polypoid mass ➡ expanding endometrial cavity in a patient with endometrial cancer. *(Right)* Axial CECT shows recurrent endometrial cancer ➡ invading the sigmoid colon ➡. Note that fat plane between the mass and the urinary bladder is intact ➡.

ENDOMETRIAL CANCER, EARLY STAGE

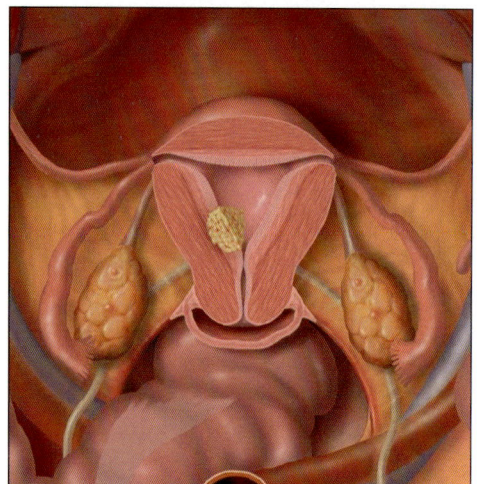

Graphic shows a small mass arising from the right aspect of the endometrium. The mass extends to the inner half of the myometrium consistent with a stage IB endometrial carcinoma.

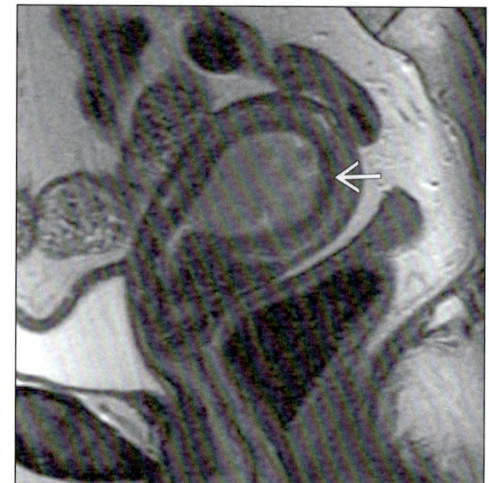

Sagittal T2WI MR shows a relatively homogeneous endometrial mass. The mass is confined to the endometrium, aside from a focus of early myometrial invasion dorsally ➡ (stage IB).

TERMINOLOGY

Abbreviations and Synonyms
- Uterine carcinoma, endometrial carcinoma

Definitions
- Endometrial cancer confined to endometrium (FIGO stage IA) or inner half (< 50% thickness) of myometrium (FIGO stage IB)

IMAGING FINDINGS

General Features
- Best diagnostic clue
  - FIGO stage IA: Diffuse/focal widening of endometrial complex > 5 mm in postmenopausal woman with bleeding
    - Smooth endometrial-myometrial interface
    - Intact subendometrial halo/junctional zone
  - FIGO stage IB: Endometrial-based mass invading inner half of myometrium (< 50% thickness)
    - Irregular inner myometrium
    - Partial or complete disruption of subendometrial halo/junctional zone
- Location: Endometrium or inner half of myometrium
- Size: Microscopic to several centimeters
- Morphology: Typically homogeneous
- CT/MR modalities of choice for detection of lymphadenopathy (accuracy 60-90%)
  - Rounded lymph nodes ≥ 0.8 cm defined as pathologic
  - Oval lymph nodes ≥ 1.0 cm short-axis defined as pathologic
  - Node signal/enhancement not predictive of metastatic involvement
  - Skip metastasis to paraaortic nodes without pelvic lymphadenopathy via ovarian lymphatics
- Staging errors: Adenomyosis, leiomyomas, hematometra, bulky tumors, microscopic disease

Ultrasonographic Findings
- Grayscale Ultrasound
  - Stage IA: Variable and nonspecific appearance
    - Thickened, hyperechoic endometrial complex with well-defined borders

DDx: Endometrial Thickening

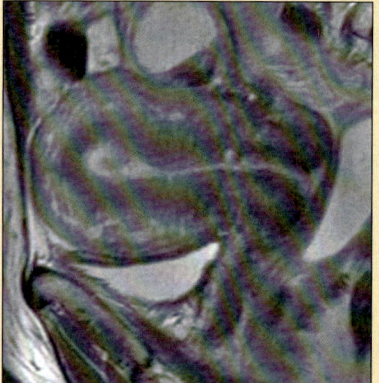

Endometrial Polyp

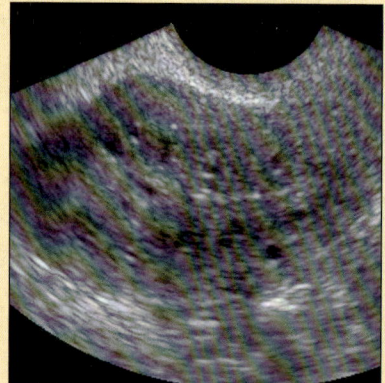

Adenomyosis

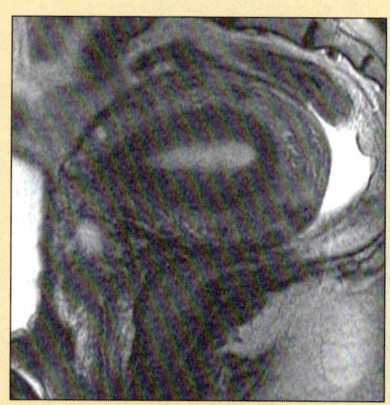

Endometrial Hyperplasia

ENDOMETRIAL CANCER, EARLY STAGE

Key Facts

Terminology
- Endometrial cancer confined to endometrium (FIGO stage IA) or inner half (< 50% thickness) of myometrium (FIGO stage IB)

Imaging Findings
- FIGO stage IA: Diffuse/focal widening of endometrial complex > 5 mm in postmenopausal woman with bleeding
- FIGO stage IB: Endometrial-based mass invading inner half of myometrium (< 50% thickness)
- Staging errors: Adenomyosis, leiomyomas, hematometra, bulky tumors, microscopic disease
- MR accuracy 80-95%: Loss of uterine zonal anatomy in postmenopausal women a potential pitfall

Top Differential Diagnoses
- Endometrial Hyperplasia
- Endometrial Polyp
- Adenomyosis
- Premenstrual Endometrium
- Uterine Sarcomas

Pathology
- Adenocarcinoma most common histological type
- Worse prognosis with papillary serous and clear-cell carcinomas
- Low incidence of malignant lymphadenopathy

Diagnostic Checklist
- Critical to differentiate from advanced disease
- Intact subendometrial halo/junctional zone excludes deep myometrial invasion (FIGO stage IC)

- Areas of decreased echogenicity within thickened endometrial complex
- Heterogeneous/homogeneous mass-like lesion
- Intact subendometrial halo
  - Stage IB: Tumor echogenicity parallels stage IA, but margins irregular or poorly defined
    - Abnormal echogenicity extends into inner myometrium
    - Focal/diffuse disruption of subendometrial halo
  - Accuracy 65-85%: Highest in early stage with small tumors, overstaging in large polypoid tumors
- Pulsed Doppler: Significant overlap in pulsatility and resistive index between benign and malignant endometrial thickening
- Color Doppler: Mild to moderate vascularity with multiple feeding vessels

CT Findings
- CECT
  - Focal/diffuse endometrial thickening
  - Centrally located mass hypodense to myometrium
  - Low accuracy (65-75%) due to lack of zonal anatomy
    - Intact band of early subendometrial enhancement in absence of myometrial invasion
  - Detection of lymphadenopathy

MR Findings
- T1WI
  - Hypointense to isointense relative to endometrium/myometrium
  - Detection of hematometra and lymphadenopathy
- T2WI
  - Hypointense/isointense relative to endometrium (100%)
  - Isointense/hyperintense relative to outer myometrium (70%)
  - Stage IA: Junctional zone intact (excludes deep myometrial invasion)
  - Stage IB: Partial/complete disruption of junctional zone
- DWI
  - Increased tumor cellularity results in greater water restriction in tumors relative to myometrium
  - Lower apparent diffusion coefficient (ADC) values, corresponding to high signal intensity on magnitude high b-value images
- T1 C+ FS
  - Improved detection, assessment of myometrial invasion, differentiation from retained debris/hematometra
    - Hypointense relative to myometrium in early and equilibrium phase (75%)
  - Stage IA: Intact band of early subendometrial enhancement
  - Stage IB: Disrupted band of early subendometrial enhancement
- MR accuracy 80-95%: Loss of uterine zonal anatomy in postmenopausal women a potential pitfall

Nuclear Medicine Findings
- PET: Nonspecific elevation of standard uptake value of primary and metastatic tumor on F-18 FDG PET

Imaging Recommendations
- Best imaging tool
  - Transvaginal ultrasound (TVS) most common detection modality
    - Postmenopausal bleeding with endometrial complex > 5 mm → endometrial sampling
  - High-resolution T2WI MR and C+ MR most accurate for local staging and treatment planning
  - CT and MR equally accurate for assessment of pelvic and paraaortic lymph nodes
    - Improved sensitivity for lymph node metastases with ultrasmall superparamagnetic iron oxide (USPIO) enhanced MR or F-18 FDG PET
- Protocol advice
  - High-resolution pelvic MR with phased-array coil and 4-5 mm slice thickness
    - Axial T1WI with larger field-of-view (FOV) extending from pelvis to renal hila for lymph nodes
    - Axial, sagittal and coronal (short-axis) T2WI with small FOV
    - Sagittal and coronal (short-axis) dynamic T1WI C+ FS with small FOV (optimal contrast at 2 minutes)

ENDOMETRIAL CANCER, EARLY STAGE

DIFFERENTIAL DIAGNOSIS

Endometrial Hyperplasia
- Significant overlap of imaging findings with stage IA carcinoma
- Typically iso- or hyperintense to myometrium on delayed C+ MR

Endometrial Polyp
- Single feeding vessel on Doppler ultrasound
- Small polyps frequently isointense on T2WI with early enhancement on C+ MR
- Fibrous core may be visible on T2WI

Adenomyosis
- Can mimic stage IB carcinoma with direct extension of the endometrium into the myometrium

Premenstrual Endometrium
- Diffuse low signal intensity endometrium on T2WI

Uterine Sarcomas
- Larger, heterogeneous and more aggressive at presentation

PATHOLOGY

General Features
- Genetics
  - Rare hereditary form: Lynch II family cancer syndrome
    - Nonpolyposis colorectal cancer, ovarian, and endometrial cancer
- Etiology
  - Unopposed estrogen action on hormonally responsive endometrium
  - Endometrial hyperplasia-carcinoma sequence
- Epidemiology
  - Most common invasive gynecological malignancy
    - 75% present with stage I disease
- Associated abnormalities: Endometrial hyperplasia (20-40%)

Gross Pathologic & Surgical Features
- Adenocarcinoma most common histological type
- Tumor confined to endometrium or inner half of myometrium

Microscopic Features
- 75% endometrioid; serous, mucinous, clear cell, squamous less common
  - Worse prognosis with papillary serous and clear-cell carcinomas
    - Peritoneal spread and lymphovascular space invasion more common

Staging, Grading or Classification Criteria
- Well-differentiated (grade I) to anaplastic (grade III)
- Early stage: Tumor confined to corpus
  - Stage IA: Limited to endometrium
  - Stage IB: Invasion < 50% of myometrium
- Low incidence of malignant lymphadenopathy
  - 1-5% with grade 1-2 adenocarcinomas
  - 10% with grade 3 adenocarcinomas

CLINICAL ISSUES

Presentation
- Most common signs/symptoms: 75-90% present with postmenopausal bleeding, 10% with leukorrhea
- Clinical Profile: Obesity, altered menstruation, low fertility index, late menopause, anovulation, and postmenopausal bleeding, tamoxifen use

Demographics
- Age: 6th to 7th decade, post-menopausal
- Ethnicity: Common in Eastern Europe and the United States; uncommon in Asia

Natural History & Prognosis
- 90-100% 5 year survival

Treatment
- Differentiation between stage IA and IB not clinically relevant
  - Exception: Progesterone therapy for stage IA disease (uterine conserving therapy)
- Multidisciplinary approach depending on tumor stage and histology
  - Total abdominal hysterectomy and bilateral salpingo-oophorectomy
  - Periaortic node dissection in tumors with poor histology
  - Adjuvant radiation/chemotherapy in the setting of poor prognostic indicators

DIAGNOSTIC CHECKLIST

Consider
- MR for local staging and treatment planning

Image Interpretation Pearls
- Critical to differentiate from advanced disease
  - Intact subendometrial halo/junctional zone excludes deep myometrial invasion (FIGO stage IC)
  - Irregular endometrial-myometrial interface suggestive of early myometrial invasion

SELECTED REFERENCES

1. Chao A et al: 18F-FDG PET in the management of endometrial cancer. Eur J Nucl Med Mol Imaging. 33(1):36-44, 2006
2. Kinkel K: Pitfalls in staging uterine neoplasm with imaging: a review. Abdom Imaging. 31(2):164-73, 2006
3. Nakao Y et al: MR imaging in endometrial carcinoma as a diagnostic tool for the absence of myometrial invasion. Gynecologic Oncology. 102:343-7, 2006
4. Chaudhry S et al: Benign and malignant diseases of the endometrium. Top Magn Reson Imaging. 2003
5. Reinhold C et al: Postmenopausal bleeding: Value of imaging. RCNA. 40:527-62, 2002
6. Hardesty LA et al: The ability of helical CT to preoperatively stage endometrial carcinoma. AJR. 176(3):603-6, 2001
7. Frei KA et al: Prediction of deep myometrial invasion in patients with endometrial cancer: Clinical utility of contrast-enhanced MR imaging-A meta-analysis and Bayesian analysis. Radiology. 216:444-9, 2000

ENDOMETRIAL CANCER, EARLY STAGE

IMAGE GALLERY

Typical

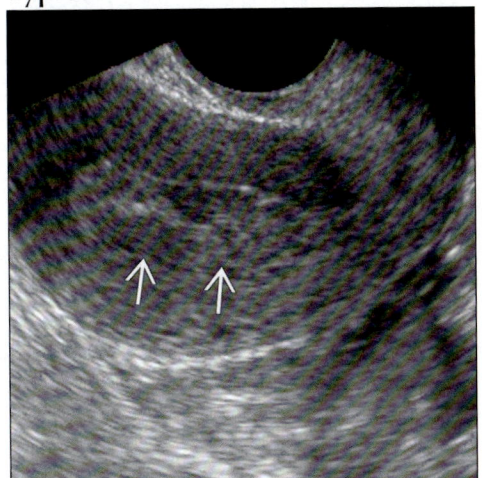
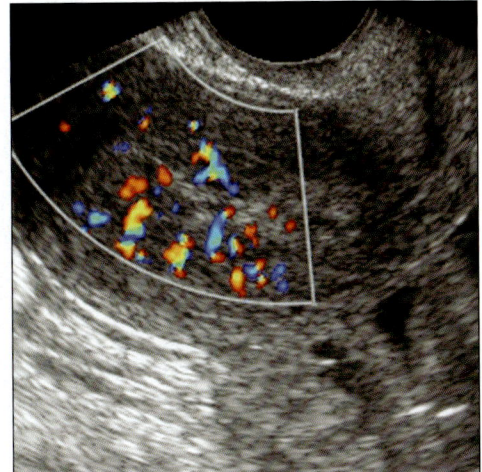

(Left) Sagittal transvaginal ultrasound shows a heterogeneous, polypoid mass distending the endometrial cavity. The tumor arises from the dorsal endometrium ➡ and does not invade the myometrium. *(Right)* Sagittal color Doppler ultrasound shows moderate vascularity of the endometrial-based mass with multiple dorsal feeding vessels.

Typical

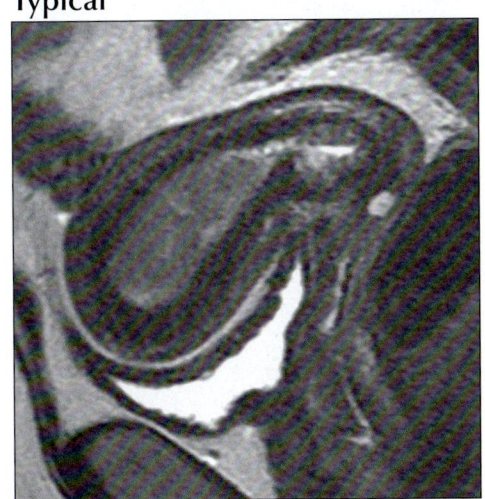
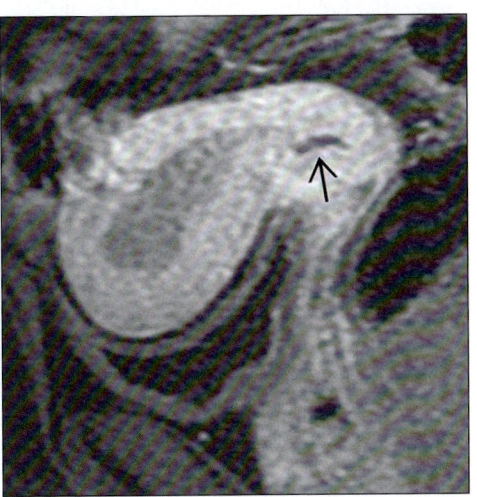

(Left) Sagittal T2WI MR shows an intermediate signal intensity mass within the endometrial cavity. The junctional zone is intact and the inner border smooth consistent with a stage IA carcinoma. *(Right)* Sagittal T1 C+ FS MR in the same patient as previous image shows the endometrial carcinoma to be hypointense relative to the myometrium. The normal cervical enhancement ➡ excludes cervical invasion.

Typical

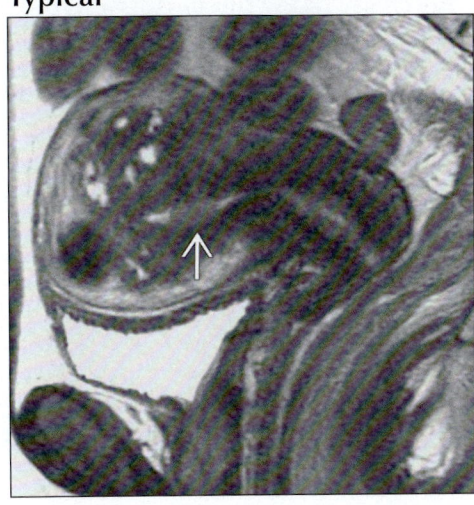
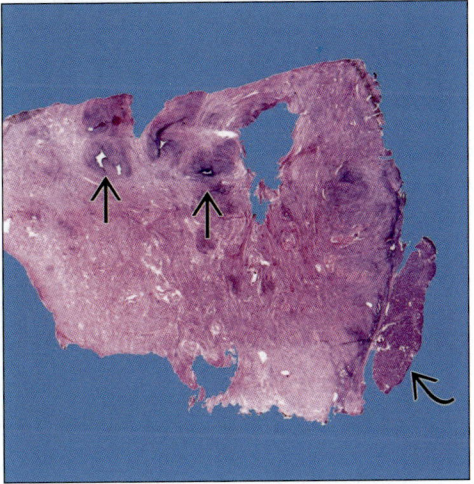

(Left) Sagittal T2WI MR shows as a polypoid endometrial carcinoma which appears confined to the endometrium, although minimal myometrial invasion ventrally ➡ cannot be completely excluded. *(Right)* Sagittal micropathology of the same patient as previous image shows the polypoid endometrial carcinoma ➡ confined to the endometrium. Incidentally there is extensive uterine adenomyosis ➡.

ENDOMETRIAL CANCER, EARLY STAGE

(Left) Sagittal T2WI MR shows an endometrial mass with an irregular endo-myometrial border consistent with a stage IB carcinoma ➡. (Right) Sagittal T1 C+ FS MR in the same patient as previous image shows normal enhancement of the endocervical mucosa ➡.

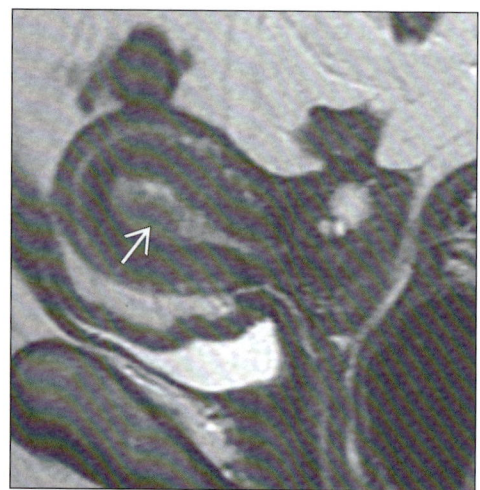 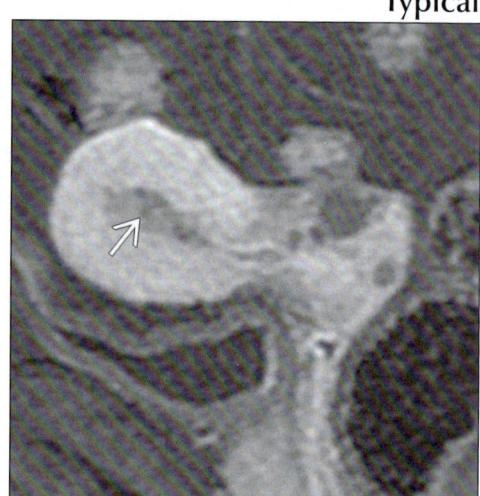

Typical

(Left) Coronal intra-operative photograph of the preceding patient shows the endometrial cancer with superficial myometrial invasion ➡. Note that the carcinoma does not extend to the cervix. (Right) Sagittal T2WI MR shows a small, intermediate signal intensity mass ➡ at the level of the fundus consistent with a stage IA carcinoma, in a background of endometrial hyperplasia.

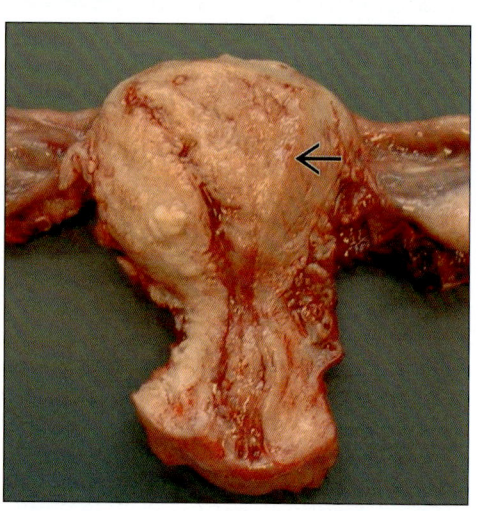 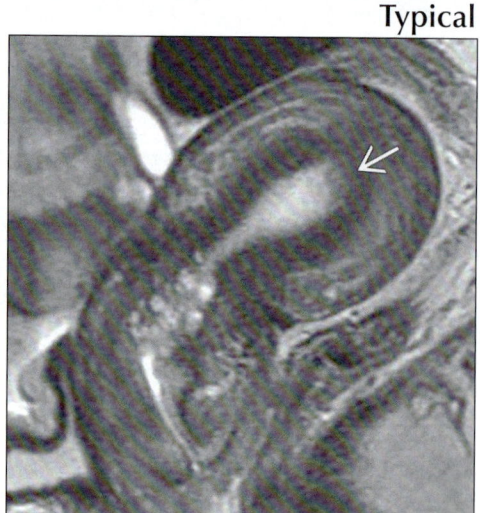

Typical

(Left) Sagittal T1 C+ FS MR (early) in the same patient as previous image shows mild enhancement ➡ of the carcinoma. The hyperintense subendometrial line ➡ is intact indicating absence of myometrial invasion. (Right) Sagittal T1 C+ FS MR (delayed) in the same patient as left shows uniform enhancement of the myometrium and hyperplastic endometrium. The small cancer ➡ remains relatively hypointense.

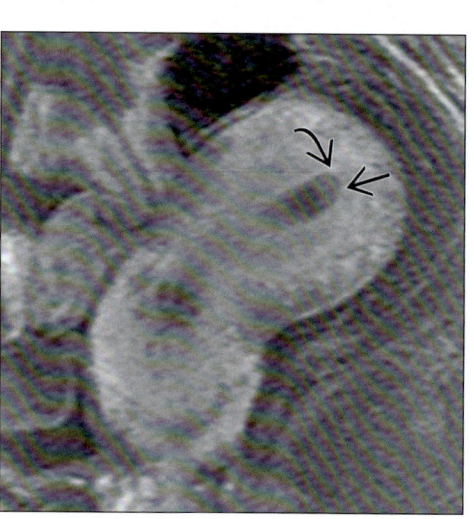 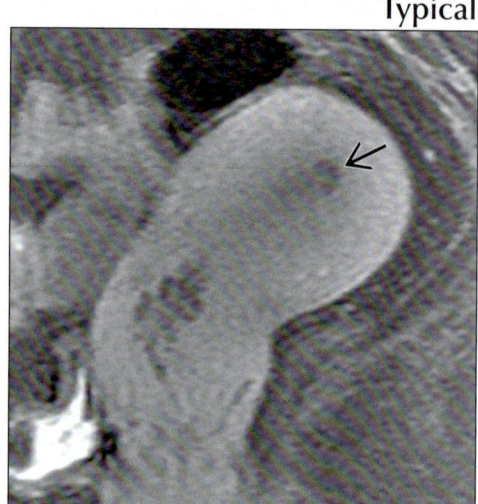

Typical

ENDOMETRIAL CANCER, EARLY STAGE

Typical

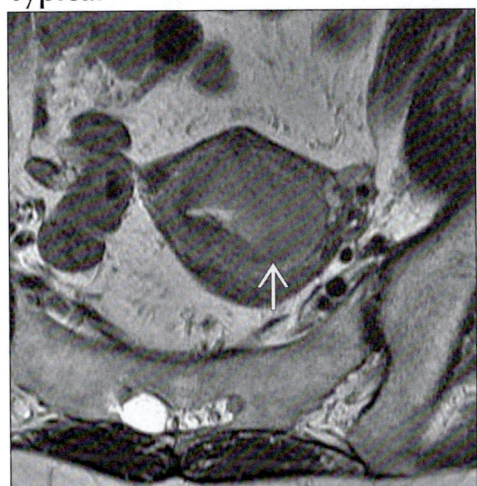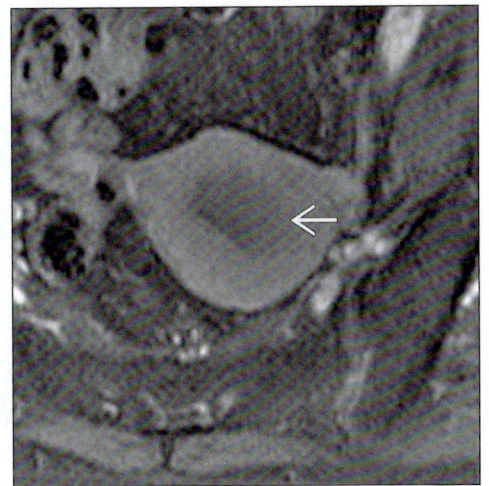

(Left) Coronal oblique T2WI MR shows a mass expanding the endometrial cavity and invading the inner half of the myometrium on the left ➡. (Right) Coronal oblique T1 C+ FS MR in the same patient as left confirms that the tumor is confined to the inner half ➡ of the myometrium (stage IB).

Typical

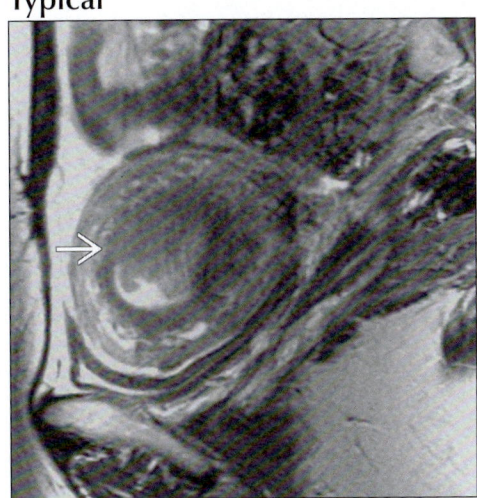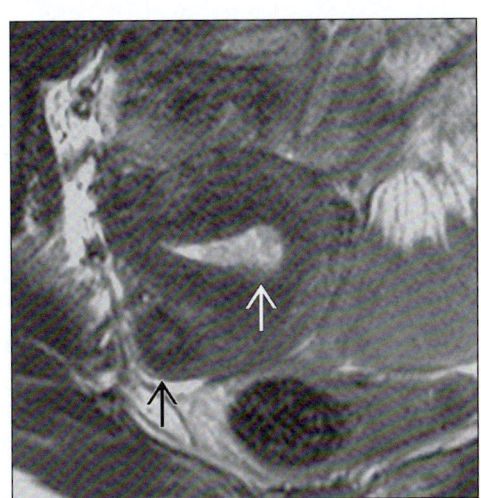

(Left) Sagittal T2WI MR shows an endometrial mass invading the inner half of the dorsal myometrium. The junctional zone is completely disrupted ➡. (Right) Axial T2WI MR shows a lobulated endometrial mass with invasion of the inner myometrium dorsally ➡ (stage IB). There is a small myometrial leiomyoma ➡. (Courtesy A. Padhani, MD).

Typical

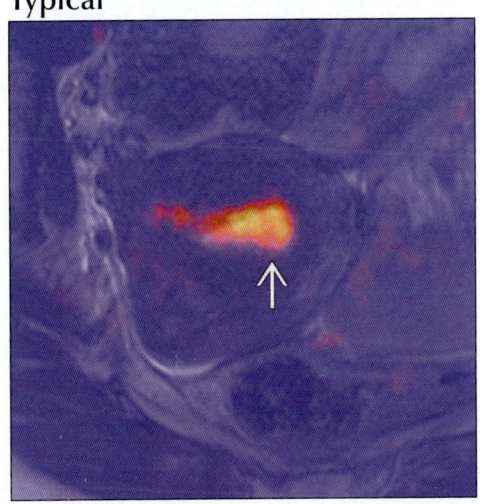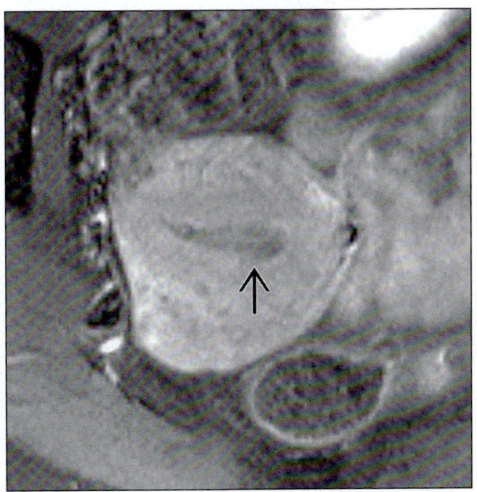

(Left) Axial DWI B800 image fused with the T2WI at the same level as previous image indicates highly cellular tissue penetrating into the inner myometrium dorsally ➡. (Courtesy A. Padhani, MD). (Right) Axial T1 C+ FS MR in the same patient shows the endometrial carcinoma with superficial myometrial invasion dorsally ➡. (Courtesy A. Padhani, MD).

ENDOMETRIAL CANCER, LATE STAGE

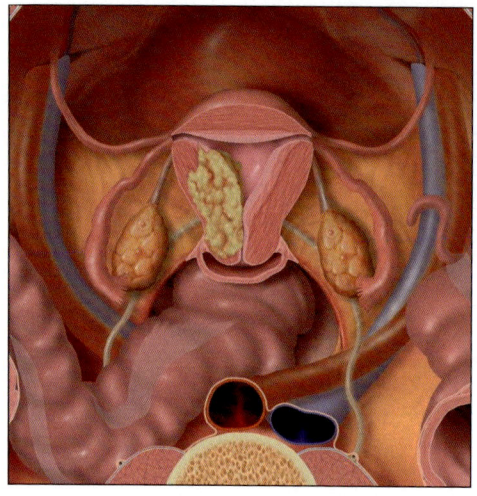

Coronal graphic shows a mass arising from the endometrium. The mass extends to the outer half of the myometrium and involves the cervical stroma, consistent with a stage IIB carcinoma.

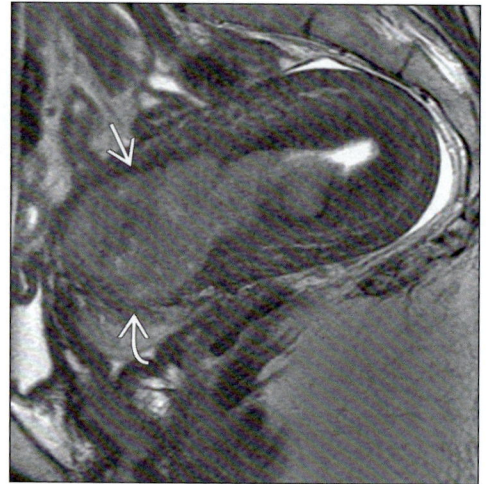

Sagittal T2WI MR shows a lobulated endometrial mass invading the outer half of the myometrium ➡ in the lower uterine segment as well as the cervical stroma ➡ (stage IIB carcinoma).

TERMINOLOGY

Abbreviations and Synonyms
- Uterine carcinoma, endometrial carcinoma

Definitions
- Endometrial carcinoma extending to outer half of myometrium (FIGO stage IC), cervix (FIGO stage II) or beyond uterus (FIGO stage III/IV)

IMAGING FINDINGS

General Features
- Best diagnostic clue: Endometrial mass involving outer half of myometrium (≥ 50% thickness), cervix, or extending beyond uterus
- Morphology: Homogeneous, infiltrative mass
- Critical to differentiate early endometrial carcinoma (stage IA/IB) from late disease (stage IC and beyond)
- Significant risk of malignant lymphadenopathy
  - 10-20% with grade 1-2 adenocarcinoma
  - 40% with grade 3 adenocarcinoma

- CT/MR modalities of choice for detection of lymphadenopathy (accuracy 60-90%)
  - Lymph nodes defined as pathologic as follows
    - Oval nodes ≥ 1.0 cm short-axis
    - Round nodes ≥ 0.8 cm diameter
    - Node signal/enhancement not predictive of metastatic involvement
    - Skip metastases to paraaortic nodes without pelvic lymphadenopathy via ovarian lymphatics

Ultrasonographic Findings
- Grayscale Ultrasound
  - Accuracy for predicting stage IC: 65-85% using transvaginal ultrasound (TVS)
    - Tendency to overstage
    - Decreased accuracy with advanced disease and bulky tumors
  - Accuracy for predicting stage II: 30-75%
    - Able to differentiate cervical stromal invasion from polypoid extension into endocervical canal
    - Tendency to understage
    - Best accuracy with dedicated TVS and/or transrectal ultrasound of cervix

DDx: Endometrial Carcinoma Staging Errors

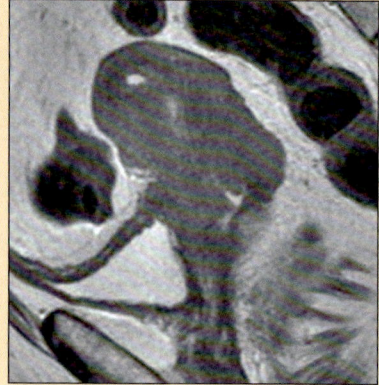

Cervical Carcinoma

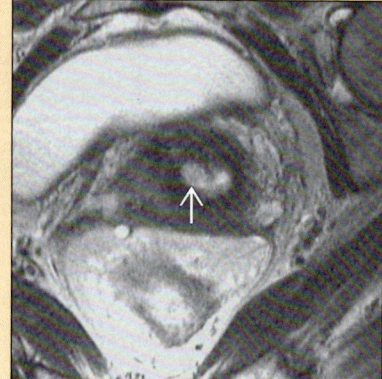

Cervical Polyp

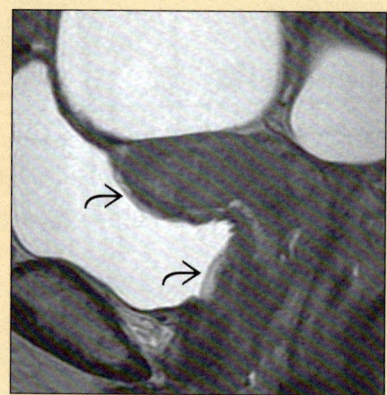

Bullous Edema

ENDOMETRIAL CANCER, LATE STAGE

Key Facts

Terminology
- Endometrial carcinoma extending to outer half of myometrium (FIGO stage IC), cervix (FIGO stage II) or beyond uterus (FIGO stage III/IV)

Imaging Findings
- Best diagnostic clue: Endometrial mass involving outer half of myometrium (≥ 50% thickness), cervix, or extending beyond uterus
- Critical to differentiate early endometrial carcinoma (stage IA/IB) from late disease (stage IC and beyond)
- Significant risk of malignant lymphadenopathy
- High resolution T2WI MR and C+ MR most accurate for local staging and treatment planning
- CT and MR equally accurate for assessment of pelvic and paraaortic lymph nodes

Top Differential Diagnoses
- Uterine Sarcomas
- Cervical Carcinoma
- Staging Errors

Pathology
- Worse prognosis with grade III endometrioid, papillary serous and clear cell carcinomas

Diagnostic Checklist
- Tumor extending to outer myometrium with complete disruption of JZ indicates stage IC disease
- Disruption of normal low SI of cervical fibrous stroma indicates stage IIB disease

---

- ○ Accuracy for predicting stage III: TVS limited for detection of extension beyond uterus

CT Findings
- CECT
  - ○ Low accuracy (45-75%) for stage IC/II
  - ○ Non-specific hypodense uterine-based mass
  - ○ Intact band of subendometrial enhancement on arterial phase excludes deep myometrial invasion
  - ○ Loss of fat planes with extra-uterine extension
  - ○ Adnexal enlargement
  - ○ Useful for detection of lymphadenopathy, peritoneal or distant metastases

MR Findings
- T1WI
  - ○ Detection of hematometra and lymphadenopathy
  - ○ Loss of fat planes with extra-uterine extension
- T2WI
  - ○ Stage IC: Tumor extends into myometrium ≥ 50%
    - Full thickness disruption of junctional zone (JZ)
    - Intact JZ excludes deep myometrial invasion
    - Intact stripe of normal outer myometrium
    - Accuracy: 80-95%
  - ○ Stage II: Tumor extends to cervix
    - IIA: Widening of internal os and endocervical canal
    - IIB: Disruption of normal low signal intensity (SI) cervical fibrous stroma
    - Accuracy: 75-95%
  - ○ Stage III/IV: Extension beyond uterus
    - IIIA: Irregular uterine contour, disruption of low SI serosa by high signal intensity tumor, heterogeneous ± enlarged adnexa
    - IIIB: Segmental loss of hypointense vaginal wall
    - IIIC: Pelvic and/or para-aortic lymphadenopathy
    - IVA: Disruption of normal low SI of bladder or rectal wall, destruction of mucosa with intraluminal mass
- DWI
  - ○ Increased tumor cellularity results in greater water restriction relative to myometrium
    - Lower apparent diffusion coefficient (ADC) values, corresponding to high signal intensity on magnitude high b-value images
- T1 C+ FS
  - ○ Stage IC: Band of early subendometrial enhancement excludes deep myometrial invasion (FIGO stage IC)
  - ○ Stage II: Disruption of normal enhancement of cervical mucosa by low SI tumor on early dynamic C+ MR

Nuclear Medicine Findings
- PET: F-18 FDG PET is useful in detecting metastases and surveillance for recurrent disease

Imaging Recommendations
- Best imaging tool
  - ○ High resolution T2WI MR and C+ MR most accurate for local staging and treatment planning
  - ○ CT and MR equally accurate for assessment of pelvic and paraaortic lymph nodes
    - Improved sensitivity for lymph node metastases with USPIO (ultrasmall superparamagnetic iron oxide)-enhanced MR or F-18 FDG PET
- Protocol advice
  - ○ High-resolution pelvic MR with phased-array coil, 4-5 mm slice thickness
    - Axial T1WI with larger field-of-view (FOV) from pelvis to renal hila for lymph nodes
    - Axial, sagittal and coronal (short-axis) T2WI with small FOV
    - Sagittal and coronal (short-axis) dynamic T1WI C+ FS with small FOV (optimal contrast at 2 minutes)

DIFFERENTIAL DIAGNOSIS

Uterine Sarcomas
- Typically more heterogeneous, large and aggressive
- May contain microscopic fat
- Gross intravascular tumor extension, and spread along ligaments and fallopian tubes

ENDOMETRIAL CANCER, LATE STAGE

Cervical Carcinoma
- Invasion of myometrium from cervix
- Endometrial carcinoma: Invasion of myometrium from endometrium

Staging Errors
- Stage IC staging errors: JZ not visualized, bulky tumor/hematometra, adenomyosis
- Stage II staging errors: Polypoid tumor extending to endocervical canal without invasion, cervical polyp/nabothian cysts, cervical gland hyperplasia
- Stage III/IV: Disease confined to muscle layer of rectum/bladder with overlying bullous edema of mucosa

PATHOLOGY

General Features
- General path comments
  - Adenocarcinoma most common histological type
  - Prognosis varies with stage, tumor grade and histology
- Genetics
  - Rare hereditary form: Lynch II family cancer syndrome
    - Nonpolyposis colorectal cancer, ovarian and endometrial cancer
- Etiology: Unopposed estrogen action on hormonally responsive endometrium: Endometrial hyperplasia-carcinoma sequence
- Associated abnormalities: Endometrial hyperplasia (20-40%)

Gross Pathologic & Surgical Features
- Accuracy of predicting deep myometrial invasion on gross inspection: 75-85%; accuracy falls to 30% with grade III tumors

Microscopic Features
- 75% endometrioid; serous, mucinous, clear cell, squamous less common
  - Worse prognosis with grade III endometrioid, papillary serous and clear cell carcinomas
    - Peritoneal spread and lymphovascular space invasion more common

Staging, Grading or Classification Criteria
- Grade I-III: Well, moderate and poorly-differentiated
- Stage IC: Invasion of outer half of myometrium (≥ 50% thickness)
- Stage II: Tumor invading cervix
  - IIA: Endocervical glandular involvement
  - IIB: Cervical stromal involvement
- Stage III: Tumor extending beyond uterus but not outside true pelvis
  - IIIA: Invasion of serosa, adnexa or positive peritoneal cytology
  - IIIB: Vaginal involvement
  - IIIC: Metastases to pelvic or paraaortic lymph nodes
- Stage IV: Adjacent organ invasion or distant metastases
  - IVA: Invasion of bladder or bowel mucosa
  - IVB: Distant metastases including intraabdominal and inguinal lymph nodes

CLINICAL ISSUES

Presentation
- Most common signs/symptoms: Postmenopausal bleeding

Demographics
- Age: 6th to 7th decade, postmenopausal

Natural History & Prognosis
- 5-yr survival: 80-85% stage IC, 70-80% stage II, 15-40% stage III-IV
- Papillary serous and clear-cell carcinomas most commonly related to peritoneal spread
- Lung most common site for hematogenous metastases

Treatment
- Multidisciplinary approach depending on stage and histology
  - Total abdominal hysterectomy, bilateral salpingo-oophorectomy, and lymph node sampling
  - Radiation ± chemotherapy

DIAGNOSTIC CHECKLIST

Consider
- MR for local staging and treatment planning
- CT for advanced cases with distant metastases
- Imaging studies should be directed to determine the following prognostic factors
  - Depth of myometrial invasion
  - Stage of disease
  - Presence of lymphadenopathy

Image Interpretation Pearls
- Tumor extending to outer myometrium with complete disruption of JZ indicates stage IC disease
- Disruption of normal low SI of cervical fibrous stroma indicates stage IIB disease

SELECTED REFERENCES

1. Chao A et al: 18F-FDG PET in the management of endometrial cancer. Eur J Nucl Med Mol Imaging. 33(1):36-44, 2006
2. Nakao Y et al: MR imaging in endometrial carcinoma as a diagnostic tool for the absence of myometrial invasion. Gynecol Oncol. 102(2):343-7, 2006
3. Chaudhry S et al: Benign and malignant diseases of the endometrium. Top Magn Reson Imaging. 14(4):339-57, 2003
4. Ascher SM et al: Imaging of cancer of the endometrium. Radiol Clin North Am. 40(3):563-76, 2002
5. Hernandez E: Endometrial adenocarcinoma: a primer for the generalist. Obstet Gynecol Clin North Am. 28(4):743-57, 2001
6. Hardesty LA et al: Use of preoperative MR imaging in the management of endometrial carcinoma: cost analysis. Radiology. 215(1):45-9, 2000

ENDOMETRIAL CANCER, LATE STAGE

IMAGE GALLERY

Typical

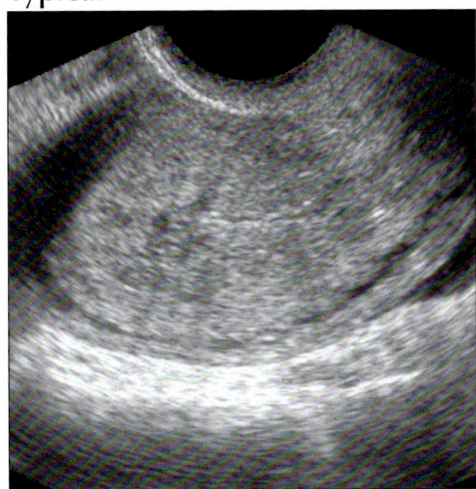
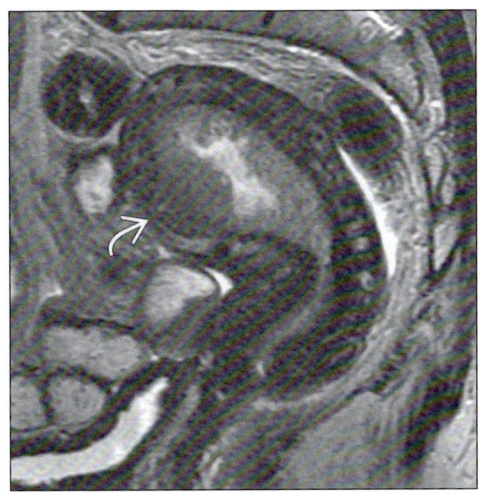

(Left) Sagittal transvaginal ultrasound shows a slightly heterogeneous echogenic mass. The depth of myometrial invasion is difficult to ascertain but the appearance is suspicious for deep invasion. (Right) Sagittal T2WI MR in the same patient as previous image, shows no or minimal myometrial invasion dorsally, while a focus of deep myometrial invasion � (stage IC) is present ventrally.

Typical

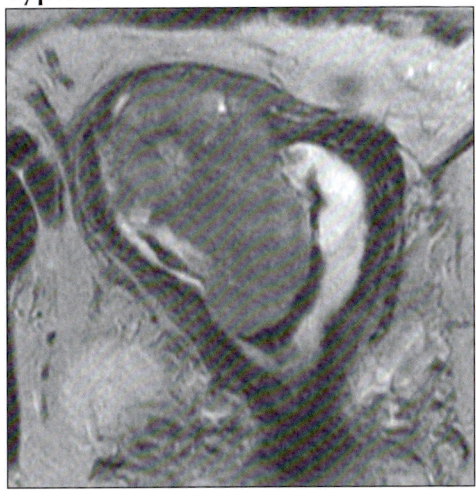
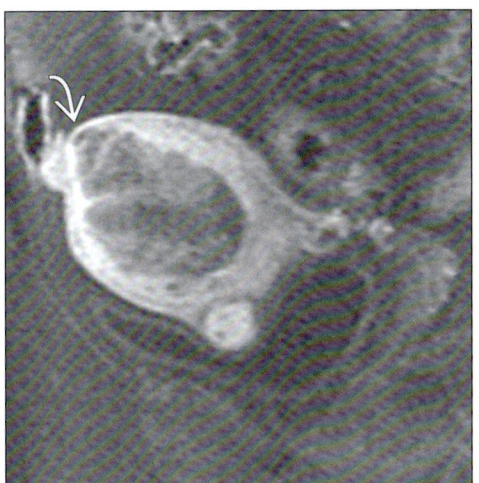

(Left) Axial T2WI MR shows a large mass filling the right horn of a subseptate uterus. Due to compression of the myometrium it is difficult to distinguish between a stage IB or IC tumor. (Right) Sagittal T1 C+ FS MR in the same patient as previous image, shows to better advantage the extension of the tumor to the outer half � (stage IC), with only a thin rim of intact overlying myometrium.

Typical

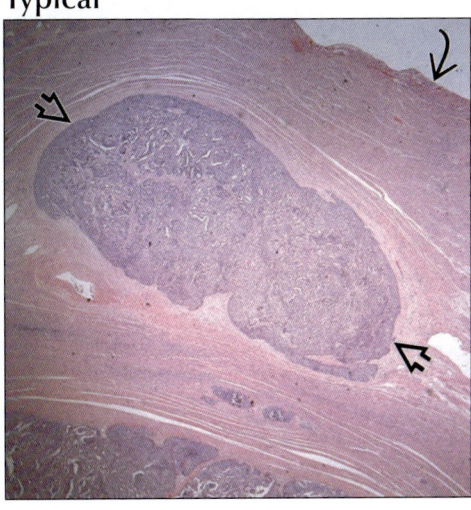
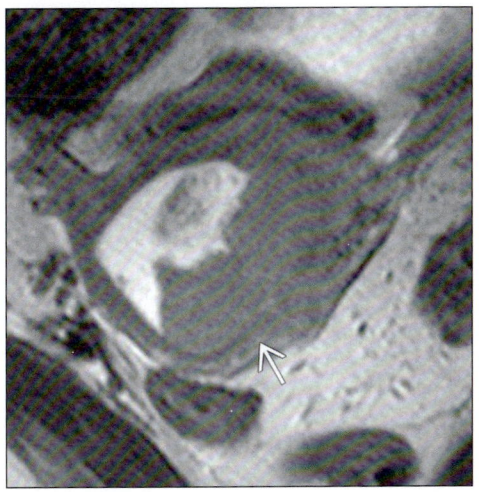

(Left) Micropathology of the hysterectomy specimen of the previous image, shows deep myometrial invasion by the endometrial carcinoma � to within 2 mm of the serosal surface �. (Right) Axial T2WI MR shows an endometrial mass with complete disruption of the junctional zone � (stage IC tumor). The exact extent of tumor invasion remains unclear. (Courtesy A. Padhani, MD).

ENDOMETRIAL CANCER, LATE STAGE

(Left) Axial DWI B800 image fused with the T2WI at the same level indicates highly cellular tissue penetrating almost to the level of the serosa posterolateral. Same patient as previous image. (Courtesy A. Padhani, MD). (Right) Axial T1 C+ FS MR in the same patient as previous image confirms the deep myometrial penetration with a rim of intact overlying myometrium ➔. (Courtesy A. Padhani, MD).

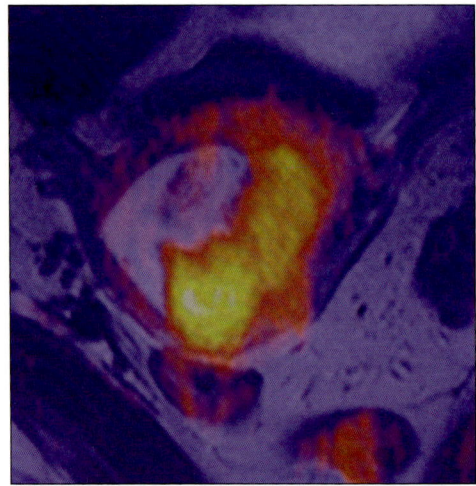
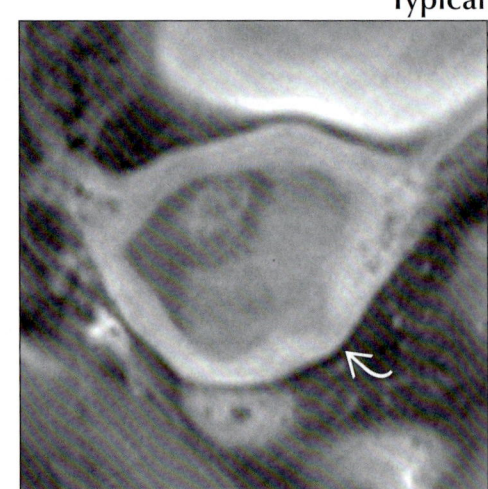

Typical

(Left) Sagittal T2WI MR shows an endometrial-based mass extending into the outer half of the myometrium ➔. A nonspecific area of intermediate signal is present within the cervical canal ➔. (Right) Sagittal T1 C+ FS MR in the same patient as previous image, shows the normal enhancing cervical mucosa ➔ thereby excluding invasion of the endocervix. Note again the deep myometrial invasion.

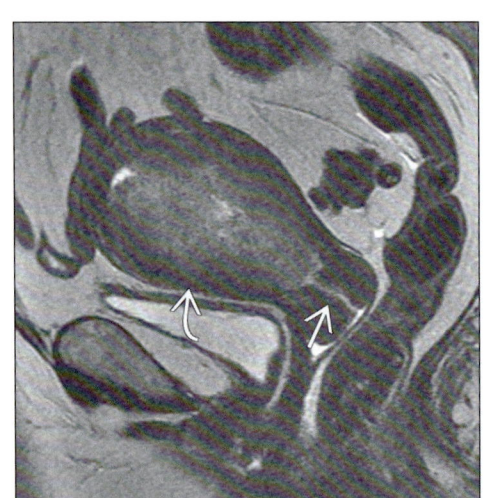
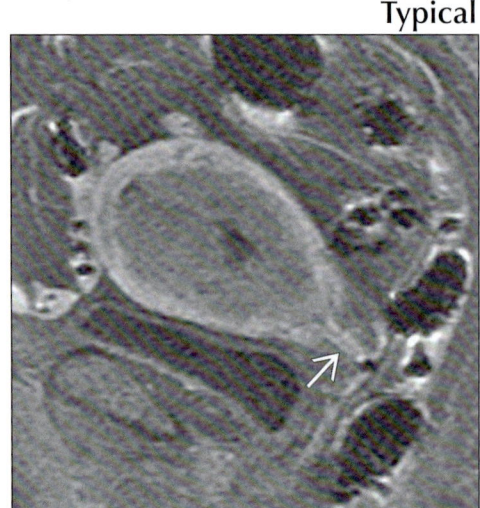

Typical

(Left) Sagittal T2WI MR shows focal endometrial thickening with abnormal hypointense signal in the lower uterine segment. The abnormal signal appears to extend into the upper cervix ➔. (Right) Sagittal T1 C+ FS MR in the same patient as previous image, shows interruption ➔ of the enhancing endocervical mucosa ➔ consistent with cervical invasion (proven stage IIB).

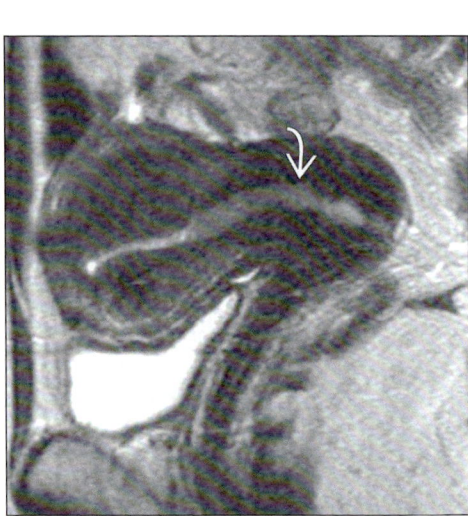
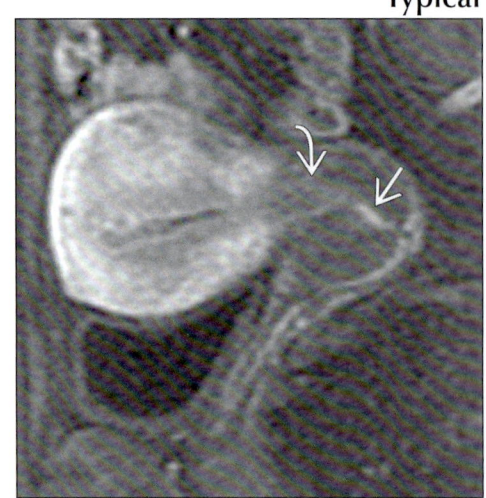

Typical

ENDOMETRIAL CANCER, LATE STAGE

Typical

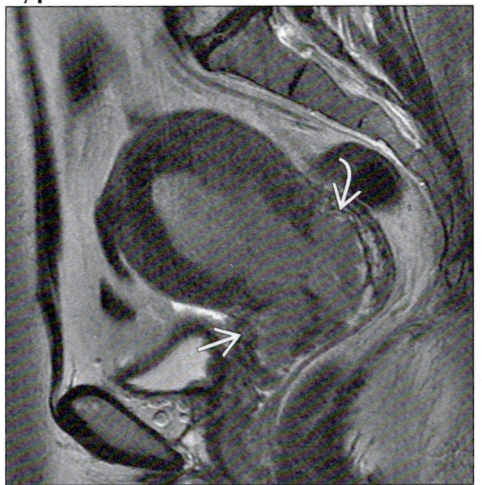
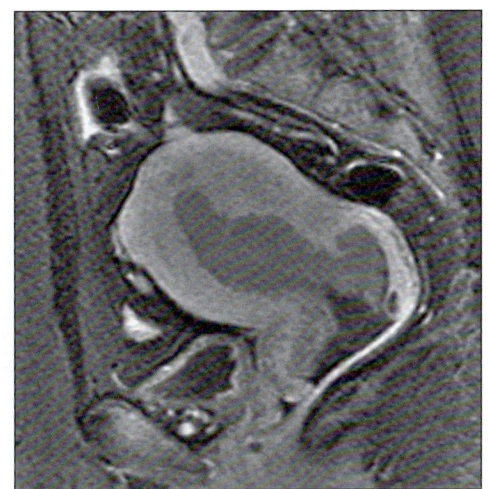

(Left) Sagittal T2WI MR shows an endometrial mass confined to the inner half of the myometrium with invasion of the cervical fibrous stroma ventrally ➔ and dorsally ➔ (proven stage IIB). *(Right)* Sagittal T1 C+ FS MR in the same patient as previous image, shows again the invasion of the ventral and dorsal cervix.

Typical

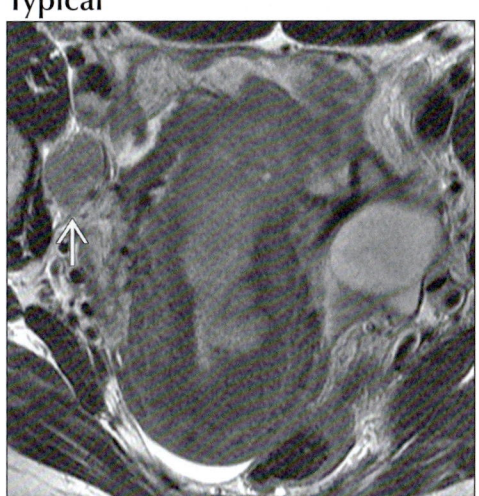
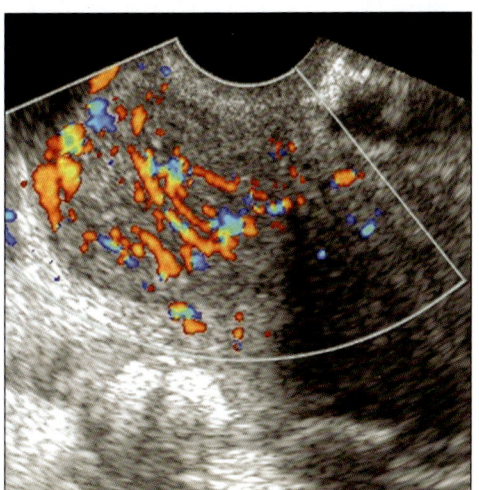

(Left) Axial T2WI MR shows an enlarged right external iliac lymph node ➔ in a patient with a stage IIIC endometrial carcinoma also invading the cervix. *(Right)* Sagittal oblique color Doppler ultrasound in the same patient as previous image, shows marked vascularity of the cervical mass secondary to cervical invasion of the endometrial carcinoma.

Typical

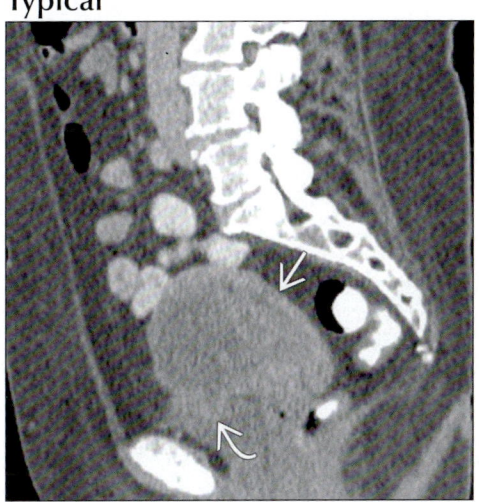
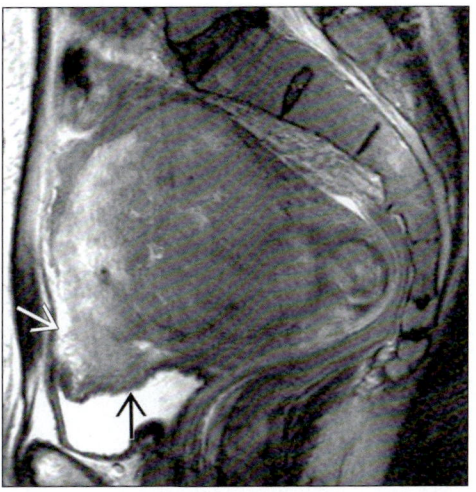

(Left) Sagittal CECT shows a large, heterogeneous, hypodense mass ➔ replacing the uterus with direct invasion into the urinary bladder resulting in a polypoid intraluminal mass ➔ (stage IVA). *(Right)* Sagittal T2WI MR shows a large mass extending beyond the serosal surface of the uterus ➔. There is invasion of the muscular layer ➔ of the urinary bladder but no mucosal involvement.

ENDOMETRIAL CANCER, RECURRENCE

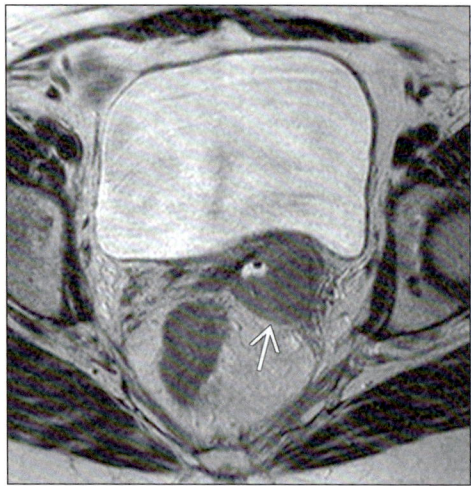

Axial T2WI MR shows a vaginal vault mass ➡ of intermediate signal intensity in a patient with previous hysterectomy for endometrial carcinoma. This mass was proven to be a recurrence.

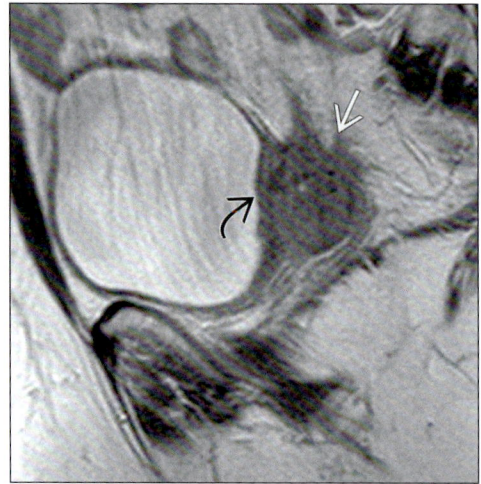

Sagittal T2WI MR in the same patient shows the spiculated ➡ superior border of the mass, as well as absence of a fat plane ➡ between the recurrence and the bladder wall indicating bladder wall invasion.

TERMINOLOGY

Abbreviations and Synonyms
- Endometrial carcinoma recurrence, uterine carcinoma recurrence, endometrial cancer relapse

Definitions
- Regrowth of endometrial carcinoma after apparent complete remission for at least 6 months following primary treatment
- Local recurrence: Tumor regrowth anywhere in the pelvis or lymph nodes below pelvic brim
- Distant metastases: Tumor regrowth anywhere else

IMAGING FINDINGS

General Features
- Best diagnostic clue: Growing pelvic mass in a patient with prior endometrial carcinoma
- Location
  - Most common sites of local recurrence
    - Vaginal vault
    - Central pelvic mass
    - Pelvic lymph nodes (pelvic sidewall mass)
    - Abdominal wall incision
  - Most common sites of distant recurrence
    - Lung
    - Liver
    - Omentum
    - Peritoneum
    - Gastrointestinal tract
    - Extra-pelvic lymph nodes (para-aortic, groin, mediastinal, axillary, supraclavicular)
    - Rarely adrenals, breast, brain, bone, skin, spleen
  - If uterus still present, parenchymal mass ± enlarged fluid-filled uterus (hematometra or hydrometra)
- Size: Variable
- Morphology
  - Well-defined focal or ill-defined infiltrative mass
  - Variable amount of necrosis

Ultrasonographic Findings
- Grayscale Ultrasound
  - TVS may demonstrate vaginal vault recurrence
  - Hypoechogenic solid mass

DDx: Endometrial Carcinoma Recurrence

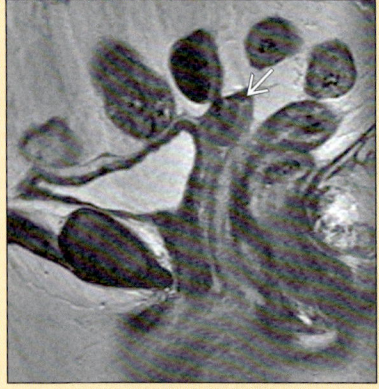

Post-Surgical Granuloma

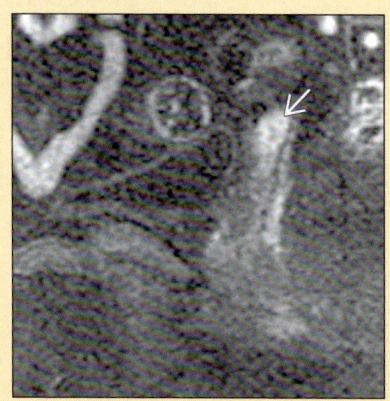

Post-Surgical Granuloma

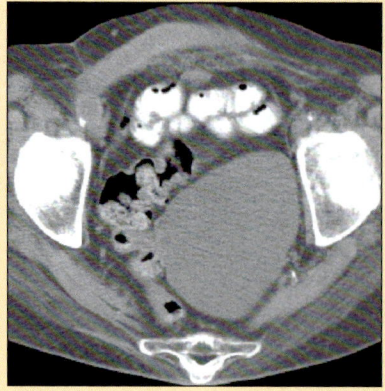

Pelvic Lymphocele

ENDOMETRIAL CANCER, RECURRENCE

Key Facts

Terminology
- Regrowth of endometrial carcinoma after apparent complete remission for at least 6 months following primary treatment
- Local recurrence: Tumor regrowth anywhere in the pelvis or lymph nodes below pelvic brim
- Distant metastases: Tumor regrowth anywhere else

Imaging Findings
- Best diagnostic clue: Growing pelvic mass in a patient with prior endometrial carcinoma
- Intermediate/high signal intensity of recurrent mass
- Areas of very bright signal corresponding to underlying necrosis

Top Differential Diagnoses
- Post-Surgical Changes
- Post-Radiation Therapy Changes
- Lymphocele

Diagnostic Checklist
- FDG PET most sensitive post-therapy surveillance modality
- For suspected local recurrence, MR is the most accurate modality
- Any nodular or irregular thickening of vaginal vault after surgery or newly appearing soft tissue mass is suspicious for recurrence
- CT should be obtained in all patients with local recurrence to look for concomitant distant disease or complications associated with recurrence

---

  - Less sensitive than CT and MR for deep pelvic recurrence, lymph node recurrence, peritoneal or omental recurrence

CT Findings
- Well defined or ill-defined, central soft tissue density pelvic mass
- On CECT, mass can be partly hypodense in keeping with foci of necrosis
- Lymph node enlargement, either pelvic or para-aortic
- Additional findings: Liver metastases, omental cake, ascites, peritoneal implants
- Chest CT: Lung metastases, mediastinal, axillary or supraclavicular lymph nodes
- CT also useful in demonstrating complications associated with recurrence
  - Hydronephrosis due to ureteral encasement
  - Small or large bowel obstruction
  - Fistulae
  - Vascular invasion/encasement

MR Findings
- T1WI
  - Intermediate signal intensity mass
  - Well-defined or infiltrative
- T2WI
  - Intermediate/high signal intensity of recurrent mass
  - Areas of very bright signal corresponding to underlying necrosis
  - Intermediate signal intensity septations, mural nodules, in partially necrotic recurrences
- T1 C+
  - Variable degree of enhancement, similar to primary tumor
  - Usually mildly vascular mass on early arterial phase, shows progressive enhancement
  - Absence of enhancement in necrotic areas

Nuclear Medicine Findings
- PET
  - Increased uptake of recurrent endometrial carcinoma on FDG PET, either local or distant
  - F18-FDG sensitivity 96-100%, specificity 78-88%

Imaging Recommendations
- Best imaging tool
  - MR excellent imaging modality when suspicion of local recurrence after surgery
  - MR most accurate modality to differentiate post-surgical changes from recurrence
  - CT best imaging modality for distant metastases
  - FDG PET highly sensitive for post-therapy surveillance

DIFFERENTIAL DIAGNOSIS

Post-Surgical Changes
- Late fibrosis (≥ 1 year after treatment): Low signal intensity on T1WI and T2WI, hypovascular
- Early fibrosis (≤ 6 months after treatment) may be high signal intensity on T2WI and be indistinguishable from recurrence; intense early enhancement favors granulation tissue

Post-Radiation Therapy Changes
- Often linear rather than nodular soft tissue stranding
- Mass with concave outer borders
- Low signal intensity T2WI and T1 C+ in late fibrosis
- T2WI higher signal intensity in early fibrosis can mimic recurrence, owing to inflammatory reaction and necrosis

Lymphocele
- Fluid signal intensity mass
- Can mimic cystic recurrence
- No enhancement, thin wall, absence of enhancing wall/nodularity

PATHOLOGY

General Features
- General path comments
  - Risk factors for recurrence
    - Age ≥ 60

ENDOMETRIAL CANCER, RECURRENCE

- High histologic grade of primary tumor
- Papillary serous and clear cell histologic subtypes (non-endometrioid)
- Lymphovascular invasion
- Extension to cervix
- Deep myometrial invasion (≥ 50%)
- Lymph node involvement
- Positive peritoneal cytology
- Local recurrence itself is a risk factor for distant metastases
  - Four patterns of recurrence
    - Direct extension
    - Lymphatic invasion
    - Peritoneal metastases (transtubal egress)
    - Hematogenous metastases (lungs)
  - Vaginal recurrence more frequent when primary treatment was surgery only
  - Distant recurrence most common in patients treated primarily by surgery and radiation therapy
  - The earlier a local recurrence, the more likely a distant metastasis will occur
- Etiology
  - Implantation of neoplastic cells in the vaginal vault at time of surgery
  - Retrograde lymphatic spread
  - Venous spread
- Epidemiology
  - 15-20% of patients treated for endometrial carcinoma eventually develop recurrence
  - Incidence decreasing with adjuvant radiation therapy, mostly with brachytherapy
  - 90% of recurrences occur within 3 years of primary therapy
    - 50% pelvic, 50% distant

CLINICAL ISSUES

Presentation
- Most common signs/symptoms
  - Asymptomatic
  - Vaginal bleeding
  - Pelvic or low back pain

Natural History & Prognosis
- Depends on type of recurrence, tumor volume, disease-free interval and treatment
- Best prognosis for isolated vaginal cuff recurrence treated with radiotherapy: 60-70% 5 year survival rate
- Other pelvic or distant recurrence: 8-14% 5 year survival rate

Treatment
- External beam radiation therapy for loco-regional recurrence, vaginal brachytherapy or both
- Targeted radiation therapy and cytotoxic chemotherapy for systemic recurrence
- Pelvic exenteration if previous irradiation, or cytoreduction surgery
- Progestagens for palliative purposes (mean duration of response 10-12 months)

DIAGNOSTIC CHECKLIST

Consider
- FDG PET most sensitive post-therapy surveillance modality
- For suspected local recurrence, MR is the most accurate modality
- Any nodular or irregular thickening of vaginal vault after surgery or newly appearing soft tissue mass is suspicious for recurrence
- CT should be obtained in all patients with local recurrence to look for concomitant distant disease or complications associated with recurrence

Image Interpretation Pearls
- MR highly accurate for differentiating recurrence from late fibrosis
- Early (≤ 6 months) post-surgical or post-radiation fibrosis can mimic recurrence

SELECTED REFERENCES

1. Chao A et al: 18F-FDG PET in the management of endometrial cancer. Eur J Nucl Med Mol Imaging. 33(1):36-44, 2006
2. Kinkel K: Pitfalls in staging uterine neoplasm with imaging: a review. Abdom Imaging. 31(2):164-73, 2006
3. Lin LL et al: Definitive radiotherapy in the management of isolated vaginal recurrences of endometrial cancer. Int J Radiat Oncol Biol Phys. 63(2):500-4, 2005
4. Manfredi R et al: Endometrial cancer: magnetic resonance imaging. Abdom Imaging. 30(5):626-36, 2005
5. Mariani A et al: Predictors of vaginal relapse in stage I endometrial cancer. Gynecol Oncol. 97(3):820-7, 2005
6. Shah C et al: Does size matter? Tumor size and morphology as predictors of nodal status and recurrence in endometrial cancer. Gynecol Oncol. 99(3):564-70, 2005
7. Kao MS: Management of recurrent endometrial carcinoma. Chang Gung Med J. 27(9):639-45, 2004
8. Saga T et al: Clinical value of FDG-PET in the follow up of post-operative patients with endometrial cancer. Ann Nucl Med. 17(3):197-203, 2003
9. Mariani A et al: Hematogenous dissemination in corpus cancer. Gynecol Oncol. 80(2):233-8, 2001
10. Kinkel K et al: Differentiation between recurrent tumor and benign conditions after treatment of gynecologic pelvic carcinoma: value of dynamic contrast-enhanced subtraction MR imaging. Radiology. 204(1):55-63, 1997
11. Mayr NA et al: Postoperative radiation therapy in clinical stage I endometrial cancer: corpus, cervical, and lower uterine segment involvement--patterns of failure. Radiology. 196(2):323-8, 1995
12. Morgan JD 3rd et al: Isolated vaginal recurrences of endometrial carcinoma. Radiology. 189(2):609-13, 1993
13. Ebner F et al: Tumor recurrence versus fibrosis in the female pelvis: differentiation with MR imaging at 1.5 T. Radiology. 166(2):333-40, 1988
14. Walsh JW et al: Computed tomography of primary, persistent, and recurrent endometrial malignancy. AJR Am J Roentgenol. 139(6):1149-54, 1982
15. Reddy S et al: Pattern of recurrences in endometrial carcinoma and their management. Radiology. 133(3 Pt 1):737-40, 1979

ENDOMETRIAL CANCER, RECURRENCE

IMAGE GALLERY

Typical

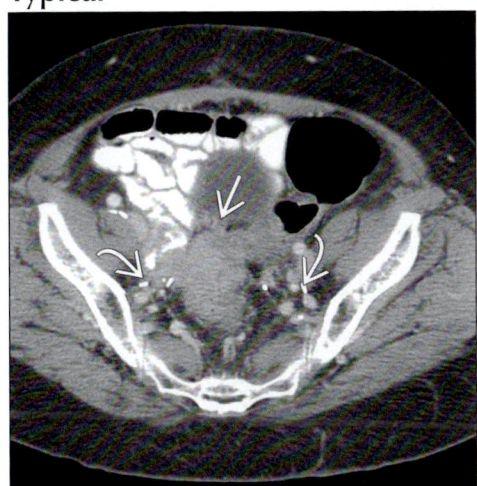 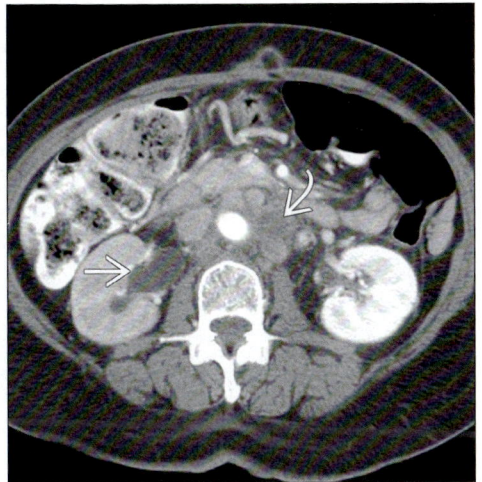

(Left) Axial CECT shows an ill-defined infiltrative central pelvic mass ➔ extending towards the right iliac vessels and ureter. There are iliac clips from a previous iliac lymphadenectomy ➔. (Right) Axial CECT shows multiple enlarged paraaortic lymph nodes, one of them being necrotic ➔. There is right hydronephrosis ➔ secondary to ureteral invasion by the pelvic mass.

Variant

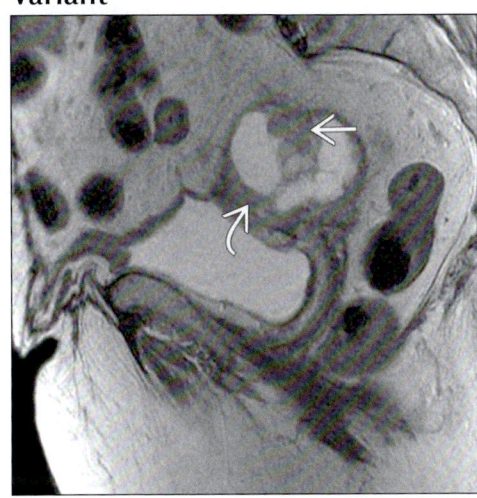 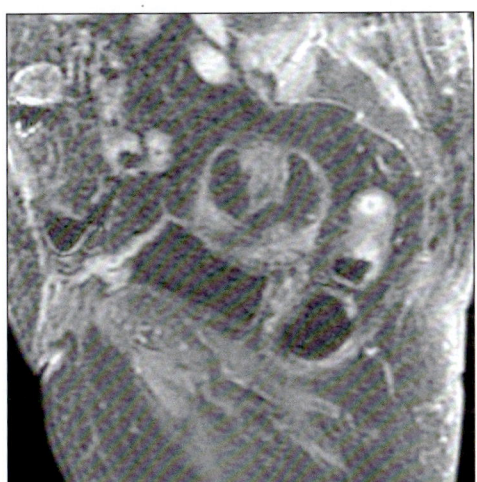

(Left) Sagittal T2WI MR shows a high signal intensity vaginal vault mass with a thick, irregular inferior wall ➔ and internal nodularities of intermediate signal intensity ➔. (Right) Sagittal T1 C+ FS MR shows enhancement of the mural nodules and wall of the mass, the center being necrotic. This is consistent with a partly necrotic endometrial carcinoma recurrence.

Variant

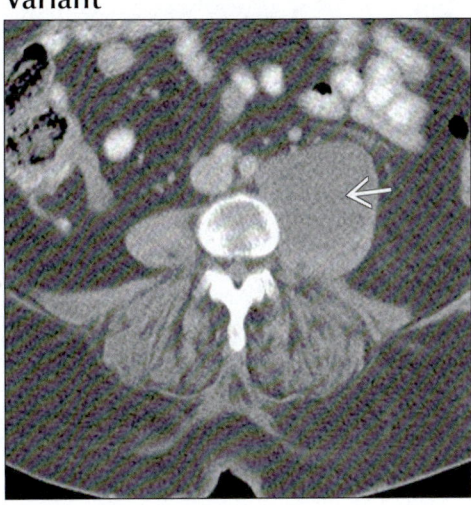 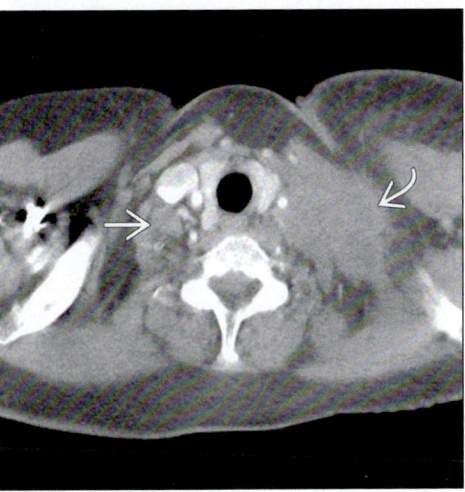

(Left) Axial CECT shows a large hypodense psoas mass ➔ in a patient with previous endometrial carcinoma which proved to be a recurrence. (Right) Axial CECT shows an infiltrating left supraclavicular mass ➔ encasing the left common carotid artery associated with enlarged right internal jugular nodes ➔.

ENDOMETRIAL CANCER, RECURRENCE

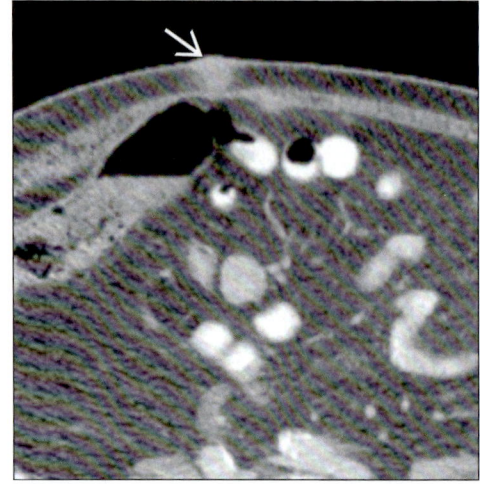 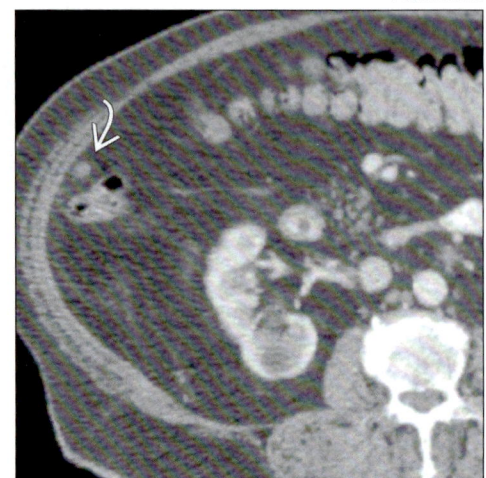

(Left) Axial CECT shows a soft tissue nodule in the umbilicus ➡ which was biopsied and proved to be an endometrial carcinoma recurrence (Sister Marie Joseph nodule). (Right) Axial CECT in the same patient as previous image shows a small right paracolic gutter peritoneal implant ➡.

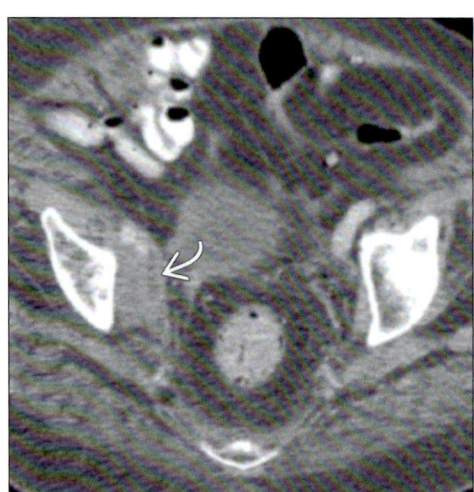 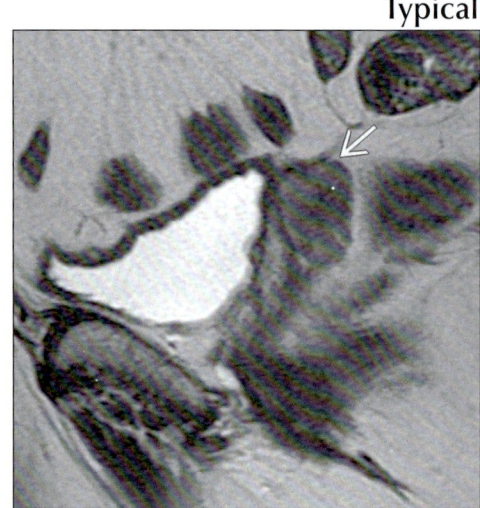

(Left) Axial CECT in the same patient as previous image shows a right pelvic sidewall mass ➡ which proved to be a local recurrence. The mass is encasing the right iliac vessels as well as ureter. (Right) Sagittal T2WI MR shows an intermediate signal intensity vaginal vault mass ➡ in a patient who had a previous hysterectomy for endometrial carcinoma. It proved to be a pelvic recurrence.

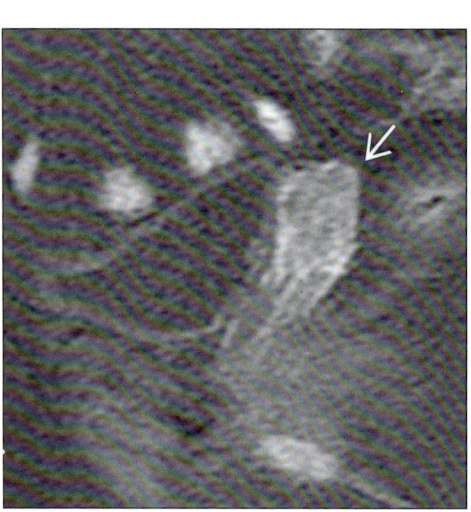 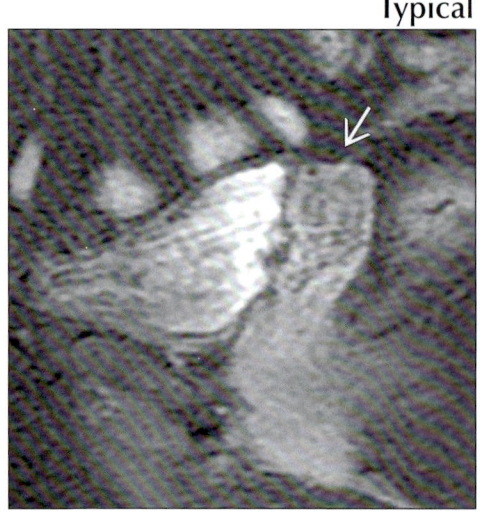

(Left) Sagittal T1 C+ FS MR acquired early after contrast injection in the same patient as previous image shows that the vaginal vault mass is enhancing but hypovascular ➡. (Right) Sagittal T1 C+ FS MR in the same patient as previous image shows that the mass ➡ enhances more intensely on delayed imaging. It was proven to be an endometrial carcinoma recurrence.

ENDOMETRIAL CANCER, RECURRENCE

Typical

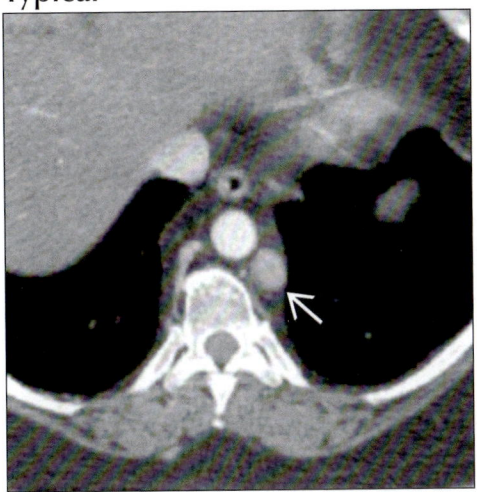
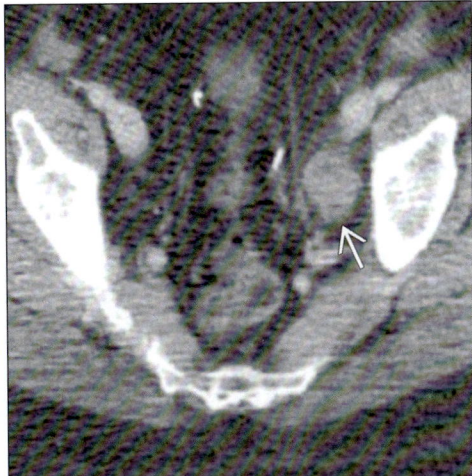

(Left) Axial CECT shows an enlarged left retrocrural lymph node ➔, proven to be recurrent endometrial carcinoma. *(Right)* Axial CECT in the same patient as previous image shows an enlarged, partially necrotic, left external iliac lymph node ➔, also from recurrent endometrial carcinoma.

Typical

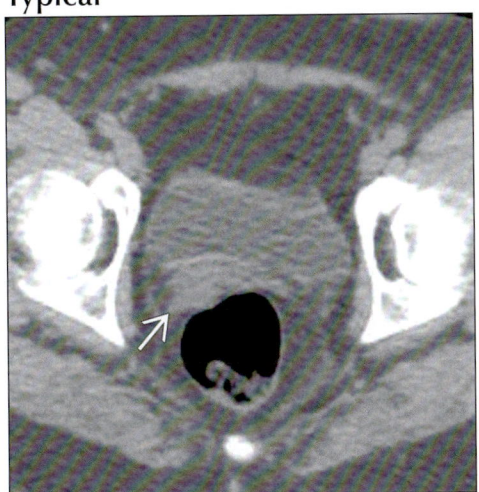
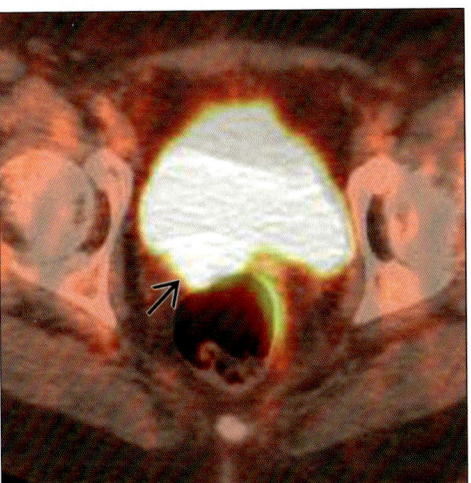

(Left) Axial NECT shows a vaginal cuff mass ➔ in a patient with previous endometrial carcinoma. This acquisition is performed at the same time as the PET scan. *(Right)* Axial fused PET/CT in the same patient as previous image shows hypermetabolic activity of the vaginal cuff mass ➔ consistent with recurrent endometrial carcinoma.

Typical

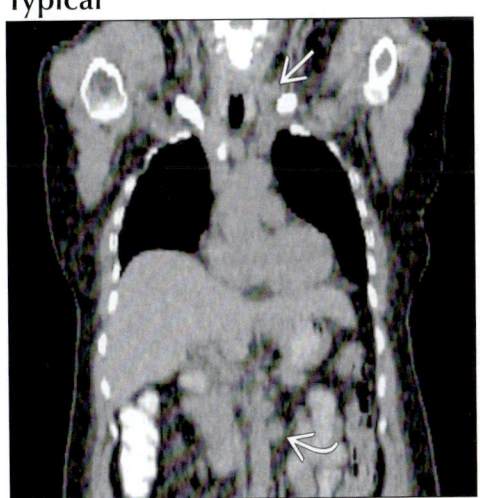
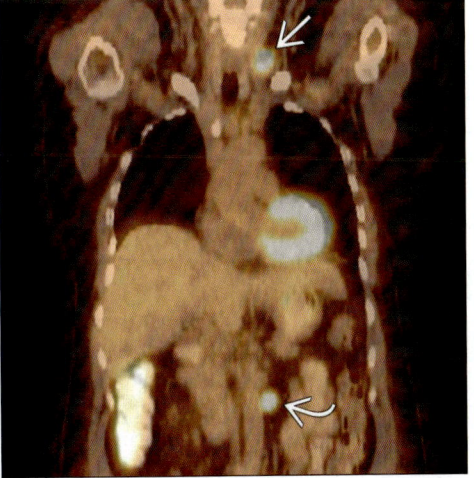

(Left) Coronal NECT shows a left internal jugular node ➔ and a left para-aortic node ➔ in a patient previously treated for endometrial carcinoma. *(Right)* Coronal fused PET/CT in the same patient as previous image shows intense hypermetabolic activity corresponding to the level of the left internal jugular ➔ and left para-aortic node ➔.

ENDOMETRIAL STROMAL SARCOMA

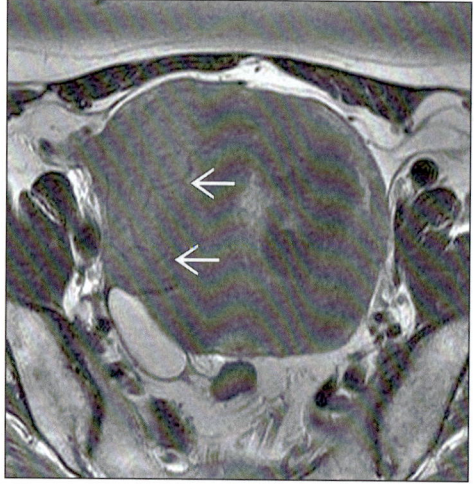

Axial T2WI MR shows an intermediate signal intensity (SI) mass replacing the normal uterus. There are low SI myometrial bands ➔ characteristic of a low grade stromal sarcoma (LGSS).

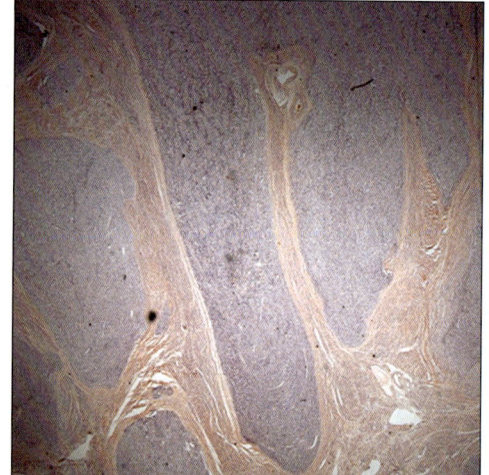

Micropathology of the hysterectomy specimen shows worm-like plugs of tumor (purple) separated by preserved muscle bundles (pink) corresponding to the low signal intensity bands on the T2WI.

TERMINOLOGY

Abbreviations and Synonyms
- Type of a uterine sarcoma

Definitions
- Malignant mesenchymal tumor of endometrium

IMAGING FINDINGS

General Features
- Best diagnostic clue
  - Large, heterogeneous, endometrial-based mass with a predominant myometrial component
  - Spread along fallopian tubes, uterine ligaments and gross intravascular extension
  - Low grade stromal sarcoma (LGSS): Bands of low signal intensity (SI) on T2WI within the area of myometrial invasion
  - High-grade (HGSS): Infiltrative borders with nodular lesions at tumor margin, intramyometrial nodular masses, areas of hemorrhage and necrosis
- Location
  - Arise from the endometrium
  - May be entirely intramyometrial
  - Rarely originate from foci of adenomyosis or endometriosis
- Size: Large, mean size 9 cm
- Morphology
  - Larger and more heterogeneous than endometrial carcinomas
  - Endometrial thickening/polypoid intrauterine mass
  - Ill-defined endo-myometrial junction
  - Myometrial component may be well-circumscribed or infiltrative
  - Overlap between imaging findings of low and high grade tumors
    - LGSS: Tumor confined to endometrium in 50%; myometrial invasion presents as worm-like plugs of tumor separated by preserved muscle bundles (low SI bands on T2WI); cystic degeneration uncommon
    - HGSS: Infiltrative lesions with necrosis and hemorrhage, marginal nodularity and intramyometrial nodules representing intravascular/lymphatic tumor spread

DDx: Uterine Mass

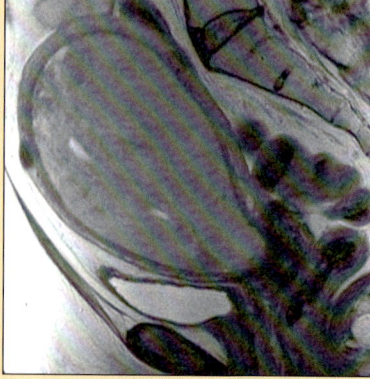

Adenosarcoma

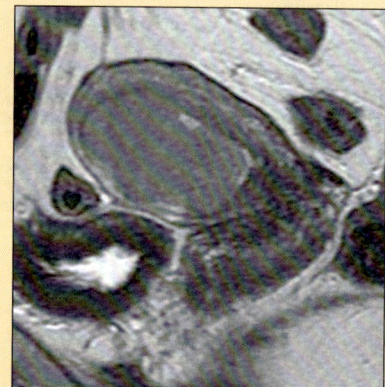

Endometrial Carcinoma

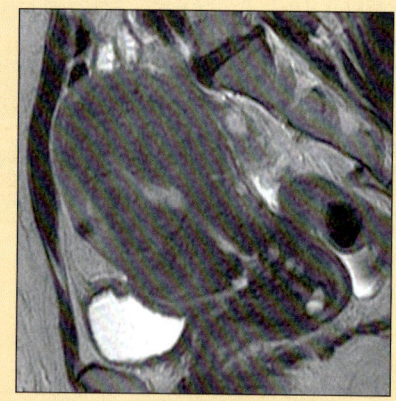

Adenomyosis

ENDOMETRIAL STROMAL SARCOMA

Key Facts

Terminology
- Malignant mesenchymal tumor of endometrium

Imaging Findings
- Large, heterogeneous, endometrial-based mass with a predominant myometrial component
- Spread along fallopian tubes, uterine ligaments and gross intravascular extension
- Low grade stromal sarcoma (LGSS): Bands of low signal intensity (SI) on T2WI within the area of myometrial invasion
- High-grade (HGSS): Infiltrative borders with nodular lesions at tumor margin, intramyometrial nodular masses, areas of hemorrhage and necrosis
- Arise from the endometrium
- Rarely originate from foci of adenomyosis or endometriosis
- High-resolution pelvic MR is modality of choice for diagnosis and local staging

Top Differential Diagnoses
- Endometrial Carcinoma
- Other Uterine Sarcomas
- Degenerated Leiomyoma
- Adenomyosis

Clinical Issues
- Most common between 35-55 years of age

Diagnostic Checklist
- Consider endometrial stromal sarcoma in the differential diagnosis of a heterogeneous, endometrial-based mass with a significant myometrial component

Ultrasonographic Findings
- Grayscale Ultrasound
  - Transvaginal ultrasound (TVS) nonspecific
    - Heterogeneous, mixed echogenicity endometrial-based mass, endo-myometrial thickening, and adnexal masses
- Pulsed Doppler: Low impedance flow
- Color Doppler: Increased vascularity

CT Findings
- NECT
  - Uterine enlargement
  - Spontaneously dense hemorrhagic areas
- CECT
  - Frequently a nonspecific appearance
  - Heterogeneously enhancing mass causing uterine enlargement
    - Strongly enhancing components common
    - Occasional cystic centers in enhancing nodules
  - Loss of pelvic fat planes with extra-uterine extension
  - Useful for detection of lymphadenopathy and distant metastases

MR Findings
- T1WI
  - Homogeneous, low to intermediate SI mass
    - High SI hemorrhagic areas
  - Useful for detection of lymphadenopathy
- T2WI
  - Heterogeneous mass, iso- or slightly hypointense relative to normal endometrium
  - LGSS: Low SI bands reflecting preserved bundles of myometrium between worm-like tumor plugs
  - HGSS: Frequently a nonspecific appearance
    - May present as high SI nodular lesions at tumor margin and myometrial nodules
- T1 C+
  - Heterogeneous enhancement less avid than myometrium
    - Portions of tumor may demonstrate marked enhancement (greater than myometrium)

Imaging Recommendations
- Best imaging tool
  - Role of imaging is to suggest the diagnosis; define disease extent for treatment planning
  - High-resolution pelvic MR is modality of choice for diagnosis and local staging
  - CT can be used in advanced disease with distant spread
- Protocol advice
  - Pelvic MR with phased-array coil, 4-5 mm slice thickness
    - Axial T1WI with larger field-of-view (FOV) from pelvis to renal hila for lymph nodes
    - Axial, sagittal and coronal (short-axis) T2WI with small FOV
    - Sagittal and coronal (short-axis) dynamic T1WI C+ FS with small FOV

DIFFERENTIAL DIAGNOSIS

Endometrial Carcinoma
- Typically smaller than endometrial stromal sarcomas
- More homogeneous with absence of necrosis

Other Uterine Sarcomas
- Difficult to differentiate from endometrial stromal sarcoma

Degenerated Leiomyoma
- Heterogeneous SI and enhancement, with cystic changes
- Persistent areas of low SI intensity on T2WI
- Well-defined borders, absence of invasion

Adenomyosis
- Diffuse or focal thickening of junctional zone
- Bulk of lesion is of low SI on T2WI
  - Small foci of high SI on T2WI are common

Benign Endometrial Stromal Nodule
- Well-circumscribed, expansile neoplasm
- No invasive features

ENDOMETRIAL STROMAL SARCOMA

Intravenous Leiomyomatosis
- Low SI uterine mass with worm-like tubular projections (representing gross intravascular extension) involving the myometrium and extending beyond the uterus
- Tumor may extend into IVC and heart

PATHOLOGY

General Features
- Etiology
  - No association with unopposed estrogen, or prior pelvic radiation
  - Originates from endometrial tissue, rarely from adenomyosis or endometriosis
- Epidemiology: 1% of uterine malignancies, 10-25% of primary uterine sarcomas

Gross Pathologic & Surgical Features
- Fungating/papillary mass filling endometrial cavity or infiltrating myometrium and adjacent structures
- Myometrial involvement presents as worm-like plugs of tumor invading the myometrium
- Hemorrhage and necrosis are frequently present, particularly in HGSS

Microscopic Features
- LGSS: Uniform cells nearly identical to proliferative phase endometrial stromal cells
  - Little pleomorphism, low mitotic rates
  - Lymphatic and vascular space invasion
- HGSS: Nuclear pleomorphism and high mitotic rates
  - Destructive myometrial invasion, in contrast to permeative invasion of LGSS

Staging, Grading or Classification Criteria
- Classified as low and high grade tumors
- Modified FIGO staging system for endometrial carcinoma is applicable
  - Stage I: Tumor confined to uterine corpus
  - Stage II: Tumor invading cervix
  - Stage III: Tumor extending beyond uterus but confined to pelvis
  - Stage IV: Bladder/rectal mucosa or distant metastases

CLINICAL ISSUES

Presentation
- Most common signs/symptoms: Abnormal vaginal bleeding
- Other signs/symptoms
  - Abdominal pain or mass
  - Related to metastases in advanced cases
- Clinical Profile
  - LGSS: Due to young age at presentation, clinical diagnosis is typically leiomyoma or adenomyosis with an unusual degree of bleeding
  - Diagnosis of HGSS is readily made at dilatation and curettage (D & C)
  - D&C may not be diagnostic in the following instances
    - LGSS cells mimic normal endometrial tissue
    - Lesions that are almost entirely intramyometrial

Demographics
- Age
  - Most common between 35-55 years of age
    - LGSS: Young premenopausal women (mean, 40 years)
    - HGSS: Postmenopausal women (mean, 60 years)

Natural History & Prognosis
- Most important prognostic factors
  - Histologic grade of tumor (DNA index)
  - Stage of disease
  - Size, cut off value 5 cm
- Lung and liver most common site of distant metastases
- 5 year survival rates
  - LGSS: Stage I > 80%
  - HGSS: Stage I 50%
  - All tumor grades: Stage II 30%, stage III-IV 10%

Treatment
- Total abdominal hysterectomy, bilateral salpingo-oophorectomy and lymph node sampling
- Radiation therapy for local control in the setting of poor prognostic markers

DIAGNOSTIC CHECKLIST

Consider
- Consider endometrial stromal sarcoma in the differential diagnosis of a heterogeneous, endometrial-based mass with a significant myometrial component

Image Interpretation Pearls
- Bands of low signal intensity (SI) on T2WI within the myometrium
- Spread along fallopian tubes, uterine ligaments and gross intravascular extension

SELECTED REFERENCES

1. Kusaka M et al: A case of high-grade endometrial stromal sarcoma arising from endometriosis in the cul-de-sac. Int J Gynecol Cancer. 16(2):895-9, 2006
2. Takeuchi M et al: Pathologies of the uterine endometrial cavity: usual and unusual manifestations and pitfalls on magnetic resonance imaging. Eur Radiol. 15(11):2244-55, 2005
3. Chaudhry S et al: Benign and malignant diseases of the endometrium. Top Magn Reson Imaging. 2003
4. Rha SE et al: CT and MRI of uterine sarcomas and their mimickers. AJR Am J Roentgenol. 181(5):1369-74, 2003
5. Sahdev A et al: MR imaging of uterine sarcomas. AJR Am J Roentgenol. 177(6):1307-11, 2001
6. Ueda M et al: MR imaging findings of uterine endometrial stromal sarcoma: differentiation from endometrial carcinoma. Eur Radiol. 11(1):28-33, 2001
7. Gandolfo N et al: Endometrial stromal sarcoma of the uterus: MR and US findings. Eur Radiol. 10(5):776-9, 2000
8. Koyama T et al: MR imaging of endometrial stromal sarcoma: correlation with pathologic findings. AJR Am J Roentgenol. 173(3):767-72, 1999

ENDOMETRIAL STROMAL SARCOMA

IMAGE GALLERY

Typical

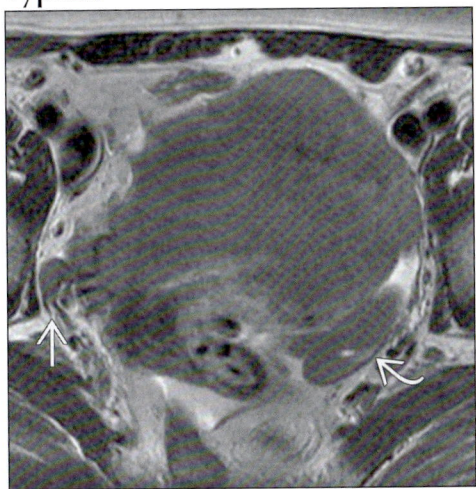
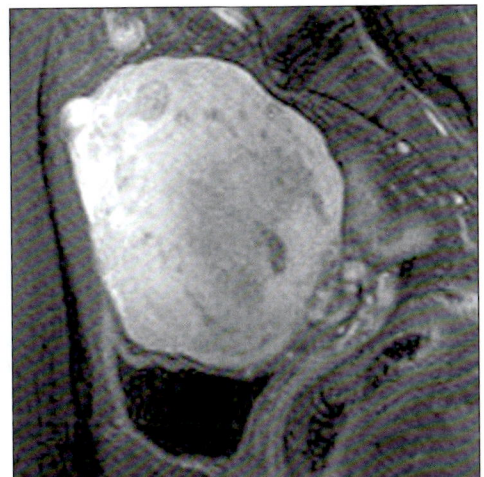

(Left) Axial T2WI MR of the same patient as previous image, shows gross intravascular extension into the periuterine vessels ➔ and spread along the left fallopian tube ➔. (Right) Sagittal T1 C+ FS MR in the same patient as previous image, shows marked enhancement of the mass during the capillary phase. Note that the contours of the uterus are lobulated.

Typical

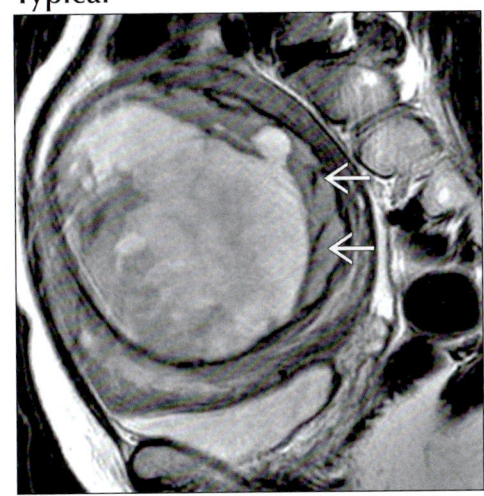
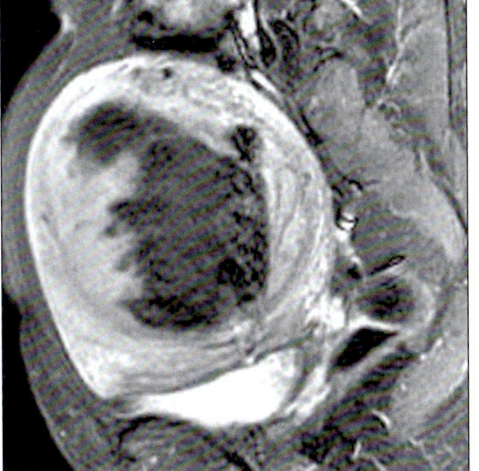

(Left) Sagittal T2WI MR shows a hyperintense endometrial mass invading the myometrium. There are low SI bands ➔ corresponding to preserved muscle bundles characteristic of a LGSS. (Right) Sagittal T1 C+ FS MR in the same patient as previous image, shows intense enhancement of the periphery of the mass.

Typical

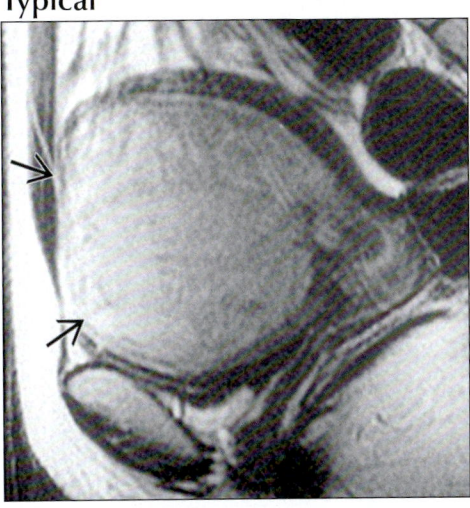
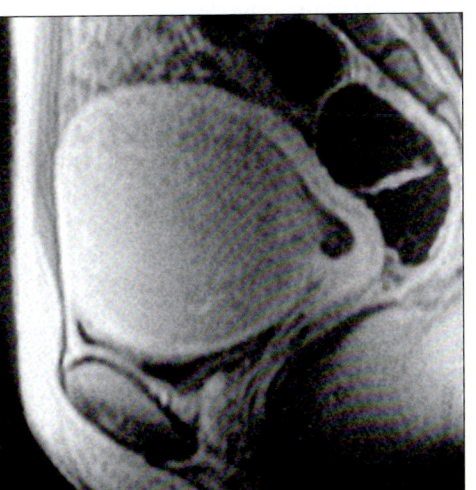

(Left) Sagittal T2WI MR of endometrial stromal sarcoma (low grade), depicts a large high signal intensity mass causing deep myometrial invasion ➔ anteriorly. (Right) Sagittal T1WI MR of endometrial stromal sarcoma (low grade). Mass enhances less than myometrium on contrast-enhanced T1WI MR.

ADENOSARCOMA

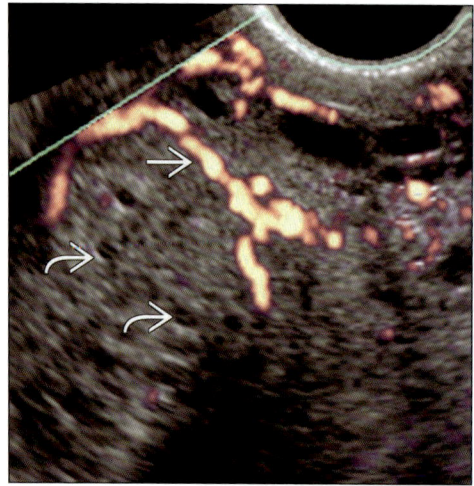

Longitudinal power Doppler ultrasound shows a large mixed echogenicity solid mass distending the uterine cavity. Note the presence of small cystic areas ➥ and a large branching feeding vessel ➔.

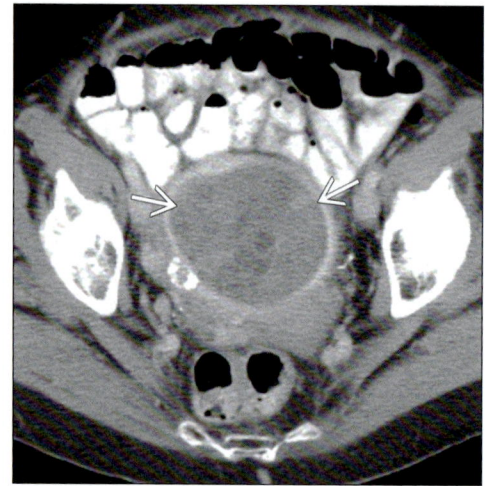

Axial CECT in the same patient as previous image shows a heterogeneous low density mass distending the endometrial cavity ➔. Pathology: Adenosarcoma.

TERMINOLOGY

Abbreviations and Synonyms
- Müllerian adenosarcoma of the uterus

Definitions
- Biphasic uterine tumor composed of benign glandular elements (epithelium) and malignant stroma (sarcoma)

IMAGING FINDINGS

General Features
- Best diagnostic clue: Heterogeneous, polypoid mass containing numerous thin septa creating a lattice-like appearance and expanding the endometrial cavity
- Location
  - 90% endometrial; 10% endocervical
  - May sometimes originate from foci of adenomyosis if arising from myometrium (very rare)
- Size: Variable, but often large reaching up to 9 cm
- Morphology: Heterogeneous polypoid mass causing expansion the endometrial cavity and protruding through a dilated cervical canal

Ultrasonographic Findings
- Grayscale Ultrasound
  - Expansion of the endometrial cavity
  - Thickened heterogeneous endometrium
  - Small hypoechoic cystic areas are present
  - Poorly defined tumor/myometrium interface
- Color Doppler: Vascular pedicle entering the mass may be seen in cases of adenosarcoma arising from an adenomatous polyp

CT Findings
- NECT
  - Uterine enlargement
  - Areas of necrosis
- CECT
  - Large uterine mass or multiple solid masses
  - Heterogeneous enhancement
  - Areas of necrosis

MR Findings
- T1WI

DDx: Uterine Masses

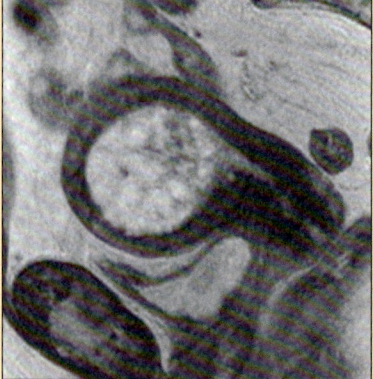

Endometrial Polyp

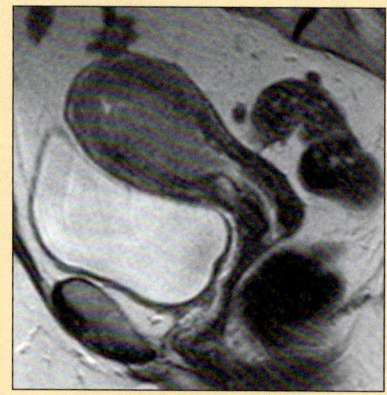

Endometrial Cancer

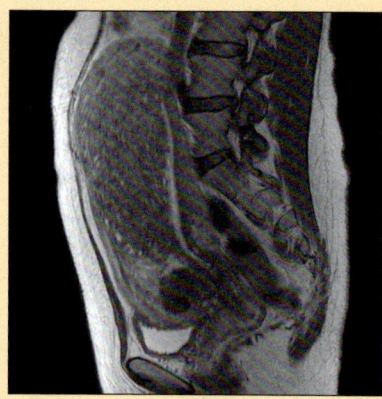

Adenomyosis

ADENOSARCOMA

Key Facts

Imaging Findings
- Best diagnostic clue: Heterogeneous, polypoid mass containing numerous thin septa creating a lattice-like appearance and expanding the endometrial cavity
- Heterogeneous mass of high signal intensity
- Single or multiple polypoid masses of heterogeneous signal intensity
- Disruption of subendometrial enhancement band indicates myometrial invasion

Top Differential Diagnoses
- Adenomatous Polyp
- Endometrial Carcinoma
- Malignant Mixed Müllerian Tumor
- Other Uterine Sarcomas
- Adenomyosis

Pathology
- Association with tamoxifen therapy for breast cancer
- Biphasic tumor composed of benign glands (epithelium) set in a malignant stroma (sarcoma)
- Myometrial invasion is seen in approximately 15% and is usually superficial (confined to inner half) in 80%
- 10% of cases show overgrowth of more than 25% of the tumor by a pure sarcoma (sarcomatous overgrowth), giving a worse prognosis

Clinical Issues
- Most common signs/symptoms: Postmenopausal bleeding
- Local recurrence in 25% of cases

  - Enlarged uterus
  - Heterogeneous mass of intermediate signal intensity
  - Areas of high signal intensity representing hemorrhage within the tumor may be present
- T2WI
  - Expansion of the endometrial cavity
  - Enhanced endometrial-myometrial interface
  - Heterogeneous mass of high signal intensity
  - Single or multiple polypoid masses of heterogeneous signal intensity
  - Mass can protrude through the the cervical os
  - May contain multiple cystic areas
  - Loss of low signal intensity junctional zone indicates myometrial invasion
- T1 C+ FS
  - Single or multiple polypoid masses that show strong enhancement
  - Enhancement of solid components and thin septa traversing the endometrial canal, creating a lattice-like appearance
  - Disruption of subendometrial enhancement band indicates myometrial invasion
  - Presence of peritoneal implants

Imaging Recommendations
- Best imaging tool
  - TVS should be used for initial investigation of women who present with postmenopausal bleeding especially if they are on long term tamoxifen treatment for breast cancer
  - MR is the most accurate imaging technique for evaluation of myometrial invasion
- Protocol advice: DCE-MRI in sagittal and axial planes to accurately demonstrate the presence of myometrial invasion

DIFFERENTIAL DIAGNOSIS

Adenomatous Polyp
- Can be indistinguishable from adenosarcoma, however presence of myometrial invasion indicates adenosarcoma

Endometrial Carcinoma
- Thickened endometrium of intermediate signal intensity on T2WI

Malignant Mixed Müllerian Tumor
- Large solid mass replacing the endometrial cavity; necrosis and hemorrhage are prominent features
- Lymph node metastases and peritoneal seeding are common

Other Uterine Sarcomas
- Uterine sarcomas tend to be larger, heterogeneous and more aggressive

Adenomyosis
- Diffuse or focal involvement of the myometrium, containing
  - Ill-defined low signal intensity with multifocal high signal intensity foci on T2WI

PATHOLOGY

General Features
- Etiology
  - Association with tamoxifen therapy for breast cancer
  - May be associated with long term use of oral contraceptives
- Epidemiology
  - Accounts for only 8% of all uterine sarcomas
  - Patients with adenosarcoma have a higher incidence of thyroid cancer, benign ovarian cyst and polycystic ovarian disease compared to the general population
  - Previous pelvic radiation has been reported
- Associated abnormalities: Endometrial polyps

Gross Pathologic & Surgical Features
- Polypoid endometrial neoplasm which grows into the uterine cavity
- Sectioned surface is frequently spongy, containing cystic spaces filled with fluid with surrounding white/tan tissue

ADENOSARCOMA

Microscopic Features
- Biphasic tumor composed of benign glands (epithelium) set in a malignant stroma (sarcoma)
- Glands are often cystically dilated or form cleft-like spaces
- Glands can be endometrial (proliferative or secretory), endocervical, tubal or hobnail in type
- One third show some epithelial atypia
- Mesenchymal component consists of malignant spindle or round cells and tends to show a greater cellularity around glands (glandular cuffing)
- 20% have heterologous elements i.e., tissue types not normally found in the uterus (e.g., fat, cartilage, rhabdomyoblasts)
- Myometrial invasion is seen in approximately 15% and is usually superficial (confined to inner half) in 80%
- Myometrial vessel invasion is rare
- 10% of cases show overgrowth of more than 25% of the tumor by a pure sarcoma (sarcomatous overgrowth), giving a worse prognosis

CLINICAL ISSUES

Presentation
- Most common signs/symptoms: Postmenopausal bleeding
- Other signs/symptoms
  - Pelvic mass
  - Pelvic pain

Demographics
- Age: Range from 13-67 years

Natural History & Prognosis
- Hematogenous metastases are extremely rare
- Increased risk of recurrence if sarcomatous overgrowth and myometrial invasion are present
- Local recurrence in 25% of cases
- Recurrence is mainly in the vagina and pelvis (60%)
- Tumor recurrence carries a bad prognosis

Treatment
- Hysterectomy, bilateral oophorectomy and lymph node sampling
- Chemotherapy and radiotherapy may be used if there is deep myometrial invasion or extrauterine spread

DIAGNOSTIC CHECKLIST

Consider
- TVS as initial imaging test in women with abnormal uterine bleeding
- MR for local staging and treatment planning

Image Interpretation Pearls
- Heterogeneous mass causing expansion of the endometrial cavity
- Disruption of the junctional zone and an irregular tumor-myometrium interface suggest myometrial invasion

SELECTED REFERENCES
1. Tjalma WA et al: Mullerian adenosarcoma of the uterus associated with long-term oral contraceptive use. Eur J Obstet Gynecol Reprod Biol. 119(2):253-4, 2005
2. Crade M et al: Pedicle sign and diagnosis of endometrial adenosarcoma. J Ultrasound Med. 23(9):1217-9, 2004
3. Lee EJ et al: Polypoid adenomyomas: sonohysterographic and color Doppler findings with histopathologic correlation. J Ultrasound Med. 23(11):1421-9; quiz 1431, 2004
4. Tinar S et al: Adenosarcoma of the uterus: a case report. MedGenMed. 6(1):51, 2004
5. Chourmouzi D et al: Sonography and MRI of tamoxifen-associated mullerian adenosarcoma of the uterus. AJR Am J Roentgenol. 181(6):1673-5, 2003
6. Rha SE et al: CT and MRI of uterine sarcomas and their mimickers. AJR Am J Roentgenol. 181(5):1369-74, 2003
7. Fong K et al: Endometrial evaluation with transvaginal US and hysterosonography in asymptomatic postmenopausal women with breast cancer receiving tamoxifen. Radiology. 220(3):765-73, 2001
8. Hann LE et al: Sonohysterography for evaluation of the endometrium in women treated with tamoxifen. AJR Am J Roentgenol. 177(2):337-42, 2001
9. Jorizzo JR et al: Endometrial polyps: sonohysterographic evaluation. AJR Am J Roentgenol. 176(3):617-21, 2001
10. Krivak TC et al: Uterine adenosarcoma with sarcomatous overgrowth versus uterine carcinosarcoma: comparison of treatment and survival. Gynecol Oncol. 83(1):89-94, 2001
11. Arici DS et al: Mullerian adenosarcoma of the uterus associated with tamoxifen therapy. Arch Gynecol Obstet. 264(2):105-7, 2000
12. Ascher SM et al: Tamoxifen-induced uterine abnormalities: the role of imaging. Radiology. 214(1):29-38, 2000
13. Grasel RP et al: Endometrial polyps: MR imaging features and distinction from endometrial carcinoma. Radiology. 214(1):47-52, 2000
14. Piura B et al: Mullerian adenosarcoma of the uterus: case report and review of literature. Eur J Gynaecol Oncol. 21(4):387-90, 2000
15. Lee HK et al: Uterine adenofibroma and adenosarcoma: CT and MR findings. J Comput Assist Tomogr. 22(2):314-6, 1998
16. Verschraegen CF et al: Clinicopathologic analysis of mullerian adenosarcoma: the M.D. Anderson Cancer Center experience. Oncol Rep. 5(4):939-44, 1998
17. Ascher SM et al: MR imaging appearance of the uterus in postmenopausal women receiving tamoxifen therapy for breast cancer: histopathologic correlation. Radiology. 200(1):105-10, 1996
18. Kaku T et al: Adenosarcoma of the uterus: a Gynecologic Oncology Group clinicopathologic study of 31 cases. Int J Gynecol Pathol. 11(2):75-88, 1992
19. Clement PB et al: Mullerian adenosarcoma of the uterus: a clinicopathologic analysis of 100 cases with a review of the literature. Hum Pathol. 21(4):363-81, 1990
20. Clement PB: Mullerian adenosarcomas of the uterus with sarcomatous overgrowth. A clinicopathological analysis of 10 cases. Am J Surg Pathol. 13(1):28-38, 1989

ADENOSARCOMA

IMAGE GALLERY

Typical

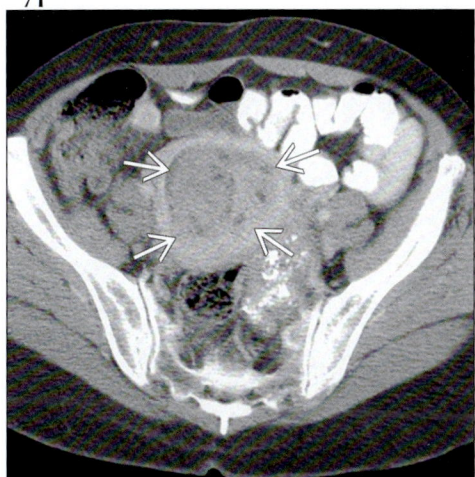
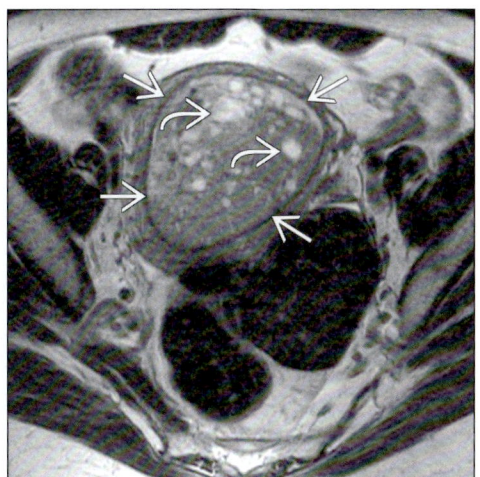

(Left) Axial CECT shows a heterogeneous low attenuation mass distending the endometrial cavity ➡. *(Right)* Axial T2WI MR in same patient as previous image shows a large mass of intermediate signal intensity distending the endometrial cavity. It contains clusters of cystic spaces ➡. The intact junctional zone excludes myometrial invasion ➡.

Typical

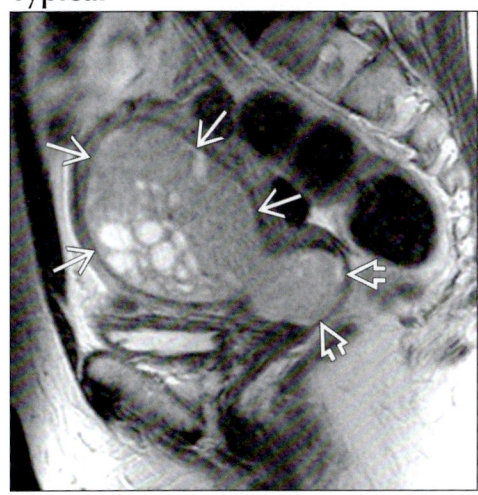
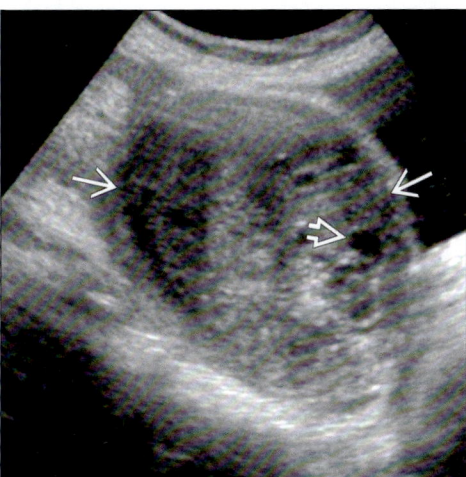

(Left) Sagittal T2WI MR of same patient as previous image shows the heterogeneous ➡ mass protruding into cervix ➡. Pathology: Adenosarcoma. *(Right)* Longitudinal transvaginal ultrasound of a different patient shows a large mixed echogenicity solid mass distending the uterine cavity ➡. Small cystic areas are also evident ➡.

Typical

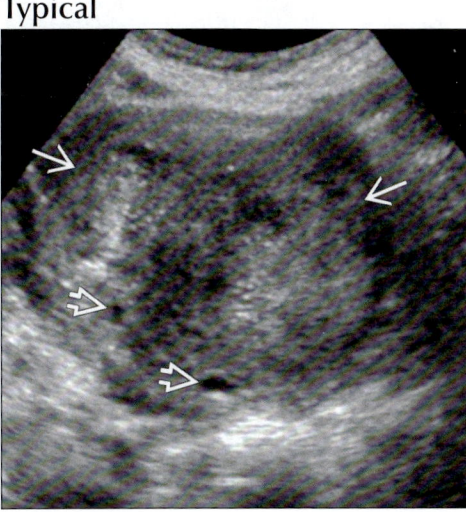
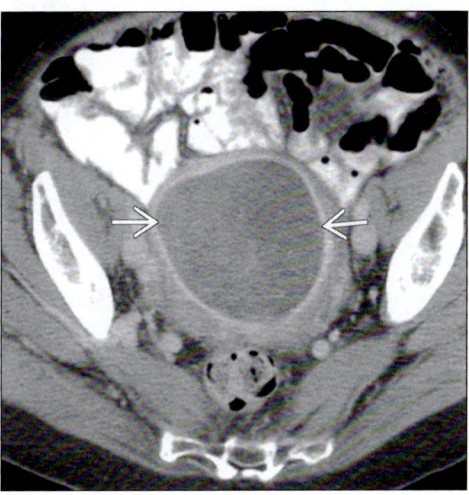

(Left) Transverse transvaginal ultrasound in the same patient as previous image again demonstrating an heterogeneous mass ➡ containing small cystic spaces ➡. *(Right)* Axial CECT in the same patient confirms the presence of a heterogeneous low density mass in the endometrial cavity ➡. Pathology: Adenosarcoma.

ADENOSARCOMA

Typical

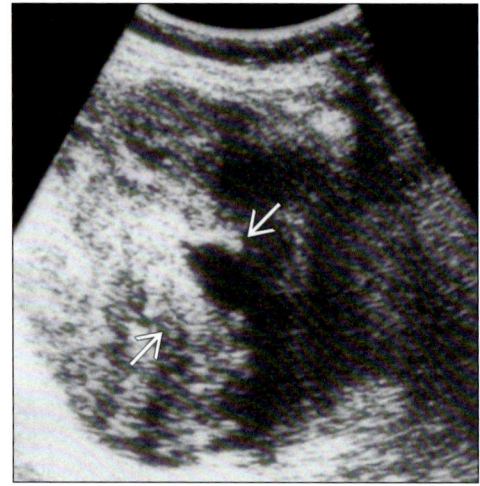
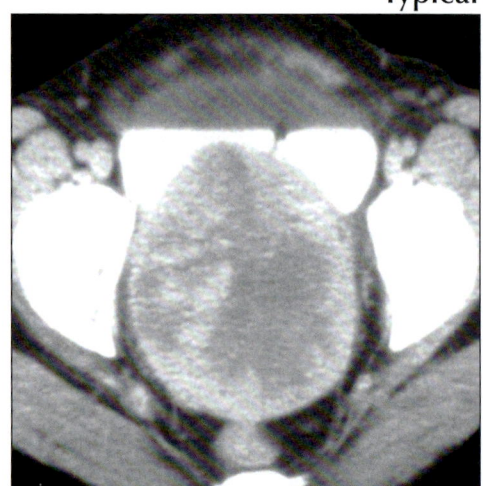

(Left) Transverse transvaginal ultrasound shows a distended endometrial cavity by an heterogeneous mass ➡ in a patient on long term tamoxifen treatment for breast cancer. (Right) Axial CECT in the same patient as previous image shows a 12 cm heterogeneous mass which has more than 50% necrosis.

Variant

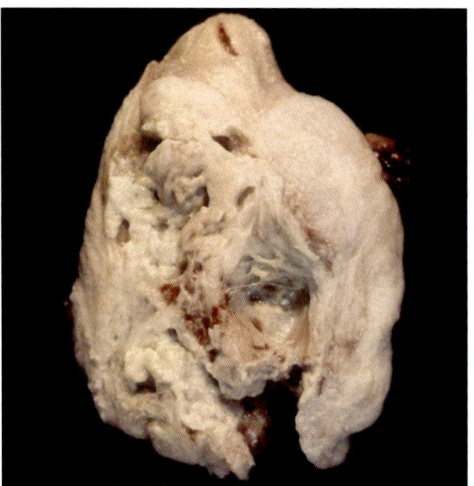
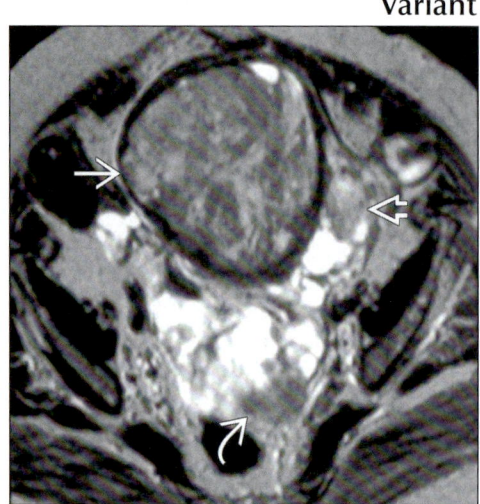

(Left) Gross pathology of same patient as previous image and histopathology confirm diagnosis of adenosarcoma with sarcomatous overgrowth. (Courtesy T. Cunha, MD). (Right) Axial T2WI MR shows a polypoid tumor of heterogeneous signal intensity distending endometrial canal. Note focal myometrial invasion ➡ and presence of metastases to left ovary ➡ and to peritoneum (Pouch of Douglas) ➡.

Variant

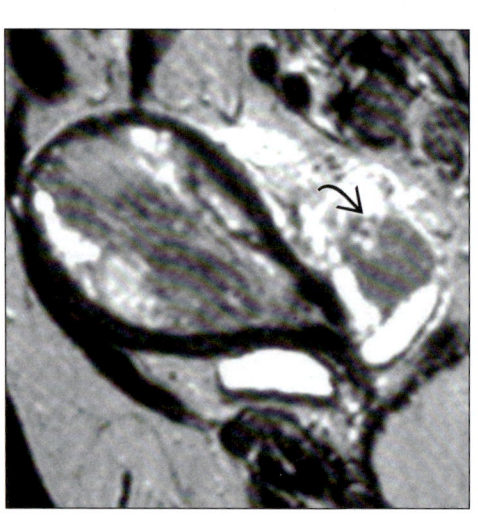
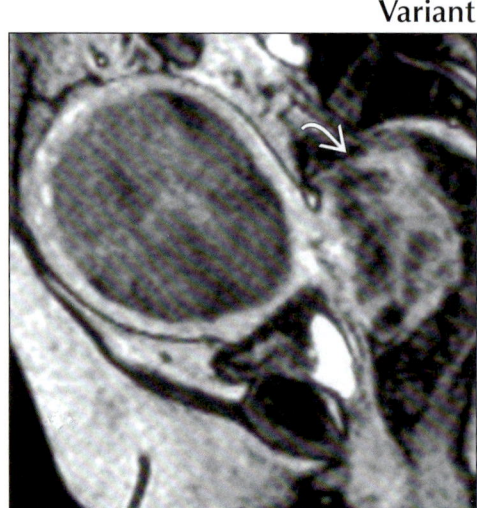

(Left) Sagittal T2WI MR in same patient as previous image confirms presence of polypoid mass and peritoneal deposit in Pouch of Douglas ➡. (Right) Sagittal T1 C+ MR shows heterogeneously enhancing mass distending endometrial cavity. Also note enhancing peritoneal deposit in Pouch of Douglas ➡. Pathology: Adenosarcoma with metastases to left ovary and Pouch of Douglas. (Courtesy T. Cunha, MD).

ADENOSARCOMA

Typical

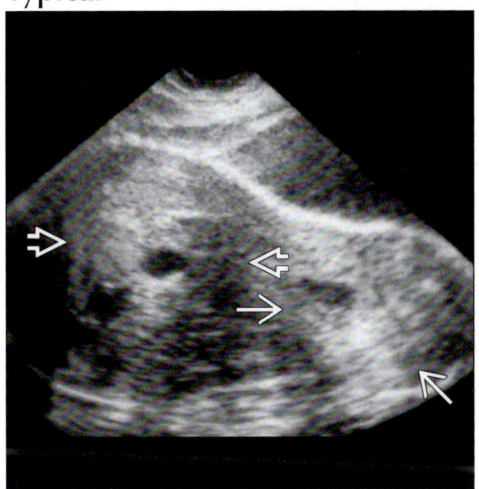 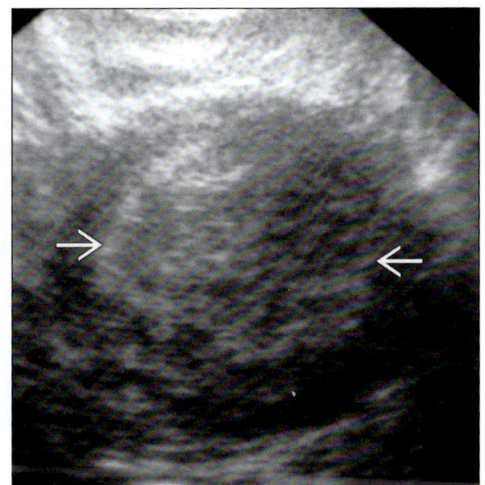

(Left) Longitudinal transvaginal ultrasound shows 2 polypoid tumors inserting in the uterine fundus ▷ and posterior wall ➡ measuring 15 cm and 3.5 cm respectively. *(Right)* Transverse transvaginal ultrasound shows the polypoid heterogeneous fundal mass ➡.

Typical

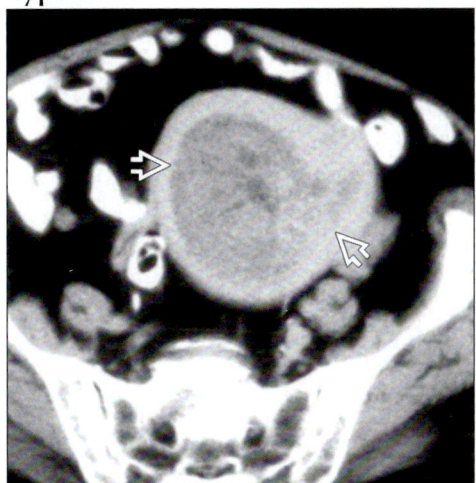 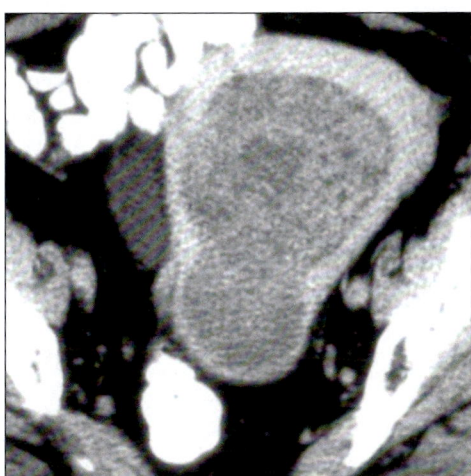

(Left) Axial CECT demonstrates the presence of the fundal mass ➡ containing areas of necrosis. *(Right)* Axial CECT shows both polypoid masses which have more then 50% necrosis.

Typical

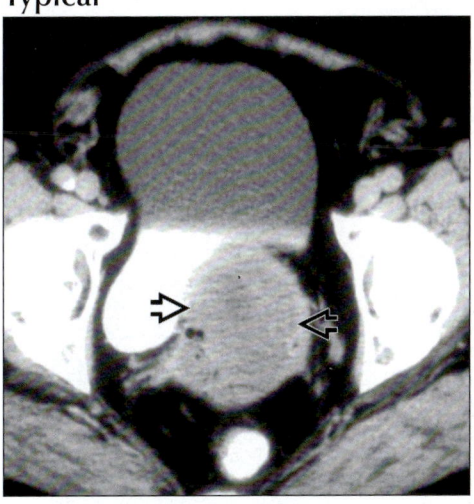 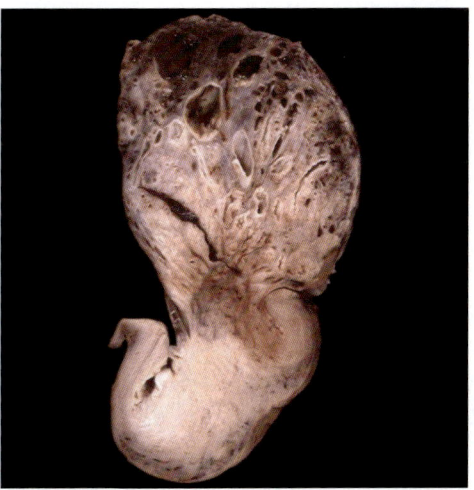

(Left) Axial CECT shows the polypoid mass prolapsing into the cervical canal ➡. *(Right)* Gross pathology confirms presence of two polypoid masses which are spongeous in appearance and have more then 50% of necrosis. Pathology: Adenosarcoma. (Courtesy T. Cunha, MD).

MALIGNANT MIXED MESODERMAL TUMOR

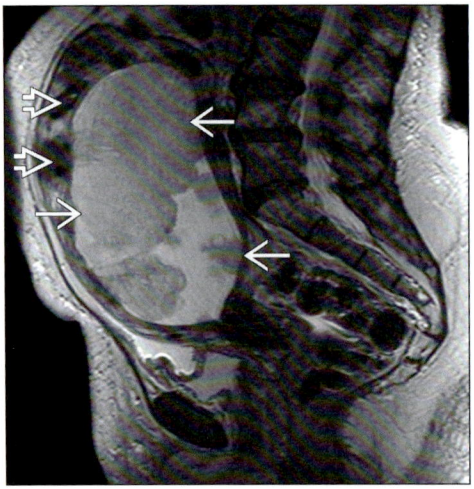 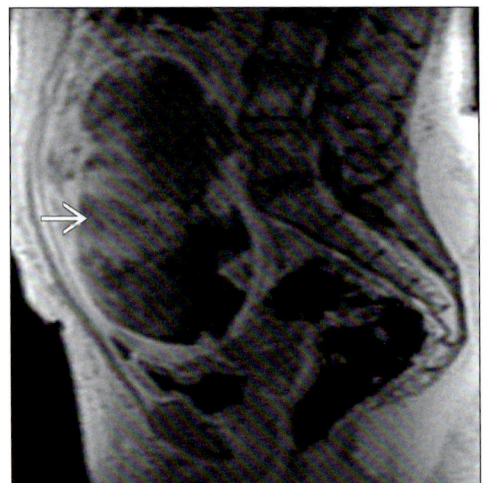

Sagittal T2WI MR shows markedly enlarged uterus with high signal intensity multifocal mass ➡ within the endometrial cavity. Small leiomyomas are also seen ➡.

Sagittal T1 C+ MR shows heterogeneous enhancement of the mass ➡.

TERMINOLOGY

Abbreviations and Synonyms
- Malignant mixed Müllerian tumor (MMMT), carcinosarcoma

Definitions
- Malignant neoplasms of uterus composed of tissues differentiating both as carcinoma and sarcoma

IMAGING FINDINGS

General Features
- Best diagnostic clue: Broad-based large uterine mass with aggressive myometrial invasion
- Location: They may arise anywhere in lower genital tract but involvement of uterine corpus is most common site
- Size: MMMTs are seen often as very large masses
- Morphology
  ○ Heterogeneous masses expanding the uterus
  ○ They may protrude through cervical os

Ultrasonographic Findings
- Grayscale Ultrasound
  ○ Appear as heterogeneous uterine mass with various echogenicity
  ○ US is limited for staging of tumor especially when mass is very large
- Color Doppler: Tumor vascularity could be detected
- Power Doppler: More sensitive to detect tumor vascularity

CT Findings
- NECT
  ○ Difficult to differentiate mass from normal uterus
  ○ Areas of hemorrhage within mass demonstrate high attenuation
- CECT
  ○ Heterogeneously-enhancing large uterine mass with marked myometrial invasion
  ○ Areas of necrosis in mass do not demonstrate enhancement

MR Findings
- T1WI
  ○ Predominantly low signal intensity uterine mass

DDx: Uterine Masses

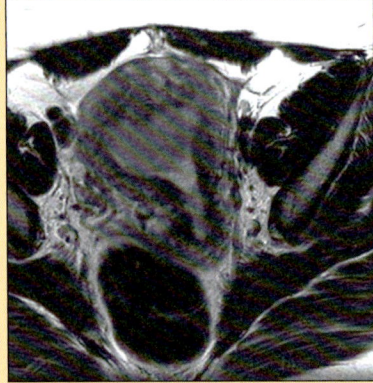 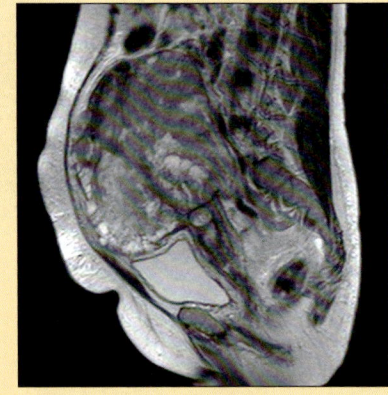 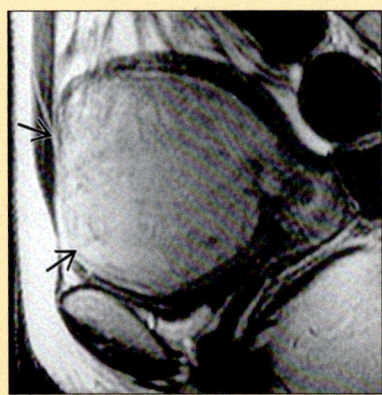

Endometrial Carcinoma

Leiomyosarcoma

Endometrial Stromal Sarcoma

MALIGNANT MIXED MESODERMAL TUMOR

Key Facts

Terminology
- Malignant mixed Müllerian tumor (MMMT), carcinosarcoma
- Malignant neoplasms of uterus composed of tissues differentiating both as carcinoma and sarcoma

Imaging Findings
- Best diagnostic clue: Broad-based large uterine mass with aggressive myometrial invasion
- Location: They may arise anywhere in lower genital tract but involvement of uterine corpus is most common site
- Size: MMMTs are seen often as very large masses
- Role of imaging is to define local extent and distant metastases of disease for treatment planning
- MR is method of choice for evaluation of local extent of disease
- CT could be used in advanced cases with distant spread

Top Differential Diagnoses
- Endometrial Carcinoma
- Leiomyosarcoma
- Endometrial Stromal Sarcoma
- Adenomyosis
- Leiomyoma

Clinical Issues
- Most common signs/symptoms: Abnormal vaginal bleeding

Diagnostic Checklist
- Any of the uterine sarcomas could appear as a large, heterogeneous and aggressive mass in uterus

---

- Areas of hemorrhage within mass demonstrate high signal intensity
- T2WI
  - Heterogeneous medium to high signal intensity uterine mass
  - Areas necrosis could be seen as high signal intensity regions within mass
- T1 C+
  - Heterogeneous enhancement of mass is lower than that of normal myometrium
  - Sagittal dynamic post-contrast images are very useful in assessment of depth of myometrial invasion

Imaging Recommendations
- Best imaging tool
  - Role of imaging is to define local extent and distant metastases of disease for treatment planning
  - MR is method of choice for evaluation of local extent of disease
  - CT could be used in advanced cases with distant spread
- Protocol advice
  - T1WI: Entire pelvis with large field of view
  - T2WI: Transverse, sagittal and coronal planes with small field of view
  - T1 C+: Dynamic post-contrast images in sagittal plane

DIFFERENTIAL DIAGNOSIS

Endometrial Carcinoma
- Difficult to differentiate from malignant mixed mesodermal tumor based on imaging
- Malignant mixed mesodermal tumors tend to be larger, heterogeneous and more aggressive

Leiomyosarcoma
- Difficult to differentiate from malignant mixed mesodermal tumor based on imaging
- Both leiomyosarcomas and malignant mixed mesodermal tumors are usually large and aggressive

Endometrial Stromal Sarcoma
- Difficult to differentiate from malignant mixed mesodermal tumor based on imaging
- Both endometrial stromal sarcomas and malignant mixed mesodermal tumors are usually large and aggressive

Adenomyosis
- Adenomyosis infiltrates myometrium without displacing endometrium
- Junctional zone is thickened in adenomyosis
- Heterotopic endometrial tissue in adenomyosis has characteristic appearance of hyperechoic foci on US and hyperintense foci on T2WI MR

Leiomyoma
- Leiomyomas typically show homogeneously low signal intensity on T2WI
- Degenerated leiomyomas with heterogeneous appearance may mimic uterine sarcomas

PATHOLOGY

General Features
- General path comments
  - Malignant mixed Müllerian tumors
    - Often large, bulky neoplasms
    - Spread extensively through endometrium and deeply invade myometrium in their early course
    - Lymph node involvement and serosal and peritoneal extension are common
    - Distant metastases commonly occur to lungs, liver and bone
- Etiology
  - Risk factors similar to endometrial carcinoma including obesity, hypertension and diabetes mellitus
  - 10-30% of cases associated with history of prior pelvic radiation treatment
- Epidemiology: Uncommon tumors representing less than 5% of all malignant uterine tumors

MALIGNANT MIXED MESODERMAL TUMOR

Gross Pathologic & Surgical Features
- Soft, polypoid, large masses invading into myometrium
- Hemorrhage and necrosis are usually present

Microscopic Features
- Spectacular array of different and bizarre malignant cells differentiating both as carcinoma and sarcoma
- Classified as homologous (tissue indigenous to uterus) or heterologous (tissue foreign to uterus) based on the nature of their sarcomatous element
- Either carcinomatous or sarcomatous component may predominate
- Mixed tumors with homologous elements have a better prognosis than those with heterologous elements
- Other types of endometrial sarcomas
  - Adenosarcomas contain benign epithelial components and sarcomatous stroma
  - Endometrial stromal sarcomas contain proliferative-phase stromal cells

Staging, Grading or Classification Criteria
- According to modification of the FIGO staging system for endometrial cancer
  - Stage I: Tumor is confined to uterine corpus
  - Stage II: Tumor is confined to corpus and cervix
  - Stage III: Extrauterine disease is confined to pelvis
  - Stage IV: Abdominal and distant disease is present

CLINICAL ISSUES

Presentation
- Most common signs/symptoms: Abnormal vaginal bleeding
- Other signs/symptoms
  - Pelvic pain
  - Vaginal discharge
- Clinical Profile
  - Mass protruding through cervix is a frequent finding at physical examination
  - Advanced cases may present with signs secondary to metastases

Demographics
- Age: More common in postmenopausal women

Natural History & Prognosis
- Most important prognostic factors
  - Stage of disease
  - Advanced age
  - Depth of myometrial invasion
  - Residual tumor after primary surgery
- 5 year survival rate: 25-30%

Treatment
- Surgery: Total abdominal hysterectomy and bilateral salpingo-oophorectomy, pelvic and para-aortic lymph node sampling
- Pre-operative and post-operative radiation treatment could be of benefit
- Chemotherapy

DIAGNOSTIC CHECKLIST

Consider
- MR for the evaluation of large uterine masses

Image Interpretation Pearls
- Any of the uterine sarcomas could appear as a large, heterogeneous and aggressive mass in uterus

SELECTED REFERENCES
1. Takeuchi M et al: Pathologies of the uterine endometrial cavity: usual and unusual manifestations and pitfalls on magnetic resonance imaging. Eur Radiol. 15(11):2244-55, 2005
2. Callister M et al: Malignant mixed Mullerian tumors of the uterus: analysis of patterns of failure, prognostic factors, and treatment outcome. Int J Radiat Oncol Biol Phys. 58(3):786-96, 2004
3. Chaudhry S et al: Benign and malignant diseases of the endometrium. Top Magn Reson Imaging. 14(4):339-57, 2003
4. Kido A et al: Diffusely enlarged uterus: evaluation with MR imaging. Radiographics. 23(6):1423-39, 2003
5. Rha SE et al: CT and MRI of uterine sarcomas and their mimickers. AJR Am J Roentgenol. 181(5):1369-74, 2003
6. Szklaruk J et al: MR imaging of common and uncommon large pelvic masses. Radiographics. 23(2):403-24, 2003
7. Inthasorn P et al: Analysis of clinicopathologic factors in malignant mixed Mullerian tumors of the uterine corpus. Int J Gynecol Cancer. 12(4):348-53, 2002
8. Ohguri T et al: MRI findings including gadolinium-enhanced dynamic studies of malignant, mixed mesodermal tumors of the uterus: differentiation from endometrial carcinomas. Eur Radiol. 12(11):2737-42, 2002
9. Sahdev A et al: MR imaging of uterine sarcomas. AJR Am J Roentgenol. 177(6):1307-11, 2001
10. To WW et al: Malignant mixed Mullerian tumors of the uterus. Int J Gynaecol Obstet. 47(1):39-44, 1994
11. Larson B et al: Mixed mullerian tumours of the uterus--prognostic factors: a clinical and histopathologic study of 147 cases. Radiother Oncol. 17(2):123-32, 1990
12. Dinh TV et al: Mixed mullerian tumors of the uterus: a clinicopathologic study. Obstet Gynecol. 74(3 Pt 1):388-92, 1989
13. Nielsen SN et al: Clinicopathologic analysis of uterine malignant mixed mullerian tumors. Gynecol Oncol. 34(3):372-8, 1989
14. Shapeero LG et al: Mixed mullerian sarcoma of the uterus: MR imaging findings. AJR Am J Roentgenol. 153(2):317-9, 1989
15. Peters WA 3rd et al: Prognostic features of sarcomas and mixed tumors of the endometrium. Obstet Gynecol. 63(4):550-6, 1984

MALIGNANT MIXED MESODERMAL TUMOR

IMAGE GALLERY

Typical

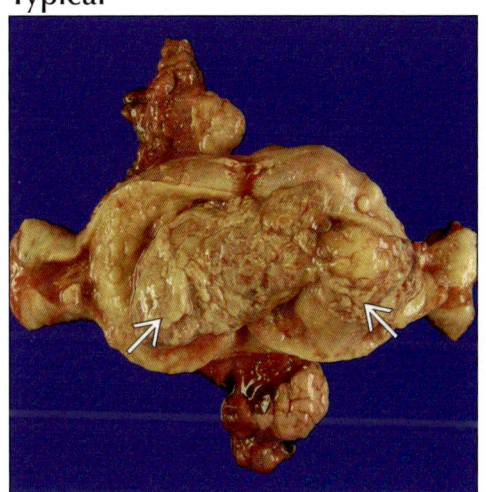
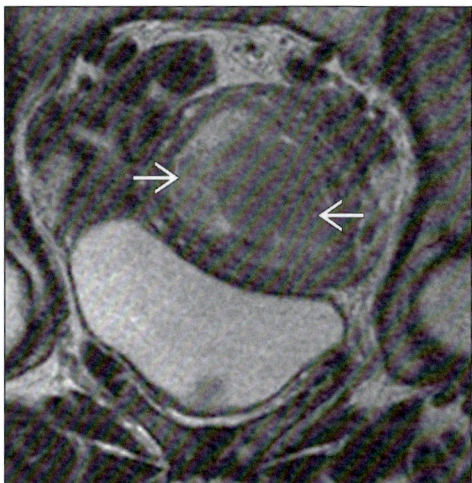

(Left) Gross pathology shows a large polypoid mass ➡ invading myometrium in a patient with malignant mixed mesodermal tumor. *(Right)* Coronal T2WI MR shows a heterogeneous high signal intensity mass ➡ in the endometrium.

Typical

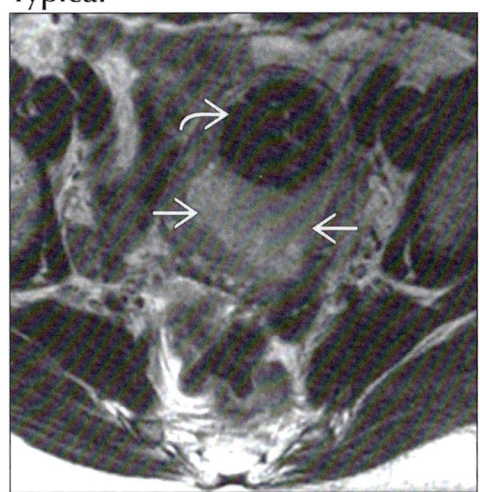
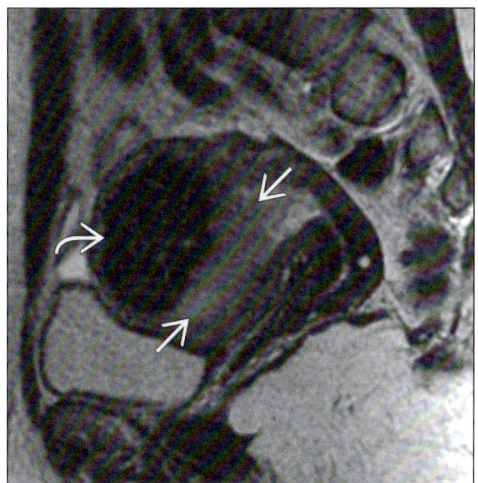

(Left) Axial T2WI MR shows a high signal intensity mass ➡ in the endometrial cavity. Note a low signal intensity leiomyoma ➡ is also seen anteriorly. *(Right)* Sagittal T2WI MR shows high signal intensity mass ➡ in the endometrial cavity. A low signal intensity leiomyoma ➡ is again seen.

Typical

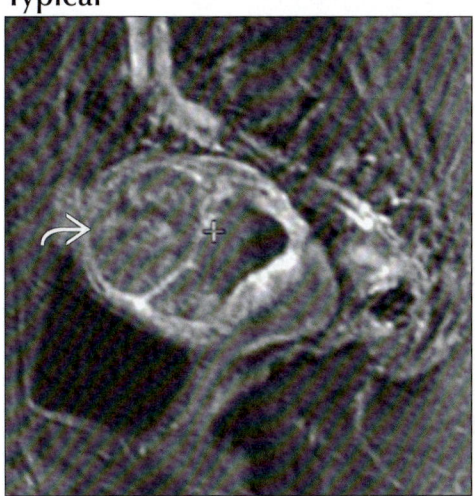
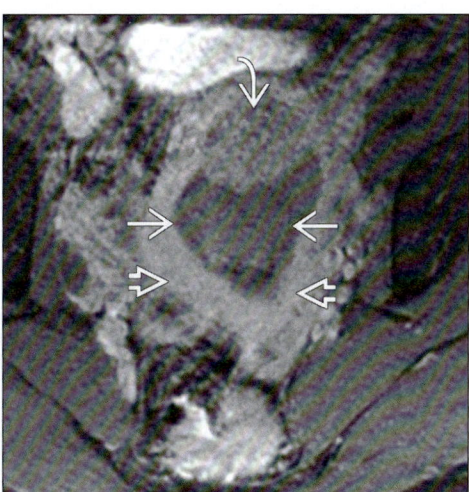

(Left) Sagittal T1 C+ FS MR shows that the mass (+) enhances heterogeneously. The leiomyoma ➡ also enhances heterogeneously during this early phase. *(Right)* Axial T1 C+ FS MR shows that the mass ➡ shows less enhancement relative to the myometrium ➡ and the leiomyoma ➡. Note that there is no deep myometrial invasion.

LEIOMYOSARCOMA, UTERUS

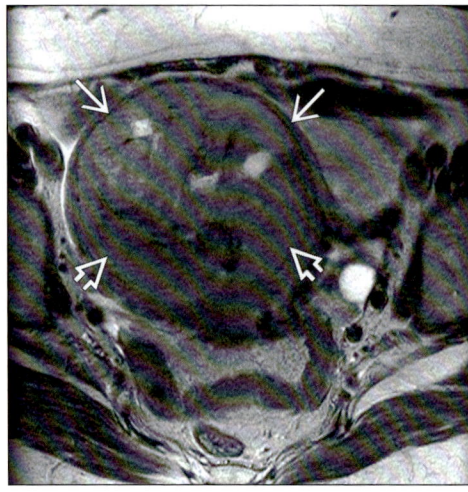

Axial T2WI MR shows a large heterogeneous mass ➡ in the uterus. Note that thinned but intact myometrium around the mass ➡ indicates that the mass is confined in the uterus.

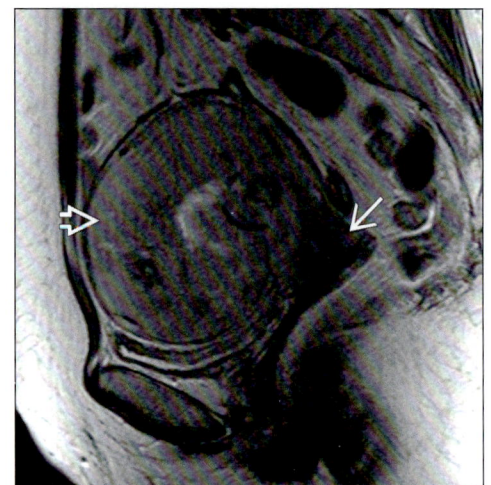

Sagittal T2WI MR shows a large heterogeneous mass ➡ in the uterine corpus. Note that the low signal intensity in the cervix ➡ is preserved which indicates it is not involved.

TERMINOLOGY

Abbreviations and Synonyms
- Uterine leiomyosarcoma

Definitions
- Malignant smooth muscle tumor of the uterus arising from myometrium itself or smooth muscle of myometrial vessels

IMAGING FINDINGS

General Features
- Best diagnostic clue: Solitary, heterogeneous, poorly-demarcated, intramural mass with areas of hemorrhage and necrosis
- Location: Myometrium, but large masses could extend into adjacent structures
- Size: They are often large (6-10 cm)
- Morphology: Well-defined or ill-defined heterogeneous masses causing uterine enlargement

Ultrasonographic Findings
- Grayscale Ultrasound
  - US is limited in evaluation of local extent of disease especially when mass is large
  - Heterogeneous echo pattern in mass due to its solid, necrotic and/or hemorrhagic regions
  - Leiomyosarcoma may be indistinguishable from a leiomyoma on US but a rapid increase in size of a mass suggests leiomyosarcoma
- Color Doppler: Shows increased vascularity in leiomyosarcomas unlike benign leiomyomas
- Power Doppler: More sensitive to detect tumor vascularity

CT Findings
- NECT
  - Difficult to differentiate mass from normal uterus
  - Areas of hemorrhage may appear as high-attenuation regions within mass
  - Areas of necrosis are seen as low-attenuation regions within mass
- CECT
  - Heterogeneously enhancing, low-attenuation mass relative to homogeneously enhancing myometrium

DDx: Uterine Masses

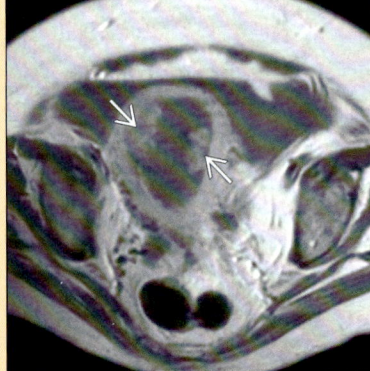

Endometrial Cancer

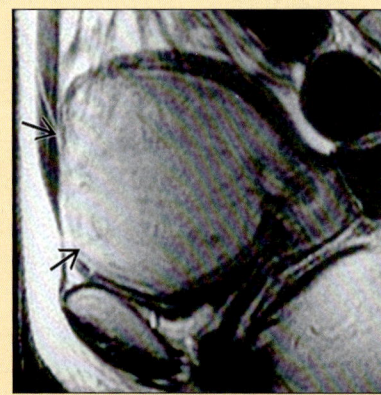

Endometrial Stromal Sarcoma

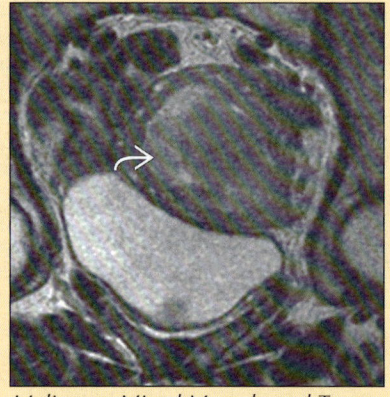

Malignant Mixed Mesodermal Tumor

LEIOMYOSARCOMA, UTERUS

Key Facts

Terminology
- Malignant smooth muscle tumor of the uterus arising from myometrium itself or smooth muscle of myometrial vessels

Imaging Findings
- Best diagnostic clue: Solitary, heterogeneous, poorly-demarcated, intramural mass with areas of hemorrhage and necrosis
- Size: They are often large (6-10 cm)
- Role of imaging is to define local extent and distant metastases of disease for treatment planning
- MR is method of choice for assessment of local extent of tumor due to its superior soft tissue resolution
- MR may be helpful to differentiate leiomyomas from leiomyosarcomas
- CT is helpful in the assessment of extent of adjacent organ invasion and distant metastases

Top Differential Diagnoses
- Leiomyoma
- Adenomyosis
- Endometrial Cancer
- Other Uterine Sarcomas

Pathology
- Arise from myometrium itself or smooth muscle of myometrial vessels
- Rare uterine tumor (< 1%)

Diagnostic Checklist
- Leiomyosarcoma may be confused with leiomyoma on imaging but a rapid increase in size of a mass suggests leiomyosarcoma

---

- Areas of necrosis do not enhance and often demonstrate irregular margins
- Uterus is often enlarged by mass

MR Findings
- T1WI
  - Low or intermediate signal intensity mass
  - Areas of hemorrhage demonstrate high signal intensity
- T2WI
  - Intermediate signal intensity heterogeneous mass relative to myometrium
  - Necrotic areas in the mass demonstrate high signal intensity
  - Uterus is often enlarged by mass
- T1 C+
  - Leiomyosarcomas demonstrate heterogeneous enhancement
  - They demonstrate less enhancement compared to normal myometrium which enhances homogeneously
  - Areas of necrosis do not enhance and often demonstrate irregular margins

Imaging Recommendations
- Best imaging tool
  - Role of imaging is to define local extent and distant metastases of disease for treatment planning
  - MR is method of choice for assessment of local extent of tumor due to its superior soft tissue resolution
  - MR may be helpful to differentiate leiomyomas from leiomyosarcomas
  - CT is helpful in the assessment of extent of adjacent organ invasion and distant metastases
- Protocol advice
  - T1WI: Entire pelvis with large field of view
  - T2WI: Transverse, sagittal and coronal planes with small field of view
  - T1 C+: Dynamic post-contrast images in sagittal plane

DIFFERENTIAL DIAGNOSIS

Leiomyoma
- Homogeneously low signal intensity on T2WI
- Degenerated leiomyomas have heterogeneous appearance and may be confused with leiomyosarcoma
- Absence of metastasis is an important clue in differential diagnosis

Adenomyosis
- Adenomyosis infiltrates myometrium without displacing the endometrium
- Junctional zone is thickened in adenomyosis
- Heterotopic endometrial tissue in adenomyosis has characteristic appearance of hyperechoic foci on US and hyperintense foci on T2WI MR

Endometrial Cancer
- Located in the endometrial cavity but may invade into myometrium
- Leiomyosarcomas are located in myometrium and often displace the endometrial cavity rather than expanding it

Other Uterine Sarcomas
- Any of the uterine sarcomas could appear as a large, heterogeneous and aggressive mass in uterus
- Difficult to differentiate different types of uterine sarcomas based on imaging

PATHOLOGY

General Features
- General path comments
  - Arise from myometrium itself or smooth muscle of myometrial vessels
  - Large size of tumor at presentation (6-10 cm)
  - Spread: Local extension, peritoneal implantation, lymphatic or hematogenous spread
  - Distant metastases: Lung, liver, brain, kidney, bone
- Epidemiology

LEIOMYOSARCOMA, UTERUS

- Rare uterine tumor (< 1%)
- Accounts for 15-40% of all uterine sarcomas

Gross Pathologic & Surgical Features
- Soft fleshy tumors containing areas of hemorrhage and necrosis

Microscopic Features
- Pleomorphic spindle-shaped muscle cells with hyperchromatic nuclei, high number of abnormal mitoses
- Irregular and extensive invasion to myometrium

Staging, Grading or Classification Criteria
- According to modification of FIGO staging system for endometrial cancer
  - Stage I: Tumor is confined to uterine corpus
  - Stage II: Tumor involves corpus and cervix
  - Stage III: Spread outside uterus but confined to pelvis
  - Stage IV: Spread outside true pelvis or into mucosa of bladder or rectum

CLINICAL ISSUES

Presentation
- Most common signs/symptoms
  - Pelvic pain
  - Vaginal bleeding
- Other signs/symptoms: Advanced cases may present with symptoms related to metastases
- Clinical Profile: Rapidly enlarging pelvic mass

Demographics
- Age: Most commonly affects women in 5th decade

Natural History & Prognosis
- Favorable prognostic factors
  - Early stage
  - Low grade
  - Premenopausal age
  - Size less than 5 cm
- 5-year overall survival ranges from 50-65%
- Recurrences occur in 45-73% of patients

Treatment
- Surgery: Total abdominal hysterectomy (TAH) and bilateral salpingo-oophorectomy (BSO)
- Adjuvant chemotherapy
- Adjuvant radiotherapy could reduce local recurrence

DIAGNOSTIC CHECKLIST

Consider
- MR for the evaluation of large uterine masses

Image Interpretation Pearls
- Leiomyosarcoma may be confused with leiomyoma on imaging but a rapid increase in size of a mass suggests leiomyosarcoma
- Any of the uterine sarcomas could appear as a large, heterogeneous and aggressive mass in the uterus

SELECTED REFERENCES

1. Wu TI et al: Prognostic factors and impact of adjuvant chemotherapy for uterine leiomyosarcoma. Gynecol Oncol. 100(1):166-72, 2006
2. Acharya S et al: Rare uterine cancers. Lancet Oncol. 6(12):961-71, 2005
3. Livi L et al: Treatment of uterine sarcoma at the Royal Marsden Hospital from 1974 to 1998. Clin Oncol (R Coll Radiol). 16(4):261-8, 2004
4. Tanaka YO et al: Smooth muscle tumors of uncertain malignant potential and leiomyosarcomas of the uterus: MR findings. J Magn Reson Imaging. 20(6):998-1007, 2004
5. Cantisani V et al: Vaginal metastasis from uterine leiomyosarcoma. Magnetic resonance imaging features with pathological correlation. J Comput Assist Tomogr. 27(5):805-9, 2003
6. Kido A et al: Diffusely enlarged uterus: evaluation with MR imaging. Radiographics. 23(6):1423-39, 2003
7. Rha SE et al: CT and MRI of uterine sarcomas and their mimickers. AJR Am J Roentgenol. 181(5):1369-74, 2003
8. Szklaruk J et al: MR imaging of common and uncommon large pelvic masses. Radiographics. 23(2):403-24, 2003
9. Goto A et al: Usefulness of Gd-DTPA contrast-enhanced dynamic MRI and serum determination of LDH and its isozymes in the differential diagnosis of leiomyosarcoma from degenerated leiomyoma of the uterus. Int J Gynecol Cancer. 12(4):354-61, 2002
10. Ohara N. Related Articles et al: A comparison of MRI findings of uterine leiomyosarcoma before surgery and at recurrence. J Obstet Gynaecol. 22(1):99, 2002
11. Sahdev A et al: MR imaging of uterine sarcomas. AJR Am J Roentgenol. 177(6):1307-11, 2001
12. Umesaki N et al: Positron emission tomography with (18)F-fluorodeoxyglucose of uterine sarcoma: a comparison with magnetic resonance imaging and power Doppler imaging. Gynecol Oncol. 80(3):372-7, 2001
13. Curtin JP et al: Corpus mesenchymal tumors. In: Principles and Practice of Gynecologic Oncology. Philadelphia, Lippincott Williams & Wilkins. 961-79, 2000
14. Murase E et al: Uterine leiomyomas: histopathologic features, MR imaging findings, differential diagnosis, and treatment. Radiographics. 19(5):1179-97, 1999

LEIOMYOSARCOMA, UTERUS

IMAGE GALLERY

Typical

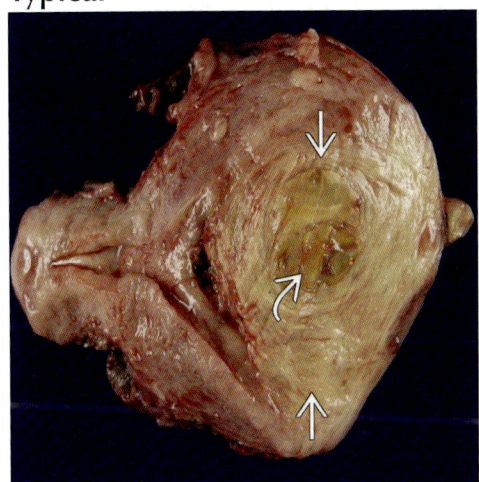
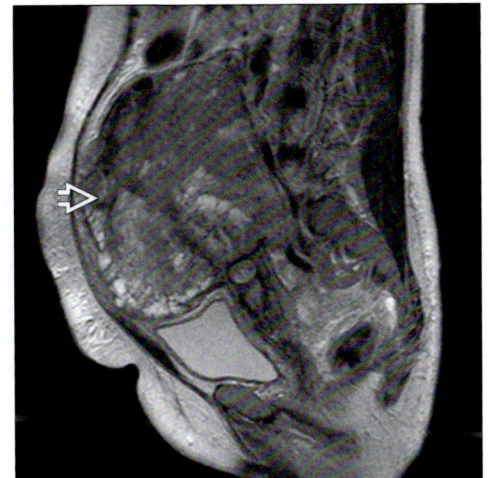

(Left) Gross pathology shows heterogeneous, poorly-demarcated, myometrial mass ➡ with central necrosis ➡ in a patient with uterine leiomyosarcoma. (Right) Sagittal T2WI MR shows a large heterogeneous mass ➡ with cystic and solid components replacing the entire uterus.

Typical

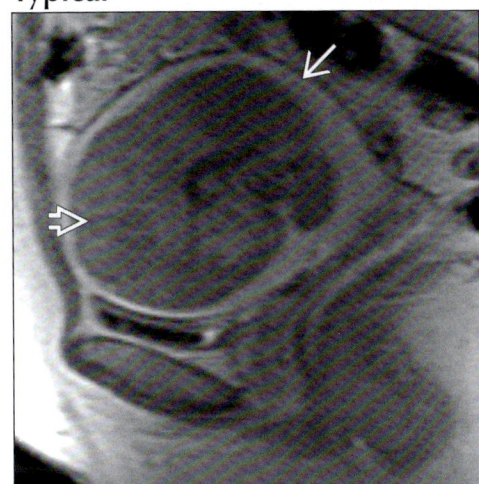
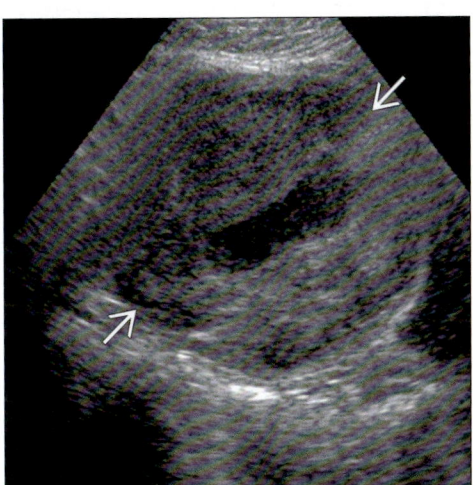

(Left) Sagittal T1 C+ MR shows another patient with a uterine mass ➡ that enhances less compared with the normal myometrium ➡ which is homogeneously enhancing. (Right) Sagittal transabdominal ultrasound shows a large leiomyosarcoma ➡ seen as a heterogeneous mass in a patient who presented with a rapidly enlarging pelvic mass.

Typical

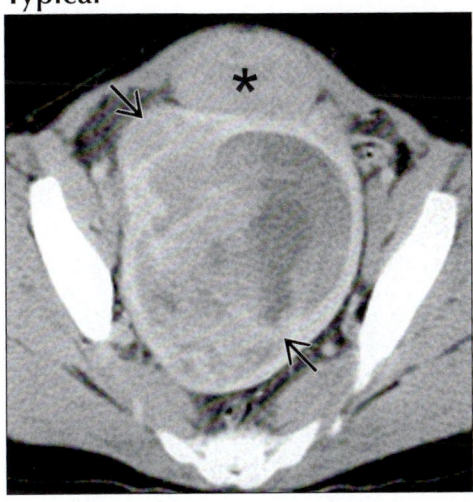
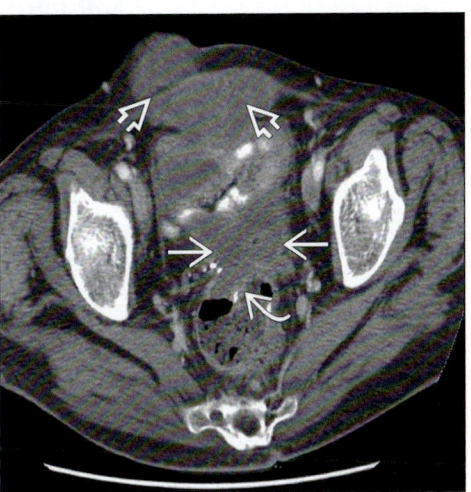

(Left) Axial CECT shows a heterogeneous uterine mass ➡ with an anterior pelvic tumor implant (*). (Right) Axial CECT shows a recurrent leiomyosarcoma ➡ invading adjacent sigmoid colon ➡. Another recurrent mass ➡ is seen in the anterior pelvic wall.

LYMPHOMA, UTERUS

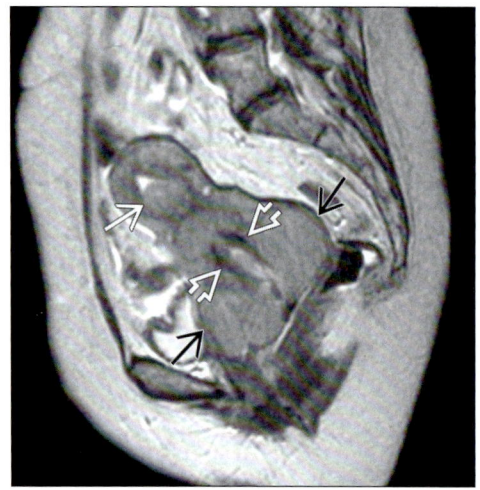

Sagittal T2WI MR shows a bulky mass of high signal intensity involving the uterine corpus ➔ and cervix ➔. Note the endocervical canal ➔ is preserved.

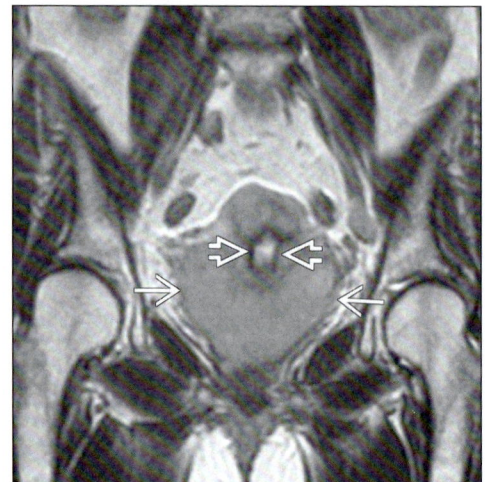

Coronal T2WI MR shows the mass ➔ with circumferential involvement of the cervix. Again noted is preservation of the endocervical canal ➔. Pathology confirmed lymphoma.

TERMINOLOGY

Abbreviations and Synonyms
- Lymphoma involving uterus

Definitions
- Primary uterine lymphoma (PUL): Extra-nodal non-Hodgkin lymphoma (NHL), confined to uterus (including the cervix and/or corpus) without evidence of other sites involvement at time of initial presentation
- Secondary uterine lymphoma: Uterine involvement is part of a generalized process (40-50% of patients with lymphoma at autopsy)

IMAGING FINDINGS

General Features
- Best diagnostic clue
  - Homogeneous myometrial mass/masses with moderate contrast-enhancement
  - Diffuse infiltration of uterus
- Location
  - Uterine corpus
    - May involve both endometrium and myometrium
    - Concomitant cervical lesions may coexist
  - Cervix is more often site of initial manifestation rather than uterine corpus
- Size: Ranges from small masses to diffuse involvement of the uterus
- Morphology: Densely packed cells gives lymphoma a uniform appearance, regardless of imaging modality

Ultrasonographic Findings
- Enlarged globular-shaped uterus
- Myometrial ill-defined hypoechoic masses
- Occasionally polypoid endometrial mass

CT Findings
- Uterine enlargement
- No associated pelvic lymphadenopathy or distant metastasis

MR Findings
- T1WI
  - Mass or masses isointense to muscle
  - Enlarged lymph nodes in case of secondary involvement by lymphoma

DDx: Uterine Masses

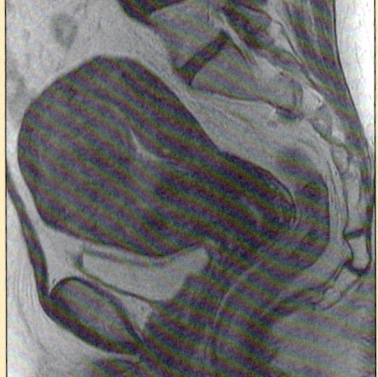

Multiple Leiomyomas

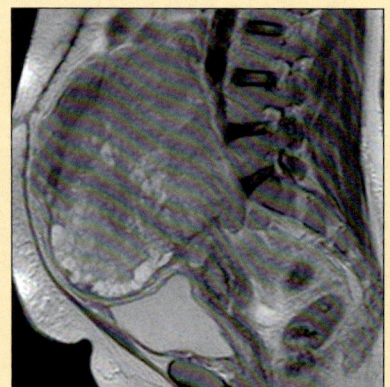

Leiomyosarcoma

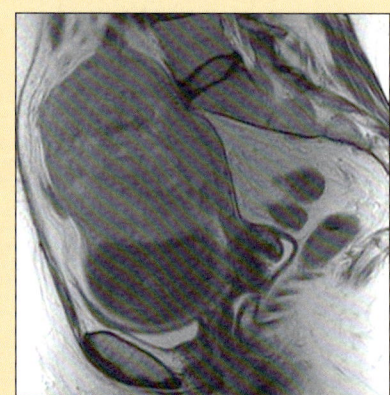

Endometrial Carcinoma

LYMPHOMA, UTERUS

Key Facts

Terminology
- Primary uterine lymphoma (PUL): Extra-nodal non-Hodgkin lymphoma (NHL), confined to uterus (including the cervix and/or corpus) without evidence of other sites involvement at time of initial presentation
- Secondary uterine lymphoma: Uterine involvement is part of a generalized process (40-50% of patients with lymphoma at autopsy)

Imaging Findings
- Morphology: Densely packed cells gives lymphoma a uniform appearance, regardless of imaging modality
- MR is modality of choice to detect multiple lesions within the uterus
- PET/CT can be performed for staging and to exclude other sites of lymphoma

Top Differential Diagnoses
- Leiomyoma
- Endometrial Carcinoma
- Uterine Sarcomas

Pathology
- Most are diffuse large B cell non-Hodgkin lymphomas
- Infiltration of vessels is typical
- Flow cytometry demonstrates a monoclonal B cell population and cell surface antigens

Clinical Issues
- Vaginal bleeding and discharge
- Patients with primary uterine lymphoma generally have intermediate or high grade lymphoma and poorer prognosis than patients with secondary lymphoma of the uterus

---

- T2WI
  - Diffusely enlarged uterus with a somewhat lobular contour
  - Single or multiple homogeneous masses
  - Slightly hyperintense to muscle
  - Coexistent cervical involvement typically preserves high-signal endocervical canal
- T1 C+: Moderate homogeneous enhancement

Imaging Recommendations
- Best imaging tool
  - MR is modality of choice to detect multiple lesions within the uterus
  - PET/CT can be performed for staging and to exclude other sites of lymphoma
- Protocol advice: T1WI, T2WI and T1WI C+ MR

DIFFERENTIAL DIAGNOSIS

Leiomyoma
- Very common
- Benign solitary/or multiple intramural, subserosal or submucosal solid masses
- Low signal intensity on all MR sequences

Endometrial Carcinoma
- Tumor of endometrial origin with possible myometrial invasion and spread to the regional lymph nodes
- MR demonstrates diffuse or polypoid thickening of endometrium with/or without invasion of the junctional zone

Uterine Sarcomas
- Leiomyosarcoma
  - Relatively rare, aggressive, malignant neoplasm arising from smooth muscle cells of the myometrium
  - Diffusely enlarged uterus with distorted zonal anatomy
  - Generally associated with bad prognosis due to widespread metastatic disease
- Rhabdosarcoma
  - Aggressive malignant pediatric tumor
  - Arises from the upper vagina and uterus
- Other uterine sarcomas
  - Mixed Müllerian tumor
  - Endometrial stromal sarcoma

PATHOLOGY

General Features
- Genetics
  - Primary Burkitt lymphoma of the uterus is extremely rare; seen in children and adolescents
  - Characterized by translocation of c-myc gene on chromosome 8 and immunoglobulin heavy chain (IgH) on chromosome 14
- Etiology: Chronic polyclonal activation of B-cells due to long-standing infections may be one of the etiologic factors
- Epidemiology
  - Initial uterine involvement occurs in only 1% of patients with lymphoma
  - Secondary involvement by lymphoma is much more common than PUL and has been seen in up to 10% of women with documented lymphoma
- Associated abnormalities
  - Can be associated with HIV infection
  - Ovaries are often involved in cases of secondary lymphoma

Gross Pathologic & Surgical Features
- Uterus may be normal in size or moderately enlarged
- Uterine corpus lesions can form polypoid masses or diffusely replace with endometrium
- Cut surface is fleshy, rubbery, white or tan and may have areas of hemorrhage or necrosis

Microscopic Features
- Most are diffuse large B cell non-Hodgkin lymphomas
- Occasional follicular lymphomas are seen
- Infiltration of vessels is typical
- Rare types include
  - Burkitt lymphoma

LYMPHOMA, UTERUS

- ○ Marginal zone lymphoma
- ○ T cell lymphoma
- Immunohistochemistry is positive for
  - ○ CD 45: Lymphoid cells
  - ○ CD 20 and CD 79a: B cell lymphoma
  - ○ CD 3: T cell lymphoma
- Flow cytometry demonstrates a monoclonal B cell population and cell surface antigens
- Must distinguish it histologically from
  - ○ Benign lymphoma-like lesion
    - ▪ Demonstrates polyclonality
  - ○ Small cell carcinoma
    - ▪ Immunoreactivity for synaptophysin, CD 56, chromogranin
  - ○ Endometrial stromal sarcoma
    - ▪ Immunoreactivity for CD 10, actin and vimentin, negative for CD45

Staging, Grading or Classification Criteria

- Ann Arbor and American Joint Committee on Cancer (AJCC)
  - ○ Stage Ie: Single extralymphatic organ or site (i.e. uterus)
    - ▪ "E" is for extranodal
  - ○ Stage IIe: Localized involvement of one extralymphatic organ and its regional lymph nodes with or without other nodes on same side of diaphragm
  - ○ Stage III: Involvement of lymph node regions on both sides of diaphragm
  - ○ Stage IV: Diffuse or disseminated involvement of one or more extralymphatic organs or tissues (e.g., bone marrow, liver) with or without associated node enlargement

CLINICAL ISSUES

Presentation

- Most common signs/symptoms
  - ○ Vaginal bleeding and discharge
  - ○ Pelvic pain
- Other signs/symptoms
  - ○ Rarely systemic symptoms such as fever and weight loss (B symptoms)
  - ○ Can be asymptomatic and discovered incidentally by abnormal cytology on routine pelvic

Demographics

- Age: Mean 53 (range 8-85)

Natural History & Prognosis

- Patients with primary uterine lymphoma generally have intermediate or high grade lymphoma and poorer prognosis than patients with secondary lymphoma of the uterus
- There is an interval of several months between detection of the uterine lesion and the appearance of any secondary lesions

Treatment

- Primary uterine lymphoma is treated with chemotherapy and radiotherapy, therefore differentiation from surgically treated uterine malignancies is crucial

DIAGNOSTIC CHECKLIST

Consider

- NHL in a work-up of uterine neoplasms even without evidence of extrauterine lymphoma involvement

Image Interpretation Pearls

- Lymphoma typically remains homogeneous by imaging even when large

SELECTED REFERENCES

1. Hamadani M et al: Marginal zone B-cell lymphoma of the uterus: a case report and review of the literature. J Okla State Med Assoc. 99(4):154-6, 2006
2. Keller C et al: Primary Burkitt lymphoma of the uterine corpus. Leuk Lymphoma. 47(1):141-5, 2006
3. Lagoo AS et al: Lymphoma of the female genital tract: current status. Int J Gynecol Pathol. 25(1):1-21, 2006
4. Nomura S et al: Burkitt lymphoma of the uterus in a human T lymphotropic virus type-1 carrier. Intern Med. 45(4):215-7, 2006
5. Agaoglu FY et al: Primary uterine lymphoma: case report and literature review. Aust N Z J Obstet Gynaecol. 45(1):88-9, 2005
6. Rittenbach J et al: Primary diffuse large B-cell lymphoma of the uterus presenting solely as an endometrial polyp. Int J Gynecol Pathol. 24(4):347-51, 2005
7. Agrawal A et al: Malignant lymphoma of uterus: a case report with a review of the literature. Aust N Z J Obstet Gynaecol. 40(3):358-60, 2000
8. Cheong IJ et al: Primary uterine lymphoma: a case report. Korean J Radiol. 1(4):223-5, 2000
9. Suzuki Y et al: Magnetic resonance images of primary malignant lymphoma of the uterine body: a case report. Jpn J Clin Oncol. 30(11):519-21, 2000
10. Vang R et al: Non-Hodgkin's lymphomas involving the uterus: a clinicopathologic analysis of 26 cases. Mod Pathol. 13(1):19-28, 2000
11. Ferry J et al: Malignant lymphoma of the genitourinary tract. Current Diagnostic Pathol. 4:145-69, 1997
12. Kim YS et al: MR imaging of primary uterine lymphoma. Abdom Imaging. 22(4):441-4, 1997
13. Kawakami S et al: MR appearance of malignant lymphoma of the uterus. J Comput Assist Tomogr. 19(2):238-42, 1995
14. Lien HH et al: Lymphoma of the uterus: findings on MR imaging. AJR Am J Roentgenol. 163(4):996, 1994
15. Young RH et al: Lymphoma-like lesions of the lower female genital tract: a report of 16 cases. Int J Gynecol Pathol. 4(4):289-99, 1985
16. Glazer HS et al: Non-Hodgkin lymphoma: computed tomographic demonstration of unusual extranodal involvement. Radiology. 149(1):211-7, 1983

LYMPHOMA, UTERUS

IMAGE GALLERY

Typical

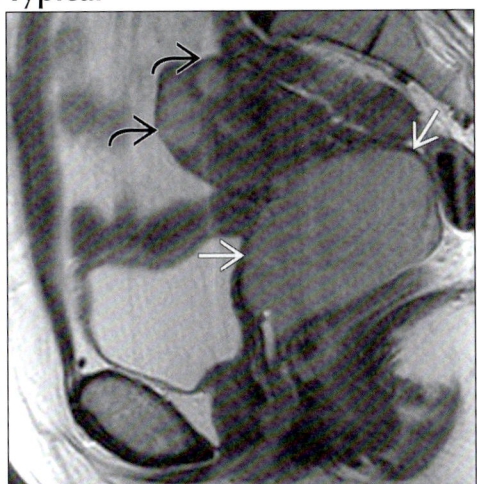
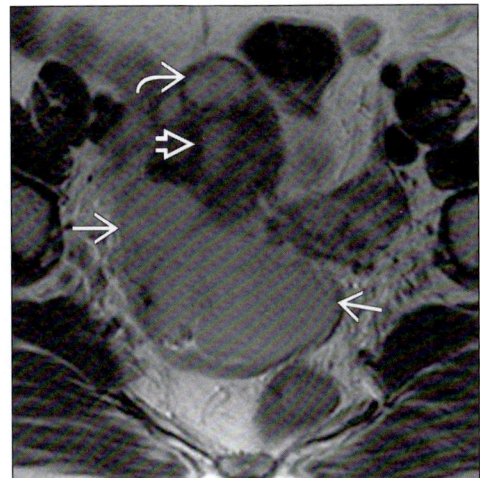

(Left) Sagittal T2WI MR shows a large cervical mass ➡ of high signal intensity and associated smaller masses of similar signal intensity within the myometrium ➡. Note the preservation of normal uterine architecture. *(Right)* Coronal oblique T2WI MR confirms the presence of the cervical ➡ and myometrial ➡ masses. Note the preservation of the normal junctional zone ➡ and the endometrium.

Typical

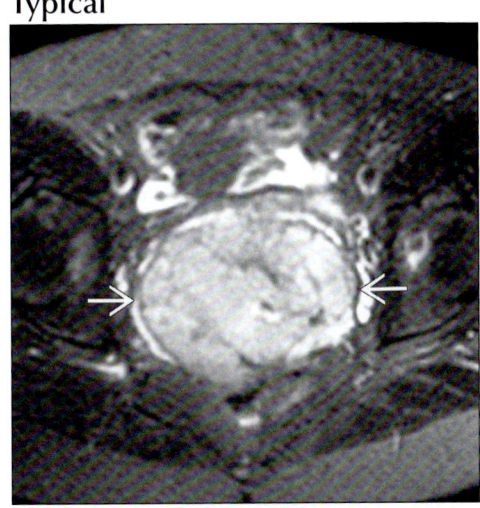
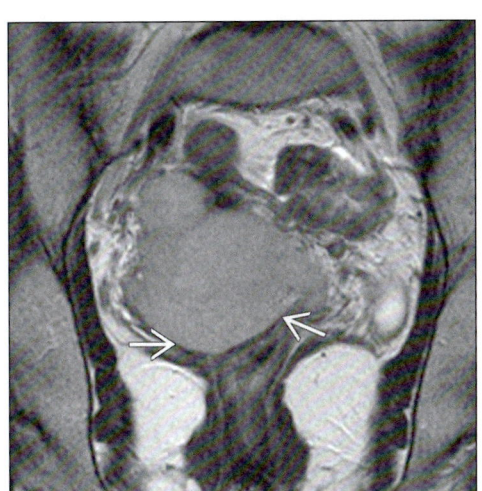

(Left) Axial T2WI FS MR of the same patient as previous image demonstrates the large heterogeneous high signal intensity cervical mass ➡. *(Right)* Coronal T2WI MR confirms the presence of the large cervical mass extending to involve the upper vagina ➡. Pathology: Primary uterine lymphoma.

Other

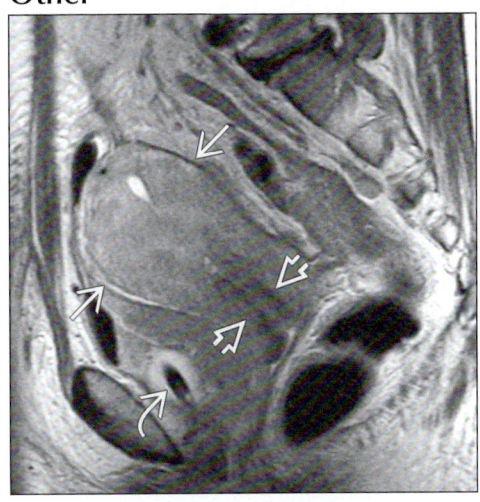
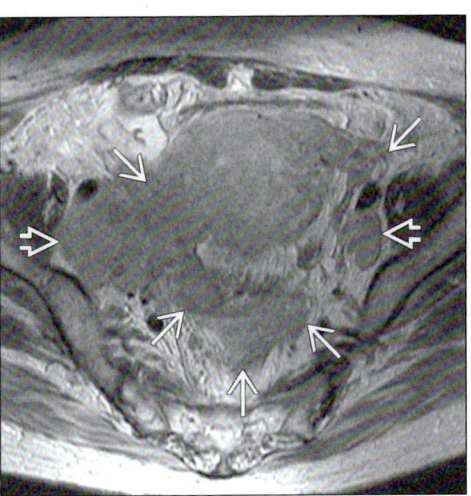

(Left) Sagittal T2WI MR shows diffuse heterogeneous appearances of uterine corpus ➡. Note preservation of normal uterine contour as well as normal low signal intensity cervical stroma ➡. Note catheter ➡ within empty bladder. *(Right)* Axial T2WI MR shows tumor extension beyond uterus ➡. There is also enlargement of external iliac nodes ➡ bilaterally. This case represents secondary involvement of uterus and pelvic lymph nodes by lymphoma.

CHORIOCARCINOMA, UTERUS

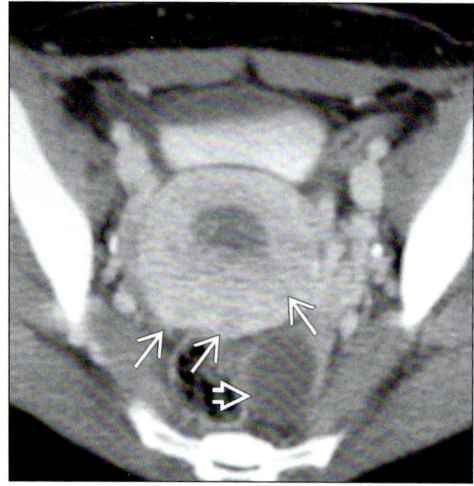

Axial CECT of uterus shows invasive molar tissue within posterior uterine wall extending to serosa ➡. Note theca lutein cyst in left ovary ➡.

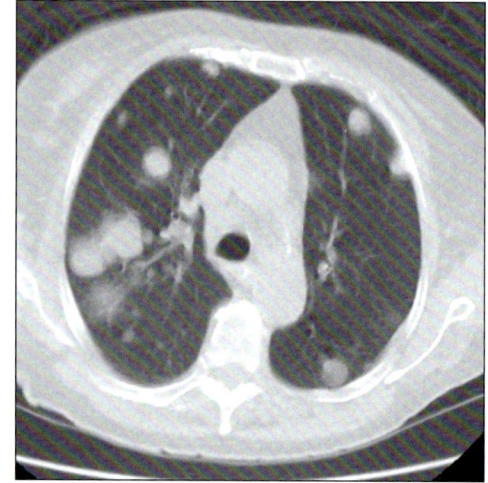

Axial NECT shows multiple round lesions in the lungs in a patient with metastatic choriocarcinoma.

TERMINOLOGY

Abbreviations and Synonyms
- Gestational trophoblastic tumor

Definitions
- Carcinoma of chorionic epithelium secondary to invasive growth of trophoblast and erosion of blood vessels

IMAGING FINDINGS

General Features
- Best diagnostic clue: Invasive endometrial process in patient with elevated human chorionic gonadotropin (hCG) with extrauterine and extrapelvic metastases
- Location
  - Localized to placenta in rare cases
  - Invasive into myometrium
  - Blood borne metastases due to affinity of trophoblast for blood vessels
    - 44% go to lungs as primary metastatic site with eventual involvement in 94%
    - 31% go to vagina as primary metastatic site with eventual involvement in 44%
    - Other sites: Brain, vulva, kidneys, liver, ovaries, bowel
- Size
  - Placental choriocarcinoma
    - Primary tumor is usually small (2.5-8 mm)
    - Extensive search of placenta often required to find tumor
  - Non-gestational primary ovarian carcinoma appears as a solid tumor
  - Uterine choriocarcinoma appears as an invasive endometrial mass
- Morphology
  - Uterine choriocarcinoma
    - Absence of villous patterns in contrast to hydatidiform or invasive mole
    - Distinguished from invasive mole by its tendency to metastasize

Ultrasonographic Findings
- Can appear similar to a complete molar pregnancy
- May have obvious extension beyond the endometrial cavity

DDx: Choriocarcinoma

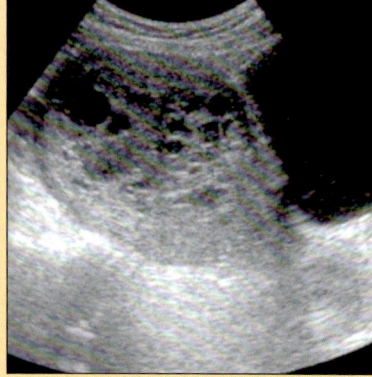
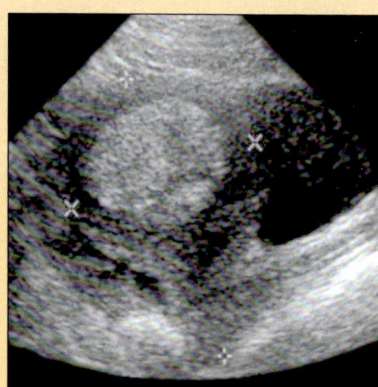
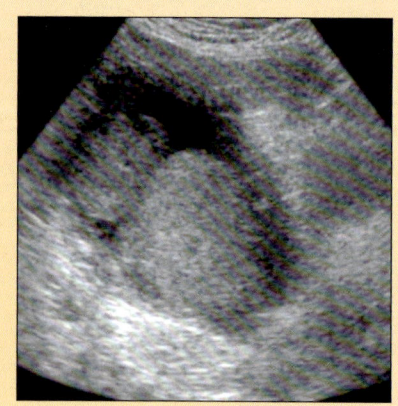

Molar Pregnancy   *Retained Products of Conception*   *Endometrial Carcinoma*

CHORIOCARCINOMA, UTERUS

Key Facts

Imaging Findings
- Best diagnostic clue: Invasive endometrial process in patient with elevated human chorionic gonadotropin (hCG) with extrauterine and extrapelvic metastases
- Absence of villous patterns in contrast to hydatidiform or invasive mole
- Distinguished from invasive mole by its tendency to metastasize
- Irregular pulmonary nodules with surrounding halo of ground glass secondary to hemorrhage
- MR better demonstrates the boundaries of myometrium and tumor than does CT

Pathology
- Etiology: Diagnostic curettage for treatment of moles may lead to dissemination of malignant trophoblast with villous tissue
- Gestation-related choriocarcinoma occurs 1/20,000-1/30,000 pregnancies in United States
- 50% follow molar pregnancy
- 18.5% of hydatidiform moles terminate with choriocarcinoma
- If presents as a primary ovarian malignancy, typical age is < 20 years old

Clinical Issues
- Rising β-hCG levels in absence or following evacuation of a pregnancy
- Clinical course depends on metastatic involvement
- Worst prognosis with nongestational choriocarcinoma
- Monitor hCG until none is detected for 3 consecutive weeks after initial treatment of complete moles

---

- Nongestational choriocarcinoma may appear as a mass with hemorrhage and necrosis

CT Findings
- Enlarged uterus
- Cystic material within endometrial cavity
- Invasion into myometrium
- Irregular pulmonary nodules with surrounding halo of ground glass secondary to hemorrhage

MR Findings
- Similar findings to CT
- MR better demonstrates the boundaries of myometrium and tumor than does CT

Imaging Recommendations
- Best imaging tool
  - Ultrasound to show the uterine tumor
  - CT and MR to evaluate metastases to lungs, brain, liver, and pelvis
    - MR better shows boundaries of myometrium and tumor involvement in pelvis than does CT
  - CXR to assess for pulmonary metastases
    - Fluoroscopy can show pulsation of nodules due to vascularity

DIFFERENTIAL DIAGNOSIS

Invasive Mole
- Excessive trophoblastic overgrowth and penetration by trophoblastic elements deep into myometrium
- Locally invasive but no distant metastases
- Villous pattern present, not seen with choriocarcinoma
- β-hCG value high (> 100,000)
- Theca lutein cysts may be present in the ovaries

Retained Products of Conception
- Mass with blood flow within the uterus after pregnancy
- Elevated hCG, but not as high as with molar pregnancy

Endometrial Cancer
- Endometrial lesion ± invasion
- β-hCG levels will not be elevated

PATHOLOGY

General Features
- Etiology: Diagnostic curettage for treatment of moles may lead to dissemination of malignant trophoblast with villous tissue
- Epidemiology
  - Gestation-related choriocarcinoma occurs 1/20,000-1/30,000 pregnancies in United States
    - 50% follow molar pregnancy
    - 25% follow miscarriage
    - 22.5% after apparently normal pregnancy may appear as infarcts on gross placental inspection
    - 2.5% after ectopic pregnancy
  - Incidence varies in different regions 1/912 pregnancies in India to 1/49,000 in Denmark
  - 18.5% of hydatidiform moles terminate with choriocarcinoma
  - If presents as a primary ovarian malignancy, typical age is < 20 years old
    - Ovarian choriocarcinomas often exist in combination with other germ cell tumors
    - Pure ovarian choriocarcinomas are rare
- Associated abnormalities
  - When choriocarcinoma follows a normal pregnancy
    - Patient and infant may be asymptomatic
    - Infant may be anemic
    - Mother may have metastases
    - Fetus may die in utero

Gross Pathologic & Surgical Features
- Distinguished from invasive mole by its pronounced tendency to metastasize
- Soft fleshy yellow-white tumor
- Large pale areas of ischemic necrosis
- Extensive hemorrhage

CHORIOCARCINOMA, UTERUS

- Rapidly growing mass invading both uterine myometrium and blood vessels with associated hemorrhage and necrosis

Microscopic Features
- Biphasic tumor composed of mononuclear cells (cytotrophoblast and intermediate trophoblast) and syncytiotrophoblast (multinucleated pleomorphic large cells)
- Large areas of hemorrhage and necrosis
- Cytotrophoblast is positive for cytokeratin immunohistochemistry
- Syncytiotrophoblast is positive for β-hCG and cytokeratin immunohistochemistry
- If villous structures are present this is referred to as invasive mole or chorioadenoma destruens

CLINICAL ISSUES

Presentation
- Most common signs/symptoms
  - Rising β-hCG levels in absence or following evacuation of a pregnancy
  - When gestationally related, can produce clinical picture similar to acute pulmonary embolism
  - Abnormal CXR following recent abortion or pregnancy in presence of elevated hCG levels
  - Hemoptysis due to pulmonary hemorrhage
  - Abnormal uterine bleeding
  - Intraplacental choriocarcinoma can present as metastases during the course of pregnancy

Demographics
- Age
  - Ovarian primary tumors in < 20 year old age group
  - Pregnancy related tumors in women on menstrual age
- Gender: Female

Natural History & Prognosis
- Metastases develop early and are generally blood borne
  - Clinical course depends on metastatic involvement
    - Metastases may disappear spontaneously
    - Metastases may disappear weeks or months after uterine evacuation
    - Metastases may proliferate and prove fatal
- Therapy usually leads to complete regression of parenchymal nodules
- Overall survival: About 90%
- Worse prognosis with solid tumor nests, high pleomorphism and high mitotic activity
- Worst prognosis with nongestational choriocarcinoma
- Better prognosis with fibrin deposits at interface between tumor and host tissues

Treatment
- Depends on type and stage
- Evacuation of uterine contents
- Monitor hCG until none is detected for 3 consecutive weeks after initial treatment of complete moles
  - Usually hCG becomes undetectable with 8-173 days
  - Monitor levels for 1 year after evacuation of a mole
  - Later recurrences can occur
- Surgery
- Chemotherapy
  - Methotrexate
  - Actinomycin D
  - Etoposide

DIAGNOSTIC CHECKLIST

Consider
- Choriocarcinoma when hCG fails to return to normal after normal or abnormal pregnancy
- Choriocarcinoma when lung metastasis are present in women after recent pregnancy

SELECTED REFERENCES

1. Kumar V: Robbins and Cotran Pathologic Basis of Disease. Philadelphia, Elsevier. 1101-13, 2005
2. Benirschke K: Pathology of the Human Placenta. 4th ed. New York, Springer-Verlag. 754-77, 2000
3. Kalir T et al: Endometrial adenocarcinoma with choriocarcinomatous differentiation in an elderly virginal woman. Int J Gynecol Pathol. 14(3):266-9, 1995
4. Redline RW et al: Pathology of gestational trophoblastic disease. Semin Oncol. 22(2):96-108, 1995
5. Brinton LA et al: Choriocarcinoma incidence in the United States. Am J Epidemiol. 123(6):1094-100, 1986
6. Bracken MB et al: Epidemiology of hydatidiform mole and choriocarcinoma. Epidemiol Rev. 6:52-75, 1984
7. Deligdisch L: Trophoblastic disease, a bridge between pregnancy and malignancy. Mt Sinai J Med. 47(5):521-7, 1980
8. Yuen BH et al: Plasma beta-subunit human chorionic gonadotropin assay in molar pregnancy and choriocarcinoma. Am J Obstet Gynecol. 127(7):711-2, 1977
9. Elston CW: The histopathology of trophoblastic tumours. J Clin Pathol Suppl (R Coll Pathol). 10:111-31, 1976
10. Mogensen B et al: Gestational choriocarcinoma in Denmark 1940-1969. A reappraisal based on modern histologic criteria. Acta Obstet Gynecol Scand. 51(1):63-9, 1972
11. Elston CW: Cellular reaction to choriocarcinoma. J Pathol. 97(2):261-8, 1969
12. Wei PY et al: The use of methotrexate in the treatment of trophoblastic diseases, especially choriocarcinoma. Am J Obstet Gynecol. 98(1):79-84, 1967
13. Lewis J Jr et al: Treatment of trophoblastic disease. With rationale for the use of adjunctive chemotherapy at the time of indicated operation. Am J Obstet Gynecol. 96(5):710-22, 1966
14. ACOSTA-SISON H: Choriocarcinoma. Philipp J Cancer. 4:122-6, 1962
15. ACOSTA-SISON H: The importance of the early diagnosis of choriocarcinoma. J Philipp Med Assoc. 38:887-9, 1962
16. BUR GE et al: Histochemical aspects of hydatidiform mole and choriocarcinoma. Obstet Gynecol. 19:156-82, 1962
17. ACOSTA-SISON H: Should one expect cure of the patient after the spontaneous regression of metastatic choriocarcinoma? Philipp J Surg. 15:86-7, 1960
18. BARDAWIL WA et al: The natural history of choriocarcinoma: problems of immunity and spontaneous regression. Ann N Y Acad Sci. 80:197-261, 1959
19. ACOSTA-SISON H: Cases of microscopically diagnosed choriocarcinoma that recovered. Philipp J Surg. 13(2):162-7, 1958

CHORIOCARCINOMA, UTERUS

IMAGE GALLERY

Typical

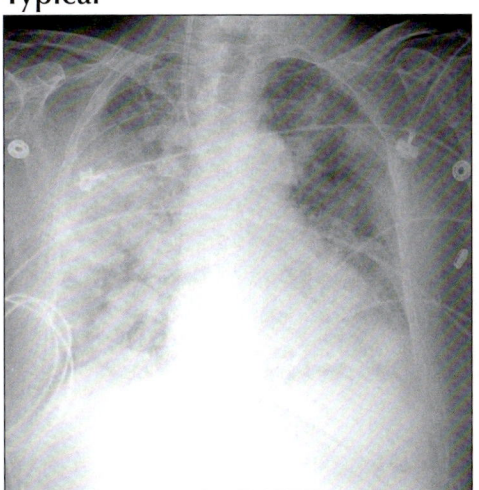
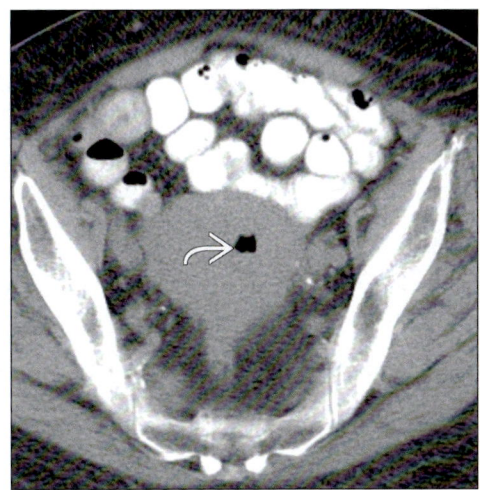

(Left) Frontal CXR shows multiple masses of varying sizes, some of which are confluent, in a patient with metastatic choriocarcinoma. *(Right)* Axial NECT shows area of necrosis ➡ within the uterus.

Typical

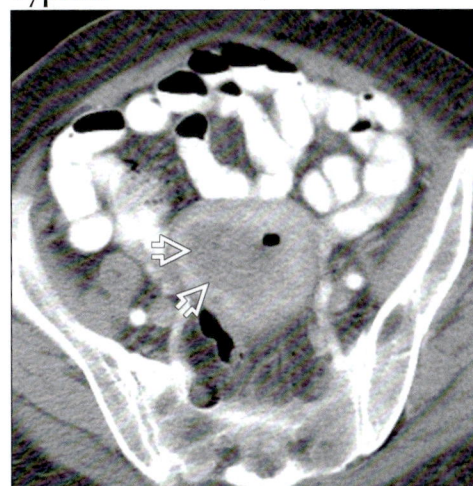
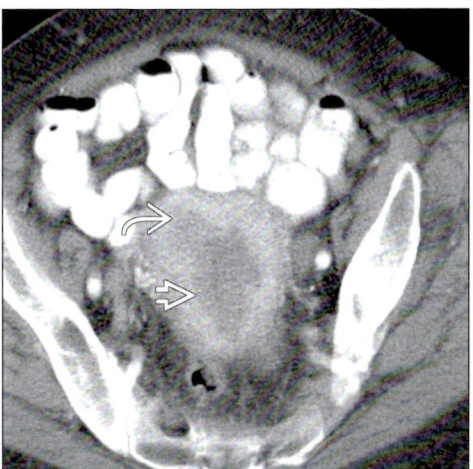

(Left) Axial CECT in same patient as previous image, shows infiltrating mass ➡ in the uterus that enhances to a lesser degree than the surrounding myometrium. *(Right)* Axial CECT shows irregular mass ➡ in the endometrial cavity with poorly defined hypodensity extending into myometrium ➡.

Typical

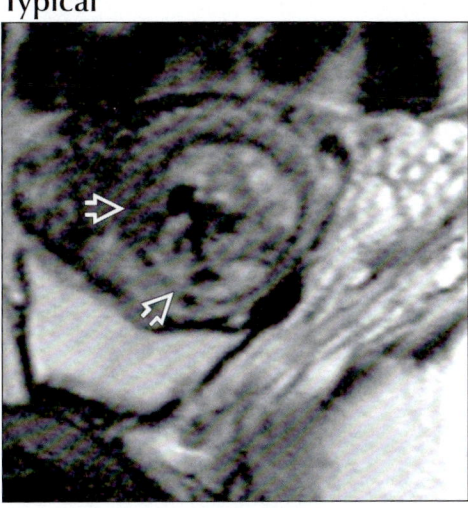
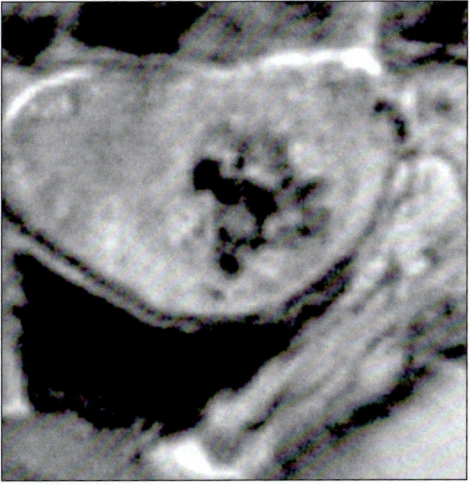

(Left) Sagittal T2WI MR shows heterogeneous mass ➡ in endometrium, extending into myometrium. *(Right)* Sagittal T1 C+ MR in same patient as previous image, shows heterogeneous enhancement of the mass.

METASTASES, UTERUS

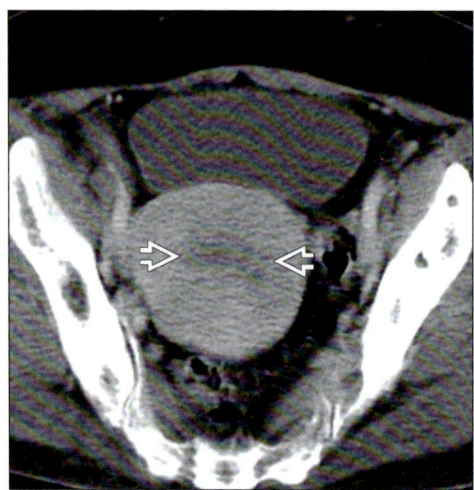

Axial CECT in a patient with past history of breast cancer shows nonspecific, irregular thickening of the endometrium ➡.

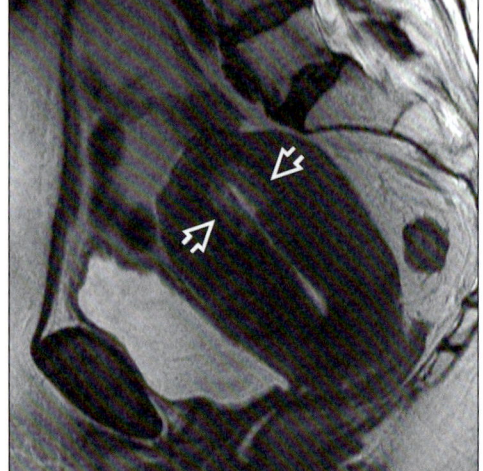

Sagittal T2WI MR shows an enlarged uterus with diffuse broadening of the myometrium and thickened irregular endometrium ➡ at the fundus. Pathology: Diffuse breast cancer metastases.

TERMINOLOGY

Abbreviations and Synonyms
- Noncontiguous secondary tumor involvement of the uterine body

Definitions
- Metastasis to the uterine body from non-uterine tumors

IMAGING FINDINGS

General Features
- Best diagnostic clue: Abnormal signal intensity mass in a preserved uterine body in patients with known malignancy such as breast or stomach cancer
- Location: More common in the myometrium, but usually concomitant involvement of both myometrium and endometrium
- Size: Usually small but can be large and cause distortion of the uterine shape

Ultrasonographic Findings
- Grayscale Ultrasound
  - Uterine shape is usually preserved
  - Uterus may be enlarged
  - Hyperechoic irregular endometrium
  - Heterogeneous myometrium or myometrial ill-defined hypoechoic lesions
- Color Doppler: Increased blood flow within the endometrial and/or myometrial lesions

CT Findings
- NECT: Enlarged uterus of preserved shape
- CECT
  - Non-specific, irregular thickening of the endometrium
  - Discrete enhancing endometrial lesions/nodules
  - Heterogeneously enhancing myometrium
  - Primary tumor such as stomach cancer may be identified

MR Findings
- T1WI
  - Usually enlarged uterus or preserved configuration
  - Mass or masses isointense to muscle

DDx: Uterine Masses

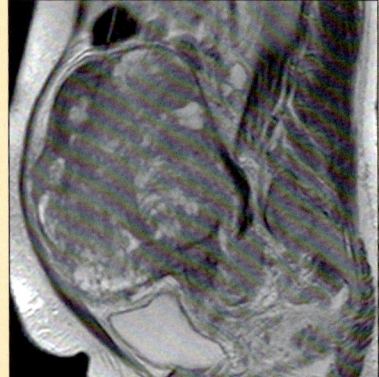
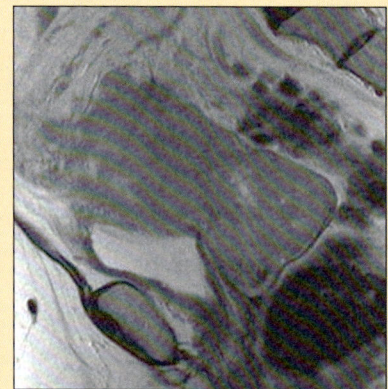
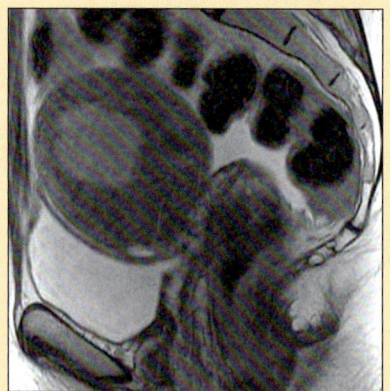

Leiomyosarcoma | Mixed Müllerian Tumor | Endometrial Carcinoma

METASTASES, UTERUS

Key Facts

Terminology
- Noncontiguous secondary tumor involvement of the uterine body

Imaging Findings
- Best diagnostic clue: Abnormal signal intensity mass in a preserved uterine body in patients with known malignancy such as breast or stomach cancer
- Location: More common in the myometrium, but usually concomitant involvement of both myometrium and endometrium
- Preservation of normal uterine shape
- Uterus frequently enlarged but may be of normal size
- Diffuse irregular infiltration of the myometrium by tumor
- Delayed DCE-MR best demonstrates heterogeneous enhancement of infiltrative tumor involving myometrium or/and endometrium

Top Differential Diagnoses
- Uterine Sarcomas (Leiomyosarcoma, MMT)
- Endometrial Carcinoma
- Leiomyoma
- Lymphoma

Diagnostic Checklist
- Infiltrative breast (invasive lobular) and stomach cancer (linitis plastica) cause diffuse infiltration of uterine body
- Invasive ductal breast cancer and melanoma cause nodular metastases to the endometrium

---

- T2WI
  - Preservation of normal uterine shape
    - Uterine shape may not be preserved with large masses
  - Uterus frequently enlarged but may be of normal size
  - Nodular irregular endometrium of intermediate signal intensity
  - Diffuse irregular infiltration of the myometrium by tumor
  - Total or partial loss of the low signal intensity junctional zone
- T1 C+ FS: Heterogeneous enhancement of the endometrial and/or myometrial lesions

Imaging Recommendations
- Best imaging tool: Gadolinium-enhanced MR is the modality of choice to detect multiple lesions within the uterus
- Protocol advice
  - T1WI, T2WI and T1WI C+ MR
  - Delayed DCE-MR best demonstrates heterogeneous enhancement of infiltrative tumor involving myometrium or/and endometrium

DIFFERENTIAL DIAGNOSIS

Uterine Sarcomas (Leiomyosarcoma, MMT)
- Lack of preservation of normal uterine shape and zonal anatomy

Endometrial Carcinoma
- Tumor of endometrial origin with possible myometrial invasion and spread to the regional lymph nodes
- MR shows diffuse or polypoid thickening of endometrium with or without invasion of junctional zone
- No evidence of primary tumor elsewhere

Leiomyoma
- Very common
- Benign solitary or multiple submucosal, intramural or subserosal solid masses
- Low signal intensity on all MR sequences

Lymphoma
- Diffusely enlarged uterus with a somewhat lobular contour
- Relative preservation of the normal T2 zonal anatomy of the uterus
- Enlarged lymph nodes in case of secondary uterine involvement by lymphoma

PATHOLOGY

General Features
- Etiology
  - Generally when tumors metastasize to the uterine body there is usually clear evidence of a primary elsewhere
  - Very rarely an occult tumor may be first identified as a metastasis in endometrial curetting
- Epidemiology
  - Breast cancer is the most primary site to metastasize to uterine body (43%)
  - Gastrointestinal tract (29%)
  - Other less common primary tumors include ovary, pancreas, lung, melanoma and kidney

Microscopic Features
- Metastases to the endometrium infiltrate diffusely, but frequently spare the endometrial glands
- Diffuse tumor infiltration or metastatic nodules in the myometrium

CLINICAL ISSUES

Presentation
- Most common signs/symptoms: Vaginal bleeding
- Other signs/symptoms: Symptoms related to known primary tumor often precede those related to the metastases to the uterus

METASTASES, UTERUS

Demographics
- Gender: Female

Natural History & Prognosis
- Patients with metastases to the uterus generally have very poor prognosis due to concomitant widespread metastatic disease

Treatment
- Chemotherapy
- Radiotherapy
- Hysterectomy if vaginal bleeding can not be controlled
- Hormone therapy
- Palliative treatment for symptom relief

DIAGNOSTIC CHECKLIST

Consider
- Metastases to uterus in a patient with
  - History of primary breast or stomach cancer
  - Vaginal bleeding
  - And abnormal signal intensity in a preserved uterine body on MR imaging

Image Interpretation Pearls
- Infiltrative breast (invasive lobular) and stomach cancer (linitis plastica) cause diffuse infiltration of uterine body
- Invasive ductal breast cancer and melanoma cause nodular metastases to the endometrium

SELECTED REFERENCES

1. Tsoi D et al: Gastric adenocarcinoma presenting as uterine metastasis--a case report. Gynecol Oncol. 97(3):932-4, 2005
2. Metser U et al: MR imaging findings and patterns of spread in secondary tumor involvement of the uterine body and cervix. AJR Am J Roentgenol. 180(3):765-9, 2003
3. Deguchi M et al: Magnetic resonance imaging diagnosis of metastasis of chronic myelocytic leukemia to the uterus. Gynecol Obstet Invest. 49(2):143-4, 2000
4. Kawakami S et al: MR appearance of malignant lymphoma of the uterus. J Comput Assist Tomogr. 19(2):238-42, 1995
5. Mambrini P et al: [Uterine metastasis revealing gastric adenocarcinoma] Gastroenterol Clin Biol. 19(8-9):725-8, 1995
6. Caskey CI et al: Distribution of metastases in breast carcinoma: CT evaluation of the abdomen. Clin Imaging. 15(3):166-71, 1991
7. Mazur MT et al: Metastases to the female genital tract. Analysis of 325 cases. Cancer. 53(9):1978-84, 1984
8. Kumar NB et al: Metastases to the uterine corpus from extragenital cancers. A clinicopathologic study of 63 cases. Cancer. 50(10):2163-9, 1982
9. Stemmermann GN: Extrapelvic carcinoma metastatic to the uterus. Am J Obstet Gynecol. 82:1261-6, 1961
10. Weingold AB et al: Extragenital metastases to the uterus. Am J Obstet Gynecol. 82:1267-72, 1961

METASTASES, UTERUS

IMAGE GALLERY

Typical

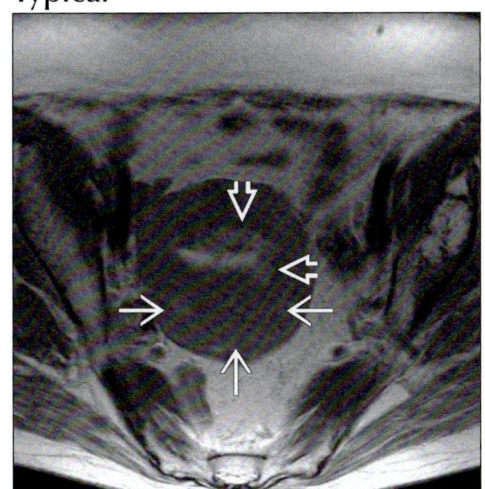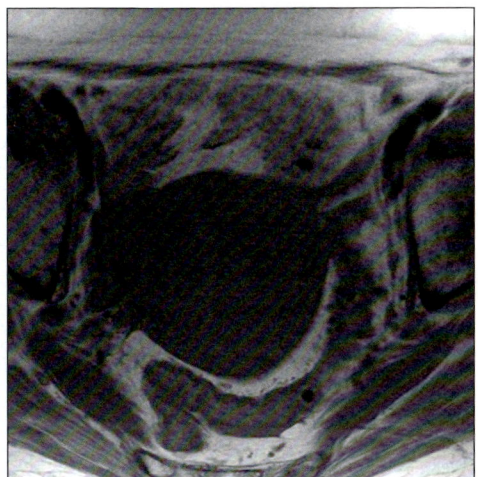

(Left) Axial T2WI MR of a patient with previous history of invasive lobular carcinoma of the breast, shows irregularities at the endometrial-myometrial junction ⇨ and diffuse broadening of the myometrium →. *(Right)* Axial T1WI MR of the same patient as previous image shows an enlarged uterus.

Typical

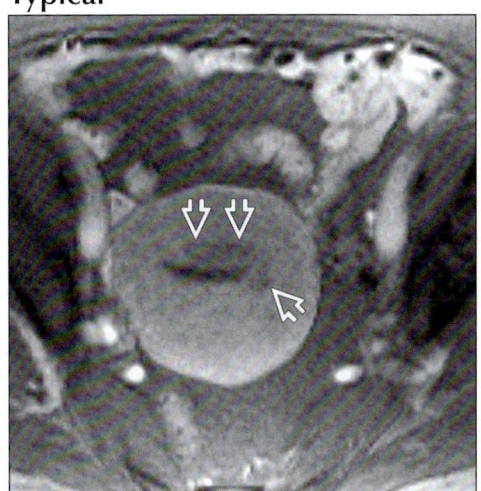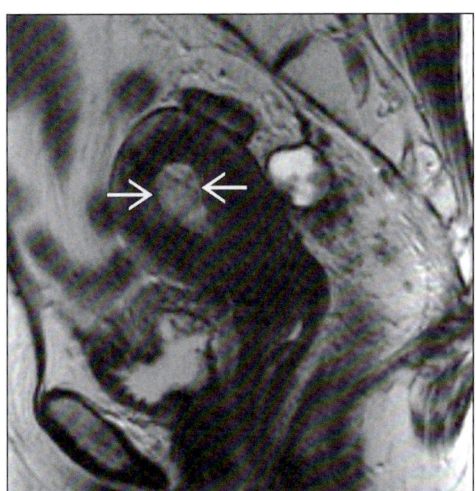

(Left) Axial T1 C+ FS MR shows irregular enhancement of the endometrial myometrial junction ⇨. At surgery, the uterus was hard. Pathology: Diffuse metastases to endometrium and myometrium. *(Right)* Sagittal T2WI MR shows nodular thickening of the endometrium → in a patient with colon cancer. Note preservation of the normal uterine shape.

Typical

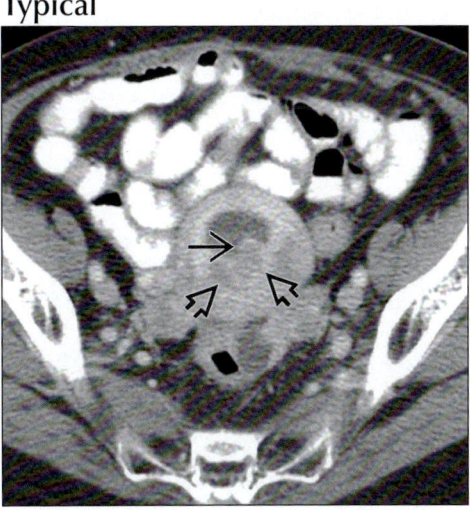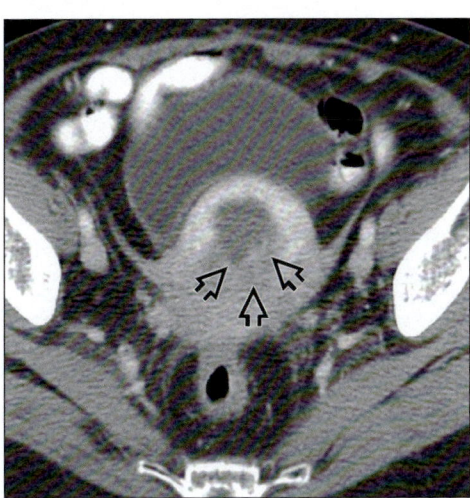

(Left) Axial CECT in the same patient as previous image shows an enhancing endometrial nodule → which is infiltrating into the myometrium ⇨. *(Right)* Axial CECT in the same patient as previous image shows irregular infiltration of the myometrium ⇨. Pathology: Nodular metastases to the endometrium and diffuse infiltration of the myometrium from colon cancer.

ADENOMYOSIS

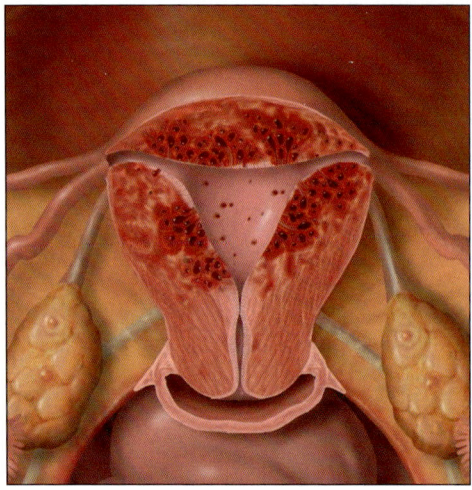

Coronal graphic shows diffuse uterine adenomyosis. The borders with the unaffected myometrium are ill-defined.

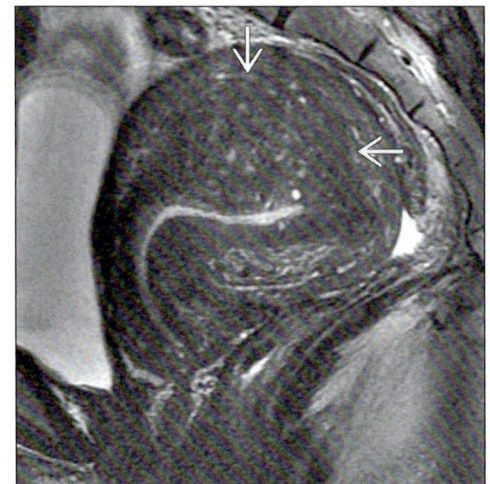

Sagittal T2WI MR shows thickening of the junctional zone (JZ), most marked at the fundus and ventral myometrium with multiple bright foci. The borders ➡ of the lesion are poorly defined.

TERMINOLOGY

Definitions
- Presence of heterotopic endometrial glands and stroma in myometrium with adjacent smooth muscle hypertrophy

IMAGING FINDINGS

General Features
- Best diagnostic clue
  - Uterine enlargement without well-defined mass ± segmental thickening of myometrial wall
  - US: Ill-defined areas of myometrial heterogeneity with decreased echogenicity ± small myometrial cysts
  - MR: Segmental/diffuse thickening of junctional zone (JZ ≥ 12 mm) ± hyperintense foci
- Morphology
  - No predilection for ventral or dorsal myometrium
    - Involvement may be diffuse or segmental
  - Elliptical rather than round myometrial abnormality
  - Poor definition of lesion borders
  - Poor definition of endo-myometrial junction
  - Relative absence of mass effect given size of lesion
  - Appearance related to distribution and amount of heterotopic endometrial tissue relative to muscular hypertrophy

Ultrasonographic Findings
- Grayscale Ultrasound
  - Poorly marginated areas of heterogeneous myometrial echotexture
    - Hypoechoic 75%
    - Isoechoic/hyperechoic 25%
  - Multiple, fine, linear areas of attenuation throughout lesion (rain shower appearance)
  - Myometrial cysts (2-6 mm) in 50%, highly specific for diagnosis
  - Subendometrial echogenic nodules or linear striations
  - Poor definition of endo-myometrial junction
  - Endometrial pseudowidening
  - Accuracy of transvaginal ultrasound (TVS): 68-86%
- Color Doppler: Speckled pattern of increased vascularity, without large peripheral vessels

DDx: Adenomyosis

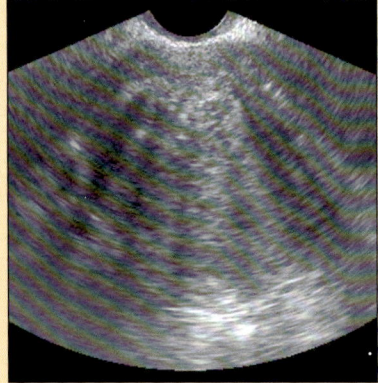

Leiomyoma

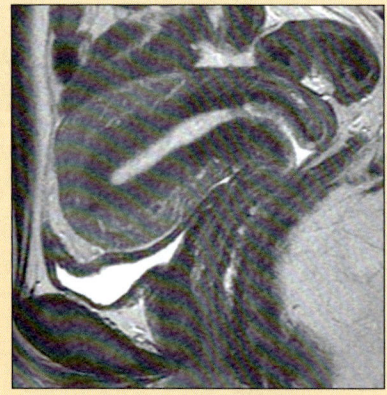

Uterine Peristalsis

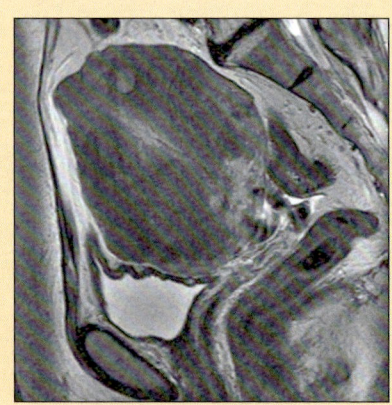

Endometrial Stromal Sarcoma

ADENOMYOSIS

Key Facts

Terminology
- Presence of heterotopic endometrial glands and stroma in myometrium with adjacent smooth muscle hypertrophy

Imaging Findings
- Uterine enlargement without well-defined mass ± segmental thickening of myometrial wall
- US: Ill-defined areas of myometrial heterogeneity with decreased echogenicity ± small myometrial cysts
- MR: Segmental/diffuse thickening of junctional zone (JZ ≥ 12 mm) ± hyperintense foci
- Relative absence of mass effect given size of lesion
- Margins of JZ ill-defined
- Color Doppler: Speckled pattern of increased vascularity, without large peripheral vessels

Top Differential Diagnoses
- Leiomyoma
- Myometrial Contraction/Peristalsis
- Diffuse Myometrial Hypertrophy
- Adenomyoma
- Uterine Malignancy
- Metastasis to Uterine Corpus

Pathology
- Epidemiology: 20-60% of hysterectomy specimens

Diagnostic Checklist
- Differentiation from leiomyoma critical due to divergent management (uterine conservation for leiomyoma vs. hysterectomy for adenomyosis)

CT Findings
- CECT
  - Not a useful diagnostic tool, findings nonspecific
  - Multidetector CECT: Early arterial enhancement of thickened JZ during menstrual phase, with punctate hypodense foci

MR Findings
- T1WI FS: High signal intensity (SI) foci representing hemorrhage of heterotopic endometrial tissue (20%)
- T2WI
  - Diffuse and symmetric thickening of JZ
    - JZ ≥ 12 mm highly predictive of adenomyosis
    - JZ ≤ 8 mm essentially excludes adenomyosis
    - JZ between 8-12 mm indeterminate, consider ancillary criteria
  - Segmental, asymmetric thickening of JZ
    - Consider adenomyosis once a myometrial contraction is excluded
    - Lesion often forms obtuse angles with JZ
  - Ancillary criteria
    - Margins of JZ ill-defined
    - High SI foci (2-6 mm) present within thickened JZ in 50%
    - Occasional fluctuation in appearance and number of high SI foci during menstrual phase
    - High SI linear striations (finger-like projections) radiating out from endometrium into myometrium
  - Post GnRH therapy changes
    - Decrease in junctional zone width
    - Decrease or resolution of high SI foci
  - Accuracy of MR: 85-90%
- T1 C+
  - No increase in diagnostic accuracy
  - Early-phase perfusion abnormalities
  - Swiss cheese appearance due to signal void of dilated glands within enhancing myometrium

Imaging Recommendations
- Best imaging tool
  - TVS initial imaging modality
  - MR as problem solving modality
    - Reserved for indeterminate cases, or for treatment planning (uterus sparing options)
- Protocol advice
  - Diagnosis with TVS must be made in real-time
  - MR: T2WI needed for diagnosis
    - Sagittal, axial and/or short-axis view
    - High-resolution imaging may increase diagnostic accuracy
    - Confirm JZ thickness when imaging during menstrual/periovulatory phases with cine MR to exclude pseudothickening from uterine peristalsis

DIFFERENTIAL DIAGNOSIS

Leiomyoma
- Well-defined, hypoechoic, myometrial-based mass
- Whorled appearance with edge shadowing
- Large vessels at periphery of lesion on color Doppler
- Hypointense to myometrium on T2WI, areas of high SI with cystic degeneration
- Mass effect on surrounding structures

Myometrial Contraction/Peristalsis
- Transient, ill-defined or sharply marginated, elliptical mass involving inner myometrium ± distortion of endometrial cavity
- Diagnose with cine MR using multiphase RARE (Rapid Acquisition with Relaxation Enhancement) sequence

Diffuse Myometrial Hypertrophy
- Diffuse, mild uterine enlargement
- Proportional and symmetric widening of JZ
  - Borders remain well-defined
  - Absence of hyperintense foci

Adenomyoma
- Mass effect on surrounding structures
- Lesion frequently discontinuous with endometrial complex
  - When continuous, forms acute angles with JZ

ADENOMYOSIS

Uterine Malignancy
- Intermediate to high SI on T2WI
- Staging errors increased with co-existing adenomyosis

Metastasis to Uterine Corpus
- Diffuse hypointense area in myometrium with uterine enlargement
- Rare, most common from breast (invasive lobular carcinoma) and gastrointestinal tract

PATHOLOGY

General Features
- General path comments
  - Heterotopic endometrial glands and stroma in myometrium with adjacent smooth muscle hypertrophy
    - Heterotopic glands must be at least 2 mm below endometrial-myometrial junction
    - Smooth muscle hypertrophy forms bulk of lesion
- Etiology
  - Unknown, likely multifactorial with hereditary component
    - Postulated endometrial migration via basement membrane defect or lymphatic/vascular channels
    - Uterine trauma from childbirth or abortion, chronic endometritis, hyperestrogenemia (Tamoxifen) are risk factors
- Epidemiology: 20-60% of hysterectomy specimens
- Associated abnormalities: Frequent association with leiomyomas, endometriosis or endometrial polyps; increased risk of endometrial carcinoma

Gross Pathologic & Surgical Features
- Firm, large and globular uterus
- Hypertrophy of myometrial smooth muscle surrounding foci of heterotopic endometrial tissue
  - Hypertrophy represented by low SI on T2WI, heterogeneity and decreased echogenicity on TVS
- Direct invasion of the endometrial zona basalis into the underlying myometrium
  - Presents as high SI or hyperechoic, finger-like projections extending out from endometrium into myometrium
- Ectopic endometrium, cystically dilated endometrial glands, and/or hemorrhage
  - Corresponding to high SI foci on T2WI
  - Ectopic endometrium: High SI foci on T2WI, echogenic nodules on TVS
  - Cystically dilated endometrial glands: High SI foci on T2WI, anechoic areas on TVS

Microscopic Features
- Endometrial glands and stroma resembling endometrial zona basalis
  - Relatively insensitive to cyclical hormonal milieu, cyclical bleeding infrequent
- Rare feature: Adenomyosis with sparse glands
  - Pathologically mimicking low-grade endometrial stromal sarcoma

Staging, Grading or Classification Criteria
- Superficial adenomyosis confined to inner myometrium (≤ 30%)
- Deep adenomyosis extends to mid and outer myometrium (> 30%)

CLINICAL ISSUES

Presentation
- Most common signs/symptoms
  - Dysmenorrhea (30%), menorrhagia (50%), metrorrhagia (20%)
  - Superficial form usually asymptomatic
- Other signs/symptoms: Pelvic pain, infertility
- Clinical Profile: 90% cases in multiparous women

Demographics
- Age: 5th and 6th decade

Natural History & Prognosis
- Rare malignant degeneration to adenocarcinoma

Treatment
- Favorable response to GnRH therapy in asymmetric adenomyosis with high SI foci on MR
- Uterine sparing therapies: Variable results
  - Superficial adenomyosis: Endometrial ablation
  - Deep adenomyosis: Myometrial excision, uterine artery embolization
- Definitive treatment: Hysterectomy

DIAGNOSTIC CHECKLIST

Consider
- Differentiation from leiomyoma critical due to divergent management (uterine conservation for leiomyoma vs. hysterectomy for adenomyosis)

Image Interpretation Pearls
- Poorly marginated, elliptical, myometrial lesion without significant mass effect
- TVS: Rain shower pattern
- MR: Low SI lesion ± multiple bright foci

SELECTED REFERENCES

1. Bergeron C et al: Pathology and physiopathology of adenomyosis. Best Pract Res Clin Obstet Gynaecol. 20(4):511-21, 2006
2. Kuligowska E et al: Pelvic pain: overlooked and underdiagnosed gynecologic conditions. Radiographics. 25(1):3-20, 2005
3. Tamai K et al: MR imaging findings of adenomyosis: correlation with histopathologic features and diagnostic pitfalls. Radiographics. 25(1):21-40, 2005
4. Atri M et al: Adenomyosis: US features with histologic correlation in an in-vitro study. Radiology. 215(3):783-90, 2000
5. Reinhold C et al: Uterine adenomyosis: endovaginal US and MR imaging features with histopathologic correlation. Radiographics. 19 Spec No:S147-60, 1999
6. Ferenczy A: Pathophysiology of adenomyosis. Hum Reprod Update. 4(4):312-22, 1998

ADENOMYOSIS

IMAGE GALLERY

Typical

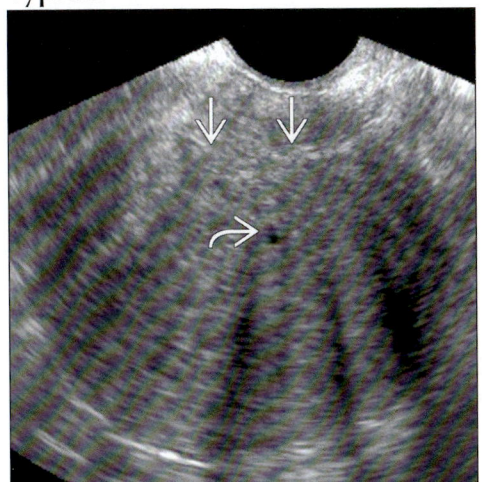
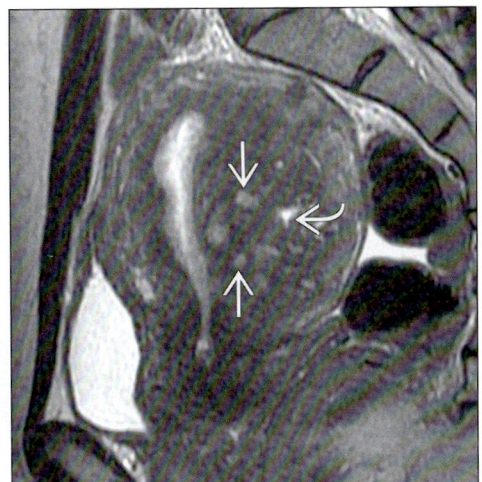

(Left) Sagittal transvaginal ultrasound shows a "rain shower" appearance of the dorsal myometrium with a 4 mm myometrial cyst ➔. The endometrium ➔ is obscured due to the adjacent adenomyosis. *(Right)* Sagittal T2WI MR in the same patient as previous image, shows the thickened JZ with foci of heterotopic endometrial tissue ➔ present in the dorsal myometrium including the small cyst ➔. Note absence of mass effect on the endometrium.

Typical

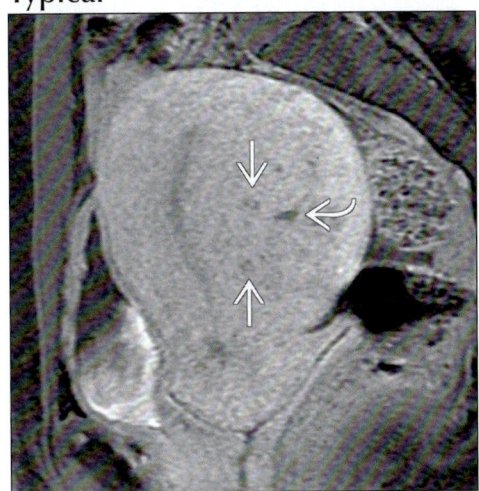
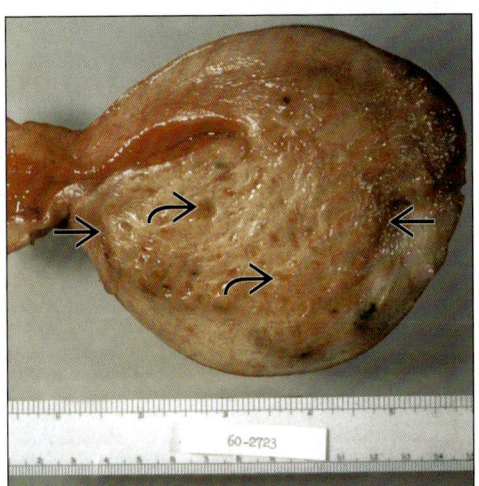

(Left) Sagittal T1 C+ FS MR shows a "swiss-cheese" appearance of the dorsal myometrium. The foci of heterotopic endometria ➔ show enhancement while the myometrial cyst ➔ remains avascular. *(Right)* Gross pathology shows segmental adenomyosis ➔ with coarsely trabeculated, hypertrophied myometrium, stippled with foci of heterotopic endometrium ➔. (Courtesy reference 8).

Typical

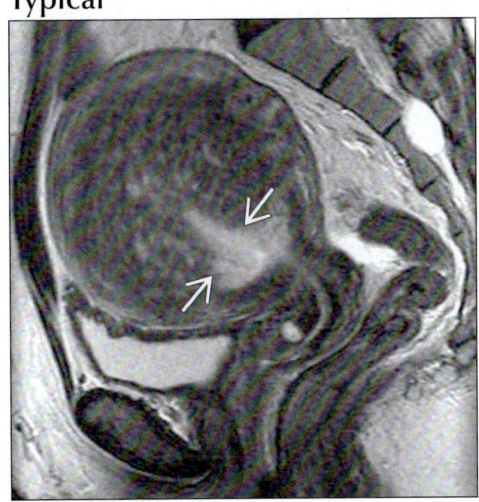
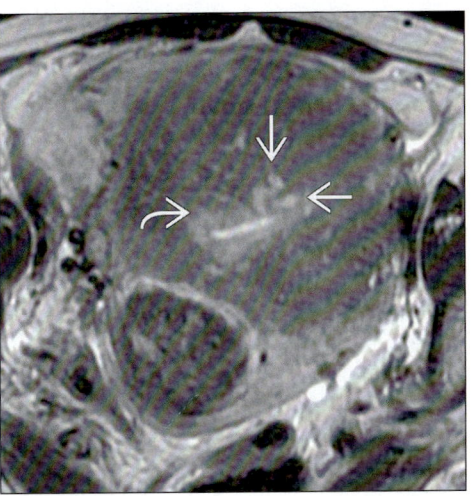

(Left) Sagittal T2WI MR shows a globular uterus with diffuse thickening of the JZ. There is pseudowidening of the endometrium ➔ due to direct extension of the endometrium into the myometrium. *(Right)* Coronal oblique T2WI MR shows linear striations of heterotopic endometrium ➔ extending into the inner myometrium, when confluent these present as endometrial pseudowidening ➔.

ADENOMYOSIS

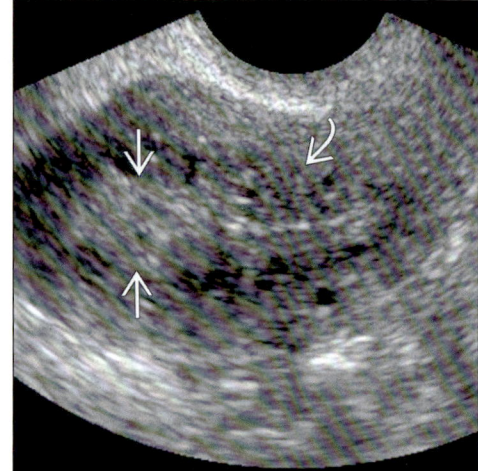
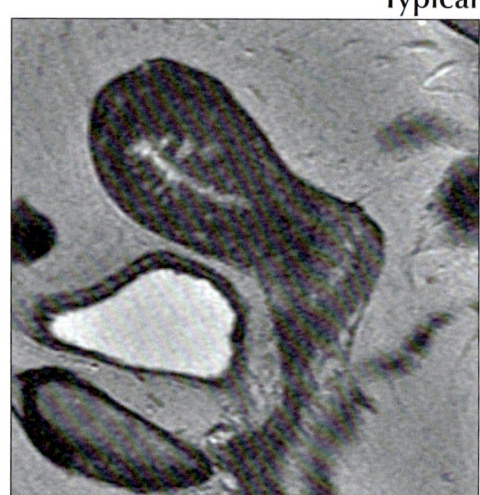

(Left) Sagittal transvaginal ultrasound shows endometrial pseudowidening ➡ in a patient with adenomyosis on Tamoxifen. The inner myometrium is of decreased echogenicity ➡ with multiple cysts. *(Right)* Sagittal T2WI MR in the same patient as previous image, shows foci of heterotopic endometrium within the inner myometrium, without the presence of endometrial thickening.

Typical

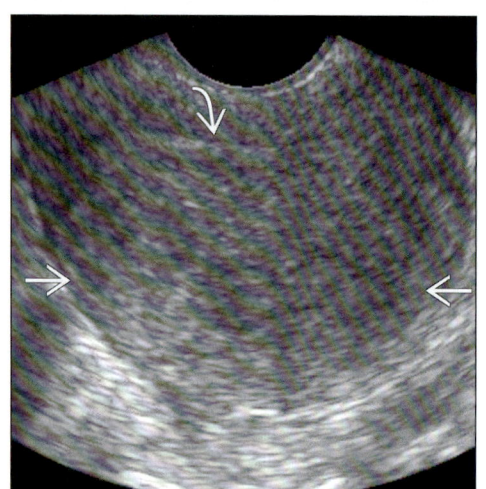
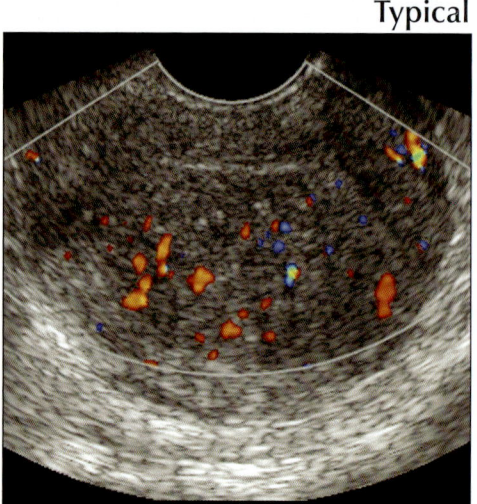

(Left) Axial transvaginal ultrasound shows asymmetric thickening of the dorsal myometrium ➡ without mass effect on the endometrium ➡. The involved myometrium is heterogeneous and hypoechoic. *(Right)* Axial color Doppler ultrasound in the same patient as previous image, shows a speckled pattern of increased vascularity in the dorsal myometrium without peripheral draping vessels seen in leiomyomas.

Typical

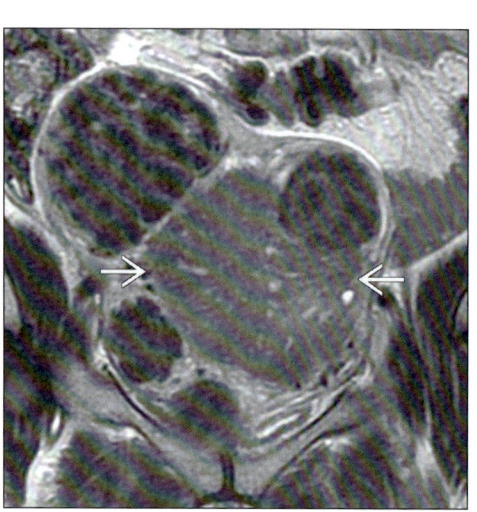
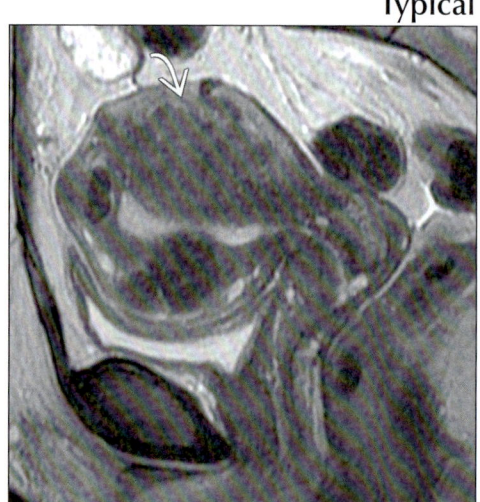

(Left) Coronal T2WI MR shows adenomyosis ➡ coexisting with uterine leiomyomas. Note the absence of mass effect by the adenomyotic lesion compared to the leiomyomas (bulging of outer contour). *(Right)* Sagittal T2WI MR shows thickening of the JZ dorsally ➡ with ill-defined borders consistent with segmental adenomyosis. Note the absence of mass effect on the endometrial lining in contradistinction to the ventral leiomyoma.

Typical

ADENOMYOSIS

Typical

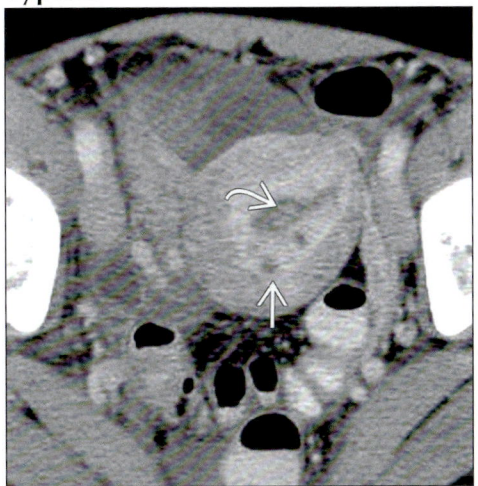
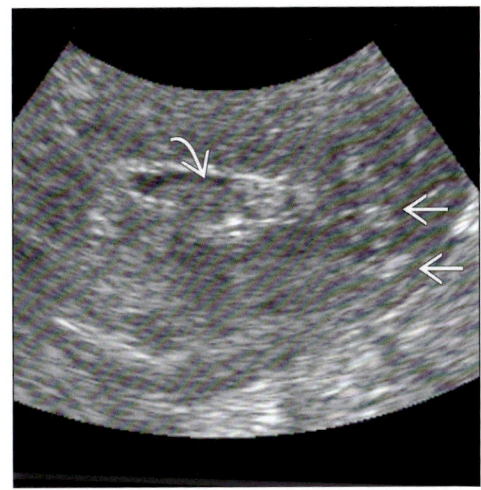

(Left) Axial CECT shows increased enhancement of a thickened JZ with hypodense foci consistent with heterotopic endometrial glands ➡. There is associated focal endometrial thickening ➡. *(Right)* Axial transvaginal ultrasound in the same patient as previous image, shows a heterogeneous myometrium of decreased echogenicity with hyperechoic foci ➡. Endometrial polyps are present ➡.

Typical

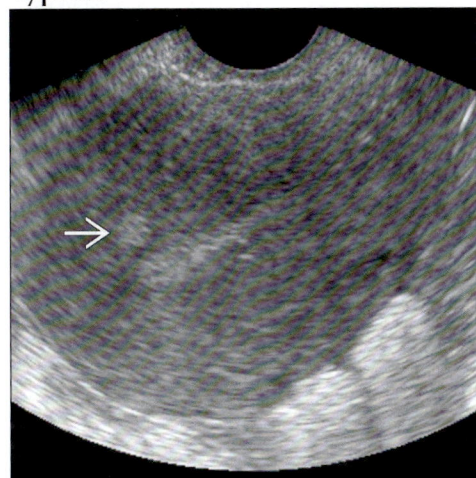
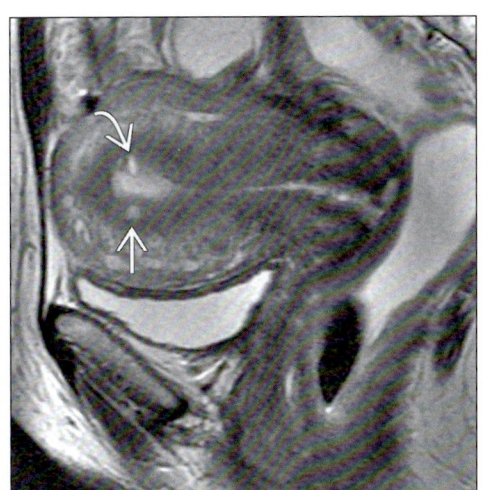

(Left) Sagittal transvaginal ultrasound shows a large hyperechoic nodule ➡ in the inner aspect of the ventral myometrium corresponding to heterotopic endometrial tissue. *(Right)* Sagittal T2WI MR in the same patient as previous image, shows the ventral nodule ➡ to be isointense to endometrium. There is a myometrial cyst ➡ dorsally that is of greater signal intensity (SI).

Typical

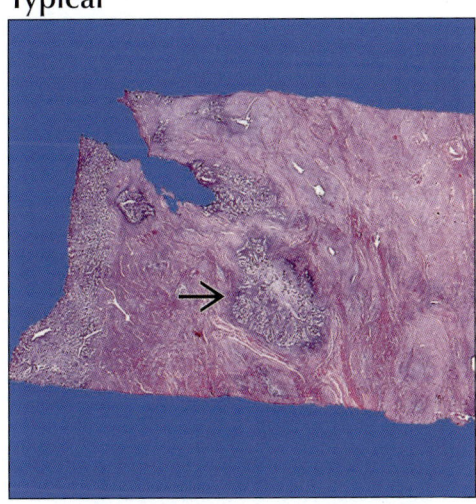
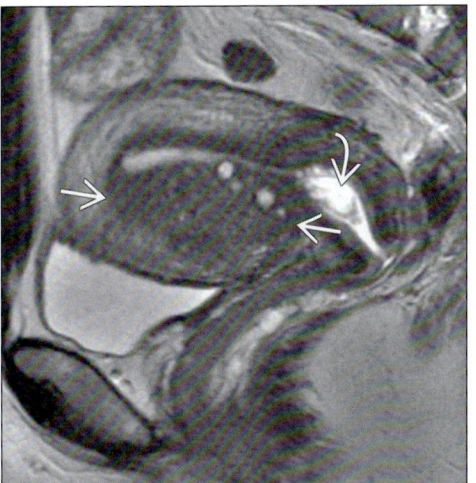

(Left) Micropathology shows the island of heterotopic endometrial tissue ➡ in the inner myometrium. There is associated muscular hypertrophy which results in the low SI of adenomyosis on T2WI. *(Right)* Sagittal T2WI MR shows thickening of the JZ ventrally resulting in an elliptical-shaped myometrial mass ➡ with multiple bright foci. Incidentally a cervical polyp is present ➡. These findings are consistent with segmental adenomyosis of the ventral myometrium.

ADENOMYOMA

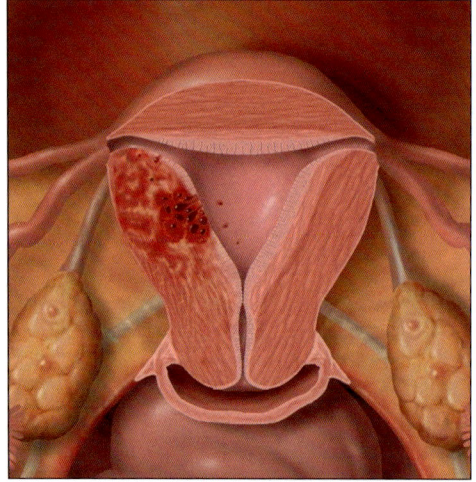

Graphic shows an adenomyoma in the right aspect of the uterus. Note although the lesion is well-circumscribed it blends into the surrounding myometrium.

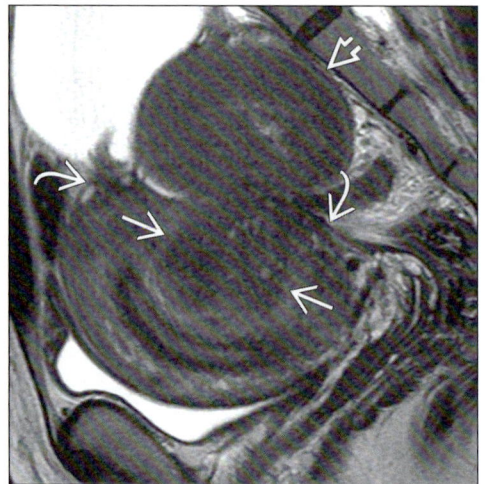

Sagittal T2WI MR shows a circumscribed hypointense myometrial mass ➡ will ill-defined borders proven to be an adenomyoma. Note the endometrioma ➡ and subserosal endometriosis ➡.

TERMINOLOGY

Definitions
- Circumscribed mass of adenomyosis in myometrium
- Distinct from segmental adenomyosis which represents a localized region of adenomyosis

IMAGING FINDINGS

General Features
- Best diagnostic clue: Circumscribed, myometrial mass with ill-defined margins and mass effect
- Location
  - Usually myometrial, most commonly corpus uteri
  - Occasionally involving or originating from endometrium to grow as a polypoid mass
  - Rarely subserosal pedunculated mass
- Morphology
  - Appearance related to distribution and amount of heterotopic endometrial tissue relative to muscular hypertrophy
  - Lesion frequently discontinuous with endometrial complex
  - Poor definition of endo-myometrial junction in lesions abutting endometrial complex
  - Elliptical or round configuration
  - Typically less mass effect on endometrium or serosa than leiomyomas, but greater than adenomyosis

Radiographic Findings
- Hysterosalpingography (HSG)
  - Has no role in diagnosing adenomyoma
    - Low sensitivity due to majority of lesions not communicating with endometrial cavity
  - Multiple spicules, 1-4 mm in length extending from endometrium into myometrium, ending in small sacs

Ultrasonographic Findings
- Grayscale Ultrasound
  - Hypoechoic, heterogeneous myometrial mass with ill-defined borders is typical
  - Internal echogenic nodules or linear striations, less commonly seen with adenomyoma than adenomyosis
  - Myometrial cysts 50%, 2-6 mm
    - Representing hemorrhagic foci ± endometrial cysts within heterotopic endometrial tissue

DDx: Adenomyoma

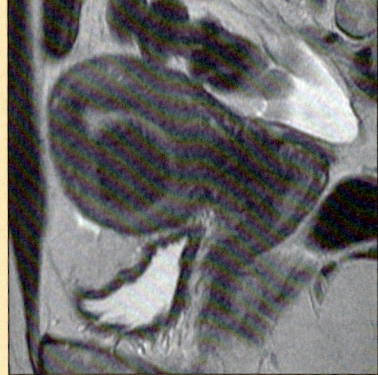

Leiomyoma

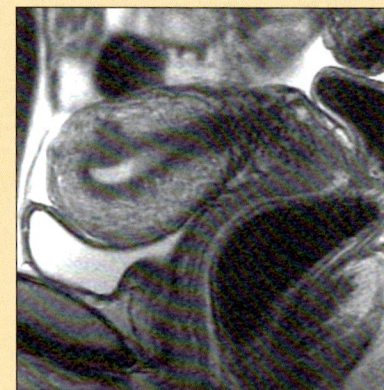

Myometrial Contraction

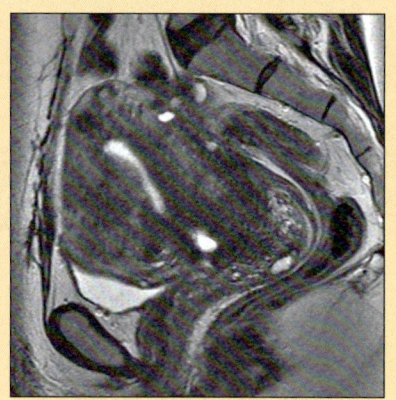

Subserosal Endometriosis

ADENOMYOMA

Key Facts

Terminology
- Circumscribed mass of adenomyosis in myometrium

Imaging Findings
- Best diagnostic clue: Circumscribed, myometrial mass with ill-defined margins and mass effect
- Occasionally involving or originating from endometrium to grow as a polypoid mass
- Lesion frequently discontinuous with endometrial complex

Top Differential Diagnoses
- Leiomyoma
- Adenomyosis
- Myometrial Contraction
- Subserosal Endometriosis
- Endometrial Polyp

Pathology
- Infiltrating into surrounding normal tissues, in contradistinction to leiomyoma which displaces normal tissues
- Gross impression frequently is leiomyoma or endometrial polyp

Diagnostic Checklist
- Differentiation from leiomyoma critical due to divergent management (uterine conservation for leiomyoma vs. hysterectomy for adenomyoma)
- Circumscribed myometrial-based mass with ill-defined borders and evidence of mass effect
- Penetrating vs. draping vascular pattern for differentiation from leiomyoma

---

- Accuracy of ultrasound not well-studied
- Color Doppler
  - "Penetrating" vascular pattern within the mass
    - Speckled pattern of increased vascularity
  - Absence of large vessels at periphery of lesion

CT Findings
- CECT
  - Variable non specific appearance
    - "Swiss cheese" appearance due to signal voids of dilated glands within enhancing myometrium

MR Findings
- T1WI FS: Occult except for occasional high signal intensity (SI) foci due to small areas of hemorrhage
- T2WI
  - Circumscribed ill-defined, low SI myometrial mass
  - Foci of high signal within low SI mass: 50%
    - Representing heterotopic endometrial tissue, hemorrhagic foci and/or endometrial cysts
  - Lesions abutting endometrial complex present as focal widening of junctional zone (JZ), typically ≥ 12 mm
    - Angle between adenomyoma and junctional zone frequently acute
    - High SI linear striations extending out from endometrium into myometrium, seen less commonly with adenomyoma than adenomyosis
  - Accuracy of MR not well-studied
    - Strongly dependent on selection criteria for patient population
- T1 C+
  - Variable, not helpful for diagnosis
  - Early-phase hypoperfusion abnormalities with dynamic T1 C+
  - "Swiss cheese" appearance due to signal void of cysts within enhancing myometrium
  - Delayed T1 C+ images show enhancement of heterotopic endometrial foci (become iso- or slightly hyperintense to adjacent myometrium)

Imaging Recommendations
- Best imaging tool
  - Transvaginal ultrasound (TVS) initial imaging modality
    - Color Doppler optimization for slow flow facilitates differentiation from leiomyoma
  - MR a problem solving modality
    - Reserved for indeterminate cases at TVS
    - Patients undergoing uterus sparing surgery
- Protocol advice
  - Diagnosis with TVS must be made in real-time
  - High-resolution fast spin echo (FSE) T2WI
    - Sagittal, axial and/or short-axis view
  - Routine acquisition of cine MR using multiphase RARE (Rapid Acquisition with Relaxation Enhancement) during menstrual phase avoids mistaking a myometrial contraction for a true lesion

DIFFERENTIAL DIAGNOSIS

Leiomyoma
- Homogeneous or heterogeneous hypoechoic mass ± calcification
- Whorled appearance and edge shadowing on TVS
- Hypointense to myometrium on T2WI, occasional peripheral cystic degeneration
- Mass effect on surrounding structures
- Large vessels at periphery of lesion (draping vs. penetrating pattern)
- May be indistinguishable from adenomyoma

Adenomyosis
- Segmental adenomyosis may be difficult to differentiate from an adenomyoma
- Poorly circumscribed, ill-defined borders and absence of mass effect
- Usually abuts endometrial complex
- Typically forms obtuse angles with junctional zone

Myometrial Contraction
- Transient, ill-defined or sharply marginated elliptical mass in inner myometrium with distortion of endometrial cavity
- Less commonly transmural

ADENOMYOMA

- Hypoechoic on TVS and hypointense on T2WI
- Diagnosis with multiphase RARE sequence

Subserosal Endometriosis
- Lesion originates from serosal surface of uterus and secondarily involves outer myometrium
- Discontinuous with junctional zone
- Associated findings of endometriosis: Solid plaque between uterus and rectum, endometriomas, ovaries tethered to uterine surface, adhesions
- Morphology indistinguishable from adenomyoma
  - Bright foci on T2 and T1 weighted images common

Endometrial Polyp
- True adenomyomas can appear identical to endometrial polyps

PATHOLOGY

General Features
- General path comments
  - Nodular aggregate of benign endometrial glands surrounded by endometrial stroma with smooth muscle bordering the endometrial stromal component
    - Lesion border merging to some degree with adjacent myometrium
    - Adjacent smooth muscle hypertrophy
  - Infiltrating into surrounding normal tissues, in contradistinction to leiomyoma which displaces normal tissues
  - Infrequent menstrual-type changes in heterotopic endometrium
- Etiology
  - Histogenesis poorly understood
  - Postulated endometrial migration via basement membrane defect or lymphatic/vascular channels
- Epidemiology: 2% of endometrial polyps are adenomyomas
- Associated abnormalities: Diffuse adenomyosis (30%), leiomyomas (50%)

Gross Pathologic & Surgical Features
- Gross impression frequently is leiomyoma or endometrial polyp
- Firm in consistency with gray-white surface on cut section
- Cystic spaces filled with dark brown material (30%)

Microscopic Features
- Nodular aggregate of benign endometrial glands surrounded by endometrial stroma and smooth muscle
- Margin indistinct from surrounding normal myometrium
- Must distinguish histologically from adenofibroma and adenosarcoma
- Atypical polypoid adenomyoma
  - Rare variant of adenomyomatous polyp
  - Atypical hyperplastic glands with foci of squamous metaplasia

CLINICAL ISSUES

Presentation
- Most common signs/symptoms: Abnormal vaginal bleeding
- Other signs/symptoms
  - Dysmenorrhea, pelvic pain, pelvic mass, infertility and anemia
  - Prolapsing mass visible at the external os
- Clinical Profile: 90% cases in multiparous women

Demographics
- Age: 5th and 6th decade

Treatment
- Hysterectomy definitive treatment
- Polypectomy and myomectomy successful without recurrence

DIAGNOSTIC CHECKLIST

Consider
- Differentiation from leiomyoma critical due to divergent management (uterine conservation for leiomyoma vs. hysterectomy for adenomyoma)

Image Interpretation Pearls
- Circumscribed myometrial-based mass with ill-defined borders and evidence of mass effect
- Penetrating vs. draping vascular pattern for differentiation from leiomyoma

SELECTED REFERENCES

1. Tahlan A et al: Uterine adenomyoma: a clinicopathologic review of 26 cases and a review of the literature. Int J Gynecol Pathol. 25(4):361-5, 2006
2. Andreotti RF et al: The sonographic diagnosis of adenomyosis. Ultrasound Q. 21(3):167-70, 2005
3. Kuligowska E et al: Pelvic pain: overlooked and underdiagnosed gynecologic conditions. Radiographics. 25(1):3-20, 2005
4. Tamai K et al: MR imaging findings of adenomyosis: correlation with histopathologic features and diagnostic pitfalls. Radiographics. 25(1):21-40, 2005
5. Matalliotakis IM et al: Adenomyosis. Obstet Gynecol Clin North Am. 30(1):63-82, viii, 2003
6. Reinhold C et al: Uterine adenomyosis: endovaginal US and MR imaging features with histopathologic correlation. Radiographics. 19 Spec No:S147-60, 1999
7. Ferenczy A: Pathophysiology of adenomyosis. Hum Reprod Update. 4(4):312-22, 1998
8. Fedele L et al: Transvaginal ultrasonography in the differential diagnosis of adenomyoma versus leiomyoma. Am J Obstet Gynecol. 167(3):603-6, 1992

ADENOMYOMA

IMAGE GALLERY

Typical

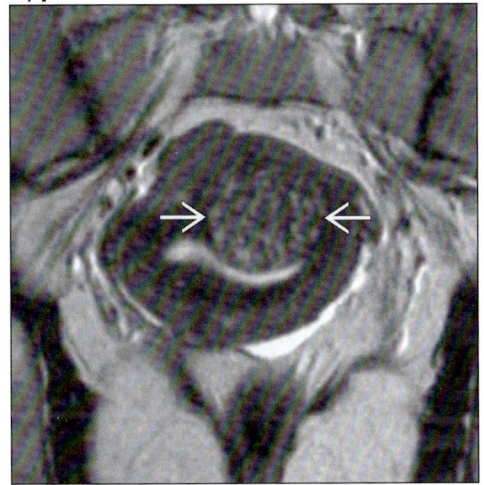 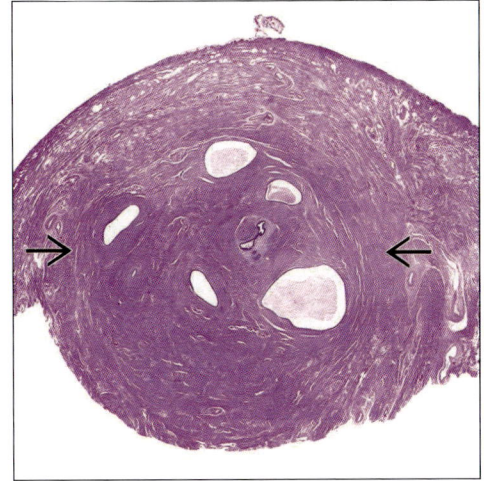

(Left) Coronal T2WI MR shows a well-circumscribed mass ➡ with ill-defined borders that blend into the surrounding myometrium. Note the mass effect on the endometrium and multiple bright foci. (Right) Micropathology shows a nodular aggregate of benign endometrial glands surrounded by smooth muscle ➡. The margin is indistinct from the surrounding myometrium. (Courtesy reference 7).

Typical

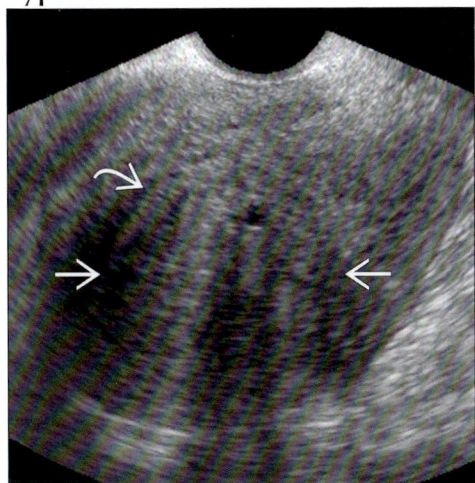 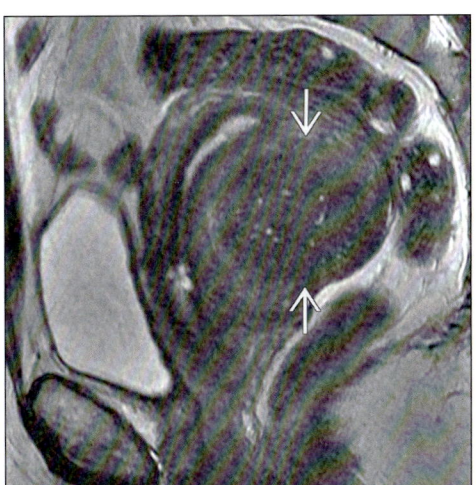

(Left) Sagittal transvaginal ultrasound shows a hypoechoic and heterogeneous mass ➡ with a small anechoic cyst in the dorsal myometrium. Note the mass effect on the endometrial lining ➡. (Right) Sagittal T2WI MR shows a circumscribed, ill-defined myometrial mass ➡ with multiple bright foci. The mass effect favors an adenomyoma (proven at surgery) over segmental adenomyosis.

Typical

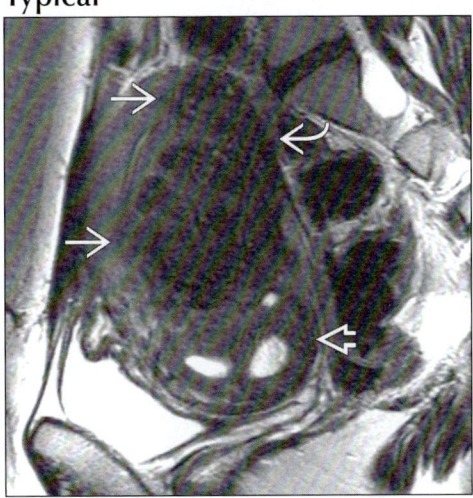 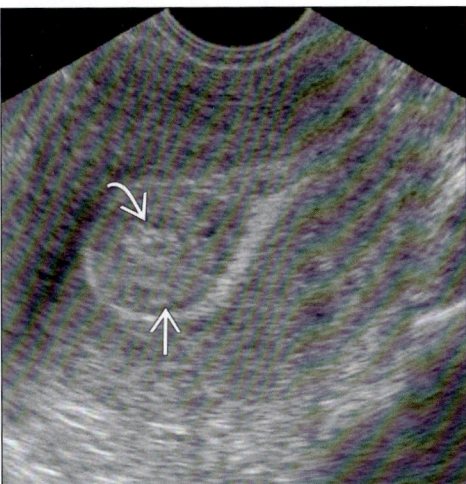

(Left) Sagittal T2WI MR shows two circumscribed myometrial masses ➡ with ill-defined borders proven to be adenomyomas. There is co-existing cystic adenomyosis ➡ and subserosal endometriosis ➡. (Right) Sagittal transvaginal ultrasound shows a focal endometrial lesion ➡ proven to be an adenomyoma. There is an echogenic nodule ➡ consistent with heterotopic endometrial tissue.

CYSTIC ADENOMYOSIS

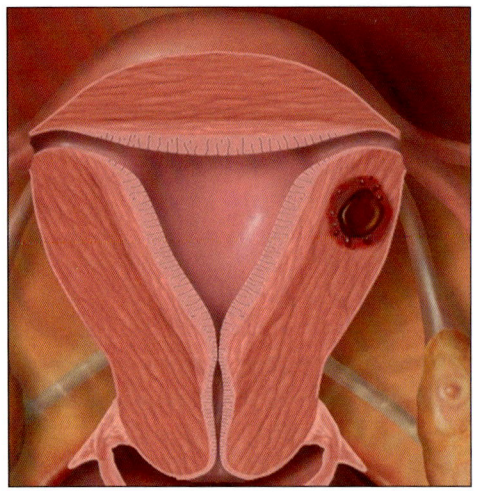

Graphic shows a hemorrhagic area in the left aspect of the myometrium consistent with cystic adenomyosis. Note that both cornua can be identified separately.

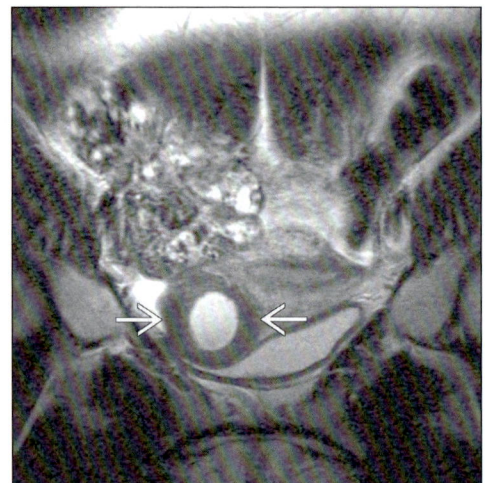

Coronal T2WI MR shows a thick-walled, cystic mass ➡ arising from the outer myometrium. Note the low signal intensity of the rim and the hyperintense central contents.

TERMINOLOGY

Definitions
- Extensive hemorrhage within ectopic endometrial glands of focal or diffuse adenomyosis

IMAGING FINDINGS

General Features
- Best diagnostic clue
  - Well-circumscribed, thick-walled, complex cystic mass of myometrial origin
  - Separate endometrial cavity with a normal configuration (both cornua present)
- Location
  - Most frequently intramural
    - Typically involves outer myometrium
  - Occasionally subserosal, rarely submucosal
- Size: Variable, 2-22 cm
- Morphology
  - Primarily round, ovoid or lobulated, less commonly multicystic
  - Well-defined margins with peripheral solid rim
  - Central cystic component with blood products in different stages of organization
    - Fluid-fluid level may be present
  - Lesion demonstrates mass effect
  - Potential for rupture into endometrial cavity
  - Associated adenomyosis in the remaining myometrium present in some cases

Ultrasonographic Findings
- Grayscale Ultrasound
  - Thick-walled, cystic, myometrial mass
  - Central cystic portion: Variable appearance depending on the degree and age of hemorrhage
    - Low to intermediate level echoes
    - Less commonly hyperechoic
    - May have a solid appearance
  - Peripheral rim: Ranges from slightly hypo- to slightly hyperechoic relative to myometrium
- Color Doppler
  - Wall shows increased vascularity
  - Central portion is avascular confirming cystic nature

CT Findings
- NECT: Well-defined myometrial mass with internal hemorrhage

DDx: Cystic Myometrial Mass

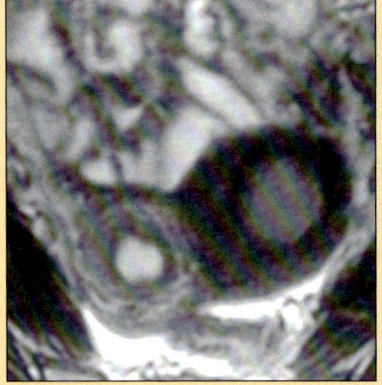

Hematometra

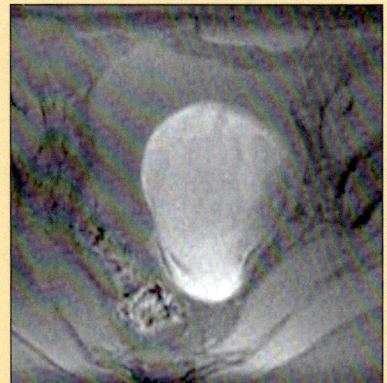

Hemorrhagic Leiomyoma

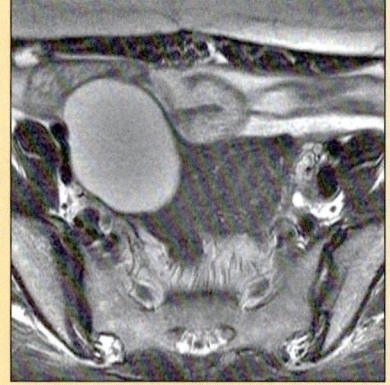

Gartner Duct Cyst

CYSTIC ADENOMYOSIS

Key Facts

Terminology
- Extensive hemorrhage within ectopic endometrial glands of focal or diffuse adenomyosis

Imaging Findings
- Well-circumscribed, thick-walled, complex cystic mass of myometrial origin
- Separate endometrial cavity with a normal configuration (both cornua present)
- Typically involves outer myometrium
- Well-defined margins with peripheral solid rim
- Central cystic component with blood products in different stages of organization
- Lesion demonstrates mass effect

Top Differential Diagnoses
- Leiomyoma with Hemorrhagic Degeneration
- Leiomyoma with Fatty Degeneration
- Hematometra
- Miscellaneous Uterine Cysts

Clinical Issues
- Progressive increase in size due to periodic intracystic secretion and bleeding
- Initial medical management: Danazol, GnRH agonist
- Myometrial excision of affected area with failure of medical treatment

Diagnostic Checklist
- Thick-walled cystic myometrial mass with internal hemorrhage
- Normal uterine configuration with presence of both cornua

- CECT
  - High density nonenhancing central cystic portion
  - Thick enhancing wall

MR Findings
- T1WI FS
  - Well-defined hyperintense myometrial mass
    - Homogeneous high signal intensity represents subacute blood
    - No signal loss with fat-suppression
  - Rim isointense to myometrium
- T2WI
  - Well-circumscribed, cystic myometrial mass
  - Central cystic portion: Appearance variable depending on the degree and age of hemorrhage
    - Intermediate to high signal intensity most common appearance
    - Less frequently hypointense relative to myometrium
    - Typically homogeneous
  - Peripheral rim: Low signal intensity due to hemosiderin deposition
- CEMR
  - Central portion nonenhancing
  - Rim-enhancement relative to normal myometrium
    - Slightly hypointense on early CE images
    - Isointense on delayed scans

Imaging Recommendations
- Best imaging tool
  - Transvaginal US initial modality
  - MR highly accurate for making the diagnosis and planning therapy
- Protocol advice
  - High-resolution fast spin echo (FSE) T2WI acquired in sagittal, axial and/or short-axis view
  - T1WI ± fat suppression in an appropriate plane

DIFFERENTIAL DIAGNOSIS

Leiomyoma with Hemorrhagic Degeneration
- Imaging findings overlap
- Appearance typically more heterogeneous
- Rim or wall less prominent

Leiomyoma with Fatty Degeneration
- Signal loss on fat-suppressed T1WI
- Chemical shift artifact on in- and opposed-phase imaging

Hematometra
- Presence of noncommunicating uterine horn
- Only one cornua identified in dominant horn

Miscellaneous Uterine Cysts
- Congenital cysts (mesonephric/paramesonephric), cervical nabothian cyst, echinococcal cyst
  - Simple cysts with thin wall

PATHOLOGY

General Features
- General path comments: Blood-filled cysts surrounded by focal myometrial hypertrophy
- Etiology
  - Not well understood
  - Hemorrhage mostly in deeply located foci of adenomyosis
    - Unclear whether hemorrhage within implants of cystic adenomyosis represents sequela of cyclic hormonal changes, or is result of spontaneous hemorrhage
    - Hormonal receptors exhibiting some degree of proliferative and secretory changes have been identified in adenomyotic implants
- Epidemiology: Rare

Gross Pathologic & Surgical Features
- Well-defined intramyometrial mass, with smooth or trabeculated white surface
- Exophytic cystic polypoid mass connected to uterus
- Thick-walled cavities with brown staining of wall and surrounding myometrium, representing hemosiderin and hemolyzed blood

CYSTIC ADENOMYOSIS

Microscopic Features
- Single dominant cyst or multiple > 5 mm clefts filled with blood
- Endometrial glands lining cyst wall
  - Main differentiating feature of cystic adenomyosis from cystic degeneration of leiomyomas
  - Smooth muscle and hyaline degeneration may occur, mimicking leiomyomas
  - Uncommonly focal squamous or mucinous epithelial metaplasia
- Hemosiderin-laden macrophages around cyst wall corresponding to low signal intensity on T2WI

CLINICAL ISSUES

Presentation
- Most common signs/symptoms: Pelvic pain ± palpable mass
- Other signs/symptoms
  - Menorrhagia, dysmenorrhea, and abdominal cramps
  - Abdominal distention and lower back pain during or after menstrual period

Demographics
- Age: More commonly seen in premenopausal women

Natural History & Prognosis
- Progressive increase in size due to periodic intracystic secretion and bleeding
- Favorable prognosis

Treatment
- Initial medical management: Danazol, GnRH agonist
  - Variable results from symptomatic relief to reduction in cyst size
- Myometrial excision of affected area with failure of medical treatment
  - Occasionally supplemented with post-excision hormonal therapy
- Successful radiofrequency ablation reported
- Definitive treatment: Hysterectomy

DIAGNOSTIC CHECKLIST

Consider
- Cystic adenomyosis in the differential diagnosis of a well-defined, cystic myometrial mass, with hemorrhagic central contents

Image Interpretation Pearls
- Thick-walled cystic myometrial mass with internal hemorrhage
- Typically occur in outer myometrium
- Normal uterine configuration with presence of both cornua

SELECTED REFERENCES
1. Fisseha S et al: Cystic myometrial lesion in the uterus of an adolescent girl. Fertil Steril. 86(3):716-8, 2006
2. Koga K et al: Images in reproductive medicine. A case of giant cystic adenomyosis. Fertil Steril. 85(3):748-9, 2006
3. Ryo E et al: Radiofrequency ablation for cystic adenomyosis: a case report. J Reprod Med. 51(5):427-30, 2006
4. Imaoka I et al: Cystic adenomyosis with florid glandular differentiation mimicking ovarian malignancy. Br J Radiol. 78(930):558-61, 2005
5. Sakai Y et al: Large cystic uterine adenomyoma showing marked epithelial metaplasia and exophytic polypoid growth. Arch Gynecol Obstet. 269(1):74-6, 2003
6. Reinhold C et al: Uterine adenomyosis: endovaginal US and MR imaging features with histopathologic correlation. Radiographics. 19 Spec No:S147-60, 1999
7. Kataoka ML et al: MRI of adenomyotic cyst of the uterus. J Comput Assist Tomogr. 22(4):555-9, 1998
8. Troiano RN et al: Cystic adenomyosis of the uterus: MRI. J Magn Reson Imaging. 8(6):1198-202, 1998
9. Iribarne C et al: Intramyometrial cystic adenomyosis. J Clin Ultrasound. 22(5):348-50, 1994

CYSTIC ADENOMYOSIS

IMAGE GALLERY

Typical

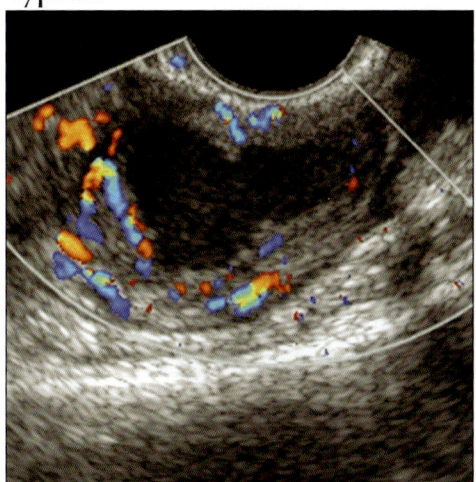 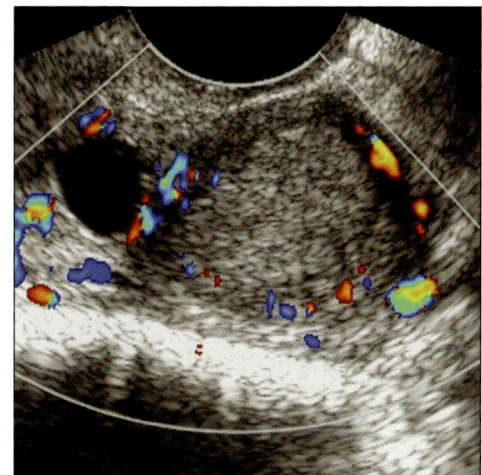

(Left) Sagittal color Doppler ultrasound shows an oblong-shaped subserosal mass, with a thick-walled rim and central cystic component containing low-level echoes. The rim shows moderate vascularity. *(Right)* Axial color Doppler ultrasound obtained two months later in the same patient as previous image, shows increased echogenicity of the central contents, which remain avascular, due to recent hemorrhage.

Typical

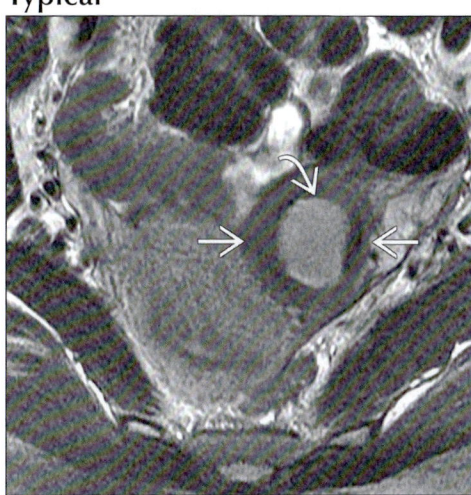 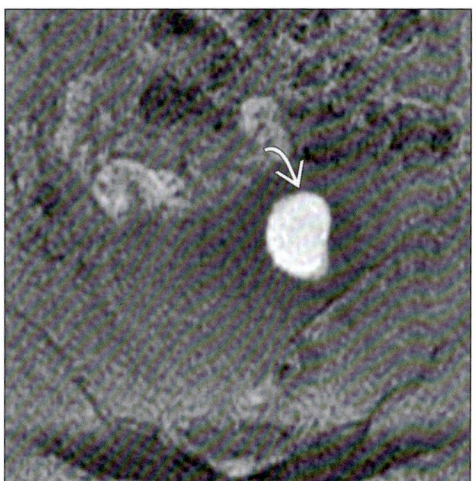

(Left) Axial T2WI MR of the same patient as previous image, shows a subserosal, thick-walled cystic mass ➡. The wall is hypointense and the cyst contents of intermediate signal intensity ➡. *(Right)* Axial T1WI FS MR in the same patient as previous image, shows homogeneous high signal intensity of the cyst contents ➡, corresponding to hemorrhage.

Typical

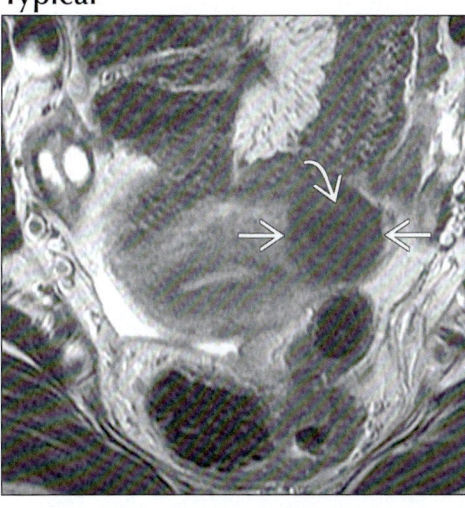 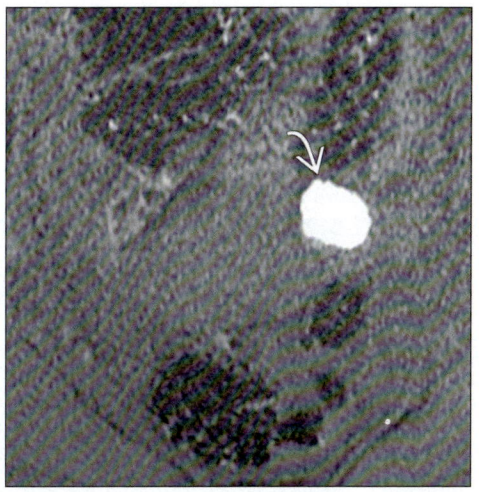

(Left) Axial T2WI MR shows a hypointense mass ➡ arising from the outer myometrium. The central component ➡ appears slightly darker than the peripheral rim. *(Right)* Axial T1WI FS MR in the same patient as previous image, shows a hyperintense mass ➡ corresponding to the markedly hypointense central component on the T2WI, indicating the presence of hemorrhage.

UTERINE AVM

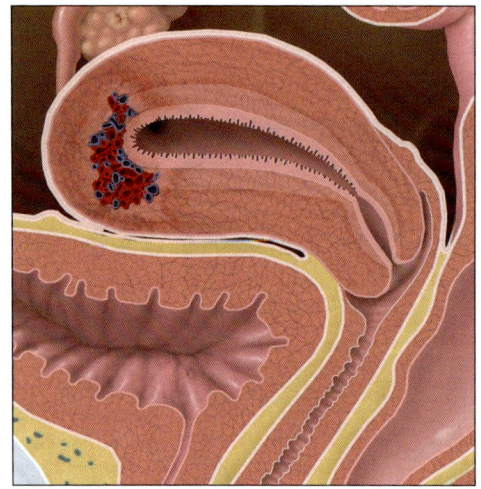

Sagittal graphic shows a uterine arteriovenous malformation (AVM) at the level of the fundus of the uterus. Note the "spongy" appearance of involved myometrium.

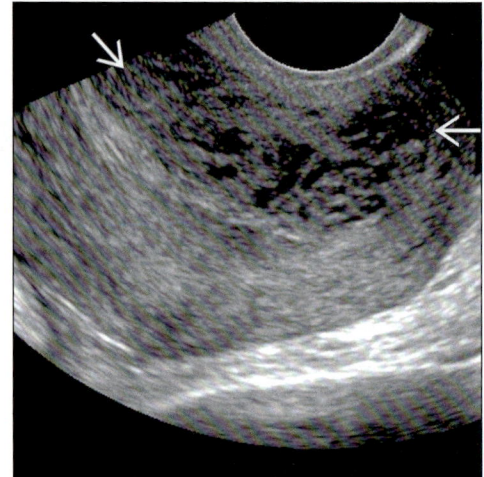

Sagittal transvaginal ultrasound shows replacement of the ventral myometrium with multiple serpiginous anechoic areas ➡. There is no mass effect. (Courtesy J. Pellerito, MD).

TERMINOLOGY

Abbreviations and Synonyms
- Uterine arteriovenous malformation (AVM), uterine arteriovenous fistula (AVF), uterine cirsoid aneurysm

Definitions
- True uterine AVM: Single or multiple arteriovenous connections between intramural arterial branches and myometrial venous plexus without intervening capillary network
- Uterine non-AVM: Arise from failure of obliteration of placental bed vessels in the absence of retained placental tissue after cessation of pregnancy, or after abortion

IMAGING FINDINGS

General Features
- Best diagnostic clue
  - Doppler US: Mosaic color pattern with aliasing and low-resistance, high-velocity flow within abnormal areas of myometrium, no intervening tissue
  - Contrast-enhanced MR: Complex, serpentine, abnormal vessels within myometrium with early venous return
- Location
  - Myometrium, localized or more extensive
  - May protrude into endometrial cavity
- Morphology: Myometrial vascular abnormality without mass effect, prominent parametrial vessels

Ultrasonographic Findings
- Grayscale Ultrasound
  - Variable and non-specific appearance
    - Classical findings: Multiple, tubular, anechoic spaces within myometrium resulting in "spongy" myometrial echotexture
    - Visible flow/pulsatility in cystic spaces
    - Generally no soft tissue interposed between vascular spaces
    - Subtle myometrial inhomogeneity
    - Normal-appearing endometrium
  - Uncommon sonographic appearances: Focal intramural mass resembling leiomyoma, endometrial mass mimicking endometrial polyp
- Pulsed Doppler

DDx: Hypervascular Uterine Mass

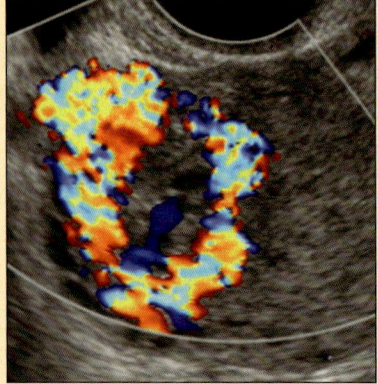
Choriocarcinoma

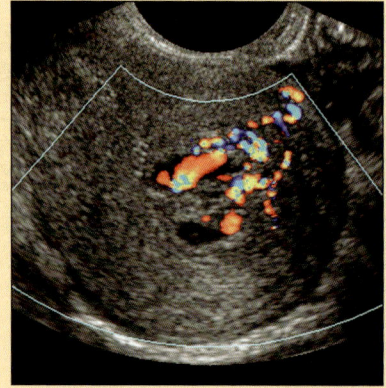
Retained Products of Conception

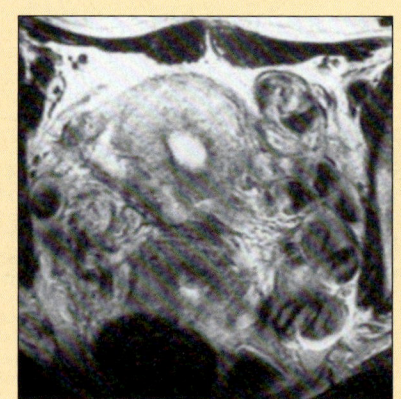
Pelvic Congestion Syndrome

UTERINE AVM

Key Facts

Terminology
- True uterine AVM: Single or multiple arteriovenous connections between intramural arterial branches and myometrial venous plexus without intervening capillary network
- Uterine non-AVM: Arise from failure of obliteration of placental bed vessels in the absence of retained placental tissue after cessation of pregnancy, or after abortion

Imaging Findings
- Doppler US: Mosaic color pattern with aliasing and low-resistance, high-velocity flow within abnormal areas of myometrium, no intervening tissue
- Contrast-enhanced MR: Complex, serpentine, abnormal vessels within myometrium with early venous return

Top Differential Diagnoses
- Gestational Trophoblastic Disease (GTD)
- Retained Products of Conception
- Pelvic Varicosities
- Uterine Hemangiomas

Clinical Issues
- Potential for life threatening vaginal bleeding, mandating early diagnosis and treatment
- In stable patients, expectant management has a role
- Fertility conserving treatment with transcatheter arterial embolization

Diagnostic Checklist
- Consider uterine AVM in a patient with a vascular uterine mass and unexpected bleeding, in the setting of recent pregnancy, D&C or other intervention

---

- High flow, low-resistance arterial flow (resistive index: 0.1-0.6; pulsatility index: 0.3-0.6)
- Typically high peak systolic velocity (PSV): > 100 cm/sec, occasionally lower PSV 20-100 cm/sec
  - PSV may correlate with need for intervention
- Pulsatile high-velocity venous waveform with low to high variation in systolic-diastolic velocities
  - Pelvic veins distal to AVM demonstrate pulsatile flow in contrast to normal monophasic flow
- Color Doppler
  - Modality of choice for diagnosis
    - Mosaic pattern of color signals within myometrial cystic spaces, due to color aliasing associated with high velocity flow
    - Apparent flow reversal of juxtaposed reds and blues indicating vessels of varying orientation with different flow directions
  - Limited in delineating extent of lesion
  - Cannot reliably differentiate true AVMs from non-arteriovenous vascular malformations (non-AVMs); seen in the same clinical setting
- Power Doppler: All cystic spaces filled with flow

CT Findings
- CTA
  - Noninvasive modality for diagnosis, evaluation, and treatment planning
  - Dual-phase intravenous CT angiography with 3-dimensional rendering
    - Hypervascular, arterial-dominant lesion with large vascular channels
    - Early filling of dilated veins diagnostic of AVM

MR Findings
- T1WI
  - Multiple, serpentine flow-related signal voids
  - Hemorrhage: Hyperintense areas with mass effect
- T2WI
  - Bulky appearance of involved myometrium
  - Distortion of uterine zonal anatomy with disruption of junctional zone
  - Multiple, serpentine flow-related signal voids
- T1 C+ FS
  - Useful for delineating extent of malformation, treatment planning and post-embolization follow-up
  - Complex, serpentine, abnormal vasculature enhancing as intensely as normal vessels
- MRA: Enlarged feeding arteries supplying a vascular network ± early venous filling

Angiographic Findings
- Historical gold standard, reserved for transcatheter embolization or surgical intervention
- True AVM (high-flow malformation)
  - Hypertrophied uterine arteries (single or bilateral)
  - Complex tangle of vessels with early venous filling
  - Direct communication between artery and vein
- Non AVM (low-flow malformation)
  - Hypertrophied uterine arteries
  - Rapid opacification of uterine parenchyma
  - Normal filling of large pelvic veins
  - No direct communication between artery and vein

Imaging Recommendations
- Protocol advice
  - Doppler US modality of choice for initial diagnosis and follow-up
  - Contrast-enhanced T1WI/MRA for confirmation and assessment of disease extent
  - Doppler US coupled with MR imaging can substitute for diagnostic angiography
  - Angiography to delineate feeding arteries and draining veins for treatment planning

DIFFERENTIAL DIAGNOSIS

Gestational Trophoblastic Disease (GTD)
- Overlapping imaging/Doppler features, positive β-hCG
- May coexist with uterine AVM

Retained Products of Conception
- Endometrial-based mass with overlapping Doppler characteristics, positive β-hCG

UTERINE AVM

- Uncommonly β-hCG can be negative with cystic degeneration of retained products

Pelvic Varicosities
- Prominent parametrial vessels with normal venous spectral waveforms

Uterine Hemangiomas
- Complex mass with acoustic shadowing due to phleboliths

PATHOLOGY

General Features
- Etiology
  - Rare in women without history of pregnancy
  - Risk factors: Dilatation and curettage (D&C), intrauterine devices, pelvic surgery, infection, GTD, endometrial/cervical carcinoma, diethylstilbestrol exposure

Gross Pathologic & Surgical Features
- Congenital (rare): Anomalous differentiation of primitive capillary plexus with small vascular connections
  - Growth in pregnancy
- Acquired (most cases): Post-traumatic or post-infectious
  - High-flow AVM: True arteriovenous malformation with hemodynamic characteristics of fistula
    - Single abnormal vascular communication between artery and vein without nidus
  - Low-flow AVM ("non-AVM"): Subinvolution of placental bed
    - Failure of obliteration of placental bed vessels in absence of retained placental tissue

Microscopic Features
- Muscular and thin-walled capillary-like vessels in varying proportions, with characteristics of both vein and artery
- Prominent intimal fibrous thickening with some elastin in walls

Staging, Grading or Classification Criteria
- Congenital vs. acquired
- High-flow AVM vs. low-flow AVM (non-AVM)

CLINICAL ISSUES

Presentation
- Most common signs/symptoms
  - Unexpected, intermittent and torrential bleeding, suggestive of arterial source
    - Particularly after delivery, miscarriage or surgical procedures on uterus
    - Hormonal changes (pregnancy, menstruation, high-dose estrogen & progestin) as bleeding trigger
    - Potentially life-threatening hemorrhage with diagnostic D&C (if AVM not suspected)
- Other signs/symptoms: Lower abdominal pain, dyspareunia, anemia, high-output cardiac failure
- Clinical Profile
  - Negative serum β-hCG
  - Refractory menometrorrhagia (requiring blood transfusion in 30% of cases)

Demographics
- Age: Between 20 and 40

Natural History & Prognosis
- Potential for life threatening vaginal bleeding, mandating early diagnosis and treatment
  - High index of suspicion to prevent diagnostic D&C
- In stable patients, expectant management has a role
  - Spontaneous resolution is common

Treatment
- Fertility conserving treatment with transcatheter arterial embolization
- Hysterectomy uncommonly performed
- Stable patients without spontaneous resolution may respond to course of medical therapy

DIAGNOSTIC CHECKLIST

Consider
- Consider uterine AVM in a patient with a vascular uterine mass and unexpected bleeding, in the setting of recent pregnancy, D&C or other intervention

Image Interpretation Pearls
- Doppler US: Mosaic color pattern with aliasing and low-resistance, high-velocity flow in an area of multiple, tubular, anechoic spaces within the myometrium
- True arteriovenous malformation (AVM): Early venous filling of a uterine vascular network with enlarged feeding arteries

SELECTED REFERENCES

1. Maleux G et al: Acquired uterine vascular malformations: radiological and clinical outcome after transcatheter embolotherapy. Eur Radiol. 16(2):299-306, 2006
2. Grivell RM et al: Uterine arteriovenous malformations: a review of the current literature. Obstet Gynecol Surv. 60(11):761-7, 2005
3. Timmerman D et al: Color Doppler imaging is a valuable tool for the diagnosis and management of uterine vascular malformations. Ultrasound Obstet Gynecol. 21(6):570-7, 2003
4. Kwon JH et al: Obstetric iatrogenic arterial injuries of the uterus: diagnosis with US and treatment with transcatheter arterial embolization. Radiographics. 22(1):35-46, 2002
5. Nagayama M et al: Fast MR imaging in obstetrics. Radiographics. 22(3):563-80; discussion 580-2, 2002
6. Nasu K et al: Uterine arteriovenous malformation: ultrasonographic, magnetic resonance and radiological findings. Gynecol Obstet Invest. 53(3):191-4, 2002
7. Polat P et al: Color Doppler US in the evaluation of uterine vascular abnormalities. Radiographics. 22(1):47-53, 2002
8. Huang MW et al: Uterine arteriovenous malformations: gray-scale and Doppler US features with MR imaging correlation. Radiology. 206(1):115-23, 1998

UTERINE AVM

IMAGE GALLERY

Typical

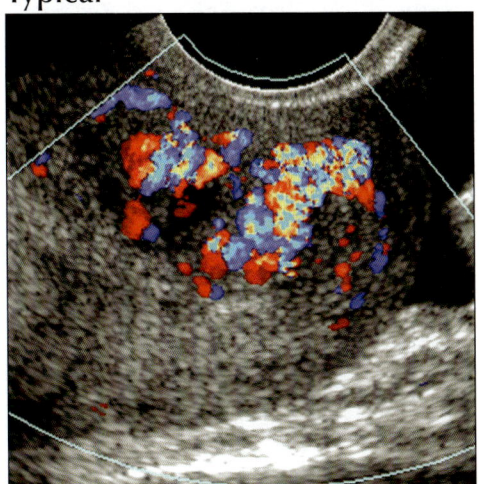
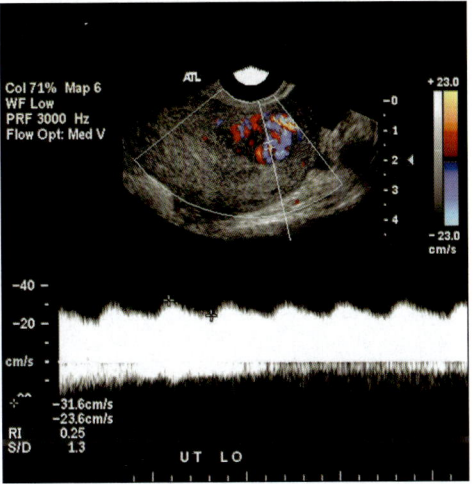

(Left) Sagittal oblique color Doppler ultrasound shows a mosaic pattern of color signal with aliasing filling the myometrial cystic spaces. (Courtesy J. Pellerito, MD). *(Right)* Sagittal transvaginal ultrasound with color and pulsed Doppler in the same patient as previous image, shows low impedance flow (RI = 0.25), as well as spectral broadening. (Courtesy J. Pellerito, MD).

Typical

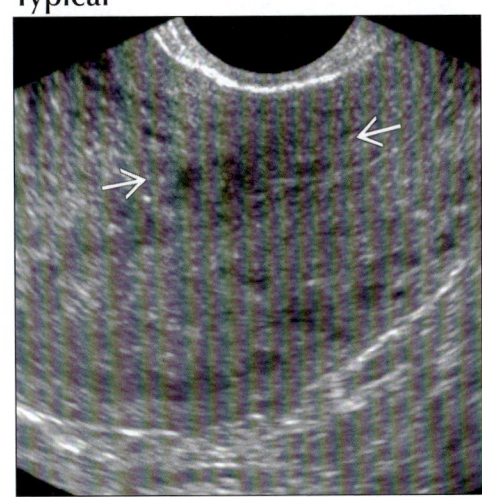
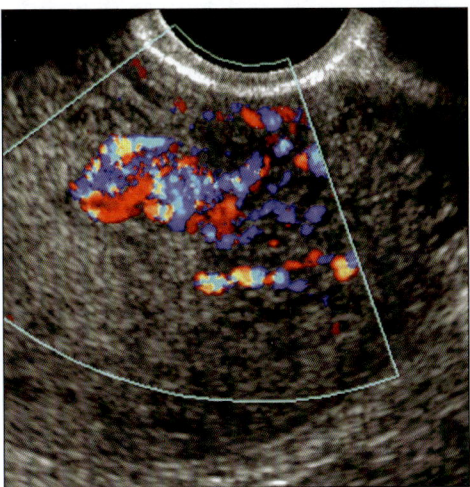

(Left) Sagittal transvaginal ultrasound shows a subtle area of heterogeneity within the inner ventral myometrium ➡. Note the absence of mass effect on the endometrial lining. *(Right)* Sagittal oblique color Doppler ultrasound in the same patient as previous image, shows apparent flow reversal of juxtaposed reds and blues indicating vessels of varying orientation and flow directions.

Typical

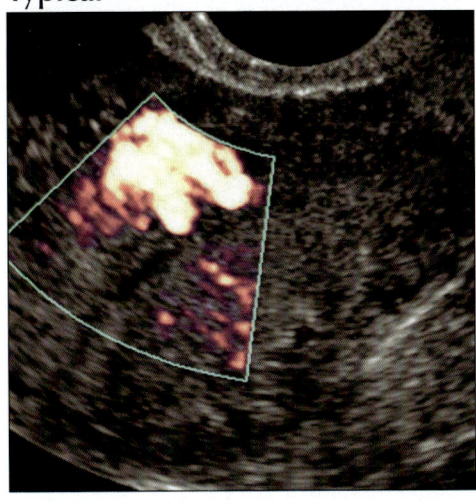
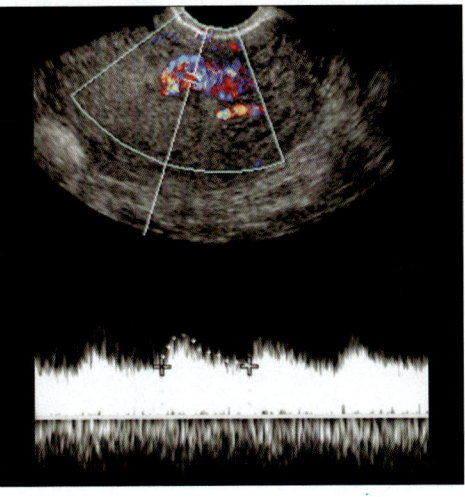

(Left) Sagittal power Doppler ultrasound in the same patient as previous image, shows the tangle of vessels consistent with an arteriovenous malformation. *(Right)* Sagittal oblique transvaginal ultrasound with color and pulsed Doppler in the same patient as previous image, shows a high peak systolic velocity (PSV) > 100 cm/sec, and low impedance.

UTERINE AVM

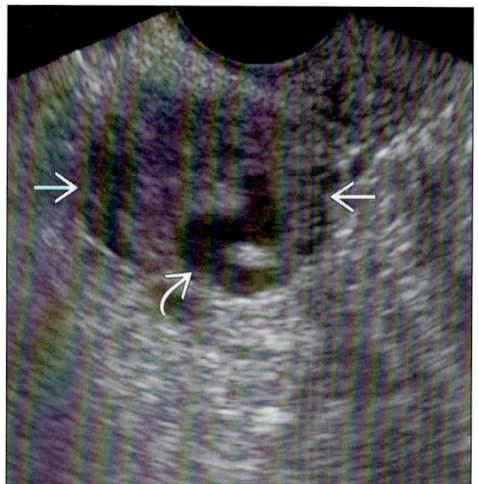 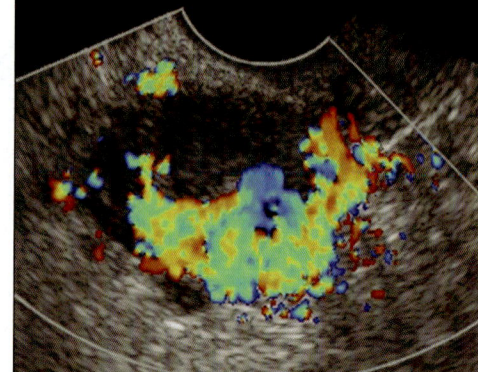

(Left) Sagittal transvaginal ultrasound shows a solid mass ➡ with a central anechoic tubular component in the right lateral aspect of the uterus ➡. *(Right)* Sagittal color Doppler ultrasound shows color mosaic and aliasing in the tubular component in this high flow arteriovenous malformation.

Typical

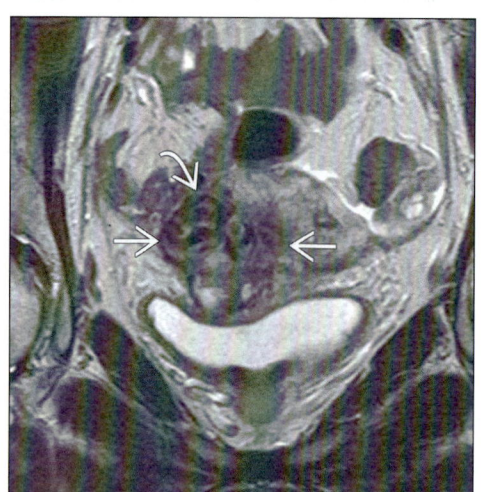 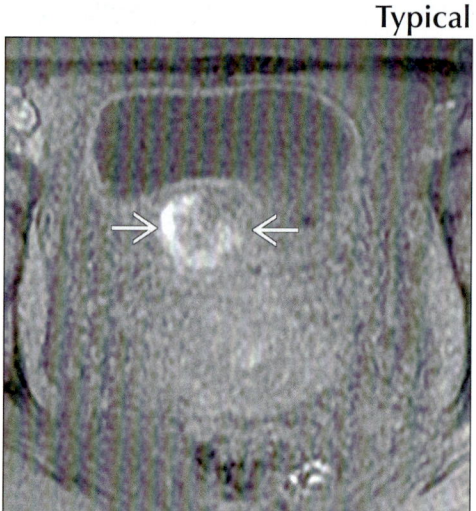

(Left) Coronal T2WI MR of the preceding patient shows a heterogeneous mass ➡ arising from the right myometrium with multiple, serpentine flow-related signal voids ➡. *(Right)* Axial T1WI FS MR in the same patient as left shows an area of high signal intensity ➡ consistent with hemorrhage. This hematoma accounts for the observed mass effect.

Typical

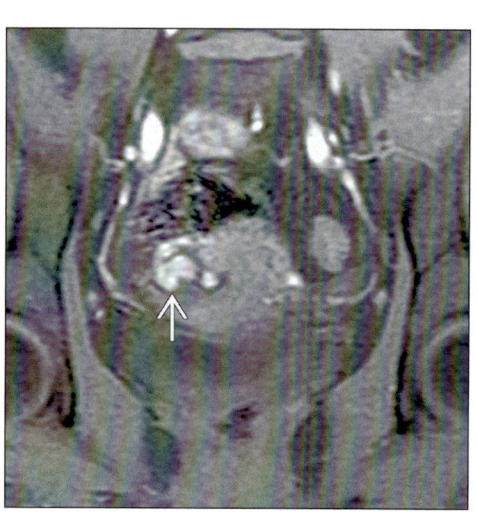 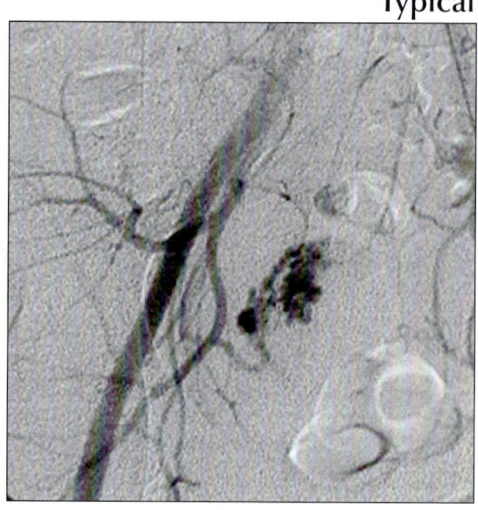

(Left) Coronal T1 C+ FS MR of the preceding patient shows dilated vascular channels ➡ in the right aspect of the myometrium. *(Right)* Frontal angiographic image of a nonselective catheterization in the same patient as left shows filling of the right-sided uterine arteriovenous malformation. (Courtesy F. Côté, MD).

Typical

UTERINE AVM

Typical

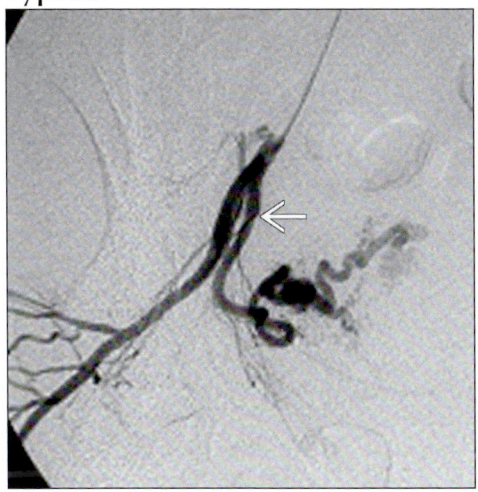 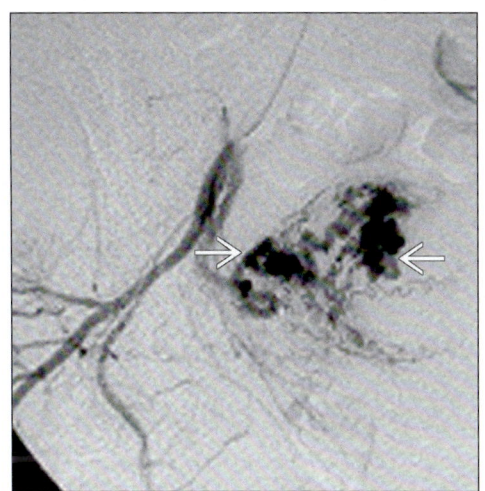

(Left) Frontal angiographic image of a selective right internal iliac catheterization in the preceding patient shows hypertrophy of the right uterine artery ➡. *(Courtesy F. Côté, MD).* *(Right)* Frontal angiographic image of a selective right internal iliac catheterization in the same patient as left shows progressive filling of the uterine AVM ➡. *(Courtesy F. Côté, MD).*

Typical

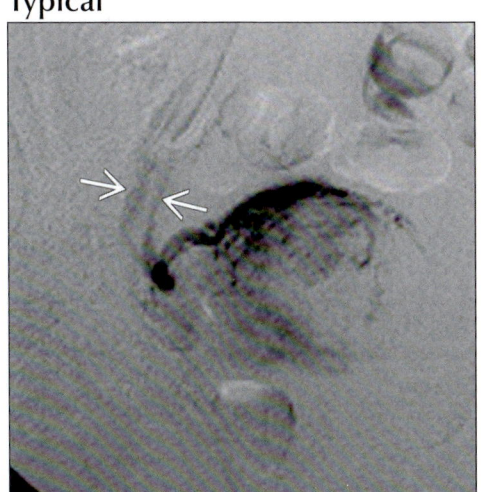 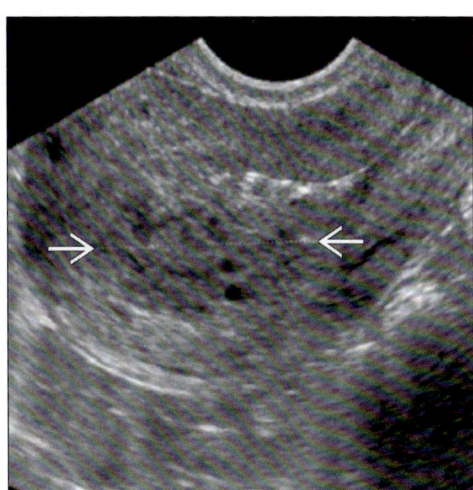

(Left) Frontal angiographic image of a selective right internal iliac catheterization in the preceding patient shows filling of the true AVM with early draining veins ➡. *(Courtesy F. Côté, MD).* *(Right)* Sagittal transvaginal ultrasound shows a heterogeneous inner myometrial mass ➡ with multiple anechoic spaces.

Typical

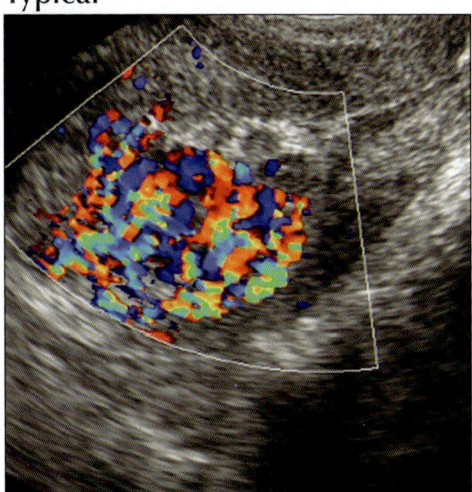 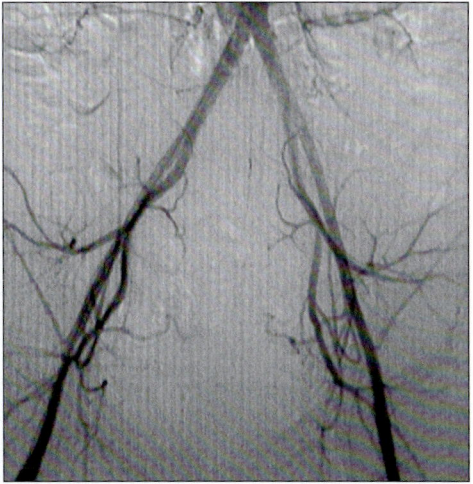

(Left) Sagittal color Doppler ultrasound in the preceding patient shows a markedly hypervascular mass in the dorsal myometrium with color mosaic. *(Right)* Frontal aortogram in the same patient as left shows spontaneous resolution of the probable low-flow malformation. Ultrasound confirmed the normal uterine appearance. *(Courtesy F. Côté, MD).*

UTERINE ARTERY EMBOLIZATION IMAGING

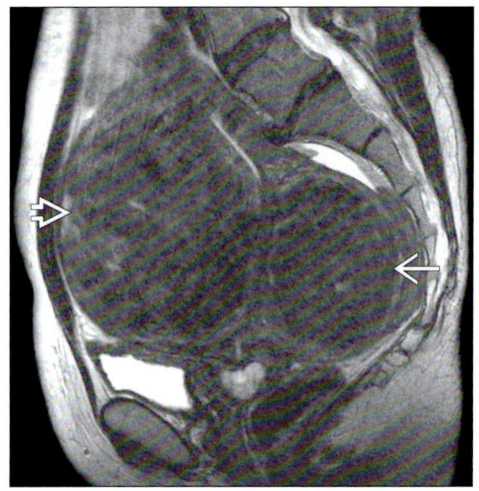

Sagittal T2WI MR pre-UAE shows an enlarged uterus with anterior ⇨ and posterior ➡ intramural leiomyomas.

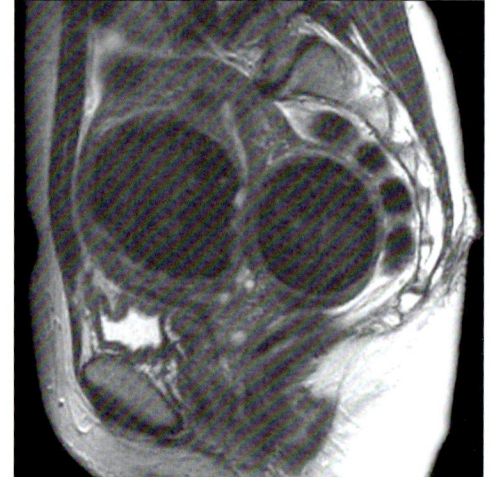

Sagittal T2WI MR in the same patient post-UAE shows interval decrease in the size of the uterus and leiomyomas. The leiomyomas are now homogeneously low in signal intensity.

TERMINOLOGY

Abbreviations and Synonyms
- UAE, Uterine leiomyoma embolization (UFE)

Definitions
- Hemorrhagic infarction & shrinkage of leiomyomas following successful UAE

IMAGING FINDINGS

General Features
- Best diagnostic clue
  - Imaging is important before and after UAE
    - Pre-UAE imaging: May help select appropriate patients
    - Post-UAE imaging: Surveillance & evaluate complications
  - Post-UAE: Devascularized, hemorrhagic & well-defined leiomyoma
    - Significant decrease (40-60%) in uterine volume
    - Significant decrease (40-70%) in dominant leiomyoma volume
- Location: Submucosal, intramural and subserosal (may be intracavitary if leiomyoma is passing)
- Size: Variable
- Morphology: Round or ovoid

Ultrasonographic Findings
- Grayscale Ultrasound
  - Transvaginal US (TVS): Post-UAE
    - Decrease in uterine and leiomyoma size & volume
    - Dominant leiomyoma may no longer be visualized
- Color Doppler
  - 44% decrease in vascularity compared to myometrial vascularity
  - May show collateral flow in treatment failures

CT Findings
- CTA: Can potentially identify ovarian artery collateral
- NECT
  - Pre-UAE
    - Similar attenuation as myometrium if simple
    - +/- Calcification
  - Post-UAE
    - May see high attenuation of hemorrhagic infarction

DDx: Uterine Artery Embolization Imaging

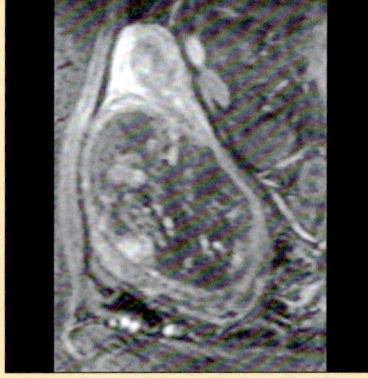
Leiomyosarcoma

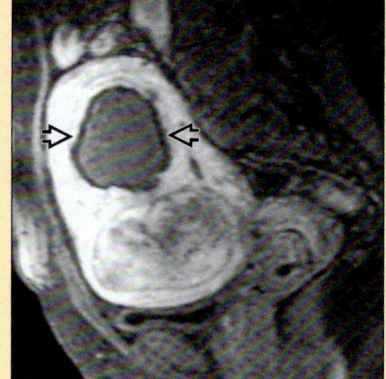
Leiomyoma Autoinfarction

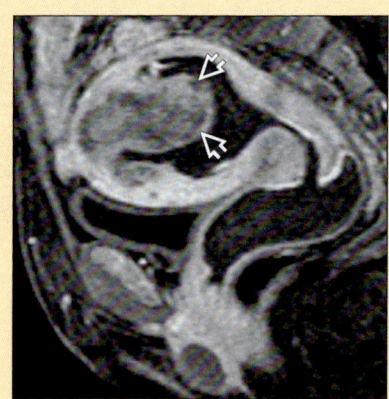
Treatment Failure

UTERINE ARTERY EMBOLIZATION IMAGING

Key Facts

Terminology
- UAE, Uterine leiomyoma embolization (UFE)
- Hemorrhagic infarction & shrinkage of leiomyomas following successful UAE

Imaging Findings
- Post-UAE: Devascularized, hemorrhagic & well-defined leiomyoma
- Significant decrease (40-60%) in uterine volume
- Significant decrease (40-70%) in dominant leiomyoma volume
- **MR/MRA for pre-UAE evaluation**
- Diagnose leiomyoma to include size, number and location
- Identify ovarian-uterine artery anastomoses
- Identify alternative and co-morbid conditions
- **MR/MRA for post-UAE**
- Monitor treatment response
- Evaluate potential complications (identify intracavitary sloughed leiomyomas, identify presence of viable uterine attachment of passing leiomyoma)

Top Differential Diagnoses
- Leiomyosarcoma
- Leiomyoma Autoinfarction
- Unsuccessful Uterine Artery Embolization

Clinical Issues
- Significant improvement in health-related quality of life
- **Significant improvement in leiomyoma specific symptoms**
- Bleeding (menorrhagia, menometrorrhagia): 81-100%
- Bulk-related symptoms: 64-96%

- CECT
  - Pre-UAE
    - Leiomyomas with variable enhancement: Less than, equal to, or more than myometrium
  - Post-UAE
    - Infarcted leiomyomas do not enhance

MR Findings
- T1WI
  - Pre-UAE
    - Isointense to myometrium
    - May have areas of low & high signal intensity (SI) if degenerated
    - If homogeneous high SI: Think hemorrhagic degeneration (autoinfarction) - will not respond further to UAE
    - Calcifications image as punctate signal voids
  - Post-UAE
    - Infarcted leiomyomas with high SI compared to myometrium
- T2WI
  - Pre-UAE
    - Low SI compared to myometrium
    - Heterogeneous SI if degenerated
  - Post-UAE
    - Infarcted leiomyomas with low SI
    - May have slighter higher SI center
- T1 C+
  - Pre-UAE
    - Leiomyomas with variable enhancement
  - Post-UAE
    - Infarcted leiomyomas do not enhance
    - Incompletely infarcted leiomyomas with variable degrees of enhancing tissue
- MRA
  - Helpful for identifying ovarian arterial collateral circulation to the uterus
    - Presence of ovarian collaterals may lead to incomplete or non-durable results and/or early menopause with amenorrhea

Angiographic Findings
- Conventional
  - Pre-UAE: Rich vascular arterial network supplying leiomyoma
  - Post-UAE: Vessels to leiomyomas embolized to near stasis with preservation of main uterine artery trunk

Imaging Recommendations
- Best imaging tool
  - MR/MRA for pre-UAE evaluation
    - Diagnose leiomyoma to include size, number and location
    - Identify ovarian-uterine artery anastomoses
    - Identify alternative and co-morbid conditions
  - MR/MRA for post-UAE
    - Monitor treatment response
    - Evaluate potential complications (identify intracavitary sloughed leiomyomas, identify presence of viable uterine attachment of passing leiomyoma)
  - In single institution study, MR provided considerable additional information compared with US & affected clinical decision making
- Protocol advice
  - Leiomyomas are common, need to look for comorbid conditions which may be causing patient's symptoms
  - Have patient void prior to scan

DIFFERENTIAL DIAGNOSIS

Leiomyosarcoma
- No specific imaging findings to diagnose leiomyosarcoma
- Diagnosis is suggested if unexpected rapid growth in leiomyoma

Leiomyoma Autoinfarction
- Commonly occurs during pregnancy
  - Estrogen promotes leiomyoma growth
  - Leiomyoma may outgrow blood supply and infarct
  - May cause acute pain

UTERINE ARTERY EMBOLIZATION IMAGING

Unsuccessful Uterine Artery Embolization
- No imaging evidence of hemorrhagic infarction & preserved vascularity

PATHOLOGY

General Features
- General path comments
  - UAE target vessels: Pre-leiomyoma vascular plexus
  - Embolize to near stasis
- Etiology: Infarct leiomyoma while preserving myometrial/endometrial perfusion
- Associated abnormalities: Co-morbid conditions often exist (adenomyosis, endometriosis)

Gross Pathologic & Surgical Features
- Soft on sectioning, may be pale if hyaline degeneration

Microscopic Features
- Hyaline degeneration
- Massive necrosis
- Dystrophic calcification
- Vascular thrombosis
- Intravascular foreign material: Histiocytic & giant cell reaction

Staging, Grading or Classification Criteria
- Pre- and post: Leiomyoma classification
  - Submucosal, intramural and subserosal
    - Submucosal: Prone to passage
    - Subserosal: If large may parasitize extrauterine vessels & may lead to treatment failure
- Ovarian artery collateral classification
  - Type I: Flow from the ovarian artery to the uterus through anastomoses with main uterine artery
  - Type II: Ovarian artery directly supplies leiomyomas (may predispose to treatment failure)
  - Type III: Uterine artery is the major arterial supply to the ovary (may predispose to ovarian failure)

CLINICAL ISSUES

Presentation
- Clinical Profile
  - Pre-UAE: Patient selection
    - Gynecologic evaluation
    - Must assess if the patient's symptoms are attributable to leiomyomas and if warrant treatment
    - Pre-UAE predictors of success: Hypervascularity, submucosal location & smaller size
    - Some patients may be better served by other therapies: Hysteroscopic resection for pedunculated submucosal leiomyomas; myomectomy for large pedunculated subserosal leiomyomas; hysterectomy for massively enlarged uterus (> 22-24 cm in length)
  - Post-UAE: Surveillance
    - Peak pain 24-48 hours post-UAE: Opioids & nonsteroidal anti-inflammatory agents successful for pain management
    - Post-embolization syndrome (severe in up to 34%): Pain, fever, elevated white blood cell count

Demographics
- Age: Premenopausal women

Natural History & Prognosis
- > 25,000 procedures performed world wide
  - Significant improvement in health-related quality of life
  - **Significant improvement in leiomyoma specific symptoms**
    - Bleeding (menorrhagia, menometrorrhagia): 81-100%
    - Bulk-related symptoms: 64-96%
  - Shorter hospital stay compared with hysterectomy (1.71 vs 5.85 days)
  - Anecdotal reports of successful pregnancy post-UAE
- Technical success rate: 84-100%
- Clinical success rate: 85-90%
- Long term (5 year) outcome
  - 73% with continued symptom control
  - Long term failure more likely in women not improved at 1 year
- Complications
  - Prolonged amenorrhea: < 5%
    - Incidence increases with advancing age
  - Leiomyoma passage: Up to 5%
  - Endometritis and pyometra necessitating hysterectomy: < 1%
  - Pulmonary embolus
  - Estimated mortality rate: 2 per 10,000 cases
- Randomized trial of UAE versus surgery for symptomatic leiomyomas
  - No significant difference in SF 36 scores between the two groups
  - Embolization group with a shorter mean hospital stay (1 day vs 5 days, p < 001)
  - 10 patients in embolization group required repeat embolization or hysterectomy
  - Conclusion: Faster recovery time after embolization must be weighed against need for further treatment in the minority of patients

SELECTED REFERENCES

1. Edwards RD et al: Uterine-artery embolization versus surgery for symptomatic uterine fibroids. N Engl J Med. 356(4):360-70, 2007
2. Spielmann AL et al: Comparison of MRI and sonography in the preliminary evaluation for fibroid embolization. AJR Am J Roentgenol. 187(6):1499-504, 2006
3. Spies JB et al: Long-term outcome of uterine artery embolization of leiomyomata. Obstet Gynecol. 106(5 Pt 1):933-9, 2005
4. Spies JB et al: Leiomyomata treated with uterine artery embolization: Factors associated with successful symptom and imaging outcome. Radiology. 222:45-52, 2002
5. Jha RC et al: Symptomatic fibroleiomyomata: MR imaging of the uterus before and after uterine artery embolization. Radiology. 217:228-35, 2000

UTERINE ARTERY EMBOLIZATION IMAGING

IMAGE GALLERY

Typical

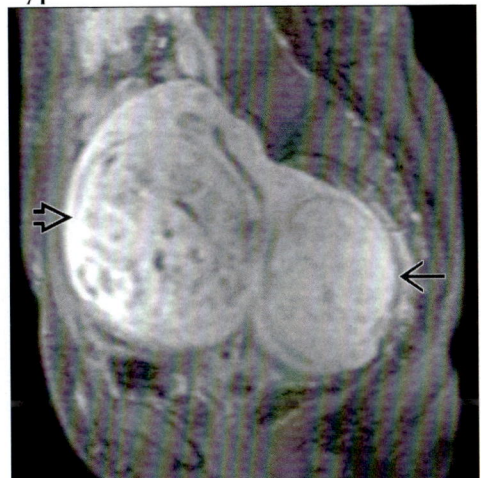
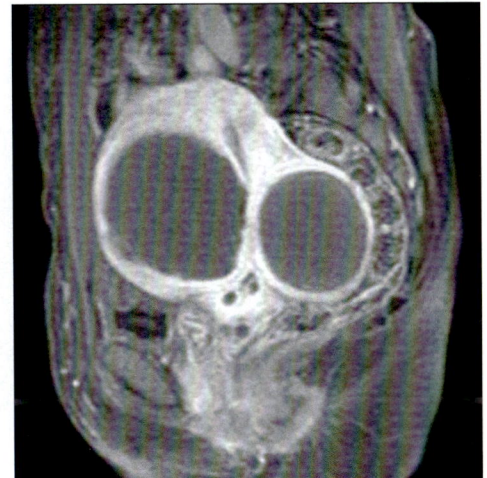

(Left) Sagittal T1 C+ FS MR in the same patient as first two images pre-UAE shows the anterior ⇨ and posterior ⇨ leiomyomas enhance and are viable. *(Right)* Sagittal T1 C+ FS MR in the same patient post-UAE shows interval hemorrhagic infarction--the leiomyomas no longer enhance. This is the characteristic imaging finding following successful UAE.

Typical

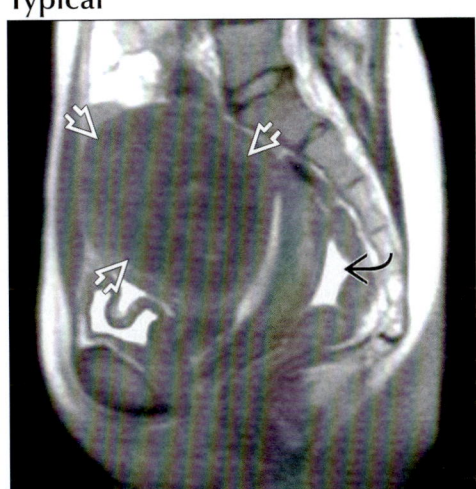
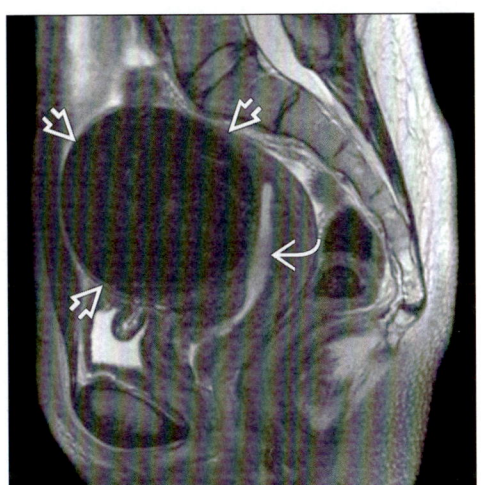

(Left) Sagittal T2WI MR pre-UAE shows a large leiomyoma ⇨. Note physiologic free fluid ⇨. *(Right)* Sagittal T2WI MR in the same patient shows interval decrease in size and signal intensity of the leiomyoma ⇨. Note some high signal intensity distending the endometrial canal ⇨.

Typical

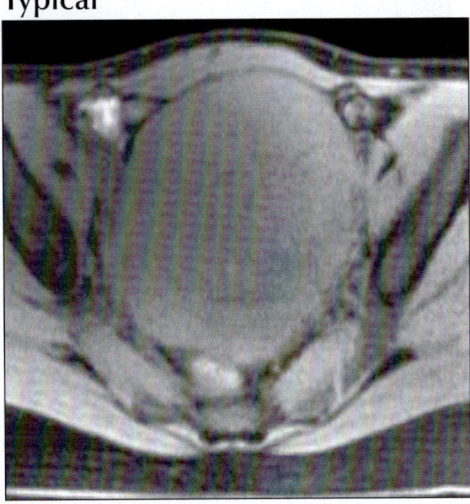
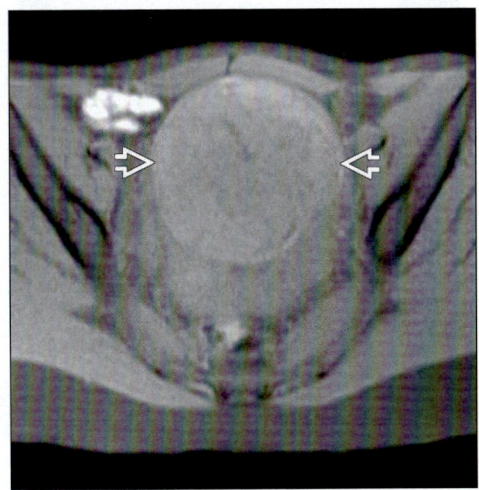

(Left) Axial T1WI FS MR in the same patient as previous image pre-UAE shows the leiomyoma is isointense to myometrium. *(Right)* Axial T1WI FS MR in the same patient post-UAE shows interval increase in leiomyoma signal intensity ⇨ suggesting hemorrhagic infarction.

UTERINE ARTERY EMBOLIZATION IMAGING

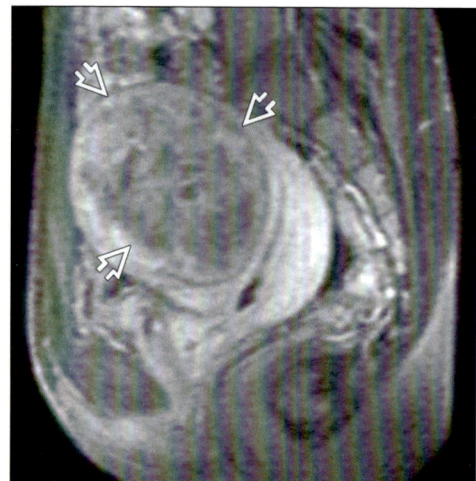

Typical

(Left) Sagittal T1 C+ FS MR in the same patient as previous image pre-UAE shows enhancement of the leiomyoma ⮕. (Right) Sagittal T1 C+ FS MR in the same patient post-UAE shows the leiomyoma ⮕ is no longer viable, consistent with hemorrhagic infarction. Enhancing endometrial tissue ➔ was a benign polyp.

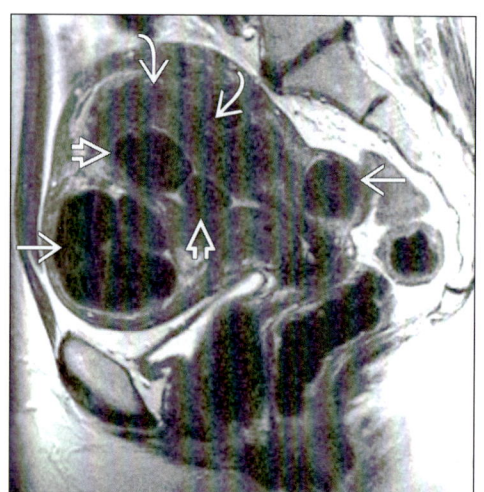

Variant

(Left) Sagittal T2WI MR pre-UAE shows multiple leiomyomas to the submucosal ⮕ and intramural ⮕ locations. Adenomyosis is also present in the posterior uterine corpus ➔. (Right) Sagittal T2WI MR in the same patient post-UAE shows interval decrease in size of the submucosal ⮕ and anterior intramural ⮕ leiomyomas. The region of adenomyosis ➔ has increased in signal intensity.

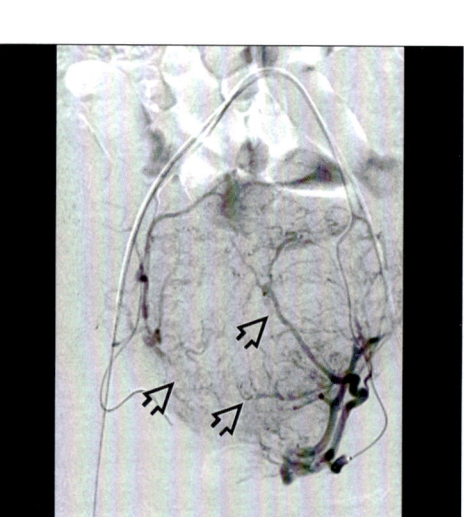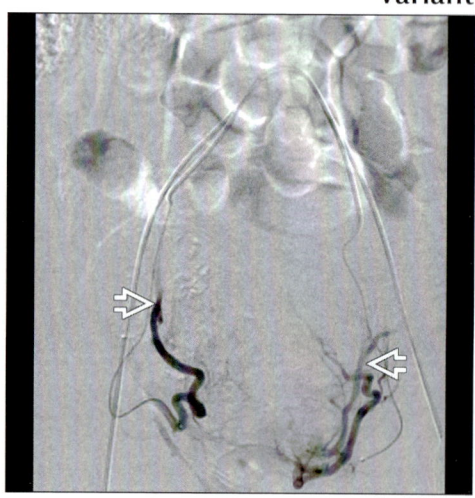

Variant

(Left) Anteroposterior conventional angiogram in the same patient as previous image before UAE shows the neovascularity ⮕ and "blush" associated with leiomyomas. (Right) Anteroposterior conventional angiogram in the same patient post-UAE shows subtotal occlusion of the bilateral uterine arteries ⮕.

UTERINE ARTERY EMBOLIZATION IMAGING

Variant

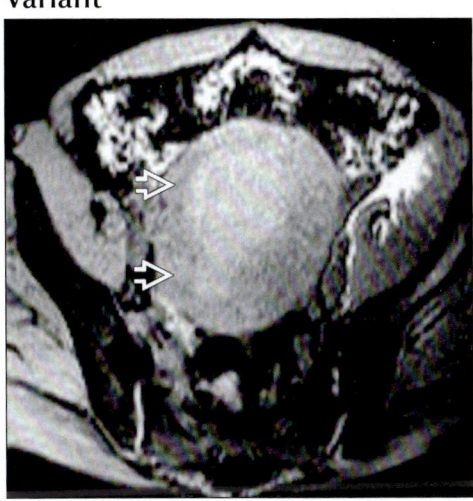
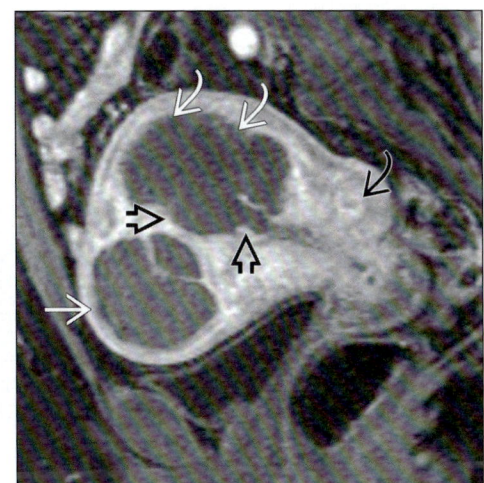

(Left) Axial T1WI FS MR in the same patient as previous image shows high signal intensity of hemorrhagic infarction ➡ within the uterus. *(Right)* Sagittal T1 C+ FS MR in the same patient post-UAE shows no enhancement of the submucosal ➡ and anterior intramural ➡ leiomyomas and area of adenomyosis ➡. Note that the posterior intramural ➡ leiomyoma remains viable.

Variant

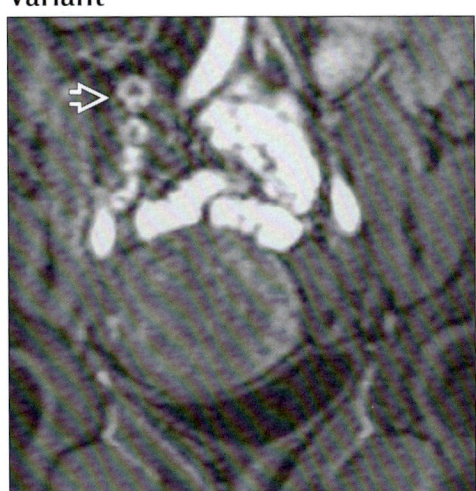
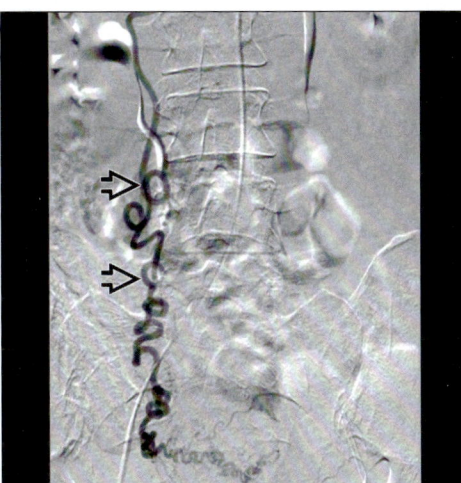

(Left) Coronal MRA pre-UAE shows an enlarged right ovarian artery ➡. Ovarian arterial supply to the uterus may lead to treatment failure, non-durable response or premature menopause. *(Right)* Coronal conventional angiogram in the same patient during UAE confirms the presence of an enlarged right ovarian artery ➡ supplying the uterus.

Typical

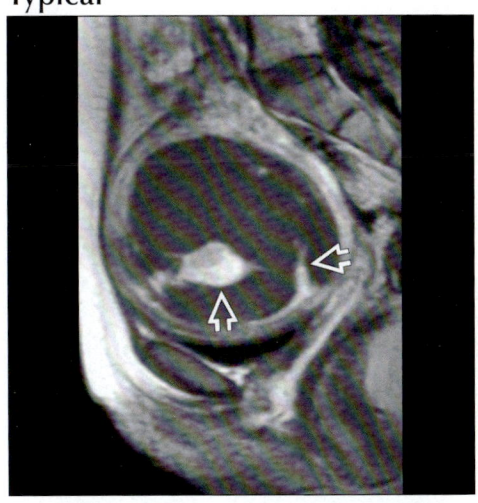
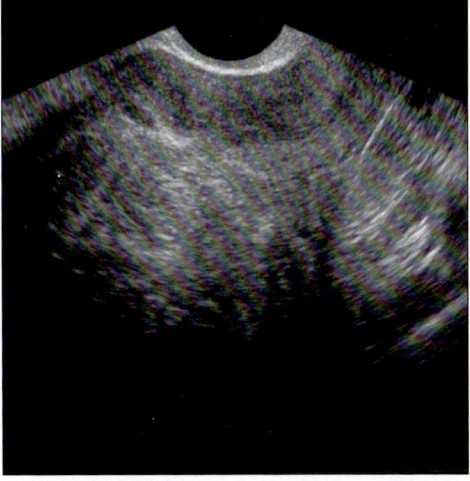

(Left) Sagittal T1 C+ FS MR post-UAE shows a persistent foci enhancement within an embolized leiomyoma ➡ consistent with incomplete infarction. *(Right)* Sagittal transvaginal ultrasound in a patient considering UAE. The uterus is incompletely imaged uterus due to leiomyomas. TVS has a limited field of view which can limit its usefulness for evaluating patients for UAE.

FAILED UTERINE ARTERY EMBOLIZATION

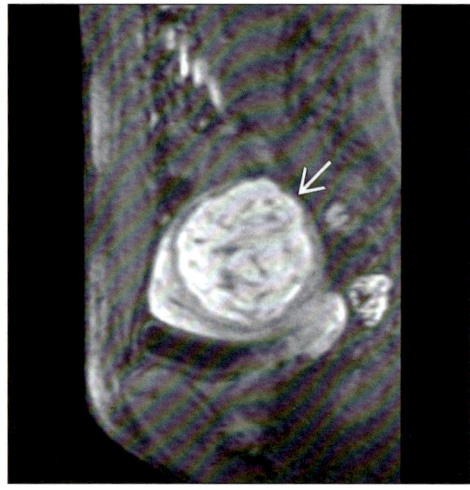

Sagittal T1 C+ FS MR shows a large enhancing intramural leiomyoma ➡. This is the pre-UAE image. (Courtesy J. Spies, MD).

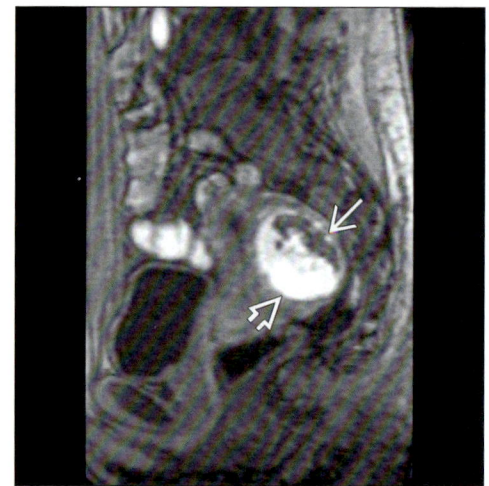

Sagittal T1 C+ FS MR shows overall volume decrease of the leiomyoma ➡ after UAE. However there is still significant enhancement of the leiomyoma ➡. (Courtesy J. Spies, MD).

TERMINOLOGY

Abbreviations and Synonyms
- Unsuccessful uterine artery embolization (UAE)

Definitions
- Failure of leiomyomas to infarct after UAE
- Failure to achieve symptom control after UAE
- Failure to perform UAE
- Leiomyoma regrowth has also been described as UAE failure

IMAGING FINDINGS

General Features
- Best diagnostic clue: Continued symptoms after UAE
- Location
  - Intramural and subserosal leiomyomas are associated with lower rates of UAE success
    - Smaller portion of embolic material is distributed to outer myometrium
- Size: Leiomyomas can range greatly in size
- Morphology: Rounded, well-circumscribed uterine masses

Ultrasonographic Findings
- Ultrasound is limited in evaluating efficacy of UAE
- Leiomyomas are evident on ultrasound; however no reproducible accurate method of evaluating perfusion

CT Findings
- CECT
  - Rounded enhancing uterine masses consistent with leiomyomas
  - Continued enlargement of non-infarcted leiomyomas
  - Not modality of choice; MR is superior in evaluating uterine pathology

MR Findings
- T1WI
  - Absence of increased T1 weighted signal intensity (SI) within the leiomyomas
    - Versus, increased T1 SI of hemorrhagic infarction after successful UAE
- T1 C+ FS
  - Persistent enhancement of leiomyomas

DDx: Failed Uterine Artery Embolization

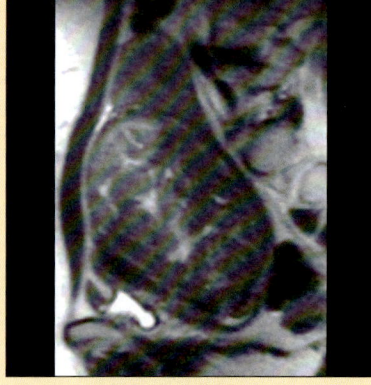
Leiomyosarcoma

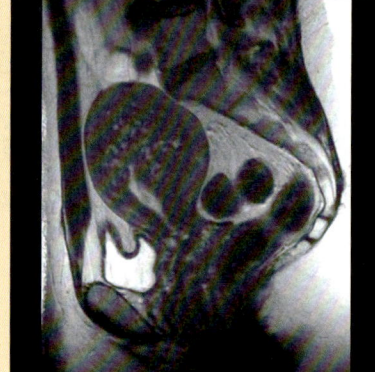
Adenomyosis

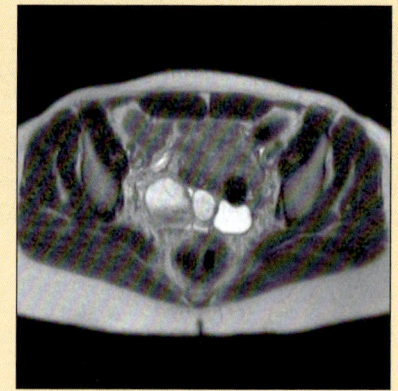
Endometriosis

FAILED UTERINE ARTERY EMBOLIZATION

Key Facts

Terminology
- Failure of leiomyomas to infarct after UAE
- Failure to achieve symptom control after UAE
- Failure to perform UAE
- Leiomyoma regrowth has also been described as UAE failure

Imaging Findings
- Intramural and subserosal leiomyomas are associated with lower rates of UAE success
- Absence of increased T1 weighted signal intensity (SI) within the leiomyomas
- Persistent enhancement of leiomyomas

Pathology
- Multifactorial

- Variant anatomy: Absent uterine artery, multiple uterine arteries, ovarian arterial collaterals
- Catheter-induced spasm
- Technical failure due to operator inexperience or too small or angled uterine artery
- Redistribution of embolization material causing recanalization of artery
- Use of spherical PVA
- Co-incident adenomyosis

Diagnostic Checklist
- Viable tissue post UAE may be present even when there has been an overall decrease in uterine volume
- Degree of leiomyoma enhancement/perfusion is better measure of success

---

- Continued growth and enhancement of untreated leiomyomas
- MRA
  - Dilated tortuous ovarian arterial collaterals may be seen
  - Maximum intensity projection (MIP) of the source images may be helpful
  - Under normal circumstances, ovarian arteries are too small to be detected
    - Ability to identify ovarian arteries suggests they are dilated providing collateral flow to uterus/leiomyomas

Angiographic Findings
- Absent uterine artery
  - This can be iatrogenic in patients with history of myomectomy
  - Uterine artery normally originates from internal iliac artery
- Multiple small uterine arteries
- Uterine artery too small or angled, preventing catheterization
- Failure to detect additional blood supply: Ovarian arterial collaterals
  - Ovarian arteries are tortuous corkscrew arteries
    - These arteries usually arise from aorta anteriorly just below level of renal hila and course retroperitoneally to ovaries through the suspensory ligament
  - Types of ovarian artery-to-uterine artery anastomoses
    - Type 1a: Ovarian artery connects to intramural uterine artery before leiomyoma supply via tubo-ovarian segment; flow in tubal artery is toward uterus, without retrograde reflux into ovary
    - Type 1b: Ovarian artery connects to intramural uterine artery before leiomyoma supply via tubo-ovarian segment; flow in the tubal artery is toward the uterus, with retrograde reflux into the ovary
    - Type 2: Ovarian artery supplies the leiomyoma directly, without connection to the uterine artery
    - Type 3: Uterine arterial supply to the ovary via the tubo-ovarian segment
  - Aortography can be performed to exclude presence of these collateral vessels
  - Arterial collaterals may be too small to be detected at the time of UAE
    - It is hypothesized that after UAE, there is compensatory enlargement of these vessels due to the loss of the main vascular supply
  - Collateral supply can also be from the round ligament artery which arise from either the inferior epigastric artery or the external iliac artery
- Arterial spasm caused by catheter
- Recanalization of artery due to redistribution of embolization material
- Spherical polyvinyl alcohol (PVA) associated with higher rates of failure when compared with tris-acryl gelatin microspheres
  - Postulated that spherical PVA redistributes more distally within uterine artery or leiomyoma, thereby allowing some revascularization

DIFFERENTIAL DIAGNOSIS

Leiomyosarcoma
- Malignant sarcoma arising from the smooth muscle cells of the myometrium

Adenomyosis
- Ectopic endometrial tissue within myometrium
- Recent study however has shown morphologic and symptomatic improvement of adenomyosis after UAE

Endometriosis
- Ectopic growth of endometrial tissue within the pelvis

PATHOLOGY

General Features
- Etiology
  - Multifactorial

FAILED UTERINE ARTERY EMBOLIZATION

- Variant anatomy: Absent uterine artery, multiple uterine arteries, ovarian arterial collaterals
- Catheter-induced spasm
- Technical failure due to operator inexperience or too small or angled uterine artery
- Redistribution of embolization material causing recanalization of artery
- Use of spherical PVA
- Co-incident adenomyosis
- Location of leiomyomas: Intramural and subserosal leiomyomas fail more often than submucosal leiomyomas
- Larger leiomyomas are associated with larger percentage of volume reduction post UAE
- Epidemiology: Technical failure ranges from 1-2%

Microscopic Features
- Less embolic material located within leiomyomas which have failed to respond to UAE
  - Versus successful leiomyoma infarction demonstrated granulomatous foreign body reaction near embolization material followed by vessel destruction
- Lack of hyaline necrosis

CLINICAL ISSUES

Presentation
- Most common signs/symptoms: Heavy menstrual bleeding, pelvic pain
- Other signs/symptoms
  - Urinary incontinence and urgency
  - Constipation
  - Interestingly lack of pelvic pain immediately following UAE can be an indicator of failure
    - Ischemia and infarction of the leiomyomas causes pelvic pain in most patients for the first few days post UAE

Demographics
- Age: Middle-aged
- Gender: Females

Treatment
- Re-embolization may be helpful
  - Aortogram recommended on repeat UAE to evaluate for presence of ovarian arterial collaterals
    - Embolization of these collaterals carry risk of ovarian dysfunction
- Hysterectomy

DIAGNOSTIC CHECKLIST

Image Interpretation Pearls
- Viable tissue post UAE may be present even when there has been an overall decrease in uterine volume
- Degree of leiomyoma enhancement/perfusion is better measure of success

SELECTED REFERENCES

1. Kitamura Y et al: MRI of adenomyosis: changes with uterine artery embolization. AJR Am J Roentgenol. 186(3):855-64, 2006
2. Spies JB et al: Spherical polyvinyl alcohol versus tris-acryl gelatin microspheres for uterine artery embolization for leiomyomas: results of a limited randomized comparative study. J Vasc Interv Radiol. 16(11):1431-7, 2005
3. Spies JB et al: Spherical polyvinyl alcohol versus tris-acryl gelatin microspheres for uterine artery embolization for leiomyomas: results of a limited randomized comparative study. J Vasc Interv Radiol. 16(11):1431-7, 2005
4. Weichert W et al: Uterine arterial embolization with tris-acryl gelatin microspheres: a histopathologic evaluation. Am J Surg Pathol. 29(7):955-61, 2005
5. Pelage JP et al: Uterine fibroid tumors: long-term MR imaging outcome after embolization. Radiology. 230(3):803-9, 2004
6. Banovac F et al: Magnetic resonance imaging outcome after uterine artery embolization for leiomyomata with use of tris-acryl gelatin microspheres. J Vasc Interv Radiol. 13(7):681-8, 2002
7. deSouza NM et al: Uterine arterial embolization for leiomyomas: perfusion and volume changes at MR imaging and relation to clinical outcome. Radiology. 222(2):367-74, 2002
8. Razavi MK et al: Angiographic classification of ovarian artery-to-uterine artery anastomoses: initial observations in uterine fibroid embolization. Radiology. 224(3):707-12, 2002
9. Spies JB et al: Leiomyomata treated with uterine artery embolization: factors associated with successful symptom and imaging outcome. Radiology. 222(1):45-52, 2002
10. Binkert CA et al: Utility of nonselective abdominal aortography in demonstrating ovarian artery collaterals in patients undergoing uterine artery embolization for fibroids. J Vasc Interv Radiol. 12(7):841-5, 2001
11. Keyoung JA et al: Intraarterial lidocaine for pain control after uterine artery embolization for leiomyomata. J Vasc Interv Radiol. 12(9):1065-9, 2001
12. Andrews RT et al: Successful embolization of collaterals from the ovarian artery during uterine artery embolization for fibroids: a case report. J Vasc Interv Radiol. 11(5):607-10, 2000
13. Burn PR et al: Uterine fibroleiomyoma: MR imaging appearances before and after embolization of uterine arteries. Radiology. 214(3):729-34, 2000
14. Jha RC et al: Symptomatic fibroleiomyomata: MR imaging of the uterus before and after uterine arterial embolization. Radiology. 217(1):228-35, 2000
15. Nikolic B et al: Ovarian artery supply of uterine fibroids as a cause of treatment failure after uterine artery embolization: a case report. J Vasc Interv Radiol. 10(9):1167-70, 1999
16. Pelage JP et al: Arterial anatomy of the female genital tract: variations and relevance to transcatheter embolization of the uterus. AJR Am J Roentgenol. 172(4):989-94, 1999
17. Aziz A et al: Transarterial embolization of the uterine arteries: patient reactions and effects on uterine vasculature. Acta Obstet Gynecol Scand. 77(3):334-40, 1998

FAILED UTERINE ARTERY EMBOLIZATION

IMAGE GALLERY

Typical

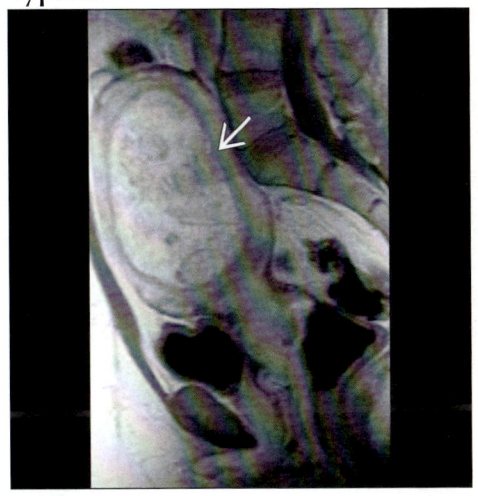
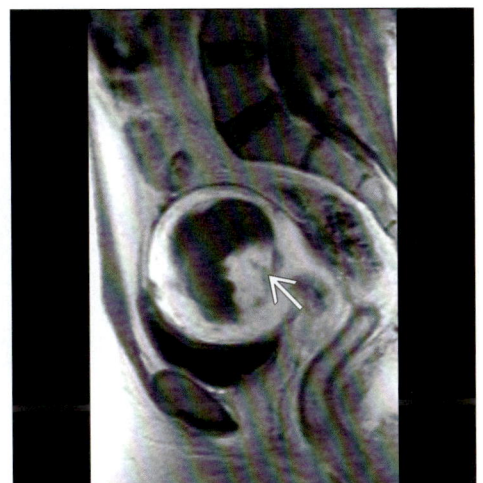

(Left) Sagittal T1WI MR shows a large intramural leiomyoma ➡ in this pre-embolization image. *(Courtesy J. Spies, MD).* *(Right)* Sagittal T1 C+ MR shows significant size decrease in the leiomyoma post UAE. However there is persistent mural nodular enhancement ➡. *(Courtesy J. Spies, MD).*

Typical

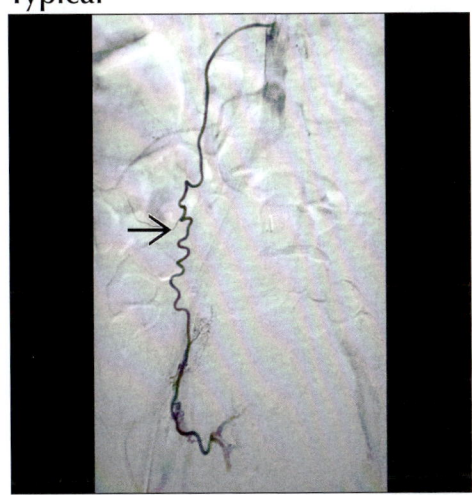
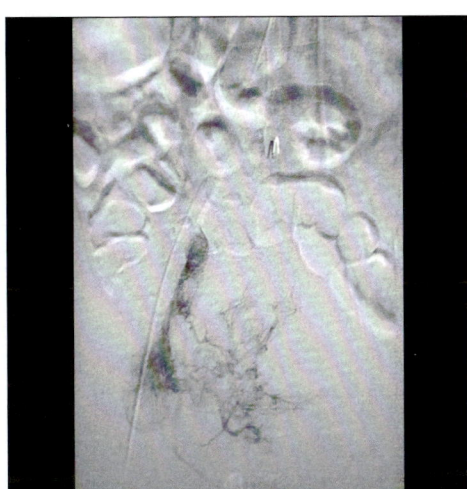

(Left) Frontal radiograph shows a right-sided ovarian arterial collateral ➡ arising from the aorta. Note the typical corkscrew appearance. *(Courtesy J. Spies, MD).* *(Right)* Frontal radiograph of the same patient as previous image, demonstrates the uterine arterial supply from the ovarian arterial collateral. *(Courtesy J. Spies, MD).*

Variant

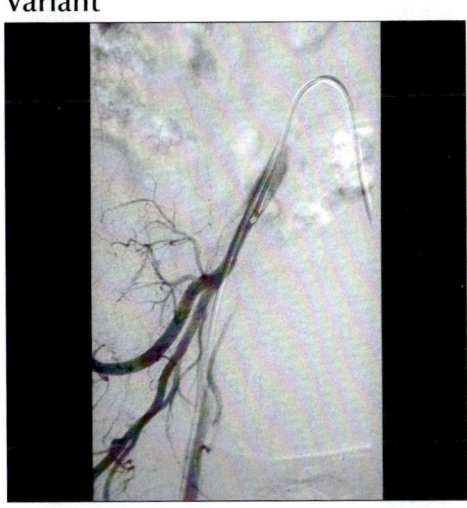
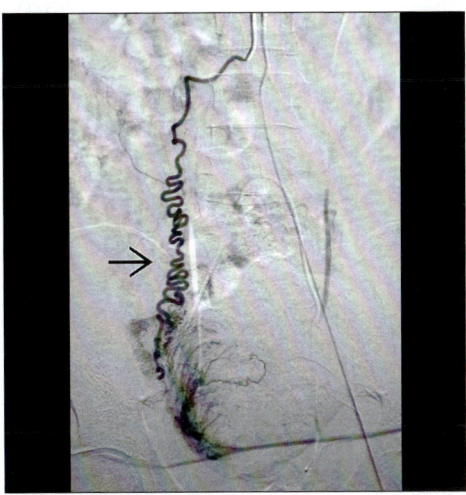

(Left) Frontal radiograph shows an angiogram of the right common iliac artery. No uterine artery is identified. *(Courtesy J. Spies, MD).* *(Right)* Frontal radiograph shows an angiogram of the same patient as previous image, that demonstrates complete replacement of the uterine artery by the right ovarian artery ➡.

COMPLICATIONS, UTERINE ARTERY EMBOLIZATION

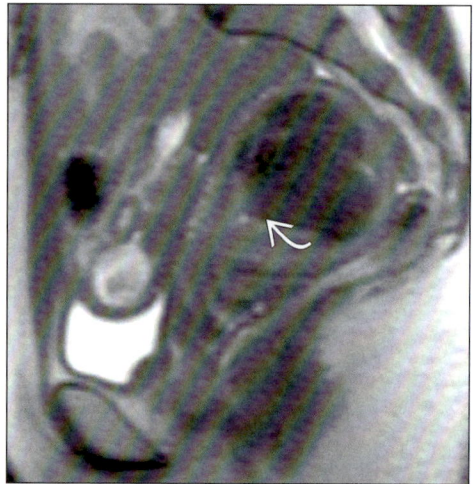

Sagittal T2WI MR post-UAE shows an infarcted leiomyoma distending the endometrial canal & "pointing" ➥ towards the cervix. Reprinted with permission from ref. 4.

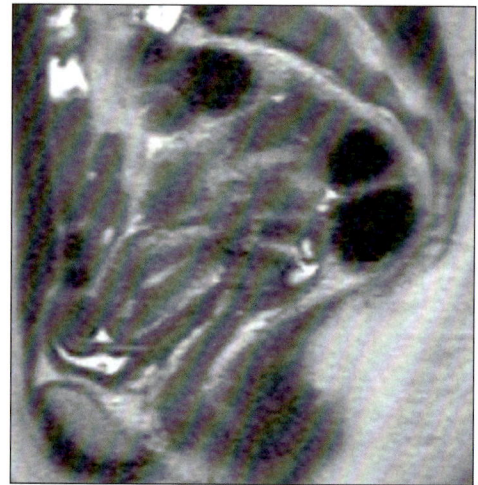

Sagittal T2WI MR in the same patient after spontaneous leiomyoma delivery, shows the uterus is now normal. Reprinted with permission from ref. 4.

TERMINOLOGY

Abbreviations and Synonyms
- Uterine artery embolization (UAE) associated complications (e.g. leiomyoma passage)
  - May occur months after UAE

Definitions
- Unexpected and unintended sequelae of UAE
- Rates vary depending on definition
  - Society of Interventional Radiology (SIR)
    - 8.5% short term complication rate
    - 1.25% serious complication rate
- Practical approach: Minor and major complications
  - Minor: Patients require only mild supportive care (e.g., over-the-counter analgesics or careful observation)
    - Puncture site hematoma
    - Urinary retention
    - Transient pain
    - Transient vessel or nerve injury at puncture site
  - Major: Patients require additional therapy beyond over-the-counter analgesics or careful observation
    - Leiomyoma passage: Most common reported major complication (2.5% of cases in largest series to date)
    - Endometritis
    - Pelvic inflammatory disease (PID)
    - Pyomyoma
    - Deep vein thrombosis
    - Pulmonary embolism
    - Ovarian dysfunction
    - Leiomyoma regrowth
    - Uterine necrosis
    - Sarcomatous degeneration of a leiomyosarcoma
    - Death

IMAGING FINDINGS

General Features
- Best diagnostic clue: Completely or partially infarcted leiomyoma that migrates toward the cervix and vagina
- Location
  - Leiomyomas in contact with the endometrial surface are at increased risk for leiomyoma passage
    - Submucosal leiomyomas

DDx: Leiomyoma Passage

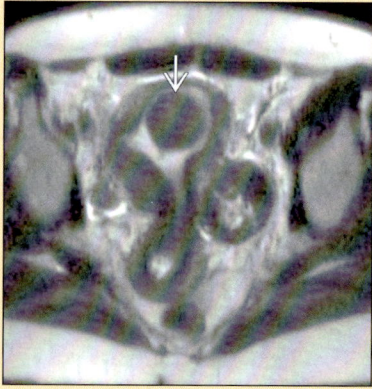

Submucosal Leiomyoma

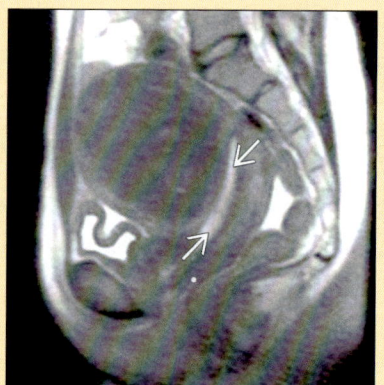

Endometrial Polyp

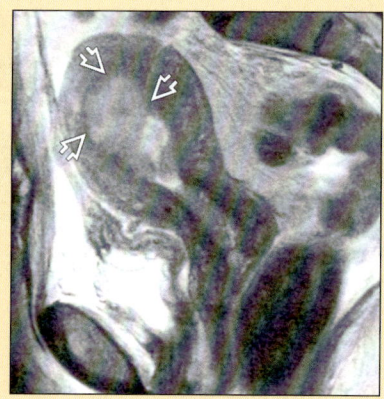

Endometrial Cancer

COMPLICATIONS, UTERINE ARTERY EMBOLIZATION

Key Facts

Terminology
- Unexpected and unintended sequelae of UAE
- Major: Patients require additional therapy beyond over-the-counter analgesics or careful observation
- Leiomyoma passage: Most common reported major complication (2.5% of cases in largest series to date)

Imaging Findings
- Best diagnostic clue: Completely or partially infarcted leiomyoma that migrates toward cervix & vagina
- Leiomyomas in contact with the endometrial surface are at increased risk for leiomyoma passage

Top Differential Diagnoses
- Submucosal Leiomyoma
- Endometrial Polyp
- Endometrial Carcinoma

Clinical Issues
- Abdominal or pelvic pain
- Vaginal discharge
- No treatment needed if leiomyoma spontaneously passes and patient's symptoms resolve
- Hysteroscopic resection is reserved for select cases
- Patient remains symptomatic
- Leiomyoma is only partially infarcted and is attached to the uterine wall

Diagnostic Checklist
- Infarcted leiomyoma with increased SI on T1, decreased SI on T2 and no enhancement on T1 C+ sequences that distend the endometrial canal and migrate towards the cervix and/or vagina
- Partially infarcted leiomyoma will have viable uterine wall attachment on T1 C+ sequences

---

- Intramural leiomyomas with a submucosal component
- Depends on time course, passing leiomyoma may involve one, two or all 3 locations
  - Endometrial canal
  - Endocervical canal
  - Endovaginal canal
- Size: Variable
- Morphology: Usually a cast of endometrial, and/or endocervical, and/or endovaginal canal

Ultrasonographic Findings
- Grayscale Ultrasound
  - Varied and complex appearance: Heterogeneous increase in echogenicity
    - Distends endometrial, and/or endocervical, and/or endovaginal canal
    - Intraparenchymal gas (the result of gas filling potential spaces left by tissue infarction/desiccation; does not imply superinfection) multiple echogenic foci with reverberation
- Color Doppler
  - If completely infarcted: Absence of intrafibroid vascularity
  - If partially infarcted: May see intrafibroid vascularity

MR Findings
- T1WI
  - If completely infarcted: High signal intensity (SI) distending endometrial, and/or endocervical, and/or endovaginal canal
  - If partially infarcted, viable regions: Isointense to myometrium
- T2WI
  - If completely infarcted: Homogeneous low SI relative to myometrium
  - If partially infarcted: May be heterogeneous relative to myometrium
- T1 C+
  - If completely infarcted: No enhancement
  - If partially infarcted: Viable components (e.g., stalk) enhance
- T1 C+ FS
  - If completely infarcted: No enhancement
  - If partially infarcted: Viable component (e.g., stalk) enhances

Imaging Recommendations
- Best imaging tool: MR
- Protocol advice: Contrast is mandatory to assess potential viable uterine attachment

DIFFERENTIAL DIAGNOSIS

Submucosal Leiomyoma
- Leiomyoma that originates from myometrium underlying the endometrium
- Best imaging clue: Subendometrial solid mass indenting or stretching endometrium
  - Transvaginal ultrasound (TVS): Well-defined, hypoechoic, subendometrial mass
  - Sonohysterography: Sessile or pedunculated, hypoechoic mass
  - T2WI MR: Well-defined hypointense mass
- May be cavitary
- Viable (majority without history of UAE)

Endometrial Polyp
- Focal endometrial hyperplasia
- Best imaging clue: Visualization of a separate endometrial lining
  - TVS: Focal endometrial thickening or mass with partial or complete separate endometrial stripe; stalk flow on color Doppler
  - Sonohysterography: Sessile or pedunculated endometrial mass and intact underlying endometrium
  - T2WI MR: Isointense to endometrium, cystic change, hypointense central fibrous core
  - T1 C+ MR: Early arterial enhancement
- Viable (majority without history of UAE)

Endometrial Carcinoma
- Malignant neoplasm of the endometrium

COMPLICATIONS, UTERINE ARTERY EMBOLIZATION

- Best imaging clue: Polypoid masses with superficial attachment to the endometrium; ± invasion
  - TVS: Polypoid mass or diffuse endometrial thickening
  - T2WI MR: Heterogeneous relative to normal endometrium; C+ MR: Helpful to depict myometrial invasion
- Viable (majority without history of UAE)

PATHOLOGY

General Features
- Epidemiology: Increased incidence of leiomyomas in African-American women

Gross Pathologic & Surgical Features
- Expelled pieces of infarcted leiomyoma and blood clots

Microscopic Features
- Hyaline necrosis (most common)
- Coagulative tumor cell necrosis
- Acute suppurative necrosis

CLINICAL ISSUES

Presentation
- Most common signs/symptoms
  - Abdominal or pelvic pain
  - Vaginal discharge
  - Fever
  - Leukocytosis
- Other signs/symptoms: May have signs and symptoms of superinfection

Demographics
- Age: Reproductive age women
- Gender: Female

Natural History & Prognosis
- May expel spontaneously
- Regardless of spontaneous or assisted expulsion, overall prognosis is excellent

Treatment
- No treatment needed if leiomyoma spontaneously passes and patient's symptoms resolve
- Hysteroscopic resection is reserved for select cases
  - Patient remains symptomatic
  - Leiomyoma is only partially infarcted and is attached to the uterine wall

DIAGNOSTIC CHECKLIST

Consider
- History and physical exam often suggestive, but imaging makes diagnosis and directs treatment

Image Interpretation Pearls
- Infarcted leiomyoma with increased SI on T1, decreased SI on T2 and no enhancement on T1 C+ sequences that distend the endometrial canal and migrate towards the cervix and/or vagina
- Partially infarcted leiomyoma will have viable uterine wall attachment on T1 C+ sequences

SELECTED REFERENCES

1. Volkers NA et al: Uterine Artery Embolization in the Treatment of Symptomatic Uterine Fibroid Tumors (EMMY Trial): Periprocedural Results and Complications. J Vasc Interv Radiol. 17(3):471-80, 2006
2. Ghai S et al: Uterine artery embolization for leiomyomas: pre- and postprocedural evaluation with US. Radiographics. 25(5):1159-72; discussion 1173-6, 2005
3. Hehenkamp WJ et al: Uterine artery embolization versus hysterectomy in the treatment of symptomatic uterine fibroids (EMMY trial): peri- and postprocedural results from a randomized controlled trial. Am J Obstet Gynecol. 193(5):1618-29, 2005
4. Kitamura Y et al: Imaging manifestations of complications associated with uterine artery embolization. Radiographics. 25 Suppl 1:S119-32, 2005
5. Ogliari KS et al: A uterine cavity-myoma communication after uterine artery embolization: two case reports. Fertil Steril. 83(1):220-2, 2005
6. Park HR et al: Uterine restoration after repeated sloughing of fibroids or vaginal expulsion following uterine artery embolization. Eur Radiol. 15(9):1850-4, 2005
7. Torigian DA et al: MRI of uterine necrosis after uterine artery embolization for treatment of uterine leiomyomata. AJR Am J Roentgenol. 184(2):555-9, 2005
8. Aungst M et al: Necrotic leiomyoma and gram-negative sepsis eight weeks after uterine artery embolization. Obstet Gynecol. 104(5 Pt 2):1161-4, 2004
9. Hascalik S et al: Transient ovarian failure: a rare complication of uterine fibroid embolization. Acta Obstet Gynecol Scand. 83(7):682-5, 2004
10. Nikolic B et al: Pyosalpinx developing from a preexisting hydrosalpinx after uterine artery embolization. J Vasc Interv Radiol. 15(3):297-301, 2004
11. Rajan DK et al: Risk of intrauterine infectious complications after uterine artery embolization. J Vasc Interv Radiol. 15(12):1415-21, 2004
12. Spies JB et al: Outcome of uterine embolization and hysterectomy for leiomyomas: results of a multicenter study. Am J Obstet Gynecol. 191(1):22-31, 2004
13. de Blok S et al: Fatal sepsis after uterine artery embolization with microspheres. J Vasc Interv Radiol. 14(6):779-83, 2003
14. Payne JF et al: Serious complications of uterine artery embolization for conservative treatment of fibroids. Fertil Steril. 79(1):128-31, 2003
15. Pron G et al: Hysterectomy for complications after uterine artery embolization for leiomyoma: results of a Canadian multicenter clinical trial. J Am Assoc Gynecol Laparosc. 10(1):99-106, 2003
16. Mehta H et al: Review of readmissions due to complications from uterine fibroid embolization. Clin Radiol. 57(12):1122-4, 2002
17. Shashoua AR et al: Ischemic uterine rupture and hysterectomy 3 months after uterine artery embolization. J Am Assoc Gynecol Laparosc. 9(2):217-20, 2002
18. Spies JB et al: Complications after uterine artery embolization for leiomyomas. Obstet Gynecol. 100(5 Pt 1):873-80, 2002

COMPLICATIONS, UTERINE ARTERY EMBOLIZATION

IMAGE GALLERY

Typical

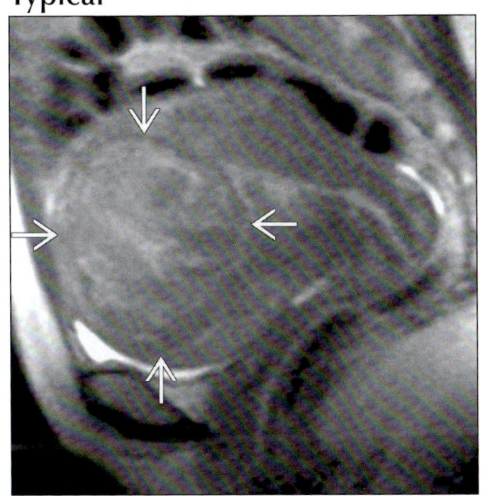
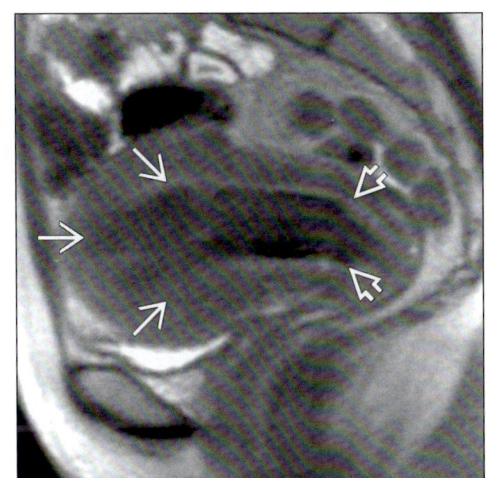

(Left) Sagittal T2WI MR pre-UAE shows an intramural leiomyoma with a submucosal component ➡. *(Right)* Sagittal T2WI MR 3 months post-UAE shows low signal intensity, infarcted leiomyoma, distending the endometrial ➡ and endocervical ➡ canals.

Typical

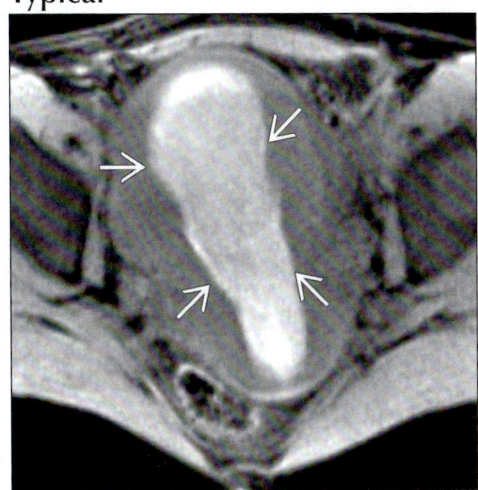
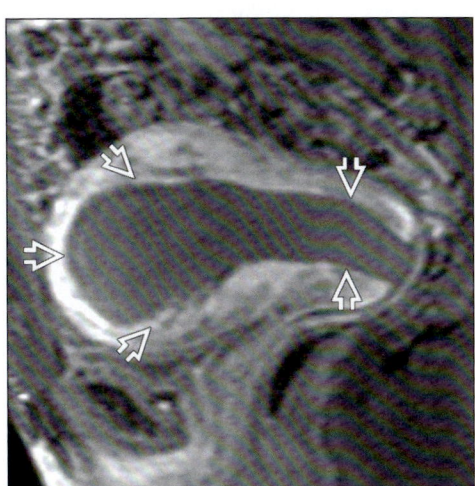

(Left) Axial T1WI FS MR post-UAE in the same patient, shows high signal intensity within the intraluminal leiomyoma ➡, consistent with hemorrhage. *(Right)* Sagittal T1 C+ FS MR post-UAE in the same patient, shows the delivering leiomyoma to be avascular ➡, consistent with hemorrhagic infarction.

Typical

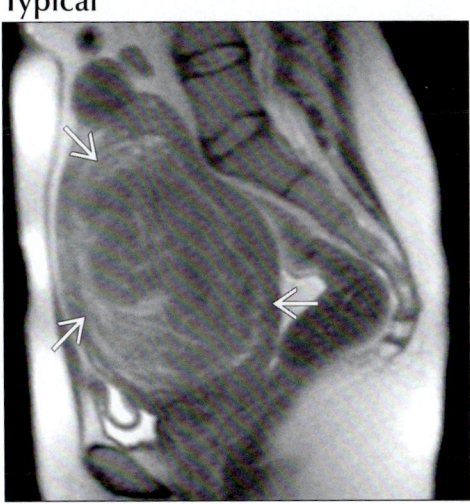
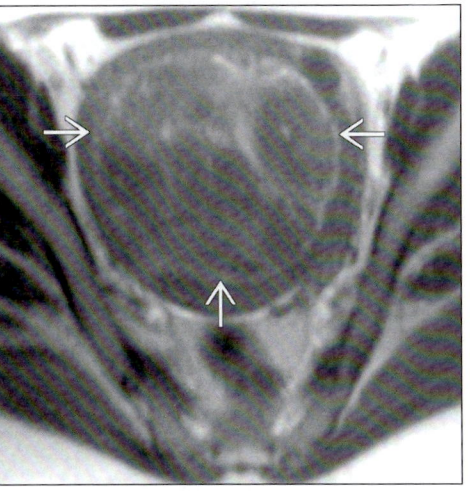

(Left) Sagittal T2WI MR pre-UAE shows a large leiomyoma distorting the uterine zonal anatomy ➡. Reprinted with permission from Kitamura Y, et al. RadioGraphics 2005; 25:S119-32. *(Right)* Axial T2WI MR pre-UAE in the same patient shows the large leiomyoma ➡.

COMPLICATIONS, UTERINE ARTERY EMBOLIZATION

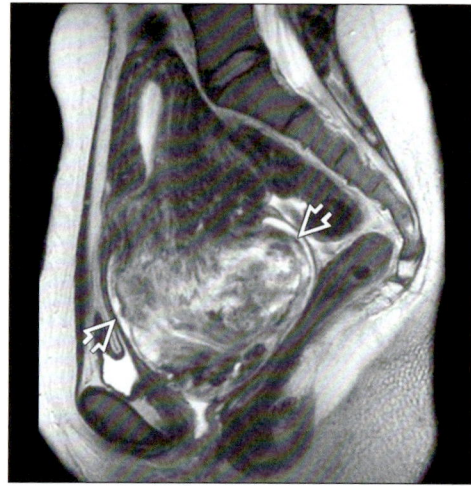
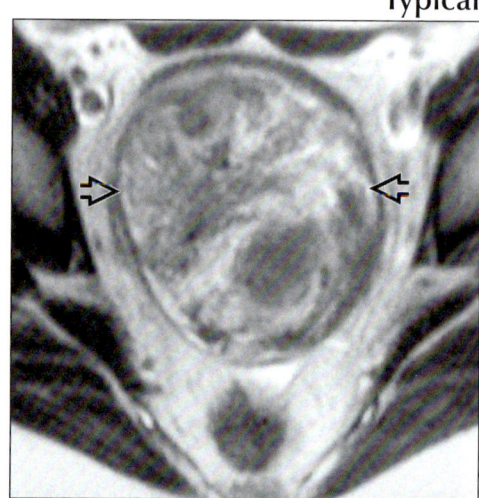

(Left) Sagittal T2WI MR 27 days post-UAE in the same patient, shows the partially embolized leiomyoma protruding down and distending the endocervical & endovaginal canals. Note the splayed vaginal walls ➡. (Right) Axial T2WI MR post-UAE in the same patient, shows the partially infarcted leiomyoma ➡ within the endovaginal canal. Reprinted with permission from Kitamura Y, et al. RadioGraphics 2005; 25:S119-32.

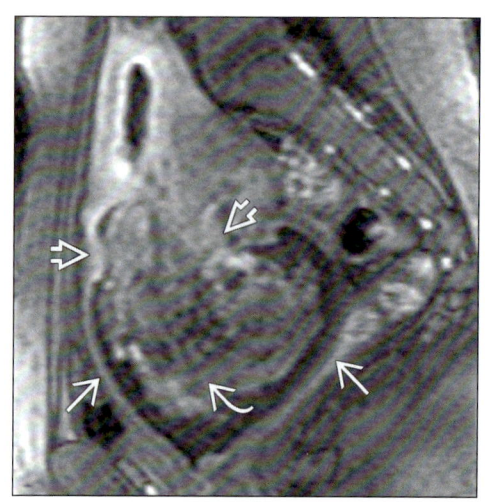
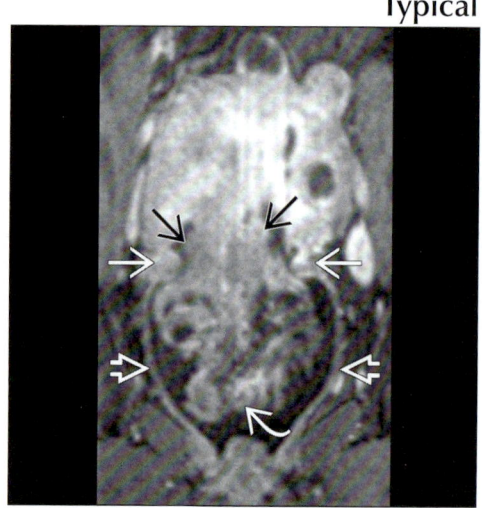

(Left) Sagittal T1 C+ FS MR post-UAE in the same patient, shows partially infarcted leiomyoma ➡, splaying the cervical ➡ & vaginal ➡ walls. Viable leiomyoma is attached to the corpus. Reprinted with permission from ref. 4. (Right) Coronal T1 C+ FS MR post-UAE in the same patient, shows the partially embolized leiomyoma ➡ attached to the posterior uterine corpus via a viable pedicle ➡. The cervix ➡ and vagina ➡ enhance.

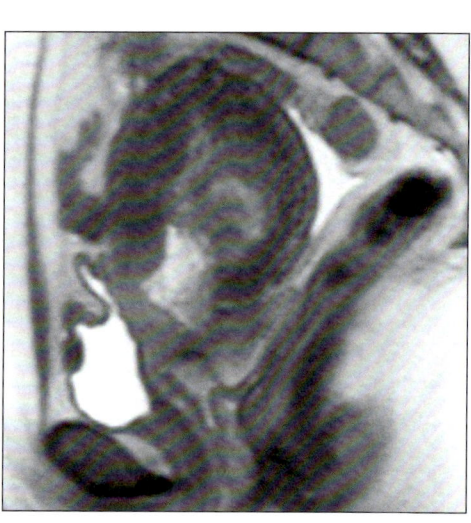
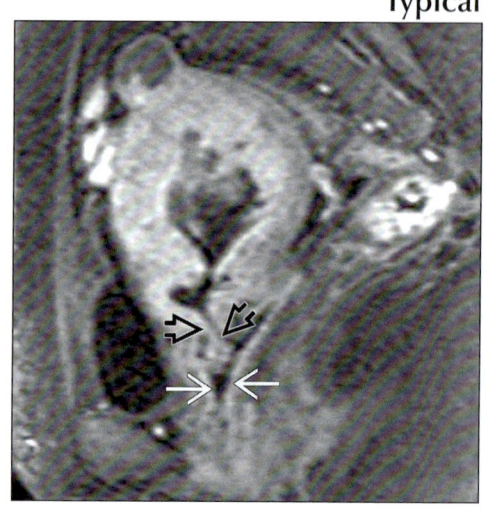

(Left) Sagittal T2WI MR 2 days post hysteroscopic resection in the same patient, shows interval near disappearance of the partially embolized leiomyoma. (Right) Sagittal T1 C+ FS MR post hysteroscopic resection in the same patient, shows the endocervical ➡ & endovaginal ➡ canals almost reapproximated. Reprinted with permission from Kitamura Y, et al. RadioGraphics 2005; 25:S119-32.

COMPLICATIONS, UTERINE ARTERY EMBOLIZATION

Typical

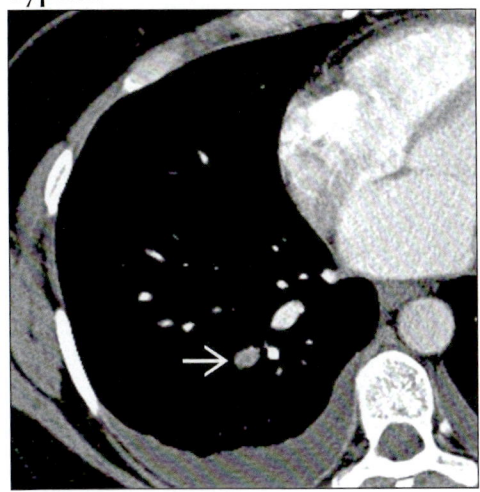 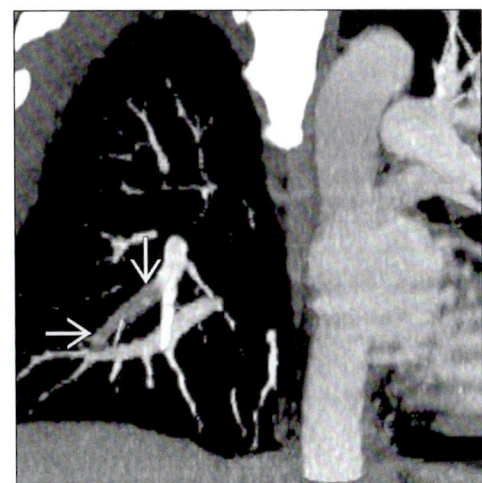

(Left) Axial CECT 4 days post-UAE, shows a filling defect ➡ within a lower lobe pulmonary artery branch diagnostic of a pulmonary embolus. Reprinted with permission from Kitamura Y, et al. RadioGraphics 2005; 25:S119-32. *(Right)* Coronal CECT post-UAE in the same patient, shows the extent of the filling defect ➡. Reprinted with permission from Kitamura Y, et al. RadioGraphics 2005; 25:S119-32.

Typical

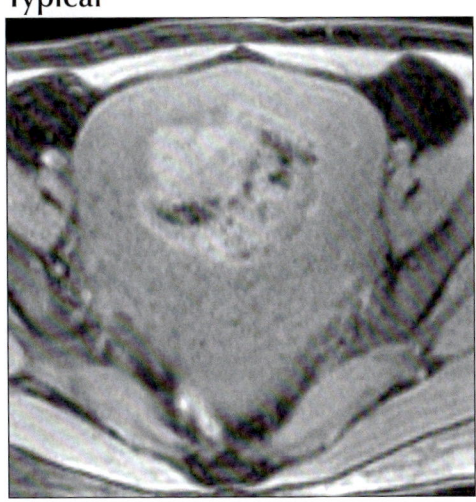 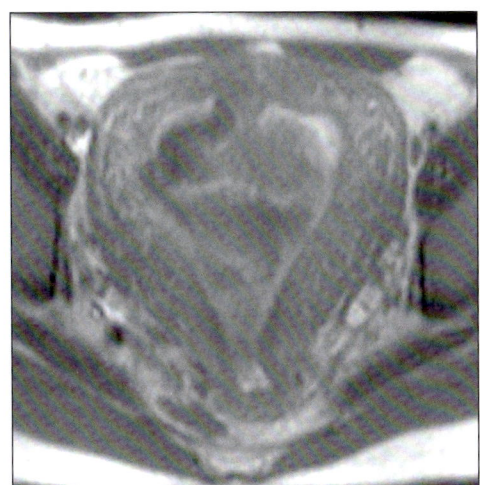

(Left) Axial T1WI FS MR 2 months post-UAE shows a hemorrhagic leiomyoma in a patient with vaginal discharge and fever. Foci of gas within the endometrium are consistent with endometritis. Reprinted with permission from Kitamura Y, et al. RadioGrahics 2005; 25:S119-32. *(Right)* Axial T2WI MR in the same patient shows heterogeneous signal of the infarcted leiomyoma. Reprinted with permission from Kitamura Y, et al. RadioGraphics 2005; 25:S119-32.

Typical

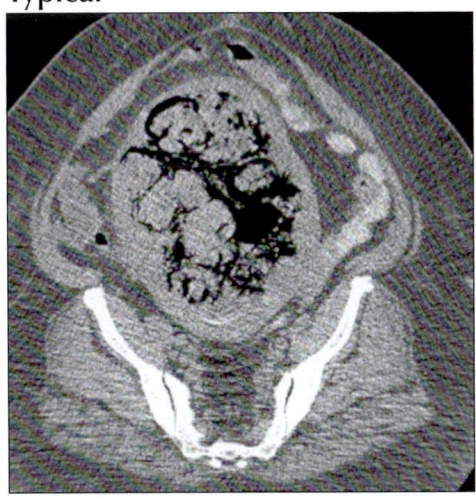 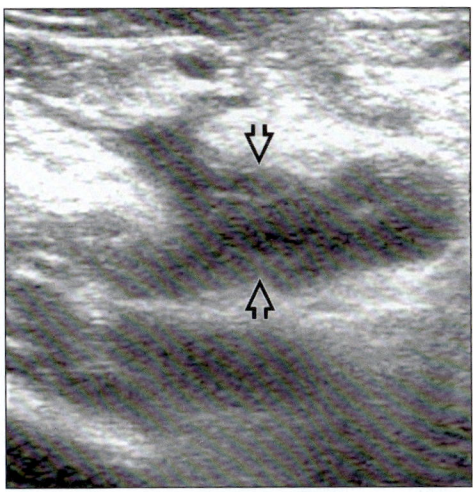

(Left) Axial NECT 10 days post-UAE, shows gas within a pyomyoma and myometrium in a septic patient. Reprinted with permission from Kitamura Y, et al. RadioGraphics 2005; 25:S119-32. *(Right)* Axial ultrasound post-UAE, shows a subtle, non-compressible ➡, echogenic thrombus in the left common femoral vein. Reprinted with permission from Kitamura Y, et al. RadioGraphics 2005; 25:S119-32.

UTERINE RUPTURE

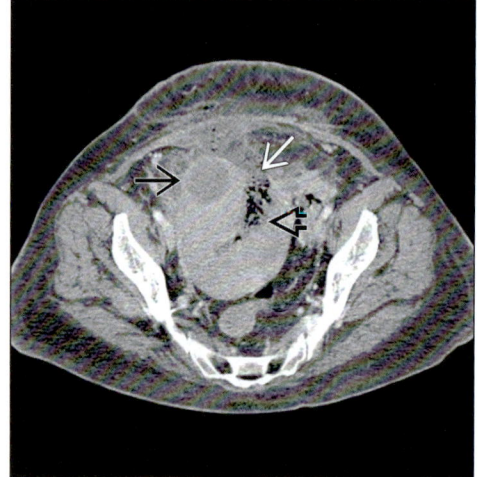

Axial CECT shows air and fluid ⇒ extending from the endometrial cavity into the peritoneal cavity through the myometrial defect ➡. A low attenuation leiomyoma ➡ is incidentally noted.

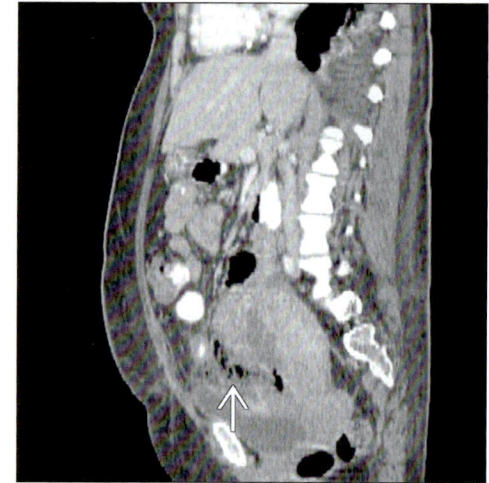

Sagittal CECT shows air and fluid tracking through the anterior myometrial defect ➡.

TERMINOLOGY

Abbreviations and Synonyms
- Uterine dehiscence, uterine perforation

Definitions
- Disruption of uterine wall
- Transmural gap in uterine wall

IMAGING FINDINGS

General Features
- Best diagnostic clue
  - Postpartum bleeding that does not respond to oxytocin & uterine massage
  - Persistent pain & fever in postpartum state
- Location
  - If rupture occurs before labor, usually in uterine body
  - If patient is in labor, usually in lower uterine segment
    - More often on left side of lower uterine segment
  - May rupture at site of previous cesarian section
    - Classic cesarian section (c-section) or high-flap operations often rupture before onset of labor
    - Low uterine incisions tend to be stronger
- Size: Can range from small to massive
- Morphology
  - Can vary from linear to stellate-like
  - Partial dehiscence can occur

Ultrasonographic Findings
- Discontinuity of myometrium
- Amniotic sac herniating through ruptured uterine wall
- Empty uterine sac
- Hemorrhagic free fluid
- Entire abdomen should be scanned for possible extruded fetal parts
- In cases of intrauterine device (IUD) related rupture
  - IUD may be seen outside the uterus
  - Eccentric location of IUD should raise suspicion of partial perforation
- Prenatal sonographic measurement of lower uterine segment thickness in post cesarian patients may be able to predict risk of rupture

CT Findings
- CT defect through uterine wall

DDx: Uterine Rupture Mimics

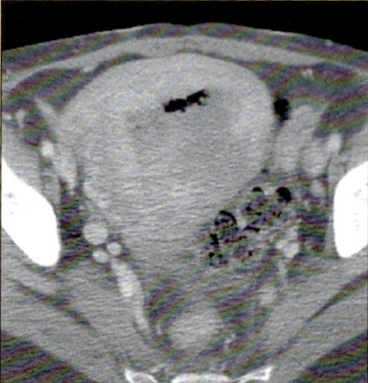

Endometritis

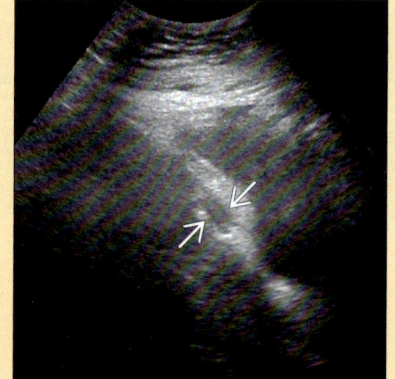

Bladder Flap Hematoma

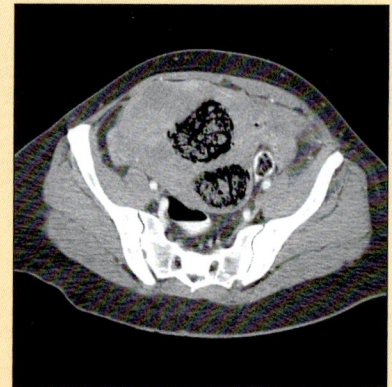

Pyomyomata

UTERINE RUPTURE

Key Facts

Terminology
- Uterine dehiscence, uterine perforation

Imaging Findings
- If rupture occurs before labor, usually in uterine body
- If patient is in labor, usually in lower uterine segment
- May rupture at site of previous cesarian section
- Size: Can range from small to massive
- Can vary from linear to stellate-like
- CT defect through uterine wall
- T1WI: High signal intensity (SI) defect through myometrium
- T2WI: High SI myometrial defect
- Best imaging tool: MR may be superior because of multiplanar capabilities but CT more available
- Imaging plane perpendicular to the line of rupture increases conspicuity

Top Differential Diagnoses
- Endometritis
- Bladder Flap Hematoma
- Air Within Leiomyoma
- Normal Cesarian Section Incision
- Failed Termination of Pregnancy

Pathology
- Postpartum
- Surgery/instrumentation
- Dilatation and curettage
- Pyometra perforation
- Transmigrated intrauterine device
- Blunt trauma

Diagnostic Checklist
- Rupture in post c-section patient with fever & pain

- Gas bubbles often seen tracking through the defect in setting of infection
- If the patient is pregnant, can see expulsion of fetus into maternal abdominal cavity
- Complications
  - Hematoma: Intraperitoneal, bladder flap
  - Abscess
  - Vesicouterine fistula
    - Fetal parts have been seen in the urinary bladder

MR Findings
- T1WI: High signal intensity (SI) defect through myometrium
- T2WI: High SI myometrial defect
- Presence of bladder flap hematoma larger than 5 cm has higher association with uterine dehiscence
- Must be distinguished from normal post c-section incision site
  - Normal incision site demonstrates hematoma within myometrium and perhaps extending to bladder flap hematoma, but size of defect will decrease over time
- May also see high T1 & T2 SI in the endometrial cavity signifying hematoma

Fluoroscopic Findings
- Hysterography
  - Extravasation of contrast from uterine cavity

Imaging Recommendations
- Best imaging tool: MR may be superior because of multiplanar capabilities but CT more available
- Protocol advice
  - Imaging plane perpendicular to the line of rupture increases conspicuity
    - Sagittal MR best for ruptures at site of previous c-section scar

DIFFERENTIAL DIAGNOSIS

Endometritis
- Infection of endometrium, often manifesting with air in the cavity

Bladder Flap Hematoma
- Hematoma between uterus and bladder

Air within Leiomyoma
- Can be due to necrosis caused by uterine artery embolization and/or infection (pyomyomata)

Normal Cesarian Section Incision
- Normal incision will demonstrate high T1 & T2 SI through the myometrium and perhaps extending to bladder flap hematoma, but size of defect will decrease over time

Failed Termination of Pregnancy
- Potassium chloride injected into myometrium may inadvertently create intramural fluid collection

Placental Abruption
- Retroplacental hematoma can be seen

Urachal Pathology
- Inflammatory phlegmon from uterine rupture has been reported to mimic urachal carcinoma

PATHOLOGY

General Features
- Etiology
  - Postpartum
    - Particularly long or difficult labor
    - Rare in primipara
  - Surgery/instrumentation
    - Prior c-section
    - Dilatation and curettage
  - Pyometra perforation
  - Transmigrated intrauterine device
    - Perforation in these cases is often silent
    - Majority of perforations are diagnosed after time of insertion
  - Blunt trauma
  - Placenta percreta
  - Choriocarcinoma

UTERINE RUPTURE

- Epidemiology
  - 3-5% of classic c-sections
  - 1-2% of lower segment c-sections
- Associated abnormalities
  - Hematoma in endometrial cavity
  - Bladder flap hematoma
  - Hemorrhagic fluid in peritoneal cavity
  - Abscesses

Gross Pathologic & Surgical Features
- Transmural myometrial necrosis
- Loss of myometrial continuity

Microscopic Features
- Myometrial defect
- Hemorrhage
- Necrosis

Staging, Grading or Classification Criteria
- Classification
  - Spontaneous rupture during labor
  - Traumatic rupture during delivery
  - Rupture due to previous myometrial scars or disease

CLINICAL ISSUES

Presentation
- Most common signs/symptoms: Pelvic pain and bleeding
- Other signs/symptoms: Fever

Demographics
- Age: Child-bearing years

Natural History & Prognosis
- Maternal death rate: 2-20%
- Fetal mortality: 10-25%
- Long term complication can include vesicouterine fistula

Treatment
- Surgical: Hysterectomy or repair of myometrial defect
- Conservative: Antibiotic therapy, drainage of abscesses if any
- If partial perforation, management is usually conservative

DIAGNOSTIC CHECKLIST

Consider
- Rupture in post c-section patient with fever & pain

Image Interpretation Pearls
- Defect through uterine wall
- May see gas bubbles extending through the defect in patients who are infected or recently post-op

SELECTED REFERENCES

1. Atug F et al: Delivery of dead fetus from inside urinary bladder with uterine perforation: case report and review of literature. Urology. 65(4):797, 2005
2. Daskalakis G et al: Sonographic findings and surgical management of a uterine rupture associated with the use of misoprostol during second-trimester abortion. J Ultrasound Med. 24(11):1565-8, 2005
3. Levsky JM et al: Incidental detection of a transmigrated intrauterine device. Emerg Radiol. 11(5):312-4, 2005
4. Smayra T et al: Vesicouterine fistulas: imaging findings in three cases. AJR Am J Roentgenol. 184(1):139-42, 2005
5. Baruah S et al: Spontaneous rupture of unscarred uterus at early mid-trimester due to placenta percreta. J Obstet Gynaecol. 24(6):705, 2004
6. Leyendecker JR et al: MR imaging of maternal diseases of the abdomen and pelvis during pregnancy and the immediate postpartum period. Radiographics. 24(5):1301-16, 2004
7. Harrison-Woolrych M et al: Uterine perforation on intrauterine device insertion: is the incidence higher than previously reported? Contraception. 67(1):53-6, 2003
8. Gotoh H et al: Predicting incomplete uterine rupture with vaginal sonography during the late second trimester in women with prior cesarean. Obstet Gynecol. 95(4):596-600, 2000
9. Lowdermilk C et al: Screening helical CT for evaluation of blunt traumatic injury in the pregnant patient. Radiographics. 19 Spec No:S243-55; discussion S256-8, 1999
10. Maldjian C et al: MR appearance of uterine dehiscence in the post-cesarean section patient. J Comput Assist Tomogr. 22(5):738-41, 1998
11. Dicle O et al: Magnetic resonance imaging evaluation of incision healing after cesarean sections. Eur Radiol. 7(1):31-4, 1997
12. Okamoto T et al: A case of uterine choriocarcinoma with spontaneous rupture twenty-three years following the antecedent pregnancy. J Obstet Gynaecol Res. 23(2):189-95, 1997
13. Rooholamini SA et al: Imaging of pregnancy-related complications. Radiographics. 13(4):753-70, 1993
14. Woo GM et al: The pelvis after cesarean section and vaginal delivery: normal MR findings. AJR Am J Roentgenol. 161(6):1249-52, 1993
15. Jones RO et al: Rupture of low transverse cesarean scars during trial of labor. Obstet Gynecol. 77(6):815-7, 1991
16. Kronthal AJ et al: Uterine perforation simulating urachal carcinoma: CT diagnosis. AJR Am J Roentgenol. 154(4):741-3, 1990
17. Rosenblatt R et al: Uterine perforation and embedding by intrauterine device: evaluation by US and hysterography. Radiology. 157(3):765-70, 1985
18. Degesys GE et al: Ultrasonographic evaluation of uterine perforation by an intrauterine device. J Ultrasound Med. 1(9):375, 1982

UTERINE RUPTURE

IMAGE GALLERY

Typical

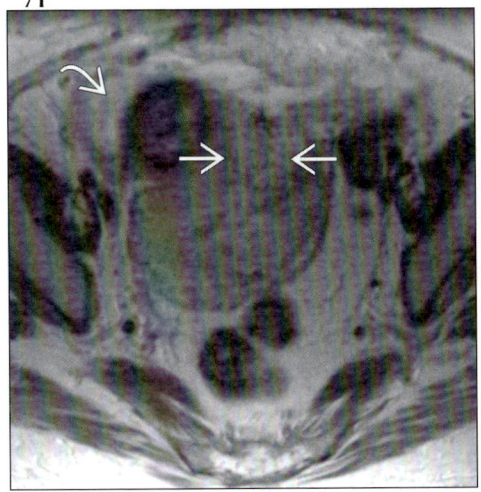
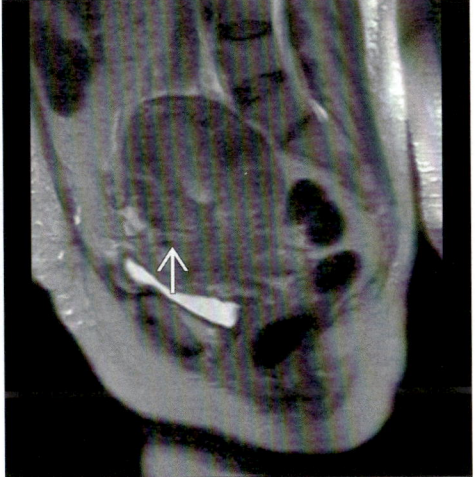

(Left) Axial T2WI MR shows the defect ➡ along the anterior myometrial margin containing air and fluid. Additional fluid ➡ is noted in the peritoneal space. *(Right)* Sagittal T2WI MR shows a track of high signal intensity fluid ➡ extending from the endometrial cavity into the peritoneal space.

Typical

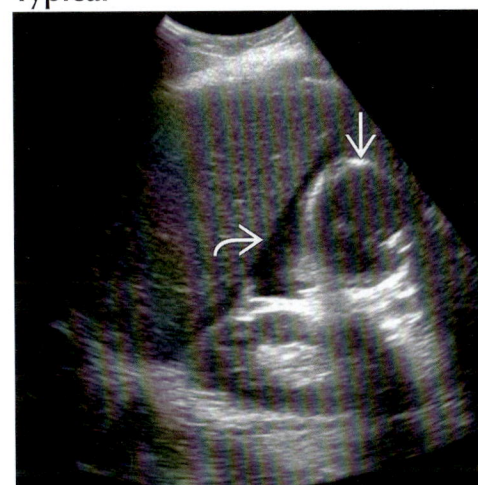
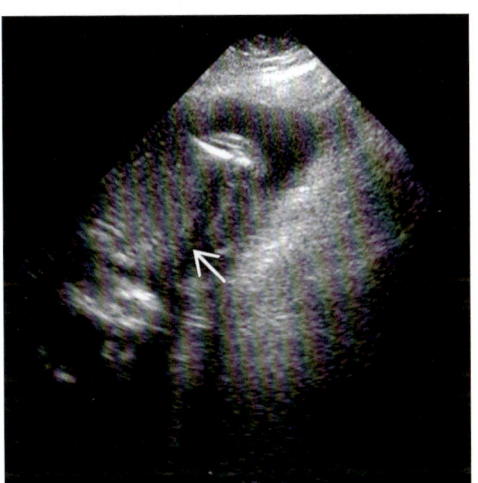

(Left) Longitudinal transabdominal ultrasound shows free fluid ➡ around the liver and a fetal head ➡ in the right upper quadrant. *(Right)* Longitudinal transabdominal ultrasound shows a fetus ➡ within the peritoneal cavity, outside the uterus.

Other

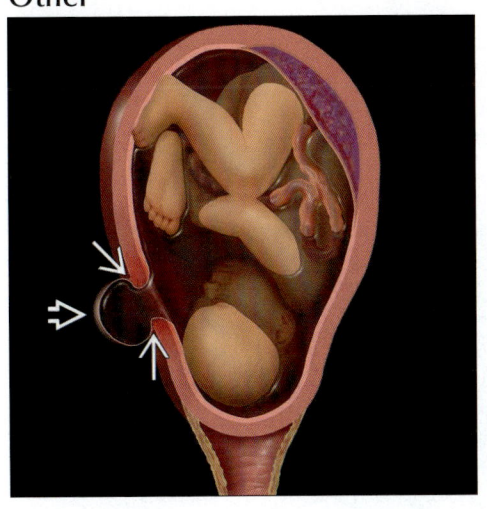
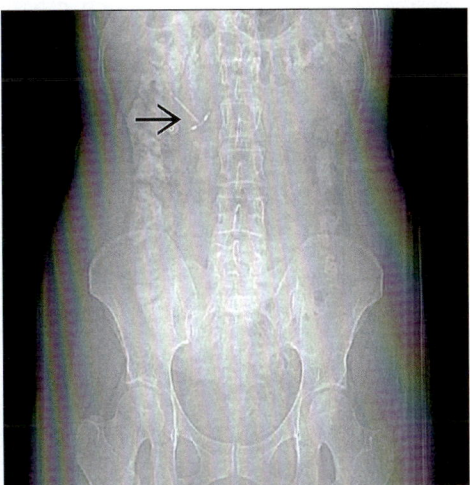

(Left) Coronal graphic shows loss of uterine wall integrity ➡ with herniation of amniotic fluid ➡. *(Right)* Coronal radiograph shows an intrauterine device ➡ in the right upper quadrant, consistent with a migrated IUD due to uterine rupture. (Courtesy B. Friedman, MD).

RETAINED PRODUCTS OF CONCEPTION

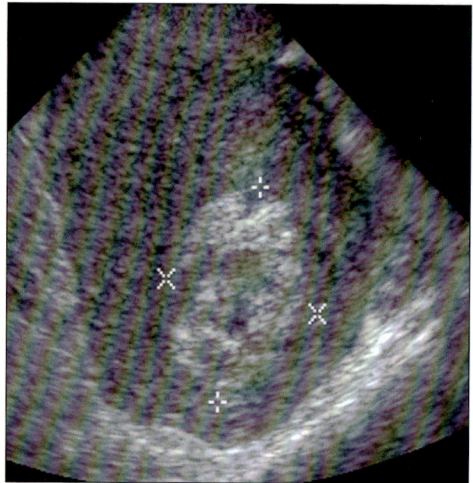

Sagittal transvaginal ultrasound shows heterogeneous echogenic mass (calipers) with calcifications.

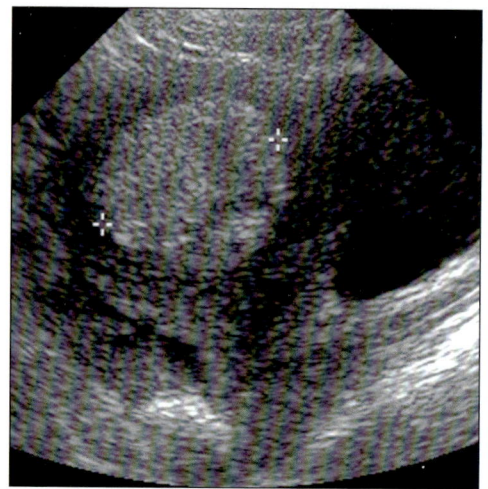

Sagittal transabdominal ultrasound shows echogenic mass (calipers) in endometrium.

TERMINOLOGY

Abbreviations and Synonyms
- Retained products of conception (RPOC)

Definitions
- Retained placental tissue after miscarriage, termination procedure, or delivery

IMAGING FINDINGS

General Features
- Best diagnostic clue: Echogenic material in the endometrial cavity with blood flow
- Location: Eccentrically located in endometrial cavity
- Size: Variable
- Morphology: Ill-defined margin with region of myometrium where placenta inserts

Ultrasonographic Findings
- Classic appearance is heterogeneous echogenic material in endometrial cavity with blood flow
- Irregular interface between endometrium and myometrium
- Calcifications with cotyledon appearance
- Calcified mass with shadowing
- Histologic RPOC can be present with sonographic appearance of normal endometrial cavity or endometrial fluid without mass
- Saline infused sonohysterography can aid in diagnosis
- Increased blood flow can be seen in region of retained tissue and in diffuse areas of myometrium
- Blood flow may simulate arteriovenous malformation
- Absence of blood flow does not exclude RPOC
- Thin myometrium suggests placenta accreta

CT Findings
- Endometrial mass
- Variable enhancement
- Ill definition with myometrium
- If myometrium is very thin, consider placenta accreta

MR Findings
- Intracavitary uterine soft-tissue mass
- Variable amounts of enhancing tissue
- Variable degree of myometrial thinning
- Obliteration of junctional zone

DDx: Retained Products of Conception

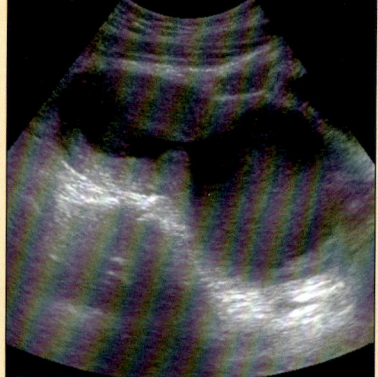

Cervical Stenosis

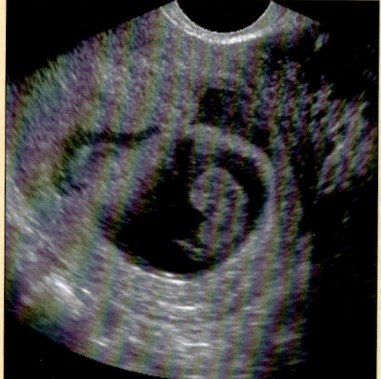

Missed Abortion

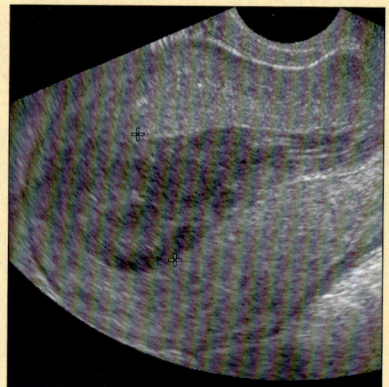

Blood Clot

RETAINED PRODUCTS OF CONCEPTION

Key Facts

Terminology
- Retained placental tissue after miscarriage, termination procedure, or delivery

Imaging Findings
- Best diagnostic clue: Echogenic material in the endometrial cavity with blood flow
- Morphology: Ill-defined margin with region of myometrium where placenta inserts
- Calcifications with cotyledon appearance
- Calcified mass with shadowing
- Saline infused sonohysterography can aid in diagnosis
- Increased blood flow can be seen in region of retained tissue and in diffuse areas of myometrium
- Blood flow may simulate arteriovenous malformation
- Absence of blood flow does not exclude RPOC
- Thin myometrium suggests placenta accreta
- Best imaging tool: Transvaginal ultrasound
- Color Doppler to assess for vascularity

Pathology
- Etiology: Adherent placental tissue not evacuated during miscarriage, D&C, vaginal birth or cesarian section
- Post-traumatic arteriovenous fistula may develop either within retained products or after instrumentation for retained products
- Color Doppler will show tangle of vessels
- Life-threatening hemorrhage can occur
- Persistent RPOC with elevated hCG can be due to invasive molar pregnancy

- If myometrium very thin, consider placenta accreta

Imaging Recommendations
- Best imaging tool: Transvaginal ultrasound
- Protocol advice
  - Transabdominal ultrasound to assess uterine size, ovaries, free fluid
  - Transvaginal ultrasound to assess material in endometrial cavity
  - Color Doppler to assess for vascularity

DIFFERENTIAL DIAGNOSIS

Blood Clot
- Heterogeneous material without blood flow
- Centrally located in endometrial cavity

Endometritis
- Heterogeneous infected material in endometrial cavity with or without RPOC
- Amount of heterogeneous material increases on follow-up imaging
- Focal tenderness to examination over uterus

Normal Postpartum
- Gas in endometrial cavity can have echogenic appearance
- Amount of gas will decrease on follow-up imaging

Gas in Endometrial Cavity After Instrumention
- Instrumentation introduces gas in endometrial cavity that can simulate mass
- Amount of gas should decrease on follow-up examination

Molar Pregnancy
- Persistent elevated human chorionic gonadotroph (hCG)
- May appear as an invasive mass

Missed Abortion
- Embryonic or fetal tissue still present in gestational sac
- Lack of cardiac activity in embryonic pole of 5 mm or greater

Cervical Stenosis
- Fluid with debris distends endometrial cavity
- Fluid with debris distends endocervical canal

PATHOLOGY

General Features
- Etiology: Adherent placental tissue not evacuated during miscarriage, D&C, vaginal birth or cesarian section
- Epidemiology
  - Within the week after first trimester spontaneous miscarriage, material seen in endometrial cavity in majority of cases
  - After vaginal delivery RPOC present in 20% of cases
  - Even after cesarian section RPOC can be present
- Associated abnormalities
  - Post-traumatic arteriovenous fistula may develop either within retained products or after instrumentation for retained products
    - Color Doppler will show tangle of vessels
    - Pulsed Doppler will show high diastolic flow
    - Life-threatening hemorrhage can occur
  - Persistent RPOC with elevated hCG can be due to invasive molar pregnancy

Gross Pathologic & Surgical Features
- Heterogeneous mass with appearance of placenta or retained fetal parts

Microscopic Features
- Chorionic villi present

CLINICAL ISSUES

Presentation
- Most common signs/symptoms
  - Bleeding

RETAINED PRODUCTS OF CONCEPTION

   - Persistent enlarged uterus
   - Vaginal pain
   - Fever
  - Other signs/symptoms: Infection

Demographics
- Age: Reproductive age
- Gender: Female

Natural History & Prognosis
- Tissue may pass on its own
  - Follow-up sonography after next menstrual cycle can be performed, rather than D&C, to confirm passage of tissue in patients who are asymptomatic
  - Low impedance flow may be present, but does not necessarily indicated clinically important RPOC
  - Follow-up hCG will demonstrate decreasing values
- Continued elevated hCG values suggest RPOC
- May act as nidus for infection
- Infected RPOC may lead to adhesions and Asherman syndrome

Treatment
- Ultrasound guidance helpful for dilatation and curettage in difficult cases (fibroids, duplication anomalies, uterine retroversion, lack of tissue at time of D&C)
- D&C can lead to uterine perforation
- Misoprostol can aid in non-surgical passage of tissue
- Small areas of RPOC (less than 1 cm) may pass spontaneously
- Larger areas of RPOC frequently necessitate D&C

DIAGNOSTIC CHECKLIST

Consider
- If large endometrial mass with no flow, consider hematoma or devascularized area of RPOC
- If thin myometrium, placenta accreta may be present
- If very vascular, D&C can lead to life-threatening hemorrhage
- If hCG is markedly elevated, molar pregnancy may be present

Image Interpretation Pearls
- Heterogeneous endometrial mass with blood flow in recently pregnant patient consistent with RPOC

SELECTED REFERENCES

1. Debby A et al: Transvaginal ultrasound after first-trimester uterine evacuation reduces the incidence of retained products of conception. Ultrasound Obstet Gynecol. 27(1):61-4, 2006
2. Brown DL: Pelvic ultrasound in the postabortion and postpartum patient. Ultrasound Q. 21(1):27-37, 2005
3. Durfee SM et al: The sonographic and color Doppler features of retained products of conception. J Ultrasound Med. 24(9):1181-6; quiz 1188-9, 2005
4. Jauniaux E et al: The role of ultrasound imaging in diagnosing and investigating early pregnancy failure. Ultrasound Obstet Gynecol. 25(6):613-24, 2005
5. Aziz N et al: Postpartum uterine arteriovenous fistula. Obstet Gynecol. 103(5 Pt 2):1076-8, 2004
6. Bhatia K et al: Intramural molar pregnancy: a case report. J Reprod Med. 49(8):689-92, 2004
7. Leyendecker JR et al: MR imaging of maternal diseases of the abdomen and pelvis during pregnancy and the immediate postpartum period. Radiographics. 24(5):1301-16, 2004
8. Maslovitz S et al: Accuracy of diagnosis of retained products of conception after dilation and evacuation. J Ultrasound Med. 23(6):749-56; quiz 758-9, 2004
9. Sadan O et al: Role of sonography in the diagnosis of retained products of conception. J Ultrasound Med. 23(3):371-4, 2004
10. Kido A et al: Retained products of conception masquerading as acquired arteriovenous malformation. J Comput Assist Tomogr. 27(1):88-92, 2003
11. Noonan JB et al: MR imaging of retained products of conception. AJR Am J Roentgenol. 181(2):435-9, 2003
12. Van den Bosch T et al: Color Doppler and gray-scale ultrasound evaluation of the postpartum uterus. Ultrasound Obstet Gynecol. 20(6):586-91, 2002
13. Wong SF et al: Transvaginal sonography in the detection of retained products of conception after first-trimester spontaneous abortion. J Clin Ultrasound. 30(7):428-32, 2002
14. Wolman I et al: Transvaginal sonohysterography for the evaluation and treatment of retained products of conception. Gynecol Obstet Invest. 50(2):73-6, 2000
15. Chung TK et al: Evaluation of the accuracy of transvaginal sonography for the assessment of retained products of conception after spontaneous abortion. Gynecol Obstet Invest. 45(3):190-3, 1998
16. Carlan SJ et al: Appearance of the uterus by ultrasound immediately after placental delivery with pathologic correlation. J Clin Ultrasound. 25(6):301-8, 1997
17. Chung T et al: A medical approach to management of spontaneous abortion using misoprostol. Extending misoprostol treatment to a maximum of 48 hours can further improve evacuation of retained products of conception in spontaneous abortion. Acta Obstet Gynecol Scand. 76(3):248-51, 1997
18. Kohlenberg CF et al: The use of intraoperative ultrasound in the management of a perforated uterus with retained products of conception. Aust N Z J Obstet Gynaecol. 36(4):482-4, 1996
19. Haines CJ et al: Transvaginal sonography and the conservative management of spontaneous abortion. Gynecol Obstet Invest. 37(1):14-7, 1994
20. Hertzberg BS et al: Ultrasound of the postpartum uterus. Prediction of retained placental tissue. J Ultrasound Med. 10(8):451-6, 1991
21. Chung T et al: A medical approach to management of spontaneous abortion using misoprostol. Extending misoprostol treatment to a maximum of 48 hours can further improve evacuation of retained products of conception in spontaneous abortion.

RETAINED PRODUCTS OF CONCEPTION

IMAGE GALLERY

Typical

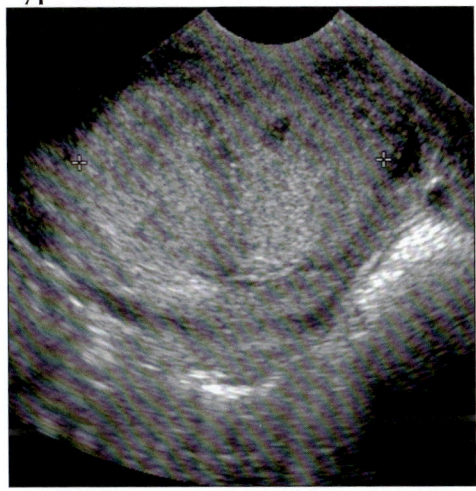
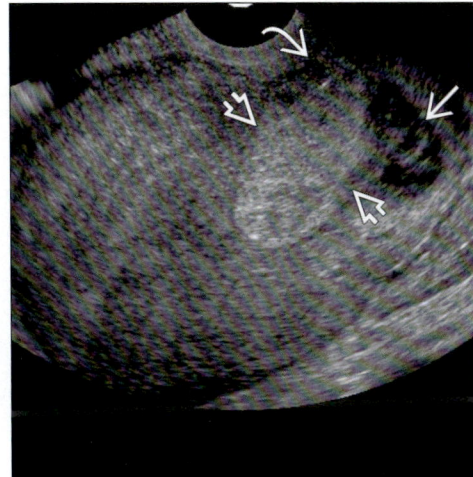

(Left) Coronal transvaginal ultrasound shows heterogeneous echogenic mass (calipers) in endometrium. *(Right)* Sagittal transvaginal ultrasound shows heterogeneous echogenic material ➡ eccentrically located in lower endometrium, extending into myometrium ➡, suggesting placenta accreta. Note blood clot ➡.

Typical

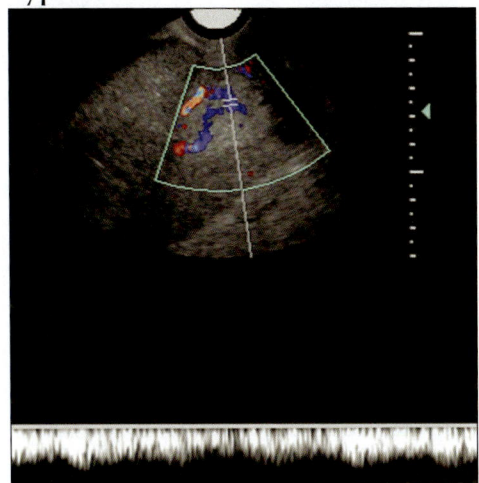
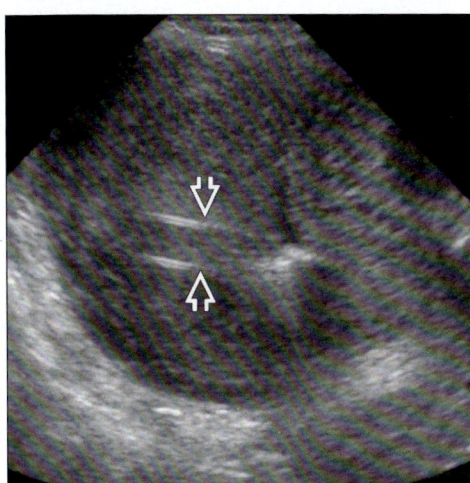

(Left) Sagittal transvaginal ultrasound in same patient as previous image shows flow in the echogenic mass. *(Right)* Sagittal transabdominal ultrasound during D&C shows catheter ➡ in endometrial cavity.

Typical

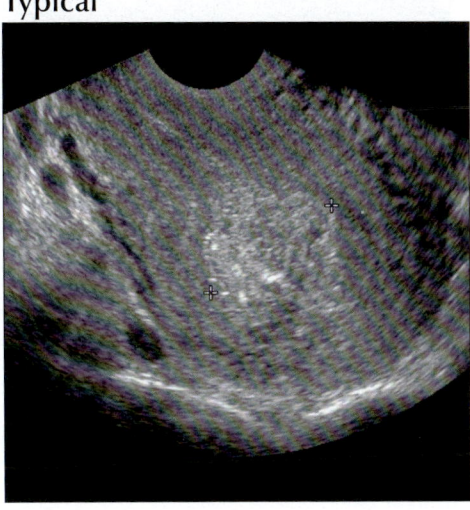
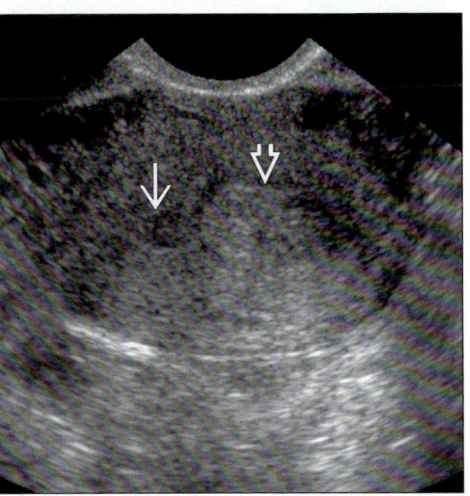

(Left) Sagittal transvaginal ultrasound shows heterogeneous material (calipers) with calcifications in endometrial cavity. Note ill-defined margins with myometrium. *(Right)* Coronal oblique transvaginal ultrasound shows echogenic material ➡ in left portion of endometrial cavity in patient with septate uterus. Note empty right endometrial cavity ➡.

RETAINED PRODUCTS OF CONCEPTION

(Left) Coronal oblique color Doppler ultrasound shows blood flow in area of RPOC extending into myometrium. *(Right)* Coronal oblique transvaginal ultrasound shows calcified mass ➡ with shadowing ➡ in endometrial cavity.

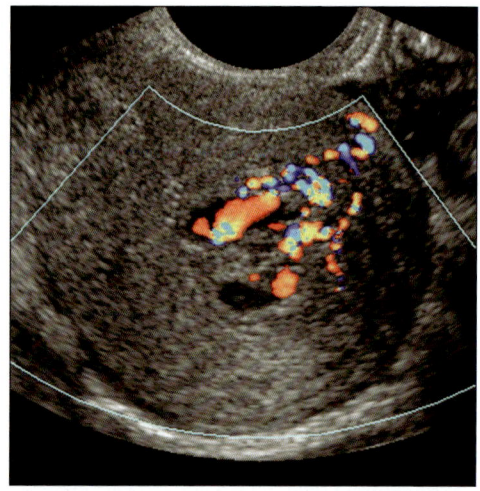
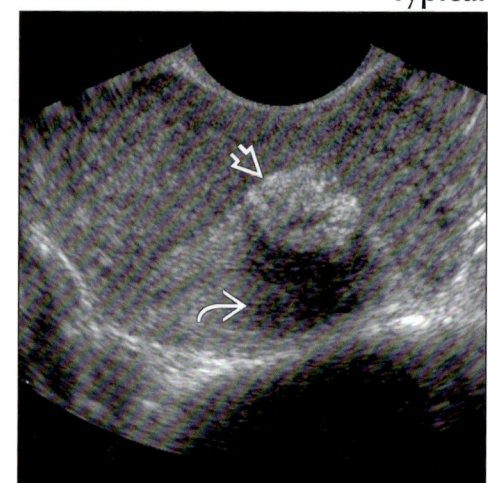

Typical

(Left) Sagittal oblique transvaginal ultrasound shows heterogeneous echogenic mass ➡ in endometrial cavity with ill-defined margins with myometrium. *(Right)* Coronal oblique transvaginal ultrasound shows heterogeneous material ➡ in endometrial cavity.

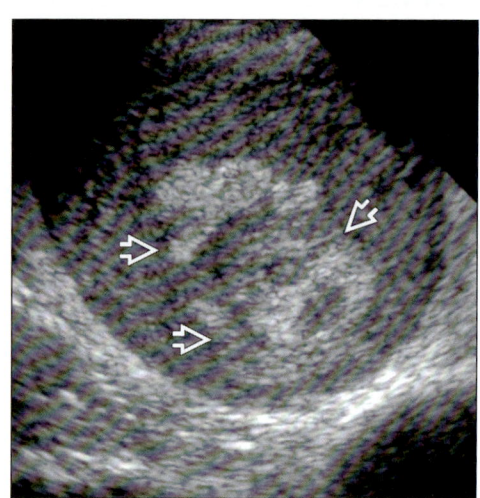
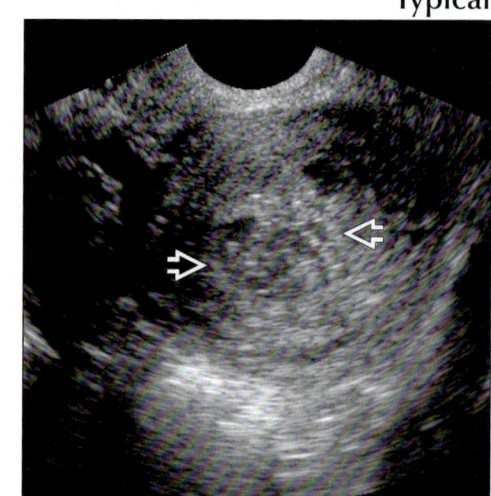

Typical

(Left) Coronal power Doppler ultrasound shows increased blood flow in endometrium extending to myometrium. *(Right)* Sagittal transvaginal ultrasound shows heterogeneous material (calipers) in endocervical canal. Other images (not shown) demonstrated flow to the more echogenic area.

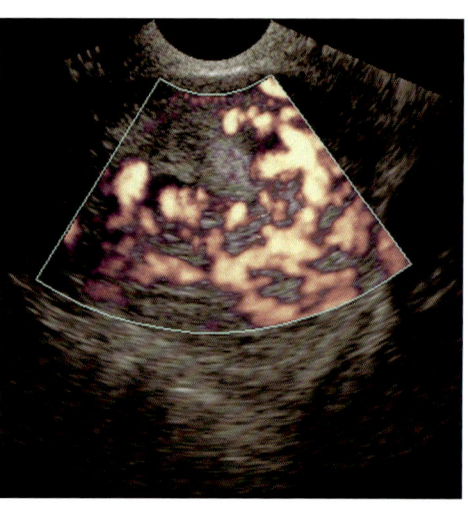
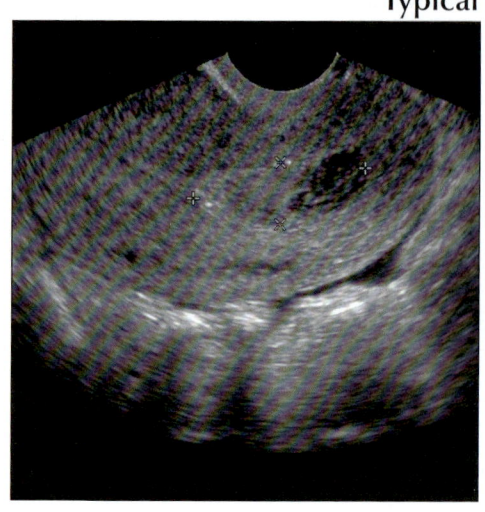

Typical

RETAINED PRODUCTS OF CONCEPTION

Typical

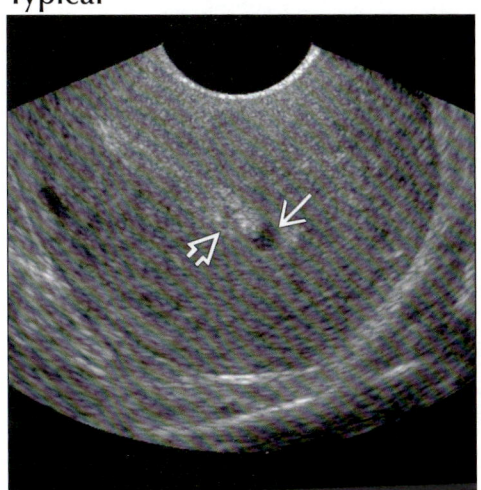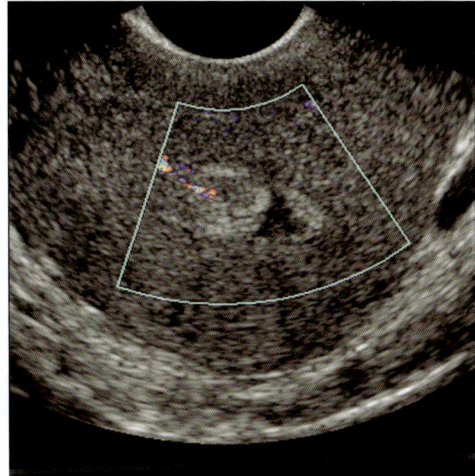

(Left) Sagittal transvaginal ultrasound shows a small amount of echogenic material ⇨ and debris ➔ in the endometrial cavity. *(Right)* Coronal color Doppler ultrasound in same case as previous image shows blood flow extending from myometrium into region of RPOC.

Typical

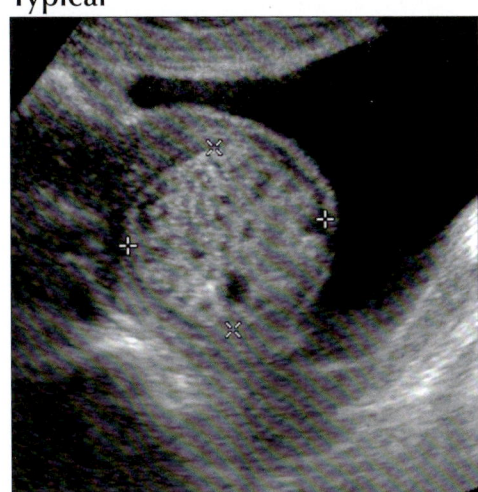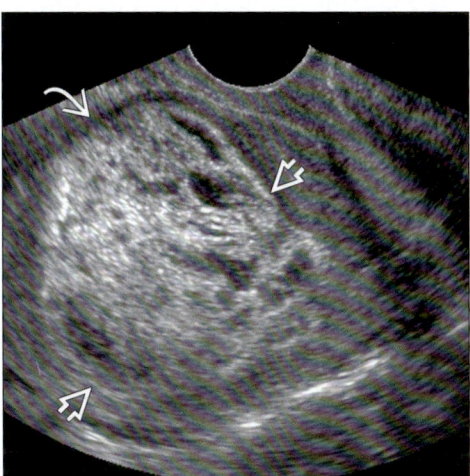

(Left) Sagittal transabdominal ultrasound shows heterogeneous material (calipers) in endometrial cavity extending to myometrium in patient with placenta accreta. *(Right)* Sagittal transvaginal ultrasound in same patient as previous image shows heterogeneous echogenic mass ➔ consistent with RPOC. The extremely thin myometrium anteriorly ➔ suggests placenta accreta.

Typical

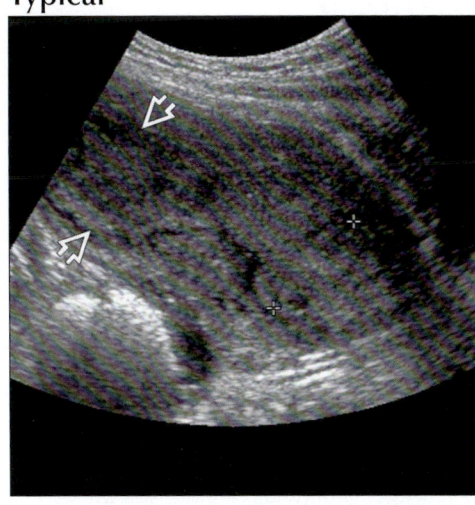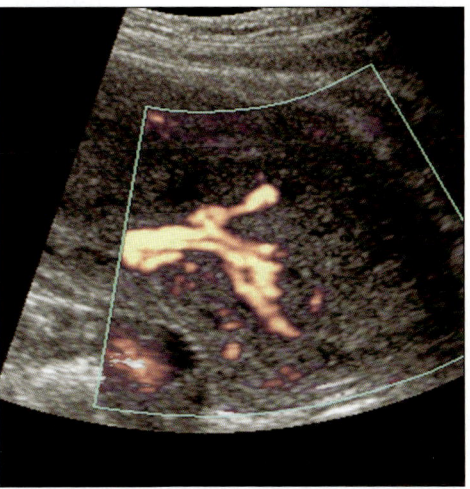

(Left) Sagittal transabdominal ultrasound shows a large amount of heterogeneous material distending the endometrial cavity (calipers and ➔). *(Right)* Sagittal power Doppler ultrasound in same patient as previous image shows blood flow to the region of RPOC.

TAMOXIFEN-INDUCED CHANGES

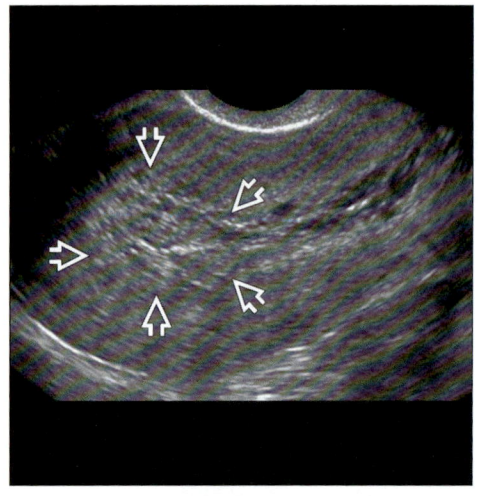

Sagittal transvaginal ultrasound shows endometrial widening ⇨ punctuated by small cysts. (Courtesy MR Reiser, (ed), Screening & Preventative Diagnosis with Radiological Imaging, Springer-Verlag, Berlin, in press).

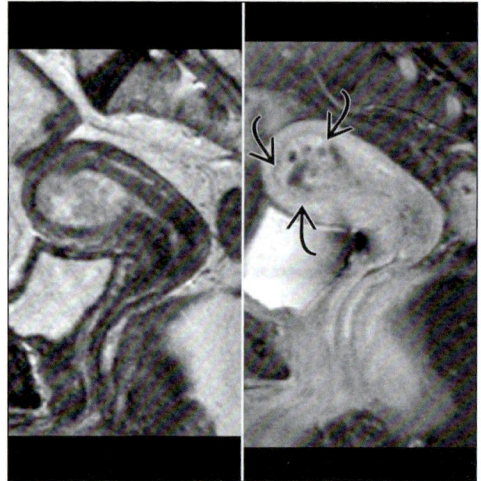

Sagittal T2WI (left) shows a heterogeneous mass distending endometrial canal. T1 C+ (right) confirms enhancing solid mass with cystic changes without myometrial invasion ⇨. Pathology: Benign polyp.

TERMINOLOGY

Definitions
- Tamoxifen-induced endometrial abnormalities include polyps, hyperplasia, cystic atrophy, adenomyosis and endometrial carcinoma
- Tamoxifen-induced abnormalities may coexist

IMAGING FINDINGS

General Features
- Best diagnostic clue: Soft tissue mass with cystic changes distending endometrial canal
- Location
  - Endometrium
  - Other abnormalities: Myometrium (leiomyomas) and ovary (cysts)
- Size: Variable: Tamoxifen polyps tend to be larger than polyps in the general female population
- Morphology: Variable: Polypoid, diffuse or focal

Ultrasonographic Findings
- Grayscale Ultrasound
  - **Cutoff value for normal endometrial thickness in asymptomatic women on tamoxifen is controversial**
    - \> 5 mm: Untreated women with postmenopausal bleeding
    - \> 8 mm for women on hormone replacement therapy
    - \> 6 mm: Study of 100+ asymptomatic women on tamoxifen (84.1% sensitivity and 58.2% specificity)
  - Polyp
    - Non-specific thickening of the endometrium
    - Hyperechoic endometrium with multiple small cystic spaces
    - Homogeneous or heterogeneous solid endometrial mass
    - Separate endometrial lining
  - Endometrial hyperplasia
    - Well-defined endometrial thickening with or without cysts
    - If focal or asymmetric, cannot exclude malignancy
  - Cystic atrophy
    - Irregular cystic endometrium, may lead to spuriously thickened endometrial measurement

DDx: Tamoxifen Associated Abnormalities

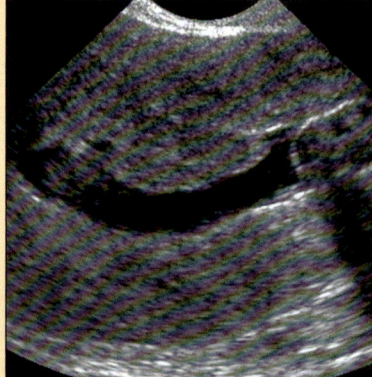
Submucosal Leiomyomas

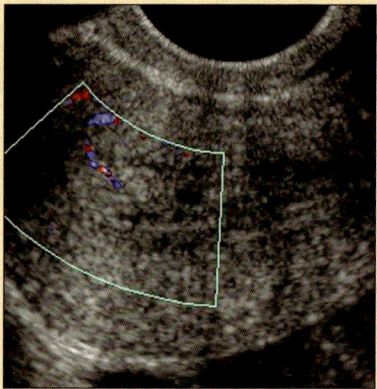
Generic Polyp

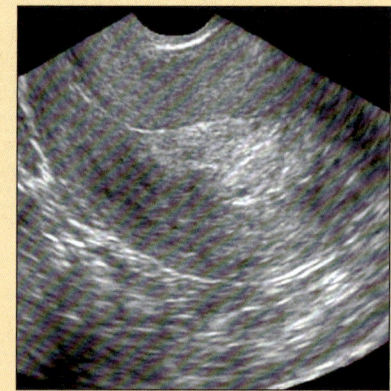
Generic Endometrial Cancer

TAMOXIFEN-INDUCED CHANGES

Key Facts

Terminology
- Tamoxifen-induced endometrial abnormalities include polyps, hyperplasia, cystic atrophy, adenomyosis and endometrial carcinoma
- Tamoxifen-induced abnormalities may coexist

Imaging Findings
- Soft tissue mass with cystic changes distending endometrial canal
- **Cutoff value for normal endometrial thickness in asymptomatic women on tamoxifen is controversial**
- > 6 mm: Study of 100+ asymptomatic women on tamoxifen (84.1% sensitivity and 58.2% specificity)
- Transvaginal ultrasound for initial imaging
- Sonohysterography should be performed if transvaginal sonography (TVS) is non-diagnostic or there is non-specific endometrial thickening
- MR if sonohysterography unable to be performed

Top Differential Diagnoses
- Submucosal Leiomyoma
- Generic Endometrial Cancer
- Generic Endometrial Polyp

Pathology
- Tamoxifen-induced endometrial polyps: 8-36%
- Tamoxifen-induced endometrial hyperplasia: 1.3-20%
- Tamoxifen-induced cystic atrophy
- Adenomyosis

Diagnostic Checklist
- Endometrial polypoid mass with cystic spaces

  - Adenomyosis
    - Heterogeneous myometrium
    - Myometrial cysts
    - Poor endometrial definition
  - Cancer
    - Diffusely or partially echogenic endometrium
    - Endometrial thickening may be well-defined or ill-defined
- Color Doppler
  - Polyp: May show feeding vessel in pedicle
  - Hyperplasia: Multiple feeding vessels; sparse vascularity

MR Findings
- Benign polyp (mean endometrial width is 1.8 cm)
  - T1WI: Isointense mass in endometrial canal
  - T2WI: Heterogeneous mass in endometrial canal
  - Usually lower in signal intensity compared to normal endometrium
  - If cancer, may see invasion into underlying myometrium
  - T1 C+: Enhancing, solid, soft tissue mass or solid mass with cystic changes (lattice-like enhancement) in endometrial canal
  - Usually enhance less than normal endometrium
- Endometrial hyperplasia
  - MR may be normal
  - T1WI: Isointense mass in endometrial canal
  - T2WI: Diffuse widening of endometrium
  - Isointense or slightly hypointense to normal endometrium
  - T1 C+: Diffuse enhancement
- Cystic atrophy
  - T1WI: Normal
  - T2WI: Endometrial/subendometrial high signal intensity cysts
  - T1 C+: Signal void endometrial/subendometrial cysts
- Adenomyosis
  - T1WI: Isointense to myometrium
    - May see foci of high signal intensity scattered in adenomyotic tissue
  - T2WI: Focal or diffuse widening of the junctional zone ≥ 12 mm
    - May see high signal intensity foci scattered in adenomyotic tissue
  - T1 C+: Variable
- Endometrial cancer
  - May be indistinguishable from a benign polyp
  - Myometrial invasion is diagnostic

Other Modality Findings
- Sonohysterography
  - Polyp: Echogenic mass, smooth margins, most with cystic spaces
  - Hyperplasia: Differentiates diffuse vs. focal abnormality
  - Cystic atrophy: Small subendometrial anechoic spaces
  - Adenomyosis: Small inner myometrial cysts
  - Cancer: Irregular heterogeneous mass or focally thickened endometrium

Imaging Recommendations
- Best imaging tool
  - Transvaginal ultrasound for initial imaging
  - Sonohysterography should be performed if transvaginal sonography (TVS) is non-diagnostic or there is non-specific endometrial thickening
    - Women on tamoxifen may require cervical dilation for sonohysterography
  - MR if sonohysterography unable to be performed
    - 8-37% sonohysterography failure rate for postmenopausal women on tamoxifen
- Protocol advice: Oral analgesics may be given prior to sonohysterography to decrease discomfort

DIFFERENTIAL DIAGNOSIS

Submucosal Leiomyoma
- Myometrial origin; T2WI: Low signal

TAMOXIFEN-INDUCED CHANGES

Generic Endometrial Cancer
- Cannot be distinguished on imaging from tamoxifen-induced cancer

Generic Endometrial Polyp
- Cannot be distinguished on imaging from tamoxifen-induced polyp

PATHOLOGY

General Features
- General path comments
  - Spectrum of endometrial abnormalities: Up to 50% of women develop abnormalities
  - Tamoxifen-induced endometrial polyps: 8-36%
    - Versus 0-10% untreated women
  - Tamoxifen-induced endometrial hyperplasia: 1.3-20%
    - Versus 0-10% untreated women
  - Tamoxifen-induced cystic atrophy
  - Adenomyosis
  - Tamoxifen-induced endometrial carcinoma: 1.3-7.5x increase in risk
  - National Breast Cancer Prevention Trial: Benefits of therapy outweigh increased risk of carcinoma
  - No analyses to support routine screening
  - Imaging findings may direct biopsy and treatment
- Etiology
  - Anti-estrogen that binds to estrogen receptors
  - May have paradoxical effects at uterine level
- Epidemiology: Up to 50% develop abnormalities by 36 months
- Associated abnormalities: Ovarian cysts

Gross Pathologic & Surgical Features
- Polyps: Large, mean diameter of 5 cm, may have stalk
- Cystic atrophy: Smooth, white, hyper-vascularized endometrium
- Cancer: Often polypoid morphology

Microscopic Features
- Polyps: Combination of proliferative activity, aberrant epithelial differentiation and focal periglandular stromal condensation
- Hyperplasia: Morphologically abnormal proliferative-type endometrium ± cytologic atypica and ± cystic dilation of glands
- Cystic atrophy: Cysts lined by atrophic endometrium
- Adenomyosis: Heterotopic endometrial glands and stroma in myometrium with surrounding smooth muscle hypertrophy/hyperplasia
- Cancer: Most are endometrioid adenocarcinomas

Staging, Grading or Classification Criteria
- See FIGO staging for endometrial carcinoma

CLINICAL ISSUES

Presentation
- Most common signs/symptoms: Abnormal uterine bleeding
- Clinical Profile: Postmenopausal breast cancer patient or high risk woman receiving tamoxifen

Demographics
- Gender: Female

Natural History & Prognosis
- Cancer: Controversy over whether tamoxifen-induced carcinomas are more aggressive than those in general female population
  - Overall prognosis is good if diagnosed early with prompt therapy
- Benign polyps and hyperplasia: Good with appropriate treatment

Treatment
- American college of obstetricians and gynecologists: Recommendations
  - Polyp: Remove
  - Atypical hyperplasia: Discontinue tamoxifen and dilatation and curettage (D&C) (if tamoxifen must be continued, consider hysterectomy)
  - Cancer: Treatment appropriate to stage of disease

DIAGNOSTIC CHECKLIST

Consider
- Tamoxifen-induced change in a patient with breast cancer and endometrial abnormality
- Must always exclude unrelated primary cancer or metastases

Image Interpretation Pearls
- Endometrial polypoid mass with cystic spaces

SELECTED REFERENCES

1. Weaver J et al: Accuracy of transvaginal ultrasound in diagnosing endometrial pathology in women with post-menopausal bleeding on tamoxifen. Br J Radiol. 78(929):394-7, 2005
2. Develioglu OH et al: The endometrium in asymptomatic breast cancer patients on tamoxifen: value of transvaginal ultrasonography with saline infusion and Doppler flow. Gynecol Oncol. 93(2):328-35, 2004
3. Markovitch O et al: The value of sonohysterography in the prediction of endometrial pathologies in asymptomatic postmenopausal breast cancer tamoxifen-treated patients. Gynecol Oncol. 94(3):754-9, 2004
4. Markovitch O et al: The value of transvaginal ultrasonography in the prediction of endometrial pathologies in asymptomatic postmenopausal breast cancer tamoxifen-treated patients. Gynecol Oncol. 95(3):456-62, 2004
5. Fong K et al: Transvaginal US and hysterosonography in postmenopausal women with breast cancer receiving tamoxifen: correlation with hysteroscopy and pathologic study. Radiographics. 23(1):137-50; discussion 151-5, 2003
6. Fung MF et al: Prospective longitudinal study of ultrasound screening for endometrial abnormalities in women with breast cancer receiving tamoxifen. Gynecol Oncol. 91(1):154-9, 2003
7. Ascher SM et al: Tamoxifen-induced uterine abnormalities: the role of imaging. Radiology. 214(1):29-38, 2000

TAMOXIFEN-INDUCED CHANGES

IMAGE GALLERY

Typical

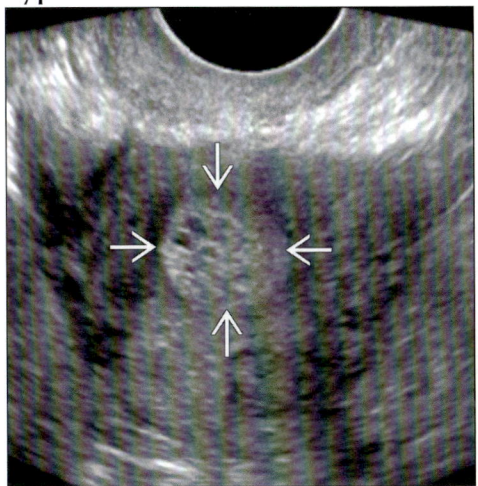 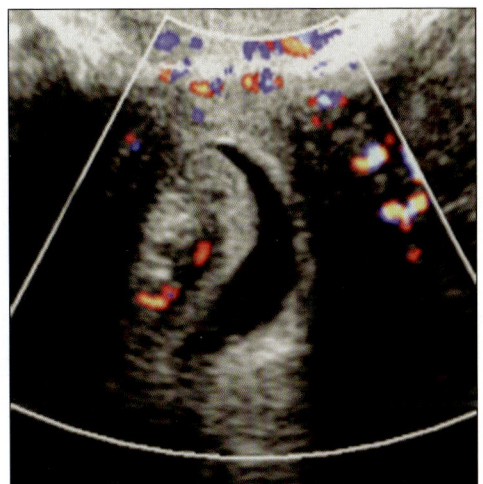

(Left) Axial transvaginal ultrasound shows the endometrial canal is expanded ➡ by an echogenic mass with small cysts. This is a typical appearance of a tamoxifen associated polyp. *(Right)* Axial color Doppler ultrasound shows feeding artery within polyp in the same patient as previous image during sonohysterography. Pathology: Benign polyp.

Typical

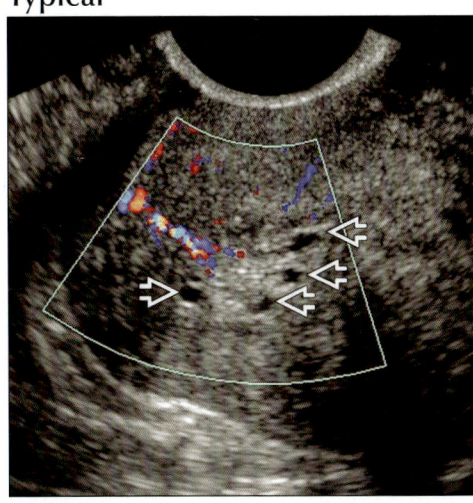 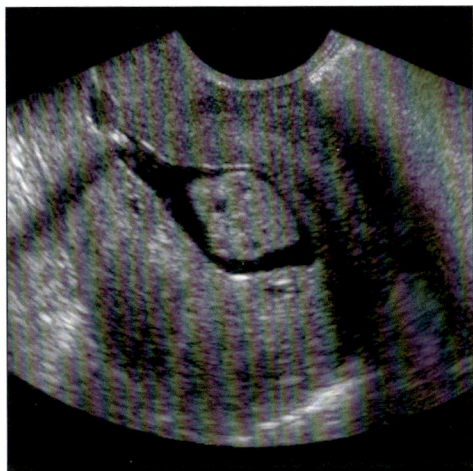

(Left) Axial color Doppler ultrasound shows endometrial canal expanded by mass with small cysts ➡. Single feeding artery seen in pedicle of this tamoxifen polyp. (Courtesy reference 6). *(Right)* Sagittal transvaginal ultrasound shows intracavitary mass surrounded by fluid following infusion of saline in same patient as previous. Pathology: Benign polyp. (Courtesy reference 6).

Typical

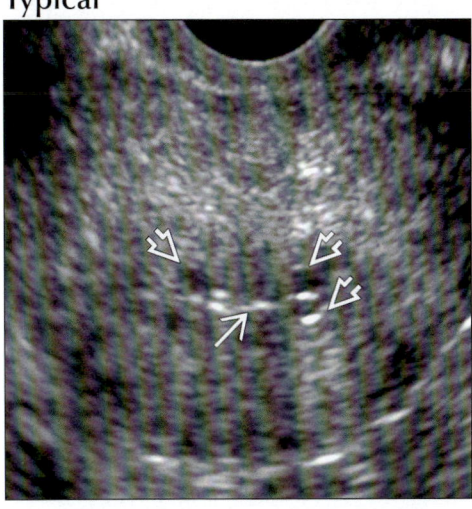 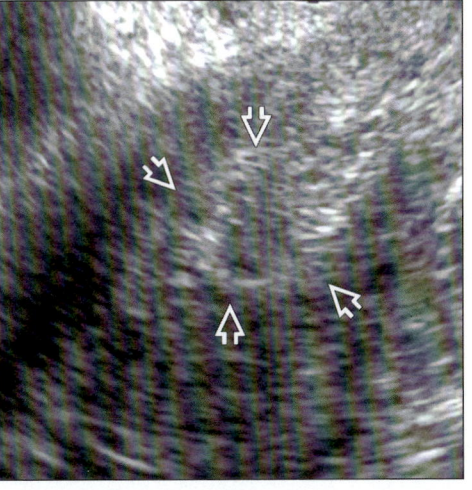

(Left) Axial transvaginal ultrasound shows small cysts ➡ flanking endometrial echo complex ➡. This appearance may lead to spuriously widened endometrial measurement. *(Right)* Sagittal transvaginal ultrasound shows expanded heterogeneous echogenic endometrium ➡. Pathology: Endometrial carcinoma.

INTRAUTERINE DEVICE EVALUATION

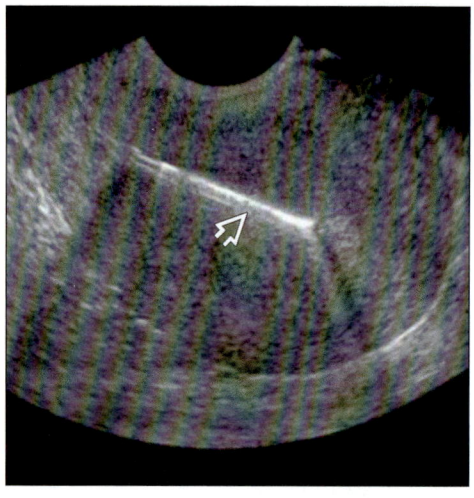

Sagittal transvaginal ultrasound shows retroflexed uterus with IUD ➡ in good position, centrally located in endometrial cavity.

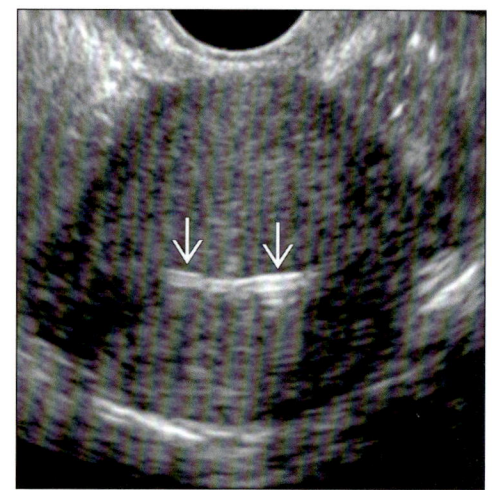

Coronal oblique transvaginal ultrasound shows fundus of the uterus with IUD cross bars ➡ in appropriate location.

TERMINOLOGY

Abbreviations and Synonyms
- Intrauterine device (IUD)
- Intrauterine contraceptive device (IUCD)

Definitions
- Device inserted into the endometrial cavity typically to prevent pregnancy
- Certain types of IUDs also release hormones such as levonorgestrel or progesterone
  - Mirena (levonorgestrel-20 IUD, Shering, AG Pharmaceutical, Germany)
  - Levonorgestrel-releasing intrauterine system (LNG-IUS)
- Copper devices cause increased copper levels
  - Copper-380 IUD (Paragard T380 A; Ortho-McNeil Pharmaceutical, Inc, Raritan, NJ)
  - Leads to changes in cervical mucus that affect sperm motility and irritate endometrium

IMAGING FINDINGS

General Features
- Best diagnostic clue: Echogenic object in the endometrial cavity
- Location
  - Endometrial cavity when normally positioned
  - Expulsion of IUD will lead to nonvisualization on imaging studies
- Morphology
  - Straight shaft (Copper T 380A, Mirena) IUD: Linear bright echo aligned with endometrial cavity with cross bars in fundal endometrium
    - Early versions of the Mirena IUD were very difficult to visualize sonographically
    - String of the Mirena IUD is very echogenic, seen as a linear bright echo in the cervix
  - Older versions of IUDs less frequently seen
    - Plastic IUDs have entrance-exit echoes in all scan planes
    - Lippes loop IUD: Seen in longitudinal plane as interrupted bright areas with shadowing
  - Round IUD

DDx: Intrauterine Device

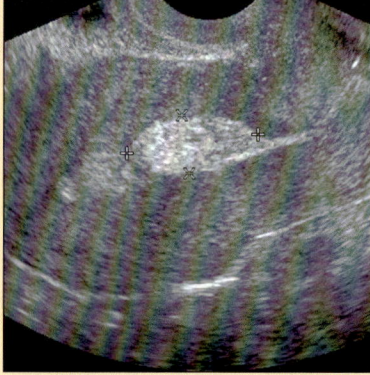

Retained Products of Conception

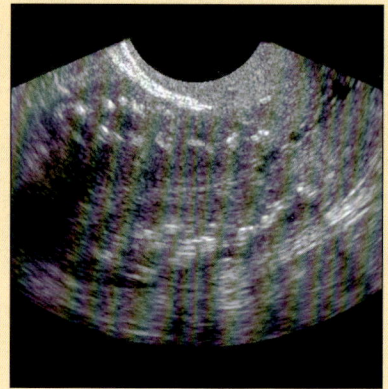

Arcuate Artery Calcifications

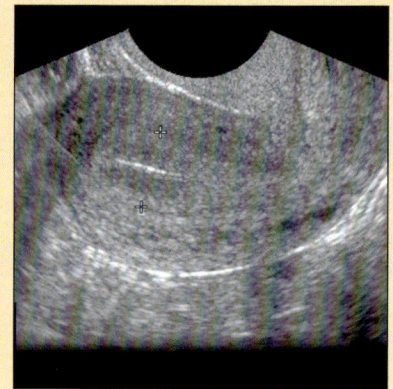

Normal Endometrial Stripe

INTRAUTERINE DEVICE EVALUATION

Key Facts

Terminology
- Device inserted into the endometrial cavity typically to prevent pregnancy

Imaging Findings
- Best diagnostic clue: Echogenic object in the endometrial cavity
- Straight shaft (Copper T 380A, Mirena) IUD: Linear bright echo aligned with endometrial cavity with cross bars in fundal endometrium
- Early versions of the Mirena IUD were very difficult to visualize sonographically
- String of the Mirena IUD is very echogenic, seen as a linear bright echo in the cervix
- Lippes loop IUD: Seen in longitudinal plane as interrupted bright areas with shadowing
- Stainless steel ring in fundus with straight shaft in lower endometrium commonly used in China
- Best imaging tool: Transvaginal ultrasound
- If an IUD is difficult to visualize sonographically, look for shadowing
- If IUD cannot be visualized, a plain film of the abdomen may show extrauterine location

Clinical Issues
- If malpositioned may cause pain, especially during intercourse
- Uterine perforation may be symptomatic or asymptomatic
- Perforated IUD should be removed laparoscopically
- IUD in pelvis can perforate into any organ including bowel, ovary, or bladder

- Stainless steel ring in fundus with straight shaft in lower endometrium commonly used in China

Imaging Recommendations
- Best imaging tool: Transvaginal ultrasound
- Protocol advice
  - Ultrasound
    - If an IUD is difficult to visualize sonographically, look for shadowing
    - Posterior shadowing best visualized when scanning perpendicular to the long axis of the IUD
    - Volume contrast imaging with 2-4 mm slice thickness can aid in IUD detection
    - IUD tip should be within 5 mm of tip of endometrial echo
    - Low IUDs may spontaneously migrate into more appropriate position
    - Cross bars of IUD should be in region of fundal endometrium
    - If cross bars extend anteriorly and/or posteriorly, this is a malpositioned IUD
  - Radiography
    - If IUD cannot be visualized, a plain film of the abdomen may show extrauterine location
  - Computed tomography
    - IUD appears of high attenuation
  - Magnetic resonance imaging
    - IUD appears as signal void
    - MR at 1.5T is safe with IUD however MR at 3.0T is not yet proven safe for use with IUD

DIFFERENTIAL DIAGNOSIS

Retained Products of Conception
- Mass with calcifications
- Calcifications not linear like IUD

Endometrial Calcifications of Dystrophic Nature
- Punctate or oblong calcifications at endometrial myometrial interface
- Likely of no clinical consequence

Bright Echo of Normal Interface of Endometrial Lining
- Very thin echogenic area at endometrial interface without shadowing

Arcuate Artery Calcifications
- In outer 1/3 of myometrium

PATHOLOGY

General Features
- Epidemiology
  - Intrauterine contraception is the most cost-effective reversible method of contraception
  - Used by 130 million women worldwide

CLINICAL ISSUES

Presentation
- Most common signs/symptoms
  - If string is not visualized outside of cervix IUD may be
    - In place, but with absent/malpositioned string
    - Malpositioned, but still in uterus
    - Perforated, outside of uterus
    - Expulsed vaginally and no longer present
    - Expulsion rate highest if IUD inserted in the immediate postpartum period after vaginal delivery
  - If malpositioned may cause pain, especially during intercourse
    - Malpositioned IUD may lead to decreased efficacy in preventing pregnancy
    - Cervical position can lead to cervical motion tenderness
    - Myometrial position of the cross bars may lead to pelvic pain
    - Malpositioned IUD should be removed & replaced

INTRAUTERINE DEVICE EVALUATION

- Uterine perforation may be symptomatic or asymptomatic
  - Perforated IUD should be removed laparoscopically
  - IUD in pelvis can perforate into any organ including bowel, ovary, or bladder
- Intraperitoneal position of LNG-IUS results in plasma LNG levels 10x higher than the plasma level of LNG observed with LNG-IUS placed in utero
  - High plasma LNG level suppresses ovulation
  - Misplaced LNG-IUS should be removed when pregnancy is desired
- Other signs/symptoms
  - Irregular menses
  - Dysmenorrhea
  - Infection
  - Ectopic pregnancy
    - If patient gets pregnant while using an IUD, likelihood of ectopic pregnancy is increased, since IUD prevents implantation in the uterus
  - LNG-IUS associated with steroidal side effects: Mood changes, oily skin, acne

Demographics
- Age: Reproductive age
- Gender: Female

Natural History & Prognosis
- IUDs aid in prevention of intrauterine pregnancy with the following mechanisms of action
  - Pre-fertilization
    - Inhibition of sperm migration and viability
    - Alteration of speed of transport of the ovum in the fallopian tube
    - Damage of ovum
  - Post-fertilization
    - Alteration of speed of transport of fertilized ovum
    - Damage to early embryo
    - Suppress endometrium
    - Prevention of pregnancy implantation
- If intrauterine pregnancy occurs with IUD in place, & patient desires to continue pregnancy, IUD should be removed
  - IUD left in place during pregnancy, increases risk of
    - Miscarriage in 50%
    - Premature rupture of membranes
    - Septic complications of chorioamnionitis, fetal infection, maternal septicemia
    - Premature delivery
  - IUD removal during pregnancy is associated with high success rate
    - Miscarriage rate of 22%, live birth 77%, preterm delivery 13.5%
    - IUD removal should be performed under sonographic guidance
- Women with chlamydial infection or gonorrhea at time of IUD insertion are at increased risk of pelvic inflammatory disease relative to women without infection at time of insertion
- Non-contraceptive health benefits
  - LNG-IUS decreases abnormal bleeding in patients with leiomyomas
  - LNG-IUS decreases dysmenorrhea in patients with symptomatic endometriosis
  - Copper and plastic IUD are associated with decreased risk of endometrial cancer
- IUD insertion can be used as a form of emergency contraception
- Perforation rate 1-2/1,000 with highest rates with
  - Placement by inexperienced operators
  - Placement < 3 months postpartum
  - Placed while patient breastfeeding
  - Placed in nulliparous patient

Treatment
- Perforated IUD treated with laparoscopic removal
- Pregnancy with IUD in place treated with sonographic guided removal
- Infection with IUD in place treated with removal of IUD, drainage of abscess if needed, antibiotics

DIAGNOSTIC CHECKLIST

Consider
- Plain film of abdomen to visualize IUD not seen sonographically

Image Interpretation Pearls
- Entire IUD should be visualized within endometrial cavity with cross bars in appropriate orientation

SELECTED REFERENCES

1. Muhler M et al: [How safe is magnetic resonance imaging in patients with contraceptive implants?] Radiologe. 46(7):574-8, 2006
2. Valsky DV et al: The shadow of the intrauterine device. J Ultrasound Med. 25(5):613-6, 2006
3. Letti Muller AL et al: Transvaginal ultrasonographic assessment of the expulsion rate of intrauterine devices inserted in the immediate postpartum period: a pilot study. Contraception. 72(3):192-5, 2005
4. Morales-Rosello J: Spontaneous upward movement of lowly placed T-shaped IUDs. Contraception. 72(6):430-1, 2005
5. Schiesser M et al: Lost intrauterine devices during pregnancy: maternal and fetal outcome after ultrasound-guided extraction. An analysis of 82 cases. Ultrasound Obstet Gynecol. 23(5):486-9, 2004
6. Caliskan E et al: Analysis of risk factors associated with uterine perforation by intrauterine devices. Eur J Contracept Reprod Health Care. 8(3):150-5, 2003
7. Hubacher D et al: Noncontraceptive health benefits of intrauterine devices: a systematic review. Obstet Gynecol Surv. 57(2):120-8, 2002
8. Stanford JB et al: Mechanisms of action of intrauterine devices: update and estimation of postfertilization effects. Am J Obstet Gynecol. 187(6):1699-708, 2002
9. Thonneau P et al: Risk factors for intrauterine device failure: a review. Contraception. 64(1):33-7, 2001
10. Tatum HJ et al: Management and outcome of pregnancies associated with the Copper T intrauterine contraceptive device. Am J Obstet Gynecol. 126(7):869-79, 1976

INTRAUTERINE DEVICE EVALUATION

IMAGE GALLERY

Other

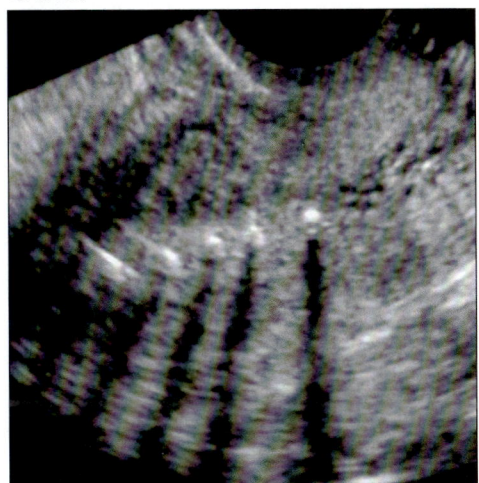
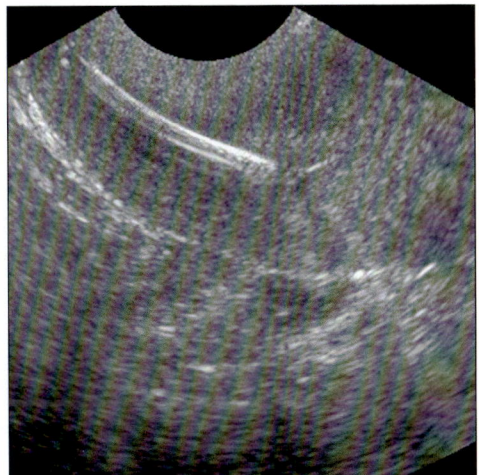

(Left) Sagittal transvaginal ultrasound shows Lippes loop IUD with multiple shadowing echogenicities, in line with the endometrial cavity. *(Right)* Sagittal transvaginal ultrasound shows low position of IUD, extending from the cervix into the lower uterus. This type of position can be associated with pelvic pain, and is not sufficient for birth control.

Typical

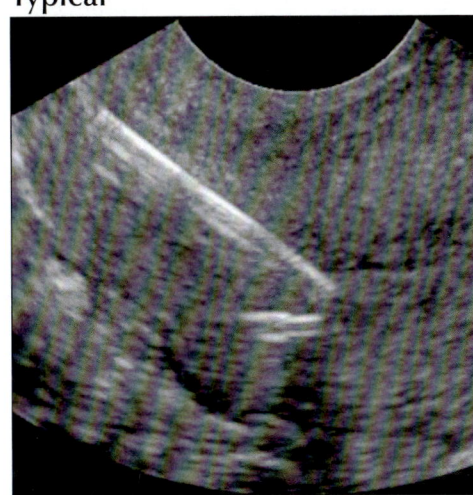
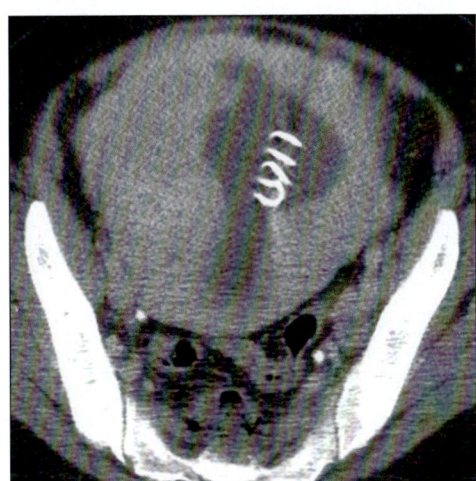

(Left) Sagittal transvaginal ultrasound shows IUD in abnormal position with cross bar extending into the myometrium. This type of placement is associated with pelvic pain, and may not prevent pregnancy implantation. *(Right)* Transverse NECT shows IUD in the endometrial cavity filled with fluid in a patient with squamous cell carcinoma.

Typical

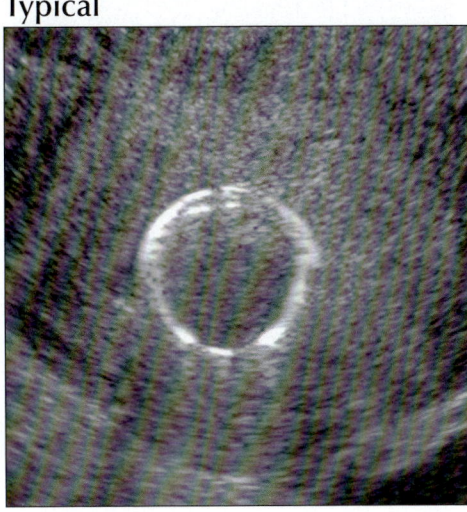
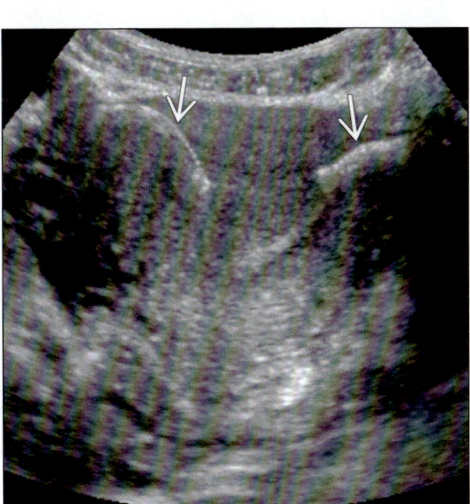

(Left) Coronal transvaginal ultrasound shows a ring-like IUD. This type of IUD is frequently seen in women from China. *(Right)* Coronal shows ESSURE devices ➡ located in the interstitial portions of the tubes. This is a relatively new device for permanent sterilization.

INTRAUTERINE DEVICE EVALUATION

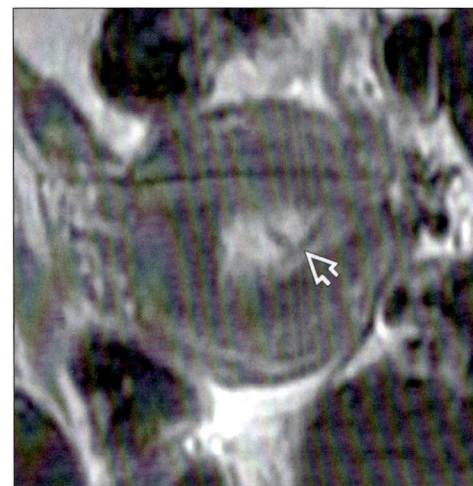 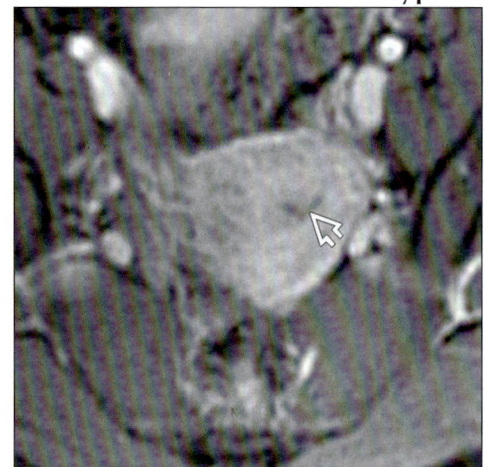

(Left) Coronal oblique T2WI MR shows cross bar of IUD ➡ in the fundal portion of the endometrium. *(Right)* Coronal oblique T1WI FS MR shows cross bar of IUD ➡ in the fundal portion of the endometrium.

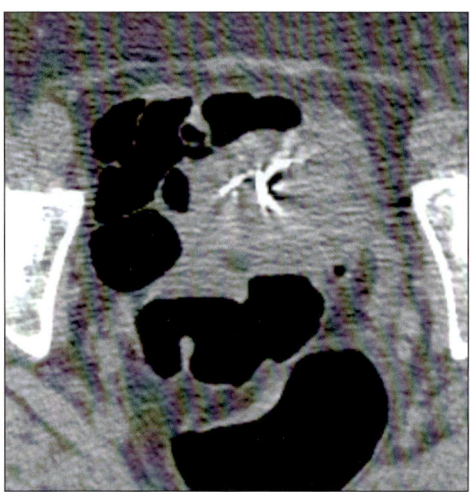 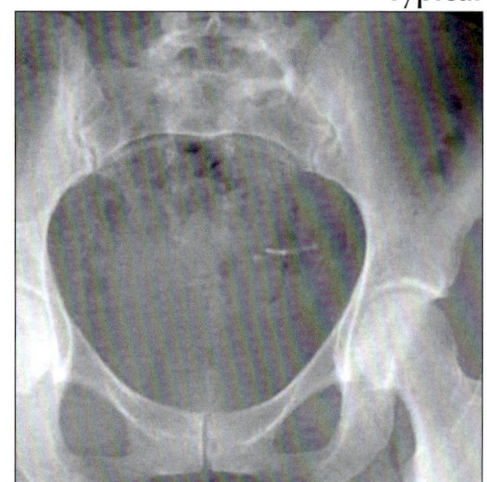

(Left) Axial NECT shows IUD in uterus. *(Right)* Frontal radiograph shows IUD in the left side of the pelvis in a patient with non-visualized IUD on ultrasound.

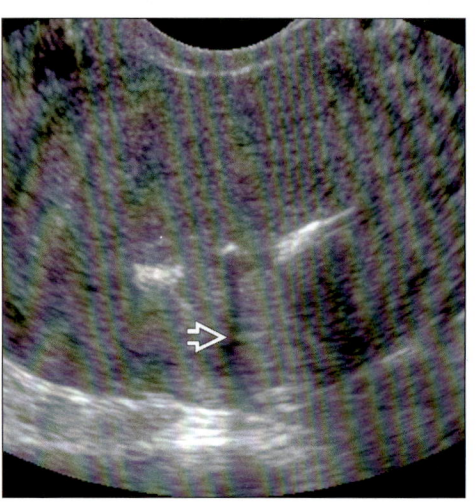 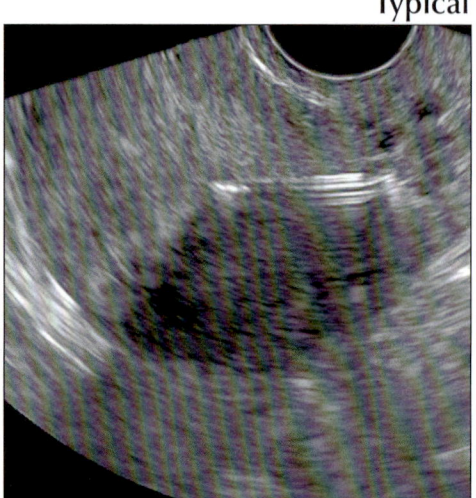

(Left) Axial transvaginal ultrasound shows shadow ➡ behind the shaft of an IUD with cross bars extending laterally in the fundal portion of the endometrium. *(Right)* Sagittal transvaginal ultrasound shows IUD in low position in the uterus.

INTRAUTERINE DEVICE EVALUATION

Typical

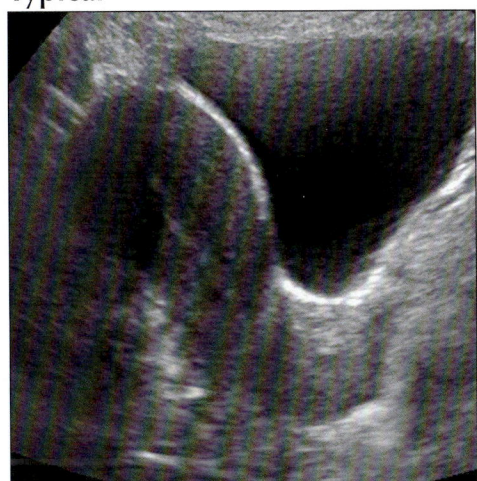
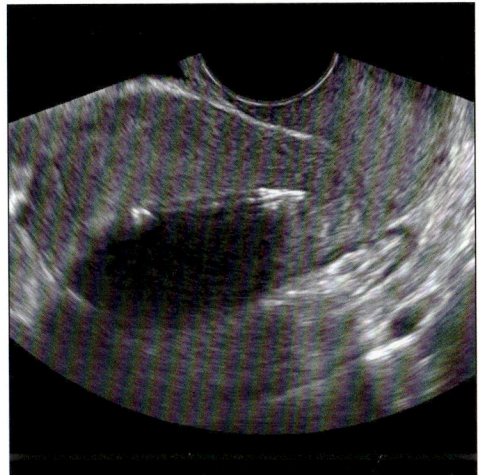

(Left) Sagittal transabdominal ultrasound shows normal appearance to the uterus in a patient with an IUD. Some IUDs are difficult to visualize. *(Right)* Sagittal transvaginal ultrasound in the same patient as previous image, shows the IUD in the endometrial cavity. The entire length of the IUD is not visualized, but the shadow is seen.

Variant

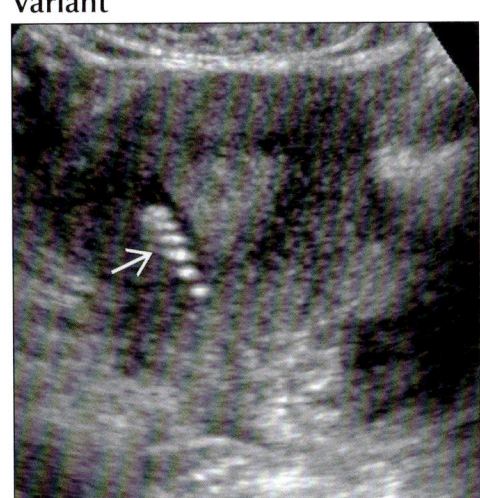
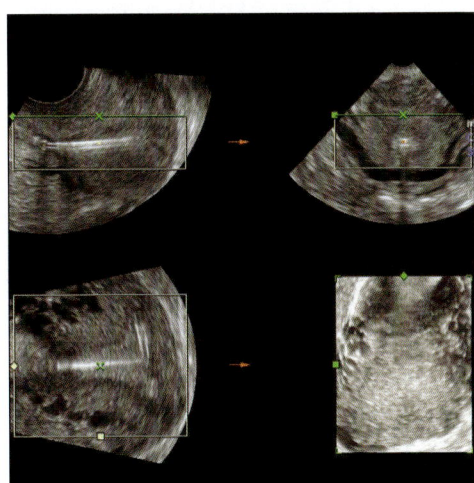

(Left) Coronal oblique transabdominal ultrasound shows fragment of an IUD ➡ embedded in the myometrium. *(Right)* 3D ultrasound shows the method of reconstructing the uterus in a coronal plane to visualize the location of an IUD.

Typical

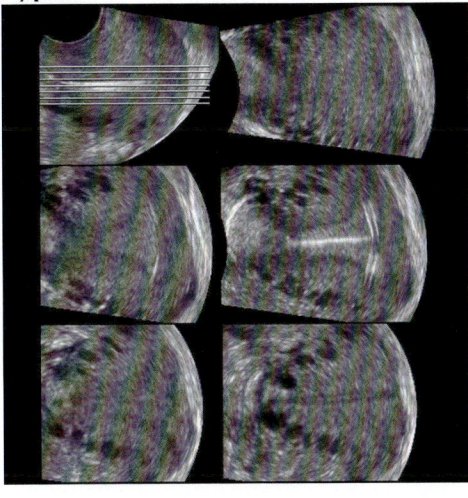
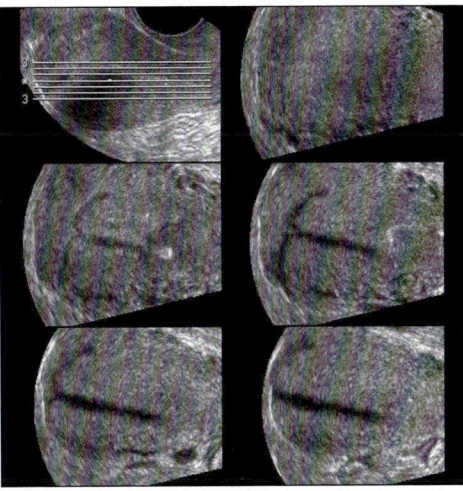

(Left) Coronal transvaginal ultrasound using "tomographic ultrasound" shows an IUD in good position in the endometrial cavity. *(Right)* Coronal oblique transvaginal ultrasound using "tomographic ultrasound" shows reconstructed planes showing the shadow of a difficult to visualize IUD.

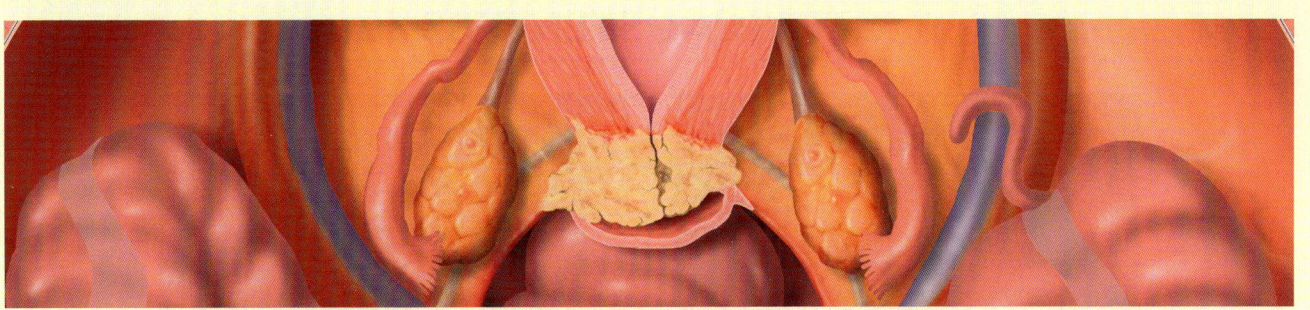

SECTION 3: Uterus-Cervix

Inflammation/Infection

Cervical Stenosis	3-2

Neoplasm, Benign

Endocervical Polyp	3-6
Leiomyoma, Cervix	3-10

Neoplasm, Malignant

Cervical Cancer, Characterization	3-14
Cervical Cancer, Stage IB-IIA	3-20
Cervical Cancer, Stage IIB-IVB	3-22
Cervical Adenocarcinoma	3-26
Small Cell Carcinoma, Cervix	3-30
Cervical Cancer, Recurrence	3-34
Adenoma Malignum	3-38
Lymphoma, Cervix	3-40
Sarcoma, Cervix	3-44
Endometrioid Cervical Adenocarcinoma	3-48
Melanoma, Cervix	3-52
Metastasis, Cervix	3-56

Miscellaneous

Nabothian Cysts	3-60
Cervical Glandular Hyperplasia	3-64
Cervical Incompetence	3-68
Post Trachelectomy Appearances	3-72
Post-Radiation Cervix	3-76

CERVICAL STENOSIS

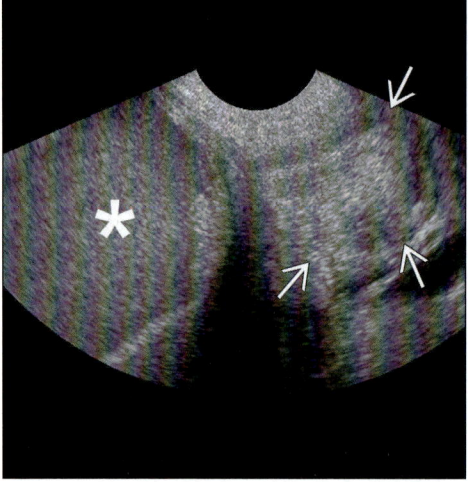

Sagittal transvaginal ultrasound shows a normal-appearing cervix ➔ in a patient with cervical stenosis secondary to endometriosis. Hematometra is present (*) because the stenosis is severe.

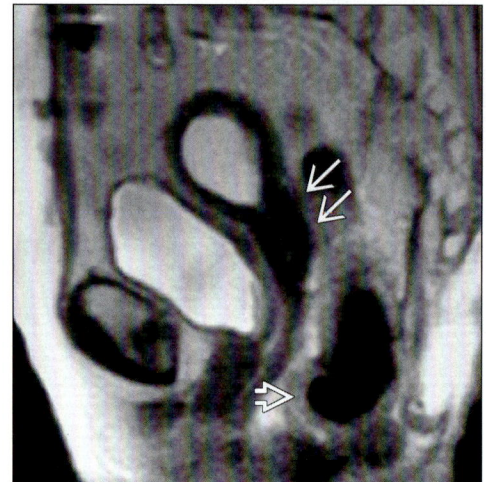

Sagittal T2WI MR shows a dilated endometrial canal and normal cervix ➔ in a patient with cervical stenosis from pelvic radiation for colon cancer. Post-radiation bowel wall thickening is also present ➔.

TERMINOLOGY

Definitions
- Cervical narrowing from an organic or iatrogenic process, when severe, results in hydrometra, pyometra or hematometra
- Recognized common complication following cone biopsy & cervical amputations and has been reported after radical trachelectomy
- Cervical canal narrowing less than 2.5-3 mm
- Defined in the literature as the inability to pass a 2.5-4.5 mm probe through the cervical os

IMAGING FINDINGS

Ultrasonographic Findings
- Transvaginal Ultrasound (TVS) Findings
  - Normal-appearing cervix
  - Uterus may or may not be distended
  - If uterus is distended, may contain
    - Anechoic/hypoechoic fluid: Hydrometra
    - Echogenic fluid: Pyometra and/or hydrometra
  - May present with inability to pass catheter during sonohysterography
  - If hematosalpinges are present, see bilateral dilated adnexal masses with convoluted tubular configuration, separate from the ovaries
    - Dilated tubes contain low level internal echoes compatible with blood

CT Findings
- Normal-appearing cervix & uterus distended with simple fluid or blood
- May see ancillary signs to suggest etiology of cervical stenosis (e.g., thickened bowel associated with radiation therapy)
- May see cystic adnexal masses representing dilated blood-filled fallopian tubes

MR Findings
- T1WI
  - Cervix: Normal morphology & signal intensity (SI) (isointense to myometrium)
  - Uterine corpus: Enlarged; SI of cavity reflects contents
    - Simple fluid: Low SI

DDx: Cervical Stenosis

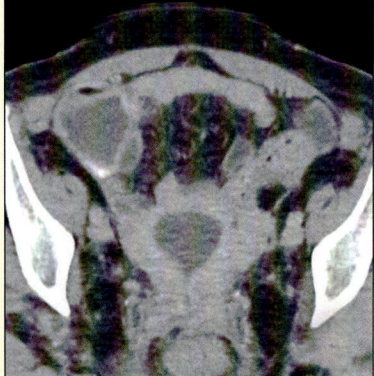
Endometritis

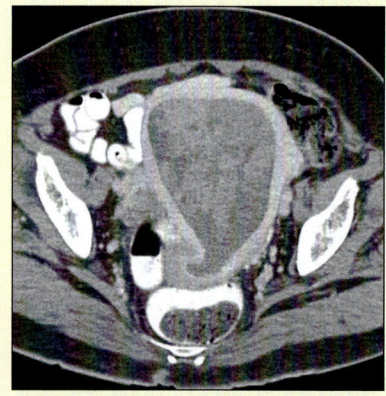
Lower Uterine Segment Cancer

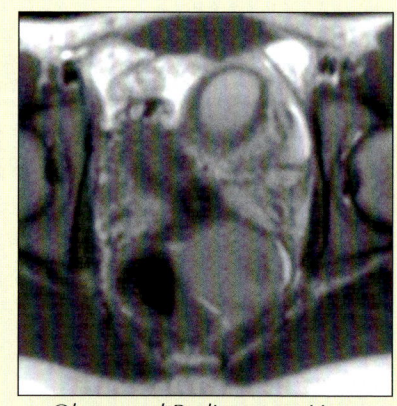
Obstructed Rudimentary Horn

CERVICAL STENOSIS

Key Facts

Terminology
- Cervical narrowing from an organic or iatrogenic process, when severe, results in hydrometra, pyometra or hematometra

Imaging Findings
- Transvaginal sonography is initial modality to evaluate pelvic pathology
- MR or CT for ancillary findings to suggest cervical stenosis etiology

Top Differential Diagnoses
- Obstructed Uterus Secondary to Malignancy
- Obstructed Uterus Secondary to Mass Effect
- Congenital Anomalies

Pathology
- Any process(es) that cause inflammation, erosion, repair & regeneration of cervical mucosa
- Organic causes: Senile atrophy; chronic infection; tumor (there is controversy whether term "cervical stenosis" should be reserved for cases of cervical narrowing that are not the result of mass effect by tumor upon endocervical canal)
- Iatrogenic causes: Radiation therapy; laser or cryosurgery; loop electrocautery excision, cervical endometriosis (most frequently seen after combined cervical conization & endometrial curettage); other types of cervical intervention

Diagnostic Checklist
- Cervix appears normal

- Proteinaceous fluid (which includes blood): Intermediate to high SI
- T2WI
  - Cervix: Loss of normal zonal architecture if cervix has been irradiated or the patient is post menopausal (e.g., atrophy)
  - Uterine corpus: Myometrium & junctional zone may be thinned by distended endometrial canal - fluid may vary in SI depending on type of fluid
    - Simple fluid: High SI
    - Proteinaceous fluid (to include blood): Intermediate to low SI

Imaging Recommendations
- Transvaginal sonography is initial modality to evaluate pelvic pathology
- MR or CT for ancillary findings to suggest cervical stenosis etiology

DIFFERENTIAL DIAGNOSIS

Obstructed Uterus Secondary to Malignancy
- Tumor of lower uterine segment or cervix
- Must always exclude tumor before ascribing cervical stenosis to postmenopausal atrophy or other non-malignant etiologies in cases of a thickened endometrium

Obstructed Uterus Secondary to Mass Effect
- Cervical or submucosal leiomyoma or other pelvic mass causing compression/obstruction of endocervical canal
- Mass effect may be due to inflammation in the lower uterine tract or cervix in the case of infection

Congenital Anomalies
- Includes imperforate hymen, complete transverse vaginal septum, cervical atresia, vaginal atresia
- In the case of uterine duplication anomalies with an obstructed horn, the blood filled horn may be mistaken for the uterus & the other horn missed

- May have associated hematocolpos, hematotrachelos & hematometra
- Kidneys should also be evaluated for associated anomalies

PATHOLOGY

General Features
- General path comments
  - Pathology reflects etiology (e.g., atrophy vs. post-instrumentation)
  - It is believed that the physical action of blood passing through endocervical canal helps prevent obliteration of the canal after cone biopsy, hence stenosis more common in the nonmenstruating patient
  - In postmenopausal patients, atrophy related decrease in endocervical glands results in decreased secretion of mucus which is also thought to help keep canal open (similar mechanism is implicated in endocervical gland removal after cone biopsy or surgery)
  - Stenosis occurs at least partially as a consequence of juxtapositioning & adherence of the exposed stromal surfaces of residual cervix after conization
- Etiology
  - Any process(es) that cause inflammation, erosion, repair & regeneration of cervical mucosa
  - Organic causes: Senile atrophy; chronic infection; tumor (there is controversy whether term "cervical stenosis" should be reserved for cases of cervical narrowing that are not the result of mass effect by tumor upon endocervical canal)
  - In postmenopausal women, cervical stenosis is not uncommon and is usually due to atrophy or uterine leiomyomata
  - Iatrogenic causes: Radiation therapy; laser or cryosurgery; loop electrocautery excision, cervical endometriosis (most frequently seen after combined cervical conization & endometrial curettage); other types of cervical intervention

CERVICAL STENOSIS

- Epidemiology
  - 20% of patients with history of in utero exposure to diethylstilbestrol
  - Endometriosis is diagnosed commonly in women with stenosis & pelvic pain

Microscopic Features
- Inflammation, erosion, repair & regeneration share histologic features
- Collapse & juxtaposition of exposed cervical stroma is at increased risk adhesion; lack of structural integrity is more pronounced as the length of central tissue removed increases

CLINICAL ISSUES

Presentation
- Most common signs/symptoms
  - Dysmenorrhea in up to 50%
  - Menstrual disturbance
  - Cyclical pain if causing hematometra & bilateral hematosalpinx
  - Presents with inability to pass catheter, dilator or probe during sonohysterogram or biopsy
- Other signs/symptoms: Infection due to fluid collection of mucus and/or blood
- Pain & cramping from uterine dilatation
- Pain is usually lower abdominal or pelvic radiating to the lower back
- May present with sense of fullness in pelvis, or with suprapubic palpable tender mass
- Urinary retention & constipation may occur because of compression of the distended uterus
- In women of reproductive age, may have retrograde menses if patent fallopian tubes leading to endometriosis and hemoperitoneum
- May lead to inadequate follow up after surgery resulting in an increased risk of recurrent dysplasia or cancer
- May lead to problems with endometrial sampling in patients with dysfunctional uterine bleeding
- May lead to in vitro fertilization failure
- Precludes most major procedures that the require the use of scopes (> 9 mm) resectoscope
- May lead to uterine infections

Natural History & Prognosis
- If not severe, egress of endometrial fluids is not hampered
- If severe, progressive uterine obstruction with endometrial cavity dilation
- Some cases resolve spontaneously

Treatment
- Dilation & evacuation of dilated endometrial canal
  - Sampling is mandatory in postmenopausal women with thickened peripheral endometrium (controversy exists over the need to always sample peripheral endometrium regardless of thickness)
  - Can be performed with successively larger dilators of with dilation with angioplasty balloon under fluoroscopic guidance
- Catheter placement if long-term drainage is required
- Laminaria tent (seaweed derivative; natural cervical dilator) is inserted into cervix
- Hysteroscopic excision of cervical tissue
- Hysterectomy is considered in following circumstances
  - Interruption of uterine flow with resultant secondary complications from fluid collection
  - Inability to pass an endometrial biopsy catheter to obtain an endometrial sample for cancer screening
  - Inability to assess the endocervix by Papanicolaou smear in patients with a previous history of cervical dysplasia

DIAGNOSTIC CHECKLIST

Image Interpretation Pearls
- Cervix appears normal
- With severe stenosis, endometrial cavity is dilated with marked hydrometra, pyometra or hematometra

SELECTED REFERENCES

1. Di Spiezio Sardo A et al: Use of office hysteroscopy to empty a very large hematometra in a young virgin patient with mosaic Turner's syndrome. Fertil Steril. 87(2):417, 2007
2. Grund D et al: A new approach to preserve fertility by using a coated nitinol stent in a patient with recurrent cervical stenosis. Fertil Steril. 87(5):1212, 2007
3. Hammoud AO et al: Ultrasonography-guided transvaginal endometrial biopsy: a useful technique in patients with cervical stenosis. Obstet Gynecol. 107(2 Pt 2):518-20, 2006
4. Newman C et al: Hysterectomy in women with cervical stenosis. Surgical indications and pathology. J Reprod Med. 48(9):672-6, 2003
5. Houlard S et al: Risk factors for cervical stenosis after laser cone biopsy. Eur J Obstet Gynecol Reprod Biol. 104(2):144-7, 2002
6. Ohara N: Acute onset of hematometra associated with endometritis and cervical stenosis. A case report. Clin Exp Obstet Gynecol. 29(1):23-4, 2002
7. Barbieri RL: Stenosis of the external cervical os: an association with endometriosis in women with chronic pelvic pain. Fertil Steril. 70(3):571-3, 1998
8. Scheerer LJ et al: Transvaginal sonography in the evaluation of hematometra. A report of two cases. J Reprod Med. 41(3):205-6, 1996
9. Zalel Y et al: Clinical significance of endometrial fluid collections in asymptomatic postmenopausal women. J Ultrasound Med. 15(7):513-5, 1996
10. C. Gompel & SG Silverberg (eds): The Cervix. In: Pathology in Gynecology & Obstetrics. Philadelphia, PA: J.B. Lippincott Company. 71-162, 1994
11. Goldstein SR: Postmenopausal endometrial fluid collections revisited: look at the doughnut rather than the hole. Obstet Gynecol. 83(5 Pt 1):738-40, 1994
12. Spitzer M et al: Cervical os obliteration after laser surgery in patients with amenorrhea. Obstet Gynecol. 76(1):97-100, 1990
13. Moncrieff D et al: Cervical stenosis after cone biopsy during post-pregnancy amenorrhoea. Case reports. Br J Obstet Gynaecol. 95(6):628-9, 1988

CERVICAL STENOSIS

IMAGE GALLERY

Typical

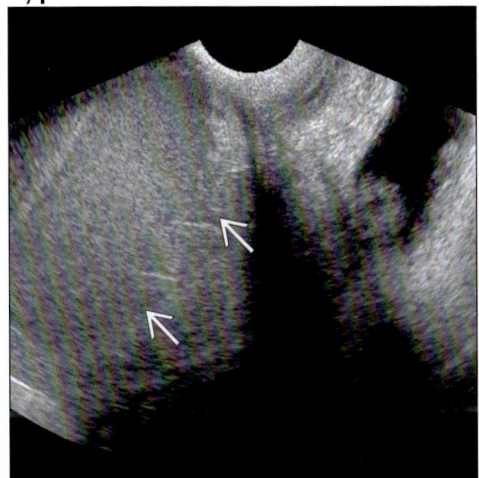 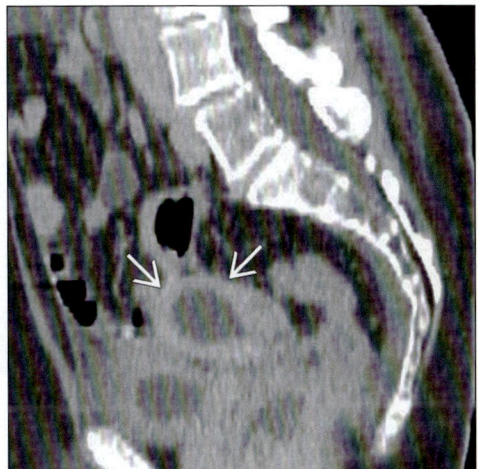

(Left) Sagittal transvaginal ultrasound shows uterus with distended cavity ➔ and normal appearing cervix. This patient presented to the ER with monthly pain corresponding to her menstrual cycle. (Right) Sagittal CECT shows fluid-filled uterus ➔ in a patient with cervical stenosis after radiation for cervical cancer.

Typical

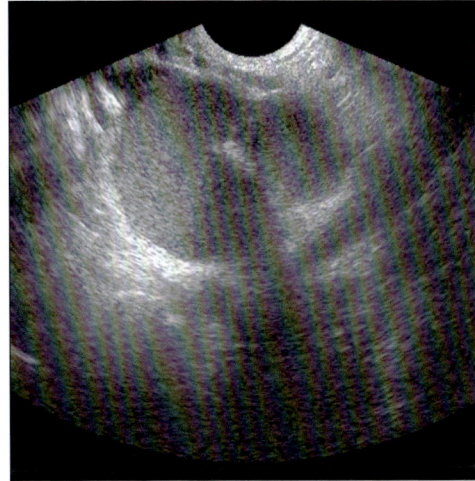 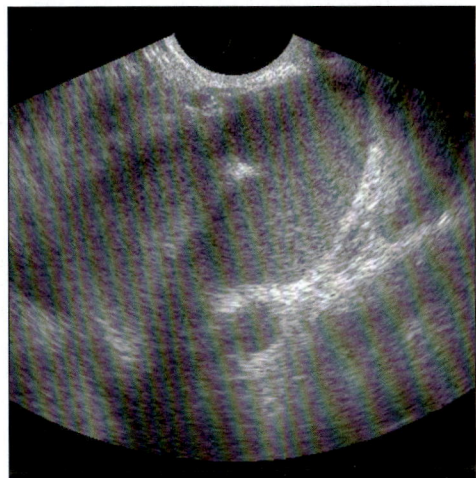

(Left) Coronal transvaginal ultrasound shows dilated tubular adnexal structures in a patient with known cervical stenosis suggestive of hemato or pyosalpinx. (Right) Coronal transvaginal ultrasound in the same patient as previous image, shows similar finding in the contralateral adnexa. The diffuse homogeneous echoes within the dilated fallopian tube represents blood.

Typical

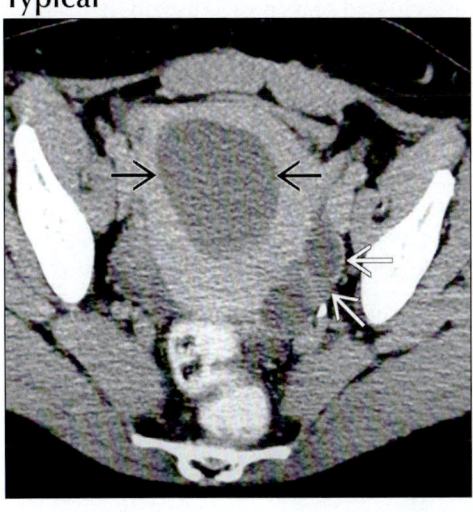 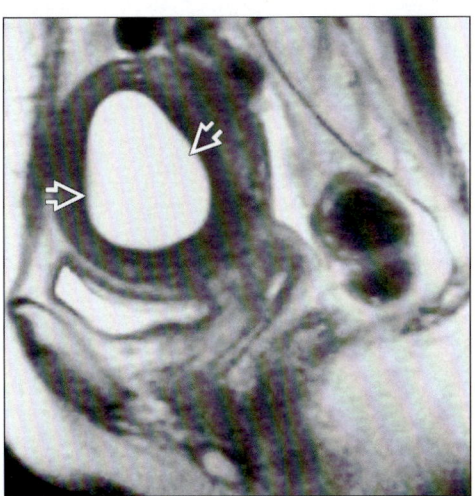

(Left) Axial CECT of the same patient as previous image, shows fluid-filled uterine cavity ➔ and left fallopian tube ➔ compatible with hematometra and hematosalpinx. (Right) Sagittal T2WI MR shows a distended endometrial canal ➔ in a patient with cervical stenosis.

ENDOCERVICAL POLYP

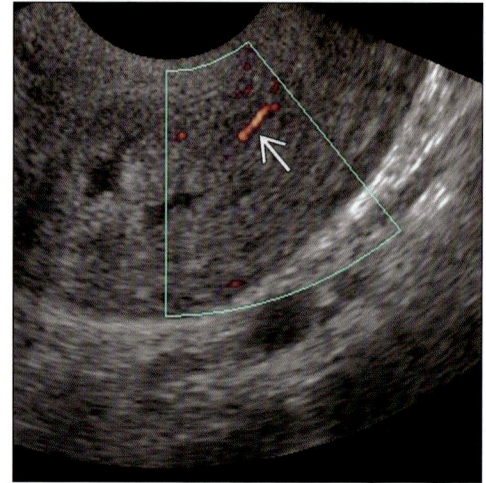

Sagittal transvaginal ultrasound shows endocervical echogenic structure ➡ surrounded by fluid in a postmenopausal patient with a history of spotting.

Axial transvaginal ultrasound through the cervix, utilizing color Doppler imaging, shows a feeding vessel characteristic of a polyp ➡.

TERMINOLOGY

Abbreviations and Synonyms
- Cervical polyp

IMAGING FINDINGS

General Features
- Best diagnostic clue
  - Small pearl-shaped mass
  - Feeding vessel in stalk demonstrated with color flow imaging
- Location: Originates from the cervical canal and may protrude through the external os
- Size
  - Measure between 2-30 mm but can reach larger sizes and protrude beyond the vulva
  - Gigantic polyps are rare
    - No demonstrated correlation with gravidity or age in the eight reported cases
- Morphology: Usually pedunculated

Ultrasonographic Findings
- Grayscale Ultrasound
  - Echogenic mass within endocervical canal
  - Often difficult to detect sonographically because endocervical polyps are indistinguishable from cervical mucus
- Transvaginal ultrasound (TVS)
  - Central feeding vessel in stalk on color flow imaging
  - Well-defined echogenic structure in endocervix
  - May or may not prolapse through external os into vaginal canal
  - May be surrounded by fluid
  - May contain cystic spaces
  - May not be visualized due to coaptation of cervix; applying moderate amount of gel to transducer may be useful as "contrast" agent
- Sonohysterography
  - May be outlined by fluid
  - Smoothly marginated mass projecting off of a stalk

MR Findings
- T1WI: Low-signal intensity fluid within cystic spaces of polyp
- T2WI

DDx: Endocervical Polyp

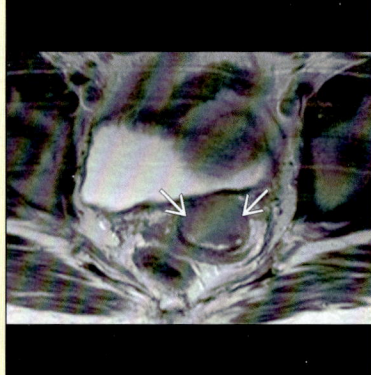
Cervical Carcinoma

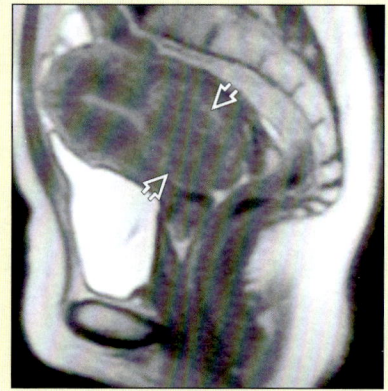
Cervical Leiomyoma

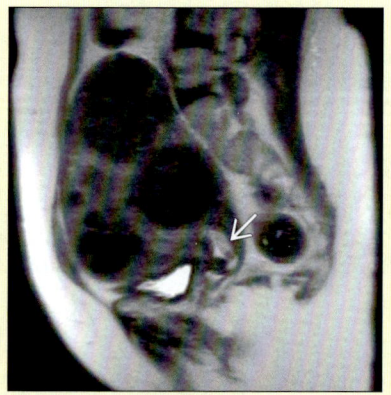
Blood Clot

ENDOCERVICAL POLYP

Key Facts

Imaging Findings
- Small pearl-shaped mass
- Central feeding vessel in stalk on color flow imaging
- Well-defined echogenic structure in endocervix
- May or may not prolapse through external os into vaginal canal
- May be surrounded by fluid
- May contain cystic spaces
- Applying generous amount of gel to transducer may be useful as a "contrast agent"

Pathology
- May be related to tamoxifen use
- Other suggested etiological factors in the development of cervical polyps include
- Chronic cervicitis
- Foreign bodies
- Estrogen secretion

Clinical Issues
- Generally asymptomatic
- 40% are symptomatic, with spotting most common
- One of the most common causes of inter-menstrual vaginal bleeding
- Common cause of postmenopausal bleeding and frequently seen in patients taking tamoxifen
- Atypical hyperplasia and endometrial adenocarcinoma has been found in cervical polyps, usually symptomatic

Diagnostic Checklist
- Must always consider endometrial polyp prolapsing through cervix

---

  - Low-signal intensity endocervical mass surrounded by high-signal intensity fluid, or
  - Large multicystic mass with high-signal intensity fluid, filling endocervical canal
- T1 C+: Brisk enhancement

Imaging Recommendations
- Best imaging tool: TVS
- Protocol advice
  - Use color flow to look for central vessel in stalk
  - Applying generous amount of gel to transducer may be useful as a "contrast agent"

DIFFERENTIAL DIAGNOSIS

Cervical Malignancy
- Cannot differentiate a cervical polyp harboring a non-invasive cancer from a purely benign polyp
- May invade underlying cervical tissue versus a benign polyp without invasion

Cervical Leiomyoma
- 10% of leiomyomas
- Usually grows submucosally or subserosally but may be polypoid

Blood Clot
- No internal vascularity, will not enhance following contrast
- Transvaginal passage of blood clot over short period of time

Endometrial Polyp or Leiomyoma
- Large enough to prolapse through external cervical os
- These tend to be polypoid
- Doppler imaging may be useful to detect and demonstrate feeding vessel and thus the stalk extending through endocervical canal and originating from intrauterine location

Sarcoma Botryoides
- Cervical involvement is exceedingly rare with the majority reported in adolescents

Müllerian Adenosarcoma
- Extremely rare aggressive variant of Müllerian mixed mesodermal tumor of the uterus
- When it presents with sarcomatous overgrowth of the cervix it can present clinically as tissue protruding through the cervical os and mimic a benign cervical polyp

Uterine Epithelioid Endometrial Stromal Sarcoma
- Rare

PATHOLOGY

General Features
- General path comments
  - Focal, hyperplastic protrusions of endocervical folds (epithelium and substantia propria)
  - Develop dysplasia and in situ or invasive carcinoma in < 1%
  - Malignancy usually found incidentally: Must differentiate from polypoid adenocarcinoma and polyp with metastatic adenocarcinoma
- Etiology
  - May be related to tamoxifen use
  - Other suggested etiological factors in the development of cervical polyps include
    - Multiparity
    - Chronic cervicitis
    - Foreign bodies
    - Estrogen secretion
- Epidemiology: Constitute 4-10% of all cervical lesions

Gross Pathologic & Surgical Features
- Usually pedunculated with pedicle of varying length
- May be sessile
- Soft, smooth red or purple, few millimeters to 3 cm

Microscopic Features
- Variety of patterns that are classified according to preponderance of tissue component

ENDOCERVICAL POLYP

- ○ Endocervical mucosal: Most common polyp, comprised of hyperplastic endocervical epithelium
- ○ Fibrous
- ○ Vascular
- ○ Mixed endocervical and endometrial
- ○ Mesodermal stromal
- Cystically dilated glands
- Large number of blood vessels at surface
- Inflammatory infiltrate in 80% of cases
- Appear edematous

CLINICAL ISSUES

Presentation
- Most common signs/symptoms
  - ○ Generally asymptomatic
  - ○ 40% are symptomatic, with spotting most common
- Other signs/symptoms
  - ○ Menometrorrhagia
  - ○ Contact bleeding
  - ○ Vaginal discharge
  - ○ Leukorrhea
  - ○ Can be misdiagnosed in early pregnancy when significant bleeding can lead to misdiagnosis of miscarriage
  - ○ Can grow significantly in pregnancy and even increase massively intrapartum
  - ○ Bleeding in the postpartum period can be a problem due to their vascularity and can be misdiagnosed for retained products
- Clinical Profile
  - ○ One of the most common causes of inter-menstrual vaginal bleeding
    - Common cause of postmenopausal bleeding and frequently seen in patients taking tamoxifen
    - Accounts for 60% of endocervical polypoid lesions
  - ○ Can be seen on speculum examination when protruding through the external os and may even be palpated on vaginal examination

Demographics
- Age: Found in peri-menopausal (4th-5th decades) multiparous women

Natural History & Prognosis
- Excellent, even if polyp harbors a carcinoma that is confined to polyp
  - ○ Carcinomatous changes reported in 1.7% of cervical polyps
- Atypical hyperplasia and endometrial adenocarcinoma has been found in cervical polyps, usually symptomatic

Treatment
- Hysteroscopy and curettage for treatment

DIAGNOSTIC CHECKLIST

Consider
- Must always consider endometrial polyp prolapsing through cervix

Image Interpretation Pearls
- Isoechoic to endometrium with feeding vessel demonstrated on color Doppler imaging
- May contain cysts

SELECTED REFERENCES

1. Goh SG et al: Uterine epithelioid endometrial stromal sarcoma presenting as a "cervical polyp". Ann Diagn Pathol. 9(2):101-5, 2005
2. Robertson M et al: Endocervical polyp in pregnancy: gray scale and color Doppler images and essential considerations in pregnancy. Ultrasound Obstet Gynecol. 26(5):583-4, 2005
3. Bernal KL et al: Embryonal rhabdomyosarcoma (sarcoma botryoides) of the cervix presenting as a cervical polyp treated with fertility-sparing surgery and adjuvant chemotherapy. Gynecol Oncol. 95(1):243-6, 2004
4. Park HM et al: Mullerian adenosarcoma with sarcomatous overgrowth of the cervix presenting as cervical polyp: a case report and review of the literature. Int J Gynecol Cancer. 14(5):1024-9, 2004
5. Tang H et al: An intrapartum giant cervical polyp. N Z Med J. 117(1206):U1181, 2004
6. Okamoto Y et al: MR imaging of the uterine cervix: imaging-pathologic correlation. Radiographics. 23(2):425-45; quiz 534-5, 2003
7. Williams PL et al: US of abnormal uterine bleeding. Radiographics. 23(3):703-18, 2003
8. Nalaboff KM et al: Imaging the endometrium: disease and normal variants. Radiographics. 21(6):1409-24, 2001
9. Al-Mulhim AA et al: Sarcoma botyroides-an unusual case of a cervical polyp. J Obstet Gynaecol. 19(5):555-6, 1999
10. Golan A et al: Cervical polyp: evaluation of current treatment. Gynecol Obstet Invest. 37(1):56-8, 1994
11. Duckman S et al: Giant cervical polyp. Am J Obstet Gynecol. 159(4):852-4, 1988

ENDOCERVICAL POLYP

IMAGE GALLERY

Typical

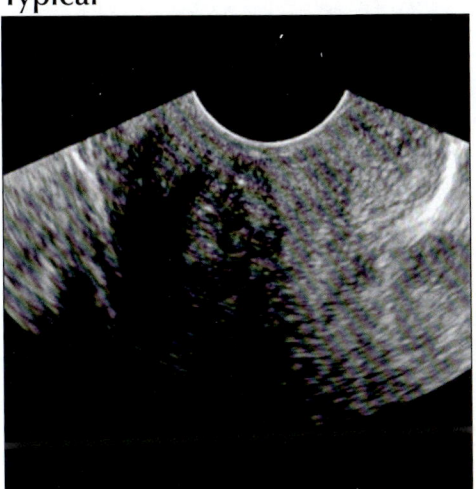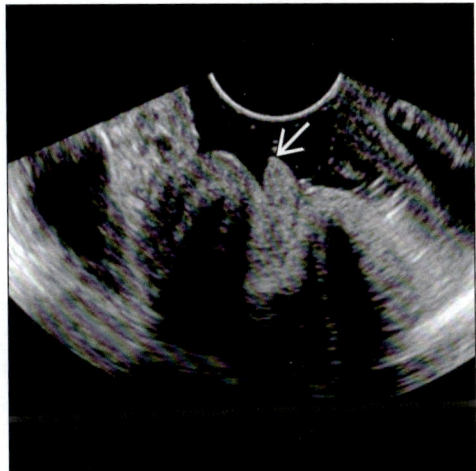

(Left) Sagittal transvaginal ultrasound shows the endocervical polyp, visible on physical examination, is not obvious. *(Right)* Sagittal transvaginal ultrasound during sonohysterography in the same patient as previous image, shows that fluid in the vagina helps delineate the polyp ➡ protruding through the cervical lips.

Typical

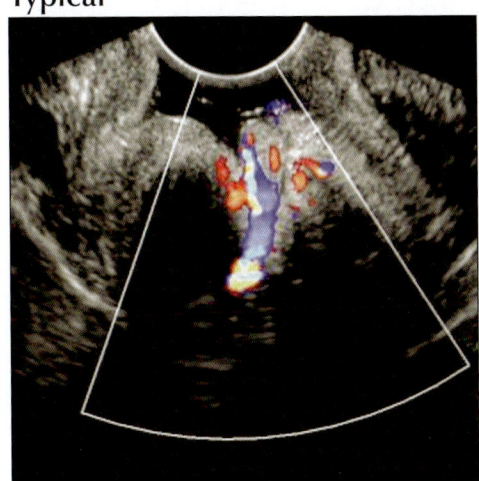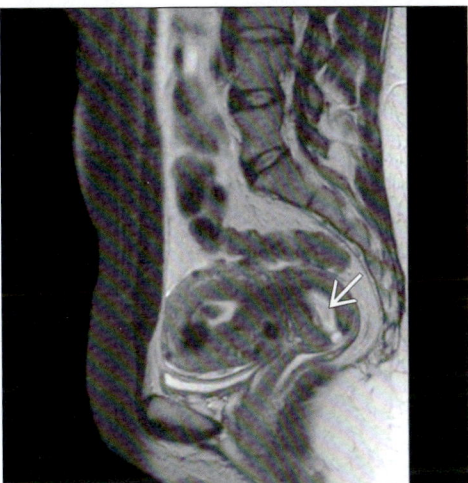

(Left) Sagittal color Doppler ultrasound in the same patient as previous image, shows the feeding vessel and site of attachment. *(Right)* Sagittal T2WI MR shows a subtle lesion ➡ within the endocervical canal.

Typical

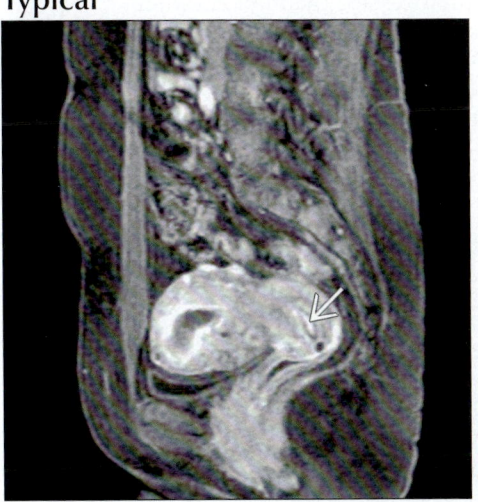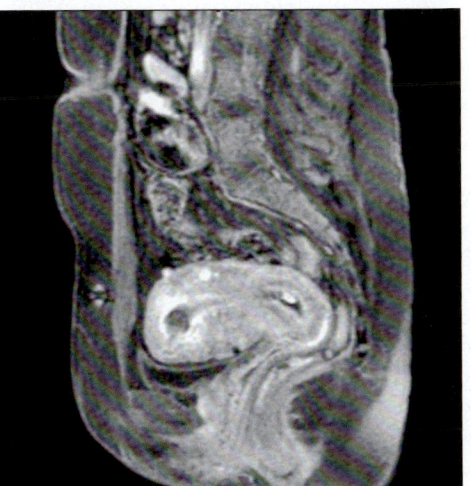

(Left) Sagittal T1 C+ FS MR in the same patient as previous image, shows enhancement of the lesion ➡ compatible with endocervical polyp. *(Right)* Sagittal T1 C+ FS MR in the same patient as previous image, shows the same enhancing structure within the endocervical canal. No intrauterine extension is seen.

LEIOMYOMA, CERVIX

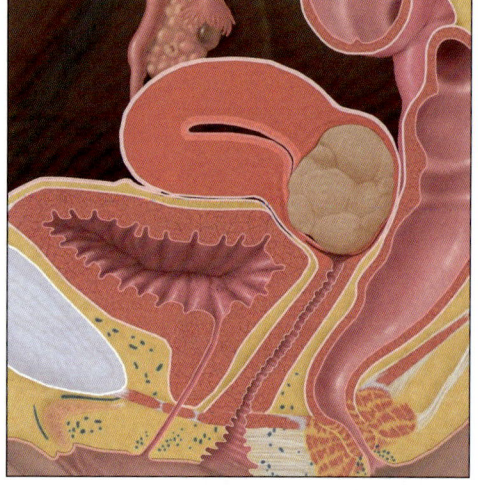

Sagittal graphic shows well-defined lobulated mass arising from posterior cervix causing mass effect on endocervical canal.

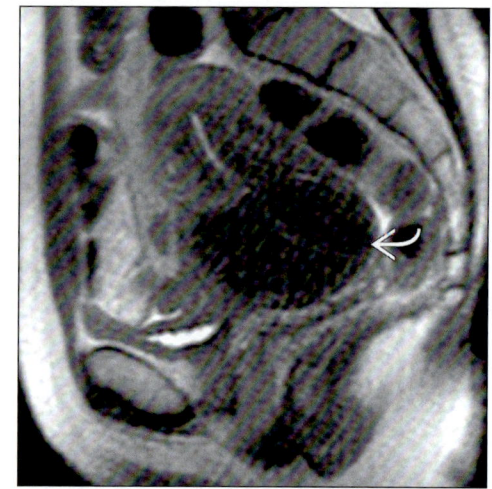

Sagittal T2WI MR shows a rounded, homogeneous, low signal intensity mass expanding the cervix ⮞. Normal cervical zonal anatomy is not discretely identified.

TERMINOLOGY

Abbreviations and Synonyms
- Cervical fibroid, fibroleiomyoma, myoma

Definitions
- Benign smooth muscle tumor of cervix

IMAGING FINDINGS

General Features
- Best diagnostic clue: Homogeneous, round, well-defined cervical mass
- Location
  - Arises within or from cervix
  - May be submucosal, intramural or subserosal
  - When large, submucosal and pedunculated, may prolapse into vagina or into uterine cavity
- Rarely, cervical canal may be "folded" into leiomyoma

Radiographic Findings
- Radiography: Coarse calcifications visible if degenerated

Ultrasonographic Findings
- Transvaginal ultrasound (TVS) findings
  - Homogeneous hypoechoic mass if not degenerated
  - May or may not cause posterior attenuation of sound
  - Heterogeneous with or without calcification if degenerated
  - Relatively avascular on Doppler or color flow US
  - Color Doppler demonstrates the "draping vessel" pattern with vessels surrounding and penetrating leiomyoma and relative lack of central vascularity
  - Feeding vessel can be traced to cervix when pedunculated

CT Findings
- NECT: Homogeneous attenuation similar to myometrium
- CECT
  - Initially enhances less than myometrium
  - May be isodense to myometrium on delayed images
- May see calcifications and/or cystic necrosis if degenerated

DDx: Cervical Leiomyoma

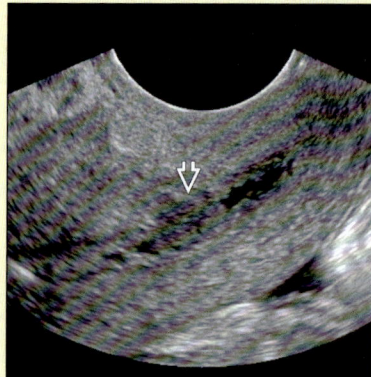

Endocervical Polyp

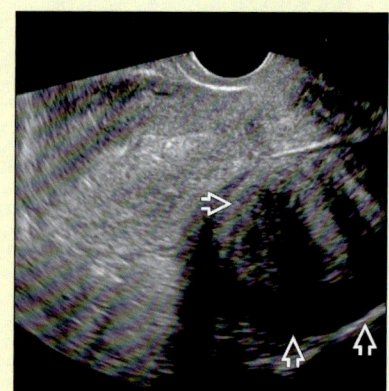

Uterine Subserosal Leiomyoma

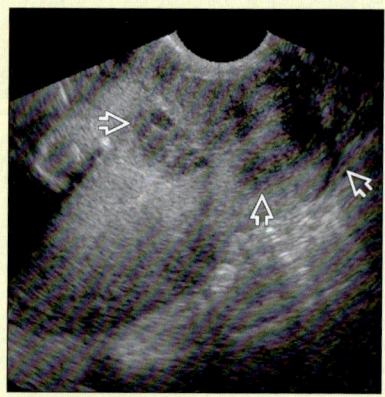

Cervical Cancer

LEIOMYOMA, CERVIX

Key Facts

Terminology
- Cervical fibroid, fibroleiomyoma, myoma
- Benign smooth muscle tumor of cervix

Imaging Findings
- Best diagnostic clue: Homogeneous, round, well-defined cervical mass
- Ultrasound is primary modality to diagnose & evaluate
- May miss cervical leiomyoma if US transducer is positioned too far anteriorly

Top Differential Diagnoses
- Malignant Cervical Neoplasms
- Endocervical Polyp
- Pedunculated Uterine Leiomyoma

Pathology
- Leiomyomas: Most common uterine neoplasm
- Cervical leiomyomas are uncommon: 8-10% of all leiomyomas
- Estrogen stimulates, often increase in size during pregnancy and with birth control pills
- Progesterone inhibits, often decrease in size with menopause

Clinical Issues
- Most leiomyomas are asymptomatic
- Often degenerated if > 5-8 cm (carneous, hyaline, fatty, cystic, calcific)
- Debilitating leiomyomas account for 1/3-1/2 of hysterectomies
- Imaging helpful to direct therapy (hysterectomy vs. uterine-sparing treatments)

MR Findings
- T1WI: Hypo- or isointense to smooth muscle (unless degenerated)
- T1WI FS: Isointense; hyperintense if hemorrhagic degeneration
- T2WI
  - Homogeneous & hypointense to cervical smooth muscle
    - Degenerated: Heterogeneous with high signal intensity (SI) areas
    - Pseudocapsule of compressed normal smooth muscle
    - Hyperintense rim of edema and dilated lymphatics & veins
    - If cellular histology may have high SI
- T1 C+
  - Most leiomyomas enhance less than smooth muscle
    - Degenerated areas may not enhance

Other Modality Findings
- Hysterosalpingogram: No findings unless there is mass effect on endocervical canal

Imaging Recommendations
- Ultrasound is primary modality to diagnose & evaluate
- May miss cervical leiomyoma if US transducer is positioned too far anteriorly
- MR reserved for equivocal or non-diagnostic cases
  - Establish diagnosis, size, number & location of leiomyoma
  - Help select patients for invasive treatment
  - Used for monitoring

DIFFERENTIAL DIAGNOSIS

Malignant Cervical Neoplasms
- Irregular morphology and not well-demarcated, especially if invasive
- May see extension beyond confines of cervix into lower uterine segment, bladder or rectum
- Heterogeneous echogenicity or signal intensity
- Increased vascularity centrally

Endocervical Polyp
- Protrude into endocervical canal & may mimic pedunculated, submucosal, cervical leiomyoma
- Usually isoechoic to endometrium
- Often have cystic spaces, must be differentiated from cervical leiomyoma with cystic degeneration
- May see feeding vessel

Pedunculated Uterine Leiomyoma
- If subserosal, may extend posterior to cervix
- If submucosal, may prolapse into endocervical canal
- Evaluation of vascular supply or identification of stalk/pedicle may help determine origin

PATHOLOGY

General Features
- General path comments
  - Leiomyomas: Most common uterine neoplasm
  - Cervical leiomyomas are uncommon: 8-10% of all leiomyomas
  - Well-defined, pseudoencapsulated mass of cervix
  - Grossly and histologically identical to those found in uterine corpus
  - Hormonally responsive
    - Estrogen stimulates, often increase in size during pregnancy and with birth control pills
    - Progesterone inhibits, often decrease in size with menopause
- Genetics: No hereditary factor clearly identified
- Etiology
  - Etiology unclear
  - Sex steroid hormones influence growth
    - Estrogen stimulates; progesterone inhibits
- Epidemiology
  - Cervical leiomyomas comprise up to 10% of all leiomyomas
  - Increased incidence in African-Americans
  - Incidence between 0.6% and 2%

LEIOMYOMA, CERVIX

Gross Pathologic & Surgical Features
- Spherical, firm, white and elastic in consistency
- Whorled bundles of smooth muscle separated by connective tissue stroma

Microscopic Features
- Uniform, anastomosed & whorled smooth muscle cells
- Variable amounts of fibrous connective tissue & small, rare blood vessels

Staging, Grading or Classification Criteria
- Leiomyomas are classified according to location

CLINICAL ISSUES

Presentation
- Most common signs/symptoms
  - Most leiomyomas are asymptomatic
  - When symptomatic, 4 major types of symptoms
    - Bleeding
    - Pressure on adjacent organs
    - Pain
    - Infertility
  - Cervical leiomyomas associated with habitual abortion
  - Rare complications
    - Torsion
    - Infection
    - Malignant degeneration
  - Often degenerated if > 5-8 cm (carneous, hyaline, fatty, cystic, calcific)
  - Debilitating leiomyomas account for 1/3-1/2 of hysterectomies
  - Imaging helpful to direct therapy (hysterectomy vs. uterine-sparing treatments)
- In pregnant patients, may cause
  - Spontaneous abortion
  - Premature labor
  - Obstructed labor necessitating cesarean section
- Meno- and/or metrorrhagia
- Anemia
- Pain
- Pelvic mass
- If exerting enough mass effect on lower uterine segment, may cause obstruction with resulting hematometra or hydrometra

Natural History & Prognosis
- Hormonally responsive
  - Grow during reproductive years, especially pregnancy
  - Shrink with menopause or induced hypoestrogenic state
  - Rapid unexpected growth may indicate malignant transformation
  - Otherwise, excessive growth is uncommon
- Good, most women are asymptomatic
- If symptomatic, most women benefit from treatment

Treatment
- Definitive: Hysterectomy
- Uterine sparing alternatives
  - Medical therapy: Gonadotropin-releasing hormone analog
    - Regrowth after cessation of treatment
  - Myomectomy: Up to 15% may recur
    - Increased surgical difficulty because of proximity to bladder & relative inaccessibility
  - Uterine artery embolization: Cervical leiomyomas tend to be refractory

DIAGNOSTIC CHECKLIST

Consider
- Mass arising from bladder, rectum or lower uterine segment

Image Interpretation Pearls
- Should search for point of origin to establish whether cervical or uterine
- Doppler may assist with search for vascular supply

SELECTED REFERENCES
1. Suneja A et al: Incarcerated procedentia due to cervical fibroid: an unusual presentation. Aus New Zeal J Obstet Gyn. 43:252-3, 2003
2. Varras M et al: Clinical considerations and sonographic findings of a large nonpedunculated primary cervical leiomyoma complicated by heavy vaginal hemorrhage: a case report and review of the literature. Clin Exp Obst Gyn. 30 (2-3):144-6, 2003
3. Bajo J et al: Contribution of transvaginal sonography to the evaluation of benign cervical conditions. J Clin Ultrasound. 27:61-4, 1999
4. Murase E et al: Uterine leiomyomas: histopathologic features, MR imaging findings, differential diagnosis and treatment. Radiographics. 19:1179-97, 1999
5. Tiltman AJ: Leiomyomas of the uterine cervix: a study of frequency. In J Gyn Path. 17:231-4, 1998
6. Mayer DP et al: Ultrasonography and magnetic resonance imaging of uterine fibroids. Obstetrics and Gynecology Clinics of North America. 22:667-725, 1995
7. Ascher SM et al: Benign myometrial conditions: leiomyomas and adenomyosis. TMRI. (In press)

LEIOMYOMA, CERVIX

IMAGE GALLERY

Typical

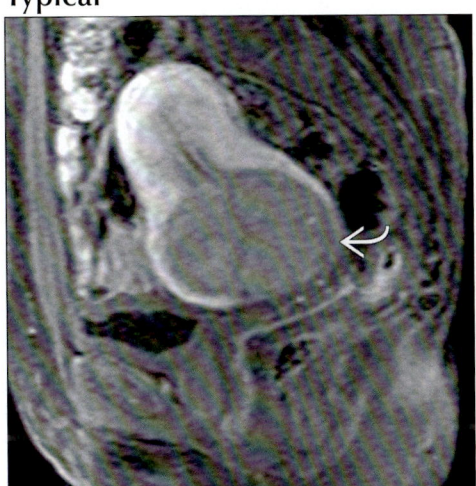
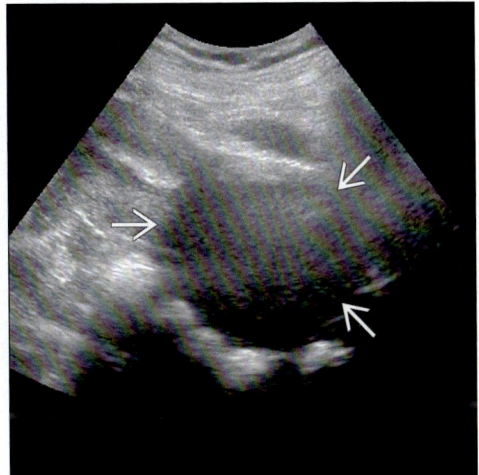

(Left) Sagittal T1 C+ FS MR in the same patient as previous images shows homogeneous enhancement of the cervical leiomyoma ➡. The leiomyoma enhances less than the myometrium. *(Right)* Sagittal transabdominal ultrasound shows a hypoechoic, large mass ➡ that appears to arise from the cervix. A transvaginal study could be performed to confirm origin.

Typical

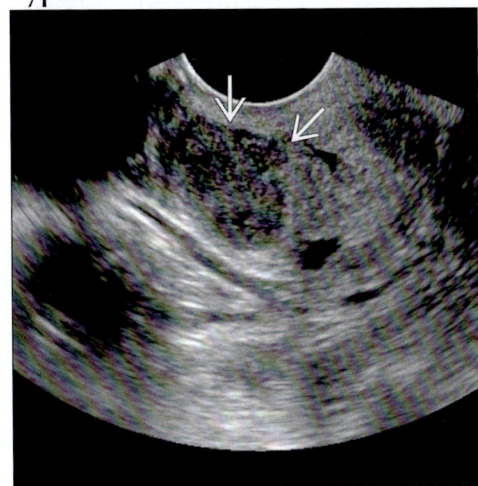
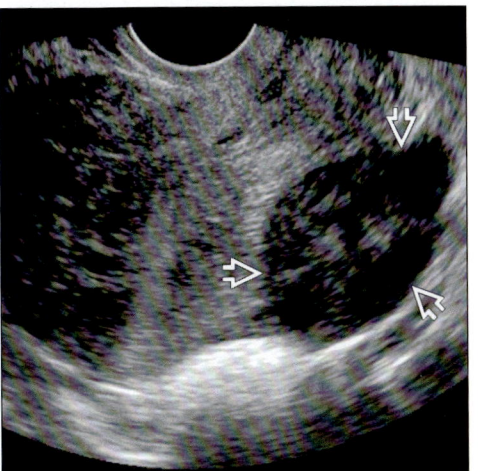

(Left) Transverse transvaginal ultrasound shows intramural, well-defined, hypoechoic mass ➡ in cervix. Enhanced sound through transmission suggested a cystic nature however biopsy confirmed diagnosis of leiomyoma. *(Right)* Sagittal transvaginal ultrasound shows well-defined hypoechoic mass ➡ posterior to the cervix. Color Doppler sonography demonstrated cervical origin of blood supply and not uterine.

Typical

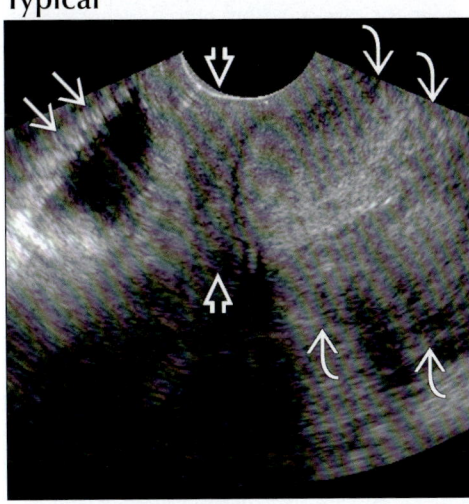
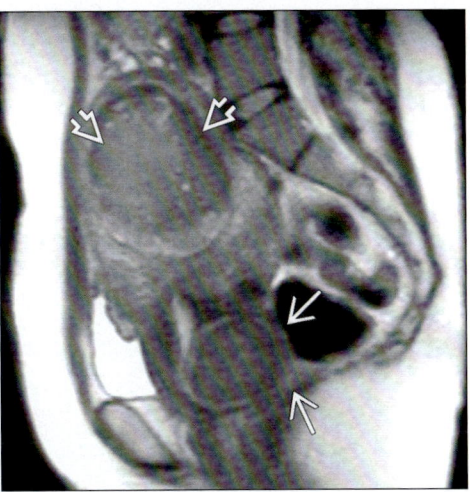

(Left) Sagittal transvaginal ultrasound shows cervix ➡ sandwiched between bladder ➡ and large subserosal leiomyoma ➡. *(Right)* Sagittal T2WI MR shows large, low-signal intensity, posterior cervical leiomyoma ➡ that causes mass effect upon endocervical canal and sigmoid colon. Note the uterine corpus intramural leiomyoma ➡.

CERVICAL CANCER, CHARACTERIZATION

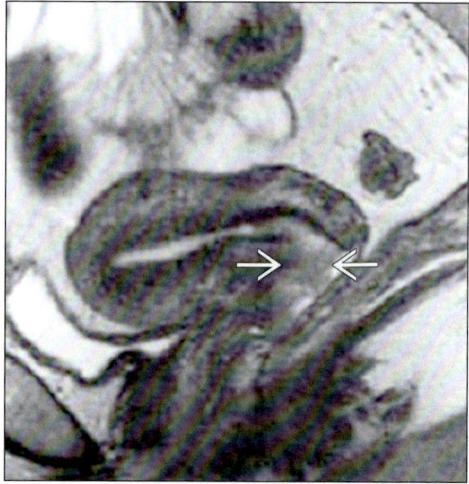

Sagittal T2WI MR shows high signal intensity mass ➡ in the cervix.

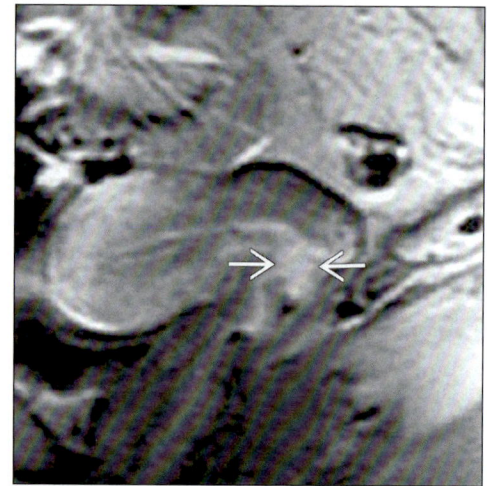

Sagittal T1 C+ FS MR shows prominent enhancement ➡ of the mass during early phase of dynamic contrast-enhanced study.

TERMINOLOGY

Abbreviations and Synonyms
- Carcinoma of cervix

Definitions
- Primary malignant tumor of uterine cervix

IMAGING FINDINGS

General Features
- Best diagnostic clue: Solid mass arising from uterine cervix
- Location
  - Cervical cancer originates from endocervical canal and invades the cervical stroma
  - In advanced cases uterus, vagina and/or adjacent organs may be involved
- Size
  - Many cases are diagnosed when the tumor is small
  - However, advanced cases may present as bulky masses

Ultrasonographic Findings
- Transvaginal ultrasound (TVS) findings
  - Cervical cancer appears as a hypoechoic mass on US
  - Transvaginal US can be used in the assessment of local extent of disease but is inadequate for detection of pelvic sidewall involvement and lymph node metastases

CT Findings
- NECT: Cervical cancer is of iso-attenuation relative to cervical stroma
- CECT: Usually iso- or hypoattenuation relative to cervical stroma

MR Findings
- T1WI: Cervical cancer is iso-intense to cervical stroma
- T2WI
  - T2WI is the most useful sequence in tumor depiction and staging
  - Cervical cancer appears as a high signal intensity mass within low signal intensity cervical stroma
    - In cervical cancers confined to the stroma, the low signal intensity stromal ring surrounding the high signal intensity tumor is completely intact

DDx: Cervical Masses

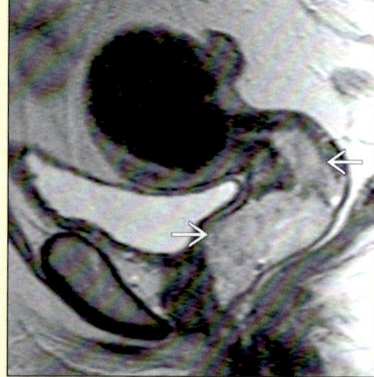

Benign Cervical Polyp

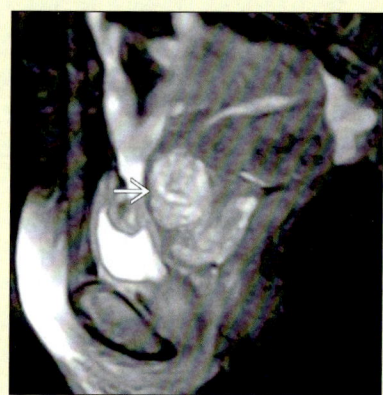

Adenoma Malignum

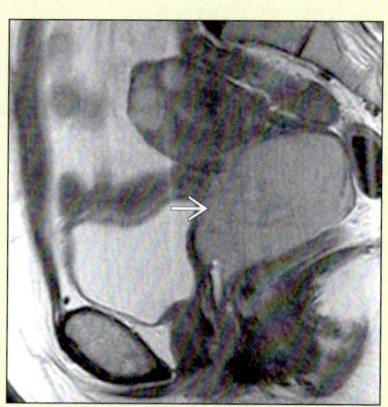

Cervical Lymphoma

CERVICAL CANCER, CHARACTERIZATION

Key Facts

Imaging Findings
- Best diagnostic clue: Solid mass arising from uterine cervix
- T2WI is the most useful sequence in tumor depiction and staging
- Cervical cancer appears as a high signal intensity mass within low signal intensity cervical stroma
- In cervical cancers confined to the stroma, the low signal intensity stromal ring surrounding the high signal intensity tumor is completely intact
- In the case of full thickness stromal invasion, the low signal intensity stroma is completely replaced by high signal intensity tumor; and a smooth tumor-parametrial interface excludes parametrial invasion
- Disruption of the stromal ring with nodular or irregular tumor signal intensity extending into the parametrium indicates parametrial invasion

Top Differential Diagnoses
- Nabothian Cysts
- Benign Cervical Polyp
- Adenoma Malignum
- Cervical Lymphoma or Metastasis

Clinical Issues
- Most important prognostic factors are:
- Histologic grade of tumor
- Tumor volume
- Depth of stromal invasion
- Adjacent organ invasion
- Lymph node involvement

  - In the case of full thickness stromal invasion, the low signal intensity stroma is completely replaced by high signal intensity tumor; and a smooth tumor-parametrial interface excludes parametrial invasion
  - Disruption of the stromal ring with nodular or irregular tumor signal intensity extending into the parametrium indicates parametrial invasion
- T1 C+
  - Cervical cancer demonstrates variable contrast-enhancement
  - Use of contrast may help detection of adjacent organ or pelvic wall invasion

Nuclear Medicine Findings
- PET
  - Can be used as an effective adjunct to CT and MR imaging in the evaluation of
    - Lymph node involvement
    - Detecting distant metastases
    - Evaluating treatment response

Imaging Recommendations
- Best imaging tool
  - Role of imaging is to define local staging in tumors > 2 cm in size
  - MR imaging is the method of choice for tumor staging and treatment planning
  - CT is mainly used in the detection of lymphadenopathy and the detection of advanced disease (such as distant metastasis), and for guiding percutaneous biopsies and planning radiation treatment
- Protocol advice
  - MR imaging protocol should include
    - T1WI; axial, large FOV including entire pelvis
    - T2WI; axial, coronal and sagittal small FOV
    - Dynamic CEMR; optional, used not for staging but for demonstrating adjacent organ invasion or fistulas

DIFFERENTIAL DIAGNOSIS

Nabothian Cysts
- Superficial epithelial cysts of variable sizes
- Nabothian cysts do not enhance

Benign Cervical Polyp
- Benign cervical polyp does not invade the stroma
- Imaging can not differentiate a benign cervical polyp from cervical cancer not invading the stroma

Adenoma Malignum
- Enlarged cervix with multiple grape-like cysts within the cervical stroma

Cervical Lymphoma or Metastasis
- Involves cervical stroma diffusely and cervical canal is intact

PATHOLOGY

General Features
- General path comments
  - Cervical cancer arises from squamocolumnar junction
    - Squamocolumnar junction is exophytic in young women and is located in endocervical canal in older women
  - Most common histologic types
    - Squamous cell carcinoma (80-90%)
    - Adenocarcinoma (worse prognosis)
- Etiology
  - Cervical intraepithelial neoplasia (CIN) is considered a precursor lesion of cervical cancer
  - Risk factors for developing cervical cancer include
    - Infection with certain types of human papilloma virus (HPV)
    - Early age at first sexual intercourse
    - Multiple sexual partners
    - Multiparity
    - History of sexually transmitted diseases
    - Low socioeconomic status

CERVICAL CANCER, CHARACTERIZATION

- Epidemiology
  - 3rd most common gynecologic malignancy
  - More frequent in young women with low socioeconomic status

Staging, Grading or Classification Criteria

- FIGO staging system
  - 0: Carcinoma in situ
  - I: Confined to cervix
    - IA: Microscopic
    - IB: Clinically visible (> 5 mm depth, > 7 mm width)
  - II: Extension beyond uterus but not reaching lateral pelvic wall
    - IIA: Extension up to upper 2/3 of vagina
    - IIB: Parametrial invasion
  - III: Extension to lower 1/3 of vagina or pelvic wall invasion
    - IIIA: Extension to lower 1/3 of vagina
    - IIIB: Pelvic wall invasion and/or hydronephrosis
  - IV: Located outside true pelvis or bladder and/or rectal invasion
    - IVA: Bladder or rectal mucosa
    - IVB: Distant metastasis

CLINICAL ISSUES

Presentation

- Most common signs/symptoms
  - Abnormal vaginal bleeding
  - Vaginal discharge
  - Pelvic pain
  - Urinary symptoms
- Other signs/symptoms: Carcinoma in situ is usually asymptomatic and discovered by abnormal Pap smear

Natural History & Prognosis

- Most important prognostic factors are:
  - Histologic grade of tumor
  - Tumor volume
  - Depth of stromal invasion
  - Adjacent organ invasion
  - Lymph node involvement
- 5 yr survival rates: 80-90% for stage I, 50-65% for stage II, 25-35% for stage III, and 0-15% for stage IV

Treatment

- Pre-invasive lesions (i.e., lesions that have not yet transgressed the basement membrane) can be treated with electrocoagulation, cryotherapy, laser ablation or local surgery
- Invasive cervical cancers are treated with surgery, radiation, or chemotherapy, or a combination of these three methods depending on tumor stage

DIAGNOSTIC CHECKLIST

Consider

- Modern cross-sectional imaging has not been incorporated into the official FIGO guidelines for routine pretreatment diagnostic evaluation of cervical cancer
- However, there is evidence that cross-sectional imaging is superior to clinical staging
- Tumor size, parametrial invasion, and lymph node status, which are all critical prognostic factors in staging and treatment planning, are well-evaluated with CT and MR imaging
- Therefore, extended clinical staging incorporating findings from CT and/or MR imaging has become common practice

Image Interpretation Pearls

- Most important issue in the staging of cervical cancer is to distinguish early disease that can be treated with surgery from advanced disease that must be treated with radiation, alone or combined with chemotherapy

SELECTED REFERENCES

1. Akin O et al: Imaging of uterine cancer. Radiol Clin North Am. 45(1):167-82, 2007
2. Choi HJ et al: Comparison of the accuracy of magnetic resonance imaging and positron emission tomography/computed tomography in the presurgical detection of lymph node metastases in patients with uterine cervical carcinoma: a prospective study. Cancer. 106(4):914-22, 2006
3. Engin G: Cervical cancer: MR imaging findings before, during, and after radiation therapy. Eur Radiol. 16(2):313-24, 2006
4. Moore DH: Cervical cancer. Obstet Gynecol. 107(5):1152-61, 2006
5. Yen TC et al: Positron emission tomography in gynecologic cancer. Semin Nucl Med. 36(1):93-104, 2006
6. Amendola MA et al: Utilization of diagnostic studies in the pretreatment evaluation of invasive cervical cancer in the United States: results of intergroup protocol ACRIN 6651/GOG 183. J Clin Oncol. 23(30):7454-9, 2005
7. Hricak H et al: Role of imaging in pretreatment evaluation of early invasive cervical cancer: results of the intergroup study American College of Radiology Imaging Network 6651-Gynecologic Oncology Group 183. J Clin Oncol. 23(36):9329-37, 2005
8. Macapinlac HA: FDG-PET in the evaluation of cervical cancer. Gynecol Oncol. 99(3 Suppl 1):S171-2, 2005
9. Ozsarlak O et al: The correlation of preoperative CT, MR imaging, and clinical staging (FIGO) with histopathology findings in primary cervical carcinoma. Eur Radiol. 13(10):2338-45, 2003
10. Pecorelli S et al: Cervical cancer staging. Cancer J. 9(5):390-4, 2003
11. Scheidler J et al: Imaging of cancer of the cervix. Radiol Clin North Am. 40(3):577-90, vii, 2002
12. Sheu MH et al: Preoperative staging of cervical carcinoma with MR imaging: a reappraisal of diagnostic accuracy and pitfalls. Eur Radiol. 11(9):1828-33, 2001
13. Nicolet V et al: MR imaging of cervical carcinoma: a practical staging approach. Radiographics. 20(6):1539-49, 2000
14. Stehman FB et al: Uterine cervix. In: Hoskins WJ, Perez CA, Young RC (eds). Principles and practice of gynecologic oncology, Lippincott Williams & Wilkins, Philadelphia. 841-918, 2000

CERVICAL CANCER, CHARACTERIZATION

IMAGE GALLERY

Typical

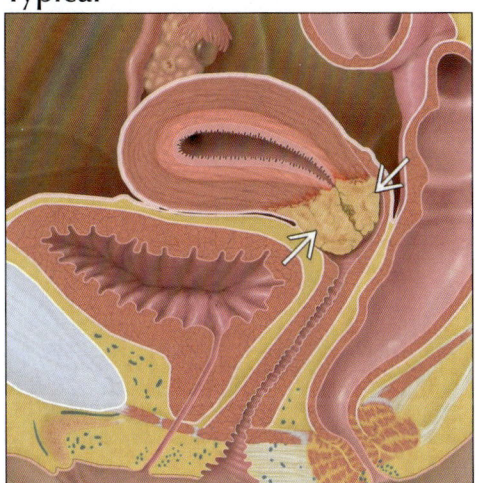
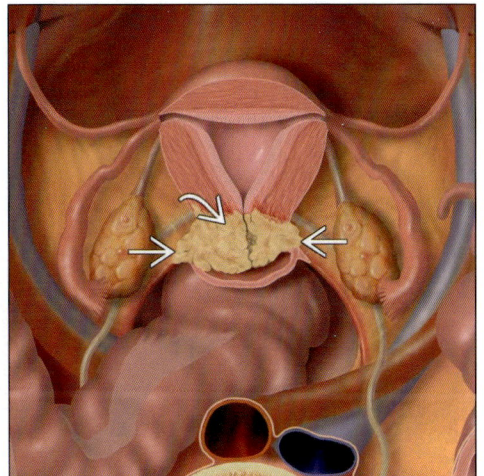

(Left) Graphic shows cervical cancer seen as a mass lesion ➡ in the cervix. There is full thickness cervical stromal invasion. *(Right)* Graphic shows cervical cancer ➡ with bilateral parametrial invasion ➡. Note that the mass extends beyond confines of the cervical stroma on both sides.

Typical

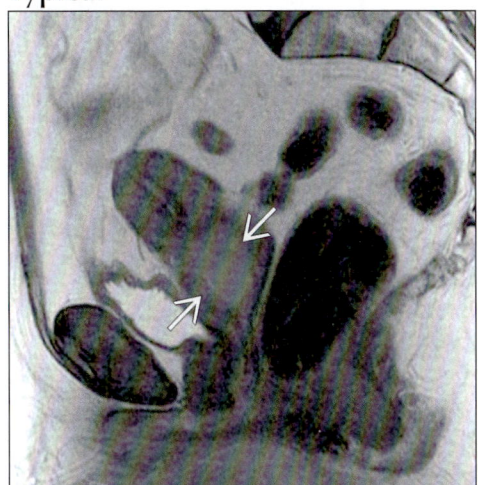
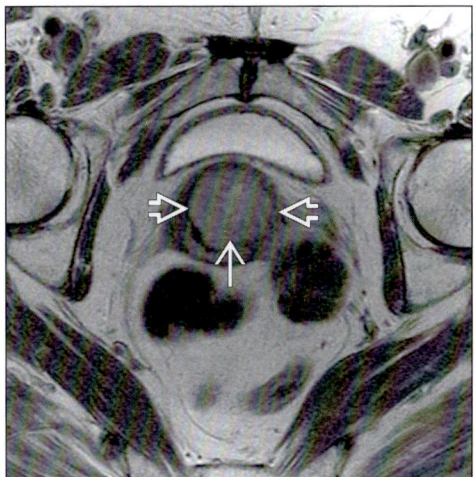

(Left) Sagittal T2WI MR shows a large high signal intensity tumor ➡ in the cervix. *(Right)* Axial T2WI MR shows intact low signal intensity cervical stromal ring ➡ indicating that the tumor ➡ is confined within the cervix.

Typical

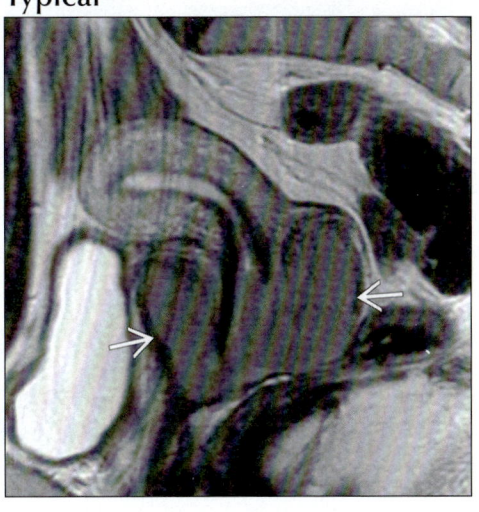
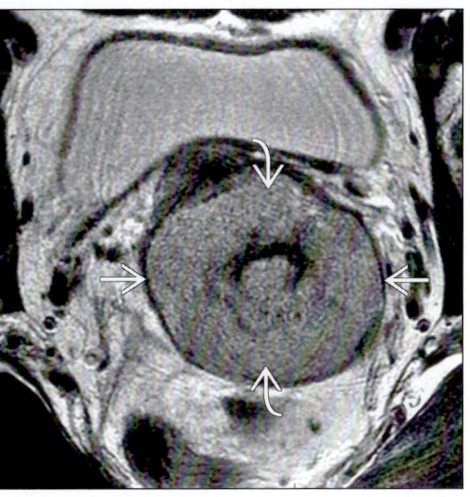

(Left) Sagittal T2WI MR shows a large cervical cancer ➡ that protrudes into and expands the upper vagina. *(Right)* Axial T2WI MR shows that the outer cervical stromal ring ➡ is intact despite the large size of the cervical mass ➡.

CERVICAL CANCER, CHARACTERIZATION

Typical

(Left) Axial CECT shows a large cervical cancer seen as a low attenuation mass ➡. Enhancing cervical stromal ring ➡ around the mass is intact indicating that the mass is confined within the cervix. *(Right)* Axial CECT shows a heterogeneous cervical mass ➡ with obvious right parametrial invasion ➡ and extension towards the right pelvic side wall.

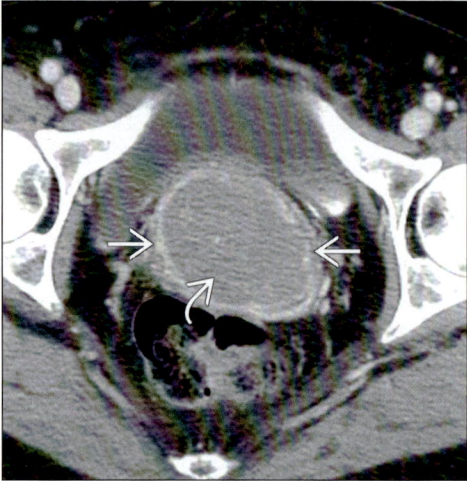 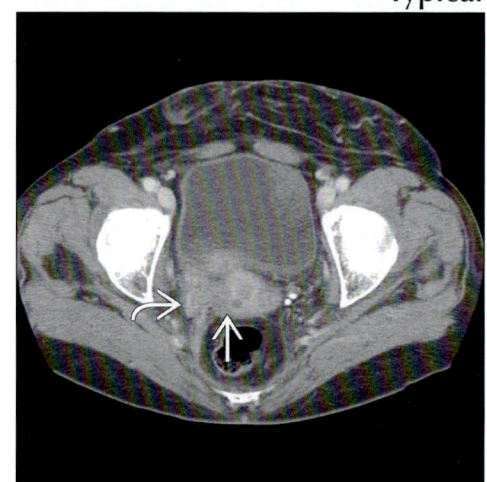

Typical

(Left) Sagittal T2WI MR shows a large cervical cancer ➡ that extends to lower uterine segment ➡ and upper vagina ➡. *(Right)* Coronal oblique T2WI MR shows that cervical stroma is completely replaced by high signal intensity tumor ➡ indicating full thickness cervical stromal invasion. Irregular tumor-parametrial interface on the right indicates parametrial invasion ➡.

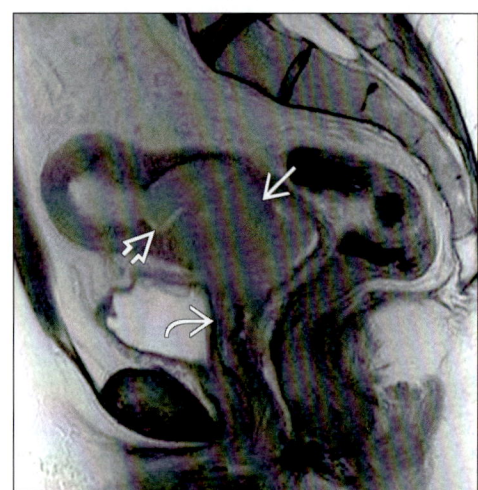 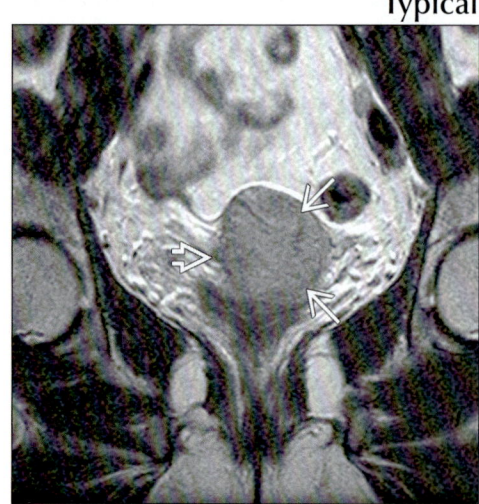

Typical

(Left) Sagittal T2WI MR shows a large cervical mass ➡ that extends to the lower uterine segment. *(Right)* Axial oblique T2WI MR shows that the mass ➡ invades the full thickness of the cervical stroma. Irregular tumor-parametrial interface on the right indicates parametrial invasion ➡.

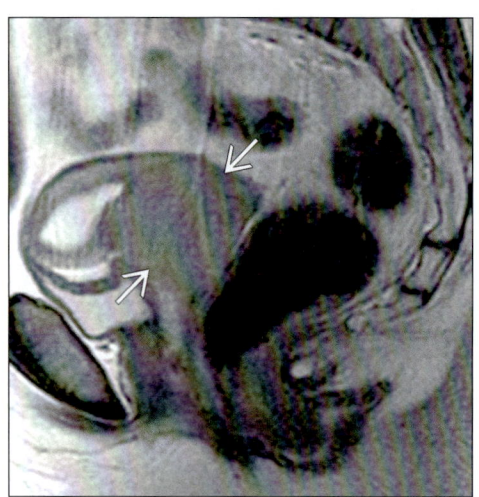 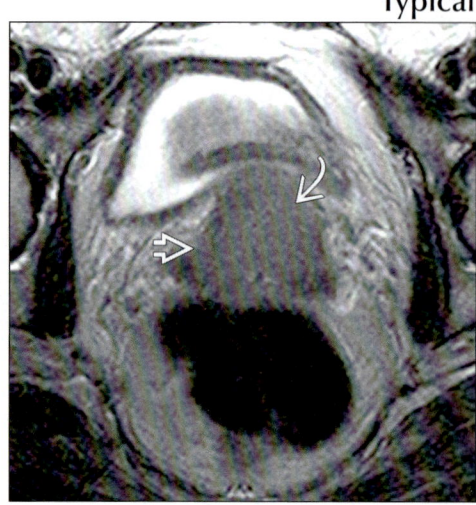

CERVICAL CANCER, CHARACTERIZATION

Typical

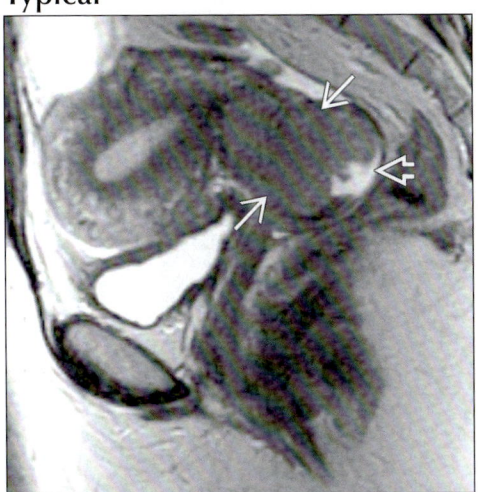
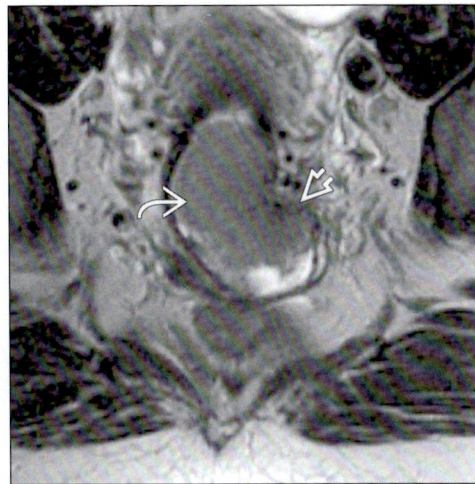

(Left) Sagittal T2WI MR shows a large cervical mass ➡ protruding into the vagina ➡. *(Right)* Axial T2WI MR shows that the large cervical mass ➡ has parametrial invasion ➡ on the left.

Typical

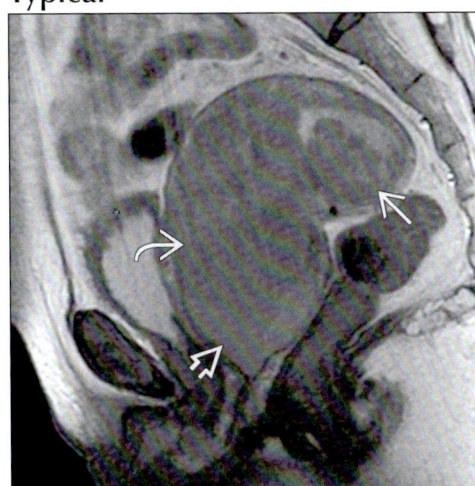
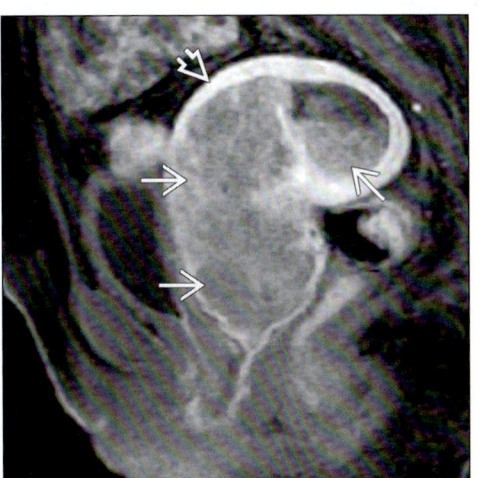

(Left) Sagittal T2WI MR shows a very large cervical mass ➡ that invades the uterus ➡ and upper vagina ➡. *(Right)* Sagittal T1 C+ FS MR shows that the cervical cancer ➡ enhances less intensely than the myometrium ➡ does.

Typical

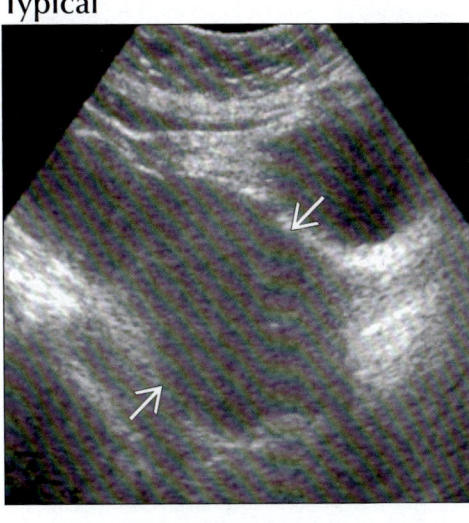
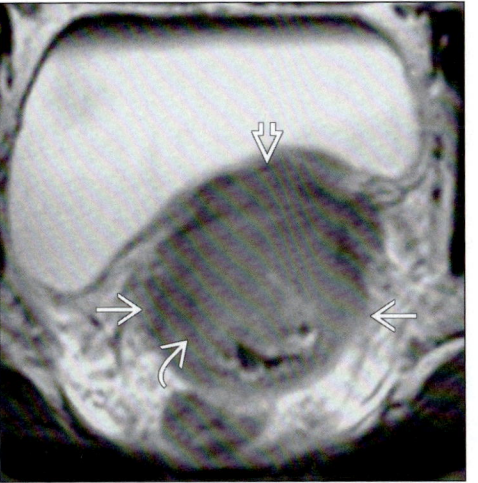

(Left) Sagittal transvaginal ultrasound shows cervical cancer ➡ seen as a hypoechoic mass in the cervix. *(Right)* Axial T2WI MR shows bilateral parametrial extension ➡ and urinary bladder wall invasion ➡ by the large cervical mass ➡.

CERVICAL CANCER, STAGE IB-IIA

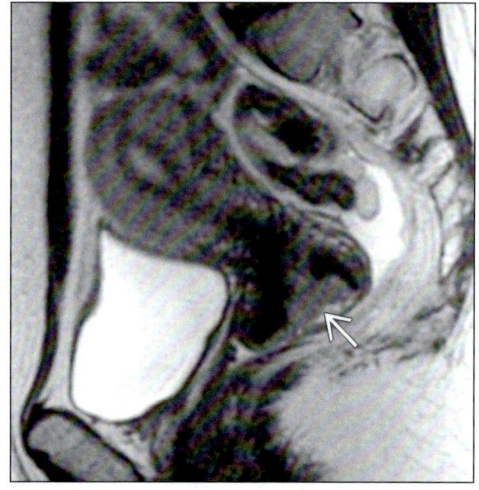

Sagittal T2WI MR shows cervical cancer seen as a high signal intensity mass ➡ in the cervix.

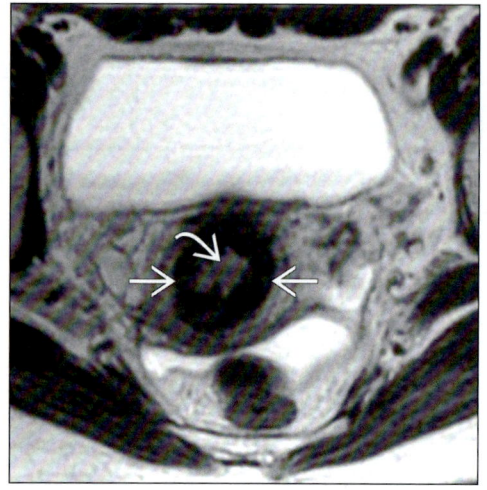

Axial T2WI MR shows that the tumor ➡ is confined within the cervix. Note that the low signal intensity cervical stroma ➡ is intact.

TERMINOLOGY

Definitions
- Clinically visible cervical cancer amenable to surgical resection

IMAGING FINDINGS

General Features
- Best diagnostic clue: Solid mass arising from uterine cervix
- Location
  - Stage IB is confined within the cervix
  - Stage IIA extends to upper 2/3 of vagina

Ultrasonographic Findings
- Poor soft tissue contrast limits tumor detection and determining stromal invasion or parametrial extension

CT Findings
- CECT: Cervical cancer is usually iso- or hypoattenuation relative to cervical stroma

MR Findings
- T1WI: Cervical cancer is iso-intense to cervical stroma
- T2WI
  - T2WI is the most useful sequence in tumor depiction and staging
  - In cervical cancers confined to the stroma, the low signal intensity stromal ring surrounding the high signal intensity tumor is completely intact
  - In the case of full thickness stromal invasion, the low signal intensity stroma is completely replaced by high signal intensity tumor; and a smooth tumor-parametrial interface excludes parametrial invasion
  - When tumor extends the vagina, normal low signal intensity of vaginal wall is replaced by high signal intensity of the tumor
- T1 C+: Cervical cancer demonstrates variable contrast-enhancement

Nuclear Medicine Findings
- PET
  - Can be used as an effective adjunct to CT and MR imaging in the evaluation of
    - Lymph node involvement

DDx: Cervical Masses

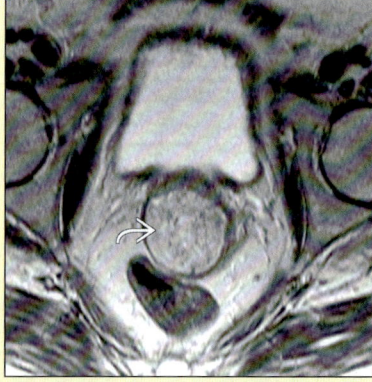

Benign Cervical Polyp

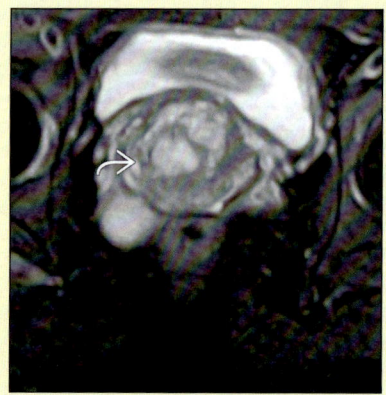

Adenoma Malignum

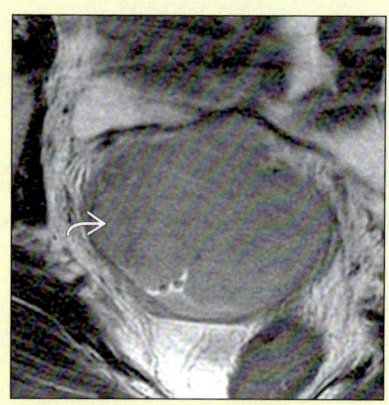

Cervical Lymphoma

CERVICAL CANCER, STAGE IB-IIA

Key Facts

Terminology
- Clinically visible cervical cancer amenable to surgical resection

Imaging Findings
- Stage IB is confined within the cervix
- Stage IIA extends to upper 2/3 of vagina
- In cervical cancers confined to the stroma, the low signal intensity stromal ring surrounding the high signal intensity tumor is completely intact
- In the case of full thickness stromal invasion, the low signal intensity stroma is completely replaced by high signal intensity tumor; and a smooth tumor-parametrial interface excludes parametrial invasion
- When tumor extends the vagina, normal low signal intensity of vaginal wall is replaced by high signal intensity of the tumor

- Detecting distant metastases
- Evaluating treatment response

Imaging Recommendations
- Best imaging tool
  - MR is the imaging method of choice
  - MR can accurately determine tumor size, tumor location (exophytic or endocervical), depth of stromal invasion and extension to vagina

DIFFERENTIAL DIAGNOSIS

Benign Cervical Polyp
- Benign cervical polyp does not invade the stroma
- Imaging can not differentiate a benign cervical polyp from cervical cancer not invading the stroma

Adenoma Malignum
- Enlarged cervix with multiple grape-like cysts within the cervical stroma

Cervical Lymphoma or Metastasis
- Involves cervical stroma diffusely and cervical canal is intact

CLINICAL ISSUES

Presentation
- Most common signs/symptoms
  - Abnormal vaginal bleeding
  - Vaginal discharge
  - Pelvic pain
  - Urinary symptoms

Treatment
- Surgery

DIAGNOSTIC CHECKLIST

Image Interpretation Pearls
- Role of imaging is to distinguish early disease that can be treated with surgery from advanced disease that must be treated with radiation, alone or combined with chemotherapy

SELECTED REFERENCES

1. Akin O et al: Imaging of uterine cancer. Radiol Clin North Am. 45(1):167-82, 2007
2. Dimopoulos JC et al: Systematic evaluation of MRI findings in different stages of treatment of cervical cancer: potential of MRI on delineation of target, pathoanatomic structures, and organs at risk. Int J Radiat Oncol Biol Phys. 64(5):1380-8, 2006
3. Engin G: Cervical cancer: MR imaging findings before, during, and after radiation therapy. Eur Radiol. 16(2):313-24, 2006
4. Moore DH: Cervical cancer. Obstet Gynecol. 107(5):1152-61, 2006
5. Narayan K: Arguments for a magnetic resonance imaging-assisted FIGO staging system for cervical cancer. Int J Gynecol Cancer. 15(4):573-82, 2005

IMAGE GALLERY

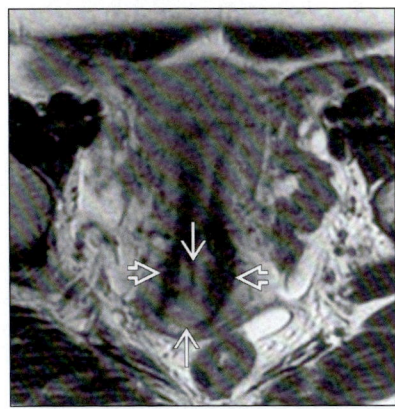 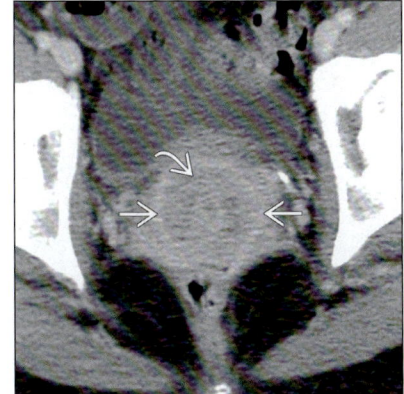 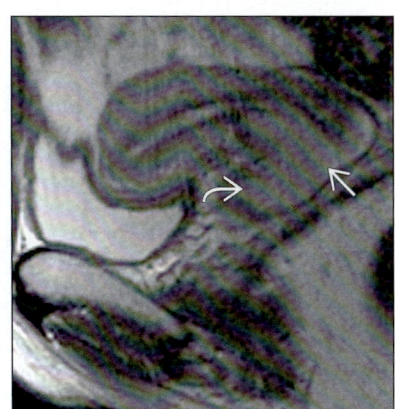

(Left) Axial T2WI MR shows a small cervical cancer ➡ confined within the cervical stroma ➡. (Center) Axial CECT shows heterogeneous tumor ➡ confined in the cervix. Note that cervical stromal ring ➡ is intact. (Right) Sagittal T2WI MR shows that cervical mass ➡ involves the upper 2/3 of the vagina ➡.

CERVICAL CANCER, STAGE IIB-IVB

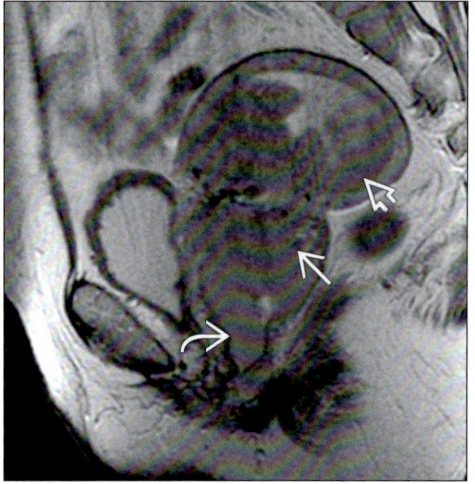

Sagittal T2WI MR shows a large cervical mass ➡ that invades the uterus ➡ and lower vagina ➡.

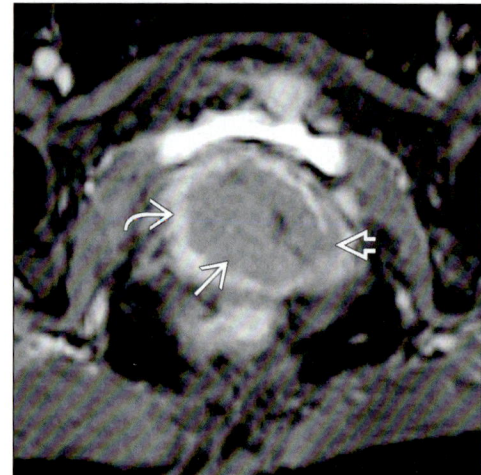

Axial T1 C+ FS MR shows that the mass ➡ enhances less than the cervical stroma ➡. Note that the cervical stromal ring is disrupted and there is obvious parametrial invasion ➡ on the left.

TERMINOLOGY

Definitions
- Advanced cervical cancer which is not amenable to surgical treatment alone

IMAGING FINDINGS

General Features
- Best diagnostic clue: Solid cervical mass that extends beyond the cervix
- Location
  - IIB: Tumor invades parametrium
  - IIIA: Tumor extends to lower 1/3 of vagina
  - IIIB: Tumor extends to pelvic wall with or without hydronephrosis
  - IVA: Tumor invades bladder or rectal mucosa
  - IVB: Tumor shows distant metastasis
- Size: Advanced cases present as large masses

Ultrasonographic Findings
- Although, hydronephrosis can be depicted, US is inadequate for detection of pelvic sidewall involvement and lymph node metastases

CT Findings
- NECT: Cervical cancer is isointense to cervical stroma
- CECT
  - Usually iso- or hypoattenuation relative to cervical stroma
  - Soft tissue density tumor invasion in fat around cervix can be seen

MR Findings
- T1WI: Cervical cancer is isointense to cervical stroma
- T2WI
  - T2WI is the most useful sequence in tumor depiction and staging
  - Parametrial invasion: Disruption of the stromal ring with nodular or irregular tumor signal intensity extending into parametrium
  - Vaginal invasion: Disruption of low signal intensity vaginal wall with high signal intensity tumor

DDx: Cervical Masses

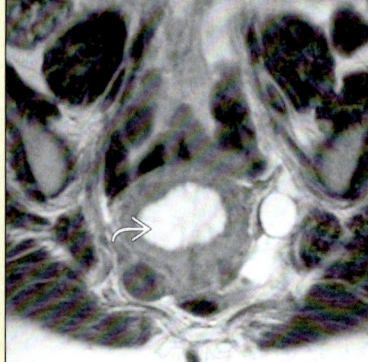

Benign Cervical Polyp

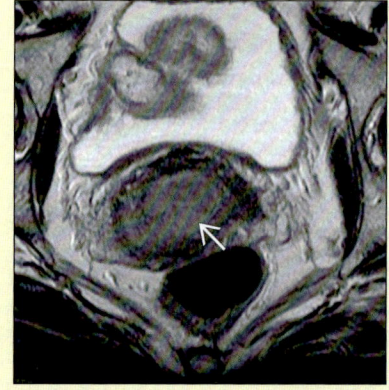

Cervical Cancer, Early Stage

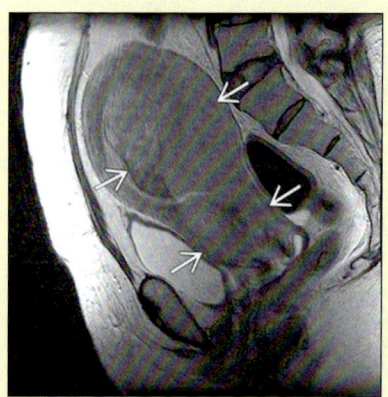

Endometrial Cancer Invading Cervix

CERVICAL CANCER, STAGE IIB-IVB

Key Facts

Terminology
- Advanced cervical cancer which is not amenable to surgical treatment alone

Imaging Findings
- Parametrial invasion: Disruption of the stromal ring with nodular or irregular tumor signal intensity extending into parametrium
- Vaginal invasion: Disruption of low signal intensity vaginal wall with high signal intensity tumor
- Pelvic side-wall invasion: Tumor extends within 3 mm of pelvic side-wall
- Hydronephrosis is an indication of ureteral invasion
- Bladder or rectal invasion: Disruption of their normal low signal intensity walls
- MR imaging is method of choice
- CT can also be used in demonstrating adjacent organ invasion, lymph node involvement or distant metastases
- PET is useful in staging especially in cases with equivocal findings on MR or CT

Diagnostic Checklist
- Cross-sectional imaging is superior to clinical staging
- Tumor size, parametrial invasion, and lymph node status, which are all critical prognostic factors in staging and treatment planning, are well-evaluated with CT and MR imaging
- Role of imaging is to distinguish early disease that can be treated with surgery from advanced disease that must be treated with radiation and/or chemotherapy

---

- Pelvic side-wall invasion: Tumor extends within 3 mm of pelvic side-wall
- Hydronephrosis is an indication of ureteral invasion
- Bladder or rectal invasion: Disruption of their normal low signal intensity walls
- T1 C+
  - Cervical cancer demonstrates variable contrast-enhancement
  - Use of contrast may help detection of adjacent organ or pelvic side-wall invasion

Nuclear Medicine Findings
- PET
  - Can be used as an effective adjunct to CT and MR imaging in the evaluation of
    - Lymph node involvement
    - Detecting distant metastases
    - Evaluating treatment response

Imaging Recommendations
- Best imaging tool
  - MR imaging is method of choice
  - CT can also be used in demonstrating adjacent organ invasion, lymph node involvement or distant metastases
  - PET is useful in staging especially in cases with equivocal findings on MR or CT
- Protocol advice
  - MR imaging protocol should include
    - T1WI; axial, large FOV including entire pelvis
    - T2WI; axial, coronal and sagittal small FOV
    - Dynamic CEMR; optional, used not for staging but for demonstrating adjacent organ invasion or fistulas

DIFFERENTIAL DIAGNOSIS

Benign Cervical Polyp
- Benign cervical polyp does not invade the stroma
- Imaging can not differentiate a benign cervical polyp from cervical cancer not invading the stroma

Cervical Cancer; Early Stages
- Cervical cancer that is confined within cervix or that extends to upper 2/3 of vagina
- Can be treated with surgery alone

Adenoma Malignum
- Enlarged cervix with multiple grape-like cysts within the cervical stroma

Cervical Lymphoma or Metastasis
- Involves stroma diffusely and cervical canal is intact

Pelvic Malignancies Secondarily Involving Cervix
- Cancers of endometrium, ovary, rectum, and urinary bladder may secondarily involve uterine cervix
- When a large pelvic mass is seen, it may be difficult to determine primary site of tumor
- Location of epicenter of tumor may be helpful in determining its origin

PATHOLOGY

General Features
- General path comments
  - Cervical cancer arises from squamocolumnar junction
  - Then, invades into cervical stroma and adjacent structures in advanced cases
  - Most common histologic types
    - Squamous cell carcinoma (80-90%)
    - Adenocarcinoma (worse prognosis)
- Etiology
  - Cervical intraepithelial neoplasia (CIN) is considered a precursor lesion of cervical cancer
  - Risk factors for developing cervical cancer include
    - Infection with certain types of human papilloma virus (HPV)
    - Early age at first sexual intercourse
    - Multiple sexual partners
    - Multiparity

CERVICAL CANCER, STAGE IIB-IVB

- History of sexually transmitted diseases
- Low socioeconomic status
- Epidemiology
  - 3rd most common gynecologic malignancy
  - More frequent in young women with low socioeconomic status

Gross Pathologic & Surgical Features
- Solid cervical mass with parametrial, lower vaginal, pelvic wall, bladder or rectum invasion

Staging, Grading or Classification Criteria
- FIGO staging system
  - 0: Carcinoma in situ
  - I: Confined to cervix
    - IA: Microscopic
    - IB: Clinically visible (> 5 mm depth; > 7 mm width)
  - II: Extension beyond uterus
    - IIA: Extension up to upper 2/3 of vagina
    - IIB: Parametrial invasion
  - III: Extension to lower 1/3 of vagina or pelvic wall invasion
    - IIIA: Extension to lower 1/3 of vagina
    - IIIB: Pelvic wall invasion and/or hydronephrosis
  - IV: Located outside true pelvis or bladder and/or rectal invasion
    - IVA: Bladder or rectal mucosa
    - IVB: Distant metastasis

CLINICAL ISSUES

Presentation
- Most common signs/symptoms
  - Abnormal vaginal bleeding
  - Vaginal discharge
  - Pelvic pain
  - Urinary symptoms
- Other signs/symptoms
  - Signs and symptoms related to invasion of adjacent organs and structures
    - Hydronephrosis
    - Hematuria
    - Rectal pain or bleeding

Natural History & Prognosis
- Most important prognostic factors
  - Histologic grade of tumor
  - Tumor volume
  - Depth of stromal invasion
  - Adjacent organ invasion
  - Lymph node involvement
- 5 yr survival rates: 80-90% for stage I, 50-65% for stage II, 25-35% for stage III, and 0-15% for stage IV

Treatment
- Radiation treatment alone or combined with chemotherapy

DIAGNOSTIC CHECKLIST

Consider
- Cross-sectional imaging is superior to clinical staging
- Tumor size, parametrial invasion, and lymph node status, which are all critical prognostic factors in staging and treatment planning, are well-evaluated with CT and MR imaging
- Therefore, extended clinical staging incorporating findings from CT and/or MR imaging has become common practice

Image Interpretation Pearls
- Role of imaging is to distinguish early disease that can be treated with surgery from advanced disease that must be treated with radiation and/or chemotherapy

SELECTED REFERENCES

1. Akin O et al: Imaging of uterine cancer. Radiol Clin North Am. 45(1):167-82, 2007
2. Sala E et al: MRI of malignant neoplasms of the uterine corpus and cervix. AJR Am J Roentgenol. 188(6):1577-87, 2007
3. Zand KR et al: Magnetic resonance imaging of the cervix. Cancer Imaging. 7:69-76, 2007
4. Brown MA et al: MR imaging of malignant uterine disease. Magn Reson Imaging Clin N Am. 14(4):455-69, v-vi, 2006
5. Engin G: Cervical cancer: MR imaging findings before, during, and after radiation therapy. Eur Radiol. 16(2):313-24, 2006
6. Kinkel K: Pitfalls in staging uterine neoplasm with imaging: a review. Abdom Imaging. 31(2):164-73, 2006
7. Rockall AG et al: Can MRI rule out bladder and rectal invasion in cervical cancer to help select patients for limited EUA? Gynecol Oncol. 101(2):244-9, 2006
8. Hricak H et al: Role of imaging in pretreatment evaluation of early invasive cervical cancer: results of the intergroup study American College of Radiology Imaging Network 6651-Gynecologic Oncology Group 183. J Clin Oncol. 23(36):9329-37, 2005
9. Jena A et al: Parametrial invasion in carcinoma of cervix: role of MRI measured tumour volume. Br J Radiol. 78(936):1075-7, 2005
10. Okamoto Y et al: MR imaging of the uterine cervix: imaging-pathologic correlation. Radiographics. 23(2):425-45; quiz 534-5, 2003
11. Ascher SM et al: Staging of gynecologic malignancies. Top Magn Reson Imaging. 12(2):105-29, 2001
12. Togashi K et al: Cervical cancer. J Magn Reson Imaging. 8(2):391-7, 1998

CERVICAL CANCER, STAGE IIB-IVB

IMAGE GALLERY

Typical

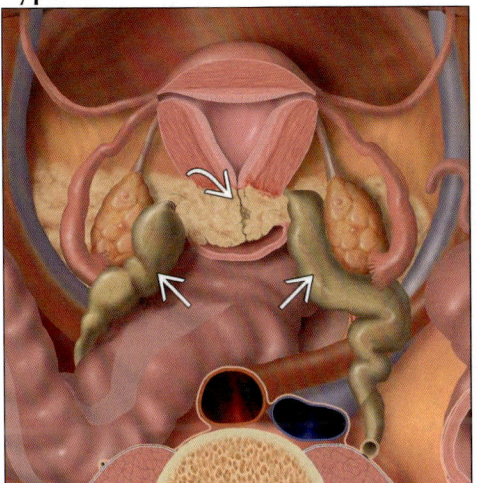
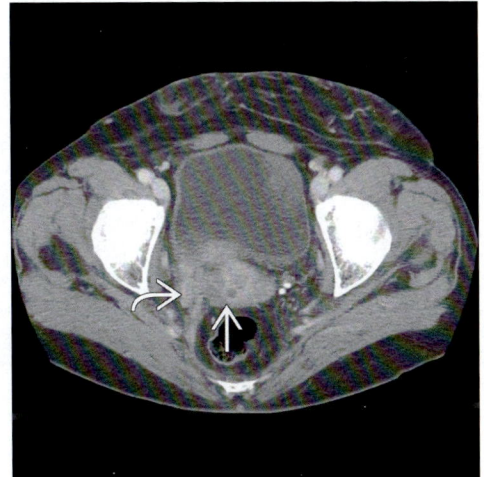

(Left) Graphic shows cervical cancer ➡ with bilateral parametrial and ureteral invasion. Dilated ureters ➡ are depicted. *(Right)* Axial CECT shows a cervical mass ➡ with right parametrial invasion ➡ and extension towards the right pelvic side-wall.

Typical

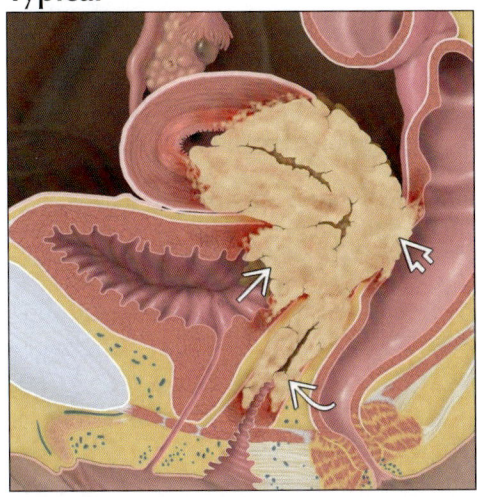
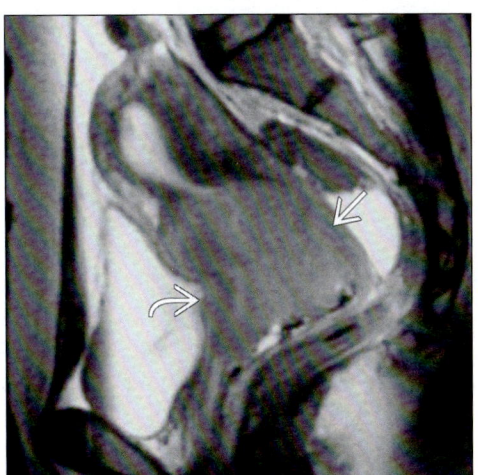

(Left) Graphic shows cervical cancer seen as a large mass invading urinary bladder ➡, rectum ➡ and lower vagina ➡. *(Right)* Sagittal T2WI MR shows a large cervical cancer ➡ invading the posterior urinary bladder wall ➡.

Typical

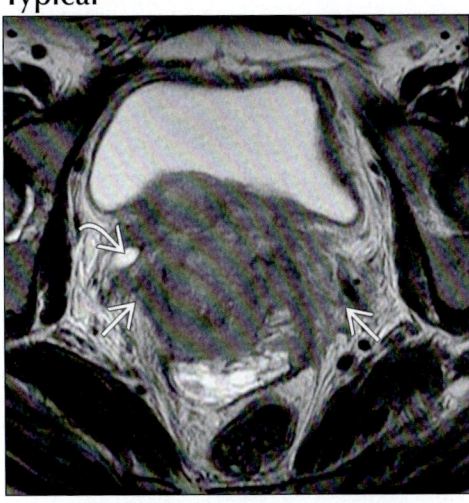
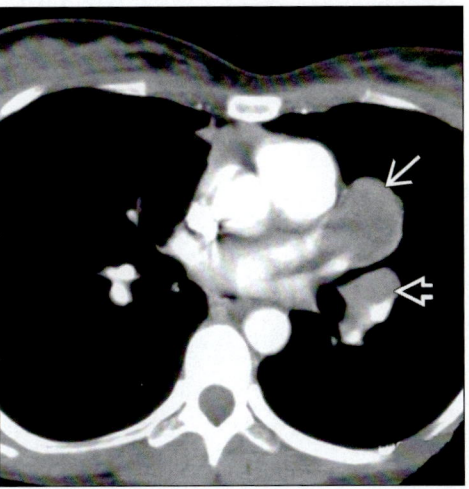

(Left) Axial T2WI MR shows cervical cancer with bilateral parametrial invasion ➡. Note that the right distal ureter ➡ is invaded and dilated. *(Right)* Axial CECT shows mediastinal ➡ and left hilar ➡ metastatic lymphadenopathy in a patient with cervical cancer.

CERVICAL ADENOCARCINOMA

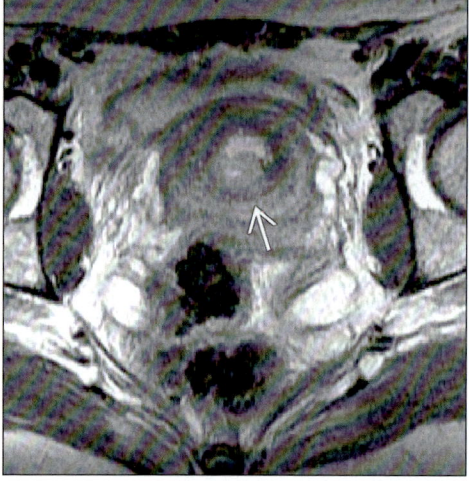

Axial T2WI MR shows a hyperintense lesion ➡ arising from the posterior lip of the cervix with effacement of the hypointense fibrous stroma. Proven cervical adenocarcinoma glassy-cell type, stage IB1.

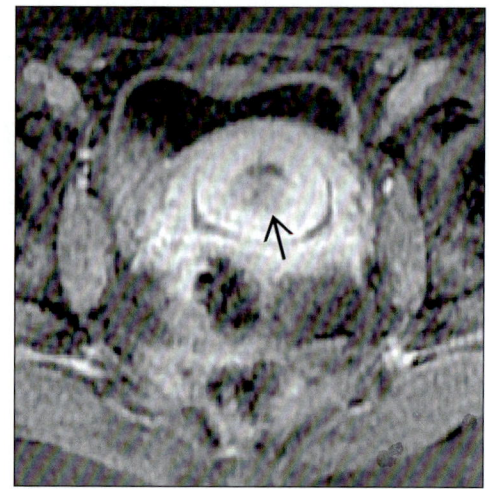

Axial T1 C+ FS MR in the same patient as previous image, shows the cervical mass ➡ to be hypovascular relative to the cervical stroma.

TERMINOLOGY

Definitions
- Subtype of cervical carcinoma arising from columnar epithelium of endocervical glands
- Comprises several histological subtypes, among them adenoma malignum

IMAGING FINDINGS

General Features
- Best diagnostic clue: High signal intensity (SI) solid, or mixed cystic/solid cervical mass on T2WI
- Location: Endocervical canal
- Size: Variable
- Morphology
  o Typically barrel-shaped mass
  o "Cervical canal" sign on T1 C+ FS owing to preservation of endocervical epithelium even in presence of large tumors
  o Adenoma malignum: Rare subtype of cervical adenocarcinoma
    ▪ Multiple grape-like cysts within cervical stroma

Ultrasonographic Findings
- Grayscale Ultrasound
  o Enlarged cervix
  o Ill-defined, iso- to hypoechoic mass, difficult to differentiate from surrounding normal cervical tissue
    ▪ Hyperechoic areas if necrosis or air present
  o Adenoma malignum
    ▪ Hyperechoic mass with hypoechoic cystic components
  o Limited evaluation of pelvic lymphadenopathy and peritoneal disease

CT Findings
- CECT
  o Iso- or hypodense cervical mass
  o Adenoma malignum
    ▪ Low attenuation mass with thin enhancing septae

MR Findings
- T1WI: Intermediate SI mass, isointense to cervical stroma
- T2WI
  o Hyperintense cervical mass

DDx: Cervical Masses

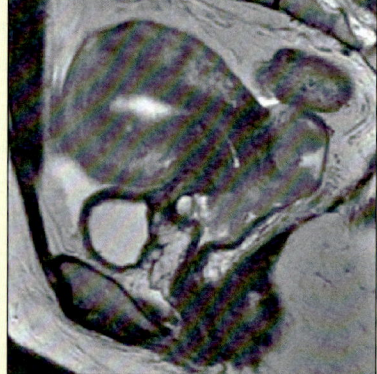

Cervical Squamous Cell Carcinoma

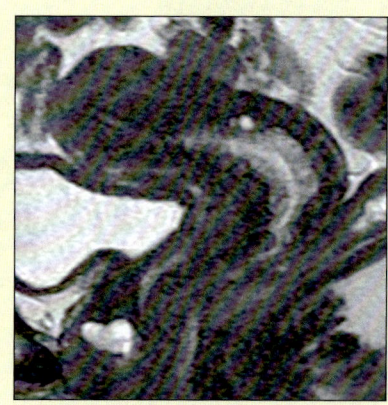

Endocervical Glandular Hyperplasia

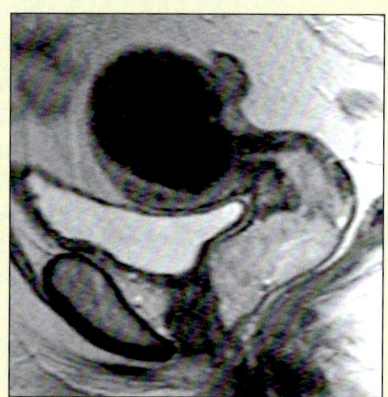

Cervical Polyp

CERVICAL ADENOCARCINOMA

Key Facts

Terminology
- Subtype of cervical carcinoma arising from columnar epithelium of endocervical glands

Imaging Findings
- Best diagnostic clue: High signal intensity (SI) solid, or mixed cystic/solid cervical mass on T2WI
- Location: Endocervical canal
- Typically barrel-shaped mass
- Preservation of endocervical epithelium due to submucosal location of tumor
- Helps differentiate from SCC which disrupts epithelium
- Overall staging accuracy less than with SCC
- Frequent understaging of advanced disease due to microscopic parametrial invasion

Top Differential Diagnoses
- Squamous Cell Carcinoma
- Nabothian Cysts
- Endocervical Glandular Hyperplasia

Pathology
- Accounts for 10-15% of cervical cancers

Clinical Issues
- Poor prognosis, lower survival rates than with SCC

Diagnostic Checklist
- Consider cervical adenocarcinoma in the setting of a large barrel-shaped cervical mass with preservation of endocervical epithelium
- "Cervical canal" sign

- Typically higher SI than SCC
- Can present as multicystic mass in cervical stroma
  - Adenoma malignum
    - Combination of few large cysts and smaller vesicles: Grape-like mass
    - Cyst contents hyperintense with solid parts of intermediate SI
    - Located deep in cervical stroma
    - Fluid accumulation (mucin) within uterus and/or vagina may be present
- T1 C+ FS
  - Hypovascular relative to cervical stroma
    - Enhancement less than with SCC
    - Enhancement often peripheral
    - Mucinous subtypes (including adenoma malignum), enhance less than other cervical adenocarcinomas
  - Thin, central band of mucosal enhancement: "Cervical canal" sign
    - Preservation of endocervical epithelium due to submucosal location of tumor
    - Helps differentiate from SCC which disrupts epithelium
  - Adenoma malignum
    - Variable enhancement
    - Avascular cysts embedded in enhancing stroma
    - Enhancement of nodules and septae

Imaging Recommendations
- Best imaging tool
  - MR is the imaging modality of choice for staging
    - Overall staging accuracy less than with SCC
    - Frequent understaging of advanced disease due to microscopic parametrial invasion
    - Small tumors (stage IB or less) may be invisible on all imaging modalities, due to their infiltrative nature and poor contrast between tumor and cervical stroma
- Protocol advice
  - T1 C+ FS sequences important for staging cervical adenocarcinoma
    - Greater contrast between tumor and cervical stroma than on T2WI
- "Cervical canal" sign

DIFFERENTIAL DIAGNOSIS

Squamous Cell Carcinoma
- Often indistinguishable from adenocarcinoma
- SI lower than adenocarcinoma on T2WI
- Hypervascular lesion typically showing homogeneous enhancement
  - Disruption of enhancing endocervical epithelium

Nabothian Cysts
- Cystically dilated endocervical glands
- Low SI on T1WI, high SI on T2WI
- Sharp margins against surrounding cervical stroma
- Typically situated superficially within cervical wall
  - Deep-seated cysts can mimic adenoma malignum
  - Adenoma malignum usually has ill-defined margins with adjacent stroma
  - Enhancing nodules, thick walls between cysts

Endocervical Glandular Hyperplasia
- Thickening of endocervical mucosa with preservation of architecture
- Can sometimes mimic cervical adenocarcinoma
- May need tissue diagnosis to make distinction

Cervical Polyp
- Pedunculated mass projecting into cervical lumen
- Vascular pedicle
- No stromal invasion

PATHOLOGY

General Features
- Etiology
  - Major etiological factor: Infection with human papillomavirus types 16 and 18
  - Precursors
    - Endocervical glandular dysplasia
    - Atypical tubal metaplasia

CERVICAL ADENOCARCINOMA

- Increased incidence in long time oral contraceptive pill users
- Risk factors: Same as SCC
  - Young age at first intercourse
  - Elevated number of sexual partners
  - Nulliparity
  - Diabetes, obesity
  - DES in utero exposure in the rare sub-type of clear cell carcinoma
- Epidemiology
  - Second most common type of cervical carcinoma after SCC
    - Accounts for 10-15% of cervical cancers
    - SCC accounts for 80%
  - Increasing incidence because of lower sensitivity of this subtype by Pap test

Gross Pathologic & Surgical Features
- Cervical mass with endophytic growth pattern
- Nearly 15% of patients have no gross lesion, since adenocarcinoma located deep within endocervical clefts

Microscopic Features
- Adenocarcinoma
  - Arises from columnar epithelium of endocervical canal
  - Abnormal glands of different sizes and shapes
  - Moderately to well-differentiated endocervical glands: Mucin-rich cystic spaces
  - Extend from surface to deeper portions of cervical wall
- Adenoma malignum (minimal deviation adenocarcinoma)
  - Well-differentiated cervical glands that produce mucin
  - Invasion into deep cervical stroma where normal glands are usually not seen
  - Minimal histological atypia

Staging, Grading or Classification Criteria
- Several subtypes identified
  - Endocervical adenocarcinoma: Most common type (70%)
    - Mucinous, intestinal, signet-ring cell type
    - Uncommon variant: Adenoma malignum (5%)
  - Endometrioid adenocarcinoma (20-25%)
  - Several rare subtypes: Clear-cell carcinoma, adenosquamous, adenoid cystic carcinoma, glassy cell carcinoma, mixed-cell type, etc.
- FIGO staging: Same as for SCC

CLINICAL ISSUES

Presentation
- Most common signs/symptoms
  - Often asymptomatic
  - If symptomatic
    - Spontaneous or postcoital bleeding
    - Pelvic pain, flank pain, lymphedema

Demographics
- Age
  - Mean age 56 years old
  - Slightly older age group than SCC

Natural History & Prognosis
- Poor prognosis, lower survival rates than with SCC
  - 5-year survival rates: 79% stage I, 64% stage II, 22% stage III, 11% stage IV
  - Detection delayed because of endocervical location
  - Early lymphatic dissemination
  - Higher incidence of ascites and para-aortic spread
  - Hematogenous metastases late in disease course: Lung, bone, adrenal gland, pancreas, liver
  - Resistant to radiotherapy and chemotherapy
- Adenoma malignum
  - Poor prognosis even if very well-differentiated adenocarcinoma
  - Early peritoneal dissemination
  - Poor response to radiation and chemotherapy

Treatment
- Depends on stage of disease, age of patient and co-morbidity
- Surgery for stages 0-IIA
- Radiotherapy for more advanced disease
- Radiosensitizing chemotherapy

DIAGNOSTIC CHECKLIST

Consider
- Consider cervical adenocarcinoma in the setting of a large barrel-shaped cervical mass with preservation of endocervical epithelium

Image Interpretation Pearls
- High SI mass on T2WI
- Hypovascular relative to cervical stroma
- "Cervical canal" sign

SELECTED REFERENCES

1. Okamoto Y et al: Pelvic imaging: multicystic uterine cervical lesions. Can magnetic resonance imaging differentiate benignancy from malignancy? Acta Radiol. 45(1):102-8, 2004
2. Matsushita M et al: MR imaging underestimates stromal invasion in patients with adenocarcinoma of the uterine cervix. Eur J Gynaecol Oncol. 22(3):201-3, 2001
3. Itoh K et al: A comparative analysis of cross sectional imaging techniques in minimal deviation adenocarcinoma of the uterine cervix. BJOG. 107(9):1158-63, 2000
4. Chung JJ et al: T2-weighted fast spin-echo MR findings of adenocarcinoma of the uterine cervix: comparison with squamous cell carcinoma. Yonsei Med J. 40(3):226-31, 1999
5. Takamura M et al: MRI of cervical adenocarcinoma with cystic components. Clin Imaging. 23(1):40-3, 1999
6. Torashima M et al: Invasive adenocarcinoma of the uterine cervix: MR imaging. Comput Med Imaging Graph. 21(4):253-60, 1997
7. Yu KK et al: Cervical carcinoma: role of imaging. Abdom Imaging. 22(2):208-15, 1997

CERVICAL ADENOCARCINOMA

IMAGE GALLERY

Typical

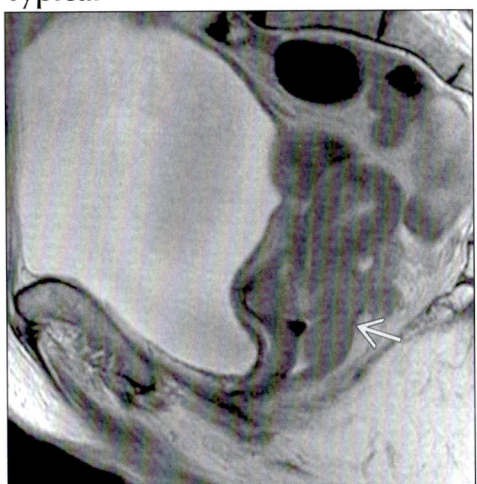
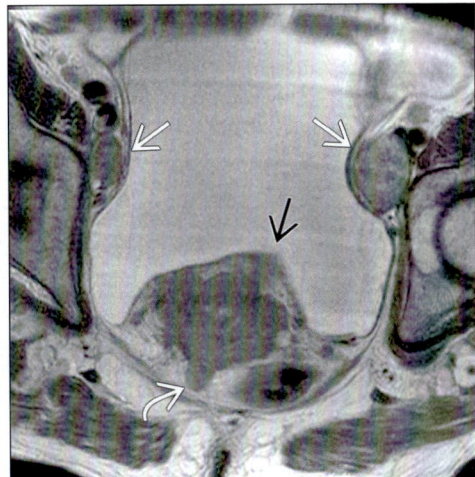

(Left) Sagittal T2WI MR shows a heterogeneous, infiltrating cervical mass ➡ which proved to be cervical adenocarcinoma. *(Right)* Axial T2WI MR in the same patient as previous image, shows that the mass is infiltrating the bladder wall ➡ (stage IVA), and extending posteriorly into the cul-de-sac ➡. There is bilateral external iliac lymphadenopathy ➡.

Variant

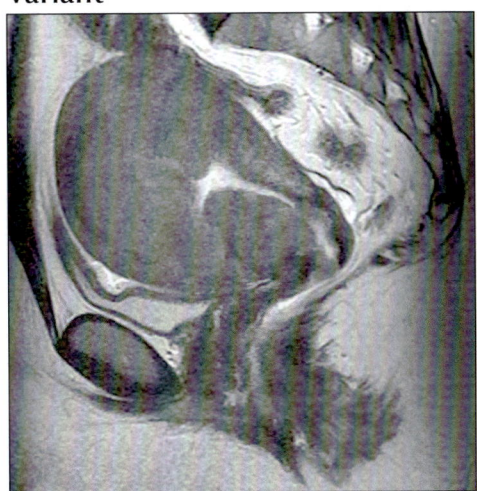
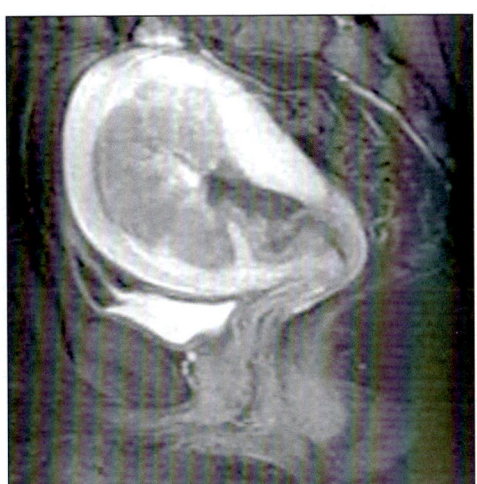

(Left) Sagittal T2WI MR in a 31 year old patient shows a large mass distending both the endocervical canal, as well as the endometrial cavity, with myometrial invasion. At histopathology the mass proved to be adenocarcinoma of cervical origin. *(Right)* Sagittal T1 C+ FS MR shows the mass to be hypovascular compared to the cervical stroma and myometrium.

Variant

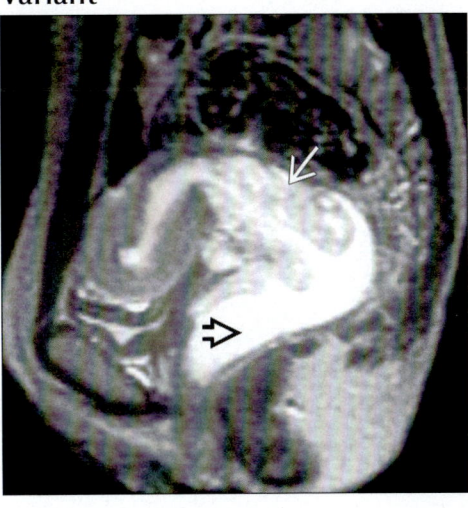
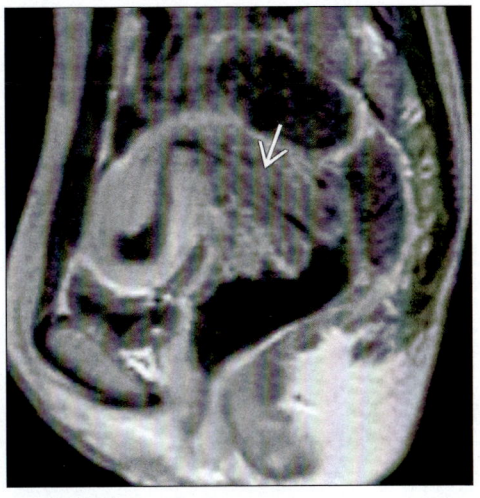

(Left) Sagittal T2WI MR shows a high signal intensity cervical mass ➡, associated with fluid distension of the vagina & endometrial cavity ➡, consistent with an adenoma malignum. Note that the lesion extends deep into the cervical stroma. *(Right)* Sagittal T1 C+ FS MR in same patient as previous image, shows no enhancement of the cystic locules within the lesion. There is, however, enhancement of multiple thin septae ➡ between the locules.

SMALL CELL CARCINOMA, CERVIX

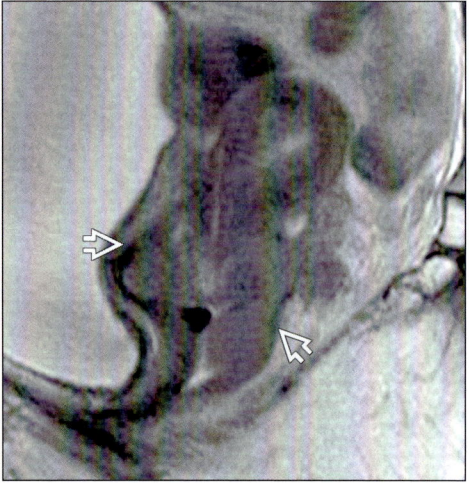

Sagittal T2WI MR shows a lobulated cervical mass of intermediate SI ➡ in a 42 year old female patient. Pathology: Small cell carcinoma of the cervix.

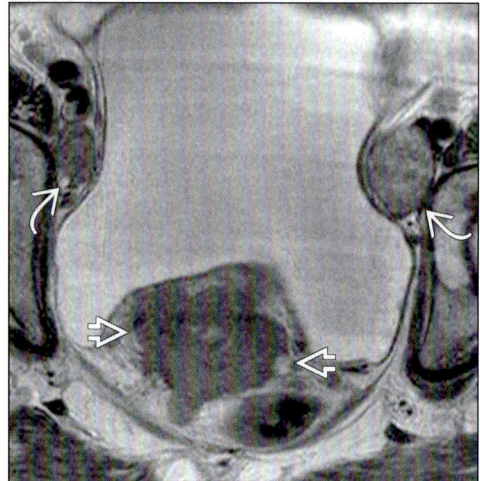

Axial oblique T2WI MR in same patient shows a large cervical tumor ➡ extending to both parametria. Note the presence of external iliac lymphadenopathy of the same signal intensity as the primary tumor ➡.

TERMINOLOGY

Abbreviations and Synonyms
- Carcinoid
- Small cell undifferentiated carcinoma
- Argyrophil cell carcinoma
- Small cell tumor with neuroendocrine feature
- Neuroendocrine carcinoma

Definitions
- Rare aggressive primary neuroendocrine tumor of the cervix

IMAGING FINDINGS

General Features
- Best diagnostic clue: Cervical mass with frequent extensive lymphadenopathy and parametrial invasion
- Location
  ○ Cervix
  ○ In advanced cases, uterus, vagina and/or adjacent organs may be involved
- Size: Variable; up to 10 cm

Ultrasonographic Findings
- Transvaginal US (TVS) findings: Tumor appears as hypoechoic mass on US

CT Findings
- CECT
  ○ Tumor of iso- or hypoattenuation relative to cervical stroma
  ○ Pelvic lymphadenopathy frequent finding
    ▪ Involves obturator, internal and external iliac lymph nodes and common iliac lymph nodes
    ▪ +/- Para-aortic lymph nodes
  ○ Hematogenous metastases may be seen in advanced cases
    ▪ E.g., liver, bone, lung, brain

MR Findings
- T1WI: Tumor is iso-intense to cervical stroma
- T2WI
  ○ Homogeneous, lobulated mass of intermediate SI (higher SI compare to the cervical stroma)
  ○ Parametrial invasion is indicated by full stromal invasion (loss of low SI cervical stroma) and
    ▪ Spiculated tumor/parametrial interface

DDx: Cervical Masses

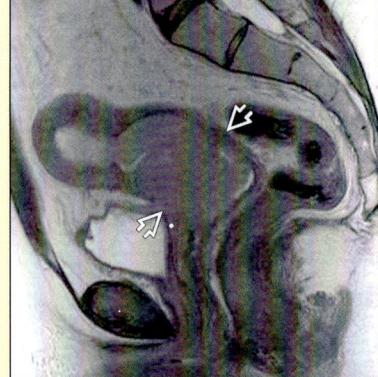

Cervical Cancer

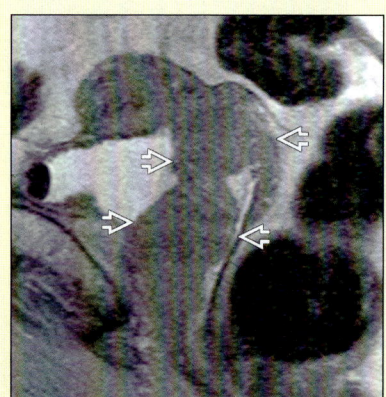

Metastasis to Cervix and Vagina

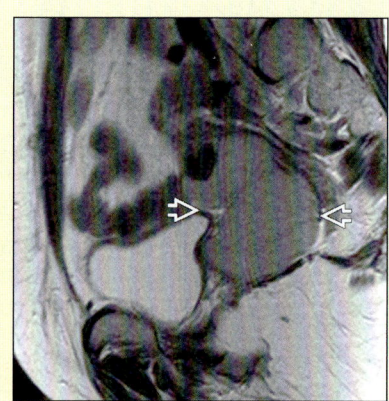

Cervical Lymphoma

SMALL CELL CARCINOMA, CERVIX

Key Facts

Terminology
- Rare aggressive primary neuroendocrine tumor of the cervix

Imaging Findings
- Best diagnostic clue: Cervical mass with frequent extensive lymphadenopathy and parametrial invasion
- Homogeneous, lobulated mass of intermediate SI (higher SI compare to the cervical stroma)
- MR imaging is method of choice for local staging
- CECT is used to assess for distant metastases

Top Differential Diagnoses
- Cervical Carcinoma
- Cervical Lymphoma
- Cervical Metastasis

Pathology
- Accounts for 0.5-2% of all uterine cervical cancers
- Immunohistochemistry necessary for diagnosis
- **Staging classification: FIGO staging system** (same for non-small cell cervical carcinoma)

Clinical Issues
- Most common signs/symptoms: Abnormal vaginal bleeding
- Regarded as systemic disease with poor prognosis due to high rate of lymph node metastasis and early systemic metastases
- Radical hysterectomy and bilateral salpingo-oophorectomy with pelvic lymphadenectomy
- +/- Radiotherapy
- + Adjuvant chemotherapy

            - Soft tissue extension into parametria
            - Encasement of periuterine vessels
        o Beware of overestimation of parametrial invasion with large tumors (PPV 70%) due to stromal edema
        o Vaginal involvement is indicated by loss of low SI anterior vaginal wall
        o Presence of hydronephrosis indicates pelvic side wall invasion
        o Bladder wall invasion is indicated by loss of low SI bladder wall
            - MR had a NPV of 100% for excluding bladder invasion
        o Regional lymphadenopathy with pelvic lymph nodes of intermediate signal intensity; greater than 8 mm in short axis diameter
- T1 C+: Tumor demonstrates variable enhancement

Imaging Recommendations
- Best imaging tool
    o MR imaging is method of choice for local staging
    o CECT is used to assess for distant metastases
- Protocol advice: MR: Axial T1WI (pelvis and upper abdomen); axial, sagittal, coronal T2WI

DIFFERENTIAL DIAGNOSIS

Cervical Carcinoma
- Imaging cannot distinguish reliably between small cell carcinoma and non-small cell carcinoma of the cervix

Cervical Lymphoma
- Diffuse involvement of the cervical stroma in lymphoma
- Possible presence of widespread lymphadenopathy and splenomegaly

Cervical Metastasis
- History of primary carcinoma

PATHOLOGY

General Features
- Etiology: History of smoking in approximately 60% of patients, although no definite correlation established
- Epidemiology
    o Accounts for 0.5-2% of all uterine cervical cancers
    o Diagnosis of primary small cell carcinoma of the cervix established by absence of concurrent small cell carcinoma elsewhere and no history of small cell carcinoma in the lung

Gross Pathologic & Surgical Features
- Lobulated mass demonstrating necrosis

Microscopic Features
- Papanicolaou cervical smear not sensitive for the diagnosis of small cell carcinoma of the cervix; punch biopsy may aid pre-operative diagnosis
- Tumor cells are small, round or fusiform with scanty cytoplasm
- Nuclear chromatin is hyperchromatic and finely granular
    o Nucleoli are inconspicuous with nuclear moulding
- Neoplastic cells grow in a diffuse manner or may be arranged in nests, trabeculae or cords
    o Peripheral palisading and a prominent perivascular concentration of cells often seen
- Necrosis is a constant feature
- Adenocarcinoma or squamous cell carcinoma co-exists in 21-77% of cases
- Immunohistochemistry necessary for diagnosis
    o Tumor cells are positive for one or more neuroendocrine markers e.g., NSE, NCAM, PGP9.5, chromogranin A, synaptophysin
- **Staging classification: FIGO staging system** (same for non-small cell cervical carcinoma)
    o 0: Carcinoma in situ
    o I: Confined to cervix
        - IA: Microscopic
        - IB: Clinically visible (> 5 mm)
    o II: Extension beyond uterus

SMALL CELL CARCINOMA, CERVIX

- IIA: Extension up to upper 2/3 of vagina
- IIB: Parametrial invasion
- III: Extension to lower 1/3 of vagina or pelvic wall invasion
  - IIIA: Extension to lower 1/4 of vagina
  - IIIB: Pelvic wall invasion and/or hydronephrosis
- IV: Located outside true pelvis or bladder and/or rectal invasion
  - IVA: Bladder or rectal mucosa
  - IVB: Distant metastasis

CLINICAL ISSUES

Presentation
- Most common signs/symptoms: Abnormal vaginal bleeding
- Other signs/symptoms
  - Vaginal discharge
  - Pelvic pain
  - Urinary symptoms

Demographics
- Age: Wide age range: 2nd to 10th decade of life; mean approximately 45 years

Natural History & Prognosis
- Regarded as systemic disease with poor prognosis due to high rate of lymph node metastasis and early systemic metastases
- 66% recurrence rate; median time to 1st relapse 8.4 months (3.6-28 months)
- Relapse occurs
  - In lymph nodes outside the original radiation field
  - Brain; several authors report an increased predilection for this site in metastatic small cell cervical carcinoma
  - Lung, liver, bone
- Overall 3 year survival rate of 60%; overall 5 year survival rate of 29-37%
- 0% 5 year survival rate reported for patients with disease greater than stage IB1
- Radiologic stage is the only independent predictor for disease free survival
  - 80% recurrence rate at 3 years for stage I and II patients versus 38% at 3 years for stage III and IV
- Other poor prognostic factors
  - Tumor size > 2 cm
  - Involved surgical margins
  - Pure versus a mixed histological pattern
  - Smoking

Treatment
- Localized disease
  - Radical hysterectomy and bilateral salpingo-oophorectomy with pelvic lymphadenectomy
  - +/- Radiotherapy
  - + Adjuvant chemotherapy
- Extensive disease
  - Neo-adjuvant chemotherapy +/- palliative surgery or radiotherapy

DIAGNOSTIC CHECKLIST

Consider
- MR for staging of local extent
- CECT for staging of distant metastases

Image Interpretation Pearls
- Often a large cervical mass with local extension, pelvic lymphadenopathy ± intra-abdominal adenopathy and distant hematogenous metastases at presentation

SELECTED REFERENCES

1. Kim KO et al: Clinical overview of extrapulmonary small cell carcinoma. J Korean Med Sci. 21(5):833-7, 2006
2. Wang KL et al: Neuroendocrine carcinoma of the uterine cervix: A clinicopathologic retrospective study of 31 cases with prognostic implications. J Chemother. 18(2):209-16, 2006
3. Tsunoda S et al: Small-cell carcinoma of the uterine cervix: a clinicopathologic study of 11 cases. Int J Gynecol Cancer. 15(2):295-300, 2005
4. Kim JH et al: Extrapulmonary small-cell carcinoma: a single-institution experience. Jpn J Clin Oncol. 34(5):250-4, 2004
5. Viswanathan AN et al: Small cell neuroendocrine carcinoma of the cervix: outcome and patterns of recurrence. Gynecol Oncol. 93(1):27-33, 2004
6. Yang DH et al: MRI of small cell carcinoma of the uterine cervix with pathologic correlation. AJR Am J Roentgenol. 182(5):1255-8, 2004
7. Chan JK et al: Prognostic factors in neuroendocrine small cell cervical carcinoma: a multivariate analysis. Cancer. 97(3):568-74, 2003
8. Hoskins PJ et al: Small-cell carcinoma of the cervix: fourteen years of experience at a single institution using a combined-modality regimen of involved-field irradiation and platinum-based combination chemotherapy. J Clin Oncol. 21(18):3495-501, 2003
9. Weed JC Jr et al: Small cell undifferentiated (neuroendocrine) carcinoma of the uterine cervix. J Am Coll Surg. 197(1):44-51, 2003
10. Nakata SI et al: Excellent results of radiotherapy for neuroendocrine carcinoma of the uterine cervix. Oncol Rep. 8(4):777-9, 2001
11. Straughn JM Jr et al: Predictors of outcome in small cell carcinoma of the cervix--a case series. Gynecol Oncol. 83(2):216-20, 2001
12. Collinet P et al: Neuroendocrine tumors of the uterine cervix. Clinicopathologic study of five patients. Eur J Obstet Gynecol Reprod Biol. 91(1):51-7, 2000
13. Chang TC et al: Phase II trial of neoadjuvant chemotherapy in early-stage small cell cervical cancer. Anticancer Drugs. 10(7):641-6, 1999
14. Sykes AJ et al: Small cell carcinoma of the uterine cervix: a clinicopathological review. Int J Oncol. 14(2):381-6, 1999
15. Zhou C et al: Small cell carcinoma of the uterine cervix: cytologic findings in 13 cases. Cancer. 84(5):281-8, 1998
16. Kim YB et al: Successful treatment of neuroendocrine small cell carcinoma of the cervix metastatic to regional lymph nodes. Gynecol Oncol. 62(3):411-4, 1996
17. Sevin BU et al: Efficacy of radical hysterectomy as treatment for patients with small cell carcinoma of the cervix. Cancer. 77(8):1489-93, 1996
18. Toki T et al: Small-cell neuroendocrine carcinoma of the uterine cervix associated with micro-invasive squamous cell carcinoma and adenocarcinoma in situ. Pathol Int. 46(7):520-5, 1996

SMALL CELL CARCINOMA, CERVIX

IMAGE GALLERY

Typical

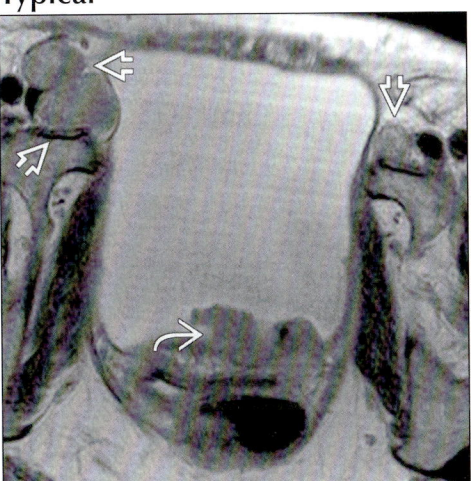
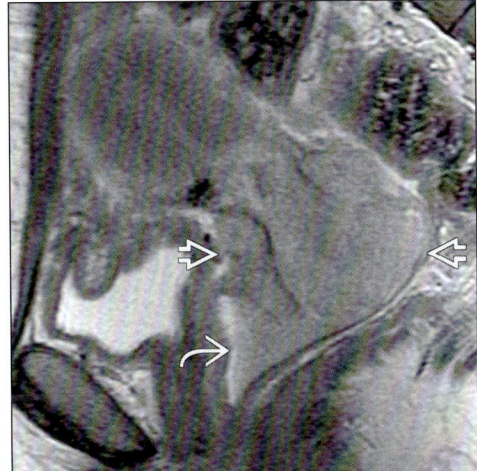

(Left) Axial oblique T2WI MR in the same patient as in the previous images shows enlarged bilateral deep inguinal lymph nodes ➡. Bladder invasion is also noted ➡ in keeping with stage IVA disease. *(Right)* Sagittal T2WI MR shows a large lobulated cervical mass of intermediate SI ➡. Note that the tumor is extending into the upper part of the vagina ➡.

Typical

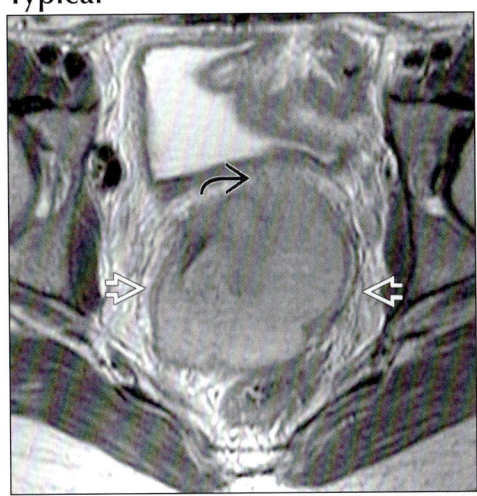
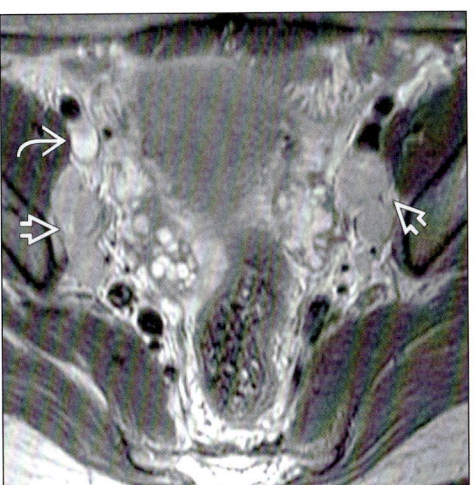

(Left) Axial oblique T2WI MR in the same patient as previous image shows a large lobulated cervical mass ➡. Note tumor extension into the paracervical fat ➡ of the utero-vesical lipoma. *(Right)* Axial T2WI MR in the same patient as previous image shows enlarged bilateral external iliac lymph nodes ➡. Also note the presence of thrombus within the right external iliac vein ➡.

Typical

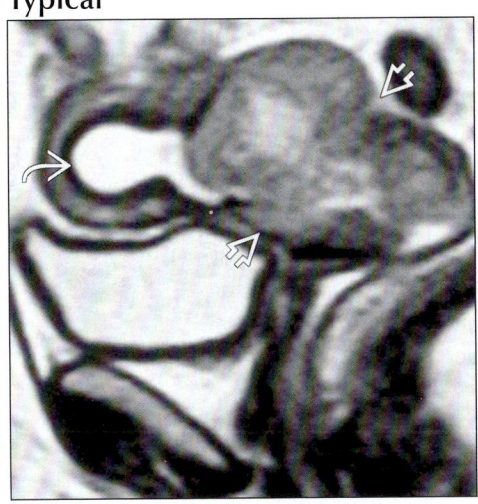
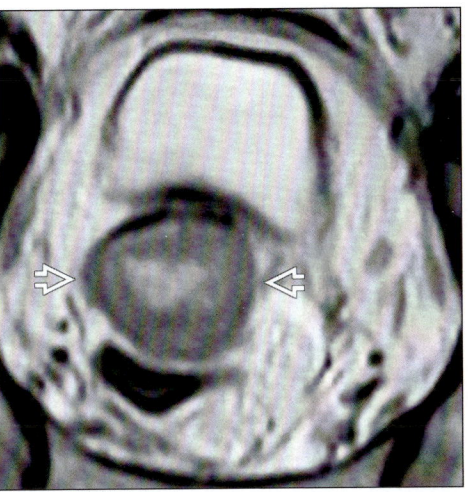

(Left) Sagittal T2WI MR shows a lobulated cervical mass ➡ of intermediate signal intensity causing fluid retention ➡ within the endometrial cavity. (Courtesy of T. Cunha, MD). *(Right)* Axial oblique T2WI MR in the same patient as previous image shows a lobulated cervical mass with bilateral parametrial invasion ➡. Pathology: Small cell carcinoma of the cervix. (Courtesy of T. Cunha, MD).

CERVICAL CANCER, RECURRENCE

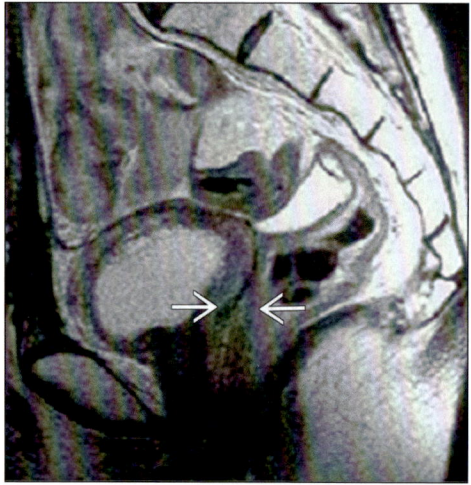

Sagittal T2WI MR shows normal vaginal cuff ➡ without evidence of recurrence. Thickening and higher than normal signal intensity of the vaginal and rectal wall represent postradiation changes.

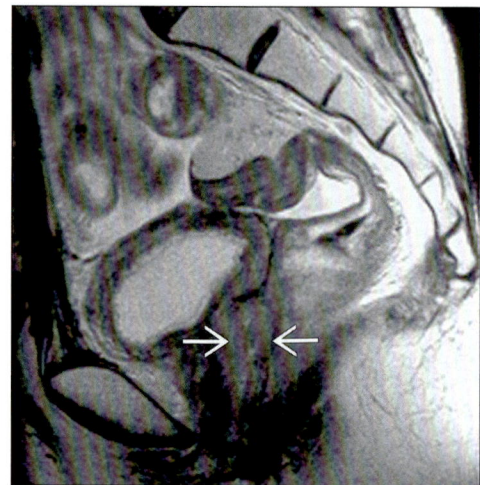

Sagittal T2WI MR shows recurrent cervical cancer seen as a high signal intensity nodular mass ➡ at the vaginal cuff on follow-up.

TERMINOLOGY

Definitions
- Recurrence is defined as local tumor re-growth or development of distant metastasis at least 6 months after the treated lesion has regressed
- Cervical cancer recurrence can be seen after radiation or surgical treatment

IMAGING FINDINGS

General Features
- Best diagnostic clue: New or enlarging heterogeneous soft tissue mass with variable amount of necrosis
- Location
  - Most common sites of local recurrence
    - Vaginal cuff
    - Cervix
    - Parametrial region
    - Pelvic side wall
    - Pelvic lymph nodes
  - Most common sites of distant recurrence
    - Extrapelvic lymph nodes
    - Peritoneum
    - Lung
    - Liver
    - Bone
- Size: Varies from small to large depending on the extent of disease
- Morphology: Recurrent cervical cancer may be seen as a well-defined focal mass or an ill-defined infiltrative mass

Ultrasonographic Findings
- Grayscale Ultrasound: US may demonstrate a soft tissue mass, but typically is not useful in further characterization of recurrent cervical cancer

CT Findings
- NECT: Recurrent cervical cancer is of iso-attenuation to cervix or soft tissues
- CECT
  - Post-radiation recurrence is usually of iso- or hypoattenuation relative to cervical stroma on CECT
  - Post surgical recurrence appears as an enhancing soft tissue mass
  - Necrosis can be seen in the recurrent mass as nonenhancing regions

DDx: Cervical Cancer: Post Treatment Appearances

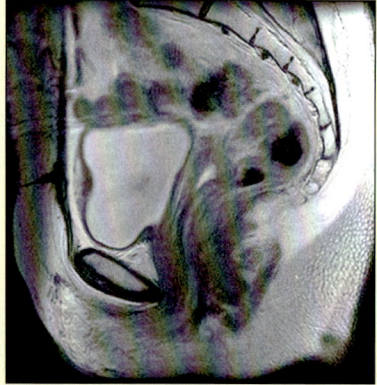
After Surgery

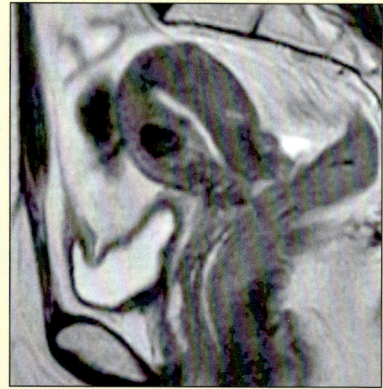
After Radiation Treatment

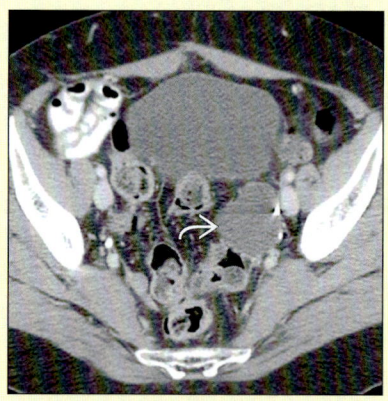
Lymphocele

CERVICAL CANCER, RECURRENCE

Key Facts

Terminology
- Recurrence is defined as local tumor re-growth or development of distant metastasis at least 6 months after the treated lesion has regressed

Imaging Findings
- Best diagnostic clue: New or enlarging heterogeneous soft tissue mass with variable amount of necrosis
- Size: Varies from small to large depending on the extent of disease
- Morphology: Recurrent cervical cancer may be seen as a well-defined focal mass or an ill-defined infiltrative mass
- CT is useful for detecting lymph node and extrauterine recurrences
- MR imaging is superior to CT for delineating local recurrences in the cervix after radiation treatment and in the vaginal cuff and pelvis after surgery
- FDG-PET is also a sensitive post-therapy surveillance modality for detection of recurrent cervical cancer

Diagnostic Checklist
- After radiation treatment, recurrence can be ruled out if reconstitution of the normal zonal anatomy of the cervix and the presence of homogeneous low signal intensity cervical stroma are seen on T2WI
- After surgery nodular or irregular thickening at the vaginal cuff or presence of a soft tissue mass in the pelvic side wall indicate recurrent disease

MR Findings
- T1WI: Recurrent cervical cancer is of intermediate signal intensity similar to the signal intensity of cervix or soft tissues
- T2WI
  - Most useful sequence in detection of tumor recurrence after radiation
  - Postradiation recurrence is seen as a high signal intensity mass within low signal intensity cervix
  - Post surgical recurrence appears as a heterogeneous high signal intensity soft tissue mass
- T1 C+
  - Recurrent cervical cancer shows varying degrees of enhancement
  - Necrosis can be seen in the recurrent mass as nonenhancing regions

Nuclear Medicine Findings
- PET
  - Recurrent cervical cancer shows increased activity on FDG-PET
  - Lymph node or distant recurrences also show increased uptake and are easily detected
  - PET may show recurrences earlier than other imaging methods do

Imaging Recommendations
- Best imaging tool
  - CT is useful for detecting lymph node and extrauterine recurrences
  - MR imaging is superior to CT for delineating local recurrences in the cervix after radiation treatment and in the vaginal cuff and pelvis after surgery
  - MR is the most accurate method to differentiate postsurgical and post-radiation changes from recurrence because of its high soft tissue contrast resolution
  - FDG-PET is also a sensitive post-therapy surveillance modality for detection of recurrent cervical cancer

DIFFERENTIAL DIAGNOSIS

Post-Surgical Changes
- Late fibrosis (> 1 year) is of low signal intensity on T2WI
- Early fibrosis may be of high signal intensity and may enhance mimicking tumor recurrence

Lymphocele
- Lymphoceles may be confused with cystic recurrences
- Lymphoceles are entirely cystic and thin-walled unless complicated with infection or hemorrhage
- Recurrent cystic masses are associated with enhancing nodular soft tissue components

Post-Radiation Changes
- Presence of uniformly low signal intensity stroma on T2WI and normal paracervical tissues exclude recurrence
- Postradiation fibrosis, inflammation, radiation necrosis show enhancement and may mimic recurrent tumor

PATHOLOGY

General Features
- General path comments
  - Most recurrences occur within first 2 years after treatment
  - Risk factors for recurrence
    - Grade and histologic type of tumor
    - Tumor size
    - Depth of stromal invasion
    - Presence of lymph node involvement

CLINICAL ISSUES

Presentation
- Most common signs/symptoms
  - Vaginal bleeding
  - Pelvic pain

CERVICAL CANCER, RECURRENCE

- Urinary symptoms
- Bowel obstruction
- Weight gain or loss
- Clinical Profile: Patients may be asymptomatic or may present with new signs/symptoms suggesting recurrence

Natural History & Prognosis
- 30% of patients with cervical carcinoma die as a result of recurrent or persistent disease

Treatment
- Therapeutic options for recurrent tumor include surgery, radiation therapy, and chemotherapy, depending on the primary tumor therapy and the location and extent of the recurrence
- Surgery: Pelvic exenteration
  - Absolute contraindications to pelvic exenteration include peritoneal metastasis and skip metastasis to bowel
  - Relative contraindications to pelvic exenteration include metastasis to retroperitoneal nodes, direct tumor invasion of adherent bowel loops, and hydroureter or hydronephrosis
- Radiation: External beam radiation therapy or brachytherapy
- Chemotherapy: Alone or in-combination with surgery/radiation

DIAGNOSTIC CHECKLIST

Consider
- Role of imaging is to detect the recurrent disease and determine its extent
- Determination of the extent of recurrent disease with imaging helps in selection of optimal therapy
  - If imaging shows locally recurrent disease, either radiation after radical hysterectomy; or pelvic exenteration after primary radiation therapy can be used
  - If imaging shows recurrent disease outside the initial treatment field, radiation to provide local control and symptomatic relief; or chemotherapy for systemic control can be used

Image Interpretation Pearls
- After radiation treatment, recurrence can be ruled out if reconstitution of the normal zonal anatomy of the cervix and the presence of homogeneous low signal intensity cervical stroma are seen on T2WI
  - However, early post-radiation changes such as a widened endocervical canal or high signal intensity cervical stroma can mimic tumor
  - Serial MR imaging is useful for distinguishing recurrent disease from radiation-induced changes, as the latter is expected to remain stable or decrease over time
- After surgery nodular or irregular thickening at the vaginal cuff or presence of a soft tissue mass in the pelvic side wall indicate recurrent disease
- Imaging is also useful in the assessment of complications related to recurrent disease such as
  - Hydronephrosis due to ureteral invasion/encasement
  - Small or large bowel obstruction
  - Rectal or vesical fistulas
  - Arterial or venous vascular invasion

SELECTED REFERENCES

1. Akin O et al: Imaging of uterine cancer. Radiol Clin North Am. 45(1):167-82, 2007
2. Chung HH et al: Clinical impact of FDG-PET imaging in post-therapy surveillance of uterine cervical cancer: from diagnosis to prognosis. Gynecol Oncol. 103(1):165-70, 2006
3. Engin G: Cervical cancer: MR imaging findings before, during, and after radiation therapy. Eur Radiol. 16(2):313-24, 2006
4. Sahdev A et al: MR imaging appearances of the female pelvis after trachelectomy. Radiographics. 25(1):41-52, 2005
5. Chang WC et al: Usefulness of FDG-PET to detect recurrent cervical cancer based on asymptomatically elevated tumor marker serum levels--a preliminary report. Cancer Invest. 22(2):180-4, 2004
6. Unger JB et al: Detection of recurrent cervical cancer by whole-body FDG PET scan in asymptomatic and symptomatic women. Gynecol Oncol. 94(1):212-6, 2004
7. Havrilesky LJ et al: The role of PET scanning in the detection of recurrent cervical cancer. Gynecol Oncol. 90(1):186-90, 2003
8. Jeong YY et al: Uterine cervical carcinoma after therapy: CT and MR imaging findings. Radiographics. 23(4):969-81; discussion 981, 2003
9. Scheidler J et al: Imaging of cancer of the cervix. Radiol Clin North Am. 40(3):577-90, vii, 2002
10. Nicolet V et al: MR imaging of cervical carcinoma: a practical staging approach. Radiographics. 20(6):1539-49, 2000
11. Stehman FB et al: Uterine cervix. In: Hoskins WJ, Perez CA, Young RC (eds). Principles and practice of gynecologic oncology, Lippincott Williams & Wilkins, Philadelphia. 841-918, 2000
12. Yamashita Y et al: Dynamic contrast-enhanced MR imaging of uterine cervical cancer: pharmacokinetic analysis with histopathologic correlation and its importance in predicting the outcome of radiation therapy. Radiology. 216(3):803-9, 2000
13. Manfredi R et al: Cervical cancer response to neoadjuvant therapy: MR imaging assessment. Radiology. 209(3):819-24, 1998
14. Blomlie V et al: Critical soft tissues of the female pelvis: serial MR imaging before, during, and after radiation therapy. Radiology. 203(2):391-7, 1997
15. Hawighorst H et al: Pelvic lesions in patients with treated cervical carcinoma: efficacy of pharmacokinetic analysis of dynamic MR images in distinguishing recurrent tumors from benign conditions. AJR Am J Roentgenol. 166(2):401-8, 1996
16. Weber TM et al: Cervical carcinoma: determination of recurrent tumor extent versus radiation changes with MR imaging. Radiology. 194(1):135-9, 1995

CERVICAL CANCER, RECURRENCE

IMAGE GALLERY

Typical

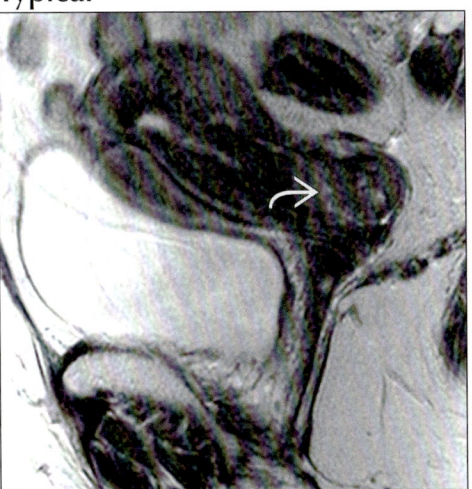
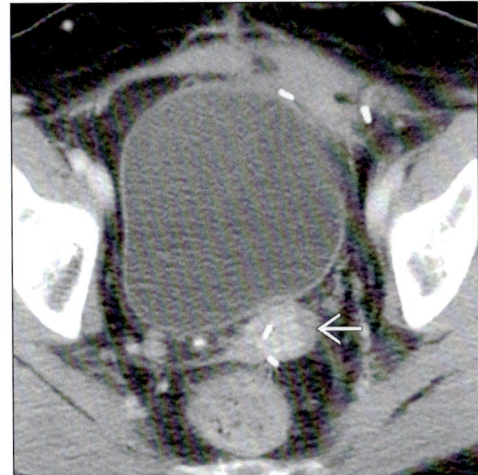

(Left) Sagittal T2WI MR shows recurrent cervical cancer after radiation treatment. Note that the mass ➔ has slightly higher signal intensity within low signal intensity cervical stoma. *(Right)* Axial CECT shows recurrent cervical cancer seen as an enhancing nodular mass ➔ at the left vaginal cuff after surgery.

Typical

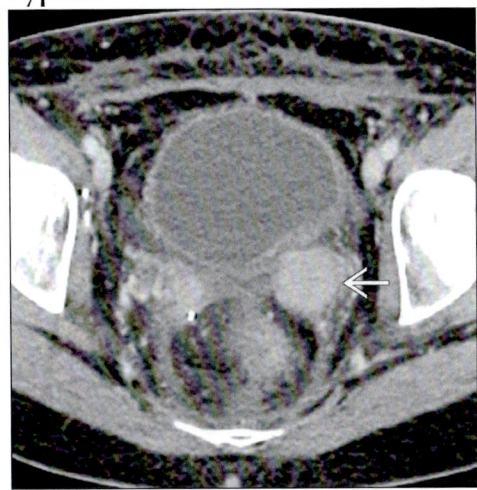
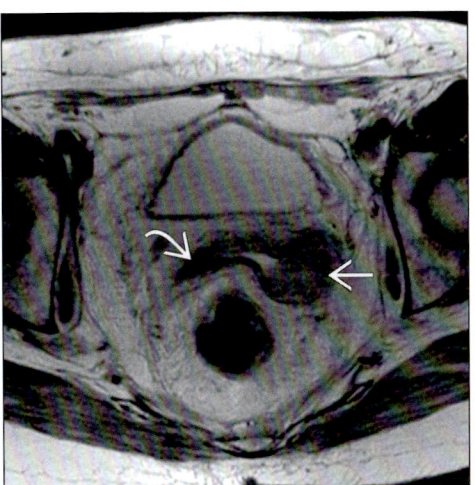

(Left) Axial CECT shows a recurrent cervical cancer seen as an enhancing mass ➔ in the left pelvis. *(Right)* Axial T2WI MR shows recurrent cervical cancer seen as a nodular mass ➔ at the left vaginal cuff. Note the normal appearance and thickness of the right vaginal cuff ➔.

Typical

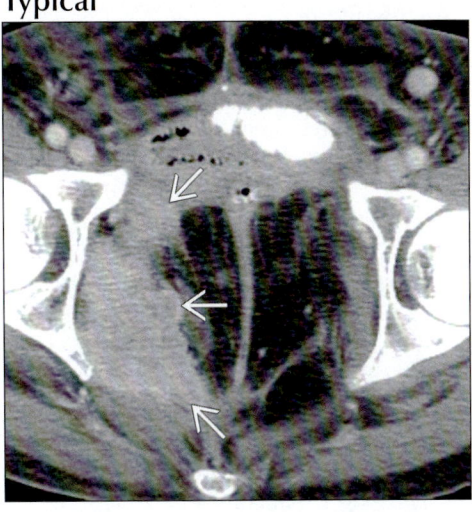
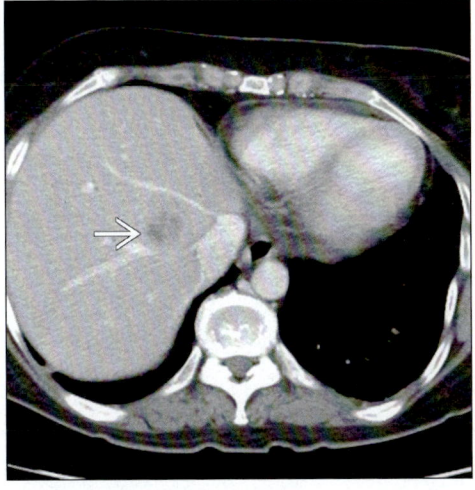

(Left) Axial CECT shows a large recurrent cervical cancer ➔ invading the right pelvic side wall. *(Right)* Axial CECT shows recurrent cervical cancer presented with liver metastasis ➔ after treatment of the primary disease.

ADENOMA MALIGNUM

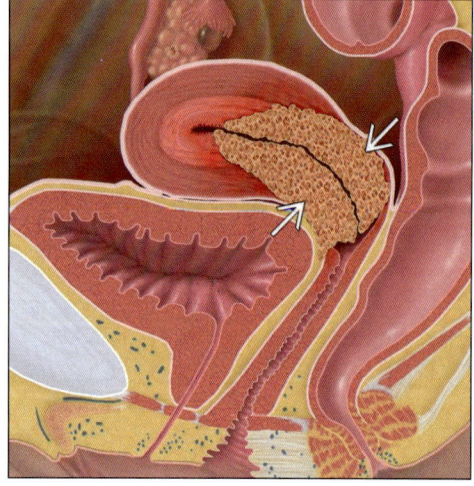

Graphic shows adenoma malignum ➔ seen as multiple grape-like cysts within the cervix.

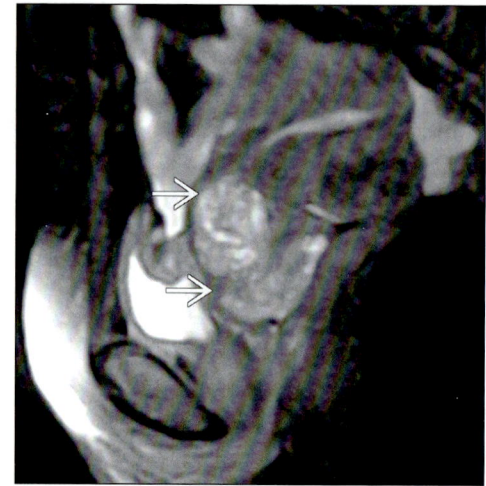

Sagittal T1WI FS MR shows an enlarged cervix with multiple cystic lesions suggesting adenoma malignum ➔.

TERMINOLOGY

Abbreviations and Synonyms
- Mucinous minimal deviation adenocarcinoma

Definitions
- Subtype of mucinous adenocarcinoma of the cervix

IMAGING FINDINGS

General Features
- Best diagnostic clue
  - Enlarged cervix: Multiple grape-like cysts within cervical stroma
  - Fluid (mucin) within uterus and/or vagina may be present

CT Findings
- Low attenuation cysts within enlarged cervix

MR Findings
- T1WI
  - Enlarged cervix with low signal intensity cysts
  - Low signal intensity fluid may be present in uterus and/or vagina
- T2WI: Multiple high signal intensity cysts within low signal intensity stroma
- T1 C+: Low signal intensity cysts embedded in enhancing stroma

DIFFERENTIAL DIAGNOSIS

Nabothian Cysts
- Cervix may be enlarged
- Superficial epithelial cysts of variable sizes
  - Deep-seated cysts are problematic

Endocervical Glandular Hyperplasia with Pyloric Gland Metaplasia
- Benign entity
- No mucoid vaginal discharge
- Does not extend into uterus

Cervical Cancer (Histology other than Adenoma Malignum)
- Invasive solid cervical mass

DDx: Cervical Masses

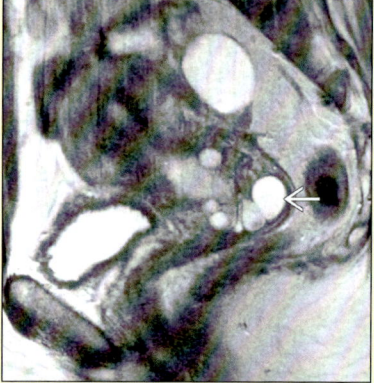

Nabothian Cysts

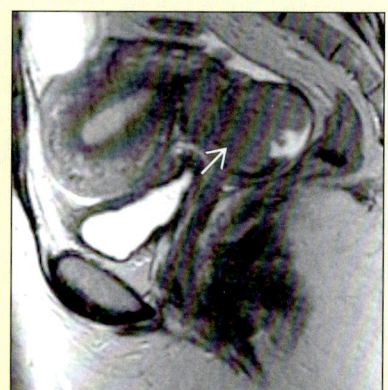

Cervical Cancer

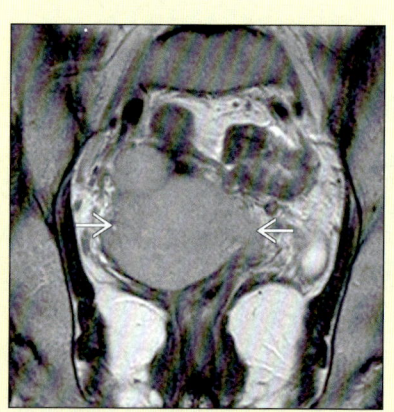

Cervical Lymphoma

ADENOMA MALIGNUM

Key Facts

Terminology
- Mucinous minimal deviation adenocarcinoma
- Subtype of mucinous adenocarcinoma of the cervix

Imaging Findings
- Enlarged cervix: Multiple grape-like cysts within cervical stroma
- Fluid (mucin) within uterus and/or vagina may be present

Pathology
- Difficult diagnosis on regular "punch" biopsy, Papanicolaou smear, or colposcopy
- Imaging findings guide deep cervical stromal biopsy
- Etiology: About 3% of all cervical adenocarcinomas

Clinical Issues
- Initial symptom is often a watery discharge

Cervical Lymphoma
- Solid mass diffusely involving the cervix

PATHOLOGY

General Features
- General path comments
  - Its deceptively benign histologic appearance occasionally leads to an incorrect diagnosis
  - Difficult diagnosis on regular "punch" biopsy, Papanicolaou smear, or colposcopy
  - Imaging findings guide deep cervical stromal biopsy
- Etiology: About 3% of all cervical adenocarcinomas
- Associated abnormalities: Peutz-Jeghers syndrome (mucocutaneous pigmentation and multiple hamartomatous polyps of the intestinal tract, mucinous tumors of the ovary)

Gross Pathologic & Surgical Features
- Cervix is enlarged, firm and indurated
- Mucosal surface may be hemorrhagic, friable, or mucoid
- Cysts are embedded deeply in cervix

Microscopic Features
- Mucinous glands the majority of which have a deceptively benign histological appearance
- Cysts are irregular in size and shape, lined by mucin-containing columnar epithelial cells

CLINICAL ISSUES

Presentation
- Most common signs/symptoms
  - Initial symptom is often a watery discharge
  - Vaginal bleeding

Demographics
- Age: Average age 25-72 years (average 42)

Natural History & Prognosis
- Prognosis is unfavorable as it disseminates into peritoneal cavity in early stage of disease
- Indolent compared to more common squamous cell cervical cancer

Treatment
- Surgery

SELECTED REFERENCES

1. Okamoto Y et al: MR imaging of the uterine cervix: imaging-pathologic correlation. Radiographics. 23(2):425-45; quiz 534-5, 2003
2. Young RH et al: Endocervical adenocarcinoma and its variants: their morphology and differential diagnosis. Histopathology. 41(3):185-207, 2002
3. Doi T et al: Adenoma malignum: MR imaging and pathologic study. Radiology. 204(1):39-42, 1997
4. Gilks CB et al: Adenoma malignum (minimal deviation adenocarcinoma) of the uterine cervix. A clinicopathological and immunohistochemical analysis of 26 cases. Am J Surg Pathol. 13(9):717-29, 1989

IMAGE GALLERY

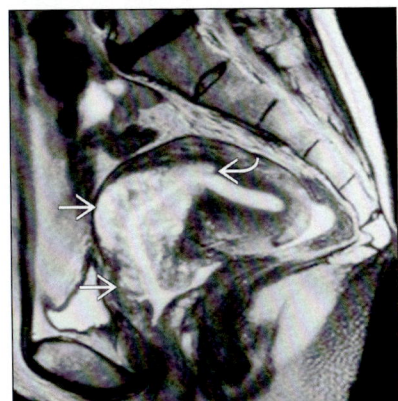
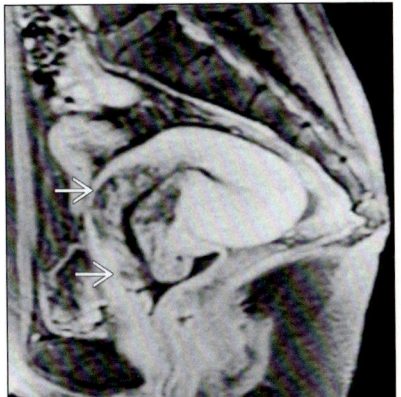
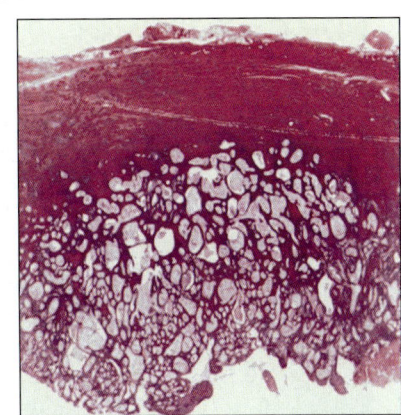

(Left) Sagittal T2WI MR shows adenoma malignum ➡ seen as grape-like cysts within enlarged cervix. Note that the lesion extends to lower uterine segment ➡. (Center) Sagittal T1 C+ FS MR shows adenoma malignum ➡. Note that the cysts do not enhance. (Right) Micropathology shows multiple cysts of various sizes within the cervical stoma.

LYMPHOMA, CERVIX

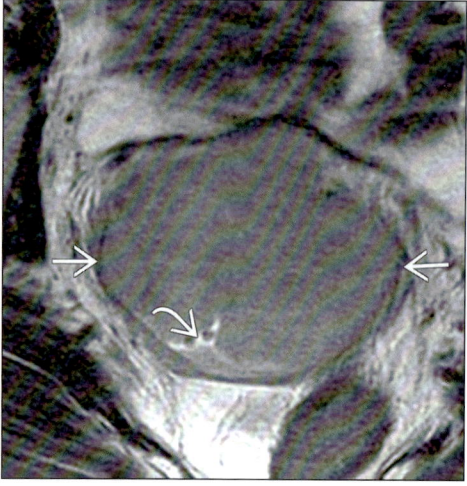

Axial oblique T2WI MR shows cervical lymphoma seen as a bulky homogeneous mass ➡ arising in the cervix. Note that the endocervical canal ➡ is intact.

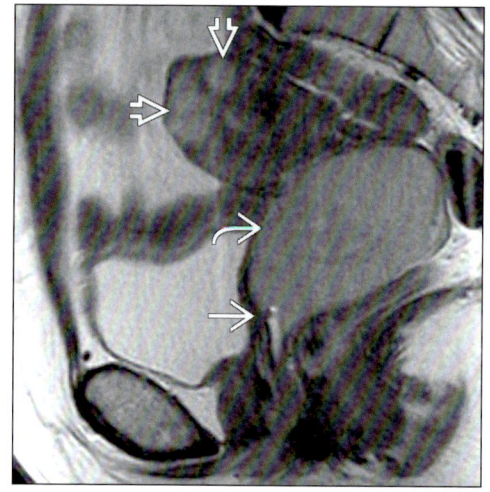

Sagittal T2WI MR shows that cervical lymphoma ➡ extends to the upper vagina ➡. Other lymphomatous lesions ➡ are also seen in the uterine fundus.

TERMINOLOGY

Definitions
- Lymphoma involving uterine cervix

IMAGING FINDINGS

General Features
- Best diagnostic clue
  - Cervical mass causing diffuse enlargement of uterine cervix is the most common finding
  - Less commonly, a polypoid or nodular mass or a submucosal mass may be seen
  - Diffuse involvement of the cervical stroma with preservation of the endocervical canal is a key finding
- Location: Cervix is the most common site of uterine lymphomas
- Size: Cervical lymphoma often presents as large mass (> 4 cm)
- Morphology: Barrel-shaped diffuse cervical stromal involvement with or without surface erosion

Ultrasonographic Findings
- Grayscale Ultrasound: US is limited in tumor depiction but a mass with uniform echogenicity causing diffuse cervical enlargement may be seen

CT Findings
- NECT: Diffuse enlargement of cervix with soft tissue attenuation
- CECT: Enhancement may be homogeneous or heterogeneous

MR Findings
- T1WI: Homogeneous mass with similar signal intensity compared to cervical stroma
- T2WI: Homogeneous mass with high signal intensity compared to cervical stroma
- T1 C+: Moderate, homogeneous or heterogeneous enhancement

Nuclear Medicine Findings
- PET
  - Lymphoma shows increased uptake on FDG PET
  - FDG PET can accurately show other sites of disease involvement

DDx: Cervical Masses

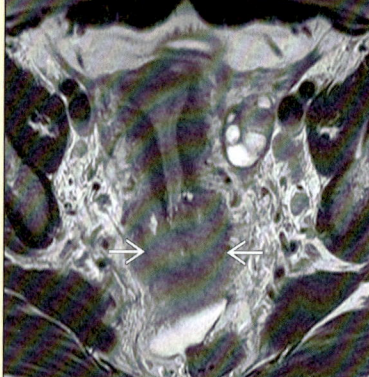

Cervical Cancer

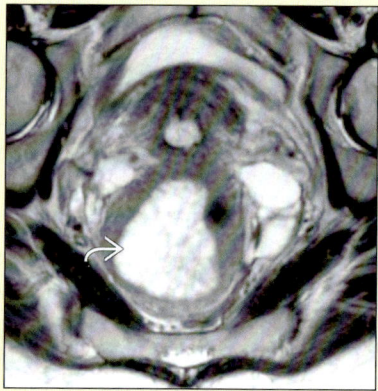

Cervical Polyp

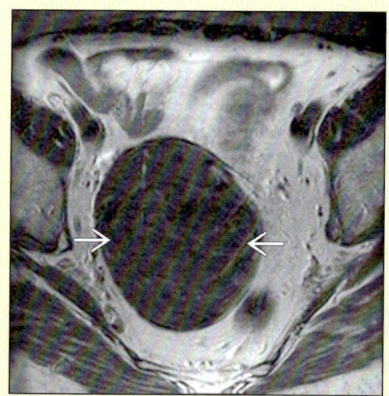

Cervical Leiomyoma

LYMPHOMA, CERVIX

Key Facts

Imaging Findings
- Cervical mass causing diffuse enlargement of uterine cervix is the most common finding
- Less commonly, a polypoid or nodular mass or a submucosal mass may be seen
- Diffuse involvement of the cervical stroma with preservation of the endocervical canal is a key finding
- Location: Cervix is the most common site of uterine lymphomas
- Size: Cervical lymphoma often presents as large mass (> 4 cm)

Pathology
- Cervical lymphomas typically originate from the cervical stroma and the superficial squamous epithelium is often preserved without ulceration
- Cervical lymphoma accounts for 2% of extranodal lymphomas in women

Diagnostic Checklist
- Because cervical lymphomas typically arise within the cervical stroma rather than the mucosa, Papanicolaou smear is not a sensitive screening tool clinically
- Imaging findings of diffuse stromal involvement can aid in the planning of deep incisional or excisional cervical biopsy to establish the diagnosis
- MR findings of a cervical mass causing diffuse enlargement of uterine cervix with preservation of endocervical canal suggests lymphoma rather than cervical cancer
- Cross-sectional imaging is also very helpful in tumor staging and follow-up of treatment response

Imaging Recommendations
- Best imaging tool
  - Cross-sectional imaging with CT or MR is used in determining the extent of disease
  - FDG PET can also be used in tumor staging and monitoring of treatment response
  - MR is the method of choice in depiction of local extent of disease
  - MR can reveal preservation of low signal intensity cervical canal, which is helpful in differential diagnosis
- Protocol advice
  - High-resolution T2WI in transverse, coronal and sagittal planes is essential
  - T1 C+ is optional

DIFFERENTIAL DIAGNOSIS

Cervical Cancer
- Cervical cancer originates in the endocervical canal and invades into the cervical stroma
- Diffuse stromal involvement and preservation of endocervical canal suggests cervical lymphoma

Cervical Polyp
- Benign cervical polyps are located in the endocervical canal and do not invade into cervical stroma

Cervical Leiomyoma
- Leiomyomas have typical low signal intensity on T2WI

Cervical Metastasis
- Cervical metastasis can occur by contiguous or non-contiguous involvement of cervical stroma

PATHOLOGY

General Features
- General path comments
  - Lymphoma rarely involves uterus
    - Cervical involvement is three times more common than endometrial involvement
  - Majority of uterine cervical lymphomas are B cell lymphomas
    - Diffuse large cell and follicular lymphomas are most common types involving cervix and uterus
  - Non-B cell lymphomas such as T lymphomas, natural killer cell lymphomas, Burkitt lymphoma also have been reported as case reports
  - Cervical lymphomas typically originate from the cervical stroma and the superficial squamous epithelium is often preserved without ulceration
    - Papanicolaou smear is negative in the majority of patients with cervical lymphoma
  - Definitive diagnosis of cervical lymphoma is usually made with histologic analysis of a deep incisional or excisional cervical biopsy
- Etiology
  - Chronic inflammation (autoimmune or not autoimmune nature) has been proposed as an etiologic factor but this has not been completely proved
  - In cervical lymphomas, the role of human papillomavirus or Epstein-Barr virus is not as clear as it is in squamous cell carcinoma or adenocarcinoma
- Epidemiology
  - Primary lymphoma of the genital tract is a very rare disease
  - Cervical lymphoma accounts for 2% of extranodal lymphomas in women

Gross Pathologic & Surgical Features
- Large tumor causing enlargement of cervix
- Endocervical canal is preserved despite large tumor size

Microscopic Features
- Lymphoma cells diffusely proliferate within cervical stroma

Staging, Grading or Classification Criteria
- Ann Arbor staging system and World Health Organization classification system are used

LYMPHOMA, CERVIX

CLINICAL ISSUES

Presentation
- Most common signs/symptoms
  - Abnormal vaginal bleeding and/or discharge
  - Pelvic discomfort or pain
  - Urinary symptoms
  - Large, bulky cervix on pelvic examination
- Other signs/symptoms
  - Weight loss
  - Weakness
  - Night sweats
  - Fever
- Clinical Profile: Primary cervical lymphomas usually grow rapidly and most patients present with a large cervical mass

Demographics
- Age
  - Age at presentation ranges from 20 years to 80 years
  - Median age varies from 40 years to 59 years

Natural History & Prognosis
- Prognosis of cervical lymphoma is better than lymphoma involving ovary
- Prognosis of cervical lymphoma is better than cervical cancer
- 89% survival rate reported in localized stages
- Prognostic factors are the same as that for other extranodal lymphomas
  - Age
  - Stage of tumor
  - Number of extranodal sites involved
  - Patient's performance status
  - Serum LDH level

Treatment
- Because cervical lymphoma is an uncommon malignancy, the standard treatment has not been established
- Chemotherapy regimen including cyclophosphamide, doxorubicin, vincristine, predninose, and bleomycin followed by pelvic radiation provides best survival rates
- Other treatment options
  - Chemotherapy alone
  - Radiation alone
  - Surgery alone

DIAGNOSTIC CHECKLIST

Consider
- Because cervical lymphomas typically arise within the cervical stroma rather than the mucosa, Papanicolaou smear is not a sensitive screening tool clinically
- Imaging findings of diffuse stromal involvement can aid in the planning of deep incisional or excisional cervical biopsy to establish the diagnosis

Image Interpretation Pearls
- MR findings of a cervical mass causing diffuse enlargement of uterine cervix with preservation of endocervical canal suggests lymphoma rather than cervical cancer
- Cross-sectional imaging is also very helpful in tumor staging and follow-up of treatment response

SELECTED REFERENCES

1. Cantu de Leon D et al: Primary malignant lymphoma of uterine cervix. Int J Gynecol Cancer. 16(2):923-7, 2006
2. Hariprasad R et al: Primary uterine lymphoma: report of 2 cases and review of literature. Am J Obstet Gynecol. 195(1):308-13, 2006
3. Semczuk A et al: Primary non-Hodgkin's lymphoma of the uterine cervix mimicking leiomyoma: case report and review of the literature. Pathol Res Pract. 202(1):61-4, 2006
4. Chan JK et al: Clinicopathologic features of six cases of primary cervical lymphoma. Am J Obstet Gynecol. 193(3 Pt 1):866-72, 2005
5. Dursun P et al: Primary cervical lymphoma: report of two cases and review of the literature. Gynecol Oncol. 98(3):484-9, 2005
6. Kosari F et al: Lymphomas of the female genital tract: a study of 186 cases and review of the literature. Am J Surg Pathol. 29(11):1512-20, 2005
7. Thyagarajan MS et al: Case report: appearance of uterine cervical lymphoma on MRI: a case report and review of the literature. Br J Radiol. 77(918):512-5, 2004
8. Au WY et al: Primary B-cell lymphoma and lymphoma-like lesions of the uterine cervix. Am J Hematol. 73(3):176-9, 2003
9. Okamoto Y et al: MR imaging of the uterine cervix: imaging-pathologic correlation. Radiographics. 23(2):425-45; quiz 534-5, 2003
10. Bode MK et al: Lymphoma of the cervix. Imaging and transcatheter arterial embolization. Acta Radiol. 43(4):431-2, 2002
11. Marin C et al: Magnetic resonance imaging of primary lymphoma of the cervix. Eur Radiol. 12(6):1541-5, 2002
12. Suzuki Y et al: Magnetic resonance images of primary malignant lymphoma of the uterine body: a case report. Jpn J Clin Oncol. 30(11):519-21, 2000
13. Bilgin T et al: Primary malignant lymphoma of the uterine cervix: difficulties in diagnosis. J Obstet Gynaecol. 19(6):671-2, 1999
14. Kim YS et al: MR imaging of primary uterine lymphoma. Abdom Imaging. 22(4):441-4, 1997
15. Kawakami S et al: MR appearance of malignant lymphoma of the uterus. J Comput Assist Tomogr. 19(2):238-42, 1995

LYMPHOMA, CERVIX

IMAGE GALLERY

Typical

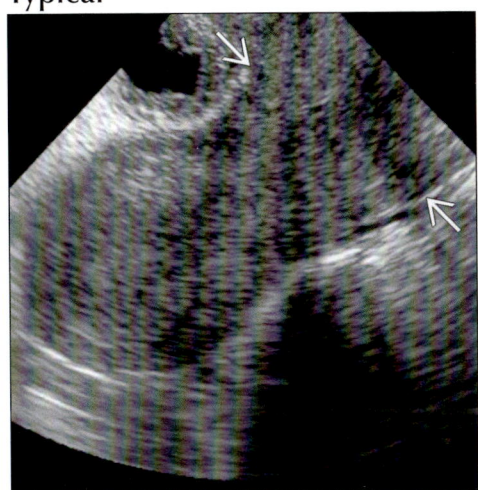
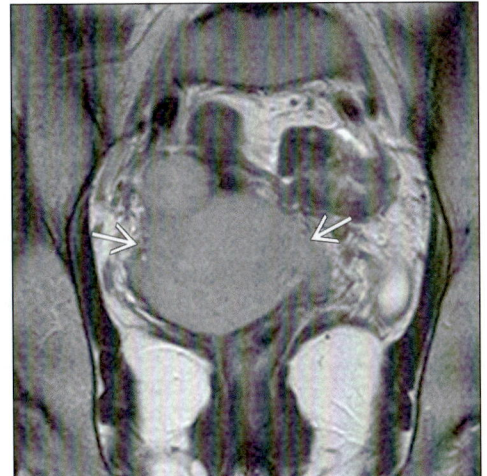

(Left) Sagittal transvaginal ultrasound shows cervical lymphoma causing diffuse enlargement of the uterine cervix ➡. *(Right)* Coronal T2WI MR shows cervical lymphoma seen as a high signal intensity mass ➡ involving the uterine cervix.

Typical

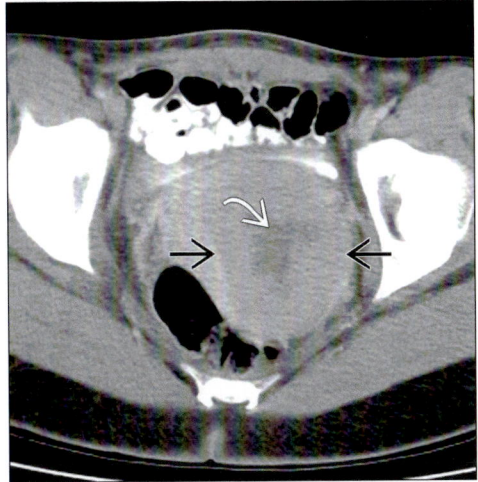
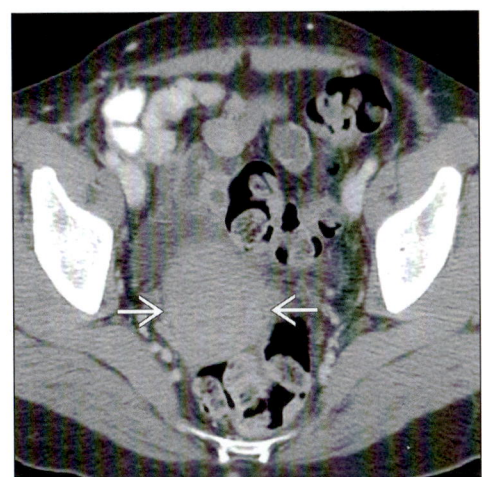

(Left) Axial CECT shows cervical lymphoma seen as a low-attenuation mass ➡ causing cervical enlargement. A central low attenuation area consistent with necrosis ➡ is also seen within the mass. *(Right)* Axial CECT shows another case of cervical lymphoma seen as a homogeneous mass ➡ in the cervix.

Typical

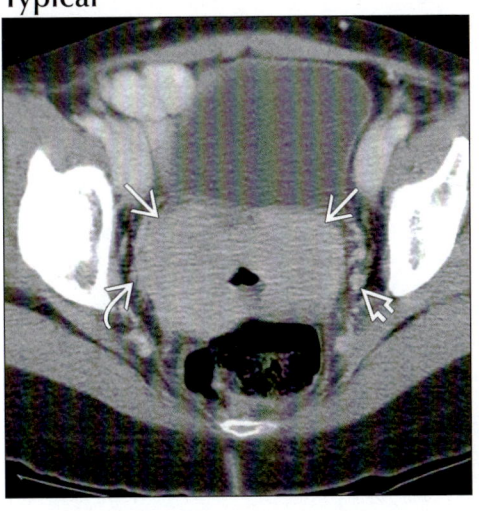
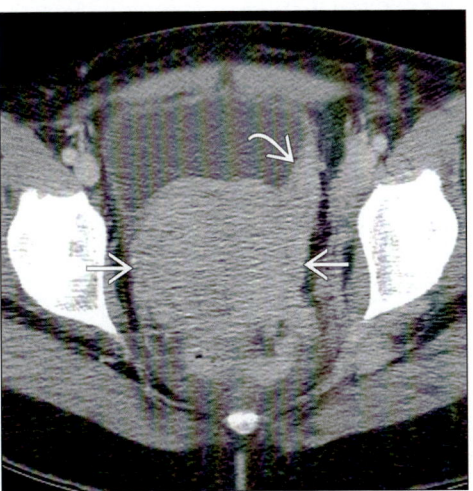

(Left) Axial CECT shows a large cervical lymphoma ➡. Note that parametrial vessels are encased on the right indicating parametrial invasion ➡. Compare to the normal parametrial vessels ➡ on the left. *(Right)* Axial CECT shows another large cervical lymphoma ➡. Note that the mass invades the urinary bladder and causes urinary bladder wall thickening ➡ on the left.

SARCOMA, CERVIX

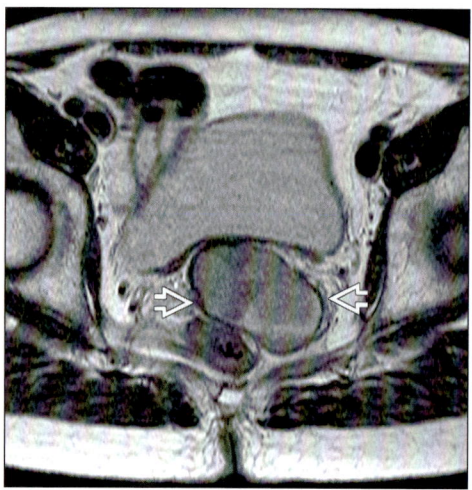

Axial T2WI MR shows an example of leiomyosarcoma with a mass of heterogeneous signal intensity arising form the cervix ➡. No parametrial extension is seen.

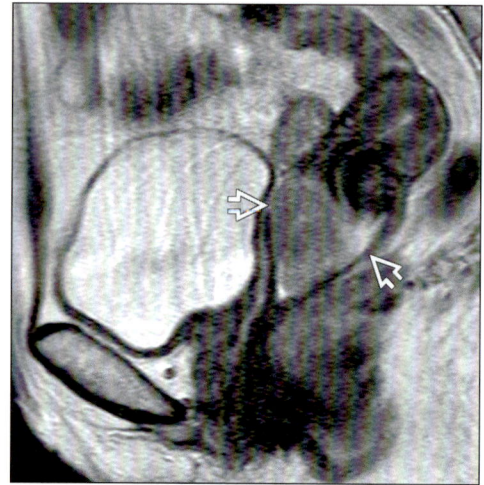

Sagittal T2WI MR shows the same patient as previous image with a bulky mass of heterogeneous signal intensity ➡ expanding the cervix. Pathology: Leiomyosarcoma.

TERMINOLOGY

Definitions
- Group of rare tumors of mesenchymal origin arising from the cervix

IMAGING FINDINGS

General Features
- Best diagnostic clue: Heterogeneous enhancing mass arising from cervix
- Location: Cervix
- Size: Variable depending on histology; can be over 10 cm
- Morphology: Diffusely infiltrating cervical tumor or polypoid mass

Ultrasonographic Findings
- Polypoid or diffusely infiltrating cervical mass of heterogeneous echotexture

CT Findings
- Heterogeneously enhancing pelvic mass
- Useful for distant staging

MR Findings
- Mass of variable size
  - May appear polypoid (e.g., botryoid subtype of embryonal rhabdomyosarcoma)
  - Heterogeneous low signal intensity on T1WI, high signal intensity on T2WI
  - Heterogeneity due to areas of hemorrhage and necrosis and presence of fat in liposarcoma
- May have low signal intensity pseudocapsule
- May extend into uterine corpus, vagina or parametria
- Demonstrates heterogeneous enhancement

Imaging Recommendations
- Best imaging tool
  - MR
    - For local staging and treatment planning
- Protocol advice
  - T1WI: Axial, large FOV
  - T2WI: Axial, sagittal, small FOV
  - T2WI: Axial oblique and coronal oblique images perpendicular and parallel to the cervix
  - T1 C+ FS: Axial, small FOV

DDx: Cervical Masses

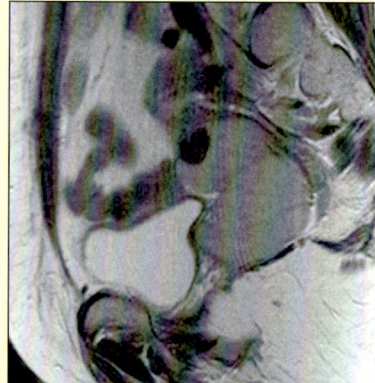
Cervical Lymphoma

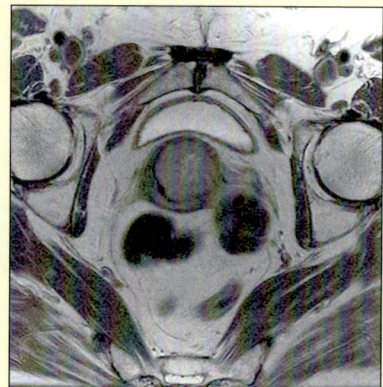
Cervical Carcinoma

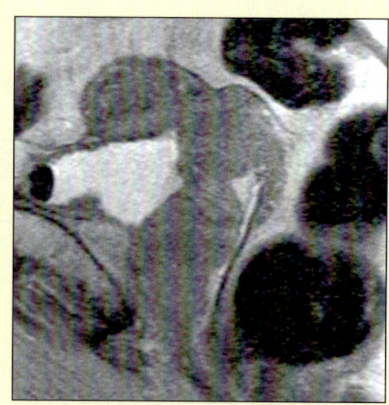
Cervical Metastasis

SARCOMA, CERVIX

Key Facts

Terminology
- Group of rare tumors of mesenchymal origin arising from the cervix

Imaging Findings
- Best diagnostic clue: Heterogeneous enhancing mass arising from cervix
- Size: Variable depending on histology; can be over 10 cm
- Morphology: Diffusely infiltrating cervical tumor or polypoid mass

Top Differential Diagnoses
- Cervical Carcinoma
- Cervical Lymphoma
- Cervical Metastasis

Pathology
- Sarcomas account for approximately 0.5% of all malignancies arising in the cervix

Clinical Issues
- Long term follow-up difficult due to rarity of sarcomas
- Patients tend to develop hematogenous metastases
- Prognosis depends on histology and is variable
- Disease free intervals between 1 year to > 8 years reported
- Multimodality treatment including surgery (total abdominal hysterectomy ± bilateral salpingo-oophorectomy ± pelvic lymphadenectomy)
- Combination chemotherapy (can be given as neoadjuvant) and radiotherapy

DIFFERENTIAL DIAGNOSIS

Cervical Carcinoma
- Carcinoma occurs much more commonly than sarcoma
- Imaging characteristics cannot reliably distinguish carcinoma from sarcoma
- Cervical carcinoma tends to be more homogeneous than cervical sarcoma

Cervical Lymphoma
- Homogeneous bulky mass of high SI on T2WI
- Enlarged lymph nodes in the case of secondary lymphoma

Cervical Metastasis
- Mass of heterogeneous high SI on T2WI
- Primary tumor may be evident

PATHOLOGY

General Features
- Epidemiology
  - Sarcomas account for approximately 0.5% of all malignancies arising in the cervix
  - Reported frequencies in the literature
    - Embryonal rhabdomyosarcoma 64%
    - Leiomyosarcoma 13%
    - Undifferentiated endocervical sarcoma 7%
    - Alveolar soft part sarcoma 5%
    - Ewing sarcoma (primitive neuroectodermal tumor) 4%
    - Malignant peripheral nerve sheath tumor 3%
    - Liposarcoma 2%
    - Others 2% e.g., myeloid (granulocytic) sarcoma, chondrosarcoma, mixed epithelial and mesenchymal tumors

Gross Pathologic & Surgical Features
- Rhabdomyosarcoma
  - Infiltrating or encapsulated tumor; may have gelatinous myxoid areas or hemorrhage and necrosis
  - Botryoid type appears as intraluminal mass composed of smooth grapelike clusters
- Leiomyosarcoma
  - Large (about 10 cm), poorly circumscribed mass that either protrudes from cervical canal or diffusely expands it circumferentially
- Malignant peripheral nerve sheath tumor
  - Polypoid masses about 3-4 cm in size
- Ewing sarcoma
  - Well-circumscribed mass of about 5-6 cm in size
- Alveolar soft part sarcoma
  - Well-circumscribed mass with mean size of approximately 2.4 cm
- Undifferentiated endocervical sarcoma
  - Variable appearance: Protruding polypoid masses, ulcerated masses, or circumferential replacement of cervix
  - Hemorrhage and necrosis is common
- Liposarcoma
  - Protuberant polypoid masses with areas of gross hemorrhage
- Malignant mixed Müllerian tumor
  - Polypoid or pedunculated mass, 1-10 cm in size, with solid and necrotic areas

Microscopic Features
- Rhabdomyosarcoma
  - Divided into embryonal (70%), alveolar (20%) and undifferentiated subtypes (10%)
    - Botryoid subtype accounts for 10% of embryonal tumors
    - Botryoid subtype arises under mucosal surface
  - Tumor cells analogous to various maturational stages of fetal muscle cells (rhabdomyoblasts)
  - Range in appearances from primitive mesenchymal tumors with stellate cells to well-differentiated lesions with myofiber-like cells and cross striations
  - Immunohistochemistry: Antibodies directed toward myoglobin, desmin, actin, and the MyoD1 gene product
- Leiomyosarcoma

SARCOMA, CERVIX

- Histological subtypes are as in the corpus uteri; includes myxoid variant, epithelioid variant with abundance of xanthomatous cells and osteoclast like giant cells
- Malignant peripheral nerve sheath tumor
  - Cells show differentiation toward cells intrinsic to the peripheral nerve sheath
  - Spindle cells may be arranged in herring bone, nodular or storiform fascicles
  - In contrast to other sarcomas, cells tend to infiltrate but not destroy native endocervical glands
  - Immunohistochemistry: Cells positive for S100 (not always) and vimentin, negative for desmin, myoglobin and actin
- Ewing sarcoma
  - Cells show varying degrees of neuroectodermal differentiation
- Alveolar soft part sarcoma
  - Comprised of large cells with eosinophilic or granular cytoplasm arranged in solid and/or alveolar nests
- Undifferentiated endocervical sarcoma
  - No specific line of differentiation
  - Moderate to high grade
- Liposarcoma
  - Includes pleomorphic, round cell and well-differentiated
- Mixed epithelial and mesenchymal tumors
  - Combination of malignant epithelial and mesenchymal components
  - Epithelial component includes squamous cell carcinoma, basaloid squamous carcinoma, adenocarcinoma, adeno-squamous carcinoma, adenoid-basal carcinoma, adenoid-cystic carcinoma and undifferentiated carcinoma
  - Sarcomatous component may be homologous (fibroblasts and smooth muscle) or heterologous (cartilage, striated muscle, bone etc.)
  - Spectrum of malignancy: Includes adenosarcoma of relatively low-grade malignancy to highly aggressive malignant mixed Müllerian tumor
  - Immunohistochemistry: Positive for cytokeratin; sarcomatous components may be positive for vimentin, desmin, muscle specific actin (SMA) and smooth muscle-specific actin (SMA)

CLINICAL ISSUES

Presentation
- Most common signs/symptoms
  - Abnormal vaginal bleeding
  - Pelvic pain
- Other signs/symptoms: Vaginal discharge

Demographics
- Age
  - Depends on histology
    - Rhabdomyosarcoma: 1st 2 decades
    - Leiomyosarcoma: 4th-6th decades
    - Undifferentiated endocervical sarcoma: 29-72 years (mean 51 years)
    - Alveolar soft part sarcoma: 8-39 years (mean 29.9 years)
    - Ewing sarcoma: 21-51 years (mean 38 years)
    - Malignant peripheral nerve sheath tumor: 25-73 years (mean 50 years)
    - Liposarcoma: 45-62 years (mean 54 years)
    - Malignant mixed Müllerian tumor: 12-93 years (mean 65 years)
- Gender: Females

Natural History & Prognosis
- Long term follow-up difficult due to rarity of sarcomas
- Patients tend to develop hematogenous metastases
- Prognosis depends on histology and is variable
- Disease free intervals between 1 year to > 8 years reported
- Rhabdomyosarcoma
  - Botryoid subtype associated with a very favorable outcome
  - Alveolar and undifferentiated associated with poor outcomes
  - 5-YSR > 50% for patients with metastatic embryonal subtype under age of 10 years
- Cervical alveolar soft part sarcoma may have better prognosis than soft tissue counterpart
  - Tends to be slow growing, can develop local and distant metastases
- Malignant mixed Müllerian tumor may have better prognosis than uterine counterpart

Treatment
- Multimodality treatment including surgery (total abdominal hysterectomy ± bilateral salpingo-oophorectomy ± pelvic lymphadenectomy)
- Combination chemotherapy (can be given as neoadjuvant) and radiotherapy

DIAGNOSTIC CHECKLIST

Consider
- Sarcoma is a rare cause of patient presenting with cervical (polypoid) mass

Image Interpretation Pearls
- Polypoid or diffusely infiltrating mass involving the cervix of heterogeneous signal intensity on T1 and T2 WI and showing heterogeneous enhancement
- May show local or distant spread

SELECTED REFERENCES
1. Fadare O: Uncommon sarcomas of the uterine cervix: a review of selected entities. Diagn Pathol. 1:30, 2006
2. Maheshwari A et al: Diagnostic dilemma in a case of malignant mixed mullerian tumor of the cervix. World J Surg Oncol. 4:36, 2006
3. Pathak B et al: Granulocytic sarcoma presenting as tumors of the cervix. Gynecol Oncol. 98(3):493-7, 2005
4. Villella JA et al: Rhabdomyosarcoma of the cervix in sisters with review of the literature. Gynecol Oncol. 99(3):742-8, 2005
5. Gotoh T et al: Epithelioid leiomyosarcoma of the uterine cervix. Gynecol Oncol. 2001

SARCOMA, CERVIX

IMAGE GALLERY

Typical

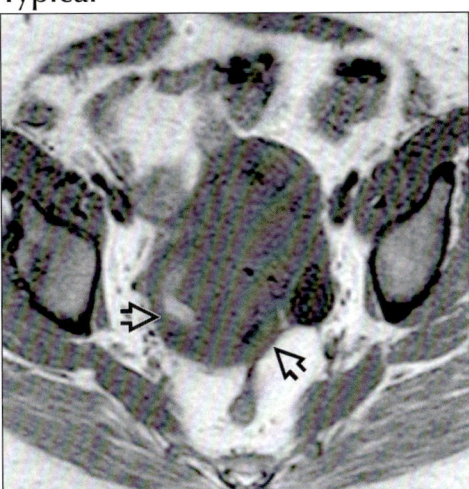
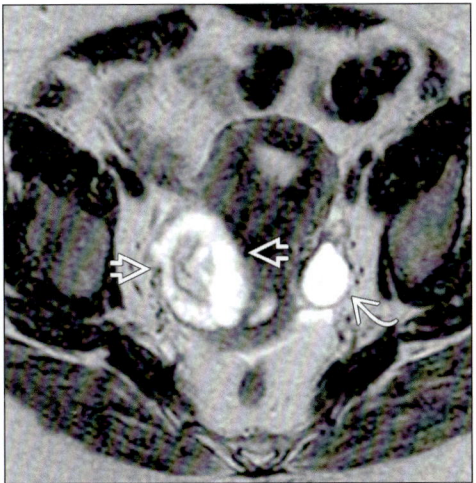

(Left) Axial T1WI MR shows an example of cervical myxoid chondrosarcoma ➡ which is predominantly low signal with central necrosis. *(Right)* Axial T2WI MR in the same patient as previous image. The cervical mass ➡ is mainly high signal on this sequence. The right ovary was seen separate to this (not shown). Left ovary was normal ➡.

Typical

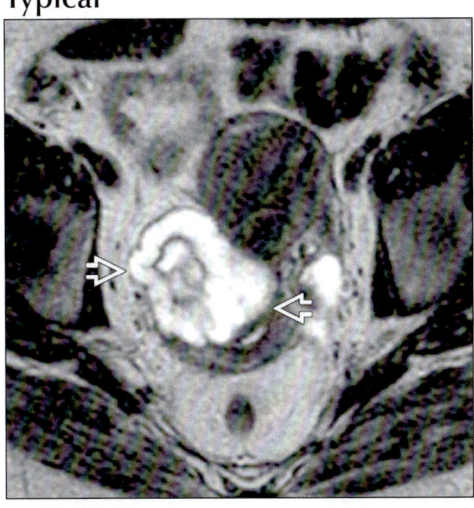
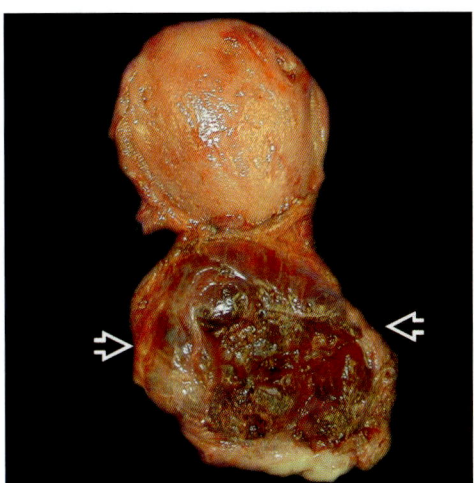

(Left) Axial T2WI MR in the same patient as previous image shows a lobulated mass of high signal intensity ➡ arising from the cervix. *(Right)* Gross pathology shows resected specimen from the same patient as previous image. The chondrosarcoma appears as a bulky cervical mass with areas of hemorrhage and necrosis ➡.

Typical

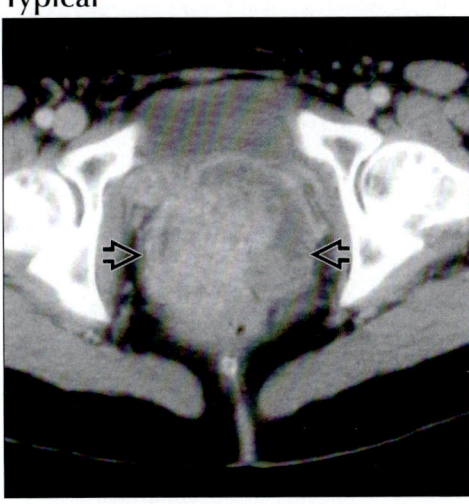
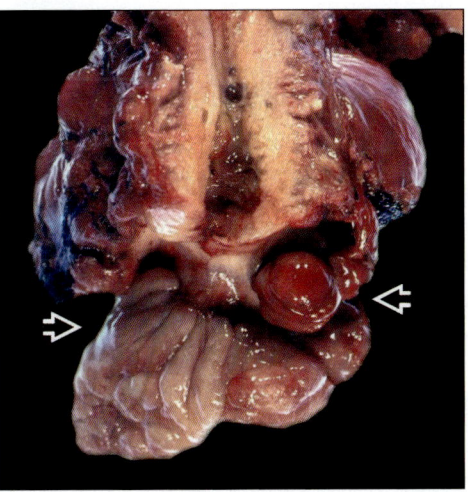

(Left) Axial CECT shows bulky cervical mass demonstrating heterogeneous enhancement ➡ in a patient with adenosarcoma. *(Right)* Gross pathology in the same patient as previous image shows a large lobulated mass arising from the cervix ➡.

ENDOMETRIOID CERVICAL ADENOCARCINOMA

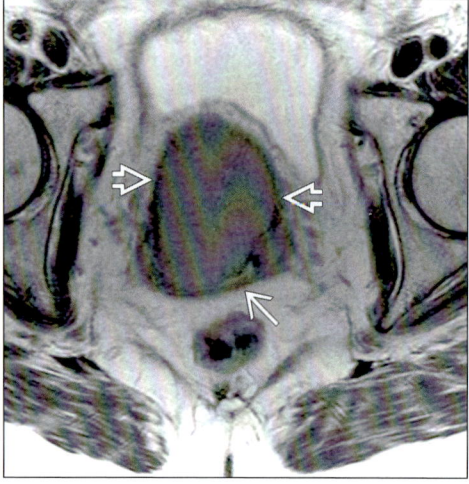 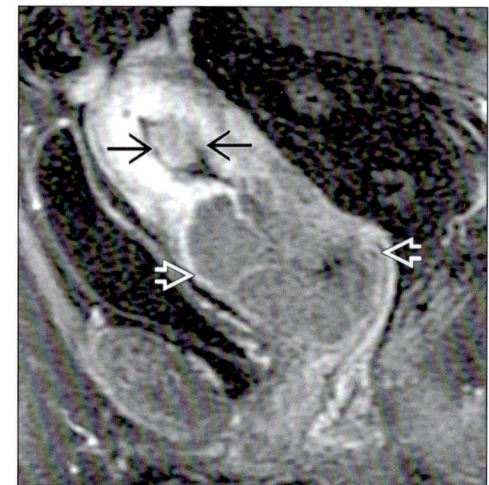

Axial oblique T2WI MR shows a large tumor of intermediate SI arising from the cervix and indenting the vagina ➡ posteriorly. Low signal intensity cervical stroma ➡ appears intact.

Sagittal T1 C+ FS MR in the same patient as previous image shows a cervical mass with rim enhancement ➡. A submucosal leiomyoma is also noted ➡. Pathology: Endometrioid cervical adenocarcinoma.

TERMINOLOGY

Definitions
- One of the major histologic subtypes of adenocarcinoma of the cervix

IMAGING FINDINGS

General Features
- Best diagnostic clue
  - High signal intensity (SI) cervical mass on T2WI in the absence of primary endometrial lesion
    - It is not usually possible to distinguish different histological subtypes of adenocarcinoma on imaging
- Location: Endocervix
- Size: Variable

Ultrasonographic Findings
- Grayscale Ultrasound
  - Transvaginal ultrasound (TVS) findings
    - Enlarged cervix or ill-defined, isoechoic mass
    - Tumors confined to the cervix are difficult to differentiate from surrounding normal cervical stroma
    - Parametrial invasion can be suspected by the presence of hypoechoic tumor extending continuously into the lateral parametrium
    - ± Hyperechoic areas if necrosis or air
  - Transrectal ultrasonography (TRUS) can also be performed
    - Findings are similar to those on transvaginal ultrasound, depending on stage of tumor
    - Useful in the pre-operative assessment of parametrial invasion
    - Less useful in the assessment of large tumors due to restricted field of view

CT Findings
- CECT
  - Normal size or enlarged cervix
  - Isodense or hypodense cervical mass
  - Irregular margins suggestive of parametrial invasion
  - ± Hydronephrosis and hydroureter if pelvic side wall involvement with tumor
  - ± Retroperitoneal or pelvic adenopathy

DDx: Cervical Masses

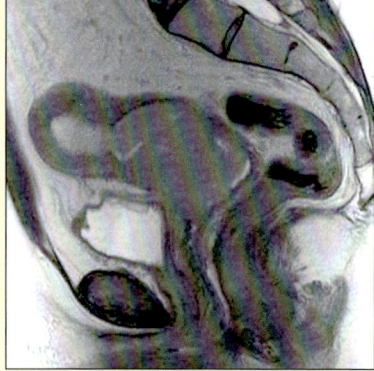 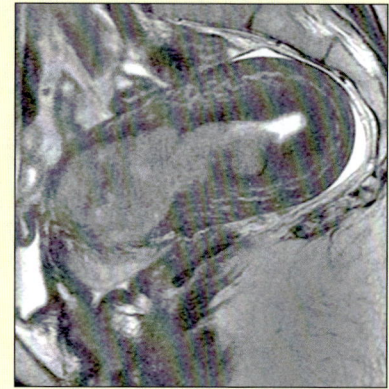 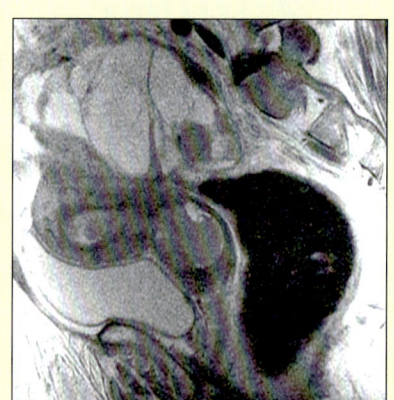

Advanced Cervical Cancer | Advanced Endometrial Cancer | Cervical Metastasis

ENDOMETRIOID CERVICAL ADENOCARCINOMA

Key Facts

Terminology
- One of the major histologic subtypes of adenocarcinoma of the cervix

Imaging Findings
- High signal intensity (SI) cervical mass on T2WI in the absence of primary endometrial lesion
- Complete disruption of low signal intensity cervical ring indicates full thickness stromal involvement

Top Differential Diagnoses
- Cervical Squamous Cell Carcinoma (SCC)
- Advanced Endometrial Adenocarcinoma
- Cervical Metastasis
- Cervical Sarcoma
- Cervical Lymphoma

Pathology
- General path comments: Tumor cells resemble primary adenocarcinoma of uterine corpus
- Human papillomavirus types 16 and 18
- Endometrioid subtype accounts for 20-25% of endocervical adenocarcinoma
- FIGO staging: Same as for cervical SCC
- FIGO grading: Similar to uterine endometrioid adenocarcinoma; based on microscopic appearance

Clinical Issues
- Often asymptomatic
- Spontaneous or postcoital bleeding
- Slightly older age group than SCC
- Cervical adenocarcinoma has worse prognosis than SCC

- ○ ± Hematogenous metastases

MR Findings
- T1WI: Intermediate SI cervical mass; isointense to cervical stroma
- T2WI
  - High SI cervical mass compared to cervical stroma
    - High SI tumor may extend into lower uterine segment
    - Tumor may extend into upper vagina with loss of normal low SI or may demonstrate hyperintense thickening of vagina
    - Complete disruption of low signal intensity cervical ring indicates full thickness stromal involvement
    - Tumor may extend into parametria and adjacent structures
- T1 C+ FS
  - Compared to squamous cell carcinoma (SCC), adenocarcinoma may show
    - Preservation of endocervical epithelium due to submucosal location
    - Less contrast-enhancement
    - Peripheral rim-enhancement compared to heterogeneous enhancement throughout tumor in SCC

Imaging Recommendations
- Best imaging tool
  - MR imaging method of choice
    - Defines local staging and treatment planning
  - CT used for distant staging
- Protocol advice
  - T1WI: Axial, large FOV
  - T2WI: Axial, sagittal; small FOV
  - T2WI: Axial or coronal oblique; small FOV
  - T1 C + FS: Optional

DIFFERENTIAL DIAGNOSIS

Cervical Squamous Cell Carcinoma (SCC)
- Higher signal on T2WI in SCC
- Greater and more heterogeneous enhancement throughout tumor

Advanced Endometrial Adenocarcinoma
- Presence of endometrial thickening ± mass
- Distension of endometrial cavity by mass
- Invasion of myometrium from endometrium
- Bulk of tumor centered on endometrial cavity

Cervical Metastasis
- ± Presence of primary tumor

Cervical Sarcoma
- Bulky mass of heterogeneous SI on T2WI

Cervical Lymphoma
- Cervical mass of homogeneous high SI on T2WI
- Associated lymphadenopathy in secondary lymphoma

PATHOLOGY

General Features
- General path comments: Tumor cells resemble primary adenocarcinoma of uterine corpus
- Etiology
  - Human papillomavirus types 16 and 18
  - Precursor: Endocervical glandular dysplasia
  - Risk factors for adenocarcinoma
    - Nulliparity
    - Diabetes
    - Young age at 1st sexual intercourse
    - Many sexual partners
    - Obesity
- Epidemiology
  - Endometrioid subtype accounts for 20-25% of endocervical adenocarcinoma
    - Three fold increase in incidence rate in all ages from 1966 to 1990
- Associated abnormalities: May arise from areas of endometriosis

Gross Pathologic & Surgical Features
- Mass in cervix

ENDOMETRIOID CERVICAL ADENOCARCINOMA

- Likely primary cervix if
  - Bulk of tumor concentrated on the cervix with little corpus enlargement

Microscopic Features
- Glands, islands and sheets of columnar cells with round nuclei
- Mucin is not a feature
- Frequently contains foci of squamous differentiation
- May be difficult to determine if primary endometrial or primary endocervical
- Likely primary cervix if
  - Areas of cervical adenocarcinoma in situ (AIS) or squamous intraepithelial lesion (SIL)

Staging, Grading or Classification Criteria
- FIGO staging: Same as for cervical SCC
- FIGO grading: Similar to uterine endometrioid adenocarcinoma; based on the microscopic appearance
  - Grade 1 = < 5% solid component
  - Grade 2 = 5-50% solid component
  - Grade 3 = > 50% solid component

CLINICAL ISSUES

Presentation
- Most common signs/symptoms
  - Often asymptomatic
  - Spontaneous or postcoital bleeding
- Other signs/symptoms: Pelvic pain

Demographics
- Age
  - Mean age 56 years
  - Slightly older age group than SCC

Natural History & Prognosis
- Cervical adenocarcinoma has worse prognosis than SCC
- 5 yr survival rates for cervical adenocarcinoma
  - 79% for stage I
  - 64% for stage II
  - 22% for stage III
  - 11% for stage IV

Treatment
- Surgery ± radiotherapy for stages I-IIA
- Chemoradiation for stages IIB-IVA
- Palliative chemotherapy and radiotherapy for stage IVB
- Total pelvic exenteration in patients with isolated pelvic recurrence

DIAGNOSTIC CHECKLIST

Consider
- Endometrioid cervical adenocarcinoma is difficult to distinguish clinically from endometrial carcinoma
  - Imaging, especially MR, is of value in determining the site of origin of the tumor
  - Biopsy of cervical mass confirms endometrioid histology

Image Interpretation Pearls
- Bulk of tumor centered in the cervix rather than endometrium

SELECTED REFERENCES

1. Chargui R et al: Prognostic factors and clinicopathologic characteristics of invasive adenocarcinoma of the uterine cervix. Am J Obstet Gynecol. 194(1):43-8, 2006
2. Sherman ME et al: Mortality trends for cervical squamous and adenocarcinoma in the United States. Relation to incidence and survival. Cancer. 15;103(6):1258-64, 2005
3. Wang SS et al: Cervical adenocarcinoma and squamous cell carcinoma incidence trends among white women and black women in the United States for 1976-2000. Cancer. 1;100(5):1035-44, 2004
4. Alfsen GC et al: Reproducibility of classification in non-squamous cell carcinomas of the uterine cervix. Gynecol Oncol. 90(2):282-9, 2003
5. Andersson S et al: Types of human papillomavirus revealed in cervical adenocarcinomas after DNA sequencing. Oncol Rep. 10(1):175-9, 2003
6. Okamoto Y et al: MR imaging of the uterine cervix: imaging-pathologic correlation. Radiographics. 23(2):425-5, 2003
7. Scheidler J et al: Imaging of cancer of the cervix. Radiol Clin North Am. 40(3):577-90, 2002
8. Young RH et al: Endocervical adenocarcinoma and its variants: their morphology and differential diagnosis. Histopathology. 41(3):185-207, 2002
9. Alfsen GC et al: Histologic subtype has minor importance for overall survival in patients with adenocarcinoma of the uterine cervix: a population-based study of prognostic factors in 505 patients with nonsquamous cell carcinomas of the cervix. Cancer. 1;92(9):2471-83, 2001
10. Grisaru D et al: Does histology influence prognosis in patients with early-stage cervical carcinoma? Cancer. 15;92(12):2999-3004, 2001
11. Alfsen GC et al: Histopathologic subtyping of cervical adenocarcinoma reveals increasing incidence rates of endometrioid tumors in all age groups: a population based study with review of all nonsquamous cervical carcinomas in Norway from 1966 to 1970, 1976 to 1980, and 1986 to 1990. Cancer. 15;89(6):1291-9, 2000
12. Palit A et al: Endometroid adenocarcinoma of the cervix in a 9-year-old girl. Br J Radiol. 71(850):1093-5, 1998
13. Torashima M et al: Invasive adenocarcinoma of the uterine cervix: MR imaging. Comput Med Imaging Graph. 21(4):253-60, 1997
14. Anton-Culver H et al: Comparison of adenocarcinoma and squamous cell carcinoma of the uterine cervix: a population-based epidemiologic study. Am J Obstet Gynecol. 166(5):1507-14, 1992
15. Innocenti P et al: Staging of cervical cancer: reliability of transrectal US. Radiology. 185(1):201-5, 1992

ENDOMETRIOID CERVICAL ADENOCARCINOMA

IMAGE GALLERY

Typical

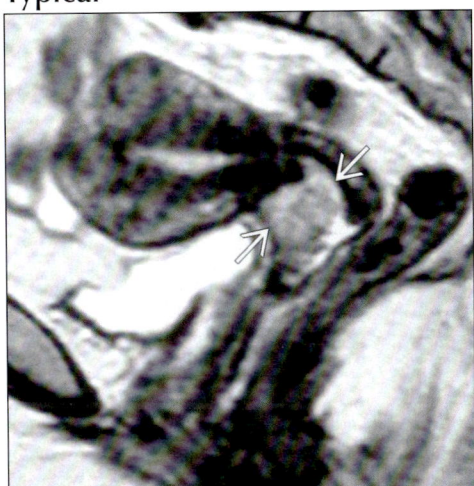
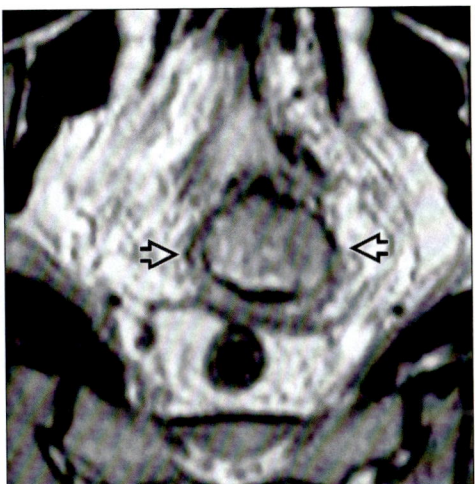

(Left) Sagittal T2WI MR shows high SI cervical mass ➡. *(Right)* Coronal oblique T2WI MR in same patient as previous image, again demonstrates cervical mass ➡. There is preservation of low SI cervical stroma excluding parametrial invasion. Pathology: Endometroid cervical adenocarcinoma.

Typical

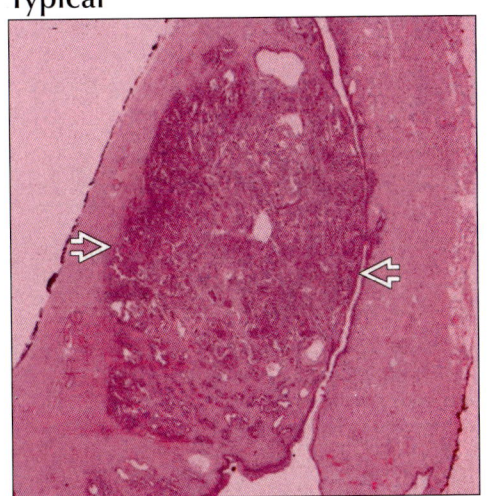
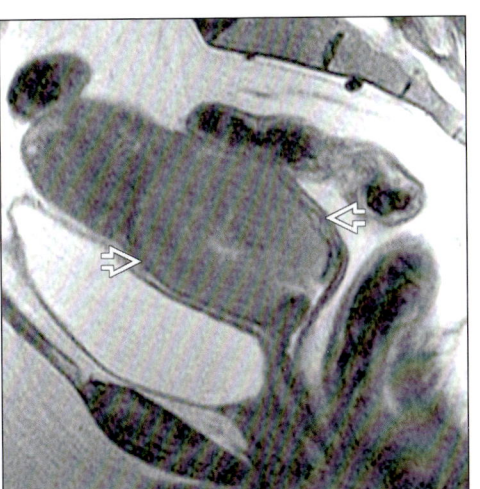

(Left) Micropathology in same patient as previous image shows irregular glands and solid sheets of malignant cells at the squamocolumnar junction ➡; no mucin is demonstrated. Pathology: Endometroid cervical adenocarcinoma. *(Right)* Sagittal T2WI MR shows a large round intermediate SI mass arising from the cervix ➡ and extending into the lower uterine segment. Pathology: Endometroid adenocarcinoma of the cervix.

Typical

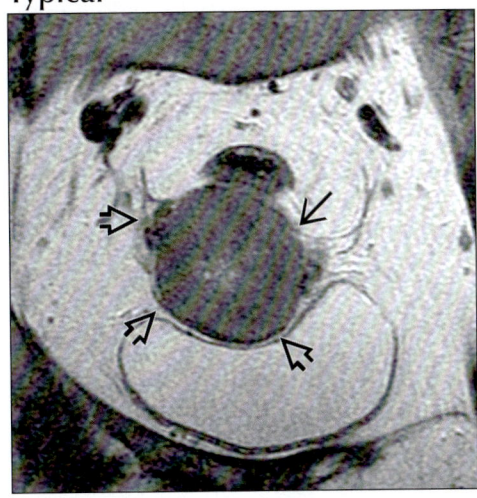
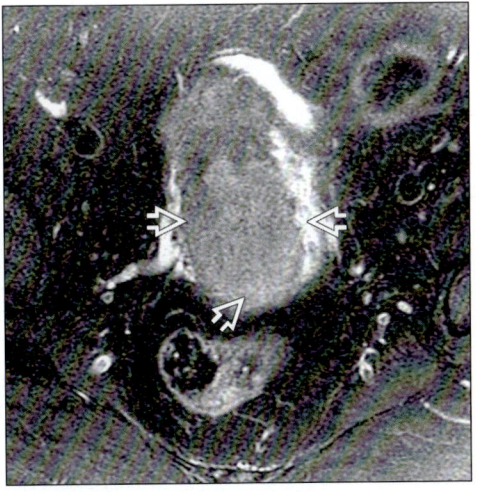

(Left) Axial oblique T2WI MR in the same patient as previous image, again demonstrates a large mass ➡ expanding the cervix of intermediate SI. There is full thickness stromal involvement ➡. No parametrial extension is seen. *(Right)* Axial T2WI FS MR in the same patient as previous image shows the intermediate signal intensity cervical mass ➡ with full thickness stromal involvement again demonstrated.

MELANOMA, CERVIX

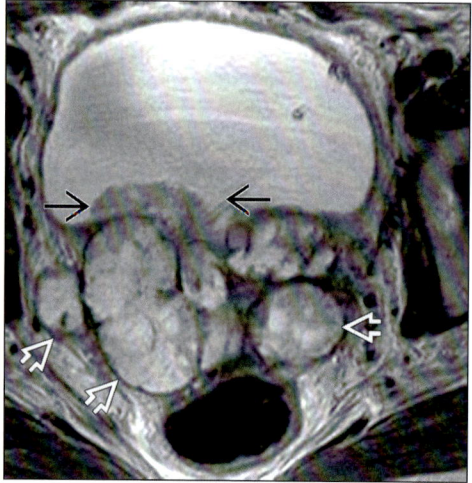

Axial T2WI MR shows a patient with recurrent cervical melanoma presenting with a large cervical mass of heterogeneous high signal intensity ➡ extending into the bladder ➡.

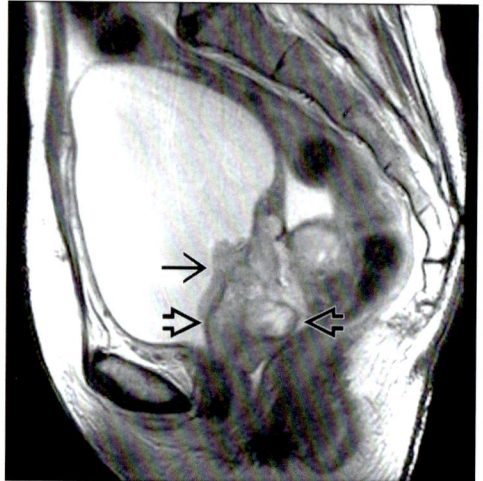

Sagittal T2WI MR in the same patient as previous image, shows recurrent tumor ➡ involving the cervix and extending into the bladder base ➡, causing bladder outlet obstruction.

TERMINOLOGY

Definitions
- Melanoma of cervix is a rare tumor
- Can be melanotic or amelanotic

IMAGING FINDINGS

General Features
- Best diagnostic clue: Cervical mass of high signal intensity on T1WI and low signal intensity on T2WI in melanotic type
- Location: Uterine cervix
- Size: Variable
- Morphology
  - Polypoid exophytic mass
  - Ulcerative
  - Infiltrative

Ultrasonographic Findings
- Grayscale Ultrasound
  - TVUS
    - Cervical mass of heterogeneous echogenicity
- Color Doppler: Cervical mass demonstrates variable vascularity

CT Findings
- Heterogeneously enhancing cervical mass
- ± Enlarged pelvic or paraaortic nodes
- ± Disseminated hematogenous metastases

MR Findings
- T1WI
  - Melanotic type: Cervical mass of high signal intensity (SI)
    - Due to paramagnetic effects of stable free radicals within melanin granules or methemoglobin within area of intratumoral hemorrhage
  - Amelanotic type: Cervical mass of intermediate to low SI
- T2WI
  - Melanotic type: Cervical mass of low SI
  - Amelanotic type: Cervical mass of intermediate to high SI
- T1 C+ FS: Heterogeneous enhancement demonstrated

Nuclear Medicine Findings
- PET

DDx: Cervical Masses

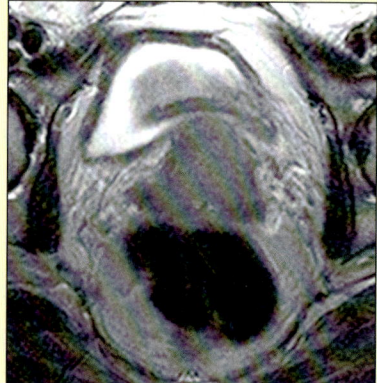

Squamous Carcinoma

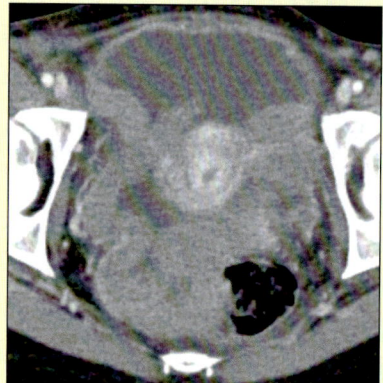

Metastatic Melanoma

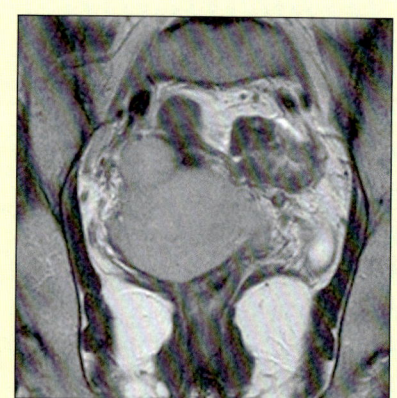

Lymphoma

MELANOMA, CERVIX

Key Facts

Terminology
- Melanoma of cervix is a rare tumor
- Can be melanotic or amelanotic

Imaging Findings
- Best diagnostic clue: Cervical mass of high signal intensity on T1WI and low signal intensity on T2WI in melanotic type
- MR for detection of tumor and local staging
- CT used to demonstrate presence of lymphatic or hematogenous metastases

Top Differential Diagnoses
- Squamous Carcinoma
- Metastatic Malignant Melanoma
- Lymphoma
- Sarcoma

Pathology
- Approximately 60 cases of primary melanoma of the female genital tract in the literature
- Arises from melanotic cells of the cervix
- Nerve tissue protein S-100 positive in most cases
- Monoclonal antibodies HMB-45 and melan A positive in most cases

Clinical Issues
- Most common signs/symptoms: Vaginal bleeding/discharge
- Age: 3rd to 8th decade; average 5th decade
- Most patients die within 3 years
- Radical hysterectomy
- External or intracavitary radiotherapy or both
- Chemotherapy combined with dimethyl triazeno imidazole carboximide (DTIC)

- Can be used for staging in recurrent melanoma
- Complements CT and MR
- Sensitivity, specificity and accuracy ranges from 70-100%
- Sensitive for soft tissue and lymph node metastases
- False negatives with lesions ≤ 1 cm in size

Imaging Recommendations
- Best imaging tool
  - MR for detection of tumor and local staging
  - CT used to demonstrate presence of lymphatic or hematogenous metastases
- Protocol advice
  - T1WI: Axial, large FOV
  - T2WI: Axial, sagittal, small FOV
  - T2WI: Axial and coronal oblique images perpendicular and parallel to long axis of the cervix
  - T1 C+ FS: Axial, small FOV

DIFFERENTIAL DIAGNOSIS

Squamous Carcinoma
- Cervical mass of heterogeneous low SI on T1WI and high SI on T2WI
- Heterogeneous enhancement

Metastatic Malignant Melanoma
- Cervical mass of high SI on T1WI, low SI on T2WI (in melanotic type)
- Presence or history of cutaneous melanoma
- ± Disseminated metastases
- Absence of junctional activity on histology, neoplastic cells localized below basement membrane

Lymphoma
- Homogeneous bulky mass of low SI on T1WI and high SI on T2WI
- Associated lymphadenopathy if secondary involvement with lymphoma

Sarcoma
- Heterogeneous enhancing cervical mass of variable SI

PATHOLOGY

General Features
- Epidemiology
  - Rare tumor, mainly reported as case reports
  - Melanoma of the female genital tract accounts for 1-5% of all melanoma cases; of this 9-13% involve the cervix
  - 5x more rare than primary melanoma of the vagina and vulva
  - Approximately 60 cases of primary melanoma of the female genital tract in the literature

Gross Pathologic & Surgical Features
- Exophytic friable polypoid mass
- Areas of ulceration and hemorrhage
- Blue/black/red/brown/grey discoloration in melanotic form
- Colorless in amelanotic form (about 50% of total)

Microscopic Features
- Arises from melanotic cells of the cervix
- Diagnosis made on having following 4 criteria
  - Presence of melanin in normal cervical epithelium
  - Absence of melanoma elsewhere in the body
  - Demonstration of junctional change in the cervix
    - May be absent if surface ulceration
  - Metastasizes according to pattern of cervical carcinoma
- Variable degree of pleomorphism; prominent nucleoli
- Electron microscopy
  - Premelanosomes and mature melanosomes present
  - No epithelial structural differentiation
- Immunohistochemistry
  - Nerve tissue protein S-100 positive in most cases
  - Monoclonal antibodies HMB-45 and melan A positive in most cases
  - Negative for epithelial markers
- FIGO staging system used rather than Clark or Breslow staging classification

MELANOMA, CERVIX

CLINICAL ISSUES

Presentation
- Most common signs/symptoms: Vaginal bleeding/discharge
- Other signs/symptoms
  - Post-coital bleeding
  - Asymptomatic; detected on routine screening

Demographics
- Age: 3rd to 8th decade; average 5th decade
- Gender: Female

Natural History & Prognosis
- 50% of all cases show vaginal involvement (stage II)
- Recurs early after treatment
- 5-YRS: Stage I 25%, stage II 14%, stage III and IV 0%
- Average survival 6 months to 14 years
- Most patients die within 3 years

Treatment
- Radical hysterectomy
- ± Para-aortic and pelvic lymphadenectomy if enlarged nodes
- External or intracavitary radiotherapy or both
- Chemotherapy combined with dimethyl triazeno imidazole carboximide (DTIC)
  - Dacarbazine shown to give response rates of 15-20%
- Immuno/biological therapy
  - Interleukin-2 and gamma interferon, bacille-calmette-gurin (BCG) or activated lymphocyte transfusion

DIAGNOSTIC CHECKLIST

Consider
- Primary melanoma of the cervix when pigmented tumor mass seen arising from cervix on speculum examination
  - In absence of melanoma elsewhere
  - Junctional change present in the cervix
  - Metastatic spread follows pattern for cervical carcinoma

Image Interpretation Pearls
- Classically, melanotic type cervical melanoma demonstrates high signal on T1WI and low SI on T2

SELECTED REFERENCES

1. Jin B et al: Primary melanoma of the uterine cervix after supracervical hysterectomy. A case report. Acta Cytol. 51(1):86-8, 2007
2. Belhocine TZ et al: Role of nuclear medicine in the management of cutaneous malignant melanoma. J Nucl Med. 47(6):957-67, 2006
3. Mousavi AS et al: Primary malignant melanoma of the uterine cervix: case report and review of the literature. J Low Genit Tract Dis. 10(4):258-63, 2006
4. Wydra D et al: Malignant melanoma of the uterine cervix. Eur J Obstet Gynecol Reprod Biol. 124(2):257-8, 2006
5. Gupta R et al: Primary malignant melanoma of cervix - a case report. Indian J Cancer. 42(4):201-4, 2005
6. Ma SQ et al: Clinical analysis of primary malignant melanoma of the cervix. Chin Med Sci J. 20(4):257-60, 2005
7. Siozos C et al: Malignant melanoma of the uterine cervix. J Obstet Gynaecol. 25(8):826-7, 2005
8. Kudrimoti J et al: Primary malignant melanoma of cervix: a case report. Indian J Pathol Microbiol. 47(2):257-8, 2004
9. Saikia UN et al: Melanin containing cells of the uterine cervix and a possible histogenesis--a case report. Indian J Pathol Microbiol. 47(1):22-3, 2004
10. Makovitzky J et al: Primary malignant melanoma of the cervix uteri: a case report of a rare tumor. Anticancer Res. 23(2A):1063-7, 2003
11. Okamoto Y et al: MR imaging of the uterine cervix: imaging-pathologic correlation. Radiographics. 2003
12. Deshpande AH et al: Primary malignant melanoma of the uterine cervix: report of a case diagnosed by cervical scrape cytology and review of the literature. Diagn Cytopathol. 25(2):108-11, 2001
13. Furuya M et al: Clear cell variant of malignant melanoma of the uterine cervix: a case report and review of the literature. Gynecol Oncol. 80(3):409-12, 2001
14. Clark KC et al: Primary malignant melanoma of the uterine cervix: case report with world literature review. Int J Gynecol Pathol. 18(3):265-73, 1999
15. Takehara M et al: Primary malignant melanoma of the uterine cervix: a case report. J Obstet Gynaecol Res. 25(2):129-32, 1999
16. Wasef WR et al: Primary malignant melanoma of the cervix uteri. J Obstet Gynaecol. 19(6):673-4, 1999
17. Teixeira JC et al: Primary melanoma of the uterine cervix figo stage III B. Sao Paulo Med J. 116(4):1778-80, 1998
18. Chang SC et al: Primary malignant melanoma of the vagina and cervix uteri: case report and literature review. Zhonghua Yi Xue Za Zhi (Taipei). 50(4):341-6, 1992
19. Yu HC et al: Detection of malignant melanoma of the uterine cervix from Papanicolaou smears. A case report. Acta Cytol. 31(1):73-6, 1987

MELANOMA, CERVIX

IMAGE GALLERY

Typical

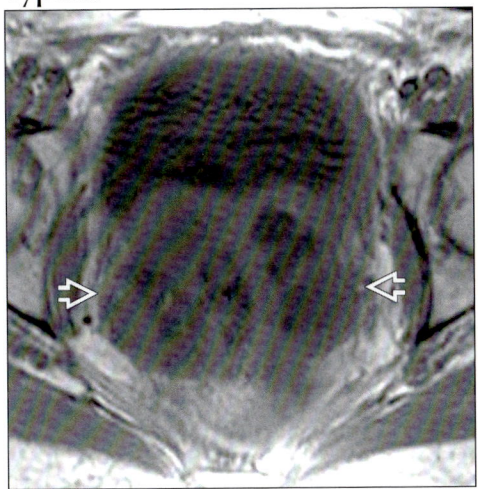
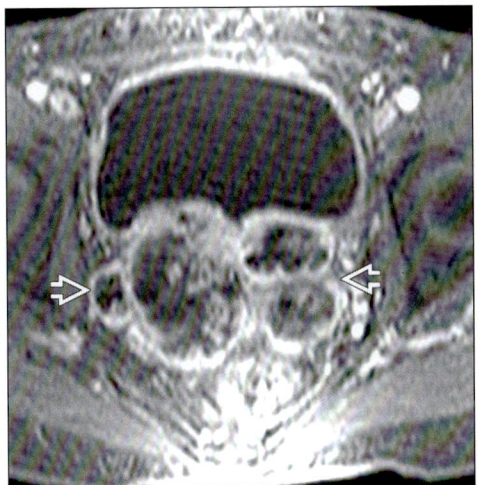

(Left) Axial T1WI MR in the same patient as the first two images shows a cervical mass of heterogeneous intermediate signal intensity ⇒. Typically a primary tumor of the melanocytic type would be of high signal intensity. *(Right)* Axial T1 C+ FS MR in same patient as previous image demonstrates a cervical mass showing rim-enhancement ⇒. Central areas of necrosis are also present. Pathology: Recurrent melanoma.

Typical

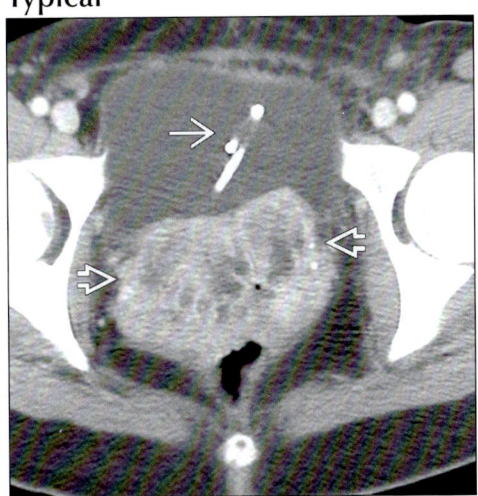
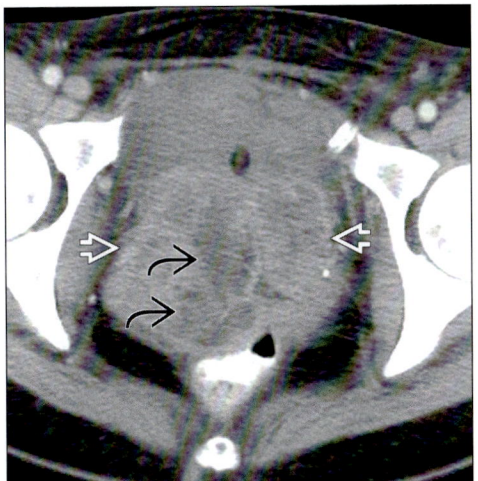

(Left) Axial CECT in the same patient as previous image shows avid enhancement in the arterial phase ⇒. Note the tip of a ureteric stent ⇒ within the bladder due to concomitant renal tract obstruction secondary to the mass. *(Right)* Axial CECT shows same patient as previous image with recurrent cervical melanoma. Less avid enhancement is shown in the portal venous phase ⇒. Areas of necrosis are demonstrated as low attenuation foci ⇒.

Typical

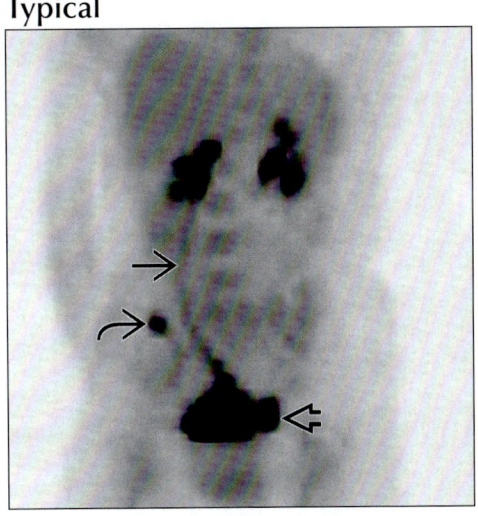
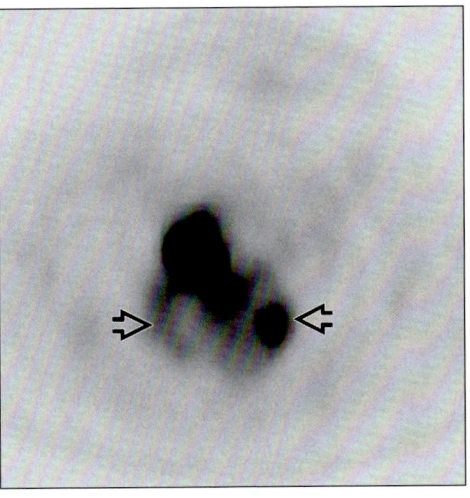

(Left) Anteroposterior PET shows avid uptake of FDG within the pelvis, corresponding to the recurrent cervical melanoma ⇒. The obstructed right kidney and ureter ⇒ is seen. Note the metastatic deposit in the bony pelvis ⇒. *(Right)* Anteroposterior PET in the same patient as previous image shows intense uptake of FDG within the pelvis corresponding to the recurrent cervical melanoma ⇒.

METASTASIS, CERVIX

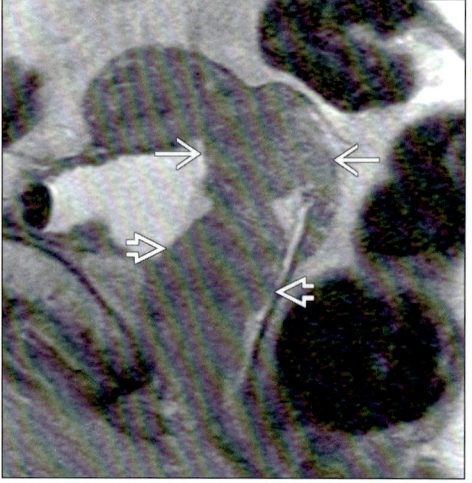

Sagittal T2WI MR shows a large cervical mass ➡ extending to involve the entire anterior vaginal wall ⬌, in a patient with a previous history of transitional cell carcinoma of the bladder.

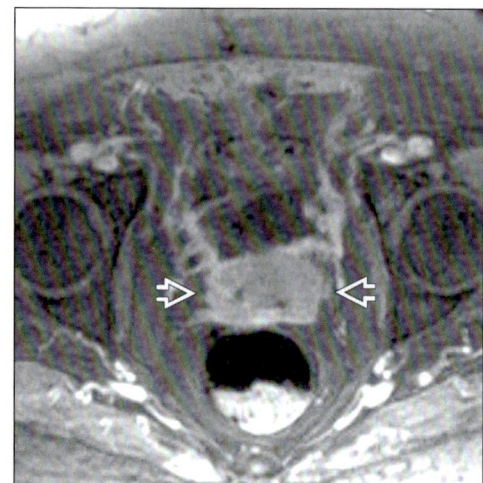

Axial T1 C+ FS MR in the same patient as previous image demonstrates an enhancing cervical mass ➡. Pathology: Metastatic transitional cell carcinoma of the bladder.

TERMINOLOGY

Definitions
- Metastasis to the cervix from a primary neoplasm arising elsewhere
- May occur at time of initial presentation or years later, possibly as part of disseminated disease
- Either by hematogenous or lymphatic spread

IMAGING FINDINGS

General Features
- Best diagnostic clue
  - Cervical mass of intermediate/high signal intensity on T2WI
  - History or concomitant presence of primary tumor elsewhere
- Location: Cervix
- Size: Variable - several centimeters

Ultrasonographic Findings
- Grayscale Ultrasound
  - TVUS
    - Cervical mass appears hypoechoic or of mixed echogenicity
- Color Doppler: Cervical mass demonstrates variable vascularity

CT Findings
- Bulky cervix
- Cervical mass demonstrating heterogeneous enhancement
- Primary tumor may be visible e.g., bowel, ovary, bladder
- ± Lymphadenopathy
  - e.g., Pelvic, retroperitoneal, mediastinal
- ± Distant metastases
  - e.g., Liver, lung, bone

MR Findings
- T1WI
  - Cervical mass of low signal intensity (SI)
  - High SI corresponds to
    - Areas of hemorrhage or melanin in the case of a melanoma primary
- T2WI
  - Cervical mass of intermediate/high SI

DDx: Cervical Masses

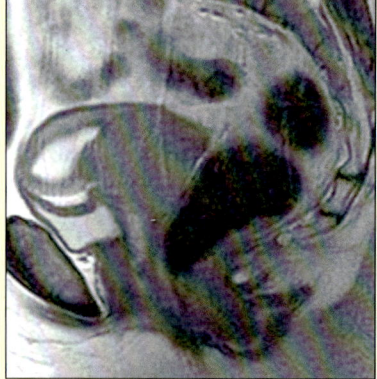

Cervical Carcinoma

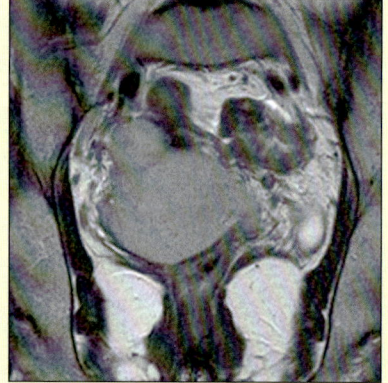

Cervical Lymphoma

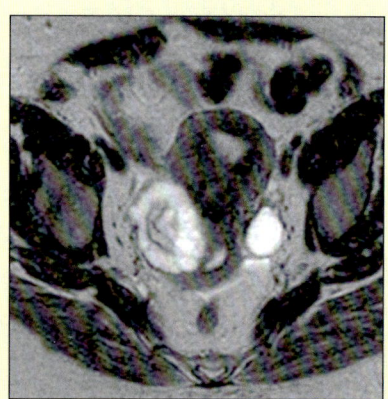

Cervical Chondrosarcoma

METASTASIS, CERVIX

Key Facts

Terminology
- Metastasis to the cervix from a primary neoplasm arising elsewhere

Imaging Findings
- Cervical mass of intermediate/high signal intensity on T2WI
- History or concomitant presence of primary tumor elsewhere
- MR is method of choice for detecting presence of cervical metastasis

Top Differential Diagnoses
- Cervical Carcinoma
- Cervical Lymphoma
- Cervical Sarcoma
- Cervical Melanoma

Pathology
- Metastases to cervix are rare
- < 5% of all cases to the female genital tract from extragenital cancers
- Endometrial carcinoma commonest primary tumor; skip lesions occur in the endocervical canal
- Histopathology and immunohistochemistry of the cervical metastasis reflects the histopathology of the primary tumor

Clinical Issues
- Most common signs/symptoms: Vaginal bleeding
- Chemotherapy ± radiotherapy
- Hormone therapy (e.g., tamoxifen in metastatic breast cancer)
- Total abdominal hysterectomy and bilateral salpingo-oophorectomy in selected cases

---

  ○ Total or partial replacement of normal low signal intensity stromal ring with high signal intensity tumor if full thickness stromal involvement
- T1 C+: Cervical mass demonstrates variable contrast-enhancement

Nuclear Medicine Findings
- PET
  ○ Can be used as an adjunct to CT and MR in the evaluation of
    ▪ Metastases to the cervix and elsewhere
    ▪ Lymph node metastases
    ▪ Treatment response

Imaging Recommendations
- Best imaging tool
  ○ MR is method of choice for detecting presence of cervical metastasis
    ▪ May not always demonstrate a small or diffusely infiltrating lesion
- Protocol advice
  ○ T1WI: Axial, large FOV
  ○ T2WI: Axial, sagittal, small FOV
  ○ T2WI: Axial oblique and coronal oblique images perpendicular and parallel to the cervix
  ○ T1 C+ FS: Axial, small FOV

DIFFERENTIAL DIAGNOSIS

Cervical Carcinoma
- Mass of heterogeneous high SI on T2WI
- Heterogeneous enhancement

Cervical Lymphoma
- Homogeneous bulky mass of high SI on T2WI

Cervical Sarcoma
- Rare cause of cervical mass
- Polypoid or diffusely infiltrating mass of heterogeneous SI on T1WI and T2WI

Cervical Melanoma
- Classically, cervical mass of high SI on T1WI and low SI on T2WI

PATHOLOGY

General Features
- Epidemiology
  ○ Metastases to cervix are rare
    ▪ < 5% of all cases to the female genital tract from extragenital cancers
  ○ Rarity due to
    ▪ Centrifugal drainage of lymphatics to cervix
    ▪ Fibrous nature of cervical stroma
    ▪ Incidence may be underestimated due to lack of routine microscopic examination at autopsy
  ○ Endometrial carcinoma commonest primary tumor; skip lesions occur in the endocervical canal
  ○ Commonest distant primaries are breast (usually lobular carcinoma) and gastrointestinal tract (stomach)
  ○ Other primary sites
    ▪ Ovary
    ▪ Skin (malignant melanoma)
    ▪ Genitourinary tract
    ▪ Gallbladder
    ▪ Pancreas
    ▪ Thyroid
    ▪ Choriocarcinoma
    ▪ Leukanemia/lymphoma

Gross Pathologic & Surgical Features
- Diffusely infiltrating tumor or bulky mass of variable size
- Areas of hemorrhage and necrosis

Microscopic Features
- Histopathology and immunohistochemistry of the cervical metastasis reflects the histopathology of the primary tumor

METASTASIS, CERVIX

- Metastatic lobular breast carcinoma may have a distinctive "indian file" histological pattern
- Metastatic endometrial carcinoma is morphologically identical to endometrioid carcinoma of the cervix
  - Distinction is made on the location of bulk of the tumor and presence of carcinoma in situ in either location
  - Only 8% of metastatic endometrial adenocarcinomas demonstrate carcinoembryonic antigen (CEA) by immunoperoxidase technique, compared to 80% of regular endocervical adenocarcinomas
- Metastatic colo-rectal carcinoma
  - Immunohistochemistry for cytokeratin 20 is positive and cytokeratin 7 is negative
- Metastatic gastric carcinoma
  - May show a signet ring pattern
- Metastatic ovarian carcinoma may resemble a papillary adenocarcinoma of the cervix

CLINICAL ISSUES

Presentation
- Most common signs/symptoms: Vaginal bleeding
- Other signs/symptoms
  - Pelvic pain
  - Asymptomatic
    - Detected on staging for primary tumor or on cervical smear

Demographics
- Age: Wide age range
- Gender: Female

Natural History & Prognosis
- Poor prognosis as usually reflects a disseminated metastatic process

Treatment
- Chemotherapy ± radiotherapy
- Hormone therapy (e.g., tamoxifen in metastatic breast cancer)
- Total abdominal hysterectomy and bilateral salpingo-oophorectomy in selected cases

DIAGNOSTIC CHECKLIST

Consider
- Metastasis to the cervix in a patient presenting with a cervical mass and history of a primary tumor elsewhere

Image Interpretation Pearls
- Heterogeneous enhancing cervical mass in the presence of a known primary tumor

SELECTED REFERENCES

1. Martinez-Roman S et al: Metastatic carcinoma of the gallbladder mimicking an advanced cervical carcinoma. Gynecol Oncol. 97(3):942-5, 2005
2. Sozen I et al: Adenocarcinoma of the cervix metastatic from a colon primary and diagnosed from a routine pap smear in a 17-year-old woman: a case report. J Reprod Med. 50(10):793-5, 2005
3. Green AE et al: Isolated cervical metastasis of breast cancer: a case report and review of the literature. Gynecol Oncol. 95(1):267-9, 2004
4. Metser U et al: MR imaging findings and patterns of spread in secondary tumor involvement of the uterine body and cervix. AJR Am J Roentgenol. 180(3):765-9, 2003
5. Ogino A et al: A case of breast cancer metastasizing to cervix after resection of pancreatic metastasis. Breast Cancer. 10(3):284-8, 2003
6. Kesavan S et al: An unusual tumour metastasis to the cervix. Ann Acad Med Singapore. 29(6):780-2, 2000
7. Yokoyama Y et al: Solitary metastasis to the uterine cervix from the early gastric cancer: a case report. Eur J Gynaecol Oncol. 21(5):469-71, 2000
8. Hepp HH et al: Breast cancer metastatic to the uterine cervix: analysis of a rare event. Cancer Invest. 17(7):468-73, 1999
9. Kennebeck CH et al: Signet ring breast carcinoma metastases limited to the endometrium and cervix. Gynecol Oncol. 71(3):461-4, 1998
10. Campora E et al: Endocervical metastases secondary to breast carcinoma. A case report. Eur J Gynaecol Oncol. 12(2):103-6, 1991
11. Yazigi R et al: Breast cancer metastasizing to the uterine cervix. Cancer. 61(12):2558-60, 1988
12. Kumar A et al: Metastases to the uterus from extrapelvic primary tumors. Int J Gynecol Pathol. 2(2):134-40, 1983

METASTASIS, CERVIX

IMAGE GALLERY

Typical

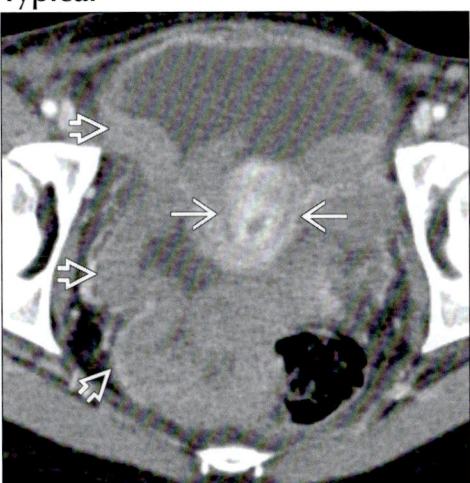 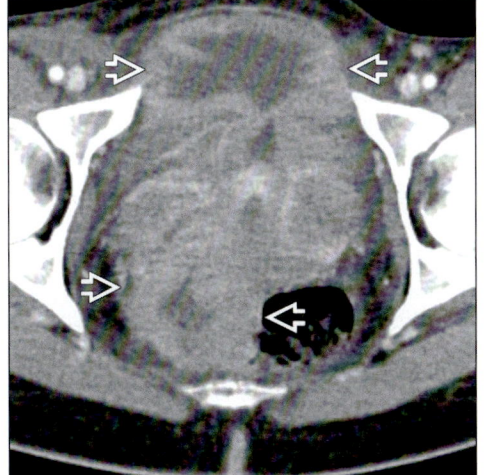

(Left) Axial CECT in a patient with extensive peritoneal carcinomatosis secondary to melanoma. Diffuse peritoneal thickening ➡ and an enhancing cervical mass is seen ➡. *(Right)* Axial CECT in the same patient as previous image, again demonstrating extensive peritoneal thickening and enhancement ➡ secondary to metastatic melanoma.

Typical

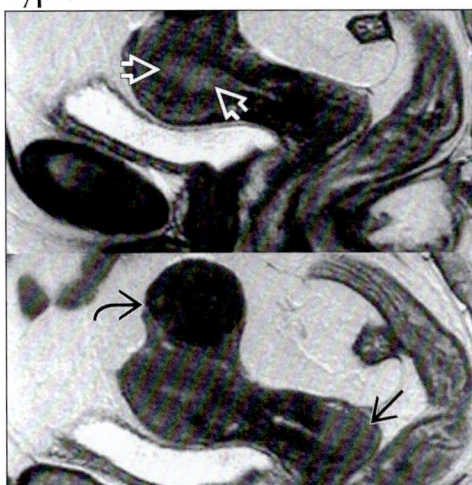 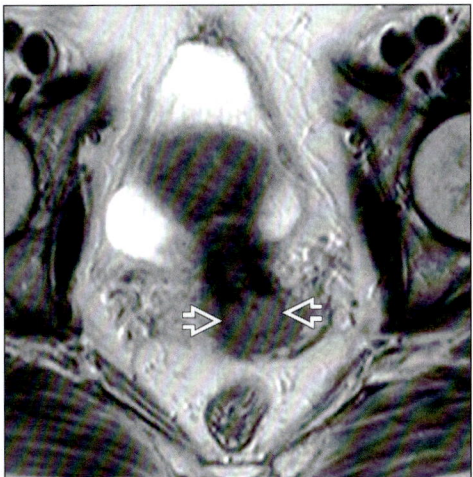

(Left) Sagittal T2WI MR images show an endometrial tumor ➡ on the midline sagittal image and skip a lesion within the cervix ➡ on the parasagittal image. Both lesions are of intermediate SI. Note incidental subserosal leiomyoma ➡. *(Right)* Axial T2WI MR in the same patient, shows a cervical lesion of intermediate SI ➡. Pathology confirmed the presence of a skip lesion within the cervix from a stage IIB endometrial carcinoma.

Typical

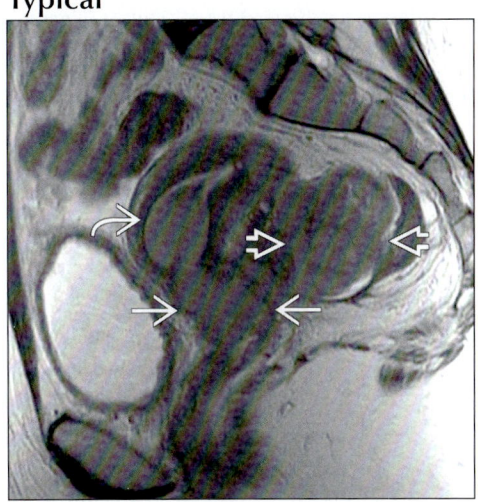 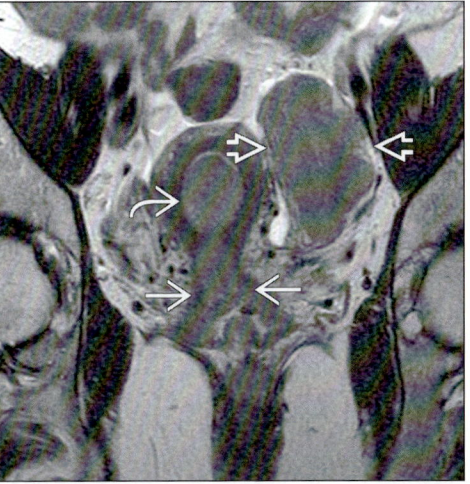

(Left) Sagittal T2WI MR shows a large cervical mass of intermediate SI ➡. The mass is extending into the lower uterine segment ➡. Note the presence of a large heterogeneous mass in the pouch of Douglas ➡. *(Right)* Coronal T2WI MR in the same patient as previous image confirms the presence of the cervical mass ➡ extending into the uterine cavity ➡. Again, note the left adnexal mass ➡. Pathology: Metastatic undifferentiated ovarian carcinoma.

NABOTHIAN CYSTS

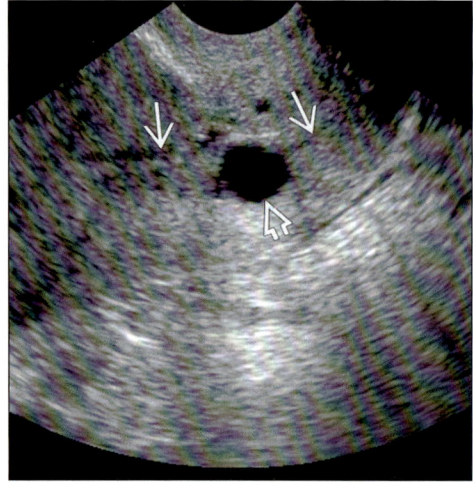

Sagittal transvaginal ultrasound through the lower uterine segment and cervix, shows a well-defined, anechoic cyst ⇨ adjacent to the endocervical canal ➡.

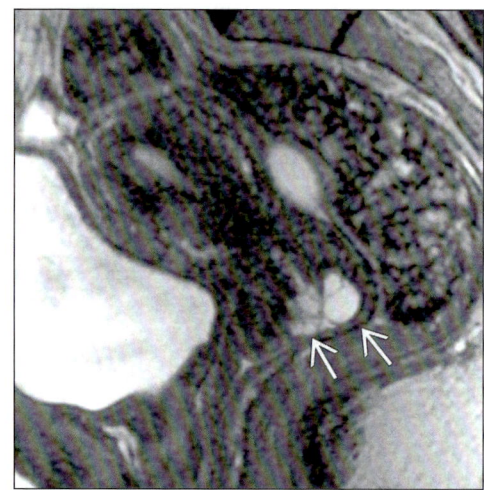

Sagittal T2WI MR shows several nabothian cysts ➡ in the cervical lips. Uncomplicated cysts are high signal intensity.

TERMINOLOGY

Abbreviations and Synonyms
- Tunnel clusters, endocervical gland cysts, retention cysts of cervix

Definitions
- Nabothian cysts and endocervical gland cysts are lined with mucin-producing epithelium and arise from glands that occur in cervix
- Tunnel cluster cysts are a specific type of nabothian cyst
  - Characterized by complex multicystic dilation of the endocervical glands

IMAGING FINDINGS

General Features
- Best diagnostic clue: Single or multiple, round, well-defined, unilocular, cystic lesions on cervical surface or in inner portion of cervical stroma near endocervical canal
- Location
  - Occur on the endocervical portion of the cervix
  - Usually seen at colposcopic examination on surface of ectocervix
    - Protrusions at the squamocolumnar transition zone
  - Usually are multiple
- Size
  - Range in size
    - Most are a few mm in diameter
    - May reach 4 cm on occasion
    - Extensive cyst formation may result in enlargement of the cervix
- Morphology
  - Round or oval
  - Smooth wall
- Anatomy
  - Nabothian cysts represent mucinous cysts at ectocervix obstructed by overgrowth of squamous epithelium at their neck
  - Tunnel clusters are distended glands located deep to endocervical canal

Ultrasonographic Findings
- Color Doppler: No color flow

DDx: Nabothian Cyst

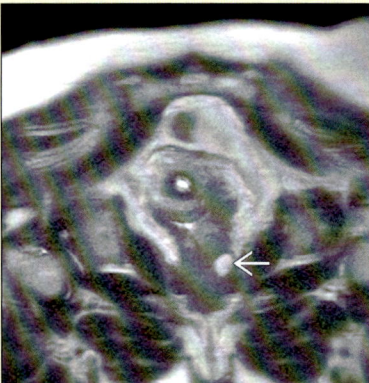

Gartner Duct Cyst

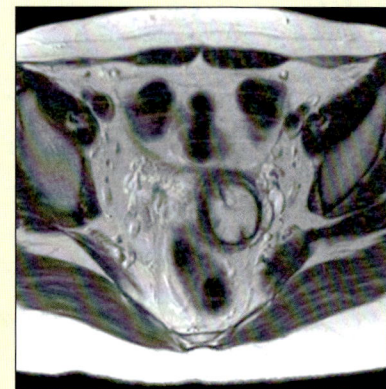

Cervical Cancer

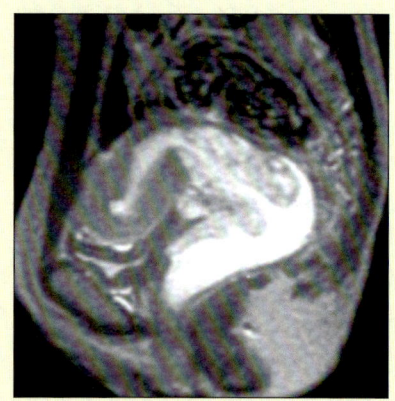

Adenoma Malignum

NABOTHIAN CYSTS

Key Facts

Terminology
- Tunnel clusters, endocervical gland cysts, retention cysts of cervix
- Nabothian cysts and endocervical gland cysts are lined with mucin-producing epithelium and arise from glands that occur in cervix

Imaging Findings
- Best diagnostic clue: Single or multiple, round, well-defined, unilocular, cystic lesions on cervical surface or in inner portion of cervical stroma near endocervical canal
- Most are a few mm in diameter
- May reach 4 cm on occasion
- Nabothian cysts represent mucinous cysts at ectocervix obstructed by overgrowth of squamous epithelium at their neck
- Very conspicuous on MR as well-defined cysts located in cervix

Top Differential Diagnoses
- Adenoma Malignum
- Gartner Duct Cyst
- Squamous Cell Carcinoma of the Cervix

Pathology
- May be seen in postpartum cervix with ectropion
- May form as a result of the healing process of chronic cervicitis

Clinical Issues
- Most common signs/symptoms: Usually asymptomatic incidental finding
- Majority require no specific treatment

- Power Doppler
  - Helps to differentiate nabothian cysts from more aggressive lesions
  - Power Doppler imaging may be useful for distinguishing nabothian cysts from carcinoma
    - Nabothian cysts show no flow whereas flow may be seen within wall of cystic portion of adenoma malignum
- Transvaginal ultrasound (TVS) findings
  - Well-defined anechoic cystic lesion(s) on cervical surface or in inner portion of cervical stroma near endocervical canal
  - Minority with mucinous contents may be hypoechoic or contain debris

CT Findings
- NECT
  - If uncomplicated, same or lower attenuation than cervix
    - If complicated, may have slightly higher attenuation than cervix
- CECT
  - Rounded low attenuation regions in cervix
  - Cysts do not enhance
- When large may simulate an endocervical gland tumor or cystic adnexal mass

MR Findings
- T1WI
  - Cysts are low or isointense in signal intensity to cervix
    - Minority with mucinous contents will show high signal intensity
- T2WI
  - Cysts are very high in signal intensity
    - If mucinous, may have lower signal intensity than simple cysts
- T1 C+: Cysts do not enhance
- Very conspicuous on MR as well-defined cysts located in cervix
- May be single or multiple and are not infrequently numerous in number
- Most often very small, measuring less than 1 cm

Imaging Recommendations
- Best imaging tool: Transvaginal ultrasound
- Protocol advice
  - Features that warrant further evaluation
    - Large
    - Multiloculated
    - Any solid elements within cysts
- Vast majority require no further evaluation

DIFFERENTIAL DIAGNOSIS

Adenoma Malignum
- Also known as mucinous minimal deviation adenocarcinoma
- Low grade mucinous carcinoma affecting deep endocervical glands
- Forms multilocular cystic masses in cervix, similar to very large tunnel clusters or endocervical gland cysts
- Any enhancement, large size, or solid components of endocervical gland cysts, suggests adenoma malignum
- Patients may present with watery vaginal discharge

Gartner Duct Cyst
- Arise in the anterolateral wall of the vagina
- If large, extend into ischiorectal fossa

Squamous Cell Carcinoma of the Cervix
- Solid mass of the cervix
- May have areas of necrosis, but solid elements predominate

Adenomyosis
- Punctate high signal intensity foci on T2WI in uterine corpus myometrium

Cystic Adnexal Mass
- Mass originates in adnexa and mimics nabothian cysts

Post-Conization Defect
- Patient history makes diagnosis
- Shortened cervical length

NABOTHIAN CYSTS

PATHOLOGY

General Features
- Etiology
  - May be seen in postpartum cervix with ectropion
  - May form as a result of the healing process of chronic cervicitis
    - Squamous epithelium grows back over the ectocervix
    - Underlying columnar cells of the endocervical glands become obstructed
    - Columnar epithelium beneath the squamous layer continues to secrete mucus and the trapped secretions result in cyst formation
  - May be seen with patients on progestogenic therapy: There is failure of the cyclic flow of the cervical mucus
- Epidemiology
  - Appear to increase in prevalence with increasing age
  - Detected in 8% of adult women & 13% of postmenopausal women

Gross Pathologic & Surgical Features
- Yellow or white cysts on surface of cervix
- Frequently multiple
- Size ranges from a few mm to 4 cm at colposcopy
- Tunnel clusters are only seen upon sectioning of cervix
- Appear as rounded cysts filled with clear fluid

Microscopic Features
- Cysts are lined by low columnar endocervical cells

CLINICAL ISSUES

Presentation
- Most common signs/symptoms: Usually asymptomatic incidental finding
- Other signs/symptoms: Rarely may become infected
- Must be differentiated from adenoma malignum

Demographics
- Age: Increasing prevalence with increasing age

Natural History & Prognosis
- Slow growing

Treatment
- Majority require no specific treatment
- Cases of symptomatic, unremitting, chronic cervicitis may benefit from
  - Cyst drainage
  - Cryosurgery
  - Conization

DIAGNOSTIC CHECKLIST

Consider
- Nabothian cysts when incidental simple cystic regions are seen either on or near the endocervical canal

Image Interpretation Pearls
- Well-defined, small, simple cysts on cervical surface or inner portion cervical stroma near the endocervical canal

SELECTED REFERENCES

1. Oguri H et al: MRI of endocervical glandular disorders: three cases of a deep nabothian cyst and three cases of a minimal-deviation adenocarcinoma. Magn Reson Imaging. 22(9):1333-7, 2004
2. Okamoto Y et al: MR imaging of the uterine cervix: imaging-pathologic correlation. Radiographics. 23(2):425-45; quiz 534-5, 2003
3. Gousse AE et al: Dynamic half Fourier acquisition, single shot turbo spin-echo magnetic resonance imaging for evaluating the female pelvis. J Urol. 164(5):1606-13, 2000
4. Li H et al: Markedly high signal intensity lesions in the uterine cervix on T2-weighted imaging: differentiation between mucin-producing carcinomas and nabothian cysts. Radiat Med. 17(2):137-43, 1999
5. Pelosi MA 3rd et al: Symptomatic cervical macrocyst as a late complication of subtotal hysterectomy. A case report. J Reprod Med. 44(6):567-70, 1999
6. Umesaki N et al: Power Doppler findings of adenoma malignum of uterine cervix. Gynecol Obstet Invest. 45(3):213-6, 1998
7. Daya D et al: Florid deep glands of the uterine cervix. Another mimic of adenoma malignum. Am J Clin Pathol. 103(5):614-7, 1995
8. Yamashita Y et al: Adenoma malignum: MR appearances mimicking nabothian cysts. AJR Am J Roentgenol. 162(3):649-50, 1994
9. Togashi K et al: CT and MR demonstration of nabothian cysts mimicking a cystic adnexal mass. J Comput Assist Tomogr. 11(6):1091-2, 1987
10. Fogel SR et al: Sonography of Nabothian cysts. AJR Am J Roentgenol. 138(5):927-30, 1982

NABOTHIAN CYSTS

IMAGE GALLERY

Typical

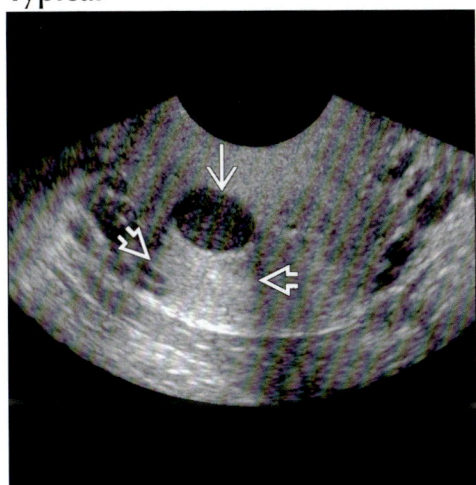
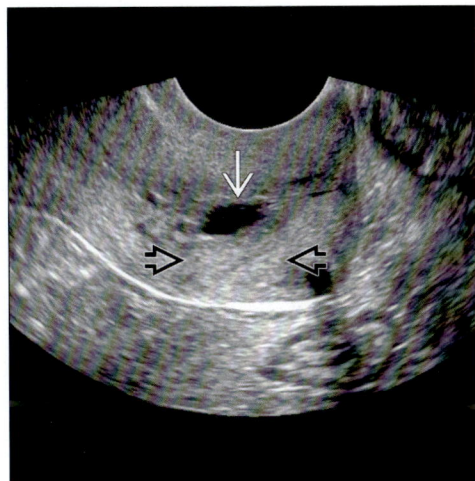

(Left) Axial transvaginal ultrasound shows an ovoid cyst with low level echoes ➡ and posterior acoustic shadowing ➡ in the cervix. Complicated nabothian cysts may have proteinaceous contents. *(Right)* Sagittal transvaginal ultrasound shows an ovoid nabothian cyst ➡ paralleling the endocervical canal. Note the posterior acoustic enhancement ➡.

Typical

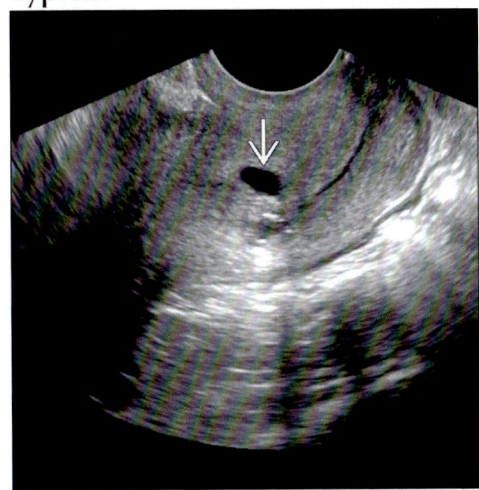
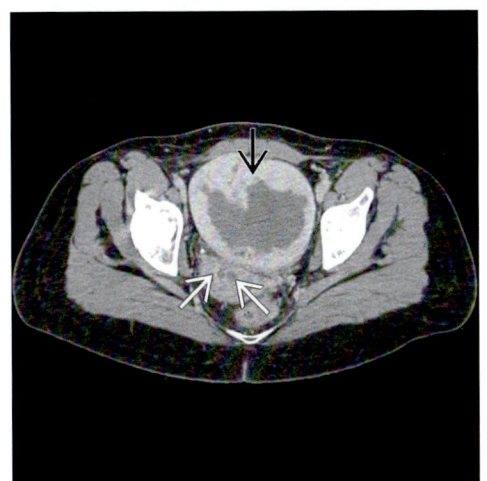

(Left) Sagittal transvaginal ultrasound shows an ovoid anechoic cyst ➡ in the anterior cervix. *(Right)* Axial CECT shows two round, low attenuation cysts ➡ within the cervix in a patient post-uterine artery embolization. Note the partially infarcted leiomyoma ➡.

Typical

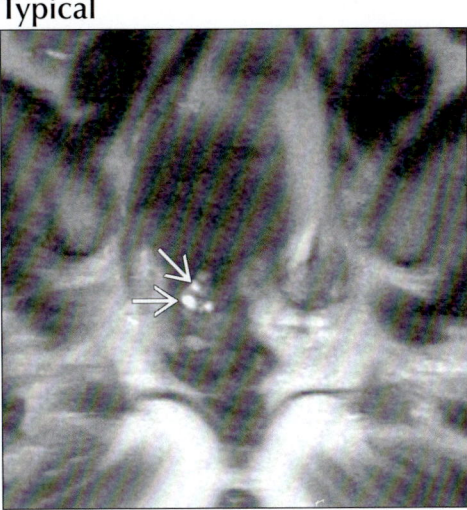
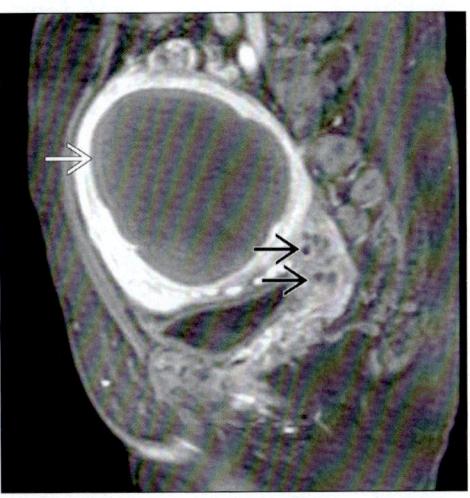

(Left) Coronal T2WI MR shows multiple high signal intensity foci ➡ within the cervix. *(Right)* Sagittal T1 C+ FS MR in the same patient as previous image, shows that the foci do not enhance ➡, consistent with cervical nabothian cysts. Also note the low signal intensity embolized leiomyoma ➡.

CERVICAL GLANDULAR HYPERPLASIA

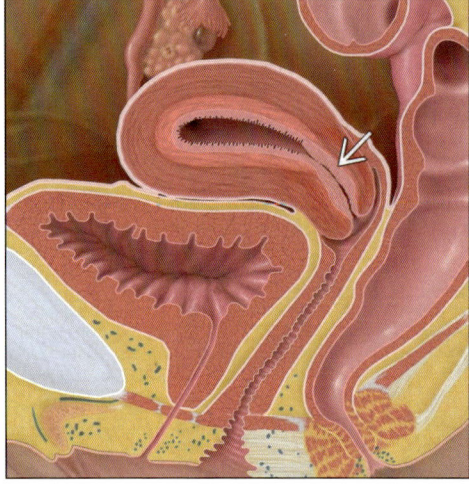

Sagittal graphic shows thickening of the endocervical mucosa ➡ with preservation of the underlying architecture in endocervical glandular hyperplasia.

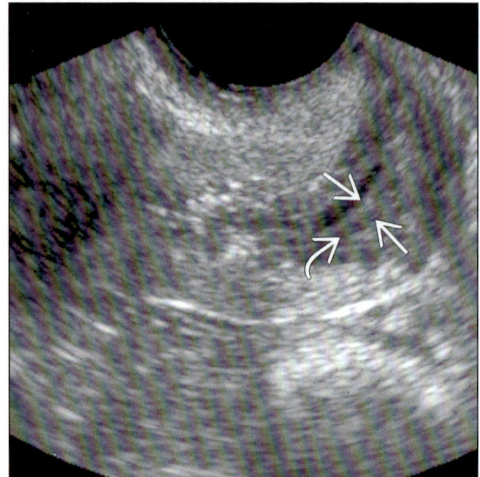

Sagittal transvaginal ultrasound shows a thickened endocervical mucosa ➡. The hypoechoic areas ➡ represent tiny cysts within the mucosa. There is a sliver of fluid in the endocervical canal.

TERMINOLOGY

Abbreviations and Synonyms
- Diffuse laminar endocervical glandular hyperplasia, microglandular hyperplasia, hyperplasia of mesonephric remnants, hyperplasia not otherwise specified

Definitions
- Benign proliferation of endocervical mucosal glandular elements
- Comprise several different histological entities

IMAGING FINDINGS

General Features
- Best diagnostic clue
  - Often undetectable on imaging
  - Thickening of endocervical mucosa ± cystic change
- Location: Superficial (inner) layer of cervical wall
- Size: Variable
- Morphology
  - "Solid" component homogeneous
  - Heterogeneity due to cystic change
  - Border with stroma well-defined
- Paucity of data in imaging literature
  - Reported cases are biased towards lesions with atypical imaging features mimicking adenoma malignum

Ultrasonographic Findings
- Grayscale Ultrasound
  - Thickened hyperechoic mucosal layer of endocervix
  - When hyperplasia: Cystic
    - Small, thin-walled anechoic cysts with posterior acoustic enhancement

CT Findings
- CECT
  - Usually no significant abnormality
  - If associated with cystic change, may show hypodense foci

MR Findings
- T1WI
  - Cervix of diffuse intermediate signal intensity (SI)
    - No zonal anatomy depicted

DDx: Cervical Gland Hyperplasia

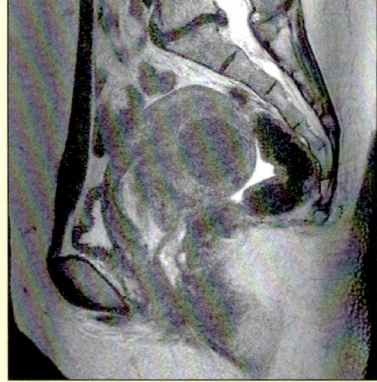

Cervical Adenocarcinoma

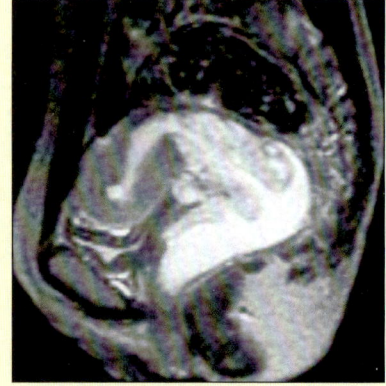

Adenoma Malignum

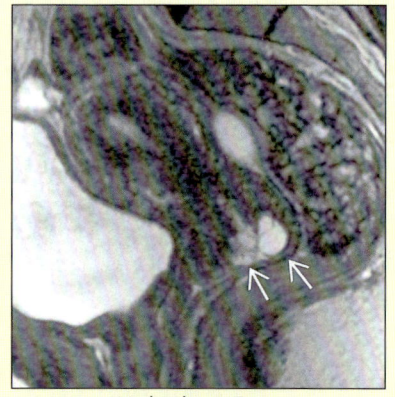

Nabothian Cysts

CERVICAL GLANDULAR HYPERPLASIA

Key Facts

Terminology
- Benign proliferation of endocervical mucosal glandular elements
- Comprise several different histological entities

Imaging Findings
- Often undetectable on imaging
- Thickening of endocervical mucosa ± cystic change
- Location: Superficial (inner) layer of cervical wall
- "Solid" component homogeneous
- Heterogeneity due to cystic change
- Reported cases are biased towards lesions with atypical imaging features mimicking adenoma malignum
- Best imaging tool: MR imaging modality of choice to demonstrate homogeneous mucosal thickening and lack of stromal or deep involvement

Top Differential Diagnoses
- Cervical Adenocarcinoma
- Nabothian Cysts
- Other Pseudoneoplastic Glandular Lesions

Pathology
- Very common, especially in reproductive age women
- Associated abnormalities: No proven evolution towards adenoma malignum or adenocarcinoma

Diagnostic Checklist
- Consider cervical gland hyperplasia in the setting of a homogeneously thickened endocervical mucosa ± cystic change
- To differentiate from adenoma malignum assess for deeply seated cysts with complex features

---

- If associated with cystic change, low SI lesions in superficial layer of cervix (endocervix)
  - Cysts may be hyperintense if high mucin content
- T2WI
  - Often no abnormality of endocervical mucosa
  - May manifest as thickening of mucosal layer
    - Maintains the normal hyperintense SI
    - Small, round cysts of high SI may coexist with mucosal thickening
- T1 C+ FS
  - Enhancement pattern ranges from normal to hypovascular
    - Early enhancement compared to cervical stroma
  - No enhancement of cysts if present
    - Thin walls, absence of mural nodules

Imaging Recommendations
- Best imaging tool: MR imaging modality of choice to demonstrate homogeneous mucosal thickening and lack of stromal or deep involvement
- Protocol advice
  - Sagittal T2WI offers best depiction of cervical zonal anatomy
  - Dynamic T1 C+ FS images exclude wall thickening or mural nodules when cystic changes present

DIFFERENTIAL DIAGNOSIS

Cervical Adenocarcinoma
- Early stage can look like cervical gland hyperplasia
- Stromal invasion and deep location of cystic lesions are suspicious for adenocarcinoma/adenoma malignum
- Ill-defined margins with adjacent stroma favors neoplasm

Nabothian Cysts
- Superficial cystic structures usually seen at squamocolumnar transition zone
- Tend to be more focal and sparse, whereas hyperplasia is more diffuse and regular

Other Pseudoneoplastic Glandular Lesions
- Papillary endocervicitis, tunnel clusters, cervical endometriosis, Arias-Stella reaction, infectious processes and reactive atypias
  - No specific imaging criteria
  - Endocervical mucosa may appear normal or present as thickening

Cervical Pregnancy
- Gestational sac distending endocervical canal
- Usually excentrically located
- Yolk sac or embryonic pole ± cardiac activity may be identified

Cervical Stenosis
- Distension of cervical lumen with fluid
  - Fluid may be simple or complex (hematometra)
- No mucosal thickening

Gartner Duct Cyst
- Arise from anterolateral wall of vagina
- Distinct from cervix

PATHOLOGY

General Features
- Epidemiology
  - Very common, especially in reproductive age women
    - Oral contraceptive pill (progesterone stimulation)
    - Pregnancy (microglandular hyperplasia)
- Associated abnormalities: No proven evolution towards adenoma malignum or adenocarcinoma

Gross Pathologic & Surgical Features
- Often no abnormality visible
- Some subtypes may be associated with erosions of friable polypoid lesions

Microscopic Features
- Diffuse laminar endocervical glandular hyperplasia

CERVICAL GLANDULAR HYPERPLASIA

- Proliferation of moderately sized, evenly spaced, endocervical glands within inner-third of cervical wall
- Discrete layer sharply demarcated from underlying cervical stroma
- Reactive cytologic atypia may be present, which is not significant
- Hyperplasia of mesonephric remnants
  - Main mesonephric duct surrounded by variable number of small, round, and occasionally cystically dilated tubules
  - Lined by non mucinous cuboidal cells
  - May develop florid hyperplasia
  - No associated stromal reaction
- Glandular hyperplasia (not otherwise specified)
  - Hyperplasia of endocervical epithelium, sometimes florid
  - Lack of deep invasion, well-demarcated margin with adjacent cervical stroma, lobular grouping, lack of stromal reaction, bland nuclear features indicate absence of neoplasia
- Microglandular hyperplasia
  - Closely packed glands
    - Lined by columnar, cuboidal or flat cells
  - Range from small and round to large, irregular and cystically dilated
  - Basophilic or eosinophilic reaction that stains for mucin
  - Many acute inflammatory cells
  - Stroma occasionally hyalinized
- Florid endocervical glandular hyperplasia with intestinal or pyloric gland metaplasia
  - Proliferating endocervical glands surrounded by clusters of smaller glands resembling pyloric glands of stomach
  - Occasional intestinal metaplasia
  - Bland nuclear features
  - Predominantly PAS-positive neutral mucin in glandular epithelium
- All glands lined by single layer of columnar mucin secreting epithelium, except for hyperplasia of mesonephric remnants

CLINICAL ISSUES

Presentation
- Most common signs/symptoms
  - Most often asymptomatic
  - May be associated with abnormal vaginal bleeding or vaginal discharge

Demographics
- Age: Reproductive age women, less commonly postmenopausal women

Natural History & Prognosis
- Often incidentally discovered on hysterectomy or cone biopsy specimen
- May be diagnosed during the work-up of a multicystic cervical mass
- Usually not identified on pap test

Treatment
- No treatment required
- Hysterectomy performed when adenoma malignum or other aggressive lesion cannot be excluded

DIAGNOSTIC CHECKLIST

Consider
- Consider cervical gland hyperplasia in the setting of a homogeneously thickened endocervical mucosa ± cystic change
- To differentiate from adenoma malignum assess for deeply seated cysts with complex features

Image Interpretation Pearls
- Thickened endocervical mucosa ± superficial cysts showing thin walls and absence of mural nodules

SELECTED REFERENCES

1. Oguri H et al: MRI of endocervical glandular disorders: three cases of a deep nabothian cyst and three cases of a minimal-deviation adenocarcinoma. Magn Reson Imaging. 22(9):1333-7, 2004
2. Okamoto Y et al: Pelvic imaging: multicystic uterine cervical lesions. Can magnetic resonance imaging differentiate benignancy from malignancy? Acta Radiol. 45(1):102-8, 2004
3. Mikami Y et al: Lobular endocervical glandular hyperplasia is a metaplastic process with a pyloric gland phenotype. Histopathology. 39(4):364-72, 2001
4. Yoden E et al: Florid endocervical glandular hyperplasia with pyloric gland metaplasia: a radiologic pitfall. J Comput Assist Tomogr. 25(1):94-7, 2001
5. Itoh K et al: A comparative analysis of cross sectional imaging techniques in minimal deviation adenocarcinoma of the uterine cervix. BJOG. 107(9):1158-63, 2000
6. Mikami Y et al: Florid endocervical glandular hyperplasia with intestinal and pyloric gland metaplasia: worrisome benign mimic of "adenoma malignum". Gynecol Oncol. 74(3):504-11, 1999
7. Nucci MR et al: Lobular endocervical glandular hyperplasia, not otherwise specified: a clinicopathologic analysis of thirteen cases of a distinctive pseudoneoplastic lesion and comparison with fourteen cases of adenoma malignum. Am J Surg Pathol. 23(8):886-91, 1999
8. Young RH et al: Pseudoneoplastic glandular lesions of the uterine cervix. Semin Diagn Pathol. 8(4):234-49, 1991

CERVICAL GLANDULAR HYPERPLASIA

IMAGE GALLERY

Typical

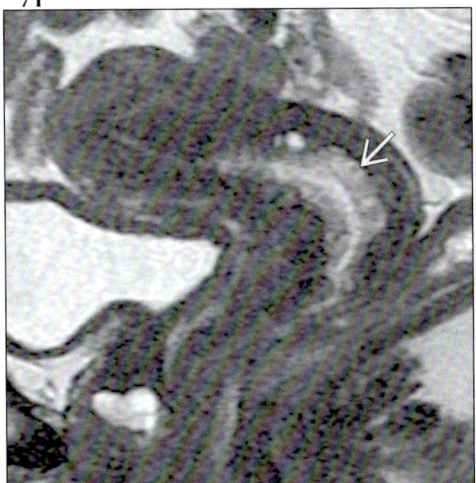
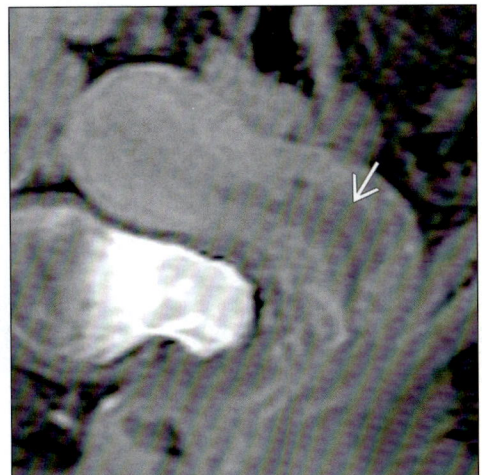

(Left) Sagittal T2WI MR shows diffuse and regular thickening of the hyperintense endocervical mucosa ➡ in keeping with glandular hyperplasia. Tiny cysts give the mucosa a slightly heterogeneous appearance. *(Right)* Sagittal T1 C+ FS MR in the same patient as previous image, shows the thickened mucosa remaining hypointense ➡ relative to the cervical stroma on the delayed post-contrast images.

Typical

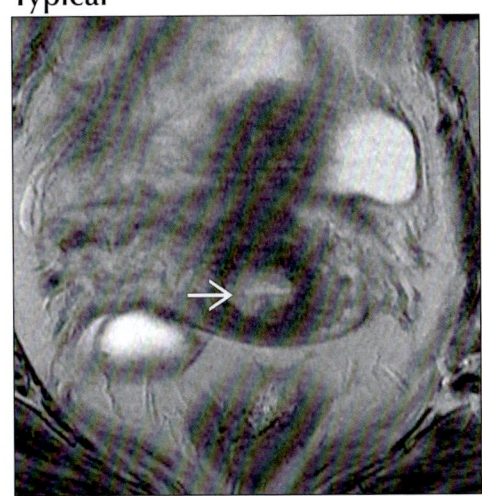
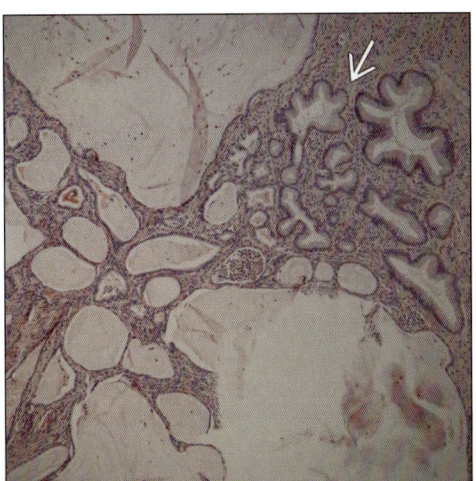

(Left) Axial T2WI MR (same patient as previous) shows good delineation of the zonal anatomy of the cervix. The hyperintense endocervical mucosa appears homogeneously thickened ➡ aside from punctate foci of cystic change. *(Right)* Micropathology (same patient as previous) shows grouped endocervical glands ➡ with dilated lumen giving the appearance of small cysts at imaging. They are lined by benign columnar epithelium. (Courtesy A. Mehio, MD).

Variant

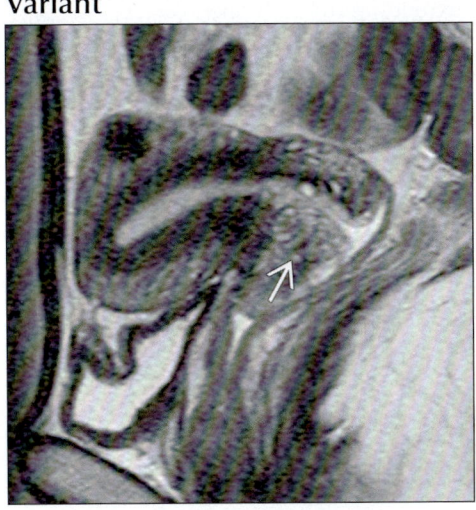
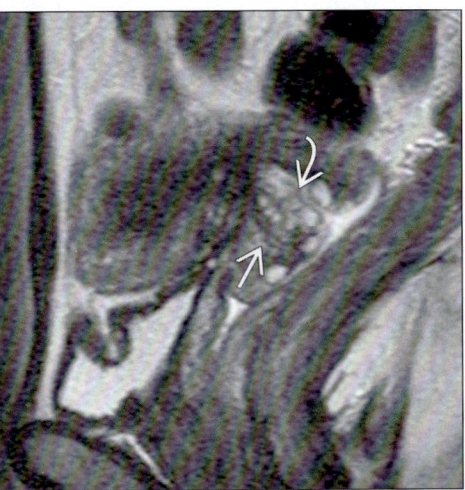

(Left) Sagittal T2WI MR shows thickening of the endocervical mucosa with multiple hyperintense foci ➡ compatible with cysts. Apparent deep extension of the cysts raised suspicion for adenoma malignum. *(Right)* Parasagittal T2WI MR in the same patient as previous image, shows preservation of the cervical stroma. Less hyperintense areas ➡ are interspersed between the cysts ➡. Histopathology confirmed the presence of lobular endocervical glandular hyperplasia.

CERVICAL INCOMPETENCE

Sagittal transvaginal ultrasound shows cervical incompetence. There is funneling of the internal os and a short cervical length (1.4 mm) indicated by the calipers.

Sagittal transabdominal ultrasound in same patient as previous image, shows importance of emptying bladder prior to measuring cervical length. Cervical length is falsely elongated.

TERMINOLOGY

Abbreviations and Synonyms
- Cervical insufficiency, cervical effacement

Definitions
- Shortening of cervix
  - Cervical length is distance between internal and external os
  - False positives possible if measure transabdominally and/or with an overdistended bladder

IMAGING FINDINGS

General Features
- Best diagnostic clue: Short cervix
- Location: Internal os is affected first
- Size: Length less than 3 cm
- Morphology
  - Open internal os
  - Funneling of membranes into endocervical canal
  - In extreme cases, see presentation of fetal parts through dilated open cervix

Ultrasonographic Findings
- Grayscale Ultrasound
  - Transabdominal scanning will demonstrate the same findings as transvaginal ultrasound (see below)
  - When cervix is obscured by presenting part, do transvaginal or translabial US for optimal visualization
- Transvaginal ultrasound (TVS) findings
  - Short cervix (< 30 mm); (normal cervical length: 3.0-4.5 cm)
  - Funneling of internal os, not significant if length > 3 cm
  - Wide internal os diameter (funnel width) > 1 cm
  - Percentage of funneling (funnel length divided by the sum of funnel length and functional length) > 50%
  - Hourglass herniation of membranes through incompetent cervix
  - Fetal parts extending through open cervix
  - Rapid dynamic changes in dilatation of cervical canal has been observed during sonography
    - It is necessary to observe cervix and lower uterine segment several times throughout exam

DDx: Cervical Incompetence Mimics

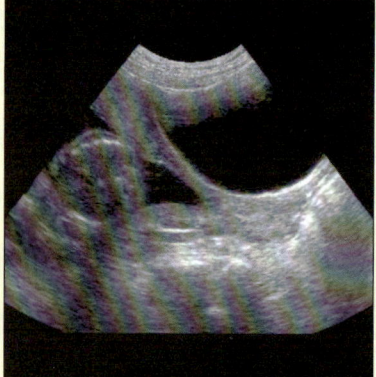
Overdistended Bladder

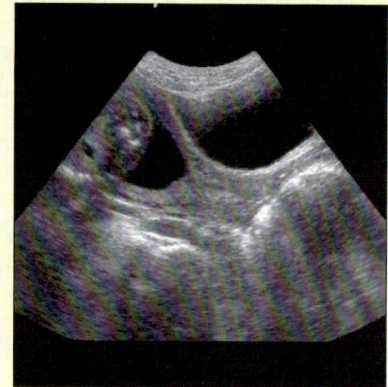
Overdistended Bladder

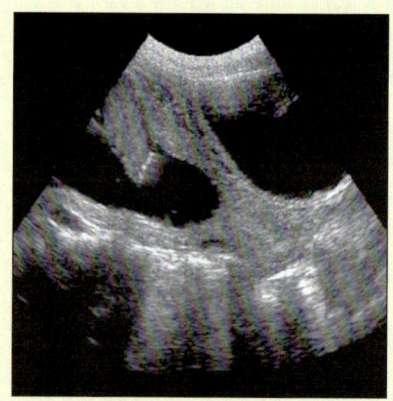
Muscle Contraction

CERVICAL INCOMPETENCE

Key Facts

Terminology
- Shortening of cervix
- Cervical length is distance between internal and external os

Imaging Findings
- Best diagnostic clue: Short cervix
- Short cervix (< 30 mm); (normal cervical length: 3.0-4.5 cm)
- Best imaging tool: Ultrasound can detect changes of incompetence before they are evident on digital examination
- TVS is the method most amenable to standardization and provides highest degree of consistency for cervical measurement

Top Differential Diagnoses
- Normal Cervical Effacement
- Placental Abruption
- Subclinical Chorioamnionitis
- Pseudodilatation/Pseudofunneling

Clinical Issues
- Affects approximately 1% of pregnant patients
- Cause of recurrent pregnancy loss
- Standard therapy is cervical cerclage

Diagnostic Checklist
- Can be missed due to compression by overdistended bladder, intermittent changes in configuration of the cervix and suboptimal visualization

MR Findings
- Findings are suggestive, not diagnostic
- Cervical length < 3.0 cm
- Internal os wider than 4.2 mm
- Asymmetric widening of endocervical canal
- Thinning or absence of low signal intensity cervical stroma
- Abnormal signal intensity of cervical stroma

Imaging Recommendations
- Best imaging tool: Ultrasound can detect changes of incompetence before they are evident on digital examination
- Protocol advice
  o Make sure whole length of cervix is visualized when scanning, external os appears symmetric, and distance from surface of posterior lip to cervical canal is equal to distance from surface of anterior lip to cervical canal
  o TVS is the method most amenable to standardization and provides highest degree of consistency for cervical measurement
  o Empty bladder prior to imaging: Full bladder may falsely elongate cervix
  o Surveillance of patients at risk should begin at 15 weeks gestation
  o Recommend assessment several times during course of exam as changes can occur during scanning
    ▪ Cervix should be observed for several minutes at a time as dynamic changes of cervix can take place in a short time period
  o Transfundal pressure, valsalva, postural challenge
    ▪ Indicated for patients at risk who have a cervical length above threshold value for diagnosis of incompetence
  o Transperineal scanning may be performed in situation when transvaginal scanning is contraindicated
  o Early manifestation of incompetent cervix may become inapparent after assuming the supine position
    ▪ May be useful to examine cervix at beginning of obstetrical exam rather than at end
    ▪ If exam is negative (regardless of whether evaluation for incompetence is done at beginning or end of exam), can have the patient stand for 15 minutes and re-evaluate

DIFFERENTIAL DIAGNOSIS

Normal Cervical Effacement
- Occurs at term gestation

Placental Abruption
- May present with cervical shortening

Subclinical Chorioamnionitis
- May present with cervical shortening

Pseudodilatation/Pseudofunneling
- Due to lower uterine segment contractions, overdistended bladder, and with undue pressure on cervix during TVS
- Apparent cervical length greater than 5 cm
- Demonstration of normal appearing cervical tissue distal to apparently dilated region
- Rounding of myometrium surrounding the apparently dilated area

PATHOLOGY

General Features
- Etiology
  o Risk factors include
    ▪ In utero exposure to diethylstilbestrol (DES)
    ▪ Congenital uterine malformations
    ▪ Cervical trauma from laceration and/or cone biopsy
    ▪ History of previous second trimester loss
    ▪ History of precipitous labor or advanced dilation before labor onset

CERVICAL INCOMPETENCE

- History of recurrent spontaneous and therapeutic abortions
- Epidemiology: Responsible for 15% of second and third trimester abortions

Gross Pathologic & Surgical Features
- Change from closed cervix to wedge shaped opening of internal os followed by progressive cervical shortening craniocaudally

CLINICAL ISSUES

Presentation
- Most common signs/symptoms
  - Vaginal spotting in second or third trimester
  - Normal appearing cervix at physical examination
  - May be asymptomatic
- Other signs/symptoms
  - Clinical diagnosed by abnormal digital cervical examination
  - May present with increased painful and/or persistent uterine contractions
- Clinical Profile
  - Painless dilatation followed by fetal expulsion that occurs in second trimester
  - Can present without identifiable risk factors

Demographics
- Age: Affects approximately 1% of pregnant patients

Natural History & Prognosis
- Early cervical effacement changes start at level of internal os which precede clinically detectable changes by 4-9 weeks
- True premature labor is preceded by several weeks of clinically detectable cervical shortening
- If untreated results in premature delivery and increased risk of pregnancy loss
- Cause of recurrent pregnancy loss

Treatment
- Standard therapy is cervical cerclage
- Decisions on placement of cerclage are based on sonographic findings rather than on clinical history or physical examination
- May perform cerclage emergently at diagnosis
- May prophylactically perform cerclage at 12-15 weeks for patients with classic history of incompetence
- Other treatments include pessary, uterine relaxation and bed rest after 24 weeks
- Bed rest and tocolytics preferred after 24 weeks

DIAGNOSTIC CHECKLIST

Image Interpretation Pearls
- Can be missed due to compression by overdistended bladder, intermittent changes in configuration of the cervix and suboptimal visualization
- Women at risk for cervical incompetency showed a high rate of dilation of the internal os with descent of the fetal membranes during transfundal pressure
  - Some women had a normal appearing internal os and cervical length before application of transfundal pressure

SELECTED REFERENCES

1. Scheerer L J et al: Ultrasound evaluation of the cervix. In: Callen PW, ed. Ultrasonography in Obstetrics and Gynecology. 4th ed. Philadelphia, PA, Saunders. 577-96, 2000
2. Leitich H et al: Cervical length and dilatation of the internal cervical os detected by vaginal ultrasonography as markers for preterm delivery: A systematic review. Am J Obstet Gynecol. 181(6):1465-72, 1999
3. Wong G et al: Maternal postural challenge as a functional test for cervical incompetence. J Ultrasound Med. 16(3):169-75, 1997
4. Iams JD et al: The length of the cervix and the risk of spontaneous premature delivery. National Institute of Child Health and Human Development Maternal Fetal Medicine Unit Network. N Engl J Med. 334(9):567-72, 1996
5. Guzman ER et al: A new method using vaginal ultrasound and transfundal pressure to evaluate the asymptomatic incompetent cervix. Obstet Gynecol. 83(2):248-52, 1994
6. Riley L et al: The implications of sonographically identified cervical changes in patients not necessarily at risk for preterm birth. J Ultrasound Med. 11(3):75-9, 1992
7. Karis JP et al: Sonographic diagnosis of premature cervical dilatation. Potential pitfall due to lower uterine segment contractions. J Ultrasound Med. 10(2):83-7, 1991
8. Hricak H et al: Cervical incompetence: preliminary evaluation with MR imaging. Radiology. 174(3 Pt 1):821-6, 1990
9. Mahony BS et al: Translabial ultrasound of the third-trimester uterine cervix. Correlation with digital examination. J Ultrasound Med. 9(12):717-23, 1990
10. Roberts WE et al: The incidence of preterm labor and specific risk factors. Obstet Gynecol. 76(1 Suppl):85S-89S, 1990
11. Ayers JW et al: Sonographic evaluation of cervical length in pregnancy: diagnosis and management of preterm cervical effacement in patients at risk for premature delivery. Obstet Gynecol. 71(6 Pt 1):939-44, 1988
12. Parulekar SG et al: Dynamic incompetent cervix uteri. Sonographic observations. J Ultrasound Med. 7(9):481-5, 1988

CERVICAL INCOMPETENCE

IMAGE GALLERY

Typical

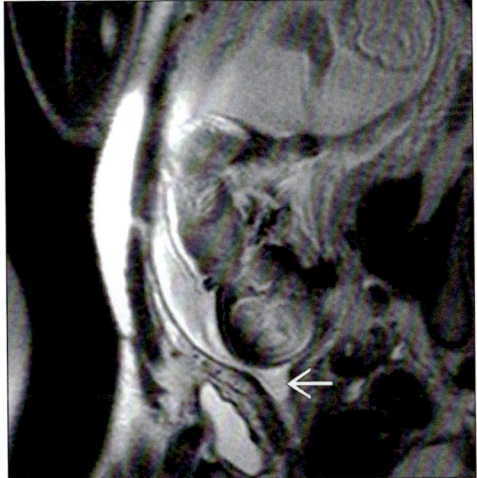
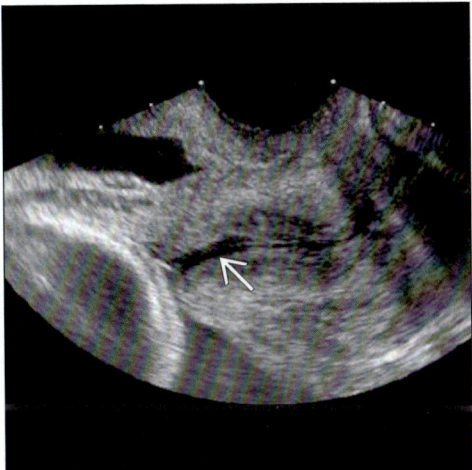

(Left) Sagittal T2WI MR shows funneling at the internal cervical os and shortening of the cervical length. The fetal membranes appear to be bulging into the incompetent internal os ➡. *(Right)* Longitudinal transvaginal ultrasound shows mild funneling at the internal cervical os ➡ not seen on the transabdominal scan. (Courtesy O. Baltarowich, MD).

Typical

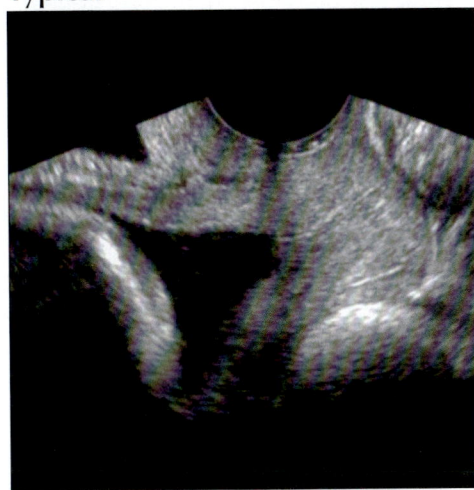
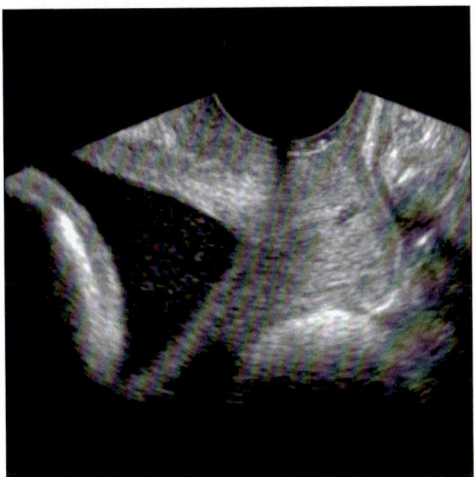

(Left) Sagittal transvaginal ultrasound shows cervical shortening and funneling at the internal os. (Courtesy O. Baltarowich, MD). *(Right)* Sagittal transvaginal ultrasound shows progression of both cervical shortening and funneling. (Courtesy O. Baltarowich, MD).

Typical

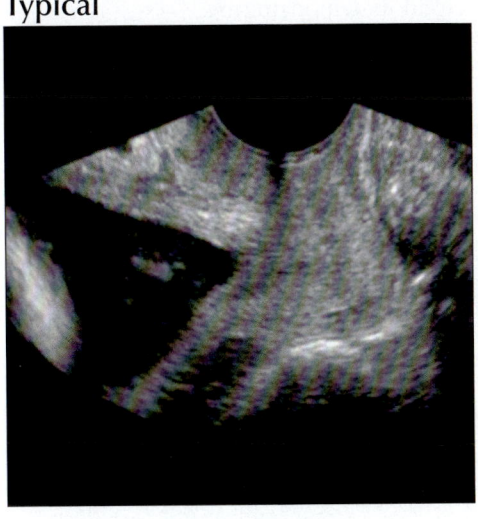
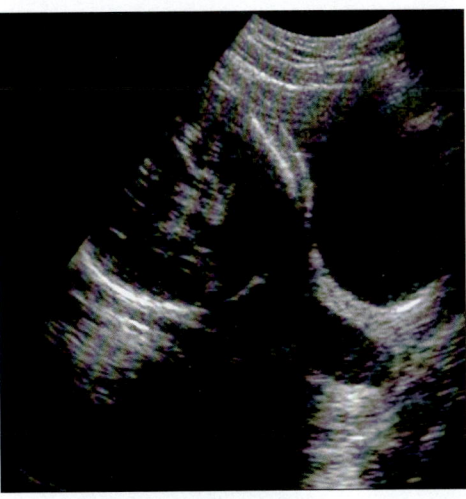

(Left) Sagittal transvaginal ultrasound obtained 5 minutes after the previous image shows dynamic changes in the cervical length and degree of funneling. (Courtesy O. Baltarowich, MD). *(Right)* Sagittal transabdominal ultrasound shows near complete cervical effacement. (Courtesy O. Baltarowich, MD).

POST TRACHELECTOMY APPEARANCES

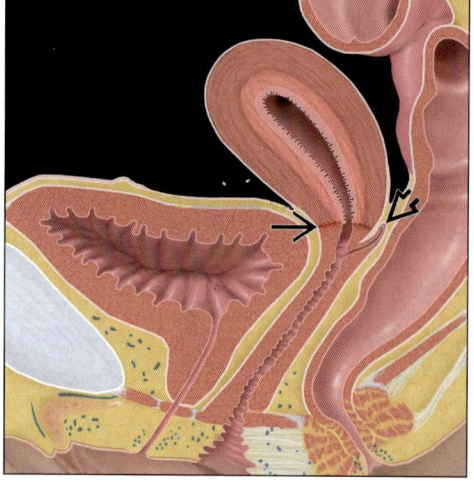

Graphic (sagittal midline section) shows post trachelectomy appearances with end to end anastomosis between corpus uteri and vagina. Note the presence of suture line ➡ and vaginal neofornix ➡.

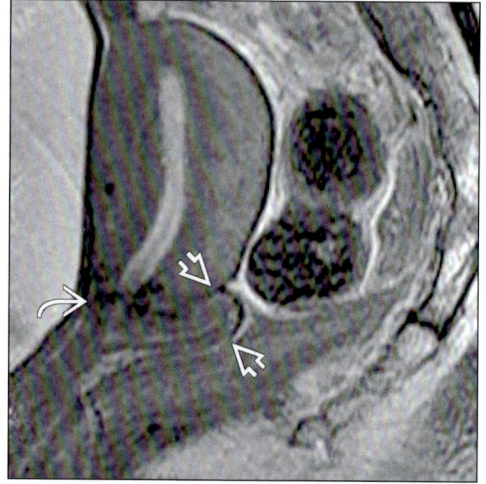

Sagittal T2WI MR shows post-trachelectomy appearances with end to end anastomosis between corpus uteri and vaginal vault (note artifact from sutures) ➡, and appearance of a vaginal neofornix ➡.

TERMINOLOGY

Definitions
- Trachelectomy is a curative surgical procedure performed for early (stage IB1 or lower) carcinoma of the cervix
- Performed as an alternative to radical hysterectomy in women wishing to preserve fertility
- First developed in 1987 by French surgeon, Daniel Dargent
- Involves
  - Surgical resection of upper vagina, affected cervix, and surrounding parametria
  - Resection is usually performed via a vaginal approach
  - End to end anastomosis performed between lower vagina and corpus uteri
- Procedure always combined with a laparoscopic bilateral pelvic lymph node dissection

IMAGING FINDINGS

General Features
- Best diagnostic clue: Surgical anastomosis between corpus uteri and vaginal vault

Ultrasonographic Findings
- Not helpful in demonstrating post-trachelectomy appearances or early recurrent disease
- May identify complications such as lymphoceles

CT Findings
- CECT
  - Not helpful in demonstrating post-trachelectomy appearances or early recurrent disease
  - May identify complications such as vaginal wall hematoma or lymphoceles

MR Findings
- T1WI: Not helpful in demonstrating post-trachelectomy appearances, recurrent disease or complications
- T2WI
  - **Normal post-operative appearances**

DDx: Other Cervical Lesions

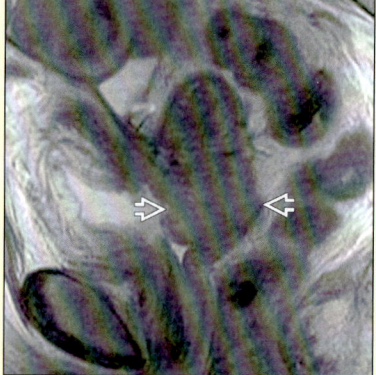

Recurrent Cervical Cancer (Post RT)

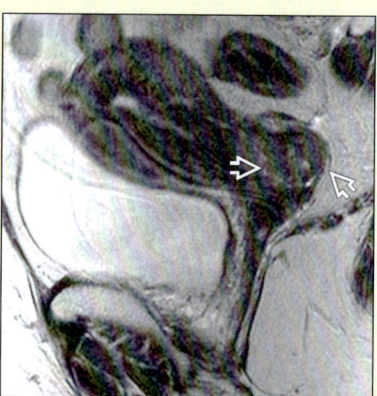

Recurrent Cervical Cancer (Post RT)

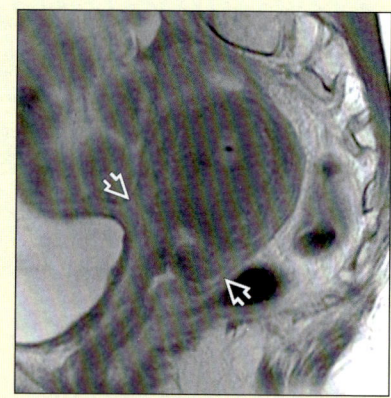

Radiation Necrosis of the Cervix

POST TRACHELECTOMY APPEARANCES

Key Facts

Terminology
- Trachelectomy is a curative surgical procedure performed for early (stage IB1 or lower) carcinoma of the cervix
- Performed as an alternative to radical hysterectomy in women wishing to preserve fertility

Imaging Findings
- Best diagnostic clue: Surgical anastomosis between corpus uteri and vaginal vault
- **Normal post-operative appearances**
- End to end surgical anastomosis between corpus uteri and vaginal vault
- Neofornix of vagina formed by closure of lateral fornices
- Suture susceptibility artifacts
- **Post-operative complications**
  - Isthmic stenosis
  - Vaginal wall hematoma
  - Lymphoceles
- Best imaging tool: MR

Top Differential Diagnoses
- Recurrent Tumor
- Radiation Necrosis

Clinical Issues
- Normal post-trachelectomy appearances to the pelvis on MR should remain stable or improve with time

Diagnostic Checklist
- Baseline MR study following trachelectomy for cervical carcinoma; regular interval MR following baseline study

---

- End to end surgical anastomosis between corpus uteri and vaginal vault
  - Seen in approximately 45%
- Neofornix of vagina formed by closure of lateral fornices
  - Seen in approximately 50%
  - Formed by surgical closure of lateral fornices
  - Appears as a posterior extension of vaginal wall at site of utero-vaginal anastomosis
  - Appearances remain stable with time
- Suture susceptibility artifacts
  - Seen in approximately 20%
  - Artifact due to the anastomotic sutures and the cerclage suture placed around corpus uteri to preserve competence in pregnancy
  - Artifact more pronounced on FSE T2WI
- Diffuse vaginal wall thickening with abnormal high signal intensity
  - Seen in between 5-10%
  - Represents post-surgical change which gradually resolves by 1 year
  - Biopsy may be needed to exclude recurrence
- Exaggeration of pelvic venous plexuses
  - Seen in approximately 10%
  - Irreversible and usually asymptomatic
  - No cause identified
- **Post-operative complications**
- Isthmic stenosis
  - Seen in 2%
  - Occurs as early as 3 months post-operatively
- Vaginal wall hematoma
  - Seen in approximately 5%
  - Appears as high signal intensity on T2WI and T1WI FS
  - Persists up to 1 year
- Lymphoceles
  - Seen in approximately 25%
  - Appear as uni/bilateral cystic lesions in obturator or external iliac distributions
  - Demonstrate high signal intensity on T2WI
  - Can persist for several years
- **Unexpected findings**
- Recurrent disease
  - Occurs in approximately 4% of patients
  - Usually occurs at the site of the surgical anastomosis
  - Appears as an enhancing soft tissue mass of intermediate to high signal intensity on T2WI
- Other incidental findings
  - Leiomyomas
  - Adenomyosis
  - Endometriomas

Imaging Recommendations
- Best imaging tool: MR
- Protocol advice
  - Axial T1WI
  - Axial, coronal and sagittal T2WI
  - Axial and sagittal T1WI FS C+ images
    - If recurrent disease is suspected

DIFFERENTIAL DIAGNOSIS

Recurrent Tumor
- Appears as intermediate to high signal on T2
- Demonstrates similar signal intensity to original tumor
- Enhances on T1 C+
- Biopsy may be required for diagnosis as may be difficult to distinguish from normal post-operative change

Radiation Necrosis
- History of pelvic irradiation
- Fluid distended endometrial cavity in approximately 50%
- High signal on T2 with variable enhancement
- Increase in SI of bone marrow in irradiated field

PATHOLOGY

General Features
- Epidemiology
  - Trachelectomy performed in premenopausal females

POST TRACHELECTOMY APPEARANCES

- With stage IB1 or lower carcinoma of the cervix
- Patient needs to be of reproductive age
- Patient wishes to remain fertile
- Preferably has a cervical lesion ≤ 2 cm
- Disease located primarily on the ectocervix
- No evidence of pelvic lymph node metastases or distant metastases
- Exclusion of unfavorable histology (e.g., neuroendocrine carcinoma)

CLINICAL ISSUES

Demographics
- Age: Premenopausal
- Gender: Females

Natural History & Prognosis
- Normal post-trachelectomy appearances to the pelvis on MR should remain stable or improve with time
- Recurrent tumor
  - In a total of 319 patients reported in the literature by 2004, overall recurrence following trachelectomy was 4.2% with a median followup of 44 months
  - Greatest risk if original tumor size > than 2 cm with depth of invasion > 1 cm
  - Other risk factors: Lymphovascular space involvement, deep stromal invasion, unfavorable histology
  - 97% 5-year survival rate reported
  - Overall death rate 2.8%
  - Recurrence and death rates comparable to classical radical abdominal hysterectomy
- Successful pregnancy rates of between 40-70% reported
  - Overall 13% 1st trimester miscarriage rate reported
  - Overall 19% 2nd trimester miscarriage rate reported
  - Risk of pre-term delivery; approximately 60% deliver > 37 weeks

DIAGNOSTIC CHECKLIST

Consider
- Baseline MR study following trachelectomy for cervical carcinoma; regular interval MR following baseline study

Image Interpretation Pearls
- End to end surgical anastomosis between corpus uteri and vaginal vault with suture susceptibility artifacts

SELECTED REFERENCES

1. Dursun P et al: Radical vaginal trachelectomy (Dargent's operation): A critical review of the literature. Eur J Surg Oncol. 2007
2. Sonoda Y et al: Radical vaginal trachelectomy and laparoscopic pelvic lymphadenectomy for early-stage cervical cancer in patients who desire to preserve fertility. Gynecol Oncol. 104(2 Suppl):50-5, 2007
3. Abu-Rustum NR et al: Fertility-sparing radical abdominal trachelectomy for cervical carcinoma: technique and review of the literature. Gynecol Oncol. 103(3):807-13, 2006
4. Hatami M et al: Preserving fertility in invasive cervical adenocarcinoma by abdominal radical trachelectomy and pelvic lymphadenectomy. Arch Iran Med. 9(4):413-6, 2006
5. Hertel H et al: Radical vaginal trachelectomy (RVT) combined with laparoscopic pelvic lymphadenectomy: prospective multicenter study of 100 patients with early cervical cancer. Gynecol Oncol. 103(2):506-11, 2006
6. Schlaerth AC et al: Role of minimally invasive surgery in gynecologic cancers. Oncologist. 11(8):895-901, 2006
7. Shepherd JH et al: Radical vaginal trachelectomy as a fertility-sparing procedure in women with early-stage cervical cancer-cumulative pregnancy rate in a series of 123 women. BJOG. 113(6):719-24, 2006
8. Plante M et al: Vaginal radical trachelectomy: a valuable fertility-preserving option in the management of early-stage cervical cancer. A series of 50 pregnancies and review of the literature. Gynecol Oncol. 98(1):3-10, 2005
9. Sahdev A et al: MR imaging appearances of the female pelvis after trachelectomy. Radiographics. 25(1):41-52, 2005
10. Ungar L et al: Abdominal radical trachelectomy: a fertility-preserving option for women with early cervical cancer. BJOG. 112(3):366-9, 2005
11. Plante M et al: Vaginal radical trachelectomy: an oncologically safe fertility-preserving surgery. An updated series of 72 cases and review of the literature. Gynecol Oncol. 94(3):614-23, 2004
12. Burnett AF et al: Radical vaginal trachelectomy and pelvic lymphadenectomy for preservation of fertility in early cervical carcinoma. Gynecol Oncol. 88(3):419-23, 2003
13. Rodriguez M et al: Radical abdominal trachelectomy and pelvic lymphadenectomy with uterine conservation and subsequent pregnancy in the treatment of early invasive cervical cancer. Am J Obstet Gynecol. 185(2):370-4, 2001
14. Dargent D et al: Laparoscopic vaginal radical trachelectomy: a treatment to preserve the fertility of cervical carcinoma patients. Cancer. 88(8):1877-82, 2000
15. Covens A et al: Is radical trachelectomy a safe alternative to radical hysterectomy for patients with stage IA-B carcinoma of the cervix? Cancer. 86(11):2273-9, 1999

POST TRACHELECTOMY APPEARANCES

IMAGE GALLERY

Typical

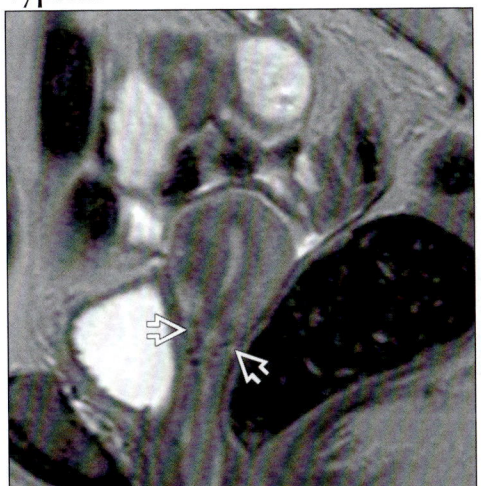
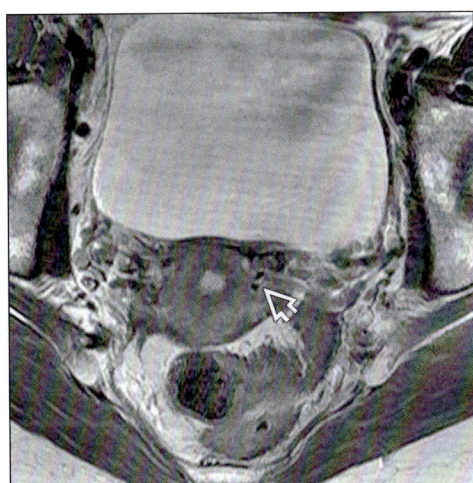

(Left) Sagittal T2WI MR shows post-trachelectomy appearances with end to end anastomosis between corpus uteri and vaginal vault (note artifact from sutures) ➤. (Courtesy B. Hamm, MD). *(Right)* Axial oblique T2WI MR in the same patient as previous image, shows typical post-trachelectomy appearances. Artifacts from sutures are again noted ➤.

Typical

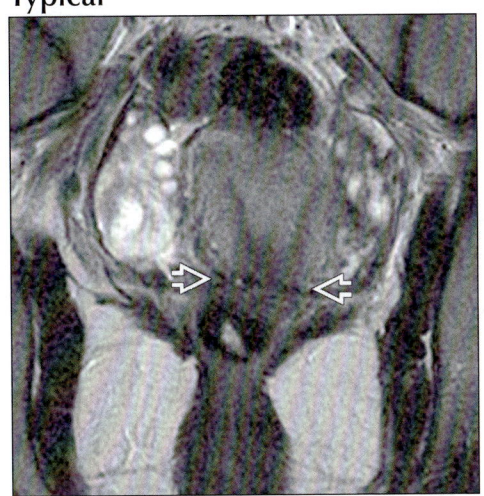
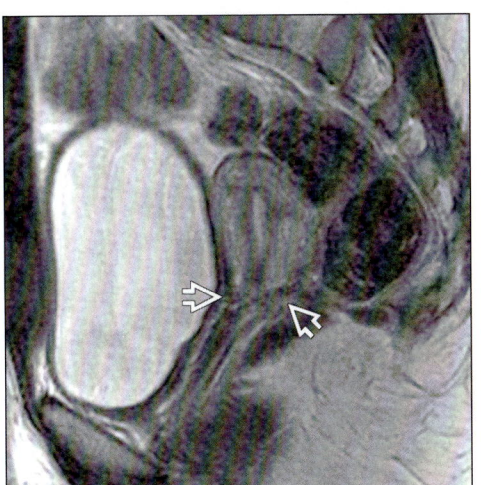

(Left) Coronal T2WI MR shows typical post-trachelectomy appearances with surgical anastomosis demonstrated between corpus uteri and vaginal vault ➤. *(Right)* Sagittal T2WI MR in the same patient as previous image, shows typical post-trachelectomy appearances with end to end surgical anastomosis between the uterine corpus and the vaginal vault ➤.

Typical

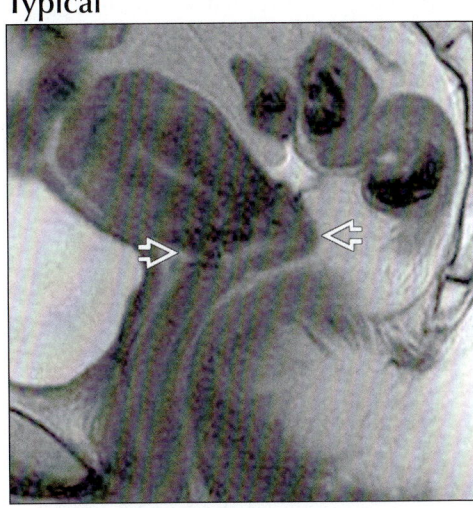
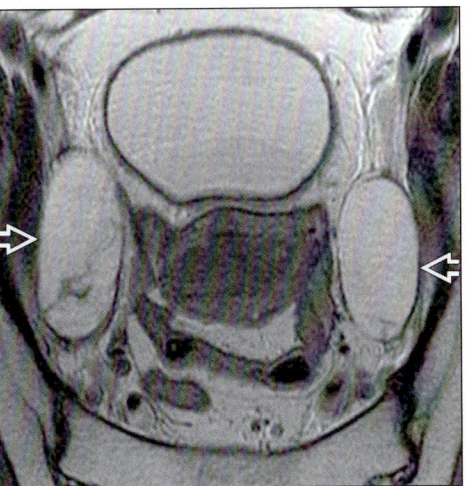

(Left) Sagittal T2WI MR shows another example of typical post-trachelectomy appearances to the vaginal vault ➤. *(Right)* Axial oblique T2WI MR in the same patient as previous image, shows development of bilateral pelvic side wall lymphoceles ➤ as a complication following trachelectomy.

POST-RADIATION CERVIX

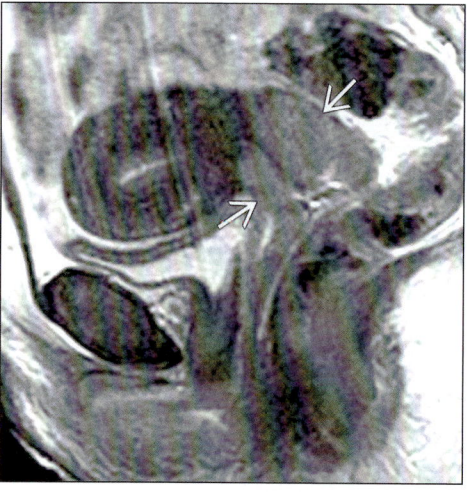

Sagittal T2WI MR shows cervical cancer ➡ seen as a large mass with high signal intensity.

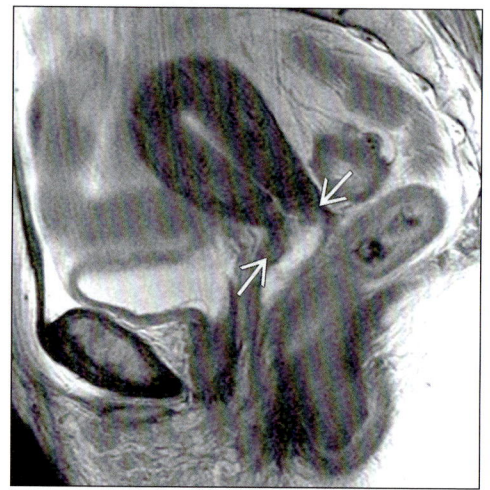

Sagittal T2WI MR shows complete tumor response. There is reconstitution of the cervical anatomy; the cervix is small and demonstrates diffuse low signal intensity ➡.

TERMINOLOGY

Abbreviations and Synonyms
- Post-RT changes

Definitions
- Radiation induced changes after external beam radiation or placement of radiation implants

IMAGING FINDINGS

General Features
- Best diagnostic clue
  - Decreased volume/size of cervical cancer
  - Decreased volume/size of uterus and cervix
  - Diffuse low signal intensity in uterus and cervix
  - Reconstitution of normal cervical anatomy
- Location: Post-radiation changes are observed in cervical cancer, cervix itself and surrounding tissues in pelvis
- Size: Cervical cancer and cervix itself decrease in size compared to their pretreatment sizes

Ultrasonographic Findings
- Grayscale Ultrasound
  - US is limited in assessment of cervical cancer after radiation treatment
  - However, it can show decrease in size of cervical mass

CT Findings
- NECT
  - It is limited in assessment of residual or recurrent tumor which is of iso attenuation to cervical stroma
  - However, it can show decrease in size of cervical mass
- CECT
  - Residual or recurrent tumor is of iso- or hypo attenuation relative to cervical stoma
  - Exact size measurement may be limited even on CECT
  - Small cervix, infiltrative postradiation changes in pelvic fat, adjacent bowel and bladder can be seen

MR Findings
- T1WI

DDx: Cervical Cancer - Post Treatment Appearances

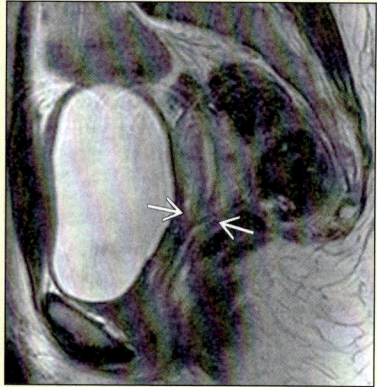

Post Trachelectomy

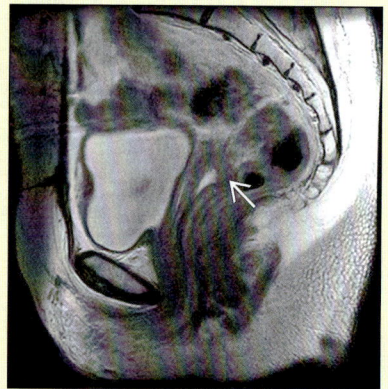

Post Hysterectomy

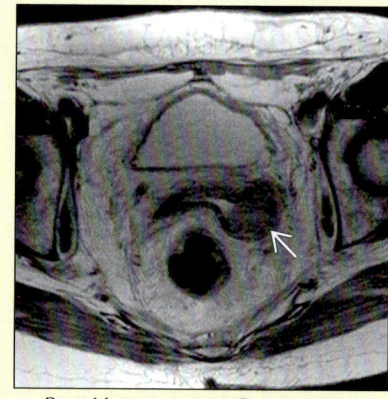

Post Hysterectomy Recurrence

POST-RADIATION CERVIX

Key Facts

Terminology
- Radiation induced changes after external beam radiation or placement of radiation implants

Imaging Findings
- Decreased volume/size of cervical cancer
- Decreased volume/size of uterus and cervix
- Diffuse low signal intensity in uterus and cervix
- Reconstitution of normal cervical anatomy
- Location: Post-radiation changes are observed in cervical cancer, cervix itself and surrounding tissues in pelvis
- MR is most commonly used for assessment of temporal changes in tumor size after radiation treatment
- T2WI is best to demonstrate post-radiation reconstitution of cervix
- PET can also be used to assess tumor response after radiation treatment
- Advantage of PET is whole-body imaging for distant metastases

Pathology
- Radiation treatment uses high-energy photons to destroy cancer cells
- Mechanism of radiation treatment is by induction of cellular death

Diagnostic Checklist
- Imaging provides important information on temporal changes in tumor volume/size after radiation treatment
- Tumor shrinkage is an important parameter indicating treatment response

---

- It is limited in assessment of residual or recurrent tumor which is isointense to cervical stroma
- Small cervix, infiltrative post-radiation changes in pelvic fat and fatty replacement in bone marrow can be seen
- T2WI
  - Best sequence to assess cervical cancer after radiation treatment
  - During first 6-12 months after radiation treatment, cervix may have high signal intensity due to edema and inflammation
  - After 12 months, cervix demonstrates uniformly low signal intensity due to fibrosis
  - Residual or recurrent cervical cancer appears as a nodular high signal intensity mass
- T1 C+
  - Contrast-enhancement is nonspecific and may be observed in both post-radiation necrosis and recurrent tumor
  - Contrast-enhancement is useful in assessment of possible complications such as vesicovaginal or rectovaginal fistula

Nuclear Medicine Findings
- PET
  - Tumor response can be assessed by FDG uptake on PET after radiation treatment
  - PET is also useful in assessing lymph nodes and distant metastases
  - PET may detect recurrences earlier than other methods do

Imaging Recommendations
- Best imaging tool
  - MR is most commonly used for assessment of temporal changes in tumor size after radiation treatment
    - T2WI is best to demonstrate post-radiation reconstitution of cervix
  - PET can also be used to assess tumor response after radiation treatment
    - Advantage of PET is whole-body imaging for distant metastases

DIFFERENTIAL DIAGNOSIS

Post Trachelectomy Changes
- Trachelectomy is surgical removal of cervix only
- It is an alternative surgical technique to preserve fertility in young women with early stages of cervical cancer
- After trachelectomy, uterine corpus remains intact with normal appearance on imaging

Post Hysterectomy Changes
- Radical hysterectomy is surgical removal of uterus, cervix, fallopian tubes, ovaries and upper vagina
- Pelvic lymph node resection is also performed during radical hysterectomy
- After radical hysterectomy only vaginal cuff remains
- Normal vaginal cuff has smooth, thin walls on imaging

Residual or Recurrent Cervical Carcinoma
- Nodular mass with high signal intensity in surgical bed after surgery or in cervical stroma after radiation treatment
- Benign conditions such as edema, inflammation, and necrosis may also have high signal on T2WI and mimic tumor
  - In such cases, biopsy is recommended to rule out residual or recurrent tumor

PATHOLOGY

General Features
- General path comments
  - After radiation treatment the cervix demonstrates
    - Fibrosis
    - Low cellularity
    - Hemosiderin deposits in the necrotic tissue
- Etiology
  - Radiation treatment uses high-energy photons to destroy cancer cells
  - Mechanism of radiation treatment is by induction of cellular death

POST-RADIATION CERVIX

Microscopic Features
- Cytology is a valuable tool for the detection of locally recurrent cervical cancer after radiation treatment
- Benign radiation changes, post-irradiation dysplasia, repair cells and active stromal cells can also be seen

CLINICAL ISSUES

Presentation
- Most common signs/symptoms
  - After radiation treatment following signs and symptoms can be observed
    - Fatigue
    - Diarrhea
    - Frequent or painful urination
    - Vaginal dryness
  - Major complications of radiation treatment include
    - Proctitis
    - Cystitis
    - Vesicovaginal fistula
    - Rectovaginal fistula
    - Vaginal scarring
    - Infection
    - Cervical stenosis

Natural History & Prognosis
- An early and marked decrease in tumor size/volume indicates favorable response to treatment
- Prognosis is good if no tumor recurrence occurs

Treatment
- Radiation treatment can be applied as external beam radiation, radioactive implants, or a combination of these
- Radiation therapy can be combined with surgery or chemotherapy depending on extent of disease
- After radiation treatment, persistent or recurrent tumor and radiation related complications can occur
- Residual or recurrent tumor and post-radiation complications are treated as appropriately

DIAGNOSTIC CHECKLIST

Consider
- Imaging provides important information on temporal changes in tumor volume/size after radiation treatment
  - Tumor shrinkage is an important parameter indicating treatment response
- Imaging is useful in detection of recurrences and complications after radiation treatment
- Imaging is also useful in treatment planning for recurrences and complications

Image Interpretation Pearls
- After radiation treatment, it is important to distinguish post-radiation changes from recurrent tumor
  - Both tumor and cervix decrease in size
  - Cervical stroma displays low signal intensity on T2WI
- Residual or recurrent tumor shows high signal intensity on T2WI
  - However, benign conditions such as edema, inflammation, and necrosis may also have high signal on T2WI mimicking tumor
- PET imaging is very useful in assessment of tumor response
  - However, radiation induced inflammatory changes may show uptake and mimic tumor

SELECTED REFERENCES

1. Akin O et al: Imaging of uterine cancer. Radiol Clin North Am. 45(1):167-82, 2007
2. Adhya AK et al: Radiation therapy induced changes in apoptosis and its major regulatory proteins, Bcl-2, Bcl-XL, and Bax, in locally advanced invasive squamous cell carcinoma of the cervix. Int J Gynecol Pathol. 25(3):281-7, 2006
3. Engin G: Cervical cancer: MR imaging findings before, during, and after radiation therapy. Eur Radiol. 16(2):313-24, 2006
4. Kerimoglu U et al: Evaluation of radiotherapy response of cervical carcinoma with gray scale and color Doppler ultrasonography: resistive index correlation with magnetic resonance findings. Diagn Interv Radiol. 12(3):155-60, 2006
5. Mayr NA et al: Serial therapy-induced changes in tumor shape in cervical cancer and their impact on assessing tumor volume and treatment response. AJR Am J Roentgenol. 187(1):65-72, 2006
6. Macapinlac HA: FDG-PET in the evaluation of cervical cancer. Gynecol Oncol. 99(3 Suppl 1):S171-2, 2005
7. Belhocine TZ: 18F-FDG PET imaging in posttherapy monitoring of cervical cancers: from diagnosis to prognosis. J Nucl Med. 45(10):1602-4, 2004
8. Follen M et al: Imaging in cervical cancer. Cancer. 98(9 Suppl):2028-38, 2003
9. Miller TR et al: Measurement of tumor volume by PET to evaluate prognosis in patients with advanced cervical cancer treated by radiation therapy. Int J Radiat Oncol Biol Phys. 53(2):353-9, 2002
10. Yamashita Y et al: Dynamic contrast-enhanced MR imaging of uterine cervical cancer: pharmacokinetic analysis with histopathologic correlation and its importance in predicting the outcome of radiation therapy. Radiology. 216(3):803-9, 2000
11. Hatano K et al: Evaluation of the therapeutic effect of radiotherapy on cervical cancer using magnetic resonance imaging. Int J Radiat Oncol Biol Phys. 45(3):639-44, 1999

POST-RADIATION CERVIX

IMAGE GALLERY

Typical

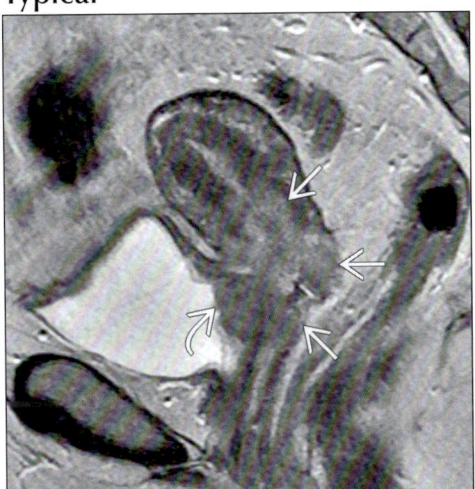
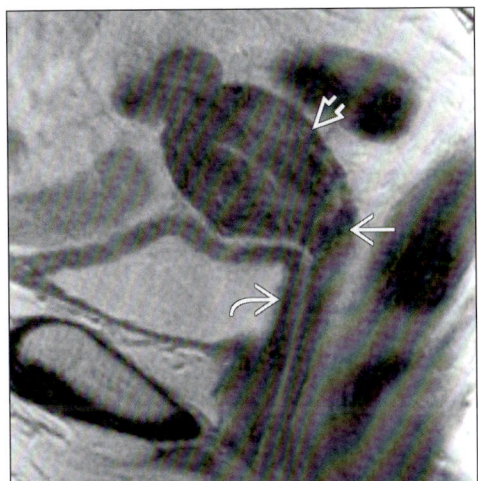

(Left) Sagittal T2WI MR shows a large cervical cancer ➡ involving the lower uterine segment and the upper vagina. Urinary bladder is also invaded ➡. *(Right)* Sagittal T2WI MR shows that the mass entirely resolved after radiation treatment. Note the normal low signal intensity in the urinary bladder wall ➡, uterus ➡ and small cervix ➡.

Typical

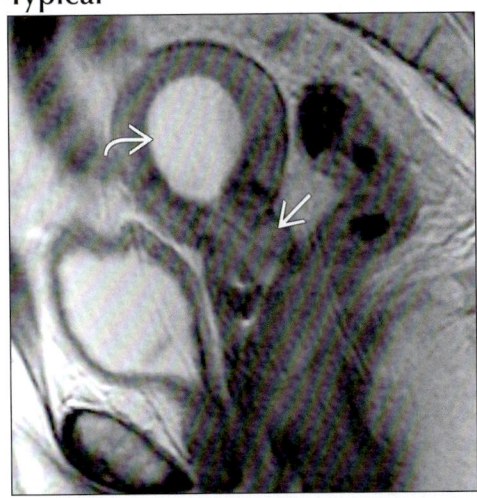
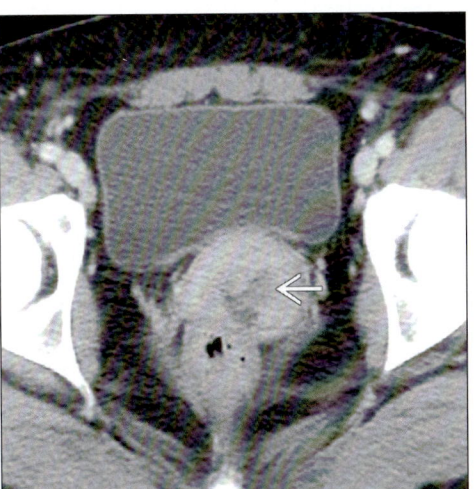

(Left) Sagittal T2WI MR shows a nodular high signal intensity lesion consistent with residual cervical cancer ➡ after radiation treatment. Dilatation in the endometrial cavity ➡ is due to cervical stenosis. *(Right)* Axial CECT shows an ill-defined low attenuation lesion ➡ in the cervix representing the residual tumor after radiation treatment.

Typical

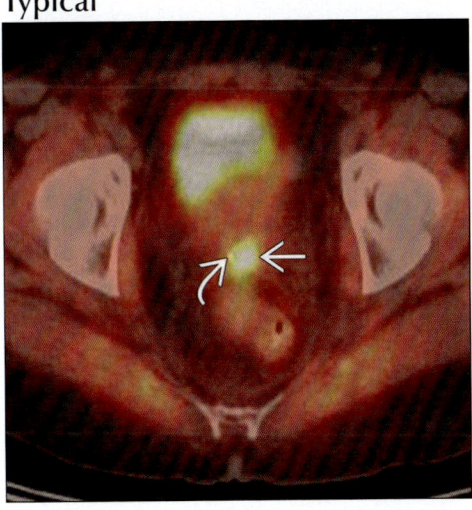
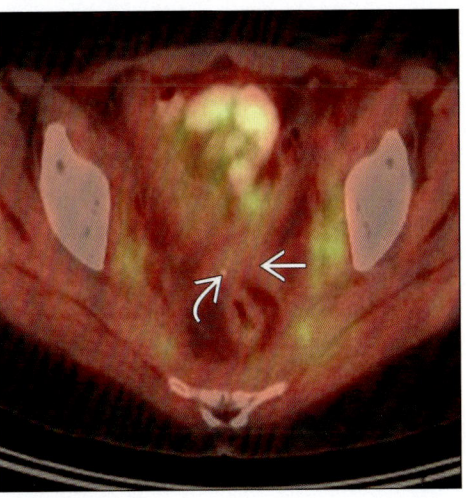

(Left) Axial fused PET/CT shows intense uptake representing cervical cancer ➡ in a patient before treatment. Note the surgical clip ➡ in the cervix used as a marker. *(Right)* Axial fused PET/CT shows no uptake in the cervix ➡ consistent with resolution of cervical cancer after radiation treatment. Note the surgical clip ➡ used as a marker confirms the location of the previously seen mass.

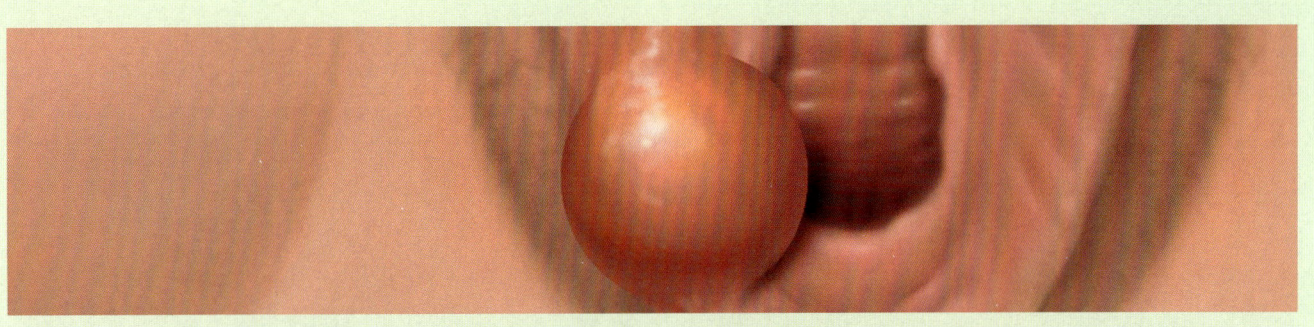

SECTION 4: Vagina

Introduction and Overview
Vaginal Anatomy & Imaging Issues   4-2

Congenital
MRKH Syndrome   4-4
Vaginal Atresia   4-8
Imperforate Hymen   4-10
Vaginal Septae   4-12
Androgen Insensitivity Syndrome   4-14
Ambiguous Genitalia   4-18
Gonadal Dysgenesis   4-22
Gartner Duct Cysts   4-26

Inflammation/Infection
Bartholinitis   4-30
Vaginal Fistula   4-32

Neoplasm, Benign
Leiomyoma, Vagina   4-38

Neoplasm, Malignant
Vaginal Carcinoma   4-40
Lymphoma, Vagina   4-46
Leiomyosarcoma, Vagina   4-48
Embryonal Rhabdomyosarcoma, Vagina   4-50
Yolk Sac Tumor, Vagina   4-52
Bartholin Gland Cancer   4-54
Metastasis, Vagina   4-56

Miscellaneous
Bartholin Cysts   4-58
Foreign Bodies, Vagina   4-62

VAGINAL ANATOMY & IMAGING ISSUES

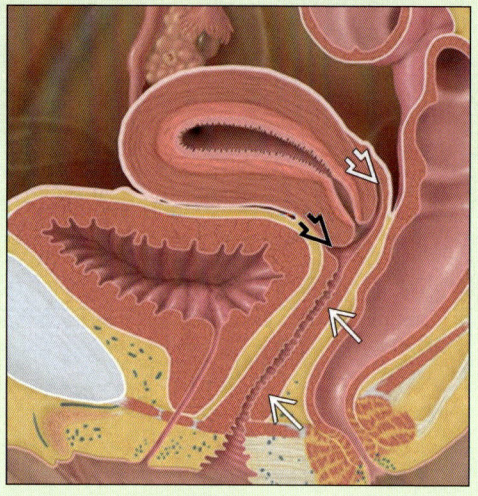

Graphic shows vagina ➡, anterior ▷ and posterior ▶ vaginal fornices. Note the relationships of vagina with urinary bladder and urethra anteriorly; and rectum posteriorly.

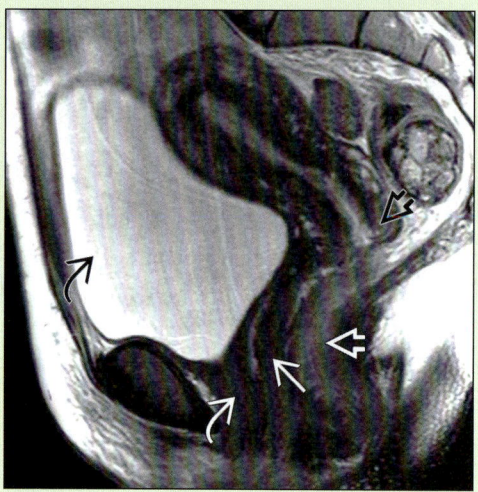

Sagittal T2WI MR shows vagina ➡, urinary bladder ▷, urethra ➡, rectum ▶, and cervix ▷.

TERMINOLOGY

Definitions
- Vagina is a fibromuscular tube that extends from vestibule to uterus
- It functions as female receptive organ during coitus and as birth canal during parturition

IMAGING ANATOMY

General Anatomic Considerations
- **Introitus** refers to external opening located between labia minora
- **Vaginal fornices** refer to vaginal recesses related to cervix
  - **Posterior fornix** (deepest) is behind cervix
  - **Anterior fornix** is in front of cervix
  - **Lateral fornices** are on both sides of cervix

Critical Anatomic Structures
- Vagina is divided into three portions
  - **Upper third** is at the level of lateral vaginal fornices and contains uterine cervix
  - **Middle third** is at the level of base of urinary bladder
  - **Lower third** is parallel to urethra
- Vagina consists of three layers which are discernible on imaging
  - Innermost **mucosal** layer
  - Middle **muscular** layer
  - Outer **adventitial** layer
- Vagina has a rich blood supply formed by branches derived from internal iliac arteries
  - Vaginal and uterine arteries in upper vagina
  - Middle rectal artery in mid-vagina
  - Internal pudendal artery in lower vagina

Anatomic Relationships
- Vagina is positioned between urethra and urinary bladder anteriorly; and anus and rectum posteriorly
- Levator ani muscles are lateral to vagina on both sides
- Distal ureters run close to lateral vaginal fornices
- Ureters enter urinary bladder slightly in front of anterior vaginal fornix

ANATOMY-BASED IMAGING ISSUES

Key Concepts or Questions
- On US, vaginal mucosa is seen as a thin hyperechoic line with adjacent medium echogenicity vaginal wall
- On CT, vagina is seen as a soft tissue density structure
  - Discrimination of cervix and adjacent soft tissue structures may be difficult on CT
- Vaginal anatomy is best depicted on MR
  - Mucosal layer and intraluminal secretions are seen as a high signal intensity stripe on T2WI and low signal intensity on T1WI
  - Muscular layer is of low signal on both T1WI and T2WI
  - Outer adventitial layer is of high signal intensity on T2WI
- Vagina may have **H**- or **W**-shaped appearance on transverse images
- Premenopausal females have many vaginal mucosal infoldings called **rugae**
- Postmenopausal women have flattened vaginal walls without distinguishable mucosal rugae or clearly separate vaginal layers due to atrophy

Imaging Approaches
- MR offers superior soft tissue resolution and multiplanar views
- MR is method of choice in imaging vagina and its pathologies

Imaging Protocols
- Recommended MR imaging protocol
  - T2WI: Transverse, sagittal, coronal planes; small field-of-view; high resolution images
  - T1WI: Transverse plane
  - T1 C+ FS: Transverse and sagittal planes; dynamic images can be obtained

VAGINAL ANATOMY & IMAGING ISSUES

Key Facts

Normal Measurements
- Vagina measures 6 to 7.5 cm along its anterior wall; and 9 cm along its posterior wall in length
- Transverse vaginal diameter increases from introitus (mean 2.6 cm) to fornices (mean 4.2 cm)

Imaging Anatomy
- Mucosal layer and intraluminal secretions are seen as a high SI stripe on T2WI and low SI on T1WI
- Muscular layer is of low SI on both T1WI and T2WI
- Outer adventitial layer is of high SI on T2WI

Age Related Changes
- Premenopausal females have many vaginal mucosal infoldings called rugae
- Postmenopausal women have flattened vaginal walls without distinguishable mucosal rugae or clearly separate vaginal layers due to atrophy

Imaging Pitfalls
- Collapsed vaginal walls limit evaluation of small vaginal lesions on cross sectional imaging
  - Filling of vagina with gel expands vaginal lumen and aids in lesion detection in these cases
- Enhancement of perivaginal venous plexus may limit assessment of tumor extension on T1 C+ because tumor also enhances
  - Careful evaluation of T2WI images are often useful in these cases

Normal Measurements
- Vagina measures 6 to 7.5 cm along its anterior wall; and 9 cm along its posterior wall in length
  - No significant difference in vaginal length has been found between pre- and postmenopausal women
  - Decreased vaginal wall thickness is observed following the menopause
- Transverse vaginal diameter increases from introitus (mean 2.6 cm) to fornices (mean 4.2 cm)

EMBRYOLOGY

Embryologic Events
- Vagina is derived from two mesodermal sources
  - Upper two thirds is of Müllerian origin and initially lined by columnar epithelium
  - Lower third is derived from urogenital sinus and lined by squamous epithelium
- Squamous epithelium migrates superiorly to line entire vagina, completed by 18th gestational week

Practical Implications
- Lymphatic drainage parallels embryological origin
  - Upper two-thirds drain to internal and external iliac lymph node chains
  - Lower third drains to inguinal region

CLINICAL IMPLICATIONS

Clinical Importance
- Most vaginal disorders are diagnosed clinically
- Imaging plays an important role in assessment of
  - Congenital malformations and associated anomalies
  - Functional vaginal disorders such as pelvic floor descent, vaginocele, etc.
  - Enterovaginal and vesicovaginal fistulas
  - Benign and malignant vaginal neoplasms

RELATED REFERENCES
1. Barnhart KT et al: Baseline dimensions of the human vagina. Hum Reprod. 21(6):1618-22, 2006
2. Lopez C et al: MRI of vaginal conditions. Clin Radiol. 60(6):648-62, 2005
3. Suh DD et al: Magnetic resonance imaging anatomy of the female genitalia in premenopausal and postmenopausal women. J Urol. 170(1):138-44, 2003
4. Chang SD: Imaging of the vagina and vulva. Radiol Clin North Am. 40(3):637-58, 2002

IMAGE GALLERY

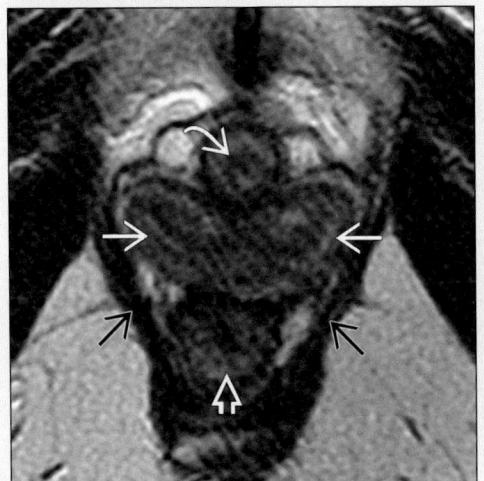
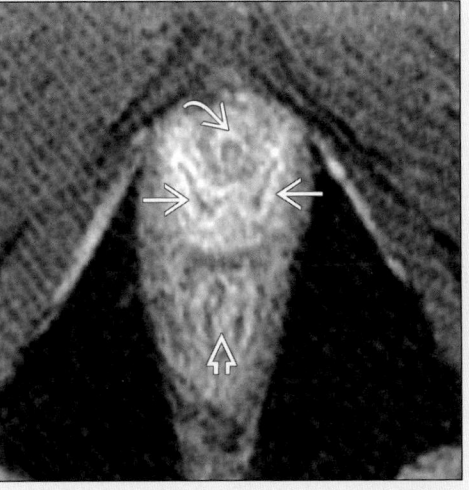

(Left) Axial T2WI MR shows the normal transverse appearance of the lower third of vagina ⇨ between the urethra ⇨ anteriorly; rectum ⇨ posteriorly; and levator ani muscles ⇨ laterally on both sides. (Right) Axial T1 C+ FS MR shows the typical "W"-shaped configuration of the lower third of vagina ⇨ between the urethra ⇨ anteriorly and rectum ⇨ posteriorly. Note the marked enhancement of the normal vaginal mucosa.

MRKH SYNDROME

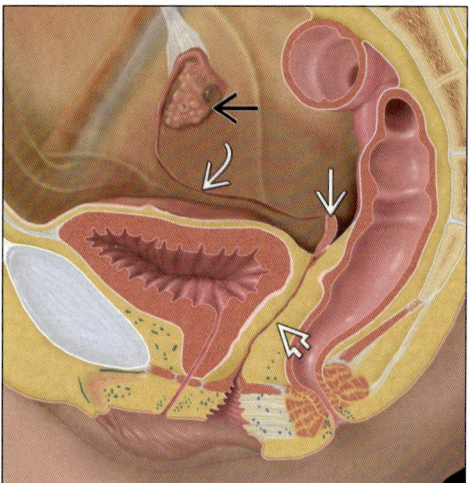

Graphic shows that the vagina, the uterus and the fallopian tube are all hypoplastic. Note that the ovary is normal.

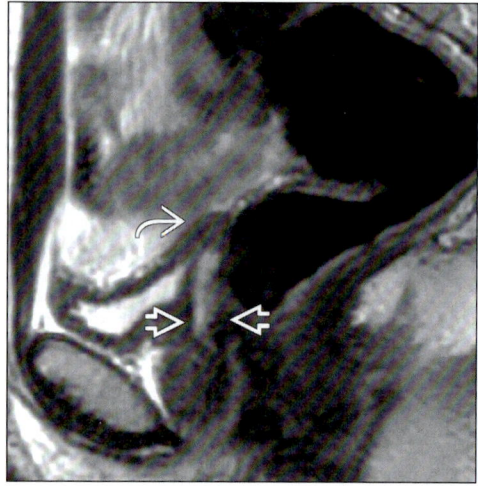

Sagittal T2WI MR shows a patient with MRKH syndrome. Note the absence of vagina and uterus with a soft tissue remnant demonstrated in the expected location of the uterus.

TERMINOLOGY

Abbreviations and Synonyms
- Congenital absence of the uterus and vagina (CAUV)
- Müllerian aplasia (MA)
- Genital renal ear syndrome (GRES)
- Müllerian duct aplasia, renal dysplasia and cervical somite anomalies (MURCS association)
- Mayer-Rokitansky-Kuster-Hauser (MRKH) syndrome

Definitions
- Most common type of class I Müllerian anomaly based on Buttram & Gibbons/American Fertility Society (AFS) classification
- Absence of the uterus, upper vagina ± fallopian tubes due to variable failure of Müllerian ducts to develop prior to fusion

IMAGING FINDINGS

General Features
- Best diagnostic clue
  - Type 1: Vaginal hypoplasia or agenesis
    - Associated uterine agenesis in 90% of cases
    - Fallopian tubes usually normal
    - Isolated with no associated anomalies
  - Type 2: Vaginal hypoplasia or agenesis
    - Associated uterine hypoplasia in 10% of cases
    - Uterine hypoplasia can be symmetric or asymmetric; rarely associated with functioning endometrial tissue
    - Hematometra in presence of functioning endometrial tissue
    - ± Hypoplasia/aplasia of one or both fallopian tubes
    - Often associated anomalies (see below)
  - Ovaries normal in majority of patients
    - Often situated more cranially in lower quadrants of abdomen
  - Normal external genitalia
- Morphology: Variable degrees of early failure of Müllerian ducts to develop prior to fusion

Ultrasonographic Findings
- Grayscale Ultrasound
  - Assessment often difficult secondary to acoustic window and peristalsing bowel loops

DDx: Absent Uterus

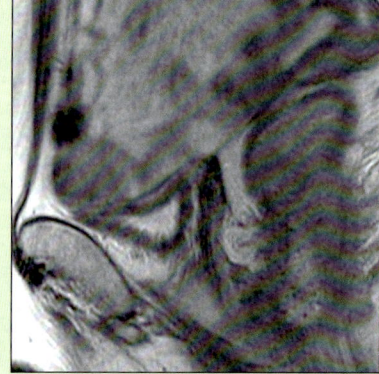
Hysterectomy

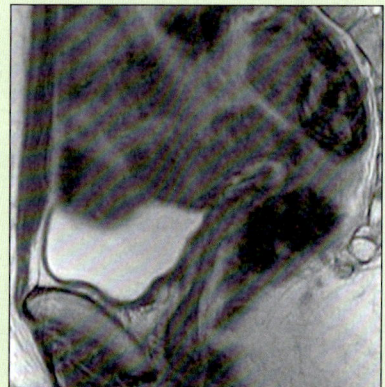
Androgen Insensitivity Syndrome

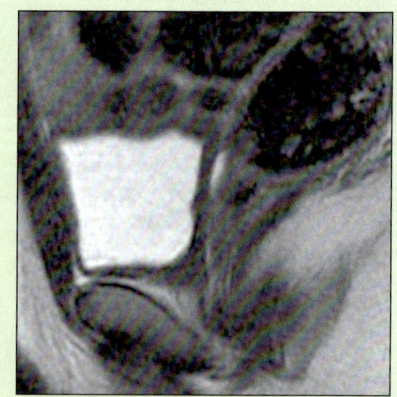
Male Pseudohermaphrodite

MRKH SYNDROME

Key Facts

Terminology
- Most common type of class I Müllerian anomaly based on Buttram & Gibbons/American Fertility Society (AFS) classification
- Absence of the uterus, upper vagina ± fallopian tubes due to variable failure of Müllerian ducts to develop prior to fusion

Imaging Findings
- Ultrasound and MR provide complimentary information

Top Differential Diagnoses
- Pseudohermaphrodite (Male)
- Androgen Insensitivity Syndrome
- Gonadal Dysgenesis
- Total Hysterectomy

Pathology
- Polygenic multifactorial inheritance with a 1-2% recurrence risk
- 1:5,000 female births
- Upper urinary tract malformations in 40-50%
- Skeletal anomalies
- Auditory defects (10-25%)
- Congenital heart defects

Clinical Issues
- Presents with primary amenorrhea
- No reproductive potential
- Secondary sexual characteristics are present with normal ovarian function
- In patients with vaginal agenesis; vaginal dilatation or reconstruction performed to allow normal sexual functioning

---

  - Uterine agenesis: No identifiable uterus at anticipated level of vaginal apex
  - Uterine hypoplasia: Small uterus typically without echogenic endometrial complex
    - Endometrial complex rarely present, results in distension of endometrial cavity with low level echoes at menarche
  - Vaginal agenesis: Echogenic connective tissue in the expected location of vagina between urethra and rectum
  - Vaginal hypoplasia/atresia: Thin hypoechoic band in expected location of vagina without normal zonal anatomy

CT Findings
- No role in evaluation of MRKH syndrome

MR Findings
- T1WI
  - Uterine agenesis: No identifiable uterus at anticipated level of vaginal apex
  - Uterine hypoplasia: Small uterus present
- T1WI FS: Hematometra presents as high signal intensity (SI) fluid within endometrial cavity
- T2WI
  - Uterine agenesis: No identifiable uterus at anticipated level of vaginal apex
    - Important not to mistake connective tissue veins around a tiny fibrous remnant as uterus
  - Uterine hypoplasia
    - Abnormal low signal intensity myometrium with poorly delineated zonal anatomy
    - Endometrial cavity (if present) and myometrium reduced in size
    - May have a unicornuate or bicornuate configuration
  - Vaginal agenesis: Absent normal vaginal zonal anatomy between urethra and rectum
    - Only veins and connective tissue demonstrated in expected location
  - Vaginal hypoplasia/atresia: Low signal intensity (SI) band in the expected location of the vagina without normal zonal anatomy

Imaging Recommendations
- Best imaging tool
  - Ultrasound and MR provide complimentary information
  - MR modality of choice for complete mapping of anatomy
- Protocol advice
  - Transabdominal ultrasound used to screen for renal tract abnormalities and to locate ovaries
    - Provides limited information regarding uterine agenesis/hypoplasia
  - Vaginal agenesis with US best assessed using a transrectal/transperineal approach
  - MR: Phased array body coil
    - Single shot fast spin echo (SS FSE) T2 coronal image through the abdomen and pelvis for renal tract anomalies
    - High resolution FSE T2WI, ≤ 4 mm slice thickness; axial, sagittal and coronal
    - Hypoplastic uterus best visualized on sagittal imaging with mildly distended urinary bladder
    - Vaginal agenesis best visualized on axial images
    - Axial T1WI ± FS to confirm hematometra

DIFFERENTIAL DIAGNOSIS

Pseudohermaphrodite (Male)
- Variable development of uterus, upper 2/3 vagina
- Partial masculinization of external genitalia
- Male karyotype (46 XY)

Androgen Insensitivity Syndrome
- Androgen insensitivity
- No uterus, upper 2/3 vagina, ovaries
- Testes (usually undescended)
- Male karyotype (46 XY)

Gonadal Dysgenesis
- Hypoplastic uterus with atrophic vagina; streak gonads

DES Exposure
- Hypoplastic uterus with T-shaped endometrial cavity

MRKH SYNDROME

- Myometrial constriction bands
- Vagina present

Total Hysterectomy
- Absent uterus
- Vagina present with normal zonal anatomy

PATHOLOGY

General Features
- Genetics
  - Polygenic multifactorial inheritance with a 1-2% recurrence risk
  - In familial cases syndrome transmitted as autosomal dominant with incomplete penetrance and variable expressivity
  - Associated with HNF-1β gene mutations in conjunction with renal anomalies and diabetes
  - Female karyotype (46 XX)
- Epidemiology
  - 1:5,000 female births
  - Approximately 5-10% of Müllerian duct anomalies (MDAs)
- Associated abnormalities
  - **Occur in type 2 MRKH syndrome**
  - Upper urinary tract malformations in 40-50%
    - Renal agenesis (23-28%)
    - Renal ectopia (17%)
    - Renal hypoplasia (4%)
    - Horseshoe kidney
    - Hydronephrosis
  - Skeletal anomalies
    - Usually involves spine (30-40%)
    - e.g., Scoliosis, isolated vertebral anomalies, spina bifida
    - Klippel-Feil association
    - Sprengel deformity
    - Rib malformation or agenesis
    - Face and limb malformations e.g., brachymesophalangy, ectrodactyly, duplicated thumb, absent radius, Holt-Oram-like syndrome, facial asymmetry
  - Auditory defects (10-25%)
    - Conductive or sensorineural deafness, dysplasia of auditory meatus, malformed ears
  - Congenital heart defects
    - e.g., Atrial septal defect, tetralogy of Fallot

CLINICAL ISSUES

Presentation
- Most common signs/symptoms
  - Primary amenorrhea
    - MRKH syndrome is the second most common cause of primary amenorrhea after gonadal dysgenesis
- Other signs/symptoms: Rarely cyclic pelvic pain
- Clinical Profile
  - Vaginal agenesis associated with complete uterine agenesis or uterine hypoplasia without functioning endometrium
    - Presents with primary amenorrhea
    - No reproductive potential
  - Vaginal agenesis associated with uterine hypoplasia with functioning endometrium
    - Primary amenorrhea with severe cyclic pain; results in hematometra
  - Secondary sexual characteristics are present with normal ovarian function
  - Normal external genitalia

Demographics
- Age: Developmental abnormality that remains undiagnosed until puberty or early adulthood

Natural History & Prognosis
- Little or no reproductive potential

Treatment
- In patients with vaginal agenesis; vaginal dilatation or reconstruction performed to allow normal sexual functioning
  - Vaginal dilatation (Frank's method)
  - Skin graft (McIndoe procedure)
  - Laparoscopic creation of neovagina (modified Vecchietti technique)
  - Construction of neovagina with segment of sigmoid colon

DIAGNOSTIC CHECKLIST

Consider
- MRKH syndrome in a young woman presenting with
  - Primary amenorrhea with normal secondary sexual characteristics
  - Associated renal, hearing, skeletal or cardiac anomalies

Image Interpretation Pearls
- Vaginal agenesis associated with uterine agenesis or hypoplasia; best demonstrated on TVS and MR

SELECTED REFERENCES

1. Fedele L et al: Laparoscopic findings and pelvic anatomy in Mayer-Rokitansky-Kuster-Hauser syndrome. Obstet Gynecol. 109(5):1111-5, 2007
2. Pizzo A et al: Syndrome of Rokitansky-Kunster-Hauser-Mayer: a description of four cases. Minerva Ginecol. 59(1):95, 2007
3. Chandiramani M et al: Mayer - Rokitansky - Kuster - Hauser syndrome. J Obstet Gynaecol. 26(7):603-6, 2006
4. Guerrier D et al: The Mayer-Rokitansky-Kuster-Hauser syndrome (congenital absence of uterus and vagina)--phenotypic manifestations and genetic approaches. J Negat Results Biomed. 5:1, 2006
5. Jurkiewicz B et al: Rokitansky-Kustner-Hauser syndrome - a case report. Eur J Pediatr Surg. 2006
6. Griesinger G et al: Mayer-Rokitansky-Kuster-Hauser syndrome associated with thrombocytopenia-absent radius syndrome. Fertil Steril. 83(2):452-4, 2005
7. Abdel-Fattah MS et al: Meyer-Rokitansky-Kuster-Hauser syndrome diagnosed in a postmenopausal woman. J Obstet Gynaecol. 24(2):198-9, 2004
8. Kula S et al: Mayer-Rokitansky-Kuster-Hauser syndrome associated with pulmonary stenosis. Acta Paediatr. 93(4):570-2, 2004

MRKH SYNDROME

IMAGE GALLERY

Typical

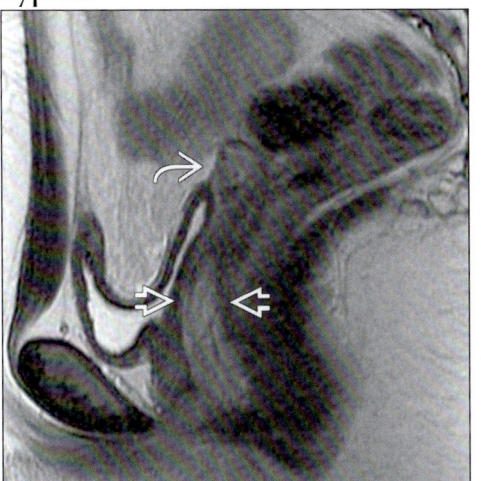
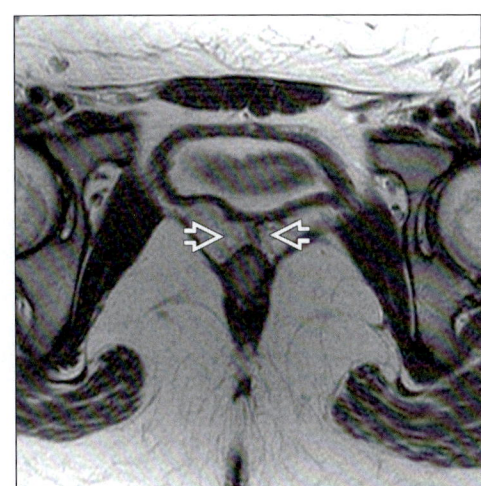

(Left) Sagittal T2WI MR shows a patient with MRKH syndrome demonstrating vaginal ⇨ and uterine agenesis with a small soft tissue remnant in the expected location of the uterus ➘. *(Right)* Axial T2WI MR shows same patient as previous image, with absent vagina ⇨.

Typical

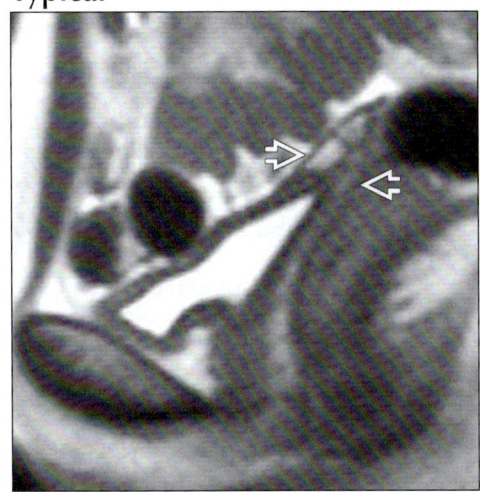
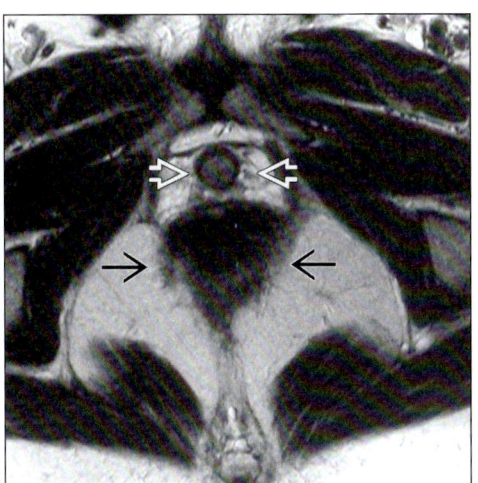

(Left) Sagittal T2WI MR shows another example of MRKH syndrome with vaginal and uterine agenesis. Connective tissue and veins are noted in the expected location of the uterus ⇨. *(Right)* Axial T2WI MR shows the same patient as previous image. Again no vagina is demonstrated in between the urethra ⇨ and rectum ⇨.

Typical

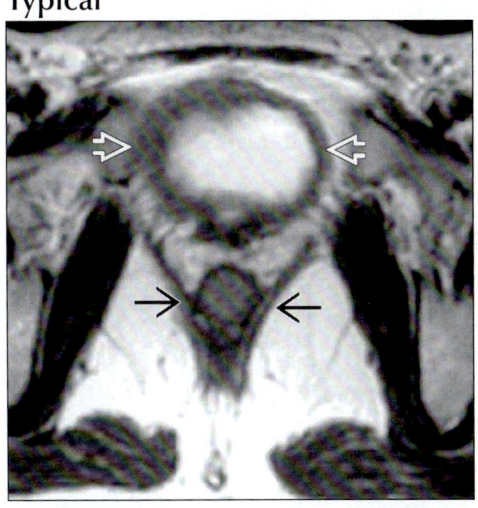
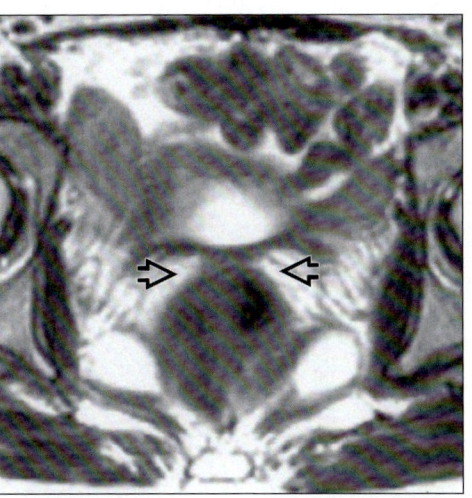

(Left) Axial T2WI MR shows a patient with MRKH syndrome with vaginal agenesis. Note the absence of vagina between bladder ⇨ and rectum ⇨. *(Right)* Coronal T2WI MR shows same patient as previous image. Again vaginal agenesis is demonstrated with no vagina ⇨ seen in relation to the bladder and rectum.

VAGINAL ATRESIA

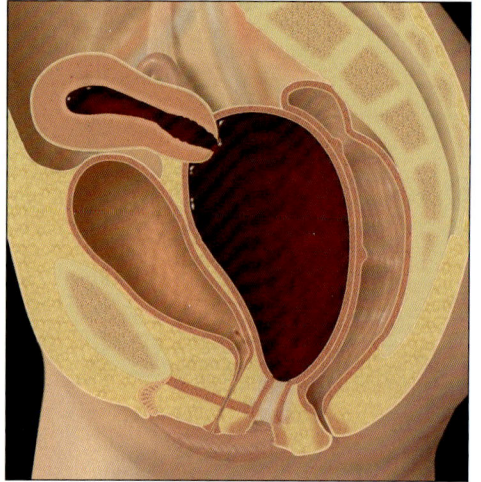

Graphic depicting vaginal atresia shows a low vaginal obstruction with secondary hematometrocolpos. The lower vagina is replaced by fibrotic tissue.

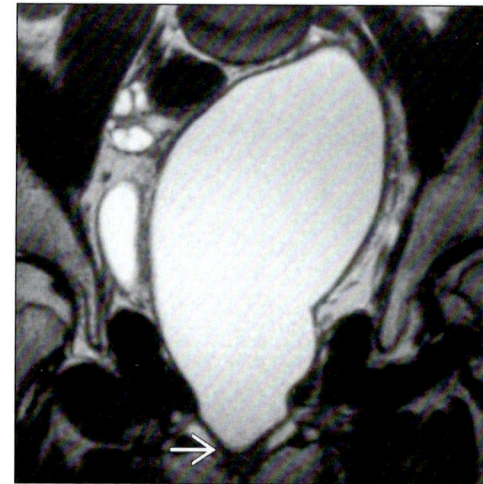

Coronal T2WI MR shows a dilated vagina with complex fluid consistent with a hematocolpos due to a low vaginal obstruction ➡.

TERMINOLOGY

Definitions
- Failure of primitive urogenital sinus to develop which gives rise to lower 1/3 of vagina
- Not considered an anomaly of Müllerian duct origin, differentiating it from vaginal agenesis
  - Müllerian structures normal

IMAGING FINDINGS

General Features
- Best diagnostic clue
  - Low vaginal obstruction with fibrotic tissue replacing zonal anatomy of lower 1/3 of vagina
  - Secondary hematometrocolpos
  - Normal uterus, upper 2/3 of vagina, and ovaries

Ultrasonographic Findings
- Distended, tubular cystic structure ending in blind pouch at lower margin of vagina
  - Intraluminal fluid contents variable: Anechoic, hypoechoic with low-level echoes, or echogenic
  - Vagina shows greater degree of distention than endometrial cavity
  - Normal zonal anatomy of lower vagina replaced by hypoechoic fibrous band

MR Findings
- T1WI FS
  - Confirms blood products in hematometrocolpos
  - Associated complications: Endometriosis
- T2WI
  - Dilatation of vagina and/or endometrial cavity
    - Intraluminal fluid of intermediate or high signal intensity
    - Occasionally fluid/debris levels
  - Vagina of greater distensibility than endometrial cavity
    - Distention of endometrial cavity usually < 1.0 cm
  - Lower margin of vagina replaced by low signal intensity fibrous tissue with loss of normal zonal anatomy extending to introitus

Imaging Recommendations
- Best imaging tool
  - Transabdominal and transperineal ultrasound can be used as initial imaging modality

DDx: Vaginal Atresia

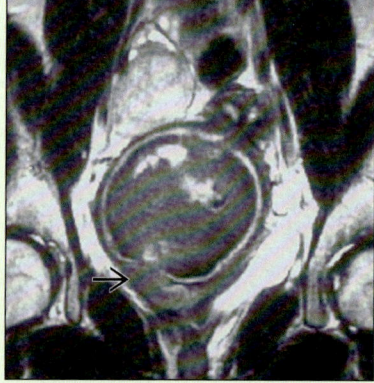

Transverse Vaginal Septum

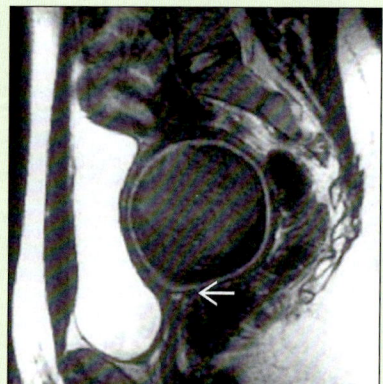

Transverse Vaginal Septum

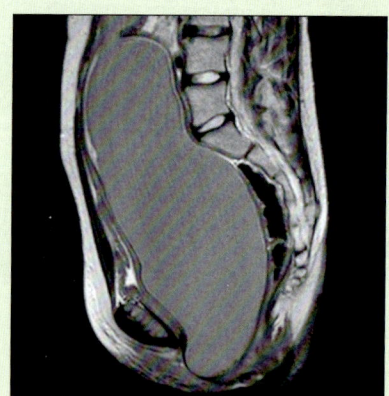

Imperforate Hymen

VAGINAL ATRESIA

Key Facts

Terminology
- Failure of primitive urogenital sinus to develop which gives rise to lower 1/3 of vagina
- Not considered an anomaly of Müllerian duct origin, differentiating it from vaginal agenesis

Imaging Findings
- Low vaginal obstruction with fibrotic tissue replacing zonal anatomy of lower 1/3 of vagina
- Secondary hematometrocolpos
- Normal uterus, upper 2/3 of vagina, and ovaries

Top Differential Diagnoses
- Transverse Vaginal Septum
- Imperforate Hymen
- Vaginal Agenesis with Uterine Hypoplasia

Clinical Issues
- Usual presentation at menarche with primary amenorrhea and cyclic abdominopelvic pain

---

  - Pelvic MR modality of choice
- Protocol advice
  - Phased-array body coil
  - High-resolution fast spin-echo (FSE) T2WI
    - ≤ 4 mm slice thickness
    - Axial and coronal/sagittal multiplanar imaging
  - T1WI ± FS: Confirms presence of blood products

DIFFERENTIAL DIAGNOSIS

Transverse Vaginal Septum
- Fibrous septum at junction of middle and upper third of vagina with hematometrocolpos
  - Isolated or in association with vertical vaginal septa of Müllerian duct anomalies (MDAs)
- Normal vaginal zonal anatomy preserved

Imperforate Hymen
- Distal vaginal obstruction associated with hematometrocolpos
- Normal uterus with preserved vaginal length

Vaginal Agenesis with Uterine Hypoplasia
- Absent normal zonal anatomy of upper 2/3 of vagina
  - Variable degree of upper vaginal distension if residual preserved segment
- Lower vagina typically preserved
- Rudimentary uterus with distended endometrial cavity

PATHOLOGY

Gross Pathologic & Surgical Features
- Not considered in spectrum of MDAs
  - Failure of canalization of urogenital sinus

CLINICAL ISSUES

Presentation
- Most common signs/symptoms
  - Usual presentation at menarche with primary amenorrhea and cyclic abdominopelvic pain
  - Progressive degree of hematometrocolpos depending on time of diagnosis following menarche

Natural History & Prognosis
- Normal reproductive outcomes after correction

Treatment
- In patients with a dimple at the introitus long term dilation is a consideration
- Vaginoplasty reserved for failed dilations

SELECTED REFERENCES
1. Lindenman E et al: Mullerian agenesis: an update. Obstet Gynecol. 90(2):307-12, 1997
2. Scanlan KA et al: Value of transperineal sonography in the assessment of vaginal atresia. AJR. 154(3):545-8, 1990
3. Togashi K et al: Vaginal agenesis: classification by MR imaging. Radiology. 162(3):675-7, 1987

IMAGE GALLERY

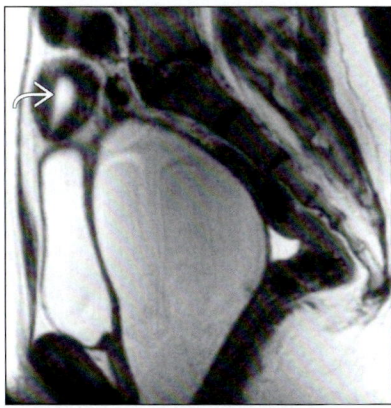 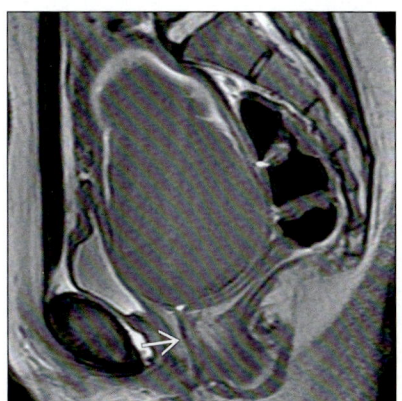 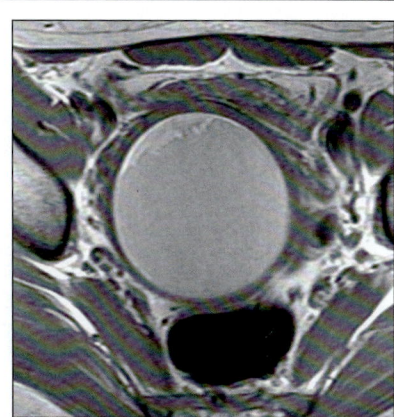

(Left) Sagittal T2WI MR in the same patient as the previous image shows the hematometrocolpos. Note the lesser distention of the endometrial cavity ➪. (Center) Sagittal T2WI MR shows obstruction at the junction of the middle and lower 1/3 of the vagina with a hematocolpos. The lower vaginal segment is atretic ➪ and without normal zonal anatomy. (Right) Axial T1WI MR in the same patient as the previous image shows the high signal intensity of the hematocolpos.

IMPERFORATE HYMEN

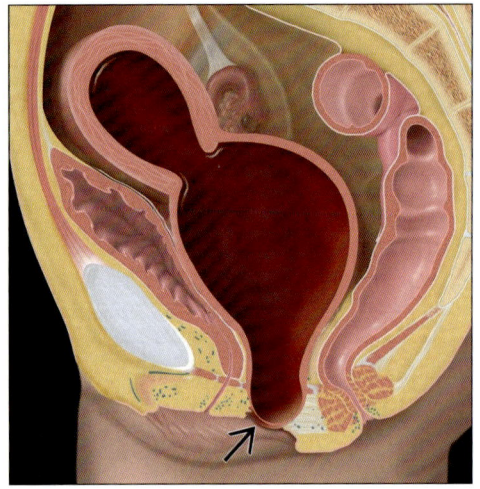
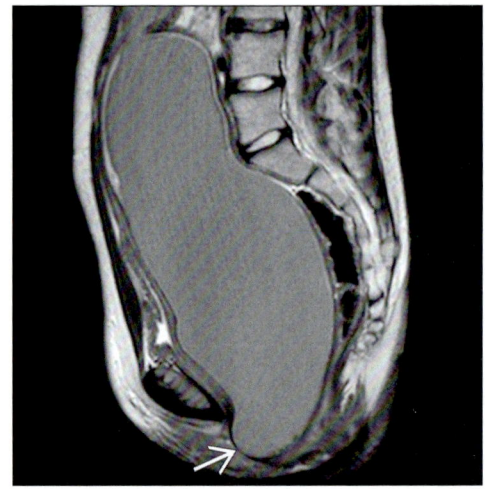

Graphic shows the presence of a thin transverse membrane ➔ with bulging at the level of the introitus and associated hematometrocolpos. These findings are consistent with an imperforate hymen.

Sagittal T2WI MR shows a hematocolpos with a thin bulging membrane ➔ at the level of the introitus. (Courtesy M. Hall-Craggs, MD).

TERMINOLOGY

Abbreviations and Synonyms
- Hymenal obstruction

Definitions
- Distal vaginal obstruction by a thin endodermal membrane at the level of the introitus
- Not considered an anomaly of Müllerian duct origin, represents failure of the sino-vaginal bulbs to completely canalize

IMAGING FINDINGS

General Features
- Best diagnostic clue
  - Very low vaginal obstruction with preservation of vaginal length
  - "Bulging" at introitus
  - Associated hematometrocolpos
  - Normal uterus, vagina and ovaries
  - Variable appearance if imperforate hymen incomplete

Ultrasonographic Findings
- Distended, tubular cystic structure throughout length of vagina ± endometrial cavity
  - Intraluminal fluid contents variable: Anechoic, hypoechoic with low-level echoes, or echogenic
  - Vagina shows greater degree of distention than endometrial cavity

MR Findings
- T1WI FS
  - Confirms high signal intensity (SI) blood products in hematometrocolpos
  - Associated complications: Endometriosis
- T2WI
  - Dilatation of vagina along its entire length ± dilatation of endometrial cavity
    - Intraluminal fluid of intermediate to high SI
    - Greater distensibility of vagina compared to endometrial cavity
  - Lower margin of vagina ends at introitus, membrane often imperceptible and difficult to delineate

Imaging Recommendations
- Best imaging tool

DDx: Imperforate Hymen

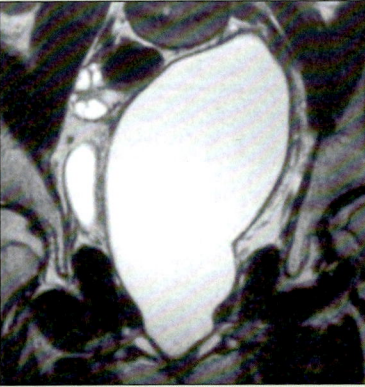
Vaginal Atresia

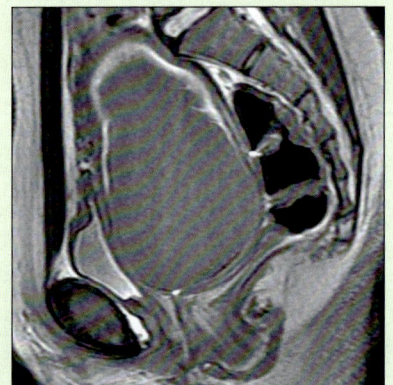
Vaginal Atresia

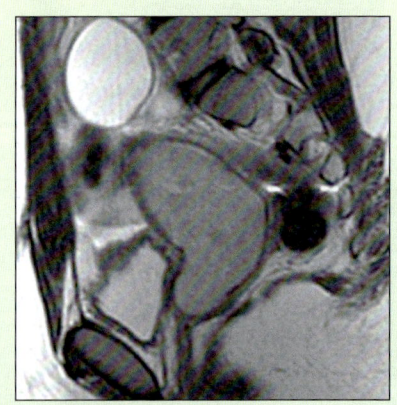
Transverse Vaginal Septum

IMPERFORATE HYMEN

Key Facts

Terminology
- Distal vaginal obstruction by a thin endodermal membrane at the level of the introitus

Imaging Findings
- Very low vaginal obstruction with preservation of vaginal length
- Associated hematometrocolpos
- Normal uterus, vagina and ovaries
- Variable appearance if imperforate hymen incomplete

Top Differential Diagnoses
- Transverse Vaginal Septum
- Vaginal Atresia

Clinical Issues
- If complete, symptoms of hematocolpos typically manifest at menarche
- If incomplete, may be associated with excessive vaginal secretions and secondary infection

○ Transabdominal and transperineal ultrasound to be used as initial imaging modality
○ MR can be used as problem solving modality
- Protocol advice
  ○ High resolution fast spin echo (FSE) T2WI with multi-planar imaging
  ○ T1WI with fat suppression

DIFFERENTIAL DIAGNOSIS

Transverse Vaginal Septum
- Fibrous septum at junction of middle and upper third of vagina with hematometrocolpos
  ○ Isolated or in association with vertical vaginal septa of Müllerian duct anomalies (MDAs)

Vaginal Atresia
- Lower 1/3 of vagina replaced by fibrous tissue with associated hematometrocolpos
  ○ Imperforate hymen always present
- Normal uterus, ovaries and upper 2/3 of vagina

Labial Adhesions
- Level of obstruction is superficial at level of labia, which may be fenestrated

Vaginal Agenesis with Uterine Hypoplasia
- Absent normal zonal anatomy of upper 2/3 of vagina
  ○ Lower vagina typically preserved
- Rudimentary uterus with distended endometrial cavity

CLINICAL ISSUES

Presentation
- Most common signs/symptoms
  ○ Most frequent obstructive anomaly of the vagina
  ○ If complete, symptoms of hematocolpos typically manifest at menarche
    ▪ May present with bladder outlet obstruction 2° to compression and mass effect by the hematocolpos
  ○ If incomplete, may be associated with excessive vaginal secretions and secondary infection

Treatment
- Surgical hymenotomy at puberty, as onset of estrogenization aids in prevention of adhesions

SELECTED REFERENCES
1. Reinhold C et al: Primary amenorrhea: evaluation with MR imaging. Radiology. 203(2):383-90, 1997
2. Blask AR et al: Obstructed uterovaginal anomalies: demonstration with sonography. Part II. Teenagers. Radiology. 179(1):84-8, 1991
3. Shaw LM et al: Imperforate hymen and vaginal atresia and their associated anomalies. J R Soc Med. 76(7):560-6, 1983

IMAGE GALLERY

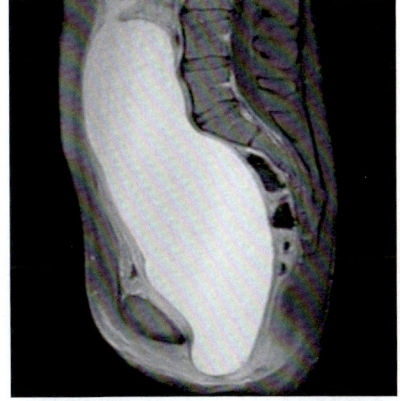
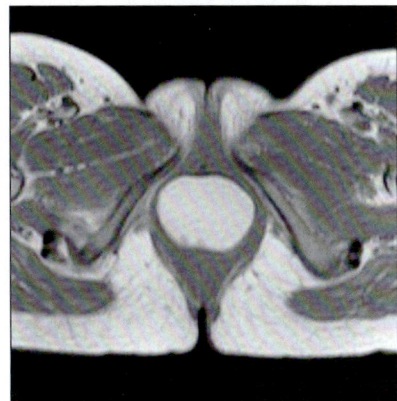
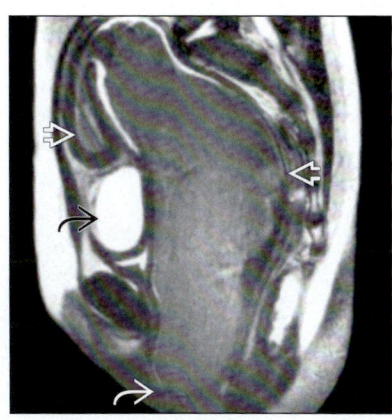

(Left) Sagittal T1 C+ FS MR in the same patient shows vaginal distention to the introitus with a high signal intensity collection consistent with hematocolpos. (Courtesy M. Hall-Craggs, MD). (Center) Axial T1WI MR shows the hematocolpos with distention of the vagina immediately above the level of the introitus. (Courtesy M. Hall-Craggs, MD). (Right) Sagittal T2WI MR shows a hematometrocolpos ➔ with a thin bulging membrane ➔ at the level of the introitus. There is a loculated, ventral hemoperitoneum ➔ compressing the urinary bladder.

VAGINAL SEPTAE

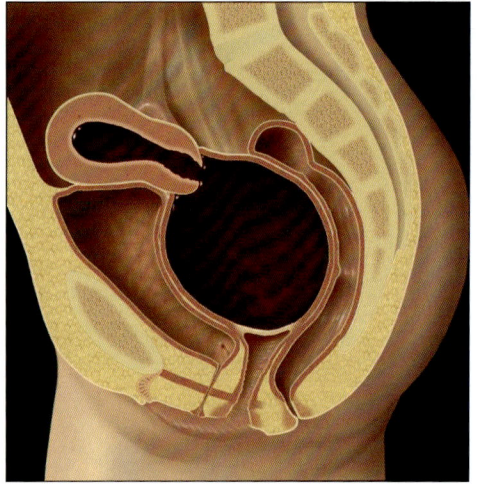

Graphic shows a transverse vaginal septum at the junction of the middle and upper 1/3 of the vagina with secondary hematometrocolpos.

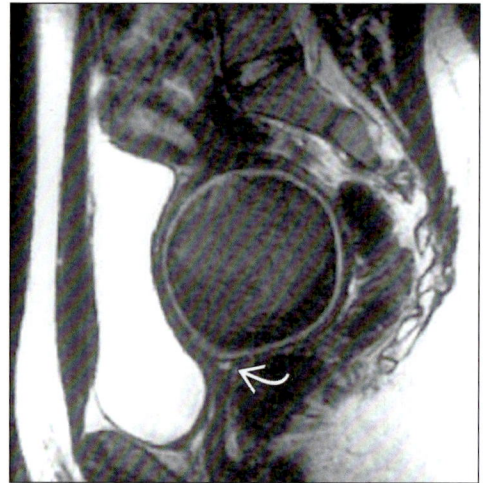

Sagittal T2WI MR shows complete obstruction ➢ at the junction of the middle and upper 1/3 of the vagina resulting in hematometrocolpos. The lower vagina demonstrates normal zonal anatomy.

TERMINOLOGY

Definitions
- Incomplete canalization of uterovaginal canal with urogenital sinus which forms lower third of vagina
- Transverse vaginal septum

IMAGING FINDINGS

General Features
- Best diagnostic clue: Distention of vagina superior to septum (hematocolpos) with lesser degree of distention of endometrium (hematometrocolpos)
- Location
  - Junction of middle and upper third of vagina
    - Inferior vaginal septum in 15%
- Morphology: Isolated or in association with vertical vaginal septa of Müllerian duct anomalies (MDAs)

Ultrasonographic Findings
- Midline, tubular, cystic structure consisting of upper vagina ± endometrial cavity between urinary bladder and rectum
  - Intraluminal fluid contents variable: Anechoic, hypoechoic with low-level echoes, or echogenic

MR Findings
- T1WI FS
  - Confirms blood products in hematometrocolpos
  - Associated complications: Endometriosis
- T2WI
  - Dilation of upper vagina ± endometrial cavity
    - Intraluminal fluid of intermediate or high signal intensity
    - Occasionally fluid/debris levels
    - Dilation unilateral in setting of obstructed complex anomalies
  - Vagina more distensible than endometrial cavity
    - Lesser distention of endometrial cavity (usually 1.0 cm) secondary to thicker muscular wall of myometrium
  - Septum can be thick and extensive
    - Thickness of septum must be reported as it may alter surgical approach

Imaging Recommendations
- Best imaging tool: MR imaging modality of choice
- Protocol advice

DDx: Vaginal Septae

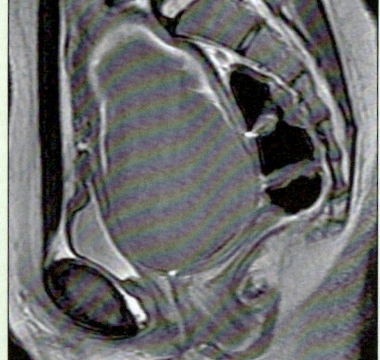

Vaginal Atresia

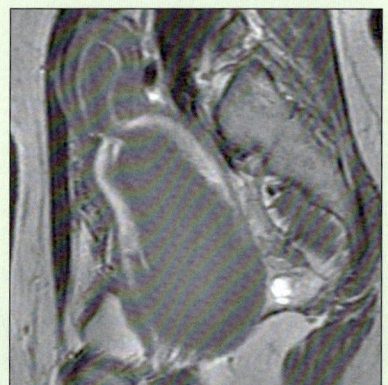

Vaginal Atresia

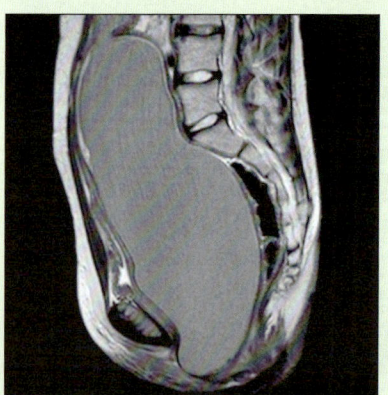

Imperforate Hymen

VAGINAL SEPTAE

Key Facts

Terminology
- Transverse vaginal septum

Imaging Findings
- Best diagnostic clue: Distention of vagina superior to septum (hematocolpos) with lesser degree of distention of endometrium (hematometrocolpos)
- Junction of middle and upper third of vagina
- Morphology: Isolated or in association with vertical vaginal septa of Müllerian duct anomalies (MDAs)

Top Differential Diagnoses
- Vaginal Agenesis with Uterine Hypoplasia
- Imperforate Hymen
- Vaginal Atresia

Clinical Issues
- Complete septum: Cyclic abdominopelvic pain with enlarging pelvic mass
- Vaginoplasty may be required if septum thick and extensive

○ High-resolution fast spin-echo (FSE) T2WI
  ▪ Axial and coronal/sagittal multiplanar imaging
○ T1WI with fat-suppression

DIFFERENTIAL DIAGNOSIS

Vaginal Agenesis with Uterine Hypoplasia
- Absent normal zonal anatomy of upper 2/3 of vagina
  ○ Variable degree of upper vaginal distension if residual preserved segment
- Lower vagina typically preserved
- Rudimentary uterus with distended endometrial cavity

Imperforate Hymen
- Distal vaginal obstruction associated with hematometrocolpos
- Normal uterus with preserved vaginal length

Vaginal Atresia
- Lower 1/3 of vagina replaced by fibrous tissue with associated hematometrocolpos
- Normal uterus, ovaries and upper 2/3 of vagina

CLINICAL ISSUES

Presentation
- Most common signs/symptoms
  ○ Presentation most often at menarche with symptoms depending on partial or complete configuration
  ○ Complete septum: Cyclic abdominopelvic pain with enlarging pelvic mass
  ○ Partial septum or unilateral septum associated with duplication anomaly
    ▪ Variable cyclic pain, progressive development of hematocolpos/hematometrocolpos
    ▪ May be asymptomatic if partial

Natural History & Prognosis
- Degree of distention of vagina and endometrial cavity related to extent of obstruction and time of diagnosis following menarche
- Associated with genitourinary, skeletal, cardiovascular and gastrointestinal anomalies

Treatment
- Surgical resection of septum
- Vaginoplasty may be required if septum thick and extensive

SELECTED REFERENCES
1. Arnold BW et al: Müllerian duct anomalies complicated by obstruction. Evaluation with pelvic magnetic resonance imaging. J Women's Imaging 3:146-52, 2001
2. Blask AR et al: Obstructed uterovaginal anomalies: demonstration with sonography. Part I. Neonates and infants. Radiology. 179:79-83, 1991
3. Blask AR et al: Obstructed uterovaginal anomalies: demonstration with sonography. Part II. Teenagers. Radiology. 179:84-8, 1991

IMAGE GALLERY

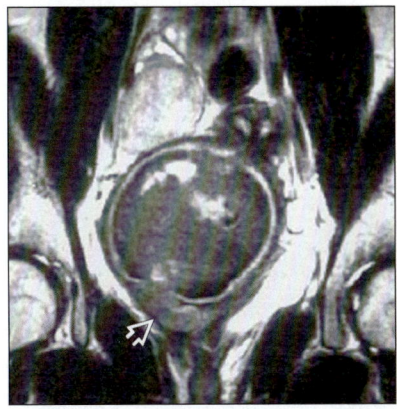
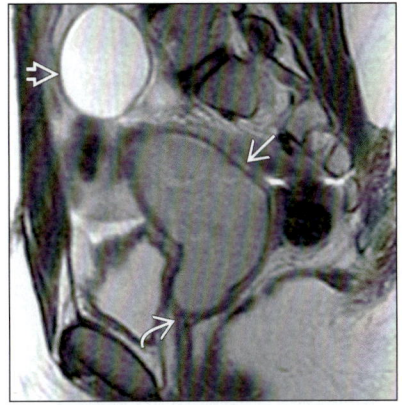
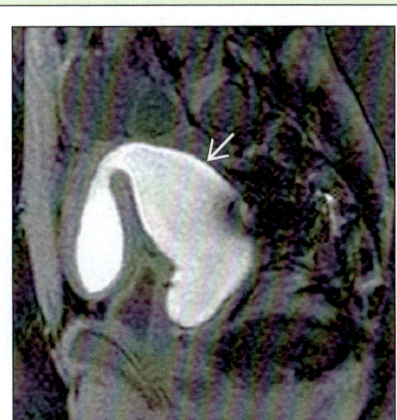

(Left) Coronal T2WI MR in the same patient as previous image shows a thick septum ➡ resulting in unilateral hematocolpos in this complex duplication anomaly. *(Center)* Sagittal T2WI MR in a patient with uterine duplication anomaly shows distention of the right hemivagina ➡ due to a transverse vaginal septum ➡. A functional ovarian cyst ➡ is noted. (Courtesy E. Siegelman, MD). *(Right)* Sagittal T1WI FS MR in the same patient as previous image shows the increased signal intensity ➡ consistent with a hematometrocolpos. (Courtesy E. Siegelman, MD).

ANDROGEN INSENSITIVITY SYNDROME

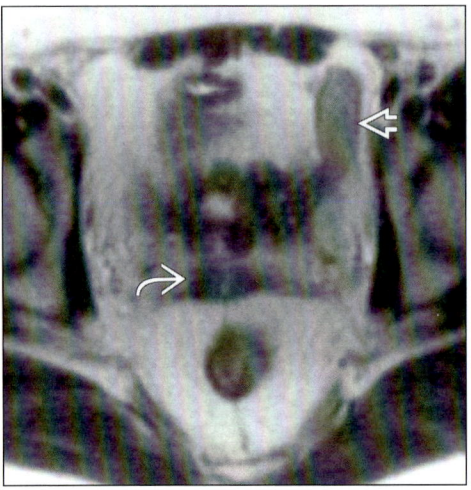

Axial T2WI MR in a patient with primary amenorrhea shows the presence of an undescended left testis ➡ that is hyperintense to muscle but hypointense relative to fat. A rudimentary uterus ➡ is present.

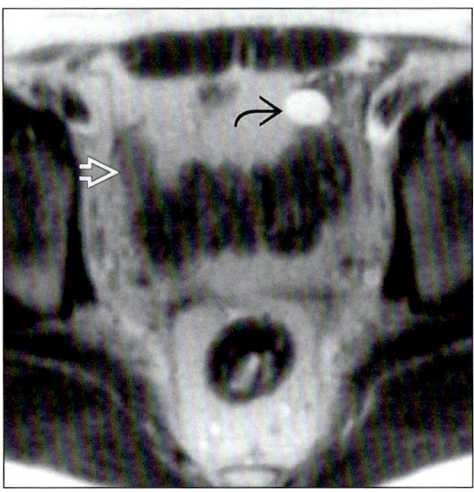

Axial T2WI MR in the same patient as previous image, shows an undescended right testis ➡. Note the unilocular cyst at the superior pole of the left testis ➡.

TERMINOLOGY

Abbreviations and Synonyms
- Complete androgen insensitivity syndrome (CAIS), testicular feminization

Definitions
- End-organ resistance to androgens
- 46,XY karyotype with female phenotype and functioning testes
- Distinct from partial androgen insensitivity syndromes

IMAGING FINDINGS

General Features
- Best diagnostic clue
  - Absence of all Müllerian derivatives: Uterus, upper 2/3 of vagina, fallopian tubes
  - Bilateral undescended testes
- Morphology
  - Müllerian derivatives
    - Absent or rudimentary uterus/fallopian tube
    - Agenesis of upper 2/3 of vagina
  - Bilateral undescended testes
    - Testes located most frequently along common or external iliac chain (70%)
    - Less common sites: Inguinal canal (25%), retroperitoneum (5%)
    - May be associated with indirect inguinal hernias
  - Cysts located at lateral poles of testes in 50%
    - Cysts are simple with thin walls
    - Represent remnants of Müllerian or Wolffian ducts
  - Secondary germ cell tumors in testes (2.5%)
    - Risk increased to 30% by 50 years of age
    - Most commonly seminoma or gonadoblastoma

Ultrasonographic Findings
- Grayscale Ultrasound
  - Absent or rudimentary uterus, fallopian tube and upper vagina
    - No identifiable uterus at anticipated level of vaginal apex
    - Echogenic connective tissue in the expected location of vagina between urethra and rectum
  - Undescended testes
    - Oval, hypoechoic to echogenic masses

DDx: Androgen Insensitivity Syndrome

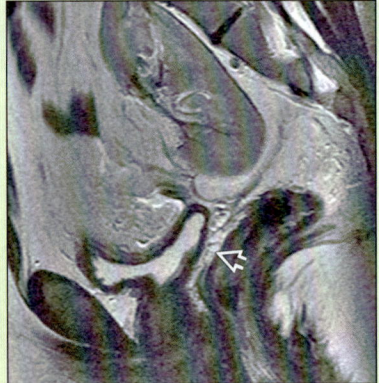

MRKH Syndrome

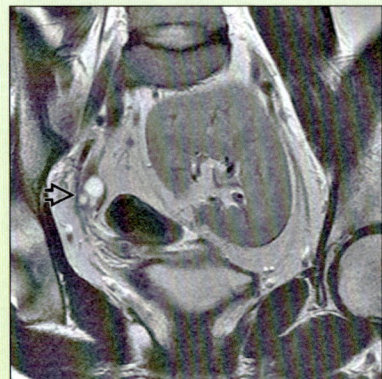

MRKH Syndrome

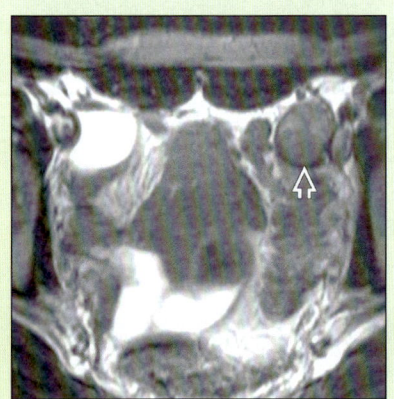

True Hermaphrodite

ANDROGEN INSENSITIVITY SYNDROME

Key Facts

Terminology
- Complete androgen insensitivity syndrome (CAIS), testicular feminization
- 46,XY karyotype with female phenotype and functioning testes

Imaging Findings
- Absence of all Müllerian derivatives: Uterus, upper 2/3 of vagina, fallopian tubes
- Bilateral undescended testes
- Testes located most frequently along common or external iliac chain (70%)
- Cysts located at lateral poles of testes in 50%
- Low SI rim of testes on T2WI helpful in distinction from lymph nodes

Top Differential Diagnoses
- Vaginal Agenesis
- Gonadal Dysgenesis
- Other Disorders of Intersexuality

Clinical Issues
- Primary amenorrhea
- Unambiguous female phenotype at birth and puberty

Diagnostic Checklist
- Consider CAIS in patients presenting with primary amenorrhea
- Search for undescended testes in all cases of abnormal internal genitalia
- Risk of secondary testicular tumor increases to 10% after puberty

---

- Accuracy of US for identifying testes in lower pelvis or inguinal canal: 85-90% (limited data)
  - Secondary germ cell tumors
    - Variable appearance, depending on histological type and background echotexture of gonad
    - Hypoechoic to hyperechoic mass with calcification

CT Findings
- NECT
  - Not well-suited to confirm absence of Müllerian derivatives
  - Undescended testes
    - Oval-shaped pelvic soft tissue density, mimicking lymph node
    - May be associated with indirect inguinal hernias

MR Findings
- T1WI
  - Undescended testes
    - Signal intensity (SI) ranging from slightly lower to slightly higher than muscle
    - SI identical to non-cystic immature ovaries
- T2WI
  - Absent or rudimentary uterus, fallopian tube and upper vagina
    - No identifiable uterus at anticipated level of vaginal apex
    - Important not to mistake connective tissue/veins around a tiny fibrous remnant as uterus
    - Only veins and connective tissue demonstrated in expected location of vagina
  - Undescended testes
    - Typically hyperintense to muscle, hypointense relative to fat
    - SI identical to non-cystic immature ovaries
    - SI typically lower than normal gonads
    - Low SI rim of testes on T2WI helpful in distinction from lymph nodes
    - Accuracy of MR for identifying testes: 55-80% (limited data)
  - Secondary germ cell tumors in testes
    - Signal intensity depending on histological type and background signal of gonad

Imaging Recommendations
- Best imaging tool
  - US: Initial method of investigation
    - Screening for presence of Müllerian derivatives, undescended testes in inguinal canal
  - MR more accurate for confirming absence of Müllerian derivatives and location of undescended testes
- Protocol advice
  - MR: Phased array body coil
  - High-resolution T1WI and fast spin echo (FSE) T2WI
  - Slice thickness ≤ 4 mm
  - Axial, sagittal and coronal images
    - Uterine agenesis best visualized on sagittal images
    - Vaginal agenesis best visualized on axial images
    - Axial and coronal images optimal for detecting undescended testes

DIFFERENTIAL DIAGNOSIS

Vaginal Agenesis
- Mayer-Rokitansky-Küster-Hauser (MRKH) syndrome
- Absent or rudimentary uterus and upper vagina
- Normal ovaries, may be located more cranially

Gonadal Dysgenesis
- Streak gonads
- Uterus usually present but hypoplastic

Other Disorders of Intersexuality
- Chromosomal and biochemical profile needed for differentiation among various entities
- In addition to gonadal dysgenesis includes
  - Female pseudohermaphrodite → two ovaries
  - Male pseudohermaphrodite → two testes
  - True hermaphrodite → ovary and testis, or ovotestis

ANDROGEN INSENSITIVITY SYNDROME

PATHOLOGY

General Features
- General path comments
  - Normal gonadal differentiation to testes due to presence of H-Y antigen
  - Absent or rudimentary uterus/fallopian tube
  - Agenesis of upper 2/3 of vagina
- Genetics
  - 46,XY karyotype
  - X-linked recessive (androgen receptor gene on X chromosome)
- Etiology
  - Androgen resistance due to absence of receptor protein, changes in receptor protein structure (receptor-negative) or post-receptor defect (receptor-positive)
    - Androgen receptor defect → no response to testosterone signal → lack of masculinization of external genitalia in utero and deficient virilization at puberty
  - Müllerian regression factor produced by testes → absent or rudimentary Müllerian derivatives (uterus, upper 2/3 of vagina, fallopian tubes)
- Epidemiology
  - Rare
  - Most common form of male pseudohermaphroditism

Gross Pathologic & Surgical Features
- Tan or white nodules within testes corresponding to hamartomas (60%)
- Cysts of Müllerian or Wolffian duct origin, located at lateral poles of testes (50%)

Microscopic Features
- Histologic gonadal characterization necessary, as gross appearance identical in testes and non-cystic immature ovaries

CLINICAL ISSUES

Presentation
- Most common signs/symptoms
  - Primary amenorrhea
    - Third most common cause after Turner syndrome and MRKH
  - Inguinal hernias at birth
    - Bilateral inguinal hernias rare in girls; 1-2% will have CAIS
    - Consider CAIS in girls presenting with bilateral inguinal hernias
- Other signs/symptoms: Abdominopelvic mass arising from intra-abdominal gonads
- Clinical Profile
  - Unambiguous female phenotype at birth and puberty
    - Normal breast development at puberty due to elevated estrogen from testes
  - Occasional incomplete forms with varying degrees of genital ambiguity and virilization/feminization
  - Usually diagnosed in perimenarchal stage

Natural History & Prognosis
- Most functioning as normal sterile females
- Increased risk of secondary testicular tumor
  - Seminoma or gonadoblastoma
    - Risk low in first two decades: 2-5%
    - Increasing after puberty: 10%
    - Peaking to 30% by 50 years of age

Treatment
- Testes left in situ (as source of estradiol) until completion of puberty and feminization, with prompt removal thereafter
- Prepubertal inguinal herniorrhaphy in 35-50%

DIAGNOSTIC CHECKLIST

Consider
- Consider CAIS in patients presenting with primary amenorrhea
- Search for undescended testes in all cases of abnormal internal genitalia

Image Interpretation Pearls
- Low SI rim of testes on T2WI helpful in distinction from lymph nodes
- Risk of secondary testicular tumor increases to 10% after puberty

SELECTED REFERENCES

1. Wein D et al: DA: Campbell-Walsh Urology: Sexual differentiation: Normal and abnormal. vol 4. 9th ed. Philadelphia, Elsevier: 3799-3829, 2007
2. Hughes IA et al: Androgen resistance. Best Pract Res Clin Endocrinol Metab. 20(4):577-98, 2006
3. Hyun G et al: A practical approach to intersex in the newborn period. Urol Clin North Am. 31(3):435-43, viii, 2004
4. Choi HK et al: MR imaging of intersexuality. Radiographics. 18(1):83-96, 1998
5. Reinhold C et al: Primary amenorrhea: evaluation with MR imaging. Radiology. 203(2):383-90, 1997
6. Gambino J et al: Congenital disorders of sexual differentiation: MR findings. AJR Am J Roentgenol. 158(2):363-7, 1992

ANDROGEN INSENSITIVITY SYNDROME

IMAGE GALLERY

Typical

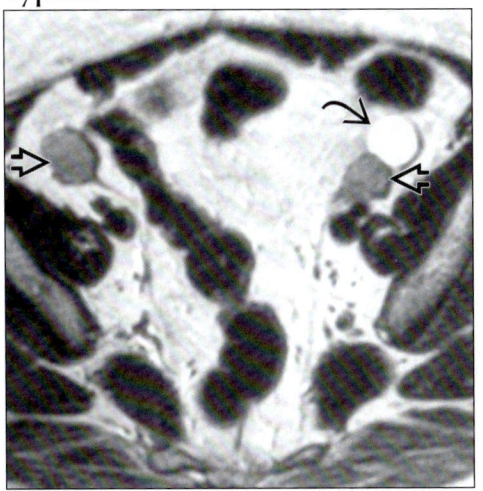
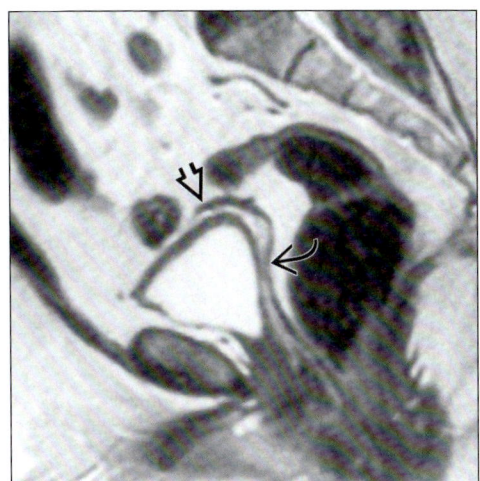

(Left) Axial T2WI MR shows bilateral ovoid masses ➔ consistent with undescended testes. The small size and low signal intensity indicate atrophy. At pathology a left inclusion cyst ➔ was present adjacent to the left testis. (Courtesy reference 5). *(Right)* Sagittal T2WI MR in the same patient as previous image, shows a fibrous band ➔ without zonal anatomy in the expected location of the vagina and a small uterine remnant ➔. (Courtesy reference 5).

Typical

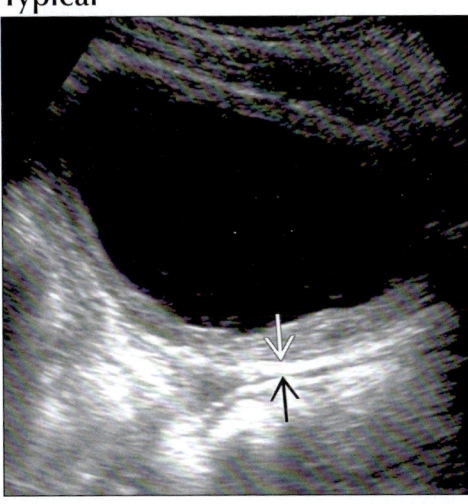
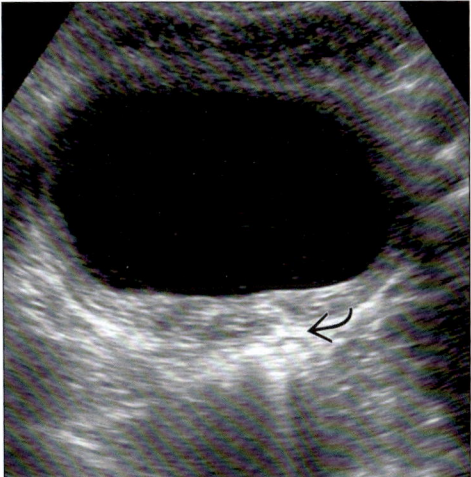

(Left) Sagittal transabdominal ultrasound shows echogenic connective tissue in the expected location of the upper 2/3 of the vagina, between the posterior bladder ➔ and anterior rectal ➔ wall. There is complete uterine agenesis. *(Right)* Axial transabdominal ultrasound in the same patient as previous image, shows upper vaginal agenesis ➔ in this patient with primary amenorrhea. The anterior wall of the rectum apposes the posterior bladder wall.

Typical

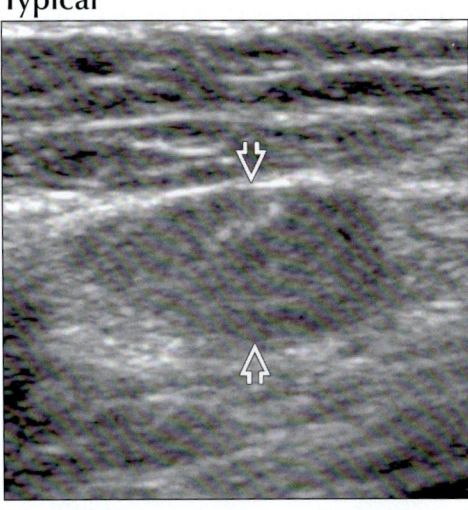
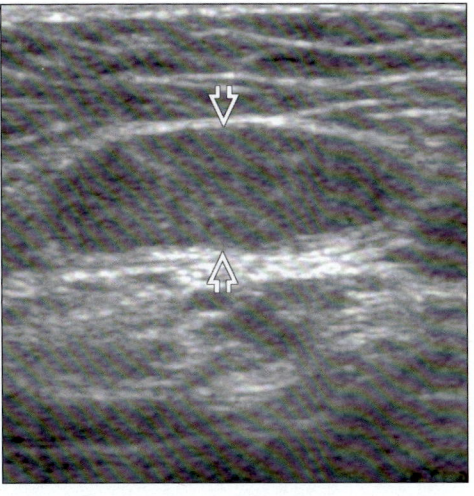

(Left) Sagittal ultrasound in the preceding patient at the level of the right inguinal region shows a hypoechoic ovoid mass ➔ consistent with an undescended testis. *(Right)* Sagittal oblique ultrasound at the level of the left inguinal region shows a hypoechoic ovoid mass ➔ consistent with an undescended testis. Note the absence of a fatty hilum.

AMBIGUOUS GENITALIA

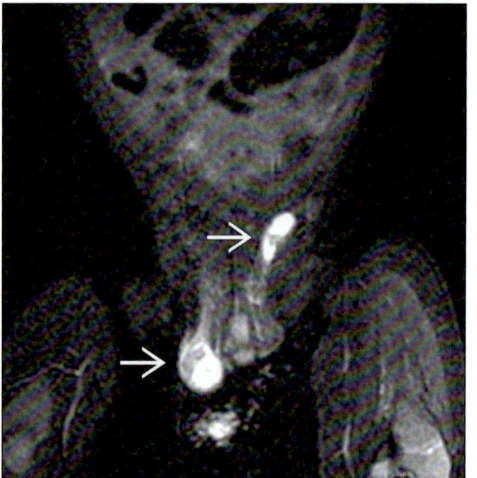

Coronal T2WI FS MR shows bilateral testes ➔, the left in the scrotum and the right in the inguinal canal, in a 2 month old baby with ambiguous genitalia.

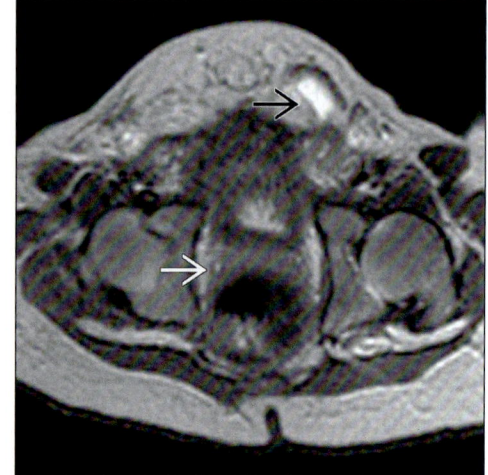

Axial T2WI MR in the same baby as previous image, shows the right inguinal testis ➔. A vagina is also demonstrated ➔, confirming internal genital organs of both genders.

TERMINOLOGY

Abbreviations and Synonyms
- Anomalies of sexual differentiation, pseudohermaphroditism, hermaphroditism, intersex conditions
- Includes: Congenital adrenal hyperplasia (CAH), congenital androgen insensitivity syndrome (CAIS), testicular feminization

Definitions
- Birth defect where the outer genitals do not have the typical appearance of the gender

IMAGING FINDINGS

General Features
- Best diagnostic clue
  - Inconsistency between the appearance of the outer genitalia and the internal genital organs
  - Main role of radiology is to demonstrate the anatomy of the genito-urinary tract, not to determine the sex
  - Evaluating the adrenal glands is necessary to exclude congenital adrenal hyperplasia or adrenal neoplasm as a cause
- Location
  - Pelvis
  - Intra-abdominal
  - Perineal and inguinal regions
  - Adrenals
- Size
  - Ovaries, uterus, testes, may be fully developed for age, rudimentary, or anywhere in between
  - Congenital adrenal hyperplasia: Enlarged adrenal glands, limb length over 20 mm and width over 4 mm in a newborn; normal adrenal size does not exclude CAH
- Morphology
  - Internal genital organs may include ovaries, testes or ovotestes, parts of the müllerian structures (uterus, fallopian tubes and upper third of vagina) or parts of the Wolffian structures (vas deferens, epididymis and seminal vesicles) in various combinations
  - May be associated with anomalies of the urinary tract
  - Female pseudohermaphroditism

DDx: Ambiguous Genitalia

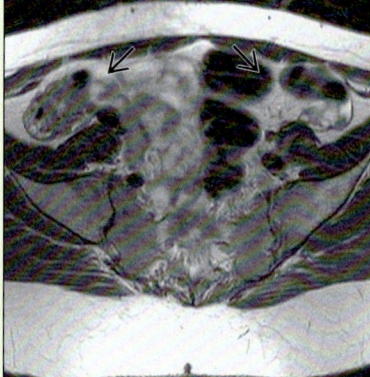

MRKH Syndrome (Normal Ovaries)

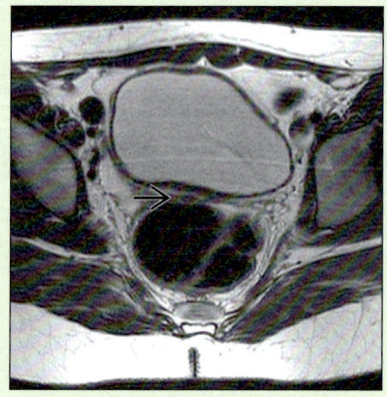

MRKH (Rudimentary Uterus)

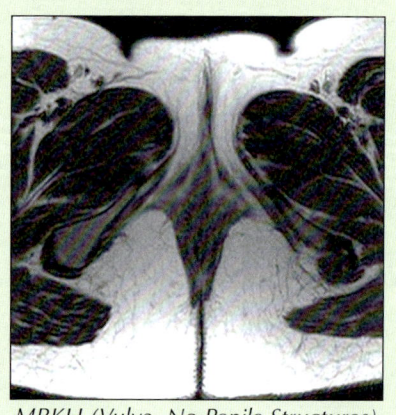

MRKH (Vulva, No Penile Structures)

AMBIGUOUS GENITALIA

Key Facts

Terminology
- Anomalies of sexual differentiation, pseudohermaphroditism, hermaphroditism, intersex conditions
- Birth defect where the outer genitals do not have the typical appearance of the gender

Imaging Findings
- Inconsistency between the appearance of the outer genitalia and the internal genital organs
- Main role of radiology is to demonstrate the anatomy of the genito-urinary tract, not to determine the sex
- Testes and ovaries best imaged on T2WI sequences; generally high signal intensity on T2WI, with intermediate signal intensity on T1WI
- T2WI helps differentiate between a penis and a hypertrophied clitoris
- Main purpose of the examination is to identify the presence or absence of testes, ovaries and uterus
- US plays a key role in detecting the gonads, including undescended testes
- MR is the most sensitive modality to visualize the ovaries and uterus and to evaluate undescended testes
- US and MR protocols should include examination of the kidneys, urinary tract and adrenal glands as well

Clinical Issues
- May be evident in the newborn or detected only later in life presenting as delayed menarche or infertility
- In CAH, associated mineralocorticoid deficiency may cause salt wasting, a true medical emergency in the newborn!

- Possess ovaries, uterus and fallopian tubes, with no testes
- Virilization of external genitalia and general phenotype
- Male pseudohermaphroditism
  - Possess testes which may be in scrotum or maldescendant
  - Absence of internal female genital tract organs (testes synthesize müllerian inhibiting substance)
  - External genitalia completely feminized in testicular feminization, with varying degrees incomplete virilization in other disorders
- True hermaphroditism
  - Possess both ovaries and testes in separate gonads or in the same gonad (ovotestis)
  - May have a testis on one side and an ovary on the other
  - Various features of both male and female external genitalia as well as internal sex organs, dependent on the amount of androgens produced by gonads
  - 75% have dominant masculine features and are raised as males

Ultrasonographic Findings
- Main purpose of the examination is to identify the presence or absence of testes, ovaries and uterus
- Optimally performed in the newborn period when maternal hormones cause the uterus and ovaries to be prominent
- Assessment of the inguinal and perineal regions necessary to evaluate for ectopic testicular tissue or an ovotestis
- In normal infants only one ovary detected in about 40% and neither ovary detected in 16%, thus non-visualization of an ovary on US does not completely exclude its existence
- 3D US may facilitate intra-uterine evaluation of ambiguous genitalia

MR Findings
- Testes and ovaries best imaged on T2WI sequences; generally high signal intensity on T2WI, with intermediate signal intensity on T1WI
- On T2WI gonads may have an outer intermediate signal intensity rim; distinguishes them from lymph nodes
- Immature ovaries lack follicles and may be very similar to small testes or ovotestes
- Dysgenetic gonads may appear as streak gonads, identified on T2WI as thin low intensity stripes
- Coronal plane helps assess position of a maldescendant testis (from the abdomen through the perineum)
- T2WI helps differentiate between a penis and a hypertrophied clitoris

Imaging Recommendations
- Best imaging tool
  - US plays a key role in detecting the gonads, including undescended testes
  - MR is the most sensitive modality to visualize the ovaries and uterus and to evaluate undescended testes
  - US and MR may also accurately assess associated anomalies of the urinary tract or adrenal gland
- Protocol advice
  - US should include the abdomen and pelvis to detect possible intra-abdominal undescended testes or ovotestes, the pelvis to detect an immature uterus, and the inguinal canals and perineum to detect possible cryptorchidism
  - MR should include axial and coronal T2WI of the abdomen and pelvis to detect high signal gonads
  - MR scanning performed in thin contiguous sections (3 mm); infantile or rudimentary uterus may be very small
  - US and MR protocols should include examination of the kidneys, urinary tract and adrenal glands as well

AMBIGUOUS GENITALIA

DIFFERENTIAL DIAGNOSIS

Agenesis of Uterus
- Most common form is the Mayer-Rokitansky-Kuster-Hauser syndrome, which is combined agenesis of the uterus, cervix, and upper portion of the vagina
- Usually normal ovaries, therefore normal female maturation and phenotype, but absence of menses

Cryptorchidism
- Children will present with absence of palpable testes in the scrotum; normal male phenotype, external and internal male genital organs

PATHOLOGY

General Features
- Genetics
  - Female pseudohermaphroditism: Karyotype 46XX
  - Male pseudohermaphroditism: Karyotype 46XY
  - True hermaphroditism: Karyotype is 46XX in 80%, 46XY in 10%, and mosaics in 10%
  - True hermaphroditism is the most likely intersex state after CAH in a 46XX child
- Etiology
  - Female pseudohermaphroditism
    - Congenital adrenal hyperplasia in over 80%, deficiency in 21-hydroxylase causes inability to produce cortisol, with elevated ACTH, resulting in increased production of 17-hydroxyprogesterone, progestins and androgen precursors
    - Additional rare causes: Maternal drug ingestion (synthetic progestins) during the first trimester of pregnancy and adrenal or ovarian androgen producing tumors (very rare)
  - Male pseudohermaphroditism
    - Inability of the testes to respond to gonadotropin stimulation
    - Congenital errors in the biosynthesis of testosterone or inability to convert testosterone to dihydrotestosterone
    - Androgen insensitivity of target organs, known also as "congenital androgen insensitivity syndrome" (CAIS) or "testicular feminization"
  - True hermaphroditism
    - Dysgenetic gonad development
- Associated abnormalities: Congenital abnormalities of the kidneys and urinary tract

CLINICAL ISSUES

Presentation
- Most common signs/symptoms
  - External appearance varies between genetically defined XX babies and XY babies
  - May be evident in the newborn or detected only later in life presenting as delayed menarche or infertility
- Other signs/symptoms: Salt wasting in a newborn may be associated with CAH and female pseudohermaphroditism

Demographics
- Age: Most commonly diagnosed in newborns
- Gender: Gender often unclear

Natural History & Prognosis
- Ambiguous genitalia is generally not a life threatening condition, however, it may cause social problems as well as infertility
- Determination of the true sex of the child with genetic testing may not always be possible
- Gender may be chosen for the child, based on the external appearance or the more dominant internal genital organs
- In CAH, associated mineralocorticoid deficiency may cause salt wasting, a true medical emergency in the newborn!
- If undescended testes are detected, surgical removal is advised to prevent development of testicular tumors

Treatment
- Treatment combines hormonal manipulation and cosmetic surgery to achieve the desired phenotype

DIAGNOSTIC CHECKLIST

Consider
- Do external and internal genital organs match karyotype and correlate with each other?
- Are there palpable testes in the scrotum? If so, karyotype is almost indefinitely XY
- When female karyotype with muscularization present, check adrenal glands for hyperplasia

Image Interpretation Pearls
- Role of radiology is to define the anatomy of the genital organs and the urinary tract, and not to determine the sex
- US and MR play an important role in identifying gonads and internal sex organs
- Basic evaluation includes identifying the absence or presence of ovaries, testes, uterus and vagina
- Testes and ovotestes may be located anywhere from the abdomen down to the perineum
- Recommend T2WI thin-section axial, coronal and sagittal imaging from the abdomen through the perineum

SELECTED REFERENCES
1. Frimberger D et al: Ambiguous genitalia and intersex. Urol Int. 75(4):291-7, 2005
2. Wright NB et al: Imaging children with ambiguous genitalia and intersex states. Clin Radiol. 50(12):823-9, 1995
3. Secaf E et al: Role of MRI in the evaluation of ambiguous genitalia. Pediatr Radiol. 24(4):231-5, 1994
4. Gambino J et al: Congenital disorders of sexual differentiation: MR findings. AJR Am J Roentgenol. 158(2):363-7, 1992

AMBIGUOUS GENITALIA

IMAGE GALLERY

Typical

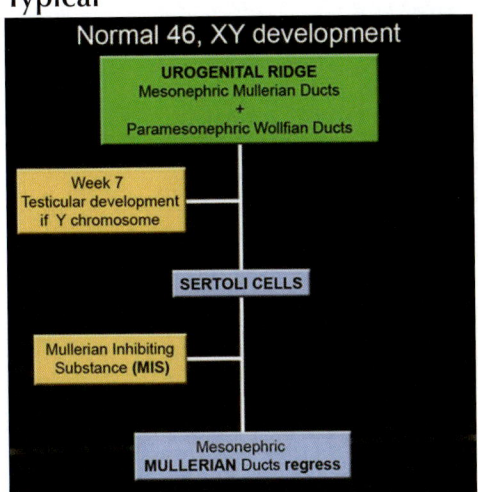
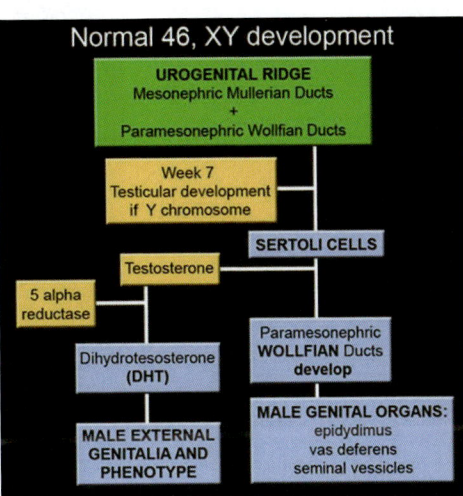

(Left) Diagram of normal male gender development. Internal male genitalia and external phenotype are dependent on development of Sertoli and Leydig cells in the testes. *(Right)* Diagram of normal male gender development (cont.). Internal male genitalia and external phenotype are dependent on development of Sertoli and Leydig cells in the testes.

Typical

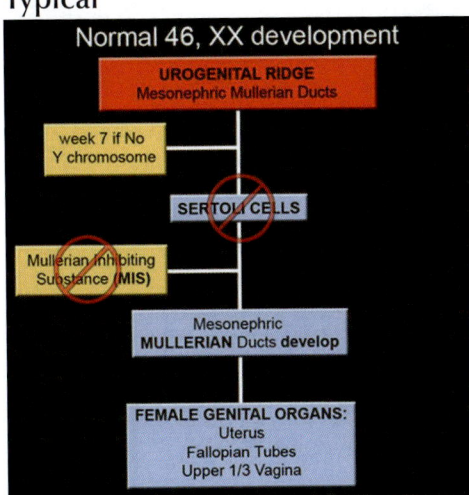
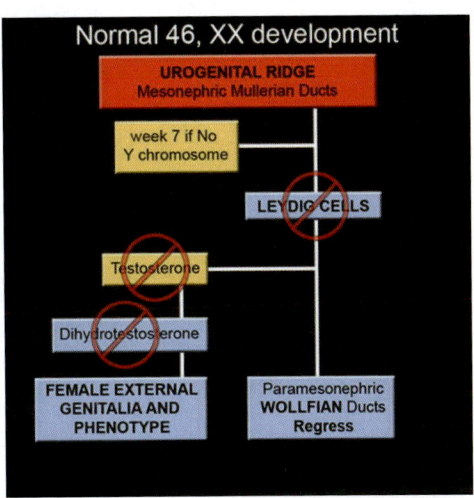

(Left) Diagram of normal female gender development. In the absence of Sertoli and Leydig cells, müllerian inhibiting substance and testosterone are not secreted, enabling female genitalia and phenotype formation. *(Right)* Diagram of normal female gender development (cont.). In the absence of Sertoli and Leydig cells, müllerian inhibiting substance and testosterone are not secreted, enabling female genitalia and phenotype formation.

Typical

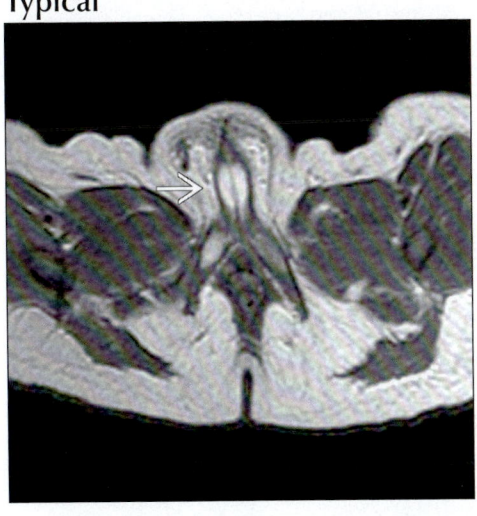
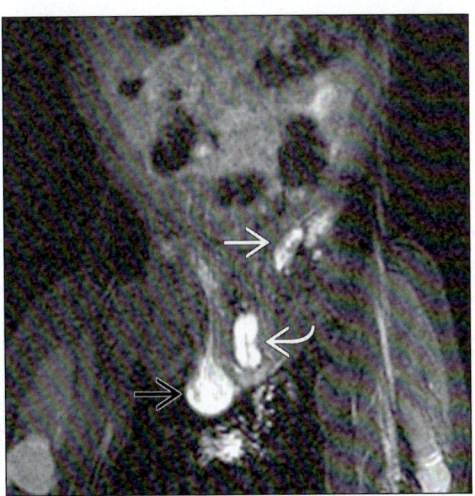

(Left) Axial T2WI MR in the same baby as first image on the first page, shows development of male external genitalia with penile corpora cavernosa ➔. *(Right)* Coronal T2WI FS MR shows bilateral testes, in the scrotum on the right ➔ and in the inguinal canal on the left ➔. Penile corpora are also noted ➔. No ovaries or uterus were seen, however, a vagina was present (second image of first page).

GONADAL DYSGENESIS

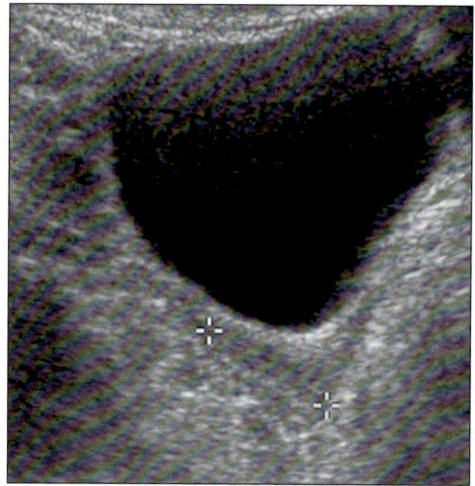

Sagittal transabdominal ultrasound in a patient presenting with primary amenorrhea shows a hypoplastic uterus (calipers). The zonal anatomy was difficult to visualize. No internal gonads were identified.

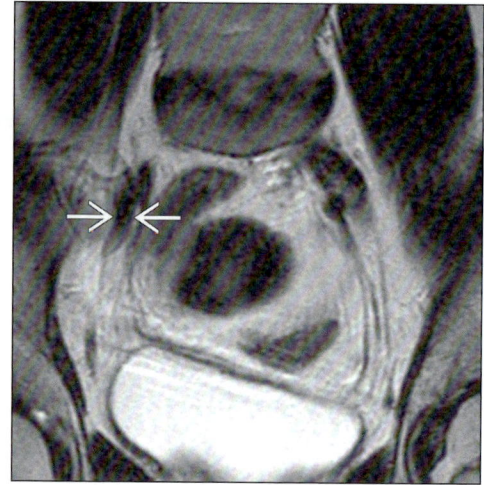

Coronal T2WI MR in the same patient as previous image, shows a right streak gonad ➡ as iso- to slightly hyperintense relative to skeletal muscle. A left streak gonad is present but not shown.

TERMINOLOGY

Definitions
- Replacement of gonads, testes or ovaries, by fibrous tissue, devoid of germ cells
- Range of abnormalities of gonads and internal genitalia with variable karyotypes
  - 45,X Turner syndrome: Most common karyotype (50%)
  - 46,XX "pure" gonadal dysgenesis (GD)
  - 46,XY "complete" GD including
    - 46,XY embryonic testicular regression (ETR)
    - 46,XY bilateral vanishing testes syndrome (BVTS)
  - 45,XO/46,XY mosaic ("mixed") GD
- Confusing use of terms "pure" and "complete" in literature; best replaced by specification of karyotype

IMAGING FINDINGS

General Features
- Best diagnostic clue
  - Unilateral or bilateral streak gonads: 2-3 cm long and 0.5 cm wide
  - Müllerian derivatives typically present but most commonly hypoplastic
- Gonads
  - Bilateral streak gonads
    - 45,X Turner syndrome, 46,XX "pure" GD and 46,XY "complete" GD
  - Asymmetric combinations of streak gonad, testis and dysgenetic gonads
    - Unique to 45,XO/46,XY mosaic GD
  - No gonads (neither testes nor ovaries)
    - Unique to 46,XY ETR-BVTS
- Müllerian derivatives
  - Present but hypoplastic
    - 45,X Turner syndrome, 46,XX "pure" GD
    - Corpus/cervix ratio 1:1
    - Thin atrophic endometrium
    - Atrophic vagina
  - Well-developed Müllerian structures
    - 46,XY "complete" GD and BVTS
  - Asymmetric internal genitalia
    - Unique to 45,XO/46,XY mosaic GD
    - Unilateral Müllerian ducts (unicornuate uterus) with contralateral Wolffian derivatives
  - Absent internal genitalia

DDx: Gonadal Dysgenesis

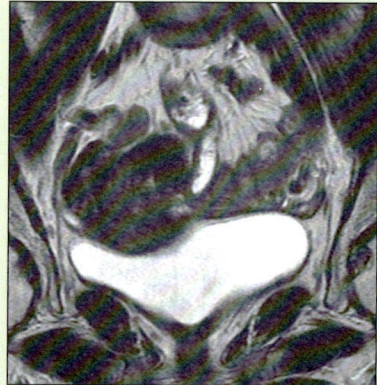

Kallmann Syndrome

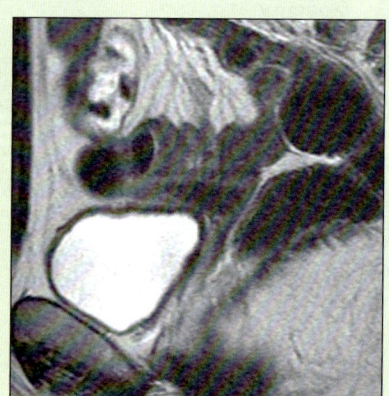

Kallmann Syndrome

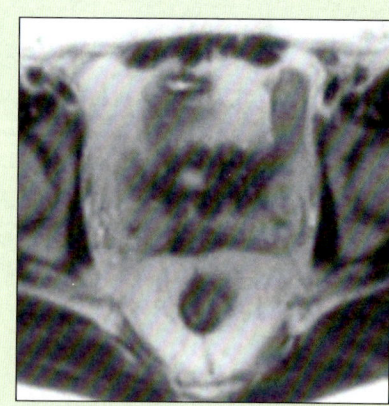

Androgen Insensitivity Syndrome

GONADAL DYSGENESIS

Key Facts

Terminology
- Replacement of gonads, testes or ovaries, by fibrous tissue, devoid of germ cells
- Range of abnormalities of gonads and internal genitalia with variable karyotypes
- 45,X Turner syndrome: Most common karyotype (50%)

Imaging Findings
- Unilateral or bilateral streak gonads: 2-3 cm long and 0.5 cm wide
- Müllerian derivatives typically present but most commonly hypoplastic
- Junctional zone anatomy more easily seen in neonate or after exogenous hormonal stimulation

Top Differential Diagnoses
- Androgen Insensitivity Syndrome
- Other Disorders of Intersexuality

Clinical Issues
- No reproductive potential
- Significant risk of malignant transformation in gonad in presence of Y chromosome
- Removal of gonads mandatory in all patients with 46,XY gonadal dysgenesis

Diagnostic Checklist
- Consider gonadal dysgenesis in patients with primary amenorrhea

---

  - Unique to 46,XY ETR

Ultrasonographic Findings
- Grayscale Ultrasound
  - Optimal evaluation in newborn due to prominence of uterus and ovaries 2° to maternal hormones
  - Mainly for identification of Müllerian derivatives
    - Hypoplastic prepubertal uterus
    - Endometrial stripe frequently not visualized
  - Streak gonads difficult to visualize
  - Undescended testes most often visualized when located in inguinal canal
    - Echogenic focus with acoustic shadowing in ectopic gonads suspicious for gonadoblastoma (frequent calcification)

CT Findings
- Not well-suited to evaluate Müllerian derivatives or identification of gonads

MR Findings
- T1WI
  - Streak gonads slightly hypointense or isointense relative to muscle on T1WI
  - Testes ranging from slightly hypointense to slightly hyperintense relative to muscle
- T2WI
  - Streak gonads: 2-3 cm long and 0.5 cm wide
    - SI lower than normal gonads
    - Isointense or slightly hyperintense to muscle
    - Typically located in the broad ligament
    - Correctly identified in 40-65% (limited data)
  - Testes
    - Typically undescended
    - SI lower than normal gonads
    - Hyperintense to muscle, hypointense relative to fat
    - Low SI rim on T2WI helpful in distinction from lymph nodes
    - Correctly identified in 55-80% (limited data)
  - Hypoplastic uterus
    - Junctional zone anatomy more easily seen in neonate or after exogenous hormonal stimulation
    - Thin endometrial complex with high SI
    - Hypointense myometrium
    - Uterus correctly identified in 93% (limited data)
  - Germ cell tumors
    - Signal dependent on histological type and background signal of gonad
    - High SI in dysgenetic gonads suspicious for secondary malignancy

Imaging Recommendations
- Best imaging tool
  - Ultrasound (US)
    - Screening for presence of Müllerian derivatives, undescended testes in inguinal canal, renal anomalies
    - Screening for gonadoblastoma for testes brought to scrotum
  - MR
    - To locate streak gonads and undescended testes
    - To document presence of Müllerian derivatives
- Protocol advice
  - MR: Phased array body coil
  - High-resolution T1WI and FSE T2WI
    - Slice thickness ≤ 4 mm
    - Transverse, sagittal and coronal images

DIFFERENTIAL DIAGNOSIS

Androgen Insensitivity Syndrome
- 46,XY karyotype with female phenotype
- Bilateral undescended testes
- Absence of upper 2/3 of vagina and uterus

Other Disorders of Intersexuality
- Chromosomal and biochemical profile needed for differentiation among various entities

Hypogonadotropic Hypogonadism (HH)
- Idiopathic HH and Kallmann syndrome (anosmia)
- Normal prepubertal gonads/internal genitalia

GONADAL DYSGENESIS

PATHOLOGY

General Features
- General path comments
  - Deficient Müllerian regression due to inadequate Müllerian inhibitory substance from dysgenetic testis
  - Lack of normal endometrial and myometrial definition with streak ovaries due to lack of estrogen
- Genetics
  - Variable karyotypes
  - Turner syndrome most common (50%)
    - Most common Turner karyotypes 45,XO (50%) and 45,XO/46,XX (15-20%)
- Epidemiology: Turner syndrome: 1 in 2500 live births
- Associated abnormalities: Turner syndrome
  - Cubitus valgus, medial tibial spur, short fourth metacarpal bone
  - Renal anomalies (horseshoe kidney, duplication, agenesis, malrotation)
  - Coarctation of aorta, multiple renal arteries (90%)

Gross Pathologic & Surgical Features
- 46,X (Turner syndrome)
  - Female external genitalia
  - Bilateral streak gonads typically in the broad ligament
    - White, fibrous structures, 2-3 cm x 0.5 cm
  - Hypoplastic prepubertal uterus/vagina
- 46,XX (pure) gonadal dysgenesis
  - Closely related to Turner syndrome
  - Lacks somatic stigmata of Turner syndrome, entailing GD only, hence the term "pure"
- 46,XY (complete) GD
  - "Complete" absence of testicular differentiation, "complete" failure to masculinize
  - Female external genitalia
  - Bilateral streak gonads
  - Well-developed Müllerian structures
- 46,XY ETR and BVTS
  - Represent a variant of 46,XY (complete) GD
  - Phenotype spectrum from complete female to normal male, dependent on timing of testicular loss
  - Absent gonads common feature of all forms
- 45,XO/46,XY mosaic (mixed) GD
  - Phenotype ranging from female with Turner syndrome (25%) to those with predominantly male ambiguous genitalia (70%), rarely normal male phenotype
  - Similar spectrum in gonadal differentiation: Bilateral streak gonads to asymmetric combinations of streak gonad, testis and dysgenetic gonads
    - Dysgenetic/streak gonad associated with ipsilateral Müllerian derivatives (unicornuate uterus, fallopian tube)
    - Well-differentiated testes with functional Sertoli and Leydig cells with ipsilateral Wolffian ducts but no Müllerian ducts

Microscopic Features
- Streak ovaries: Interlacing waves of dense fibrous stroma
  - Devoid of oocytes, otherwise indistinguishable from normal ovarian stroma
- Dysgenetic testes composed of immature hypoplastic seminiferous tubules and persistent stroma resembling that of streak gonads
  - Testes lack germinal elements: Patients infertile
- Rudimentary cords without recognizable testicular tissue in ETR and BVTS

CLINICAL ISSUES

Presentation
- Most common signs/symptoms: Amenorrhea with normal external genitalia
- 45,X (Turner syndrome)
  - Four classic features: Female phenotype, short stature, absence of secondary sexual characteristics, somatic abnormalities (protean manifestations)
  - External genitalia remaining infantile at puberty

Natural History & Prognosis
- No reproductive potential
- Significant risk of malignant transformation in gonad in presence of Y chromosome
  - Usually in first two decades of life
  - Gonadoblastoma most common, followed by dysgerminoma or seminoma
  - Very high risk (30% by age of 30) in 46,XY (complete) GD
    - Frequently bilateral gonadoblastomas

Treatment
- Removal of gonads mandatory in all patients with 46,XY gonadal dysgenesis
- Sex assignment based on external genitalia

DIAGNOSTIC CHECKLIST

Consider
- Consider gonadal dysgenesis in patients with primary amenorrhea

Image Interpretation Pearls
- Secondary malignancy with high SI in dysgenetic gonads

SELECTED REFERENCES
1. Wein D et al: DA: Campbell-Walsh Urology: Sexual differentiation: Normal and abnormal. vol 4. 9th ed. Philadelphia, Elsevier: 3799-3829, 2007
2. Choi HK et al: MR imaging of intersexuality. Radiographics. 18(1):83-96, 1998
3. Reinhold C et al: Primary amenorrhea: evaluation with MR imaging. Radiology. 203(2):383-90, 1997
4. Wright NB et al: Imaging children with ambiguous genitalia and intersex states. Clin Radiol. 50(12):823-9, 1995
5. Gambino J et al: Congenital disorders of sexual differentiation: MR findings. AJR Am J Roentgenol. 158(2):363-7, 1992

GONADAL DYSGENESIS

IMAGE GALLERY

Typical

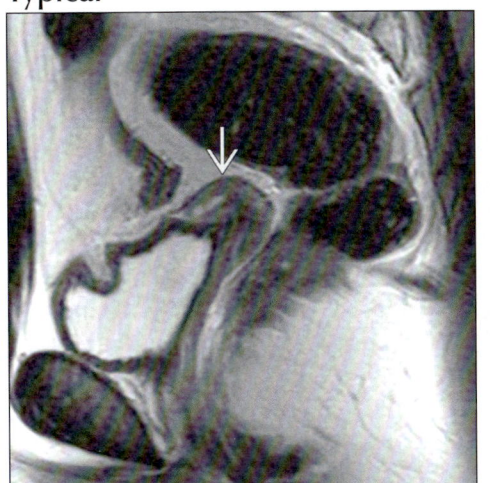
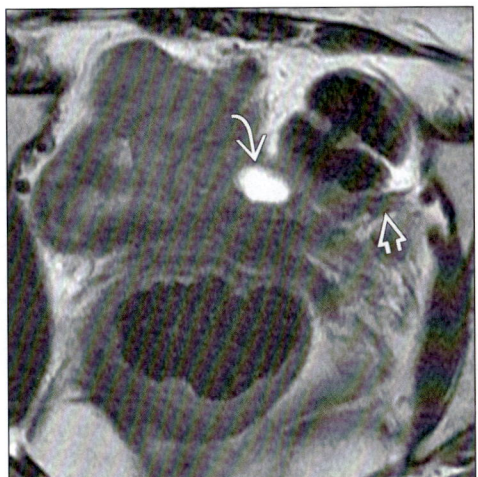

(Left) Sagittal T2WI MR in the same patient as previous image, shows to better advantage the hypoplastic uterus ➡ with preserved zonal anatomy. The outer myometrium is of decreased signal intensity. The patient was proven to have 46,XX pure gonadal dysgenesis (GD). *(Right)* Axial T2WI MR in a patient with Turner syndrome shows a left-sided streak gonad ➡. The high signal intensity area ➡ seen in the midline represents a hematometra.

Typical

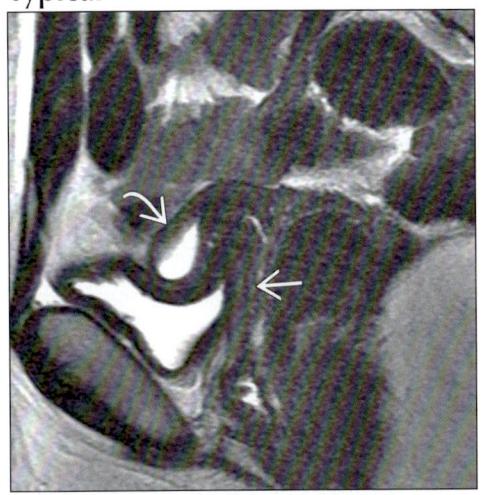
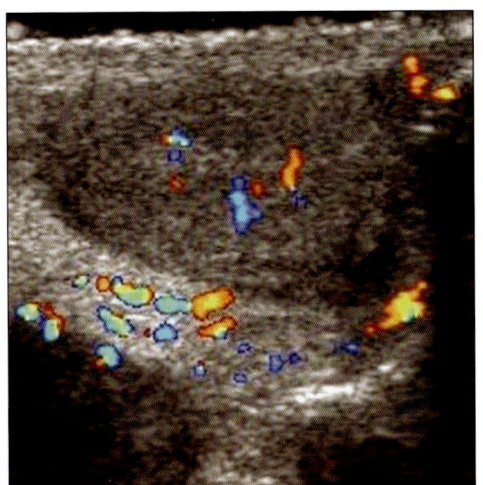

(Left) Sagittal T2WI MR in the same patient as previous image, shows a hypoplastic uterus ➡ and vagina ➡. There is a hematometra distending the endometrial cavity without a uterine anomaly. *(Right)* Sagittal oblique ultrasound in a newborn with male ambiguous genitalia shows a left gonad proven to be a testes at biopsy. A right streak gonad was present (not shown) in this patient with 45,XO/46,XY mosaic (mixed) GD. (Courtesy K. Oudjane, MD).

Typical

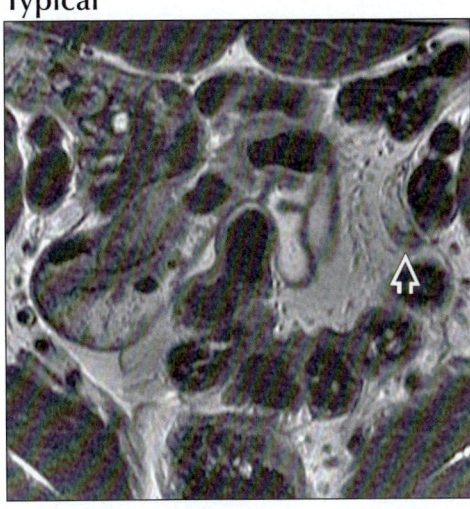
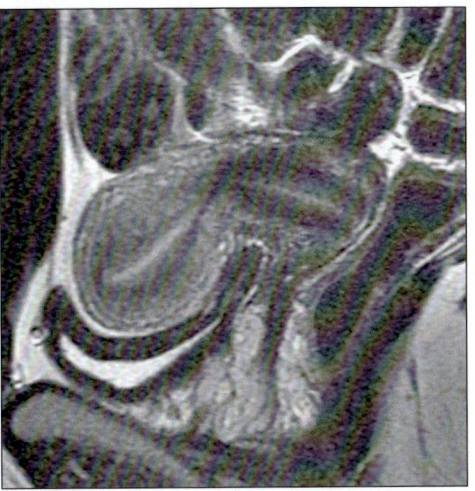

(Left) Axial T2WI MR in a patient with 46,XX "pure" gonadal dysgenesis shows a left streak gonad ➡. The signal intensity is slightly hyperintense to muscle. *(Right)* Sagittal T2WI MR in the same patient as previous image, shows a uterus of normal volume with some zonal differentiation. The corpus/cervix ratio, however, remains almost 1:1. The patient is receiving exogenous hormones.

GARTNER DUCT CYSTS

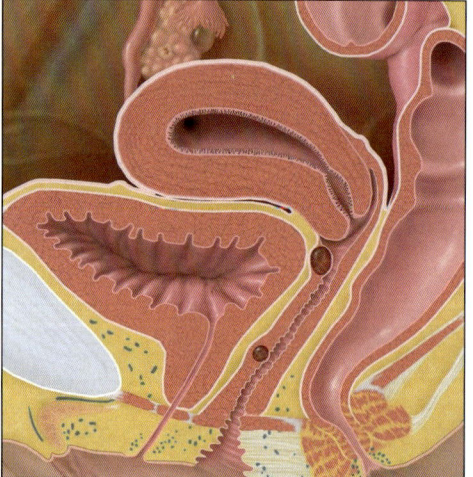
Gartner duct cysts can be found along the anterolateral wall of the vagina as depicted in this graphic.

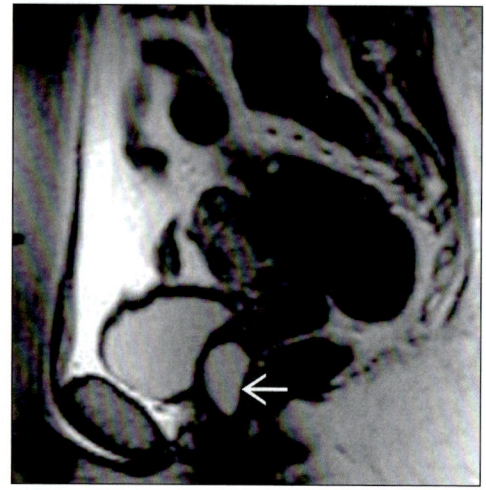
Sagittal T2WI MR shows a large ovoid Gartner duct cyst ➡. (Courtesy G. Israel, MD).

TERMINOLOGY

Definitions
- Embryologic remnant of caudal end of mesonephric/Wolffian duct

IMAGING FINDINGS

General Features
- Best diagnostic clue: Rounded cystic structure arising from vaginal wall
- Location
  ○ Anterolateral wall of vagina
  ○ Typically located above level of pubic symphysis
- Size
  ○ Usually less than 2 cm
  ○ May extend out into the ischiorectal fossa when large
  ○ Case report of 16 cm cyst resulting in asymmetry of buttocks
- Morphology
  ○ Small
  ○ Round
  ○ Sharply marginated

Ultrasonographic Findings
- Grayscale Ultrasound
  ○ Anechoic or hypoechoic, well-circumscribed mass within the vagina
  ○ Less commonly, cysts can be echogenic due to hemorrhage or protein content
  ○ Separate from the cervix
  ○ Sometimes multiple cysts
- Color Doppler: No flow

CT Findings
- NECT
  ○ Well-defined round mass with low attenuation similar to water
    ▪ If proteinaceous, contents may be higher attenuation
  ○ Arise from anterolateral vaginal wall
- CECT: Do not enhance

MR Findings
- T1WI
  ○ Most are low in signal intensity (SI) on T1WI similar to simple fluid

DDx: Gartner Duct Cyst

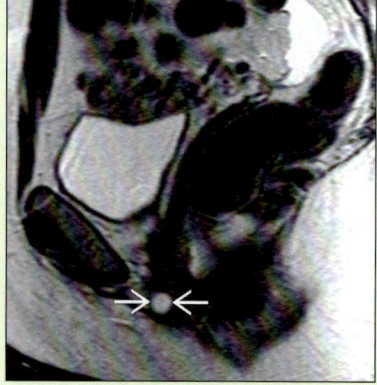
Bartholin Gland Cyst

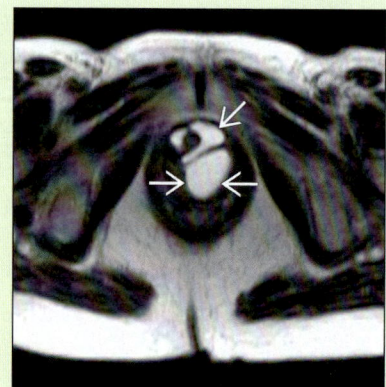
Urethral Diverticulum

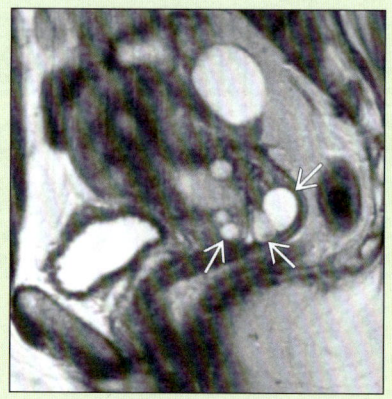
Nabothian Cysts

GARTNER DUCT CYSTS

Key Facts

Terminology
- Embryologic remnant of caudal end of mesonephric/Wolffian duct

Imaging Findings
- Best diagnostic clue: Rounded cystic structure arising from vaginal wall
- Anterolateral wall of vagina
- Typically located above level of pubic symphysis
- May extend out into the ischiorectal fossa when large
- Most are low in signal intensity (SI) on T1WI similar to simple fluid
- T1WI SI can be variable if proteinaceous
- Very high T2WI SI
- T1 C+: No enhancement
- Axial, coronal & sagittal T2WI are key in determining vaginal location

Top Differential Diagnoses
- Bartholin Duct Cyst
- Urethral Diverticulum
- Nabothian Cyst
- Skene Gland Cyst
- Uterus Didelphys with Obstructed Hemivagina

Pathology
- Most common benign cystic lesion of vagina

Clinical Issues
- Most common signs/symptoms: Majority are asymptomatic and incidental findings
- Excellent prognosis
- If symptomatic, marsupialization of cyst into vagina
- Must evaluate for associated ureteral, renal & genital tract anomalies

---

- T1WI SI can be variable if proteinaceous
- T2WI
  - Very high T2WI SI
    - May be slightly lower if proteinaceous
  - Coronal & sagittal planes are helpful for localizing vaginal wall location
  - May be septated
  - Separate from the urethra & cervix
- T1 C+: No enhancement

Imaging Recommendations
- Best imaging tool
  - Typically ultrasound is used to localize and characterize vaginal cysts
  - MR reserved for complicated cases
  - Advantages of MR
    - Multiplanar capabilities
    - Lack of ionizing radiation (especially important for women of reproductive age)
- Protocol advice
  - Axial, coronal & sagittal T2WI are key in determining vaginal location
  - Perform ultrasound with transvaginal probe at introitus or slightly inserted into the vagina to visualize vaginal cyst

DIFFERENTIAL DIAGNOSIS

Bartholin Duct Cyst
- Cystic lesion located in posterolateral inferior third of the vagina
- Associated with labia majora
- Typically images as simple fluid
  - Complex (proteinaceous) imaging characteristics when complicated by infection and/or hemorrhage

Urethral Diverticulum
- Usually located in the mid urethra (at the level of the pubic symphysis)
- Typically involve the posterolateral wall of the urethra

Nabothian Cyst
- Located within cervix, often multiple
- May be large with proteinaceous contents

Skene Gland Cyst
- Located just lateral to the external urethral meatus

Uterus Didelphys with Obstructed Hemivagina
- Not true cystic lesion - distended uterus
- Endometrial cavity distended with menstrual blood & debris
- Symptomatic with primary dysmenorrhea

Cyst of Müllerian Origin
- Identical in gross appearance to Gartner duct cyst

Vaginal Leiomyoma
- Rare, solid mass of vaginal wall

Periurethral Collagen Injections
- Periurethral collagen is used to treat female stress urinary incontinence
- Note that collagen injections can migrate and have variable appearances

Imperforate Hymen
- Results in hematocolpos

PATHOLOGY

General Features
- General path comments: True cyst within anterolateral vaginal wall
- Etiology
  - Embryology: Incomplete regression of mesonephric/Wolffian duct
  - Arise in lower remnants of mesonephric duct
- Epidemiology
  - Most common benign cystic lesion of vagina
  - Up to 1% of women
- Associated abnormalities

GARTNER DUCT CYSTS

- Ipsilateral renal dysplasia or agenesis
- Ipsilateral Müllerian duct obstruction
- Crossed, fused renal ectopia
- Ectopic ureter
- Bicornuate uterus
- Uterus didelphys
- Diverticulosis of fallopian tubes

Gross Pathologic & Surgical Features
- Cyst located within anterolateral vaginal wall

Microscopic Features
- Lined by nonciliated, nonmucinous cuboidal or columnar epithelium
- Large pale nuclei
- May have foci of squamous metaplasia
- Smooth muscle fibers may be present in wall

CLINICAL ISSUES

Presentation
- Most common signs/symptoms: Majority are asymptomatic and incidental findings
- Other signs/symptoms
  - Palpable mass
  - Mass effect on urethra, resulting in urinary tract symptoms
  - Pelvic pain
  - Dyspareunia
  - May even interfere with the birth process

Demographics
- Age: Extremely rare in infants

Natural History & Prognosis
- Excellent prognosis
- Typically do not enlarge
- Usually remain asymptomatic
- Rarely can become infected & form an abscess

Treatment
- Most require no treatment
- If symptomatic, marsupialization of cyst into vagina
- Must evaluate for associated ureteral, renal & genital tract anomalies

DIAGNOSTIC CHECKLIST

Consider
- Gartner duct cyst when vaginal cyst is anterolateral & above pubic symphysis

SELECTED REFERENCES

1. Binsaleh S et al: Gartner duct cyst simplified treatment approach. Int Urol Nephrol. 21, 2006
2. Dwyer PL et al: Congenital urogenital anomalies that are associated with the persistence of Gartner's duct: a review. Am J Obstet Gynecol. 185:354-9, 2006
3. Hahn WY et al: MRI of female urethral and periurethral disorders. AJR. 182:677-82, 2004
4. Ohya T et al: Diagnosis and treatment for persistent Gartner duct cyst in an infant: a case report. J Pediatr Surg. 37:E4, 2002
5. Sherer DM et al: Transvaginal ultrasonographic depiction of a Gartner Duct Cyst. J Ultrasound Med. 20:1253-5, 2001
6. Corcos J et al: Periurethral collagen injection for the treatment of female stress urinary incontinence: 4-year follow-up results. Urology. 54:815-8, 1999
7. Llauger J et al: The normal and pathologic ischiorectal fossa at CT and MR imaging. Radiographics. 18:61-82, 1998
8. Sheih CP et al: Diagnosing the combination of renal dysgenesis, Gartner's duct cyst, and ipsilateral Mullerian duct obstruction. J Urol. 159:217-21, 1998
9. Leonovicz PF et al: Vaginal ectopic ureter with Gartner's duct cyst. J Urol. 158:2235, 1997
10. Siegelman ES et al: Multicoil MR imaging of symptomatic female urethral and periurethral disease. Radiographics. 17:349-65, 1997
11. Hagspiel KD: Giant Gartner duct cyst: magnetic resonance imaging findings. Abdom Imaging. 20:566-8, 1995
12. Koroku M et al: A case of Gartner's duct cyst with a right aplastic kidney. Int J Urol. 2:211-3, 1995
13. Gompel C et al: The Vagina. In: Pathology in Gynecology and Obstetrics. J.G. Lippincott Company. Philadelphia 46-71, 1994
14. Kim B et al: Diagnosis of urethral diverticula in women: value of MR imaging. AJR. 161:809-15, 1993
15. Rosenfeld DL et al: Gartner's duct cyst with a single vaginal ectopic ureter and associated renal dysplasia or agenesis. J Ultrasound Med. 12:775-8, 1993
16. Kier R: Nonovarian gynecologic cysts: MR imaging findings. AJR. 158:1265-9, 1992
17. Kier R: Nonovarian gynecologic cysts: MR imaging findings. AJR. 158:1265-9, 1992
18. Rabinerson D et al: Combined anomalies of the Müllerian and Wolffian systems. Acta Obstet Gynecol Scand. 71:156-7, 1992
19. Hricak H et al: Female urethra: MR imaging. Radiology. 178:527-35, 1991
20. Lee MJ et al: Large Gartner duct cyst associated with a solitary crossed ectopic kidney: imaging features. JCAT. 15:145-51, 1991
21. Lee MJ et al: Large Gartner's duct cyst associated with a solitary crossed ectopic kidney: imaging features. J Comput Assist Tomogr. 15:149-51, 1991
22. Dodd GD et al: Lipomatous tumors of the pelvis in women: spectrum of imaging findings. AJR. 155:317-22, 1989
23. Muram D et al: Urinary retention secondary to a Gartner's duct cyst. Obstet Gynecol. 72:51-1, 1988
24. Naisby GP: Gartner's duct associated with diverticulosis of the fallopian tubes. Clin Radiol. 38:207-8, 1987
25. Miller EV et al: Skene's duct cyst. J Urol. 131:966-7, 1984
26. McCarthy S et al: Sonography of vaginal masses. AJR. 140:1005-8, 1983
27. Little HK et al: Hematocolpos: diagnosis made by ultrasound. J Clin Ultrasound. 6:341-2, 1978
28. Scheible FW: Ultrasonographic features of Gartner's duct cyst. J Clin Ultrasound. 6:438-9, 1978
29. Beresford JM et al: Abscess formation in Gartner's duct cysts associated with ipsilateral renal agenesis. A report of two cases. Obstet Gynecol. 49:28-30, 1977

GARTNER DUCT CYSTS

IMAGE GALLERY

Typical

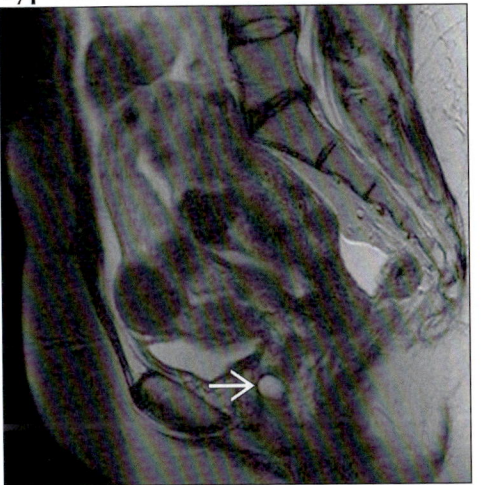
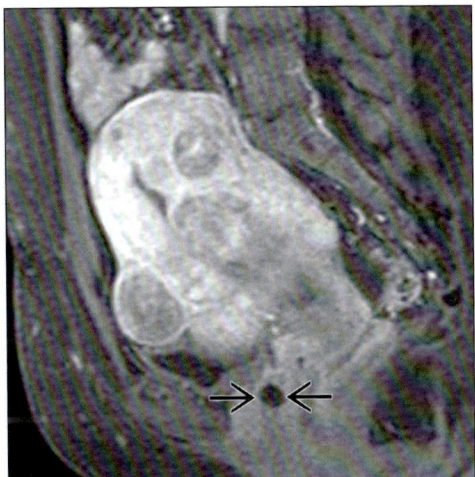

(Left) Sagittal T1WI MR shows a small cyst ➡ located in the vaginal wall. Note the location above the level of the pubic symphysis. *(Right)* Sagittal T1 C+ FS MR in the same patient as previous image shows no enhancement of the same cyst ➡.

Typical

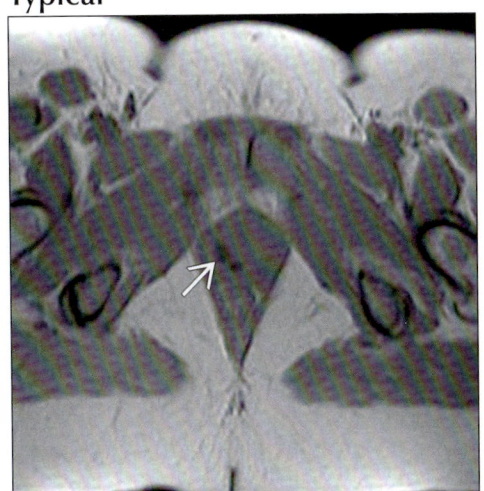
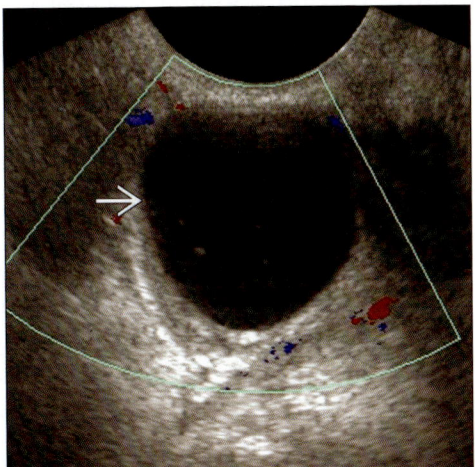

(Left) Axial T1WI MR shows an ovoid T1 hypointense lesion ➡ in the left vaginal wall. *(Right)* Axial transvaginal ultrasound shows an avascular cyst in the vaginal wall ➡.

Variant

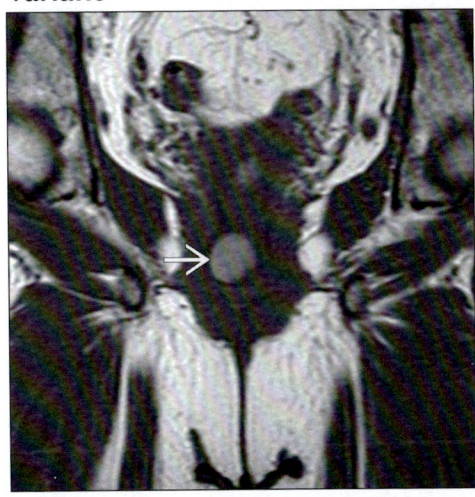
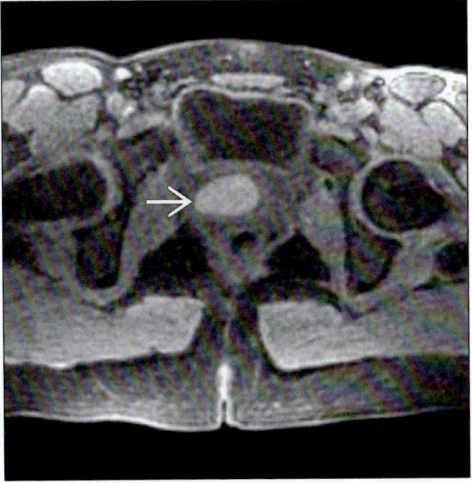

(Left) Coronal T1WI MR shows a hyperintense lesion ➡ in the vaginal wall, consistent with a proteinaceous vs. hemorrhagic Gartner duct cyst. *(Right)* Axial T1WI FS MR shows hyperintense Gartner dust cyst ➡, signifying presence of proteinaceous material or hemorrhage.

BARTHOLINITIS

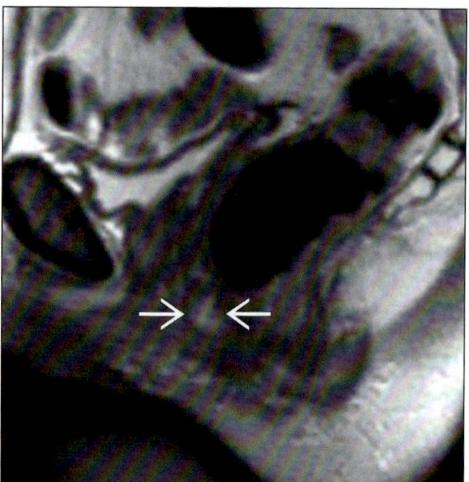

Sagittal T2WI MR shows an irregular, thick-wall, high SI lesion ➡ in the posterolateral vaginal wall in a 44 year old patient presenting with perineal pain and swelling.

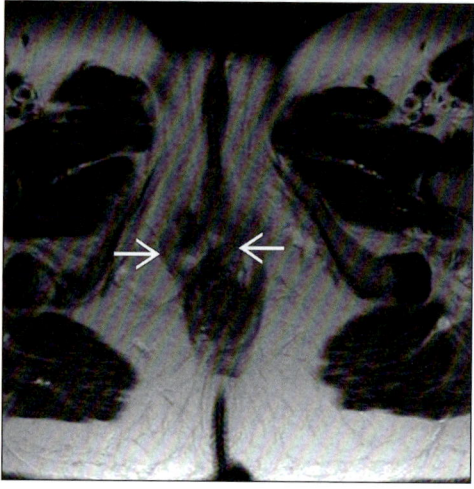

Axial T2WI MR in the same patient confirms the presence of an irregular, high SI perineal lesion ➡. Pathology: Chronic bartholinitis.

TERMINOLOGY

Definitions
- Infection of one or both Bartholin glands or their ducts

IMAGING FINDINGS

General Features
- Location
  o Bartholin glands located bilaterally at the posterior introitus at base of labia minora
    ▪ Glands drain into ducts approximately 2.5 cm long
    ▪ Bartholin gland ducts empty into vestibule at 4 and 8 o'clock positions

Ultrasonographic Findings
- Unilocular, thick-walled cyst in the posterolateral portion of the lower vagina on perineal ultrasound
- May see induration of tissues as surrounding edema

CT Findings
- CECT: Cystic lesion in the lower vagina/perineum ± rim-enhancement

MR Findings
- T1WI: Variable SI depending on amount of protein and/or hemorrhage
- T2WI: High SI well-circumscribed cystic lesion in posterolateral distal vagina/perineum± air-fluid level; high SI surrounding tissues indicated edema
- T1 C+FS: Irregular rim-enhancement

Imaging Recommendations
- Best imaging tool
  o Bartholinitis is a clinical diagnosis
  o MR indicated to establish diagnosis if in doubt and to detect complications (e.g., abscess)

DIFFERENTIAL DIAGNOSIS

Bartholin Gland Carcinoma
- Significant soft-tissue component; can be difficult to differentiate from chronic Bartholinitis

DDx: Perineal Masses

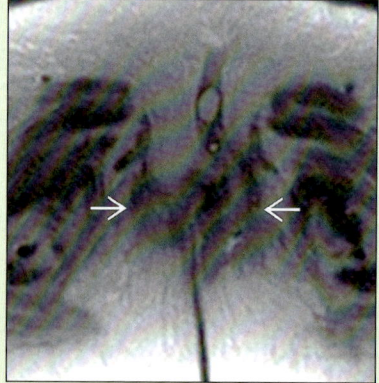

Vulval Carcinoma

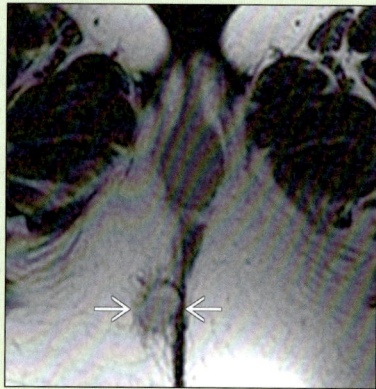

Bartholin Gland Carcinoma

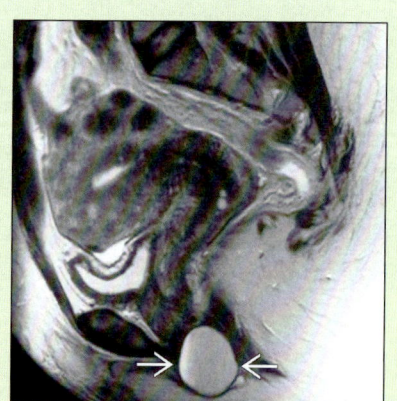

Bartholin Cyst

BARTHOLINITIS

Key Facts

Terminology
- Infection of one or both Bartholin glands or their ducts

Imaging Findings
- CECT: Cystic lesion in the lower vagina/perineum ± rim-enhancement
- T1WI: Variable SI depending on amount of protein and/or hemorrhage
- T2WI: High SI well-circumscribed cystic lesion in posterolateral distal vagina/perineum ± air-fluid level; high SI surrounding tissues indicated edema
- T1 C+FS: Irregular rim-enhancement
- Unilocular, thick-walled cyst in the posterolateral portion of the lower vagina on perineal ultrasound
- Bartholinitis is a clinical diagnosis
- MR indicated to establish diagnosis if in doubt and to detect complications (e.g., abscess)

Vulval Carcinoma
- Older age group; locally aggressive soft tissue mass ± inguinal lymphadenopathy

Perineal Cysts
- Bartholin cyst: Well-defined, thin wall cyst with no rim-enhancement
- Gartner duct cyst: Located more medially and cranially
- Epidermal inclusion cyst: Mobile and non tender, caused by trauma or surgery

PATHOLOGY

General Features
- Etiology
  - Obstruction of a distal duct → retention of secretions → cyst formation → secondary infection
  - May be secondary to sexually transmitted disease
  - May be result of vulvovaginal surgery
  - Polymicrobial: Anaerobes, Neisseria Gonorrhea, Chlamydia Trachomatis
- Epidemiology: 2% women will develop bartholinitis or a Bartholin abscess in their lifetime

CLINICAL ISSUES

Presentation
- Most common signs/symptoms
  - May be asymptomatic
  - Pain on walking or sitting, dyspareunia
  - Usually unilateral involvement as a small cyst as a medially protruding mass in the posterior introitus

Demographics
- Age
  - Most common in the reproductive years
  - Bartholin glands gradually involute after the age of 30

Treatment
- Antibiotic treatment
- Incision and drainage for a Bartholin gland abscess
- Marsupialization for Bartholin duct cyst
- Placement of word catheter
  - Can be used for gland abscess or duct cysts
  - Tip of catheter left into incised cyst or abscess for 3-4 weeks to allow epithelization of the surgically created tract
- Cauterization

SELECTED REFERENCES
1. Omole F et al: Management of Bartholin's duct cyst and gland abscess. Am Fam Physician. 68(1):135-40, 2003
2. Siegelman ES et al: High-resolution MR imaging of the vagina. Radiographics. 17(5):1183-203, 1997
3. Moulopoulos LA et al: Magnetic resonance imaging and computed tomography appearance of asymptomatic paravaginal cysts. Clin Imaging. 17(2):126-32, 1993

IMAGE GALLERY

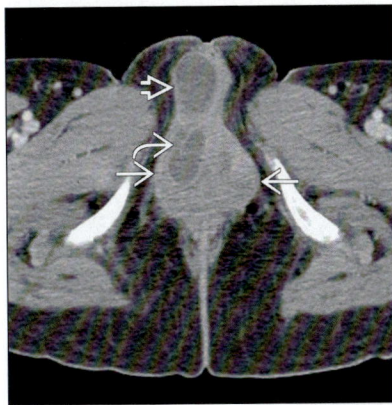 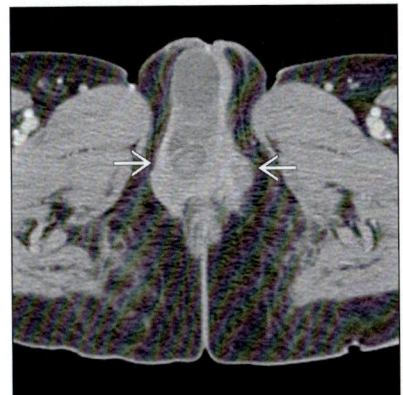 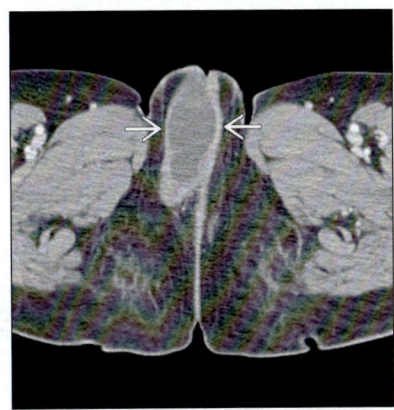

(Left) Axial CECT in an immunosuppressed patient post heart and lung transplant shows a complex cystic mass ➡ centered in the lower vagina and extending to the right labia ➡. Internal septations and rim-enhancement ➡ is noted. *(Center)* Axial CECT in the same patient as the image on the left shows the extent of bilateral cystic lesions ➡ (smaller on the left). *(Right)* Axial CECT in the same patient as the previous two images, shows the anterior extent of the cystic lesion ➡ into the right labia. Pathology: Bilateral Bartholin gland abscesses.

VAGINAL FISTULA

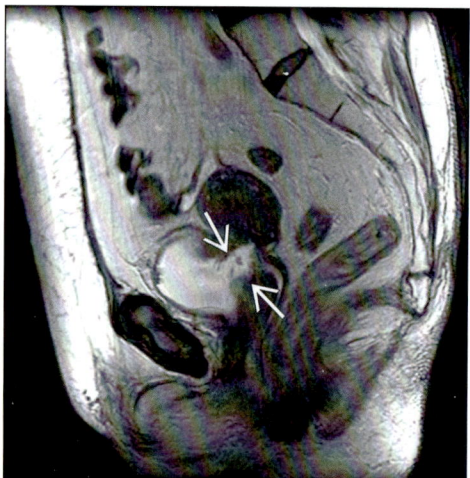

Sagittal T2WI MR shows a fistula tract ➡ between urinary bladder and upper vagina.

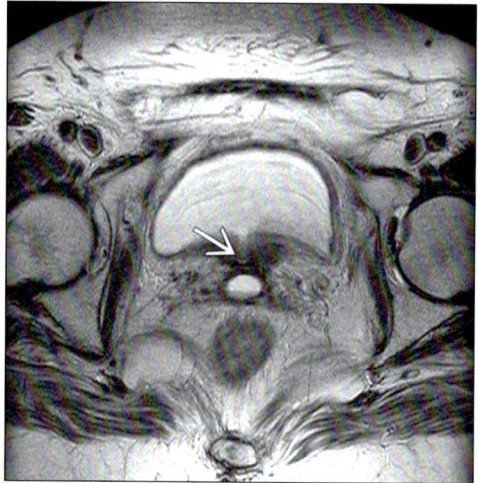

Axial T2WI MR in the same patient previous image shows a fistula tract ➡ between urinary bladder and fluid-filled vagina.

TERMINOLOGY

Definitions
- Epithelium-lined passageway permitting abnormal communication between vagina and other pelvic organs

IMAGING FINDINGS

General Features
- Best diagnostic clue: CEMR images most accurately demonstrate fistulous tract wall-enhancement and low signal intensity fluid within the fistula
- Location
  - Exact location is difficult to determine by physical examination and conventional techniques (vaginoscopy, methylene blue test, IVP, fistulography)
  - MR most useful in determining exact location
- Types of fistula
  - Urethrovaginal
    - Co existent vesicovaginal fistulas seen
    - Fistula between urethra and neo-vagina (recognized complication of transgender surgery)
  - Vesicovaginal
    - Most common location interureteral ridge
    - Fistula involves posterior bladder wall
    - Associated with tumor recurrence in vaginal vault
  - Ureterovaginal
  - Colovaginal
    - 40% of diverticulum related fistulas
    - Sigmoid colon most commonly involved
  - Rectovaginal
    - Rare
    - Small portion of all anorectal fistulas
  - Complex
    - Fistulas involving multiple organs (e.g., vesicovaginal-rectovaginal)

Ultrasonographic Findings
- Grayscale Ultrasound
  - Difficult to diagnose
  - Fistulous tract may be seen as thin linear band of varying echogenicity
  - Vesicovaginal fistulas

DDx: More Examples of Vesicovaginal Fistulas

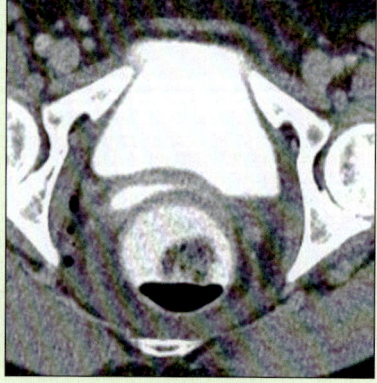

Axial CECT

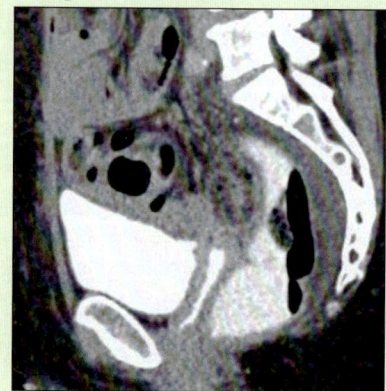

Sagittal CECT

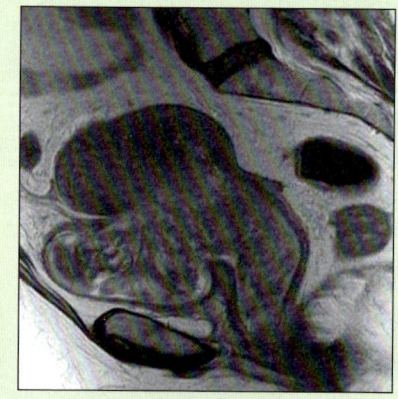

Sagittal MR

VAGINAL FISTULA

Key Facts

Imaging Findings
- **Vaginogram**
- Contrast material inserted via Foley catheter or rectal barium enema tip with balloon into vagina
- **Advantages over contrast enema**
- Vaginal contrast material is in a confined area and more likely to enter a fistulous tract
- No bowel loops filled with contrast agent to mask the tract or the contrast in the vagina
- **Cystogram**
- Commonly used in evaluating vesicovaginal fistulas
- Excretory urography may be useful to exclude concomitant ureterovaginal fistula
- **MR to evaluate**
- Vaginal fistula anatomy
- Secondary extensions or multiple fistulous tracts
- Complications of fistulas (abscesses)
- Anal sphincter anatomy and damage
- **T1WI**
- Low signal intensity tract
- **T2WI**
- High signal linear tract extending between the vagina and organ of interest (anal canal, rectum, sigmoid, bladder etc.)
- Thin low SI fibrous wall with a small amount of high SI fluid in the tract
- Low SI bubbles of air may be seen within the high SI tract
- Concomitant high SI edema or fluid collection can be demonstrated in the rectovaginal septum
- **T1 C+ FS** (early phase of contrast-enhancement) shows low signal intensity tract with enhanced tract wall

---

- Abnormal collection of air may be seen in bladder as nondependent linear echogenic focus with distal shadowing
- Endoanal ultrasound may reveal associated anal sphincter injury in anorectovaginal fistulas
- Color Doppler
  - Useful in evaluating vesicovaginal fistulas
  - US color Doppler with contrast media demonstrates jet phenomenon through bladder wall toward the vagina
    - Detects fistulous tract
    - Assesses distance from fistula to ureterovesical junction (UVJ)

CT Findings
- Larger tracts may be demonstrated as low attenuation linear regions
- Inflammatory changes with fat stranding may be demonstrated
- Vesicovaginal fistula
  - Bladder is usually collapsed because of decompression via fistula
  - Air and fluid may be present within the vagina
  - Air within the bladder may be present
  - Delayed phase of contrast-enhancement may demonstrate excreted contrast medium within the vagina

MR Findings
- **MR to evaluate**
  - Vaginal fistula anatomy
  - Secondary extensions or multiple fistulous tracts
  - Complications of fistulas (abscesses)
  - Anal sphincter anatomy and damage
- Endoanal/endoluminal coil
  - Advantages
    - Provides excellent images of the rectum, anal canal, rectovaginal septum and vagina
    - It allows identification of the smaller anovaginal fistulous tracts
    - Improves signal to noise ratio and spatial resolution
  - Disadvantages
    - It has limited field of view and may not depict the full extend of the fistulous tract
    - May not depict other types of vaginal fistulas
    - Patient discomfort at insertion or the coil
- Pelvic coil
  - Most larger fistulous tracts can be depicted
  - Large field of view, the entire pelvis imaged and other types of fistulae can be evaluated (e.g., vesicovaginal)
- **T1WI**
  - Low signal intensity tract
- **T2WI**
  - High signal linear tract extending between the vagina and organ of interest (anal canal, rectum, sigmoid, bladder etc.)
  - Thin low SI fibrous wall with a small amount of high SI fluid in the tract
  - Low SI bubbles of air may be seen within the high SI tract
  - Concomitant high SI edema or fluid collection can be demonstrated in the rectovaginal septum
- **T1 C+ FS** (early phase of contrast-enhancement) shows low signal intensity tract with enhanced tract wall

Fluoroscopic Findings
- Contrast enema
  - Conventional fluoroscopic method used to evaluate rectovaginal/colovaginal fistulas
  - Contrast material inserted via rectal tube into rectum, spot films to evaluate path of contrast medium
  - Water soluble contrast medium used as risk of leakage into peritoneal cavity
  - Contrast medium seen from the rectum/colon into vagina
  - May fail to demonstrate contrast medium in vagina as contrast medium may traverse the bowel as path of least resistance
  - Vaginal contrast may be obscured by contrast in overlapping loops of rectosigmoid
  - Fistula tract may be obscured by contrast in overlapping loops of bowel
- **Vaginogram**

VAGINAL FISTULA

- Contrast material inserted via Foley catheter or rectal barium enema tip with balloon into vagina
- Balloon inflated to seal vaginal orifice
- Water soluble contrast material used
  - Risk of leakage into peritoneal cavity via fistula
  - Risk of venous extravasation (especially if contrast medium enters the uterus)
- Spot films to evaluate fistulous tract from vagina to rectosigmoid
  - Rectosigmoid
  - Bladder
  - Ureters
- **Advantages over contrast enema**
  - Vaginal contrast material is in a confined area and more likely to enter a fistulous tract
  - No bowel loops filled with contrast agent to mask the tract or the contrast in the vagina
  - Multiple fistulas can be recognized
- Cystogram
  - Commonly used in evaluating vesicovaginal fistulas
  - Water soluble contrast medium via a Foley catheter into the bladder
  - Spot films to demonstrate tract between bladder and vagina
  - Excretory urography may be useful to exclude concomitant ureterovaginal fistula
  - Among conventional techniques cystoscopy is most accurate (92%)
    - Air within bladder is suggestive of either fistula or recent cystoscopy
    - After cystoscopy air should disappear within 3-4 micturitions
    - Gas in the irradiated bladder may be seen for more than one week after cystoscopy due to impaired emptying
- Direct visualization
  - Vaginoscopy and cystourethroscopy for urethrovaginal, vesicovaginal fistulas and some colovaginal fistulas

Imaging Recommendations
- Best imaging tool: MR is the study of choice to demonstrate a fistulous tract
- Protocol advice
  - Pelvic phase array coil used if other type of fistula or extensive anovaginal fistula
  - Endoluminal coil may be useful if anovaginal fistula suspected
  - Fat-suppressed T2WI are usually sufficient for diagnosis
  - Dynamic CEMR with fat-suppression increases the conspicuity of enhancing sinus tract

PATHOLOGY

General Features
- Etiology
  - Obstetric trauma (prolonged delivery, hysterectomy)
  - Surgery (vaginal repair, hysterectomy, urological)
  - Inflammation (diverticular disease)
  - Inflammatory bowel disease (Crohn)
  - Post-operative, perineal infection
  - Radiotherapy
  - Pelvic malignancy (bladder cancer, cervical/endometrial cancer)
  - Foreign body

Gross Pathologic & Surgical Features
- Fistulous tract which may contain fluid, urine, air, blood or pus

Microscopic Features
- Tract is lined by squamous epithelium at vaginal end and transitional epithelium or colonic mucosa depending on the organ connected
- Tract may show focal ulceration
- Acute and chronic inflammation
- Evidence of healing with fibrosis
- Tumor cells visible in malignancy
- Stromal non caseating granulomata together with background inflammation in Crohn disease
- Caseating granulomata in TB
- Dense fibrosis/sclerosis of stroma with atypical stromal cells seen with history of radiation

CLINICAL ISSUES

Presentation
- Most common signs/symptoms: Vaginal bleeding, discharge, flatus
- Other signs/symptoms
  - Day and night urinary or fecal incontinence
  - Recurrent urinary tract/vaginal infection

Natural History & Prognosis
- Good if not associated with recurrent malignancy

Treatment
- Corrective surgery

DIAGNOSTIC CHECKLIST

Image Interpretation Pearls
- Fistulous tract demonstrated as linear abnormality between the vagina and organ of interest on conventional radiography or MR

SELECTED REFERENCES
1. Dwarkasing S et al: Anovaginal fistulas: evaluation with endoanal MR imaging. Radiology. 231(1):123-8, 2004
2. Yu NC et al: Fistulas of the genitourinary tract: a radiologic review. Radiographics. 24(5):1331-52, 2004
3. Kruskal JB et al: Peroxide-enhanced anal endosonography: technique, image interpretation, and clinical applications. Radiographics. 21 Spec No:S173-89, 2001
4. Volkmer BG et al: Colour Doppler ultrasound in vesicovaginal fistulas. Ultrasound Med Biol. 26(5):771-5, 2000
5. Semelka RC et al: Pelvic fistulas: appearances on MR images. Abdom Imaging. 22(1):91-5, 1997
6. Outwater E et al: Pelvic fistulas: findings on MR images. AJR Am J Roentgenol. 160(2):327-30, 1993

VAGINAL FISTULA

IMAGE GALLERY

Typical

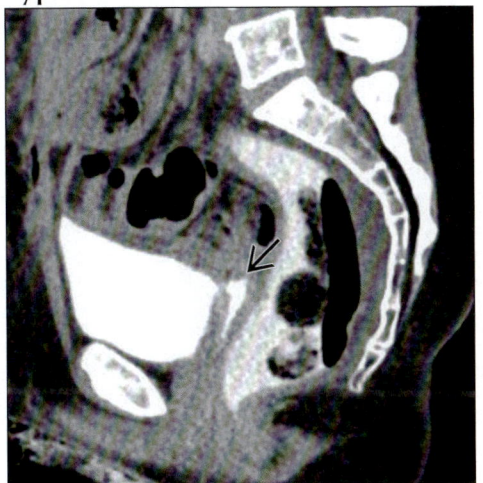
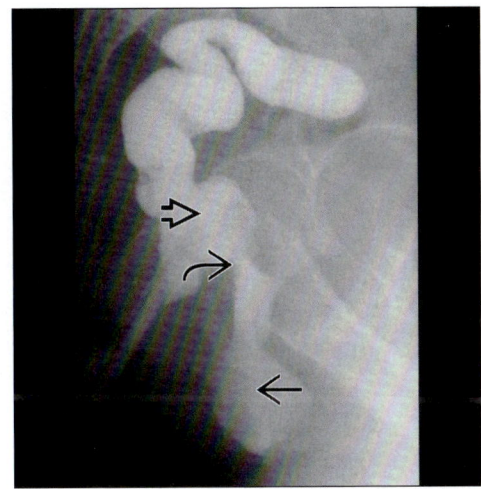

(Left) Sagittal CECT reconstructed image shows a colovaginal fistula. Contrast medium is seen within the vaginal lumen ➡. *(Right)* Lateral radiograph from a barium enema study on the same patient as previous image, shows contrast medium filling the vagina ➡ through a fistulous tract ➡ from the sigmoid colon ➡. Appearances are consistent with a colovaginal fistula.

Typical

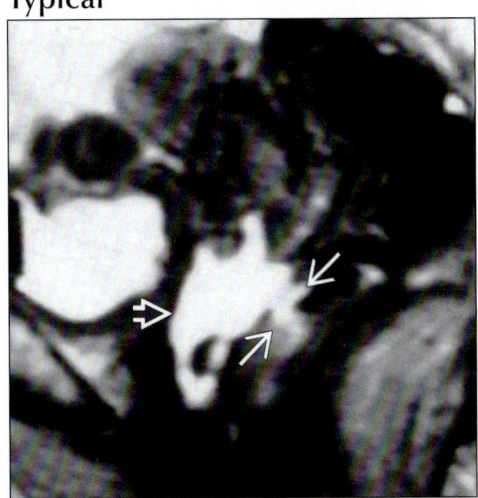
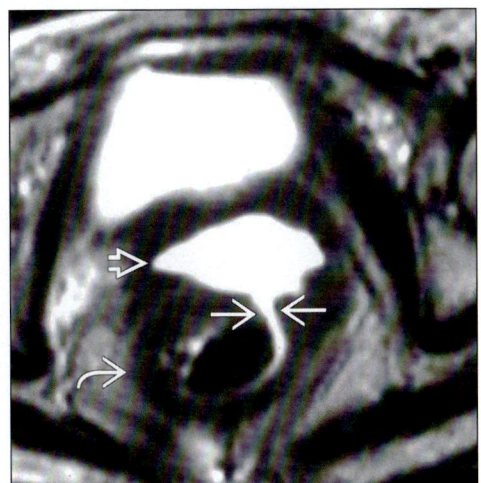

(Left) Sagittal T2WI MR in a 50 year old patient shows high SI hydrocolpos ➡ secondary to a necrotic cervical tumor invading the vagina. Note the linear high SI rectovaginal fistula tract ➡. *(Right)* Axial T2WI MR in the same patient as previous image, confirms the presence of a fistulous tract ➡ between the vagina ➡ and the rectum ➡. (Courtesy T. Cunha, MD).

Typical

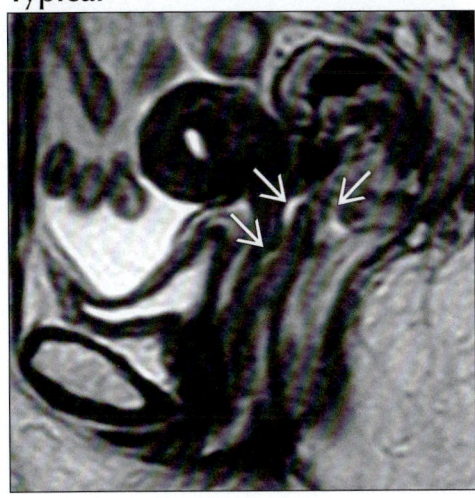
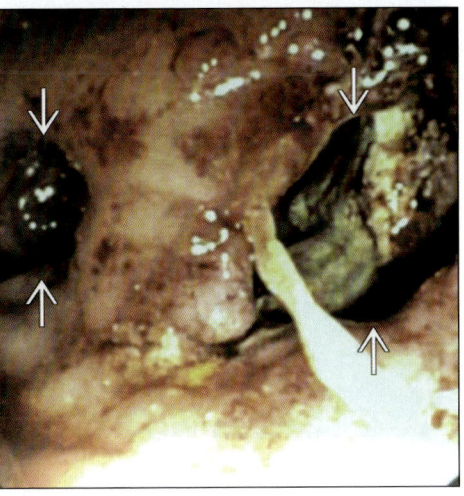

(Left) Sagittal T2WI MR shows high SI linear bands ➡ between the rectum and the vagina in a 56 year old woman following radiation therapy for cervical carcinoma. Appearances are consistent with multiple rectovaginal fistulas. *(Right)* Intra-operative photograph in the same patient as previous image, shows two fistula openings ➡ from the vagina into the rectum. (Courtesy T. Cunha, MD).

VAGINAL FISTULA

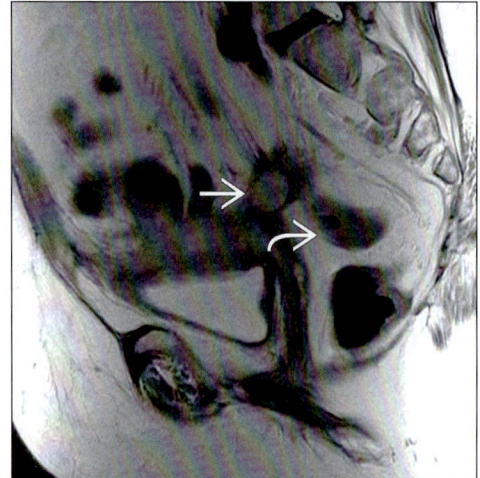

(Left) Sagittal T2WI MR shows a vaginal vault recurrence in a patient with past history of endometrial cancer. Note very close proximity of the lesion ➡ to the sigmoid colon ➡.
(Right) Axial T1 C+ FS MR in the same patient as previous image, shows the fistulous tract ➡ between the vaginal vault ➡ and sigmoid colon ➡.

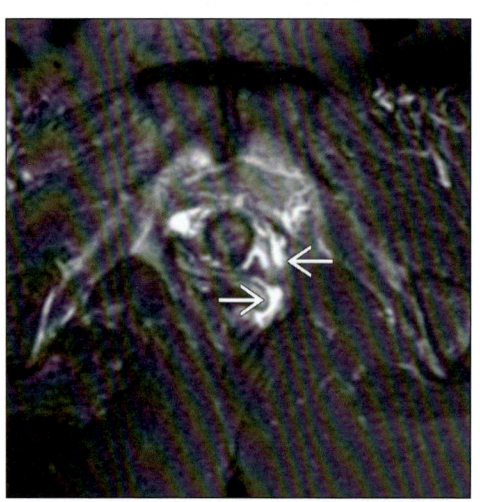 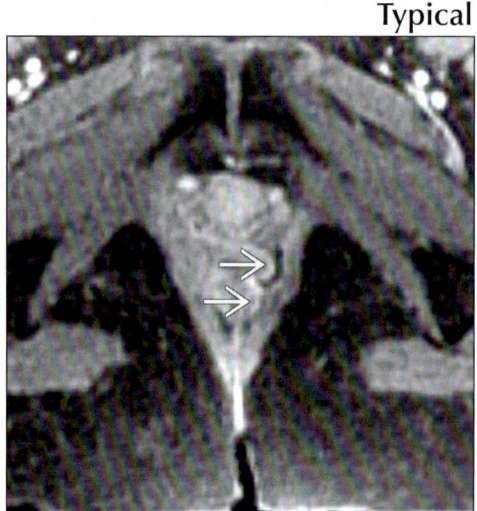

(Left) Axial T2WI FS MR shows a fistulous tract between the vagina and the anus, as linear high SI band ➡ in a patient following radiation therapy for cervical carcinoma. *(Right)* Axial T1 C+ FS MR in the same patient as previous image, confirms the presence of an anovaginal fistula. Note the low signal intensity fistulous tract ➡ which is demonstrating wall enhancement.

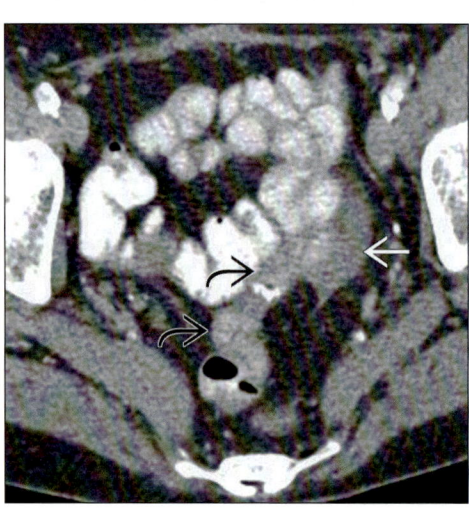 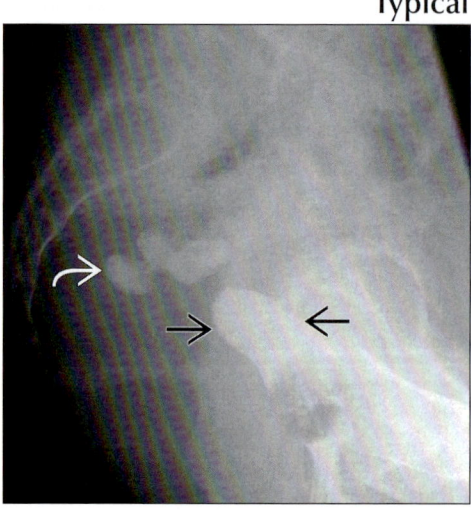

(Left) Axial CECT shows soft tissue mass in the region of the vaginal vault ➡ in close proximity to the sigmoid colon ➡ in a patient with previous endometrial carcinoma. *(Right)* Sagittal radiograph from a vaginogram in the same patient as previous image, shows contrast medium tracking from the vagina ➡ into the sigmoid colon ➡. Appearances are those of colo-vaginal fistula.

VAGINAL FISTULA

Typical

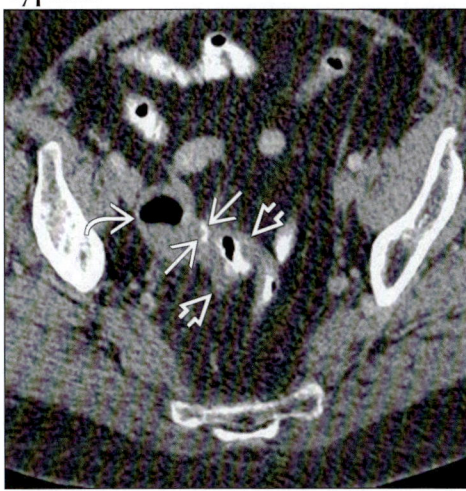
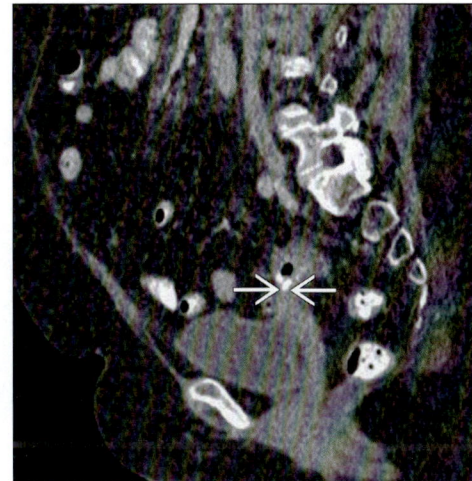

(Left) Axial CECT shows a fistula track ➡ between the sigmoid colon ➡ and the vaginal vault ➡ secondary to recurrent endometrial cancer. Note the air-fluid level ➡ within the vaginal vault. (Right) Sagittal CECT reconstructed image in the same patient as previous image, confirms the presence of a colovaginal fistula ➡.

Typical

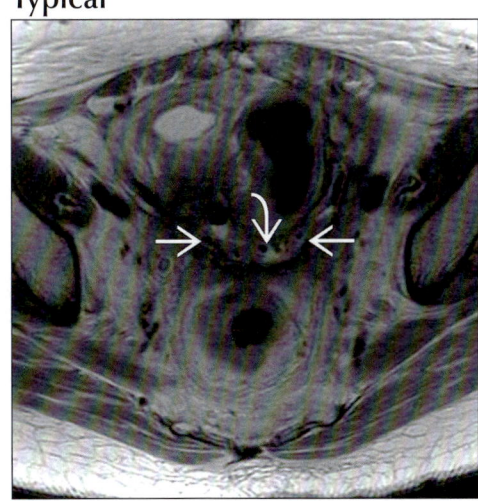
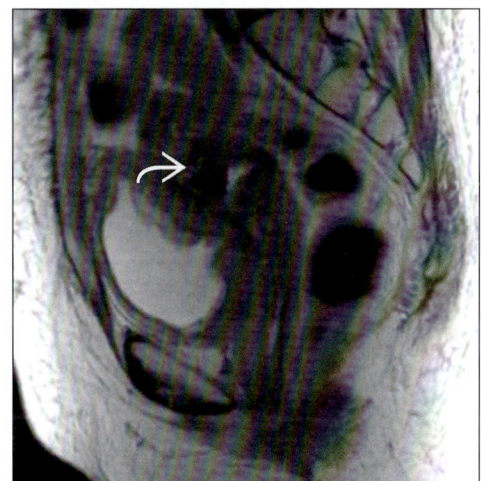

(Left) Axial T2WI MR shows bubbles of air ➡ within a fluid-filled vaginal vault ➡ in a patient after surgery & radiotherapy for cervical carcinoma. (Right) Sagittal T2WI MR (same patient as previous image) shows air & fluid within the vaginal vault ➡. Note the thickened bladder wall due to radiotherapy. Although a fistulous tract could not be demonstrated between the vaginal vault & the sigmoid colon, the clinical & imaging features were consistent with a colovaginal fistula.

Typical

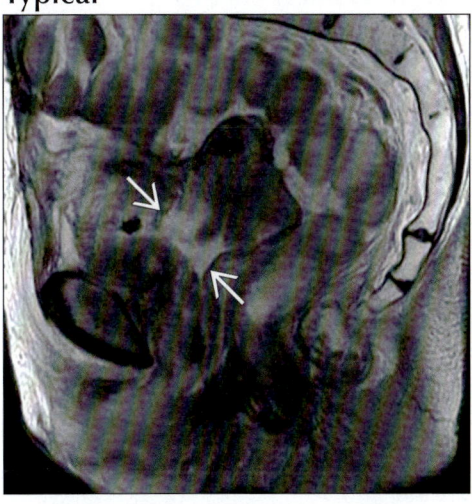
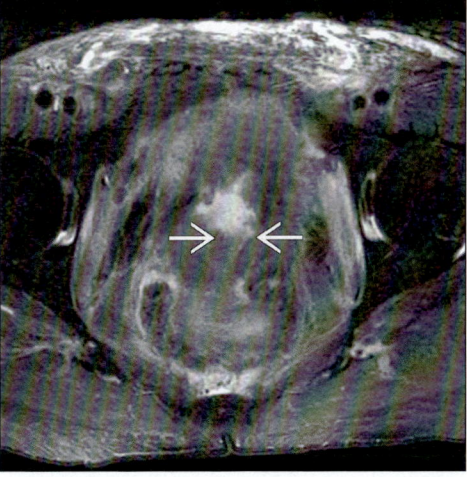

(Left) Sagittal T2WI MR shows a vesico-vaginal fistula ➡ in a patient after radio-chemotherapy for stage 4 vaginal carcinoma. (Right) Axial T2WI FS MR in the same patient as previous image, confirms the presence of a vesicovaginal fistula ➡. Note the extensive soft tissue edema within the pelvis.

LEIOMYOMA, VAGINA

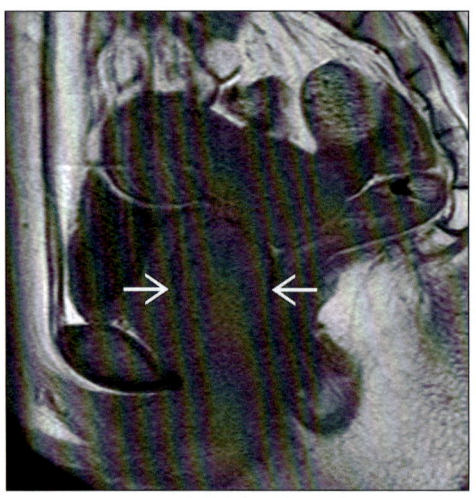

Sagittal T1WI MR shows a low SI mass ➡ arising from the anterior vaginal wall. This was found to be a leiomyoma.

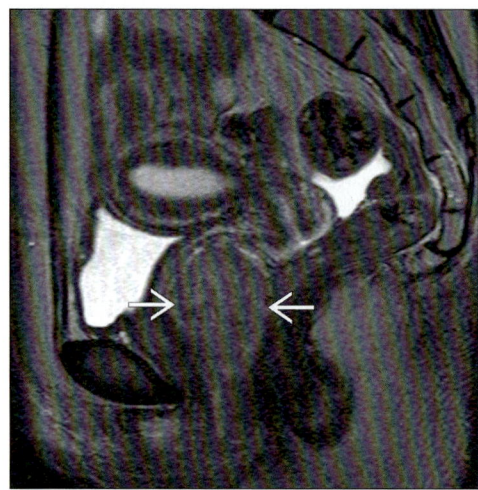

Sagittal T2WI MR shows the same tumor ➡ as in previous image, with similar SI to that of the myometrium.

TERMINOLOGY

Definitions
- Benign smooth muscle tumor of vagina

IMAGING FINDINGS

General Features
- Best diagnostic clue: Solid soft tissue mass arising from the vaginal wall
- Location: Anywhere along the vagina, but most commonly in the midline anterior wall
- Size: Between 1-5 cm

Ultrasonographic Findings
- Well-defined hypoechoic mass in the vaginal wall
- Separate from the cervix
  - May be confused for a cervical leiomyoma
- May show cystic degeneration as hypoechoic well-defined regions

MR Findings
- Similar to typical uterine leiomyoma
  - Low signal intensity (SI) on both T1WI and T2WI
  - Homogeneous SI similar to myometrium
- Some reported to show atypical features
  - High SI on T2WI
  - Marked contrast-enhancement on early dynamic phase
- May undergo degeneration with similar MR features to that of a uterine leiomyoma
  - Hyaline: Low SI on T2WI; myxoid & cystic: High SI on T2WI; hemorrhagic: High SI on T1WI & T1WI FS

Imaging Recommendations
- Best imaging tool
  - MR shows the characteristics features of leiomyoma
    - Be aware of atypical tumors (high SI on T2WI)

DIFFERENTIAL DIAGNOSIS

Vaginal Carcinoma
- Solid heterogeneous mass with features of invasion of surrounding tissues

Vaginal Leiomyosarcoma
- Bulky heterogeneous mass

DDx: Vaginal/Cervical Masses

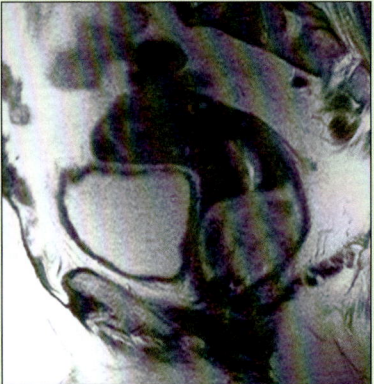

Vaginal Leiomyosarcoma

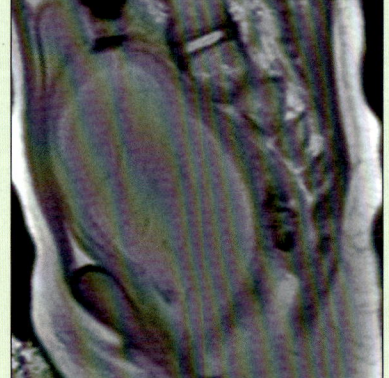

Vaginal Rhabdomyosarcoma

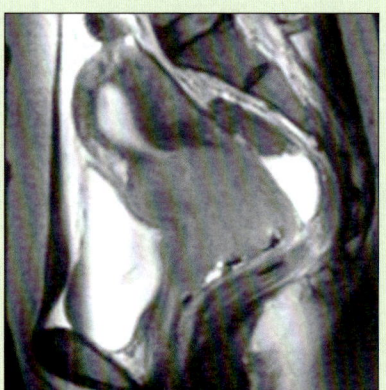

Cervical Carcinoma

LEIOMYOMA, VAGINA

Key Facts

Imaging Findings
- Best diagnostic clue: Solid soft tissue mass arising from the vaginal wall
- Location: Anywhere along the vagina, but most commonly in the midline anterior wall
- Low signal intensity (SI) on both T1WI and T2WI
- Homogeneous SI similar to myometrium
- Well-defined hypoechoic mass in the vaginal wall

Top Differential Diagnoses
- Vaginal Carcinoma
- Vaginal Leiomyosarcoma
- Vaginal Rhabdomyosarcoma
- Cervical Carcinoma

Diagnostic Checklist
- Well-defined mass, usually arising from midline anterior vaginal wall, with imaging features identical to a uterine leiomyoma

Vaginal Rhabdomyosarcoma
- Large heterogeneous mass in younger age group

Cervical Carcinoma
- Bulk of mass centered in cervix with possible extension to vagina

PATHOLOGY

Gross Pathologic & Surgical Features
- Circumscribed gray/white firm, rubbery nodule
- Average size 3 cm, range < 1-15 cm

Microscopic Features
- Mitotic counts < 1 per high high power fields indicate a benign leiomyoma
- Mitotic counts between 1-4 per 10 high power fields indicate a leiomyoma of "uncertain malignant potential"
- Mitotic counts > 5 per 10 high power fields, especially with cytological atypia indicate presence of leiomyosarcoma

CLINICAL ISSUES

Presentation
- Most common signs/symptoms: Asymptomatic when small
- Other signs/symptoms
  - Low back pain occurs due to pressure on the pelvic ligaments or lumbar plexus
  - Dysuria, dyspareunia

Demographics
- Age: 35-50 years

Natural History & Prognosis
- Regress in menopause
- Sarcomatous transformation may occur but very rare

Treatment
- Excision and enucleation, pre operative embolization for vascular tumors

DIAGNOSTIC CHECKLIST

Image Interpretation Pearls
- Well-defined mass, usually arising from midline anterior vaginal wall, with imaging features identical to a uterine leiomyoma

SELECTED REFERENCES
1. Bukhari AS et al: Vaginal fibroid--a case report. J Obstet Gynaecol. 25(1):83-4, 2005
2. Gowri R et al: Leiomyoma of the vagina: an unusual presentation. J Obstet Gynaecol Res. 29(6):395-8, 2003
3. Shimada K et al: MR imaging of an atypical vaginal leiomyoma. AJR Am J Roentgenol. 178(3):752-4, 2002

IMAGE GALLERY

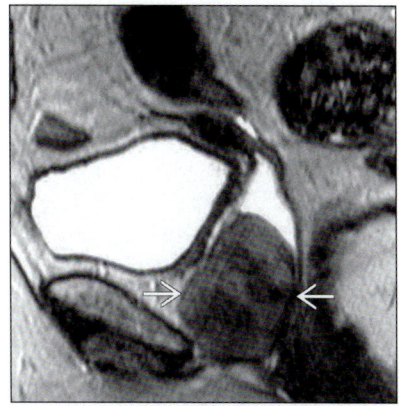 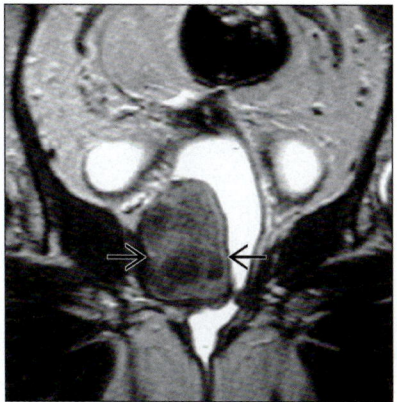 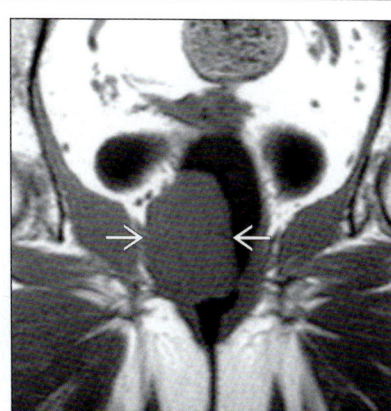

(Left) Sagittal T2WI MR shows a heterogeneous mass ➡ of intermediate SI arising from the vaginal wall on a 62 year old woman. Note presence of fluid retention in the cervix and upper vagina. (Center) Coronal T2WI MR shows the same tumor ➡ as on the previous image. This mass is centered on the right side of the vagina. (Right) Coronal T1WI MR in the same patient as previous images shows a well-defined low SI vaginal mass ➡. Pathology: Vaginal Leiomyoma.

VAGINAL CARCINOMA

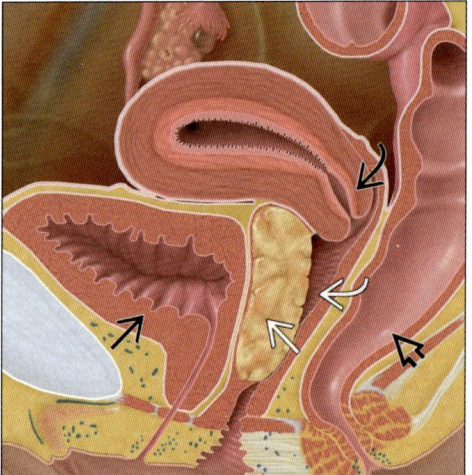

Graphic shows vaginal cancer ➡. Note close relationship of cervix ➡, bladder ➡ and rectum ➡ with vagina ➡.

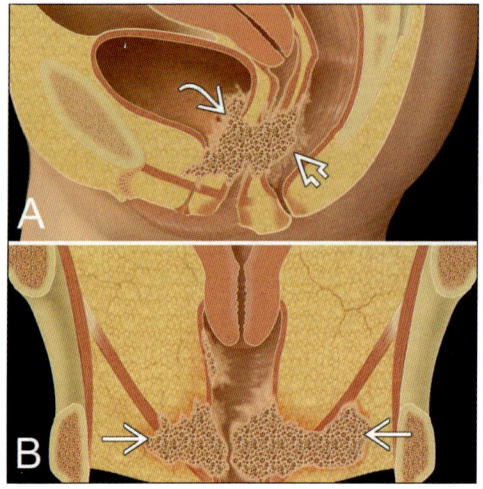

Graphic shows the most common pattern of spread of vaginal cancer by direct extension to bladder ➡ anteriorly, rectum posteriorly ➡ (A); and pelvic side wall laterally ➡ (B).

TERMINOLOGY

Definitions
- Primary malignant tumor of vagina

IMAGING FINDINGS

General Features
- Best diagnostic clue
  - Usually exophytic nodular solid mass originating from vagina
  - Alteration in vaginal contour or disruption in vaginal wall are commonly seen
- Location: Most commonly seen in upper portion of posterior wall
- Morphology: Lobulated exophytic masses or infiltrating flat lesions

Ultrasonographic Findings
- Grayscale Ultrasound
  - Homogeneous or heterogeneous soft tissue echogenicity mass in vagina
  - US is limited in local staging of vaginal cancer
- Color Doppler: Vascularity is seen in solid components of mass
- Power Doppler: Improved detection of vascularity in mass

CT Findings
- NECT: Soft-tissue attenuation mass in vagina
- CECT
  - Diffuse or heterogeneous enhancement
  - Necrotic components can be seen as non-enhancing areas
  - Useful in identification of vesicovaginal fistulas

MR Findings
- T1WI: Intermediate signal intensity masses expanding vagina
- T2WI
  - High to intermediate signal intensity mass originating from vaginal wall and expanding vagina
  - Low signal intensity vaginal wall is a very useful landmark in determining local extent of disease
  - Necrotic areas of mass may have high signal intensity
- T1 C+
  - Diffuse or heterogeneous enhancement

DDx: Vaginal Masses

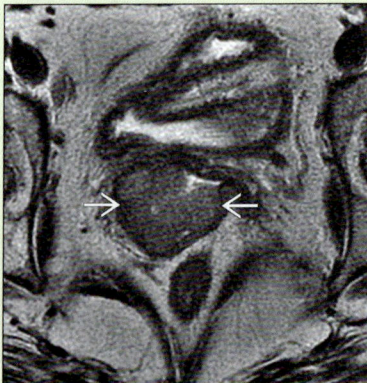
Metastasis

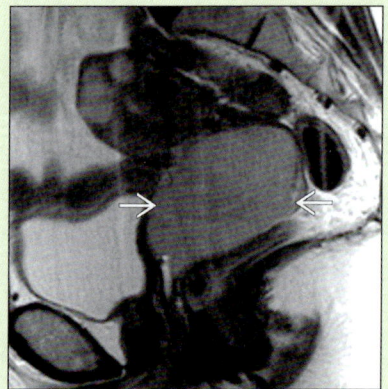
Lymphoma

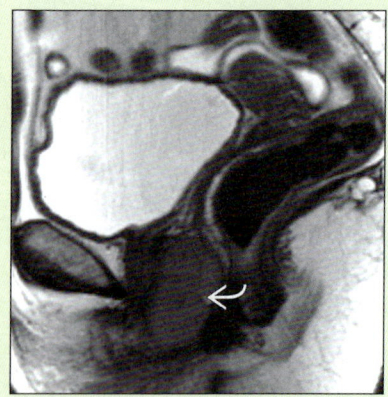
Melanoma

VAGINAL CARCINOMA

Key Facts

Terminology
- Primary malignant tumor of vagina

Imaging Findings
- Usually exophytic nodular solid mass originating from vagina
- Alteration in vaginal contour or disruption in vaginal wall are commonly seen
- MR is method of choice for local staging due to its excellent soft tissue contrast

Pathology
- Most vaginal cancers are squamous cell carcinomas (80-90%) and adenocarcinomas (5-10%)
- Vaginal cancer most commonly spreads by direct extension to adjacent organs
- Lymphatic and hematogenous spread can also be seen

Clinical Issues
- Age: Most common in postmenopausal women at 60 to 70 years of age

Diagnostic Checklist
- Disruption of low signal intensity vaginal wall on T2WI and irregular tumor-fat interface indicate invasion of paravaginal tissues
- High signal intensity tumor extension to pelvic muscles on T2WI is indication of pelvic sidewall invasion
- High signal intensity tumor in normal low signal intensity walls on T2WI indicate invasion to bladder and/or rectum

---

- Necrotic components can be seen as non-enhancing areas
- Useful in identification of vesicovaginal fistulas

Nuclear Medicine Findings
- PET
  - Vaginal cancer and its metastases show increased uptake on FDG PET
  - Urine filled bladder may obscure uptake in vaginal mass

Imaging Recommendations
- Best imaging tool
  - MR is method of choice for local staging due to its excellent soft tissue contrast
  - CT is of limited usefulness in local staging of early localized disease because of its suboptimal soft tissue contrast
  - CT is more useful in detection of advanced disease and lymphadenopathy
  - PET may be helpful in initial staging or detection of recurrences especially in cases with equivocal findings on other imaging modalities
- Protocol advice
  - T2WI: Transverse, coronal and sagittal planes; small field-of-view
  - T1 C+: Useful in characterization of mass and evaluation of complications such as fistulas
  - Intravaginal contrast (e.g., filling of vagina with US gel, saline, barium, etc.) may be helpful in assessing small lesions

DIFFERENTIAL DIAGNOSIS

Bartholin Cyst
- Well-defined cystic masses located in posterolateral aspect of lower 1/3 of vagina
- May have low to high signal intensity on T1WI depending on proteinaceous content

Cervical Cancer
- Bulk of mass is located in cervix which may extend to vagina

Vaginal Metastasis
- Vaginal metastases are much more common than primary vaginal cancers
- Vagina is most commonly affected by direct extension of primary bladder, vulval, cervical or rectal cancers
- Vagina is also a common site of recurrence in gynecologic cancers such as cervix and ovary

Vaginal Lymphoma
- Lymphoma usually causes homogeneous diffuse thickening in vaginal wall
- Vagina is often secondarily involved in lymphoma
- Presence of widespread lymphoma is helpful in differential diagnosis

Vaginal Melanoma
- Vaginal melanoma may have high signal intensity on T1WI

Infectious or Inflammatory Disease of Vagina
- Acute or chronic infectious/inflammatory conditions may cause diffuse vaginal wall thickening
- Usually clinically diagnosed and responds to appropriate treatment

PATHOLOGY

General Features
- General path comments
  - Most vaginal cancers are squamous cell carcinomas (80-90%) and adenocarcinomas (5-10%)
  - Vaginal carcinoma is usually found in association with vaginal intraepithelial carcinoma (dysplasia/carcinoma in situ)
  - Clear cell carcinoma of vagina is a subtype of adenocarcinoma associated with maternal exposure to diethylstilbestrol (DES) during pregnancy

VAGINAL CARCINOMA

- Vaginal cancer most commonly spreads by direct extension to adjacent organs
- Lymphatic and hematogenous spread can also be seen
- Epidemiology
  - Vaginal cancer is a rare malignancy
  - Accounts for 1-2% of gynecologic malignancies

Gross Pathologic & Surgical Features
- Usually exophytic mass and rarely infiltrating or flat lesion

Microscopic Features
- Neoplastic cells infiltrating stroma in cords or isolated clusters

Staging, Grading or Classification Criteria
- FIGO staging
  - Stage I: Tumor confined to vagina
  - Stage II: Tumor invades paravaginal tissues but does not extend to pelvic wall
  - Stage III: Tumor extends to pelvic wall
  - Stage IVA: Tumor invades mucosa of bladder or rectum and/or extends beyond true pelvis
  - Stage IVB: Distant metastasis

CLINICAL ISSUES

Presentation
- Most common signs/symptoms
  - Abnormal vaginal bleeding
  - Vaginal discharge
  - Pain
- Other signs/symptoms: Palpable or visible vaginal mass
- Clinical Profile
  - Risk factors include
    - Advanced age
    - Human papilloma virus infection
    - Chronic irritative vaginitis
    - Prior carcinoma involving cervix or vulva

Demographics
- Age: Most common in postmenopausal women at 60 to 70 years of age

Natural History & Prognosis
- 5 year survival rates: 76% for stage I, 44% for stage II, 31% for stage III, and 18% for stage IV

Treatment
- Early stages; surgical resection or radiation (external beam or brachytherapy)
- Advanced stages; pelvic exenteration and radiation

DIAGNOSTIC CHECKLIST

Consider
- When detected in early stages, vaginal cancer is often curable
- Cervical and vulvar cancers need to be ruled out by biopsy and clinical assessment

- Role of imaging is to determine extent of disease for treatment planning

Image Interpretation Pearls
- MR is method of choice to depict local extent of disease
  - Disruption of low signal intensity vaginal wall on T2WI and irregular tumor-fat interface indicate invasion of paravaginal tissues
  - High signal intensity tumor extension to pelvic muscles on T2WI is indication of pelvic sidewall invasion
  - High signal intensity tumor in normal low signal intensity walls on T2WI indicate invasion to bladder and/or rectum
- MR is also useful in evaluating treatment response, assessment of recurrences and treatment-related complications

SELECTED REFERENCES

1. Hellman K et al: Clinical and histopathologic factors related to prognosis in primary squamous cell carcinoma of the vagina. Int J Gynecol Cancer. 16(3):1201-11, 2006
2. Akata D et al: Efficacy of transvaginal contrast-enhanced MRI in the early staging of cervical carcinoma. Eur Radiol. 15(8):1727-33, 2005
3. Brown MA et al: MRI of the female pelvis using vaginal gel. AJR Am J Roentgenol. 185(5):1221-7, 2005
4. Creasman WT. Related Articles et al: Vaginal cancers. Curr Opin Obstet Gynecol. 17(1):71-6, 2005
5. Chang SD: Imaging of the vagina and vulva. Radiol Clin North Am. 40(3):637-58, 2002
6. Diakomanolis E et al: Primary invasive vaginal cancer. Report of 12 cases. Eur J Gynaecol Oncol. 23(6):573-4, 2002
7. Stryker JA. Related Articles et al: Radiotherapy for vaginal carcinoma: a 23-year review. Br J Radiol. 73(875):1200-5, 2000
8. Tsuda K et al: MR imaging of non-squamous vaginal tumors. Eur Radiol. 9(6):1214-8, 1999
9. Liu PF et al: MRI of the uterus, uterine cervix, and vagina: diagnostic performance of dynamic contrast-enhanced fast multiplanar gradient-echo imaging in comparison with fast spin-echo T2-weighted pulse imaging. Eur Radiol. 8(8):1433-40, 1998
10. Siegelman ES et al: High-resolution MR imaging of the vagina. Radiographics. 17(5):1183-203, 1997
11. Leminen A et al: Therapeutic and prognostic considerations in primary carcinoma of the vagina. Acta Obstet Gynecol Scand. 74(5):379-83, 1995
12. Gilles R et al: Case report: clear cell adenocarcinoma of the vagina: MR features. Br J Radiol. 66(782):168-70, 1993
13. Hata K et al: Preoperative diagnostic imaging of primary vaginal carcinoma by transvaginal color Doppler and magnetic resonance imaging. Gynecol Obstet Invest. 32(2):126-8, 1991

VAGINAL CARCINOMA

IMAGE GALLERY

Typical

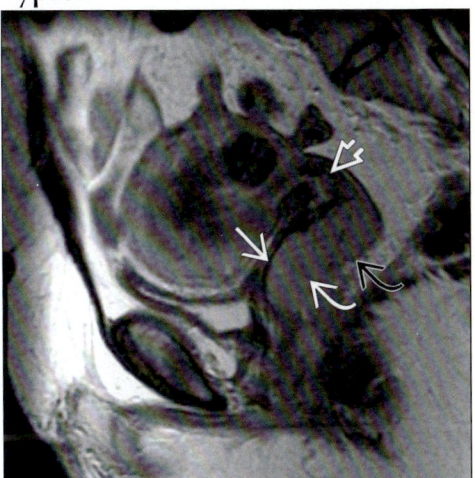
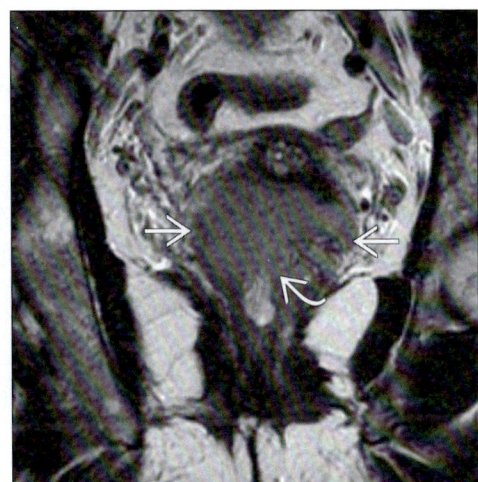

(Left) Sagittal T2WI MR shows vaginal cancer seen as a homogeneous mass ➡ expanding the vaginal lumen. Note that the cervix ➡ and the anterior vaginal wall ➡ are intact. The mass invades the posterior vaginal wall ➡. *(Right)* Coronal T2WI MR shows a large mass ➡ in the vagina. Note paravaginal extension of the mass ➡ bilaterally.

Typical

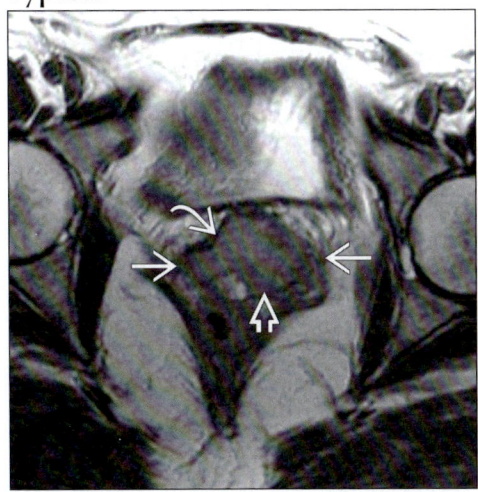
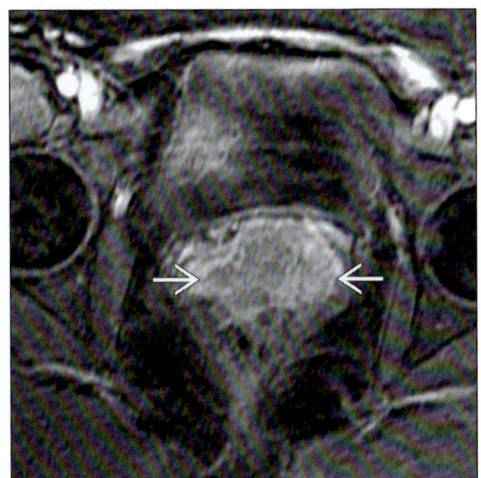

(Left) Axial T2WI MR shows a vaginal mass with bilateral paravaginal ➡ and posterior vaginal wall invasion ➡. Note that the intact anterior vaginal wall has low signal intensity ➡. *(Right)* Axial T1 C+ FS MR shows marked enhancement of the vaginal mass ➡.

Typical

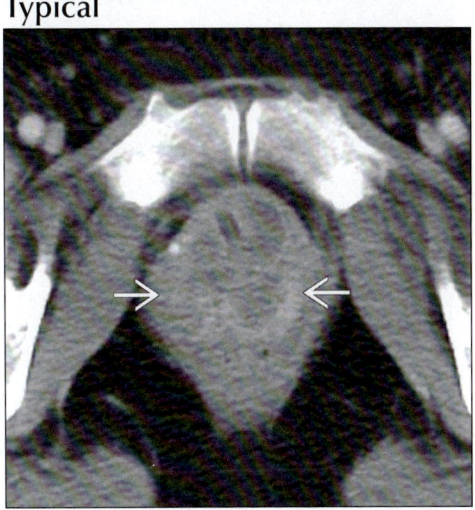
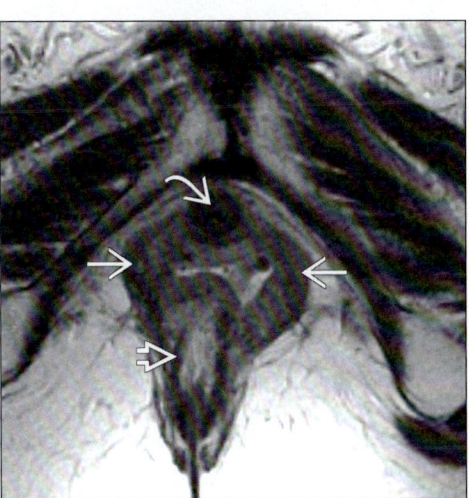

(Left) Axial CECT shows an enhancing lobulated mass ➡ in the vagina. *(Right)* Axial T2WI MR shows vaginal carcinoma seen as diffuse vaginal wall thickening ➡. The urethra ➡ anteriorly and the rectum ➡ posteriorly are intact.

VAGINAL CARCINOMA

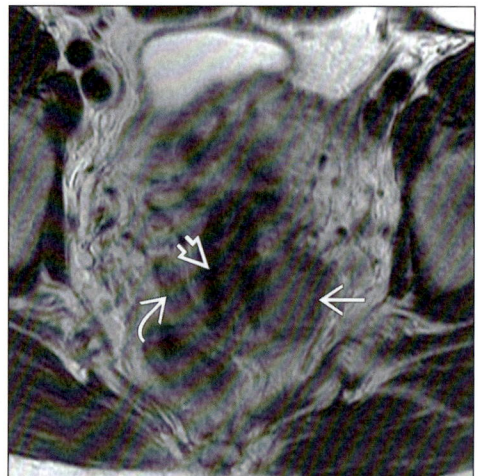

(Left) Axial T2WI MR shows vaginal cancer seen as a nodular mass ➡ in the left vaginal fornix. Note that the right vaginal fornix ➡ and the cervix ➡ are intact. (Right) Sagittal T2WI MR shows vaginal cancer ➡ in the left posterior vaginal fornix.

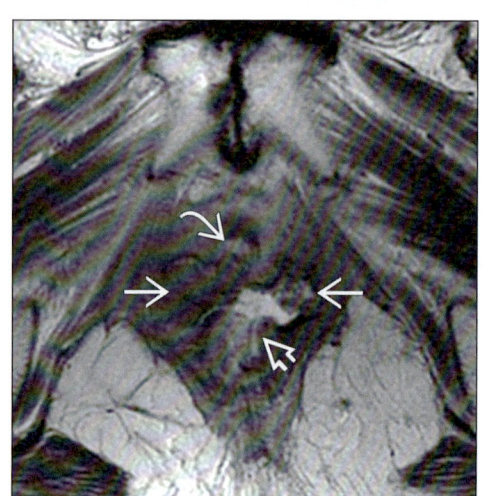 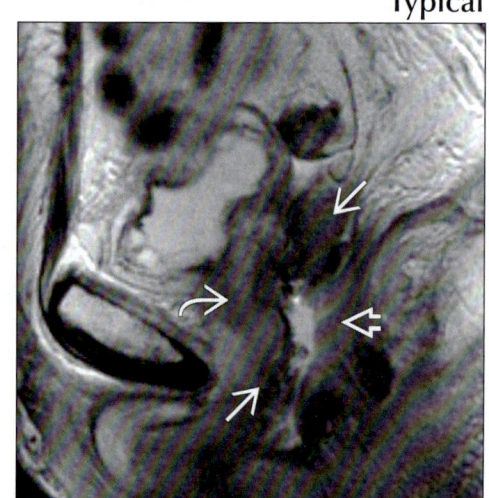

(Left) Axial T2WI MR shows vaginal cancer ➡ causing fistula formation anteriorly with the urethra ➡ and posteriorly with the rectum ➡. (Right) Sagittal T2WI MR shows vaginal cancer ➡. Anteriorly the urethra ➡ and posteriorly the rectum ➡ are invaded by the mass.

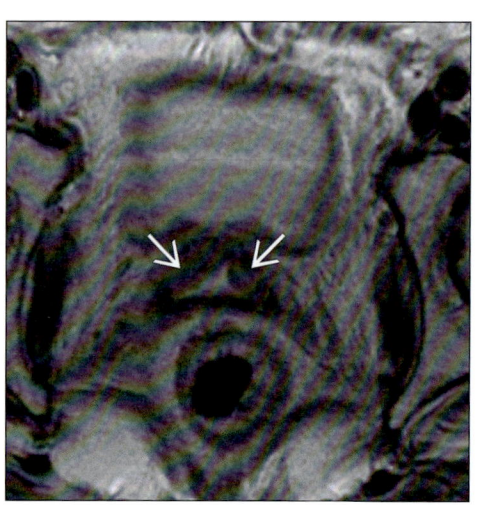 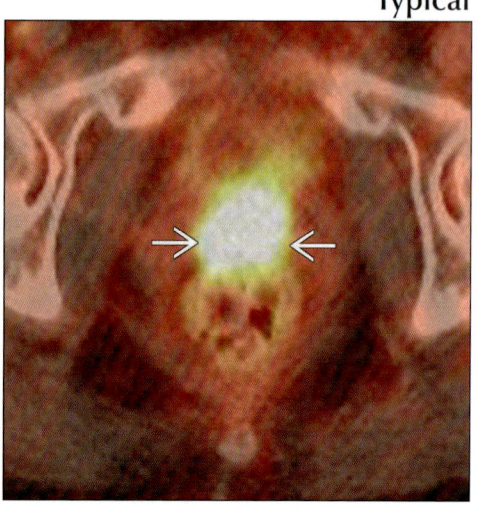

(Left) Axial T2WI MR shows vaginal cancer ➡ causing vaginal wall thickening that is especially prominent anteriorly. (Right) Axial fused PET/CT shows intense uptake ➡ in the vaginal mass in the same patient as previous image.

VAGINAL CARCINOMA

Typical

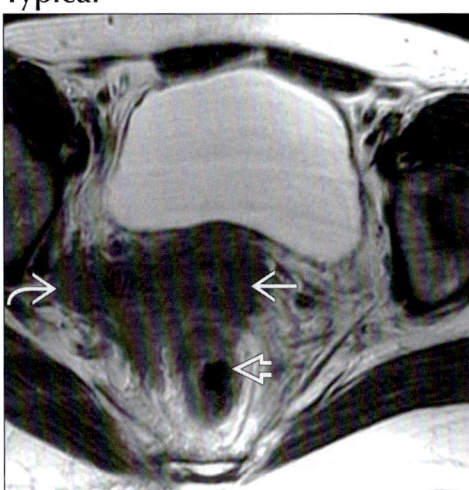
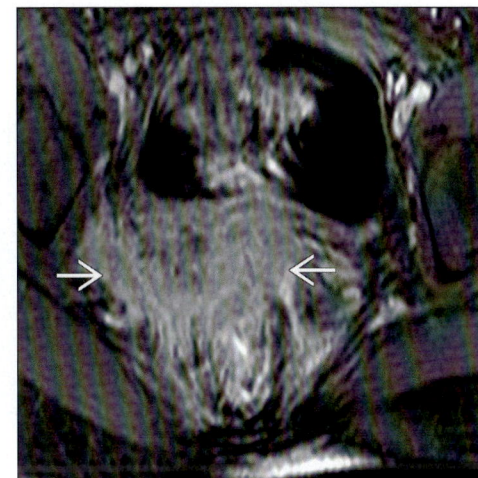

(Left) Axial T2WI MR shows vaginal cancer seen as a large mass ➡ invading the rectum ➡ posteriorly and extending to the right pelvic side wall ➡ laterally. (Right) Axial T1 C+ FS MR shows intense enhancement ➡ of the mass.

Typical

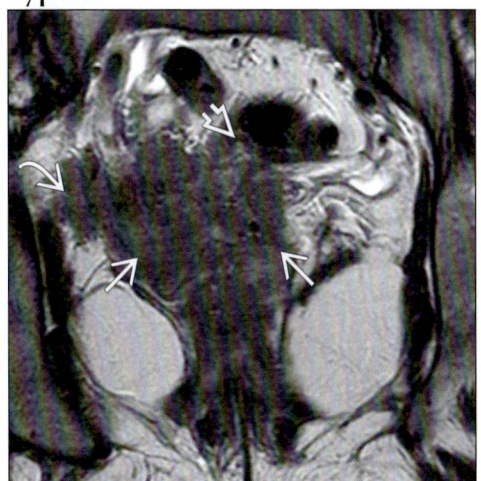
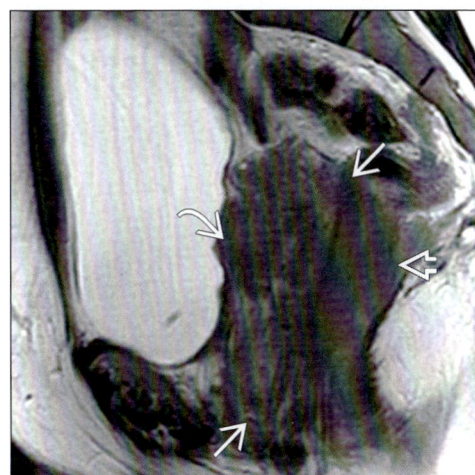

(Left) Coronal T2WI MR shows a large vaginal mass ➡ extending to the right pelvic side wall ➡ and invading the rectosigmoid ➡. (Right) Sagittal T2WI MR shows a vaginal mass ➡ invading the urinary bladder ➡ anteriorly and the rectum ➡ posteriorly.

Typical

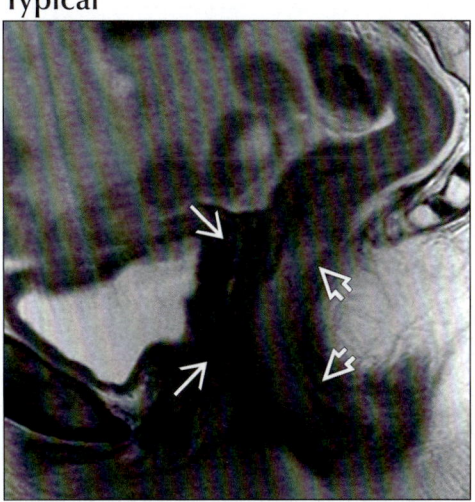
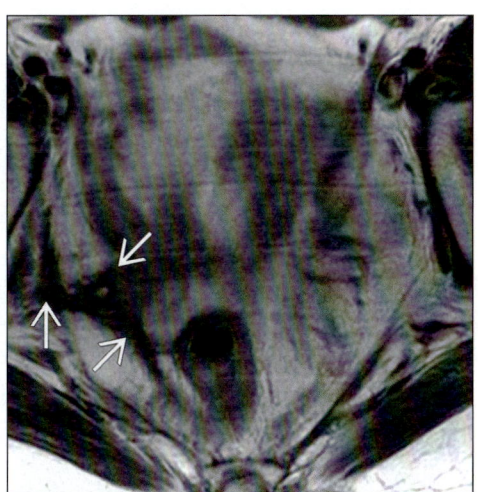

(Left) Sagittal T2WI MR shows that the vaginal mass in the same patient as previous image, resolved after radiation treatment. Normal vagina ➡ and rectum ➡ are seen. (Right) Axial T2WI MR shows an irregular low signal intensity fibrotic scar ➡ after radiation treatment in the same patient as previous image, with vaginal cancer that extended to the right pelvic side wall.

LYMPHOMA, VAGINA

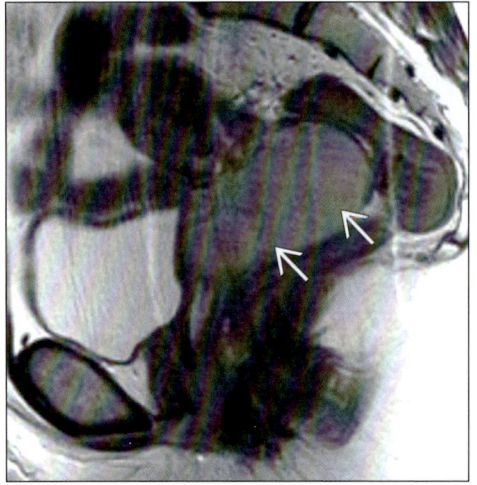

Sagittal T2WI MR shows vaginal lymphoma seen as a bulky homogeneous mass ➡ with intermediate signal intensity in the vagina.

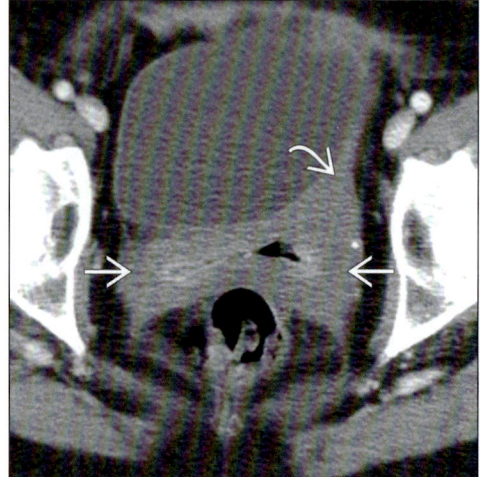

Axial CECT shows vaginal lymphoma causing diffuse wall thickening ➡ in the vagina. Note that the mass involves the urinary bladder ➡ on the left.

TERMINOLOGY

Definitions
- Primary or secondary involvement of vagina with lymphoma
  - Primary lymphoma of vagina is very rare
  - Secondary vaginal lymphoma is more common
- Most commonly non-Hodgkin lymphoma involves vagina

IMAGING FINDINGS

General Features
- Best diagnostic clue: Diffuse thickening of vaginal wall or bulky mass in vagina
- Morphology: Infiltrative or polypoid masses

Ultrasonographic Findings
- Grayscale Ultrasound: Hypoechoic homogeneous mass

CT Findings
- CECT: Homogeneous diffuse vaginal wall thickening or vaginal masses with moderate enhancement

MR Findings
- T1WI: Homogeneous signal intensity similar to muscle
- T2WI: Homogeneous intermediate signal intensity
- T1 C+: Moderate enhancement

Nuclear Medicine Findings
- PET: Lymphoma shows avid FDG uptake

Imaging Recommendations
- Best imaging tool
  - CT is most commonly used method in assessing extent of disease
  - PET is useful in assessment of extent of disease and treatment response

DIFFERENTIAL DIAGNOSIS

Vaginal Cancer
- More invasive, often heterogeneous mass

Vaginal Metastasis
- Often secondary involvement by adjacent pelvic malignancy

DDx: Vaginal Lesions

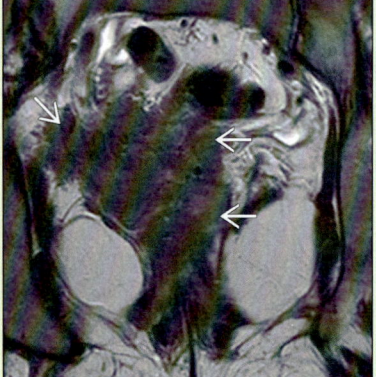

Vaginal Cancer

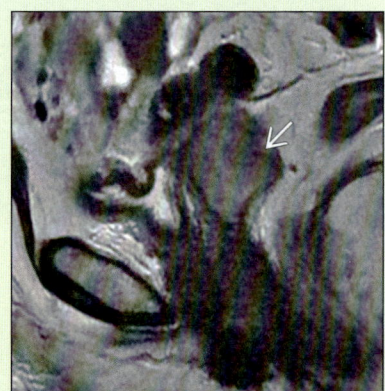

Vaginal Metastasis

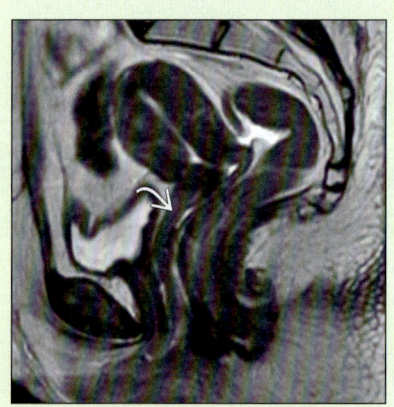

Post-Radiation Changes

LYMPHOMA, VAGINA

Key Facts

Terminology
- Primary lymphoma of vagina is very rare
- Secondary vaginal lymphoma is more common
- Most commonly non-Hodgkin lymphoma involves vagina

Imaging Findings
- Best diagnostic clue: Diffuse thickening of vaginal wall or bulky mass in vagina

Pathology
- Lymphoma infiltrates subepithelial connective tissue
- Vaginal epithelium is usually intact

Clinical Issues
- Prognosis is generally good

Diagnostic Checklist
- Role of imaging is to determine extent of disease and monitor treatment response

Post-Radiation Changes
- Mild diffuse vaginal wall thickening after radiation treatment to pelvis

PATHOLOGY

General Features
- General path comments
  - Lymphoma infiltrates subepithelial connective tissue
  - Vaginal epithelium is usually intact

Microscopic Features
- Most are diffuse large B cell lymphomas, which have large pleomorphic lymphoma cells with large vesicular nuclei, surrounded by a thin cytoplasmic rim

Staging, Grading or Classification Criteria
- Ann Arbor staging system is used for staging
- Low, intermediate, or high grade based on histopathologic features

CLINICAL ISSUES

Presentation
- Most common signs/symptoms
  - Abnormal vaginal bleeding and/or discharge
  - Dyspareunia and perineal discomfort
  - Ureteral-like colic and urinary frequency
- Other signs/symptoms: Systematic symptoms are rare in primary vaginal lymphoma but common in secondary lymphoma

Demographics
- Age: Mostly premenopausal women (mean age; 50 years)

Natural History & Prognosis
- Prognosis is generally good
- Overall 5 yr survival is 70%

Treatment
- Chemotherapy and/or radiation

DIAGNOSTIC CHECKLIST

Image Interpretation Pearls
- Diagnosis of lymphoma is made with biopsy
- Role of imaging is to determine extent of disease and monitor treatment response

SELECTED REFERENCES

1. Kosari F et al: Lymphomas of the female genital tract: a study of 186 cases and review of the literature. Am J Surg Pathol. 29(11):1512-20, 2005
2. Vang R et al: Non-Hodgkin's lymphoma involving the vagina. Am J Surg Pathol. 24(5):719-25, 2000
3. Clow WM et al: An unusual cause of postmenopausal bleeding and incontinence of urine: primary lymphoma of the vagina. Br J Obstet Gynaecol. 102(2):164-5, 1995

IMAGE GALLERY

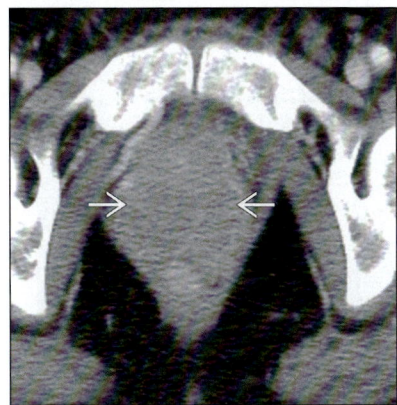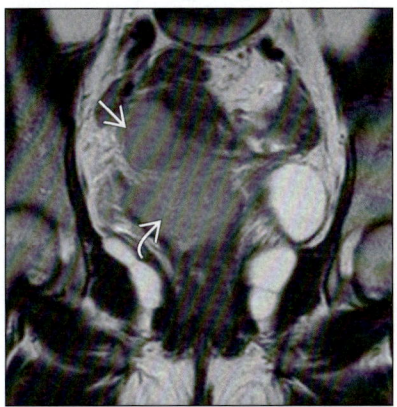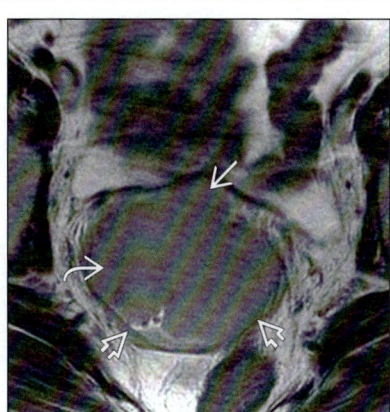

(Left) Axial CECT shows vaginal lymphoma seen as a bulky mass ➔ in the vagina. (Center) Coronal T2WI MR shows vaginal lymphoma ➔ extending to the cervix and the lower uterine segment ➔. (Right) Axial T2WI MR shows vaginal lymphoma seen as a mass ➔ expanding the vagina. Note that the posterior vaginal wall ➔ is intact but the mass extends to the vesicovaginal fat ➔ anteriorly.

LEIOMYOSARCOMA, VAGINA

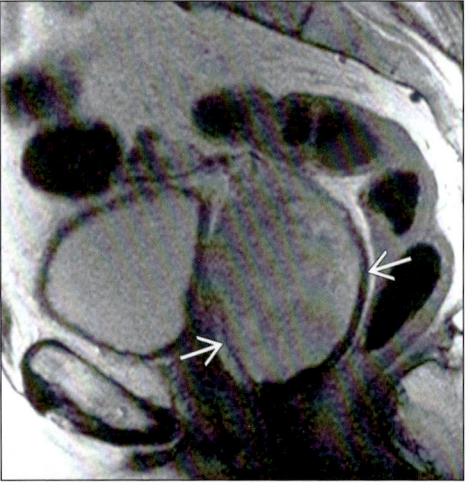

Sagittal T2WI MR shows a large, high SI exophytic mass ➡ arising from the vagina in a patient with vaginal leiomyosarcoma.

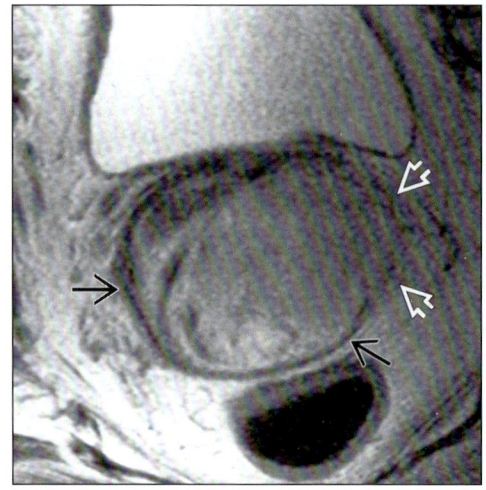

Axial T2WI MR in the same patient shows that vaginal leiomyosarcoma ➡ involves the left parametria ➡.

TERMINOLOGY

Abbreviations and Synonyms
- Primary nonsquamous vaginal sarcoma

Definitions
- Malignant vaginal lesion

IMAGING FINDINGS

General Features
- Location
  ○ Bulky lesion in the upper vagina
  ○ May invade surrounding structures: Cervix, bladder, ureter, rectum
    ▪ It can completely obstruct the cervix causing a hydrometra or the ureter causing hydroureter and hydronephrosis
- Size: Can reach large size & displace uterus superiorly
- Morphology: Friable, exophytic mass

Ultrasonographic Findings
- Heterogeneous mass with hypoechoic cystic areas indicating tumor necrosis
- May be difficult to resolve whether primary tumor lies in the vagina or cervix

CT Findings
- Heterogeneous enhancement on CECT
- Areas of low attenuation correspond to regions of tumor necrosis

MR Findings
- Heterogeneous solid mass arising from vaginal wall
- T1WI: Intermediate signal intensity (SI)
- T2WI: Moderate to high SI
  ○ Extension to the cervix and parametria, pelvic and inguinal nodes can be evaluated
  ○ If cervical extension and obstruction, high SI hydrocolpos and hydrometra
- T1 C+ FS: Avid enhancement

Imaging Recommendations
- Best imaging tool

DDx: Vaginal/Cervical Masses

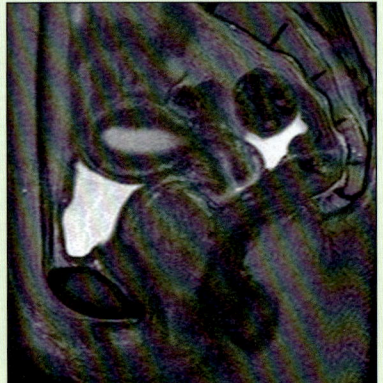

Vaginal Leiomyoma

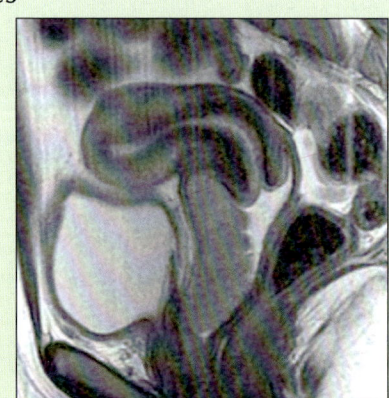

Vaginal Carcinoma

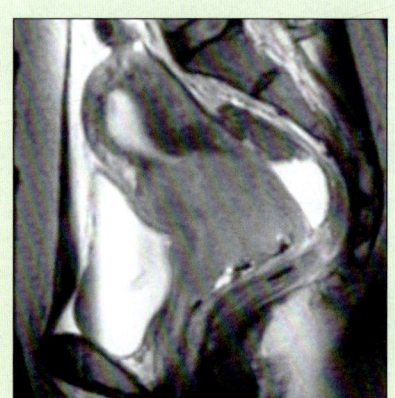

Cervical Carcinoma

LEIOMYOSARCOMA, VAGINA

Key Facts

Imaging Findings
- Bulky lesion in the upper vagina
- Heterogeneous enhancement on CECT
- Areas of low attenuation correspond to regions of tumor necrosis
- T1WI: Intermediate signal intensity (SI)
- T2WI: Moderate to high SI
- If cervical extension and obstruction, high SI hydrocolpos and hydrometra
- T1 C+ FS: Avid enhancement
- Heterogeneous mass with hypoechoic cystic areas indicating tumor necrosis
- MR for local tumor staging (extension to cervix, bladder, rectum) and evaluation of lymph nodes
- CT for evaluation of distant metastasis (lung, liver and bone)

○ MR for local tumor staging (extension to cervix, bladder, rectum) and evaluation of lymph nodes
○ CT for evaluation of distant metastasis (lung, liver and bone)

DIFFERENTIAL DIAGNOSIS

Vaginal Leiomyoma
- Well-defined vaginal mass, separate from the cervix

Vaginal Carcinoma
- Irregular exophytic mass altering vaginal contour

Cervical Carcinoma
- Heterogeneous mass centered in cervix with possible extension to vagina

PATHOLOGY

General Features
- Etiology: Association with prior pelvic irradiation has been reported
- Epidemiology: 50-55 years, uncommon in younger women

Gross Pathologic & Surgical Features
- \> 3 cm diameter pale/yellow tumor with areas of hemorrhage, necrosis ± cystic change

Microscopic Features
- Marked cytological atypia
- Mitotic counts of > 5 per 10 high power fields
- Infiltrating margins

CLINICAL ISSUES

Presentation
- Most common signs/symptoms
  ○ Protruding mass at the introitus
  ○ Vaginal bleeding and/or discharge
  ○ Vaginal pain

Natural History & Prognosis
- Early hematogenous spread
- Frequent local recurrence

Treatment
- Surgery (± pelvic exenteration) followed by adjuvant radiotherapy
- Chemotherapy for unresectable or metastatic disease

SELECTED REFERENCES
1. Ahram J et al: Leiomyosarcoma of the vagina: case report and literature review. Int J Gynecol Cancer. 16(2):884-91, 2006
2. Moller K et al: Primary leiomyosarcoma of the vagina: a case report involving a TVT allograft. Gynecol Oncol. 94(3):840-2, 2004
3. Ciaravino G et al: Primary leiomyosarcoma of the vagina. A case report and literature review. Int J Gynecol Cancer. 10(4):340-347, 2000

IMAGE GALLERY

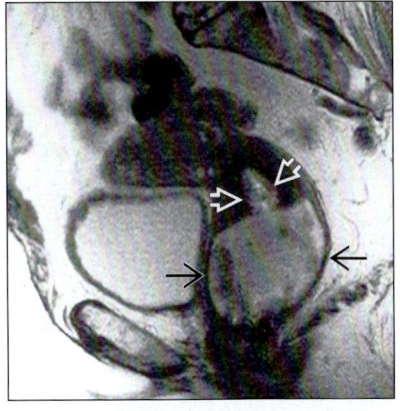 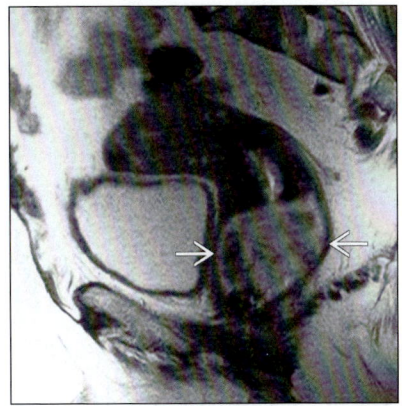 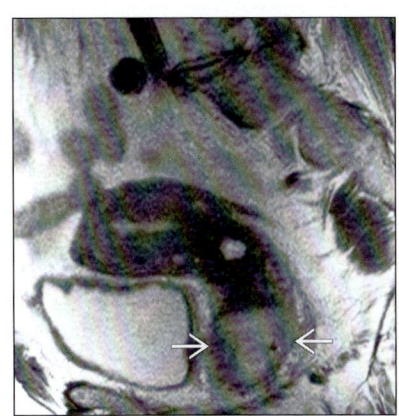

(Left) Sagittal T2WI MR shows a vaginal leiomyosarcoma ➔ extending superiorly into the endocervical canal ➔. (Center) Sagittal T2WI MR shows the same tumor as previous image as heterogeneous high SI mass ➔. (Right) Sagittal T2WI MR in the same patient as previous two images shows the exophytic leiomyosarcoma ➔ arising from the vagina.

EMBRYONAL RHABDOMYOSARCOMA, VAGINA

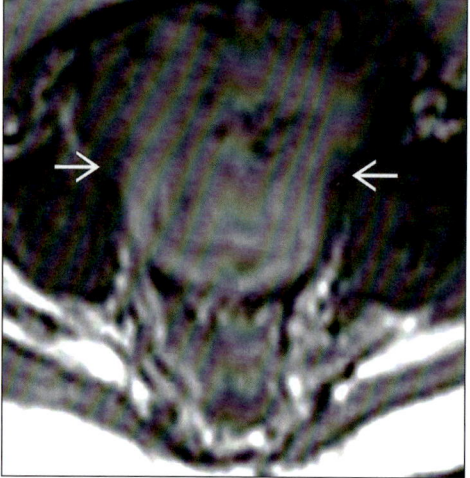

Axial T2WI MR shows a large heterogeneous soft tissue mass ➡ arising from the pelvis in a young girl with vaginal bleeding and abdominal discomfort.

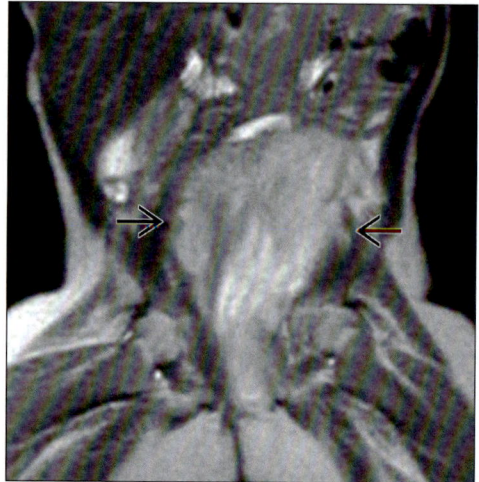

Coronal T2WI MR in the same patient shows the extent of the pelvis mass ➡ displacing abdominal organs. Pathology: Embryonal Rhabdomyosarcoma. (Courtesy P. Set, MD).

TERMINOLOGY

Definitions
- Common tumor of the lower genitourinary tract in children

IMAGING FINDINGS

General Features
- Location
  - Solid tumor originating in vagina
  - Botryoid rhabdomyosarcoma
    - Variant of embryonal rhabdomyosarcoma characteristically occurring in vagina and bladder
    - Intraluminal mass composed of smooth grape-like clusters

Ultrasonographic Findings
- Tumor may be hyperechoic, hypoechoic or mixed echogenicity
- Lucent foci represent areas of necrosis or hemorrhage
- Hypervascular mass on Doppler US
- Botryoid rhabdomyosarcoma: Polypoid intraluminal vaginal mass resembling cluster of grapes

CT Findings
- Large, heterogeneous soft tissue mass
- Heterogeneous enhancement on CECT

MR Findings
- T1WI: Low SI pelvic mass
- T2WI: Large pelvic mass of high SI; multiple thin low SI septae within the mass giving a grape-like appearance in botryoid rhabdomyosarcoma
- Areas of hemorrhage show variable SI depending on stage of evolution
- T1W C+ FS: Heterogeneous enhancement

Imaging Recommendations
- Protocol advice
  - US for screening a child with suspected pelvic mass
  - MR for accurate assessment of local tumor extent
  - CT/MR for detection of inguinal/retroperitoneal lymphadenopathy and skeletal metastases
  - CT for detection of pulmonary metastases
  - Follow up with MR for local recurrence

DDx: Vaginal Masses in Pediatric Patients

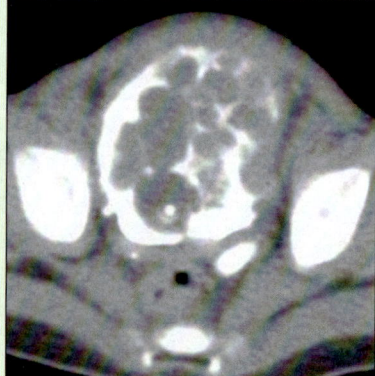

Rhabdomyosarcoma, Bladder

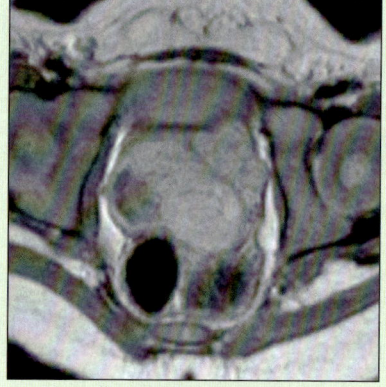

Yolk Sac Tumor, Vagina

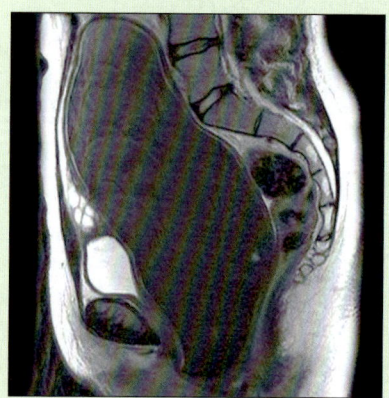

Hydrometrocolpos

EMBRYONAL RHABDOMYOSARCOMA, VAGINA

Key Facts

Terminology
- Common tumor of the lower genitourinary tract in children

Imaging Findings
- Solid tumor originating in vagina
- Large, heterogeneous soft tissue mass
- T1WI: Low SI pelvic mass
- T2WI: Large pelvic mass of high SI; multiple thin low SI septae within the mass giving a grape-like appearance in botryoid rhabdomyosarcoma
- US for screening a child with suspected pelvic mass
- MR for accurate assessment of local tumor extent
- CT/MR for detection of inguinal/retroperitoneal lymphadenopathy and skeletal metastases
- CT for detection of pulmonary metastases
- Follow up with MR for local recurrence

DIFFERENTIAL DIAGNOSIS

Bladder Rhabdomyosarcoma
- Vaginal tumors that are infiltrative, high and anteriorly placed may be indistinguishable from a bladder tumor

Yolk Sac Tumor, Vagina
- When large, indistinguishable from rhabdomyosarcoma on imaging alone
- Elevated serum levels of α-fetoprotein levels

Hydrometrocolpos
- High SI on T1WI, low SI on T2WI, associated with congenital vaginal and uterine duplication anomalies

PATHOLOGY

Microscopic Features
- Dense zone of rhabdomyoblasts (cambium layer) lies underneath the intact surface epithelium
- Immunohistochemical stains for muscle specific actin & desmin demonstrate muscle fibrils

CLINICAL ISSUES

Presentation
- Most common signs/symptoms
  - Mass in the vagina, vulva or perineum prolapsing into introitus
  - Vaginal bleeding, abdominal pain

Demographics
- Age: Infancy and early childhood

Natural History & Prognosis
- Relatively good prognosis if early detection
- Local recurrence is common

Treatment
- Neo-adjuvant chemotherapy followed by surgery

DIAGNOSTIC CHECKLIST

Consider
- Embryonal rhabdomyosarcoma in an infant or young child presenting with a large pelvic mass

Image Interpretation Pearls
- Often the exact organ of origin can not be established due to large size of the tumor at presentation

SELECTED REFERENCES

1. Agrons GA et al: From the archives of the AFIP. Genitourinary rhabdomyosarcoma in children: radiologic-pathologic correlation. Radiographics. 17(4):919-37, 1997
2. Fletcher BD et al: Magnetic resonance imaging for diagnosis and follow-up of genitourinary, pelvic, and perineal rhabdomyosarcoma. Urol Radiol. 14(4):263-72, 1992

IMAGE GALLERY

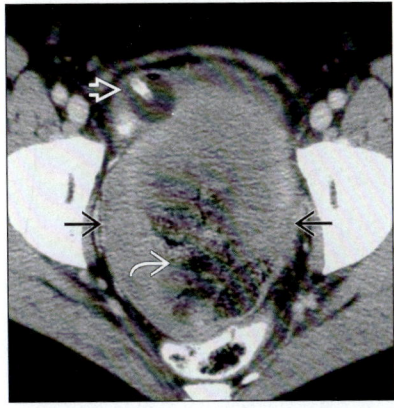 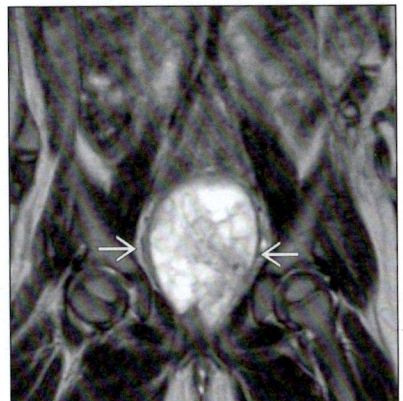 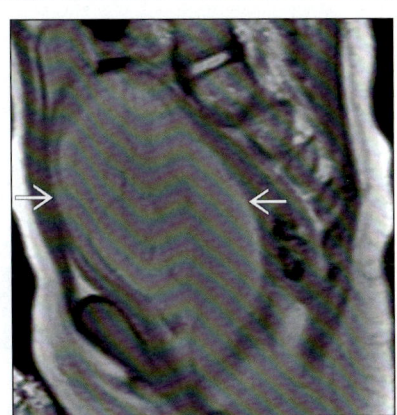

(Left) Axial CECT shows large, mixed attenuation, pelvic mass ➡ with areas of necrosis ➡. Note anterior bladder displacement ➡. Pathology: Embryonal rhabdomyosarcoma arising from the cervix/vagina. (Center) Coronal T2WI MR shows a heterogeneous, high SI, intraluminal, vaginal mass ➡ in a 2 year old girl complaining of abdominal pain. The mass is composed of smooth grape-like clusters. (Right) Sagittal T2WI MR in the same patient confirms presence of an intraluminal vaginal mass ➡. Pathology: Botryoid rhabdomyosarcoma. (Courtesy Prof. B. Hamm, MD).

YOLK SAC TUMOR, VAGINA

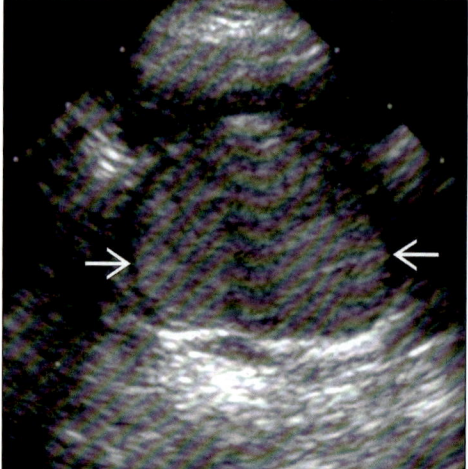

Transverse ultrasound shows a large heterogeneous vaginal mass ➔ replacing the normal vaginal canal.

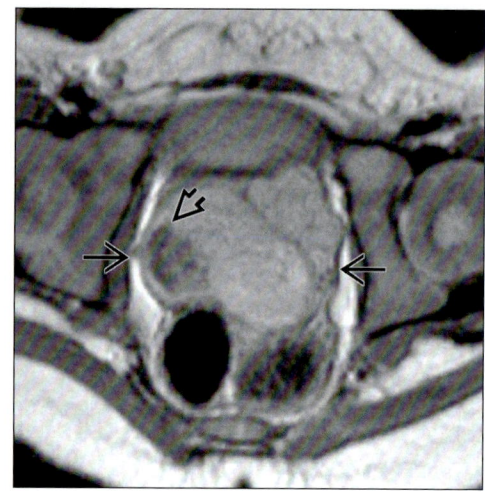

Axial PDWI MR shows an intermediate SI vaginal mass ➔ in the same patient as previous image, with necrotic areas of low SI ⇨. Pathology: Yolk sac tumor.

TERMINOLOGY

Abbreviations and Synonyms
- Endodermal sinus tumor

Definitions
- Rare primary malignant germ cell tumor of the vagina

IMAGING FINDINGS

General Features
- Best diagnostic clue
  - Solid mass arising from the vagina
  - Almost exclusively in girls less than 3 years old
- Location: Vagina

Ultrasonographic Findings
- Echogenic soft tissue mass
- Inferior to uterus and cervix
- Posterior to bladder

CT Findings
- Mixed attenuation and irregular margins
- CECT: Heterogeneous enhancement

MR Findings
- Heterogeneous mass, arising from the vagina, inferior to the cervix
- May approximate bladder anteriorly and rectum posteriorly with loss of fat planes
- Can be difficult to delineate from uterus and cervix, may extend into the uterus and fallopian tubes
- May show areas of necrosis, especially if large
- T1WI: Low signal intensity
- T2WI: High signal intensity
- T1 C+: Irregular enhancement

Imaging Recommendations
- Best imaging tool: MR imaging superior to CT for defining anatomy, tumor extent and invasion of soft tissue planes
- Protocol advice
  - US imaging of choice for screening of symptoms
  - MR or CT for tumor localization and staging

DDx: Solid Vaginal Masses in Pediatric Patients

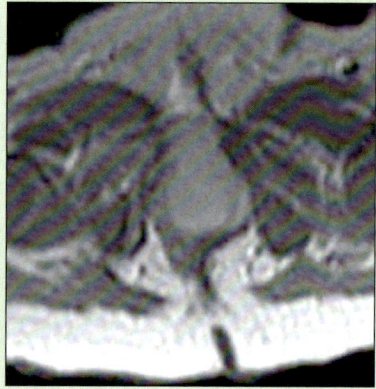

Embryonal Rhabdomyosarcoma

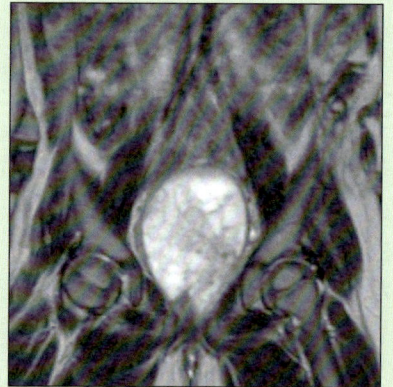

Sarcoma Botryoides

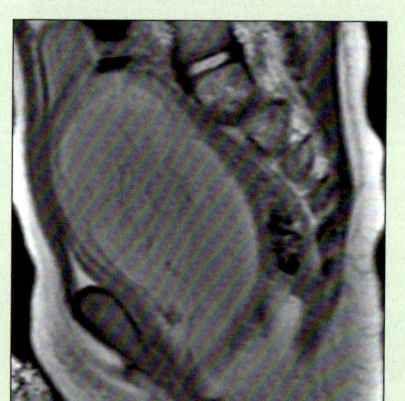

Sarcoma Botryoides

YOLK SAC TUMOR, VAGINA

Key Facts

Terminology
- Endodermal sinus tumor

Imaging Findings
- Almost exclusively in girls less than 3 years old
- Heterogeneous mass, arising from the vagina, inferior to the cervix
- Can be difficult to delineate from uterus and cervix, may extend into the uterus and fallopian tubes
- May show areas of necrosis, especially if large

- Best imaging tool: MR imaging superior to CT for defining anatomy, tumor extent and invasion of soft tissue planes

Top Differential Diagnoses
- Embryonal Rhabdomyosarcoma

Diagnostic Checklist
- Imaging features are nonspecific, final diagnosis is based on histology and raised AFP

DIFFERENTIAL DIAGNOSIS

Embryonal Rhabdomyosarcoma
- More common than yolk sac tumor, similar presentation and age group
- Characteristic grape-like clusters in sarcoma botryoides

Clear Cell Carcinoma of the Vagina
- Seen in older pediatric patients

PATHOLOGY

General Features
- Associated abnormalities
  - Raised serum alpha fetal protein
  - Serum AFP levels used in preoperative diagnosis, monitoring treatment, detecting recurrences

Gross Pathologic & Surgical Features
- Polypoid or sessile soft, tan or white vaginal masses
- 1-5 cm in diameter

Microscopic Features
- Variety of histological patterns including microcystic, reticular, papillary and solid types
- Schiller-duval bodies characteristic
- Extracellular hyaline droplets common
- Positive for alpha-fetoprotein (AFP), alpha-1-antitrypsin (A1AT), cytokeratin, and placental alkaline phosphatase
- Negative for beta subunit of human chorionic gonadotropin (βhCG)

CLINICAL ISSUES

Presentation
- Most common signs/symptoms
  - Vaginal bleeding/discharge
  - Mass effect on bladder, ureters or urethra

Natural History & Prognosis
- Vaginal subtype very aggressive

Treatment
- Surgery/combination chemotherapy

DIAGNOSTIC CHECKLIST

Image Interpretation Pearls
- Imaging features are nonspecific, final diagnosis is based on histology and raised AFP

SELECTED REFERENCES
1. Deshmukh C et al: Yolk sac tumor of vagina. Indian J Pediatr. 72(4):367, 2005
2. Kumar V et al: Vaginal endodermal sinus tumor. Indian J Pediatr. 72(9):797-8, 2005
3. Chatterjee U et al: Endodermal sinus tumor of vagina. J Indian Assoc Pediatr Surg. 8:235-8, 2003

IMAGE GALLERY

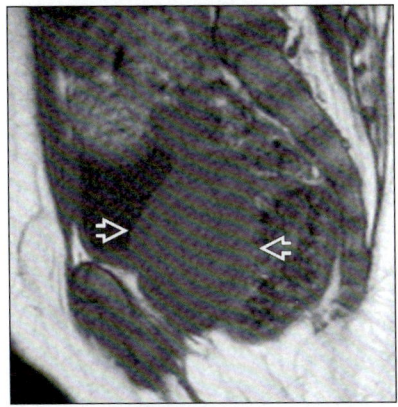 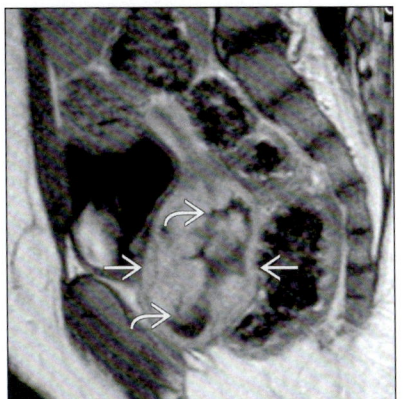 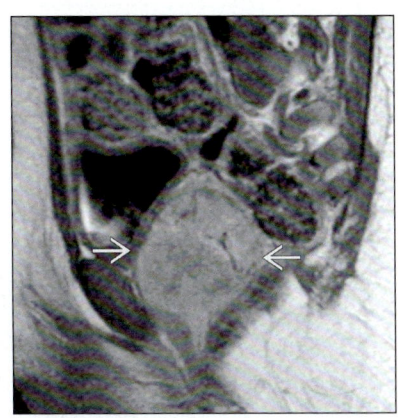

(Left) Sagittal T1WI MR shows a large low SI solid mass ⇨ arising from the vagina. (Center) Sagittal T1 C+ MR in the same patient as previous image shows avid enhancement of the solid vaginal mass ⇨ which contains multiple areas of necrosis ⇨. (Right) Sagittal T1 C+ MR in the same patient as previous image confirms the presence of an avidly enhancing vaginal mass ⇨. Pathology: Yolk sac tumor.

BARTHOLIN GLAND CANCER

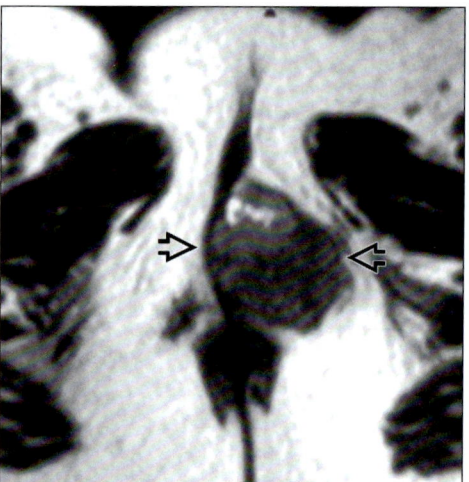

Axial T2WI MR shows a soft tissue mass ⇒ of heterogeneous signal intensity in the region of the left Bartholin gland.

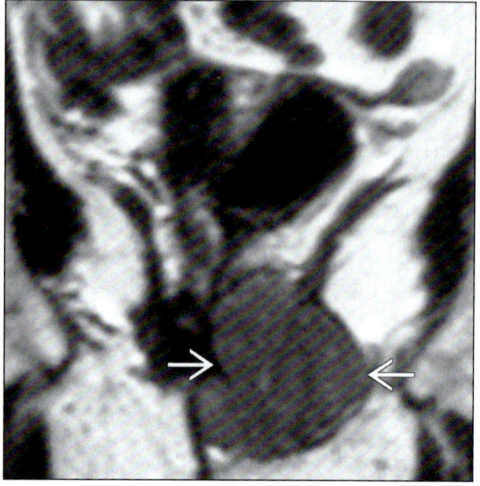

Coronal T2WI MR in the same patient confirms the presence of a soft tissue mass ⇒ in the region of the Bartholin gland. Pathology: Bartholin gland carcinoma.

TERMINOLOGY

Definitions
- Carcinoma of the Bartholin gland

IMAGING FINDINGS

General Features
- Best diagnostic clue: Mass in the region of the Bartholin gland
- Location
  - Posterolateral third of vagina, medial to labia minora
  - Paravaginal/periurethral position

Ultrasonographic Findings
- Soft tissue mass in the region of the Bartholin gland
- Enlarged inguinal lymph nodes may be present

CT Findings
- Enhancing soft tissue mass

MR Findings
- T1WI: Intermediate signal intensity
- T2WI: High signal intensity
- T1W C+: Enhancing mass
- Local lymphadenopathy/tumor extension

Imaging Recommendations
- Best imaging tool: MR
- Protocol advice
  - MR useful in treatment planning
  - MR and CT useful in evaluating deep pelvic lymphadenopathy and distant metastases

DIFFERENTIAL DIAGNOSIS

Bartholin Gland Cyst or Abscess
- Cystic mass located within the Bartholin gland

Gartner Duct Cyst
- Cyst located paravaginally

Vulva Carcinoma
- Solid mass located in the vulva

DDx: Vulvar/Bartholin Gland Masses

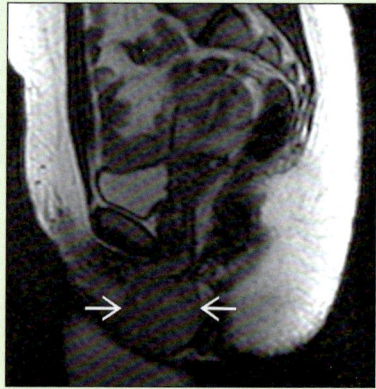

Vulvar Carcinoma

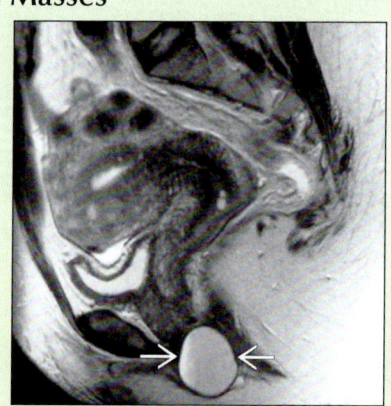

Bartholin Gland Cyst

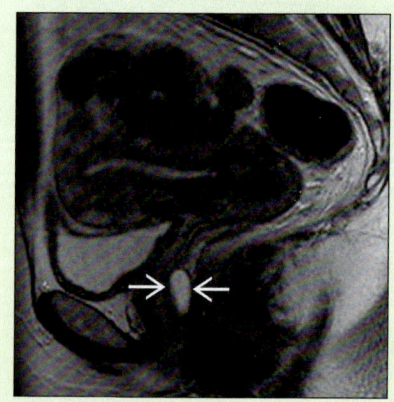

Gartner Duct Cyst

BARTHOLIN GLAND CANCER

Key Facts

Imaging Findings
- Best diagnostic clue: Mass in the region of the Bartholin gland
- Posterolateral third of vagina, medial to labia minora
- MR useful in treatment planning
- MR and CT useful in evaluating deep pelvic lymphadenopathy and distant metastases

Top Differential Diagnoses
- Bartholin Gland Cyst or Abscess
- Gartner Duct Cyst
- Vulva Carcinoma

Clinical Issues
- Solid nodules, often misdiagnosed as Bartholin gland cyst
- Painless lump in posterior half of vulva, pruritus, bleeding
- Overlying skin intact

PATHOLOGY

General Features
- Etiology: Reported association between high risk human papilloma virus (HPV) subtypes (e.g., HPV 16), squamous cell carcinoma & transitional cell carcinoma

Microscopic Features
- 40% are squamous cell carcinomas
- Mucinous tumors express carcinoembryonic antigen (CEA) and ca19-9
- 10-20% adenoid cyst carcinoma
- Rest are transitional cell carcinomas, adenosquamous carcinomas and neuroendocrine tumors (e.g., Merkel cell carcinoma)

CLINICAL ISSUES

Presentation
- Most common signs/symptoms
  - Solid nodules, often misdiagnosed as Bartholin gland cyst
  - Painless lump in posterior half of vulva, pruritus, bleeding
  - Overlying skin intact

Demographics
- Age: Average age 60 years

Natural History & Prognosis
- Approximately 7% prior bartholinitis or abscess
- 5 year survival
  - Negative inguinal femoral nodes: 52-89%
  - Multiple positive nodes: 18-20%

Treatment
- Radical vulvectomy with inguino-femoral lymphadenectomy; if tumor
  - ≤ 2 cm and not midline extension → ipsilateral lymphadenectomy adequate
  - ≥ 2 cm or midline extension → bilateral inguino-femoral lymphadenectomy and adjuvant (chemo)radiotherapy

DIAGNOSTIC CHECKLIST

Image Interpretation Pearls
- Enhancing, heterogeneous soft tissue mass in the region of the Bartholin gland

SELECTED REFERENCES
1. Yang SY et al: Adenoid cystic carcinoma of the Bartholin's gland: report of two cases and review of the literature. Gynecol Oncol. 100(2):422-5, 2006
2. Kokcu A et al: Primary-adenocarcinoma of Bartholin's gland: a case report. Eur J Gynaecol Oncol. 25(5):651-2, 2004
3. Finan MA et al: Bartholin's gland carcinoma, malignant melanoma and other rare tumours of the vulva. Best Pract Res Clin Obstet Gynaecol. 17(4):609-33, 2003

IMAGE GALLERY

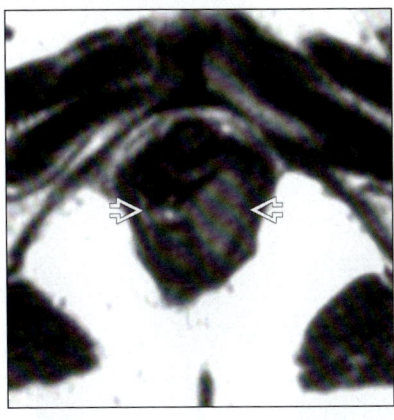 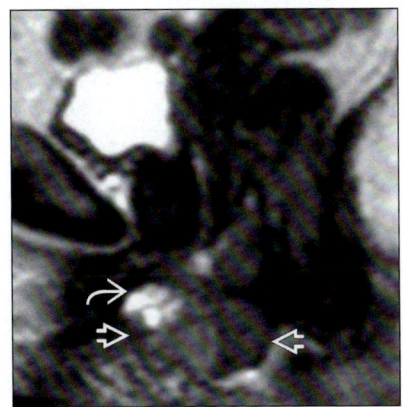 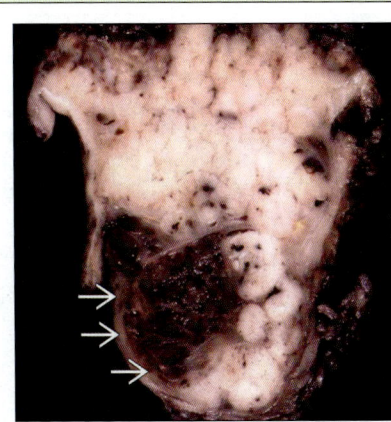

(Left) Axial T2WI MR in the same patient as previous image, shows a soft tissue mass ➡ of intermediate signal intensity in the region of the left Bartholin gland. *(Center)* Sagittal T2WI MR confirms the presence of a heterogeneous signal intensity mass ➡ which contains an area of high signal intensity ➡ in keeping with necrosis. *(Right)* Gross pathology shows the gross specimen of the Bartholin gland mass. Note the presence of a necrotic area confirming the imaging finding ➡. Pathology: Bartholin gland carcinoma.

METASTASIS, VAGINA

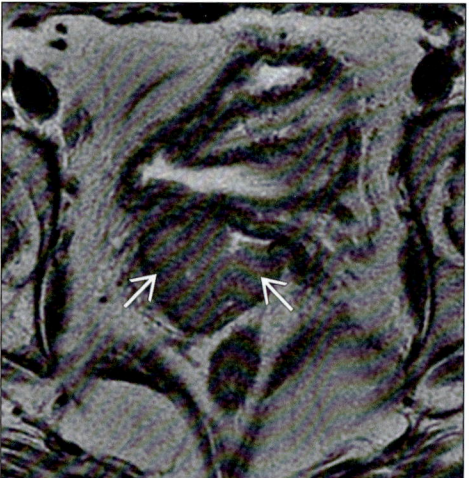

Axial T2WI MR shows metastasis seen as a polypoid mass ➡ in the vagina in a patient who had surgery for endometrial cancer in the past.

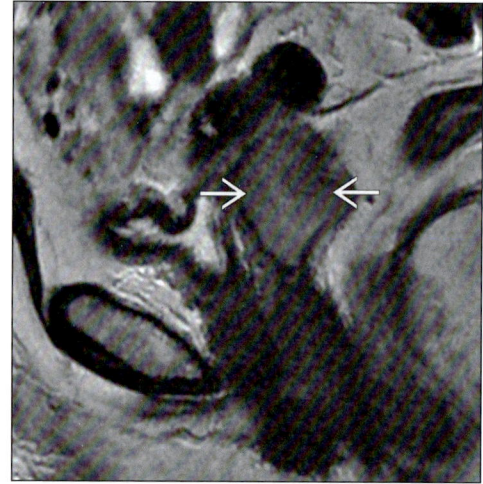

Sagittal T2WI MR shows that the mass ➡ at the vaginal cuff grows into the vaginal lumen which is expanded by the mass in the same patient.

TERMINOLOGY

Definitions
- Secondary malignancy of the vagina

IMAGING FINDINGS

General Features
- Best diagnostic clue: Solid or mixed solid and cystic mass involving the vagina
- Morphology: Sessile or polypoid mass in the vagina or diffuse vaginal wall thickening

Ultrasonographic Findings
- Grayscale Ultrasound: Echogenic vaginal mass or diffuse vaginal wall thickening
- Color Doppler: Vascularity may be detected in solid masses

CT Findings
- CECT: Mass with variable enhancement or diffuse wall thickening in the vagina

MR Findings
- T1WI: Medium signal intensity
- T2WI: Heterogeneous high signal intensity
- T1 C+: Variable enhancement

Nuclear Medicine Findings
- PET: FDG uptake in vaginal mass

Imaging Recommendations
- Best imaging tool
  - CT and MR are most commonly used to detect vaginal metastases and assess extent of disease
  - PET can be helpful in cases with equivocal findings on other imaging modalities

DIFFERENTIAL DIAGNOSIS

Primary Vaginal Malignancy
- Although less common than metastasis, primary vaginal malignancies have similar imaging characteristics and must always be considered in differential diagnosis

DDx: Vaginal Lesions

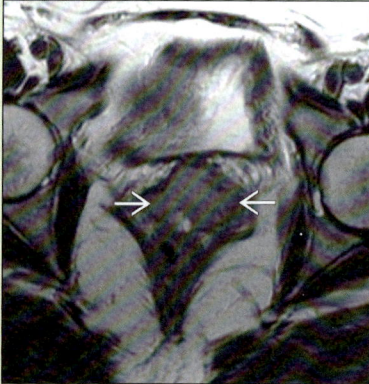

Vaginal Cancer

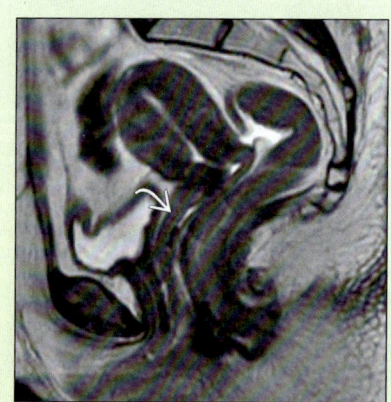

Post-Radiation Changes

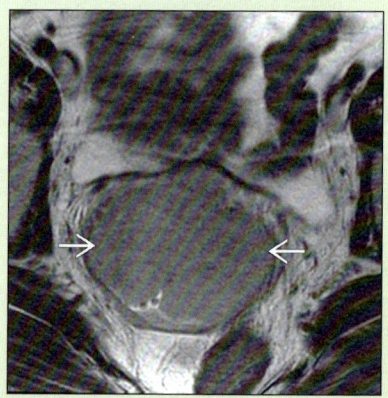

Lymphoma

METASTASIS, VAGINA

Key Facts

Terminology
- Secondary malignancy of the vagina

Imaging Findings
- Best diagnostic clue: Solid or mixed solid and cystic mass involving the vagina

Pathology
- Metastases are more common than primary malignancies of the vagina

- Often results from direct spread of cervical, endometrial or vulvar primary cancer
- Vaginal stump is most common site for local recurrence after surgery for uterine and cervical malignancies

Diagnostic Checklist
- Diagnosis is usually made clinically
- Role of imaging is to define extent of disease and differentiate radiation changes from recurrent tumor

Post-Radiation Changes
- Diffuse vaginal, rectal and bladder wall thickening can be seen after radiation treatment
- Post-radiation fibrosis is of low signal intensity on T1WI and T2WI

Vaginal Lymphoma
- Homogeneous masses or diffuse vaginal wall thickening

PATHOLOGY

General Features
- General path comments
  - Metastases are more common than primary malignancies of the vagina
  - Often results from direct spread of cervical, endometrial or vulvar primary cancer
    - Endometrium and cervix are most common sources for vaginal metastasis
    - Ovary, rectum, kidney and breast are other common primaries metastasizing to vagina
  - Vaginal stump is most common site for local recurrence after surgery for uterine and cervical malignancies

Gross Pathologic & Surgical Features
- Sessile or polypoid mass in the vagina

CLINICAL ISSUES

Presentation
- Most common signs/symptoms
  - Abnormal vaginal bleeding
  - Vaginal discharge
  - Pain

Treatment
- Surgery and/or radiation

DIAGNOSTIC CHECKLIST

Consider
- Diagnosis is usually made clinically
- Role of imaging is to define extent of disease and differentiate radiation changes from recurrent tumor

Image Interpretation Pearls
- Mass in the vagina or vaginal wall thickening in a patient with known malignancy

SELECTED REFERENCES
1. Chang SD: Imaging of the vagina and vulva. Radiol Clin North Am. 40(3):637-58, 2002
2. Siegelman ES et al: High-resolution MR imaging of the vagina. Radiographics. 17(5):1183-203, 1997
3. Chang YC et al: Vagina: evaluation with MR imaging. Part II. Neoplasms. Radiology. 169(1):175-9, 1988

IMAGE GALLERY

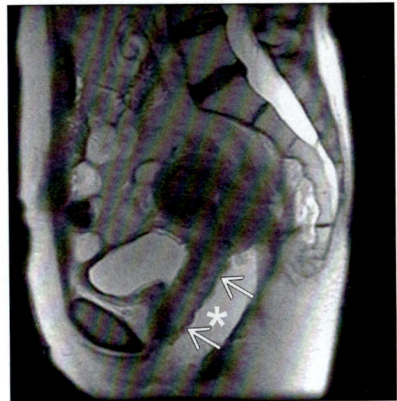
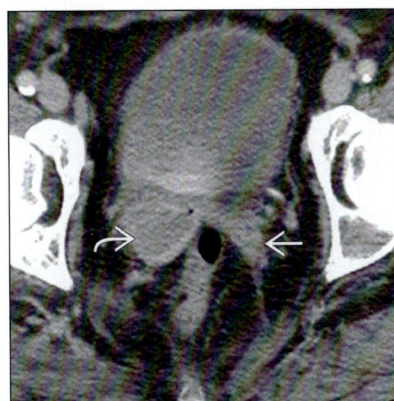
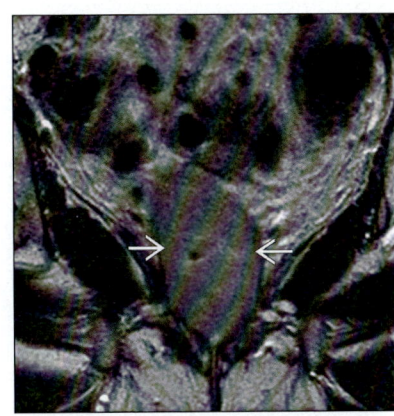

(Left) Sagittal T2WI MR shows diffuse irregular wall thickening ➡ in the anterior vaginal wall due to metastatic rectal cancer. The vagina is distended with mucin (*) secreted by the mass. Note that the rectum is surgically absent. (Center) Axial CECT shows metastatic soft tissue nodule ➡ in the vaginal cuff on the right. Note the normal appearance of the left vaginal cuff ➡ for comparison. (Right) Coronal T2WI MR shows vaginal metastasis seen as a bulky mass ➡ expanding the vaginal lumen.

BARTHOLIN CYSTS

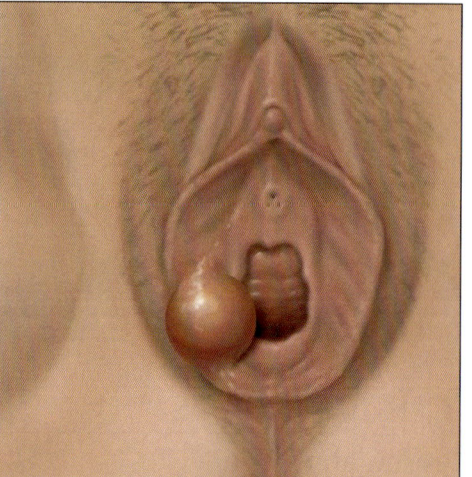

Graphic shows a labial nodule consistent with a Bartholin cyst.

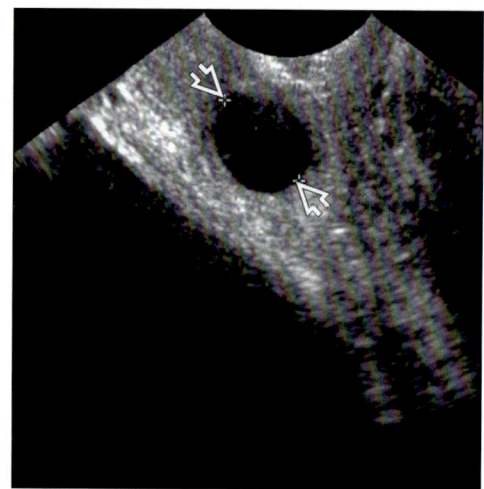

Sagittal transperineal US shows a simple Bartholin gland cyst ➡. Because they are superficial, these cysts are amenable to scanning at the vaginal introitus.

TERMINOLOGY

Definitions
- Cystic dilatation of Bartholin gland
  - Bartholin glands are bilateral mucin-secreting glands lying on posterolateral aspect of vulvar vestibule

IMAGING FINDINGS

General Features
- Best diagnostic clue: Round, well-defined, unilocular cyst lying at posterior aspect of vulva, just posterolateral to vaginal introitus
- Location
  - Posterolateral aspect of vulvar vestibule
  - Usually unilateral
- Size
  - Usually 1-4 cm in diameter
  - May grow to as large as 10 cm
- Morphology: Smoothly marginated round cysts
- Anatomy: Glands lie below the pelvic diaphragm at vaginal introitus
  - This distinguishes them from other perivaginal cysts such as Gartner duct cysts

Ultrasonographic Findings
- Grayscale Ultrasound
  - Anechoic or hypoechoic cysts with a thin or inapparent wall
    - Perineal ultrasound will demonstrate the cyst
    - Transabdominal ultrasound or transvaginal ultrasound will not visualize
- Color Doppler: No vascularity should be seen

CT Findings
- NECT
  - Solitary, round, low-attenuation cyst near vaginal introitus
  - If infected
    - Contents may be higher in attenuation
    - Wall may be thickened
- CECT
  - No enhancement
  - Rim-enhancement may be present if infected

DDx: Bartholin Cyst

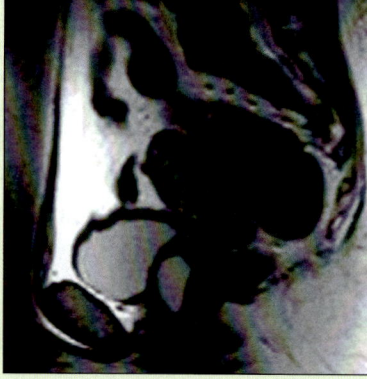

Gartner Duct Cyst

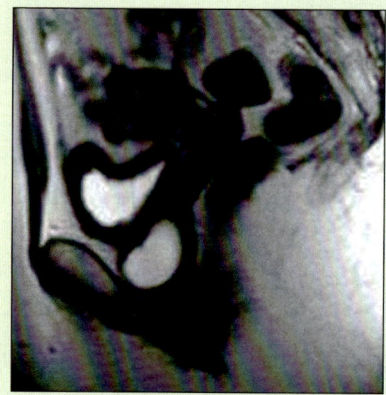

Urethral Diverticulum

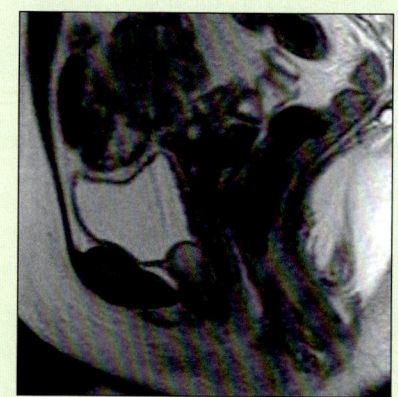

Periurethral Collagen Injection

BARTHOLIN CYSTS

Key Facts

Terminology
- Cystic dilatation of Bartholin gland
- Bartholin glands are bilateral mucin-secreting glands lying on posterolateral aspect of vulvar vestibule

Imaging Findings
- Best diagnostic clue: Round, well-defined, unilocular cyst lying at posterior aspect of vulva, just posterolateral to vaginal introitus
- Usually 1-4 cm in diameter
- Rim-enhancement may be present if infected
- T1WI: Variable T1 weighted signal intensity (SI) depending on intracystic protein content
- Very high T2WI SI
- Anechoic or hypoechoic cysts with a thin or inapparent wall
- Perineal ultrasound will demonstrate the cyst
- Multiplanar capabilities of MR make this the ideal modality

Pathology
- Bartholin glands may also give rise to abscesses, tumors and cysts
- Epidemiology: Prevalence of 2%

Clinical Issues
- Most common signs/symptoms: Most patients are asymptomatic
- May experience dyspareunia
- Palpable mass in labia majora
- Some will resolve spontaneously due to clearance of obstruction of Bartholin duct

MR Findings
- T1WI: Variable T1 weighted signal intensity (SI) depending on intracystic protein content
- T2WI
  - Very high T2WI SI
  - Cyst wall is smooth
  - Most are unilocular but septations may be seen
- T1 C+
  - No enhancement of the wall unless infected
  - If infected: Wall may be thick and enhance

Imaging Recommendations
- Best imaging tool
  - Multiplanar capabilities of MR make this the ideal modality
  - Perineal US is most cost-effective way of imaging Bartholin gland cysts
- Protocol advice: Make sure to image below pelvic diaphragm

DIFFERENTIAL DIAGNOSIS

Gartner Duct Cyst
- Also known as mesonephric cyst
- Located on anterolateral wall of vagina above pelvic diaphragm

Urethral Diverticulum
- Diverticulum communicating with urethral lumen

Periurethral Collagen Injection
- Performed to alleviate urinary incontinence

Adenocarcinoma of Bartholin Gland
- Nodular soft tissue in expected location of a Bartholin cyst

Nabothian Cyst
- Cyst in communication with endocervical canal

Squamous Inclusion Cyst
- Arise from entrapped squamous mucosa during repair of a vaginal laceration

Skene Gland Cyst
- Paired Skene glands lie lateral to the external urethral meatus

Urethral Caruncle
- Benign excrescences of urethral mucosa
- Most commonly seen in postmenopausal women

Prolapsed Ureterocele
- Presents in childhood as mass eccentric to urethral meatus

PATHOLOGY

General Features
- General path comments
  - Bartholin glands are major vestibular glands of vulva
  - Bartholin glands may also give rise to abscesses, tumors and cysts
- Etiology
  - Bartholin glands arises from urogenital sinus in the ventral division of endodermal cloaca
  - Bartholin glands are homologues of male bulbourethral glands
  - Cysts arise from obstruction of Bartholin gland
- Epidemiology: Prevalence of 2%

Gross Pathologic & Surgical Features
- Appear clinically as a focal bulging in lateral vulva

Microscopic Features
- Lining of Bartholin duct system is a continuum
  - Ductules are lined with single layer of cuboidal epithelium
  - This then transitions into a pseudostratified columnar epithelium
  - As ductules approach the main duct, the lining becomes a low stratified transitional epithelium

BARTHOLIN CYSTS

- Cytoplasm contains secretory granules and granulofibrillar bodies
- Glands are arranged in lobules

CLINICAL ISSUES

Presentation
- Most common signs/symptoms: Most patients are asymptomatic
- Other signs/symptoms
  o May experience dyspareunia
  o Palpable mass in labia majora
  o Signs of infection
    ▪ Redness
    ▪ Severe tenderness
    ▪ Fever
    ▪ Warmth over labia
- Clinical Profile: Cysts may rapidly enlarge

Natural History & Prognosis
- Some will resolve spontaneously due to clearance of obstruction of Bartholin duct
- When infected, abscesses may contain a variety of bacteria such as Neisseria gonorrhoeae or Escherichia coli
- Abscess formation causes severe tenderness and vulvar pain
- Recurrence rate of Bartholin gland cyst after marsupialization is low
- A variety of tumors can arise from Bartholin gland
  o 40% are adenocarcinomas
  o 40% are squamous cell carcinomas

Treatment
- Small asymptomatic cysts require no treatment
- If symptomatic treatment options include
  o Marsupialization of cyst or surgical excision
    ▪ Marsupialization is associated with fewer complications
  o Aspiration
  o Incision & drainage
  o Window operation: Oval opening excised from side of the lesion, allowing drainage
  o Application of silver nitrate to the abscess cavity
  o Carbon dioxide laser excision
  o Insertion of a catheter
- If cyst is discovered in a postmenopausal woman, it may contain tumor and should be excised

DIAGNOSTIC CHECKLIST

Image Interpretation Pearls
- Cysts posterolateral to the vagina below pelvic diaphragm

SELECTED REFERENCES
1. Dewdney S et al: Leiomyosarcoma of the vulva: a case report. J Reprod Med. 50(8):630-2, 2005
2. Owen JW et al: Placement of a Word catheter: a resident training model. Am J Obstet Gynecol. 192(5):1385-7, 2005
3. Gocmen A et al: Endometriosis in the Bartholin gland. Eur J Obstet Gynecol Reprod Biol. 114(1):110-1, 2004
4. Horiguchi H et al: Angiomyofibroblastoma of the vulva: report of a case with immunohistochemical and molecular analysis. Int J Gynecol Pathol. 22(3):277-84, 2003
5. Kaur A et al: Multifocal aggressive angiomyxoma: a case report. J Clin Pathol. 53(10):798-9, 2000
6. Ergeneli MH: Silver nitrate for Bartholin gland cysts. Eur J Obstet Gynecol Reprod Biol. 82(2):231-2, 1999
7. Hill DA et al: Office management of Bartholin gland cysts and abscesses. Am Fam Physician. 57(7):1611-6, 1619-20, 1998
8. Peters WA 3rd: Bartholinitis after vulvovaginal surgery. Am J Obstet Gynecol. 178(6):1143-4, 1998
9. Siegelman ES et al: High-resolution MR imaging of the vagina. Radiographics. 17(5):1183-203, 1997
10. Siegelman ES et al: Multicoil MR imaging of symptomatic female urethral and periurethral disease. Radiographics. 17(2):349-65, 1997
11. Dmochowski RR et al: Benign female periurethral masses. J Urol. 152(6 Pt 1):1943-51, 1994
12. Yuce K et al: Outpatient management of Bartholin gland abscesses and cysts with silver nitrate. Aust N Z J Obstet Gynaecol. 34(1):93-6, 1994
13. Moulopoulos LA et al: Magnetic resonance imaging and computed tomography appearance of asymptomatic paravaginal cysts. Clin Imaging. 17(2):126-32, 1993
14. Kier R: Nonovarian gynecologic cysts: MR imaging findings. AJR Am J Roentgenol. 158(6):1265-9, 1992
15. Brenner B: Laser vaporisation of Bartholin duct cysts. N Z Med J. 104(906):80-1, 1991
16. Hricak H et al: Female urethra: MR imaging. Radiology. 178(2):527-35, 1991
17. Cho JY et al: Window operation: an alternative treatment method for Bartholin gland cysts and abscesses. Obstet Gynecol. 76(5 Pt 1):886-8, 1990
18. Downs MC et al: The ambulatory surgical management of Bartholin duct cysts. J Emerg Med. 7(6):623-6, 1989
19. Kaufman R et al: Cystic tumors. Benign diseases of the vulva and vagina. Year Book Medical Publishers, Inc. Chicago IL. 269-76, 1989
20. Kaufman RH et al: Benign diseases of the vagina and vulva. Chicago: Year Book Medical. 237-85, 1989
21. Lashgari M et al: Excision of Bartholin duct cysts using the CO2 laser. Obstet Gynecol. 67(5):735-7, 1986
22. Wheelock JB et al: Primary carcinoma of the Bartholin gland: a report of ten cases. Obstet Gynecol. 63(6):820-4, 1984
23. Rorat E et al: Human bartholin gland, duct, and duct cyst. Histochemical and ultrastructural study. Arch Pathol. 99(7):367-74, 1975
24. Willis RA: The Borderland of Embryology and Pathology, ed 2. Washington, Butterworth & Co., 42, 1962

BARTHOLIN CYSTS

IMAGE GALLERY

Typical

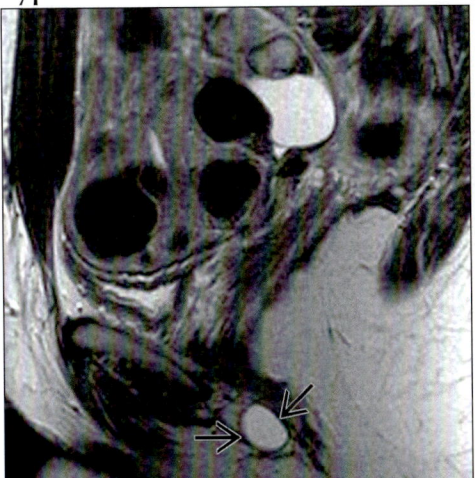
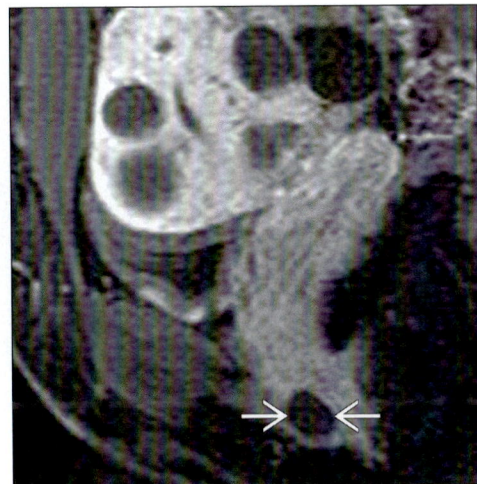

(Left) Sagittal T2WI MR shows a small round cyst ➡ in the perineum, below the pubic symphysis. *(Right)* Sagittal T1 C+ FS MR in the same patient as previous image shows no enhancement of the Bartholin gland cyst ➡.

Typical

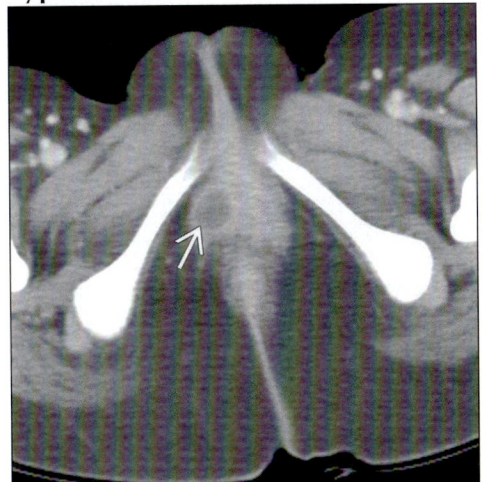
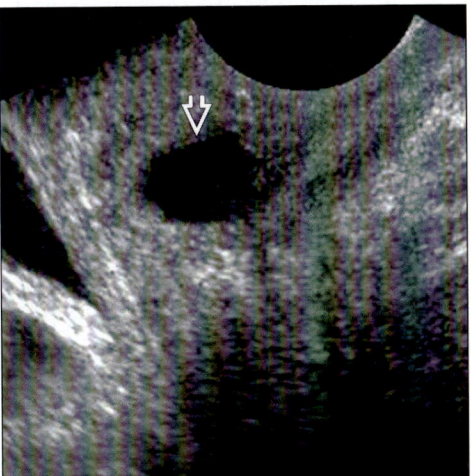

(Left) Axial CECT shows a low attenuation Bartholin gland cyst ➡ at the right side of the vaginal introitus. *(Right)* Sagittal transperineal US in the same patient at the vaginal introitus shows the cyst ➡ at the level of the vulvar vestibule.

Variant

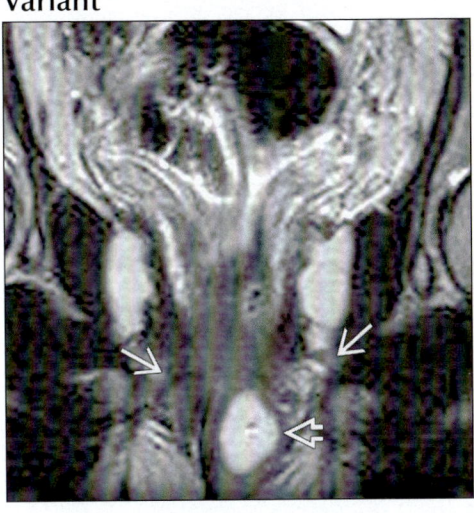
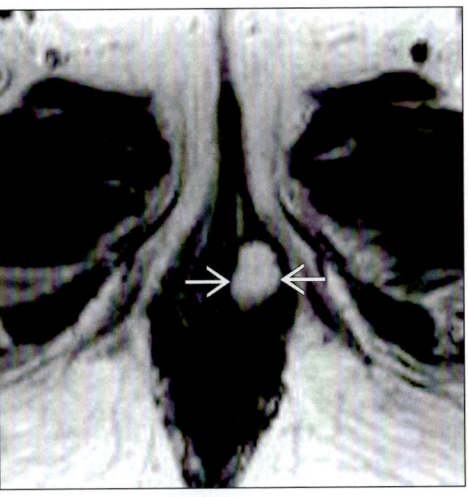

(Left) Coronal T2WI MR shows a left vulvar Bartholin gland cyst ➡. Note that the cyst lies below the pelvic diaphragm ➡. The cyst was clinically infected and contains a tiny focus of air. *(Right)* Axial T2WI MR shows a somewhat lobular cyst ➡ in the left vulvar region. Most Bartholin gland cysts are round.

FOREIGN BODIES, VAGINA

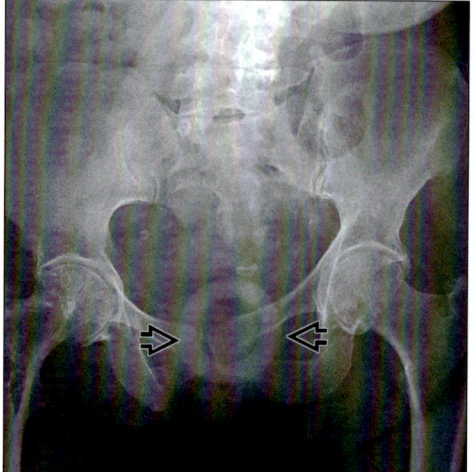

Anteroposterior radiograph shows a ring pessary ⇨ in an elderly female with uterine prolapse. Note its radiodense appearance and large diameter and width.

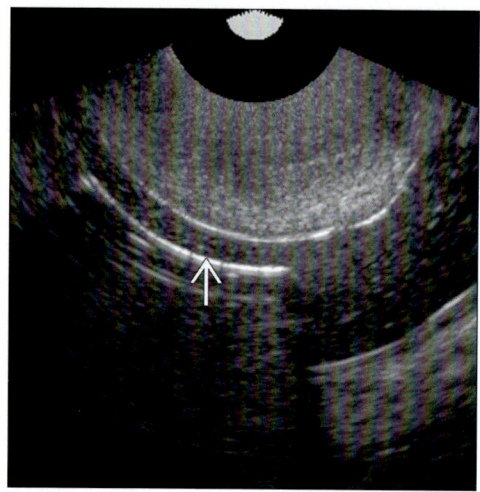

Longitudinal ultrasound shows a ring pessary in an elderly female with uterine prolapse. Note the linear echoic appearance ➡.

TERMINOLOGY

Definitions
- Device or foreign material found within the vaginal lumen
  - Iatrogenic
    - Vaginal pessary
    - Past instrumentation
    - Retained surgical swab/sponge
  - Non iatrogenic
    - Traumatic/penetrating injury
    - Intentional
    - Abuse

IMAGING FINDINGS

General Features
- Size: Inflammatory reaction may form a mass/granuloma and ↑ size with time
- Morphology
  - Metallic, wooden, plastic material
  - Vaginal tampon
    - Sufficient gas normally trapped into fibers → radiolucent object
  - Vaginal contraceptive ring
    - In women of reproductive age
    - Inserted between day 1 to 5 of menstrual cycle
    - In situ for 3 weeks, hormonal release via vaginal mucosal absorption
    - Ring removed for 1week, new ring inserted
    - Transparent flexible polymer ring
    - Radiolucent
    - Low concentration of etonogestrel and estradiol
    - Located anywhere in the vagina
    - May lie in any orientation
  - Vaginal pessary
    - In women with pelvic laxity, to support pelvic floor
    - Prevents uterine/vaginal/bladder neck prolapse
    - Similar appearances to contraceptive ring
    - Larger in diameter and width than contraceptive ring
    - May contain radiodense marker or strip
    - Positioned in most posterior aspect of vagina
  - Retained surgical swab = Gossypiboma = Textiloma

DDx: Vaginal Abnormalities that May Simulate a Foreign Body

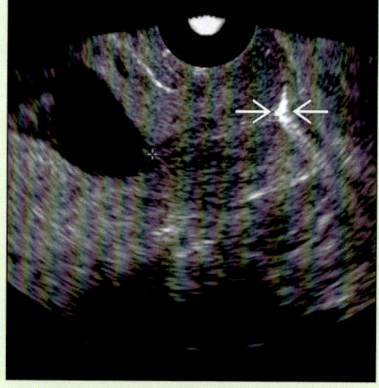

Air in the Vagina

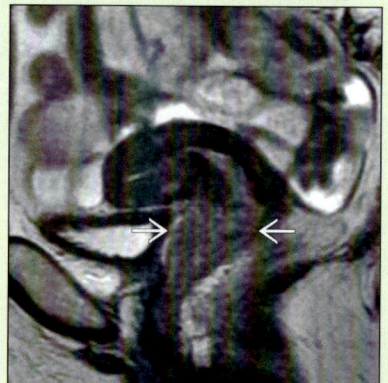

Vaginal Carcinoma

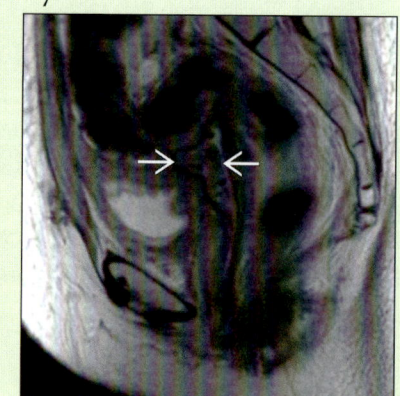

Vaginal Fistula

FOREIGN BODIES, VAGINA

Key Facts

Imaging Findings
- **Vaginal contraceptive ring**
- In women of reproductive age
- Radiolucent
- Located anywhere in the vagina
- May lie in any orientation
- **Vaginal pessary**
- In women with pelvic laxity, to support pelvic floor
- Prevents uterine/vaginal/bladder neck prolapse
- Similar appearances to contraceptive ring
- Larger in diameter and width than contraceptive ring
- May contain radiodense marker or strip
- Positioned in most posterior aspect of vagina
- **Retained swabs**
- Characteristic whirl-like appearance
- Sponge marker radiopaque and readily identifiable
- **Vaginal tampon**
- Can be utilized in CT as negative contrast to provide anatomical landmark location

Top Differential Diagnoses
- Air in the vagina
- Vaginal Clot
- Vaginal Carcinoma
- Vaginitis Emphysematosa
- Vaginal Fistula

Clinical Issues
- Removal under general anesthetic and examination under anesthesia may be necessary
- Treat complications (abscess drainage/perforated organ repair)

- Aseptic fibrous tissue reaction → adhesion, encapsulation, granuloma
- Exudative-type tissue reaction → abscess formation
- May organize and increase in size with time
- Patient may remain asymptomatic
  - Brachytherapy implants, a combination of
    - Tandem: Metal tube placed in uterus
    - Ovoids: Metal hollow holders placed in vagina, on both sides of cervix
    - Cylinders: Metal hollow holders placed in vagina

Radiographic Findings
- Supine film initially
- Oblique/lateral views may be of use
- Radiopaque objects
  - Some foods, animal bones, some fish bones
  - Some soil, gravel, mineral fragments
  - Glass
  - Metal (not aluminium)
  - Some pills and poisons
    - CHIPES: Chloral Hydrate, Iodides, Phenothiazines, Enteric coated pills, Solvents
  - Vaginal pessary with radiopaque marker
- Radiolucent objects
  - Most food, medicines, fish bones
  - Splinters, thorns and most wood
  - Most plastics, aluminium
  - Vaginal contraceptive rings and pessaries (without marker)
    - Lucent ring
  - Tampon
- **Retained swabs**
  - Characteristic whirl-like appearance
    - Gas trapped within the swab fibers
    - Not always present
  - Sponge body may be faintly visible
  - Sponge marker radiopaque and readily identifiable

Ultrasonographic Findings
- Wooden/metallic foreign bodies
  - Highly echogenic
  - Acoustic shadowing
    - May mask organs/pathology
- Pessary
  - Characteristic linear echoic lines
- Tampon
  - Variable appearance depending on amount of gas trapped in fibers
    - May appear as solid mass
    - If gas present → echogenic foci
- Retained swabs
  - Highly echogenic
  - Sharply delineated acoustic shadow
    - Present even in the absence of air or calcification
  - Less commonly
    - Cystic mass or hypoechoic mass with irregular internal echoes

CT Findings
- Scout image always interrogated
  - Some foreign bodies may not be appreciated on axial images
- Wooden foreign bodies
  - Retained wood as linear cylindric foci of increased attenuation
- Metallic foreign bodies
  - Strong artifact
- Plastic foreign bodies
  - Lucent, characteristic sharp borders
  - Ring pessary: Characteristic lucent ring
    - If radiopaque marker/strip → high attenuation ring
- Retained swabs: Variable appearance
  - Complex mass
  - Low or high density
  - Enhancing rim on CECT
  - May contain gas pockets centrally (equivalent to whirl like appearance of plain film)
  - May contain foci of calcification
- **Vaginal tampon**
  - Low attenuation
  - Can be utilized in CT as negative contrast to provide anatomical landmark location
    - Vagina low attenuation and distended

FOREIGN BODIES, VAGINA

- Cervix just above termination of low attenuation region

MR Findings
- Wooden foreign bodies
  - Variable signal intensity
  - Equal to or less than that of skeletal muscle on both T1 and T2 weighted images
  - Surrounding inflammatory response can be appreciated as enhancing region
- Metallic foreign bodies
  - Strong susceptibility artifact
- Plastic foreign bodies
  - Sharp low signal intensity margins
- Tampon
  - Signal void from air pockets within fibers
- Retained swabs
  - Hypointense on T1 weighted images
  - Very hyperintense on T2 weighted images
  - Characteristic wavy, striped or spotty appearance of gauze fibers

Imaging Recommendations
- Best imaging tool: Plain abdominal radiograph or CT scout
- Protocol advice
  - Plain abdominal radiograph initially
    - Provides diagnosis in most cases
  - CT/MR useful in
    - Foreign bodies located deep in the vagina
    - Evaluating complications (abscess/migration/organ perforation)
  - US
    - First line of investigations when presenting with vaginal bleeding
  - Detailed clinical history very relevant
  - Be aware of possible abuse especially in mentally retarded and children

DIFFERENTIAL DIAGNOSIS

Air in the Vagina
- Highly echogenic with associated posterior acoustic shadowing

Vaginal Clot
- Characteristic SI on MR indicating blood products

Vaginal Carcinoma
- Locally invasive soft tissue mass; enlarged inguinal and/or retroperitoneal lymph nodes may be present

Vaginitis Emphysematosa
- Located within vaginal wall rather than within lumen
- May create low attenuation ring around vagina

Vaginal Fistula
- Relevant clinical history is helpful; flecks of air may be present within the vagina
- MR may demonstrate the fistulous track

PATHOLOGY

Microscopic Features
- Epithelium may show reactive changes, hyperplastic features, ulceration or necrosis
- Underlying stroma may show chronic inflammation with foreign body giant cells ± granulomata

CLINICAL ISSUES

Presentation
- Most common signs/symptoms
  - Vaginal bleeding
  - Vaginal discharge
- Other signs/symptoms: Pain

Demographics
- Age
  - Children
    - Especially if personality/emotional problems
    - In cases of physical/sexual abuse
  - Adults at risk
    - Recent vaginal instrumentation/surgery
    - Emotionally disturbed/unusual sexual activities
    - Mentally retarded

Natural History & Prognosis
- Most foreign bodies do not cause significant injury
- May be encrusted in mineral salts
- Inflammatory reaction → granuloma
- Mucosal injuries
  - Mostly minor
    - Some irritation/discharge per vaginam
    - May cause edema → passage or removal of object difficult
  - Rarely may cause
    - Severe mucosal bleeding
    - Perforation through vaginal wall; migration into peritoneal cavity
    - Abscess, fistula formation

Treatment
- Removal under general anesthetic and examination under anesthesia may be necessary
- Treat complications (abscess drainage/perforated organ repair)

SELECTED REFERENCES

1. Lopez C et al: MRI of vaginal conditions. Clin Radiol. 60(6):648-62, 2005
2. Hunter TB et al: Foreign bodies. Radiographics. 23(3):731-57, 2003
3. Hunter TB: Special report: medical devices and foreign bodies: an introduction. Radiographics. 23(1):193-4, 2003
4. Jawaid: Gossypiboma – The forgotten swab. Special Communication. Pak J Med Sci. 19(2):141-3. 2003
5. Williams PL et al: US of abnormal uterine bleeding. Radiographics. 23(3):703-18, 2003
6. Van Goethem JW et al: MR and CT imaging of paraspinal textiloma (gossypiboma). J Comput Assist Tomogr. 15(6):1000-3, 1991
7. Nokes SR et al: Significance of vaginal air on computed tomography. J Comput Assist Tomogr. 10(6):997-9, 1986

FOREIGN BODIES, VAGINA

IMAGE GALLERY

Typical

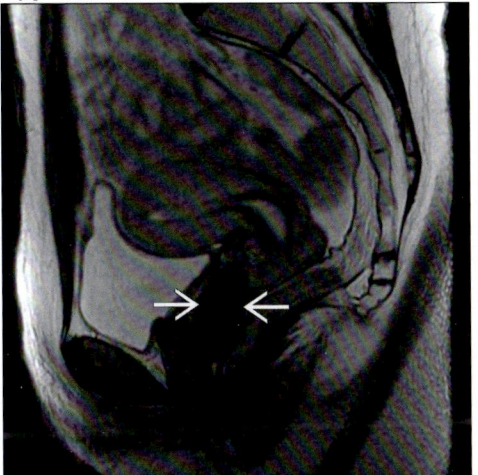
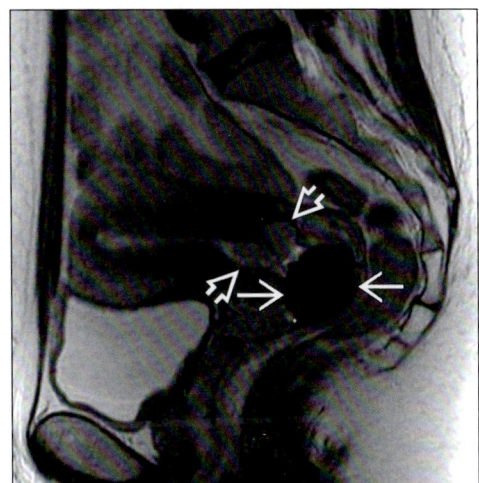

(Left) Sagittal T2WI MR shows a low signal intensity tampon ➡ in situ within the vagina. *(Right)* Sagittal T2WI MR shows a low signal intensity surgical pack ➡ impregnated with anticoagulant agents placed within the vagina to stop hemorrhage after excision biopsy in a patient with carcinoma of the cervix ➡.

Typical

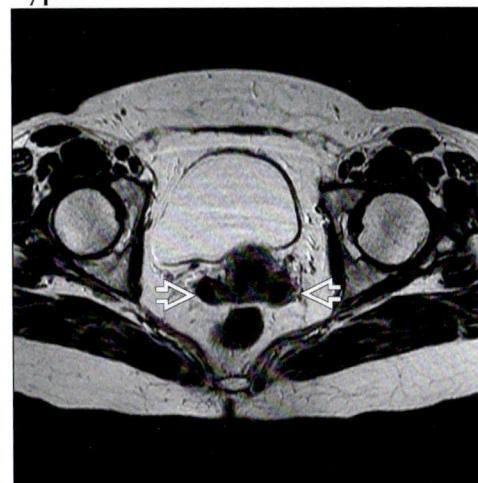
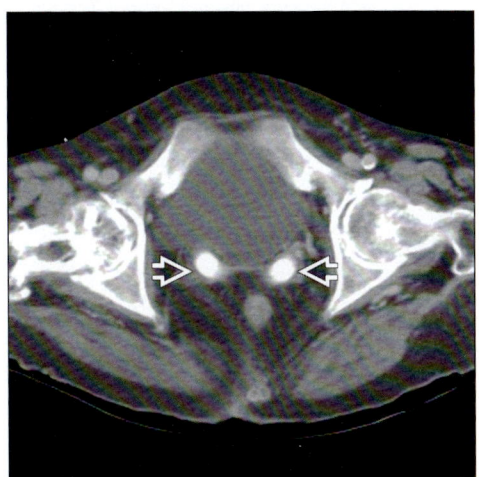

(Left) Axial T2WI FS MR shows a ring pessary within the vaginal lumen ➡. Note the signal void within the ring. *(Right)* Axial CECT shows a vaginal pessary in the same orientation as the previous image ➡.

Typical

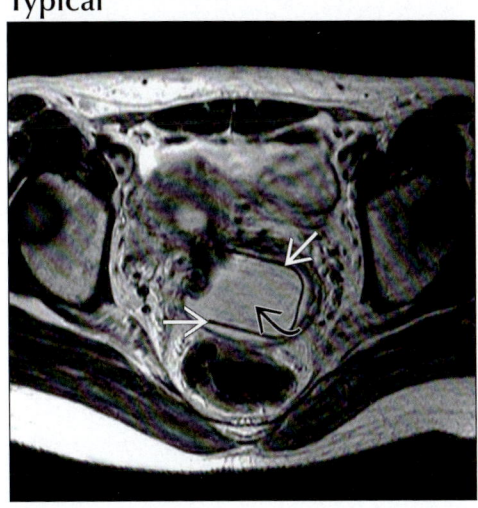
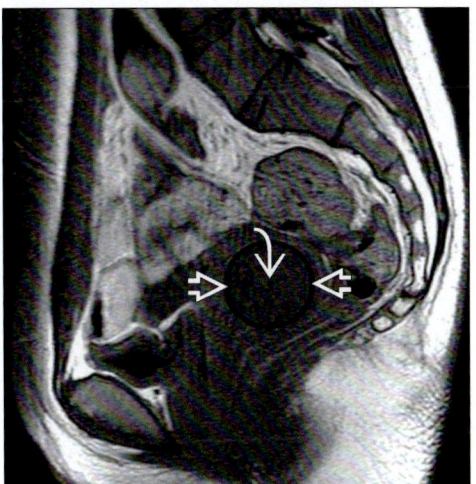

(Left) Axial T2WI FS MR shows a cross-section of a plastic bottle within the vagina. Note the low signal intensity bottle margins ➡ and the high signal fluid contents ➡. *(Right)* Sagittal T1WI MR shows the same bottle on a different orientation within the vagina ➡ containing low signal intensity fluid contents ➡.

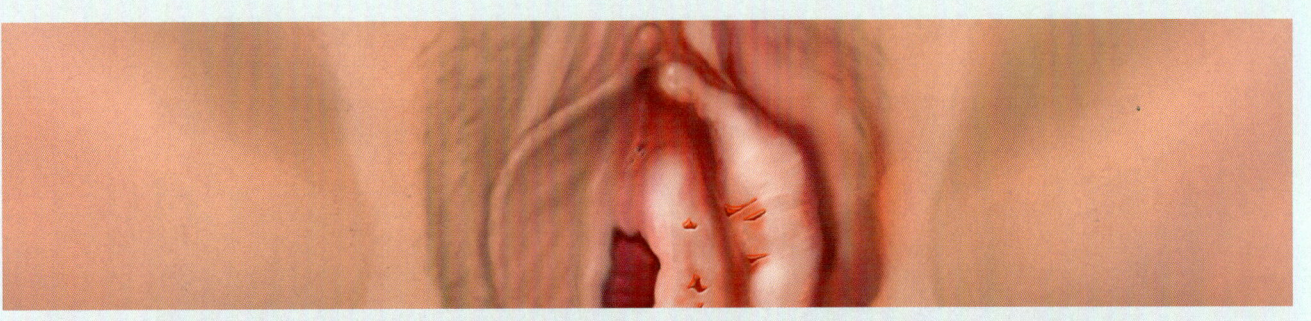

SECTION 5: Vulva

Introduction and Overview
Vulvar Anatomy & Imaging Issues   5-2

Neoplasm, Malignant
Carcinoma, Vulva   5-4
Leiomyosarcoma, Vulva   5-10
Melanoma, Vulva   5-12
Aggressive Angiomyxoma, Vulva   5-16
Lymphoma, Vulva   5-20
Merkel Cell Tumor, Vulva   5-22

Miscellaneous
Hemangioma, Vulva   5-24

VULVAR ANATOMY & IMAGING ISSUES

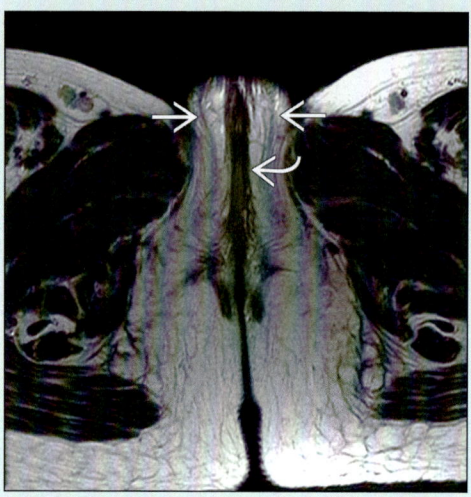

Axial T2WI MR shows labia majora ➡ composed of mounds of fatty tissue, and the labium minora ➡ as a linear hypointense midline structure.

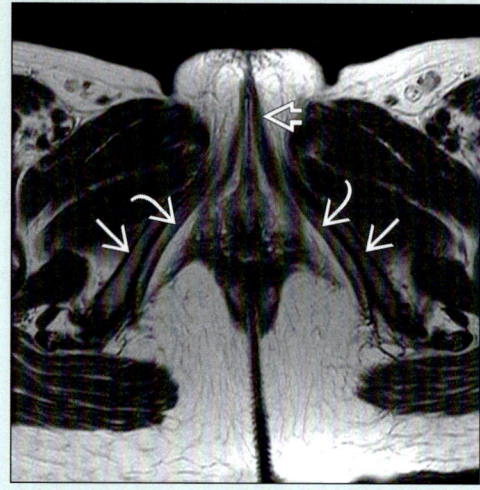

Axial T2WI MR shows ischiopubic rami ➡, crura of clitoris ➡, and labia minora ➡.

TERMINOLOGY

Definitions
- Vulva refers to external female genitalia
- Comprised of mons pubis, labia majora, labia minora, clitoris, vestibular bulb, vestibular glands and vestibule of vagina

IMAGING ANATOMY

General Anatomic Considerations
- Vulvar anatomy is not well visualized by conventional imaging techniques
- MR depicts exquisite anatomic detail of vulva with excellent soft tissue contrast

Critical Anatomic Structures
- **Labia majora** are seen as two mounds of anterior soft tissue originating at the border with medial thighs bilaterally
  - Their shape varies due to individual variation in labial height and width
- **Labia minora** surround vaginal introitus close to midline
  - They enhance greater than labia majora, and are of uniform shape
- **Clitoris** is composed of glans clitoris, clitoral body and bilateral crura
  - Clitoral body is formed by two corpora cavernosa projecting anteroinferiorly into mons pubis, separated by a fibrous septum
  - Glans clitoris is a small button-like extension of the body of the clitoris; covered by a dorsal hood derived from labia minora
  - Clitoris appears as a wishbone-shaped structure on axial MR
  - Posteriorly each crus tapers to a thin line continuous with the ischiocavernosus muscle
- **Introitus** is a linear midline slit of low signal intensity, enclosed by labia minora
- **Bartholin glands** develop within labia minora in posterolateral aspect of introitus at 4 and 8 o'clock positions posterior to vestibular bulbs
- **Vestibular bulbs** are paired paramedian elongated paravaginal erectile bodies parallel to clitoral crura, anterior and cephalad to Bartholin glands, and lateral to urethra

Anatomic Relationships
- Wishbone shape of clitoris encloses inverted V of vestibular bulbs, urethra and vagina, forming pyramid-shaped clitoro-urethrovaginal complex

ANATOMY-BASED IMAGING ISSUES

Key Concepts or Questions
- **Lymphatic drainage** of vulva is initially superficial to inguinal lymph nodes; followed by deep inguinal nodal involvement; with subsequent spread to the pelvic lymph nodes
- Vulvar lesions may have bilateral lymphatic drainage

Normal Measurements
- Labia majora measure an average of 22 mm in height and 50 mm in width
- Labia minora measure 10 mm width
- Vestibular bodies measure an average of 8 mm in premenopausal females and 5 mm in the postmenopausal
- Clitoral body width is an average of 10 mm

PATHOLOGIC ISSUES

General Pathologic Considerations
- Diseases of the vulva constitute a small fraction of gynecologic practice, and usually do not rely on radiologic imaging for diagnosis
- Benign and malignant conditions may involve the vulva

VULVAR ANATOMY & IMAGING ISSUES

Key Facts

Anatomic Variations
- Vulvar anatomy may show variations from patient to patient
- After menopause, variable degree of atrophy is seen

Best Imaging Tool
- MR provides images of vulva and adjacent structures with excellent soft tissue detail which can not be achieved by US or CT
- Other advantages of MR include lack of ionizing radiation compared with CT and nonintrusiveness compared with US

Role of Imaging
- Most vulvar pathologies are detected clinically
- Imaging plays an important role in malignant vulvar pathologies
- Imaging is used to define extent of disease and for treatment planning purposes

○ Most common benign conditions which may be diagnosed radiologically include Bartholin cyst, neurofibroma and hemangioma
○ Most common malignant conditions include vulvar cancer, melanoma, skin cancer, Bartholin gland cancer, Paget disease, Merkel cell carcinoma

- PET is useful in detecting lymph node involvement and distant metastases

Imaging Protocols
- Recommended MR imaging protocol should include
  ○ Transverse T1WI
  ○ Transverse, sagittal and coronal T2WI
  ○ Transverse T1WI FS; before and after contrast

PATHOLOGY-BASED IMAGING ISSUES

Imaging Approaches
- Chest radiograph may detect hematogenous spread of metastases from vulvar cancer
- Barium enema may be helpful in assessing rectal mucosal involvement by vulvar lesions
- Cystourethrography may be used to assess urethral mucosal involvement
- US may be used to assess soft tissues
- CECT is useful in disease staging, with limited assessment of local organ involvement, lymphadenopathy, hydronephrosis, and distant metastases
- MR offers superior local anatomic delineation, allowing accurate assessment of involvement of local structures and organ systems, thereby facilitating treatment planning
- Sentinel lymph node mapping with Tc-99m sulfur colloid is used for intraoperative evaluation of inguinal nodal chain for metastatic disease in patients with vulvar cancer

RELATED REFERENCES

1. Paramasivam S et al: Pelvic anatomy and MRI. Best Pract Res Clin Obstet Gynaecol. 20(1):3-22, 2006
2. Lloyd J et al: Female genital appearance: "normality" unfolds. BJOG. 112(5):643-6, 2005
3. O'Connell HE et al: Clitoral anatomy in nulliparous, healthy, premenopausal volunteers using unenhanced magnetic resonance imaging. J Urol. 173(6):2060-3, 2005
4. Moore RG et al: Sentinel node identification and the ability to detect metastatic tumor to inguinal lymph nodes in squamous cell cancer of the vulva. Gynecol Oncol. 89(3):475-9, 2003
5. Sohaib SA et al: Imaging in vulval cancer. Best Pract Res Clin Obstet Gynaecol. 17(4):543-56, 2003
6. Suh DD et al: Magnetic resonance imaging anatomy of the female genitalia in premenopausal and postmenopausal women. J Urol. 170(1):138-44, 2003
7. Chang SD: Imaging of the vagina and vulva. Radiol Clin North Am. 40(3):637-58, 2002

IMAGE GALLERY

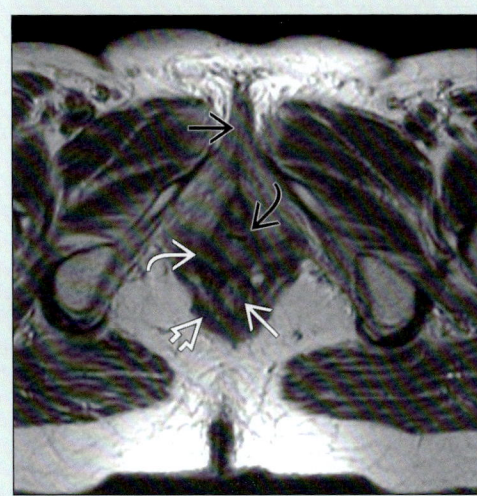
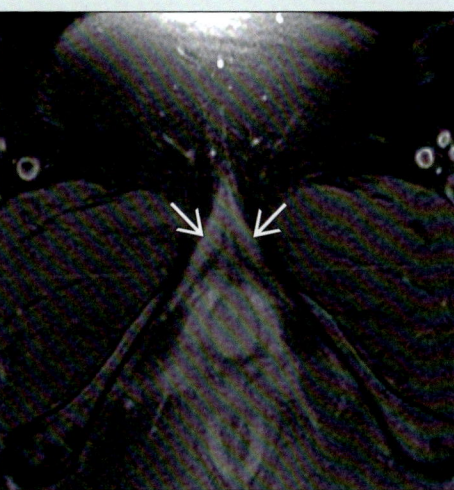

(Left) Axial T2WI MR shows puborectalis muscle ➡ forming a sling around rectum ➡ posteriorly, collapsed vagina ➡ anterior to rectum, urethra ➡ and body of clitoris ➡ most anteriorly. *(Right)* Axial T1 C+ FS MR shows diffusely enhancing crura of clitoris ➡ joining in midline forming a wishbone-shaped structure pointing anteriorly towards mons pubis.

CARCINOMA, VULVA

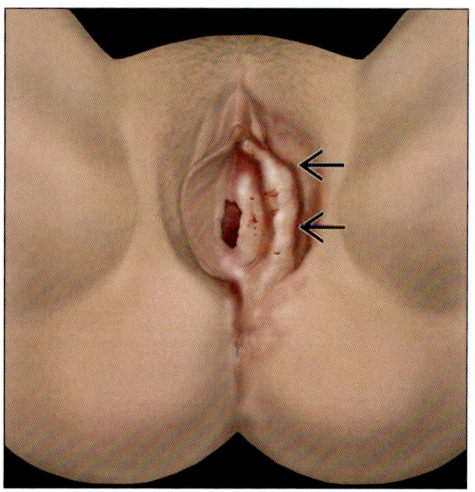

Schematic drawing of a typical case of vulvar carcinoma ➡.

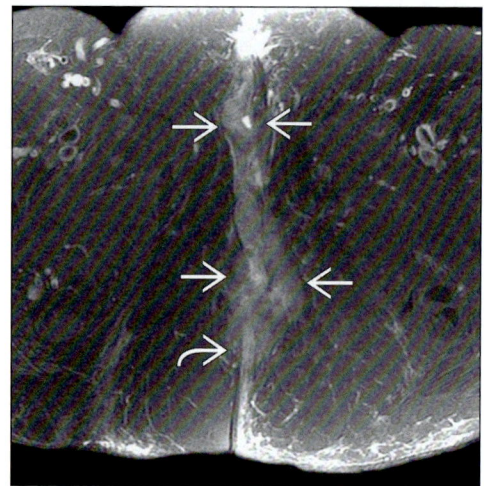

Axial T2WI FS MR shows a high signal intensity, lobulated vulva mass ➡. The mass is extending posteriorly to invade the anus ➡.

TERMINOLOGY

Definitions
- Primary malignant tumor of vulva

IMAGING FINDINGS

General Features
- Best diagnostic clue: Solid enhancing mass in vulva
- Location: Vulva lateral or close to midline, most commonly labia minora and majora (up to 70%), clitoris or perineum
- Size: Few millimeters to few centimeters
- Morphology: Fungating mass with necrosis and ulceration

Radiographic Findings
- Diagnosis of vulvar cancer and assessment of superficial lymph node involvement are done clinically
- Imaging modalities are useful in evaluating the extent of the primary tumor, deep inguinal and pelvic lymph node involvement

Ultrasonographic Findings
- Solid vulvar mass
- Useful in interrogating the groin for lymphadenopathy and guiding lymph node biopsy if required

CT Findings
- Enhancing solid mass in vulva
- Useful in evaluation of lymphadenopathy and metastatic disease

MR Findings
- T1WI: Low to intermediate signal intensity vulvar mass
- T2WI
  - Intermediate to high signal intensity vulvar mass
  - Areas heterogeneous signal intensity indicative of necrosis may be present
- T1 C+: Variable heterogeneous enhancement
- Enlarged inguinal and/or pelvic lymph nodes may be present

DDx: Vulvar Masses

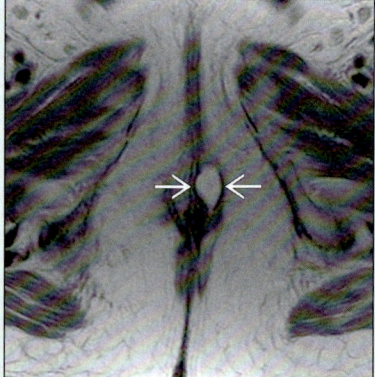

Bartholin Cyst

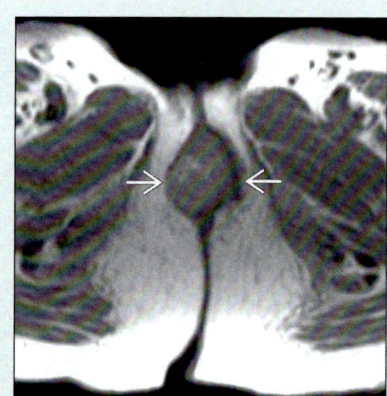

Vulva Melanoma

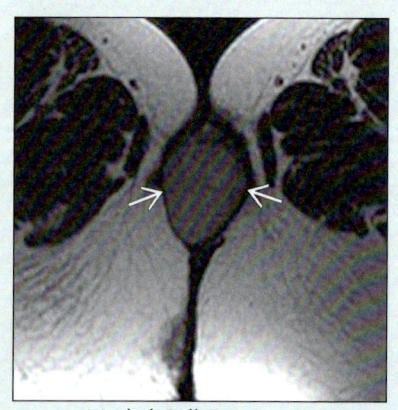

Merkel Cell Carcinoma

CARCINOMA, VULVA

Key Facts

Imaging Findings
- Best diagnostic clue: Solid enhancing mass in vulva
- Diagnosis of vulvar cancer and assessment of superficial lymph node involvement are done clinically
- Imaging modalities are useful in evaluating the extent of the primary tumor, deep inguinal and pelvic lymph node involvement
- Best imaging tool: MR is very useful in treatment planning by evaluating tumor extent to urethra, vagina, anus and periosteum as well as presence of lymphadenopathy

Top Differential Diagnoses
- Bartholin Cyst
- Bartholinitis
- Vulva Melanoma
- Merkel Cell Carcinoma

Pathology
- Most common histologic type is squamous cell carcinoma (85%)

Clinical Issues
- Most common signs/symptoms: Pruritus or irritation of vulvar area

Diagnostic Checklist
- CT or MR for nodal involvement which directly affects prognosis
- Presence of inguinal lymph nodes > 1 cm post lymph node dissection is considered abnormal and indicates local relapse which is associated with very poor prognosis

Nuclear Medicine Findings
- PET: Increased FDG uptake in the primary tumor and metastatic lymph nodes

Imaging Recommendations
- Best imaging tool: MR is very useful in treatment planning by evaluating tumor extent to urethra, vagina, anus and periosteum as well as presence of lymphadenopathy
- Protocol advice: Axial T1WI, axial, sagittal and coronal T2WI and axial and coronal T1WI FS C+ images

DIFFERENTIAL DIAGNOSIS

Bartholin Cyst
- Well-defined, non-enhancing cyst in typical location of Bartholin gland posterolateral to vaginal introitus within the labia majora

Bartholinitis
- Thick-walled cystic mass with rim-enhancement and infiltrative changes in adjacent fat suggestive of inflammation

Vulva Melanoma
- Usually of intermediate to high signal intensity on T1WI due to paramagnetic effect of melanin content

Merkel Cell Carcinoma
- Rare neuroendocrine tumor seen in younger women, frequently presents with distant metastasis and associated with poor prognosis

PATHOLOGY

General Features
- General path comments
  - Most common histologic type is squamous cell carcinoma (85%)
  - Other types are melanoma, Bartholin gland cancer, sarcomas, basal cell carcinoma, adenocarcinomas and extramammary Paget disease
  - Human papillomavirus (HPV) positive tumors occur in younger age group, may be multifocal and are associated with vulvar intraepithelial neoplasia (VIN), which is a precancerous lesion
  - HPV negative vulvar cancers are associated with vulvar inflammation or lichen sclerosis (inflammatory dermatoses)
  - Verrucous carcinoma is a distinct variety of squamous cell carcinoma
    - Well-differentiated, low grade, slow growing exophytic mass, with characteristic verrucous architecture
    - Excellent prognosis as it does not metastasize
- Genetics: Gain in chromosome 17 in lichen sclerosis and loss of chromosome 17 in HPV-related vulvar cancers
- Etiology: HPV related squamous vulva cancers are associated with HPV types 16, 18 and 33
- Epidemiology
  - Rare malignancy accounting for 5% of female genital tract cancers
  - Risk factors include multiple sexual partners, history of genital warts, pre-invasive cervical cancer and smoking
- Associated abnormalities
  - Cervical intra-epithelial neoplasia (CIN) and invasive cervical cancer, both of which are induced by HPV infection
  - Immunocompromised women (e.g., HIV infection) bear considerable risk for vulvar intra-epithelial neoplasia and invasive cancer

Gross Pathologic & Surgical Features
- Vulvar epithelial neoplasia can present as white, red or brown vulvar lesions which can be multifocal
  - White color lesions can be explained by hyperkeratosis
  - Red color lesions are usually vascular reflecting angiogenesis and increased neovascularity

CARCINOMA, VULVA

- Invasive vulvar carcinoma appears as exophytic or papillomatous mass or endophytic ulcerative lesion

Microscopic Features
- Squamous cell carcinomas of vulva show broad anastomosing masses of atypical squamous cells with prominent intercellular bridges and cytoplasmic inclusions of keratin
- Squamous carcinoma associated with inflammatory dermatoses tends to be well-differentiated with keratin pearl formation
- Squamous carcinoma associated with VIN tends to be moderate to poorly differentiated with more nuclear pleomorphism and less keratin formation

Staging, Grading or Classification Criteria
- FIGO staging
  - Stage I: Tumor 2 cm or less, confined to vulva
    - IA: Stromal invasion 1 mm or less
    - IB: Stromal invasion more than 1 mm
  - Stage II: Tumor greater than 2 cm, confined to vulva
  - Stage III: Tumor of any size invading lower urethra, vagina, perineum or anus
  - Stage IVA: Tumor of any size invading mucosa of bladder or rectum, or tumor fixed to pelvic bone
  - Stage IVB: Distant metastasis including pelvic lymph node metastasis

CLINICAL ISSUES

Presentation
- Most common signs/symptoms: Pruritus or irritation of vulvar area
- Other signs/symptoms
  - Palpable mass in vulva, ulceration, bleeding or pain
  - Vulvar cancer tends to grow locally, and voiding difficulty may develop due to urethral obstruction particularly in midline tumors

Demographics
- Age
  - Bimodal age distribution is observed
    - Incidence of HPV related vulvar cancer in younger women (< 50 years old) is increasing worldwide
    - Incidence of non-HPV related vulvar cancer in older women (< 70 years old) remains stable over the years

Natural History & Prognosis
- Most important prognostic factors are tumor size, lymph node involvement and depth of invasion
- 5-year survival rates: 90% for stage I, 80% for stage II, 50 to 60% for stage III, and 15% for stage IV
  - Distant metastases are exceedingly rare, mostly to liver and lung, predominantly in patients with long history of vulvar cancer and recurrent disease which is refractory to treatment

Treatment
- Early stage is treated with partial vulvectomy
  - 1 cm tumor-free margin is considered adequate, tumor-free margin l8 mm is associated with 50% local recurrence rate
  - Lateral tumors usually metastasizes to ipsilateral lymph nodes; therefore, unilateral inguinofemoral lymph node dissection with removal of all superficial inguinal nodes and femoral nodes medial to the femoral vein is considered adequate
  - Bilateral inguinal metastases are common in midline or close to midline (less than 1 cm) tumors, and bilateral groin dissection is optimal for medial tumors
- Advanced stages
  - Pelvic exenteration and bilateral lymph node dissection with radiation and chemotherapy
  - Chemo radiation with or without surgery should be regarded as the first choice for patients with locally advanced vulvar cancer only when primary surgery will necessitate performance of a stoma

DIAGNOSTIC CHECKLIST

Consider
- CT or MR for nodal involvement which directly affects prognosis

Image Interpretation Pearls
- Solid enhancing vulvar mass with or without lymph node involvement
- Presence of inguinal lymph nodes > 1 cm post lymph node dissection is considered abnormal and indicates local relapse which is associated with very poor prognosis

SELECTED REFERENCES

1. Jamieson DJ et al: Vulvar, vaginal, and perianal intraepithelial neoplasia in women with or at risk for human immunodeficiency virus. Obstet Gynecol. 107(5):1023-8, 2006
2. Land R et al: Routine computerized tomography scanning, groin ultrasound with or without fine needle aspiration cytology in the surgical management of primary squamous cell carcinoma of the vulva. Int J Gynecol Cancer. 16(1):312-7, 2006
3. Weikel W et al: Surgical therapy of recurrent vulvar cancer. Am J Obstet Gynecol. 195(5):1293-302, 2006
4. Woolderink JM et al: Patterns and frequency of recurrences of squamous cell carcinoma of the vulva. Gynecol Oncol. 103(1):293-9, 2006
5. Rouzier R et al: Surgery for vulvar cancer. Clin Obstet Gynecol. 48(4):869-78, 2005
6. Hall TB et al: The role of ultrasound-guided cytology of groin lymph nodes in the management of squamous cell carcinoma of the vulva: 5-year experience in 44 patients. Clin Radiol. 58(5):367-71, 2003
7. Sohaib SA et al: Imaging in vulval cancer. Best Pract Res Clin Obstet Gynaecol. 17(4):543-56, 2003
8. Chang SD: Imaging of the vagina and vulva. Radiol Clin North Am. 40(3):637-58, 2002
9. Hawnaur JM et al: Identification of inguinal lymph node metastases from vulval carcinoma by magnetic resonance imaging: an initial report. Clin Radiol. 57(11):995-1000, 2002
10. Sohaib SA et al: MR imaging of carcinoma of the vulva. AJR Am J Roentgenol. 178(2):373-7, 2002
11. Abang Mohammed DK et al: Inguinal node status by ultrasound in vulva cancer. Gynecol Oncol. 77(1):93-6, 2000

CARCINOMA, VULVA

IMAGE GALLERY

Typical

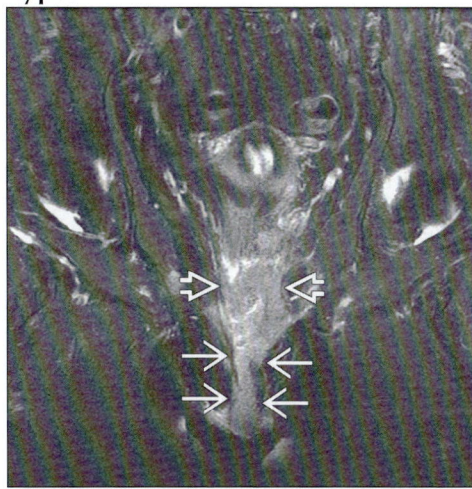
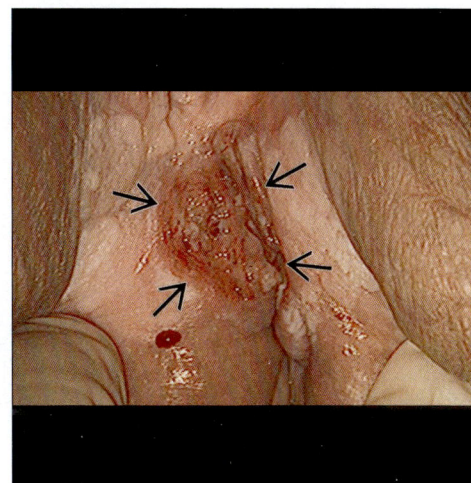

(Left) Coronal T2WI FS MR shows a high signal intensity, lobulated vulva mass ➡. The mass is extending superiorly to invade the lower vagina ➡. Pathology: Vulva carcinoma. *(Right)* Clinical photograph shows a typical case of vulvar carcinoma ➡.

Typical

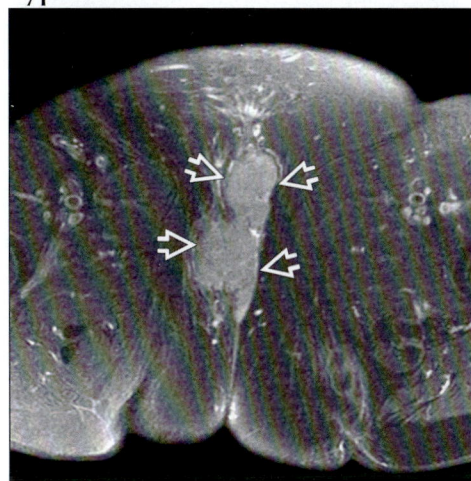
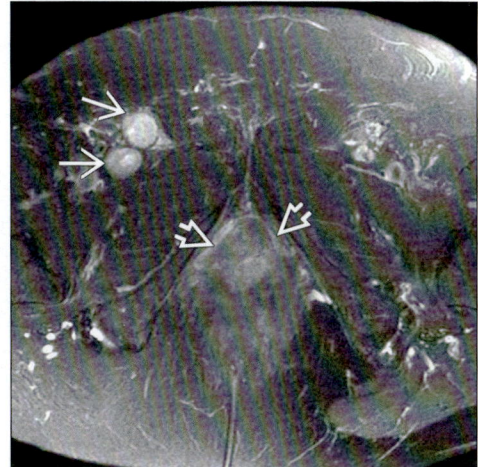

(Left) Axial T2WI FS MR in the same patient as previous image, shows an intermediate signal intensity lobulated mass ➡ in the vulva. *(Right)* Axial T2WI FS MR shows enlarged right inguinal lymph nodes ➡ (in the same patient as previous image) with vulva carcinoma ➡.

Typical

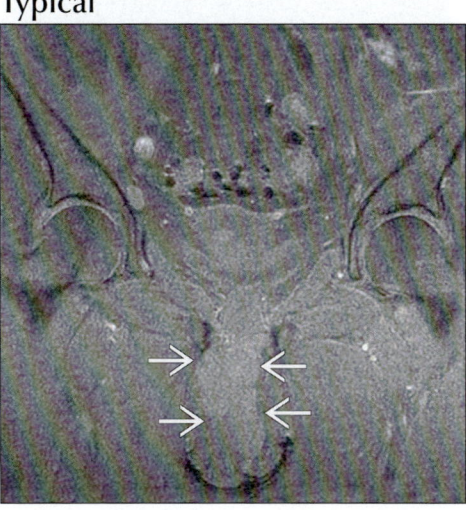
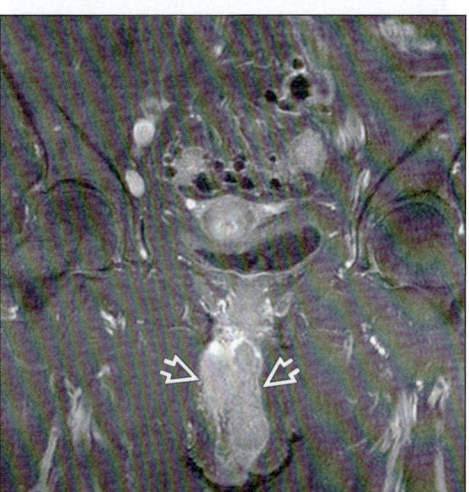

(Left) Coronal T1WI FS MR in the same patient as previous image, shows a lobulated mass ➡ of intermediate signal intensity. *(Right)* Coronal T1 C+ FS MR shows a lobulated vulva mass ➡ which enhances after administration of i/v gadolinium.

CARCINOMA, VULVA

Typical

(Left) Axial T2WI MR shows a well-defined mass ➡ of high signal intensity arising from labia major on the left side. (Right) Coronal T2WI MR in the same patient as previous image, shows the extent of the mass ➡ arising from labia majora. The mass is displacing the urethra ➡ to the right.

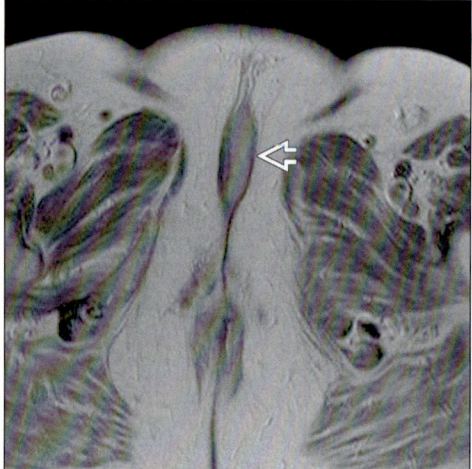

Typical

(Left) Axial T1WI FS MR in the same patient as previous image, shows a well-defined mass ➡ of intermediate signal intensity arising from left labia majora. (Right) Axial T1 C+ FS MR shows avid enhancement of the well-defined mass ➡ arising from the left labia majora.

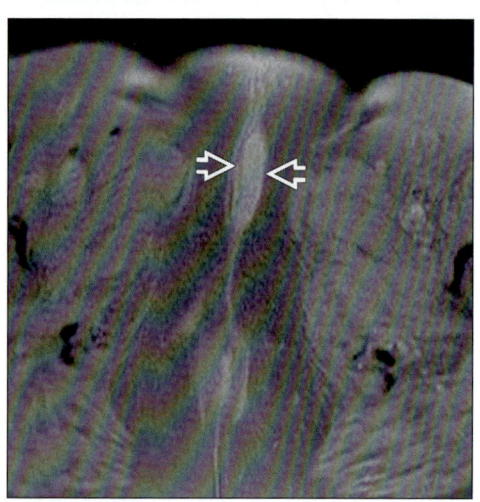 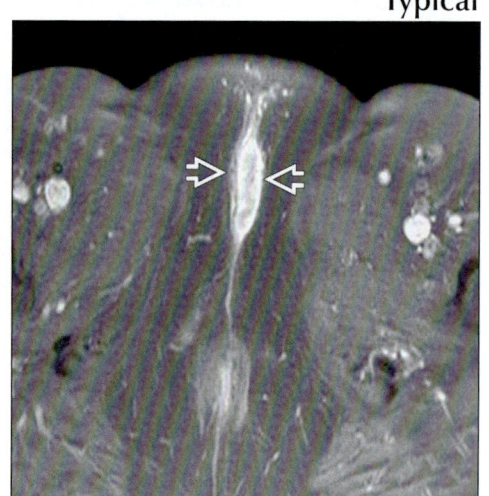

Typical

(Left) Axial NECT shows a vulva mass ➡ in a patient with vulva carcinoma. Also note the presence of a soft tissue mass in the right inguinal region ➡. (Right) Axial fused PET/CT in the same patient as previous image, shows avid FDG uptake in the vulva mass ➡. Also note the increased FDG uptake in the right inguinal lymph node mass ➡.

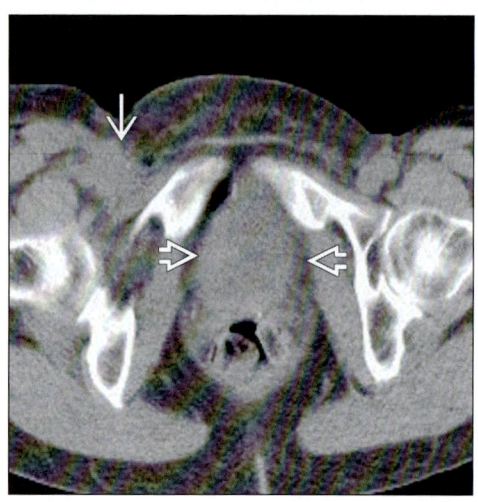 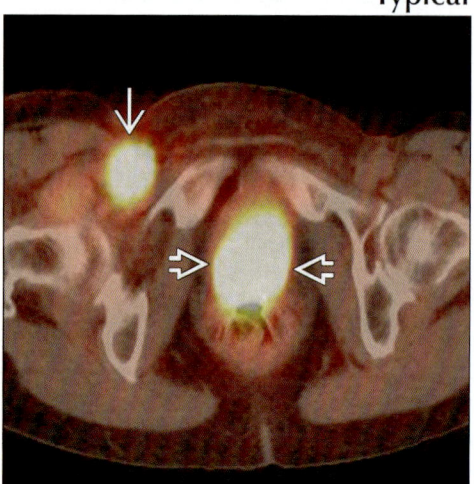

CARCINOMA, VULVA

Typical

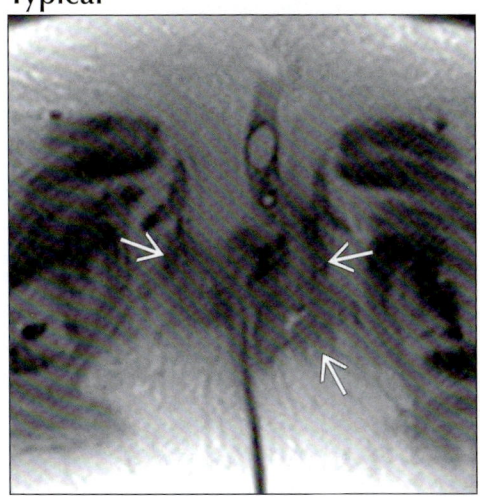
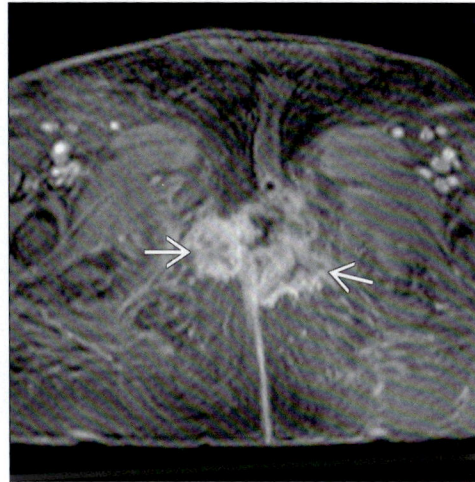

(Left) Axial T1WI MR shows typical case of recurrent squamous carcinoma of the vulva. Note the irregular intermediate signal mass in the perineum ➡. *(Right)* Axial T1 C+ FS MR in the same patient as previous image, shows an irregular enhancing mass ➡ in the perineum.

Typical

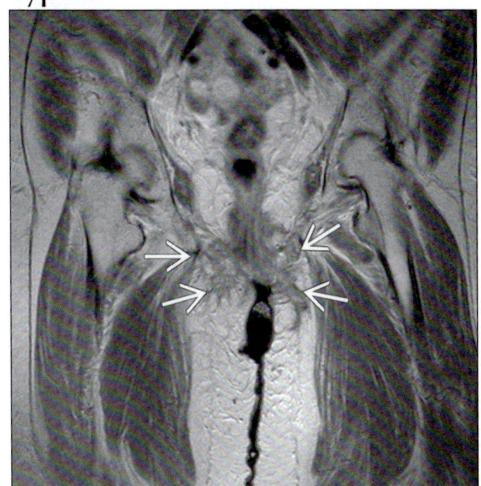
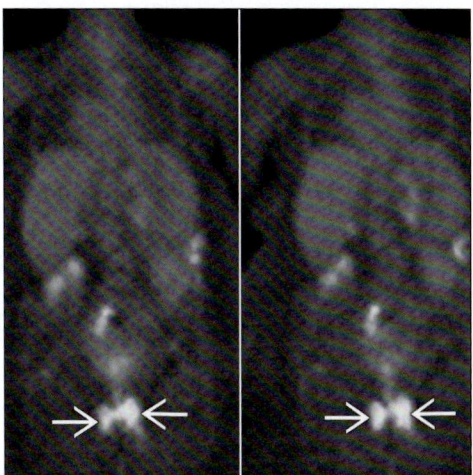

(Left) Coronal T2WI MR in the same patient as previous image, shows the extent of the recurrent vulva carcinoma ➡. *(Right)* Coronal PET in the same patient as previous image, shows an FDG avid vulva mass ➡ confirming the presence of recurrent squamous carcinoma of the vulva.

Typical

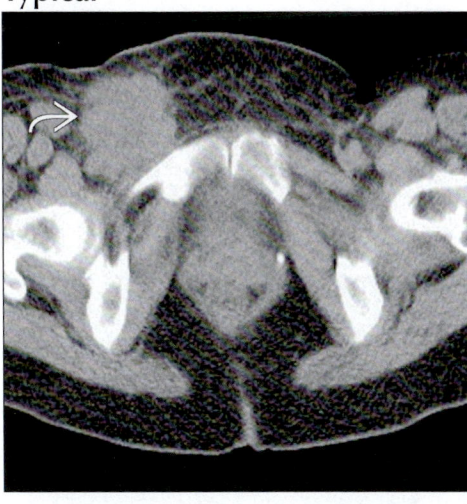
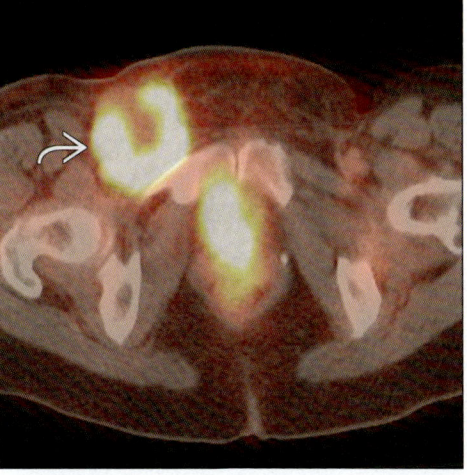

(Left) Axial NECT in a patient with known vulva carcinoma, shows a large lobulated mass in the right inguinal region ➡. Note the low attenuation center suggestive of necrosis. *(Right)* Axial fused PET/CT in the same patient as previous image, shows avid FDG uptake in the right inguinal lymph node mass ➡. Note the presence of a central photopenic area indicative of tumor necrosis. Pathology: Recurrent vulva carcinoma.

LEIOMYOSARCOMA, VULVA

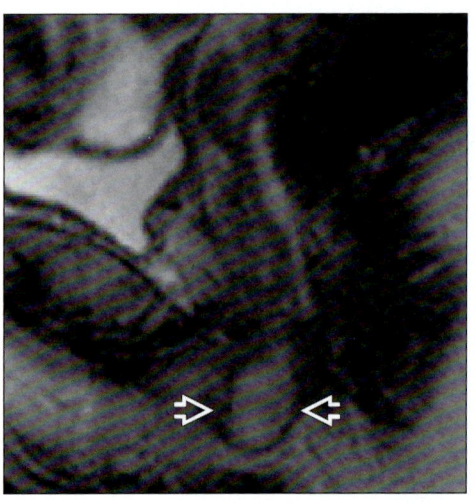

Sagittal T2WI MR shows a lobulated vulvar mass ➡ of high signal intensity.

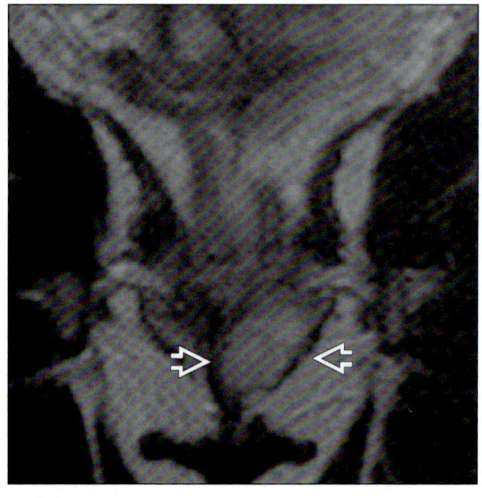

Coronal T2WI MR in the same patient, confirms the presence of a high SI, left-sided vulvar mass ➡. Pathology: Vulvar leiomyosarcoma.

TERMINOLOGY

Definitions
- Most common vulvar sarcoma arising from smooth muscle

IMAGING FINDINGS

General Features
- Best diagnostic clue: Heterogeneously enhancing vulvar mass
- Location: Vulva (labium major/minor)
- Size: Variable: Up to 10 cm
- Morphology: Vulvar mass with necrosis and ulceration

Ultrasonographic Findings
- Useful for interrogating the groin for lymphadenopathy and guiding lymph node biopsy

CT Findings
- CECT: Vulvar mass showing heterogeneous enhancement; there may be associated inguinal lymphadenopathy or hematogenous metastases

MR Findings
- T1WI: Low to intermediate signal intensity vulvar mass
- T2WI: Intermediate to high signal intensity vulvar mass
- T1 C+ FS: Variable heterogeneous enhancement

Imaging Recommendations
- Best imaging tool: MR most accurate for local staging; CECT to evaluate for distant metastases
- Protocol advice: Axial T1WI, axial, coronal, sagittal T2WI, axial and coronal T1WI FS C+ images

DIFFERENTIAL DIAGNOSIS

Other Malignant Vulvar Tumors
- e.g., squamous cell carcinoma and mesenchymal tumors; difficult to distinguish from leiomyosarcoma

Benign Conditions
- e.g., Bartholin abscess shows heterogeneous enhancement; Bartholin cyst does not enhance and is high signal on T2

DDx: Vulvar Masses

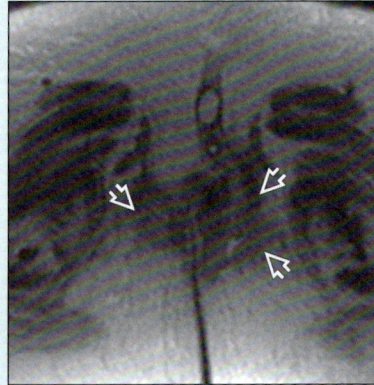

Vulvar Carcinoma

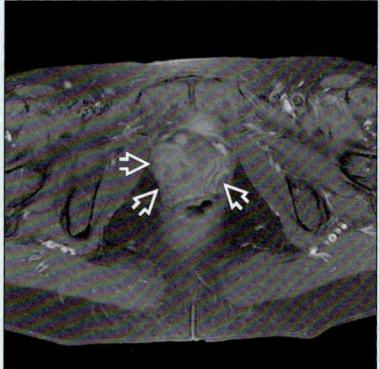

Aggressive Angiomyxoma

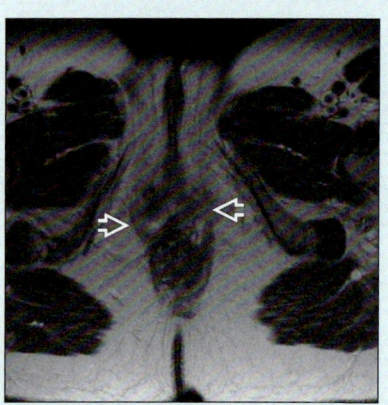

Bartholinitis

LEIOMYOSARCOMA, VULVA

Key Facts

Terminology
- Most common vulvar sarcoma arising from smooth muscle

Imaging Findings
- Best diagnostic clue: Heterogeneously enhancing vulvar mass

Clinical Issues
- Firm vulvar mass

- Slow growing neoplasm; can get hematogenous metastases and inguinal lymphadenopathy
- Grade is an important prognostic factor
- Wide local excision or radical vulvectomy ± bilateral inguinal lymph node resection

Diagnostic Checklist
- MR used for local staging, CECT used for assessment of distant metastases

PATHOLOGY

General Features
- Etiology: Possibly oestrogen dependent as may increase in size in pregnancy
- Epidemiology: Accounts for 1-3% of vulvar malignancies

Gross Pathologic & Surgical Features
- Tumors are often 5 cm or larger at presentation

Microscopic Features
- Smooth muscle tumor with three or more of the following criteria are considered malignant
  - > 5 cm in diameter; 5 or more mitoses per 10 high power fields; infiltrative margins; moderate to severe cytologic atypia
- Immunohistochemical stains are positive for smooth muscle actin, vimentin and may be positive for desmin

CLINICAL ISSUES

Presentation
- Most common signs/symptoms
  - Firm vulvar mass
  - ± Local pain and ulceration
- Other signs/symptoms: From hematogenous metastases

Demographics
- Age: Perimenopausal or postmenopausal women

Natural History & Prognosis
- Slow growing neoplasm; can get hematogenous metastases and inguinal lymphadenopathy
- Grade is an important prognostic factor

Treatment
- Wide local excision or radical vulvectomy ± bilateral inguinal lymph node resection
- Adjuvant radiotherapy for high grade tumor or locally recurrent low grade tumors
- Chemotherapy in metastatic disease

DIAGNOSTIC CHECKLIST

Consider
- MR used for local staging, CECT used for assessment of distant metastases

Image Interpretation Pearls
- Heterogeneously-enhancing vulvar mass

SELECTED REFERENCES

1. Ulutin HC et al: Soft tissue sarcoma of the vulva: A clinical study. Int J Gynecol Cancer. 13(4):528-31, 2003
2. Nielsen GP et al: Smooth-muscle tumors of the vulva. A clinicopathological study of 25 cases and review of the literature. Am J Surg Pathol. 20(7):779-93, 1996

IMAGE GALLERY

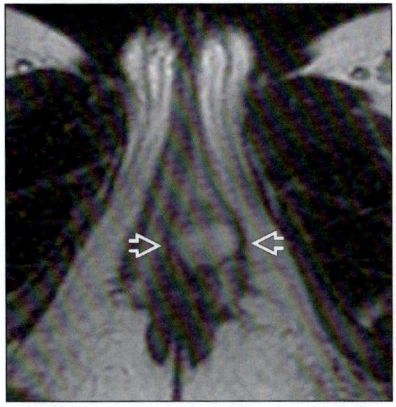 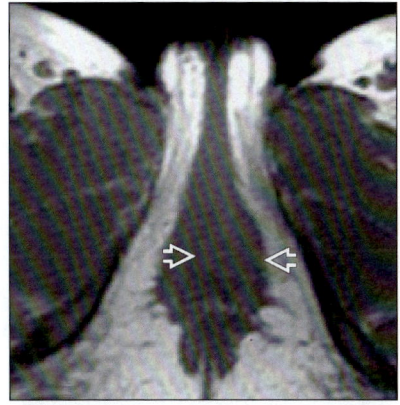 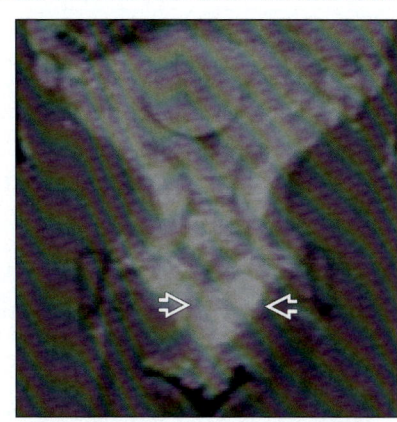

(Left) Axial T2WI MR shows left-sided, lobulated vulvar mass ➡ of high signal intensity. *(Center)* Axial T1WI MR shows vulvar asymmetry in keeping with a left-sided vulvar mass ➡. *(Right)* Coronal T1 C+ FS MR in the same patient confirms the presence of an avidly enhancing, left-sided vulvar mass ➡. Pathology: Vulvar leiomyosarcoma.

MELANOMA, VULVA

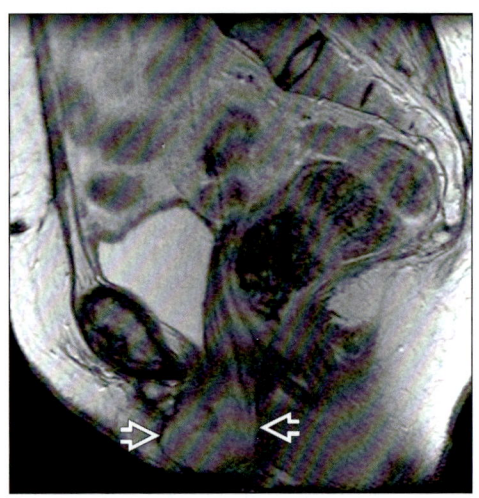

Sagittal T2WI MR shows a well-defined, relatively homogeneous, high signal intensity vulvar mass ➡.

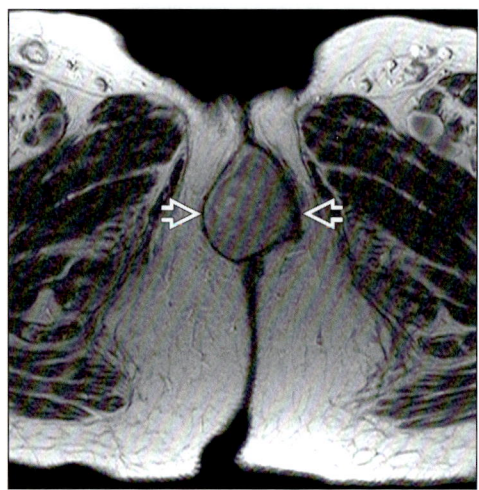

Axial T2WI MR confirms the presence of a high signal intensity vulvar mass ➡. Pathology: Vulvar melanoma.

TERMINOLOGY

Abbreviations and Synonyms
- Melanocyte malignancy

Definitions
- Subtype of cutaneous melanoma with similar prognostic and staging factors

IMAGING FINDINGS

General Features
- Best diagnostic clue: Vulvar mass with high signal on both T1WI and T2WI
- Location: Half of patients have clitoral-preclitoral lesions, another half have lesions arising from labia minora/majora
- Size: Ranges between 0.5 cm and 4 cm with mean size 1.5 cm

Ultrasonographic Findings
- High frequency US has potential role for assessing depth of invasion

CT Findings
- NECT: Isoattenuation mass relative to muscle
- CECT: Tumor enhancement allows evaluation for local invasion and metastatic disease

MR Findings
- T1WI
  - High SI consistent with paramagnetic effect of melanin may be seen
  - May demonstrate low or intermediate SI in case of low melanin content within the lesion (amelanotic melanoma)
  - Hemorrhage may be present in large lesions
- T2WI: High SI, necrosis may be present within large lesions
- T1 C+ FS
  - Tumor demonstrates homogeneous enhancement
  - No enhancement of necrotic areas

Nuclear Medicine Findings
- PET
  - FDG-avid malignancy
  - Excellent for lymph nodes and distant metastases

DDx: Vulvar Masses

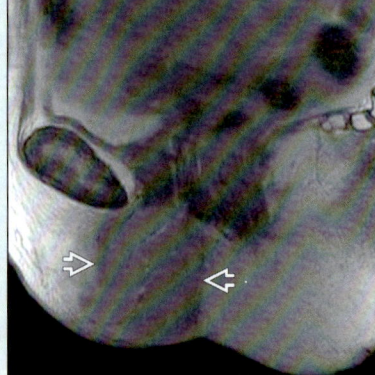

Vulvar Carcinoma

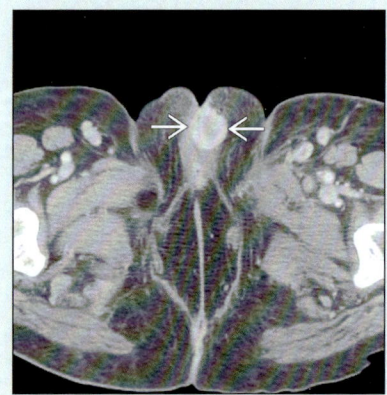

Vulvar Metastasis

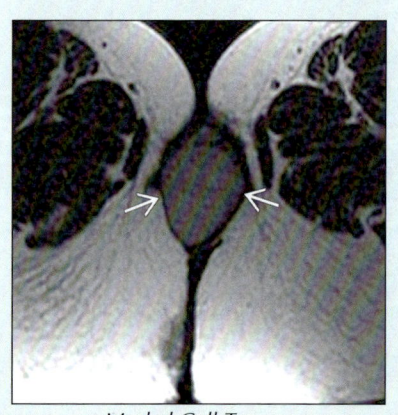

Merkel Cell Tumor

MELANOMA, VULVA

Key Facts

Terminology
- Subtype of cutaneous melanoma with similar prognostic and staging factors

Imaging Findings
- Best diagnostic clue: Vulvar mass with high signal on both T1WI and T2WI
- Best imaging tool: MR for local extent and PET for staging

Top Differential Diagnoses
- Vulvar Squamous Carcinoma
- Atypical Melanocytic Nevus, Genital Type
- Vulvar Metastases
- Merkel Cell Carcinoma
- Paget Disease

Pathology
- Immunohistochemical stains are positive for Melan A, S100, HMB45

Clinical Issues
- Lesions on the labia minora with involvement of the urethra and vagina have a worse prognosis due to technical difficulty in achieving clear margins
- Most important prognostic factors are Breslow thickness, ulceration, evidence of regression, presence of a vertical growth phase, satellite lesions and lymphovascular space invasion

Diagnostic Checklist
- High SI T1WI vulvar lesion, however amelanotic melanoma can be of low or intermediate SI on T1WI

Imaging Recommendations
- Best imaging tool: MR for local extent and PET for staging
- Protocol advice: T1WI, T2WI and T1 C+ FS

DIFFERENTIAL DIAGNOSIS

Vulvar Squamous Carcinoma
- Most common type of vulvar cancer, slow growing tumor, distant metastases are rare and mortality is low compared to vulvar melanoma

Atypical Melanocytic Nevus, Genital Type
- Benign condition seen in young women of mean age 23 years
- Typically elevated with flat or mushroom appearance

Vulvar Metastases
- Usually from adjacent organs (vagina, anus, urethra)

Merkel Cell Carcinoma
- An aggressive cutaneous neoplasm associated with grave prognosis; most patients die within one year of diagnosis from widespread metastatic disease

Paget Disease
- Usually confined to the epithelium, in general very slow-growing, non-malignant or described as carcinoma in situ
- Invasive adenocarcinoma is present in 10-20% of cases

PATHOLOGY

General Features
- Genetics
  - Personal and family history of melanoma, particularly first-degree relatives
  - Phenotype (fair skin, blonde or red hair, blue or green eyes)
- Etiology: Malignant transformation of melanocytes that arise from neural crest cells within basal layer of the epidermis
- Epidemiology
  - Vulvar melanoma is rare tumor but it is the second most common vulvar malignancy
  - Accounts for 5-10% of vulval cancers and represents 2% of all melanomas

Gross Pathologic & Surgical Features
- Pigmented vulvar mass with irregular or scalloped borders, often black with shades of red, white or blue, ulceration may be present

Microscopic Features
- In-situ malignant melanoma composed of atypical melanocytes arranged singly and in nests in the epidermis without invasion into underlying dermis
- Tumor cells may be round (epithelioid) or spindle shaped and may or may not contain melanin pigment (amelanotic melanoma)
- Malignant melanoma can show a radial (growth is in a horizontal direction) or vertical growth within the dermis
- Breslow thickness is measurement of tumor taken from the top of the granular layer overlying the tumor to the deepest melanoma cells
- Clarke level indicates the depth of the tumor
  - Level 1: Tumor confined to epidermis
  - Level 2: Tumor in papillary dermis but not filling or expanding it
  - Level 3: Tumor fills and expands papillary dermis
  - Level 4: Tumor present in reticular dermis
  - Level 5: Tumor in subcutaneous fat
- Immunohistochemical stains are positive for Melan A, S100, HMB45

CLINICAL ISSUES

Presentation
- Most common signs/symptoms: Mass with irregular border and color variegation (blue, brown, black, red)

MELANOMA, VULVA

- Other signs/symptoms: Pruritus (persistent pruritus can be the earliest symptom of the disease), bleeding, discharge, burning, ulceration

Demographics
- Age: Peak incidence in the 5th-6th decade of life, the median age at diagnosis is 66 years

Natural History & Prognosis
- Local recurrence frequent; 5 year survival rate 37-54%
- Central lesions are associated with worse prognosis than lateral lesions (37% vs 61% 10-year survival rate) due to higher risk for groin nodal involvement and local recurrence
- Lesions on the labia minora with involvement of the urethra and vagina have a worse prognosis due to technical difficulty in achieving clear margins
- Most important prognostic factors are Breslow thickness, ulceration, evidence of regression, presence of a vertical growth phase, satellite lesions and lymphovascular space invasion
- 5 year survival for tumors greater than 1.5 mm deep is 20%, compared with 69% for tumors 1.5 mm or less deep
- Melanoma is one of the few tumors that can undergo spontaneous regression
- 90-100% of patients with inguinal node disease die of the disease
- TNM staging of the American Joint Committee for cancer
  - Stage 0 Tis N0 M0: Intraepithelial/in situ melanoma
  - Stage I
    - IA: T1a N0 M0: Melanoma ≤ 1 mm in thickness, Clark's level II or III, without ulceration
    - IB: T1b N0 M0: Melanoma ≤ 1 mm in thickness, Clark's level IV or V, with ulceration
    - IB: T2a N0 M0: Melanoma 1.01-2 mm in thickness without ulceration
  - Stage II
    - IIA: T2b N0 M0: Melanoma 1.01-2 mm in thickness with ulceration
    - IIA: T3a N0 M0: Melanoma 2.01-4 mm in thickness without ulceration
    - IIB: T3b N0 M0: Melanoma 2.01-4 mm in thickness with ulceration
    - IIB: T4a N0 M0: Melanoma > 4 mm in thickness without ulceration
    - IIC: T4b N0 M0: Melanoma > 4 mm in thickness with ulceration
  - Stage III
    - IIIA: T1-4a N1a M0: Single regional nodal microscopic metastasis without ulceration of primary lesion
    - IIIA: T1-4a N2a M0: 2-3 microscopic positive regional nodes without ulceration of primary lesion
    - IIIB: T1-4bN1a M0: Single regional nodal micrometastasis, with ulceration of primary lesion
    - IIIB: T1-4bN2a M0: 2-3 macroscopic regional nodes, with ulceration of primary lesion
    - IIIB: T1-4a N1b M0: Single regional nodal macrometastasis, without ulceration of primary lesion
    - IIIB: T1-4a N2b M0: 2-3 macroscopic regional nodes, without ulceration of primary lesion
    - IIIB: T1-4a/b N2c M0: Satellite or in-transit metastasis without metastatic lymph nodes or ulceration of primary lesion
    - IIIC: T1-4b N2a M0: Single macroscopic regional node, with ulceration of primary lesion
    - IIIC: T1-4b N2b M0: 2-3 macroscopic metastatic regional nodes, with ulceration of primary lesion
    - IIIC: Any T N3 M0: 4 or more metastatic nodes, matted nodes/gross extracapsular extension, or satellite or in-transit metastasis with metastatic lymph nodes
  - Stage IV
    - Any T any N M1a: Metastasis to skin, subcutaneous tissues, or distant lymph nodes
    - Any T any N M1b: Metastasis to lung
    - Any T any N M1c: Metastasis to all other visceral sites or distant metastasis at any site associated with an elevated serum LDH

Treatment
- Surgical resection with 1 cm margins for less than 1 mm thick tumor, and 2 cm margins for 1-4 mm thick tumor
- Local excision with tumor-free margins can be performed with unilateral sentinel lymph node evaluation
- Nodal dissection with adjuvant therapy with interferon alpha 2b is reserved for patients with lymph node metastasis
- Adjuvant treatment for advanced stage disease include chemotherapy, radiation and immunotherapy

DIAGNOSTIC CHECKLIST

Consider
- Diagnosis is usually made by physical examination and biopsy
- MR is used to estimate local extent of disease in order to guide surgery
- CECT of chest, abdomen and pelvis and MR of head for presumed stage IV disease

Image Interpretation Pearls
- High SI T1WI vulvar lesion, however amelanotic melanoma can be of low or intermediate SI on T1WI

SELECTED REFERENCES

1. Wechter ME et al: Vulvar melanoma: review of diagnosis, staging, and therapy. J Low Genit Tract Dis. 8(1):58-69, 2004
2. Takehara M et al: Imaging studies in patients with malignant melanoma in the female genital tract. Int J Gynecol Cancer. 12(5):506-9, 2002
3. Irvin WP Jr et al: Vulvar melanoma: a retrospective analysis and literature review. Gynecol Oncol. 83(3):457-65, 2001
4. DeMatos P et al: Mucosal melanoma of the female genitalia: a clinicopathologic study of forty-three cases at Duke University Medical Center. Surgery. 124(1):38-48, 1998
5. Raber G et al: Malignant melanoma of the vulva. Report of 89 patients. Cancer. 78(11):2353-8, 1996

MELANOMA, VULVA

IMAGE GALLERY

Typical

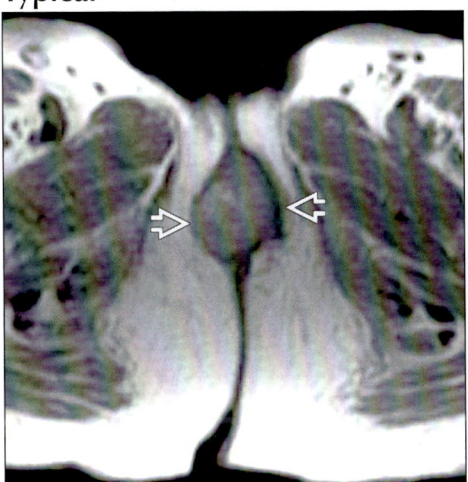
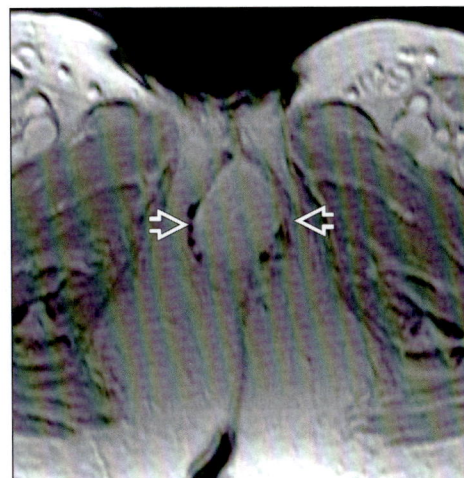

(Left) Axial T1WI MR shows a well-defined vulvar mass ➤ of high signal intensity consistent with paramagnetic effect of melanin. High signal intensity on T1WI is characteristic of melanocytic melanomas. *(Right)* Axial T1 C+ MR in the same patient as previous image shows avid, homogeneous contrast-enhancement following administration of gadolinium ➤. Pathology: Vulvar melanoma.

Typical

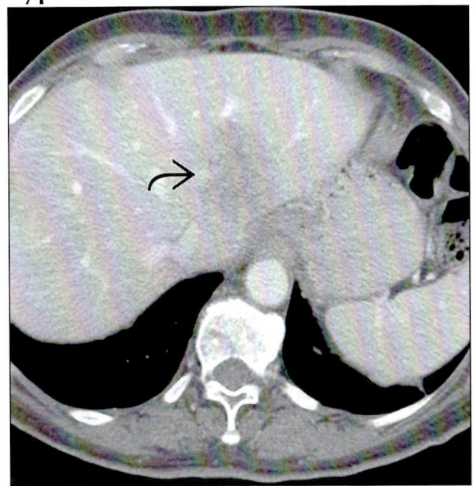
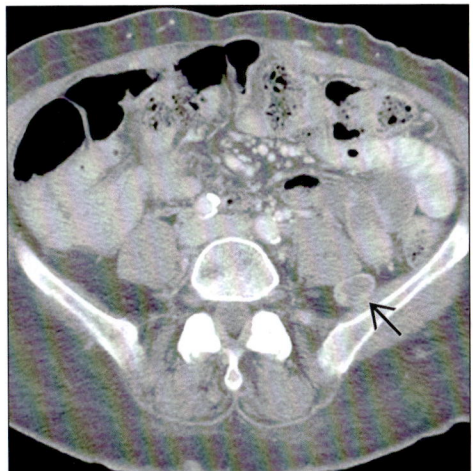

(Left) Axial CECT shows a large liver metastases ➤ in a patient with primary vulvar melanoma. *(Right)* Axial CECT in the same patient as previous image shows an enhancing soft tissue nodule ➤ just anterior to the left iliacus muscle representing another metastatic deposit.

Typical

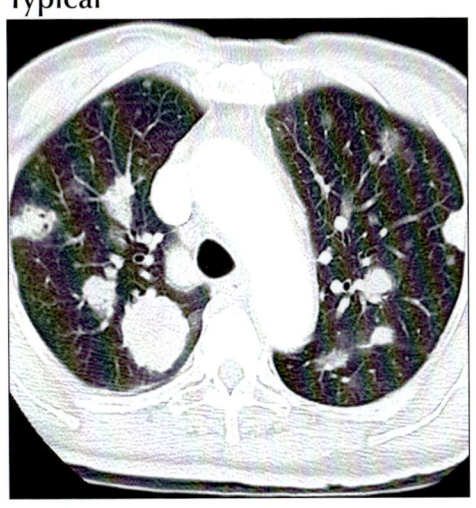
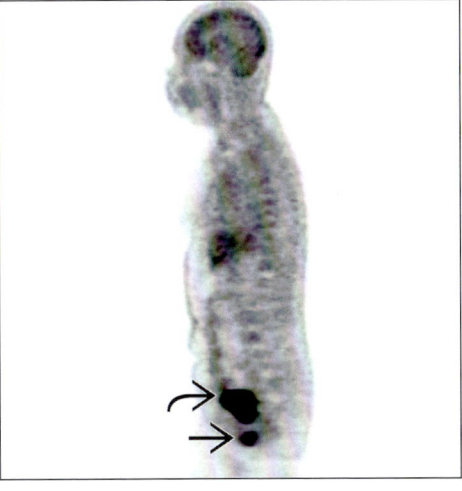

(Left) Axial CECT in the same patient as previous image shows multiple lung metastases from primary vulvar melanoma. *(Right)* Sagittal PET shows a focus of increased FDG uptake ➤ in the region of the vulva in a patient with primary vulvar melanoma. Note the presence of physiological FDG uptake within the bladder ➤.

AGGRESSIVE ANGIOMYXOMA, VULVA

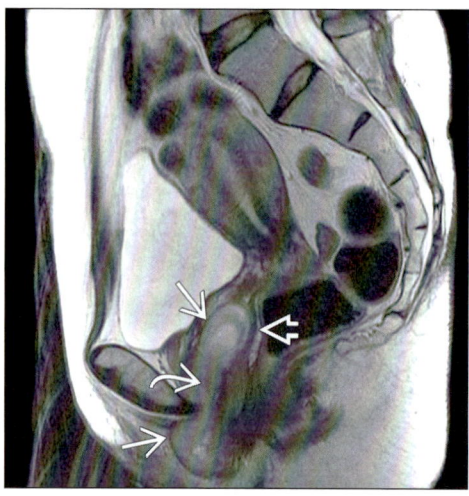

Sagittal T2WI MR shows a high signal intensity, soft tissue mass ➡ straddling the pelvic diaphragm. The mass is displacing the vagina posteriorly ➡. Note the presence of stretched fibromuscular bundles ➡.

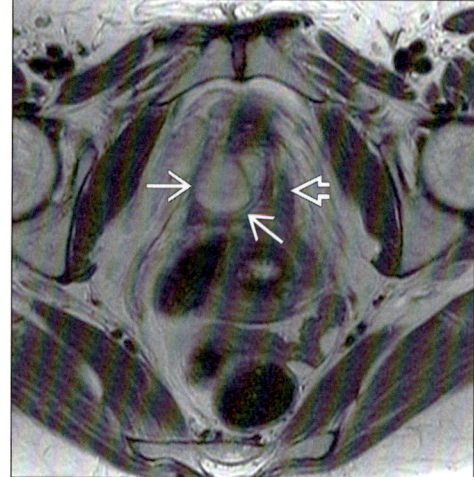

Axial oblique T2WI MR shows the intrapelvic component of the soft tissue mass ➡. Note the lateral displacement of the vagina ➡. Pathology: Aggressive angiomyxoma.

TERMINOLOGY

Abbreviations and Synonyms
- Aggressive angiomyxoma (AAM)

Definitions
- Benign mesenchymal tumor arising from connective tissues of perineum or lower pelvis, predominantly in women
  - Very rarely arises directly from any pelvic or perineal viscus
  - Tumor is not usually diagnosed before surgery and its anatomical extent is frequently not perceived

IMAGING FINDINGS

General Features
- Best diagnostic clue: Large soft tissue mass displaying unusual growth pattern of translevator extension with growth around perineal structures
- Location
  - Pelvis and perineum
    - Vulva
    - Extension to retroperitoneum
    - Extension to gluteal/thigh/inguinal region
- Size
  - Large, slow growing tumor
    - Can grow to large size
- Morphology
  - Well-defined
    - Poorly encapsulated
    - Gelatinous
  - Tendency to deviate rather than infiltrate local structures such as vagina, urethra, bladder and rectum
    - Can infiltrate local structures (very rare)

Ultrasonographic Findings
- Hypoechoic mass
- Can appear completely cystic

CT Findings
- NECT
  - Well-defined mass
  - Soft tissue attenuation less than muscle
    - May appear partly cystic
  - Deviation rather than infiltration of local structures
  - May demonstrate infiltration (very rare)

DDx: Pelvis/Perineal Masses

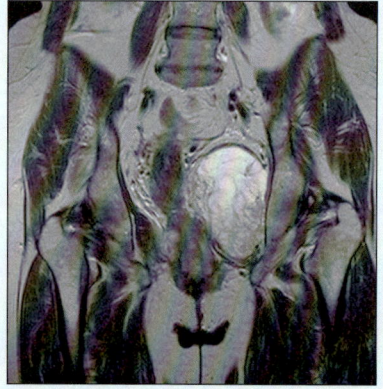

Hemangiopericytoma

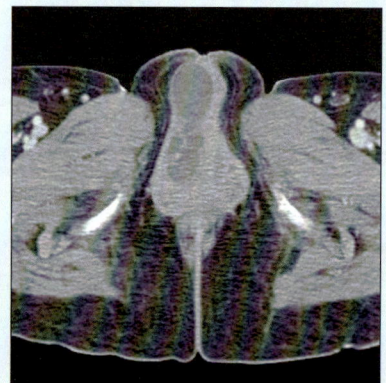

Bartholinitis

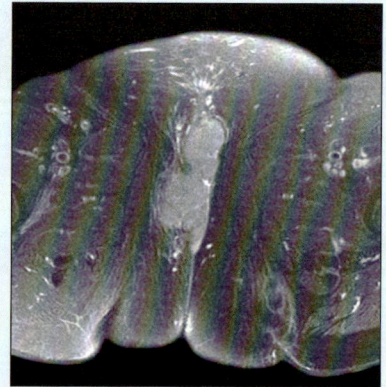

Vulval Carcinoma

AGGRESSIVE ANGIOMYXOMA, VULVA

Key Facts

Terminology
- Benign mesenchymal tumor arising from connective tissues of perineum or lower pelvis, predominantly in women
- Tumor is not usually diagnosed before surgery and its anatomical extent is frequently not perceived

Imaging Findings
- Very high signal intensity relative to muscle, related to loose myxoid matrix and high water content of the tumor
- "Swirled" low intensity bands or layered strands within very high intensity tumor
- "Swirled" enhancing bands or layered tissue within the tumor representing strands of fibrovascular tissue
- Best imaging tool: MR to determine the extent of the primary or recurrent tumor

Top Differential Diagnoses
- Hemangiopericytoma
- Bartholinitis
- Vulval Carcinoma

Pathology
- Tumor tends to grow around structures of pelvic floor without penetrating muscularis layer of vagina or rectum
- Mesenchymal stellate and spindle-shaped neoplastic cells embedded in collagenous and hyaluronic acid containing stroma with loose myxoid background

Diagnostic Checklist
- Large, relatively benign-looking mass with myxoid signal characteristics on MR and typical "swirling" pattern following intravenous contrast medium

---

- Fat planes are usually well-preserved
- Bone involvement can occur
  - Usually lytic
  - May have soft tissue component
- CECT
  - Heterogeneous IV contrast medium enhancement
  - Characteristic "swirling" internal architecture

MR Findings
- T1WI
  - Isointense to muscle
    - Less commonly hypointense
  - Relatively homogeneous
- T2WI
  - Very high signal intensity relative to muscle, related to loose myxoid matrix and high water content of the tumor
  - Relatively homogeneous
  - "Swirled" low intensity bands or layered strands within very high intensity tumor
- STIR: High signal intensity relative to muscle
- T1 C+
  - Avid heterogeneous contrast medium enhancement
  - "Swirled" enhancing bands or layered tissue within the tumor representing strands of fibrovascular tissue
    - This appearance may relate to presence of bands of fibromuscular stroma that are stretched as they protrude through the pelvic diaphragm

Angiographic Findings
- Highly vascular mass
  - Internal iliac artery supply

Other Modality Findings
- Intravenous urogram
  - Extrinsic pelvic mass
  - Deviation of bladder/ureters
  - Outflow/ureteric compression unusual

Imaging Recommendations
- Best imaging tool: MR to determine the extent of the primary or recurrent tumor
- Protocol advice
  - Multiplanar MR of the pelvis with dynamic contrast-enhancement
    - Multiple orthogonal planes are crucial to establish if tumor traverses pelvic diaphragm, essential for surgical planning and complete excision

DIFFERENTIAL DIAGNOSIS

Hemangiopericytoma
- Large expansile lobulated mass with frequent bleeding due to hypervascular nature
- Prominent serpentine intratumoral vessels
- Speckled calcifications if present are best seen on CT

Bartholinitis
- Can be clinically indistinguishable as AAM usually presents with labial swelling and Bartholinitis-like clinical features
- Thick-walled cystic mass with rim-enhancement and infiltrative changes in adjacent fat suggestive of inflammation

Vulval Carcinoma
- Soft tissue mass that invades rather than displaces the adjacent structures
- Intermediate to high SI rather than very high SI on T2WI MR
- No characteristic "swirling" pattern on CECT or MR
- Enlarged inguinal lymph nodes may be seen at presentation

Vulval Angiomyofibroblastoma
- This tends to be smaller (typically < 5 cm)
- Usually involves superficial parts of vulva unlike AAM

PATHOLOGY

General Features
- Epidemiology
  - Predominantly Caucasian

AGGRESSIVE ANGIOMYXOMA, VULVA

- Has been seen in other races

Gross Pathologic & Surgical Features
- Well-defined, lobular, gelatinous/rubbery mass
  - Can appear grayish/blue
  - May have an infiltrative edge
- Deep pelvic planes usually involved
- Tumor tends to grow around structures of pelvic floor without penetrating muscularis layer of vagina or rectum

Microscopic Features
- Mesenchymal stellate and spindle-shaped neoplastic cells embedded in collagenous and hyaluronic acid containing stroma with loose myxoid background
- Ultrastructurally resemble fibroblasts
- Hemorrhage and cysts are not a feature
- Thick-walled small vessels
- Nuclear atypia and mitosis absent
- Immunohistochemistry positive for vimentin but not desmin or myosin
- Can be estrogen and progesterone receptor positive

CLINICAL ISSUES

Presentation
- Most common signs/symptoms: Labial swelling with Bartholinitis-like clinical picture
- Other signs/symptoms
  - Genitourinary disturbance due to pressure effects (rare)
  - Bowel disturbance (rare)
  - Pain (rare)
- Imaging frequently occurs after clinical suspicion that the tumor represents lipoma, Bartholin cyst or hernia
- Pre-operative histological diagnosis can be difficult
  - Biopsy yield low
  - Often non diagnostic myxoid tissue
  - Usually requires surgical specimen

Demographics
- Age
  - Second to eighth decade
    - Most commonly second to fourth decade
- Gender: 90% female
- Ethnicity: Usually Caucasian

Natural History & Prognosis
- Slow growing with displacement rather than invasion of adjacent structures
- No distant metastasis
- High local recurrence rate of 36-72%
  - Usually due to inadequate surgical resection because of initial clinical misdiagnosis

Treatment
- Surgical resection
  - Due to risk of recurrence surgical planning critical (multidisciplinary approach)
  - Re-do surgery if inadequate initial clearance due to misdiagnosis
- Hormonal treatment with GnRH analogue
- Watchful waiting

DIAGNOSTIC CHECKLIST

Consider
- AAM in a young female patient with a large vulval mass which straddles across the pelvic diaphragm

Image Interpretation Pearls
- Large, relatively benign-looking mass with myxoid signal characteristics on MR and typical "swirling" pattern following intravenous contrast medium

SELECTED REFERENCES

1. Varras M et al: Aggressive angiomyxoma of the vulva: our experience of a rare case with review of the literature. Eur J Gynaecol Oncol. 27(2):188-92, 2006
2. Abu JI et al: Aggressive angiomyxoma of the perineum. Int J Gynecol Cancer. 15(6):1097-100, 2005
3. Alobaid A et al: Aggressive angiomyxoma of the vulva or perineum: report of three patients. J Obstet Gynaecol Can. 27(11):1023-6, 2005
4. Dragoumis K et al: Aggressive angiomyxoma of the vulva extending into the pelvis: report of two cases. J Obstet Gynaecol Res. 31(4):310-3, 2005
5. Gungor T et al: Aggressive angiomyxoma of the vulva and vagina. A common problem: misdiagnosis. Eur J Obstet Gynecol Reprod Biol. 112(1):114-6, 2004
6. Ribaldone R et al: Aggressive angiomyxoma of the vulva. Gynecol Oncol. 95(3):724-8, 2004
7. Behranwala KA et al: 'Aggressive' angiomyxoma: a distinct clinical entity. Eur J Surg Oncol. 29(7):559-63, 2003
8. Jeyadevan NN et al: Imaging features of aggressive angiomyxoma. Clin Radiol. 58(2):157-62, 2003
9. Fine BA et al: Primary medical management of recurrent aggressive angiomyxoma of the vulva with a gonadotropin-releasing hormone agonist. Gynecol Oncol. 81(1):120-2, 2001
10. Nielsen GP et al: Mesenchymal tumors and tumor-like lesions of the female genital tract: a selective review with emphasis on recently described entities. Int J Gynecol Pathol. 20(2):105-27, 2001
11. Bigotti G et al: Angiomyofibroblastoma and aggressive angiomyxoma: two benign mesenchymal neoplasms of the female genital tract. An immunohistochemical study. Pathol Res Pract. 195(1):39-44, 1999
12. Kehagias D et al: MR appearance of pelvic hemangiopericytoma. Eur Radiol. 9(1):163-5, 1999
13. Outwater EK et al: Aggressive angiomyxoma: findings on CT and MR imaging. AJR Am J Roentgenol. 172(2):435-8, 1999
14. Chien AJ et al: Aggressive angiomyxoma of the female pelvis: sonographic, CT, and MR findings. AJR Am J Roentgenol. 171(2):530-1, 1998
15. Davani M et al: Aggressive angiomyxoma of pelvic soft tissues: MR imaging appearance. AJR Am J Roentgenol. 170(4):1113-4, 1998
16. Abdel-Nabi AG et al: Aggressive angiomyxoma of the vulva. J Obstet Gynaecol. 17(3):317, 1997
17. Fetsch JF et al: Aggressive angiomyxoma: a clinicopathologic study of 29 female patients. Cancer. 78(1):79-90, 1996
18. Elchalal U et al: Aggressive angiomyxoma of the vulva. Gynecol Oncol. 47(2):260-2, 1992
19. Fletcher CD et al: Angiomyofibroblastoma of the vulva. A benign neoplasm distinct from aggressive angiomyxoma. Am J Surg Pathol. 16(4):373-82, 1992

AGGRESSIVE ANGIOMYXOMA, VULVA

IMAGE GALLERY

Typical

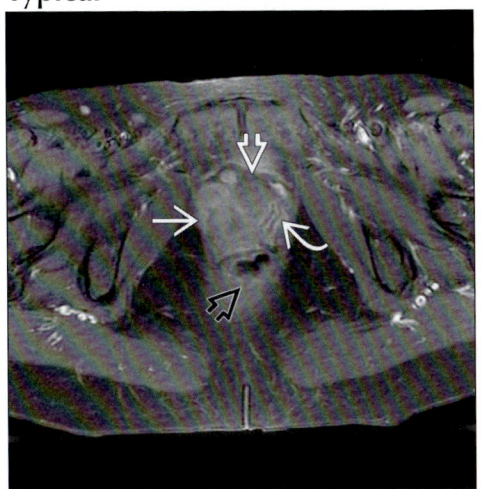 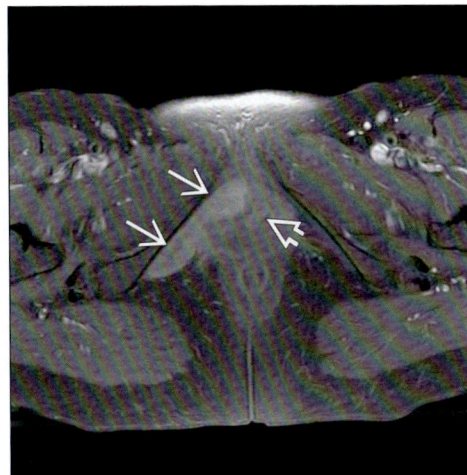

(Left) Axial T1 C+ FS MR shows an enhancing soft tissue mass ➡ encircling the urethra ➡ and displacing the rectum posteriorly ➡. Note presence of "swirled" enhancing bands within the tumor ➡. *(Right)* Axial T1 C+ FS MR demonstrates translevator extension of the tumor ➡. Tumor is causing displacement of the urethra ➡ posteriorly and to the left.

Typical

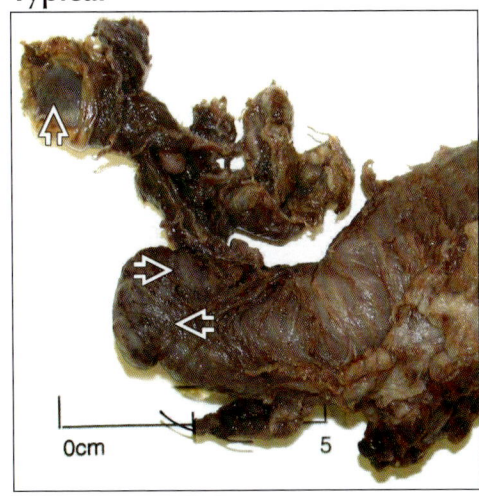 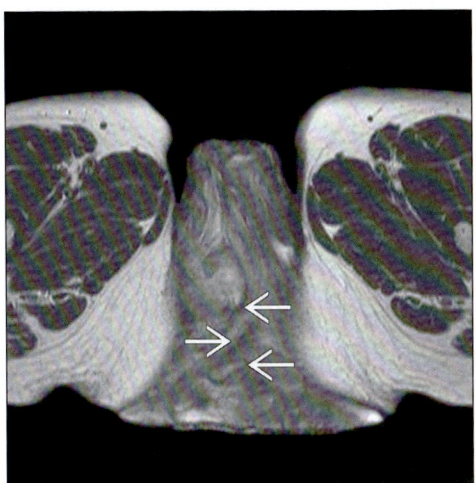

(Left) Gross pathology shows the surgical specimen (same case as previous image). Multiple areas of dark blue color ➡ represent extensive vascularity of the tumor. Pathology: Aggressive angiomyxoma. *(Right)* Axial T2WI MR shows a typical case of aggressive angiomyxoma originating from the perineum in a 35 year old female patient. Note presence of typical low-signal intensity bands within the tumor ➡.

Typical

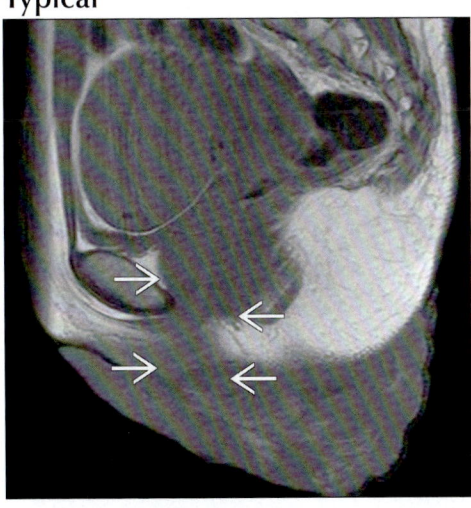 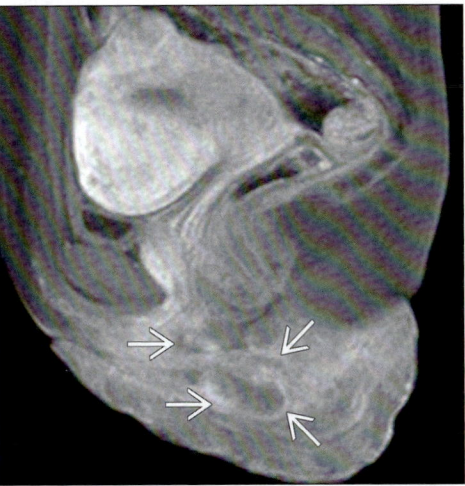

(Left) Sagittal T1WI MR (same patient as previous image) shows a large mass of homogeneous low signal intensity ➡ traversing the pelvic diaphragm. *(Right)* Sagittal T1 C+ FS MR confirms the translevator extension of the mass. Note multiple areas of "swirled" enhancing bands ➡ characteristic of aggressive angiomyxoma. Pathology: Aggressive angiomyxoma.

LYMPHOMA, VULVA

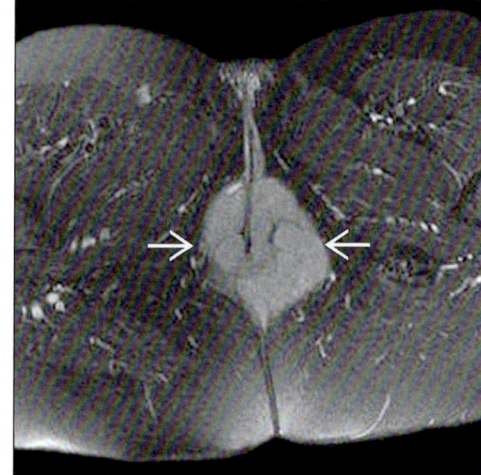

Axial T1WI MR shows a vulval mass ➡ of signal intensity isointense to muscle. No enlarged lymph nodes were present.

Axial T2WI FS MR confirms the presence of a vulval mass of homogeneous high signal intensity ➡. Pathology: Primary vulval lymphoma.

TERMINOLOGY

Definitions
- Non-Hodgkin lymphoma (NHL) of vulva with or without evidence of other sites of involvement at presentation

IMAGING FINDINGS

General Features
- Best diagnostic clue: Homogeneous vulva mass with moderate contrast medium enhancement
- Location
  - Initial vulval involvement occurs only in 4% of patients with primary NHL of the female genital tract
  - When the mass involves both vagina and vulva it can be impossible to establish the origin
- Morphology: Uniform density due to densely packed cells

Ultrasonographic Findings
- No role in evaluation of the vulva lesion
- Useful in guiding lymph node biopsy in cases of secondary involvement by lymphoma

CT Findings
- Homogeneously enhancing soft tissue mass
- May appear as thickening of the vulva rather than a discrete mass
- Enlarged lymph nodes and evidence of other sites of involvement in cases of secondary involvement by lymphoma

MR Findings
- T1WI
  - Mass isointense to muscle
  - Enlarged lymph nodes in cases of secondary involvement by lymphoma
- T2WI: High signal intensity relative to muscle
- T1 C+: Homogeneous enhancement

Nuclear Medicine Findings
- PET/CT
  - Avid FDG uptake in primary tumor and lymph nodes (in case of secondary vulval involvement)

DDx: Vulval Masses

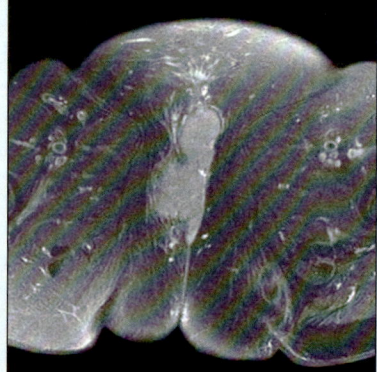
Vulval Carcinoma

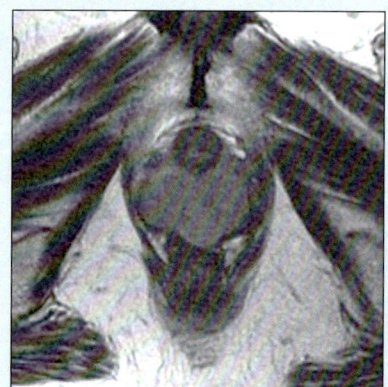
Vulval Melanoma

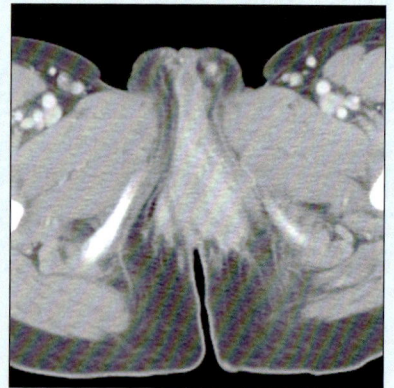
Vulval Hemangioma

LYMPHOMA, VULVA

Key Facts

Terminology
- Non-Hodgkin lymphoma (NHL) of vulva with or without evidence of other sites of involvement at presentation

Imaging Findings
- When the mass involves both vagina and vulva it can be impossible to establish the origin
- MR for evaluation of primary tumor
- CECT and PET/CT for complete lymphoma staging

Top Differential Diagnoses
- Vulval Carcinoma
- Vulva Melanoma
- Vulva Hemangioma

Diagnostic Checklist
- Both primary and secondary vulva lymphoma are treated with chemo/radiotherapy, thus differentiation from other vulval lesions is crucial

Imaging Recommendations
- Best imaging tool
  - MR for evaluation of primary tumor
  - CECT and PET/CT for complete lymphoma staging

DIFFERENTIAL DIAGNOSIS

Vulval Carcinoma
- Irregular, invasive solid mass with spread to the regional lymph nodes

Vulva Melanoma
- Typical high SI on T1WI

Vulva Hemangioma
- Marked enhancement and presence of phleboliths

PATHOLOGY

General Features
- Etiology: May occur as a consequence of immunosuppression or HIV infection

Microscopic Features
- Sheets of malignant cells, the degree of pleomorphism depends on the type of lymphoma
- Two thirds are diffuse large B cell lymphoma
- Immunohistochemical stains are positive for CD45 (lymphoid marker), CD 20 & CD 79a (B cell markers), CD 3 (T cell marker)

CLINICAL ISSUES

Natural History & Prognosis
- Aggressive disease with very poor prognosis

Treatment
- Combination of chemotherapy and radiotherapy

DIAGNOSTIC CHECKLIST

Consider
- Both primary and secondary vulva lymphoma are treated with chemo/radiotherapy, thus differentiation from other vulval lesions is crucial

Image Interpretation Pearls
- Tumor homogeneity
- Presence of other sites of involvement in case of secondary vulva lymphoma

SELECTED REFERENCES
1. Lagoo AS et al: Lymphoma of the female genital tract: current status. Int J Gynecol Pathol. 25(1):1-21, 2006
2. Vang R et al: Non-Hodgkin's lymphoma involving the vulva. Int J Gynecol Pathol. 19(3):236-42, 2000
3. Kaplan EJ et al: HIV-related primary non-Hodgkin's lymphoma of the vulva. Gynecol Oncol. 61(1):131-8, 1996

IMAGE GALLERY

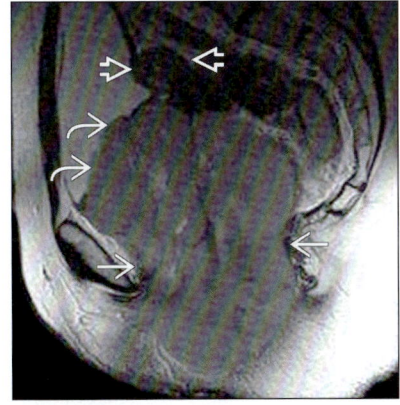
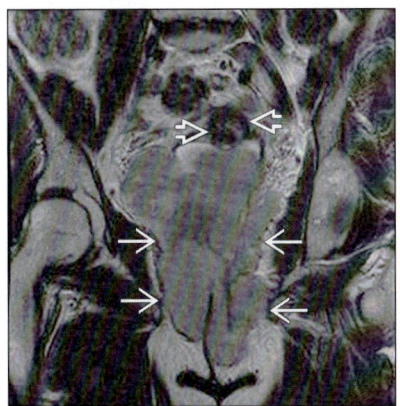
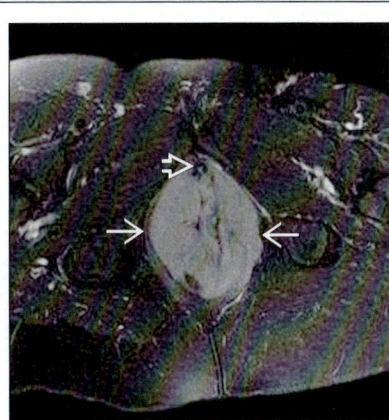

(Left) Sagittal T2WI MR shows a large mass ➡ of relatively high signal intensity centered in the vulva/vagina. The mass invades the posterior bladder wall ➡. The uterus ➡ appears intact. (Center) Coronal T2WI MR shows the presence of the vulva/vaginal mass ➡ in the same patient. Note preservation of the normal cervix ➡. (Right) Axial T2WI FS MR confirms the presence of high signal intensity vulval mass ➡. Tumor is inseparable from urethra ➡. No enlarged lymph nodes were present. Pathology: Primary lymphoma of the vulva/vagina.

MERKEL CELL TUMOR, VULVA

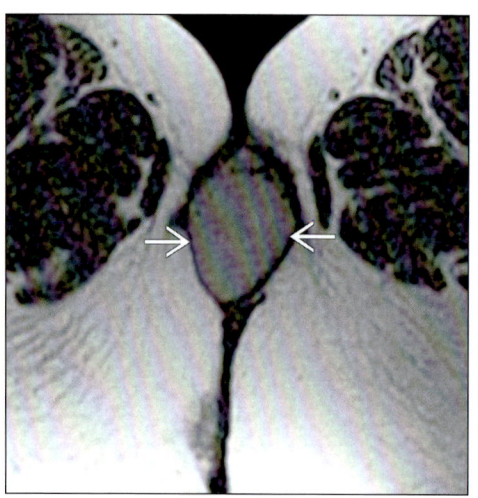

Axial T2WI MR shows Merkel cell tumor ➡ that is intermediate signal intensity in the vulva.

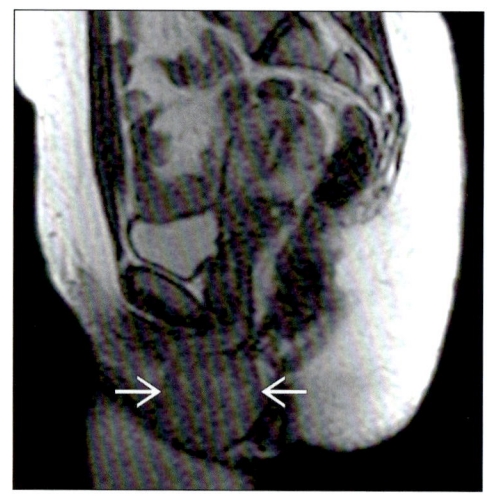

Sagittal T2WI MR shows intermediate signal intensity mass ➡ in the vulva.

TERMINOLOGY

Abbreviations and Synonyms
- Trabecular carcinoma, endocrine carcinoma, primary cutaneous neuroendocrine carcinoma

Definitions
- Malignant cutaneous neoplasm arising from Merkel cells in basal layer of the epidermis

IMAGING FINDINGS

General Features
- Best diagnostic clue: Relatively homogeneous cutaneous soft tissue masses
- Location
  - Merkel cell tumors commonly arise in the skin of face, scalp, extremities, and buttocks
  - In vulva it most commonly originates from labia majora
- Size: Ranges from 1.5-9 cm

CT Findings
- CECT: Enhancing cutaneous masses

MR Findings
- T1WI: Low signal intensity
- T2WI: Slightly hyperintense relative to muscle
- T1 C+: Moderate enhancement

Imaging Recommendations
- Best imaging tool
  - MR is method of choice for the evaluation of local extent of tumor
  - CT is performed to exclude metastatic disease

DIFFERENTIAL DIAGNOSIS

Vulvar Carcinoma
- Appears as solid mass frequently associated with inguinal or pelvic adenopathy

Vulvar Melanoma
- May demonstrate high signal intensity on T1WI

DDx: Vulvar Masses

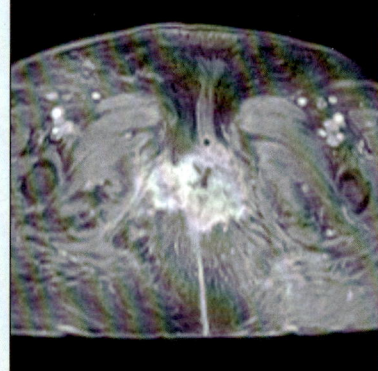

Vulvar Cancer

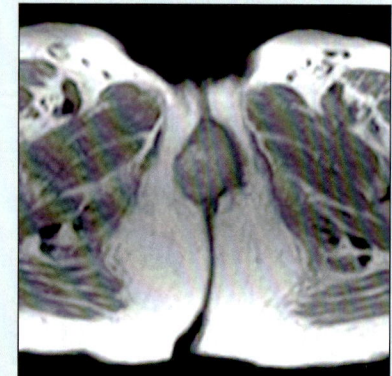

Melanoma

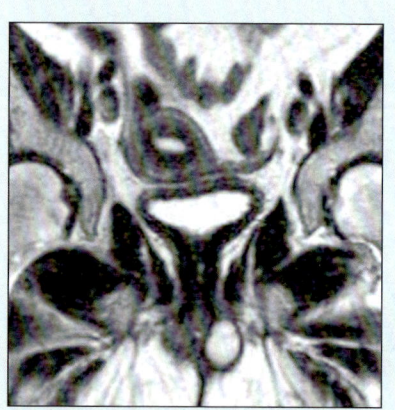

Bartholin Cyst

MERKEL CELL TUMOR, VULVA

Key Facts

Terminology
- Malignant cutaneous neoplasm arising from Merkel cells in basal layer of the epidermis

Imaging Findings
- In vulva it most commonly originates from labia majora
- MR is method of choice for the evaluation of local extent of tumor
- CT is performed to exclude metastatic disease

Clinical Issues
- Painless sessile vulvar mass, vulvar irritation and discharge
- Merkel cell carcinoma of the vulva pursues more aggressive clinical behavior than Merkel cell tumor at other locations
- Local recurrence and metastasis to lymph nodes, lungs, liver and bones are common

Bartholin Cyst
- Cystic lesion in vulva

PATHOLOGY

General Features
- General path comments: Main differences between carcinoid tumor and Merkel cell tumor (both of which are neuroendocrine neoplasms) are that in carcinoid tumor there is no necrosis or atypia and mitotic activity is low

Gross Pathologic & Surgical Features
- Gray-white rubbery mass that involves skin and subcutaneous tissue
- Areas of hemorrhage, superficial skin ulcerations and irregular infiltrative margins are typical

Microscopic Features
- Small round or cubic oat-like cells with hyperchromatic nuclei and a small amount of cytoplasm
- Clusters of tumor cells form tubules or rosettes with a distinct trabecular pattern

CLINICAL ISSUES

Presentation
- Most common signs/symptoms
  - Painless sessile vulvar mass, vulvar irritation and discharge
  - Mass can involve or originate from Bartholin gland and may mimic Bartholin abscess or cyst
- Other signs/symptoms: Malaise, fatigue and other signs of systemic manifestation are seen in cases of advanced disease

Natural History & Prognosis
- Fatality rate approaches 100%
- Merkel cell carcinoma of the vulva pursues more aggressive clinical behavior than Merkel cell tumor at other locations
- Local recurrence and metastasis to lymph nodes, lungs, liver and bones are common

Treatment
- Surgery: Vulvectomy and lymphadenectomy
- Chemotherapy: For disseminated disease
- Adjuvant radiotherapy is beneficial for pelvic lymph nodes and local recurrences

SELECTED REFERENCES
1. Khoury-Collado F et al: Merkel cell carcinoma of the Bartholin's gland. Gynecol Oncol. 97(3):928-31, 2005
2. Hierro I et al: Merkel cell (neuroendocrine) carcinoma of the vulva. A case report with immunohistochemical and ultrastructural findings and review of the literature. Pathol Res Pract. 196(7):503-9, 2000
3. Fawzi HW et al: Neuroendocrine (Merkel cell) carcinoma of the vulva. J Obstet Gynaecol. 17(1):100-1, 1997

IMAGE GALLERY

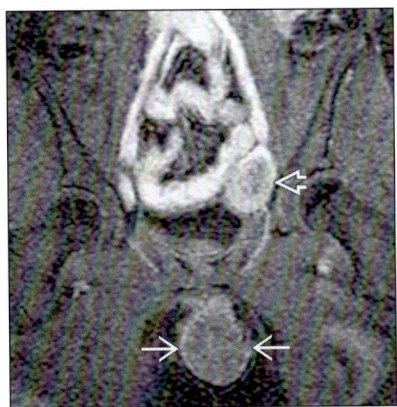 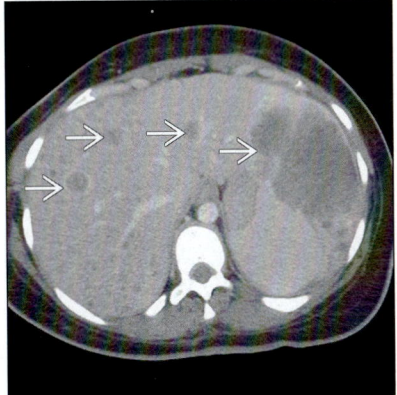 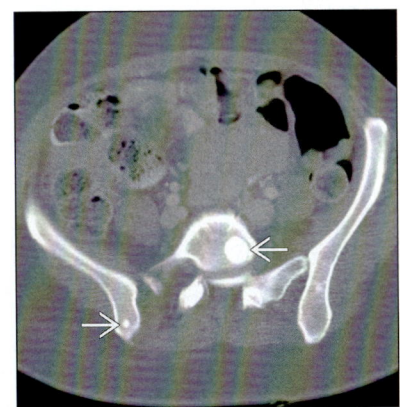

(Left) Coronal T1 C+ FS MR shows enhancing vulvar mass ➔ and left external iliac lymphadenopathy ➔. (Center) Axial CECT shows multiple metastases ➔ in the liver. (Right) Axial CECT shows bone metastases ➔.

HEMANGIOMA, VULVA

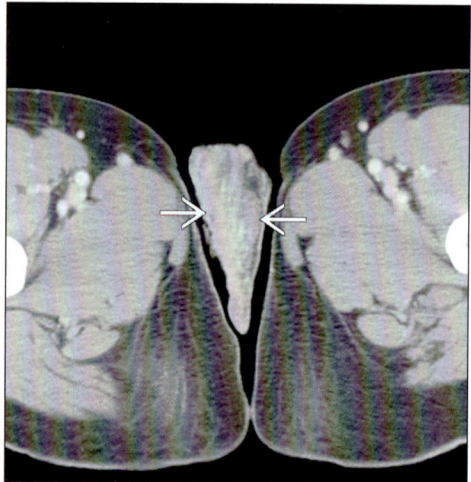

Axial CECT shows a vulvar hemangioma ➡ that enhances markedly.

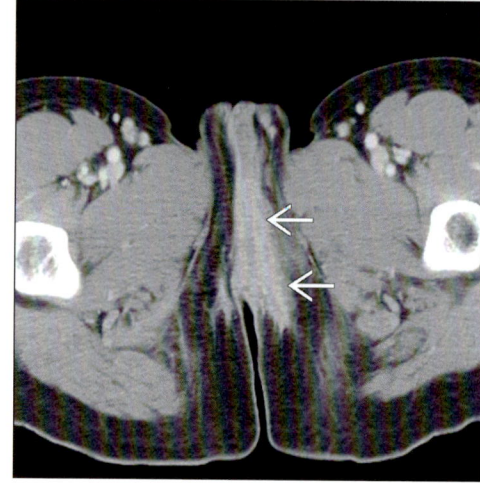

Axial CECT shows that the vulvar hemangioma ➡ extends to perineum.

IMAGING FINDINGS

General Features
- Best diagnostic clue: Lobulated, enhancing mass containing linear fatty deposits and phlebolith(s)
- Location: Vulvar hemangiomas often involve labia majora, posterior commissure and clitoris
- Size: Varies from small lesions to several centimeters

Ultrasonographic Findings
- Grayscale Ultrasound
  - Seen as complex masses
  - Phleboliths may cause acoustic shadowing
- Color Doppler: Evaluation may show low-resistance arterial flow with forward flow during both systole and diastole

CT Findings
- Hemangiomas show intense enhancement
- Phleboliths in the hemangioma can be seen

MR Findings
- T1WI
  - Hemangiomas usually demonstrate intermediate signal intensity between that of muscle and fat
  - Fatty septa between lobules of mass may be seen
- T2WI
  - Hemangiomas have extensive areas of heterogeneous multiple high signal intensity lobules
  - Central low signal areas in mass may be due to thrombi or flow
- T1 C+: Demonstrate extensive enhancement

Imaging Recommendations
- Best imaging tool: MR is most useful to characterize and determine anatomic extent due to superior contrast resolution

DIFFERENTIAL DIAGNOSIS

Vulvar Cancer
- Soft tissue mass in the vulva with necrosis, ulceration or lymphadenopathy

Plexiform Neurofibroma
- Occurs in neurofibromatosis I
- May demonstrate "target sign" on T2WI, with central low signal that enhances with gadolinium, unlike in hemangioma

DDx: Vulvar Masses

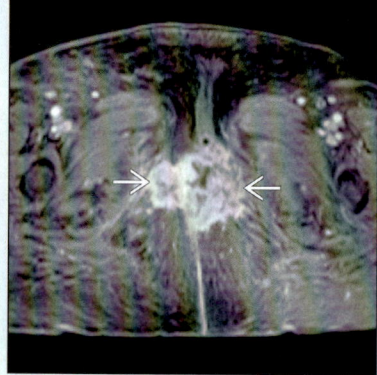

Vulvar Cancer

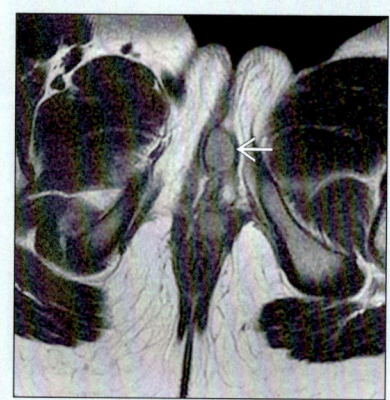

Neurofibroma

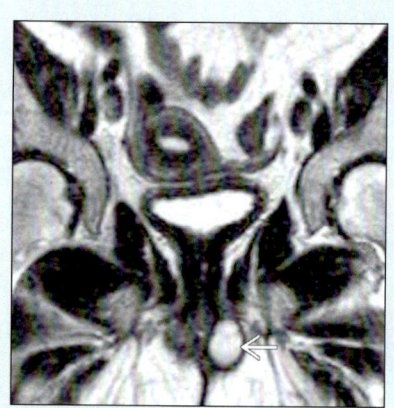

Bartholin Cyst

HEMANGIOMA, VULVA

Key Facts

Imaging Findings
- Best diagnostic clue: Lobulated, enhancing mass containing linear fatty deposits and phlebolith(s)
- Location: Vulvar hemangiomas often involve labia majora, posterior commissure and clitoris
- Size: Varies from small lesions to several centimeters
- Best imaging tool: MR is most useful to characterize and determine anatomic extent due to superior contrast resolution

Pathology
- General path comments: Benign tumor resembling normal vessels
- Hemangiomas are seen as red-blue spongy masses
- Dilated, blood-filled cystic spaces lined by flattened endothelium

Vulvar Endometriosis
- Dark red, brown or bluish papules usually located on the posterior fourchette
- Believed to be a result of surgical implantation during gynecologic surgery such as episiotomy

Bartholin Cyst
- Cystic dilatation of Bartholin gland

PATHOLOGY

General Features
- General path comments: Benign tumor resembling normal vessels

Gross Pathologic & Surgical Features
- Hemangiomas are seen as red-blue spongy masses

Microscopic Features
- Dilated, blood-filled cystic spaces lined by flattened endothelium

CLINICAL ISSUES

Presentation
- Most common signs/symptoms
  - Painless, bluish soft tissue mass in the vulva
  - Occasionally ulcerations and bleeding may be seen
  - Hemangiomas may increase in size as a result of infection, trauma or hormonal influence (menses, pregnancy)

Natural History & Prognosis
- Massive hemangiomas with extensive involvement of vulva and vagina may create a risk obstruction and bleeding during labor and delivery

Treatment
- None required if asymptomatic
- Laser therapy, embolotherapy, sclerotherapy, or surgical resection may relieve symptoms

SELECTED REFERENCES

1. Bava GL et al: Life-threatening hemorrhage from a vulvar hemangioma. J Pediatr Surg. 37(4):E6, 2002
2. Lazarou G et al: Vulvar arteriovenous hemangioma. A case report. J Reprod Med. 45(5):439-41, 2000
3. Kempinaire A et al: Capillary-venous malformation in the labia majora in a 12-year-old girl. Dermatology. 194(4):405-7, 1997
4. Tjaden BL et al: Vulvar congenital dysplastic angiopathy. Obstet Gynecol. 75(3 Pt 2):552-4, 1990
5. O'Neal MF et al: MR demonstration of extensive pelvic involvement in vulvar hemangiomas. J Comput Assist Tomogr. 12(2):219-21, 1988

IMAGE GALLERY

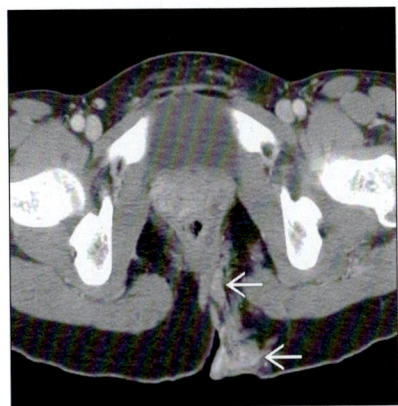 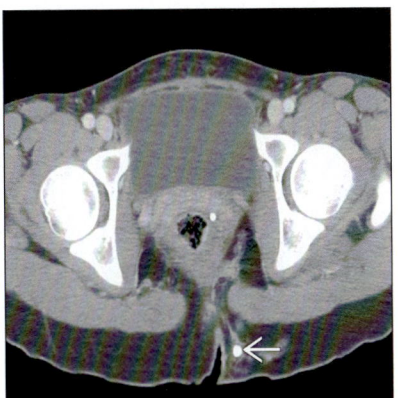 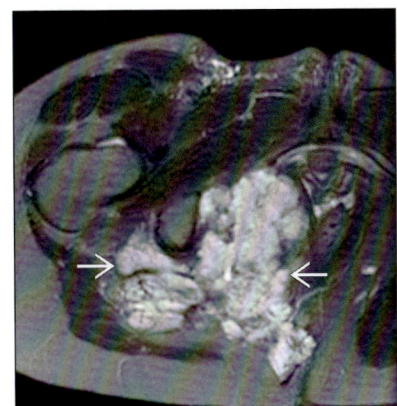

(Left) Axial CECT shows markedly enhancing hemangioma ➡ extending to gluteal region. *(Center)* Axial CECT shows a phlebolith ➡ in the superior aspect of the hemangioma. *(Right)* Axial T2WI FS MR shows a lobulated high signal intensity hemangioma ➡ in the right pelvis.

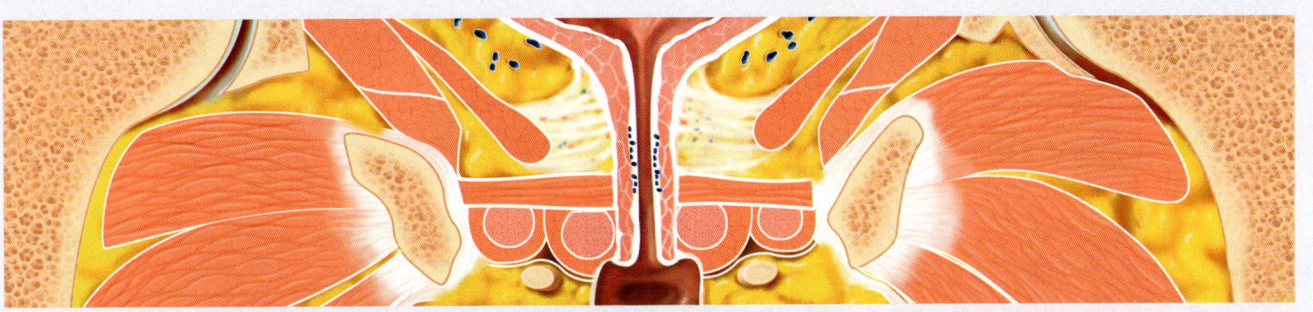

SECTION 6: Urethra

Introduction and Overview
Urethral Anatomy & Imaging Issues   6-2

Neoplasm, Benign
Leiomyoma, Urethra   6-6
Schwannoma, Urethra   6-8

Neoplasm, Malignant
Carcinoma, Urethra   6-10
Metastasis, Urethra   6-14

Miscellaneous
Diverticulum, Urethra   6-18
Prolapse, Urethra   6-22

URETHRAL ANATOMY & IMAGING ISSUES

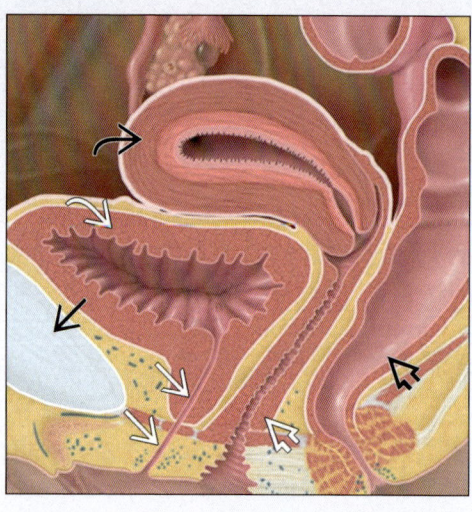

Sagittal graphic shows urethra ➡, bladder ➡, vagina ➡, rectum ➡, uterus ➡, and symphysis pubis ➡.

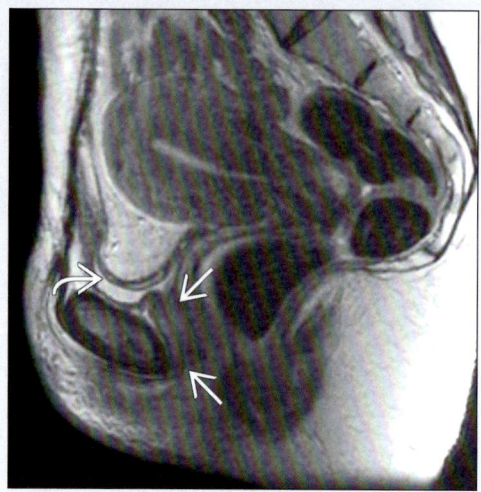

Sagittal T2WI MR shows female urethra ➡. Note bladder ➡ is not distended.

TERMINOLOGY

Definitions
- Female urethra is a tubular conduit that courses between internal urethral meatus and external urethral meatus

IMAGING ANATOMY

General Anatomic Considerations
- Female urethra is about 4 cm in length
- It is about 6 mm in diameter when not dilated
- Mucous membrane of female urethra is continuous distally with that of vulva and proximally with that of bladder
  - Proximal one-third of urethra is lined by transitional epithelium
  - Distal two-thirds is lined by stratified squamous epithelium
- Urethra contains two layers of smooth muscle
  - Inner layer of smooth muscle is longitudinal
  - Thinner outer layer of smooth muscle is circular
- Outer portion of urethra is composed of striated muscle
- Striated muscle sphincter at the orifice reinforces two concentric layers of smooth muscle
- Paraurethral glands of Skene drain into urethra
- Urethropelvic ligaments support urethra

Critical Anatomic Structures
- Female urethra is posterior to symphysis pubis and anterior to vagina

Anatomic Relationships
- Female urethra courses obliquely, caudally and anteriorly
- It perforates urogenital diaphragm and opens in front of vaginal opening and behind glans clitoridis

PATHOLOGIC ISSUES

General Pathologic Considerations
- Urethral diverticulum
  - Most commonly on posterolateral wall of midurethra
  - It is important to determine number, location, size, neck and content of diverticula on imaging
  - Complications of urethral diverticulum include
    - Infection
    - Hemorrhage
    - Stone formation
    - Development of malignancy
- Urethral neoplasm
  - Benign tumors such as leiomyoma, schwannoma, nephrogenic adenoma
  - Primary malignant tumors such as squamous cell carcinoma, transitional cell carcinoma, adenocarcinoma
  - Secondary malignant tumors
    - Most commonly by contiguous extension of malignancy from adjacent organs
    - Less commonly hematogenous spread
- Periurethral cysts
  - Vaginal cysts: Müllerian cyst, Gartner duct cyst, epidermal inclusion cyst
  - Skene duct cysts
  - Bartholin gland cysts
- Urinary anomalies
  - Ectopic ureters and ureteroceles may drain in or around urethra
- Urinary incontinence
  - Female urethra and its supporting structures work in combination to maintain urinary continence
  - Cause of incontinence is usually multifactorial
  - Simultaneous functional and morphologic assessment is necessary for correct diagnosis
- Urethral strictures and fistulas
  - Post-traumatic
  - Infectious/inflammatory
  - Neoplastic
  - Post-treatment: Surgery or radiation

URETHRAL ANATOMY & IMAGING ISSUES

Key Facts

Urethral Disorders
- Female urethra and periurethral structures may be affected by a wide variety of pathologies including congenital, neoplastic, infectious/inflammatory, and traumatic etiologies
- Urethral problems may result from both anatomic or functional disorders

Imaging of Urethra and Periurethral Structures
- Selection of imaging method depends on clinical scenario, availability of imaging resources and expertise in interpretation
- Anatomic and functional imaging or both may be necessary for correct diagnosis

- Conventional urethrography is most commonly used method and may be sufficient in many patients
- Cross-sectional imaging (especially MR) is used as problem solving tool in certain patients
- MR can provide both anatomic imaging with excellent resolution and functional imaging

Clinical and Imaging Correlation
- Clinical assessment of women with urethral symptoms is not always sufficient
- In many cases further evaluation with imaging is necessary
- Many disorders of female urethra have characteristic imaging findings
- Imaging provides useful information for diagnosis and treatment planning

---

- Post-operative changes
  - Periurethral injection of collagen for urinary stress incontinence

PATHOLOGY-BASED IMAGING ISSUES

Key Concepts or Questions
- Imaging studies are performed when patient has urethral problems such as
  - Dysuria
  - Dyspareunia
  - Dribbling
  - Recurrent urinary tract infections
  - Urethral mass
  - Urethral obstruction

Imaging Approaches
- **Voiding cystourethrography (VCUG)**
  - Most commonly used imaging method in evaluation of female urethra
  - This method can depict urethral lumen and lesions within lumen or those communicate with lumen
- **Double-balloon urethrography**
  - Double balloon (positive pressure) urethrography is more sensitive than voiding cystourethrography
    - A special catheter with two balloons is used; one balloon is inflated proximally and the other distally
  - It is technically difficult and needs expertise
  - It may be painful to patient
- **CT**
  - CT can provide information about urethra and periurethral structures
  - Dedicated thin slices and coronal & sagittal reformations are useful
- **Ultrasound**
  - US is a simple non-invasive method of imaging urethra and periurethral structures
  - Several US techniques are available to image urethra
    - High-resolution transvaginal sonography
    - Transperineal sonography
    - Transurethral sonography
    - Transrectal sonography
- **MR**
  - High-resolution, multiplanar MR provides excellent anatomic images of urethra and periurethral structures
  - Dynamic evaluation of urethra during strain is possible with MR
  - Phased-array pelvic and endovaginal or endorectal coils can be used
  - On T2WI, urethra is seen as concentric rings of different signal intensities with a typical "target" appearance
    - Outer ring of low signal intensity that corresponds to outer striated muscle
    - Middle layer of higher signal intensity that corresponds to smooth muscle and submucosa
    - Inner ring of low signal intensity with a high-signal-intensity zone in the center that correspond to mucosa

Imaging Protocols
- **Voiding cystourethrography (VCUG)**
  - Bladder is filled with contrast material via a transurethral or suprapubic catheter
  - Anterior-posterior, oblique and lateral images of bladder are obtained
  - Transurethral catheter is withdrawn and patient voids under fluoroscopic observation
  - During voiding spot radiographs of bladder and urethra are obtained
- **Double-balloon urethrography**
  - With this method contrast material can be forced into a diverticular ostium by positive pressure in relatively closed urethral lumen
- **Ultrasound**
  - 5-10-MHz probes for transperineal, transvaginal and transrectal US
    - Linear array probe for transperineal scanning and curved array probe for transvaginal scanning
    - Place probe between labia for transperineal approach

URETHRAL ANATOMY & IMAGING ISSUES

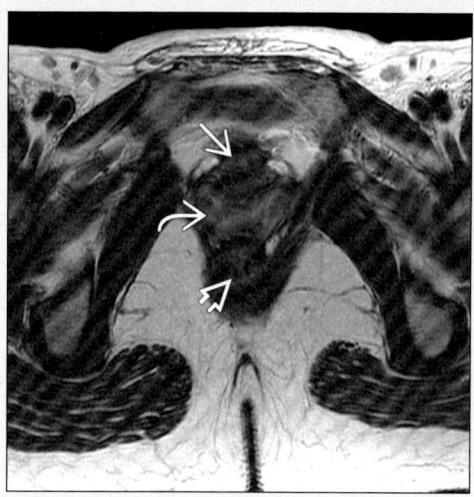

Axial T2WI MR shows female urethra ➡, vagina ➡, and rectum ➡.

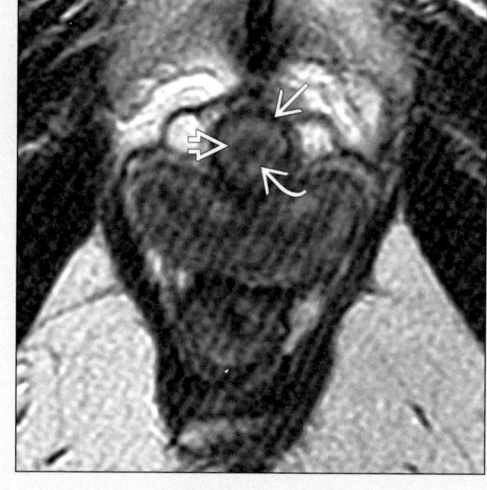

Axial T2WI MR shows "target" appearance of female urethra. Note outer low signal intensity striated muscle ➡, inner high signal intensity smooth muscle and submucosa ➡, and central mucosa ➡.

- Place probe 1-2 cm in vaginal introitus for transvaginal approach
- Place probe in rectum for transrectal approach
  - 12.5-MHz, 6.2-F, catheter-based transducer on an intravascular US machine for endourethral US
- CT
  - Pre- and post-contrast; thin-sections in transverse plane
  - Sagittal and coronal reconstructions may be obtained
- MR
  - T1WI: Pre-contrast and dynamic post-contrast
    - Focal or nodular enhancement is suspicious for tumor
  - T2WI: Small field-of-view; transverse, coronal and sagittal planes

Imaging Pitfalls
- VCUG and double-balloon urethrography can not assess periurethral structures and lesions that do not communicate with urethral lumen
- Content of a urethral diverticulum is not always simple fluid and may be complex on US, CT and MR due to hemorrhage or infection
  - This should not be confused with neoplasm

CLINICAL IMPLICATIONS

Clinical Importance
- Conventional urethrography can provide limited anatomic information
  - Urethral lumen, intraluminal lesions and lesions that communicate with lumen may be assessed
  - Nature of filling defects can not be determined except calcified stones
  - Periurethral structures can not be optimally assessed
  - Functional information can be obtained with voiding cystourethrography
- Cross-sectional imaging provide excellent images of urethra and periurethral structures
  - MR is method of choice due to its excellent soft tissue resolution
  - Various urethral and periurethral pathologies can be optimally evaluated with MR
  - MR can provide both anatomic and functional information at the same time

RELATED REFERENCES

1. Elsayes KM et al: Endovaginal magnetic resonance imaging of the female urethra. J Comput Assist Tomogr. 30(1):1-6, 2006
2. Macura KJ et al: MR imaging of the female urethra and supporting ligaments in assessment of urinary incontinence: spectrum of abnormalities. Radiographics. 26(4):1135-49, 2006
3. Prasad SR et al: Cross-sectional imaging of the female urethra: technique and results. Radiographics. 25(3):749-61, 2005
4. Macura KJ et al: Evaluation of the female urethra with intraurethral magnetic resonance imaging. J Magn Reson Imaging. 20(1):153-9, 2004
5. Kim JK et al: The urethra and its supporting structures in women with stress urinary incontinence: MR imaging using an endovaginal coil. AJR Am J Roentgenol. 180(4):1037-44, 2003
6. Siegel CL et al: Sonography of the female urethra. AJR Am J Roentgenol. 170(5):1269-74, 1998
7. Siegelman ES et al: Multicoil MR imaging of symptomatic female urethral and periurethral disease. Radiographics. 17(2):349-65, 1997
8. Kuo HC. Related Articles et al: Transrectal sonography of the female urethra in incontinence and frequency-urgency syndrome. J Ultrasound Med. 15(5):363-70, 1996

URETHRAL ANATOMY & IMAGING ISSUES

IMAGE GALLERY

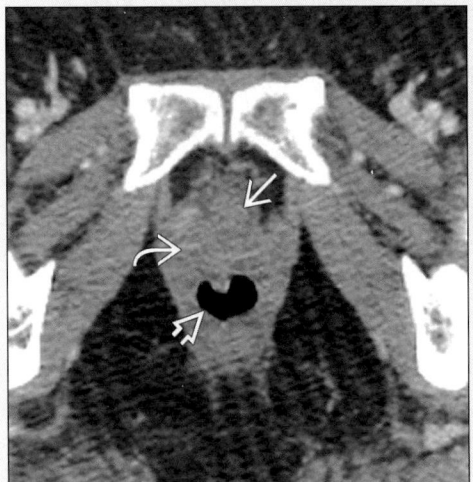
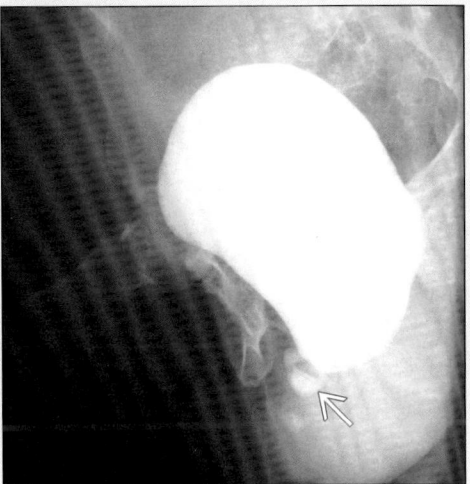

(Left) Axial CECT shows female urethra ➡, vagina ➡, and rectum ➡. *(Right)* Oblique voiding cystourethrogram shows a urethral diverticulum ➡ seen as a contrast-filled sac around the urethra.

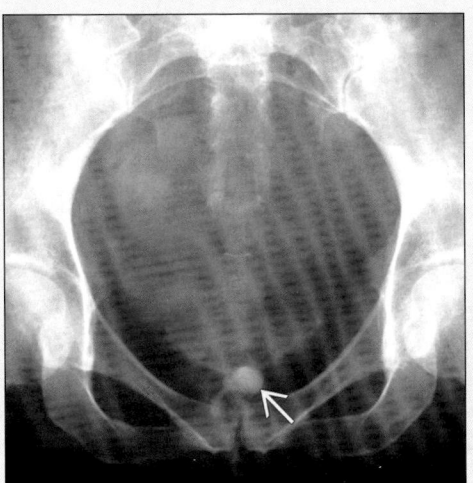
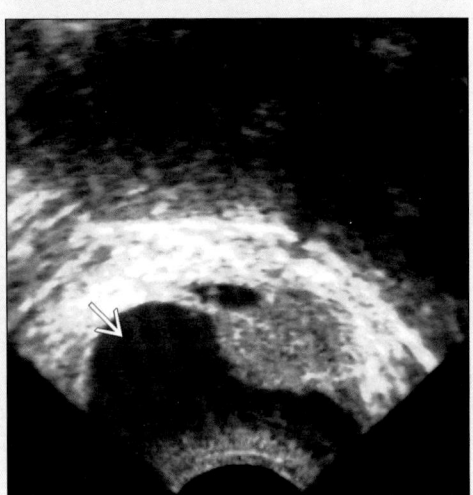

(Left) Frontal voiding cystourethrogram shows retained contrast in the urethral diverticulum ➡ on post-voiding image. *(Right)* Axial transvaginal ultrasound shows urethral diverticulum ➡.

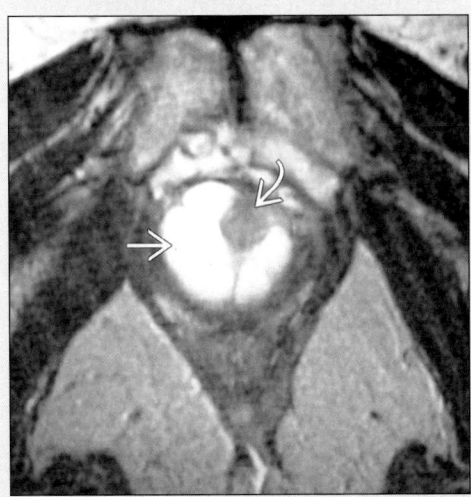
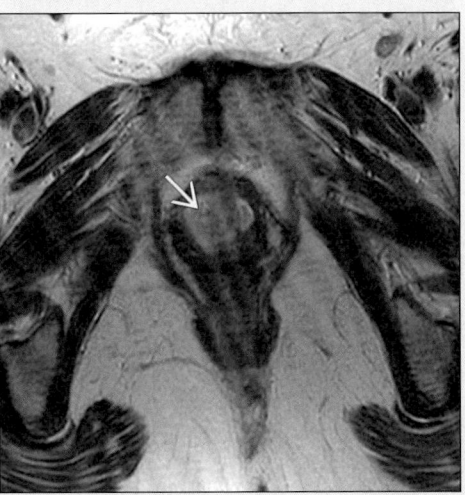

(Left) Axial T2WI MR shows a urethral diverticulum ➡ seen as a cystic lesion encasing urethra ➡ posterolaterally. *(Right)* Axial T2WI MR shows urethral cancer ➡ seen as a soft tissue mass expanding the urethra.

LEIOMYOMA, URETHRA

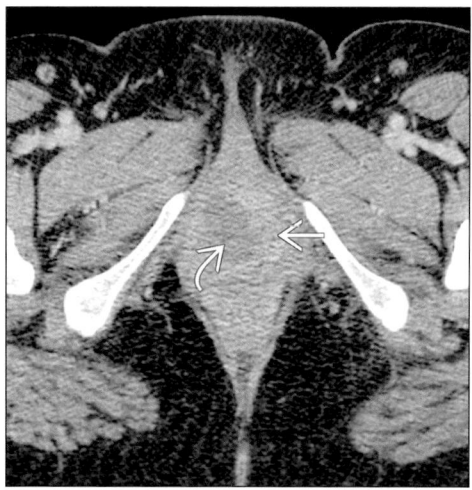

Axial CECT shows a urethral leiomyoma ➔ seen as a low-attenuation mass in the urethra ➔.

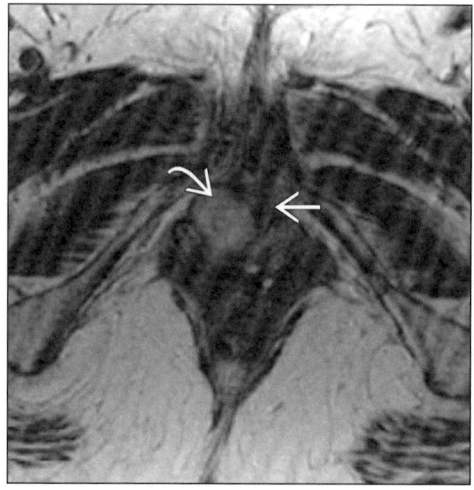

Axial T2WI MR shows a urethral leiomyoma ➔ seen as a high signal intensity mass. Note the low signal intensity of the urethra ➔.

TERMINOLOGY

Definitions
- Benign, smooth muscle tumor of female urethra

IMAGING FINDINGS

General Features
- Best diagnostic clue: Well-defined, homogeneous soft tissue mass in or around urethra
- Location
  - They can be seen in any segment of urethra
    - But most commonly proximal urethra is involved
- Size: Usually small but rarely may present as large masses
- Morphology: Well-defined, round soft tissue masses

Ultrasonographic Findings
- Grayscale Ultrasound: Well-defined masses with homogeneous echogenicity
- Color Doppler: Leiomyomas have increased vascularity

CT Findings
- NECT: Isoattenuation relative to muscle
- CECT: Iso- or slightly low-attenuation relative to muscle

MR Findings
- T1WI: Iso- to hypointense relative to muscle
- T2WI: Hyperintense relative to muscle
- T1 C+: Uniform enhancement

Imaging Recommendations
- Best imaging tool: MR is most useful in determining the location and extent of urethral leiomyoma

DIFFERENTIAL DIAGNOSIS

Urethral Diverticulum
- Urethral diverticulum is seen as a multiseptated cystic lesion unlike leiomyoma which is a solid lesion

Urethral Cancer
- Imaging methods can not always accurately differentiate urethral cancer from leiomyoma

DDx: Urethral Masses

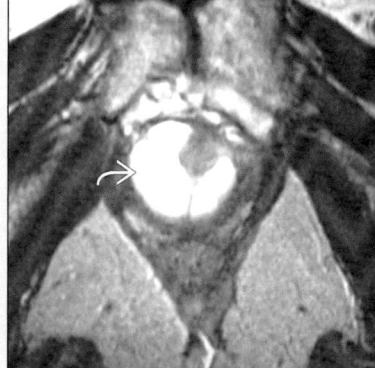

Urethral Diverticulum

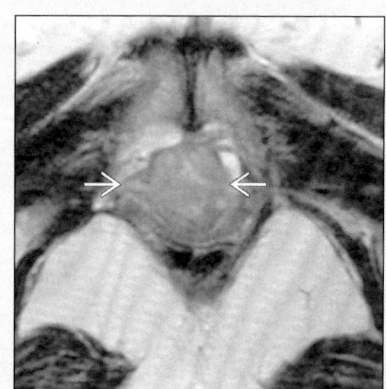

Urethral Cancer

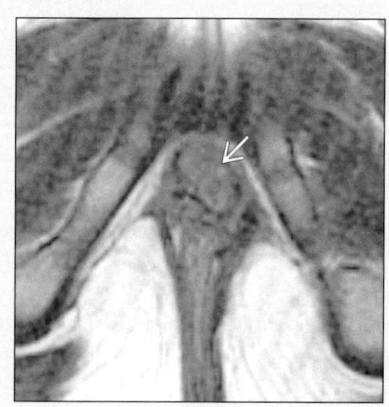

Urethral Schwannoma

LEIOMYOMA, URETHRA

Key Facts

Imaging Findings
- Best diagnostic clue: Well-defined, homogeneous soft tissue mass in or around urethra
- Best imaging tool: MR is most useful in determining the location and extent of urethral leiomyoma

Top Differential Diagnoses
- Urethral Diverticulum
- Urethral Cancer
- Urethral Schwannoma

Pathology
- Leiomyomas are benign tumors of smooth muscle origin
- They are the most common mesenchymal neoplasms of urethra

Clinical Issues
- No malignant transformation has been reported

- However, an invasive mass that disrupts urethra suggests urethral cancer

Urethral Schwannoma
- Difficult to differentiate urethral schwannoma from leiomyoma
- Diagnosis is usually made on histological examination

PATHOLOGY

General Features
- General path comments
  - Leiomyomas are benign tumors of smooth muscle origin
  - They are the most common mesenchymal neoplasms of urethra
- Epidemiology: Urethral leiomyoma is a very rare condition

CLINICAL ISSUES

Presentation
- Most common signs/symptoms
  - Urinary tract infection
  - Hematuria
  - Mass protruding through urethral orifice
- Other signs/symptoms: Obstructive symptoms are rare

Demographics
- Gender: More common in females than in males

Natural History & Prognosis
- No malignant transformation has been reported
- Recurrence may occur in cases with incomplete resection

Treatment
- Local surgical excision or transurethral excision

DIAGNOSTIC CHECKLIST

Image Interpretation Pearls
- Benign and malignant tumors of urethra may have similar appearances on imaging
  - Invasion to adjacent structures suggests urethral cancer
- Role of imaging is to define local extent of lesion for surgical planning

SELECTED REFERENCES

1. Prasad SR et al: Cross-sectional imaging of the female urethra: technique and results. Radiographics. 25(3):749-61, 2005
2. Pavlica P et al: Female paraurethral leiomyoma: ultrasonographic and magnetic resonance imaging findings. Acta Radiol. 45(7):796-8, 2004
3. Saad AG et al: Leiomyoma of the urethra: report of 3 cases of a rare entity. Int J Surg Pathol. 11(2):123-6, 2003
4. Ikeda R et al: MRI appearance of a leiomyoma of the female urethra. Clin Radiol. 56(1):76-9, 2001

IMAGE GALLERY

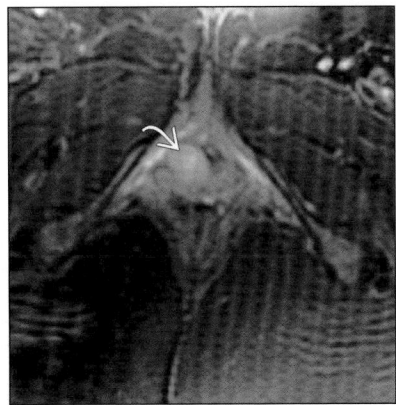
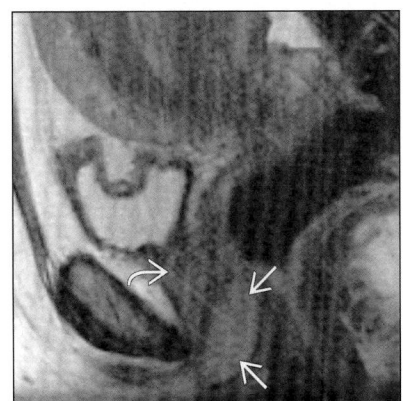
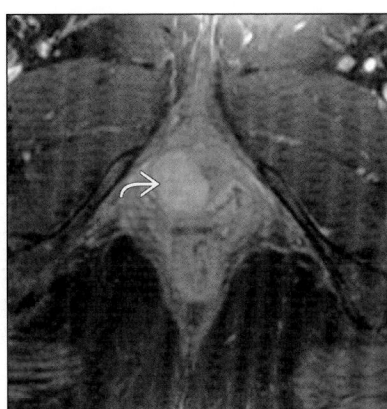

(Left) Axial T2WI FS MR shows a urethral leiomyoma ➔ seen as a high signal intensity mass. *(Center)* Sagittal T2WI MR shows a urethral leiomyoma ➔ in the lower aspect of the urethra ➔. *(Right)* Axial T1 C+ FS MR shows homogeneous enhancement in the urethral leiomyoma ➔.

SCHWANNOMA, URETHRA

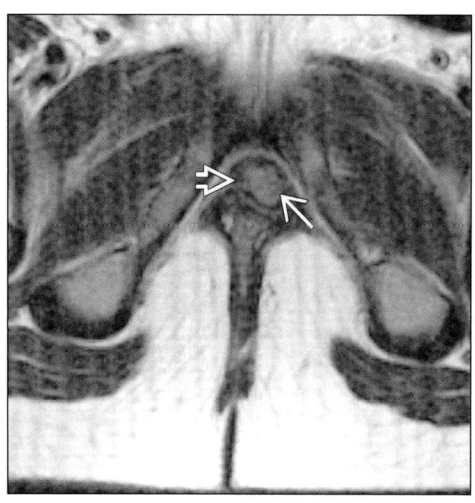

Axial T2WI MR shows schwannoma seen as a well-circumscribed, high signal intensity nodular mass ➡ displacing the urethra ➡.

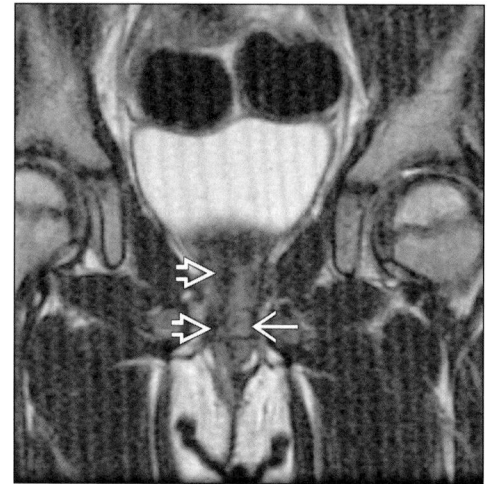

Coronal T2WI MR shows schwannoma ➡ adjacent to the distal urethra ➡.

TERMINOLOGY

Abbreviations and Synonyms
- Benign peripheral nerve sheath tumor, neurilemmoma

Definitions
- Benign neoplasm arising from Schwann cells of peripheral nerves
- They may occur as a solitary lesion or in the setting of neurofibromatosis type I
- Genitourinary tract schwannomas are extremely rare, with less than 20 cases reported

IMAGING FINDINGS

General Features
- Best diagnostic clue: Rounded fusiform well-circumscribed urethral or periurethral mass
- Morphology: Well-circumscribed, encapsulated mass attached to a peripheral nerve

CT Findings
- CECT
  - Well-defined, homogeneously enhancing mass
  - Large tumors may demonstrate heterogeneous enhancement

MR Findings
- T1WI: Signal intensity similar to muscle
- T2WI: Typical high signal intensity with low signal intensity central region (target sign)
- T1 C+
  - Homogeneous enhancement
  - Large tumors may demonstrate heterogeneous enhancement
  - Cystic nonenhancing areas con be seen

Imaging Recommendations
- Best imaging tool: MR is recommended for detection and characterization

DIFFERENTIAL DIAGNOSIS

Urethral Leiomyoma
- Leiomyoma has intermediately high signal intensity on T2WI

DDx: Urethral Lesions

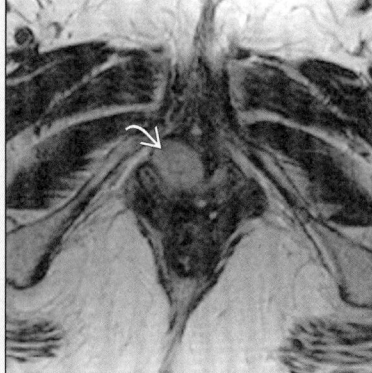
Urethral Leiomyoma

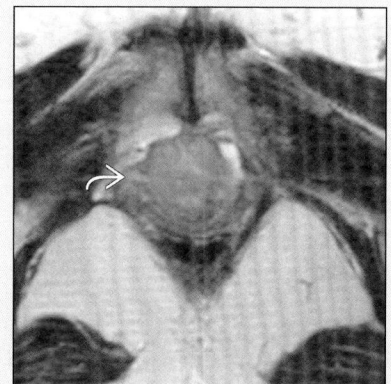
Urethral Cancer

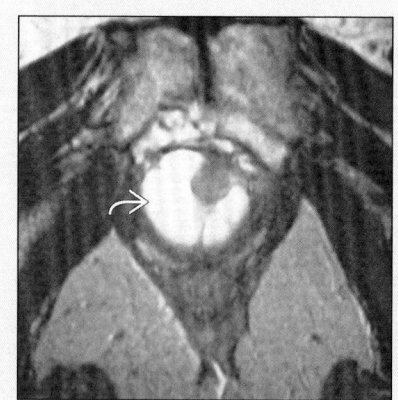
Urethral Diverticulum

SCHWANNOMA, URETHRA

Key Facts

Terminology
- Benign peripheral nerve sheath tumor, neurilemmoma
- Benign neoplasm arising from Schwann cells of peripheral nerves
- They may occur as a solitary lesion or in the setting of neurofibromatosis type I
- Genitourinary tract schwannomas are extremely rare, with less than 20 cases reported

Imaging Findings
- Best diagnostic clue: Rounded fusiform well-circumscribed urethral or periurethral mass
- T2WI: Typical high signal intensity with low signal intensity central region (target sign)

Diagnostic Checklist
- Painful or rapidly enlarging lesions should raise concern for malignant peripheral nerve sheath tumor

Urethral Cancer
- Usually irregular infiltrative, heterogeneous mass

Urethral Diverticulum
- Cystic lesion with or without septations encasing urethra

PATHOLOGY

Gross Pathologic & Surgical Features
- Firm, tan or gray masses
- May have areas of cystic or xanthomatous change

Microscopic Features
- Elongated spindle cells with Antoni A (cellular, arranged in interlacing fascicles) and Antoni B (hypocellular, myxoid matrix) growth patterns
- S-100 immunoreactivity

CLINICAL ISSUES

Presentation
- Most common signs/symptoms
  - Dysuria
  - Urinary retention
  - Recurrent urinary tract infections

Demographics
- Age: Most commonly present in adolescence or early adulthood

Treatment
- Surgical resection in symptomatic cases

DIAGNOSTIC CHECKLIST

Consider
- Painful or rapidly enlarging lesions should raise concern for malignant peripheral nerve sheath tumor

Image Interpretation Pearls
- Well-circumscribed, encapsulated mass associated with a peripheral nerve and typical target sign on T2WI

SELECTED REFERENCES
1. Hughes MJ et al: Imaging features of retroperitoneal and pelvic schwannomas. Clin Radiol. 60(8):886-93, 2005
2. Kulkarni S et al: Vaginal schwannoma. J Obstet Gynaecol. 25(1):84-5, 2005
3. Ellison DW et al: Cellular schwannoma of the vagina. Gynecol Oncol. 46(1):119-21, 1992
4. Terada S et al: Vaginal schwannoma. Arch Gynecol Obstet. 251(4):203-6, 1992

IMAGE GALLERY

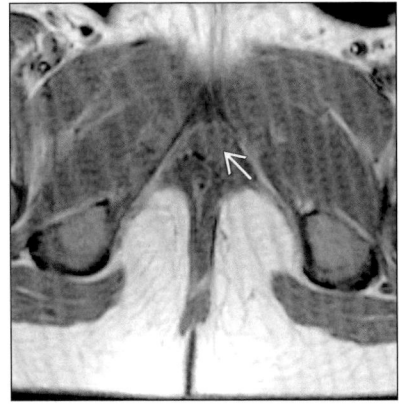 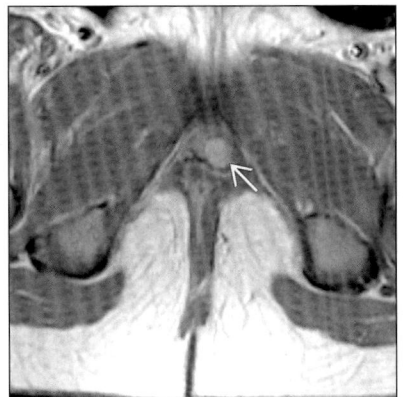 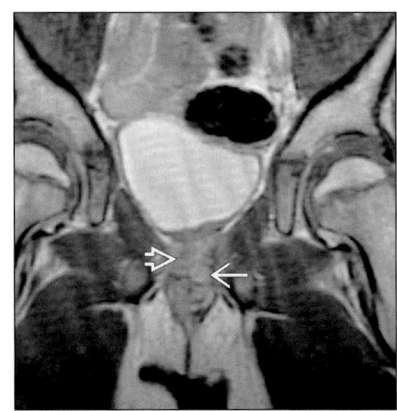

(Left) Axial T1WI MR shows schwannoma ➡ with signal intensity similar to muscle. *(Center)* Axial T1 C+ MR shows diffuse enhancement of schwannoma ➡. *(Right)* Coronal T1 C+ MR shows enhancing schwannoma ➡ adjacent to the distal urethra ➡.

CARCINOMA, URETHRA

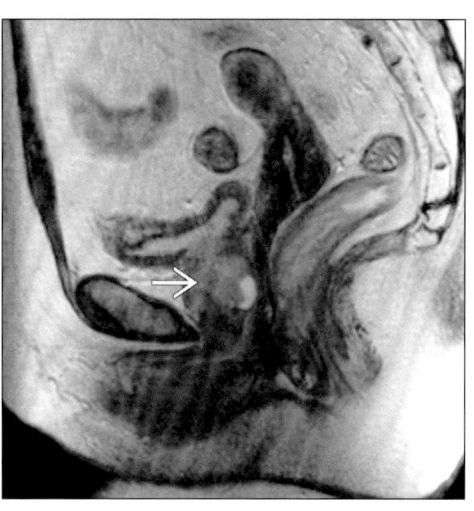

Sagittal T2WI MR shows intermediate signal intensity urethral cancer ➔ expanding the urethra.

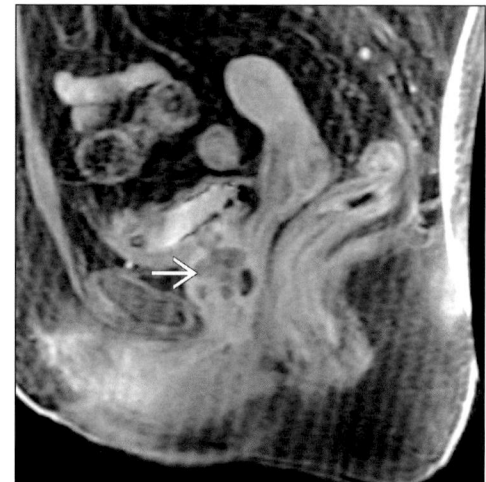

Sagittal T1 C+ FS MR shows that the urethral cancer ➔ enhances heterogeneously.

TERMINOLOGY

Definitions
- Primary malignant tumor of urethra

IMAGING FINDINGS

General Features
- Best diagnostic clue: Solid mass arising from urethra disrupting normal "target-like" appearance of urethra
- Location
  - In female patients, urethral cancer is classified as anterior or "entire"
    - Anterior tumors are located exclusively in distal third of urethra
    - Tumors are classified "entire" when any portion of urethra other than distal third is involved
- Size: Varies but usually small masses
- Morphology: They may be seen as nodular masses or as infiltrative tumors

Ultrasonographic Findings
- Grayscale Ultrasound
  - Transperineal, transvaginal, transrectal approaches can be used
  - Endourethral sonography is a special technique performed with a catheter-based transducer
  - Urethral cancers appear as hypo- to isoechoic, irregularly marginated lesions

CT Findings
- CECT
  - CT is limited in the evaluation of urethral tumors
  - Difficult to differentiate urethra from vagina and bladder base
  - Urethral cancers may be seen as homogeneously-enhancing masses

MR Findings
- T1WI: Low signal intensity mass which is difficult to differentiate from the normal urethra
- T2WI
  - Urethral wall demonstrates low signal intensity similar to muscle on T2WI
  - Urethral cancer is seen as a relatively high signal intensity mass disrupting "target-like" zonal anatomy of urethra
- T1 C+

DDx: Urethral and Periurethral Lesions

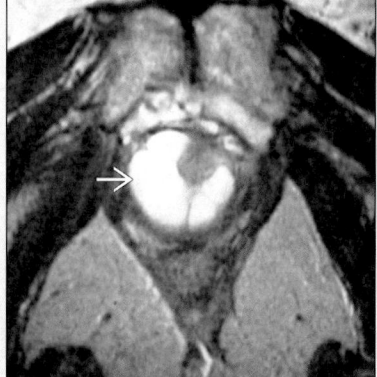

Urethral Diverticulum

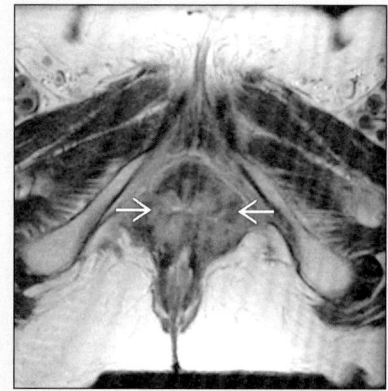

Vaginal Cancer

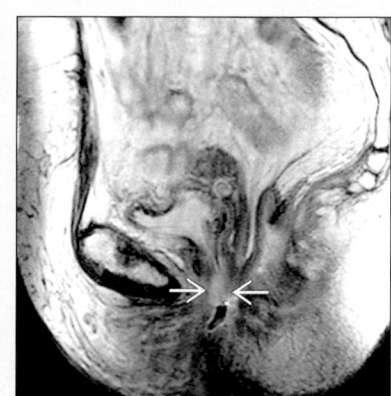

Fistula between Urethra & Vagina

CARCINOMA, URETHRA

Key Facts

Terminology
- Primary malignant tumor of urethra

Imaging Findings
- Best diagnostic clue: Solid mass arising from urethra disrupting normal "target-like" appearance of urethra
- In female patients, urethral cancer is classified as anterior or "entire"
- Anterior tumors are located exclusively in distal third of urethra
- Tumors are classified "entire" when any portion of urethra other than distal third is involved
- Best imaging tool: MR is method of choice due to its high accuracy in local staging of urethral cancers

Top Differential Diagnoses
- Benign Tumors of Urethra
- Benign mesenchymal tumors have imaging characteristics similar to those of urethral cancer
- Urethral Diverticula
- Urethral diverticula are multiseptated, entirely cystic lesions
- Markedly inflamed diverticula can be mistaken for a neoplasm at imaging studies

Pathology
- Epidemiology: Urethral cancer is a rare malignancy accounting for less than 0.02% of all malignancies in women

Diagnostic Checklist
- Size, location and local extension must be determined for treatment planning

---

  - Urethral cancers demonstrate variable enhancement
  - T1 C+ images are most useful in evaluating the urethra and periurethral tissues

Fluoroscopic Findings
- Voiding Cystourethrogram: Urethral cancers are seen as filling defects in the urethra

Imaging Recommendations
- Best imaging tool: MR is method of choice due to its high accuracy in local staging of urethral cancers
- Protocol advice
  - T2WI: Transverse, coronal and sagittal; small field of view
  - T1 C+ FS: Transverse

DIFFERENTIAL DIAGNOSIS

Benign Tumors of Urethra
- Benign mesenchymal tumors have imaging characteristics similar to those of urethral cancer
  - Such as fibrous polyp and leiomyoma of urethra

Urethral Diverticula
- Urethral diverticula are multiseptated, entirely cystic lesions
- Surround the urethra rather than expanding it as seen in urethral cancers
- Markedly inflamed diverticula can be mistaken for a neoplasm at imaging studies

Tumors of Adjacent Organs
- Tumors originating from adjacent organs and extending to urethra may mimic urethral cancer
  - Such as tumors of bladder neck and vagina

Urethral Fistulas
- Marked inflammatory changes around the fistula may mimic urethral cancer on imaging

PATHOLOGY

General Features
- General path comments
  - Urethral cancers are of epithelial origin
  - Spread is by local extension and with subsequent involvement of the bladder neck, vagina or vulva
  - Lymphatic drainage occurs to pelvic or inguinal lymph nodes
  - Most common sites of metastasis are lung, liver, bone and brain
- Etiology
  - Risk factors include
    - History of bladder cancer
    - Sexually transmitted diseases
    - Chronic urinary tract infections
    - Age over 60
    - Chronic irritation (from childbirth, sexual intercourse)
    - Smoking
- Epidemiology: Urethral cancer is a rare malignancy accounting for less than 0.02% of all malignancies in women

Gross Pathologic & Surgical Features
- Papillary mass growing within and expanding urethra
- Large lesions may demonstrate ulceration

Microscopic Features
- Histologic types are
  - Squamous cell carcinoma (60%), most common
  - Transitional cell carcinoma (20%)
  - Adenocarcinoma (10%)
- Adenocarcinoma is the most common urethral cancer associated with a urethral diverticulum

Staging, Grading or Classification Criteria
- TNM staging
- Primary tumor (T)
  - Tx: Primary tumor cannot be assessed
  - T0: No evidence of primary tumor
  - Ta: Noninvasive papillary, polypoid, or verrucous carcinoma

CARCINOMA, URETHRA

- o Tis: Carcinoma in situ
- o T1: Tumor invades subepithelial connective tissue
- o T2: Tumor invades any of the following: Corpus spongiosum, prostate, periurethral muscle
- o T3: Tumor invades any of the following: Corpus cavernosum, beyond prostate capsule, anterior vagina, bladder neck
- o T4: Tumor invades other adjacent organs
- Regional lymph nodes (N)
  - o Nx: Regional lymph nodes cannot be assessed
  - o N0: No regional lymph node metastasis
  - o N1: Metastasis in a single lymph node, 2 cm or less in greatest dimension
  - o N2: Metastasis in a single lymph node, more than 2 cm in greatest dimension, or in multiple lymph nodes
- Distant metastasis (M)
  - o Mx: Distant metastasis cannot be assessed
  - o M0: No distant metastasis
  - o M1: Distant metastasis

CLINICAL ISSUES

Presentation
- Most common signs/symptoms
  - o Urethral bleeding or gross hematuria
  - o Dysuria
  - o Dyspareunia
  - o Urinary obstruction
  - o Urethral discharge
- Other signs/symptoms
  - o Recurrent urinary tract infections
  - o Diminished urine stream and straining to void (due to urethral stricture)
  - o Palpable mass
- Clinical Profile: Clinical diagnosis is difficult and symptoms may mimic chronic urinary tract infection

Demographics
- Age: Urethral cancers are most commonly seen in postmenopausal women
- Gender: Urethral cancer is much more common in women than in men

Natural History & Prognosis
- 5 year survival rate for noninvasive urethral cancer treated surgically or with radiation is approximately 60%
- Recurrence rate for invasive urethral cancer treated with surgery, chemotherapy, and radiation combined is higher than 50%

Treatment
- Surgery
  - o Local excision in early disease
  - o Wide excision in advanced disease
- Radiotherapy
  - o Alone in early disease
  - o In combination with surgery in advanced disease
- Chemotherapy
  - o In combination with surgery and radiotherapy for advanced cases

DIAGNOSTIC CHECKLIST

Consider
- MR is method of choice due to its superior soft tissue resolution
- Local extent of disease is best depicted on MR

Image Interpretation Pearls
- Size, location and local extension must be determined for treatment planning

SELECTED REFERENCES

1. Prasad SR et al: Cross-sectional imaging of the female urethra: technique and results. Radiographics. 25(3):749-61, 2005
2. Thyavihally YB et al: Primary carcinoma of the female urethra: single center experience of 18 cases. Jpn J Clin Oncol. 35(2):84-7, 2005
3. Dimarco DS et al: Surgical treatment for local control of female urethral carcinoma. Urol Oncol. 22(5):404-9, 2004
4. Hahn WY et al: MRI of female urethral and periurethral disorders. AJR Am J Roentgenol. 182(3):677-82, 2004
5. Kawashima A et al: Imaging of urethral disease: a pictorial review. Radiographics. 24 Suppl 1:S195-216, 2004
6. Ryu JA et al: MR imaging of the male and female urethra. Radiographics. 21:1169-85, 2001
7. Milosevic MF et al: Urethral carcinoma in women: results of treatment with primary radiotherapy. Radiother Oncol. 56(1):29-35, 2000
8. Wasserman NF: Urethral neoplasm. Clinical urography. 2nd ed. Vol 2. Philadelphia, Saunders. 1699-1715, 2000
9. Chalpin DB et al: Case 2: Adenocarcinoma of the female urethra. AJR. 171:827,830-31, 1998
10. Dalbagni G et al: Female urethral carcinoma: an analysis of treatment outcome and a plea for a standardized management strategy. Br J Urol. 82(6):835-41, 1998
11. Amin MB et al: Primary carcinomas of the urethra. Semin Diagn Pathol. 14(2):147-60, 1997
12. Ampil FL. Related Articles et al: Primary malignant neoplasm of the female urethra. Obstet Gynecol. 66(6):799-804, 1985

CARCINOMA, URETHRA

IMAGE GALLERY

Typical

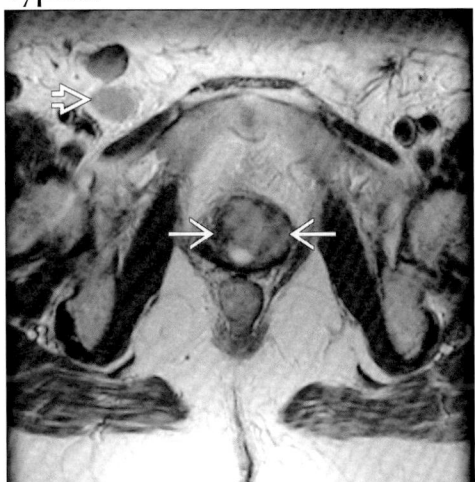
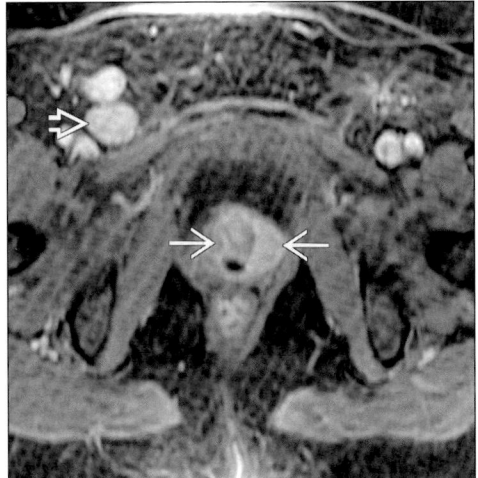

(Left) Axial T2WI MR shows intermediate signal intensity urethral mass ➔ that expands the urethra. A right inguinal lymphadenopathy ➔ is also seen. *(Right)* Axial T1 C+ FS MR shows heterogeneous enhancement of the urethral cancer ➔. Right inguinal lymphadenopathy ➔ is again seen.

Typical

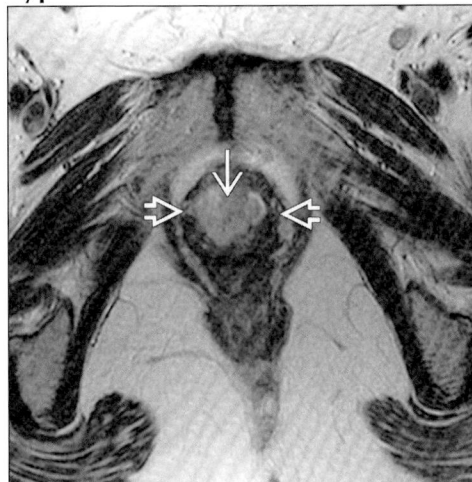
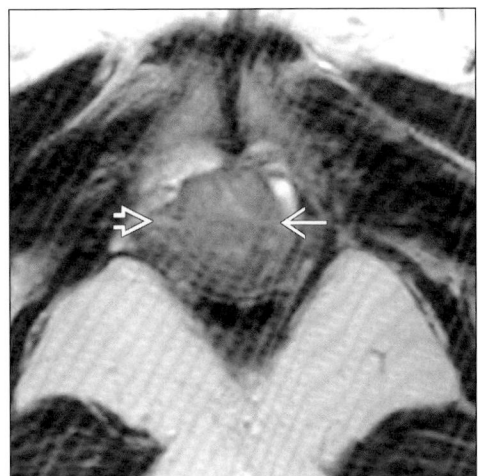

(Left) Axial T2WI MR shows intermediate signal intensity urethral mass ➔. Note that low signal intensity urethral muscular wall ➔ is preserved. *(Right)* Axial T2WI MR shows the urethral mass ➔ with periurethral extension ➔ on the right.

Typical

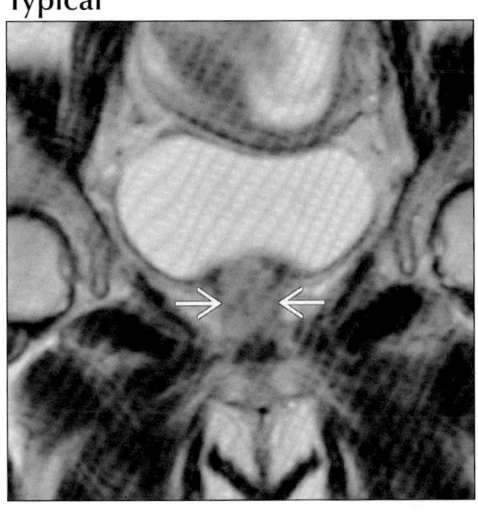
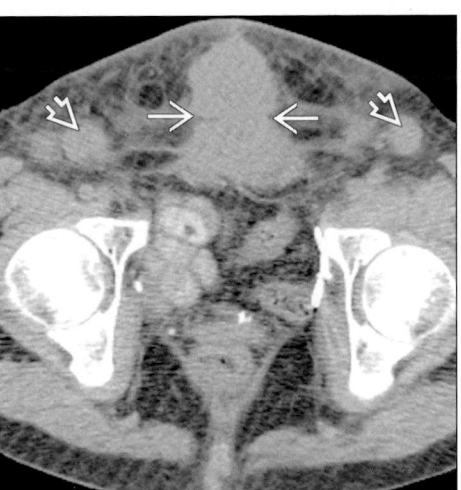

(Left) Coronal T2WI MR shows urethral mass ➔ expanding the urethra. *(Right)* Axial NECT shows recurrent mass ➔ in the anterior abdominal wall along the surgical incision line in a patient with urethral cancer. Bilateral inguinal lymphadenopathy ➔ is also seen.

METASTASIS, URETHRA

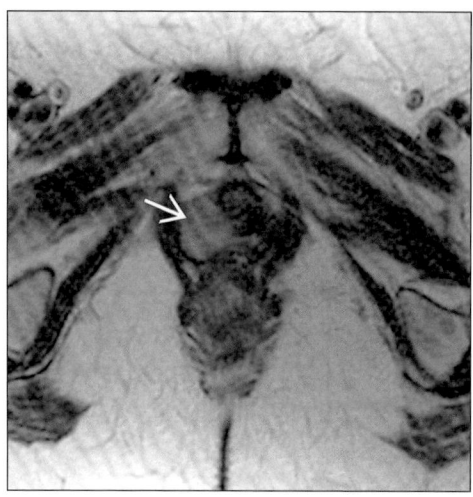

Axial T2WI MR shows a mildly hyperintense periurethral mass ➡ invading the outer muscular layer of the urethra which proved to be a metastasis from endometrial carcinoma.

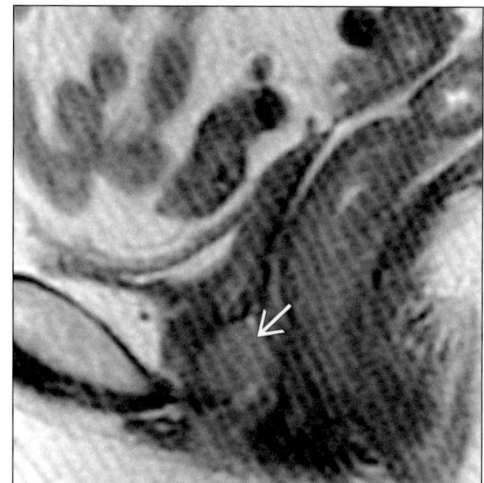

Sagittal T2WI MR in the same patient as previous image shows the mildly hyperintense periurethral mass ➡, invading the outer layer of urethra and extending posteriorly to the vaginal wall.

TERMINOLOGY

Definitions
- Urethral involvement by extraurethral malignancy
  - Hematogenous (true metastasis)
  - Direct extension from contiguous pelvic primary

IMAGING FINDINGS

General Features
- Best diagnostic clue: Solid mass arising in urethral lumen or disrupting urethral wall
- Location: Anywhere in urethra
- Size: Variable
- Morphology: Either well-defined lobulated mass or infiltrative mass

Ultrasonographic Findings
- Poor visualization with transvesical approach
- Transperineal with high-resolution linear array, transvaginal or transrectal approach can be used
- Endourethral sonography also possible in specialized centers
- Hypo- to isoechoic urethral mass
- Disruption of normal hypoechoic/hyperechoic urethral lumen/mucosa interface

CT Findings
- CECT
  - Limited utility due to lack of soft tissue differentiation
    - Difficult to differentiate urethra from vagina
    - May be difficult to know if urethra is invaded or displaced
  - Can demonstrate urethral mass with soft tissue attenuation
  - Homogeneous or heterogeneous enhancement ± necrotic hypoattenuating areas
    - Degree and type of enhancement depends on underlying primary neoplasm

MR Findings
- T1WI
  - Low or intermediate signal intensity mass
  - Difficult to differentiate from normal urethra
- T2WI
  - Relatively high signal intensity mass, may vary with primary neoplasm

DDx: Urethral and Periurethral Lesions

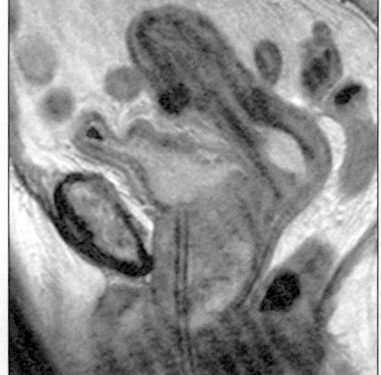

Urethral Carcinoma

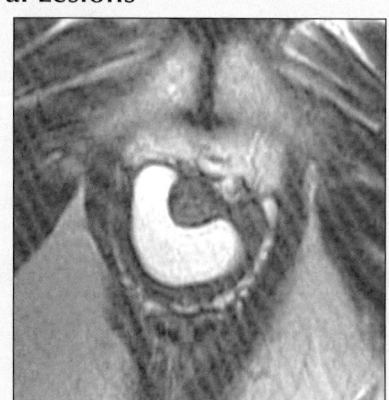

Urethral Diverticulum

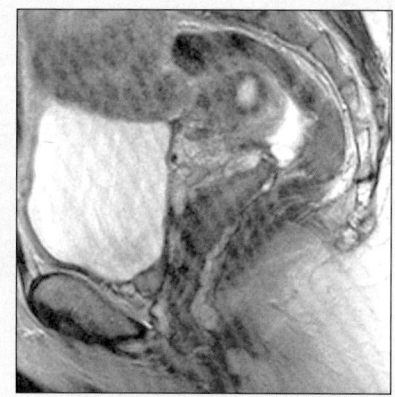

Periurethral Collagen Injection

METASTASIS, URETHRA

Key Facts

Terminology
- Urethral involvement by extraurethral malignancy

Imaging Findings
- Best diagnostic clue: Solid mass arising in urethral lumen or disrupting urethral wall
- Hematogenous metastasis: Lesion usually intraluminal with or without extension to periurethral tissues
- Disruption of "target-like" appearance of urethral wall indicates periurethral extension

Top Differential Diagnoses
- Urethral Carcinoma
- Benign Primary Urethral Mesenchymal Tumors
- Urethral Diverticulum
- Periurethral Collagen Injection

Pathology
- Most commonly contiguous extension from adjacent organs neoplasm like bladder, cervix, vagina or anus
- Hematogenous metastasis: Arise from mucosa-submucosa, malignant involvement can be transmural
- Direct extension from contiguous neoplasm: First reaches outer muscular layers, then submucosa and mucosa

Diagnostic Checklist
- MR is imaging modality of choice to determine urethral origin and local extent
- Imaging appearance mimics urethral carcinoma
- Histology is clue to diagnosis

- ○ Hematogenous metastasis: Lesion usually intraluminal with or without extension to periurethral tissues
  - ▪ Disruption of "target-like" appearance of urethral wall indicates periurethral extension
- ○ Direct extension from other pelvic malignancy manifests as an infiltrative mass
- ○ Occasionally signal abnormalities confined to periurethral tissues
- T1 C+ FS
  - ○ Variable enhancement
    - ▪ Depends on primary malignancy
  - ○ Contrast administration can help depict periurethral extension

Other Modality Findings
- Voiding cystourethrogram
  - ○ Single or multiple small mucosal nodules seen as filling defects
  - ○ Urethral narrowing and mucosal irregularity

Imaging Recommendations
- Best imaging tool
  - ○ MR offers best anatomic delineation and precise depiction of intraluminal and periurethral involvement
    - ▪ Can readily diagnose direct invasion from a contiguous organ neoplasm (bladder, vagina, cervix)
  - ○ Transperineal, transvaginal and transrectal ultrasound can also detect urethral metastases
  - ○ Endourethral sonography with catheter-based transducer offers excellent depiction of urethral anatomy and degree of invasion
- Protocol advice
  - ○ Multiplanar T2WI, high-resolution with small field-of-view (FOV)
  - ○ Contrast administration can be helpful

DIFFERENTIAL DIAGNOSIS

Urethral Carcinoma
- Imaging appearance can completely mimic urethral metastasis
- Solid urethral mass
- Disruption of normal target-like appearance of urethra
- Low signal intensity on T1WI
- Relatively high signal intensity on T2WI
- No history of primary neoplasm

Benign Primary Urethral Mesenchymal Tumors
- Usually well-defined polypoid masses
- Leiomyoma: Iso- to hypointense relative to muscle on T1WI and T2WI, intramural location
- Less commonly: Hemangioma, fibrous polyp
- Usually well-defined polypoid masses

Urethral Diverticulum
- Involve mid aspect of urethra
- Arise from posterolateral wall
- Multiseptated cystic lesion surrounding urethra
- Heterogeneous signal intensity if inflamed
- Hyperintense on T2WI, and brighter than urine on T1WI
- Fluid-fluid levels

Periurethral Collagen Injection
- Can be mistaken for a neoplasm
- US: Echogenic periurethral lesion
- T1WI: Hyperintense nodules in urethral wall
- T2WI: Iso- to hyperintense relative to urethral submucosal layer

PATHOLOGY

General Features
- Etiology
  - ○ Most commonly contiguous extension from adjacent organs neoplasm like bladder, cervix, vagina or anus

METASTASIS, URETHRA

- Hematogenous spread from distant neoplasm
  - Prostate
  - Kidney
  - Ureter
  - Testis
  - Colorectal
  - Lung
  - Melanoma
- Retrograde venous or retrograde lymphatic spread
• Epidemiology: Very rare entity

Gross Pathologic & Surgical Features
• Polypoid or infiltrative mass
• Can be ulcerated

Microscopic Features
• Depends on the primary neoplasm
• Hematogenous metastasis: Arise from mucosa-submucosa, malignant involvement can be transmural
• Direct extension from contiguous neoplasm: First reaches outer muscular layers, then submucosa and mucosa

CLINICAL ISSUES

Presentation
• Most common signs/symptoms
  - Hematuria
  - Obstruction
  - Pain
  - Dyspareunia
  - Dysuria
  - Urethral induration and nodularity
• Other signs/symptoms: May be the first presentation of unknown underlying malignancy

Demographics
• Gender: More reported cases in men than in women

Natural History & Prognosis
• Depends on the primary neoplasm and staging

Treatment
• Depends on extent of disease and symptomatology
• Surgery in resectable cases
• Chemotherapy and radiation therapy depending on underlying primary neoplasm

DIAGNOSTIC CHECKLIST

Consider
• Urethral metastasis in a patient with a known primary neoplasm presenting with hematuria or urethral mass

Image Interpretation Pearls
• MR is imaging modality of choice to determine urethral origin and local extent
• Imaging appearance mimics urethral carcinoma
• Histology is clue to diagnosis

SELECTED REFERENCES

1. Noorani S et al: Urethral metastasis: an uncommon presentation of a colonic adenocarcinoma. Int Urol Nephrol. 2007
2. Prasad SR et al: Cross-sectional imaging of the female urethra: technique and results. Radiographics. 25(3):749-61, 2005
3. Cheng CW et al: A rare cause of acute urinary retention: urethral metastasis from renal cell carcinoma. Int Urol Nephrol. 36(2):145-7, 2004
4. Hahn WY et al: MRI of female urethral and periurethral disorders. AJR Am J Roentgenol. 182(3):677-82, 2004
5. Kawashima A et al: Imaging of urethral disease: a pictorial review. Radiographics. 24 Suppl 1:S195-216, 2004
6. Tefilli MV et al: Urethral metastasis of lung carcinoma with germinative cell features. Int Braz J Urol. 29(5):431-3, 2003
7. Ryu J et al: MR imaging of the male and female urethra. Radiographics. 21(5):1169-85, 2001
8. Stragier J et al: Adenocarcinoma of the rectum with a solitary metastasis to the urethra in a female. Eur J Surg Oncol. 20(6):696-7, 1994

METASTASIS, URETHRA

IMAGE GALLERY

Typical

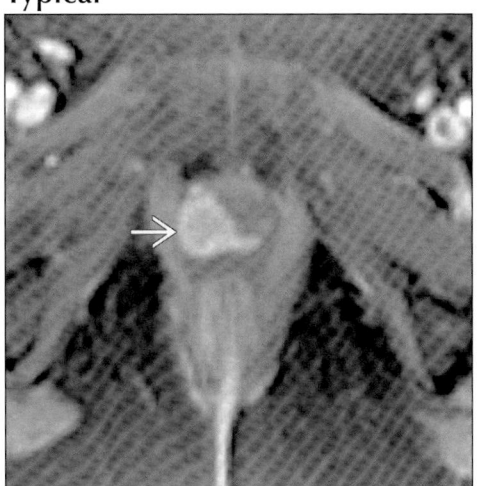

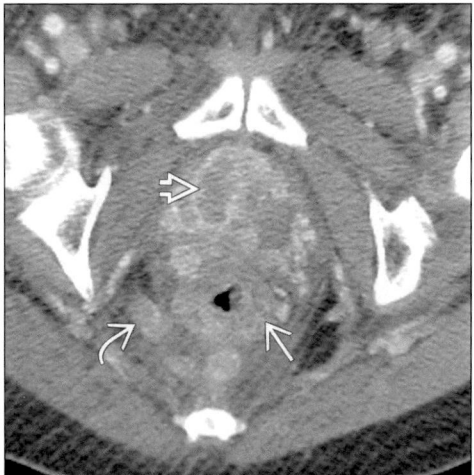

(Left) Axial T1 C+ FS MR in the preceding patient shows intense enhancement of the urethral and periurethral mass ➡. *(Right)* Axial CECT shows a vaginal vault mass from recurrent cervical carcinoma invading the urethra ➡ and rectal wall ➡. There are also enhancing perirectal nodules ➡.

Typical

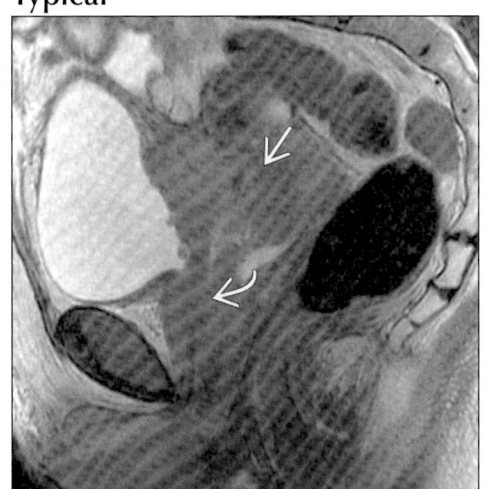

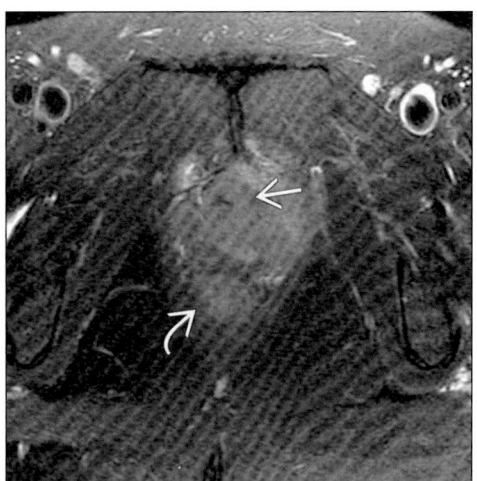

(Left) Sagittal T2WI MR shows an infiltrating upper vaginal carcinoma ➡ secondarily invading the urethra ➡ and posterior bladder wall in a 36 year old immunosuppressed woman. *(Right)* Axial T2WI FS MR in the same patient as left shows the vaginal carcinoma disrupting the normal target-like urethral appearance ➡. The mass also invades the ano-rectal junction ➡.

Typical

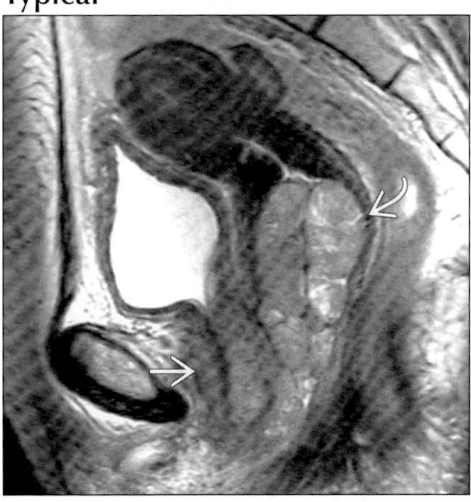

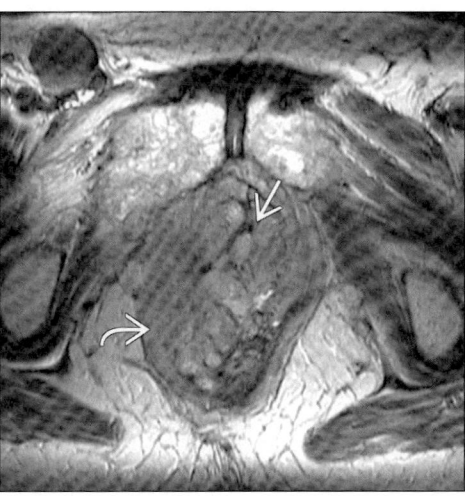

(Left) Sagittal T2WI MR shows a hyperintense mass circumferentially invading the urethra ➡ and vagina ➡ in a patient with previous renal cell carcinoma. These were proven to be metastases. *(Right)* Axial T2WI MR in the same patient as previous image shows the compressed urethral lumen ➡ due to invasion of the surrounding urethral wall by the metastasis as well as the vaginal invasion ➡.

DIVERTICULUM, URETHRA

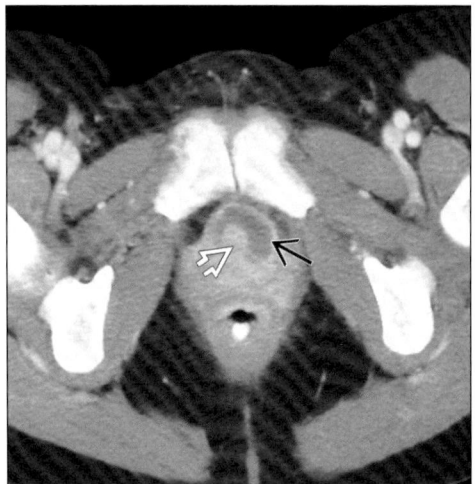
Axial CECT shows a low attenuation diverticulum ⇨ around the urethra ⇨.

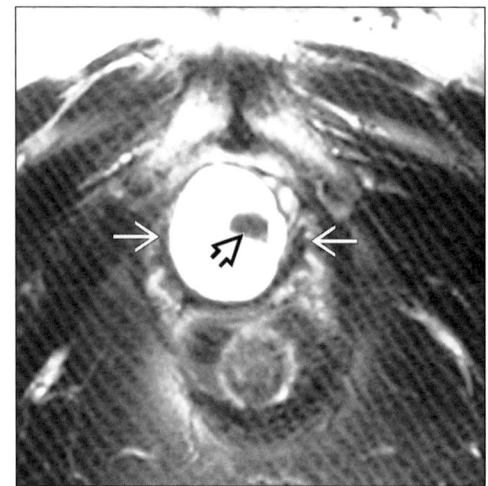
Axial T2WI FS MR demonstrates well-defined, high signal intensity diverticulum ⇨ surrounding the urethra ⇨.

TERMINOLOGY

Definitions
- Localized outpouching of urethra

IMAGING FINDINGS

General Features
- Best diagnostic clue: Multiseptated cystic lesion adjacent or surrounding urethra
- Location: Most commonly occurs in mid-urethra and on posterolateral wall rather than on anterior wall

Ultrasonographic Findings
- Grayscale Ultrasound
  - US with transvaginal or endorectal probe can demonstrate urethral diverticulum and assess the size, location, content and wall thickness of the diverticulum
  - Urethral diverticula appear as anechoic cystic lesions around the urethra

CT Findings
- CECT
  - Low attenuation nonenhancing lesion adjacent or around the urethra
  - Inflamed diverticulum may have heterogeneous density higher than simple fluid
  - Virtual CT urethroscopy which is less invasive than conventional urethroscopy can also be used to depict urethral diverticula

MR Findings
- T1WI
  - Low signal intensity lesion adjacent or around the urethra
  - Inflamed diverticulum may have heterogeneous signal intensity higher than that of urine on T1WI
- T2WI
  - High signal intensity cystic lesion with low signal intensity outer wall adjacent or around the urethra
  - Inflamed diverticulum may demonstrate fluid-fluid levels on T2WI
- T1 C+: Submucosal region may enhance; however, fluid in diverticulum does not

DDx: Urethral and Periurethral Conditions

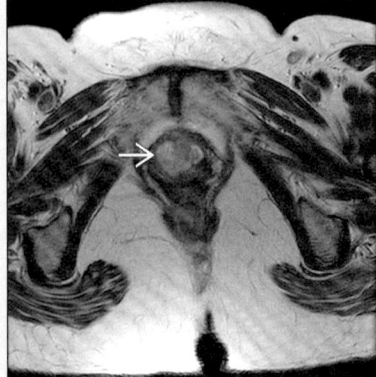
Urethral Cancer

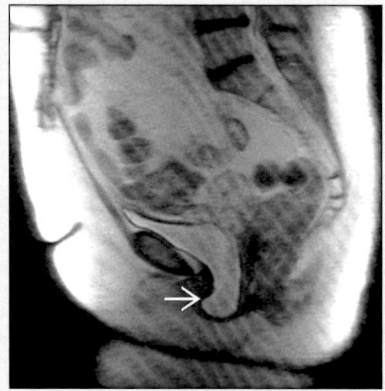
Cystocele

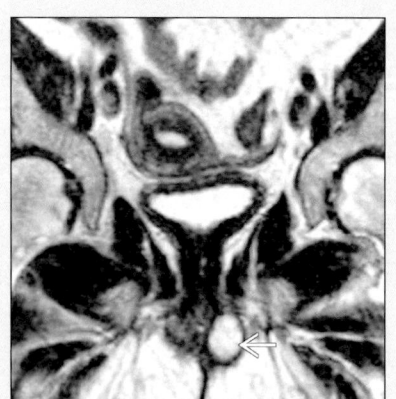
Bartholin Gland Cyst

DIVERTICULUM, URETHRA

Key Facts

Terminology
- Localized outpouching of urethra

Imaging Findings
- Best diagnostic clue: Multiseptated cystic lesion adjacent or surrounding urethra
- Location: Most commonly occurs in mid-urethra and on posterolateral wall rather than on anterior wall
- MR is superior to other imaging modalities in demonstrating urethral diverticulum because of its multiplanar capabilities and excellent soft tissue contrast
- MR allows direct visualization of diverticulum and evaluation of anatomic relationship to urethra or adjacent structures
- MR is very useful in diagnosing inflammation and tumor of diverticulum

Pathology
- Congenital urethral diverticula are rare
- Most are acquired resulting from inflammation of periurethral glands and ducts leading to local glandular dilatation and subsequent rupture into urethra
- Other etiologies include urethral injury during childbirth, surgery or catheterization

Clinical Issues
- The classical presentation of post-void dribbling, urethral pain, tender periurethral mass and/or expression of pus from the urethra on physical examination is uncommon
- Gender: More common in women than in men

Fluoroscopic Findings
- Voiding Cystourethrogram
  o Defines size, number and location of urethral diverticula
  o Presence of filling defects in urethral diverticulum may suggest the possibility of calculi or a tumor
- Retrograde Urethrogram
  o Double-balloon urethrogram is definitive for diagnosis
  o Defines size, number and location of urethral diverticula

Imaging Recommendations
- Best imaging tool
  o MR is superior to other imaging modalities in demonstrating urethral diverticulum because of its multiplanar capabilities and excellent soft tissue contrast
  o MR allows direct visualization of diverticulum and evaluation of anatomic relationship to urethra or adjacent structures
  o MR is very useful in diagnosing inflammation and tumor of diverticulum
- Protocol advice
  o T1WI: Transverse plane
  o T2WI: Transverse, coronal and sagittal planes with small field-of-view

DIFFERENTIAL DIAGNOSIS

Urethral Benign or Malignant Tumors
- Tumors are solid unlike cystic diverticulum
- They expand the urethral lumen

Urethral Duplication
- Usually associated with other genital anomalies
- Rare in women

Cystocele
- Urinary bladder descends below pubococcygeal line

Vaginal and Vulvar Cysts
- Bartholin gland cyst: Posterolateral to vaginal introitus below pelvic diaphragm
- Gartner duct cyst: Anterolateral wall of vagina above pelvic diaphragm
- Inclusion cysts

PATHOLOGY

General Features
- General path comments
  o Urethral diverticula vary in size, shape and communication with urethra
  o They may be unilocular or multilocular, spherical or horseshoe-shaped
  o Diverticular opening into urethral lumen may be narrow or wide
- Etiology
  o Congenital urethral diverticula are rare
  o Most are acquired resulting from inflammation of periurethral glands and ducts leading to local glandular dilatation and subsequent rupture into urethra
  o Other etiologies include urethral injury during childbirth, surgery or catheterization
- Epidemiology: Urethral diverticulum occurs in up to 5% of women

Gross Pathologic & Surgical Features
- Urethral diverticulum is a urethral evagination consisting of mostly fibrous tissue
- Surrounding periurethral fascia often remains intact
- Severely infected urethral diverticulum may erode into vagina

Microscopic Features
- Often an epithelial lining is absent
- Chronic inflammation within the diverticulum results in marked fibrosis and adherence of diverticular wall to neighboring structures

DIVERTICULUM, URETHRA

CLINICAL ISSUES

Presentation
- Most common signs/symptoms
  - Many urethral diverticula are asymptomatic and discovered incidentally
  - The classical presentation of post-void dribbling, urethral pain, tender periurethral mass and/or expression of pus from the urethra on physical examination is uncommon
  - Most patients present with nonspecific, refractory, lower urinary tract symptoms and undergo extensive evaluation and empirical treatments before diagnosis is made
- Other signs/symptoms: Other less frequent symptoms include hematuria and an anterior vaginal wall mass
- Clinical Profile
  - Recurrent urinary tract infections occur in approximately 40% of patients
  - Stone formation or, rarely, carcinoma or endometriosis

Demographics
- Age: Urethral diverticulum in women usually presents between the decades 3 and 5, although it has been reported in neonates and young women
- Gender: More common in women than in men

Natural History & Prognosis
- Success rate of urethral diverticulectomy is between 86-100%
- Recurrence is seen between 1-29% of cases

Treatment
- Medical treatment
  - Infected urethral diverticula are treated with appropriate antibiotics prior to surgery
- Surgery
  - Current treatment of choice
  - Surgical techniques include transurethral saucerization of the diverticulum, marsupialization of the diverticular sac into the vagina, and excision of the diverticulum

DIAGNOSTIC CHECKLIST

Consider
- Symptoms of urethral diverticulum may mimic a wide variety of conditions which can contribute to delay in diagnosis
- MR is recommended when clinical findings strongly suggest a urethral diverticulum but all other imaging modalities are nonconclusive

Image Interpretation Pearls
- Urethral diverticula appear as multiseptated cystic lesion adjacent or surrounding urethra
- Presence of filling defects within diverticulum suggests the possibility of urethral calculi or a tumor

SELECTED REFERENCES

1. Elsayes KM et al: Endovaginal magnetic resonance imaging of the female urethra. J Comput Assist Tomogr. 30(1):1-6, 2006
2. Chou CP et al: CT voiding urethrography and virtual urethroscopy: preliminary study with 16-MDCT. AJR Am J Roentgenol. 184(6):1882-8, 2005
3. Chou CP et al: Urethral diverticulum: diagnosis with virtual CT urethroscopy. AJR Am J Roentgenol. 184(6):1889-90, 2005
4. Kim SH et al: CT voiding cystourethrography using 16-MDCT for the evaluation of female urethral diverticula: initial experience. AJR Am J Roentgenol. 184(5):1594-6, 2005
5. Prasad SR et al: Cross-sectional imaging of the female urethra: technique and results. Radiographics. 25(3):749-61, 2005
6. Chowdhry AA et al: Endometriosis presenting as a urethral diverticulum: a case report. J Reprod Med. 49(4):321-3, 2004
7. Kawashima A et al: Imaging of urethral disease: a pictorial review. Radiographics. 24 Suppl 1:S195-216, 2004
8. Macura KJ et al: Evaluation of the female urethra with intraurethral magnetic resonance imaging. J Magn Reson Imaging. 20(1):153-9, 2004
9. Blander DS et al: Endoluminal magnetic resonance imaging in the evaluation of urethral diverticula in women. Urology. 57(4):660-5, 2001
10. Ryu JA et al: MR imaging of the male and female urethra. Radiographics. 21:1169-85, 2001
11. Romanzi LJ et al: Urethral diverticulum in women: diverse presentations resulting in diagnostic delay and mismanagement. J Urol. 164:428-33, 2000
12. Khati NJ et al: MR imaging diagnosis of a urethral diverticulum. Radiographics. 18(2):517-22, 1998
13. Nurenberg P et al: Role of MR imaging with transrectal coil in the evaluation of complex urethral abnormalities. AJR Am J Roentgenol. 169(5):1335-8, 1997
14. Siegelman ES et al: Multicoil MR imaging of symptomatic female urethral and periurethral disease. Radiographics. 17(2):349-65, 1997
15. Vargas-Serrano B et al: Transrectal ultrasonography in the diagnosis of urethral diverticula in women. J Clin Ultrasound. 25(1):21-8, 1997
16. Debaere C et al: MR imaging of a diverticulum in a female urethra. J Belge Radiol. 78(6):345-6, 1995
17. Hricak H et al: Female urethra: MR imaging. Radiology. 178(2):527-35, 1991

DIVERTICULUM, URETHRA

IMAGE GALLERY

Typical

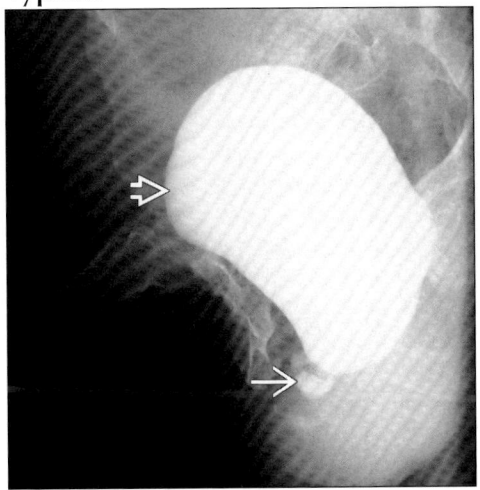
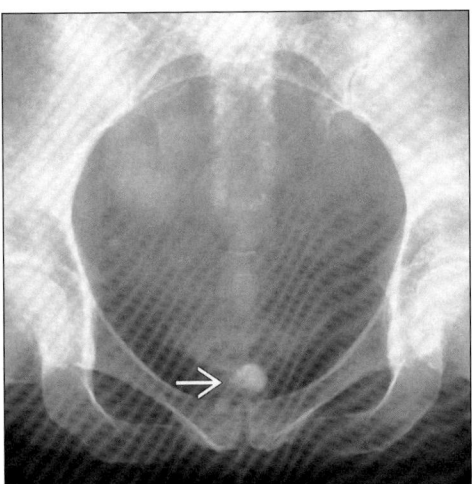

(Left) Oblique voiding cystourethrogram shows contrast filling urethral diverticulum ➡ below the urinary bladder ➡. *(Right)* Frontal voiding cystourethrogram shows retained contrast in the urethral diverticulum ➡.

Typical

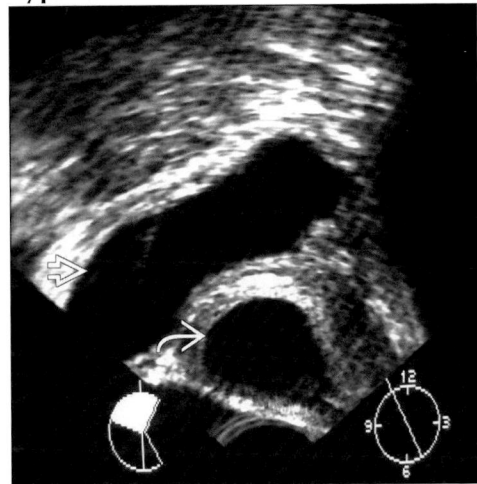
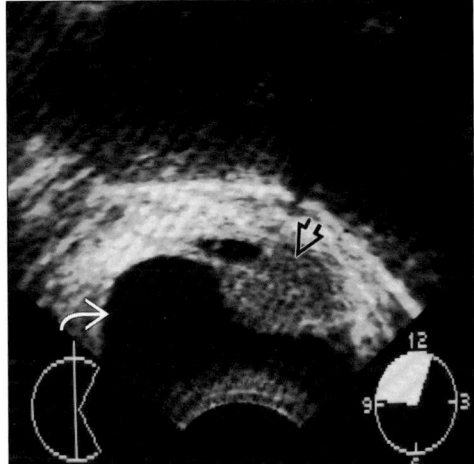

(Left) Sagittal oblique transvaginal ultrasound shows an anechoic urethral diverticulum ➡ just inferior to the urinary bladder ➡. *(Right)* Axial transvaginal ultrasound shows anechoic diverticulum ➡ around the urethra ➡.

Typical

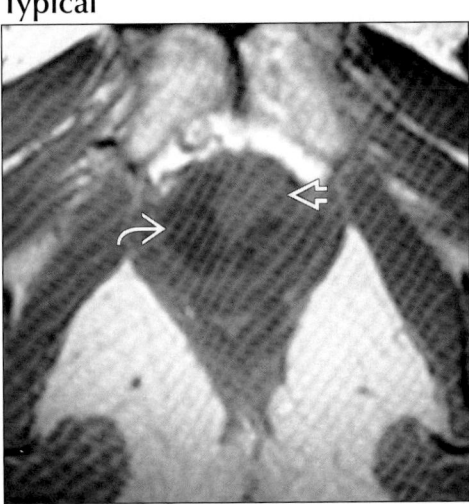
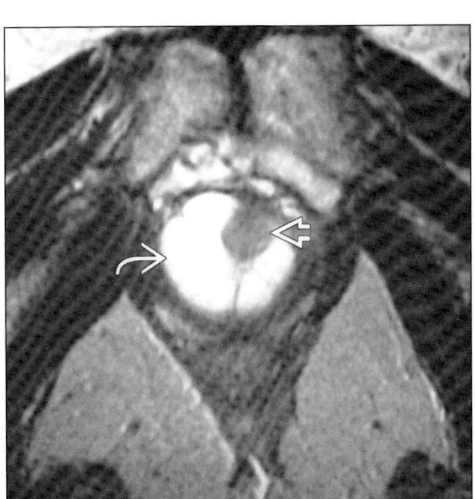

(Left) Axial T1WI MR shows low signal intensity diverticulum ➡ around the urethra ➡. *(Right)* Axial T2WI MR shows high signal intensity diverticulum ➡ around the urethra ➡.

PROLAPSE, URETHRA

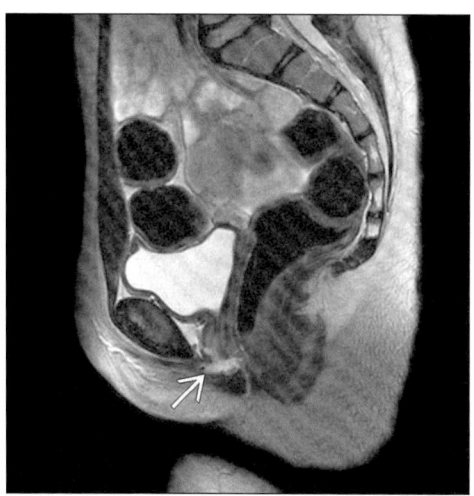

Sagittal T2WI MR shows T2 hyperintense lesion ➡, consistent with urethral prolapse, protruding through the urethral meatus.

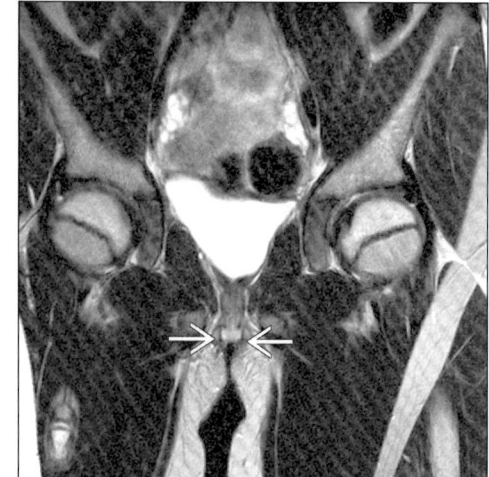

Coronal T2WI MR shows T2 hyperintense mass ➡, consistent with urethral prolapse, at the urethral meatus.

TERMINOLOGY

Abbreviations and Synonyms
- Urethral protrusion
- Urethral eversion

Definitions
- Protrusion of the urethra through the external meatus

IMAGING FINDINGS

General Features
- Best diagnostic clue: Rounded soft tissue surrounding urethral meatus
- Location: Perineal
- Size: 11 mm to 30 mm in diameter
- Morphology
  ○ Doughnut-shaped fleshy tissue with central lumen encircling the urethral meatus
  ○ Usually complete circumference eversion but partial eversion can be seen

Ultrasonographic Findings
- Grayscale Ultrasound
  ○ Transperineal approach
  ○ Clover-shaped hypoechoic mass protruding from urethral meatus
- Color Doppler
  ○ May be vascular
    ▪ Vascularity diminishes with topical estrogen and antibiotics

CT Findings
- CECT: Enhancing soft tissue protruding through urethral meatus

MR Findings
- T2WI: Protrusion of high signal intensity urethral mucosa through the urethral meatus
- T1 C+ FS: Enhancing soft tissue extending through urethral meatus

Imaging Recommendations
- Best imaging tool: MR because of its excellent spatial resolution and multiplanar capabilities
- Protocol advice

DDx: Mimics of Urethral Prolapse

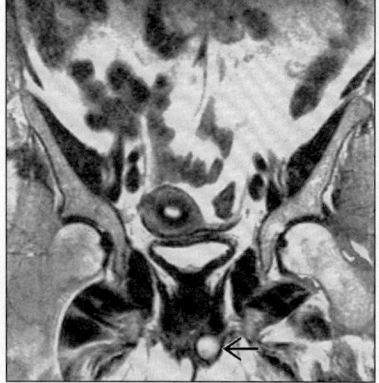
Bartholin Gland Cyst

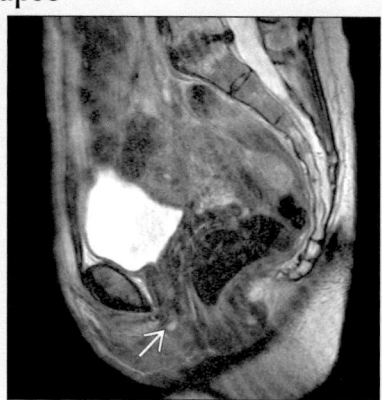
Skene Gland Cyst

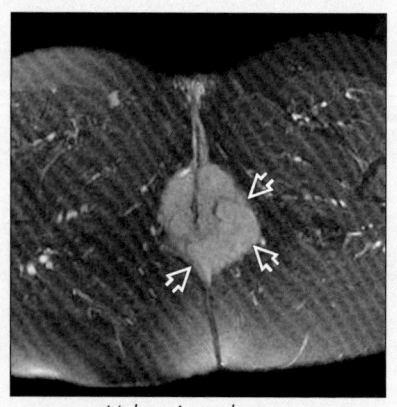
Vulvar Lymphoma

PROLAPSE, URETHRA

Key Facts

Terminology
- Urethral protrusion
- Protrusion of the urethra through the external meatus

Imaging Findings
- Best diagnostic clue: Rounded soft tissue surrounding urethral meatus
- Doughnut-shaped fleshy tissue with central lumen encircling the urethral meatus
- T2WI: Protrusion of high signal intensity urethral mucosa through the urethral meatus
- T1 C+ FS: Enhancing soft tissue extending through urethral meatus
- Best imaging tool: MR because of its excellent spatial resolution and multiplanar capabilities
- Axial T2 weighted images should extend far below the pubic symphysis

Top Differential Diagnoses
- Bartholin Gland Cyst
- Skene Gland Cyst
- Vulvar Tumor
- Vaginal Tumor
- Bulging Imperforate Hymen

Clinical Issues
- Most common signs/symptoms: Palpable mass occupying the introitus
- Vulvar bleeding, often mistaken to be early menarche
- Dysuria
- Urinary frequency
- Cured with resection

- Axial T2 weighted images should extend far below the pubic symphysis
- Sagittal and coronal T2 weighted images are helpful

DIFFERENTIAL DIAGNOSIS

Urethral Cancer
- Most commonly squamous cell carcinoma
- Enhancing soft tissue within urethra

Bartholin Gland Cyst
- Paired glands located in the posterolateral third of the vagina associated with the labia majora
- Below the level of the pubic symphysis
- Usually simple cyst imaging characteristics unless infected

Skene Gland Cyst
- Paired glands located laterally to the external urethral meatus
- Usually asymptomatic
- Typical appearance: Well-circumscribed cystic lesion rather than rosette type appearance of urethral prolapse

Urethral Diverticulum
- Cystic lesion typically emanating from posterolateral wall of the mid-urethra
- Mid-urethral location helps to differentiate this from prolapse

Vulvar Tumor
- Solid enhancing lesions arising in the vulva
  - Polyp
  - Papilloma
  - Hemangioma
  - Lymphoma

Vaginal Tumor
- Sarcoma botryoides
  - Grape-like tumor expanding vaginal cavity
- Vaginal polyp

Prolapsed Ureterocele
- Intravenous urogram can be performed to confirm this diagnosis

Bulging Imperforate Hymen
- Hydro(metro)culpos: Vagina distended with fluid and blood products

Condyloma Acuminatum
- Sexually transmitted genital warts

Perineal Trauma
- Hematoma
- History of sexual abuse

Periurethral Abscess
- Rim-enhancing periurethral fluid collection with associated inflammatory signs

PATHOLOGY

General Features
- Etiology
  - Multiple theories
    - Decreased estrogen resulting in laxity of periurethral fascia, vaginal atrophy, and mucosal redundancy
    - Urethral mal-position
    - Poor bladder support
    - Fascial defects
    - Prior pelvic surgery or trauma
    - Prior periurethral injections of bulking agents such as collagen and calcium hydroxylapatite for treatment of stress incontinence
    - Abnormal circumferential plane of cleavage between inner longitudinal and outer circular muscle layers of distal urethra
    - Muscular asynergia caused by strong detrusor and week pelvic floor muscles
    - Increased intra-abdominal pressure caused by coughing or straining
    - Excessive redundancy of urethral mucosa

PROLAPSE, URETHRA

- Epidemiology: Rare
- Associated abnormalities: Usually no associated abnormalities of the urogenital tract

Gross Pathologic & Surgical Features
- Usually polypoid, edematous, hemorrhagic, friable mass
- Often described as a rosette of tissue

Microscopic Features
- Benign polypous tissue composed of fibrovascular stroma
- Dilated and thrombosed veins in the deep layers of the urethral submucosa
- Cystic dilatation of mucosal glands
- Cleavage between inner longitudinal and outer circular smooth muscle layers

Staging, Grading or Classification Criteria
- Grade 1: Minimal or segmental prolapse without inflammation
- Grade 2: Circumferential prolapse with edema
- Grade 3: Edematous mass protruding beyond labia minora
- Grade 4: Severe hemorrhagic inflammation or necrosis or ulceration of the prolapse

CLINICAL ISSUES

Presentation
- Most common signs/symptoms: Palpable mass occupying the introitus
- Other signs/symptoms
  - Vulvar bleeding, often mistaken to be early menarche
  - Dysuria
  - Urinary frequency
  - Rarely, acute urinary retention
- Clinical Profile
  - Children usually present with vaginal bleeding, not pain
  - Adults often present with pain & urinary symptoms

Demographics
- Age
  - Most often affects two different age groups
    - Premenarchal children, ages 4 to 9 (incidence in this age group reported as 1:3,000)
    - Postmenopausal elderly women
- Ethnicity
  - In children, African American girls are more commonly affected (93%)
  - Postmenopausal patients are usually Caucasian women (86%)

Natural History & Prognosis
- Cured with resection
- Complications can arise if untreated
  - Infection
  - Ulceration
  - Necrosis
  - Gangrene
  - Urethral stenosis

Treatment
- Local treatment
  - Topical estrogen
  - Antibiotics
  - Sitz baths
  - High recurrence rate, up to 67%
  - Local therapy often reserved for children, not adults
- Surgery
  - Excision with primary closure of the urethral mucosa is treatment of choice
  - Fibrin glue injection after excision may help support remaining urethra
  - Complications of surgery are unusual
    - Recurrence
    - Meatal stenosis
    - Urethritis
    - Urinary retention
- Manual reduction is not indicated

DIAGNOSTIC CHECKLIST

Image Interpretation Pearls
- Consider diagnosis of urethral prolapse particularly in pediatric patient with history of bleeding

SELECTED REFERENCES

1. Ghoniem GM et al: Urethral prolapse after durasphere injection. Int Urogynecol J Pelvic Floor Dysfunct. 17(3):297-8, 2006
2. Palma PC et al: Massive prolapse of the urethral mucosa following periurethral injection of calcium hydroxylapatite for stress urinary incontinence. Int Urogynecol J Pelvic Floor Dysfunct. 17(6):670-1, 2006
3. Lang ME et al: Vaginal bleeding in the prepubertal child. CMAJ. 172(10):1289-90, 2005
4. Yang JM et al: Transperineal sonographic findings in a woman with urethral mucosa prolapse. J Clin Ultrasound. 32(5):261-3, 2004
5. Valerie E et al: Diagnosis and treatment of urethral prolapse in children. Urology. 54(6):1082-4, 1999
6. Harris RL et al: Urethral prolapse after collagen injection. Am J Obstet Gynecol. 178(3):614-5, 1998
7. Desai SR et al: Urethral prolapse in a premenarchal girl: case report and literature review. Aust N Z J Surg. 67(9):660-2, 1997
8. Rudin JE et al: Prolapse of urethral mucosa in white female children: experience with 58 cases. J Pediatr Surg. 32(3):423-5, 1997
9. Anveden-Hertzberg L et al: Urethral prolapse: an often misdiagnosed cause of urogenital bleeding in girls. Pediatr Emerg Care. 11(4):212-4, 1995
10. Poirier MP et al: Pediatric vaginal bleeding. Urethral prolapse. Acad Emerg Med. 2(6):527-8, 563-5, 1995
11. Fernandes ET et al: Urethral prolapse in children. Urology. 41(3):240-2, 1993
12. Lowe FC et al: Urethral prolapse in children: insights into etiology and management. J Urol. 135(1):100-3, 1986
13. Jerkins GR et al: Treatment of girls with urethral prolapse. J Urol. 132(4):732-3, 1984
14. Bullock KN: Strangulated prolapse of female urethra. Urology. 21(1):46-8, 1983
15. Nussbaum AR et al: Interlabial masses in little girls: review and imaging recommendations. AJR Am J Roentgenol. 141(1):65-71, 1983

PROLAPSE, URETHRA

IMAGE GALLERY

Typical

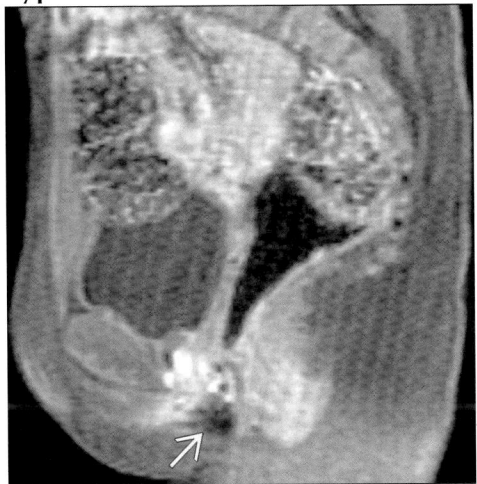
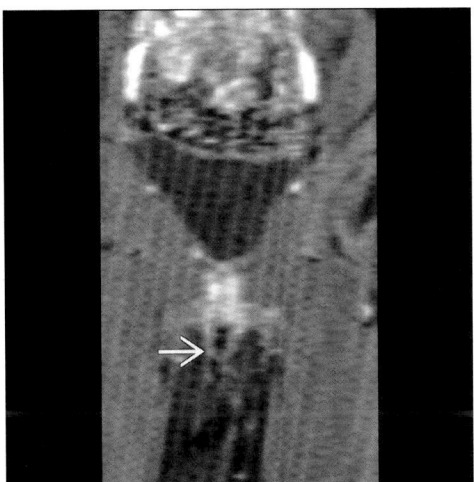

(Left) Sagittal T1 C+ FS MR shows nonenhancing T1 hypointense lesion ➡ protruding through urethral meatus. *(Right)* Coronal T1 C+ FS MR multiplanar reconstruction shows a small area of rim-enhancement ➡ just beyond the urethral meatus.

Typical

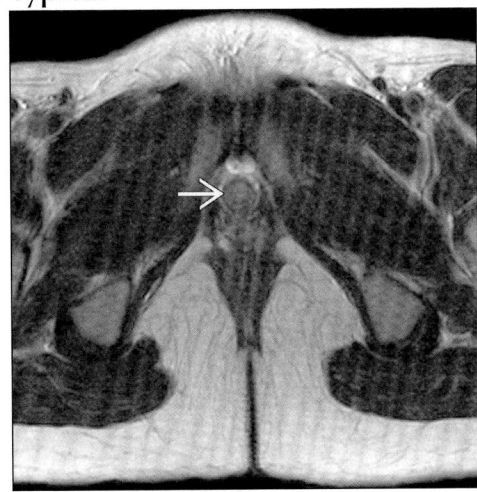
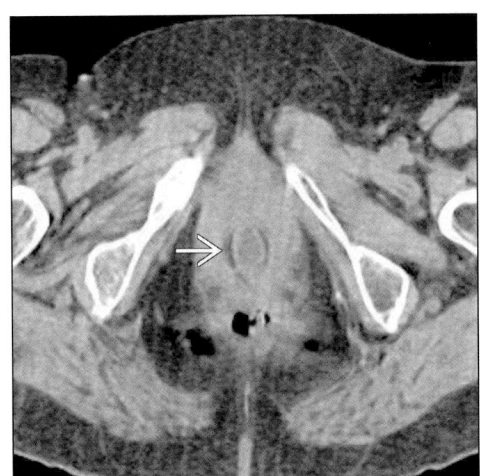

(Left) Axial T2WI MR shows loss of the normal target appearance of the distal urethra ➡, presumably due to eversion of the mucosa distally. *(Right)* Axial NECT shows a well-circumscribed fluid attenuation structure and surrounding fat ➡ within the perineum. Physical exam confirmed urethral prolapse.

Typical

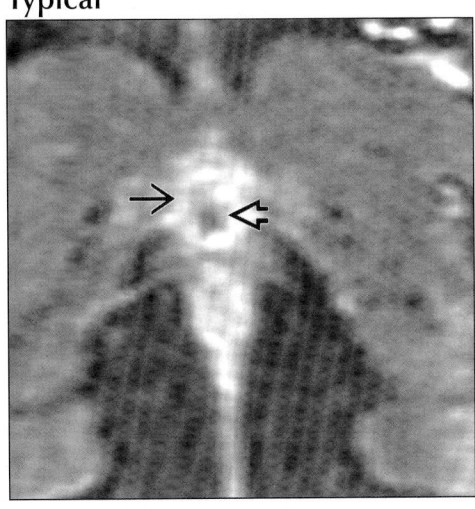
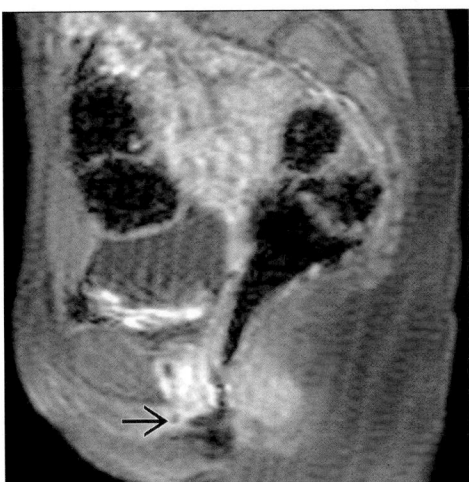

(Left) Axial T1 C+ FS MR multiplanar reconstruction shows enhancing soft tissue ➡ beyond the urethral meatus. Urethral lumen ⬅ is seen centrally. *(Right)* Sagittal T1 C+ FS MR shows protrusion of soft tissue ➡ in the anterior perineum, consistent with urethral prolapse.

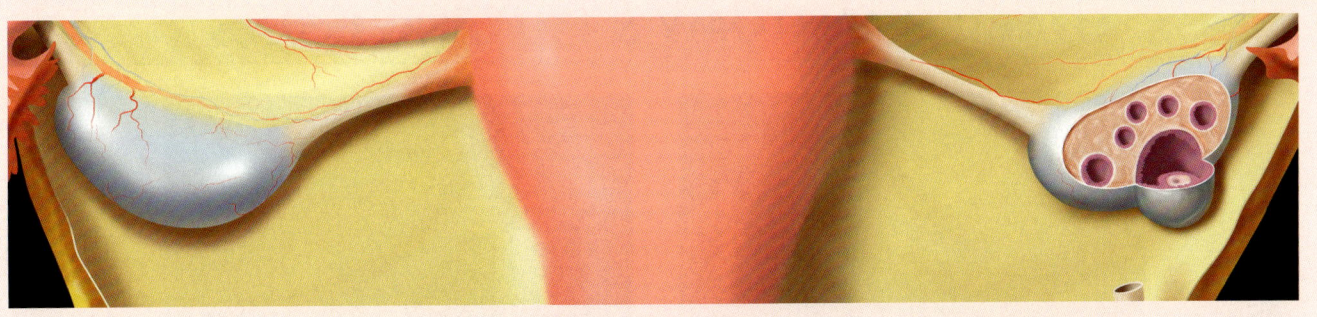

SECTION 7: Ovary

Introduction and Overview

Ovarian Anatomy & Imaging Issues	7-2

Normal Variants

Follicular Cyst	7-8
Corpus Luteal Cyst	7-12
Theca Lutein Cysts	7-16
Luteoma of Pregnancy	7-20

Neoplasm, Benign

Dermoid (Mature Teratoma)	7-22
Fibrothecoma, Ovary	7-28
Adenofibroma	7-32
Granulosa Cell Tumor	7-34
Sclerosing Stromal Tumor	7-40
Cystadenofibroma	7-44
Serous Cystadenoma	7-48
Mucinous Cystadenoma	7-54
Brenner Tumor	7-60

Neoplasm, Malignant

Mucinous Cystadenocarcinoma	7-64
Serous Cystadenocarcinoma	7-70
Endometrioid Carcinoma, Ovary	7-74
Sertoli-Leydig Cell Tumor	7-80
Dysgerminoma	7-84
Yolk Sac Tumor, Ovary	7-88
Lymphoma, Ovary	7-92
Clear Cell Carcinoma, Ovary	7-96
Immature Teratoma, Ovary	7-100
Metastases, Ovary	7-106
Ovarian Cancer, Characterization & Staging	7-112
Ovarian Cancer, Recurrent; Resectable	7-118
Ovarian Cancer, Recurrent; Unresectable	7-122
Choriocarcinoma, Ovary	7-126
Struma Ovarii	7-130
Carcinoid, Ovary	7-134
Undifferentiated Carcinoma, Ovary	7-138
Embryonal Carcinoma, Ovary	7-142
Mixed Mullerian Tumor, Ovary	7-146
Krukenberg Tumor	7-150

Miscellaneous

Inclusion Cyst, Ovary	7-154
Ovarian Hyperstimulation Syndrome	7-158
Paraovarian Cyst	7-162
Endometrioma	7-166
Endometriosis	7-170
Adnexal Torsion	7-176
Massive Ovarian Edema	7-182
Polycystic Ovary Syndrome	7-186
Fibromatosis, Ovary	7-190
Hemorrhagic Cysts, Ovary	7-192
Meigs Syndrome	7-198

OVARIAN ANATOMY & IMAGING ISSUES

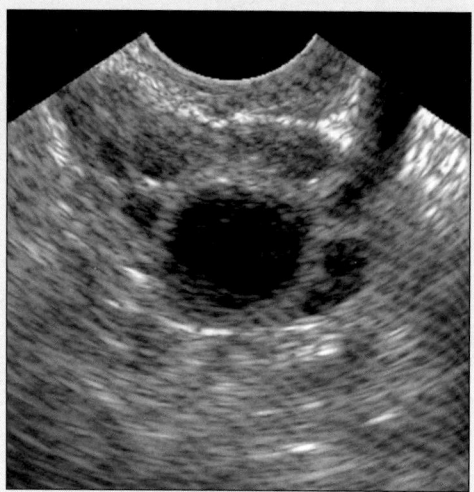

Transverse transvaginal ultrasound shows normal ovary with developing follicles and a dominant follicle.

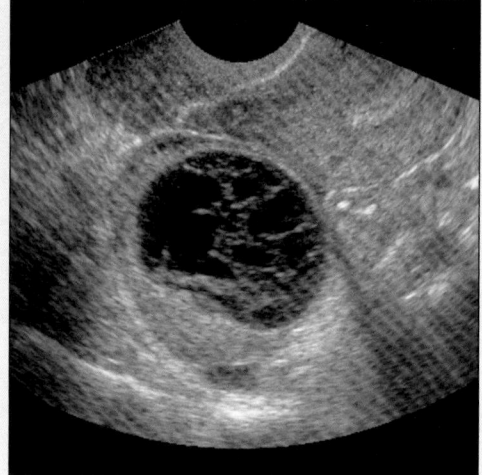

Transverse transvaginal ultrasound shows classic appearance of hemorrhagic cyst with strands of linear echoes.

TERMINOLOGY

Abbreviations
- Follicle-stimulating hormone (FSH), estradiol (E2), luteinizing hormone (LH)

IMAGING ANATOMY

General Anatomic Considerations
- Ovary consists of medulla and cortex
  - Medulla is highly vascular and receives vessels from the ovarian hilum
  - Cortex contains ovarian follicles in different stages of development and is imbedded in dense fibrocellular stroma
    - During reproductive years most of the ovary consists of cortex
  - Tunica albuginea covers the ovary
- Physiology
  - Typical menstrual cycle is 28 days & consists of follicular phase, ovulation, and luteal phase
  - Cycle ranges 23-35 days in 90% of women
  - Follicular phase
    - FSH in late luteal phase initiates development of 5-12 primary ovarian follicles
    - Developing follicles are thin-walled, anechoic, less than 1 cm in diameter
    - One follicle per cycle (typically) develops into a mature (dominant) follicle
    - Dominant follicle appears as thin-walled, anechoic, up to 2.9 cm in diameter
    - Granulosa cells in dominant follicle respond to FSH by increasing E2 production
    - E2 inhibits further production of FSH
    - E2 feeds back to pituitary resulting in LH surge
  - LH surge leads to ovulation about day 14 of cycle
  - Luteal phase
    - E2 levels decline
    - Progesterone levels from developing corpus luteum increase
    - Follicles that do not ovulate become atretic
    - Corpus luteum proliferates and becomes vascularized
    - Corpus luteum frequently contains hemorrhage and has a complex appearance
    - Corpus luteum can be thick-walled, heterogeneous, hypervascular with low impedance flow
    - If fertilization does not occur the corpus luteum regresses at about day 24
    - Regressing corpus luteum has a crenated appearance and can appear solid but will have through transmission

Anatomic Relationships
- Ovarian fossa bounded above by external iliac vessels, in front by obliterated umbilical artery, and behind by ureter
- Ovaries are displaced during the first pregnancy, and probably do not return to original position
- Long axis of ovary typically oriented in craniocaudal direction
- Suspensory ligament inserts at superior pole of ovary together with ovarian fimbria of fallopian tube
- Caudal pole of ovary is attached to uterus by the ovarian ligament
- Mesovarium is a short peritoneal fold attaching ovary to posterior surface of the broad ligament and containing the neurovascular bundle
- In patient after hysterectomy, ovaries can move high in pelvis due to loss of suspensory ligaments
- Ovary has dual arterial blood supply
  - Ovarian arteries arise laterally from aorta just distal to renal arteries and descend towards pelvis paralleling ureter
  - Ovarian arteries cross over external iliac vessels and turn medially in the suspensory ligament of ovary
  - Ovarian branches of uterine artery run in the broad ligament
  - Vascular branches enter ovary through mesovarium at ovarian hilum
- Ovarian veins form a plexus in the broad ligament that communicates with uterine venous plexus

OVARIAN ANATOMY & IMAGING ISSUES

Key Facts

Ovarian Appearance Changes with Respect to Patient Age
- Ovarian volume increases during childhood
- Even after menopause, thin-walled anechoic cysts are frequently seen

Ovarian Appearance Changes with Respect to Phase of Menstrual Cycle
- During menstrual years, cysts less than 3 cm are common

Hemorrhagic Corpus Luteum Cysts can Mimic Ovarian Pathology
- Blood clot within cyst can be mobile and will not demonstrate flow

- If a complex cyst is visualized that is not typical for a hemorrhagic cyst then follow-up is typically obtained in an interval of 6 weeks

Findings that Increase Likelihood of Malignancy Include
- Advanced age
- Thick irregular septations
- Solid elements with blood flow
- Low resistive index

MR is Helpful in Distinguishing Between Solid Ovarian Lesion and Leiomyoma
- Connection to uterus frequently better seen on MR

- Right ovarian vein drains directly into inferior vena cava caudal to right renal vein
- Left ovarian vein drains into left renal vein

ANATOMY-BASED IMAGING ISSUES

Key Concepts or Questions
- Is a cyst physiologic or neoplastic?
  - Cyst size, wall thickness, and internal appearance should be assessed
  - Small cysts less than 3 cm are likely physiologic
  - Large cysts (greater than 6 cm) if thin walled and anechoic are likely neoplastic but also likely benign
  - Postmenopausal women commonly have small thin-walled anechoic cysts
  - If cyst has thick septations or solid elements it is likely neoplastic
  - Complex cysts of uncertain etiology can be followed sonographically and should resolve over time
- What is the etiology of a "simple cyst"?
  - "Simple cyst" is thin-walled, anechoic with enhanced through transmission
  - Etiologies include functional cyst, paraovarian or paratubal cyst, hydrosalpinx, cystadenoma, peritoneal inclusion cyst, theca lutein cyst
- Is blood flow present in presumed solid elements?
  - Solid elements with blood flow increase likelihood of malignancy
  - Clot in a hemorrhagic cyst can mimic a solid nodule, but should not demonstrate flow
  - Artifactual flow on Doppler ultrasound can be seen in blood clot due to motion of clot
    - Real time scanning aids in diagnosis
  - Low resistive index (< 0.4) is associated with malignancy, but is less predictive of malignancy than are grayscale findings
- Is the ovary too large?
  - Isoechoic cysts can give the appearance of an enlarged ovary
  - If patient has acute or intermittent pain, torsion is a possibility
    - Check for arterial and venous waveforms, although these can be present in torsed ovaries
  - Solid tumors can give appearance of an enlarged ovary
    - If it is unclear if solid adnexal lesion is arising from the ovary or uterus, MR is helpful
  - In postmenopausal women an ovary twice the size of contralateral ovary is worrisome for malignancy
  - Bilateral enlarged ovaries can be due to polycystic ovarian syndrome, metastatic disease, lymphoma

Imaging Approaches
- TAS for large masses
- TVS to best characterize internal characteristics of cyst
- MR for complex lesions not completely characterized by ultrasound
- CT not recommended for characterization of cysts but is helpful in staging ovarian carcinoma

Imaging Protocols
- Functional cysts result from normal function of ovary (follicular cysts, luteal cysts, hemorrhagic cysts)
  - Most common cause of ovarian enlargement in young women
  - Typically measure less than 5 cm in diameter, but can be up to 20 cm
  - Regress during subsequent menstrual cycle
  - If less than 3 cm, benign-appearing functional cysts do not require follow-up
  - Follow-up in 6 weeks (when patient is at a different phase of menstrual cycle) if large or atypical in appearance
  - If cyst does not regress, hormonal therapy can at times suppress follicular activity
  - Persistent large cysts (> 6 cm) likely neoplastic, but if thin-walled and anechoic, are likely benign
- MR for characterization of adnexal masses not completely assessed by ultrasound
  - Simple cysts have thin wall with contents that follow signal intensity of water
  - Hemorrhagic cysts have thick irregular wall that may enhance with gadolinium, and heterogeneous internal contents

OVARIAN ANATOMY & IMAGING ISSUES

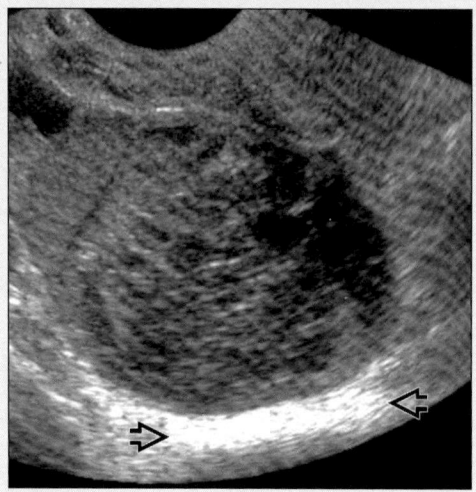

Transverse transvaginal ultrasound shows classic appearance of hemorrhagic corpus luteum cyst. Note the strands of internal echogenicity and posterior increased through transmission ⇨.

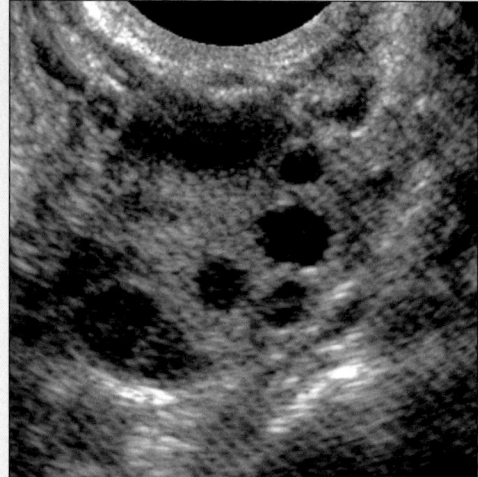

Axial oblique transvaginal ultrasound shows normal ovary with multiple developing follicles.

- Assess for connection to uterus to diagnose exophytic and pedunculated fibroids

Imaging Pitfalls
- Blood clot within a cyst can appear solid
  - Through transmission indicates cystic nature
  - Blood clot can "jiggle" when ovary pressed during transvaginal scanning
- Color Doppler can show artifactual flow in region of hemorrhage
  - Motion of clot can simulate flow
  - Pulsed Doppler will not show a venous or arterial tracing
- Hydrosalpinx can simulate a complex ovarian cyst: Oblique imaging planes can show tubular nature of cyst
- Vessels can simulate adnexal cysts: Color Doppler will show flow within vessel

Normal Measurements
- Ovaries in girls less than 2 years of age are typically less than 1 cc in volume
- Young girls can have small cysts, typically less than 5 mm
- Ovary volume increases from early childhood to approximately 16 years of age
- As menarche approaches, girls can have larger cysts
- After menarche ovaries are ovoid 3 cm x 2 cm x 2 cm
- Women of menstrual age: Mean ovarian volume of 10 cc
- Postmenopausal ovarian size decreases

PATHOLOGY-BASED IMAGING ISSUES

Key Concepts or Questions
- Adnexal mass findings that increase likelihood of malignancy
  - Larger mass size
  - Solid elements in cyst
  - Thick septations with vascular nodularity
  - Low resistive index
  - Absent diastolic notch
  - Abnormal CA-125 (not good for screening due to low specificity)
  - Older age of patient
  - Ascites
  - Metastatic disease

EMBRYOLOGY

Embryologic Events
- Wolffian ducts degenerate in normal female
- Ovaries descend from the peritoneum into pelvis to lie at superior margin of broad ligament
- At puberty ovaries descend deeper into pelvis to lie at lateral margin of uterus

Practical Implications
- Cysts in remnant of Wolffian ducts present as paraovarian cysts
- If descent of ovaries fails to occur, ovaries are in a more superior location than normal

RELATED REFERENCES

1. Holm K et al: Pubertal maturation of the internal genitalia: an ultrasound evaluation of 166 healthy girls. Ultrasound Obstet Gynecol. 6(3):175-81, 1995
2. Cohen HL et al: Ovarian cysts are common in premenarchal girls: a sonographic study of 101 children 2-12 years old. AJR Am J Roentgenol. 159(1):89-91, 1992
3. Siegel MJ: Pediatric gynecologic sonography. Radiology. 179(3):593-600, 1991
4. Cohen HL et al: Ovarian volumes measured by US: bigger than we think. Radiology. 177(1):189-92, 1990
5. Nussbaum AR et al: Neonatal ovarian cysts: sonographic-pathologic correlation. Radiology. 168(3):817-21, 1988
6. Orsini LF et al: Pelvic organs in premenarchal girls: real-time ultrasonography. Radiology. 153(1):113-6, 1984
7. Moore K: The Developing Human. 3rd ed. Philadelphia, WB Saunders, 1982

OVARIAN ANATOMY & IMAGING ISSUES

IMAGE GALLERY

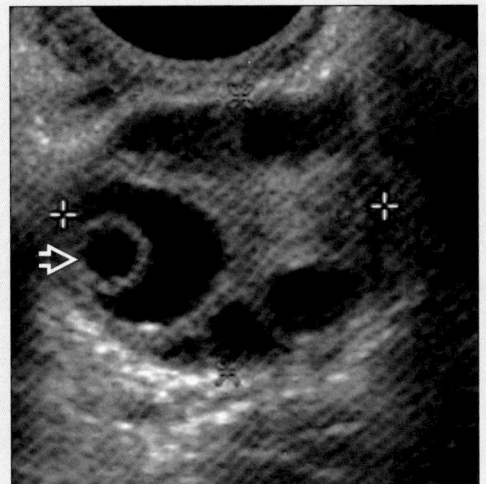
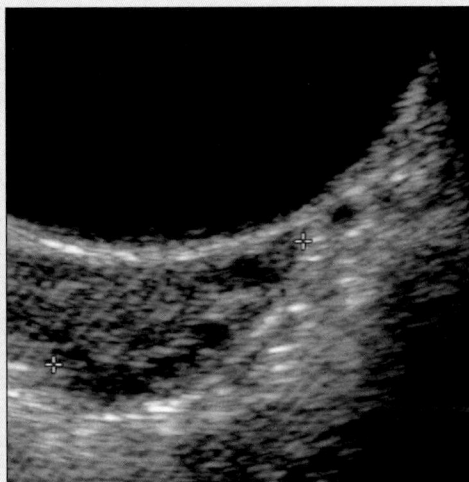

(Left) Transverse transvaginal ultrasound shows normal appearance to the ovary (calipers) with a follicle ➡ impinging on a larger cyst. This type of appearance is common and will resolve on follow-up. *(Right)* Transverse transabdominal ultrasound shows normal appearance to the ovary (calipers).

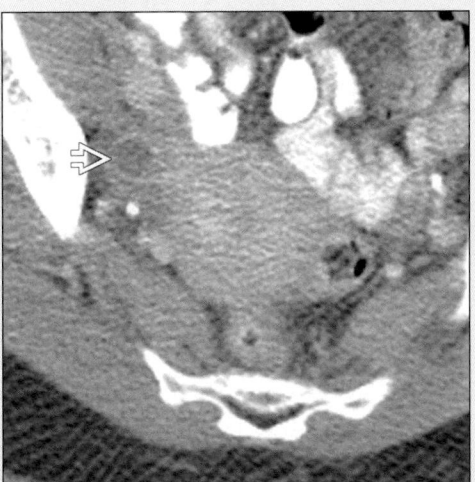
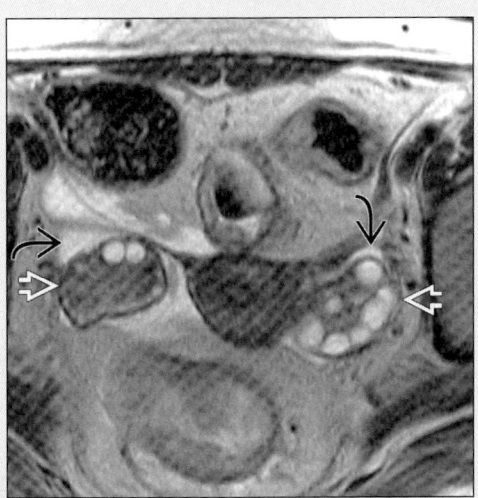

(Left) Transverse CECT shows normal appearance of ovary with small cyst ➡. *(Right)* Transverse T2WI MR shows normal appearance of ovaries ➡ with small amount of free fluid ➡ in the pelvis.

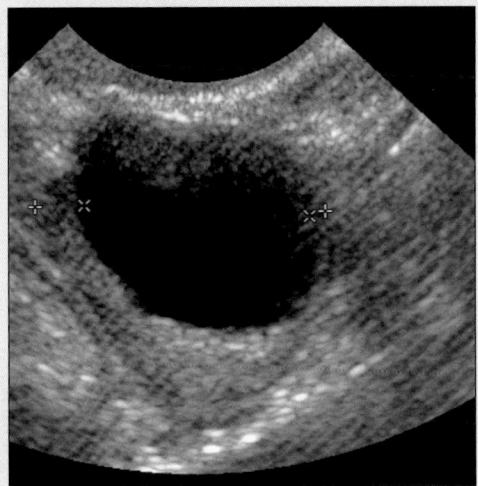
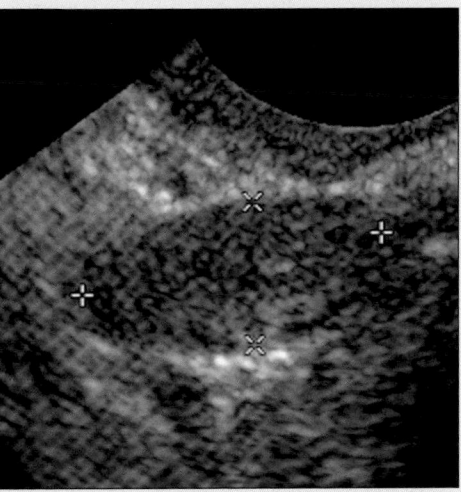

(Left) Transverse transvaginal ultrasound shows 3 cm cyst (calipers x) in ovary (calipers +) in the physiologic range. *(Right)* Transverse transvaginal ultrasound shows ovoid appearance of postmenopausal ovary (calipers). Note lack of cysts.

OVARIAN ANATOMY & IMAGING ISSUES

IMAGE GALLERY

(Left) Transverse transvaginal ultrasound shows cyst *(calipers)* with thick slightly irregular wall consistent with hemorrhagic corpus luteum. *(Right)* Axial T2WI MR shows case of corpus luteal cyst with a low signal area within the right ovary ➔.

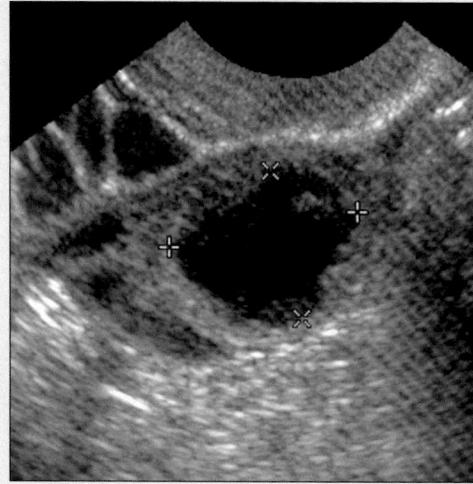 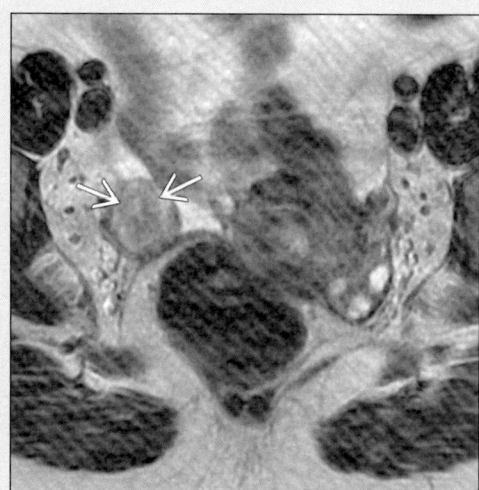

(Left) Axial T1 C+ MR in same patient as previous image shows intense peripheral enhancement post gadolinium ➔, making the diagnosis easier. *(Right)* Transverse transvaginal ultrasound shows typical case of endometrioma with layering low level internal echoes ➔.

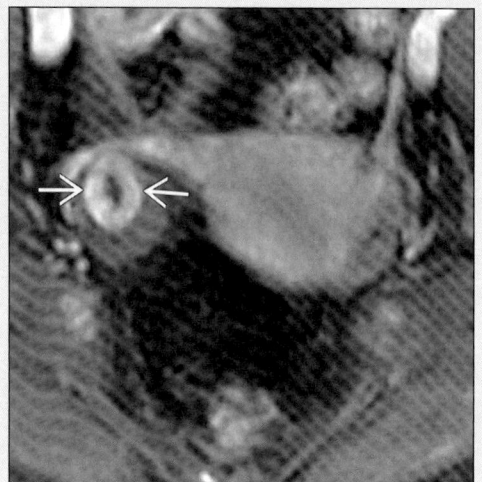 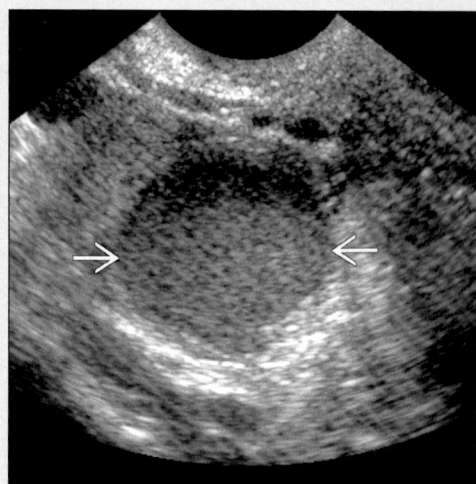

(Left) Longitudinal transvaginal ultrasound shows typical case of hydrosalpinx with an oblong cyst. This should not be mistaken for an ovarian tumor. *(Right)* Axial CECT shows typical case of bilateral tubo-ovarian abscess with multiple thick-walled low attenuation areas ➔ and free fluid ➔.

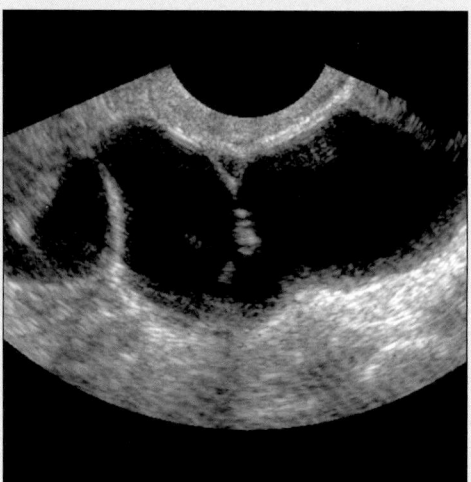 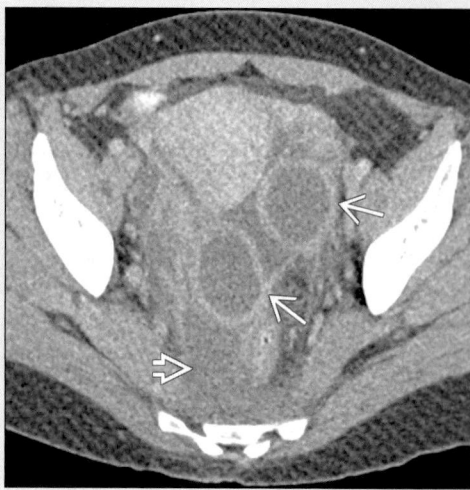

OVARIAN ANATOMY & IMAGING ISSUES

IMAGE GALLERY

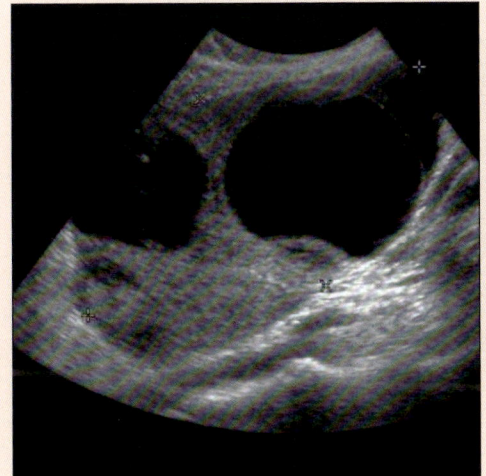
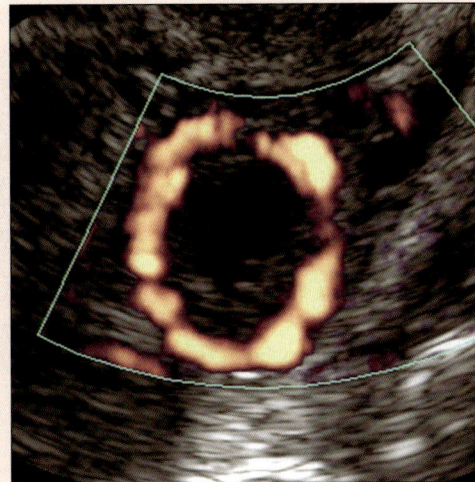

(Left) Sagittal transabdominal ultrasound shows an enlarged hyperstimulated right ovary (calipers). *(Right)* Transverse power Doppler ultrasound shows a corpus luteum cyst with hypervascular rim.

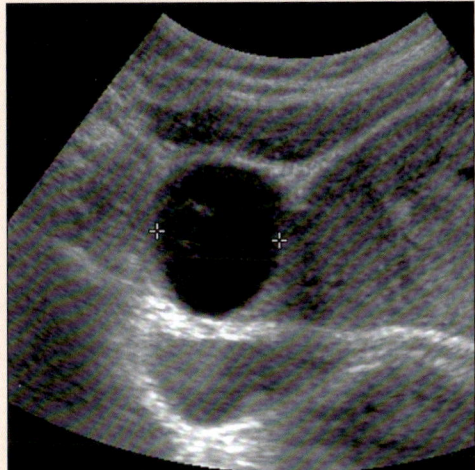
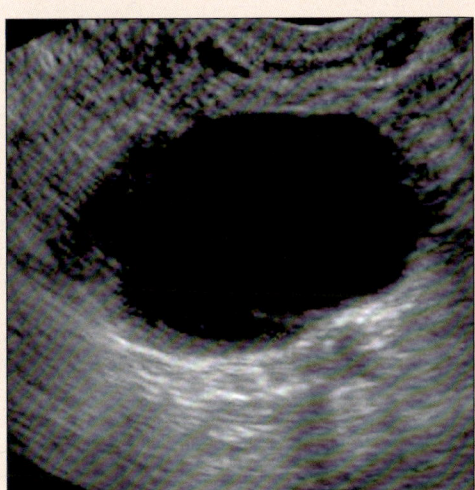

(Left) Transverse transabdominal ultrasound shows corpus luteum cyst in right ovary (calipers) in pregnant patient with intrauterine pregnancy (IUP). *(Right)* Transverse transvaginal ultrasound shows 3 cm benign-appearing adnexal cyst in 68 year old (postmenopausal) woman. Histology showed a "simple cyst."

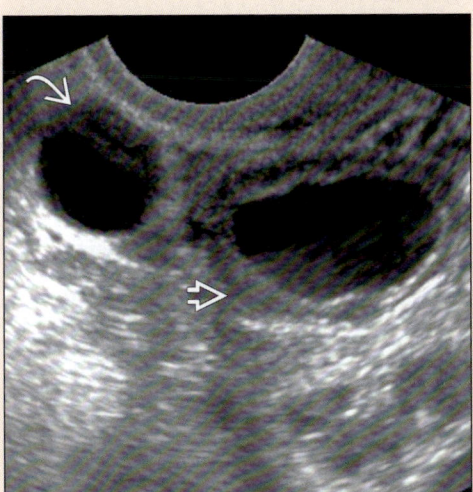
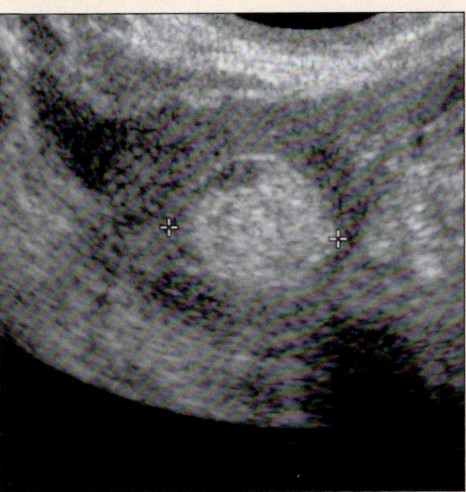

(Left) Axial oblique transvaginal ultrasound shows thick-walled corpus luteum cyst ➡ and separate from the ovary, a paraovarian or paratubal cyst ➡. *(Right)* Transverse transvaginal ultrasound shows a well-defined echogenic mass (calipers) in the ovary, consistent with a small dermoid.

FOLLICULAR CYST

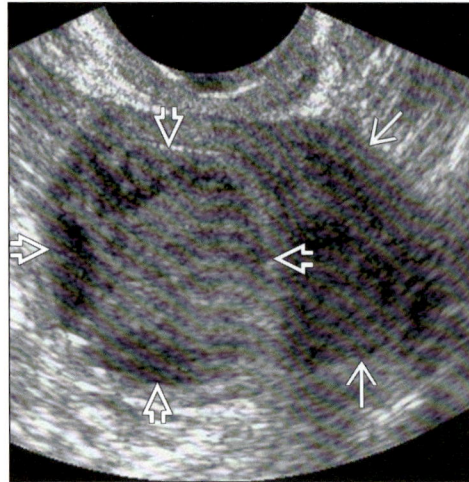

Oblique transvaginal ultrasound shows a hemorrhagic follicular cyst ⇨ within the ovary ➡.

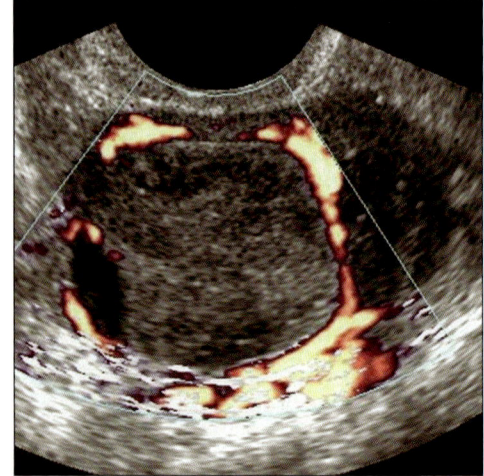

Oblique power Doppler ultrasound of the same patient as previous image, shows significant vascularity ("ring of fire") of the cyst wall pre-ovulation.

TERMINOLOGY

Abbreviations and Synonyms
- Physiologic cyst, dominant follicle

Definitions
- Hormone dependent ovarian cyst
- Occurs during follicular phase of menstrual cycle

IMAGING FINDINGS

General Features
- Best diagnostic clue
  - Simple ovarian cyst that resolves over time
  - Wall becomes thicker and more vascular approaching ovulation
- Location: Cortex of the ovary
- Size: 2 to 8 cm, rarely larger
- Morphology
  - Rounded or oval-shaped depending on number of cysts
  - May be complicated by hemorrhage

Ultrasonographic Findings
- Grayscale Ultrasound
  - Common appearance: Thin or thick-walled unilocular clear cyst
  - Less common appearance: Hemorrhagic cyst
    - Hypo- to hyperechogenic content
    - Heterogeneous echogenic content
    - Spider-web-like content
    - Retracted clot with concave or convex border
    - Solid mural nodule
    - Fluid-fluid level
    - Diffuse low-level echoes less common than endometriomas
- Pulsed Doppler: Low resistance arterial flow
- Color Doppler
  - Cyst wall highly vascular approaching ovulation: "Ring of fire"
  - Solid mural nodule avascular
  - Cyst contents do not demonstrate flow with Doppler imaging
- Power Doppler
  - Cyst wall highly vascular approaching ovulation: "Ring of fire"

DDx: Complicated Ovarian Cyst

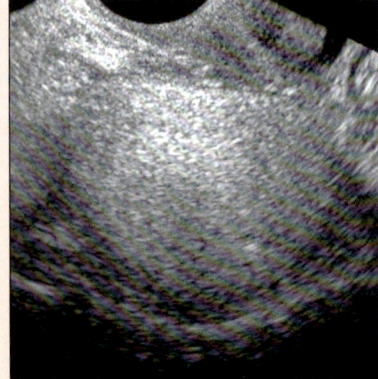

Dermoid

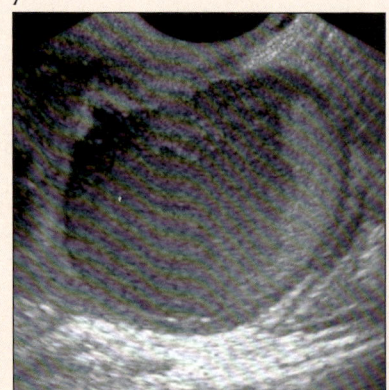

Endometrioma

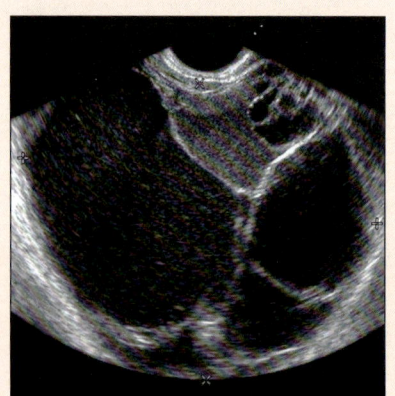

Mucinous Tumor

FOLLICULAR CYST

Key Facts

Terminology
- Physiologic cyst, dominant follicle
- Occurs during follicular phase of menstrual cycle

Imaging Findings
- Simple ovarian cyst that resolves over time
- Wall becomes thicker and more vascular approaching ovulation
- Location: Cortex of the ovary
- Common appearance: Thin or thick-walled unilocular clear cyst
- Less common appearance: Hemorrhagic cyst
- US follow-up for larger (> 3 cm) or atypical cases
- Follow-up in 6 weeks during early follicular phase

Top Differential Diagnoses
- Endometrioma
- Surface Epithelial Tumor
- Ovarian Abscess
- Ovarian Dermoid

Clinical Issues
- More commonly painful when associated with ovarian remnant syndrome
- Rupture and hemoperitoneum an uncommon presentation
- Age: Seen in the ovaries from menarche until menopause including the first year after menopause
- Majority regress spontaneously in 2 cycles

Diagnostic Checklist
- US follow-up for larger (> 3 cm) or atypical cases
- Ovarian cyst that resolves over time

  - Solid mural nodule avascular

CT Findings
- NECT
  - Most common appearance: Thin-walled cyst with fluid-density content
  - Less common appearance: Thin to thick-walled ± hemorrhagic content
- CECT: Enhancing wall

MR Findings
- T1WI
  - Simple appearing cyst in most cases
    - Cyst wall: Low signal intensity
    - Cyst content: Low signal intensity (simple fluid)
  - Cyst content may vary if complicated by hemorrhage
- T2WI
  - Simple appearing cyst in most cases
    - Cyst wall: Intermediate signal intensity
    - Cyst content: High signal intensity (simple fluid)
  - Cyst content may vary if complicated by hemorrhage
- T1 C+ FS
  - Cyst wall initially hypovascular
  - Cyst wall shows increasing enhancement close to ovulation

Imaging Recommendations
- Best imaging tool
  - Transvaginal ultrasound (TVS) with color Doppler
  - Most cases diagnosed by TVS
  - US follow-up for larger (> 3 cm) or atypical cases
    - Follow-up in 6 weeks during early follicular phase
- Protocol advice: Lowest required pulse repetition frequency (PRF) to detect significant vascularity in mural nodule and cyst wall

DIFFERENTIAL DIAGNOSIS

Endometrioma
- Hypovascular cyst wall
- Uniform low level echoes
- Hyperechoic mural foci (hemosiderin, calcification)
- High signal intensity T1WI
- Low signal intensity T2WI (shading)

Surface Epithelial Tumor
- Vascular septa
- Vascular mural nodule or solid component
- "Ring of fire" unusual

Ovarian Abscess
- Clinical and laboratory signs of infection
- Inflamed adnexal fat
- Thick-walled fallopian tube ± pyosalpinx

Ovarian Dermoid
- Fat content
- No mural vascularity

PATHOLOGY

General Features
- General path comments
  - Seen in follicular phase of cycle
  - Ruptured cyst and hemoperitoneum uncommon
- Etiology: Responds to follicle stimulating hormone (FSH) in the follicular phase
- Epidemiology: Follicular cyst seen from fetal life to early postmenopause
- Associated abnormalities: Abnormal release of anterior pituitary gonadotropins in some cases

Gross Pathologic & Surgical Features
- Thin-walled unilocular

Microscopic Features
- Inner layer granulosa cells and outer layer theca interna cells
- Content serous to serosanguineous

FOLLICULAR CYST

CLINICAL ISSUES

Presentation
- Most common signs/symptoms: Most are asymptomatic
- Other signs/symptoms
  - Pain
    - More commonly painful when associated with ovarian remnant syndrome
    - Ureteric and intestinal obstruction may occur with ovarian remnant syndrome
  - Palpable adnexal mass
  - Rupture and hemoperitoneum an uncommon presentation
- Clinical Profile
  - In patients who are on ovarian stimulation to assist reproduction, there are increased number of follicles
  - The above may result in ovarian hyperstimulation syndrome with
    - Bilaterally enlarged ovaries with prominent stroma and numerous follicles
    - Clear ascites

Demographics
- Age: Seen in the ovaries from menarche until menopause including the first year after menopause

Natural History & Prognosis
- Physiologic process with spontaneous resolution
  - Majority regress spontaneously in 2 cycles
  - Persistence in minority of cases

Treatment
- Expectant management
  - Follow-up ultrasound in 6 weeks, preferentially immediately post menstruation for larger cysts
- Estrogen-progesterone preparation for persistent follicles
- Can be aspirated transabdominally or transvaginally when symptomatic, especially in ovarian remnant syndrome, if no response to hormone therapy

DIAGNOSTIC CHECKLIST

Consider
- US follow-up for larger (> 3 cm) or atypical cases

Image Interpretation Pearls
- Ovarian cyst that resolves over time

SELECTED REFERENCES

1. Tamai K et al: MR features of physiologic and benign conditions of the ovary. Eur Radiol. 16(12):2700-11, 2006
2. Patel MD et al: The likelihood ratio of sonographic findings for the diagnosis of hemorrhagic ovarian cysts. J Ultrasound Med. 24(5):607-14; quiz 615, 2005
3. Swire MN et al: Various sonographic appearances of the hemorrhagic corpus luteum cyst. Ultrasound Q. 20(2):45-58, 2004
4. Guerriero S et al: The diagnosis of functional ovarian cysts using transvaginal ultrasound combined with clinical parameters, CA125 determinations, and color Doppler. Eur J Obstet Gynecol Reprod Biol. 110(1):83-8, 2003
5. Jain KA: Sonographic spectrum of hemorrhagic ovarian cysts. J Ultrasound Med. 21(8):879-86, 2002
6. Miele V et al: Hemoperitoneum following ovarian cyst rupture: CT usefulness in the diagnosis. Radiol Med (Torino). 104(4):316-21, 2002
7. Dill-Macky MJ et al: Ovarian sonography: In Ultrasonography in Obstetrics and Gynecology. 4th Edition. W.B.Saunders company. 863-4, 2000
8. MacKenna A et al: Clinical management of functional ovarian cysts: a prospective and randomized study. Hum Reprod. 15(12):2567-9, 2000
9. Borgfeldt C et al: Transvaginal sonographic ovarian findings in a random sample of women 25-40 years old. Ultrasound Obstet Gynecol. 13(5):345-50, 1999
10. Hertzberg BS et al: Adnexal ring sign and hemoperitoneum caused by hemorrhagic ovarian cyst: pitfall in the sonographic diagnosis of ectopic pregnancy. AJR Am J Roentgenol. 173(5):1301-2, 1999
11. Hertzberg BS et al: Ovarian cyst rupture causing hemoperitoneum: imaging features and the potential for misdiagnosis. Abdom Imaging. 24(3):304-8, 1999
12. Guerriero S et al: Sonographic differential diagnosis of persistent ovarian cysts. Ultrasound Obstet Gynecol. 12(1):74-5, 1998
13. Sickler GK et al: Free echogenic pelvic fluid: correlation with hemoperitoneum. J Ultrasound Med. 17(7):431-5, 1998
14. Outwater EK et al: Normal ovaries and functional cysts: MR appearance. Radiology. 198(2):397-402, 1996
15. Atri M et al: Endovaginal sonographic appearance of benign ovarian masses. Radiographics. 14(4):747-60; discussion 761-2, 1994
16. Okai T et al: Transvaginal sonographic appearance of hemorrhagic functional ovarian cysts and their spontaneous regression. Int J Gynaecol Obstet. 44(1):47-52, 1994
17. Bass IS et al: The sonographic appearance of the hemorrhagic ovarian cyst in adolescents. J Ultrasound Med. 3(11):509-13, 1984

FOLLICULAR CYST

IMAGE GALLERY

Typical

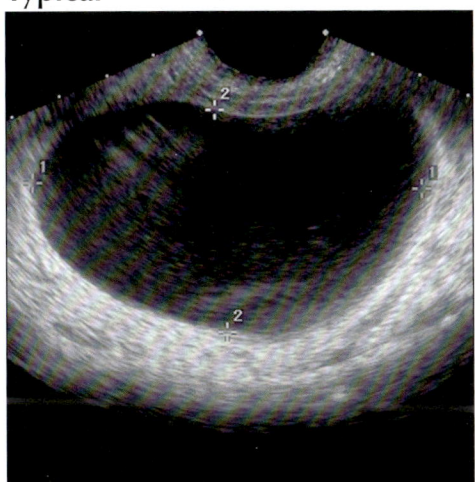 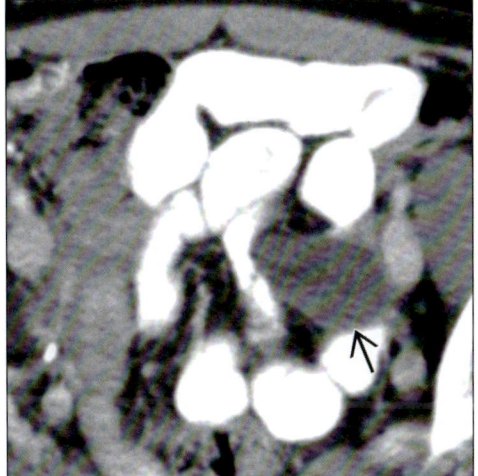

(Left) Sagittal transvaginal ultrasound shows a 7 cm thin-walled, anechoic cyst (calipers) that was a luteinized follicular cyst at pathology. (Right) Axial CECT shows a nonspecific left adnexal cyst ➡. The cyst wall is thin and region of interest measurements showed the cyst content to be fluid density. At histology this was proven to be a follicular cyst.

Typical

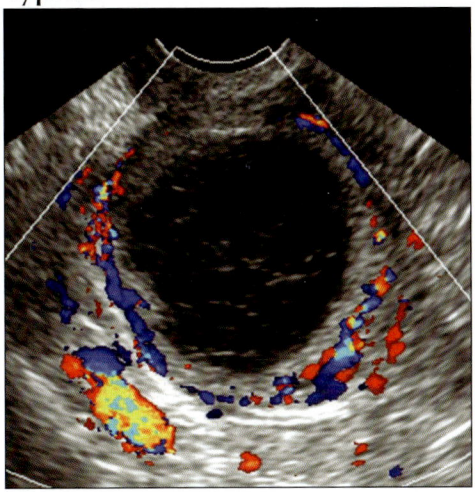 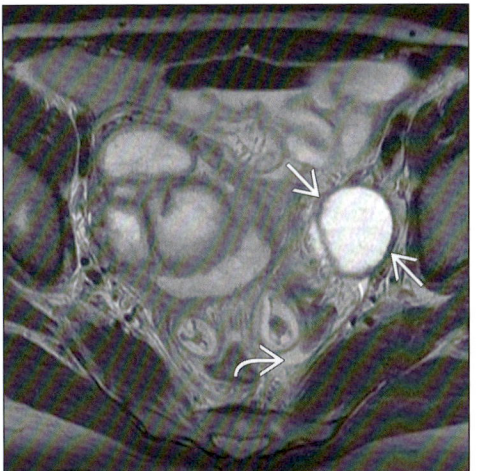

(Left) Axial color Doppler ultrasound shows significant vascularity ("ring of fire") of the wall of a hemorrhagic cyst with spider-web-like contents. (Right) Axial T2WI MR shows a thick-walled left ovarian cyst ➡ containing high signal intensity material. Note the small amount of free intra-peritoneal fluid ➡. The complex right adnexal mass is a tubo-ovarian abscess.

Typical

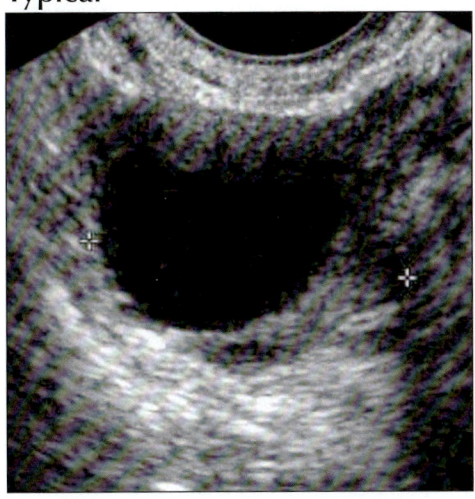 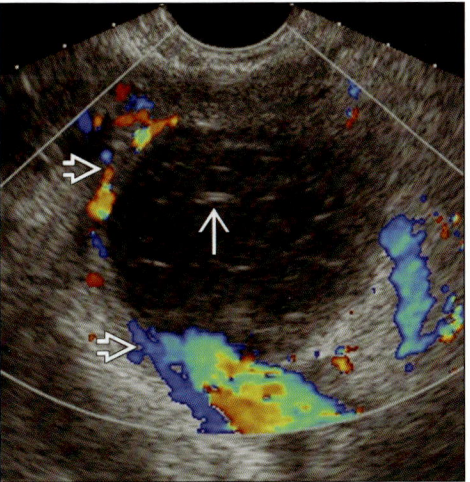

(Left) Transverse transvaginal ultrasound shows a 3 cm thin-walled, anechoic cyst within the ovary (calipers). (Right) Transverse color Doppler ultrasound of a follicular cyst shows spider-web-like content of the cyst ➡ and significant vascularity of the wall ➡ pre-ovulation.

CORPUS LUTEAL CYST

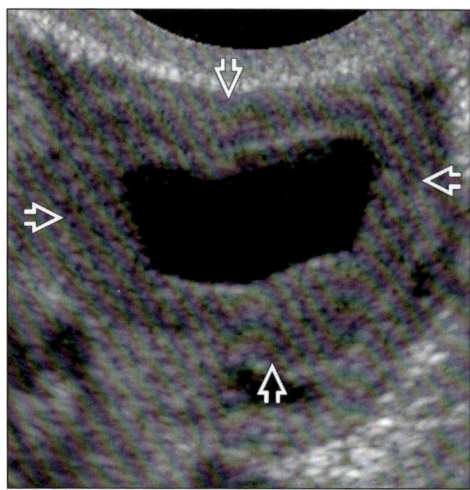

Axial transvaginal ultrasound shows a thick-walled cystic ovarian mass ➡. The cyst contents are anechoic.

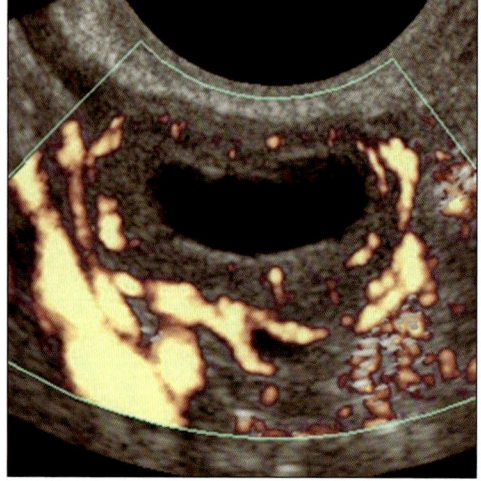

Axial power Doppler ultrasound of the same patient as previous image shows increased vascularity of the cyst wall, consistent with a corpus luteum cyst.

TERMINOLOGY

Abbreviations and Synonyms
- Corpus luteum cyst, physiologic cyst

Definitions
- Hormone dependent ovarian cyst
- Luteinized functional cyst
- Corpus luteal cyst (CLC): Seen in the secretory phase
- Corpus luteum of pregnancy: Peaks in size at 7 weeks

IMAGING FINDINGS

General Features
- Best diagnostic clue
  - Vascular corrugated thick-walled cyst
  - Vascular solid-appearing mass
- Location: Cortex of the ovary
- Size: Can rarely reach 8 cm
- Morphology: Thick-walled cyst with involuting wall ("Mercedes Benz" sign)

Ultrasonographic Findings
- Transvaginal ultrasound (TVS)
  - Thick-walled unilocular clear cyst
  - Thick-walled unilocular hemorrhagic cyst
    - Heterogeneous echogenic content
    - Spider-web-like content
    - Retracted clot with concave or convex border
    - Fluid-fluid level
    - Diffuse low level echoes less common than endometriomas
  - Thick-walled involuting cyst ± hemorrhagic content
  - Collapsed thick-walled cyst
    - Mercedes Benz sign
    - Slit-like sign
  - Solid-appearing mass
  - Hemoperitoneum due to rupture is uncommon
- Pulsed Doppler
  - Low resistance flow
- Color Doppler
  - High vascularity of cystic mass wall
  - "Ring of fire" of increased vascularity in the periphery of the mass
  - No vascular solid mural nodule

DDx: Vascular Solid Ovarian Mass

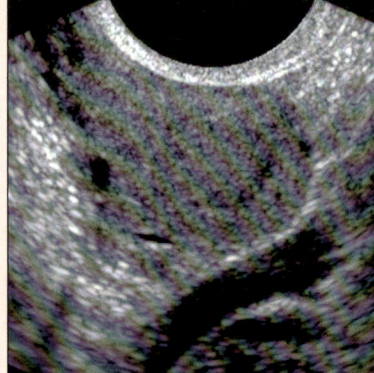

Sertoli Leydig Cell Tumor

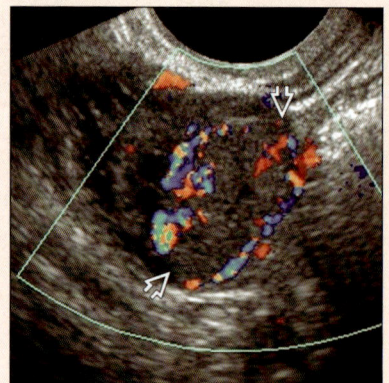

Sertoli Leydig Cell Tumor

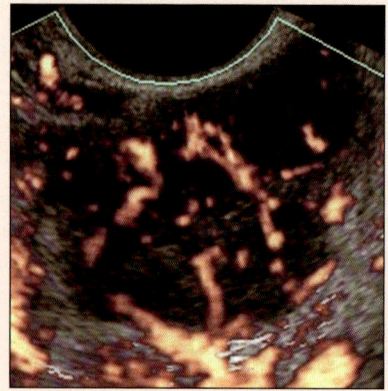

Granulosa Cell Tumor

CORPUS LUTEAL CYST

Key Facts

Terminology
- Corpus luteum cyst, physiologic cyst
- Corpus luteal cyst (CLC): Seen in the secretory phase
- Corpus luteum of pregnancy: Peaks in size at 7 weeks

Imaging Findings
- Thick-walled unilocular clear cyst
- Thick-walled unilocular hemorrhagic cyst
- Collapsed thick-walled cyst
- Solid-appearing mass
- High vascularity of cystic mass wall
- US follow-up for larger (> 4 cm) or atypical cases
- Follow-up in 6 weeks during early follicular phase

Top Differential Diagnoses
- Endometrioma
- Surface Epithelial Tumor
- Sex-Cord Stromal Tumor
- Germ Cell Tumor
- Ovarian Abscess

Clinical Issues
- Clinical Profile: Generally an asymptomatic incidental finding
- Age: CLC during reproductive years, rarely sporadic ovulation in early postmenopause
- Majority regress spontaneously in 2 months

Diagnostic Checklist
- CLC is the most likely diagnosis when a vascular cyst or solid-appearing mass is present in premenopausal women
- Ring of fire in the wall of a cyst on TVS
- Highly vascular solid-appearing mass

- Cyst contents do not demonstrate flow with Doppler imaging
- High vascularity of solid-appearing mass

CT Findings
- CECT
  - Enhancing thick-walled cyst
  - When collapsed it mimics small, solid masses
  - Hyperdense pelvic fluid in case of rupture complicated by hemorrhage (30-50 HU)

MR Findings
- T1WI
  - Cyst wall: Low signal intensity
  - Cyst contents: Low to high signal intensity
    - High signal intensity corresponds to hemorrhagic content
- T2WI
  - Cyst wall: High signal intensity
  - Cyst contents: Low to high signal intensity
    - Signal variable depending on age and degree of hemorrhage
  - Solid-appearing mass: Low to high signal intensity
- T1 C+ FS
  - Cyst wall shows intense and early enhancement
    - Collapsed thick-walled cyst (Mercedes Benz sign)
    - Collapsed thick-walled cyst (slit-like sign)
  - Intensely enhancing solid-appearing mass

Imaging Recommendations
- Best imaging tool
  - Most cases diagnosed by transvaginal US
  - US follow-up for larger (> 4 cm) or atypical cases
    - Follow-up in 6 weeks during early follicular phase
- Protocol advice: Lowest required pulse repetition frequency (PRF) to detect vascularity

DIFFERENTIAL DIAGNOSIS

Endometrioma
- Hypovascular cyst wall
- Uniform low-level echoes
- Hyperechoic mural foci (hemosiderin, calcification)
- High signal intensity T1WI
- Low signal intensity T2WI (shading)

Surface Epithelial Tumor
- Vascular septa
- Vascular mural nodule or solid component
- Ring of fire unusual

Sex-Cord Stromal Tumor
- When small, these malignant tumors can be solid and vascular mimicking a solid CLC
- Cystic changes in larger tumors
- No resolution on short term follow-up

Germ Cell Tumor
- When small, these malignant tumors can be solid and vascular mimicking a solid CLC
- Cystic changes in larger tumors
- No resolution on short term follow-up

Ovarian Abscess
- Clinical history and laboratory signs of infection
- Inflamed adnexal fat
- Thick-walled fallopian tube ± pyosalpinx

PATHOLOGY

General Features
- Theca lutein cysts
  - Variant of CLC
  - Due to overstimulation by high levels of human chorionic gonadotropin (β-hCG)
  - Seen in trophoblastic disease or exogenous β-hCG for fertility treatment
  - Multilocular bilateral

Gross Pathologic & Surgical Features
- Convoluted yellow lining in CLC
- Involuting CLC appears solid

CORPUS LUTEAL CYST

Microscopic Features
- Large luteinized granulosa and small luteinized theca interna cells
- Content serous to serosanguineous

CLINICAL ISSUES

Presentation
- Most common signs/symptoms: Pain
- Other signs/symptoms
  - Palpable adnexal mass
  - Rupture and hemoperitoneum is an uncommon presentation
- Clinical Profile: Generally an asymptomatic incidental finding

Demographics
- Age: CLC during reproductive years, rarely sporadic ovulation in early postmenopause

Natural History & Prognosis
- Majority regress spontaneously in 2 months
- Complete resolution in majority, persistence in minority
- Involuting CLC becomes corpus albicans

Treatment
- Expectant management
  - Follow-up ultrasound in 6 weeks, preferentially immediately postmenstruation
- Estrogen-progesterone preparation for persistent cysts
- No treatment for corpus luteum of pregnancy if continuous reduction after 7 weeks

DIAGNOSTIC CHECKLIST

Consider
- CLC is the most likely diagnosis when a vascular cyst or solid-appearing mass is present in premenopausal women

Image Interpretation Pearls
- Ring of fire in the wall of a cyst on TVS
- Highly vascular solid-appearing mass

SELECTED REFERENCES

1. Tamai K et al: MR features of physiologic and benign conditions of the ovary. Eur Radiol. 16(12):2700-11, 2006
2. Patel MD et al: The likelihood ratio of sonographic findings for the diagnosis of hemorrhagic ovarian cysts. J Ultrasound Med. 24(5):607-14; quiz 615, 2005
3. Stein MW et al: Sonographic comparison of the tubal ring of ectopic pregnancy with the corpus luteum. J Ultrasound Med. 23(1):57-62, 2004
4. Swire MN et al: Various sonographic appearances of the hemorrhagic corpus luteum cyst. Ultrasound Q. 20(2):45-58, 2004
5. Guerriero S et al: The diagnosis of functional ovarian cysts using transvaginal ultrasound combined with clinical parameters, CA125 determinations, and color Doppler. Eur J Obstet Gynecol Reprod Biol. 110(1):83-8, 2003
6. Jain KA: Sonographic spectrum of hemorrhagic ovarian cysts. J Ultrasound Med. 21(8):879-86, 2002
7. Dill-Macky MJ et al: Ovarian sonography: In Ultrasonography in Obstetrics and Gynecology. 4th Edition. W.B.Saunders company. 863-4, 2000
8. MacKenna A et al: Clinical management of functional ovarian cysts: a prospective and randomized study. Hum Reprod. 15(12):2567-9, 2000
9. Borgfeldt C et al: Transvaginal sonographic ovarian findings in a random sample of women 25-40 years old. Ultrasound Obstet Gynecol. 13(5):345-50, 1999
10. Hertzberg BS et al: Adnexal ring sign and hemoperitoneum caused by hemorrhagic ovarian cyst: pitfall in the sonographic diagnosis of ectopic pregnancy. AJR Am J Roentgenol. 173(5):1301-2, 1999
11. Hertzberg BS et al: Ovarian cyst rupture causing hemoperitoneum: imaging features and the potential for misdiagnosis. Abdom Imaging. 24(3):304-8, 1999
12. Ishihara K et al: Sonographic appearance of hemorrhagic ovarian cyst with acute abdomen by transvaginal scan. Nippon Ika Daigaku Zasshi. 64(5):411-5, 1997
13. Outwater EK et al: Normal ovaries and functional cysts: MR appearance. Radiology. 198(2):397-402, 1996
14. Atri M et al: Endovaginal sonographic appearance of benign ovarian masses. Radiographics. 14(4):747-60; discussion 761-2, 1994
15. Okai T et al: Transvaginal sonographic appearance of hemorrhagic functional ovarian cysts and their spontaneous regression. Int J Gynaecol Obstet. 44(1):47-52, 1994
16. Bass IS et al: The sonographic appearance of the hemorrhagic ovarian cyst in adolescents. J Ultrasound Med. 3(11):509-13, 1984

CORPUS LUTEAL CYST

IMAGE GALLERY

Typical

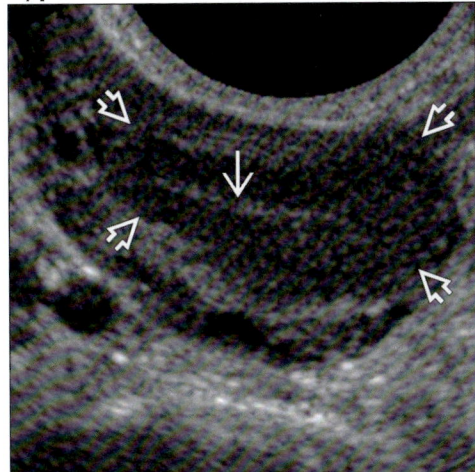
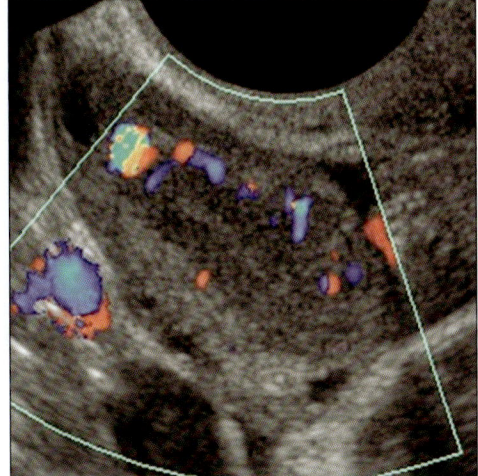

(Left) Oblique transvaginal ultrasound shows a hypoechoic solid mass ➡ with a central echogenic interface ("slit-like" sign) ➡. *(Right)* Oblique color Doppler ultrasound of the same patient as previous image shows increased vascularity of this mass.

Typical

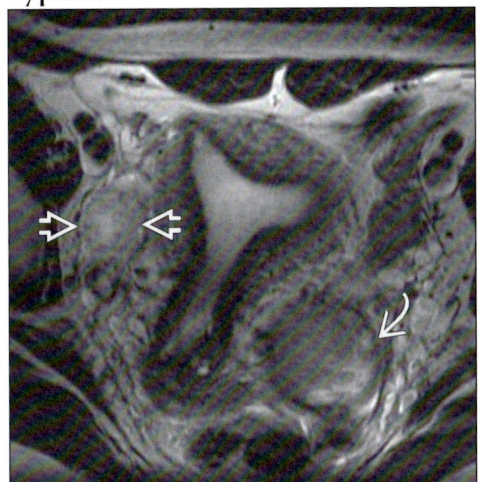
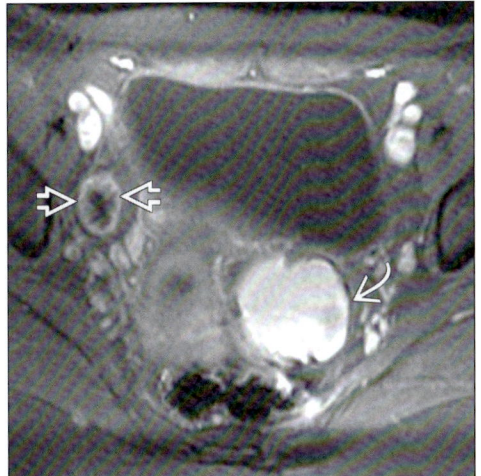

(Left) Axial T2WI MR shows a heterogeneous hyperintense mass ➡ in the right ovary. A left-sided hematosalpinx ➡ is present. *(Right)* Axial T1 C+ FS MR in the same patient as previous image shows intense enhancement of the wall ➡ of this mass consistent with a corpus luteum cyst. A left-sided hematosalpinx ➡ is present.

Typical

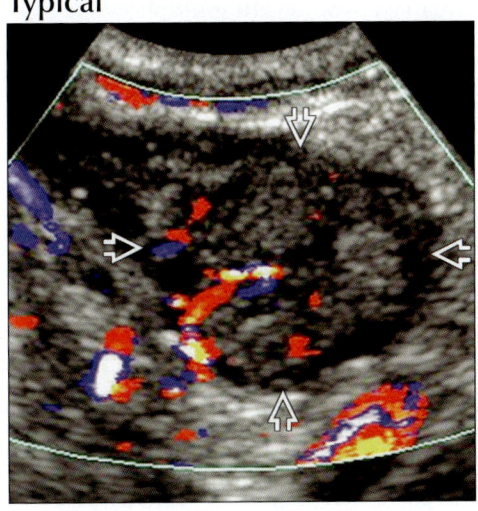
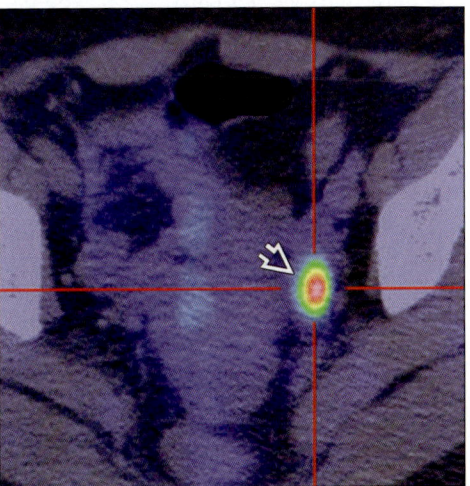

(Left) Oblique color Doppler ultrasound shows a heterogeneous solid ovarian mass ➡ with increased vascularity consistent with a collapsed corpus luteum cyst. *(Right)* Axial fused PET/CT in a premenopausal woman shows an FDG-avid lesion ➡ in the left ovary that resolved on 6 week follow-up MR and PET/CT without additional therapy consistent with a corpus luteum cyst. (Courtesy R. Hicks, MD).

THECA LUTEIN CYSTS

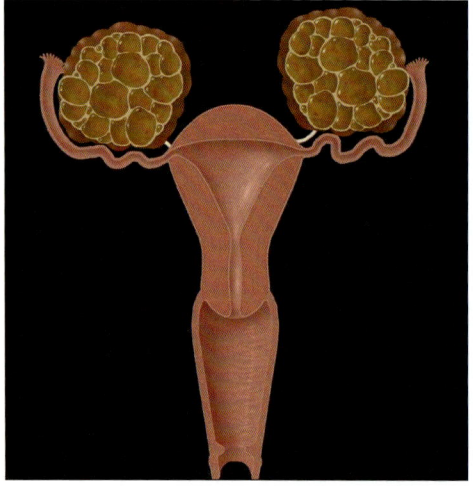

Theca lutein cysts. Graphic shows enlargement of both ovaries due to multiple cysts of varying size.

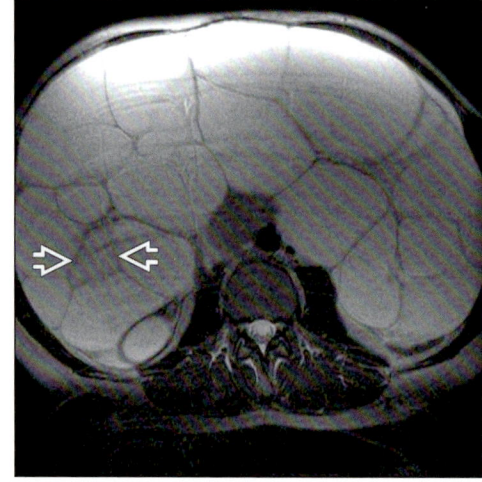

Axial T2WI MR shows marked enlargement of both ovaries due to multiple cysts of varying size. There is mild T2-shortening within a right-sided ovarian cyst ⇨ due to hemorrhage within the cyst.

TERMINOLOGY

Abbreviations and Synonyms
- Hyperreactio luteinalis

Definitions
- Multiple theca lutein cysts in association with increased levels of, or abnormal ovarian response to, human chorionic gonadotropin (β-hCG)
- Subtype of ovarian functional cysts along with follicular cysts and corpus luteum cysts

IMAGING FINDINGS

General Features
- Best diagnostic clue
  - Bilaterally enlarged ovaries with multiple cysts of varying size
  - Hypervascular central uterine mass if associated with molar pregnancy
  - Presence of simple or hemorrhagic ascites suggests ovarian hyperstimulation syndrome
- Location: Typically bilateral, rarely unilateral
- Size
  - Largest of physiologic ovarian cysts
  - Ovaries typically 6-12 cm in length, but may be as large as 20 cm
  - Individual cysts variable in size but usually measure several cms
- Morphology
  - Preservation of underlying ovarian architecture
    - "Multilocular" cysts a misnomer, since individual cysts separated by residual ovarian tissue, rather than true septations
  - Thin walled
  - No nodules or solid component
- Complications
  - Cyst rupture or hemorrhage
  - Ovarian torsion

Ultrasonographic Findings
- Grayscale Ultrasound
  - Bilaterally enlarged ovaries with multiple cysts giving the appearance of multiloculated cystic masses
    - Cysts typically anechoic

DDx: Ovarian Cystic Lesions

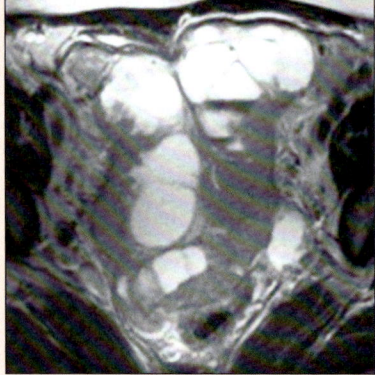
Serous Cystadenocarcinoma

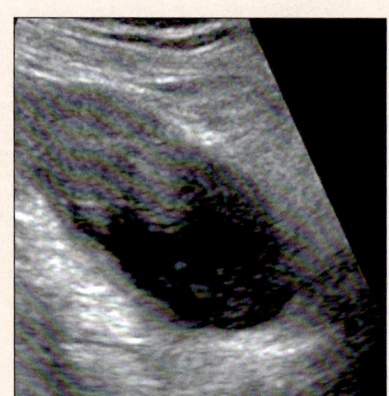
Luteoma of Pregnancy

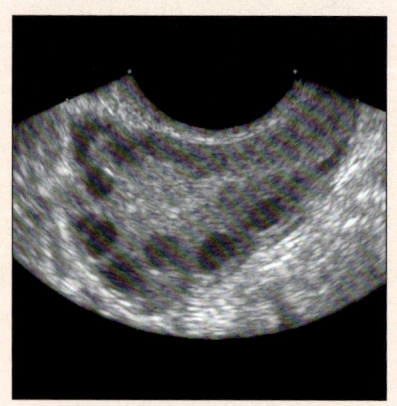
Polycystic Ovary Disease

THECA LUTEIN CYSTS

Key Facts

Terminology
- Hyperreactio luteinalis
- Multiple theca lutein cysts in association with increased levels of, or abnormal ovarian response to, human chorionic gonadotropin (β-hCG)

Imaging Findings
- Bilaterally enlarged ovaries with multiple cysts of varying size
- Hypervascular central uterine mass if associated with molar pregnancy
- Preservation of underlying ovarian architecture
- "Multilocular" cysts a misnomer, since individual cysts separated by residual ovarian tissue, rather than true septations

Top Differential Diagnoses
- Ovarian Epithelial Neoplasms
- Luteoma of Pregnancy
- Polycystic Ovary Disease (PCOD)

Clinical Issues
- Typically regress after causative factor is removed

Diagnostic Checklist
- Theca lutein cysts must be considered before ovarian neoplasm in the setting of a positive β-hCG or history of ovarian stimulation, and bilateral "multilocular" ovarian cystic masses
- Misdiagnosis can result in unnecessary surgical removal of ovaries for suspected ovarian neoplasm

---

- Cysts may contain echoes if complicated by hemorrhage
- Thin "septations" between cysts
- No wall irregularity or nodularity
  - Ascites: Anechoic or low level echoes if hemorrhagic
- Color Doppler: Normal Doppler flow or increased vascularity in surrounding ovarian parenchyma

CT Findings
- NECT
  - Multiple simple or less commonly high-attenuation ovarian cysts
  - Ascites: Simple (0-15 HU) or complex (30-50 HU) if hemorrhagic
- CECT
  - "Spoke-wheel" appearance of ovaries: Central stroma surrounded by peripheral cysts
  - Higher attenuation of stroma compared to cysts

MR Findings
- T1WI
  - Variable signal intensity (SI) of cysts
    - Most often low SI in keeping with simple cysts
    - May be intermediate to high SI when hemorrhagic
  - Ascites low SI if simple, may cause T1 shortening if hemorrhagic
- T2WI
  - Cysts typically high SI
    - SI may vary between cysts due to hemorrhage
  - T2 shortening of ascites if hemorrhagic
- T1 C+
  - No enhancement of cysts
  - Normal or increased enhancement of residual ovarian tissue between cysts mimics enhancing septations
    - "Spoke-wheel" appearance

Imaging Recommendations
- Best imaging tool
  - Ultrasound initial examination
  - MR if diagnosis uncertain or complication suggests neoplasm
- Protocol advice: Combined use of transvaginal and transabdominal approach allows complete evaluation in the setting of large lesions

DIFFERENTIAL DIAGNOSIS

Ovarian Epithelial Neoplasms
- More frequently unilateral, although may be bilateral
- Multilocular
- Mural or septal thickening may be present
- Papillary projections or solid component

Luteoma of Pregnancy
- Ovarian enlargement (up to 12 cm)
- More commonly unilateral
- Solid or predominantly vascular solid mass
- Stromal cells stimulated rather than follicles
- May cause virilization
- Most regress spontaneously

Polycystic Ovary Disease (PCOD)
- Multiple peripheral follicles
- Uniform size of cysts (usually ≤ 1 cm)
- Enlarged low SI T2WI central stroma
- Clinical signs of hyperandrogenism and chronic anovulation

Granulosa Cell Tumor
- Unilateral
- Most commonly seen in postmenopausal women
- Small masses, predominantly solid
- On T2WI, "sponge-like" appearance due to intercalated high SI intratumoral cysts and lower SI solid components
- Estrogenically active
- 10-15% associated with endometrial carcinoma

THECA LUTEIN CYSTS

PATHOLOGY

General Features
- General path comments: Subtype of functional ovarian cyst
- Etiology
  - Excessive β-hCG usually as a result of gestational trophoblastic disease (GTD): Hydatidiform mole or choriocarcinoma
  - Increased ovarian stroma sensitivity to HCG
    - Multiple pregnancy
    - Triploid gestation
    - Immune or non immune fetal hydrops with placental hydropic changes
    - Erythroblastosis foetalis
    - Pharmacologic stimulation for ovarian induction: Clomiphene, human menopausal gonadotropin
    - GnRH analogues
    - Diabetes complicating pregnancy
    - Maternal hypothyroidism: Elevated TSH shares an α-subunit with hCG
    - Very rarely normal pregnancy
- Epidemiology: 25-45% of women with GTD will have theca lutein cysts
- Associated abnormalities
  - Presence of theca lutein cysts in GTD increases probability of one of its more aggressive forms: Invasive mole or choriocarcinoma
  - Ovarian hyperstimulation syndrome
    - Ascites
    - Pleural effusion
    - Hemoconcentration
    - Oliguria
    - Theca lutein cysts

Gross Pathologic & Surgical Features
- Markedly edematous and congested ovarian parenchyma
- Numerous unilocular cysts
- Cysts contain amber colored serosanguineous fluid

Microscopic Features
- Diagnosis seldom confirmed histologically due to benign evolution of disease in most cases
- Numerous luteinized follicular cysts
- Marked luteinization of theca interna cells and, in some cases, granulosa cells
- Marked edema of theca interna layer
- Intervening stroma containing luteinized stromal cells

CLINICAL ISSUES

Presentation
- Most common signs/symptoms
  - Usually asymptomatic
  - Abdominal pain if hemorrhage, rupture or torsion occurs
- Other signs/symptoms
  - If associated with ovarian hyperstimulation syndrome
    - Pain, abdominal distention, nausea, vomiting
    - Extravascular accumulation of exudates leads to weight gain, ascites, pleural effusions, intravascular volume depletion with hemoconcentration and oliguria
  - Virilization secondary to androgen production in 15-25% of cases unassociated with GTD
    - Serum testosterone elevated in virilized as well as non-virilized patients

Demographics
- Age: Women of child-bearing age

Natural History & Prognosis
- Excellent
- Typically regress after causative factor is removed
  - When associated with GTD, disappear within 2-4 months after resolution of condition
  - Rare cases of persistence or increase in size after β-HCG regression
- In itself, presence of theca lutein cysts in GTD increases risk of post-molar trophoblastic disease, especially if bilateral

Treatment
- Conservative management recommended to avoid unnecessary oophorectomy
- Rare cases of torsion or hemorrhage, may need ovariotomy to remove infarcted tissue or to control bleeding

DIAGNOSTIC CHECKLIST

Consider
- Theca lutein cysts must be considered before ovarian neoplasm in the setting of a positive β-hCG or history of ovarian stimulation, and bilateral "multilocular" ovarian cystic masses
- Misdiagnosis can result in unnecessary surgical removal of ovaries for suspected ovarian neoplasm

Image Interpretation Pearls
- Association of molar pregnancy and enlarged multicystic ovaries is diagnostic of theca lutein cysts
- Multiple cysts of varying size with preservation of underlying ovarian architecture

SELECTED REFERENCES

1. Allen SD et al: Radiology of gestational trophoblastic neoplasia. Clin Radiol. 61(4):301-13, 2006
2. Tamai K et al: MR features of physiologic and benign conditions of the ovary. Eur Radiol. 16(12):2700-11, 2006
3. Jung SE et al: MR imaging of maternal diseases in pregnancy. AJR Am J Roentgenol. 177(6):1293-300, 2001
4. al-Harbi O et al: Recurrent bilateral theca lutein cysts in association with normal pregnancy. Ultrasound Obstet Gynecol. 11(3):222-4, 1998
5. Wagner BJ et al: From the archives of the AFIP. Gestational trophoblastic disease: radiologic-pathologic correlation. Radiographics. 16(1):131-48, 1996
6. Montz FJ et al: The natural history of theca lutein cysts. Obstet Gynecol. 72(2):247-51, 1988
7. Hricak H et al: Gestational trophoblastic neoplasm of the uterus: MR assessment. Radiology. 161(1):11-6, 1986

THECA LUTEIN CYSTS

IMAGE GALLERY

Variant

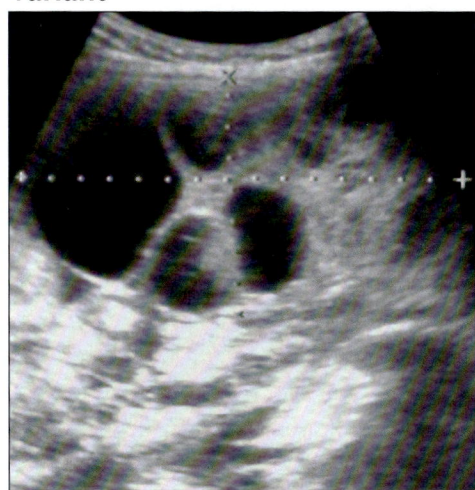
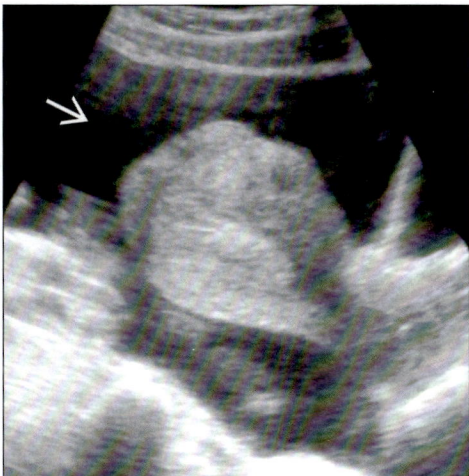

(Left) Sagittal transabdominal ultrasound in a 5 week pregnant patient who received clomiphene for infertility, shows an enlarged ovary (10 cm x 5 cm, calipers) with peripheral theca lutein cysts. *(Right)* Sagittal transabdominal ultrasound shows moderate ascites ➡ in the same patient as previous patient with ovarian hyperstimulation syndrome. The intra-uterine pregnancy is not demonstrated.

Typical

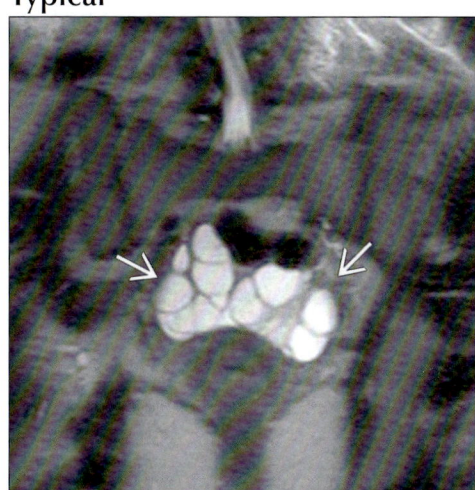
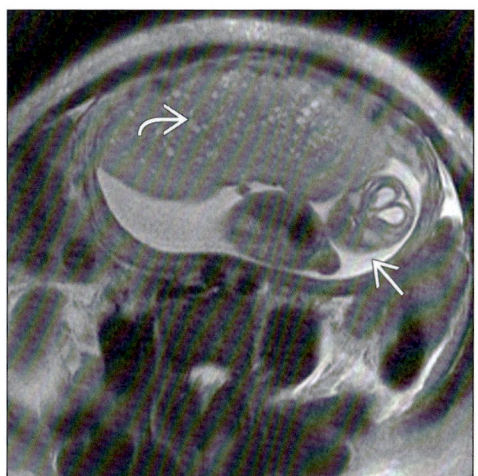

(Left) Coronal T2WI MR shows bilateral ovarian enlargement ➡ secondary to theca lutein cysts in a patient with partial molar pregnancy. *(Right)* Axial T2WI MR in the same patient as previous image, shows the intra-uterine pregnancy ➡. The placenta is heterogeneous with multiple hyperintense foci ➡ (cystic degeneration) which proved to be a partial mole.

Typical

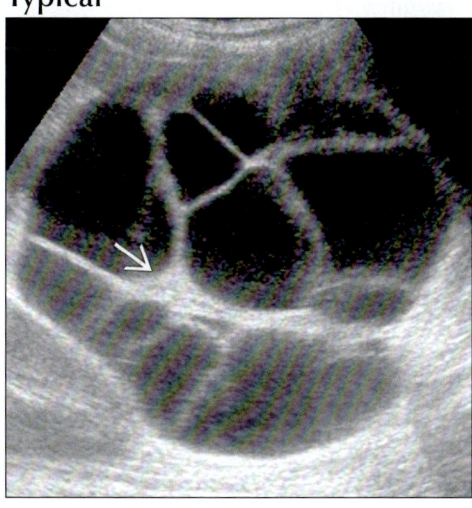
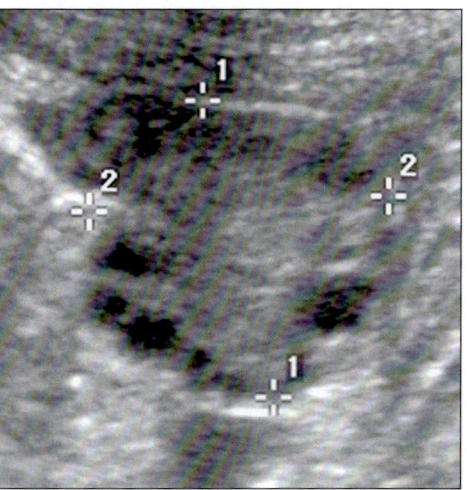

(Left) Transverse transabdominal ultrasound shows markedly enlarged ovaries with theca lutein cysts seen in the setting of spontaneous twins. Residual central ovarian stromal tissue is seen between the cysts creating a "spoke-wheel" appearance ➡. *(Right)* Transverse transabdominal ultrasound obtained two months later shows resolution of the theca lutein cysts with a normal appearance of the ovary (calipers).

LUTEOMA OF PREGNANCY

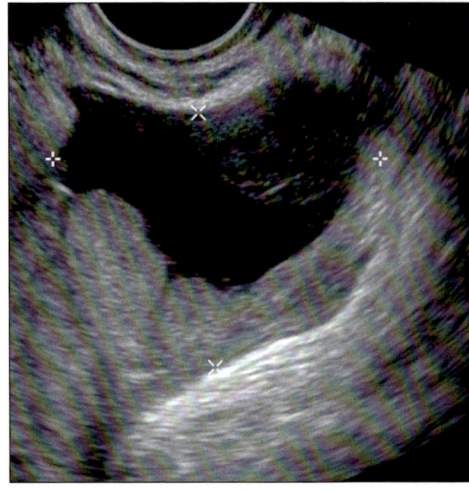 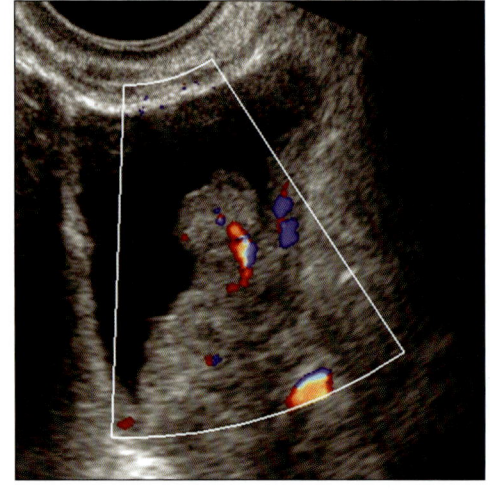

Transverse transvaginal ultrasound shows cystic mass (calipers) with solid nodular component inferiorly. Patient was 23 weeks pregnant.

Oblique color Doppler ultrasound in same patient as previous image shows nodular component with blood flow.

TERMINOLOGY

Definitions
- Solid ovarian non-neoplastic mass that occurs during pregnancy, with elevated androgen levels

IMAGING FINDINGS

General Features
- Best diagnostic clue: Solid lesion in patient with hirsutism in pregnancy
- Location: Ovary, unilateral (2/3 of cases) or bilateral (1/3 of cases)
- Size: Microscopic to 20 cm
- Morphology
  - Solid, multinodular in 50% of cases, hypervascular
  - Complex cystic appearance can be due to areas of hemorrhage

Imaging Recommendations
- Best imaging tool
  - Ultrasound
  - MR
    - Intermediate signal intensity on T1WI, marked enhancement of solid nodules, low signal intensity on T2WI
- Protocol advice: Lack of ancillary signs of malignancy (i.e., no signs of metastatic disease)

DIFFERENTIAL DIAGNOSIS

Ovarian Neoplasm
- Typically present prior to pregnancy and persists after pregnancy
- May have signs of metastatic disease

PATHOLOGY

General Features
- Epidemiology
  - Multiparous women
  - Afro-Caribbean descent
  - Pre-existing polycystic ovarian syndrome
- Associated abnormalities: Virilization

DDx: Luteoma of Pregnancy

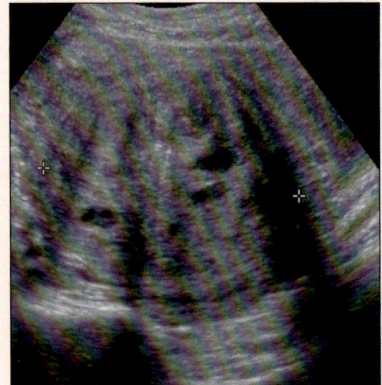 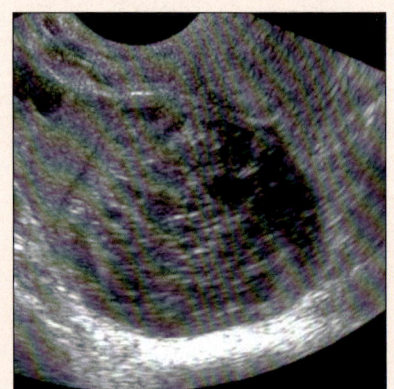 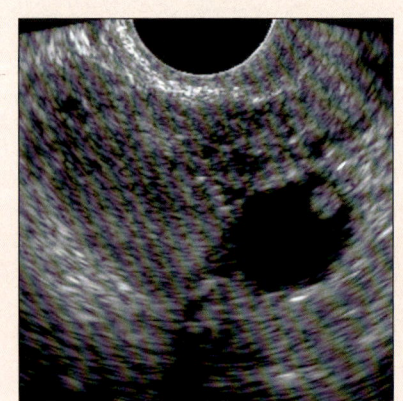

Necrotic Leiomyoma   *Hemorrhagic Cyst*   *Mucinous Cystadenoma*

LUTEOMA OF PREGNANCY

Key Facts

Terminology
- Solid ovarian non-neoplastic mass that occurs during pregnancy, with elevated androgen levels

Imaging Findings
- Complex cystic appearance can be due to areas of hemorrhage

Clinical Issues
- May be asymptomatic with ovarian enlargement seen at time of cesarian section or tubal ligation
- Most common cause of virilization in pregnancy is luteoma
- May cause clitoromegaly in female fetus/newborn
- Recognition is important to avoid oophorectomy, with concomitant risk to both the patient and the fetus

Gross Pathologic & Surgical Features
- Soft reddish tan fleshy with areas of hemorrhage

Microscopic Features
- Sharply-circumscribed, rounded masses of cells
- Eosinophilic cells surrounded by blood vessels
- On electron microscopy, cells contain abundant smooth endoplasmic reticulum, dispersed Golgi apparatus, and tubular cristae in mitochondria, similar to other steroid producing cells

CLINICAL ISSUES

Presentation
- Most common signs/symptoms
  - May be asymptomatic with ovarian enlargement seen at time of cesarian section or tubal ligation
  - 25% of luteoma cases are hormonally active, with secretion of androgens
    - Plasma testosterones (Dihydrotestosterone) are often markedly elevated (up to 70 times normal)
    - Urinary 17-ketosteroids, such as androstenedione and dehydroepiandrosterone can be elevated
  - 10-50% of mothers with elevated androgen levels are masculinized
  - Most common cause of virilization in pregnancy is luteoma
  - 60-70% of female infants born to masculinized mothers are themselves masculinized to varying degrees
- Other signs/symptoms
  - May cause clitoromegaly in female fetus/newborn
  - Rare cause of pseudohermaphrodite in female fetus (male genitalia with XX chromosomes)

Demographics
- Age: Reproductive age; third and fourth decades of life
- Gender: Female

Natural History & Prognosis
- Regress postpartum
- Rarely recur in subsequent pregnancy

Treatment
- Recognition is important to avoid oophorectomy, with concomitant risk to both the patient and the fetus
- Monitor with ultrasound and hormone levels postpartum to ensure resolution

SELECTED REFERENCES
1. Wang HK et al: Magnetic resonance imaging of pregnancy luteoma. J Comput Assist Tomogr. 27(2):155-7, 2003
2. Mazza V et al: Prenatal diagnosis of female pseudohermaphroditism associated with bilateral luteoma of pregnancy: case report. Hum Reprod. 17(3):821-4, 2002
3. Choi JR et al: Luteoma of pregnancy: sonographic findings in two cases. J Ultrasound Med. 19(12):877-81, 2000

IMAGE GALLERY

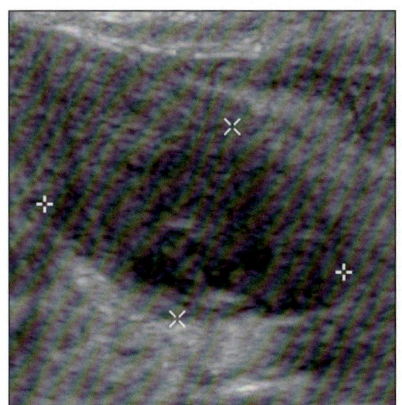
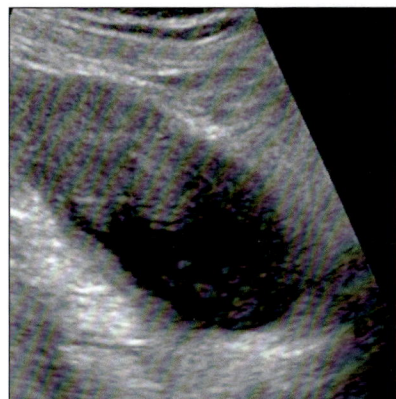
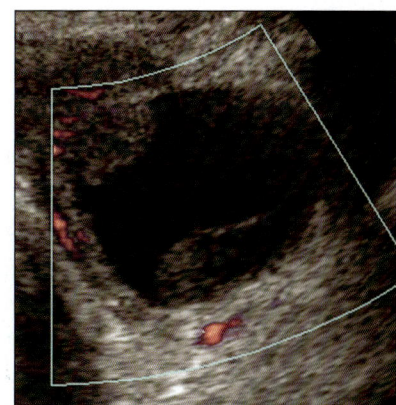

(Left) Transverse transabdominal ultrasound shows heterogeneous cystic mass (calipers) in left adnexa of pregnant patient. *(Center)* Oblique transabdominal ultrasound shows heterogeneous cystic and solid mass in adnexa of pregnant patient. *(Right)* Transverse power Doppler ultrasound shows nodular components of cyst without blood flow.

DERMOID (MATURE TERATOMA)

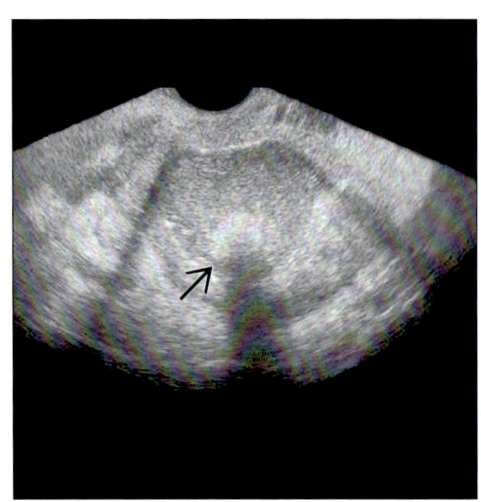

Coronal transvaginal ultrasound shows complex cystic mass with an echogenic nodule ➔ projecting in the cyst lumen. The nodule represents the Rokitansky plug.

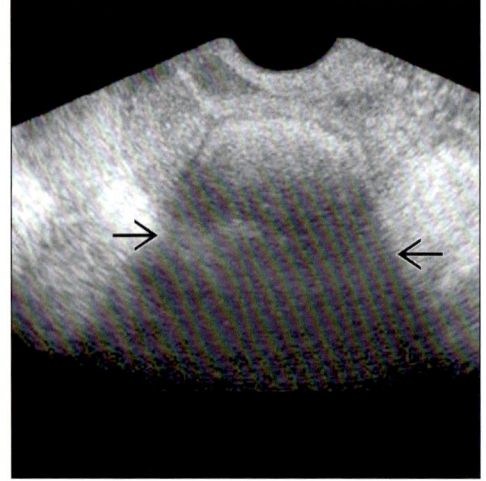

Coronal transvaginal ultrasound shows a predominantly echogenic lesion with posterior acoustic shadowing ➔. This is the "tip of the iceberg" sign.

TERMINOLOGY

Abbreviations and Synonyms
- Mature cystic teratoma of the ovary
- Dermoid cysts

Definitions
- Congenital cystic tumor composed of well-differentiated derivations from at least two of three germ cell layers

IMAGING FINDINGS

General Features
- Best diagnostic clue
  - Presence of fat on CT or MR
  - Characteristic US appearance is a cystic adnexal mass containing an echogenic focus with distal acoustic shadowing
- Location
  - Usually unilateral
  - Bilateral in 20% of patients
- Imaging accurately diagnoses dermoids
- May see several within one ovary
- Vary in size from 0.5 cm to more than 40 cm

Ultrasonographic Findings
- Grayscale Ultrasound
  - US appearance is dependent on the size of the dermoid plug, the presence and location of calcified elements, and the histologic composition of the fatty component
  - May be entirely echogenic or mostly cystic
- Transvaginal ultrasound (TVS) findings
  - Three most common US manifestations
    - Cystic lesion with densely echogenic shadowing nodule projecting into lumen (Rokitansky nodule or dermoid plug)
    - "Tip of iceberg": Diffusely or partially echogenic mass usually demonstrating sound attenuation owing to sebaceous material & hair within cyst cavity
    - "Dermoid mesh": Multiple thin, echogenic lines and dots caused by hair in the cyst cavity
  - Shadowing calcified structures such as bone and teeth
  - Fluid-fluid level: Sebum layered on serous fluid

DDx: Dermoid

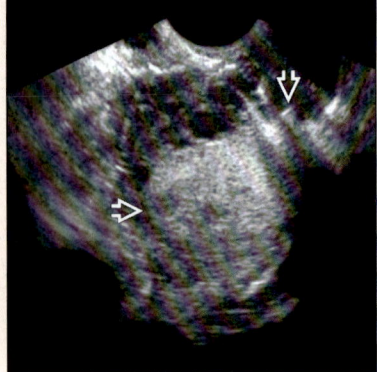

Endometrioma

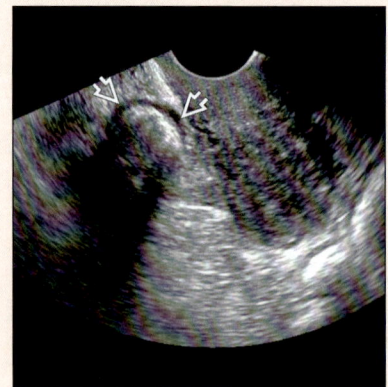

Bowel

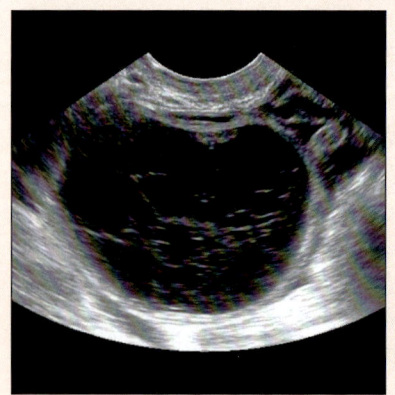

Hemorrhagic Cyst

DERMOID (MATURE TERATOMA)

Key Facts

Terminology
- Mature cystic teratoma of the ovary
- Dermoid cysts
- Congenital cystic tumor composed of well-differentiated derivations from at least two of three germ cell layers

Imaging Findings
- Presence of fat on CT or MR
- Characteristic US appearance is a cystic adnexal mass containing an echogenic focus with distal acoustic shadowing
- Usually unilateral
- Imaging accurately diagnoses dermoids
- Three most common US manifestations

- Cystic lesion with densely echogenic shadowing nodule projecting into lumen (Rokitansky nodule or dermoid plug)
- "Tip of iceberg": Diffusely or partially echogenic mass usually demonstrating sound attenuation owing to sebaceous material & hair within cyst cavity
- "Dermoid mesh": Multiple thin, echogenic lines and dots caused by hair in the cyst cavity

Pathology
- Most common benign ovarian tumor in women younger than 45 years
- Constitutes 5-25% of all ovarian neoplasms

Clinical Issues
- Nonsurgical management is advocated if less than 6 cm due to slow growth

---

- Pure sebum within the cyst may be hypoechoic or anechoic
- Echogenic focus is often associated with shadowing
  - May see progressive fading of sound beyond a moderately echogenic mass which has been shown to contain soft tissue or fat mixed with hair
  - Or may see very bright echogenic focus which casts a well-demarcated sharp acoustic shadow related to the presence of teeth or bone
- Floating nodules which include fat, hair and soft tissue: Confirm floating elements by changing patient position
- Findings suggestive of torsion
  - Uterus deviated toward side of torsion
  - Engorged blood vessels on affected side
  - Straight blood vessels that drape around mass
  - More midline position of ovary
  - If prior scan is available, change in location of ovary toward midline
- Pitfalls in US diagnosis
  - Blood clot within hemorrhagic cysts can appear echogenic
  - Echogenic bowel can frequently be mistaken for echogenic portion of teratoma
  - Perforated appendix with appendicolith has been described as a false positive finding

CT Findings
- Fat attenuation (-90 to -130 HU) within a cyst is diagnostic
- Fat has been reported in 93% of cases
- Teeth or calcifications in 56%
- May see floating mass of hair at the fat-fluid interface
- With or without calcification in wall
- May see dermoid plug in wall of cyst

MR Findings
- T1WI
  - Sebaceous/fat component very high signal intensity
  - Calcification, bone, hair and fibrous tissue are low signal intensity
- T2WI: Signal intensity of sebaceous component is variable
- T1WI with frequency selective fat-saturation: Suppression of high-signal-intensity sebum/fat is diagnostic
  - Allows differentiation from blood products in hemorrhagic cysts which do not suppress
- Chemical shift artifact in frequency encoding direction can be used to detect fat and distinguish it from hemorrhage
- Gradient echo opposed phase imaging demonstrate fat-water interfaces
- Findings that suggest torsion
  - Mass with high-signal intensity rim on T1WI
  - Absence of enhancement

DIFFERENTIAL DIAGNOSIS

Endometriomas
- Transvaginal sonography: Cystic mass with internal echoes, nodules in wall related to fibrosis or desiccated blood, may appear echogenic
- MR: Complex mass or masses
  - T1WI: High signal intensity which does not suppress with fat saturation
  - T2WI: Shading with varying degrees of intermediate to low signal intensity (a function of different stages of blood products)

Bowel
- Intraluminal gas or fecal material can mimic Rokitansky protuberance
- Observation of peristalsis helps make the diagnosis

Hemorrhagic Cyst
- Lacelike appearance can mimic dermoid mesh

Pedunculated Lipoleiomyoma
- Unusual variant of leiomyoma which contains fat
- Uterine in origin

DERMOID (MATURE TERATOMA)

PATHOLOGY

General Features
- General path comments
  - Most common benign ovarian tumor in women younger than 45 years
  - Most common ovarian neoplasm removed at surgery
  - Most common ovarian mass in children
  - Constitutes 5-25% of all ovarian neoplasms
  - Composed of well-differentiated derivatives of three germ layers: Ectoderm, mesoderm and endoderm
  - Contains mature tissues e.g., skin, brain, muscle, fat, epithelium
  - Ectodermal elements predominate
  - Always benign in pure cases
- Epidemiology
  - Occur most commonly during reproductive years: Mean age is 30 years
  - Affects a younger age group than epithelial ovarian neoplasms
  - May be encountered throughout lifespan
  - Rarely seen before puberty

Gross Pathologic & Surgical Features
- Cut surface reveals cavity filled with fatty sebaceous material which is liquid at body temperature and semisolid at room temperature
- Surrounding firm capsule of varying thickness
- Usually unilocular (88%) but may be multilocular
- Arising from cyst wall and projecting into lumen is one or more Rokitansky protuberances which may contain hair, teeth, calcification and other atypical tissues
- Most of the hair arises from the dermoid plug

Microscopic Features
- Orderly arrangement or tissues in dermoid plug - cutaneous, bronchial, gastrointestinal tissues, bone, teeth, etc.
- Squamous epithelium lines the wall of the cyst
- Compressed ovarian stroma, often hyalinized, covers the external surface
- Hair follicles, skin glands, muscle and other tissues lie within the wall
- Ectodermal tissue is invariably present
- Mesodermal tissue is present in over 90% of cases
- Endodermal tissue is seen in a majority of cases
- Adipose tissue in 67-75% of cases
- Teeth in 31% of cases
- Struma ovarii: Accounts for 3% of all cases of ovarian teratomas and is composed predominantly or solely of mature thyroid tissue

CLINICAL ISSUES

Presentation
- Usually incidentally found in asymptomatic patient
- Symptoms (when present): Abdominal pain, abdominal mass, swelling, abnormal uterine bleeding

Natural History & Prognosis
- Can be complicated by ovarian torsion, most common during pregnancy
- Dermoids involved in torsion are larger than average (approximately 11 cm on average) which may be result of torsion rather than the cause
- Other complications include rupture and chemical peritonitis (less than 1%), adhesions, infection
- Grow slowly, average rate 1.8 mm each year
- Growth stops after menopause
- Malignant degeneration in 2% is related to differentiated tissues giving rise to carcinoma or sarcoma
  - Most common type is squamous cell carcinoma arising from the squamous lining of the cyst
  - Occurs in the 6th or 7th decade of life
  - Development of cancer rarely alters symptoms in any recognizable way, exception being sudden growth
  - Preoperative diagnosis of malignant transformation is difficult
  - Other types that can occur include basal cell carcinoma, sebaceous tumor, malignant melanoma, adenocarcinoma, sarcoma, and neuroendodermal tumor
- Local recurrence in < 1% after excision

Treatment
- Uncomplicated cases: Excision with conservation of part of ovary
- Nonsurgical management is advocated if less than 6 cm due to slow growth

DIAGNOSTIC CHECKLIST

Image Interpretation Pearls
- Presence of fat is diagnostic

SELECTED REFERENCES
1. Rim SY et al: Malignant transformation of ovarian mature cystic teratoma. Int J Gynecol Cancer. 16(1):140-4, 2006
2. Yazici B et al: Floating ball appearance in ovarian cystic teratoma. Diagn Interv Radiol. 12(3):136-8, 2006
3. Zagame L et al: Growing teratoma syndrome after ovarian germ cell tumors. Obstet Gynecol. 108(3 Pt 1):509-14, 2006
4. Pereira JM et al: CT and MR imaging of extrahepatic fatty masses of the abdomen and pelvis: techniques, diagnosis, differential diagnosis, and pitfalls. Radiographics. 25(1):69-85, 2005
5. Wootton-Gorges SL et al: Giant cystic abdominal masses in children. Pediatr Radiol. 35(12):1277-88, 2005
6. Kim KA et al: Benign ovarian tumors with solid and cystic components that mimic malignancy. AJR Am J Roentgenol. 182(5):1259-65, 2004
7. Jung SE et al: CT and MR imaging of ovarian tumors with emphasis on differential diagnosis. Radiographics. 22(6):1305-25, 2002
8. Kim HC et al: Fluid-fluid levels in ovarian teratomas. Abdom Imaging. 27(1):100-5, 2002
9. Outwater EK et al: Ovarian teratomas: tumor types and imaging characteristics. Radiographics. 21(2):475-90, 2001
10. Jeong YY et al: Imaging evaluation of ovarian masses. Radiographics. 20(5):1445-70, 2000

DERMOID (MATURE TERATOMA)

IMAGE GALLERY

Typical

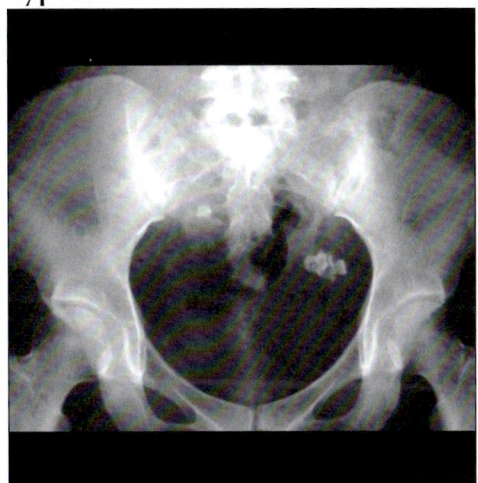
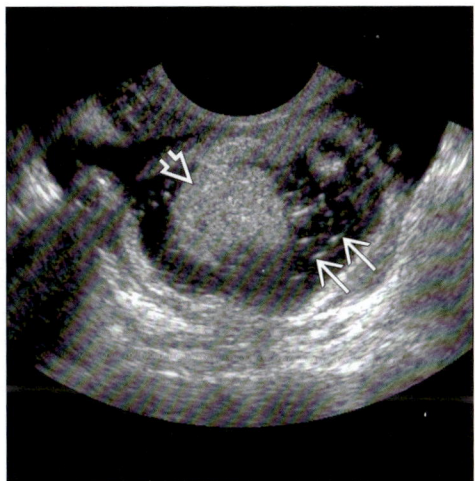

(Left) Frontal radiograph of the pelvis shows a cluster of teeth in the left hemipelvis. Note second calcification in the right pelvis overlying the sacrum. This patient had bilateral dermoid cysts. *(Right)* Sagittal transvaginal ultrasound shows a cystic adnexal mass containing an echogenic nodule ➡ and a network of fine linear echoes ➡ compatible with the "dermoid mesh". The mesh represents hair.

Typical

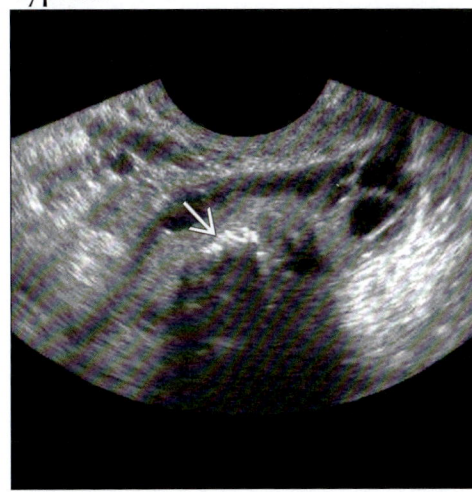
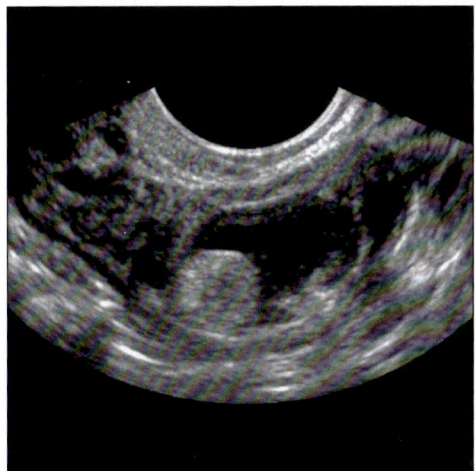

(Left) Sagittal transvaginal ultrasound shows a mass in the ovary with a predominant calcified component ➡. *(Right)* Sagittal transvaginal ultrasound shows cystic ovarian mass with a dermoid plug. Unlike the first case, this nodule does not shadow. Note dependent material in the cyst.

Typical

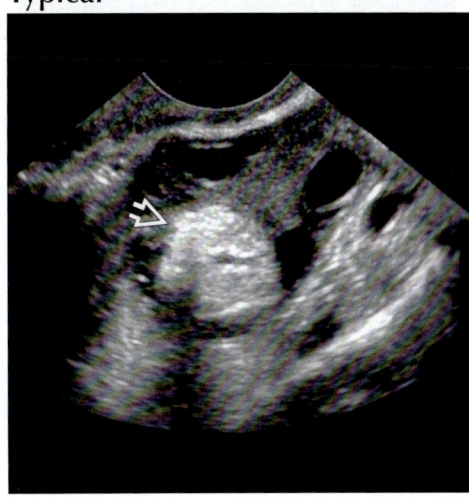
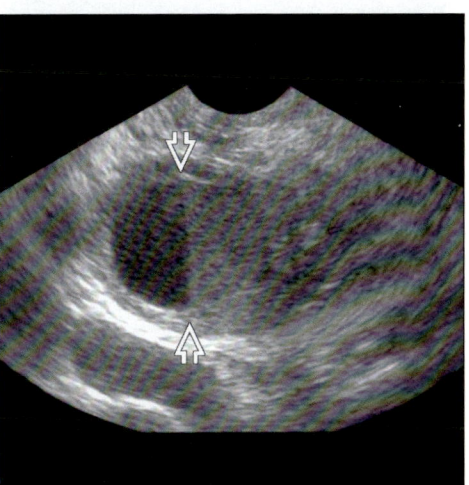

(Left) Sagittal transvaginal ultrasound shows an almost completely echogenic mass ➡ with a small shadowing focus. *(Right)* Sagittal transvaginal ultrasound shows a complex cystic ovarian lesion with a fat-fluid level ➡.

DERMOID (MATURE TERATOMA)

Typical

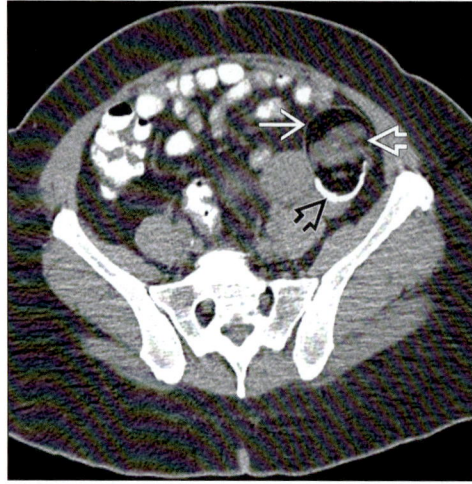 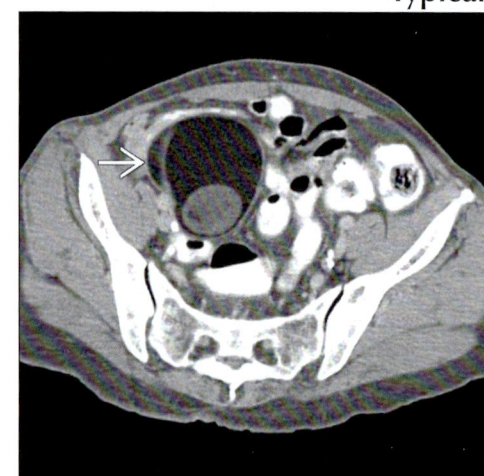

(Left) Axial NECT shows a left pelvic mass composed of fat ➡, soft tissue ➡ and calcification ➡. The fat component is diagnostic for dermoid. *(Right)* Axial CECT shows a mass with fat attenuation component ➡ in the right hemipelvis. The presence of fat is diagnostic of a dermoid cyst.

Typical

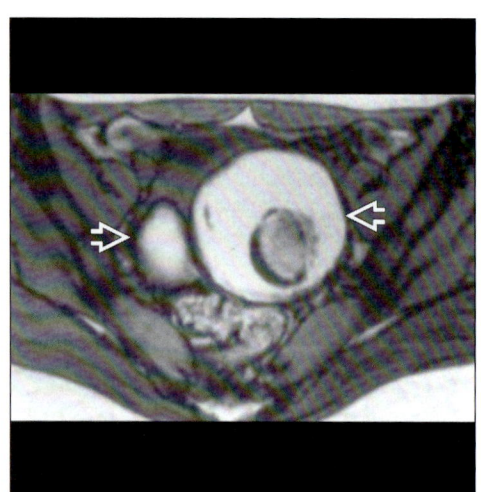 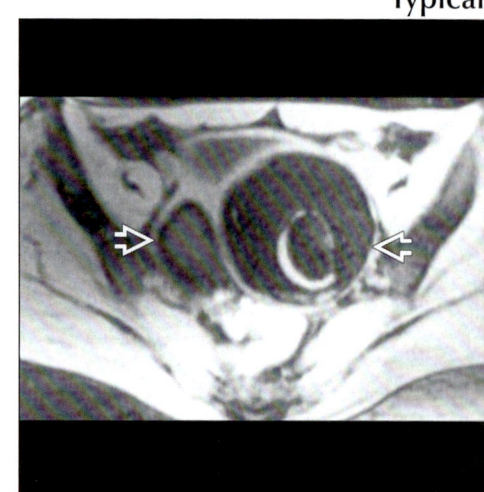

(Left) Axial T1WI MR shows bilateral high signal intensity masses ➡. The mass on the left is complex. *(Right)* Axial T1WI FS MR shows loss of high signal in the bilateral masses ➡ consistent with macroscopic fat. This constellation of findings is diagnostic for a dermoid.

Variant

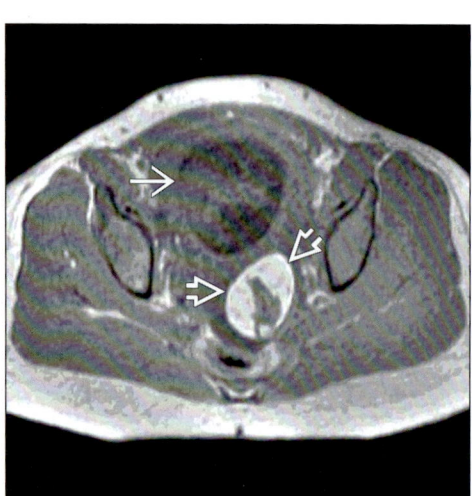 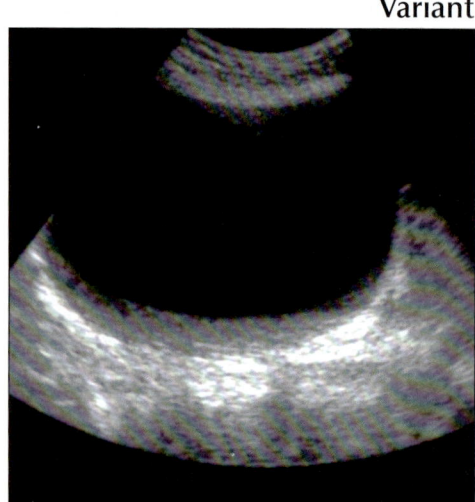

(Left) Axial T1WI MR in a pregnant patient ➡ shows a left adnexal mass with high signal intensity elements ➡. Torsion may occur during pregnancy as the ovary gets displaced by the gravid uterus. *(Right)* Sagittal transabdominal ultrasound shows a dermoid that images as an anechoic cyst.

DERMOID (MATURE TERATOMA)

Variant

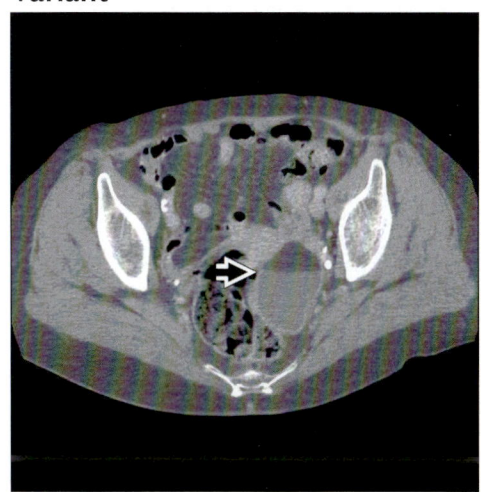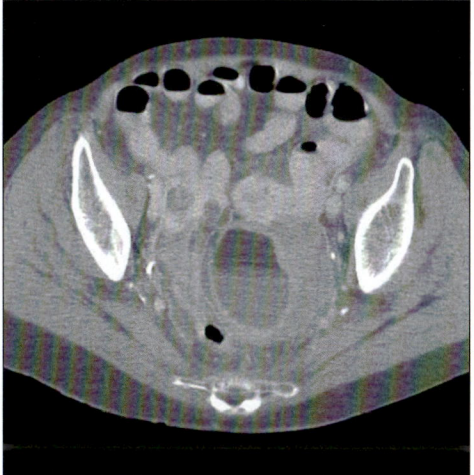

(Left) Axial CECT shows left pelvic cystic mass with a fat-fluid level ➡. The fat level is composed of sebaceous material. *(Right)* Axial CECT of the same patient, 3 months after the previous scan. She presented to the emergency room in acute pelvic pain. The dermoid cyst has shifted in location to the center of the pelvis and is now surrounded by fluid and inflammatory change. This is compatible with torsed ovary secondary to the presence of a dermoid cyst.

Typical

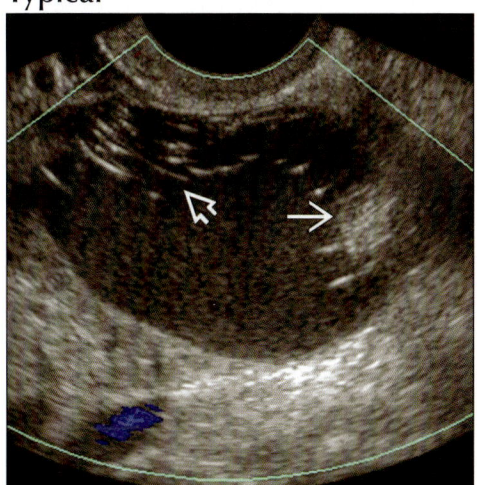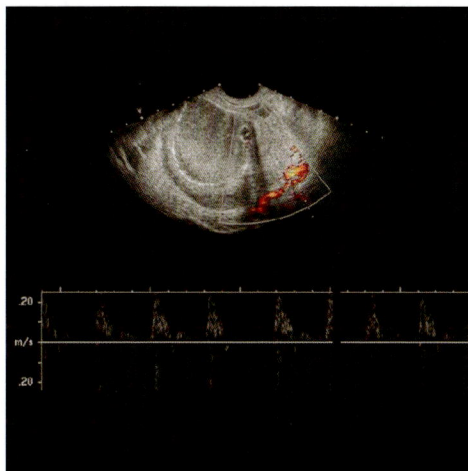

(Left) Sagittal color Doppler ultrasound shows a complex cystic mass with dermoid mesh ➡ and mural nodule ➡. Lack of detectable vascular flow led to diagnosis of torsed dermoid cyst which was confirmed in the operating room. *(Right)* Coronal pulsed Doppler ultrasound shows flow only in the periphery of this ovary, which contains a dermoid cyst. Note high resistance arterial flow which led to the diagnosis of torsion.

Typical

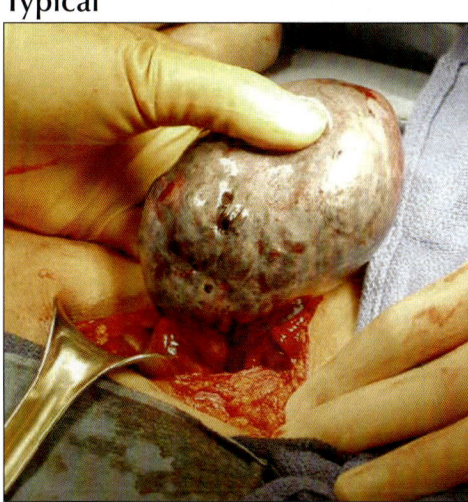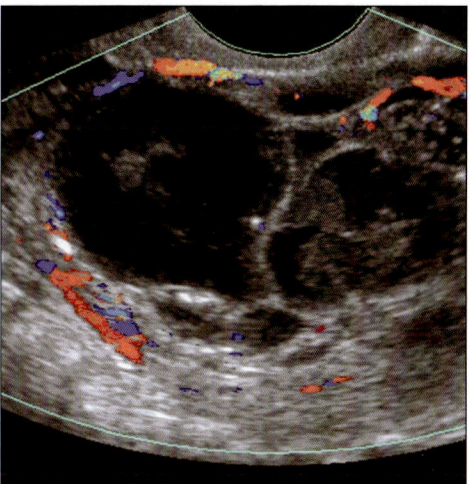

(Left) Intra-operative photograph of the same patient as previous image, shows a large adnexal mass representing a torsed ovary with a dermoid cyst. *(Right)* Sagittal color Doppler ultrasound shows a complex cystic mass. At pathology the solid tissue was thyroid type compatible with struma ovarii.

FIBROTHECOMA, OVARY

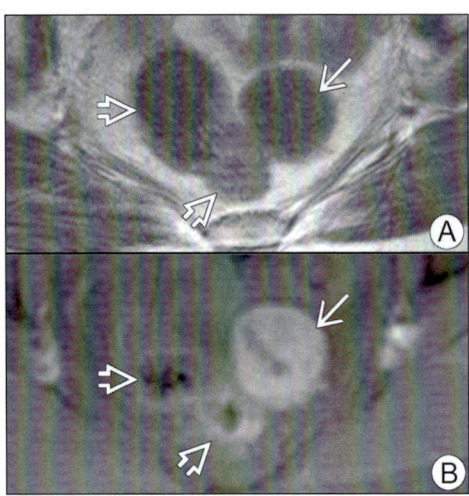

Axial (A) T2WI shows a low signal intensity mass ➡ to left of rectosigmoid ➡. (B) T1 C+ MR shows enhancement of the mass ➡ and rectosigmoid ➡.

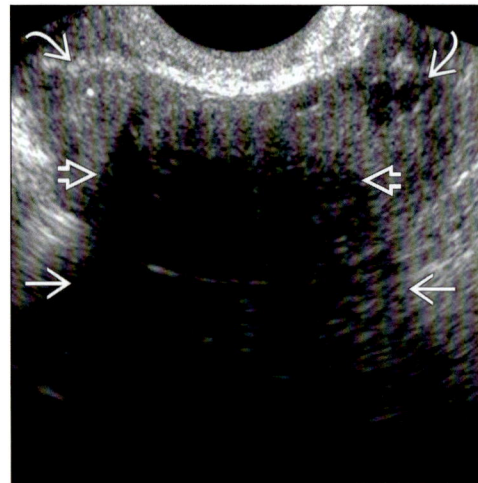

Axial transvaginal ultrasound shows a hypoechoic mass ➡ in the ovary ➡ causing significant attenuation ➡ of sound.

TERMINOLOGY

Abbreviations and Synonyms
- Fibroma; thecoma

Definitions
- Benign ovarian neoplasm
  - Spectrum including fibroma, thecoma & fibrothecoma

IMAGING FINDINGS

General Features
- Best diagnostic clue
  - Solid ovarian mass
    - Transvaginal ultrasound: Hypoechoic & attenuating
    - MR: T2WI: Low signal intensity: T1 C+: Negligible enhancement
- Location: Ovary
- Size: Median approximately 13 cm
- Morphology
  - Solid mass
    - ± Calcification
    - ± Cystic component in larger lesions

Ultrasonographic Findings
- Grayscale Ultrasound
  - Transabdominal and transvaginal US (TVS)
  - Hypoechoic mass
    - With edge shadows
    - With sound attenuation
  - Absolute lack of sound penetration in the absence of calcification or echogenic interface at the start of shadowing
  - ± Calcification
  - ± Cyst in larger lesions
  - Non-attenuating hypo/hyper/heterogeneous mass atypical
- Pulsed Doppler: Wide range of resistive indices depending on vascularity
- Color Doppler
  - Generally hypovascular
    - Occasionally may show increased vascularity
- Power Doppler
  - Generally hypovascular
    - Occasionally may show increased vascularity

DDx: Adnexal Masses

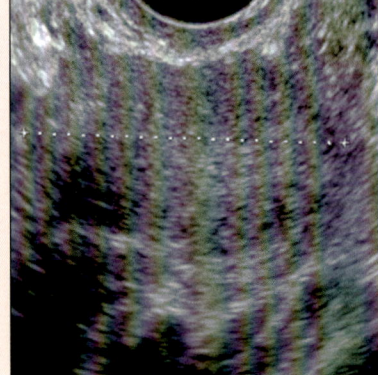

Brenner Tumor

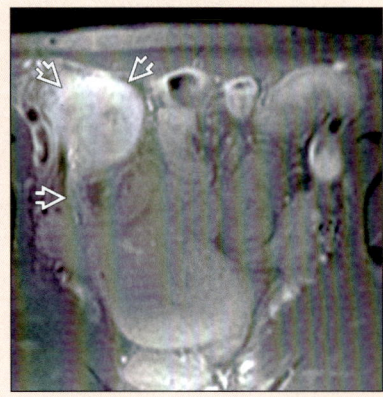

Pedunculated Leiomyoma

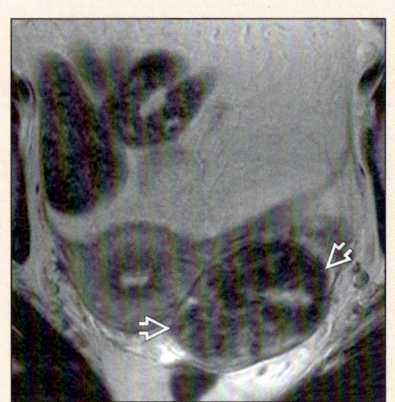

Broad Ligament Fibroma

FIBROTHECOMA, OVARY

Key Facts

Terminology
- Benign ovarian neoplasm
- Spectrum including fibroma, thecoma & fibrothecoma

Imaging Findings
- Solid ovarian mass
- Transvaginal ultrasound: Hypoechoic & attenuating
- MR: T2WI: Low signal intensity: T1 C+: Negligible enhancement
- Best imaging tool: TVS for screening, MR if a hypoechoic attenuating mass not seen on TVS or to differentiate from pedunculated leiomyoma

Top Differential Diagnoses
- Pedunculated Uterine Leiomyoma
- Brenner Tumor
- Dermoid

Pathology
- Thecoma may be associated with endometrial thickening if it secretes estrogen
- Thecoma may be associated with hirsutism and amenorrhea if it secretes androgen

Clinical Issues
- Always benign

Diagnostic Checklist
- Fibrothecoma if significant attenuation of sound on TVS in a patient with a palpable adnexal mass
- May be mistaken for gas containing bowel on TVS and T2WI

- Ascites

CT Findings
- NECT
  - Nonspecific adnexal mass isodense to the uterus
    - ± Calcification
- CECT
  - Early: Hypovascular with negligible enhancement
  - Delayed: Progressive enhancement

MR Findings
- T1WI: Low to intermediate signal intensity
- T2WI
  - Predominantly low signal intensity
    - Homogeneous or heterogeneous
  - Central high signal intensity cystic areas
  - Some edema in larger lesions
- T1 C+ FS
  - Different degrees of enhancement
    - Tends to have delayed enhancement
- Signal void foci on T1WI & T2WI if calcified
- If thecoma elements predominate
  - Fat elements can be identified
  - Fat imaged on frequency selective fat-saturation or out-of-phase gradient echo sequences
- Ascites

Imaging Recommendations
- Best imaging tool: TVS for screening, MR if a hypoechoic attenuating mass not seen on TVS or to differentiate from pedunculated leiomyoma
- Protocol advice: Highest MHz transducer to see attenuation on TVS

DIFFERENTIAL DIAGNOSIS

Pedunculated Uterine Leiomyoma
- Uterine in origin
  - Look for pedicle
- Will often see a separate ovary

Brenner Tumor
- Small tumors
- When benign, tend to be homogeneous on imaging studies
- Incidental finding when operated for other ovarian pathology

Dermoid
- TVS: 3 most common imaging features
  - Cystic lesion with densely echogenic shadowing mural nodule
  - "Tip of Iceberg" sign: Echogenic mass with sound attenuation
  - "Dermoid mesh": Multiple thin echogenic lines and dots
- MR: Presence of macroscopic fat is diagnostic

PATHOLOGY

General Features
- General path comments
  - Most common sex cord-stromal tumor
  - 1% bilateral
  - 1% associated with Meigs syndrome
    - Ascites: 10-15% with ascites; usually associated with larger tumors
    - Pleural effusion
    - Both disappear with removal of tumor
  - May be part of basal cell nevus syndrome
    - Basel cell carcinomas
    - Keratocytes of jaw
    - Calcification of dura
    - Mesenteric cysts
    - Ovarian fibromas: Usually bilateral & calcified
- Genetics: Not known
- Etiology: Not known
- Epidemiology
  - Fibroma: 4% of ovarian tumors
  - Thecoma: 1% of ovarian tumors
- Associated abnormalities
  - Thecoma may be associated with endometrial thickening if it secretes estrogen
  - Thecoma may be associated with hirsutism and amenorrhea if it secretes androgen

FIBROTHECOMA, OVARY

Gross Pathologic & Surgical Features
- Chalky-white hard surface with a whorled appearance on cross section
- Fibroma may be cystic and 10% calcified

Microscopic Features
- Fibroma: Bundles of intersecting spindle cells producing collagen
- Thecoma: Swollen lipid-laden stromal cells resembling theca cells
- Absence of lipid cells differentiates fibroma from thecoma

CLINICAL ISSUES

Presentation
- Most common signs/symptoms: Asymptomatic: Usually incidental finding
- Other signs/symptoms
  - Adnexal mass
  - Ovary torsion
  - Clinical signs of estrogenic or androgenic activity

Demographics
- Age
  - Fibroma: Mean, 48 years
  - Thecoma: Postmenopausal

Natural History & Prognosis
- Always benign

Treatment
- American College of Obstetricians and Gynecologists (ACOG) Recommendations
  - Excision of the affected ovary by laparoscopy for larger lesion

DIAGNOSTIC CHECKLIST

Consider
- Fibrothecoma if significant attenuation of sound on TVS in a patient with a palpable adnexal mass

Image Interpretation Pearls
- Hypoechoic attenuating mass on TVS
- Hypointense on T2WI with no or delayed enhancement
- May be mistaken for gas containing bowel on TVS and T2WI

SELECTED REFERENCES
1. Tanaka YO et al: MR findings of ovarian tumors with hormonal activity, with emphasis on tumors other than sex cord-stromal tumors. Eur J Radiol. 62(3):317-27, 2007
2. Kawano Y et al: Magnetic resonance imaging findings in leiomyoma of the ovary: a case report. Arch Gynecol Obstet. 273(5):298-300, 2006
3. Takeshita T et al: Ovarian fibroma (fibrothecoma) with extensive cystic degeneration: unusual MR imaging findings in two cases. Radiat Med. 23(1):70-4, 2005
4. Yoshitake T et al: Bilateral ovarian leiomyomas: CT and MRI features. Abdom Imaging. 30(1):117-9, 2005
5. Chang SD et al: Limited-sequence magnetic resonance imaging in the evaluation of the ultrasonographically indeterminate pelvic mass. Can Assoc Radiol J. 55(2):87-95, 2004
6. Cho SM et al: CT and MRI findings of cystadenofibromas of the ovary. Eur Radiol. 14(5):798-804, 2004
7. Sala EJ et al: Magnetic resonance imaging of benign adnexal disease. Top Magn Reson Imaging. 14(4):305-27, 2003
8. Jung SE et al: CT and MR imaging of ovarian tumors with emphasis on differential diagnosis. Radiographics. 22(6):1305-25, 2002
9. Schwartz RK et al: Ovarian fibroma: findings by contrast-enhanced MRI. Abdom Imaging. 22(5):535-7, 1997
10. Troiano RN et al: Fibroma and fibrothecoma of the ovary: MR imaging findings. Radiology. 204(3):795-8, 1997
11. Atri M et al: Endovaginal sonographic appearance of benign ovarian masses. Radiographics. 14(4):747-60; discussion 761-2, 1994
12. Bazot M et al: Fibrothecomas of the ovary: CT and US findings. J Comput Assist Tomogr. 17(5):754-9, 1993
13. Athey PA et al: Sonography of ovarian fibromas/thecomas. J Ultrasound Med. 6(8):431-6, 1987
14. Yaghoobian J et al: Ultrasound findings in thecoma of the ovary. J Clin Ultrasound. 11(2):91-3, 1983

FIBROTHECOMA, OVARY

IMAGE GALLERY

Typical

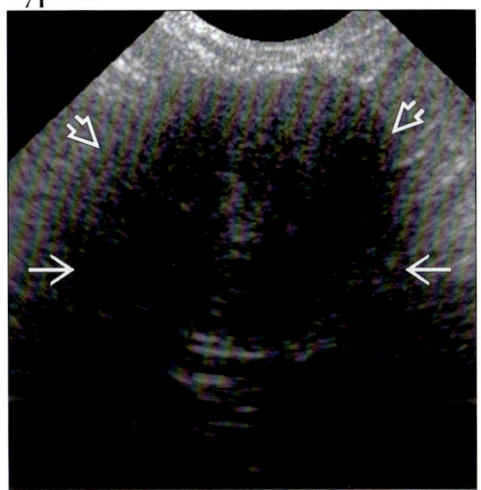
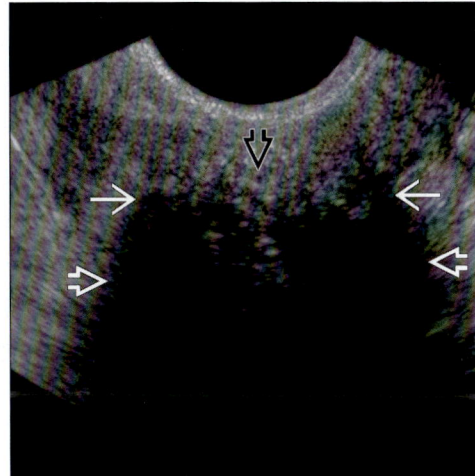

(Left) Axial transvaginal ultrasound shows a hypoechoic mass ➡ completely replacing ovary causing significant sound attenuation ➡. *(Right)* Axial transvaginal ultrasound shows a hypoechoic mass ➡ in the ovary with punctate calcifications ➡ causing significant sound attenuation ➡.

Typical

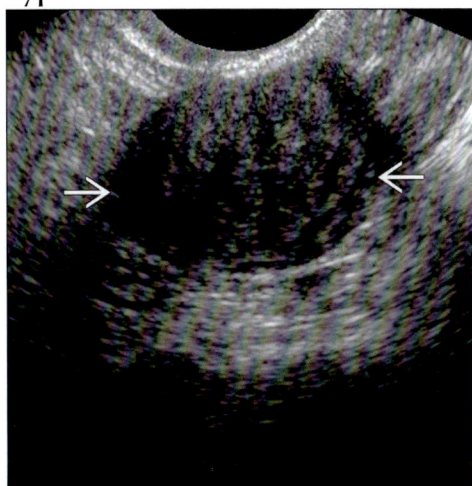
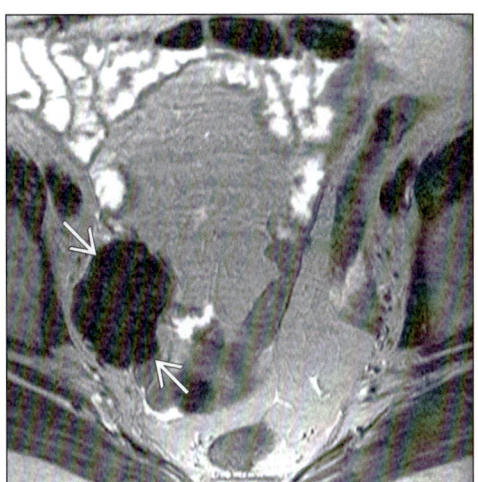

(Left) Axial transvaginal ultrasound shows a well-defined hypoechoic mass ➡ with edge shadows. *(Right)* Axial T2WI MR in the same patient as previous image, shows a hypointense mass ➡ in the right adnexa.

Typical

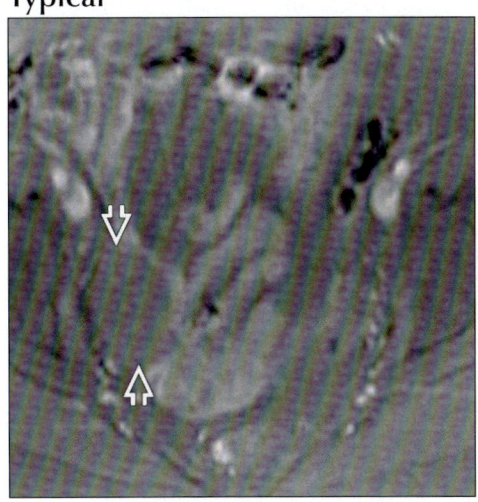
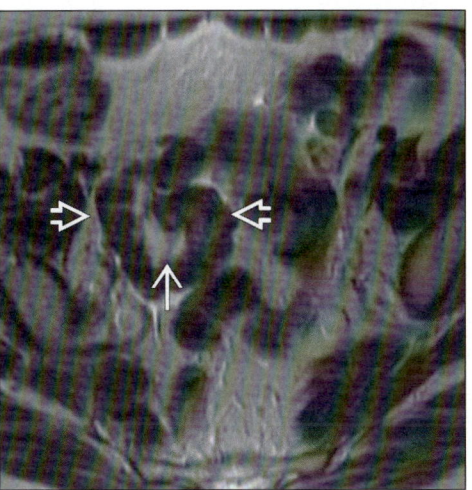

(Left) Axial T1 C+ FS MR in the same patient as previous image, shows the mass ➡ demonstrating minimal punctate enhancement. *(Right)* Axial T2WI MR shows a predominantly hypointense mass ➡ containing a central hyperintense component ➡ corresponding to edema or cystic degeneration.

ADENOFIBROMA

Axial CECT shows a slightly enlarged right ovary ➡ without a discrete mass. The patient had a surgically confirmed 2 cm adenofibroma. The fallopian tube ➡ is thickened secondary to endometriosis.

Transabdominal ultrasound in the same patient as previous image, shows a small, solid ovarian mass ➡ which is almost indistinguishable from the normal parenchyma.

TERMINOLOGY

Definitions
- Subtype of benign epithelial tumor → benign epithelial elements within a fibrous stroma

IMAGING FINDINGS

General Features
- Best diagnostic clue: Solid ovarian mass
- Location: Can be bilateral (10-20% of cases)
- Size: Variable

Ultrasonographic Findings
- Grayscale Ultrasound: Solid ovarian mass
- Color Doppler: Increased vascularity in 50% of cases

CT Findings
- CECT: Heterogeneous, solid enhancing mass

MR Findings
- T2WI: Solid mass with very low signal intensity fibrous components
- T1 C+: Heterogeneous, solid enhancing mass

Imaging Recommendations
- Best imaging tool
  - US → should be initial modality to evaluate ovarian mass
  - MR better than US to characterize fibrous component

DIFFERENTIAL DIAGNOSIS

Metastases
- Variable size; often solid, commonly cystic
- Accompanied by fluid in the pelvis

Solid Ovarian Masses with Fibrous Components
- Fibroma, fibrothecoma and Brenner tumor
- Fibrous component: Low signal intensity on T2WI
- They may be entirely solid and partially calcified

Primary Ovarian Malignancy
- More advanced stages of epithelial tumors have greater proportion of solid components and vascularity

DDx: Adenofibroma

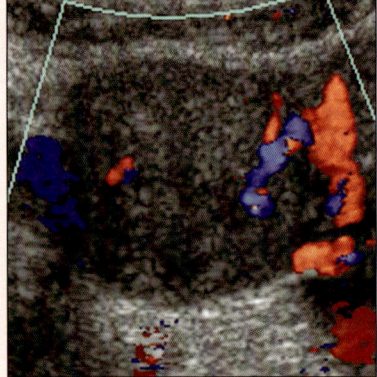
Pedunculated Leiomyoma

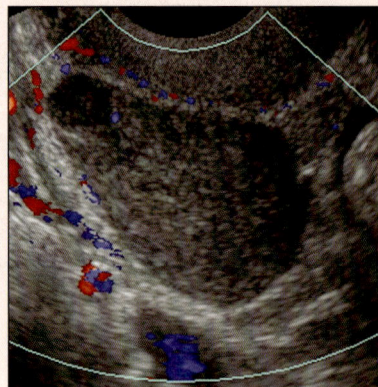
Ovarian Fibroma

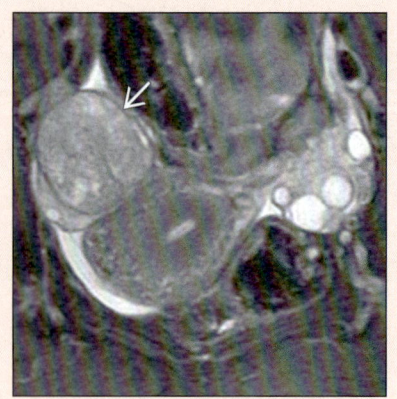
Endometrioid Carcinoma

ADENOFIBROMA

Key Facts

Terminology
- Subtype of benign epithelial tumor → benign epithelial elements within a fibrous stroma

Imaging Findings
- Location: Can be bilateral (10-20% of cases)
- T2WI: Solid mass with very low signal intensity fibrous components
- Grayscale Ultrasound: Solid ovarian mass

Pathology
- Termed cystadenofibroma or adenofibroma depending on relative amounts of cystic, solid and fibrous tissue
- Epithelial component of adenofibromas: Serous, mucinous, endometrioid, clear cell

Diagnostic Checklist
- Low T2 signal intensity aids characterization

Uterine Leiomyomas
- Attached to the uterus, separate to ovary
- Variable signal intensity on T2WI depending on degree of necrosis

PATHOLOGY

Gross Pathologic & Surgical Features
- Termed cystadenofibroma or adenofibroma depending on relative amounts of cystic, solid and fibrous tissue
- Serous adenofibroma → solid, spongy sectioned surface with minute, colorless fluid containing cysts
  - Papillary adenofibromas may have a complex surface architecture, adhere to pelvic structures and on sectioning may be confused with malignancy
- Mucinous, endometrioid and clear cell adenofibromas → gross solid stromal components

Microscopic Features
- Stroma: Fibrous appearing, variably cellular, may be focally calcified
- Epithelial component of adenofibromas: Serous, mucinous, endometrioid, clear cell
  - Serous adenofibroma → most common subtype, lined with columnar epithelium, no mitotic figures
  - Mucinous adenofibromas → contain mucinous glands and small cysts
  - Endometrioid adenofibromas → glands lined by cells resembling endometrial cells; may have mucin
  - Clear cell adenofibromas → glands lined by cuboidal cells with clear cytoplasm

CLINICAL ISSUES

Presentation
- Most common signs/symptoms
  - Abnormal vaginal bleeding
  - Pelvic pain
  - Asymptomatic pelvic mass

Demographics
- Age: Majority are postmenopausal, mean age: 57 years

DIAGNOSTIC CHECKLIST

Image Interpretation Pearls
- Low T2 signal intensity aids characterization

SELECTED REFERENCES

1. Volmar KE et al: Fine-needle aspiration cytology of endometrioid adenofibroma of the ovary. Diagn Cytopathol. 31(1):38-42, 2004
2. Alcazar JL et al: Sonographic features of ovarian cystadenofibromas: spectrum of findings. J Ultrasound Med. 20(8):915-9, 2001
3. Outwater EK et al: Ovarian fibromas and cystadenofibromas: MRI features of the fibrous component. J Magn Reson Imaging. 7(3):465-71, 1997

IMAGE GALLERY

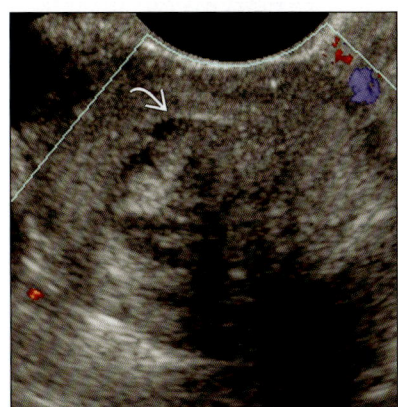
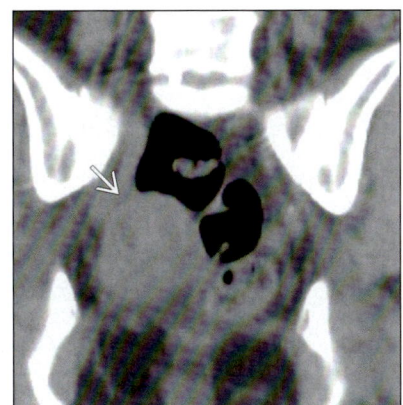
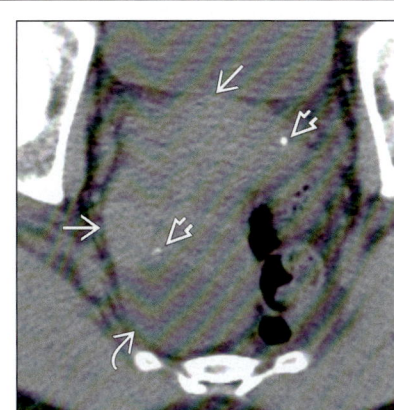

(Left) Transvaginal ultrasound with color Doppler shows heterogeneous solid component ➡ of an ovarian cystadenofibroma in a patient who presented with a torsion. *(Center)* Coronal CECT shows heterogeneous solid component of a large ovarian cystadenofibroma ➡. *(Right)* Axial CECT shows large, heterogeneous solid ➡ and cystic ➡ ovarian mass with tiny calcifications ➡, which on pathology was proven to be a cystadenofibroma.

GRANULOSA CELL TUMOR

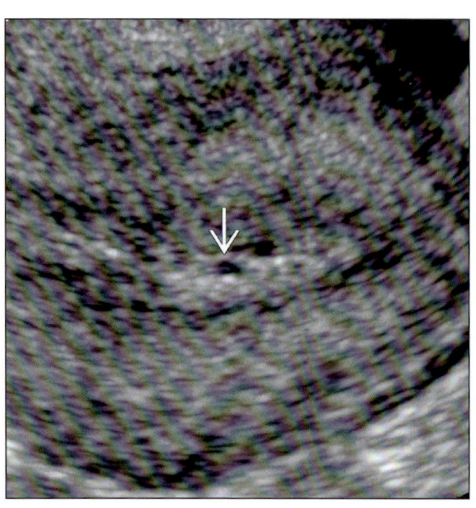

Sagittal transvaginal ultrasound shows thickened endometrial stripe with cystic changes representing cystic hyperplasia ➡ in a patient with an adult granulosa cell tumor.

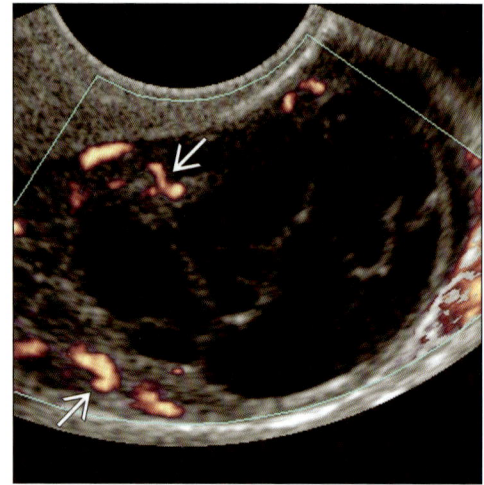

Sagittal power Doppler ultrasound in the same patient shows multilocular cystic ovarian mass with thick septations. Power Doppler demonstrated flow in the solid components ➡.

TERMINOLOGY

Abbreviations and Synonyms
- Granulosa and granulosa-theca cell tumors

Definitions
- Neoplasm composed of a pure or at least 10% population of granulosa cells often in a fibrothecomatous background
  - Major subtypes: Adult and juvenile type

IMAGING FINDINGS

General Features
- Best diagnostic clue: Large solid and cystic adnexal mass and thickened endometrial stripe
- Location
  - Almost always unilateral
  - 9% of the adult type and 2% of the juvenile type are bilateral
- Size: Average size is 12.5 cm

Ultrasonographic Findings
- Grayscale Ultrasound
  - Echogenic, solid ovarian mass with variable amount of cystic components
    - Usually multilocular with thick or thin walls and septations
    - Solid component → homogeneous or heterogeneous
    - Heterogeneous echogenicity if hemorrhage, fibrosis or necrosis
    - Unilocular and solid appearances are uncommon
  - Thickened endometrial stripe → cystic changes
- Color Doppler: Low resistance vessels in thickened septations or solid component

CT Findings
- Solid, enhancing mass with variable cystic or hemorrhagic/degenerating areas of low attenuation
- Enlarged uterus with endometrial thickening

MR Findings
- T1WI
  - Solid and cystic mass

DDx: Ovarian Mass

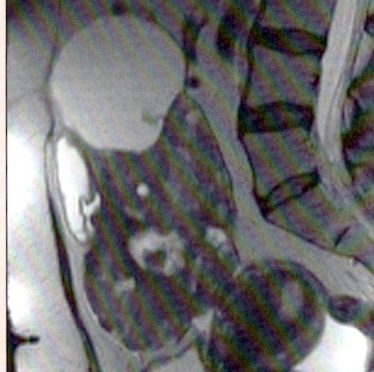
Fibroma with Focal Degeneration

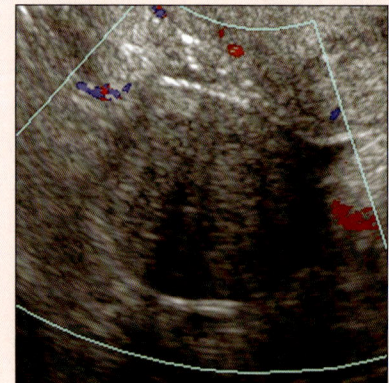
Fibrothecoma

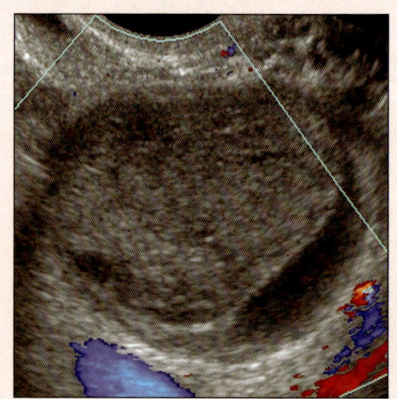
Hemorrhagic Ovarian Cyst

GRANULOSA CELL TUMOR

Key Facts

Terminology
- Neoplasm composed of a pure or at least 10% population of granulosa cells often in a fibrothecomatous background
- Major subtypes: Adult and juvenile type

Imaging Findings
- Best diagnostic clue: Large solid and cystic adnexal mass and thickened endometrial stripe
- Almost always unilateral
- Low signal on T2WI or fluid-fluid levels with intracystic hemorrhage
- Color Doppler: Low resistance vessels in thickened septations or solid component

Pathology
- Endometrial lesion: Classically described is anovulatory pattern with cystic hyperplasia
- Atypical hyperplasia or endometrial carcinomas in 5% of tumors
- Tumor cells grow in a variety of patterns, best known is microfollicular with Call-Exner bodies

Clinical Issues
- Metrorrhagia, postmenopausal bleeding
- Isosexual precocious puberty in pediatric population

Diagnostic Checklist
- Tumor secretes estrogen therefore consider when endometrial lesion is seen in association with heterogeneous solid adnexal mass

---

- Cysts may have increased signal intensity due to hemorrhage
- T2WI
  - Common appearances: Multilocular (sponge-like) cystic mass or solid mass with internal cysts
    - Uncommon appearances: Unilocular cystic mass or entirely solid mass
    - Low signal on T2WI or fluid-fluid levels with intracystic hemorrhage
    - Thick septations may have low signal intensity
  - Juvenile type usually solid mass, hyperintense signal
  - Enlarged uterus; thick and hyperintense endometrium
- T1 C+
  - Solid component enhances
  - Juvenile type → homogeneous enhancement

Imaging Recommendations
- Best imaging tool: Ultrasound to assess endometrium and adnexa

DIFFERENTIAL DIAGNOSIS

Mucinous or Serous Cystadenoma or Cystadenocarcinoma
- If tumor presents as multilocular cystic mass with thickened septations differentiation is difficult
- Unilocular cystic mass is a rare presentation of a granulosa cell tumor, more commonly seen in cystadenoma or cystadenocarcinoma
- Large granulosa cell tumors are less likely to have peritoneal spread than large epithelial tumors

Ovarian Metastasis
- Solid ovarian tumor is an uncommon presentation of granulosa cell tumor
- Metastasis are commonly bilateral, granulosa cell tumors are usually unilateral

Hemorrhagic Ovarian Cyst
- Apparent septations or retracting clot do not show flow on color Doppler
- Changes or resolves on followup

Fibroma/Fibrothecoma
- Solid ovarian mass
- May be associated with thickened endometrial stripe

Uterine Myoma
- Show attachment to uterus from a necrotic, exophytic leiomyoma

PATHOLOGY

General Features
- Etiology
  - Unknown; several studies suggest increased risk in infertile women and those exposed to ovulation induction agents
  - Estrogen stimulates proliferation of the granulosa cells of the ovary → may have a role in the pathogenesis of the tumor
    - Cells have high expression of estrogen receptor B → role is not well understood
- Epidemiology
  - Uncommon, 1-2% of all ovarian malignancies
  - 5% of granulosa cell tumors are juvenile type
  - Most common sex cord-stromal tumor after fibromas and fibrothecomas
- Associated abnormalities: Capacity to secrete estrogens and less commonly androgens and progestins

Gross Pathologic & Surgical Features
- Endometrial lesion: Classically described is anovulatory pattern with cystic hyperplasia
  - Atypical hyperplasia or endometrial carcinomas in 5% of tumors
- Gross appearance → varies depending on percentage of theca cells, degree of necrosis and hemorrhage
  - Typically solid, variably cystic, larger tumors are hemorrhagic, necrosis is focal and uncommon
  - Encapsulated with smooth or lobulated surface
  - 10-15% → tumor capsule may rupture
  - If prominent theca cells → yellow and firm

GRANULOSA CELL TUMOR

- Macroscopic appearance of the juvenile type is similar to adult type

Microscopic Features
- Adult type: Proliferation of granulosa cells, stromal component of fibroblasts, theca or luteinized cells
  - Granulosa cells: Scant cytoplasm, ovoid nucleus with longitudinal groove, rare mitotic activity
  - Tumor cells grow in a variety of patterns, best known is microfollicular with Call-Exner bodies
    - Different patterns explain variable imaging appearances: Macrofollicular pattern with cystic spaces → multilocular masses; trabecular or diffuse patterns → homogeneous solid masses; intratumoral bleeding, infarcts and fibrous degeneration → heterogeneously solid tumors
    - Different patterns mimic other tumors, other histologic and immunohistochemical characteristics aid distinction
- If granulosa and thecal cells coexist in same tumor → granulosa-theca cell tumor
- Juvenile granulosa cell tumor is a rare variant (less than 5% of all granulosa cell tumors)
  - Less well-differentiated than adult type
  - Nuclei are larger, lack groove, cytoplasm more eosinophilic and sometimes vacuolated
  - Cytologic atypia with bizarre nuclei, abundant mitotic figures (in contrast to the adult type)
- Adult and juvenile granulosa tumor cells are positive for Inhibin immunohistochemistry

CLINICAL ISSUES

Presentation
- Most common signs/symptoms
  - Abdominal mass, abdominal pain
  - Metrorrhagia, postmenopausal bleeding
  - Isosexual precocious puberty in pediatric population
  - 5-15% hemoperitoneum and acute abdominal pain secondary to rupture of cystic lesion
  - 10% ascites
  - 10% clinically occult
- Other signs/symptoms
  - 60% develop endometrial hyperplasia, 5% develop endometrial cancer
  - Increased risk of breast cancer, incidence of 3.7-20%
  - Infertility due to unregulated inhibin secretion
  - Androgenic activity may occur (virilization)

Demographics
- Age
  - Wide range (newborn to postmenopausal)
  - Adult type: Mean age 55
  - Juvenile type: 97% less than 30 years
  - 10% present during pregnancy
- Gender: Female

Natural History & Prognosis
- Hormonally active neoplasms → early diagnosis, high survival rates, slow growth, long interval to relapse
- Natural history characterized by indolent course and propensity for late recurrence
- Median time to relapse is 4-6 years after initial diagnosis, recurrence reported as late as 37 years
- Over 90% of tumors: Stage I disease at diagnosis → surgery alone achieves survival rates of 85-90% for 10 years
  - Less advanced stage → significant favorable prognostic factor for survival
  - Poor prognostic factors: Tumor size greater than 10-15 cm, high mitotic index, tumor rupture, lymphatic invasion
  - Despite atypia, mortality for juvenile type tumors is less than 3% if confined to ovary
- Advanced stage disease has a worse prognosis: Stage II → 50-65% and stages III and IV → 17-33%
- Juvenile type → high cure rate
  - Recurrences are uncommon; typically occur in first year and rarely later

Treatment
- Radical surgery (total abdominal hysterectomy and bilateral salpingo-oophorectomy) is preferable
- More conservative unilateral salpingo-oophorectomy with careful staging and endometrial biopsy is possible for early stages and those who wish to remain fertile
- Limited and inconclusive data regarding value of adjuvant radiotherapy or systemic chemotherapy due to rarity of tumors and long interval to relapse
- Management during pregnancy depends on gestational age, size of the mass and symptoms
- Hormonal therapy of recurrent granulosa cell tumors has been successfully reported
  - Important to know if the tumor has receptors for estrogen (present in 30%) or progesterone (present in most cases)
- Use of serologic tumor markers for follow-up is controversial: Include inhibin, CA-125 and estradiol levels
- Management of advanced or relapsed disease is not standard

DIAGNOSTIC CHECKLIST

Consider
- Tumor secretes estrogen therefore consider when endometrial lesion is seen in association with heterogeneous solid adnexal mass
- Tendency to recur many years after initial excision

SELECTED REFERENCES
1. Crew KD et al: Long natural history of recurrent granulosa cell tumor of the ovary 23 years after initial diagnosis: a case report and review of the literature. Gynecol Oncol. 96(1):235-40, 2005
2. Tanaka YO et al: Functioning ovarian tumors: direct and indirect findings at MR imaging. Radiographics. 24 Suppl 1:S147-66, 2004
3. Kim SH et al: Granulosa cell tumor of the ovary: common findings and unusual appearances on CT and MR. J Comput Assist Tomogr. 26(5):756-61, 2002
4. Ko SF et al: Adult ovarian granulosa cell tumors: spectrum of sonographic and CT findings with pathologic correlation. AJR Am J Roentgenol. 172(5):1227-33, 1999

GRANULOSA CELL TUMOR

IMAGE GALLERY

Typical

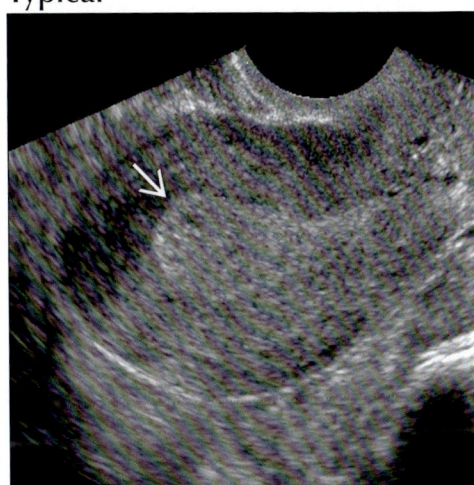
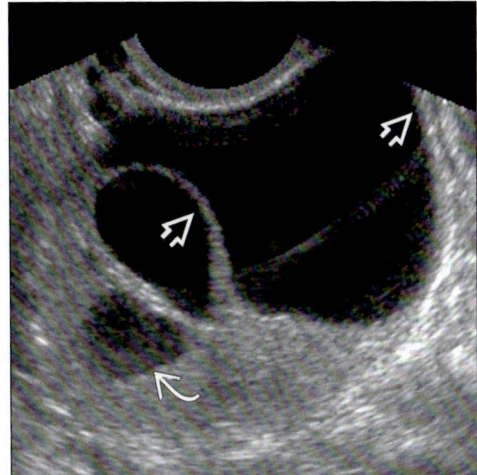

(Left) Sagittal transvaginal ultrasound in a patient with abnormal uterine bleeding, shows thickened endometrial stripe ➡ from cystic hyperplasia. *(Right)* Sagittal transvaginal ultrasound in the same patient shows large multilocular cystic ovarian mass with large cysts and thick walls ➡. Focal hemorrhage or necrosis ➡ is seen within solid component.

Typical

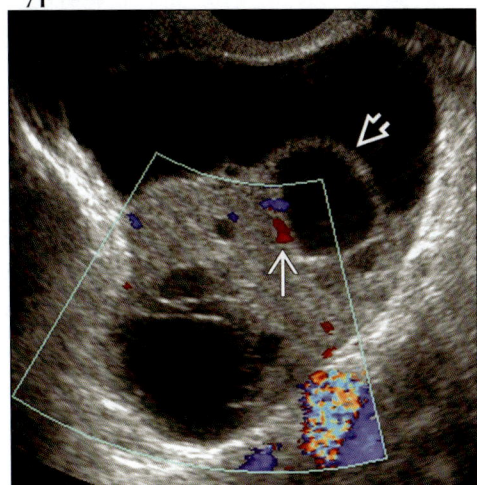
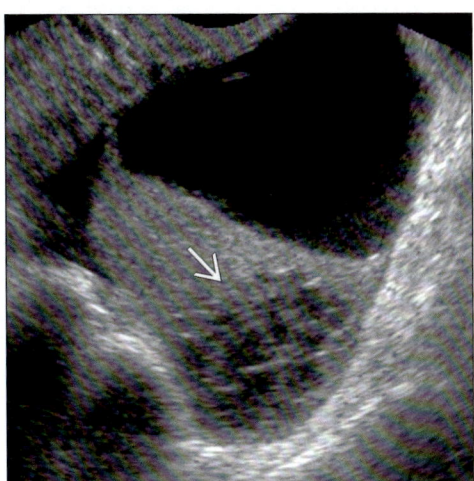

(Left) Transverse color Doppler ultrasound of an adult granulosa cell tumor shows increased flow ➡ in solid component. Cysts have variable sizes and some of them well-defined walls ➡. *(Right)* Transverse transvaginal ultrasound shows an ovarian mass with a large cyst and a heterogeneous area in the solid component likely from hemorrhage and degeneration ➡ within a granulosa cell tumor.

Typical

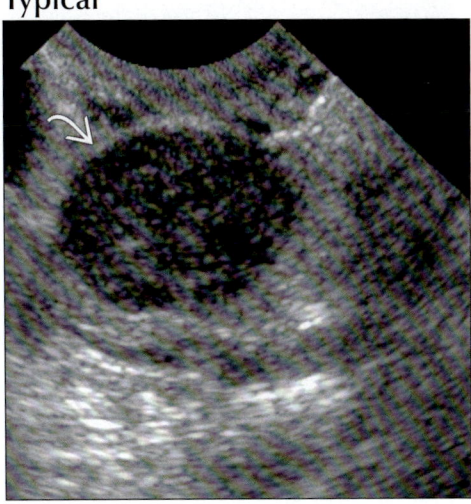
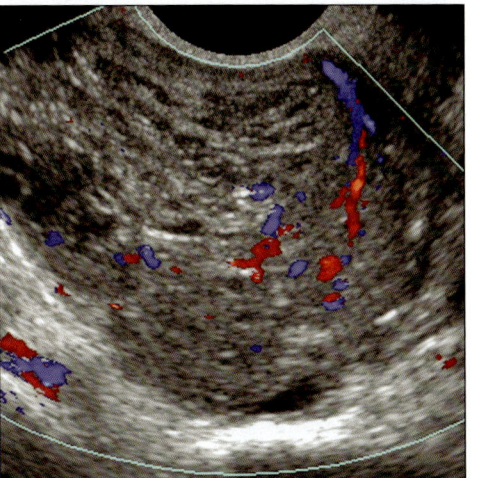

(Left) Transverse transvaginal ultrasound shows a small, solid ovarian mass ➡ in a patient who presented with abnormal uterine bleeding and a thickened endometrial stripe. *(Right)* Sagittal color Doppler ultrasound shows large predominantly solid, hypervascular ovarian mass with small internal cysts.

GRANULOSA CELL TUMOR

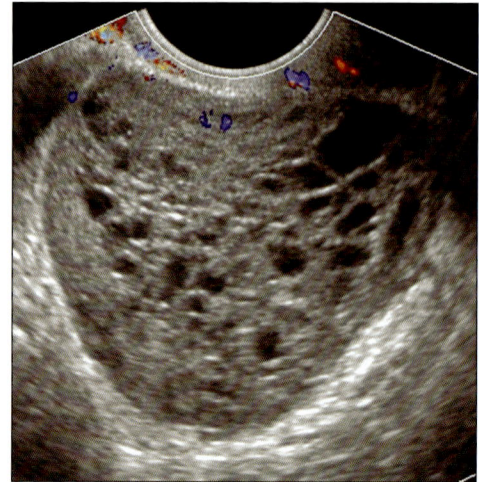

(Left) Sagittal color Doppler ultrasound shows large ovarian mass with a "sponge-like" appearance. (Right) Sagittal transvaginal ultrasound shows ovarian mass with multiple thin walled cystic spaces of variable sizes.

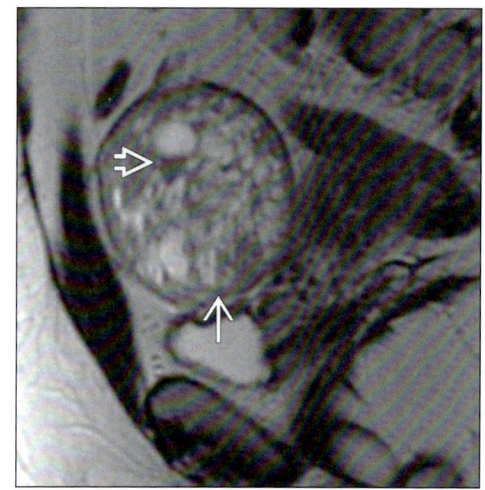 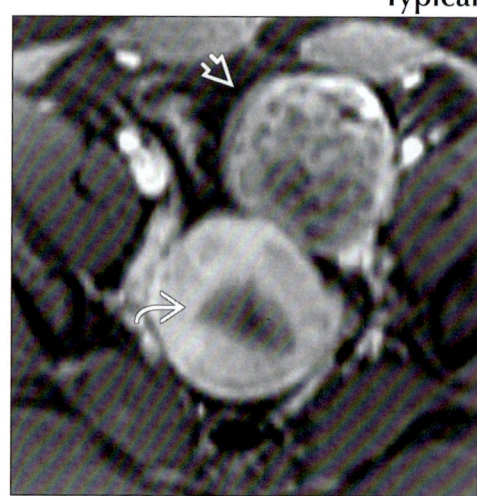

(Left) Sagittal T2WI MR shows a large multicystic ovarian mass with areas of low signal intensity ➡ and fluid-fluid levels related to hemorrhage ➡. (Right) Axial T1 C+ MR in the same patient shows enlarged uterus with thickened endometrial stripe ➡ and a left ovarian heterogeneously enhancing mass ➡ that proved to be an adult granulosa cell tumor.

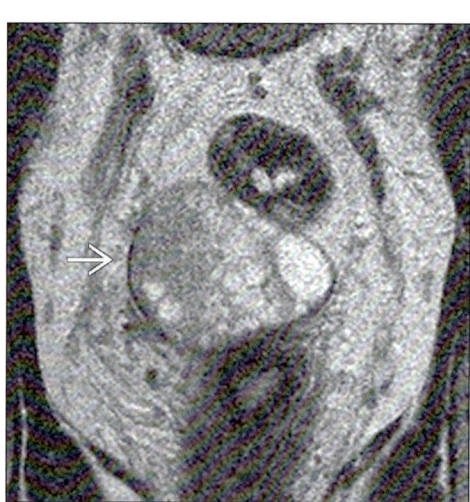 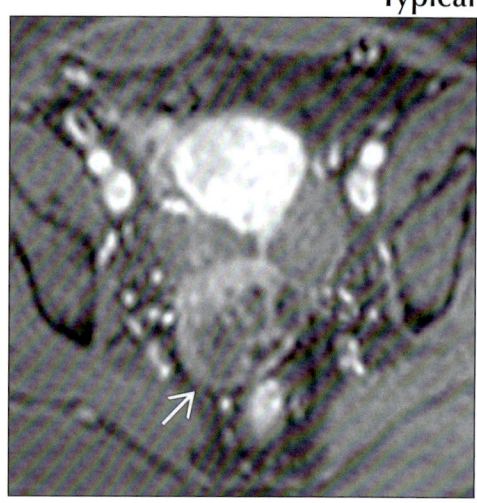

(Left) Coronal T2WI MR shows a large partially solid ovarian mass ➡ with multiple cysts of different sizes. (Right) Axial T1 C+ MR shows a heterogeneously enhancing, partially cystic ovarian mass ➡ in a patient with an adult granulosa cell tumor.

GRANULOSA CELL TUMOR

Typical

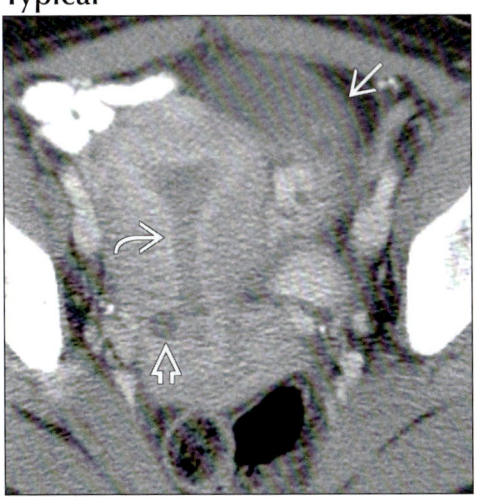
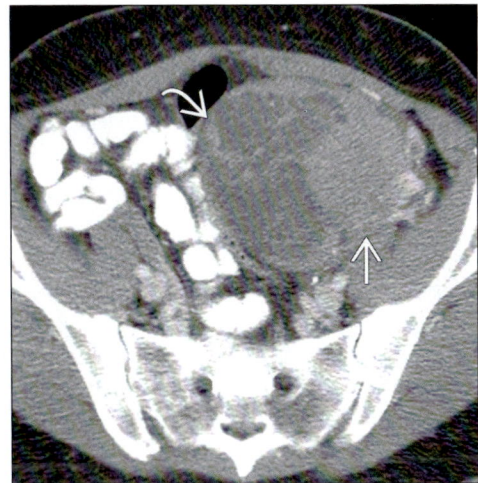

(Left) Axial CECT shows thickened endometrial stripe ➡ in a patient with a left ovarian mass ➡. There is a nabothian cyst in the cervix ➡. *(Right)* Axial CECT on the same patient shows a left ovarian heterogeneously enhancing mass with solid ➡ and cystic components and enhancing septations ➡.

Typical

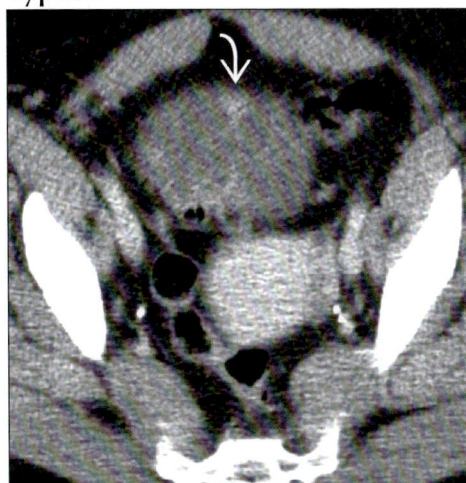
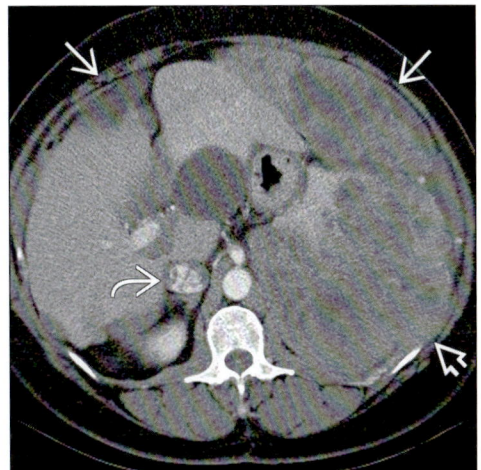

(Left) Axial CECT shows predominantly cystic ovarian mass with few ➡ enhancing components in a patient with an adult granulosa cell tumor. *(Right)* Axial CECT shows large masses in the spleen ➡, peritoneal cavity ➡ and filling defects in the inferior vena cava ➡. The patient had previous resection of a granulosa cell tumor.

Typical

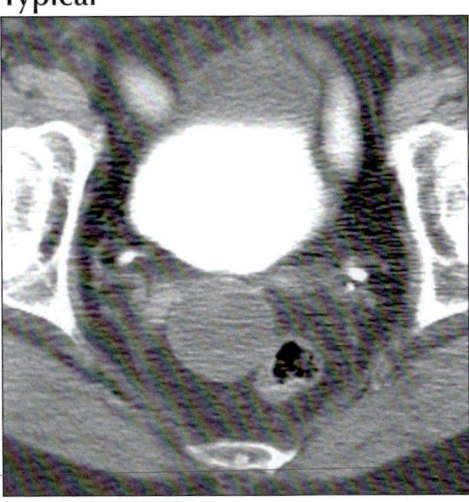
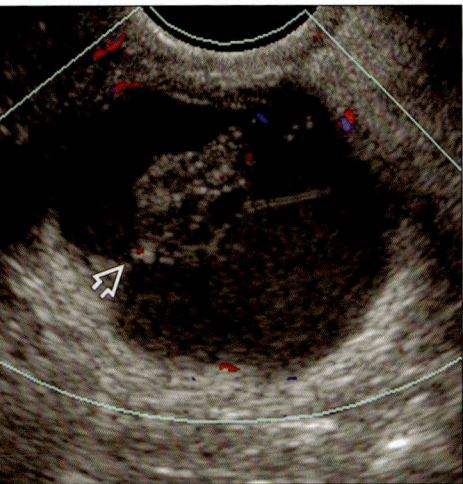

(Left) Axial CECT shows a hypodense vaginal mass in a patient with a history of prior granulosa cell tumor and elevated inhibin levels. *(Right)* Sagittal color Doppler ultrasound in the same patient shows recurrent vaginal tumor which is predominantly cystic and has a solid vascular ➡ component.

SCLEROSING STROMAL TUMOR

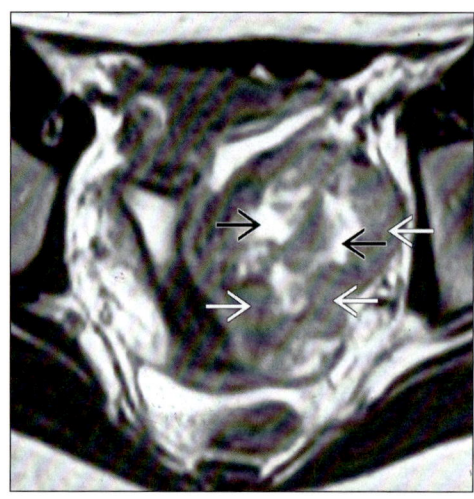

Axial T2WI MR shows a left ovarian mass. Note the pseudolobular pattern of the outer part of the lesion with intermediate signal intensity nodules ➔ interposed between high signal intensity clefts ➔.

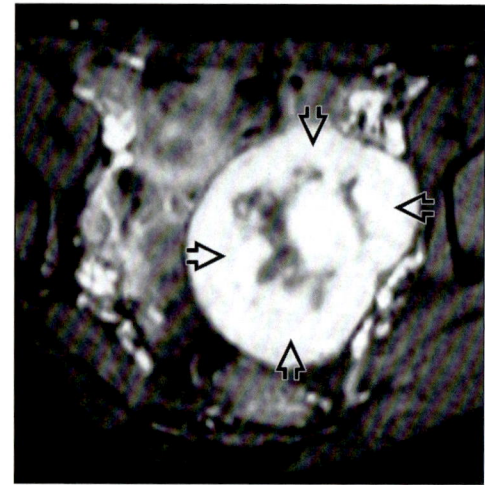

Axial T1 C+ FS MR shows avid enhancement of the outer part of the mass ➔ with a typical pseudolobular pattern. Pathology: Sclerosing stromal tumor. (Courtesy T.M. Cunha, MD).

TERMINOLOGY

Abbreviations and Synonyms
- Sclerosing stromal tumor (SST)

Definitions
- Benign sex cord stromal tumor

IMAGING FINDINGS

General Features
- Best diagnostic clue: Early and strong enhancement of peripheral tumor tissue and its centripetal progression on dynamic contrast-enhanced MR and CT
- Location: Unilateral ovarian mass
- Size: Variable, usually 3-5 cm
- Morphology: Large mass with pseudolobular pattern

Ultrasonographic Findings
- Grayscale Ultrasound
  - Multilocular cystic mass of heterogeneous echogenicity
  - Irregular thick septae and tumor wall
  - Solid mass with central hypoechoic star-shaped area
  - Mainly solid mass (rare)
  - Small amount of ascites
- Pulsed Doppler: Low-resistance flow
- Color Doppler
  - Prominent peripheral vessels
  - No arteriovenous shunting

CT Findings
- NECT
  - Mass of heterogeneous attenuation
  - Solid, nodular periphery and low attenuation irregular central area
- CECT
  - Early and strong enhancement of the periphery
  - Centripetal progression of the enhancement on delayed images

MR Findings
- T1WI
  - Thin low-signal intensity outer rim
  - Intermediate signal intensity outer part of lesion
  - Low signal intensity central area
- T2WI
  - Thin rim of low signal intensity

DDx: Ovarian Masses

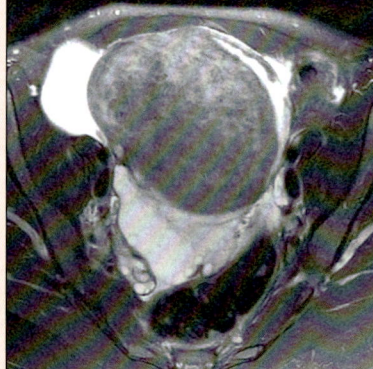
Fibroma

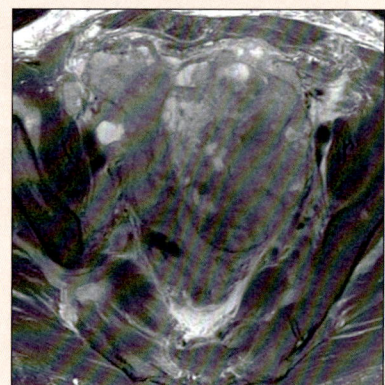
Ovarian Carcinoma

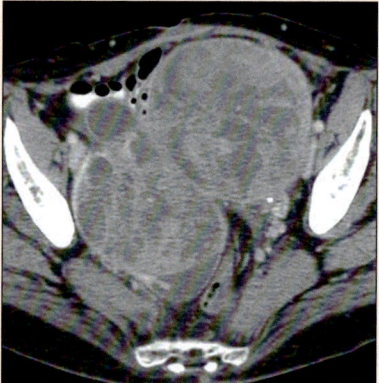
Krukenberg Tumor

SCLEROSING STROMAL TUMOR

Key Facts

Terminology
- Benign sex cord stromal tumor

Imaging Findings
- Best diagnostic clue: Early and strong enhancement of peripheral tumor tissue and its centripetal progression on dynamic contrast-enhanced MR and CT
- Best imaging tool: MR
- Protocol advice: T2WI and dynamic contrast-enhanced T1WI with fat saturation

Top Differential Diagnoses
- Ovarian Fibroma
- Ovarian Carcinoma
- Krukenberg Tumor
- Metastases to the Ovary
- Massive Ovarian Edema

Pathology
- Unilateral, firm, solid, lobulated tumor
- Pseudolobulated cellular zones alternate with acellular edematous or dense collagenous connective tissue zones
- Cellular areas contain numerous branched vessels
- Prominent sclerosis around individual cells and cell clusters

Clinical Issues
- Most common signs/symptoms: Menstrual irregularity
- Anovulation due to hormonal secretion (estrogen, progesterone, testosterone)
- Age: 80% occur under 30 years of age

  - Pseudolobular or spoke-wheel pattern of outer part of lesion
    - Intermediate to low signal intensity nodules interposed between high signal intensity septa
  - Very high signal intensity central area
- Dynamic T1 C+ FS
  - Early avid enhancement of thin surrounding rim represents compressed ovarian cortex on pathology
  - Early avid enhancement of outer part of mass with typical pseudolobular pattern representing pseudolobulated cellular areas
  - Later enhancement of intermediate part of mass with centripetal progression representing edematous ovarian stroma
  - Lack of enhancement of central area, even on delayed images representing collagenous acellular areas

Imaging Recommendations
- Best imaging tool: MR
- Protocol advice: T2WI and dynamic contrast-enhanced T1WI with fat saturation

DIFFERENTIAL DIAGNOSIS

Ovarian Fibroma
- Fibromas and thecomas are uncommon in first three decades of life
- Usually uniform low signal intensity on T2WI
- Lack of thin surrounding rim
- Mild and low enhancement on dynamic contrast-enhanced MR

Ovarian Carcinoma
- Older age group
- High values of tumor markers such as CA125 and/or CA19-9
- Signal intensity of solid components in ovarian cancer on T2WI are lower than those of SST
- Ovarian carcinoma shows early enhancement and fast wash-out on dynamic contrast-enhanced MR
- Ascites very common

Krukenberg Tumor
- Presence of primary gastrointestinal malignancy at time of diagnosis
- Usually bilateral
- Usually solid

Metastases to the Ovary
- Presence of primary tumor such as breast or endometrium
- Usually bilateral
- Cystic or solid

Massive Ovarian Edema
- Preserved ovarian follicles within edematous stroma
- Absence of lesion heterogeneity

PATHOLOGY

General Features
- Etiology: Arise from perifollicular myoid stromal cells in the theca externa
- Epidemiology: SST accounts for 6% of ovarian stromal tumors
- Associated abnormalities: Endometrial hyperplasia (rare)

Gross Pathologic & Surgical Features
- Unilateral, firm, solid, lobulated tumor
- 3-5 cm diameter
- Cut surface is pale and fleshy with white and yellow areas
- Cystic spaces may be seen occasionally
- Rarely presents as unilocular cyst

Microscopic Features
- Pseudolobulated cellular zones alternate with acellular edematous or dense collagenous connective tissue zones
- Cellular areas contain numerous branched vessels
- Tumor cells rounded with vacuolated or eosinophilic cytoplasm and spindle cells are admixed

SCLEROSING STROMAL TUMOR

- Prominent sclerosis around individual cells and cell clusters
- Immunohistochemical stains positive for desmin and smooth muscle actin in spindle cells only

CLINICAL ISSUES

Presentation
- Most common signs/symptoms: Menstrual irregularity
- Other signs/symptoms
  - Anovulation due to hormonal secretion (estrogen, progesterone, testosterone)
  - Pelvic pain
  - Palpable mass
  - Masculinization
  - Abnormal uterine bleeding
  - Ascites

Demographics
- Age: 80% occur under 30 years of age

Natural History & Prognosis
- Surgical removal of tumor is curative
- No local or distant recurrence

Treatment
- Oophorectomy

DIAGNOSTIC CHECKLIST

Consider
- SST in a young female patient presenting with prolonged menstrual irregularity and adnexal mass

Image Interpretation Pearls
- Dynamic contrast-enhanced MR findings typical for SST
  - Early striking peripheral enhancement with centripetal progression
  - Prolonged enhancement of inner portion of lesion

SELECTED REFERENCES

1. Jung SE et al: CT and MRI findings of sex cord-stromal tumor of the ovary. AJR Am J Roentgenol. 185(1):207-15, 2005
2. Calabrese M et al: Sclerosing stromal tumor of the ovary in pregnancy: clinical, ultrasonography, and magnetic resonance imaging findings. Acta Radiol. 45(2):189-92, 2004
3. Deval B et al: Sclerosing stromal tumor of the ovary: color Doppler findings. Ultrasound Obstet Gynecol. 22(5):531-4, 2003
4. Fefferman NR et al: Sclerosing stromal tumor of the ovary in a premenarchal female. Pediatr Radiol. 33(1):56-8, 2003
5. Kim JY et al: Sclerosing stromal tumor of the ovary: MR-pathologic correlation in three cases. Korean J Radiol. 4(3):194-9, 2003
6. Kuscu E et al: Sclerosing stromal tumor of the ovary: a case report. Eur J Gynaecol Oncol. 24(5):442-4, 2003
7. Mikami M et al: Magnetic resonance imaging in sclerosing stromal tumor of the ovary. Int J Gynaecol Obstet. 83(3):319-21, 2003
8. Yerli H et al: Sclerosing stromal tumor of the ovary with torsion. MRI features. Acta Radiol. 44(6):612-5, 2003
9. Torricelli P et al: Sclerosing stromal tumor of the ovary: US, CT, and MRI findings. Abdom Imaging. 27(5):588-91, 2002
10. Joja I et al: Sclerosing stromal tumor of the ovary: US, MR, and dynamic MR findings. J Comput Assist Tomogr. 25(2):201-6, 2001
11. Ihara N et al: Sclerosing stromal tumor of the ovary: MRI. J Comput Assist Tomogr. 23(4):555-7, 1999
12. Matsubayashi R et al: Sclerosing stromal tumor of the ovary: radiologic findings. Eur Radiol. 9(7):1335-8, 1999
13. Duska LR et al: Masculinizing sclerosing stromal cell tumor in pregnancy: report of a case and review of the literature. Eur J Gynaecol Oncol. 19(5):441-3, 1998
14. Kim SH et al: CT and MR findings of Krukenberg tumors: comparison with primary ovarian tumors. J Comput Assist Tomogr. 20(3):393-8, 1996
15. Ha HK et al: Krukenberg's tumor of the ovary: MR imaging features. AJR Am J Roentgenol. 164(6):1435-9, 1995
16. Hamper UM et al: Transvaginal color Doppler sonography of adnexal masses: differences in blood flow impedance in benign and malignant lesions. AJR Am J Roentgenol. 160(6):1225-8, 1993
17. Shaw JA et al: Sclerosing stromal tumor of the ovary: an ultrastructural and immunohistochemical analysis with histogenetic considerations. Ultrastruct Pathol. 16(3):363-77, 1992
18. Kawamura N et al: Sclerosing stromal tumour of the ovary. Br J Radiol. 60(718):1031-3, 1987
19. Hsu C et al: Sclerosing stromal tumor of the ovary: case report and review of the literature. Int J Gynecol Pathol. 2(2):192-200, 1983
20. Ho Yuen B et al: Sclerosing stromal tumor of the ovary. Obstet Gynecol. 60(2):252-6, 1982
21. Chalvardjian A et al: Sclerosing stromal tumors of the ovary. Cancer. 31(3):664-70, 1973

SCLEROSING STROMAL TUMOR

IMAGE GALLERY

Typical

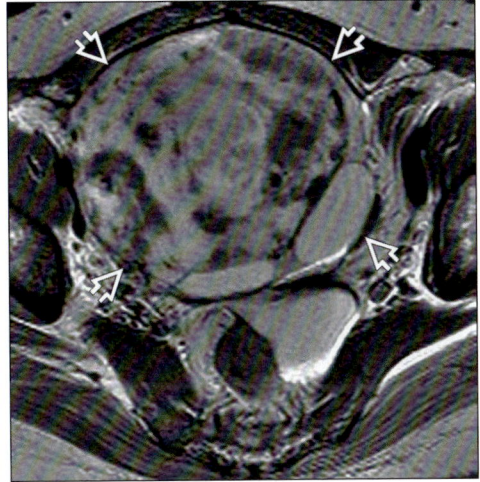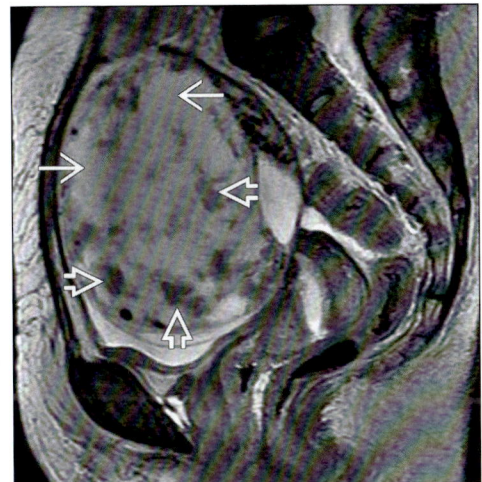

(Left) Axial T2WI MR show a sclerosing stromal tumor of the right ovary ➔ in a 38 year-old woman who had undergone subtotal hysterectomy for uterine leiomyoma 8 years earlier. (Right) Sagittal T2WI MR shows a heterogeneous signal intensity mass. The solid part of the mass has heterogeneous high signal intensity ➔ with scattered areas of low signal intensity ➔ that are distributed predominant in the peripheral portion of the mass.

Typical

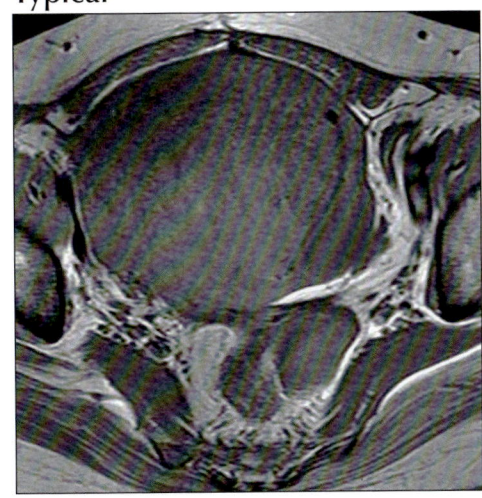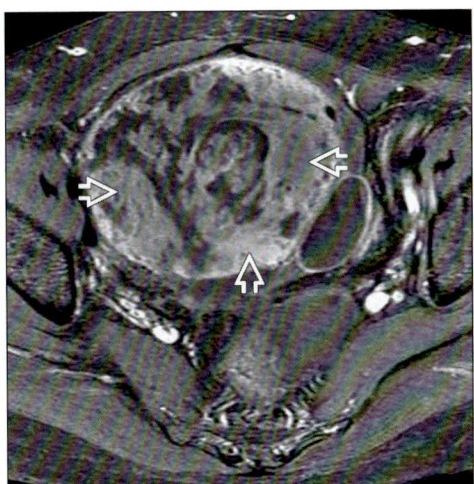

(Left) Axial T1WI MR (same patient as previous image) shows a large pelvic mass of homogeneous intermediate signal intensity. (Right) Axial T1 C+ FS MR shows avid and early nodular enhancement of predominantly the peripheral portion of the mass ➔ producing a typical pseudolobular or spoke-wheel appearance which is characteristic of sclerosing stromal tumor of the ovary.

Typical

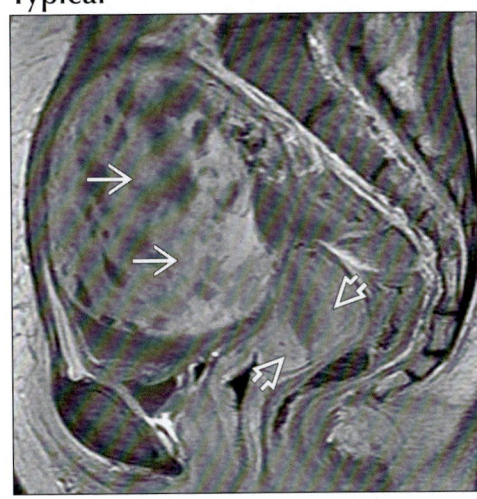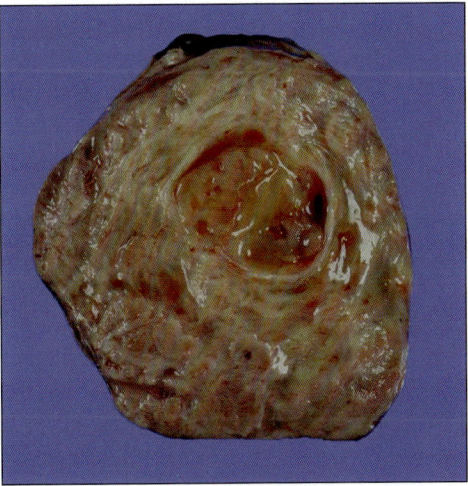

(Left) Sagittal T1 C+ MR shows persistent delayed enhancement of the intermediate part of the mass ➔ with centripetal progression representing edematous ovarian stroma. Note the presence of remnant uterine cervix ➔ after subtotal hysterectomy. (Right) Gross pathology shows a pale and fleshy cut surface with white and yellow areas. Central cystic spaces are also seen. (Courtesy S.H. Kim, MD).

CYSTADENOFIBROMA

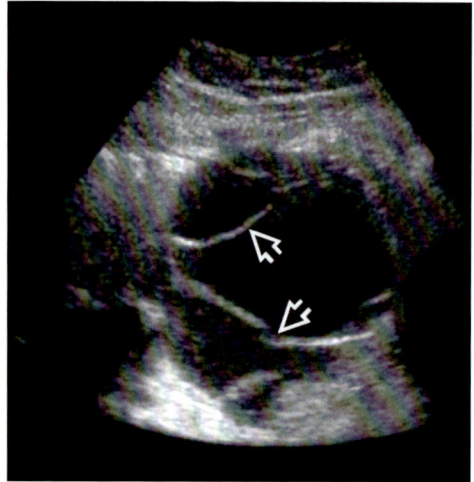

Sagittal transabdominal ultrasound shows a predominantly cystic ovarian mass with variable width septations ➡.

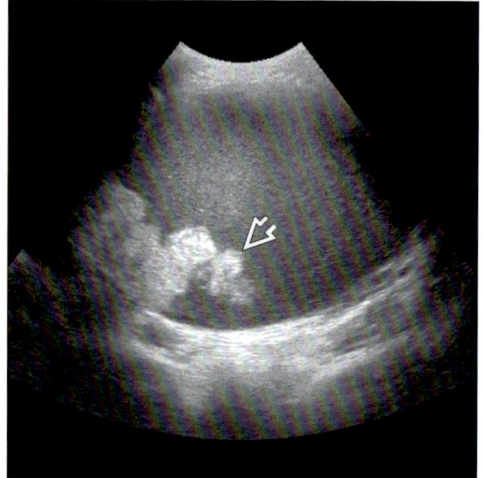

Sagittal transabdominal ultrasound shows cystic ovarian mass with a papillary projection ➡.

TERMINOLOGY

Definitions
- Subtype of ovarian serous cystadenoma, a benign tumor of epithelial origin
  - Most likely subtype of serous tumors to mimic a malignant lesion
  - Mimics malignancy because of presence of a vascular or enhancing solid component
  - Malignant gross appearance at surgery
  - Fibrous stroma is dominant component

IMAGING FINDINGS

General Features
- Best diagnostic clue
  - Complex unilocular cystic mass (nonspecific)
  - Papillary projections protrude into cyst cavity
  - Specific low T2 signal intensity of the solid portion is helpful in distinguishing cystadenofibroma from malignant ovarian tumors
- Location
  - Bilateral in 12-20%
  - One reported case of multicentric ovarian and extraovarian cystadenofibroma
  - Ovarian or paraovarian
- Size: Most are smaller than typical mucinous tumors

Ultrasonographic Findings
- Grayscale Ultrasound
  - Relatively large at diagnosis
  - Mimics a malignant lesion sonographically
- Transvaginal ultrasound (TVS) findings
  - 20-44% appear completely cystic
  - 30% with thick or thin septations
  - 83% with thin wall
  - 56-80% with solid nodule, papillary projection
  - Half are vascular on color flow imaging

CT Findings
- NECT: Heterogeneous due to solid nodules
- CECT
  - Unilocular or multilocular cystic mass with septations < 3 mm
    - May have papillary projection or small solid component
  - Solid component with marked enhancement

DDx: Cystadenofibroma

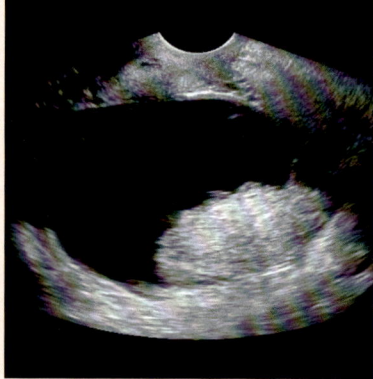

Serous Papillary Cancer

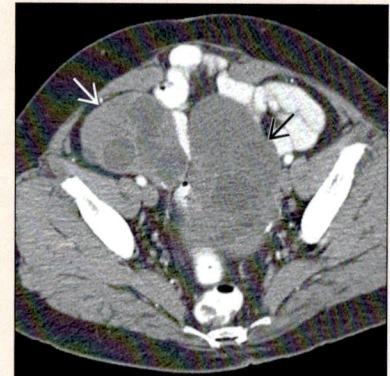

Ovarian Metastases

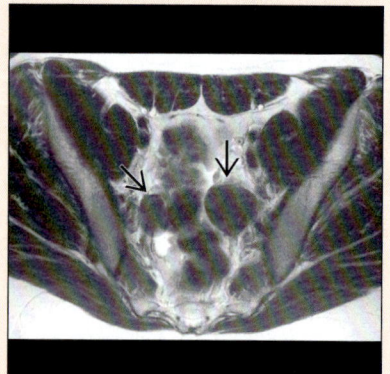

Brenner Tumors

CYSTADENOFIBROMA

Key Facts

Terminology
- Subtype of ovarian serous cystadenoma, a benign tumor of epithelial origin

Imaging Findings
- Complex unilocular cystic mass (nonspecific)
- Papillary projections protrude into cyst cavity
- Bilateral in 12-20%
- Size: Most are smaller than typical mucinous tumors
- Solid component with marked enhancement
- Unilocular or multilocular heterogeneous high signal intensity (SI) cystic mass
- Low SI small solid component or papillary projection
- MR is better than CT and US for characterization
- Presence of low SI T2WI solid components aids diagnosis

Top Differential Diagnoses
- Ovarian Cystadenocarcinoma
- Sclerosing Stromal Tumor
- Ovarian Masses with Fibrous Components
- Metastatic Ovarian Tumors
- Endometriomas

Pathology
- Differs from cystadenoma due to presence of prominent fibrous tissue component in addition to epithelial elements

Clinical Issues
- Most common signs/symptoms: May be asymptomatic and incidentally found on imaging
- Patients undergo surgical removal

MR Findings
- T2WI
  - Unilocular or multilocular heterogeneous high signal intensity (SI) cystic mass
    - Low SI small solid component or papillary projection
  - Black sponge appearance
    - Solid component of very low SI or
    - Solid component with multiple tiny high SI cysts
  - Predominantly cystic type
    - High SI cyst
    - Diffuse or partial thickening of the low SI cyst wall without any definite solid component
- T1 C+: Solid components with marked enhancement

Imaging Recommendations
- Best imaging tool
  - MR is better than CT and US for characterization
    - Presence of low SI T2WI solid components aids diagnosis
- Protocol advice
  - TVS is initial modality for evaluating adnexal mass
    - MR for lesion characterization
  - CECT or CEMR to evaluate for presence of extra-ovarian disease
    - If present, think alternative malignant process

DIFFERENTIAL DIAGNOSIS

Ovarian Cystadenocarcinoma
- Malignant
- Multilocular with thick septations, papillary projections, diameter > 4 cm
- Extension beyond ovary not seen with cystadenofibroma

Sclerosing Stromal Tumor
- Rare benign sex cord-stromal ovarian tumor in young women
- Large mass with high SI cystic components & heterogeneous solid component
- Striking early peripheral enhancement & prolonged central enhancement

Ovarian Masses with Fibrous Components
- Includes fibroma, fibrothecoma and Brenner tumor
- Fibrous component also demonstrates low signal intensity on T2WI
- Brenner tumors may have abundant fibrous stroma but manifest as multilocular cystic mass with solid component or as a small mostly solid mass
- Fibromas usually appear entirely solid
- Extensive amorphous calcification is often present within the solid component

Metastatic Ovarian Tumors
- Specifically metastases with a highly fibrous component
  - Most often from a gastrointestinal tract primary tumor
- Often demonstrate hypointense solid components on T2WI with strong enhancement
- Struma ovarii may have a multicystic tumor with solid component, multilobulated surface and low signal intensity on T2WI

Endometriomas
- Characteristically homogeneously hyperintense on the T1WI with relatively low signal intensity on T2WI
- May contain a peripheral rim of low signal intensity on T2WI representing hemosiderin and/or fibrous capsule
- TVS: Homogeneous carpeting of low level echoes with or without avascular rim nodules

PATHOLOGY

General Features
- General path comments
  - Usually unilocular cyst filled with serous fluid
  - Solid component
  - May be a thick-walled complex cyst
  - Vary in size, up to 30 cm

CYSTADENOFIBROMA

○ Lining either entirely flat or have focal, visible, coarse papillary projections

Gross Pathologic & Surgical Features
- Cystic and solid elements
- Cystic component over 1 cm in diameter
- Lining may be flat or have focal visible, coarse papillary projections
- Cut surface may demonstrate a yellowish fibrous nodule protruding into cystic lumen
- Cell type cannot be differentiated on the basis of their gross appearance
- Appears malignant at time of surgery

Microscopic Features
- Papillary projections represent folds of proliferating neoplastic epithelium growing over a stromal core
- Glandular structures scattered within dense fibrous tissue
- Those that appear purely cystic on imaging have small foci of fibrous stromas detected only microscopically
- Epithelial component is usually serous
- Differs from cystadenoma due to presence of prominent fibrous tissue component in addition to epithelial elements

Staging, Grading or Classification Criteria
- Can be classified according to epithelial cell types into
  ○ Serous
  ○ Endometrioid
  ○ Mucinous
  ○ Clear cell
  ○ Mixed
- Degree of epithelial proliferation/atypia and its relation to the stromal component is used to classify lesions
  ○ Benign (no cytological atypia or stromal invasion)
  ○ Borderline (cytological atypia, no stromal invasion)
  ○ Malignant (cystadenocarcinofibroma) (cytological atypia & stromal invasion)

CLINICAL ISSUES

Presentation
- Most common signs/symptoms: May be asymptomatic and incidentally found on imaging
- Other signs/symptoms
  ○ Palpable mass
  ○ Abdominal distension
  ○ Vague gastrointestinal symptoms
- May present with acute pain if causing ovarian torsion
- Hormonal activity rare

Demographics
- Age
  ○ Peak incidence in 4th & 5th decades
  ○ Range 15-65 years

Natural History & Prognosis
- Good: Cystadenofibroma is benign

Treatment
- Patients undergo surgical removal

○ Cannot be differentiated from malignant lesion pre-operatively
- At initial exploratory laparotomy, staging of tumor is undertaken if malignancy is found
- Frozen section intraoperatively may be useful in avoiding unnecessary resection

DIAGNOSTIC CHECKLIST

Image Interpretation Pearls
- Vascular or enhancing solid component which lends the lesion a malignant appearance
- Low T2 signal intensity of solid portion

SELECTED REFERENCES
1. Cho SM et al: CT and MRI findings of cystadenofibromas of the ovary. Eur Radiol. 14(5):798-804, 2004
2. Kim KA et al: Benign ovarian tumors with solid and cystic components that mimic malignancy. AJR Am J Roentgenol. 182(5):1259-65, 2004
3. Takeuchi M et al: Ovarian cystadenofibromas: characteristic magnetic resonance findings with pathologic correlation. J Comput Assist Tomogr. 27(6):871-3, 2003
4. Jung SE et al: CT and MR imaging of ovarian tumors with emphasis on differential diagnosis. Radiographics. 22(6):1305-25, 2002
5. Alcazar JL et al: Sonographic features of ovarian cystadenofibromas: spectrum of findings. J Ultrasound Med. 20(8):915-9, 2001
6. Fatum M et al: Papillary serous cystadenofibroma of the ovary--is it really so rare? Int J Gynaecol Obstet. 75(1):85-6, 2001
7. Gougoutas CA et al: Pelvic endometriosis: various manifestations and MR imaging findings. AJR Am J Roentgenol. 175(2):353-8, 2000
8. Hricak H et al: Complex adnexal masses: detection and characterization with MR imaging--multivariate analysis. Radiology. 214(1):39-46, 2000
9. Moon WJ et al: Brenner tumor of the ovary: CT and MR findings. J Comput Assist Tomogr. 24(1):72-6, 2000
10. Brown DL et al: Benign and malignant ovarian masses: selection of the most discriminating gray-scale and Doppler sonographic features. Radiology. 208(1):103-10, 1998
11. Korbin CD et al: Paraovarian cystadenomas and cystadenofibromas: sonographic characteristics in 14 cases. Radiology. 208(2):459-62, 1998
12. Outwater EK et al: Ovarian fibromas and cystadenofibromas: MRI features of the fibrous component. J Magn Reson Imaging. 7(3):465-71, 1997
13. Wagner BJ et al: From the archives of the AFIP. Ovarian epithelial neoplasms: radiologic-pathologic correlation. Radiographics. 14(6):1351-74; quiz 1375-6, 1994
14. Ghossain MA et al: Epithelial tumors of the ovary: comparison of MR and CT findings. Radiology. 181(3):863-70, 1991
15. Hafiz MA et al: Multicentric ovarian and extraovarian cystadenofibroma. Obstet Gynecol. 68(3 Suppl):94S-98S, 1986

CYSTADENOFIBROMA

IMAGE GALLERY

Typical

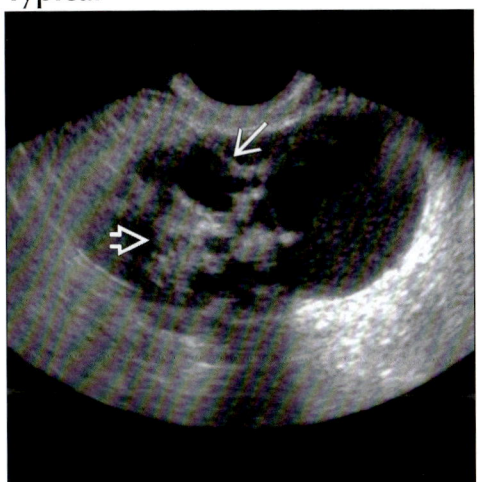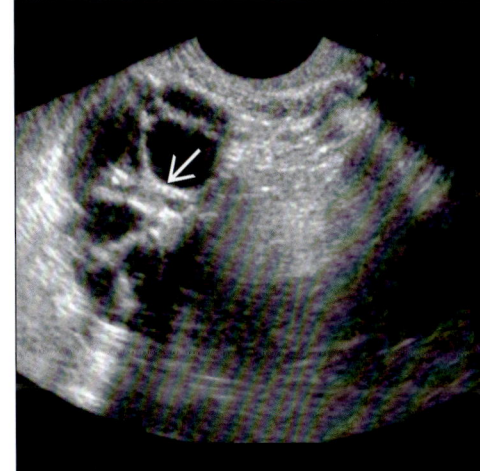

(Left) Sagittal transvaginal ultrasound shows cystic ovarian mass with thick septations ➡ and papillary solid component ➡. *(Right)* Sagittal transvaginal ultrasound shows ovarian mass with solid, and cystic component. Thick septations traverse the cystic component ➡.

Typical

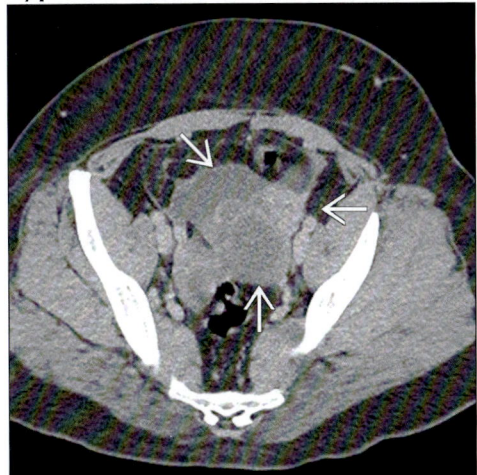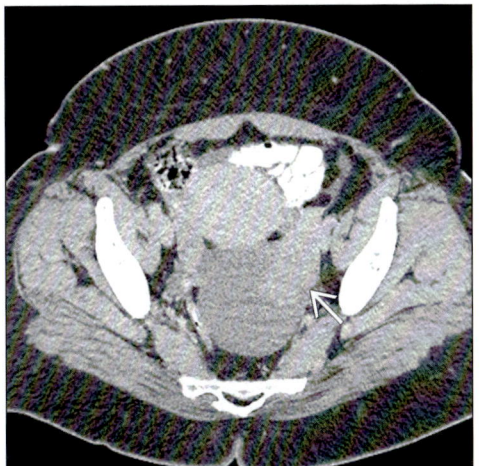

(Left) Axial CECT shows cystic ovarian mass ➡ with solid component and septations. *(Right)* Axial CECT shows cystic ovarian mass with solid component ➡. This component appeared papillary on subsequent US.

Typical

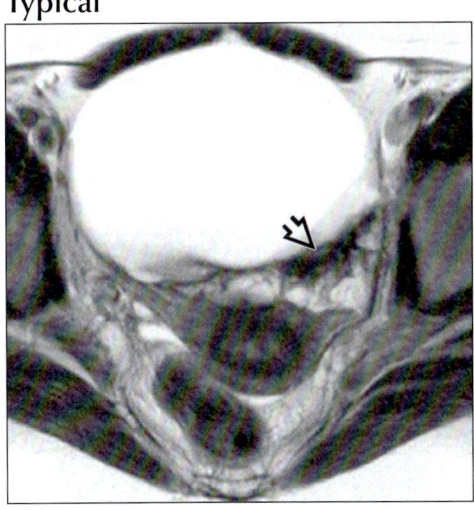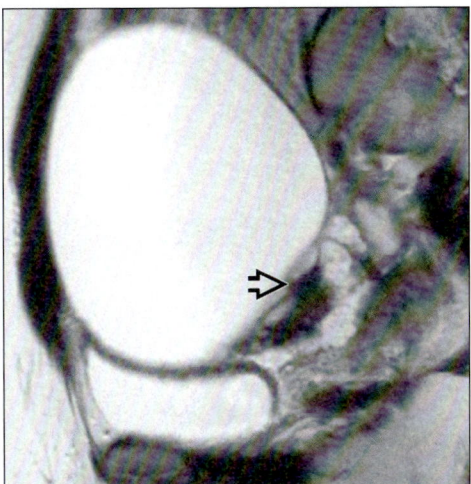

(Left) Axial T2WI MR through the pelvis demonstrates a multilocular cystic mass with a low SI solid component ➡ involving the left ovary. *(Right)* Sagittal T2WI MR of the same patient as previous image, shows multiloculated cystic left ovarian mass with a low SI component ➡.

SEROUS CYSTADENOMA

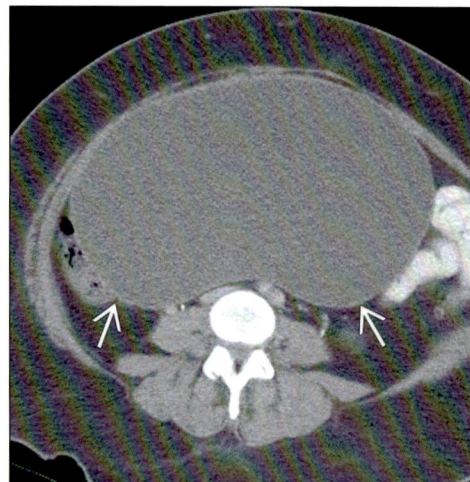

Axial CECT shows a massive unilocular cyst filling most of the abdominal cavity ➡. There are no solid components or vegetations.

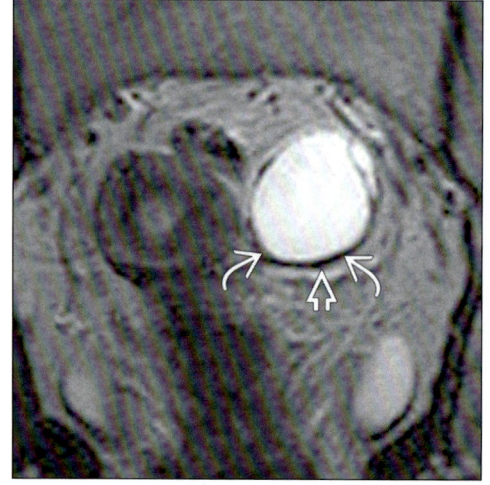

Coronal oblique T2WI MR shows a cyst in the left adnexa ➡ with a thin septation and a thin fibrous wall ➡. Note that there are no vegetations or solid components.

TERMINOLOGY

Abbreviations and Synonyms
- Benign epithelial ovarian tumor

Definitions
- Benign ovarian epithelial tumor
- Thin-walled, serous containing cyst(s), lined by single layer of epithelium
- More aggressive forms are termed borderline or malignant

IMAGING FINDINGS

General Features
- Best diagnostic clue
  - Smooth, thin-walled, unilocular ovarian cyst
    - Can be up to 30 cm
    - Average size 10 cm
  - Imaging appearance is usually indistinguishable from functional ovarian follicular cysts
- Location: Ovary
- Size: Variable, up to 30-50 cm

- Morphology: Thin walled cysts with watery, straw-colored fluid
- Usually unilocular but may be multilocular
- 12-20% of all cases are bilateral
- Vegetations or papillary projections on the interior of cyst wall appear as small nodular projections
  - Papillary projections are usually occult on gross specimen, and found only by histology

Ultrasonographic Findings
- Grayscale Ultrasound: Persistent large (> 6 cm) anechoic, thin-walled cyst
- Color Doppler: No apparent flow in cyst wall
- **Transvaginal ultrasound (TVS) findings:**
  - Anechoic with thin walls and posterior acoustic enhancement
  - Unilocular cysts which are not readily distinguishable from functional cysts
  - High resistance flow on pulsed wave Doppler imaging
    - Higher resistive indices & pulsatility indices than malignant neoplasms

DDx: Serous Cystadenoma

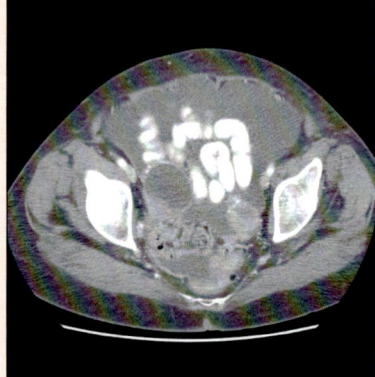

Serous Cystadenocarcinoma

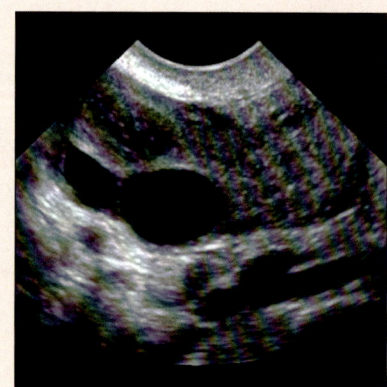

Simple Ovarian Cysts

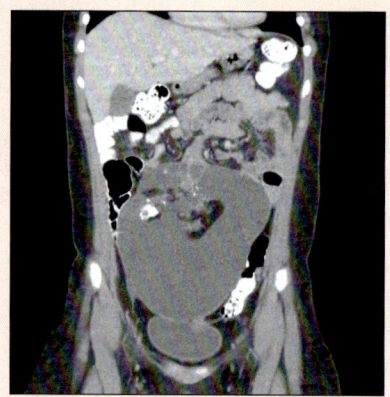

Cystic Teratoma

SEROUS CYSTADENOMA

Key Facts

Terminology
- Benign epithelial ovarian tumor
- Thin-walled, serous containing cyst(s), lined by single layer of epithelium
- More aggressive forms are termed borderline or malignant

Imaging Findings
- Smooth, thin-walled, unilocular ovarian cyst
- Imaging appearance is usually indistinguishable from functional ovarian follicular cysts
- 12-20% of all cases are bilateral
- **Transvaginal ultrasound (TVS) findings:**
- Anechoic with thin walls and posterior acoustic enhancement
- US for initial evaluation

Top Differential Diagnoses
- Functional Cysts of the Ovary
- Paratubal Cyst
- Borderline Tumors of the Ovary
- Endometrioma
- Serous Cystadenocarcinoma
- Mucinous Tumors

Pathology
- Account for 1/4 of all benign ovarian neoplasms
- Bilateral in 12-20% of all cases
- Ovarian tumor of epithelial origin

Clinical Issues
- Most common signs/symptoms: Usually asymptomatic
- Curative cystectomy or oophorectomy

- Large size & persistence of cyst increases likelihood that benign appearing cyst is a neoplasm such as cystadenoma

CT Findings
- NECT: Low attenuation
- CECT
  - Appear as nonspecific ovarian cysts
  - May be very large and protrude into abdominal cavity
  - Cyst wall is thin or inapparent (< 3 mm)
  - Fairly homogeneous & lacking internal structures
    - No septations, or solid elements

MR Findings
- T1WI
  - Cyst contents are usually low signal intensity (SI)
    - May be higher in SI if complicated
- T2WI
  - Cyst contents show high SI
  - Papillary projections image as high SI protrusions with thin fibrous low SI cores
    - Increasing complexity suggests borderline tumors with malignant potential
- T1 C+
  - Papillary projections enhance following contrast
    - Enhancing papillary projections are typical of borderline or malignant tumors

Imaging Recommendations
- Best imaging tool
  - US for initial evaluation
  - MR imaging useful adjunct to US to improve tissue characterization
  - CT more often utilized than MR for pre-operative extent of disease work-up contemplated

DIFFERENTIAL DIAGNOSIS

Functional Cysts of the Ovary
- Follicular cysts or corpus luteum cysts may mimic cystadenoma
  - Functional cysts typically resolve over 1-2 menstrual cycles whereas cystadenomas will persist unchanged or grow
  - Corpus luteum cysts tend to show observable flow in wall on color Doppler & have thicker wall than serous cystadenomas
    - Presence of papillary projections & nodular septa should suggest an ovarian neoplasm

Paratubal Cyst
- Paratubal cysts are separate from the ovary
- Benign epithelial lined cyst
- May attach to fallopian tube, broad ligament, or ovarian surface
- Usually contiguous with or adjacent to the ovary
- Rare reports of serous neoplastic conversion

Borderline Tumors of the Ovary
- Tend to have more prominent and larger papillary projections than cystadenomas
- Often seen in younger patients
- One in three cases are bilateral
- May recur even after many years (20-50)
- Occasionally display invasive behavior with progression

Endometrioma
- May appear as unilocular cysts or multilocular cysts
  - T1WI: Cyst contents show very high signal intensity
  - T2WI: Cyst contents show low signal intensity (shading); a rare pattern in serous cystadenomas
  - TVS: Classic carpeting of low level echoes with or without avascular mural nodules

Serous Cystadenocarcinoma
- May be multiloculated
- Solid elements common
- Commonly occurs in sixth decade of life
- Two thirds are bilateral
- Clinically silent until late in course, usually disseminated at presentation

Mucinous Tumors
- Less common than serous neoplasms

SEROUS CYSTADENOMA

- May be very large and tend to be multiloculated
- MR demonstrates variable signal within loculations owing to mucinous debris and hemorrhage ("stained glass" appearance)
- TVS demonstrates regions of varying echogenicity

Mature Teratoma
- Readily recognized on CT by presence of fat and calcifications
- MR
  - T1WI: High SI
  - T2WI: Intermediate SI
  - Fat-suppressed scans are diagnostic & confirm the presence of fatty elements
- TVS: Cystic adnexal mass containing an echogenic focus with distal acoustic shadowing

Fibrotic Tumors, Fibroma
- Rare, accounting for only 4% of ovarian neoplasms
- Solid, hypoechoic, hyperattenuating masses on US
- Solid and slightly hypodense on CT with poor contrast-enhancement
- T1WI: Low SI
- T2WI: Well-circumscribed, low SI and associated scattered areas of high SI internally

PATHOLOGY

General Features
- General path comments
  - Common tumor of ovary found at surgery
  - Account for 1/4 of all benign ovarian neoplasms
  - Bilateral in 12-20% of all cases
  - Ovarian tumor of epithelial origin
    - Arise from the coelomic epithelium/peritoneum covering the ovary
    - Serous tumors account for about 50% of all epithelial tumors
    - May be benign, borderline (low malignant potential), or malignant
  - Histologically, typically have two components
    - Neoplastic epithelium lines internal surface of cyst
    - Fibrous stromal component forms much of rest of cyst wall
    - When the fibrous stromal component is prominent grossly, the tumors are typically termed a cystadenofibroma or adenofibroma
  - Psammomatous calcifications are present in about 15% of benign tumors microscopically & occasionally are macroscopic
- Etiology: Arise from surface epithelium of ovary
- Epidemiology
  - Can be encountered at any age but peak incidence in 4th & 5th decades
  - Account for a significant proportion of incidental cysts in postmenopausal women
    - Up to 84% of simple adnexal cysts in postmenopausal women are serous cystadenomas at surgery
  - About 50-70% of serous tumors are benign
  - If found in younger individuals more likely benign or borderline

Gross Pathologic & Surgical Features
- Average 10 cm in diameter but may be very large and fill pelvis and abdomen
- Usually unilocular but can be multilocular
- Linings are smooth or have small papillary projections

Microscopic Features
- Cyst lining is composed of a single layer of benign epithelium
- Epithelium tends to form papillary structures
- Epithelium resembles fallopian tube mucosa
- Wall of cyst is composed of fibrous stroma

Staging, Grading or Classification Criteria
- Epithelial tumors are classified as
  - Benign
  - Borderline or low malignant potential
  - Malignant

CLINICAL ISSUES

Presentation
- Most common signs/symptoms: Usually asymptomatic
- Other signs/symptoms
  - If large, may cause bulk-related symptoms
  - Rarely, acute pelvic pain due to torsion

Natural History & Prognosis
- Believed to have no malignant potential if benign at diagnosis
- Do not recur after oophorectomy

Treatment
- Curative cystectomy or oophorectomy

DIAGNOSTIC CHECKLIST

Consider
- Serous cystadenoma for persistent simple cyst > 6 cm
  - To document persistence: Repeat US performed 6 weeks after initial observation

Image Interpretation Pearls
- Slow growing simple cyst suggests serous cystadenoma

SELECTED REFERENCES

1. Dorum A et al: Prevalence and histologic diagnosis of adnexal cysts in postmenopausal women: an autopsy study. Am J Obstet Gynecol. 192(1):48-54, 2005
2. Jung SE et al: CT and MR imaging of ovarian tumors with emphasis on differential diagnosis. Radiographics. 22(6):1305-25, 2002
3. Jeong YY et al: Imaging evaluation of ovarian masses. Radiographics. 20(5):1445-70, 2000
4. Yamashita Y et al: Adnexal masses: accuracy of characterization with transvaginal US and precontrast and postcontrast MR imaging. Radiology. 194(2):557-65, 1995
5. Kurman RJ et al: The behavior of serous tumors of low malignant potential: are they ever malignant? Int J Gynecol Pathol. 12(2):120-7, 1993

SEROUS CYSTADENOMA

IMAGE GALLERY

Typical

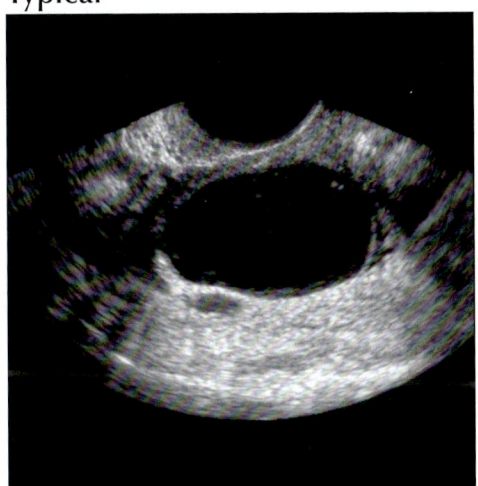
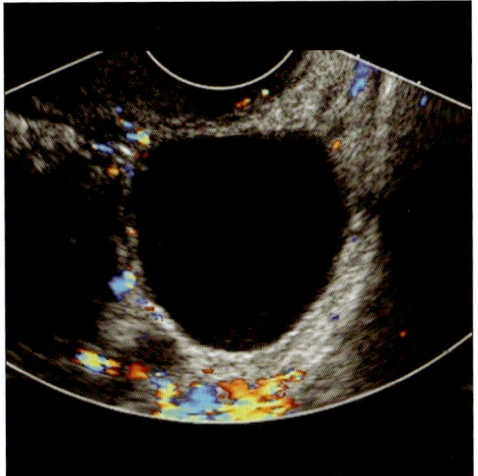

(Left) Sagittal transvaginal ultrasound shows 4 cm anechoic unilocular cystic left ovarian lesion in a postmenopausal female. *(Right)* Axial color Doppler ultrasound in the same patient as previous image, shows a thin wall and no mural flow.

Typical

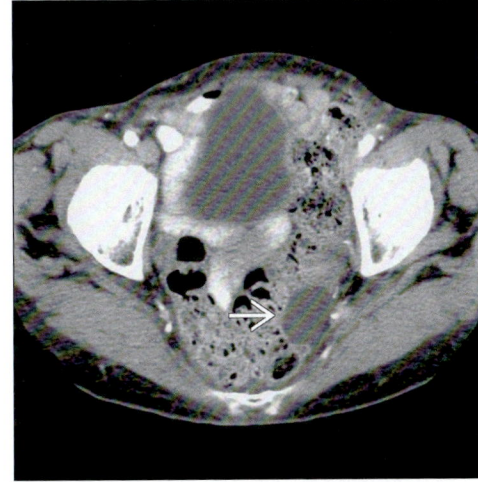
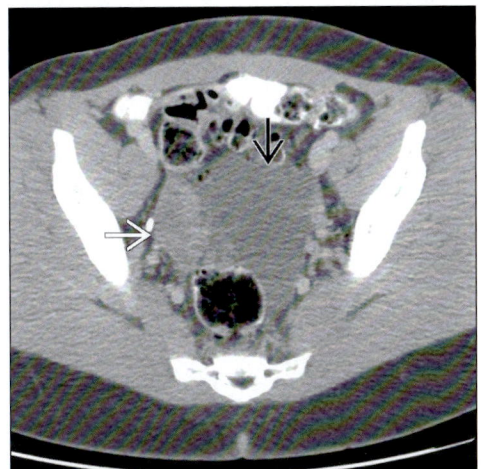

(Left) Axial CECT shows a nonenhancing, left-ovarian, unilocular, serous cystadenoma ➡. *(Right)* Axial CECT shows a left serous cystadenoma ➡. Note the normal right ovary ➡.

Typical

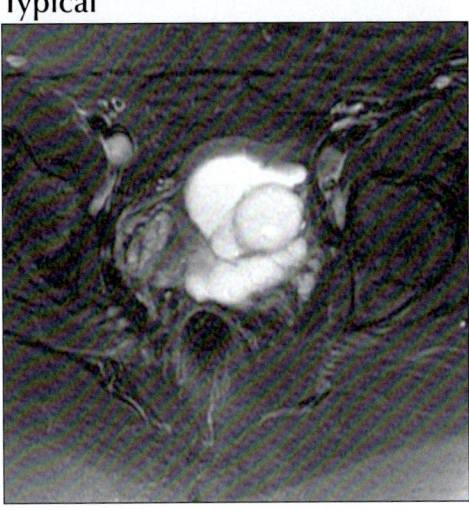
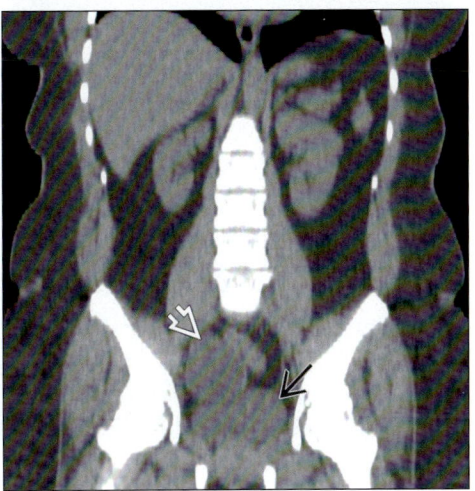

(Left) Axial T2WI FS MR shows multiseptated but thin-walled serous cystadenoma. *(Right)* Coronal non-contrast CT reformat demonstrates a cystic, thin-walled mass ➡ in the right adnexa displacing the bladder ➡ inferiorly.

SEROUS CYSTADENOMA

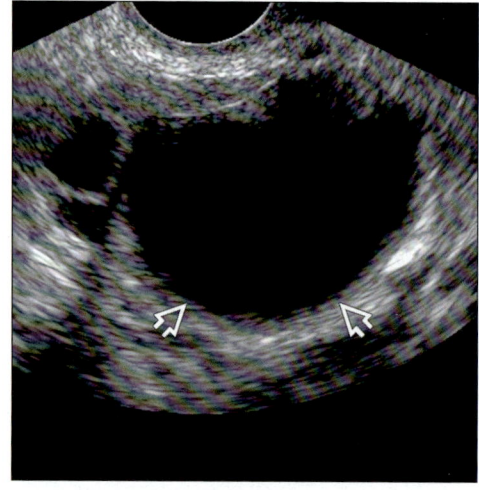
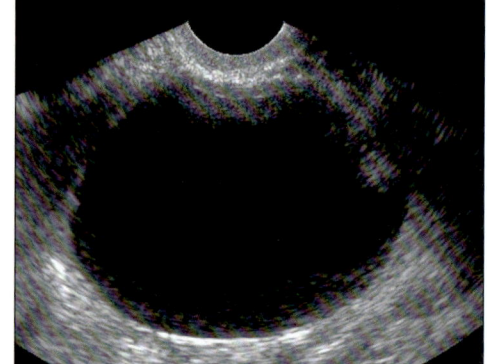

Typical

(Left) Sagittal transvaginal ultrasound shows a dominant cyst ➤ in the right ovary with adjacent physiologic follicles. *(Right)* Sagittal transvaginal ultrasound in the same patient as previous image, 5 years later, shows interval increase in size of the right anechoic cystic mass.

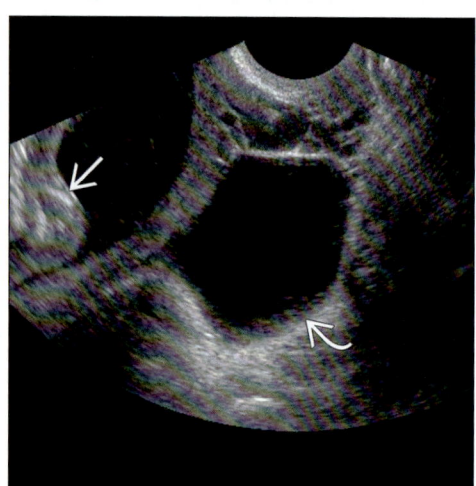
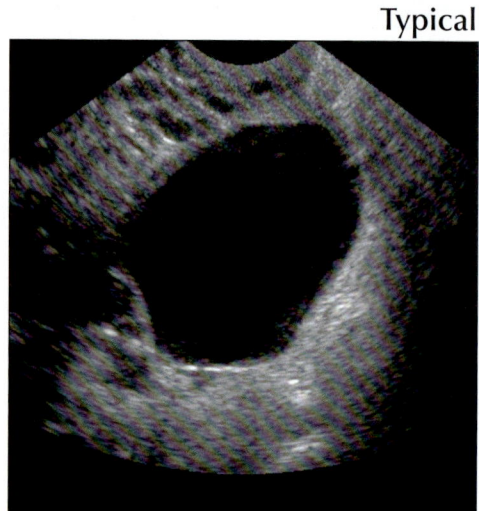

Typical

(Left) Sagittal transvaginal ultrasound in a pregnant patient, shows a polygonal, thin-walled cyst ➤. Note the fetal shoulder ➤. Most cysts in pregnant patients resolve, but if a cyst is seen in the 2nd trimester, follow up is warranted. *(Right)* Sagittal transvaginal ultrasound in the same patient as previous image, post-partum, shows the cyst is still present.

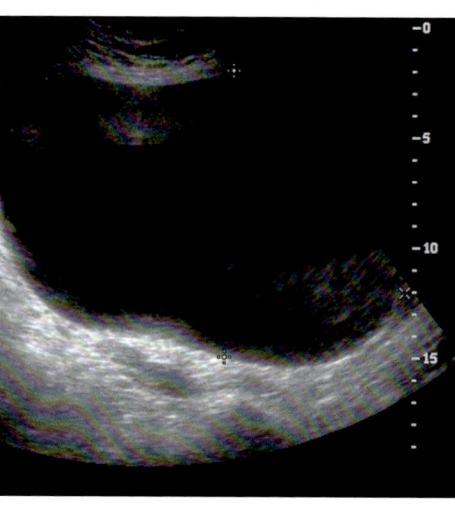
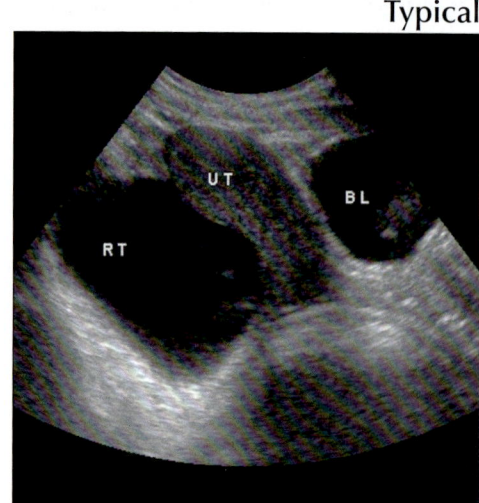

Typical

(Left) Sagittal transabdominal ultrasound shows a 20 cm cyst in an elderly postmenopausal woman. *(Right)* Sagittal oblique transabdominal ultrasound in a postpartum patient, shows a large, right, anechoic, cystic mass (RT), posterior to the uterus (UT). The distended bladder (BL) serves an acoustic window.

SEROUS CYSTADENOMA

Typical

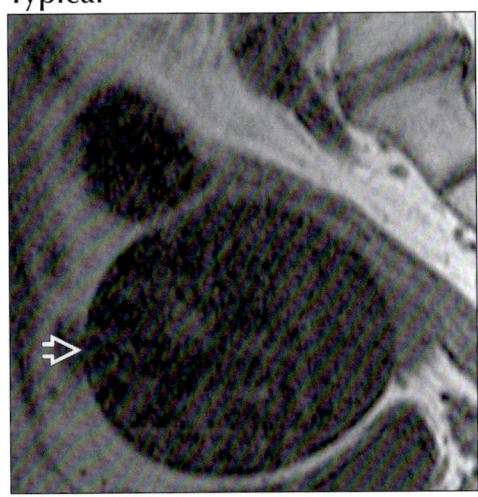
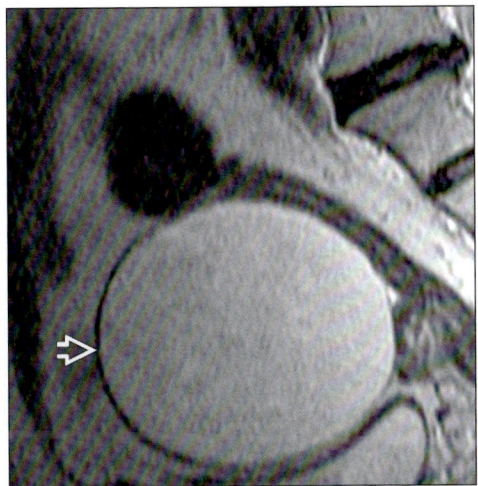

(Left) Sagittal T1WI MR shows an 8 cm, low signal intensity mass ➡ incidentally noted on a lumbar MR. *(Right)* Sagittal T2WI MR in the same patient as previous image, shows the mass becomes brighter in signal intensity ➡.

Typical

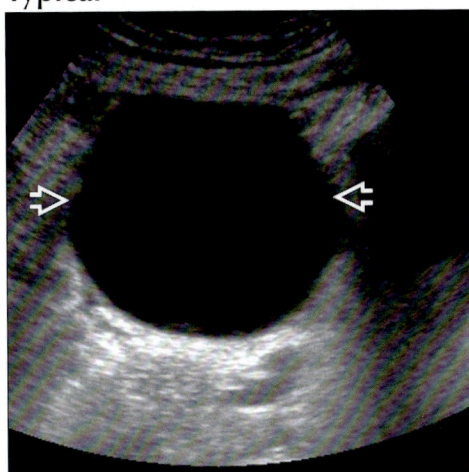
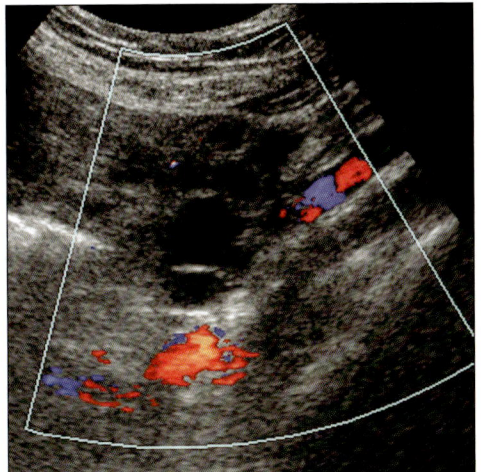

(Left) Sagittal transvaginal ultrasound shows a thin-walled, anechoic cyst ➡ in the right ovary. *(Right)* Sagittal color Doppler ultrasound in the same patient as previous image, shows a left, thin-walled, septated, avascular cyst in this patient with bilateral serous cystadenomas.

Typical

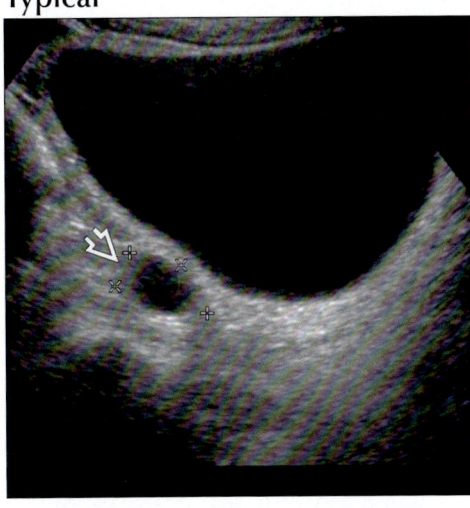
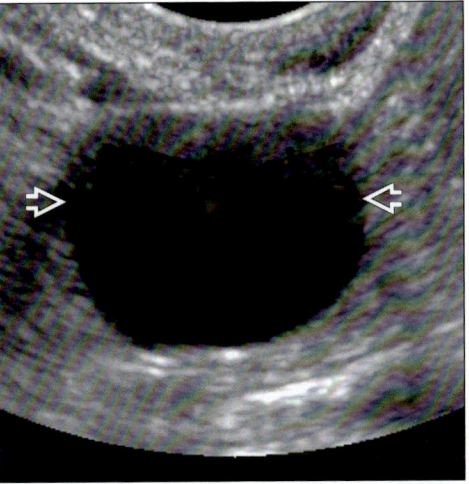

(Left) Sagittal transabdominal ultrasound shows a small cyst ➡ within the right ovary in a postmenopausal woman. *(Right)* Sagittal transvaginal ultrasound in the same patient as previous image, shows the cyst ➡ to be thin-walled and anechoic.

MUCINOUS CYSTADENOMA

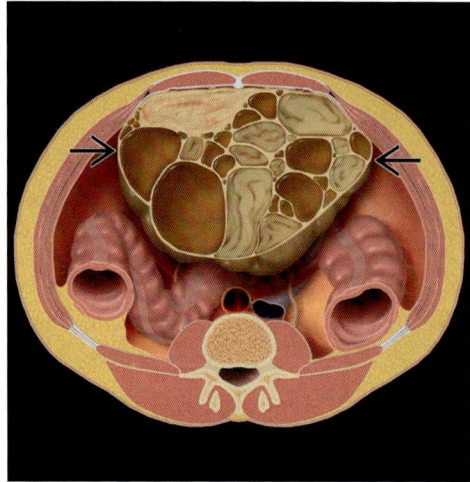

Axial graphic shows a multilocular cystic mass ➔ in the abdomen exhibiting differing densities within the locules.

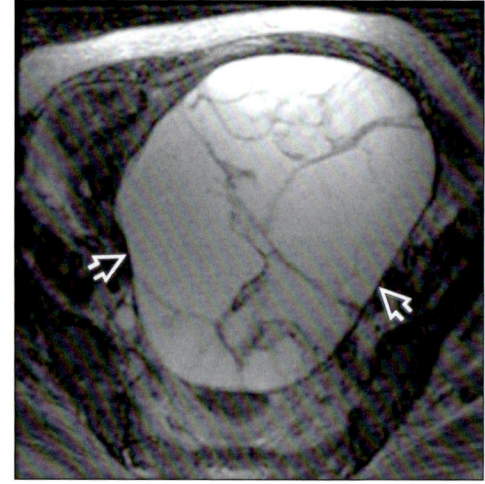

Axial T2WI MR shows a large multicystic mass ➔ with thin septations. No solid components or papillary projections are seen.

TERMINOLOGY

Abbreviations and Synonyms
- Benign mucinous tumor

Definitions
- Cystic ovarian neoplasm containing mucinous material lined by a single layer of uniform columnar cells

IMAGING FINDINGS

General Features
- Best diagnostic clue: Multilocular cyst, with septations < 3 mm, often very large without solid components
- Location
  ○ Pelvis
  ○ Usually unilateral
  ○ Bilateral in 5% of cases
- Size
  ○ Can range widely in size
  ○ Commonly large masses filling entire pelvis
- Morphology
  ○ Typically multiloculated cystic mass
  ○ Smooth walled cysts of varying sizes
  ○ Presence of solid components or papillary projections suggest borderline or malignant tumor
  ○ Bilateral mucinous tumors suggest a borderline or malignant tumor
  ○ Mucin containing cysts can be complicated by hemorrhage or cellular debris

Ultrasonographic Findings
- **Transvaginal ultrasound**
  ○ Multiloculated cystic lesion
  ○ Locules may show low-level echoes and differing echogenicity
    ▪ Potential pitfall is an echogenic locule mimicking a solid component
  ○ Pulsed-wave Doppler shows generally high-resistance waveforms with higher resistive indices and higher pulsatility indices than malignant tumors
    ▪ However, considerable overlap in Doppler findings between benign and malignant ovarian tumors
    ▪ Lack of Doppler flow does not exclude malignancy

DDx: Ovarian Mucinous Cystadenoma

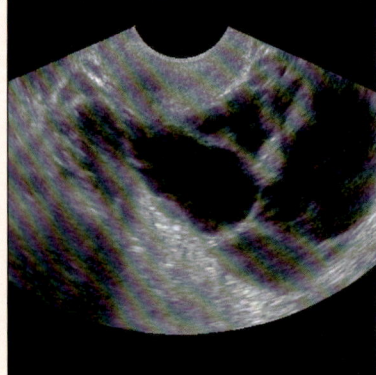

Mucinous Cystadenocarcinoma

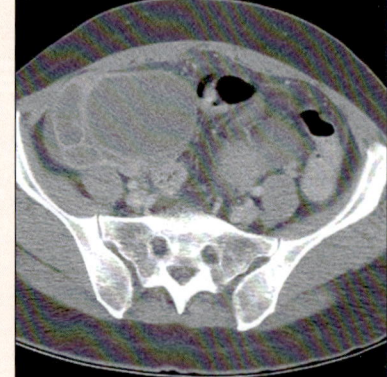

Tubo-Ovarian Abscess

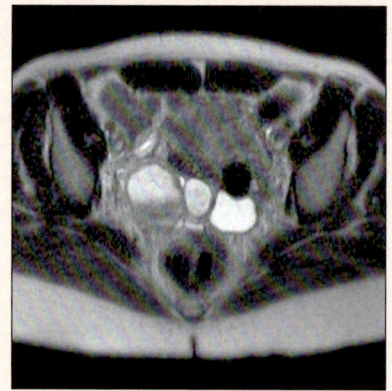

Endometriosis

MUCINOUS CYSTADENOMA

Key Facts

Terminology
- Benign mucinous tumor
- Cystic ovarian neoplasm containing mucinous material lined by a single layer of uniform columnar cells

Imaging Findings
- Best diagnostic clue: Multilocular cyst, with septations < 3 mm, often very large without solid components
- Usually unilateral
- Commonly large masses filling entire pelvis
- Mucin containing cysts can be complicated by hemorrhage or cellular debris
- **Transvaginal ultrasound**
- Multiloculated cystic lesion
- Locules may show low-level echoes and differing echogenicity
- Potential pitfall is an echogenic locule mimicking a solid component
- Transabdominal ultrasound may be necessary in evaluating full extent of larger tumors

Pathology
- Comprise 20-25% of all benign ovarian neoplasms and 75-85% of all ovarian mucinous tumors
- Bilateral in 2-3% of cases
- May be very large & fill pelvis & abdominal cavity

Clinical Issues
- Most common signs/symptoms: Palpable mass, increasing abdominal girth & pelvic pain
- Excision is curative

- Papillary projections are less common than in serous cystadenomas
- Transabdominal ultrasound may be necessary in evaluating full extent of larger tumors

CT Findings
- NECT: Mural calcifications can be seen
- CECT
  - Multilocular cystic mass with thin cyst wall and thin septations
  - Locules contain fluid of varying attenuation

MR Findings
- T1WI
  - Cyst contents are generally low signal intensity
    - Locules may show higher signal intensity from concentration of mucinous components or hemorrhage
- T2WI
  - T2 hyperintense cysts
  - "Stained glass" appearance due to varying signal intensities of the cysts
  - Thin, regular septa
  - Lack of endocystic or exocystic vegetations
- T1 C+: Cyst walls and septations demonstrate enhancement but are thin without nodularity

Imaging Recommendations
- Best imaging tool
  - Ultrasonography is often sufficient to characterize tumor
    - MR may be performed if US is equivocal or non-diagnostic
    - CT is useful for staging if malignancy is being considered
  - Extensive imaging evaluation is usually unnecessary

DIFFERENTIAL DIAGNOSIS

Serous Cystadenoma
- Tremendous overlap between imaging findings of serous and mucinous cystadenomas

Mucinous Cystadenocarcinoma
- Papillary projections or solid components within tumor suggest a borderline or malignant tumor

Functional Cyst
- Follicular cysts and corpus luteum cysts

Peritoneal Inclusion Cyst
- Peritoneal pseudocysts are loculations of fluid which occur around ovary in patients with paraovarian adhesions due to endometriosis or prior surgery
- Ovary will be intact within pseudocyst; in mucinous cystadenoma, the ovary is not distinguished from mass

Endometrioma
- T1 high signal intensity due to hemorrhage
- T2 "shading": Decrease in signal intensity

Cystic Teratoma
- Characteristically contain fat

Tubo-Ovarian Abscess
- Complex cystic lesions in pelvis due to infection

Mucocele
- Dilated appendix filled with mucin

PATHOLOGY

General Features
- General path comments
  - Comprise 20-25% of all benign ovarian neoplasms and 75-85% of all ovarian mucinous tumors
  - Bilateral in 2-3% of cases
  - May be very large & fill pelvis & abdominal cavity
  - Cyst wall is composed of a fibrous stroma
- Genetics: Two patients reported to be fumarate hydratase germline mutation carriers
- Etiology
  - Etiology of mucinous ovarian tumors is not known

MUCINOUS CYSTADENOMA

- Occasionally mucinous tumors are associated with other ovarian tumors implying a common origin
  - Teratomas, granulosa cell, carcinoid, & Brenner tumors
  - Appendiceal tumors may metastasize to ovary and cause a mucinous ovarian tumor identical to mucinous cystadenomas
- Epidemiology
  - Can occur at any age but are rare in young women and children
  - Most commonly present in 3rd to 5th decades
  - Increased incidence in Peutz-Jeghers syndrome
  - Comprise 20% of all ovarian neoplasms

Gross Pathologic & Surgical Features
- Form the largest ovarian tumors: Up to 100 kg
- Outer surface is lobulated
- Internal surface is multiseptated or has cysts within cysts
- Cyst contents are viscous material
- Wall thickness varies from very thin to a few mm in thickness

Microscopic Features
- Cysts are filled with mucinous material
- Cysts are lined with a single layer of non atypical mucin-producing epithelium
  - Similar to endocervical or intestinal epithelium
- Ovarian stroma is often very cellular and foci of luteinization can occur
- Rupture of mucinous glands results in granulomas with multiple macrophages
- Papillae are unusual

CLINICAL ISSUES

Presentation
- Most common signs/symptoms: Palpable mass, increasing abdominal girth & pelvic pain
- Clinical Profile
  - Symptoms of abdominal or pelvic pressure or bloating
  - Acute presentations due to ovarian torsion include pelvic pain and fever
  - CA-125 levels may be mildly elevated

Demographics
- Age: Present in 3rd to 5th decades

Natural History & Prognosis
- Excision is curative
- Massive tumors can result in abdominal compartment syndrome
- Pseudomyxoma peritonei thought to be a result of mucinous cystadenocarcinoma or tumor of low malignant potential rather than of mucinous cystadenoma

Treatment
- Excision of the mucinous cystadenoma
- Suspicious peritoneal areas should be biopsied to exclude peritoneal implants or microinvasion
- Because mucinous cystadenomas are frequently large when they present, surgery is indicated to exclude malignancy and to prevent torsion

DIAGNOSTIC CHECKLIST

Consider
- Mucinous cystadenoma when evaluating a large multilocular cystic mass with variable appearance of cystic material

SELECTED REFERENCES

1. Ylisaukko-oja SK et al: Germline fumarate hydratase mutations in patients with ovarian mucinous cystadenoma. Eur J Hum Genet. 14(7):880-3, 2006
2. Hart WR: Mucinous tumors of the ovary: a review. Int J Gynecol Pathol. 24(1):4-25, 2005
3. Okada S et al: Calcifications in mucinous and serous cystic ovarian tumors. J Nippon Med Sch. 72(1):29-33, 2005
4. Chao A et al: Abdominal compartment syndrome secondary to ovarian mucinous cystadenoma. Obstet Gynecol. 104(5 Pt 2):1180-2, 2004
5. Hussain SM et al: MR imaging features of pelvic mucinous carcinomas. Eur Radiol. 10(6):885-91, 2000
6. Jeong YY et al: Imaging evaluation of ovarian masses. Radiographics. 20(5):1445-70, 2000
7. Tanaka YO et al: Differential diagnosis of gynaecological "stained glass" tumours on MRI. Br J Radiol. 72(856):414-20, 1999
8. Brown DL et al: Ovarian masses: can benign and malignant lesions be differentiated with color and pulsed Doppler US? Radiology. 190(2):333-6, 1994
9. Wagner BJ et al: From the archives of the AFIP. Ovarian epithelial neoplasms: radiologic-pathologic correlation. Radiographics. 14(6):1351-74; quiz 1375-6, 1994
10. Hendrickson MR et al: Well-differentiated mucinous neoplasms of the ovary. Pathology (Phila). 1(2):307-34, 1993
11. Young RH et al: Pathology of epithelial tumors. Hematol Oncol Clin North Am. 6(4):739-60, 1992
12. Buy JN et al: Epithelial tumors of the ovary: CT findings and correlation with US. Radiology. 178(3):811-8, 1991
13. Ghossain MA et al: Epithelial tumors of the ovary: comparison of MR and CT findings. Radiology. 181(3):863-70, 1991
14. Sawyer RW et al: Computed tomography of benign ovarian masses. J Comput Assist Tomogr. 9(4):784-9, 1985

MUCINOUS CYSTADENOMA

IMAGE GALLERY

Typical

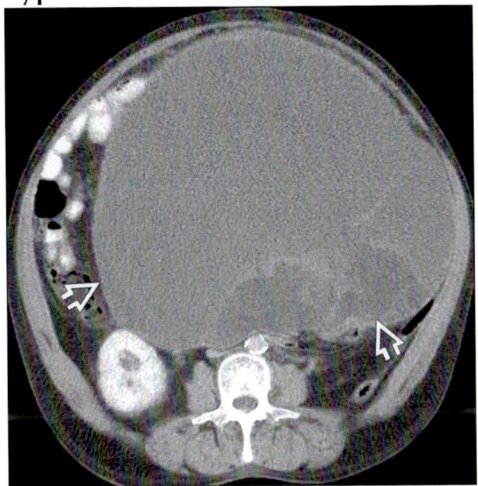
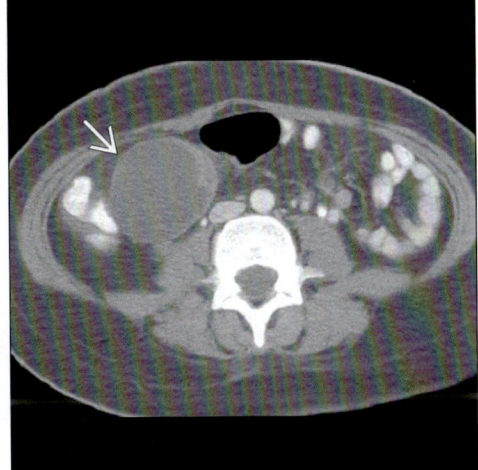

(Left) Axial CECT through the mid-abdomen shows a large, multicystic mass ➡, filling most of the abdominal cavity. Note the well-defined wall and absence of solid components. *(Right)* Axial CECT shows a well-circumscribed cystic mass ➡ in the right lower abdomen.

Typical

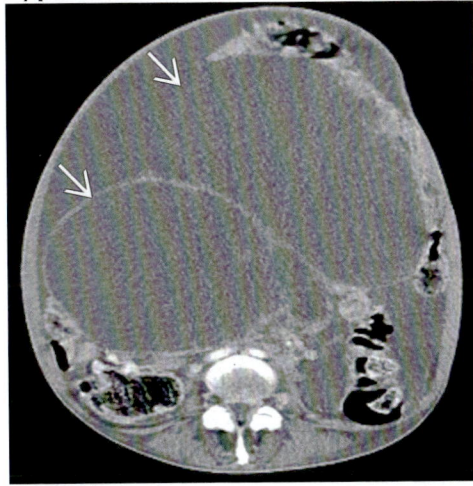
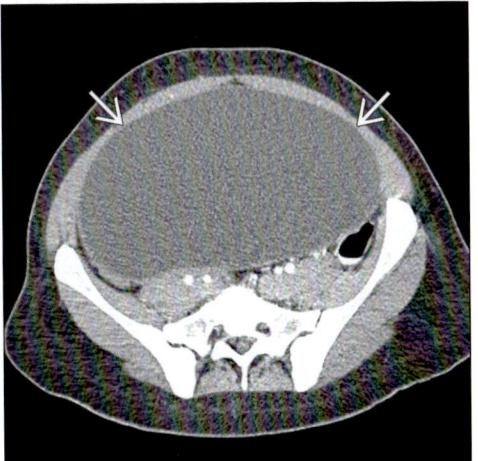

(Left) Axial CECT shows a large multiloculated cystic mass ➡ occupying most of the abdomen, causing mass effect on adjacent bowel loops and the abdominal wall. *(Right)* Axial CECT shows a unilocular cystic mass ➡ in the pelvis.

Typical

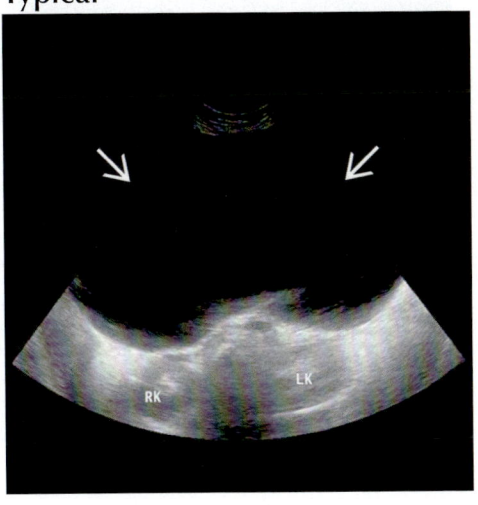
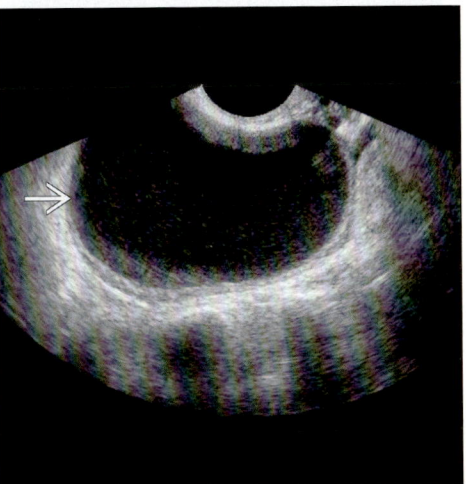

(Left) Transverse transabdominal ultrasound shows a large, anechoic mass ➡ in the abdomen. Note the lack of mural nodularity. RK and LK denote the kidneys. *(Right)* Transverse transvaginal ultrasound shows a unilocular, well-circumscribed cystic mass ➡ without septations or internal complexity.

MUCINOUS CYSTADENOMA

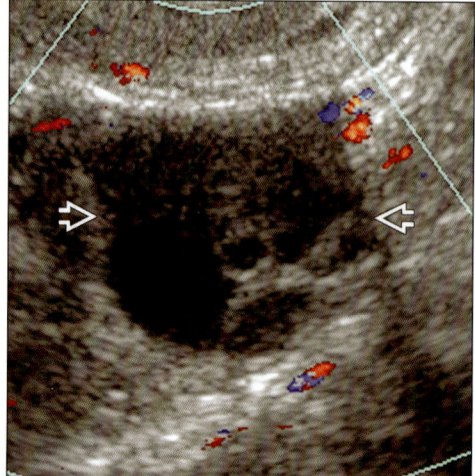 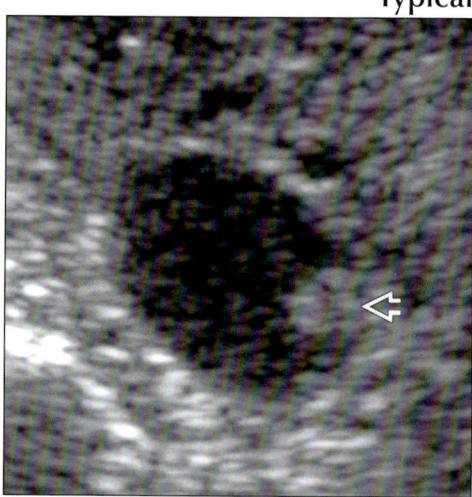

(Left) Transverse color Doppler ultrasound shows a cystic lesion ➡ with several septations. (Right) Longitudinal transvaginal ultrasound shows a cyst with a small mural nodule ➡. Although the presence of a nodule increases the likelihood of malignancy, this was a benign mucinous cystadenoma.

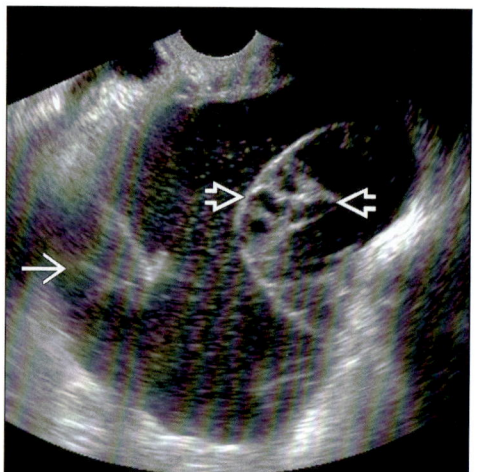 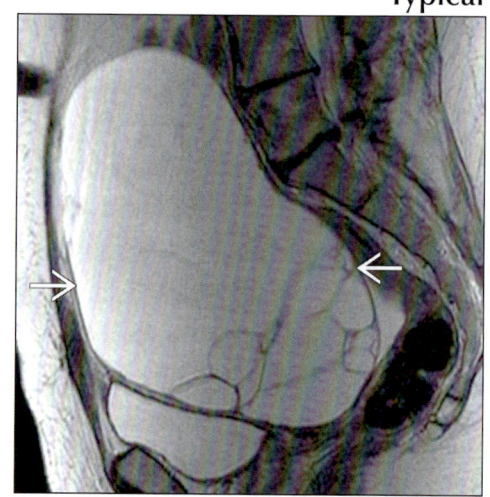

(Left) Longitudinal transvaginal ultrasound shows a cyst with echogenic material in the cystic portion ➡ and multiple septations ➡. (Right) Sagittal T2WI MR shows a large multiloculated cyst ➡.

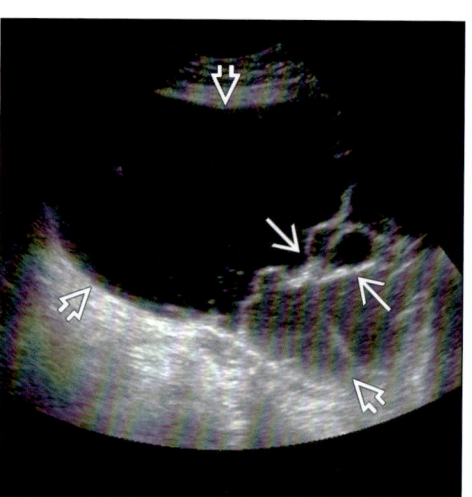 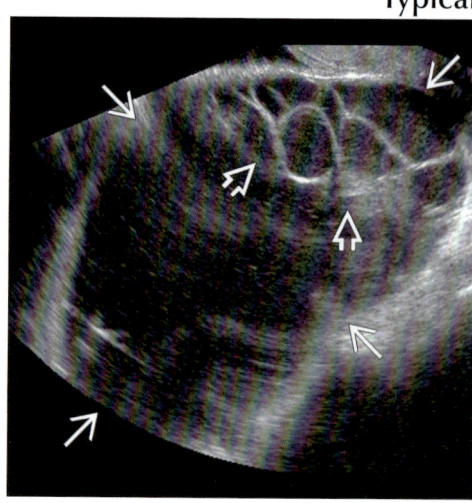

(Left) Transverse transabdominal ultrasound shows a cyst ➡ with multiple septations ➡. (Right) Transverse transvaginal ultrasound in the same patient as previous image, shows the cyst ➡ with multiple septations ➡.

MUCINOUS CYSTADENOMA

Typical

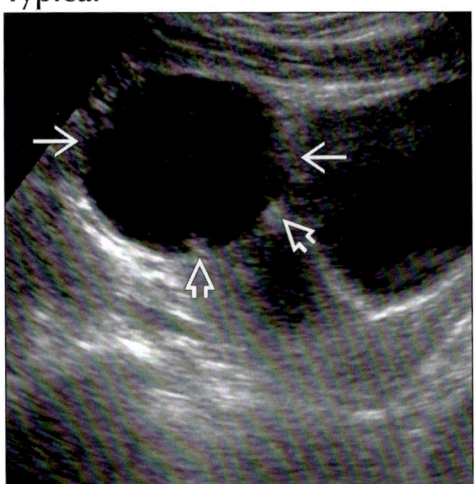
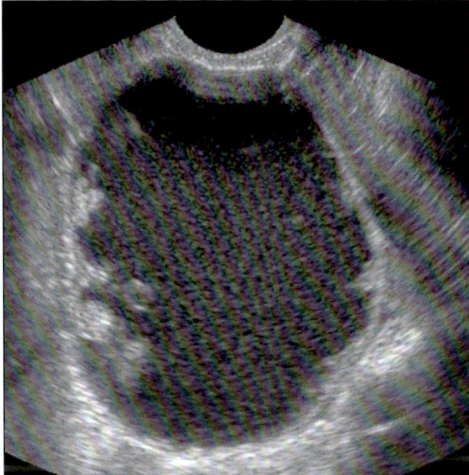

(Left) Transverse transabdominal ultrasound shows a cyst ➡ with some wall irregularities ➡. *(Right)* Transverse transvaginal ultrasound in the same patient as previous image, shows the heterogeneous material within the cyst and many more areas of mural nodularity than were shown on the TA image.

Typical

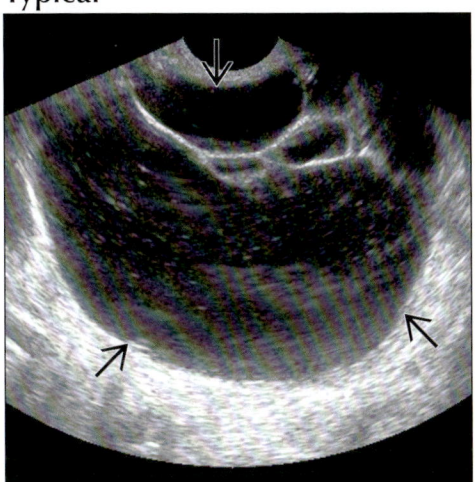
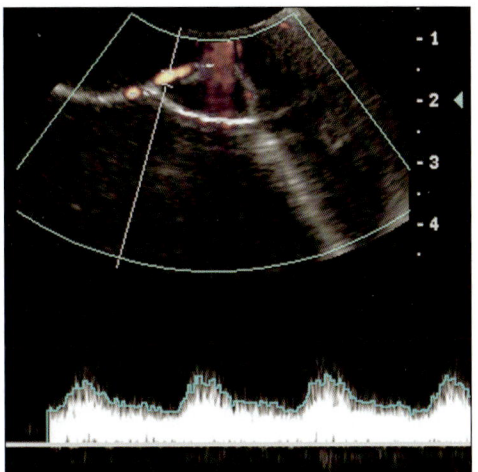

(Left) Transverse transvaginal ultrasound shows a multiseptated cyst ➡. *(Right)* Transverse pulsed Doppler ultrasound in the same patient as previous image, shows vascularity within the septations.

Typical

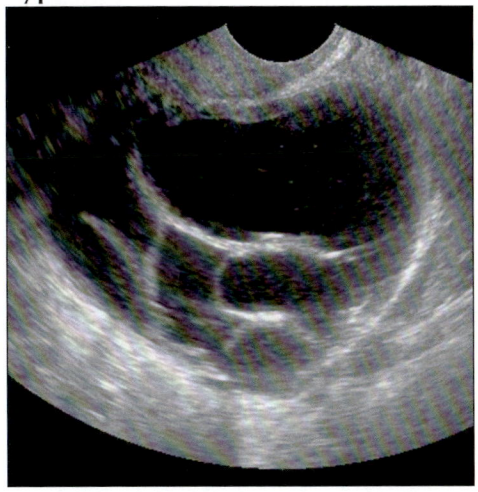
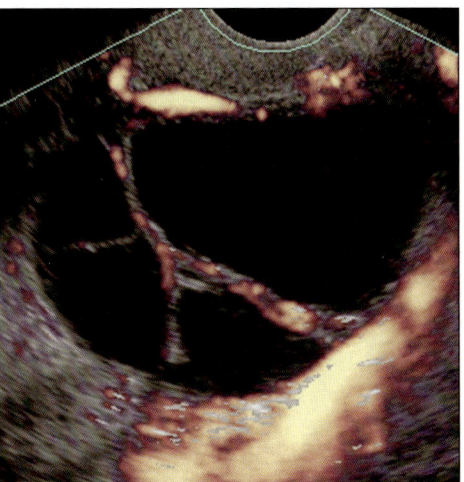

(Left) Transverse transvaginal ultrasound shows a cyst with multiple septations. *(Right)* Longitudinal power Doppler ultrasound in the same patient as previous image, shows flow within these septations.

BRENNER TUMOR

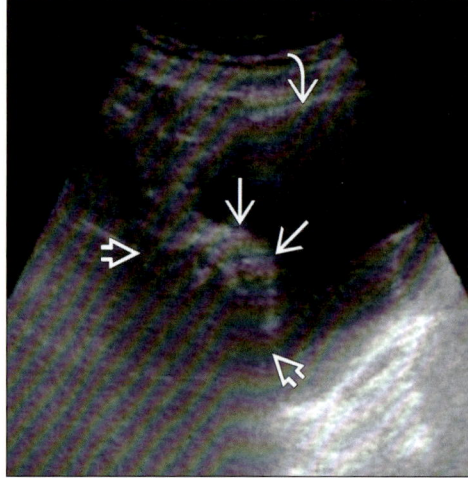

Longitudinal ultrasound shows hyperechogenicity along the anterior margin of a left adnexal mass, posterior to the bladder. Note the accompanying posterior acoustic shadowing due to calcifications.

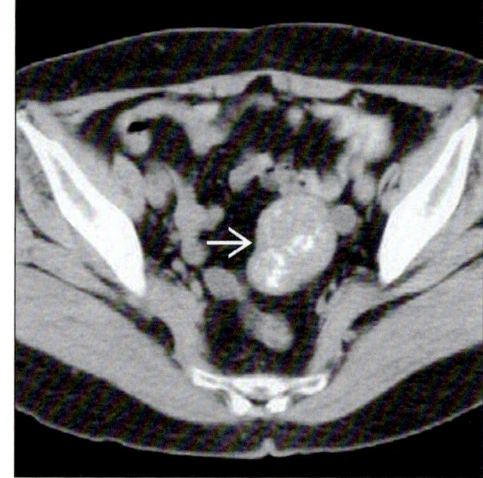

Axial NECT shows a solid left adnexal mass containing amorphous calcifications. Pathology: Benign Brenner tumor.

TERMINOLOGY

Abbreviations and Synonyms
- Transitional tumor of the ovary

Definitions
- Ovarian tumor comprising transitional type epithelium and stroma
- Three types; benign Brenner tumor, atypical proliferating transitional cell (Brenner) tumor and malignant Brenner tumor

IMAGING FINDINGS

General Features
- Best diagnostic clue: Combination of calcifications demonstrated by US or CT and low SI on T2WI MR strongly suggests the diagnosis of Brenner tumors
- Location: Usually unilateral
- Size
  - Usually small (< 5 cm)
  - Borderline and malignant Brenner tumors are larger than benign ones
- Benign Brenner tumors are usually solid: Multiloculated cystic mass with solid components on US/CT/MR is relatively common finding of benign as well as borderline & malignant Brenner tumors

Ultrasonographic Findings
- Difficult to differentiate from other adnexal lesions such as fibroma or pedunculated leiomyoma
- Benign Brenner tumor
  - Hypoechoic solid mass
  - Posterior acoustic shadowing due to presence of extensive calcifications
- Borderline and malignant Brenner tumor
  - Hypoechoic cystic mass with solid component or papillary projections

CT Findings
- Benign Brenner tumor
  - Small solid mass (usually) with extensive amorphous calcifications
- Borderline and malignant Brenner tumor
  - Multilocular cystic mass with solid components
  - Nonspecific mild to moderate enhancement of solid components on CECT

DDx: Ovarian Masses

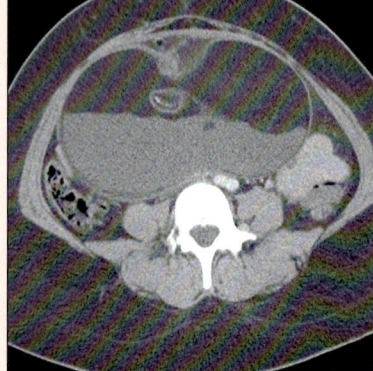

Mature Teratoma

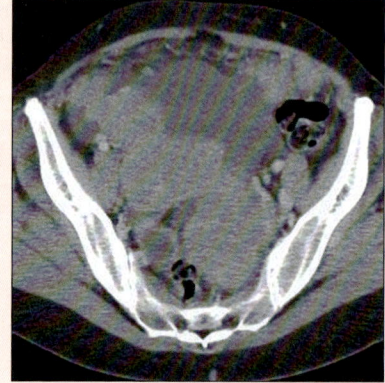

Ovarian Cancer

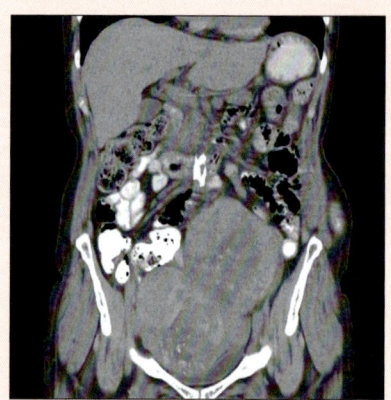

Krukenberg Tumor

BRENNER TUMOR

Key Facts

Terminology
- Three types; benign Brenner tumor, atypical proliferating transitional cell (Brenner) tumor and malignant Brenner tumor

Imaging Findings
- Best diagnostic clue: Combination of calcifications demonstrated by US or CT and low SI on T2WI MR strongly suggests the diagnosis of Brenner tumors
- Location: Usually unilateral
- Usually small (< 5 cm)
- Benign Brenner tumors are usually solid: Multiloculated cystic mass with solid components on US/CT/MR is relatively common finding of benign as well as borderline & malignant Brenner tumors

Top Differential Diagnoses
- Mature Teratoma
- Fibroma/Fibrothecoma
- Ovarian Cancer
- Krukenberg Tumor
- Subserosal Pedunculated Leiomyoma

Pathology
- Vast majority are benign, with few reports of borderline and malignant counterparts
- Other ipsilateral ovarian tumors (often mucinous cystadenomas) are present in 30% of cases

Diagnostic Checklist
- Extensive amorphous calcifications within solid component (US/CT/MR) is characteristic of Brenner tumors

MR Findings
- T1WI
  - Benign Brenner tumor
    - Usually entirely solid mass of low SI
  - Borderline and malignant Brenner tumor
    - Low SI cystic component with homogeneous intermediate SI solid component
- T2WI
  - Benign Brenner tumor
    - Usually entirely solid mass of very low SI due to the presence of dense fibrous stroma
    - Calcifications may be difficult to detect on MR
  - Borderline and malignant Brenner tumor
    - Very high SI cystic component that may contain intermediate to high SI solid component and/or low SI septae
- Contrast-enhanced MR
  - Benign Brenner tumor
    - Avid rapid homogeneous enhancement
  - Borderline and malignant Brenner tumor
    - Mild patchy enhancement of solid component and septae with persistent enhancement on delayed images

Imaging Recommendations
- Best imaging tool: CECT or MR
- Protocol advice: T1WI, T2WI and gadolinium enhanced T1WI

DIFFERENTIAL DIAGNOSIS

Mature Teratoma
- Usually contains fat density, calcifications, and/or teeth

Fibroma/Fibrothecoma
- Can be indistinguishable from a benign Brenner tumor as both are of very low SI on T2WI, however fibromas usually show internal edema and cystic changes when large
- Usually shows minimal contrast-enhancement

Ovarian Cancer
- Brenner tumors show lower mean SI on T2WI than other non-fibrous ovarian masses
- Extensive amorphous calcifications are very rare in ovarian cancer
- Diffuse peritoneal spreading and ascites is common in ovarian carcinoma, but it is not a feature of Brenner tumors

Krukenberg Tumor
- Usually bilateral with additional finding of primary malignancy

Subserosal Pedunculated Leiomyoma
- Dystrophic-type calcification in leiomyoma usually has a mottled appearance with a curvilinear rim

PATHOLOGY

General Features
- Etiology
  - Tumor derived from ovarian surface epithelium undergoing transitional cell metaplasia
  - Malignant transitional cell carcinoma differs from malignant Brenner tumor in that it does not have an associated Brenner component
- Epidemiology
  - Brenner tumors constitute 2-3% of all primary ovarian tumors
  - Vast majority are benign, with few reports of borderline and malignant counterparts
- Associated abnormalities
  - Other ipsilateral ovarian tumors (often mucinous cystadenomas) are present in 30% of cases
  - Endometrial hyperplasia in 4-14%

Gross Pathologic & Surgical Features
- Brenner tumor is a rare exception to the general rule that the presence of solid tissue within a cystic mass indicates malignancy
- Benign Brenner tumor

BRENNER TUMOR

- Most benign Brenner tumors are < 2 cm diameter, can be up to 10 cm
- Well circumscribed, unencapsulated, bosselated, firm tumor with a rubbery consistency, a reflexion of their dense fibrous stroma
- May have a cystic component
- Most frequently left-sided, bilateral in 5-7% of cases
• Atypical proliferating transitional cell (Brenner) tumor
  - Up to 23 cm diameter with smooth external surface
  - Multicystic cut surface showing polypoid or papillary areas
  - Unilateral
• Malignant Brenner tumor
  - Unilateral, partly cystic tumor

Microscopic Features
• Benign Brenner tumor
  - Circumscribed nest of benign transitional cell epithelium set in a fibrous stroma
  - No atypia
  - Hyalinization and calcification seen in 50% of cases
• Atypical proliferating transitional cell (Brenner) tumor
  - Nodules and ribbons of atypical transitional epithelium set in a fibrous stroma
  - Resembles a low grade transitional cell carcinoma of bladder
  - No stromal invasion
• Malignant Brenner tumor
  - Malignant transitional epithelium with stromal invasion
  - Foci of either benign or borderline Brenner tumor must be present for diagnosis
  - Necrosis and calcification is present in most tumors
  - May see squamous and glandular differentiation

CLINICAL ISSUES

Presentation
• Most common signs/symptoms
  - Benign Brenner tumor
    - Often incidental finding
  - Atypical proliferating transitional cell (Brenner) tumor
    - Presents with symptoms relating to size of ovarian mass such as abdominal distention and pain
  - Malignant Brenner Tumor
    - Abdominal pain, swelling, 20% have abnormal uterine bleeding
• Other signs/symptoms: Any type of Brenner tumor may produce estrogen or androgen activity and patients may present with abnormal vaginal bleeding

Demographics
• Age
  - Benign Brenner tumor = 4th-8th decade
  - Atypical proliferating transitional cell (Brenner) tumor = mean age 60 years
  - Malignant Brenner tumor = mean age 60 years

Natural History & Prognosis
• Benign Brenner tumor
  - Benign behavior
• Atypical proliferating transitional cell (Brenner) tumor
  - No convincing evidence of malignant behavior
• Malignant Brenner tumor
  - Poor prognosis as 20% present with extraovarian spread at time of diagnosis
  - Limited data suggest that the prognosis for a malignant Brenner tumor is better than that of a malignant transitional cell carcinoma

Treatment
• Benign Brenner tumors are treated with local excision
• Malignant Brenner tumors are treated like ovarian carcinoma

DIAGNOSTIC CHECKLIST

Image Interpretation Pearls
• Extensive amorphous calcifications within solid component (US/CT/MR) is characteristic of Brenner tumors

SELECTED REFERENCES

1. Tamai K et al: MR features of physiologic and benign conditions of the ovary. Eur Radiol. 2006
2. Heye S et al: Left ovarian Brenner tumor. JBR-BTR. 88(5):245-6, 2005
3. Takahama J et al: Borderline Brenner tumor of the ovary: MRI findings. Abdom Imaging. 29(4):528-30, 2004
4. Yoshida S et al: Brenner tumour. Lancet. 362(9387):858, 2003
5. Hiroi H et al: A case of estrogen-producing Brenner tumor with a stromal component as a potential source for estrogen. Oncology. 63(2):201-4, 2002
6. Jung SE et al: CT and MR imaging of ovarian tumors with emphasis on differential diagnosis. Radiographics. 22(6):1305-25, 2002
7. Robboy SJ et al: Pathology of the Female Genital Tract. 1st ed. Lon, Harcourt. 587-92, 2002
8. Ohara N et al: Magnetic resonance imaging of a benign Brenner tumor with an ipsilateral simple cyst. Arch Gynecol Obstet. 265(2):96-9, 2001
9. Hermanns B et al: Differential diagnosis, prognostic factors, and clinical treatment of proliferative Brenner tumor of the ovary. Ultrastruct Pathol. 24(3):191-6, 2000
10. Moon WJ et al: Brenner tumor of the ovary: CT and MR findings. J Comput Assist Tomogr. 24(1):72-6, 2000
11. Outwater EK et al: Ovarian Brenner tumors: MR imaging characteristics. Magn Reson Imaging. 16(10):1147-53, 1998
12. Hata K et al: Doppler ultrasound in a patient with ovarian Brenner tumor of low malignant potential: comparison with Gray-scale ultrasound, magnetic resonance imaging and tumor marker suggesting malignancy. Gynecol Obstet Invest. 43(2):135-8, 1997
13. Sugimura K et al: Malignant Brenner tumor: MR findings. AJR Am J Roentgenol. 157(6):1355-6, 1991
14. Conforti S et al: Bilateral Brenner tumor. Eur J Gynaecol Oncol. 10(6):438-41, 1989
15. Athey PA et al: Sonographic features of Brenner tumor of the ovary. J Ultrasound Med. 6(7):367-72, 1987
16. Sawyer RW et al: Computed tomography of benign ovarian masses. J Comput Assist Tomogr. 9(4):784-9, 1985
17. Williams CO: Radiologic seminar CLXXXIV: Brenner tumor of the ovary--ultrasound findings. J Miss State Med Assoc. 19(9):168-9, 1978

BRENNER TUMOR

IMAGE GALLERY

Typical

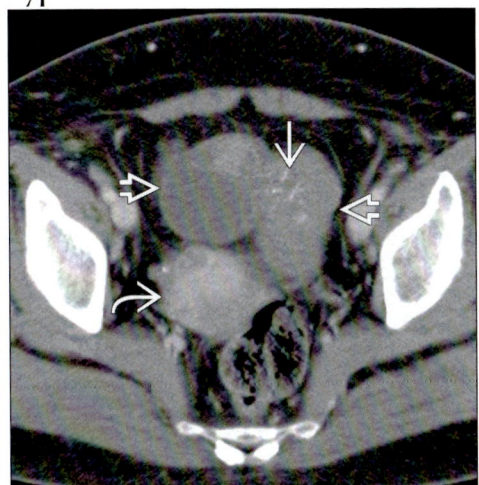 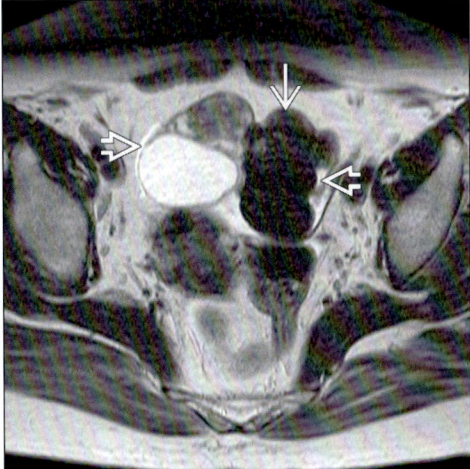

(Left) Axial CECT shows a mixed solid and cystic mass ➡ just anterior to the uterus ➡. Note presence of amorphous calcifications ➡ within the solid component of the mass. *(Right)* Axial T2WI MR confirms the presence of a mixed cystic and solid pelvic mass ➡. Note that the solid component is of very low signal intensity ➡. Pathology: Borderline Brenner tumor

Typical

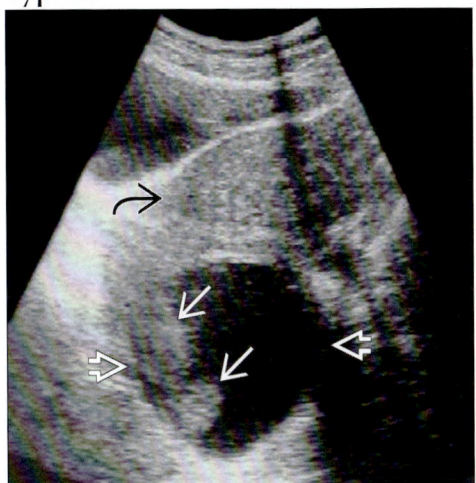 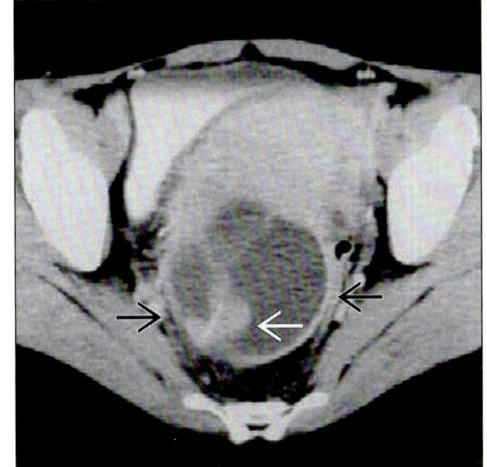

(Left) Transverse ultrasound shows a round cystic mass ➡ containing solid components ➡. The mass is located posterior to the uterus ➡. (Courtesy S.H. Kim, MD). *(Right)* Axial CECT in the same patient as previous image shows a low attenuation pelvic mass ➡ which contains an enhancing soft tissue nodule ➡. Pathology: Malignant Brenner tumor. (Courtesy S.H. Kim, MD).

Variant

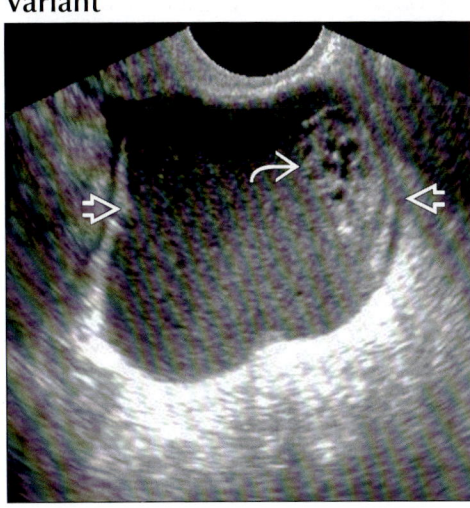 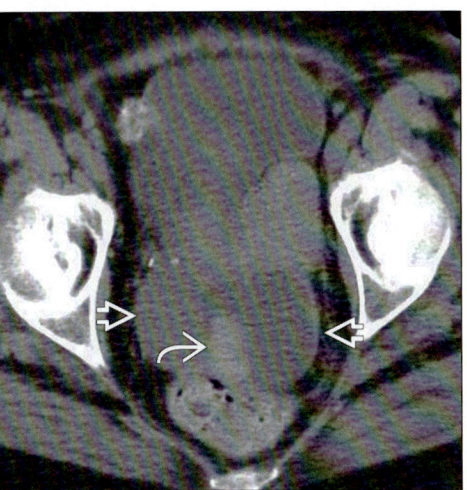

(Left) Transverse ultrasound shows a complex cystic adnexal mass ➡ which contains a heterogeneous solid nodule ➡. *(Right)* Axial NECT in the same patient as previous image confirms the presence of the complex cystic adnexal mass ➡ with solid component ➡. Pathology: Brenner tumor in mucinous cystadenocarcinoma of low malignant potential.

MUCINOUS CYSTADENOCARCINOMA

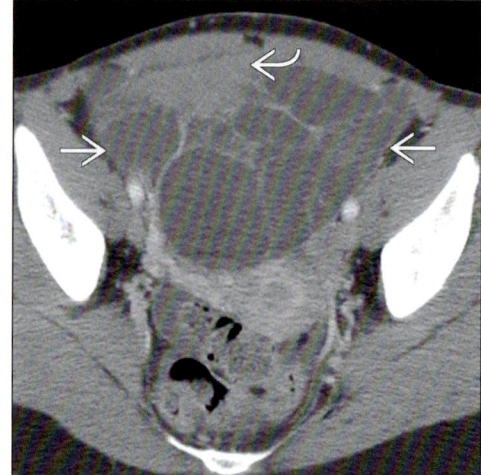

Coronal graphic shows ovarian mucinous cystadenocarcinoma with variable cystic ➡ and solid ➡ components.

Axial CECT shows an ovarian mucinous cystadenocarcinoma. A multiloculated cystic mass ➡ with a solid component ➡ is seen.

TERMINOLOGY

Abbreviations and Synonyms
- Mucinous adenocarcinoma, malignant mucinous tumor

Definitions
- Second most common type of epithelial cancer of ovary

IMAGING FINDINGS

General Features
- Best diagnostic clue
  - Multilocular cystic ovarian mass with variable appearance of cystic components on imaging studies depending on mucin content of cystic components
  - Nodules or solid components are seen associated with multilocular cystic mass
  - Pseudomyxoma peritonei may be seen in mucinous adenocarcinomas
  - Pseudomyxoma peritonei seen as diffuse intraperitoneal material that may contain septa and cause scalloping of surfaces of liver and/or spleen
- Size: Often large masses; 6-40 cm
- Morphology: Large, multilocular cystic tumors with solid mural nodules

Ultrasonographic Findings
- Grayscale Ultrasound
  - Multiloculated cystic mass containing different echogenic patterns in the cystic components
  - Solid mural nodules can be seen within cystic components
- Color Doppler: Solid components demonstrate vascularity

CT Findings
- NECT
  - Multiseptated, low attenuation cystic masses
  - High attenuation may be seen in some loculi due to high protein content of mucinous material
- CECT
  - Low-attenuation, multiloculated, cystic mass
  - Thick septae and solid mural nodules demonstrate enhancement

DDx: Ovarian Masses

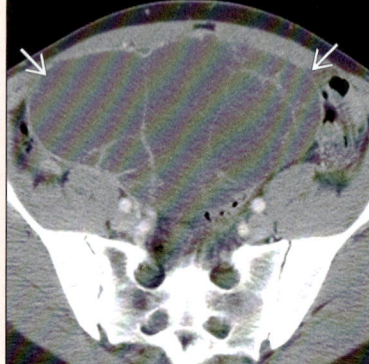
Mucinous Cystadenoma

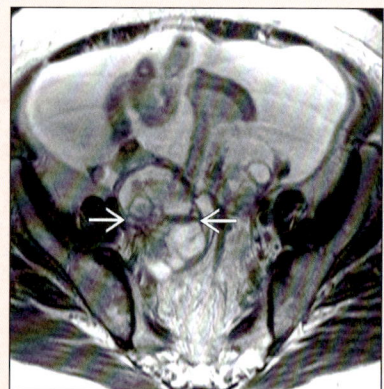
Serous Adenocarcinoma

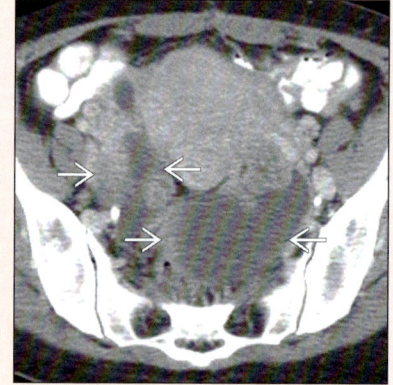
Ovarian Metastases

MUCINOUS CYSTADENOCARCINOMA

Key Facts

Terminology
- Mucinous adenocarcinoma, malignant mucinous tumor
- Second most common type of epithelial cancer of ovary

Imaging Findings
- Multilocular cystic ovarian mass with variable appearance of cystic components on imaging studies depending on mucin content of cystic components
- Nodules or solid components are seen associated with multilocular cystic mass
- Pseudomyxoma peritonei may be seen in mucinous adenocarcinomas
- Pseudomyxoma peritonei seen as diffuse intraperitoneal material that may contain septa and cause scalloping of surfaces of liver and/or spleen
- Morphology: Large, multilocular cystic tumors with solid mural nodules

Top Differential Diagnoses
- Benign Serous or Mucinous Cystadenoma of Ovary
- Serous Adenocarcinoma Of Ovary
- Ovarian Metastasis

Pathology
- Malignant mucinous tumors often demonstrate benign-appearing, borderline, and invasive patterns coexisting within the same tumor

Diagnostic Checklist
- Multilocular cystic adnexal mass with variable appearance of cystic components on imaging studies due to variable mucin content of the cystic components

MR Findings
- T1WI
  - Signal intensity varies depending on degree of mucin concentration of cystic components of mass
  - Loculi with watery mucin have lower signal intensity than loculi with thicker mucin
- T2WI
  - Signal intensity varies depending on degree of mucin concentration of cystic components of mass
  - Loculi with watery mucin have high signal intensity and loculi with thicker mucin have lower signal intensity
  - Solid mural nodules demonstrate intermediate signal intensity
- T1 C+: Thick septae and solid mural nodules demonstrate enhancement

Imaging Recommendations
- Best imaging tool
  - US is method of choice for initial characterization
  - MR may be used in cases when US is equivocal
  - CT is reserved for staging if malignancy is being considered

DIFFERENTIAL DIAGNOSIS

Benign Serous or Mucinous Cystadenoma of Ovary
- Often less than 4 cm in size
- Entirely cystic
- Wall thickness less than 3 mm
- Absence of ascites, peritoneal disease or lymphadenopathy

Serous Adenocarcinoma of Ovary
- More common than mucinous adenocarcinoma
- Mixed cystic and solid mass with papillary projections
- Psammoma bodies may be present

Ovarian Metastasis
- Most ovarian metastases are solid or a mixture of solid and cystic tumors
- Clinical presentation is often due to primary disease

PATHOLOGY

General Features
- General path comments
  - Most (90%) of ovarian cancers originate from germinal epithelium
  - Mucinous cystadenocarcinoma is the second most common type of epithelial ovarian cancer
  - Epithelial ovarian cancer subtypes
    - Serous (50%), mucinous (20%), endometrioid (20%), clear cell (10%) and undifferentiated (1%)
  - Malignant mucinous tumors often demonstrate benign-appearing, borderline, and invasive patterns coexisting within the same tumor
  - Borderline tumors have a great degree of cellular proliferation but no stromal invasion
  - Degree of malignancy of carcinomatous component may vary from noninvasive to invasive, and from well-differentiated to undifferentiated carcinoma
  - This tumor heterogeneity likely reflects the progression from benign to malignant neoplasia that occurs in the development of mucinous carcinomas
  - Methods of spread
    - Direct extension
    - Intraperitoneal implantation
    - Lymphatic dissemination in pelvis and paraaortic region
    - Less commonly, hematogenously to liver or lungs
- Genetics: It has been reported that there is an increasing frequency of codon 12/13 K-ras mutations in benign, borderline, and carcinomatous mucinous ovarian tumors, supporting the hypothesis that K-ras mutational activation is an early event in mucinous ovarian tumorigenesis

MUCINOUS CYSTADENOCARCINOMA

- Epidemiology: Malignant (15%) and borderline (10%) mucinous tumors of the ovary are less common than benign (75%) mucinous tumors

Gross Pathologic & Surgical Features
- Large, multilocular cystic masses that contain gelatinous material
- Pseudomyxoma peritonei seen as diffuse gelatinous material in peritoneal cavity

Microscopic Features
- Epithelium that characterizes mucinous tumors resembles lining of endocervix or intestine
- Benign, borderline (cytological atypia, no stromal invasion) and invasive carcinoma (stromal invasion) may be seen in different areas of same tumor
- Tumor is composed of glands, cribriform patterns and solid sheets
- Less intracytoplasmic mucin content seen in higher histologic grades
- Immunohistochemistry may help to distinguish primary ovarian mucinous tumor from metastatic colorectal adenocarcinoma
    - Ovarian mucinous cystadenocarcinoma is positive for cytokeratin 7, ± cytokeratin 20
    - Colorectal carcinoma is negative for cytokeratin 7, positive for cytokeratin 20

Staging, Grading or Classification Criteria
- FIGO staging system
    - I: Tumor confined to ovaries
        - IA: Intracapsular and unilateral
        - IB: Intracapsular and bilateral
        - IC: Ruptured capsule, tumor on ovarian capsule, malignant cells in ascites or peritoneal washings
    - II: Local extension; confined to true pelvis
        - IIA: Involvement of fallopian tubes or uterus
        - IIB: Involvement of other pelvic tissues such as sigmoid, pelvic implants
        - IIC: Pelvic extension with malignant cells in ascites or peritoneal washings
    - III: Nodal metastases or peritoneal implants outside the pelvis
        - IIIA: Microscopic abdominal implants
        - IIIB: < 2 cm abdominal implants
        - IIIC: > 2 cm abdominal implants or positive nodes
    - IV: Distant metastases (excluding peritoneal metastases); e.g., malignant pleural effusion, intrahepatic metastases

CLINICAL ISSUES

Presentation
- Most common signs/symptoms
    - Pelvic mass
    - Pelvic pain
    - Abdominal swelling due to ovarian enlargement or ascites
- Other signs/symptoms: Anemia, cachexia
- Clinical Profile
    - Many women may present with advanced-stage disease
    - May be asymptomatic until an abdominal mass is found during routine pelvic examination or until disease is advanced

Demographics
- Age: Predominantly perimenopausal and postmenopausal women

Natural History & Prognosis
- Most important prognostic factors
    - Histologic type, grade and stage of disease
    - Prognosis for patients with advanced disease is directly related to success of cytoreductive surgery
- 5 year survival rates: 80-90% for early stages and 15-20% for advanced stages

Treatment
- Cytoreductive (tumor-debulking) surgery
    - To reduce maximum diameter of remaining implants less than 1 cm
- Neoadjuvant chemotherapy
    - Preoperative and/or after surgery

DIAGNOSTIC CHECKLIST

Image Interpretation Pearls
- Mucinous cystadenocarcinoma of ovary should be considered in presence of the following
    - Multilocular cystic adnexal mass with variable appearance of cystic components on imaging studies due to variable mucin content of the cystic components
    - Presence of pseudomyxoma peritonei that causes scalloping of liver or splenic margin

SELECTED REFERENCES

1. Kikkawa F et al: Clinical characteristics and prognosis of mucinous tumors of the ovary. Gynecol Oncol. 2006
2. Togashi K. Related Articles et al: Ovarian cancer: the clinical role of US, CT, and MRI. Eur Radiol. 13 Suppl 4:L87-104, 2003
3. Jung SE et al: CT and MR imaging of ovarian tumors with emphasis on differential diagnosis. Radiographics. 22(6):1305-25, 2002
4. Rodriguez IM et al: Mucinous tumors of the ovary: a clinicopathologic analysis of 75 borderline tumors (of intestinal type) and carcinomas. Am J Surg Pathol. 26(2):139-52, 2002
5. Jeong YY et al: Imaging evaluation of ovarian masses. Radiographics. 20(5):1445-70, 2000
6. Lee KR et al: Mucinous tumors of the ovary: a clinicopathologic study of 196 borderline tumors (of intestinal type) and carcinomas, including an evaluation of 11 cases with 'pseudomyxoma peritonei'. Am J Surg Pathol. 24(11):1447-64, 2000
7. Ozols RF et al: Epithelial ovarian cancer. In: Hoskins WJ, Perez CA, Young RC (eds). Principles and practice of gynecologic oncology, Lippincott Williams & Wilkins, Philadelphia. 981-1057, 2000
8. Zissin R et al: Synchronous mucinous tumors of the ovary and the appendix associated with pseudomyxoma peritonei: CT findings. Abdom Imaging. 25(3):311-6, 2000
9. Kawamoto S et al: CT of epithelial ovarian tumors. Radiographics. 19 Spec No:S85-102; quiz S263-4, 1999

MUCINOUS CYSTADENOCARCINOMA

IMAGE GALLERY

Typical

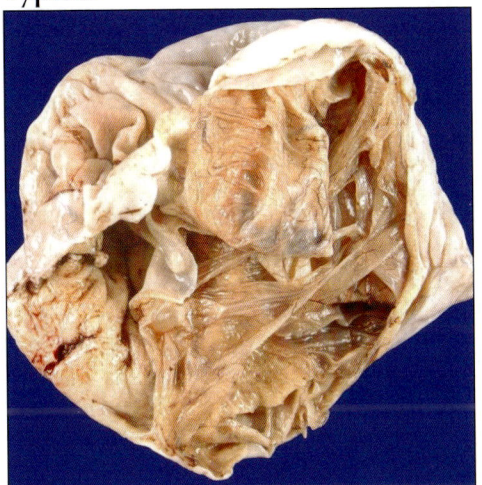
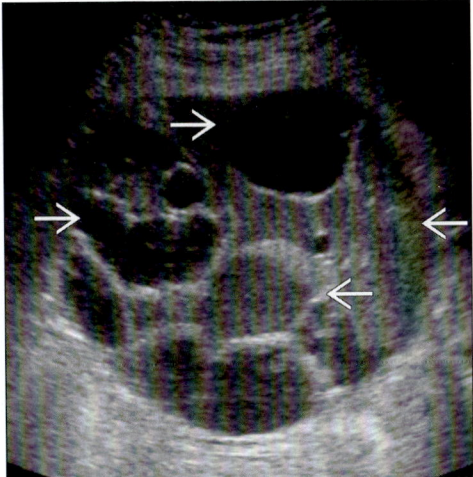

(Left) Gross pathology shows a large, multilocular cystic ovarian mass in a patient with mucinous cystadenocarcinoma. *(Right)* Axial transabdominal ultrasound shows different echogenic patterns ➡ in the cystic components of the mass due to variable mucin content.

Typical

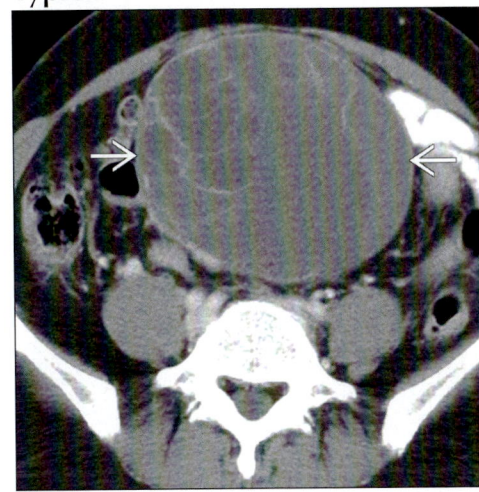
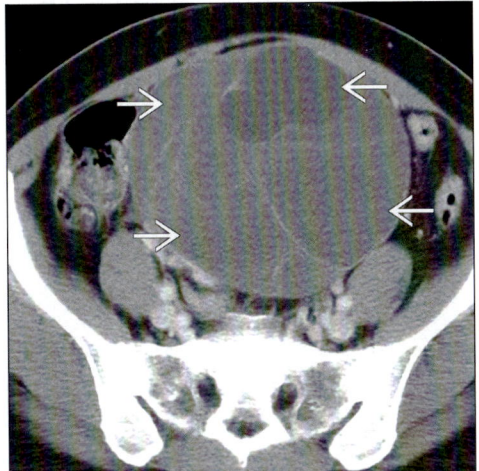

(Left) Axial CECT shows a mucinous cystadenocarcinoma of the ovary. A multiloculated cystic mass ➡ is seen. *(Right)* Axial CECT shows that multiloculated cystic mass contains different densities in the cystic components ➡ reflecting variable mucin content.

Typical

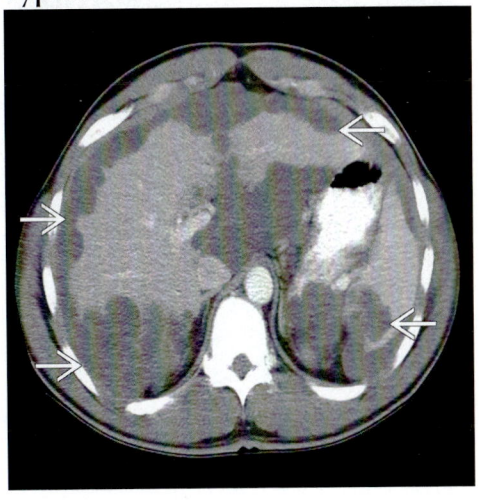
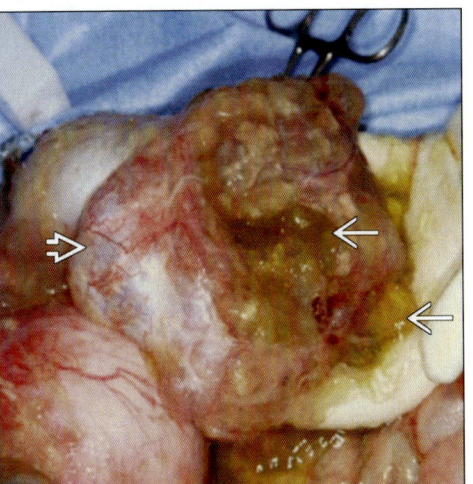

(Left) Axial CECT shows pseudomyxoma peritonei ➡ scalloping surfaces of the liver and spleen in a patient with ovarian mucinous tumor. *(Right)* Intra-operative photograph shows gelatinous material ➡ reflecting mucin content in an ovarian mucinous tumor ➡.

MUCINOUS CYSTADENOCARCINOMA

(Left) Axial oblique transabdominal ultrasound shows a borderline mucinous tumor of the ovary. Note the cystic mass ➡ contains different echogenic patterns. (Right) Axial oblique color Doppler ultrasound shows a borderline mucinous tumor of the ovary. Note vascularity ➡ in the periphery of the mass.

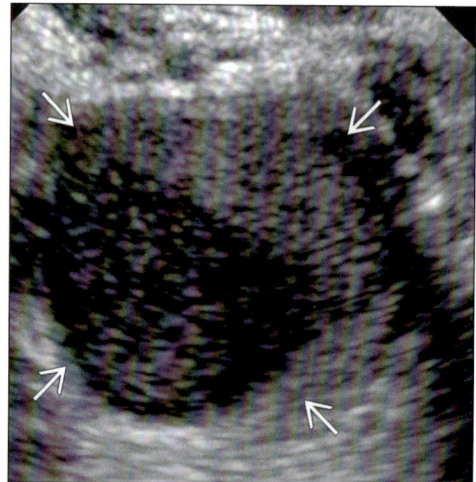

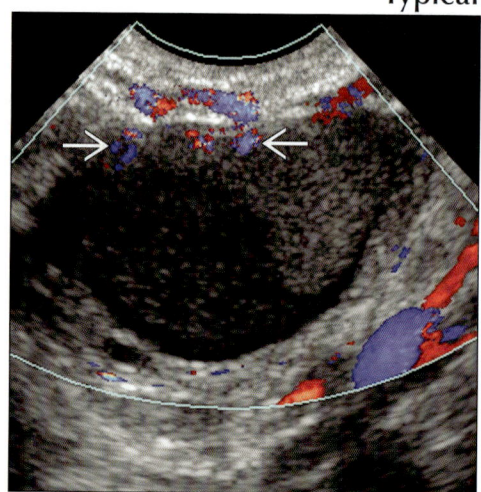
Typical

(Left) Axial oblique transvaginal ultrasound shows a borderline mucinous tumor of the ovary. Multiloculated cystic mass ➡ with various echogenic patterns is seen. (Right) Axial oblique transvaginal ultrasound shows mucinous cystadenocarcinoma seen as a complex cystic mass ➡ with solid nodular ➡ components.

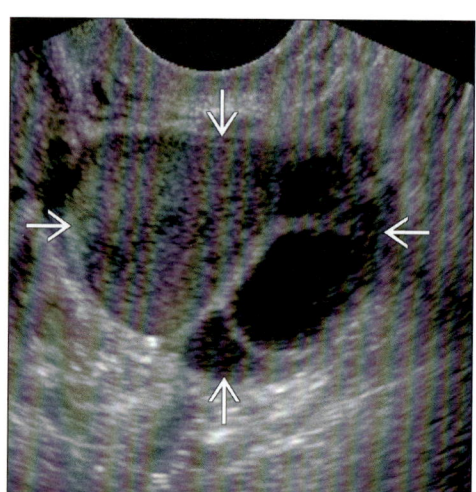

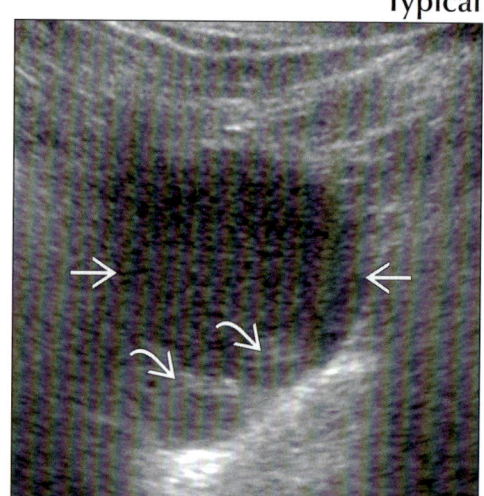
Typical

(Left) Axial oblique transvaginal ultrasound shows mucinous cystadenocarcinoma of the ovary. The mass contains a heterogeneous solid component ➡, thick septation ➡ and cystic components ➡ with echogenic contents. (Right) Axial oblique color Doppler ultrasound shows vascularity ➡ in the solid component of the mucinous cystadenocarcinoma.

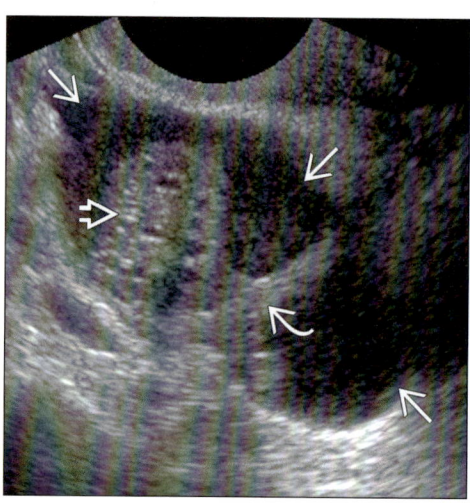

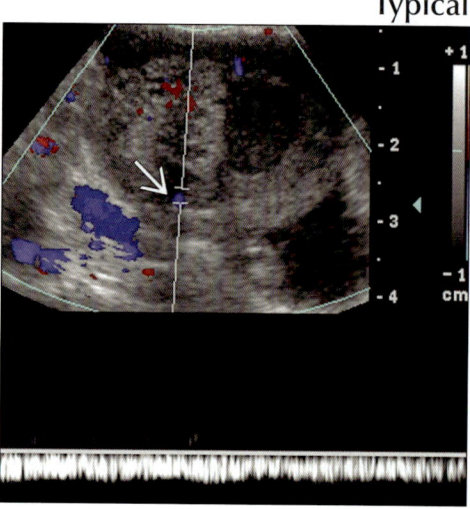
Typical

MUCINOUS CYSTADENOCARCINOMA

Typical

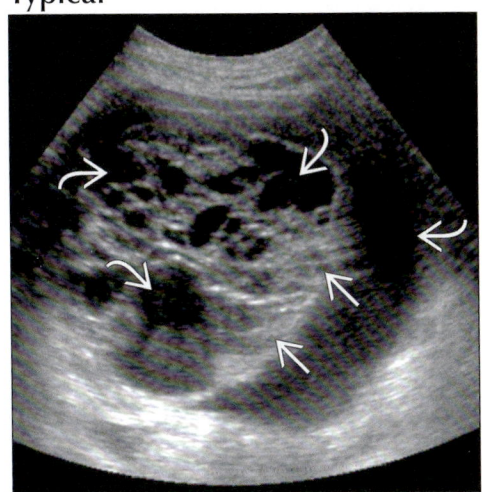 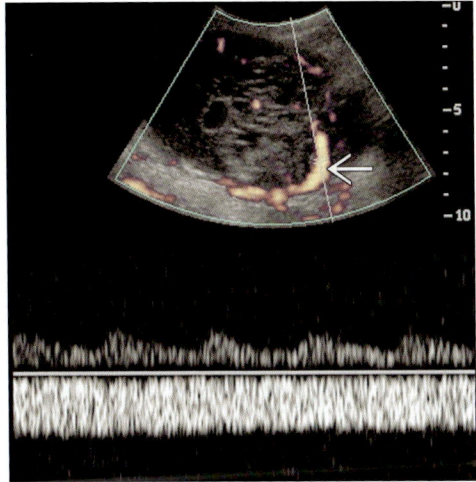

(Left) Axial oblique transabdominal ultrasound shows ovarian mucinous cystadenocarcinoma with heterogeneous solid ➡ and echogenic cystic ➡ components. *(Right)* Axial oblique power Doppler ultrasound shows vascularity ➡ in the solid component of the mucinous cystadenocarcinoma.

Typical

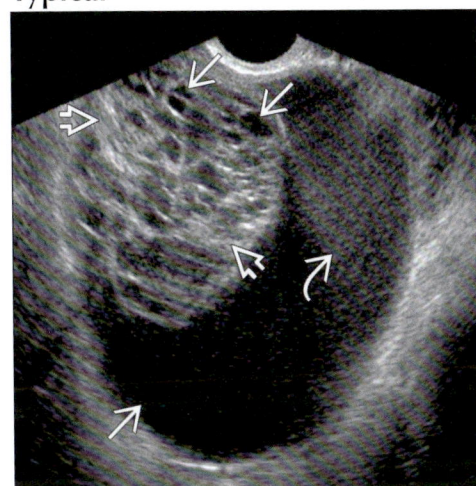 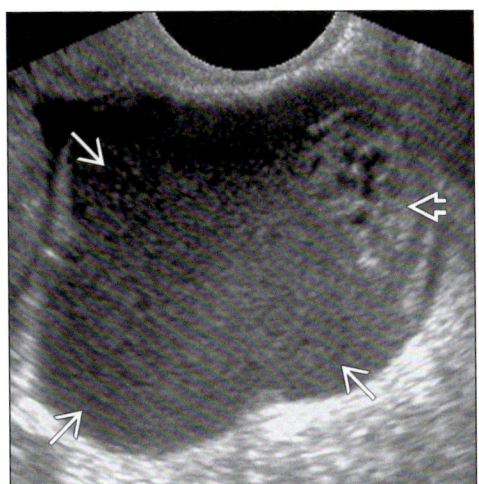

(Left) Sagittal oblique transvaginal ultrasound shows mucinous cystadenocarcinoma with solid ➡ and cystic ➡ components. Note layering echogenic material ➡ in the largest cystic component. *(Right)* Axial oblique transvaginal ultrasound shows mucinous cystadenocarcinoma with a large echogenic cystic ➡ and a smaller mixed cystic and solid ➡ components.

Typical

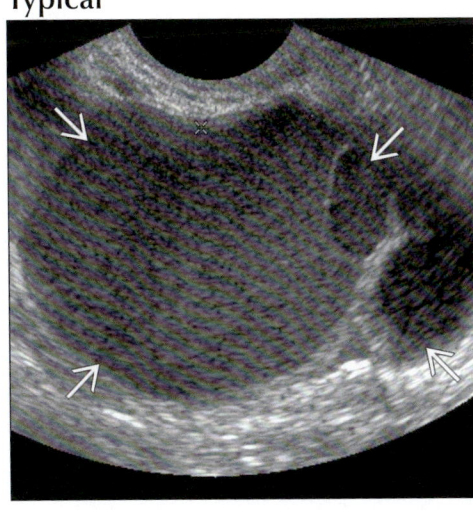 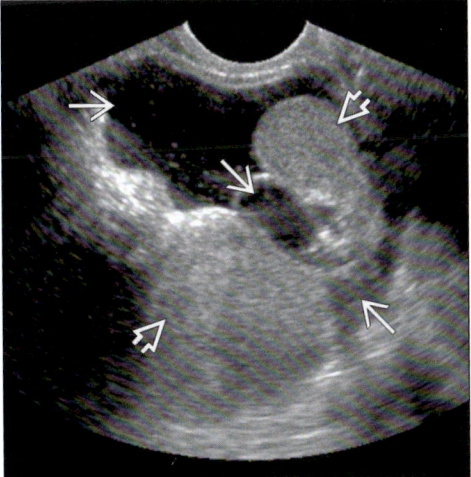

(Left) Sagittal oblique transvaginal ultrasound shows mucinous cystadenocarcinoma of the ovary seen as a lobulated multiloculated cystic mass with various echogenic patterns ➡. *(Right)* Axial oblique transvaginal ultrasound shows a large mucinous cystadenocarcinoma with solid ➡ and cystic ➡ components.

SEROUS CYSTADENOCARCINOMA

Axial T2WI MR shows bilateral ovarian serous cystadenocarcinomas with cystic and solid components. Ascites is also seen.

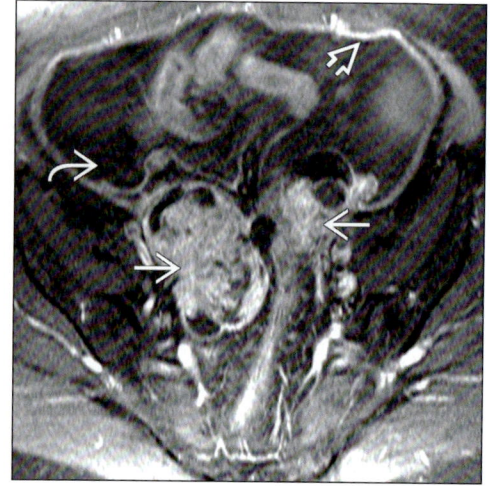

Axial T1 C+ FS MR shows that the solid components of the serous cystadenocarcinomas enhance markedly. Peritoneal enhancement and ascites reflecting peritoneal carcinomatosis are also seen.

TERMINOLOGY

Abbreviations and Synonyms
- Serous adenocarcinoma, malignant serous tumor

Definitions
- Most common type of epithelial cancer of ovary

IMAGING FINDINGS

General Features
- Best diagnostic clue: Most often seen as cystic masses with solid/papillary components in ovary
- Location: Unilateral or bilateral involvement of ovaries can be seen
- Size: Varies but may present as large masses
- Morphology
  o Predominantly cystic masses with papillary solid components
  o May also be seen as predominately solid masses

Ultrasonographic Findings
- Grayscale Ultrasound: Cystic adnexal mass containing different echogenic patterns, thick walls, septations, nodules or papillary projections
- Color Doppler: Solid components demonstrate vascularity

CT Findings
- NECT
  o Low attenuation cystic mass with soft tissue density solid components
  o Although psammoma bodies (microscopic calcifications) present in 30% of histologic specimens, they are detected only in 12% of cases with CT
- CECT
  o Low attenuation cystic mass with enhancing solid components
  o Contrast-enhancement helps to differentiate blood clot, which does not enhance, from enhancing solid components of tumor

DDx: Ovarian Masses

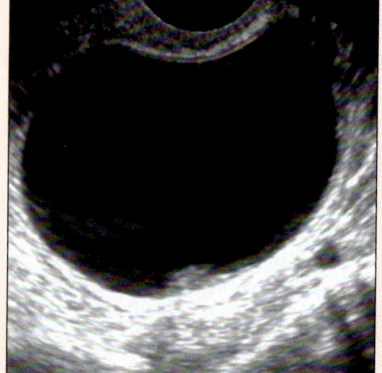
Serous Cystadenoma

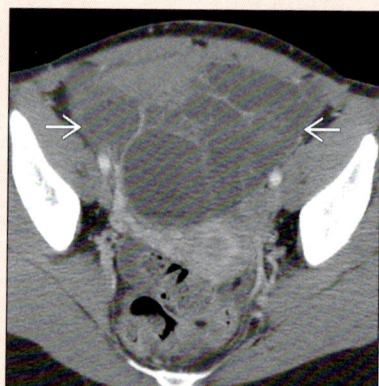
Mucinous Cystadenocarcinoma

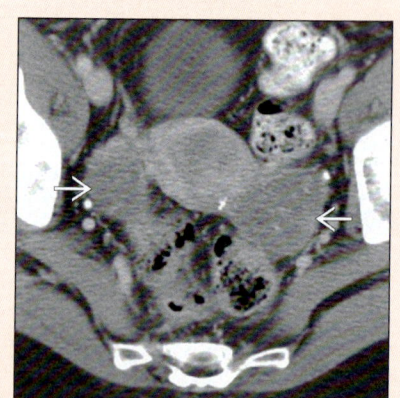
Ovarian Metastasis

SEROUS CYSTADENOCARCINOMA

Key Facts

Terminology
- Serous adenocarcinoma, malignant serous tumor
- Most common type of epithelial cancer of ovary

Imaging Findings
- Best diagnostic clue: Most often seen as cystic masses with solid/papillary components in ovary
- Location: Unilateral or bilateral involvement of ovaries can be seen
- Predominantly cystic masses with papillary solid components
- May also be seen as predominately solid masses

Top Differential Diagnoses
- Benign Serous or Mucinous Cystadenoma of Ovary
- Mucinous Cystadenocarcinoma of Ovary
- Ovarian Metastasis

Pathology
- Serous cystadenocarcinoma is most common type of epithelial ovarian cancer
- Epidemiology: Malignant (25%) and borderline (15%); serous ovarian neoplasms less common than benign (60%) serous tumors of ovary

Diagnostic Checklist
- Bilaterality and peritoneal carcinomatosis seen more frequently in serous than in mucinous cystadenocarcinomas
- Thick, irregular wall or thick septa
- Papillary projections or soft tissue components
- Ancillary findings of peritoneal implants, ascites, and lymphadenopathy

MR Findings
- T1WI: Low to intermediate signal intensity cystic mass with intermediate intensity solid components
- T2WI: High signal intensity cystic mass with heterogeneous signal intensity solid components
- T1 C+
  - Solid components of mass demonstrate marked enhancement
  - Contrast-enhancement helps to differentiate blood clot which does not enhance from enhancing mural nodules

Imaging Recommendations
- Best imaging tool
  - US, CT, or MR can be used to detect and characterize an adnexal mass
  - US is most commonly used method to detect & characterize an adnexal mass
  - MR is superior to US and CT in tumor characterization due to better soft tissue resolution
  - CT most often used in advanced disease to assess peritoneal carcinomatosis or distant metastases
- Protocol advice
  - Color Doppler is needed to assess for flow in solid appearing components on US
  - Contrast-enhancement is essential to demonstrate enhancing solid components on both CT and MR

DIFFERENTIAL DIAGNOSIS

Benign Serous or Mucinous Cystadenoma of Ovary
- Often less than 4 cm in size
- Entirely cystic
- Wall thickness less than 3 mm
- Absence of ascites, peritoneal disease or lymphadenopathy

Mucinous Cystadenocarcinoma of Ovary
- Tend to be larger and multiloculated
- Often variable echogenicity (US), density (CT) or signal intensity (MR) owing to mucinous contents of cystic components
- Pseudomyxoma peritonei may be associated with mucinous adenocarcinoma

Ovarian Metastasis
- Most ovarian metastases are solid or mixture of solid and cystic tumors
- Clinical presentation often due to primary disease

PATHOLOGY

General Features
- General path comments
  - Most (90%) of ovarian cancers originate from germinal epithelium
  - Epithelial ovarian cancer subtypes
    - Serous (50%), mucinous (20%), endometrioid (20%), clear cell (10%) and undifferentiated (1%)
  - Serous cystadenocarcinoma is most common type of epithelial ovarian cancer
  - Methods of spread
    - Direct extension
    - Intraperitoneal implantation
    - Lymphatic dissemination in pelvis and paraaortic region
    - Less commonly, hematogenously to liver or lungs
- Epidemiology: Malignant (25%) and borderline (15%); serous ovarian neoplasms less common than benign (60%) serous tumors of ovary

Gross Pathologic & Surgical Features
- Most often unilocular or septated cystic masses with papillary solid projections

Microscopic Features
- Epithelium that characterizes serous tumors resembles lining of fallopian tube
- Histologically papillary, glandular and solid pattern of growth

SEROUS CYSTADENOCARCINOMA

- Tumor usually contains glands, solid sheets of cells, or slitlike spaces
- Tumor cells often diffusely infiltrate fibrous stroma
- Laminated psammoma bodies usually present
- Features that help distinguish serous cystadenocarcinomas from borderline serous tumors include
  - Obvious stromal invasion
  - Extensive cellular budding and confluent cellular growth
  - Nuclear atypia

Staging, Grading or Classification Criteria
- FIGO staging system
  - I: Tumor confined to ovaries
    - IA: Intracapsular and unilateral
    - IB: Intracapsular and bilateral
    - IC: Ruptured capsule, tumor on ovarian capsule, malignant cells in ascites or peritoneal washings
  - II: Local extension; confined to true pelvis
    - IIA: Involvement of fallopian tubes or uterus
    - IIB: Involvement of other pelvic tissues such as sigmoid, pelvic implants
    - IIC: Pelvic extension with malignant cells in ascites or peritoneal washings
  - III: Nodal metastases or peritoneal implants outside pelvis
    - IIIA: Microscopic abdominal implants
    - IIIB: < 2 cm abdominal implants
    - IIIC: > 2 cm abdominal implants or positive nodes
  - IV: Distant metastases (excluding peritoneal metastases); e.g., malignant pleural effusion, intrahepatic metastases

CLINICAL ISSUES

Presentation
- Most common signs/symptoms
  - Pelvic mass
  - Pelvic pain
  - Abdominal swelling due to ovarian enlargement or ascites
- Other signs/symptoms: Anemia, cachexia
- Clinical Profile
  - Many women present with advanced-stage disease
    - May be asymptomatic until an abdominal mass is found during routine pelvic examination or until disease is advanced

Demographics
- Age: Predominantly perimenopausal and postmenopausal women

Natural History & Prognosis
- Most important prognostic factors
  - Histologic type, grade and stage of disease
  - Prognosis for patients with advanced disease directly related to success of cytoreductive surgery
- 5 year survival rates: 80-90% for early stages and 15-20% for advanced stages

Treatment
- Cytoreductive (tumor-debulking) surgery
  - To reduce maximum diameter of remaining implants by less than 1 cm
- Neoadjuvant chemotherapy

DIAGNOSTIC CHECKLIST

Consider
- Bilaterality and peritoneal carcinomatosis seen more frequently in serous than in mucinous cystadenocarcinomas

Image Interpretation Pearls
- Imaging findings that are suggestive of serous cystadenocarcinoma include
  - Thick, irregular wall or thick septa
  - Papillary projections or soft tissue components
  - Ancillary findings of peritoneal implants, ascites, and lymphadenopathy

SELECTED REFERENCES

1. Acs G: Serous and mucinous borderline (low malignant potential) tumors of the ovary. Am J Clin Pathol. 123 Suppl:S13-57, 2005
2. Dexeus S et al: Conservative management of epithelial ovarian cancer. Eur J Gynaecol Oncol. 26(5):473-8, 2005
3. Rabban JT et al: Current issues in the pathology of ovarian cancer. J Reprod Med. 50(6):467-74, 2005
4. Sohaib SA et al: The role of magnetic resonance imaging and ultrasound in patients with adnexal masses. Clin Radiol. 60(3):340-8, 2005
5. Kaku T et al: Histological classification of ovarian cancer. Med Electron Microsc. 36(1):9-17, 2003
6. Togashi K. Related Articles et al: Ovarian cancer: the clinical role of US, CT, and MRI. Eur Radiol. 13 Suppl 4:L87-104, 2003
7. Deavers MT et al: Micropapillary and cribriform patterns in ovarian serous tumors of low malignant potential: a study of 99 advanced stage cases. Am J Surg Pathol. 26(9):1129-41, 2002
8. Jung SE et al: CT and MR imaging of ovarian tumors with emphasis on differential diagnosis. Radiographics. 22(6):1305-25, 2002
9. Sawicki W et al: Preoperative discrimination between malignant and benign adnexal masses with transvaginal ultrasonography and colour blood flow imaging. Eur J Gynaecol Oncol. 22(2):137-42, 2001
10. Jeong YY et al: Imaging evaluation of ovarian masses. Radiographics. 20(5):1445-70, 2000
11. Ozols RF et al: Epithelial ovarian cancer. In: Hoskins WJ, Perez CA, Young RC (eds). Principles and Practice of Gynecologic Oncology, Philadelphia, Lippincott Williams & Wilkins. 981-1057, 2000
12. Kawamoto S et al: CT of epithelial ovarian tumors. Radiographics. 19 Spec No:S85-102; quiz S263-4, 1999
13. Kurtz AB et al: Diagnosis and staging of ovarian cancer: comparative values of Doppler and conventional US, CT, and MR imaging correlated with surgery and histopathologic analysis--report of the Radiology Diagnostic Oncology Group. Radiology. 212(1):19-27, 1999

SEROUS CYSTADENOCARCINOMA

IMAGE GALLERY

Typical

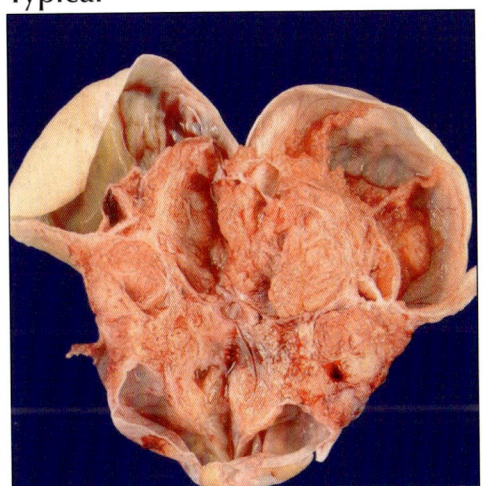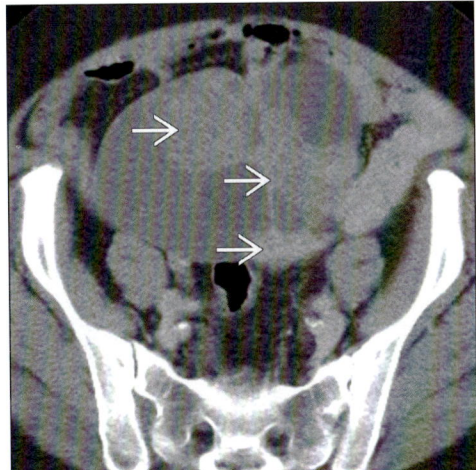

(Left) Gross pathology shows a cystic mass with septations and solid components in a patient with ovarian serous cystadenocarcinoma. *(Right)* Axial CECT shows enhancing solid components ➡ in the cystic mass.

Typical

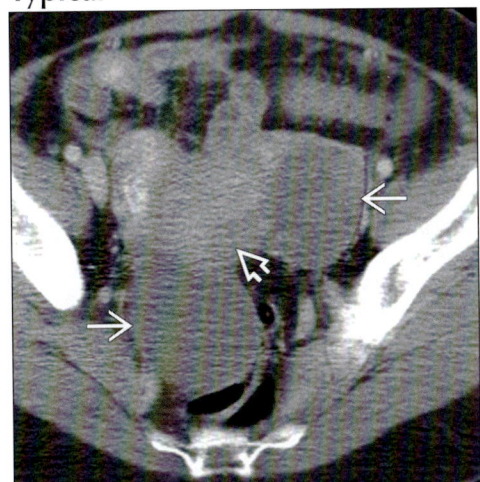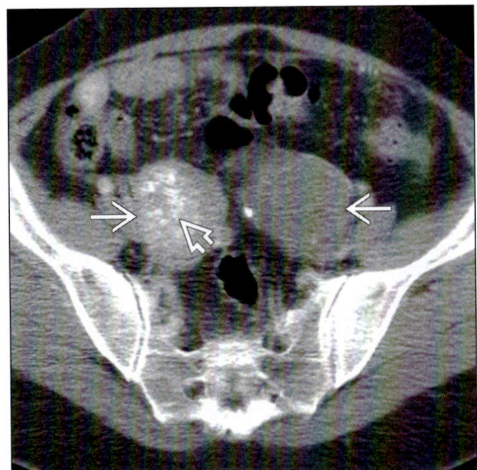

(Left) Axial CECT shows bilateral ovarian serous cystadenocarcinomas ➡. Uterus ⇨ is also seen. *(Right)* Axial CECT shows bilateral ovarian serous cystadenocarcinomas ➡. Note that calcifications ⇨ are seen in the mass on the right.

Typical

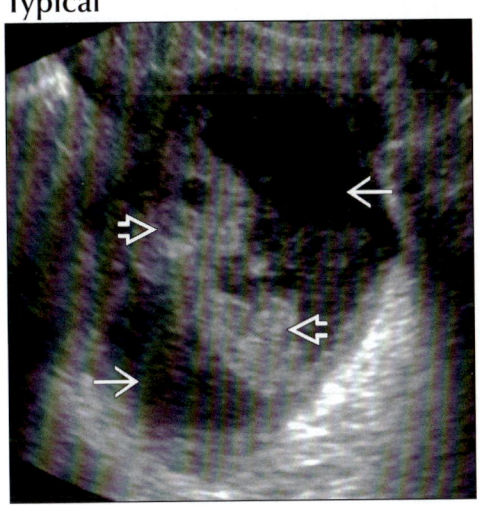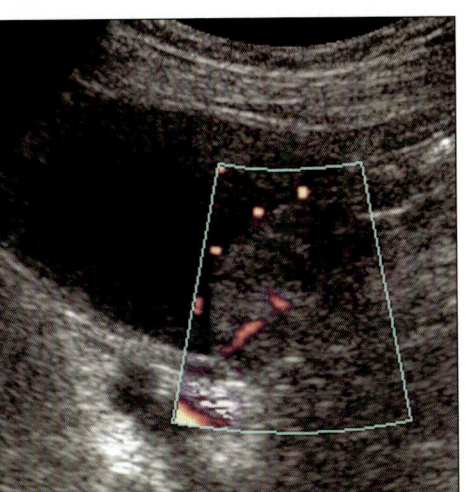

(Left) Sagittal oblique transvaginal ultrasound shows a left ovarian serous cystadenocarcinoma with hypoechoic cystic ➡ and echogenic solid ⇨ components. *(Right)* Axial oblique transabdominal power Doppler ultrasound shows flow in the solid component of an ovarian serous cystadenocarcinoma.

ENDOMETRIOID CARCINOMA, OVARY

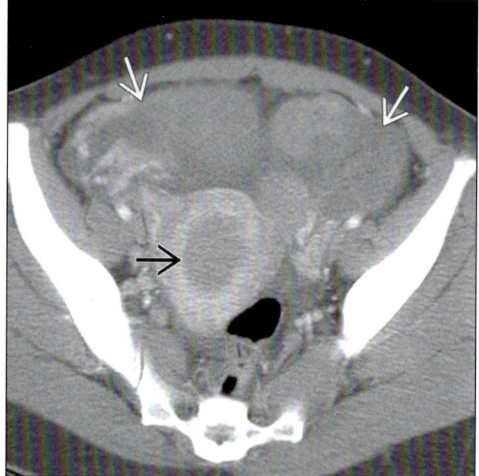

Transverse color Doppler ultrasound shows a mixed solid and cystic adnexal mass proven to be an endometrioid carcinoma. Flow is identified within thick septations ➡ confirming solid portions within the mass.

Axial CECT (same patient as previous) shows bilateral adnexal masses ➡. Endometrium is thickened ➡ in keeping with atypical complex hyperplasia with small foci of endometrioid adenocarcinoma.

TERMINOLOGY

Abbreviations and Synonyms
- Proliferative endometrioid tumor, endometrioid tumor of low malignant potential

Definitions
- Subtype of epithelial ovarian neoplasm

IMAGING FINDINGS

General Features
- Best diagnostic clue
  - Mixed solid/cystic ovarian mass
  - Endometrial thickening
- Location: 30% are bilateral
- Morphology
  - Imaging appearance nonspecific
  - Most commonly mixed solid/cystic mass
  - More often predominantly solid than other epithelial malignancies
  - Solid nodule developing within endometrioma or area of endometriosis

Ultrasonographic Findings
- Grayscale Ultrasound
  - Mixed solid/cystic mass
  - Alternating anechoic and intermediate echogenicity areas
  - Predominantly solid mass with areas of hemorrhage or necrosis
  - May demonstrate associated ascites and peritoneal implants in advanced stages
- Color Doppler: Vascularity demonstrated in solid components

CT Findings
- NECT
  - Low attenuation cystic mass
  - Solid areas present as soft tissue density
- CECT
  - Enhancing solid components
  - Mural tumoral nodules enhance
    - Allows differentiation from blood clot or debris
  - Staging of advanced disease
    - Ascites and intraperitoneal metastases (outside pelvis)
    - Retroperitoneal lymphadenopathy

DDx: Endometrioid Carcinoma

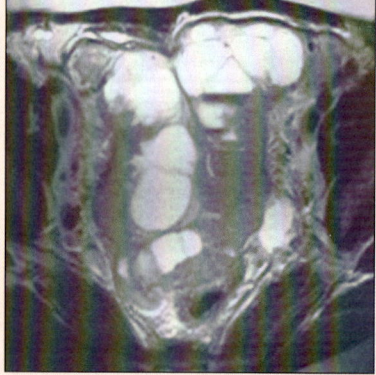

Serous Cystadenocarcinoma

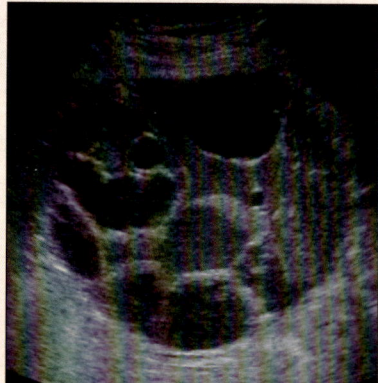

Mucinous Cystadenocarcinoma

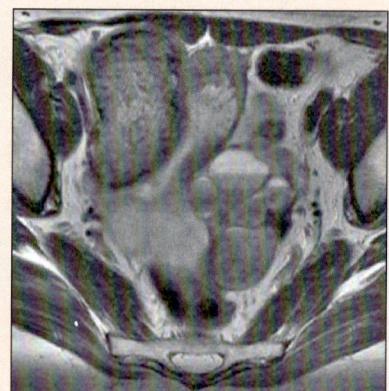

Endometrioma

ENDOMETRIOID CARCINOMA, OVARY

Key Facts

Imaging Findings
- Mixed solid/cystic ovarian mass
- Endometrial thickening
- Location: 30% are bilateral
- Imaging appearance nonspecific
- More often predominantly solid than other epithelial malignancies
- Solid nodule developing within endometrioma or area of endometriosis

Top Differential Diagnoses
- Serous Cystadenoma/Carcinoma
- Mucinous Cystadenoma/Carcinoma
- Clear Cell Carcinoma
- Endometrioma

Pathology
- Third most common malignant ovarian neoplasm after serous and mucinous cystadenocarcinomas
- 15-20% of patients have endometriosis, compared to 3-5% with mucinous/serous cystadenoma
- Endometrial hyperplasia or carcinoma in 20-35%, as an independent primary tumor rather than metastatic

Diagnostic Checklist
- Endometrioid carcinoma must be considered in presence of a pure solid ovarian mass in a postmenopausal woman with coexisting endometrial neoplasm
- Endometriotic cysts with enhancing mural nodules are very suspicious for endometrioid or clear cell carcinoma

---

- Liver and/or lung metastasis

MR Findings
- T1WI
  - Low to intermediate signal intensity (SI) cystic mass
  - Intermediate SI solid components
  - When arising from an endometrioma, may present as low or intermediate SI nodule in an otherwise high SI mass
  - In the setting of endometriosis, bright SI endometriotic foci may be seen in cul-de-sac or along utero-sacral ligaments
- T1WI FS: Confirms bright signal on T1WI is related to blood products or high mucin content, rather than fat
- T2WI
  - High SI cystic mass
  - Intermediate or heterogeneous SI solid components
  - When arising from an endometrioma, may present as an intermediate or high SI nodule in an otherwise low SI mass
  - In the setting of endometriosis, low SI endometriotic plaque may be seen in cul-de-sac or along utero-sacral ligaments
- T1 C+ FS
  - Solid components show marked enhancement
  - Subtraction views help demonstrate true enhancement when lesion is hyperintense prior to contrast administration

Imaging Recommendations
- Best imaging tool
  - Transvaginal ultrasound (TVS) is the initial modality of choice: Demonstrates cystic and solid nature of a mass
  - MR is a problem solving modality in cases of indeterminate adnexal mass on TVS
  - CT of the abdomen and pelvis is most often used for pre-operative staging and follow-up
- Protocol advice: Color Doppler and contrast-enhanced images differentiate tumoral tissue from blood clot/debris

DIFFERENTIAL DIAGNOSIS

Serous Cystadenoma/Carcinoma
- Most commonly presents as cystic mass with papillary projections
- Calcified psammoma bodies may be detected by CT

Mucinous Cystadenoma/Carcinoma
- Large, multiloculated cystic mass
- "Marble" appearance due to variable mucin content within locules

Clear Cell Carcinoma
- Almost always malignant
- 30-35% associated with endometriosis
  - May develop from an endometrioma
- Mixed solid/cystic mass
- No definite imaging criteria to differentiate from other epithelial neoplasms

Endometrioma
- Uniform high SI on T1WI
- Low SI on T2WI: Shading
- Absence of enhancing soft tissue nodule

PATHOLOGY

General Features
- Etiology
  - Most arise from ovarian surface epithelium
  - May arise from endometriosis
- Epidemiology
  - Third most common malignant ovarian neoplasm after serous and mucinous cystadenocarcinomas
    - 15-20% of epithelial ovarian cancers
    - 20-25% of all ovarian carcinomas
  - 15-20% of patients have endometriosis, compared to 3-5% with mucinous/serous cystadenoma
  - 80% of endometrioid ovarian neoplasms are malignant
  - 20% borderline

ENDOMETRIOID CARCINOMA, OVARY

- Presentation at earlier stage than other ovarian carcinomas
  - ≥ 50% of patients have stage I or II disease
- Associated abnormalities
  - Endometrial hyperplasia or carcinoma in 20-35%, as an independent primary tumor rather than metastatic
    - Cause of association not precisely known
    - Patients with synchronous endometrioid cancers tend to be younger, obese, nulliparous and premenopausal, suggesting an underlying hormonal "field effect"
  - Direct association with endometriosis in 15-20% of cases
  - 1% of patients with endometriosis will develop malignant transformation (endometrioid carcinoma, clear cell carcinoma, or both)
    - Malignant transformation most commonly in ovaries although extra-gonadal sites can be affected
    - Subgroup of postmenopausal women with a long history of endometriosis especially predisposed

Gross Pathologic & Surgical Features
- Similar to other epithelial lesions
- Mass with variable cystic and solid components
- Occasionally completely solid

Microscopic Features
- Tubular glandular pattern embedded in a fibrous, collagenized stroma
- Neoplastic cells lack mucin
- Alcian Blue-positive glycocalyx
- Mimic endometrial adenocarcinoma with pseudostratified epithelium and metastatic colon carcinoma
  - Ovary and endometrial carcinoma are positive for cytokeratin 7, negative for cytokeratin 20 immunochemistry (reverse pattern seen with metastatic colon cancer)
- Squamous differentiation in 33%
- Include malignant mixed mesodermal tumors (carcinosarcomas)
- Most commonly clearly malignant tumor, with destructive infiltrative growth pattern
- High incidence of concomitant synchronous endometrial carcinoma, as a second primary tumor rather than metastatic
  - Histologic dissimilarity of tumors
  - No evidence of spread of endometrial or ovarian cancer

Staging, Grading or Classification Criteria
- FIGO staging system for ovarian cancer

CLINICAL ISSUES

Presentation
- Most common signs/symptoms
  - Increase in abdominal girth
  - Postmenopausal vaginal bleeding
  - Hypermenorrhea
- Other signs/symptoms: Elevated CA-125

Demographics
- Age
  - 5th-6th decade
  - Younger age when associated with endometriosis

Natural History & Prognosis
- Overall better outcome than serous or mucinous carcinoma, independent of stage
  - Present at earlier stage
  - Younger patients

Treatment
- Cytoreductive surgery
- Neoadjuvant chemotherapy

DIAGNOSTIC CHECKLIST

Consider
- Endometrioid carcinoma must be considered in presence of a pure solid ovarian mass in a postmenopausal woman with coexisting endometrial neoplasm

Image Interpretation Pearls
- Endometriotic cysts with enhancing mural nodules are very suspicious for endometrioid or clear cell carcinoma

SELECTED REFERENCES

1. Imaoka I et al: Developing an MR imaging strategy for diagnosis of ovarian masses. Radiographics. 26(5):1431-48, 2006
2. Valenzuela P et al: Endometrioid adenocarcinoma of the ovary and endometriosis. Eur J Obstet Gynecol Reprod Biol. 2006
3. Soliman PT et al: Synchronous primary cancers of the endometrium and ovary: a single institution review of 84 cases. Gynecol Oncol. 94(2):456-62, 2004
4. Jung SE et al: CT and MR imaging of ovarian tumors with emphasis on differential diagnosis. Radiographics. 22(6):1305-25, 2002
5. Seidman JD et al: Blaustein's pathology of the female genital tract: Surface Epithelia Tumors of the Ovary. 5th ed. New York, Springer-Verlag. 791-904, 2002
6. Jeong YY et al: Imaging evaluation of ovarian masses. Radiographics. 20(5):1445-70, 2000
7. Wagner BJ et al: From the archives of the AFIP. Ovarian epithelial neoplasms: radiologic-pathologic correlation. Radiographics. 14(6):1351-74; quiz 1375-6, 1994
8. Norris HJ: Proliferative endometrioid tumors and endometrioid tumors of low malignant potential of the ovary. Int J Gynecol Pathol. 12(2):134-40, 1993

ENDOMETRIOID CARCINOMA, OVARY

IMAGE GALLERY

Typical

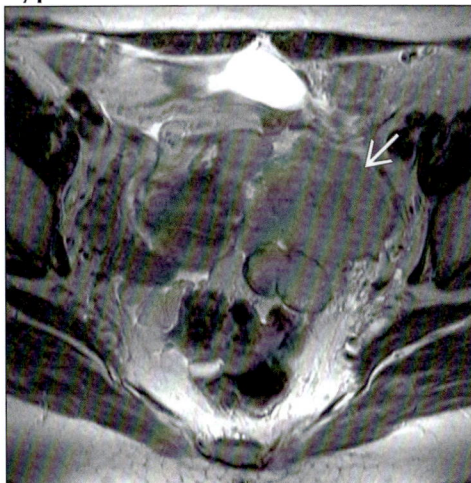
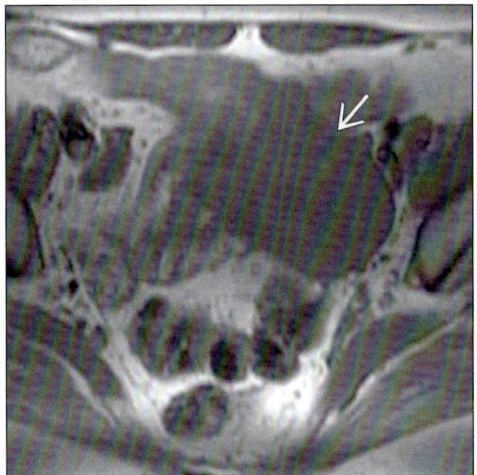

(Left) Axial T2WI MR shows a solid, lobulated, left adnexal mass ➔ of intermediate signal intensity (SI). No separate left ovary was identified. *(Right)* Axial T1WI MR in the same patient as previous image, shows the adnexal mass ➔ to be of relatively homogeneous intermediate SI.

Typical

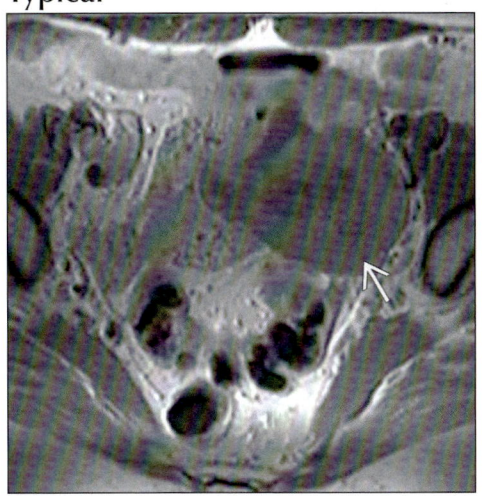
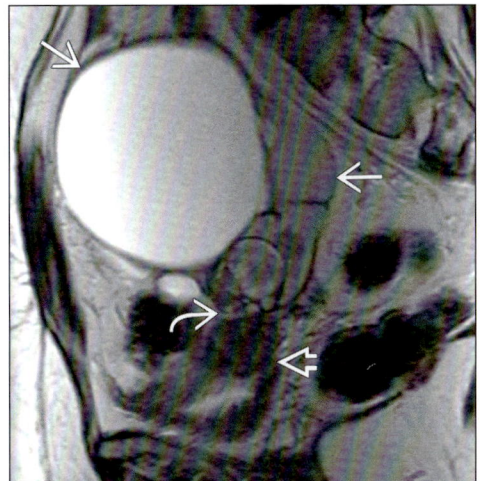

(Left) Axial T1 C+ MR (same patient as previous image) shows peripheral, heterogeneous enhancement of the left adnexal mass ➔ confirming its solid nature. *(Right)* Sagittal T2WI MR shows a complex left adnexal mass. There is a tubular component with locules of variable SI ➔, suggesting the presence of a hydro/hematosalpinx. Along the inferior portion of the mass a nodular component ➔ is suspected extending to the bladder wall ➔.

Typical

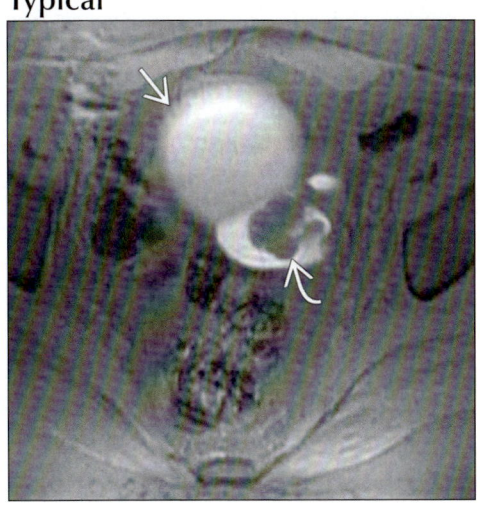
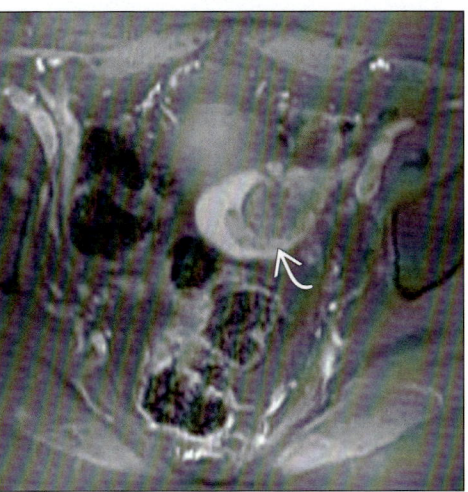

(Left) Axial T1WI FS MR (same patient as previous image) shows the cystic portion of the lesion to be hyperintense ➔ consistent with hemorrhagic products. Nodular component ➔ is of intermediate SI. *(Right)* Axial T1 C+ FS MR (same patient as previous image) shows enhancement of the nodular component ➔. The final diagnosis was endometrioid carcinoma arising from left ovarian endometriosis with secondary invasion of the left fallopian tube & bladder wall.

ENDOMETRIOID CARCINOMA, OVARY

Typical

(Left) Sagittal transabdominal ultrasound shows a large complex cyst with nodular solid component ➤. Histology was endometrioid tumor. (Right) Transverse transvaginal ultrasound in the same patient as previous image, shows the nodular solid components ➤.

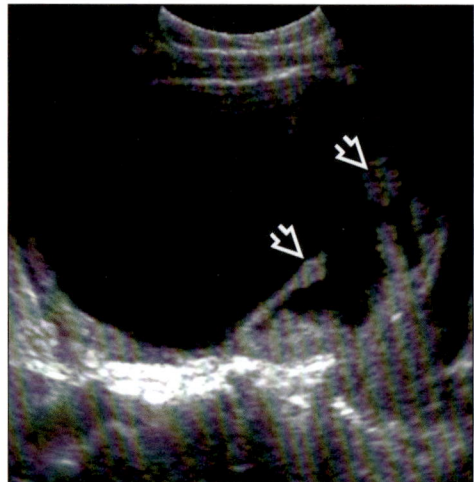
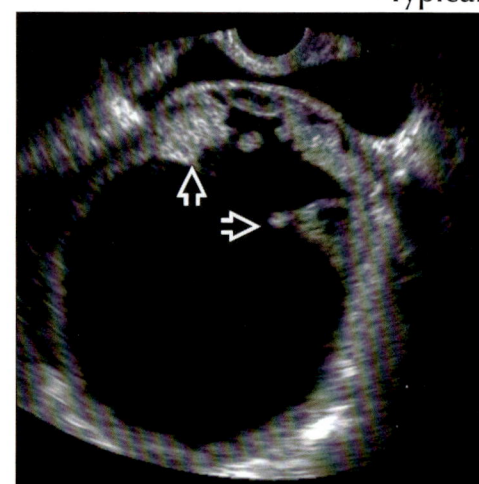

Typical

(Left) Sagittal oblique transvaginal ultrasound shows a cyst (calipers) with low level internal echoes and a solid component ➤ anteriorly. (Right) Transverse transvaginal ultrasound shows the ovary (calipers) with a cyst ➤ with scattered low level internal echoes.

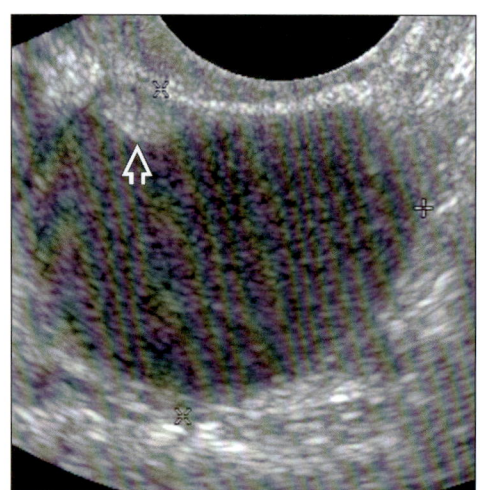
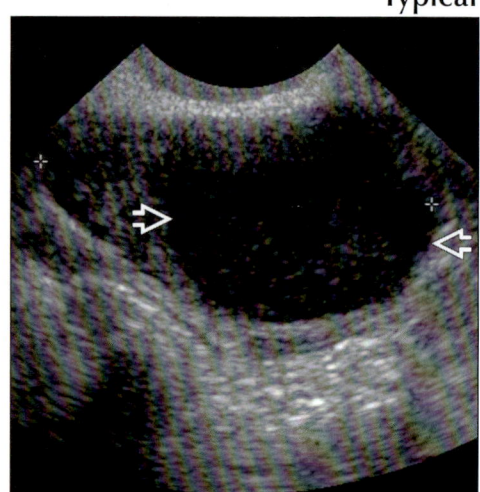

Typical

(Left) Sagittal oblique color Doppler ultrasound shows a complex cyst ➤ arising from some normal appearing ovarian tissue ➤. A complex nodule is seen inferiorly ➤. (Right) Transverse transvaginal ultrasound in the same patient as previous image, shows the heterogeneous solid component ➤ of the tumor.

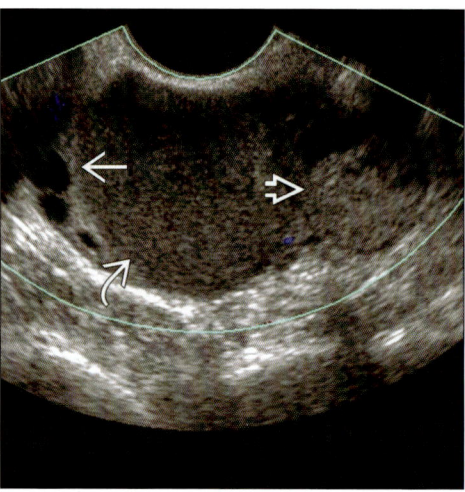
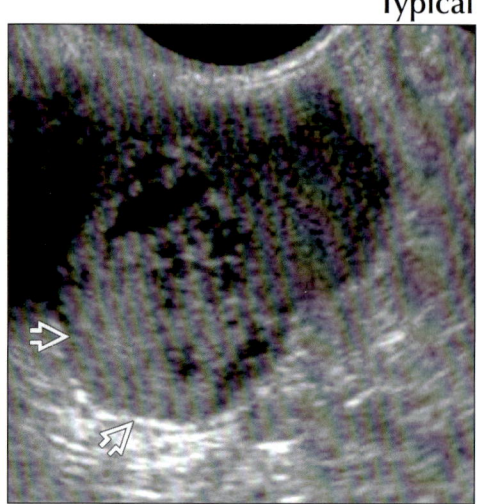

ENDOMETRIOID CARCINOMA, OVARY

Typical

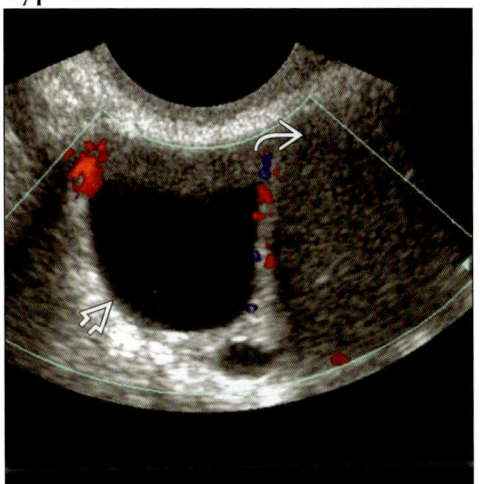
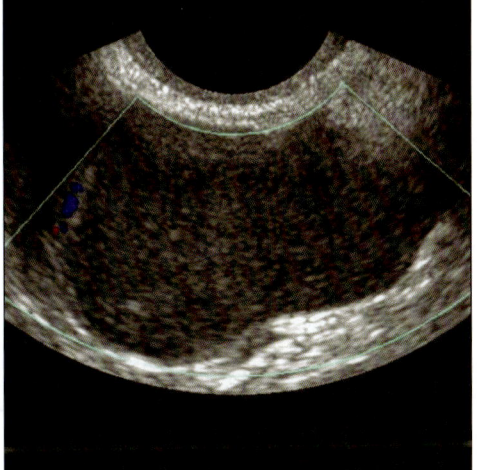

(Left) Transverse color Doppler ultrasound shows a complex mass with an anechoic cyst ➤ and a cyst with low level internal echoes ➤, suggestive on an endometrioma. *(Right)* Transverse color Doppler ultrasound in the same patient as previous image, shows a cyst with diffuse low level internal echoes. Histology showed an endometrioid tumor arising from an endometrioma.

Typical

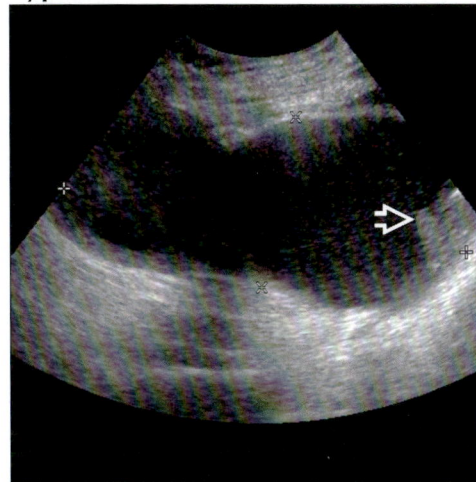
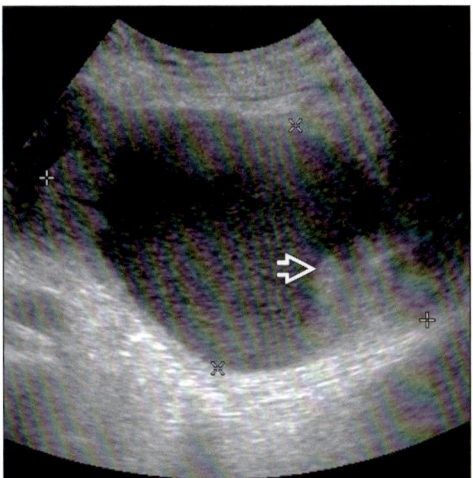

(Left) Sagittal transabdominal ultrasound shows a large bilobed cyst (calipers) with solid elements ➤. *(Right)* Sagittal transabdominal ultrasound in the same patient as previous image, shows complex cyst (calipers) with frond-like solid portion ➤ inferiorly. Low level internal echoes are seen within the cyst.

Typical

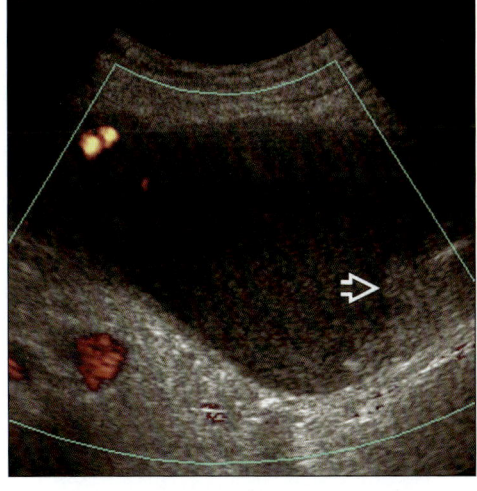
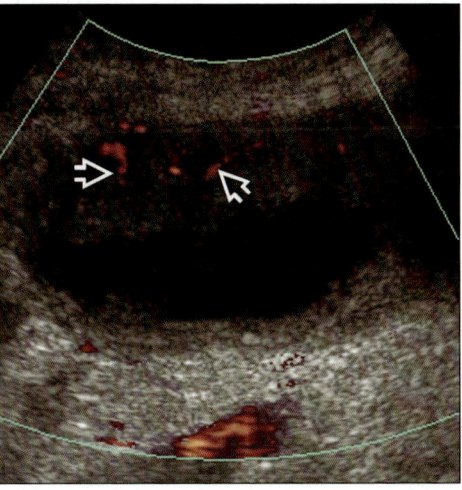

(Left) Sagittal power Doppler ultrasound in the same patient as previous image shows cyst with low level internal echoes and a solid appearing component inferiorly ➤. *(Right)* Transverse power Doppler ultrasound in the same patient as previous image, shows flow in a solid-appearing portion ➤ anteriorly. Histology was endometrioid tumor.

SERTOLI-LEYDIG CELL TUMOR

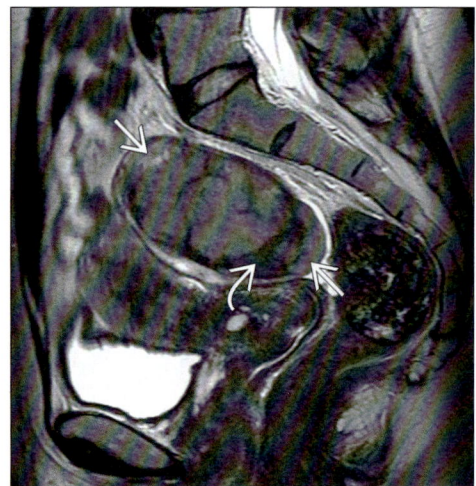

Sagittal T2WI MR shows Sertoli-Leydig cell tumor seen as an intermediate signal intensity solid mass ➡ with low signal intensity fibrous components ➚.

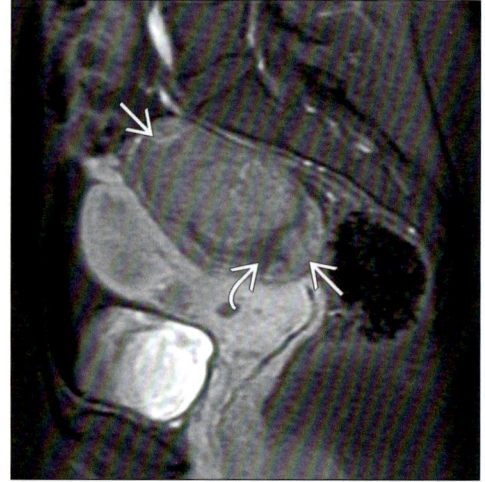

Sagittal T1 C+ FS MR shows marked enhancement in the tumor ➡. Note that fibrous components ➚ demonstrate relatively less enhancement.

TERMINOLOGY

Abbreviations and Synonyms
- Arrhenoblastoma, androblastoma, gonadal stromal tumor of android type

Definitions
- Type of sex cord-stromal tumor of ovary

IMAGING FINDINGS

General Features
- Best diagnostic clue: Well-defined, enhancing, solid mass in ovary
- Location
  - Mostly unilateral
  - Bilateral tumors are very rare
- Size
  - Tumor size varies from very small to large tumors measuring up to 5-15 cm
  - Hormonally active tumors may be small when symptomatic
- Morphology
  - Mostly nodular solid tumors
  - Cystic, necrotic, and hemorrhagic components may be present

Ultrasonographic Findings
- Grayscale Ultrasound
  - Heterogeneous echogenicity similar to soft tissue
  - Anechoic or hypoechoic cystic areas may also be seen
- Color Doppler
  - Intratumoral vascularity can be detected
  - Detection of vascularity in tumor helps in excluding a complex cyst
- Power Doppler: Provides improved detection of intratumoral vascularity

CT Findings
- NECT
  - Soft tissue attenuation lesion
  - Calcification is rare
- CECT
  - Marked enhancement in solid portion of tumor
  - Enhancement can be homogeneous or heterogeneous

DDx: Sex Cord-Stromal Tumors of Ovary

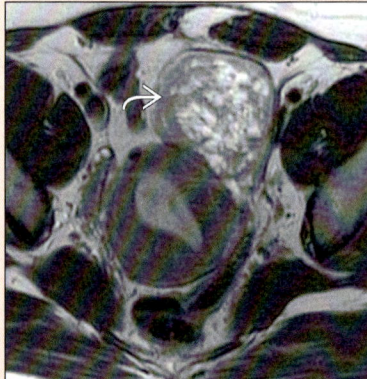

Granulosa Cell Tumor

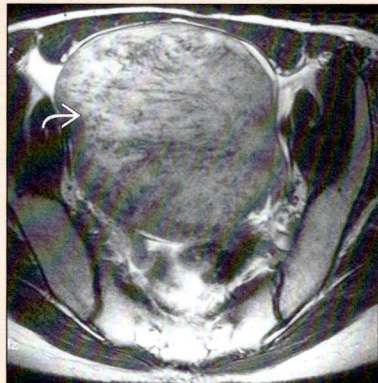

Fibrothecoma

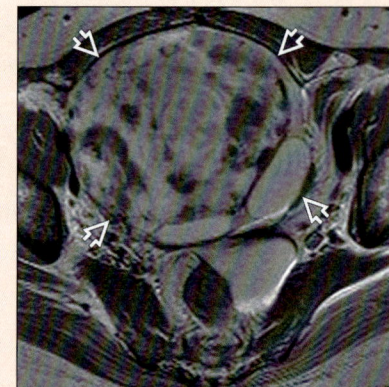

Sclerosing Stromal Tumor

SERTOLI-LEYDIG CELL TUMOR

Key Facts

Terminology
- Type of sex cord-stromal tumor of ovary

Pathology
- They contain Sertoli cells, Leydig cells, and fibroblasts
- These cellular components can be seen in varying proportions
- Varying cellular differentiation can be seen in different components of these tumors
- Sertoli-Leydig cell tumors are the most common virilizing ovarian tumors
- However, they represent less than 0.5% of all ovarian tumors
- Associated abnormalities: Virilization occurs in one-third to one-half of patients

Clinical Issues
- Most common presenting symptom is due to virilization
- Loss of female secondary sex characteristics
- Progressive masculinization
- Average age is 25 and 75% of cases are under 30
- Most of these tumors have benign clinical courses
- However, malignancy can be seen in about 20% of cases
- Preservation of fertility is important in young women with tumors confined in ovary

Diagnostic Checklist
- Most patients undergo extensive clinical, laboratory and imaging work-up for definitive diagnosis
- Predominantly solid, unilateral ovarian mass in a patient with virilization

---

  - Non-enhancing cystic or necrotic components can also be seen

MR Findings
- T1WI
  - Signal intensity similar to muscle
  - Small tumors may not be differentiated form ovarian stroma
- T2WI
  - Intermediate signal intensity in solid component
  - Low signal intensity can be seen in fibrous stroma
  - High signal intensity cystic or necrotic areas can be seen
- T1 C+
  - Marked enhancement in solid portion of tumor
  - Enhancement can be homogeneous or heterogeneous
  - Non-enhancing cystic or necrotic components can also be seen

Imaging Recommendations
- Best imaging tool
  - Transvaginal US or MR can be used to detect these tumors
  - MR with contrast may be better to detect small tumors

DIFFERENTIAL DIAGNOSIS

Granulosa Cell Tumor
- Most commonly present with estrogenic manifestations
- They can have various appearances including solid, mixed cystic and solid, or completely cystic tumors

Fibroma, Fibrothecoma, and Thecoma
- Typically low signal intensity on T2WI due to their abundant collagen and fibrous contents
- Intratumoral edema or cellular components may have intermediate to high signal intensity
- Fibroma shows no estrogenic activity
- Lipid-rich thecoma can show estrogenic activity

Sclerosing Stromal Tumor of Ovary
- Masses with cystic and heterogeneous solid components
- They demonstrate early peripheral enhancement with centripetal progression

PATHOLOGY

General Features
- General path comments
  - Sertoli-Leydig cell tumors are classified under sex cord-stromal tumors of ovary
  - They contain Sertoli cells, Leydig cells, and fibroblasts
    - These cellular components can be seen in varying proportions
    - Varying cellular differentiation can be seen in different components of these tumors
  - Subtypes of Sertoli-Leydig cell tumor are
    - Well-differentiated
    - Intermediately-differentiated
    - Poorly-differentiated
    - Retiform
- Epidemiology
  - Sertoli-Leydig cell tumors are the most common virilizing ovarian tumors
  - However, they represent less than 0.5% of all ovarian tumors
- Associated abnormalities: Virilization occurs in one-third to one-half of patients

Gross Pathologic & Surgical Features
- Yellow/tan nodular solid tumors that rarely contain cysts
- Poorly-differentiated tumors have more necrosis or hemorrhage

Microscopic Features
- Tumor cells stain positively for inhibin immunohistochemistry

SERTOLI-LEYDIG CELL TUMOR

- Generally see a combination of Sertoli and Leydig cells, although pure Leydig cell tumors may occur
- Well-differentiated
  - Cellular and acellular areas
  - Solid or tubular structures lined by Sertoli-type cells
  - Intervening stroma contains Leydig cells (polyhedral eosinophilic cells)
  - Leydig cells may contain Reinke crystals
- Moderately-differentiated
  - Cellular areas separated by loose fibrous/fibromyxoid stroma
  - Immature Sertoli cells (resembling sex cords of immature testes) form cords or sheets
  - Mature Leydig cells seen in the loose stroma
- Poorly-differentiated
  - Sheets of spindle shaped cells with occasional thin cord-like structures
  - Mitoses prominent
  - Leydig cells are more difficult to find
- Retiform (resemblance to rete testis) variant
  - Seen in 14% of moderately differentiated tumors & 30% of poorly differentiated tumors
  - Irregular network of slit-like spaces lined by cuboidal cells
  - 40% of tumors with a retiform pattern show heterologous elements (fat, cartilage, muscle, bone)

CLINICAL ISSUES

Presentation
- Most common signs/symptoms
  - Most common presenting symptom is due to virilization
  - Loss of female secondary sex characteristics
    - Oligomenorrhea
    - Amenorrhea
    - Atrophy of breasts
    - Disappearance of female body contours
  - Progressive masculinization
    - Acne
    - Increasing facial hair growth
    - Temporal balding
    - Deepening of voice
    - Enlargement of clitoris
- Other signs/symptoms
  - Increased serum testosterone and androstenedione
  - Abdominal swelling and pain
  - Increased red blood cell count

Demographics
- Age
  - They usually occur in young women
    - Average age is 25 and 75% of cases are under 30
  - Cases in older women have also been reported

Natural History & Prognosis
- Most of these tumors have benign clinical courses
- However, malignancy can be seen in about 20% of cases

Treatment
- Treatment is individualized depending on
  - Patient's age and preference
  - Tumor grade and stage
- Preservation of fertility is important in young women with tumors confined in ovary
  - Young women with stage I tumors can be treated with unilateral salpingooophorectomy
- Stage II or higher disease requires total abdominal hysterectomy and bilateral salpingooophorectomy
- Adjuvant therapy can be given with radiation or combination chemotherapy
  - In cases with tumors containing poorly differentiated elements or heterologous elements

DIAGNOSTIC CHECKLIST

Consider
- Virilization in a female can be caused by several different conditions such as
  - Cushing syndrome
  - Adrenal neoplasms
  - Ovarian neoplasms
  - Other ovarian conditions such as
    - Polycystic ovary syndrome
    - Stromal hyperplasia
    - Stromal hyperthecosis
- Most patients undergo extensive clinical, laboratory and imaging work-up for definitive diagnosis
- Imaging is indicated depending on clinical scenario
- In many cases appropriate imaging can be the problem solving tool
- Sertoli-Leydig cell tumors in some patients with virilization may be small and difficult to detect on imaging
  - Exploratory laparotomy with intraoperative selective venous blood sampling may be useful be to localize these small tumors

Image Interpretation Pearls
- Predominantly solid, unilateral ovarian mass in a patient with virilization

SELECTED REFERENCES

1. Caringella A et al: A case of Sertoli-Leydig cell tumor in a postmenopausal woman. Int J Gynecol Cancer. 16(1):435-8, 2006
2. Elbadrawy M et al: Secondary amenorrhoea due to Leydig cell tumour. J Obstet Gynaecol. 25(5):529-30, 2005
3. Jung SE et al: CT and MRI findings of sex cord-stromal tumor of the ovary. AJR Am J Roentgenol. 185(1):207-15, 2005
4. Oliva E et al: Sertoli cell tumors of the ovary: a clinicopathologic and immunohistochemical study of 54 cases. Am J Surg Pathol. 29(2):143-56, 2005
5. Appetecchia M et al: Sertoli-Leydig cell androgens-estrogens secreting tumor of the ovary: ultra-conservative surgery. Eur J Obstet Gynecol Reprod Biol. 116(1):113-6, 2004
6. Tanaka YO et al: Functioning ovarian tumors: direct and indirect findings at MR imaging. Radiographics. 24 Suppl 1:S147-66, 2004
7. Jung SE et al: CT and MR imaging of ovarian tumors with emphasis on differential diagnosis. Radiographics. 22(6):1305-25, 2002
8. Lantzsch T et al: Sertoli-Leydig cell tumor. Arch Gynecol Obstet. 264(4):206-8, 2001

SERTOLI-LEYDIG CELL TUMOR

IMAGE GALLERY

Typical

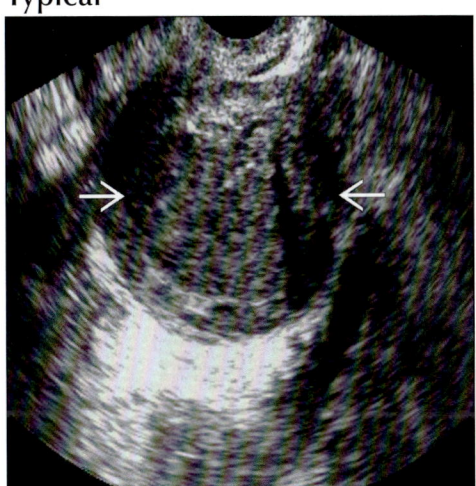
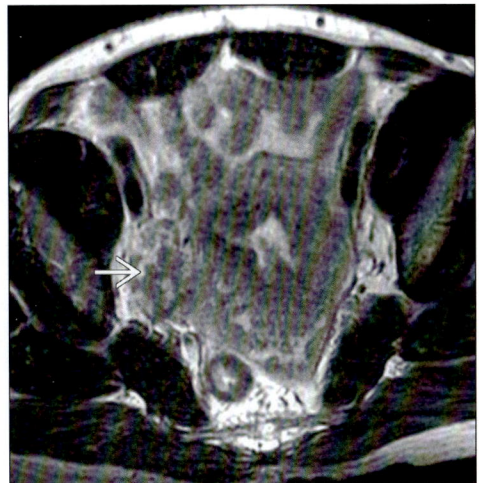

(Left) Axial oblique transabdominal ultrasound shows Sertoli-Leydig cell tumor seen as an echogenic solid mass ➡ in the ovary. *(Right)* Axial T2WI MR shows Sertoli-Leydig cell tumor seen as a heterogeneous solid mass ➡ in the right ovary in a patient with virilization. (Courtesy F. Coakley, MD).

Typical

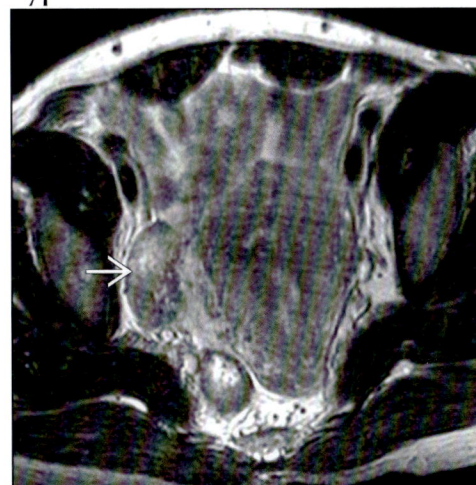
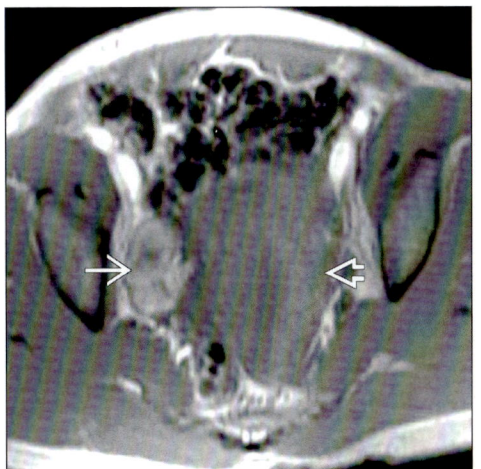

(Left) Axial T2WI MR shows Sertoli-Leydig cell tumor seen as a heterogeneous, well-defined, solid mass ➡ in the right ovary (Courtesy F. Coakley, MD). *(Right)* Axial T1 C+ MR shows that the mass ➡ has marked early enhancement during the arterial phase. Compare to enhancement in uterus ➡. (Courtesy F. Coakley, MD).

Typical

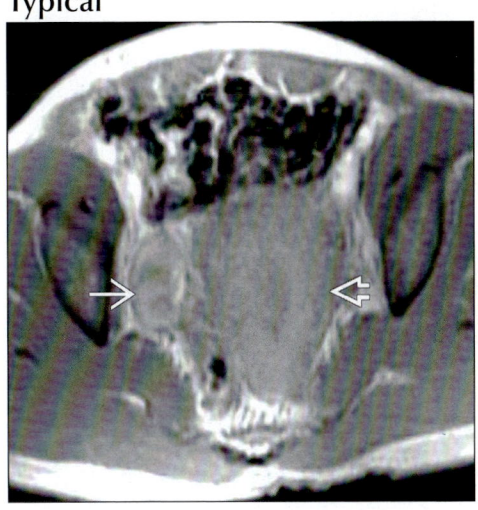
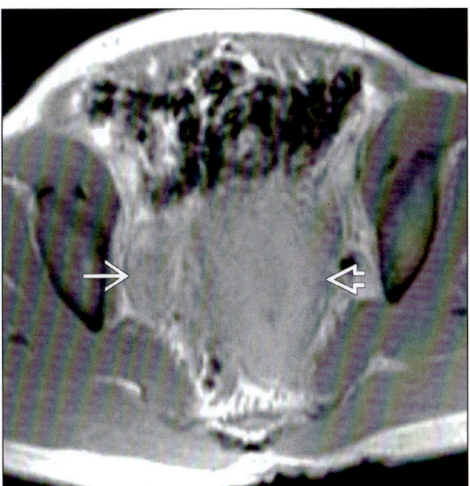

(Left) Axial T1 C+ MR shows that the mass ➡ remains slightly hyperintense compared to uterus ➡ during intermediate phase. (Courtesy F. Coakley, MD). *(Right)* Axial T1 C+ MR shows that the mass ➡ becomes isointense compared to uterus ➡ during delayed phase. (Courtesy F. Coakley, MD).

DYSGERMINOMA

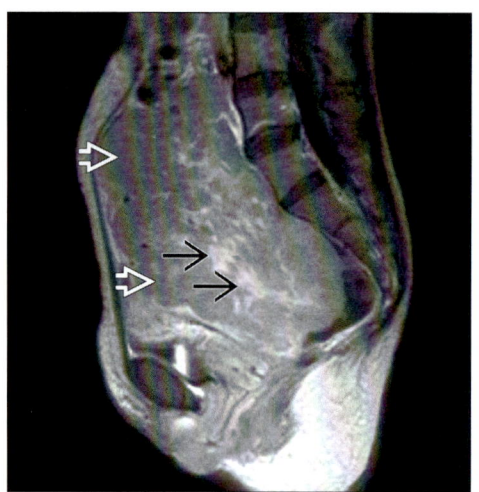

Sagittal T2WI MR shows ovarian dysgerminoma seen as lobulated, homogeneous intermediate signal intensity mass ⇨ with central high signal intensity area representing fibrovascular septa →.

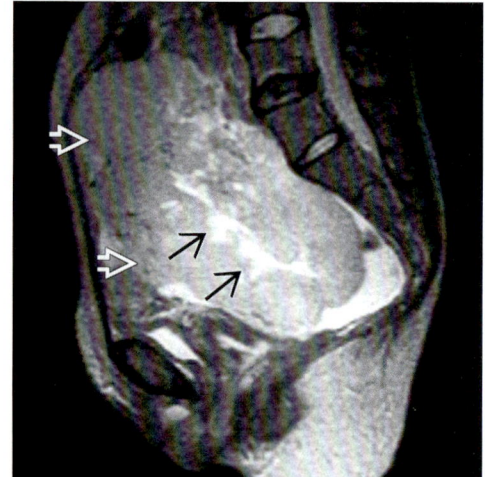

Sagittal T1 C+ MR shows that the dysgerminoma ⇨ homogeneously enhances. Note that strongly-enhancing fibrovascular septa → are seen within the mass.

TERMINOLOGY

Abbreviations and Synonyms
- Ovarian dysgerminoma

Definitions
- Type of malignant germ cell tumor of ovary
- Homologous to testicular seminoma

IMAGING FINDINGS

General Features
- Best diagnostic clue
  - Multilobulated solid adnexal mass with prominent fibrovascular septae
  - Speckled calcifications may be present
- Location: Usually unilateral ovarian involvement
- Size: Usually present as large masses
- Morphology: Large, lobulated, soft tissue masses

Ultrasonographic Findings
- Grayscale Ultrasound
  - Multilobulated solid ovarian mass with heterogeneous echogenicity
  - Necrotic/cystic portions are seen as anechoic areas
- Color Doppler: May demonstrate prominent flow in fibrovascular septae
- Power Doppler: More sensitive to flow in fibrovascular septae

CT Findings
- NECT
  - Solid components demonstrate soft tissue density
  - Necrotic areas demonstrate low attenuation
  - Areas of hemorrhage and speckled calcifications can be seen as high attenuation
- CECT
  - Multilobulated solid components demonstrate relatively homogeneous enhancement
  - Highly enhancing fibrovascular septae can be seen in mass
  - Non-enhancing areas representing necrosis may be present

MR Findings
- T1WI
  - Solid components demonstrate soft tissue intensity

DDx: Ovarian Masses

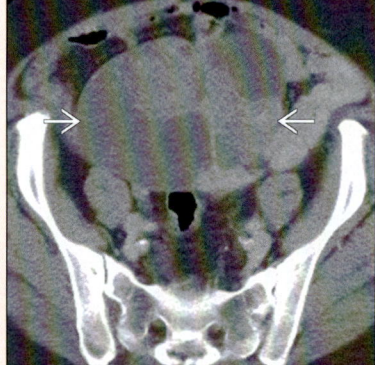

Serous Cystadenocarcinoma

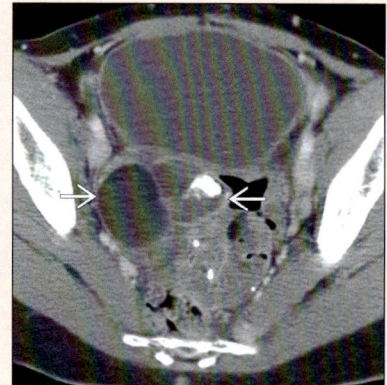

Malignant Teratoma

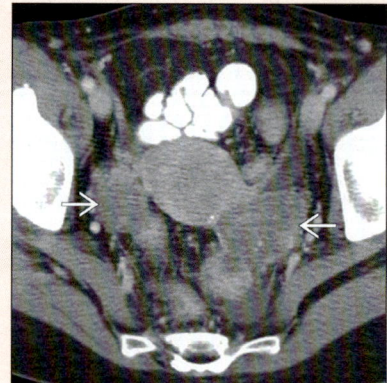

Ovarian Metastases

DYSGERMINOMA

Key Facts

Terminology
- Type of malignant germ cell tumor of ovary

Imaging Findings
- Multilobulated solid adnexal mass with prominent fibrovascular septae
- Speckled calcifications may be present
- MR is superior to US and CT in tumor characterization due to its better soft tissue resolution
- Protocol advice: Contrast-enhancement in CT and MR; and color or power Doppler in US are necessary to demonstrate fibrovascular septae within dysgerminoma

Top Differential Diagnoses
- Epithelial (Serous and Mucinous) Tumors of Ovary
- Teratoma
- Sex Cord-Stromal Tumors of Ovary
- Ovarian Metastasis

Pathology
- Germ cell tumors represent 15-20% of all ovarian tumors
- Dysgerminoma is the female equivalent of seminoma
- Dysgerminoma is the most common malignant germ cell tumor of the ovary

Diagnostic Checklist
- Dysgerminoma should be considered in differential diagnosis of young patient with pelvic mass, ascites, and pleural effusion
- Imaging findings characteristic of fibrovascular septae within large solid ovarian mass should raise possibility of dysgerminoma in young patient

---

  - Hemorrhage in mass seen as high signal intensity areas
- T2WI
  - Soft tissue components demonstrate intermediate-signal-intensity
  - Low-signal-intensity fibrovascular septae can be seen in mass
  - Necrotic areas demonstrate high-signal-intensity
- T1 C+
  - Soft tissue components demonstrate relatively homogeneous enhancement
  - Fibrovascular septae in mass demonstrate marked enhancement

Imaging Recommendations
- Best imaging tool
  - US, CT or MR can be used to detect and characterize adnexal mass
  - MR is superior to US and CT in tumor characterization due to its better soft tissue resolution
- Protocol advice: Contrast-enhancement in CT and MR; and color or power Doppler in US are necessary to demonstrate fibrovascular septae within dysgerminoma

DIFFERENTIAL DIAGNOSIS

Epithelial (Serous and Mucinous) Tumors of Ovary
- More complex, usually multiloculated masses
- Mainly cystic tumors containing solid components

Teratoma
- Complex mass with cystic and solid components
- Contain fat and calcifications

Sex Cord-Stromal Tumors of Ovary
- Typically solid ovarian masses
- Often manifest with tumor-mediated hormonal effects

Ovarian Metastasis
- Most ovarian metastases are solid or mixture of solid and cystic tumors
- Clinical presentation often due to primary disease

PATHOLOGY

General Features
- General path comments
  - Germ cell tumors represent 15-20% of all ovarian tumors
    - Germ cell tumors are the second most common ovarian tumors after epithelial ovarian neoplasms
  - Types of benign germ cell tumors
    - Mature teratoma
  - Types of malignant germ cell tumors
    - Immature teratoma
    - Dysgerminoma
    - Endodermal sinus tumor
    - Embryonal carcinoma
    - Choriocarcinoma
    - Malignant mixed germ cell tumor
  - Dysgerminoma is the female equivalent of seminoma
  - Ovarian dysgerminomas are "nonfunctional" neoplasms
    - May be accompanied by ovarian stromal luteinization and steroid hormone production; occasionally result in chemical or clinical hyperandrogenism
  - Pure dysgerminoma does not produce alpha fetoprotein (AFP)
  - Human chorionic gonadotropin (HCG) producing syncytiotrophoblastic giant cells are present in 5%
- Epidemiology
  - Dysgerminomas represent 0.5-2% of all malignant ovarian tumors
  - Dysgerminoma is the most common malignant germ cell tumor of the ovary

DYSGERMINOMA

Gross Pathologic & Surgical Features
- Lobulated, solid, soft to firm mass

Microscopic Features
- Germ cells with fibrous trabeculae infiltrated by lymphocytes and in some cases sarcoid-like granulomas

Staging, Grading or Classification Criteria
- FIGO staging system
  - Stage I: Tumor confined to ovaries
  - Stage II: Local extension; confined to true pelvis
  - Stage III: Nodal metastases or peritoneal implants outside pelvis
  - Stage IV: Distant metastases (excluding peritoneal metastases)

CLINICAL ISSUES

Presentation
- Most common signs/symptoms
  - Abdominal/pelvic pain
  - Abdominal/pelvic mass
  - Marked abdominal distension due to large mass and/or ascites
- Other signs/symptoms
  - Constipation
  - Nausea and vomiting
  - Urinary symptoms
- Clinical Profile
  - Most common presentation due to abdominal pain and/or palpable abdominal mass
  - 15-20% diagnosed during pregnancy or in postpartum period

Demographics
- Age
  - 75% occur in early reproductive years (2nd-3rd decade)
  - 10% in prepubertal girls

Natural History & Prognosis
- 5-year survival rates: 95% for early stages and 65% for advanced stages

Treatment
- Surgery: Most patients with dysgerminoma present with stage I disease and surgery is adequate
- Fertility-preserving operation can be considered in early-stage patients
- Chemotherapy: Reserved for advanced or recurrent disease
- Radiotherapy: Less commonly used in recent years in spite of radiosensitivity of dysgerminoma

DIAGNOSTIC CHECKLIST

Consider
- Dysgerminoma should be considered in differential diagnosis of young patient with pelvic mass, ascites, and pleural effusion
- In dysgerminomas nodal metastases are more likely than peritoneal metastases, which are more commonly seen in epithelial ovarian cancers

Image Interpretation Pearls
- Imaging findings characteristic of fibrovascular septae within large solid ovarian mass should raise possibility of dysgerminoma in young patient

SELECTED REFERENCES

1. De Backer A et al: Ovarian germ cell tumors in children: a clinical study of 66 patients. Pediatr Blood Cancer. 46(4):459-64, 2006
2. Boran N et al: Pregnancy outcomes and menstrual function after fertility sparing surgery for pure ovarian dysgerminomas. Arch Gynecol Obstet. 271(2):104-8, 2005
3. Gucer F et al: Ovarian dysgerminoma associated with Pseudo-Meigs' syndrome and functioning ovarian stroma: a case report. Gynecol Oncol. 97(2):681-4, 2005
4. Lu KH et al: Update on the management of ovarian germ cell tumors. J Reprod Med. 50(6):417-25, 2005
5. Guven S et al: Management of ovarian dysgerminoma during a pregnancy complicated by preeclampsia; a case report. Eur J Gynaecol Oncol. 25(6):759-60, 2004
6. Ramirez Torres N et al: [Clinical experience with chemotherapy of the malignant tumor of germinal cells (dysgerminoma) of the ovary] Ginecol Obstet Mex. 72:500-7, 2004
7. Togashi K. Related Articles et al: Ovarian cancer: the clinical role of US, CT, and MRI. Eur Radiol. 13 Suppl 4:L87-104, 2003
8. Jung SE et al: CT and MR imaging of ovarian tumors with emphasis on differential diagnosis. Radiographics. 22(6):1305-25, 2002
9. Akyuz C et al: Malignant ovarian tumors in children: 22 years of experience at a single institution. J Pediatr Hematol Oncol. 22(5):422-7, 2000
10. Ayhan A et al: Pure dysgerminoma of the ovary: a review of 45 well staged cases. Eur J Gynaecol Oncol. 21(1):98-101, 2000
11. Tewari K et al: Malignant germ cell tumors of the ovary. Obstet Gynecol. 95(1):128-33, 2000
12. Williams SD et al: Ovarian germ-cell tumors. In: Hoskins WJ, Perez CA, Young RC (eds). Principles and practice of gynecologic oncology, Lippincott Williams & Wilkins, Philadelphia. 1059-73, 2000
13. Casey AC et al: Dysgerminoma: the role of conservative surgery. Gynecol Oncol. 63(3):352-7, 1996
14. Kim SH et al: Ovarian dysgerminoma: color Doppler ultrasonographic findings and comparison with CT and MR imaging findings. J Ultrasound Med. 14(11):843-8, 1995
15. Tanaka YO et al: Ovarian dysgerminoma: MR and CT appearance. J Comput Assist Tomogr. 18(3):443-8, 1994

DYSGERMINOMA

IMAGE GALLERY

Typical

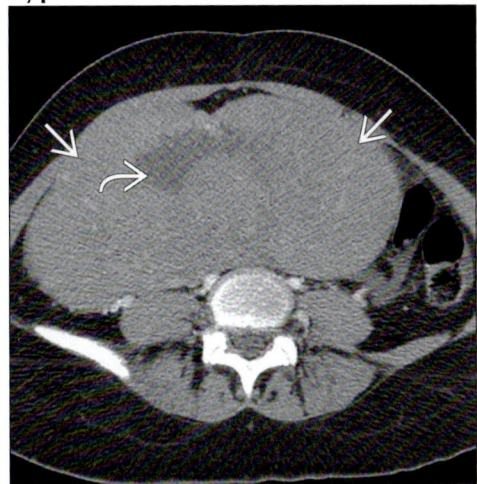
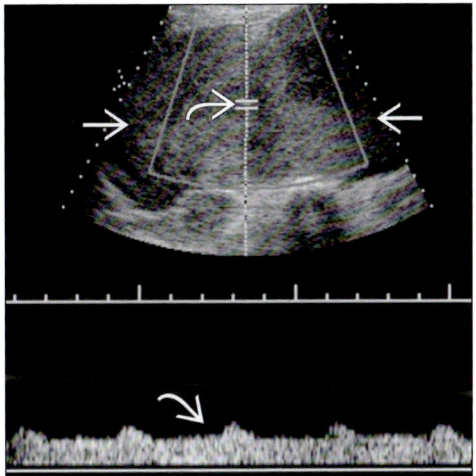

(Left) Axial CECT shows a large ovarian dysgerminoma ➔ that shows homogeneous enhancement except a central necrotic component ➔. *(Right)* Axial pulsed Doppler ultrasound shows heterogeneous echogenicity and vascular flow ➔ in a large ovarian dysgerminoma ➔.

Typical

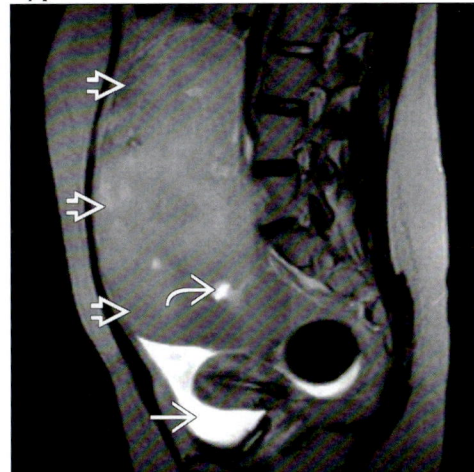
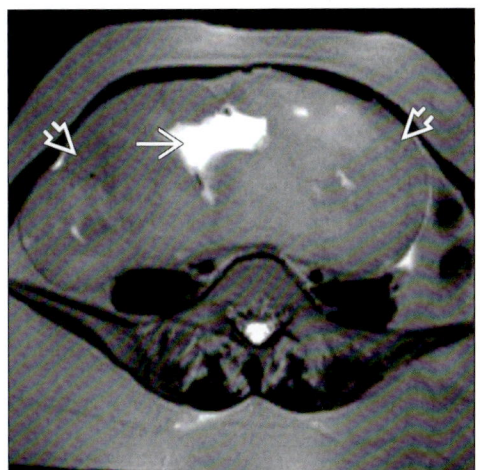

(Left) Sagittal T2WI MR shows a large ovarian dysgerminoma ➔ seen as a solid mass with a necrotic area ➔. Pelvic ascites ➔ are also seen. *(Right)* Axial T2WI MR shows a large ovarian dysgerminoma ➔ with a central necrotic area ➔.

Typical

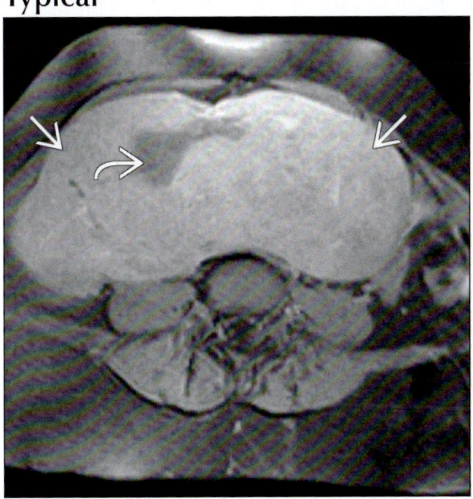
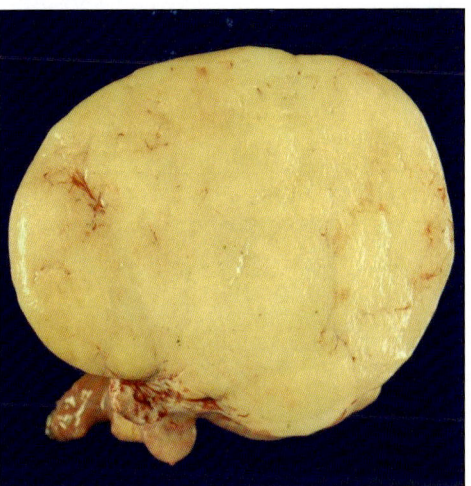

(Left) Axial T1 C+ FS MR shows that the mass shows marked homogeneous enhancement ➔ except the necrotic component ➔ which does not enhance. *(Right)* Gross pathology shows homogeneous solid ovarian mass in a patient with dysgerminoma.

YOLK SAC TUMOR, OVARY

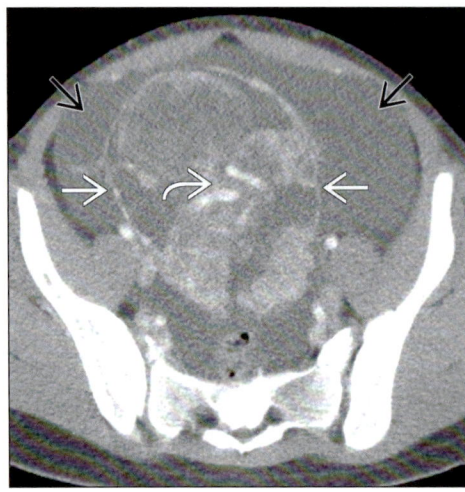

Axial CECT shows a strongly enhancing, predominantly solid pelvic mass containing necrotic areas. Note the presence of ascites and central intratumoral vessels.

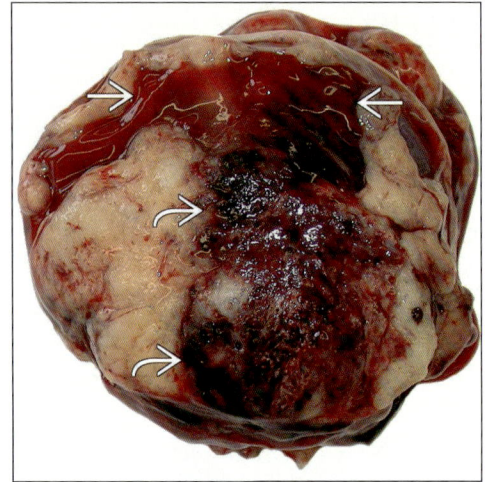

Gross pathology in the same patient as previous image, shows a large, solid, yellow tumor containing areas of hemorrhage and necrosis. Pathology: Malignant yolk sac tumor of the right ovary.

TERMINOLOGY

Abbreviations and Synonyms
- Endodermal sinus tumor

Definitions
- Type of malignant germ cell tumor

IMAGING FINDINGS

General Features
- Best diagnostic clue: Strongly enhancing solid mass with a varying amount of cystic portions and hemorrhage
- Location: Usually unilateral, with only 1% being bilateral
- Size: Mean 15 cm, ranges 7-28 cm
- Morphology: Predominantly solid mass containing irregular cystic or necrotic areas

Ultrasonographic Findings
- Predominantly solid mass
- Anechoic or hypoechoic cystic areas are usually present
- Multiple vessels may be seen within the solid mass
- Concurrent mature teratoma may be present
- Ascites and peritoneal implants may be present
- Enlarged pelvic lymph nodes and hydronephrosis may be present

CT Findings
- Complex, mainly solid adnexal mass with areas of low-attenuation representing necrosis and/or hemorrhage
- Avid peripheral enhancement and central necrosis following contrast medium administration
- Multiple intratumoral vessels can sometimes be appreciated
- Ascites and peritoneal implants may be present
- Enlarged pelvic and para-aortic lymph nodes may be present
- Co-existing mature teratoma with or without fat and calcifications may be present

MR Findings
- T1WI
  - Mainly solid mass of low signal intensity

DDx: Adnexal/Right Iliac Fossa Mass

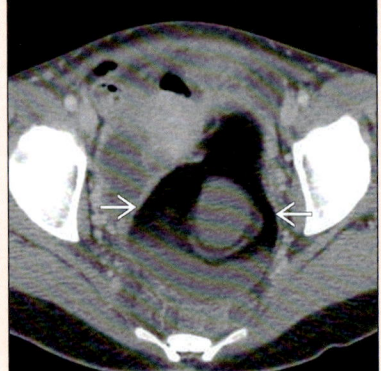

Mature Cystic Teratoma

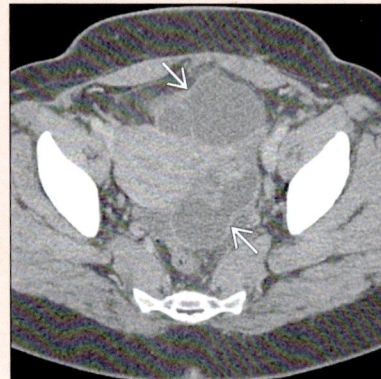

Tubo-Ovarian Abscess

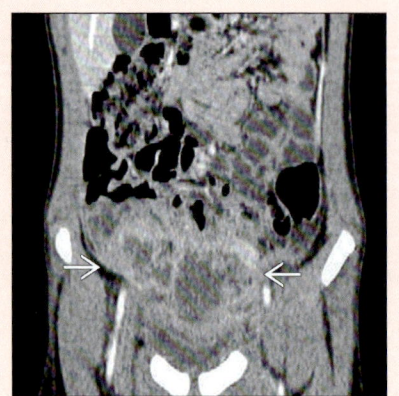

Appendicular Abscess

YOLK SAC TUMOR, OVARY

Key Facts

Terminology
- Endodermal sinus tumor
- Type of malignant germ cell tumor

Imaging Findings
- Best diagnostic clue: Strongly enhancing solid mass with a varying amount of cystic portions and hemorrhage
- Best imaging tool: CT or MR
- Protocol advice: Contrast medium administration is helpful to show enhancing solid components

Top Differential Diagnoses
- Mature Cystic Teratoma
- Tubo-Ovarian Abscess
- Appendiceal Abscess
- Other Malignant Germ Cell Tumors

Pathology
- Schiller-Duval bodies are pathognomonic but are only present in 20% of tumors

Clinical Issues
- Abdominal pain and palpable abdominal and pelvic mass
- Elevated serum α-fetoprotein in the majority of patients

Diagnostic Checklist
- Diagnosis of yolk sac tumor should be considered in a girl or young woman presenting with a large complex pelvic mass and elevated serum α-fetoprotein
- Prominent intratumoral signal voids and peripheral strong enhancement on MR

- ○ Portions of high signal intensity can be found caused by hemorrhage
- ○ Enlarged pelvic and para-aortic lymph nodes may be present
- T1WI FS
  - ○ High signal intensity areas following fat suppression indicate presence of hemorrhage
  - ○ Drop in signal intensity following fat suppression in a co-existing mature teratoma if present
- T2WI
  - ○ Heterogeneous, high signal intensity, mainly solid mass
  - ○ Areas of very high signal intensity represent hemorrhage
  - ○ Multiple signal-void structures can be seen caused by hypervascularity of the tumor
  - ○ Ascites and peritoneal deposits may be present
  - ○ Enlarged pelvic and para-aortic lymph nodes may be present
- T1 C+
  - ○ Strong peripheral enhancement due to tumor hypervascularity and irregular central necrosis
  - ○ Peritoneal deposits if present are best appreciated on delayed contrast-enhanced images

Imaging Recommendations
- Best imaging tool: CT or MR
- Protocol advice: Contrast medium administration is helpful to show enhancing solid components

DIFFERENTIAL DIAGNOSIS

Mature Cystic Teratoma
- Fat-containing mass with peripheral blood flow and avascular central solid portion (floating Rokitansky nodule on fat-fluid interface)

Tubo-Ovarian Abscess
- Raised inflammatory markers, fever, vaginal discharge
- Tubular unilateral or bilateral cystic adnexal lesions that demonstrate rim-enhancement on contrast-enhanced images

Appendiceal Abscess
- Raised inflammatory markers, fever, pain starts is epigastrium and moves into the right iliac fossa
- An appendicolith may be present
- Normal ovaries are seen separately from the inflammatory mass which is intimately related to the cecum

Other Malignant Germ Cell Tumors
- Dysgerminoma
  - ○ Usually a very large solid mass containing multiple fibrovascular septa
  - ○ Calcifications may be present
  - ○ Normal α-fetoprotein levels
- Choriocarcinoma
  - ○ History of recent intra/extrauterine pregnancy in case of gestational type
  - ○ Presence of intra/extrauterine trophoblastic disease, ovarian theca luteum cyst or corpus luteum cyst in gestational choriocarcinoma
  - ○ Normal α-fetoprotein levels
  - ○ Markedly elevated β-hCG levels
- Embryonal carcinoma
  - ○ Usually very large mass at presentation
  - ○ Serum β-hCG levels are usually elevated
- Dysgerminoma, non-gestational choriocarcinoma and embryonal carcinoma may co-exist with yolk sac tumor and can be very difficult to distinguish on imaging alone

Ovarian Carcinoma
- Usually bilateral rather than unilateral
- Older age-group
- Normal α-fetoprotein levels

PATHOLOGY

General Features
- Epidemiology
  - ○ Less than 1% of all malignant ovarian tumors

YOLK SAC TUMOR, OVARY

- Second most common malignant germ cell tumor of the ovary in children
- 9-16% of pediatric ovarian tumors
- Associated abnormalities
  - Pure yolk sac tumors are virtually always unilateral
  - Ipsilateral or contralateral mature teratomas can coexist in 14% of cases

Gross Pathologic & Surgical Features
- Large, friable, bosselated masses
- Cut surface is solid, grey/yellow with areas of hemorrhage, necrosis and cystic change

Microscopic Features
- Yolk sac tumors exhibit several distinct histological patterns, a combination of which can be seen in most tumors
- Reticular (microcystic, myxomatous), pseudopapillary (endodermal sinus), alveolar-glandular, polyvesicular vitelline and solid growth patterns
- Reticular pattern is most common forming a honeycomb network of variably sized cystic spaces lined by cells with clear cytoplasm and prominent nucleoli
- Schiller-Duval bodies are pathognomonic but are only present in 20% of tumors
- Schiller-Duval bodies are "renal glomerulus"-like structures with a central elongated capillary in a loose stroma surrounded by a single layer of cuboidal cells
- Thought to recapitulate the endodermal sinuses in the placenta
- Neoplastic cells stain positively for alpha-fetoprotein (AFP), alpha-1-antitrypsin (A1AT), cytokeratin, and placental alkaline phosphatase immunohistochemistry
- Neoplastic cells are negative for the beta subunit of human chorionic gonadotropin (B hCG)
- Many intracellular and extracellular periodic-acid Schiff (PAS) positive hyaline globules are seen
- Globules are also positive for AFP and A1AT immunohistochemistry

CLINICAL ISSUES

Presentation
- Most common signs/symptoms
  - Abdominal pain and palpable abdominal and pelvic mass
  - Short duration of symptoms (1-4 weeks) as these tumors grow rapidly
- Other signs/symptoms
  - Increasing abdominal girth, abdominal distension, weight loss
  - Acute abdominal pain in cases or tumor torsion or rupture (very rare)
  - Elevated serum α-fetoprotein in the majority of patients

Demographics
- Age: Most commonly occur in the second decade of life, rare in middle-aged or older women
- Gender: Female

Natural History & Prognosis
- Highly malignant tumors with poor prognosis
- Five-year survival rate varies according to stage at diagnosis
  - Stage I: 95%
  - Stage II: 75%
  - Stage III: 30%
  - Stage IV: 25%
- Worst prognosis is associated with residual tumor size of < 2 cm and presence of > 100 mL of ascites

Treatment
- Combination of cytoreductive surgery and chemotherapy

DIAGNOSTIC CHECKLIST

Consider
- Diagnosis of yolk sac tumor should be considered in a girl or young woman presenting with a large complex pelvic mass and elevated serum α-fetoprotein

Image Interpretation Pearls
- Prominent intratumoral signal voids and peripheral strong enhancement on MR

SELECTED REFERENCES
1. Aoki Y et al: Yolk sac tumor of the ovary during pregnancy: a case report. Gynecol Oncol. 99(2):497-9, 2005
2. Ayhan A et al: Endodermal sinus tumor of the ovary: the Hacettepe University experience. Eur J Obstet Gynecol Reprod Biol. 123(2):230-4, 2005
3. Ulbright TM: Germ cell tumors of the gonads: a selective review emphasizing problems in differential diagnosis, newly appreciated, and controversial issues. Mod Pathol. 18 Suppl 2:S61-79, 2005
4. Young RH: Sex cord-stromal tumors of the ovary and testis: their similarities and differences with consideration of selected problems. Mod Pathol. 18 Suppl 2:S81-98, 2005
5. Lopez JM et al: Ovarian yolk sac tumor associated with endometrioid carcinoma and mucinous cystadenoma of the ovary. Ann Diagn Pathol. 7(5):300-5, 2003
6. Nawa A et al: Prognostic factors of patients with yolk sac tumors of the ovary. Am J Obstet Gynecol. 184(6):1182-8, 2001
7. Oh C et al: Ovarian endodermal sinus tumor in a postmenopausal woman. Gynecol Oncol. 82(2):392-4, 2001
8. Yamaoka T et al: Yolk sac tumor of the ovary: radiologic-pathologic correlation in four cases. J Comput Assist Tomogr. 24(4):605-9, 2000

YOLK SAC TUMOR, OVARY

IMAGE GALLERY

Typical

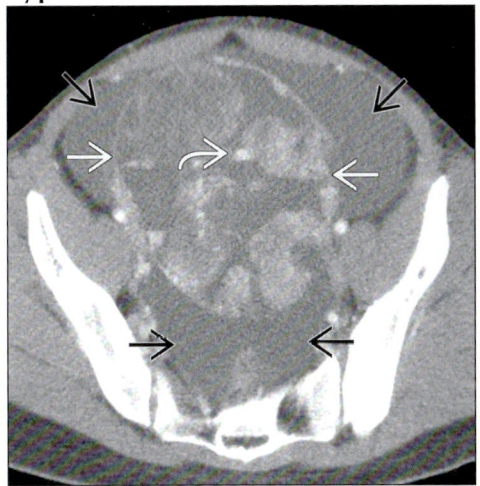
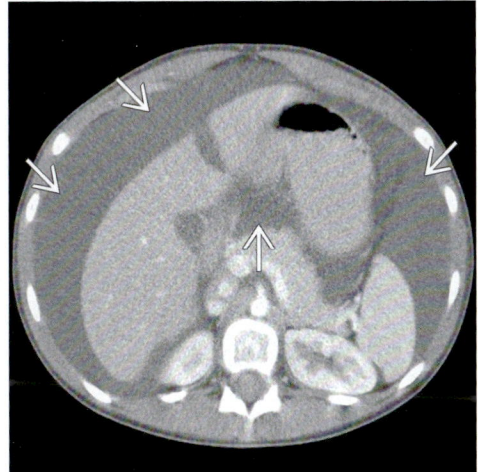

(Left) Axial CECT shows a central strongly enhancing pelvic mass ➔ in a 12 year old girl presenting with abdominal distension. Note the presence of ascites ➔ and large intratumoral vessels ➔. *(Right)* Axial CECT in the same patient as previous image, shows a large amount of ascites ➔ around the liver, spleen, in the lesser sac and in the hepatorenal fossa.

Typical

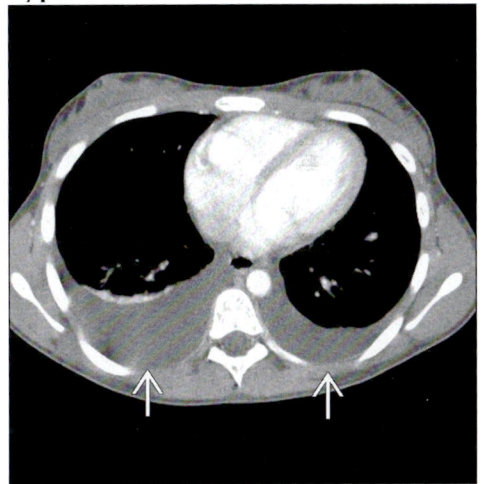
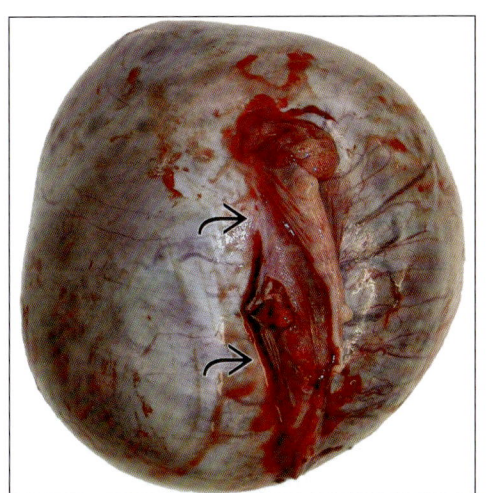

(Left) Axial CECT in the same patient as previous image, shows bilateral pleural effusions ➔, larger on the right. Cytology from pleural fluid contained malignant cells. *(Right)* Gross pathology in the same patient as previous image, shows an 8 cm solid mass. Note the presence of capsular rupture ➔. Pathology: Malignant yolk sac tumor of the right ovary.

Typical

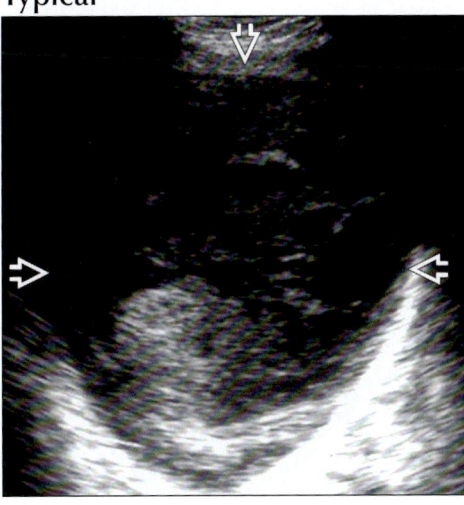
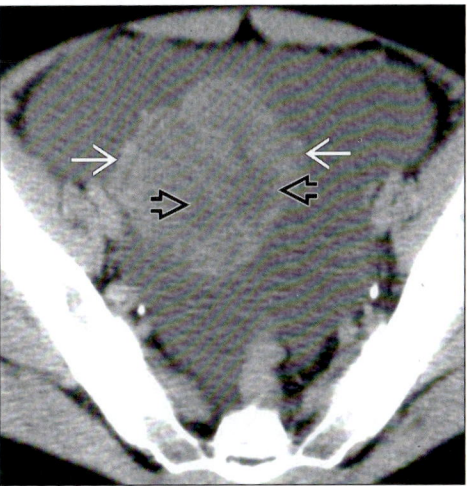

(Left) Axial transabdominal ultrasound shows a complex pelvic mass ➔ in a 21 year old female patient presenting with abdominal pain and distension. *(Right)* Axial CECT in the same patient as previous image, shows a solid right adnexal mass ➔ which contains areas of central necrosis ➔. A large amount of ascites is present. Pathology: Malignant yolk sac tumor of the right ovary. (Courtesy T.M. Cunha, MD).

LYMPHOMA, OVARY

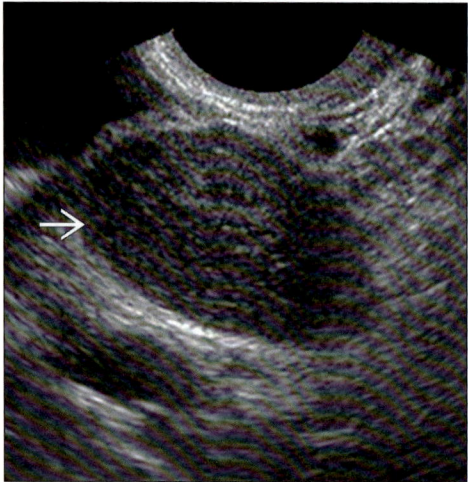

Sagittal oblique transvaginal ultrasound shows ovarian lymphoma seen as a well-defined homogeneous mass ➡ diffusely involving the right ovary.

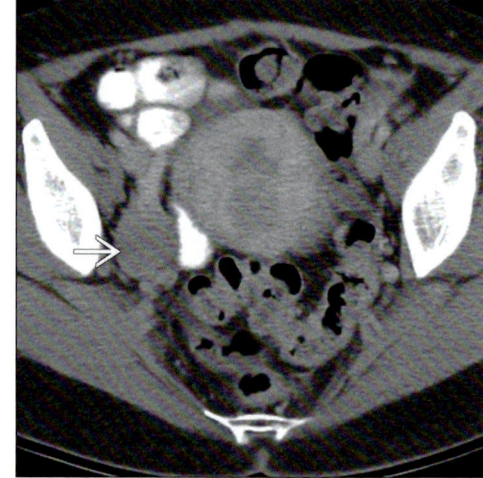

Axial CECT shows a well-defined homogeneous mass ➡ with mild enhancement in the right ovary.

TERMINOLOGY

Definitions
- Ovarian involvement by lymphoma
- Most often ovaries are secondarily involved in presence of systemic lymphoma
- Primary ovarian lymphoma without systemic disease: Extremely rare
- Criteria for diagnosis of primary ovarian lymphoma include
  - At time of diagnosis, lymphoma is clinically confined to ovary & adjacent lymph nodes and no evidence of systemic lymphoma present
  - Peripheral blood and bone marrow do not contain any abnormal cells
  - If further lymphomatous lesions occur at sites remote from ovary, then at least several months should have elapsed between appearance of ovarian and extra-ovarian lesions

IMAGING FINDINGS

General Features
- Best diagnostic clue: Homogeneous solid mass in ovary without ascites
- Location: Bilateral or unilateral ovarian involvement can be seen
- Size: Varies but may present as large ovarian masses
- Morphology: Ovaries usually diffusely involved; areas of necrosis and cysts may be found in large tumors

Ultrasonographic Findings
- Color Doppler: Shows mild vascularization
- Power Doppler: Helpful in detecting mild vascularization
- Transvaginal ultrasound (TVS) findings
  - Well-defined solid masses with homogeneous and hypoechoic echotexture in ovaries

CT Findings
- NECT: Well-defined, homogeneous low-attenuation masses
- CECT

DDx: Ovarian Masses

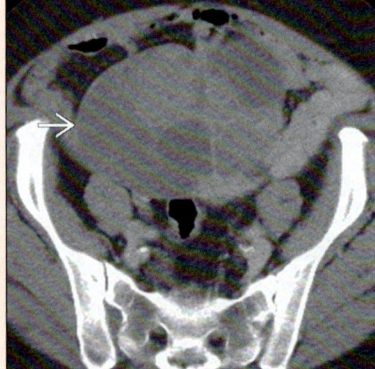

Ovarian Carcinoma

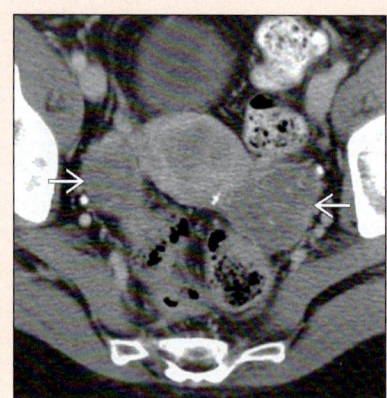

Ovarian Metastasis

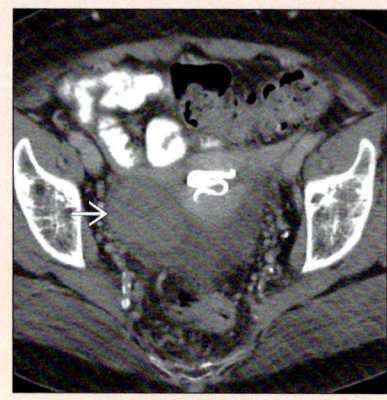

Ovarian Fibroma

LYMPHOMA, OVARY

Key Facts

Terminology
- Ovarian involvement by lymphoma
- Most often ovaries are secondarily involved in presence of systemic lymphoma
- Primary ovarian lymphoma without systemic disease: Extremely rare

Imaging Findings
- Best diagnostic clue: Homogeneous solid mass in ovary without ascites
- Location: Bilateral or unilateral ovarian involvement can be seen
- Size: Varies but may present as large ovarian masses
- Morphology: Ovaries usually diffusely involved; areas of necrosis and cysts may be found in large tumors
- CT is most commonly used imaging method in staging of lymphoma because chest, abdomen and pelvis can be scanned at same time
- FDG PET also useful method for staging and assessment of therapeutic response in lymphoma

Top Differential Diagnoses
- Ovarian Carcinomas
- Ovarian Metastasis
- Solid Ovarian Neoplasms

Pathology
- Either diffuse or nodular involvement
- Lymphomatous cells may be aggregated into islands or form thin rows of cells within ovary

---

- Mild to moderate, homogeneous contrast-enhancement
- Cystic areas and necrosis are rare

MR Findings
- T1WI: Medium signal intensity, well-defined ovarian mass
- T2WI
  - Intermediate signal intensity, well-defined ovarian mass
  - Signal intensity of ovarian lymphoma on T2WI MR lower than that of most ovarian carcinoma
- T1 C+
  - Mild to moderate, homogeneous contrast-enhancement
  - Cystic areas and necrosis are rare

Nuclear Medicine Findings
- PET: FDG PET shows marked uptake in lymphoma

Imaging Recommendations
- Best imaging tool
  - CT is most commonly used imaging method in staging of lymphoma because chest, abdomen and pelvis can be scanned at same time
  - FDG PET also useful method for staging and assessment of therapeutic response in lymphoma

DIFFERENTIAL DIAGNOSIS

Ovarian Carcinomas
- Ovarian carcinomas have complex structure with cystic or necrotic areas and solid components
- Unlike lymphoma, ascites usually present in ovarian carcinomas

Ovarian Metastasis
- Ovarian metastasis may resemble lymphoma because both cause diffuse ovarian enlargement without ascites
- However, extensive involvement of lymph node chains suggests lymphoma
- In ovarian metastasis, primary tumor usually evident on imaging or clinical history and extensive involvement of lymph node chains suggests lymphoma

Solid Ovarian Neoplasms
- Fibroma, fibrothecoma, Sertoli-Leydig cell tumor, sarcoma, dysgerminoma, granulosa cell tumor, etc.: Solid ovarian masses like lymphoma

PATHOLOGY

General Features
- General path comments
  - Ovarian lymphoma almost always part of generalized disease
  - Although very rare, primary ovarian lymphoma cases have been reported
- Epidemiology
  - Malignant lymphomas involve ovaries at necropsy or autopsy in 7-26% of patients with lymphoma
  - Primary ovarian lymphoma extremely rare, accounting for 0.5% of all non-Hodgkin lymphomas and 1.5% of all ovarian neoplasms

Gross Pathologic & Surgical Features
- Firm, rubbery or soft mass which may contain areas of necrosis and cysts when tumor is large
- Calcifications may be detected after treatment

Microscopic Features
- Either diffuse or nodular involvement
- Lymphomatous cells may be aggregated into islands or form thin rows of cells within ovary

Staging, Grading or Classification Criteria
- Staging for ovarian lymphomas is controversial
- FIGO staging for ovarian cancer or modified Ann Arbor lymphoma staging classification are used
- However, neither method is optimal because both were originally designed for other disease entities
  - FIGO system was intended for ovarian epithelial tumors

LYMPHOMA, OVARY

  ○ Ann Arbor staging system was intended for Hodgkin disease and does not address issue of bilateral ovarian involvement

CLINICAL ISSUES

Presentation
- Most common signs/symptoms
  ○ Abdominal-pelvic mass
  ○ Abdominal pain
  ○ Palpable lymphadenopathy
  ○ Vaginal bleeding
  ○ Amenorrhea, irregular menses
- Other signs/symptoms
  ○ Weight loss
  ○ Malaise
- Clinical Profile
  ○ Ovary rarely first site of detection of lymphoma
  ○ Most often patients present with signs and symptoms related to systemic lymphoma
  ○ Burkitt lymphoma, in endemic regions, most commonly presents with ovarian mass after jaw involvement

Demographics
- Age
  ○ Median age of patients is 36 years, 2/3 of cases are younger than 40 years
  ○ Peak incidence of Burkitt lymphoma is 5-10 years

Natural History & Prognosis
- Prognosis of ovarian lymphoma much better than ovarian cancer

Treatment
- Most patients with ovarian lymphomas are treated with surgery and chemotherapy; radiotherapy optional
- Because it is not possible to predict which patients will develop generalized disease; recommended that all patients be staged and treated with combination of surgery and chemotherapy regimens appropriate for their specific histology

DIAGNOSTIC CHECKLIST

Consider
- Ovarian lymphoma should be considered in patient with known lymphoma and homogeneous, solid, bilateral or unilateral ovarian mass(es)

Image Interpretation Pearls
- Imaging findings of ovarian lymphoma non-specific but features that suggest lymphoma include
  ○ Well-defined, homogeneous masses without significant necrosis, hemorrhage, or calcifications
  ○ Relatively mild enhancement after contrast administration
  ○ Frequent bilateral ovarian involvement

SELECTED REFERENCES

1. Chishima F et al: Ovarian Burkitt's lymphoma diagnosed by a combination of clinical features, morphology, immunophenotype, and molecular findings and successfully managed with surgery and chemotherapy. Int J Gynecol Cancer. 16 Suppl 1:337-43, 2006
2. Komoto D et al: A case of non-hodgkin's lymphoma of the ovary: usefulness of 18F-FDG PET for staging and assessment of the therapeutic response. Ann Nucl Med. 20(2):157-60, 2006
3. Lanjewar DN et al: HIV-associated primary non-Hodgkin's lymphoma of ovary: A case report. Gynecol Oncol. 2006
4. Koksal Y et al: A case of primary ovarian lymphoma in a child with high levels of CA125 and CA19-9. J Pediatr Hematol Oncol. 27(11):594-5, 2005
5. Yildirim Y. Related Articles et al: Primary ovarian large B-cell lymphoma in patient with juvenile rheumatoid arthritis treated with low dose Methotrexate. Gynecol Oncol. 97(1):249-52, 2005
6. Iyengar P et al: Precursor B-cell lymphoblastic lymphoma of the ovaries: an immunohistochemical study and review of the literature. Int J Gynecol Pathol. 23(2):193-7, 2004
7. Ambulkar I et al: Primary ovarian lymphoma: report of cases and review of literature. Leuk Lymphoma. 44(5):825-7, 2003
8. Rizvi AA et al: Primary ovarian lymphoma manifesting with severe hypercalcemia. Endocr Pract. 9(5):389-93, 2003
9. Yamada T et al: A case of malignant lymphoma of the ovary manifesting like an advanced ovarian cancer. Gynecol Oncol. 90(1):215-9, 2003
10. Niitsu N et al: Ovarian follicular lymphoma: a case report and review of the literature. Ann Hematol. 81(11):654-8, 2002
11. Ferrozzi F et al: Non-Hodgkin lymphomas of the ovaries: MR findings. J Comput Assist Tomogr. 24(3):416-20, 2000
12. Mansouri H et al: Primary malignant lymphoma of the ovary: an unusual presentation of a rare disease. Eur J Gynaecol Oncol. 21(6):616-8, 2000
13. Mitsumori A et al: MR appearance of non-Hodgkin's lymphoma of the ovary. AJR Am J Roentgenol. 173(1):245, 1999
14. Dao AH. Related Articles et al: Malignant lymphoma of the ovary: report of a case successfully managed with surgery and chemotherapy. Gynecol Oncol. 70(1):137-40, 1998
15. Creatsas GK et al: Non-Hodgkin's ovarian lymphoma during adolescence: report of two cases. J Pediatr Adolesc Gynecol. 10(4):219-22, 1997

LYMPHOMA, OVARY

IMAGE GALLERY

Typical

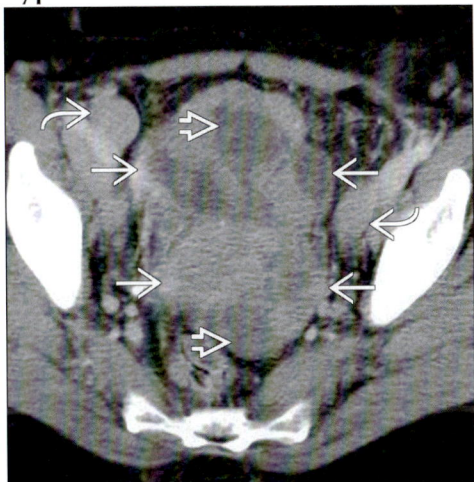
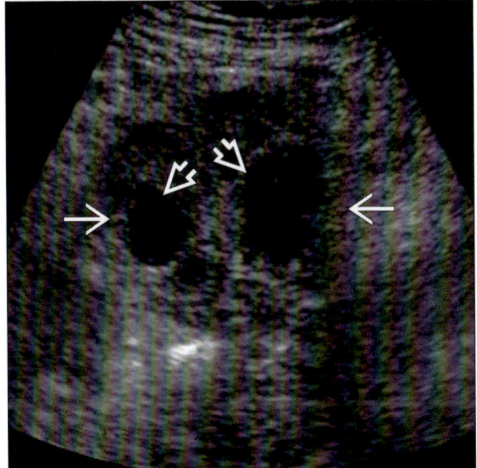

(Left) Axial CECT shows ovarian lymphoma seen as large pelvic mass ➡ with necrotic areas ➡. Bilateral external iliac lymphadenopathy ➡ is also seen. *(Right)* Axial oblique transabdominal ultrasound shows a large ovarian lymphoma seen as a heterogeneous mass ➡ in the ovary. Cystic areas ➡ are noted in the mass.

Typical

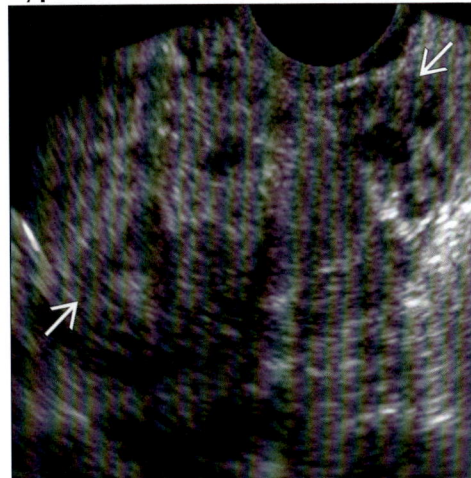
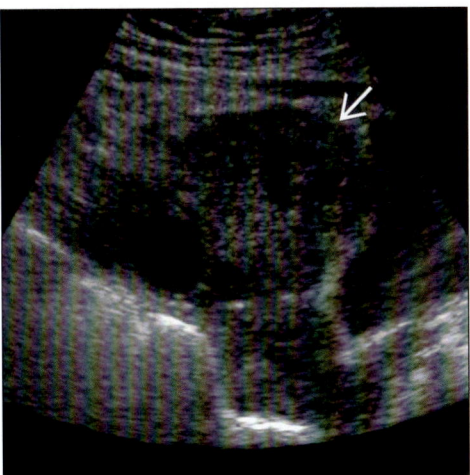

(Left) Axial oblique transvaginal ultrasound shows ovarian lymphoma seen as a mildly heterogeneous solid mass ➡ in the ovary. *(Right)* Axial oblique transabdominal ultrasound in a different patient shows ovarian lymphoma as a homogeneous mass ➡ in the ovary.

Typical

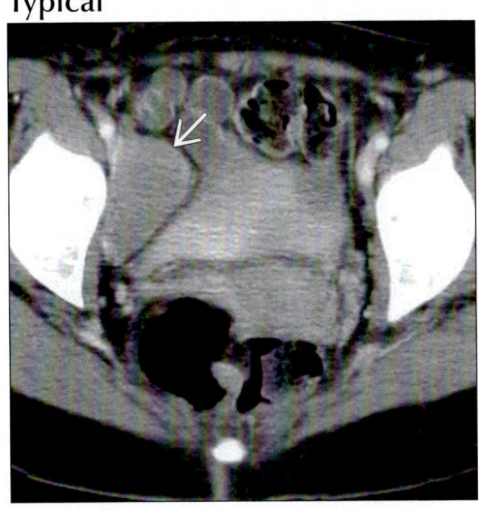
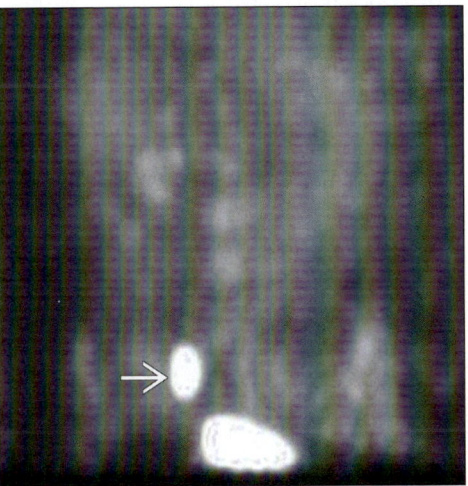

(Left) Axial CECT shows ovarian lymphoma ➡ diffusely involving the right ovary. *(Right)* Coronal PET in the same patient as in previous image shows marked uptake in the right ovary ➡ that is involved by lymphoma.

CLEAR CELL CARCINOMA, OVARY

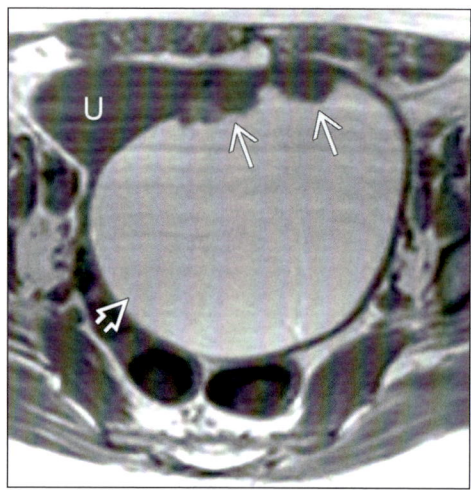

Axial T1WI MR shows left ovarian clear cell carcinoma seen as a cystic mass ➡ with solid nodular protrusions ➡. Note that cystic component is of high signal intensity due to hemorrhage. (U: Uterus).

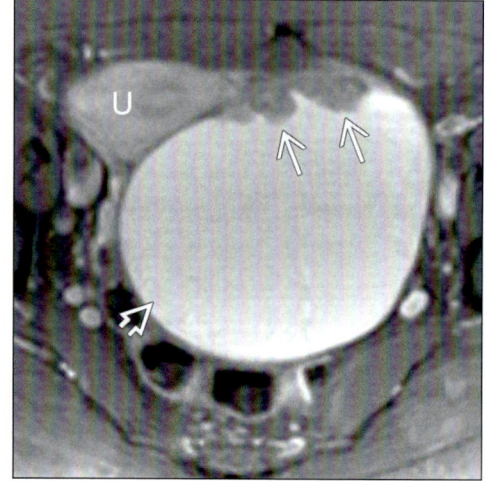

Axial T1 C+ FS MR shows that solid nodular protrusions ➡ are enhancing. Cystic component of the mass ➡ remains high signal intensity confirming presence of hemorrhage rather than fat. (U: Uterus).

TERMINOLOGY

Abbreviations and Synonyms
- Clear cell carcinoma (CCC)

Definitions
- Rare type of epithelial ovarian cancer
- First described as "mesonephroma" to describe an ovarian neoplasm composed of clear and "hobnail cells" with a pattern resembling immature glomeruli
- These ovarian tumors are strictly defined as lesions characterized by clear cells growing in solid/tubular or glandular patterns as well as hobnail cells lining tubules and cysts

IMAGING FINDINGS

General Features
- Best diagnostic clue: Large cystic adnexal mass with one or more solid protrusions
- Location: Usually unilateral ovarian involvement
- Size: Most often present as large tumors
- Morphology: Usually large cystic mass with one or more solid components protruding into cystic component

Ultrasonographic Findings
- Grayscale Ultrasound
  - Cystic adnexal mass containing solid projections
  - Cystic component may demonstrate variable echogenicity due to hemorrhage
- Color Doppler: Solid components demonstrate vascularity

CT Findings
- NECT
  - Low attenuation cystic mass with soft tissue density solid components
  - Cystic component may be of high attenuation due to hemorrhage
- CECT
  - Large unilocular cystic mass with enhancing solid protrusion(s)
  - Contrast-enhancement helps to differentiate hemorrhage from enhancing solid projections

DDx: Ovarian Masses

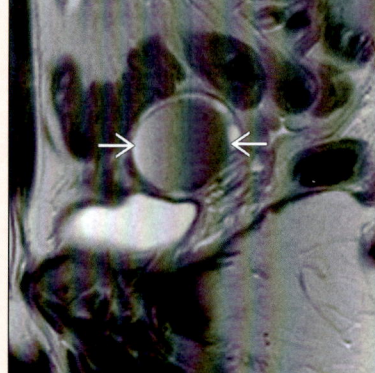
Endometrioma

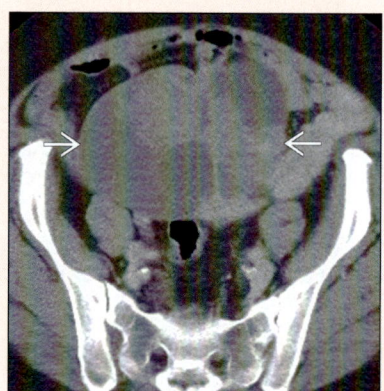
Serous Cystadenocarcinoma

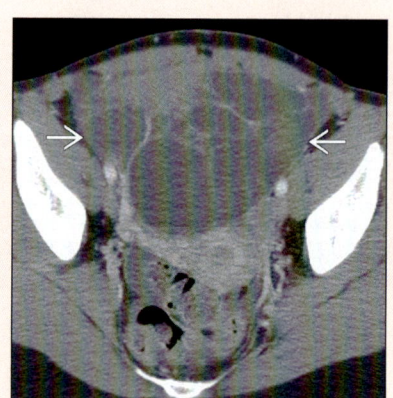
Mucinous Cystadenocarcinoma

CLEAR CELL CARCINOMA, OVARY

Key Facts

Imaging Findings
- Best diagnostic clue: Large cystic adnexal mass with one or more solid protrusions
- Morphology: Usually large cystic mass with one or more solid components protruding into cystic component

Top Differential Diagnoses
- Endometrioma
- Benign Serous or Mucinous Cystadenoma of Ovary
- Serous or Mucinous Adenocarcinoma of Ovary
- Ovarian Metastasis

Pathology
- Clear cell tumors of ovary are almost always malignant

Clinical Issues
- Although usually presents at early stages, prognosis of clear cell carcinoma is worse compared stage-by-stage to other types of ovarian cancer

Diagnostic Checklist
- Clear cell carcinoma of the ovary has certain distinct features compared to other epithelial ovarian cancers
- Frequently presents as a large pelvic mass
- Rarely occurs bilaterally
- Often associated with endometriosis
- Often accompanied by a thromboembolic complication
- Associated hypercalcemia is very common

MR Findings
- T1WI
  - Cystic component may be of varying signal intensity from low to very high intensity depending on hemorrhagic content
  - Solid components have intermediate signal intensity
- T2WI: High signal intensity cystic mass with heterogeneous signal intensity solid components
- T1 C+
  - Solid components of the mass demonstrate marked enhancement
  - Contrast-enhancement helps to differentiate blood clot which does not enhance from enhancing solid projections

Imaging Recommendations
- Best imaging tool
  - US, CT or MR can be used to detect and characterize an adnexal mass
  - US is most commonly used method to detect & characterize an adnexal mass
  - MR is superior to US and CT in tumor characterization due to its better soft tissue resolution
  - CT is most often used in advanced disease to assess peritoneal carcinomatosis or distant metastases
- Protocol advice
  - Color Doppler is needed to assess for flow in solid appearing components on US
  - Contrast-enhancement is essential to demonstrate enhancing solid components on both CT and MR

DIFFERENTIAL DIAGNOSIS

Endometrioma
- Endometriomas contain hemorrhage and may have thick, irregular walls
- However, endometriomas do not have enhancing solid projections

Benign Serous or Mucinous Cystadenoma of Ovary
- Usually less than 4 cm in size
- Entirely cystic without solid components

Serous or Mucinous Adenocarcinoma of Ovary
- More complex, usually multiloculated masses
- Tend to present at advanced stages compared to clear cell carcinoma

Ovarian Metastasis
- Most ovarian metastases are solid or a mixture of solid and cystic tumors
- Clinical presentation is often due to primary disease

PATHOLOGY

General Features
- General path comments
  - Clear cell carcinoma is a rare type of epithelial ovarian cancer
    - Serous (50%), mucinous (20%), endometrioid (20%), clear cell (10%) and undifferentiated (1%)
  - Methods of spread
    - Direct extension
    - Intraperitoneal implantation
    - Lymphatic dissemination in pelvis and paraaortic region
    - Less commonly, hematogenously to liver or lungs
- Epidemiology
  - Clear cell tumors of ovary are almost always malignant
  - Benign clear cell tumors are not reported and borderline tumors are very rare
- Associated abnormalities: Association with endometriosis (30-35%) is more common than other types of ovarian cancer (8%)

CLEAR CELL CARCINOMA, OVARY

Gross Pathologic & Surgical Features
- Large cystic mass with one or more solid nodules protruding into cyst lumen

Microscopic Features
- Polyhedral cells containing abundant clear cytoplasm with eccentric nuclei
- Cells grow in aggregates or form tubules
- "Hobnail cells" found in most tumors are characterized by prominent bulbous nuclei that protrude beyond apparent cytoplasmic limits

Staging, Grading or Classification Criteria
- FIGO staging system
  - I: Tumor confined to ovaries
    - IA: Intracapsular and unilateral
    - IB: Intracapsular and bilateral
    - IC: Ruptured capsule, tumor on ovarian capsule, malignant cells in ascites or peritoneal washings
  - II: Local extension; confined to true pelvis
    - IIA: Involvement of fallopian tubes or uterus
    - IIB: Involvement of other pelvic tissues such as sigmoid, pelvic implants
    - IIC: Pelvic extension with malignant cells in ascites or peritoneal washings
  - III: Nodal metastases or peritoneal implants outside the pelvis
    - IIIA: Microscopic abdominal implants
    - IIIB: < 2 cm abdominal implants
    - IIIC: > 2 cm abdominal implants or positive nodes
  - IV: Distant metastases (excluding peritoneal metastases); e.g., malignant pleural effusion, intrahepatic metastases

CLINICAL ISSUES

Presentation
- Most common signs/symptoms
  - Pelvic mass
  - Pelvic pain
  - Abdominal swelling due to ovarian enlargement or ascites
- Other signs/symptoms
  - Hypercalcemia (most common paraneoplastic syndrome in ovarian cancer) is more common in clear cell carcinoma than in other ovarian cancers
  - Thromboembolic complications are common in clear cell carcinoma
- Clinical Profile
  - Usually presents with stage I/II disease
  - This is likely due to slow growth of tumor and presentation of the tumors as large pelvic masses

Demographics
- Age: Occurs most frequently between ages of 40-70 years

Natural History & Prognosis
- Although usually presents at early stages, prognosis of clear cell carcinoma is worse compared stage-by-stage to other types of ovarian cancer
  - This is likely due to clear cell carcinoma's insensitivity to conventional platinum-based chemotherapy
- Patients with pure-type clear cell carcinomas have worse overall survival than those with mixed-type clear cell carcinomas

Treatment
- Cytoreductive (tumor-debulking) surgery
  - To reduce the maximum diameter of the remaining implants by less than 1 cm
- Chemotherapy: Pre-operative and/or after surgery
  - Clear cell carcinomas respond poorly to chemotherapy

DIAGNOSTIC CHECKLIST

Consider
- Clear cell carcinoma of the ovary has certain distinct features compared to other epithelial ovarian cancers
  - Frequently presents as a large pelvic mass
  - Rarely occurs bilaterally
  - Often associated with endometriosis
  - Often accompanied by a thromboembolic complication
  - Associated hypercalcemia is very common

Image Interpretation Pearls
- Large cystic adnexal mass with one or more solid protrusions
- Cystic component may contain hemorrhage

SELECTED REFERENCES
1. Takano M et al: Clear cell carcinoma of the ovary: a retrospective multicentre experience of 254 patients with complete surgical staging. Br J Cancer. 2006
2. Ho CM et al: Evaluation of complete surgical staging with pelvic and para-aortic lymphadenectomy and paclitaxel plus carboplatin chemotherapy for improvement of survival in stage I ovarian clear cell carcinoma. Gynecol Oncol. 88(3):394-9, 2003
3. Togashi K. Related Articles et al: Ovarian cancer: the clinical role of US, CT, and MRI. Eur Radiol. 13 Suppl 4:L87-104, 2003
4. Jung SE et al: CT and MR imaging of ovarian tumors with emphasis on differential diagnosis. Radiographics. 22(6):1305-25, 2002
5. Matsuoka Y et al: MR imaging of clear cell carcinoma of the ovary. Eur Radiol. 11(6):946-51, 2001
6. Kita T et al: Exploratory study of effective chemotherapy to clear cell carcinoma of the ovary. Oncol Rep. 7(2):327-31, 2000
7. Sugiyama T et al: Clinical characteristics of clear cell carcinoma of the ovary: a distinct histologic type with poor prognosis and resistance to platinum-based chemotherapy. Cancer. 88(11):2584-9, 2000
8. Behbakht K et al: Clinical characteristics of clear cell carcinoma of the ovary. Gynecol Oncol. 70(2):255-8, 1998
9. Goff BA et al: Clear cell carcinoma of the ovary: a distinct histologic type with poor prognosis and resistance to platinum-based chemotherapy in stage III disease. Gynecol Oncol. 60(3):412-7, 1996
10. Forstner R et al: CT and MRI of ovarian cancer. Abdom Imaging. 20(1):2-8, 1995

CLEAR CELL CARCINOMA, OVARY

IMAGE GALLERY

Typical

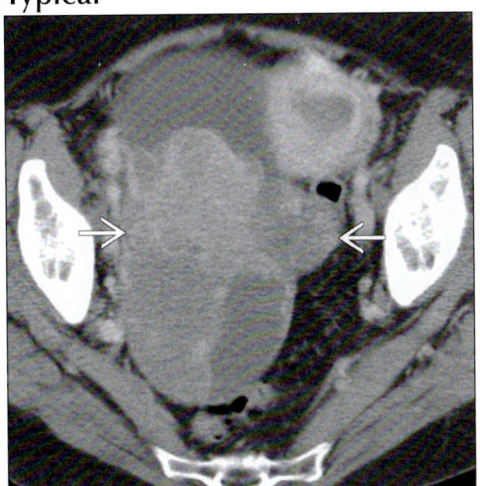 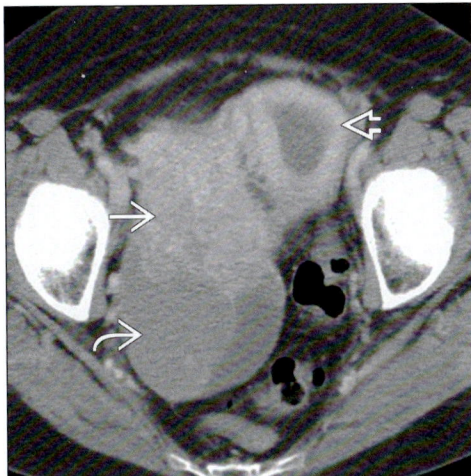

(Left) Axial CECT shows a right ovarian clear cell carcinoma seen as a complex cystic and solid mass ➡. *(Right)* Axial CECT shows that solid component ➡ is enhancing markedly. Hemorrhage ➡ is seen in the cystic component. Uterus ➡ is also seen.

Typical

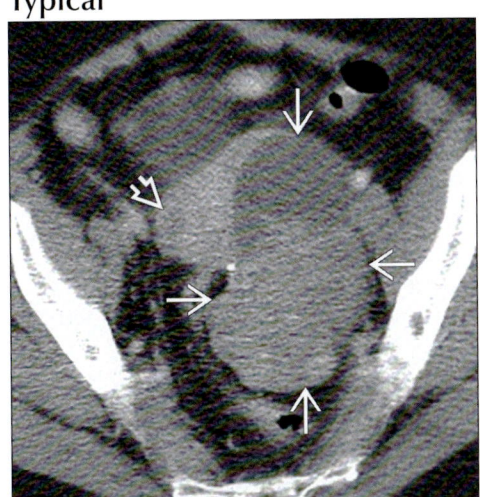 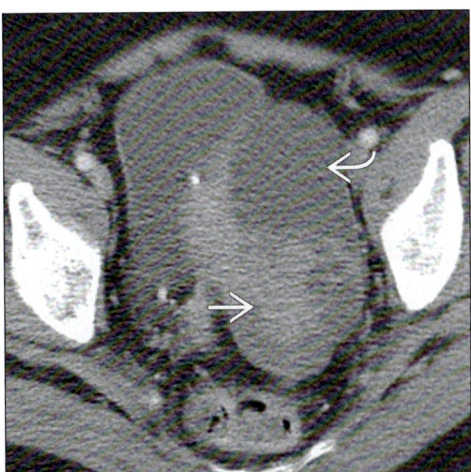

(Left) Axial CECT shows left ovarian clear cell carcinoma ➡. Uterus ➡ is also seen. *(Right)* Axial CECT shows enhancing solid ➡ and nonenhancing cystic ➡ components of the mass.

Typical

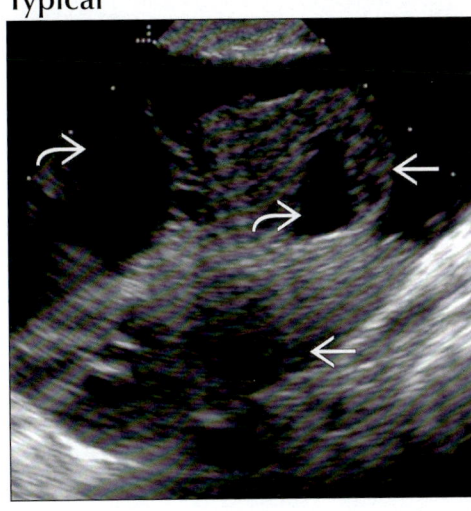 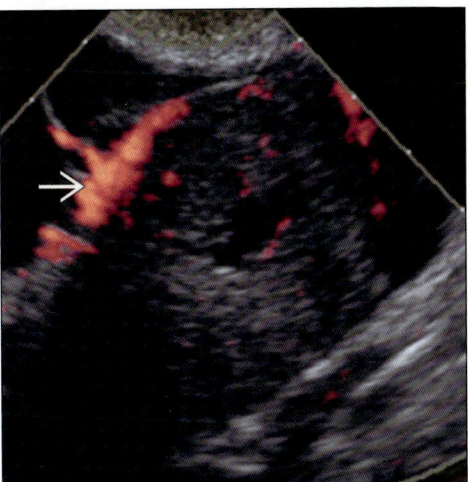

(Left) Sagittal oblique transvaginal ultrasound shows ovarian clear cell carcinoma seen as a mixed cystic ➡ and solid ➡ mass. *(Right)* Sagittal oblique power Doppler ultrasound shows marked vascularity ➡ in the solid component of the mass.

IMMATURE TERATOMA, OVARY

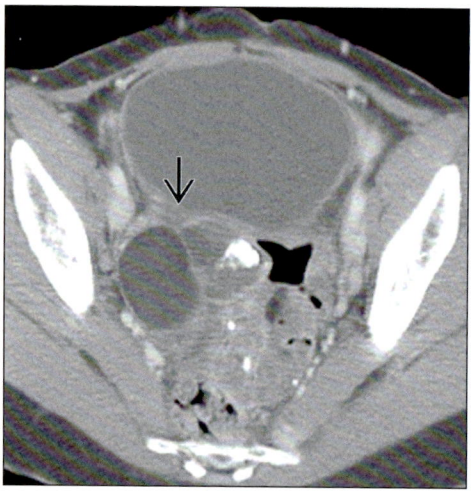

Axial CECT shows a right adnexal mass ➡ containing areas of fat, calcification and enhancing soft tissue. Pathology: Immature teratoma.

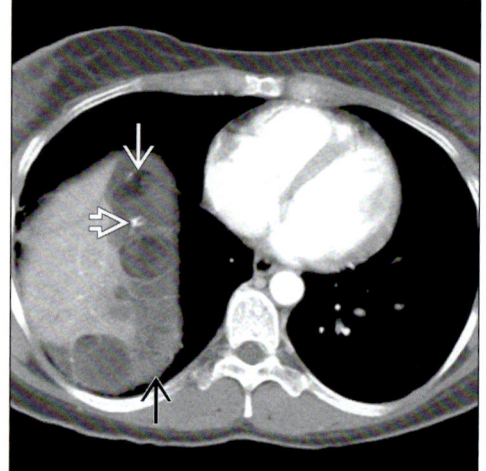

Axial CECT shows capsular implants at liver dome which contain areas of fat ➡, calcification ➡ and enhancing soft tissue ➡.

TERMINOLOGY

Abbreviations and Synonyms
- Malignant teratoma

Definitions
- Malignant form of teratoma that contains immature or embryonic tissues, thought to arise from post-meiotic germ cells

IMAGING FINDINGS

General Features
- Best diagnostic clue: Small foci of fat and scattered calcifications within predominantly solid heterogeneous mass in young female
- Location: Usually unilateral
- Size: Typically large ranging from 5-25 cm
- Morphology
  o Hemorrhage may be present
  o Tumor capsule is not always well-defined and may frequently perforate

Ultrasonographic Findings
- Heterogeneous predominantly solid ovarian mass
- Scattered calcifications are usually present, producing posterior acoustic shadowing
- Hyperechoic areas suggest the presence of fat and hemorrhage, but small foci of fat within the solid component may be difficult to appreciate

CT Findings
- Tumor has characteristic appearances
- Large solid unilateral ovarian mass with ill-defined borders
- No detectable capsule
- Tumor demonstrates areas of low-attenuation fat, enhancing soft tissue and high-attenuation calcification
- Small foci of fat and calcifications are more easily detected with CT than MR
- Advanced stages of immature teratoma may demonstrate ascites and peritoneal tumor implants

MR Findings
- Complex mass containing cystic areas, enhancing soft tissue components and fat

DDx: Ovarian Masses

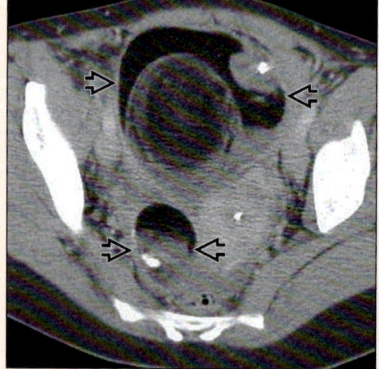
Mature Teratoma

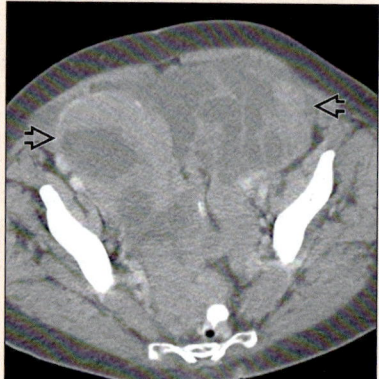
Ovarian Carcinoma

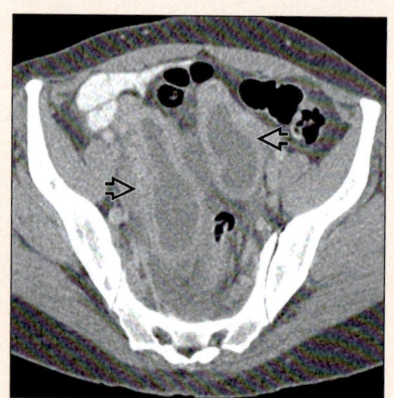
Tubo-Ovarian Abscess

IMMATURE TERATOMA, OVARY

Key Facts

Terminology
- Malignant teratoma

Imaging Findings
- Tumor demonstrates areas of low-attenuation fat, enhancing soft tissue and high-attenuation calcification
- Advanced stages of immature teratoma may demonstrate ascites and peritoneal tumor implants
- Contrast-enhanced MR: Both CT and MR perform similarly and have characteristic appearances
- Protocol advice: Fat suppression must be used in MR whenever a high-signal intensity ovarian mass is encountered on T1WI

Top Differential Diagnoses
- Mature Cystic Teratoma
- Mature Solid Teratomas
- Ovarian Cancer
- Tuboovarian Abscess

Pathology
- Contains immature structures resembling those of embryo; mature elements and other forms of germ cell tumors can be found in association with immature teratomas
- Immature teratomas usually do not produce beta-hCG but 33-65% produce alpha-fetoprotein

Clinical Issues
- Most common signs/symptoms: Asymptomatic palpable unilateral abdominal mass

---

- Fat can be diagnosed due to its high signal intensity on T1WI and T2WI
- Both fat and hemorrhage demonstrate high signal intensity on T1WI
- Fat suppression is useful for differentiating fat from hemorrhage; on T1WI FS, fat demonstrates low SI while hemorrhage remains of high SI
- Scattered calcifications may be present but could be difficult to identify on MR

Imaging Recommendations
- Best imaging tool: Contrast-enhanced MR: Both CT and MR perform similarly and have characteristic appearances
- Protocol advice: Fat suppression must be used in MR whenever a high-signal intensity ovarian mass is encountered on T1WI

DIFFERENTIAL DIAGNOSIS

Mature Cystic Teratoma
- Immature teratomas are typically larger than mature teratomas
- Mature teratomas are predominantly cystic with dense calcifications, whereas immature teratomas are predominantly solid with small foci of lipid material and scattered calcifications

Mature Solid Teratomas
- Radiologically indistinguishable from immature teratomas
- Mostly solid with no identifiable immature components
- It must be extensively sampled at biopsy to exclude an immature teratoma

Ovarian Cancer
- Most common ovarian malignancy that has tendency of early peritoneal spread, the majority of patients present with peritoneal carcinomatosis (stage III disease)
- Older patients with peak incidence in postmenopausal women
- Frequently bilateral, heterogeneous, mixed cystic and solid, adnexal, irregularly-shaped masses without detectable fat on all imaging modalities
- In general associated with poor prognosis due to presentation at advanced stages

Tubo-Ovarian Abscess
- Seen in young sexually active women
- Patients are usually very unwell with fever, pelvic/abdominal pain and vaginal discharge
- Unilateral or bilateral inflammatory cystic thick-walled masses associated with infiltrative changes in adjacent pelvic fat and loculated ascites
- No detectable fat within these lesions

PATHOLOGY

General Features
- General path comments
  - Contains immature structures resembling those of embryo; mature elements and other forms of germ cell tumors can be found in association with immature teratomas
  - Bilateral involvement less than 5%
  - Immature teratomas usually do not produce beta-hCG but 33-65% produce alpha-fetoprotein
  - Gliomatosis peritonei; presence of mature peritoneal glial implants (0.1-1.1 cm) sometimes with ascites resembling peritoneal carcinomatosis
  - Metastatic disease is usually confined to abdominal peritoneal cavity but intrahepatic and lung metastases can occur
- Epidemiology: Less than 1% of all ovarian malignant tumors
- Associated abnormalities: Mature teratoma may coexist in contralateral ovary up to 25% of cases

Gross Pathologic & Surgical Features
- Predominantly solid, lobulated mass of grey color that contains numerous cysts

IMMATURE TERATOMA, OVARY

- Hemorrhage and necrosis are relatively common
- Solid tissue may contain cartilage, bone, or immature neural tissue
- Cysts contain clear fluid, sebaceous material and hair
- Capsule may be absent and may demonstrate perforation if present

Microscopic Features
- Wide variety of tissues representing all three germ layers including immature as well as mature elements
- Diagnosis rests on presence of embryonic tissue rather than immature fetal type tissue
- Predominant tissue is neuroectodermal: Neuroepithelial rosettes, mitotically active glia, rarely areas resembling glioblastoma or neuroblastoma
- Immature epithelium of both ectodermal and endodermal types, as well as immature cartilage and muscle can frequently be seen
- Peritoneal implants are usually lower grade than the primary tumor
- Amount of yolk sac tumor is a major predictor of grade, stage and rate of recurrence
- Immunohistochemical stains for glial fibrillary acid protein (GFAP), S100 and neuron specific enolase (NSE) are positive in the neural tissue

Staging, Grading or Classification Criteria
- Grade 1: Neoplasms containing < 1 low power field of immature neuroepithelium on any one microscope section examined
- Grade 2: 1-3 low power fields of immature neuroepithelium on any one microscope section examined
- Grade 3: > 3 low power fields of immature neuroepithelium on any one microscope section examined
- Alternative proposed two tiered grading system
- Low grade (grade 1 above): Neoplasms containing < 1 low power field of immature neuroepithelium on any one microscope section examined
- High grade (grades 2 & 3 above): Neoplasms containing > 1 low power field of immature neuroepithelium on any one microscope section examined
- Staging: Same as ovarian cancer

CLINICAL ISSUES

Presentation
- Most common signs/symptoms: Asymptomatic palpable unilateral abdominal mass
- Other signs/symptoms
  - Abdominal pain, discomfort and change in bowel habit
    - Acute abdominal pain in 10% due to hemorrhage, rupture or torsion
  - Abdominal distention secondary to the presence of ascites and peritoneal implants is usually associated with higher grade and advanced stage of the tumor
  - Vaginal bleeding

Demographics
- Age: Two peaks: The first larger peak in young women in first 2 decades of life, the second smaller peak in pre- and postmenopausal women

Natural History & Prognosis
- Prognosis depends on stage and grade of tumor at presentation
- 10-year survival rates: Grade 1, 82%; grade 2, 62%; grade 3, 30%
- Post-chemotherapy differentiation of immature teratoma and peritoneal implants into more mature tumor has been described ("retroconversion phenomenon")

Treatment
- Stage I grade 1 tumor (confined to the ovary) is treated with unilateral salpingooophorectomy
- Stage I grade 2 and 3 tumors require staging procedure, adjuvant chemotherapy and continued follow-up to detect recurrence

DIAGNOSTIC CHECKLIST

Consider
- MR for evaluation of primary lesion
- CT for detection of peritoneal metastases

Image Interpretation Pearls
- Large heterogeneous usually unilateral ovarian mass with solid enhancing components, scattered calcifications and foci of fat

SELECTED REFERENCES

1. Rim SY et al: Malignant transformation of ovarian mature cystic teratoma. Int J Gynecol Cancer. 16(1):140-4, 2006
2. Papadias K et al: Teratomas of the ovary: a clinico-pathological evaluation of 87 patients from one institution during a 10-year period. Eur J Gynaecol Oncol. 26(4):446-8, 2005
3. Terzic M et al: Immature ovarian teratoma in a young girl: very short course and lethal outcome. A case report. Int J Gynecol Cancer. 15(2):382-4, 2005
4. Yamaoka T et al: Immature teratoma of the ovary: correlation of MR imaging and pathologic findings. Eur Radiol. 13(2):313-9, 2003
5. Jung SE et al: CT and MR imaging of ovarian tumors with emphasis on differential diagnosis. Radiographics. 22(6):1305-25, 2002
6. Talerman A: Blausteins Pathology of the Female Genital Tract: 5th ed. NY, Springer-Verlag. 994-7, 2002
7. Outwater EK et al: Ovarian teratomas: tumor types and imaging characteristics. Radiographics. 21(2):475-90, 2001
8. Jeong YY et al: Imaging evaluation of ovarian masses. Radiographics. 20(5):1445-70, 2000
9. O'Connor DM et al: The influence of grade on the outcome of stage I ovarian immature (malignant) teratomas and the reproducibility of grading. Int J Gynecol Pathol. 13(4):283-9, 1994

IMMATURE TERATOMA, OVARY

IMAGE GALLERY

Typical

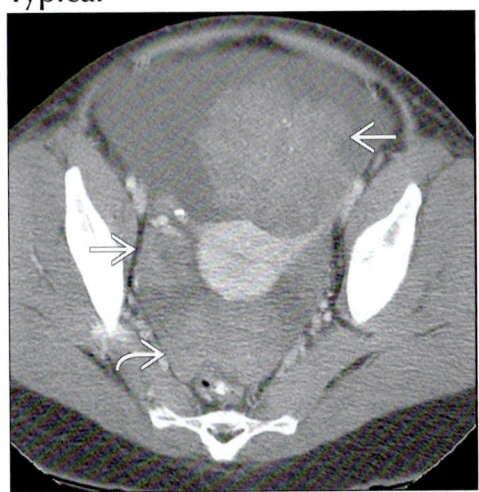 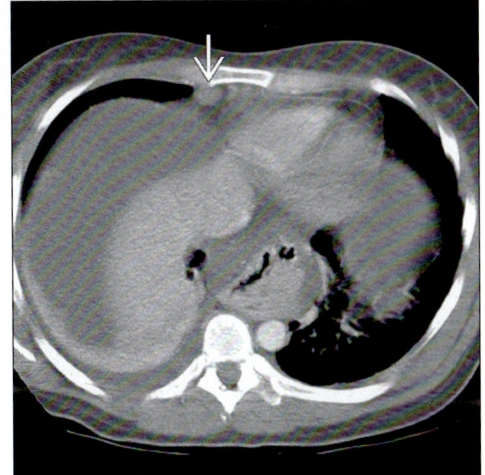

(Left) Axial CECT of a 30 year old female patient shows bilateral irregularly shaped adnexal masses ➡ with punctate calcifications and peritoneal implant in cul-de-sac ➡. (Right) Axial CECT in the same patient as previous image shows right superior diaphragmatic lymphadenopathy ➡ and ascites.

Typical

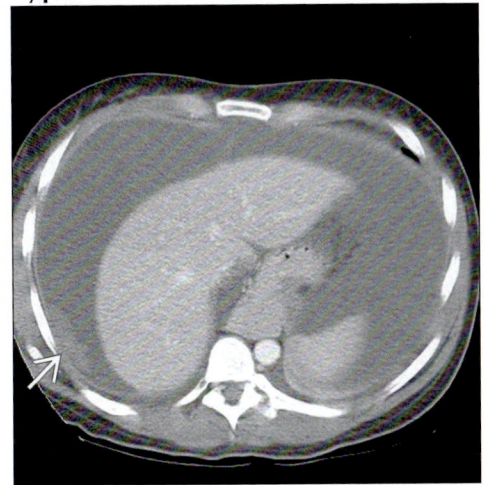 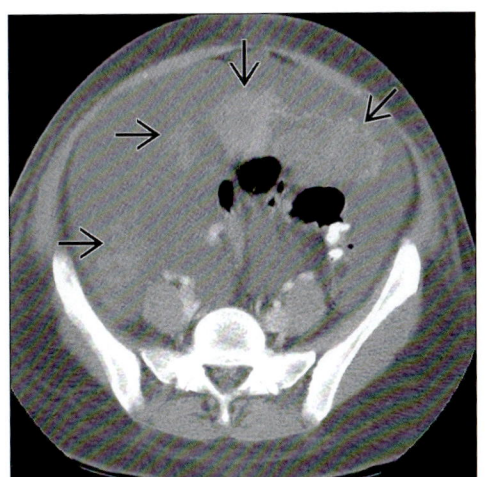

(Left) Axial CECT in the same patient as previous image shows a peritoneal tumor deposit ➡ in the perihepatic space outlined by ascites. (Right) Axial CECT in the same patient as previous image shows multiple omental masses ➡ and ascites. Pathology: Immature teratoma.

Typical

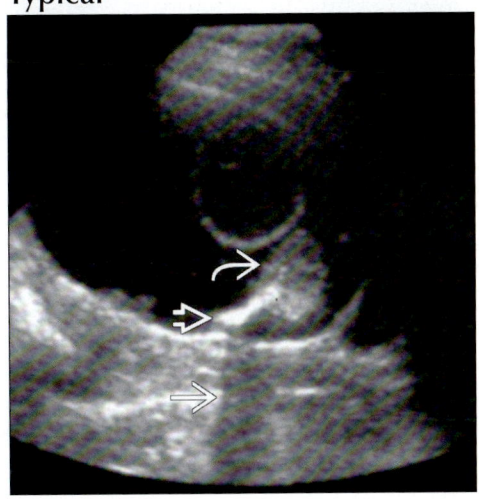 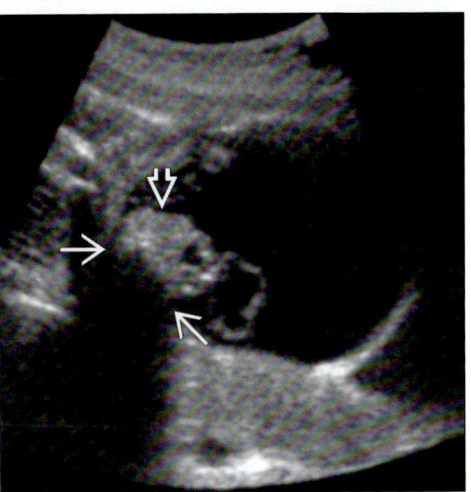

(Left) Longitudinal transabdominal US in a 15 year old girl shows a predominantly cystic mass with a solid component ➡. Note presence of highly echogenic material ➡ producing posterior acoustic shadowing ➡ suggestive of calcifications. (Right) Transverse transabdominal US (same patient as previous image) confirms presence of a cystic mass containing solid elements ➡. Presence of posterior acoustic shadowing ➡ indicates intratumoral calcification.

IMMATURE TERATOMA, OVARY

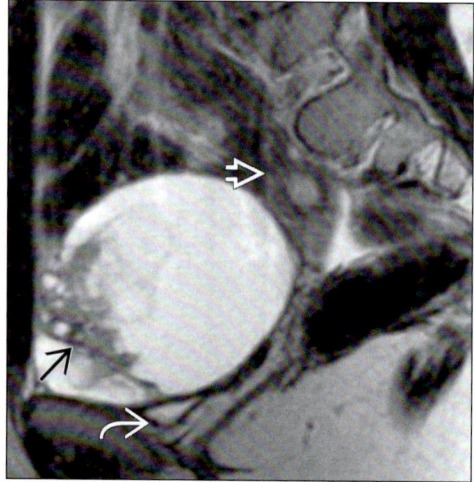
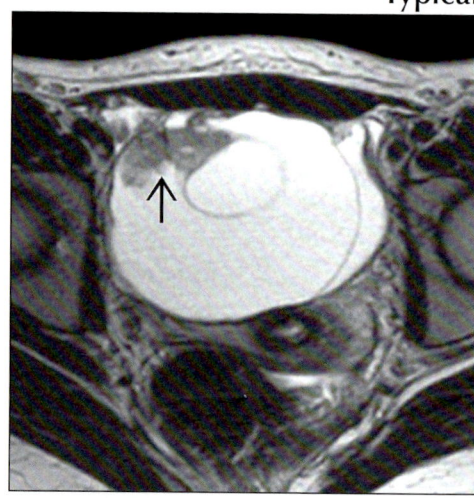

(Left) Sagittal T2WI MR in the same patient as previous image shows a predominantly cystic mass with a heterogeneous soft tissue component ➡. Note inferior displacement of the bladder ➡ and posterior displacement of the uterus ➡. (Right) Axial T2WI MR in the same patient as previous image confirms the presence of a large pelvic mass. The mass is predominantly cystic containing only a small amount of solid tissue ➡.

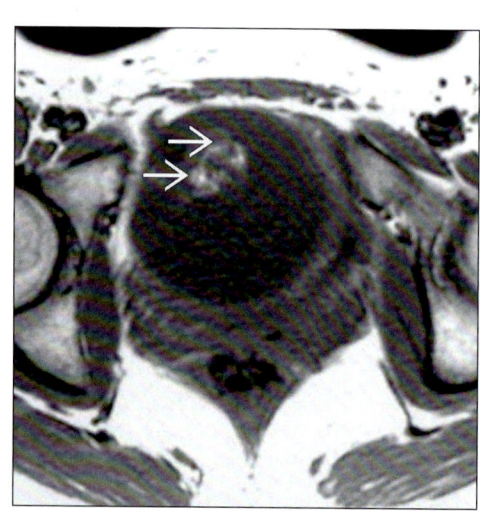
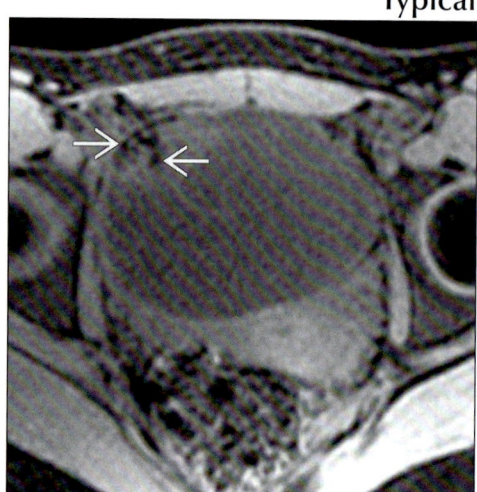

(Left) Axial T1WI MR in the same patient as previous image shows a cystic complex mass with soft tissue component that has a small amount of fat within it ➡. (Right) Axial T1WI FS MR in the same patient as previous image shows drop in signal intensity within small fatty component ➡ of the cystic mass.

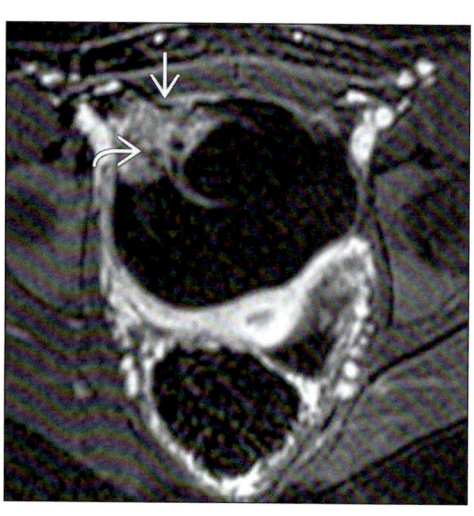
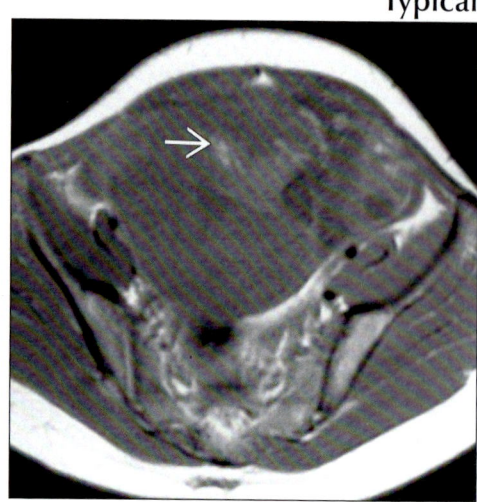

(Left) Axial T1 C+ FS MR (same patient as previous image) shows enhancing soft tissue component ➡ within cystic mass. Note the drop in SI of tiny fatty portion ➡ of the mass. Pathology: Grade 2 immature cystic teratoma. (Right) Axial T1WI MR shows a large cystic pelvic mass in the midline of a 13 yo girl. Areas of high signal on T1WI ➡ represent tiny areas of fat. Without confirmatory fat-saturated images, these high T1 signal areas could also represent hemorrhage.

IMMATURE TERATOMA, OVARY

Typical

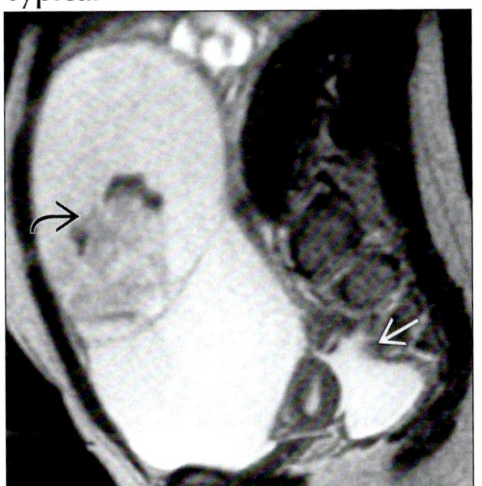
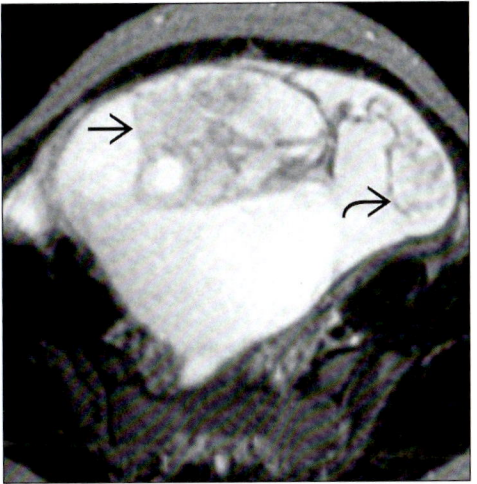

(Left) Sagittal T2WI MR in the same patient as previous image shows a large cystic pelvic mass which contains a central solid component ➔. A small amount of loculated free fluid is seen in the cul-de-sac ➔. *(Right)* Axial T2WI FS MR in the same patient as previous image, confirms the presence of a large cystic pelvic mass containing multiple internal septae ➔ and a solid component ➔.

Typical

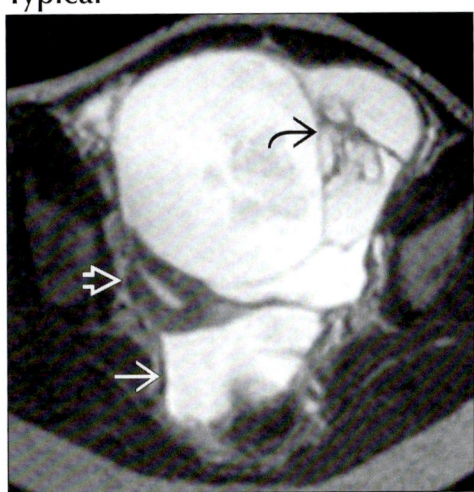
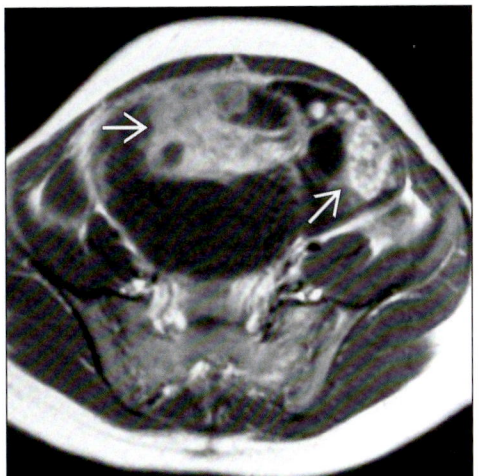

(Left) Axial T2WI FS MR in the same patient as previous image demonstrates the large midline cystic pelvic mass which contains multiple internal septae ➔. The mass is displacing the uterus ➔ posteriorly and to the right. Free fluid ➔ is seen in the cul-de-sac. *(Right)* Axial T1 C+ MR in the same patient as previous image shows the presence of the solid component ➔ which enhances after gadolinium administration.

Typical

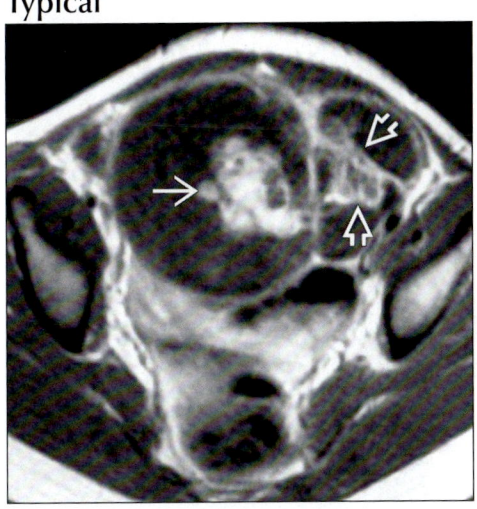
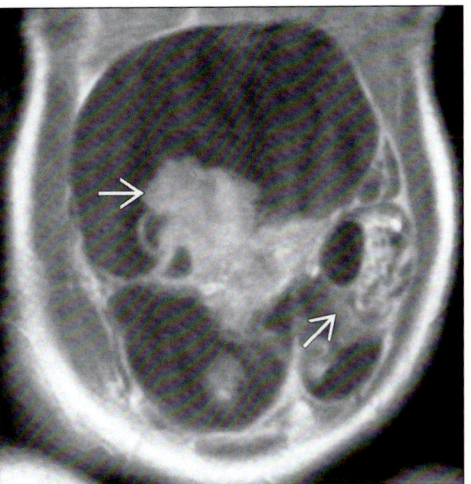

(Left) Axial T1 C+ MR in the same patient as previous image confirms the presence of enhancing soft tissue ➔ and multiple septa ➔ within the cystic mass. *(Right)* Coronal T1 C+ MR in the same patient as previous image confirms the presence of enhancing solid components ➔ within the cystic mass. Pathology: Immature teratoma.

METASTASES, OVARY

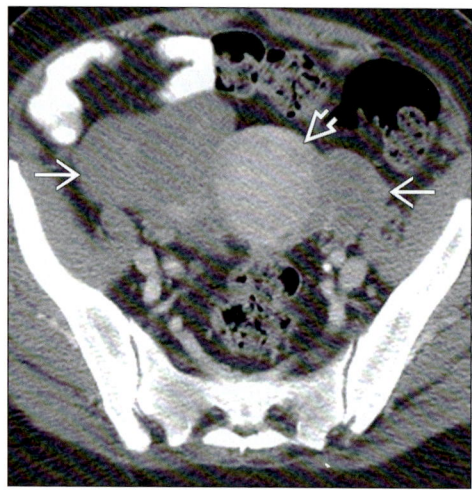

Axial CECT shows bilateral ovarian metastases ➡ from colon cancer. Uterus ⇨ is also seen.

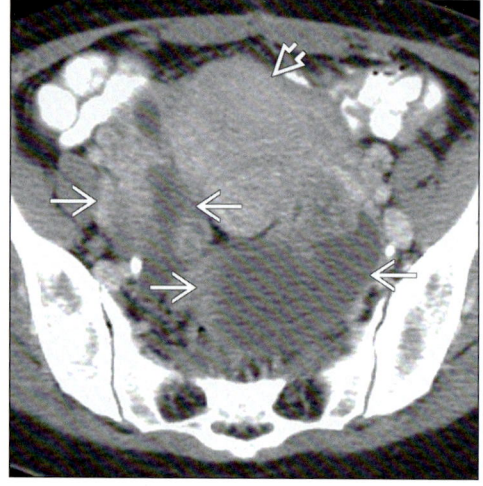

Axial CECT shows bilateral ovarian metastases ➡ with cystic and solid components. Uterus ⇨ is also seen.

TERMINOLOGY

Abbreviations and Synonyms
- Metastases to ovary, Krukenberg tumor
  - "Krukenberg tumor" is sometimes used inappropriately by some to include all metastatic ovarian carcinomas
  - Krukenberg tumor: Metastases to ovary consisting of mucin-filled signet ring cells in a cellular stroma, usually from a carcinoma of gastric antrum

Definitions
- Secondary (metastatic) neoplasms to the ovary

IMAGING FINDINGS

General Features
- Best diagnostic clue
  - Bilateral ovarian masses in a patient with known primary carcinoma
  - Metastases to ovary are usually solid masses
  - However, cystic and necrotic areas can be seen and the tumors can resemble primary ovarian cancer
- Location: Commonly both ovaries are involved
- Size: Often large masses
- Morphology: Solid, lobulated masses

Ultrasonographic Findings
- Grayscale Ultrasound: Heterogeneous echotexture
- Color Doppler: Solid components demonstrate vascularity

CT Findings
- NECT: Metastatic ovarian tumors often have soft tissue density but may demonstrate low attenuation cystic or necrotic areas
- CECT
  - Solid components often demonstrate marked inhomogeneous enhancement
  - Cystic and necrotic areas do not enhance

MR Findings
- T1WI: Solid components demonstrate medium signal intensity
- T2WI
  - Solid components demonstrate heterogeneous signal intensity

DDx: Ovarian Malignancies

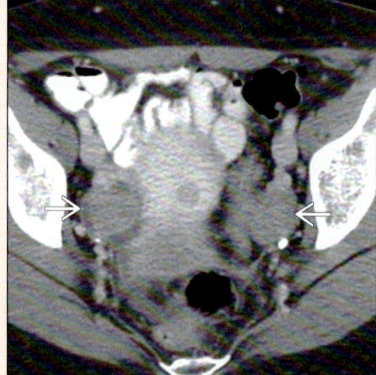

Bilateral Ovarian Cancer

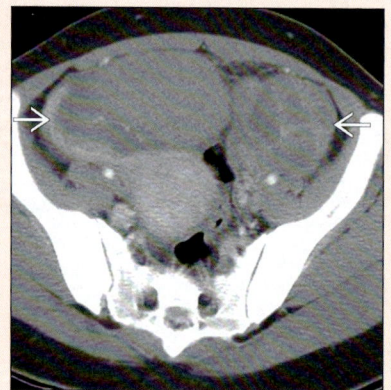

Bilateral Ovarian Cancer

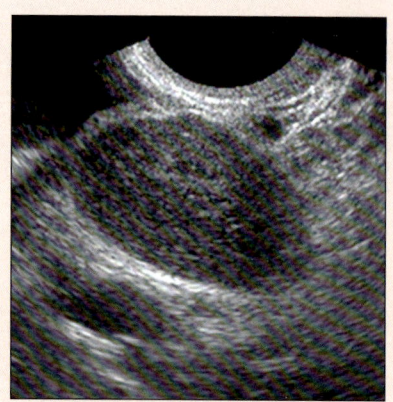

Ovarian Lymphoma

METASTASES, OVARY

Key Facts

Terminology
- Metastases to ovary, Krukenberg tumor

Imaging Findings
- Bilateral ovarian masses in a patient with known primary carcinoma
- Location: Commonly both ovaries are involved
- Ultrasound is usually the first modality to demonstrate ovarian involvement in patient with known malignancy
- CT and MR can be used to assess the extent of disease

Pathology
- Metastases to ovary occur most commonly in colon cancer, gastric cancer, breast cancer, lung cancer and contralateral ovarian cancer

- Krukenberg tumors are metastatic ovarian tumors that contain mucin-secreting signet ring cells usually originating from gastrointestinal tract (especially stomach)
- 5-15% of malignant ovarian tumors are metastatic tumors to ovary

Diagnostic Checklist
- Imaging findings of primary ovarian cancer and metastases to ovaries overlap in many cases and confident imaging distinction between the two may be challenging
- **Features more often seen in metastases to the ovary include**
- Bilateral ovarian masses
- Predominately solid appearance of the mass

---

  o Cystic and necrotic components demonstrate high signal intensity
- T1 C+: Solid components show marked heterogeneous enhancement

Imaging Recommendations
- Best imaging tool
  o Ultrasound is usually the first modality to demonstrate ovarian involvement in patient with known malignancy
  o CT and MR can be used to assess the extent of disease

DIFFERENTIAL DIAGNOSIS

Primary Ovarian Cancer
- Most primary ovarian carcinomas are predominantly cystic masses
  o Multilocularity of a cystic mass suggests primary ovarian tumor
- Whereas, most secondary malignancies of ovary are predominantly solid or a mixture of solid and cystic areas

Ovarian Lymphoma
- Ovarian lymphomas are often homogeneous solid masses
- Extensive involvement of lymph node chains is seen in lymphoma

PATHOLOGY

General Features
- General path comments
  o Metastases to ovary occur by hematogenous, lymphatic, transperitoneal or direct extension
  o Metastases to ovary occur most commonly in colon cancer, gastric cancer, breast cancer, lung cancer and contralateral ovarian cancer

  o Other rare sites include endometrial carcinoma, melanoma, pancreatic carcinoma and carcinoid tumor
  o Krukenberg tumors are metastatic ovarian tumors that contain mucin-secreting signet ring cells usually originating from gastrointestinal tract (especially stomach)
- Epidemiology
  o 5-15% of malignant ovarian tumors are metastatic tumors to ovary
  o 5-30% of cancer patients have ovarian metastases at autopsy
  o Only 30-40% of ovarian metastases are Krukenberg tumors

Gross Pathologic & Surgical Features
- Metastases to ovary are usually solid, large, kidney-shaped masses
- They have a tendency to preserve the contour of ovary
- Hemorrhage or necrosis may be present within the mass

Microscopic Features
- Hyperplasia of ovarian stromal cells with significant number of signet ring cells
- Features favoring a metastatic rather than a primary ovarian neoplasm include
  o Bilaterality
  o Nodular pattern of ovarian involvement
  o Infiltrative pattern of stromal invasion
  o Microscopic surface deposits of tumor
  o Marked lymphovascular invasion (especially in the hilum and outside the ovary)
  o Single cell infiltration and signet ring forms
  o Cells floating in mucin
  o Variation in growth pattern from one nodule to another

Staging, Grading or Classification Criteria
- Staging is based on staging system of the primary malignancy

METASTASES, OVARY

CLINICAL ISSUES

Presentation
- Most common signs/symptoms
  - Abdominal pain
  - Palpable pelvic masses
- Other signs/symptoms: Occasionally associated hormonal activity can be seen due to reactive ovarian stromal hyperplasia
- Clinical Profile
  - In many cases there is a known history of a primary neoplasm
  - Usually symptoms of primary disease precede symptoms secondary to ovarian metastasis
  - On occasions presentation is with symptoms related to an ovarian mass in a patient with no known history of malignancy

Demographics
- Age: More common in premenopausal women due to vascularity of ovaries

Natural History & Prognosis
- Poor prognosis with mortality rate of about 90% one year after ovarian metastasis is discovered

Treatment
- Radical tumor-reductive surgery
- Poor response to chemotherapy
- Due to high risk of ovarian metastasis, palliative bilateral oophorectomy may be performed during surgery for colon cancer

DIAGNOSTIC CHECKLIST

Consider
- Imaging findings of primary ovarian cancer and metastases to ovaries overlap in many cases and confident imaging distinction between the two may be challenging
- In patients with metastases to ovaries, primary tumor is often clinically overt and associated with findings of widespread metastatic disease
- Investigation of gastrointestinal tract is recommended in a patient without known primary cancer

Image Interpretation Pearls
- **Features more often seen in metastases to the ovary include**
  - Bilateral ovarian masses
  - Predominately solid appearance of the mass

SELECTED REFERENCES

1. Chang WC et al: CT and MRI of adnexal masses in patients with primary nonovarian malignancy. AJR Am J Roentgenol. 186(4):1039-45, 2006
2. Khunamornpong S et al: Primary and metastatic mucinous adenocarcinomas of the ovary: Evaluation of the diagnostic approach using tumor size and laterality. Gynecol Oncol. 101(1):152-7, 2006
3. Kiyokawa T et al: Krukenberg tumors of the ovary: a clinicopathologic analysis of 120 cases with emphasis on their variable pathologic manifestations. Am J Surg Pathol. 30(3):277-99, 2006
4. Lewis MR et al: Ovarian involvement by metastatic colorectal adenocarcinoma: still a diagnostic challenge. Am J Surg Pathol. 30(2):177-84, 2006
5. Hart WR. Related Articles et al: Diagnostic challenge of secondary (metastatic) ovarian tumors simulating primary endometrioid and mucinous neoplasms. Pathol Int. 55(5):231-43, 2005
6. Irving JA et al: Lung carcinoma metastatic to the ovary: a clinicopathologic study of 32 cases emphasizing their morphologic spectrum and problems in differential diagnosis. Am J Surg Pathol. 29(8):997-1006, 2005
7. McCluggage WG et al: Metastatic neoplasms involving the ovary: a review with an emphasis on morphological and immunohistochemical features. Histopathology. 47(3):231-47, 2005
8. Prat J. Related Articles et al: Ovarian carcinomas, including secondary tumors: diagnostically challenging areas. Mod Pathol. 18 Suppl 2:S99-111, 2005
9. Alcazar JL et al: Transvaginal gray scale and color Doppler sonography in primary ovarian cancer and metastatic tumors to the ovary. J Ultrasound Med. 22(3):243-7, 2003
10. Lee KR et al: The distinction between primary and metastatic mucinous carcinomas of the ovary: gross and histologic findings in 50 cases. Am J Surg Pathol. 27(3):281-92, 2003
11. Seidman JD et al: Primary and metastatic mucinous adenocarcinomas in the ovaries: incidence in routine practice with a new approach to improve intraoperative diagnosis. Am J Surg Pathol. 27(7):985-93, 2003
12. Jung SE et al: CT and MR imaging of ovarian tumors with emphasis on differential diagnosis. Radiographics. 22(6):1305-25, 2002
13. Brown DL et al: Primary versus secondary ovarian malignancy: imaging findings of adnexal masses in the Radiology Diagnostic Oncology Group Study. Radiology. 219(1):213-8, 2001
14. McCarville MB et al: Secondary ovarian neoplasms in children: imaging features with histopathologic correlation. Pediatr Radiol. 31(5):358-64, 2001
15. Hann LE et al: Adnexal masses in women with breast cancer: US findings with clinical and histopathologic correlation. Radiology. 216(1):242-7, 2000
16. Lindner V et al: [Ovarian metastasis of colorectal adenocarcinomas. A clinico-pathological study of 41 cases] Ann Pathol. 19(6):492-8, 1999
17. Ronnett BM et al: The morphologic spectrum of ovarian metastases of appendiceal adenocarcinomas: a clinicopathologic and immunohistochemical analysis of tumors often misinterpreted as primary ovarian tumors or metastatic tumors from other gastrointestinal sites. Am J Surg Pathol. 21(10):1144-55, 1997
18. Kim SH et al: CT and MR findings of Krukenberg tumors: comparison with primary ovarian tumors. J Comput Assist Tomogr. 20(3):393-8, 1996
19. Lash RH et al: Intestinal adenocarcinomas metastatic to the ovaries. A clinicopathologic evaluation of 22 cases. Am J Surg Pathol. 11(2):114-21, 1987

METASTASES, OVARY

IMAGE GALLERY

Typical

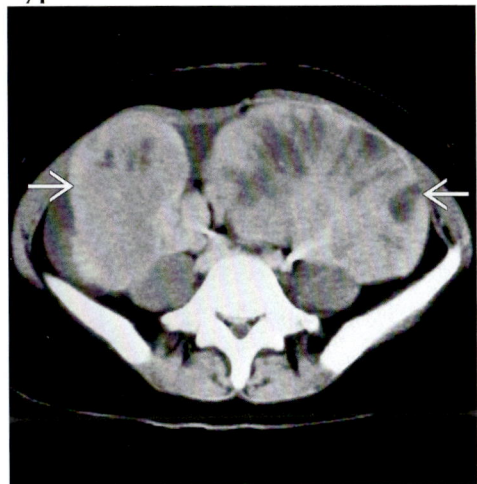
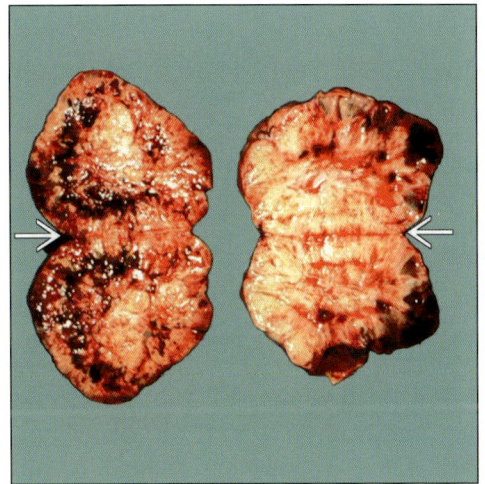

(Left) Axial CECT shows bilateral ovarian metastases from gastric cancer (Krukenberg tumor). Bilateral, heterogeneously enhancing, solid adnexal masses ➡ are seen. *(Right)* Gross pathology specimen shows ovarian metastasis from gastric cancer (Krukenberg tumor). Bilateral solid ovarian masses ➡ are depicted.

Typical

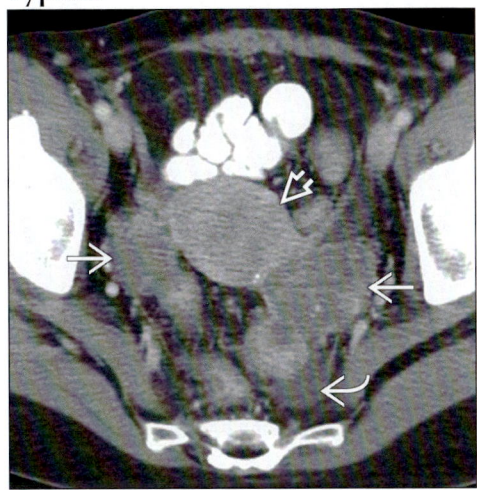
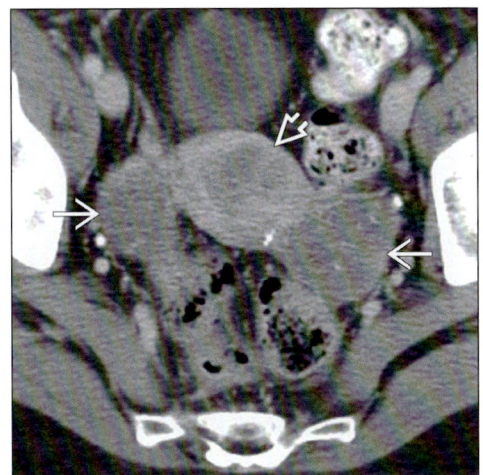

(Left) Axial CECT shows bilateral heterogeneously enhancing ovarian metastases ➡. Uterus ➡ is also seen. There is small amount of pelvic ascites ➡. *(Right)* Axial CECT shows bilateral ovarian metastases ➡ with heterogeneous enhancement. Uterus ➡ is also seen.

Typical

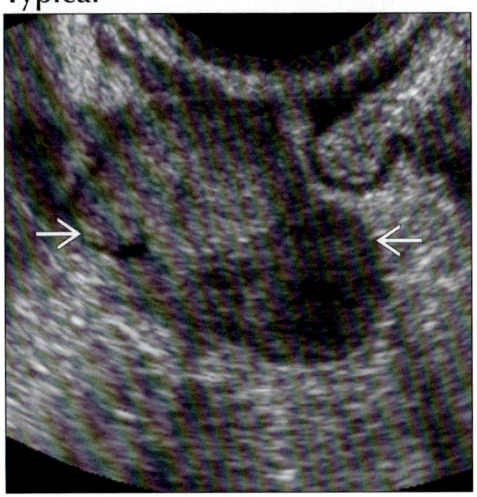
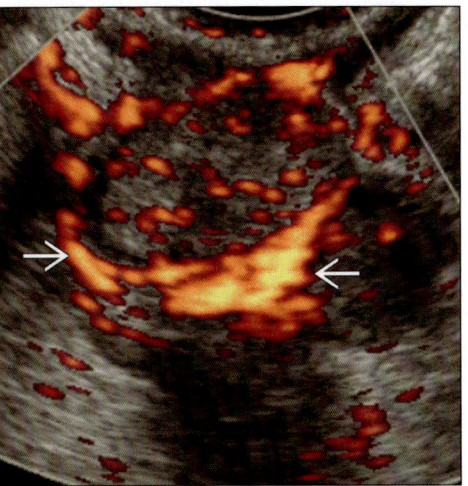

(Left) Sagittal oblique transabdominal ultrasound shows a left ovarian metastasis ➡ seen as a solid mass with heterogeneous echogenicity. *(Right)* Sagittal oblique power Doppler ultrasound shows marked vascularity ➡ in the left ovarian metastasis.

METASTASES, OVARY

Typical

(Left) Axial CECT shows a heterogeneously enhancing solid ➔ metastasis in the right ovary. (Right) Axial T2WI MR shows the same right ovarian metastasis as previous image ➔ seen as a heterogeneous solid mass.

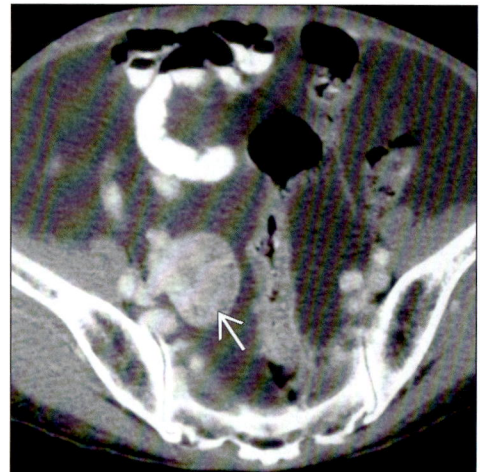
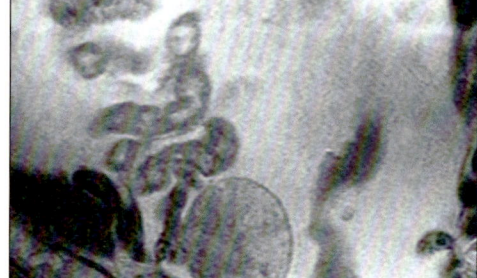

Typical

(Left) Axial T1WI MR shows an intermediate signal intensity left ovarian metastasis ➔ from adenocarcinoma of the appendix. A pelvic implant ➔ is also seen anteriorly on the right. (Right) Axial T2WI MR shows a large left ovarian metastasis ➔ with heterogeneous high signal intensity. A right pelvic implant ➔ and pelvic ascites ➔ are also seen.

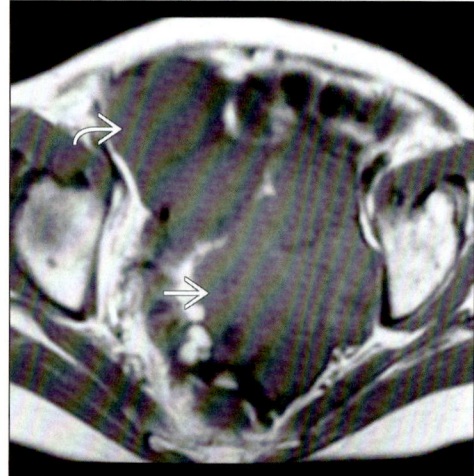
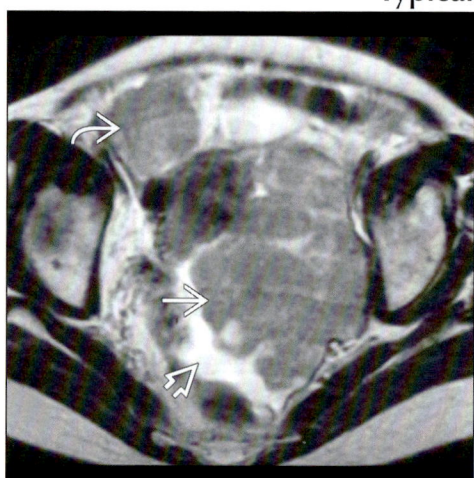

Typical

(Left) Axial CECT shows bilateral ovarian metastases ➔ that have predominantly cystic components. The uterus ➔ is also seen. (Right) Axial CECT shows enhancing solid components ➔ of the bilateral ovarian metastases ➔ in the same patient as previous image.

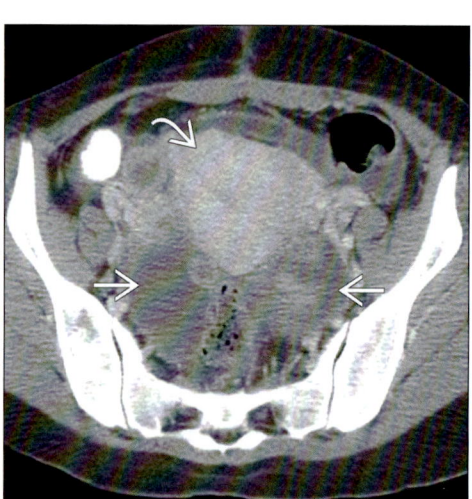
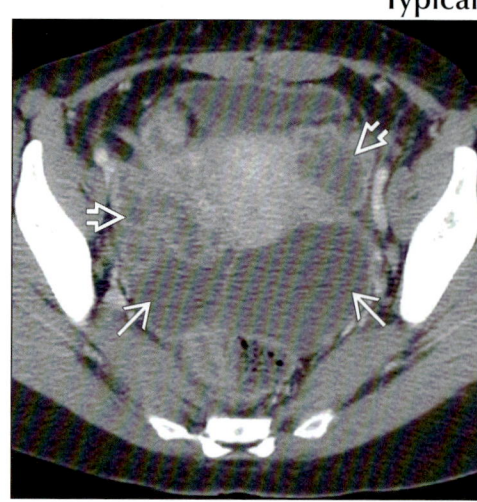

METASTASES, OVARY

Typical

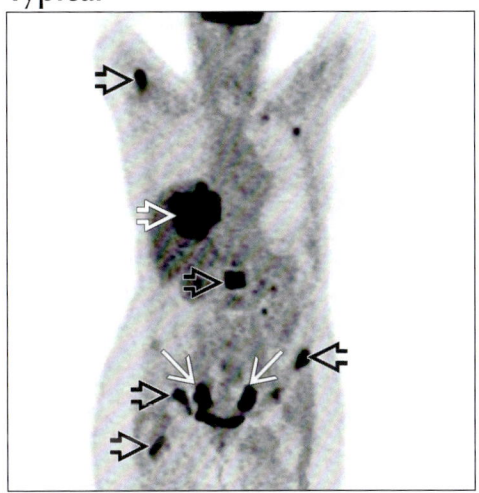 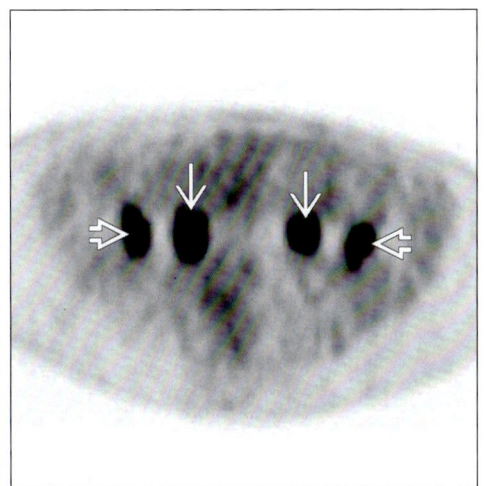

(Left) Coronal PET shows bilateral ovarian metastases ➔ in a patient with breast cancer. A large liver metastasis ➔ and multiple bone metastases ➔ are also seen. *(Right)* Axial PET shows bilateral ovarian metastases ➔ and bilateral pelvic bone metastases ➔.

Typical

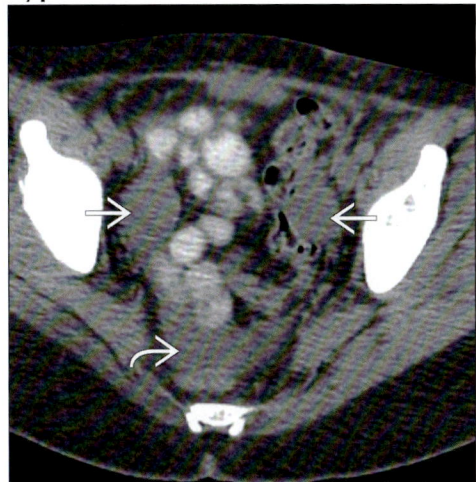 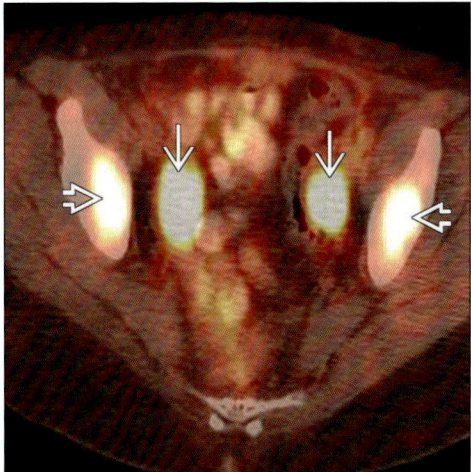

(Left) Axial NECT shows bilateral ovarian metastases ➔ and pelvic ascites ➔. *(Right)* Axial fused PET/CT shows intense uptake in the ovarian metastases ➔ and bone metastases ➔.

Typical

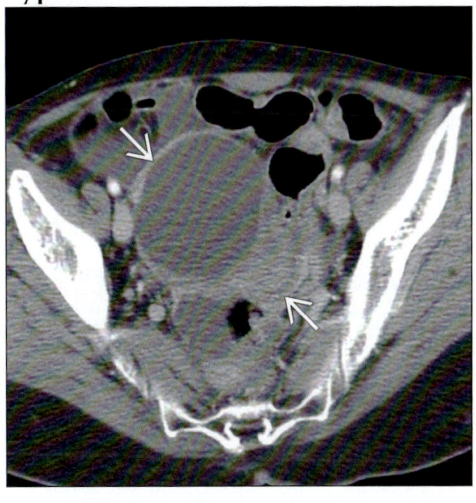 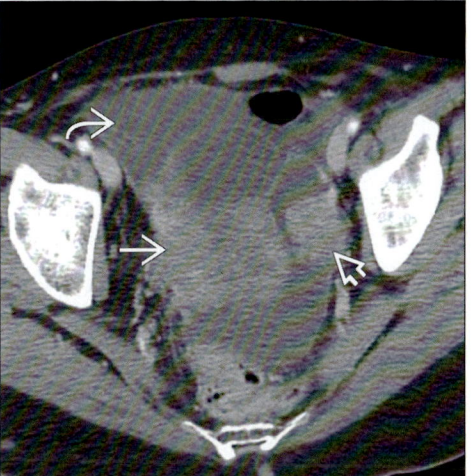

(Left) Axial CECT shows a mixed cystic and solid metastasis ➔ in the right ovary in a patient with gastric cancer. *(Right)* Axial CECT shows a solid left ovarian metastasis ➔ in addition to the right ovarian metastasis ➔ in the same patient as previous image. Pelvic ascites ➔ is also seen.

OVARIAN CANCER, CHARACTERIZATION & STAGING

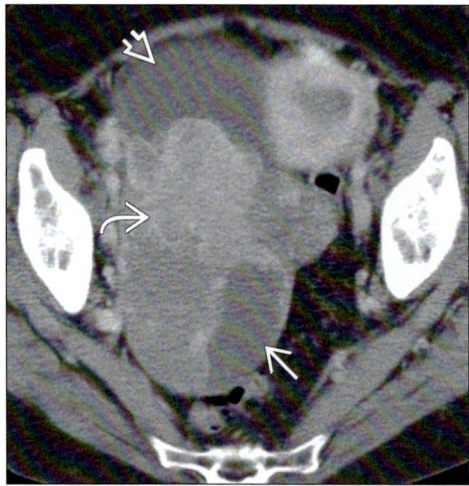

Axial CECT shows a large right ovarian cancer seen as a complex mass with cystic ➡ and solid ➡ components. Ascites ➡ is also seen.

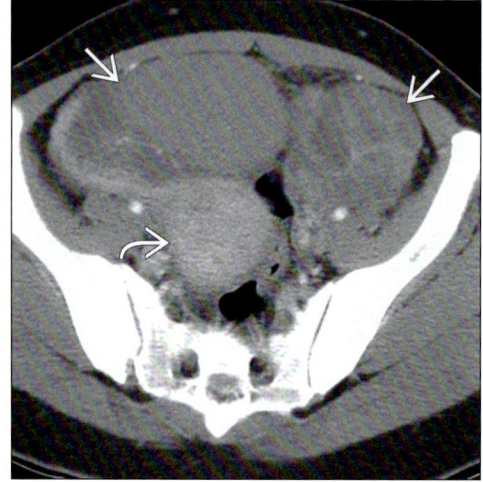

Axial CECT shows bilateral ovarian cancer seen as complex masses ➡ in the adnexal regions. Uterus ➡ is also seen.

TERMINOLOGY

Definitions
- Primary malignant neoplasm of ovary

IMAGING FINDINGS

General Features
- Best diagnostic clue
  - Unilateral or bilateral complex cystic adnexal masses with septations and papillary projections or solid adnexal masses with variable degree of necrosis
  - Advanced cases are frequently associated with ascites and peritoneal carcinomatosis
- Location: Unilateral or bilateral ovarian involvement can be seen
- Size: Often large masses at time of initial diagnosis

Ultrasonographic Findings
- Grayscale Ultrasound
  - Cystic components may be entirely anechoic or may contain low level echoes
  - Thick septations (> 3 mm), echogenic mural nodularity or papillary projections are seen in the cystic mass
  - Fibrinous debris or clot adherent to cyst wall may mimic papillary projections on grayscale ultrasound
- Color Doppler
  - Helps identifying solid components that show vascularity in a complex cystic mass
  - Central color Doppler flow within solid components of ovarian mass is a good predictor of malignancy
  - On spectral Doppler ovarian cancers generally have low resistance waveforms (RI < 0.4)

CT Findings
- NECT: Cystic adnexal mass with septations and soft tissue density papillary projections
- CECT
  - Solid mural nodules demonstrate enhancement
  - May facilitate detection of peritoneal implants and distant metastases

MR Findings
- T1WI
  - Low to intermediate signal intensity masses

DDx: Ovarian Masses

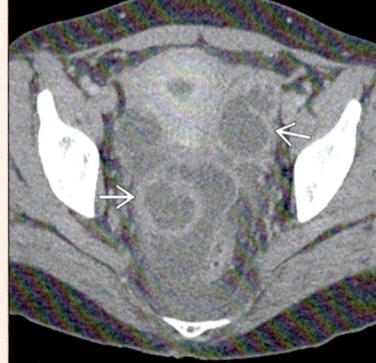

Tubo-Ovarian Abscess

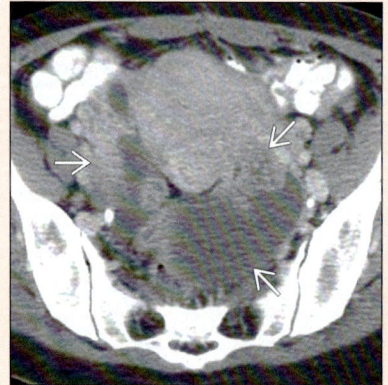

Metastases to Ovary

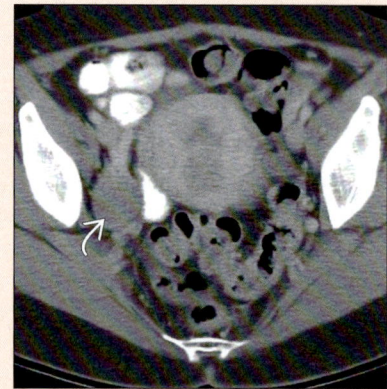

Ovarian Lymphoma

OVARIAN CANCER, CHARACTERIZATION & STAGING

Key Facts

Imaging Findings
- Unilateral or bilateral complex cystic adnexal masses with septations and papillary projections or solid adnexal masses with variable degree of necrosis
- Advanced cases are frequently associated with ascites and peritoneal carcinomatosis
- Location: Unilateral or bilateral ovarian involvement can be seen
- Size: Often large masses at time of initial diagnosis

Pathology
- Fifth most common malignancy in women
- Leading cause of death from gynecologic cancer

Clinical Issues
- Nulliparity, family history, and use of fertility drugs increase risk of ovarian cancer
- Up to 85% of patients present with peritoneal disease at time of initial presentation
- Age: Peak incidence at age 40-65 years

Diagnostic Checklist
- Role of imaging in ovarian cancer includes
- Characterization of an adnexal mass
- Imaging features associated with malignancy are solid-cystic complex mass, wall irregularity, thick septations and papillary projections in a cystic lesion, and large size of a lesion
- Pre-operative staging to determine if patients are candidates for neoadjuvant therapy prior to surgery
- Follow-up of treatment response and detection of recurrent disease

---

- High signal intensity areas due to fat or hemorrhage can be seen
- T1WI FS: Helps distinguish between fat and hemorrhage as signal from fat is suppressed
- T2WI: High signal intensity cystic masses with thick septations, and/or intermediate signal intensity mural nodules
- T1 C+: Facilitates detection of papillary projections in cystic mass, tumor necrosis and peritoneal implants

Nuclear Medicine Findings
- PET
  - FDG PET is a promising method in evaluation of recurrent or residual disease
  - Sensitivity of FDG PET in detecting small tumor implants is limited

Imaging Recommendations
- Best imaging tool
  - US is the initial modality for detection and characterization of an adnexal mass
  - MR is a problem-solving modality in cases of indeterminate adnexal mass on US
  - CT of abdomen and pelvis is most commonly used for pre-operative staging and follow-up after treatment

DIFFERENTIAL DIAGNOSIS

Tubo-Ovarian Abscess
- Acutely ill patient with fever and bilateral adnexal masses and pelvic ascites

Endometriosis
- Chronic painful pelvic masses; high signal intensity on T1WI; "shading" phenomena on T2WI

Hemorrhagic Cyst
- Unilateral adnexal cyst; high on T1WI; undergoing transformation and spontaneous resolution

Cystic Teratoma
- Cystic mass with solid nodule and fat-fluid level; best evaluated with MR

Ovarian Metastases
- Bilateral masses, frequently solid with areas of necrosis in a patient with known malignancy

Ovarian Lymphoma
- Homogeneous solid adnexal masses

PATHOLOGY

General Features
- General path comments
  - 85% ovarian malignant tumors are of surface epithelial origin, remaining 15% derived from germ and stromal cells
    - Malignant epithelial tumors are of serous, mucinous, endometrioid, clear cell, undifferentiated and Brenner types
    - Malignant germ cell tumors are of dysgerminoma, immature teratoma, endodermal sinus tumor, malignant mixed germ cell tumor, embryonal carcinoma and choriocarcinoma types
    - Sex cord-stromal tumors originate from stromal cells (granulosa and Sertoli cells) or stromal cells (fibroblasts, theca cells, Leydig cells)
- Genetics
  - 90% are sporadic
  - 10% are due to hereditary syndromes such as BRCA-1 and BRCA-2 mutation (risk of breast cancer), Lynch syndrome II (risk of colon cancer)
- Epidemiology
  - Fifth most common malignancy in women
  - Leading cause of death from gynecologic cancer

Gross Pathologic & Surgical Features
- Cystic masses with internal polypoid excrescences or solid masses with necrosis

OVARIAN CANCER, CHARACTERIZATION & STAGING

Microscopic Features
- Depends on type of ovarian cancer

Staging, Grading or Classification Criteria
- Comprehensive staging laparotomy includes
  - Total abdominal hysterectomy
  - Bilateral salpingo-oophorectomy
  - Omentectomy
  - Peritoneal washings
  - Random sampling of multiple peritoneal sites
  - Pelvic and retroperitoneal lymphadenectomy
- FIGO staging system
  - Stage I: Tumor limited to ovaries
  - Stage II: Tumor confined to pelvis
  - Stage III: Intraperitoneal metastases outside the pelvis, and/or positive retroperitoneal lymph nodes
  - Stage IV: Distant metastases

CLINICAL ISSUES

Presentation
- Most common signs/symptoms
  - Abdominal pain
  - Abdominal distention
  - Pelvic mass
  - Vaginal bleeding
- Clinical Profile
  - Nulliparity, family history, and use of fertility drugs increase risk of ovarian cancer
  - Up to 85% of patients present with peritoneal disease at time of initial presentation

Demographics
- Age: Peak incidence at age 40-65 years

Natural History & Prognosis
- Most patients present with advanced stage
- 5 year survival approaches 80-90% in patients with stage I disease
- 5 year survival ranges from 5-50% in women with stage III-IV disease

Treatment
- Surgical cytoreduction: Reduction of all tumor deposits to a maximal diameter of less than 1 cm
- Chemotherapy
- Radiation

DIAGNOSTIC CHECKLIST

Consider
- Combination of CA-125 and US screening are only justified in high-risk population (positive family history, or patients with breast cancer)

Image Interpretation Pearls
- **Role of imaging in ovarian cancer includes**
  - Characterization of an adnexal mass
    - Imaging features associated with malignancy are solid-cystic complex mass, wall irregularity, thick septations and papillary projections in a cystic lesion, and large size of a lesion
  - Pre-operative staging to determine if patients are candidates for neoadjuvant therapy prior to surgery
    - Peritoneal metastases appear as nodular or plaque-like enhancing soft tissue masses of varying sizes
    - Implants most commonly seen in cul-de-sac, paracolic gutters, subdiaphragmatic space, splenic hilum, porta hepatic, & along falciform ligament
    - Diffuse infiltration of omentum by tumor is called omental caking
    - Presence of lymph node metastases in ovarian cancer is an important prognostic feature
    - Internal iliac, obturator, external iliac, paraaortic and superior diaphragmatic lymph nodes are common sites of involvement
    - Common sites of distant metastases are liver, lung, pleura, adrenal, spleen, bone and brain
  - Follow-up of treatment response and detection of recurrent disease
    - Recurrent ovarian malignancies manifest as pelvic masses, peritoneal tumor implants, malignant ascites, lymphadenopathy, lung or pleural lesions or liver metastases
    - Two types of pelvic recurrence are described; central recurrence at vaginal cuff and pelvic sidewall recurrence
    - Recurrent disease with pelvic sidewall invasion, bulky upper abdominal disease and large bowel obstruction are non-resectable

SELECTED REFERENCES
1. Kinkel K et al: Indeterminate ovarian mass at US: incremental value of second imaging test for characterization--meta-analysis and Bayesian analysis. Radiology. 236(1):85-94, 2005
2. Smith LH et al: Ovarian cancer: can we make the clinical diagnosis earlier? Cancer. 104(7):1398-407, 2005
3. Sohaib SA et al: The role of magnetic resonance imaging and ultrasound in patients with adnexal masses. Clin Radiol. 60(3):340-8, 2005
4. Spencer JA: A multidisciplinary approach to ovarian cancer at diagnosis. Br J Radiol. 78 Spec No 2:S94-102, 2005
5. Togashi K: Ovarian cancer: the clinical role of US, CT, and MRI. Eur Radiol. 13 Suppl 4:L87-104, 2003
6. Coakley FV et al: Peritoneal metastases: detection with spiral CT in patients with ovarian cancer. Radiology. 223(2):495-9, 2002
7. Brown DL et al: Primary versus secondary ovarian malignancy: imaging findings of adnexal masses in the Radiology Diagnostic Oncology Group Study. Radiology. 219(1):213-8, 2001
8. Hricak H et al: Complex adnexal masses: detection and characterization with MR imaging--multivariate analysis. Radiology. 214(1):39-46, 2000
9. Jeong YY et al: Imaging evaluation of ovarian masses. Radiographics. 20(5):1445-70, 2000
10. Tempany CM et al: Staging of advanced ovarian cancer: comparison of imaging modalities--report from the Radiological Diagnostic Oncology Group. Radiology. 215(3):761-7, 2000
11. Kurtz AB et al: Diagnosis and staging of ovarian cancer: comparative values of Doppler and conventional US, CT, and MR imaging correlated with surgery and histopathologic analysis--report of the Radiology Diagnostic Oncology Group. Radiology. 212(1):19-27, 1999

OVARIAN CANCER, CHARACTERIZATION & STAGING

IMAGE GALLERY

Typical

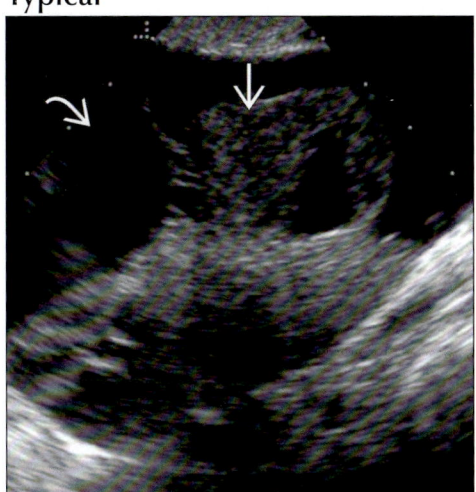
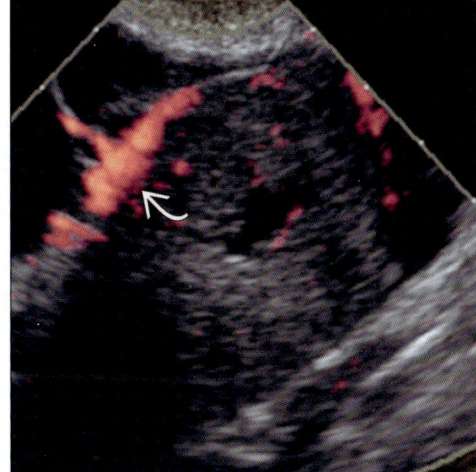

(Left) Sagittal oblique transabdominal ultrasound shows a large ovarian cancer with anechoic cystic ➡ and echogenic solid components ➡. *(Right)* Sagittal oblique power Doppler ultrasound shows marked vascularity ➡ in the solid component of the mass.

Typical

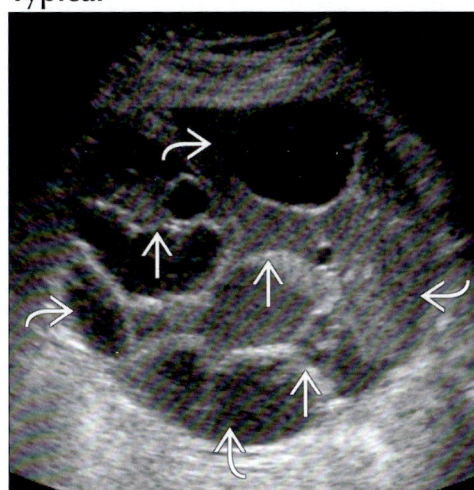
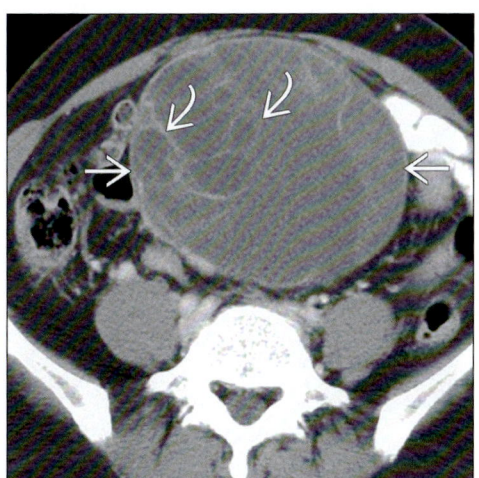

(Left) Axial oblique transabdominal ultrasound shows a large ovarian cancer seen as a complex cystic mass with various echoes in the cystic locules ➡ separated with thick septations ➡. *(Right)* Axial CECT shows an ovarian cancer seen as a complex cystic mass ➡ with enhancing septations ➡.

Typical

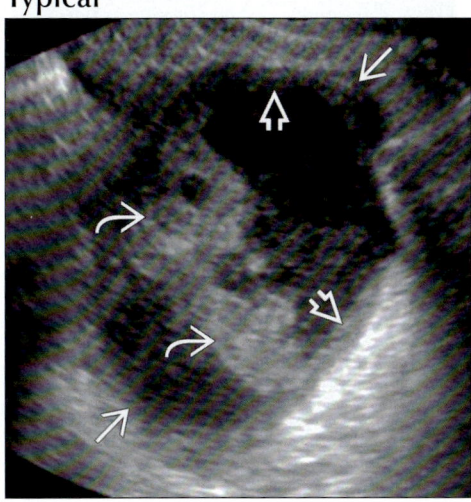
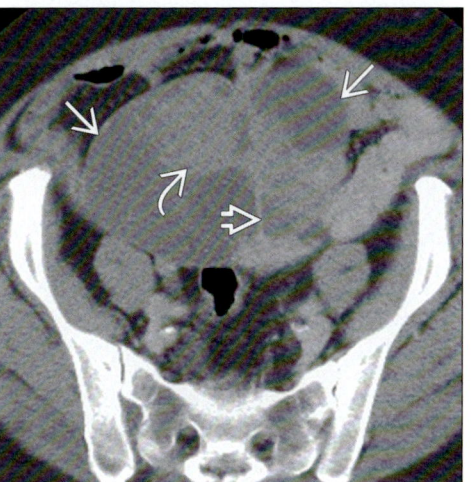

(Left) Axial oblique transabdominal ultrasound shows an ovarian cancer with a solid component ➡ projecting into complex cystic mass ➡. Note that the mass has thick walls ➡. *(Right)* Axial CECT shows a large ovarian cancer seen as a cystic mass ➡ with enhancing solid components ➡ and thick septations ➡.

OVARIAN CANCER, CHARACTERIZATION & STAGING

Typical

(Left) Axial T2WI MR shows a large ovarian cancer with high signal intensity cystic ⇨ and intermediate signal intensity solid components ⇨. Layering low signal intensity hemorrhage ⇨ is also seen in some of the cystic components. (Right) Sagittal T2WI MR shows the same tumor with cystic ⇨ and solid ⇨ components.

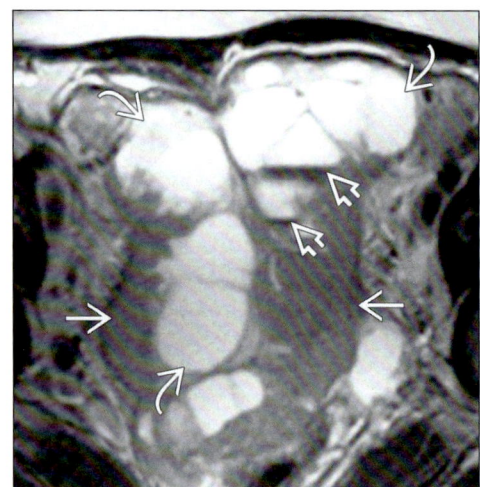
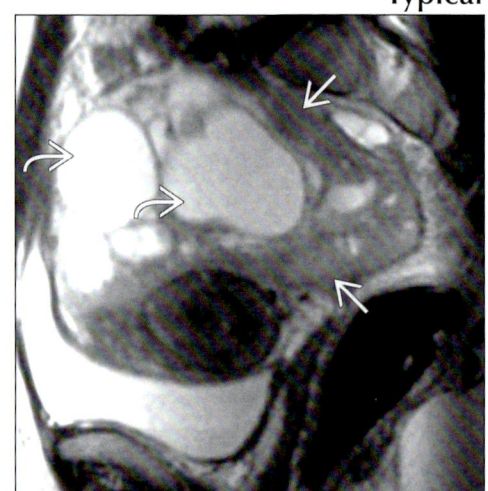

Typical

(Left) Axial T2WI MR shows a right ovarian cancer seen as a complex cystic and solid mass ⇨. Ascites ⇨ is also seen. (Right) Axial T1 C+ FS MR shows that the solid components ⇨ of the mass enhance, whereas cystic components ⇨ do not. Note the thickened and enhancing peritoneum ⇨ consistent with peritoneal carcinomatosis.

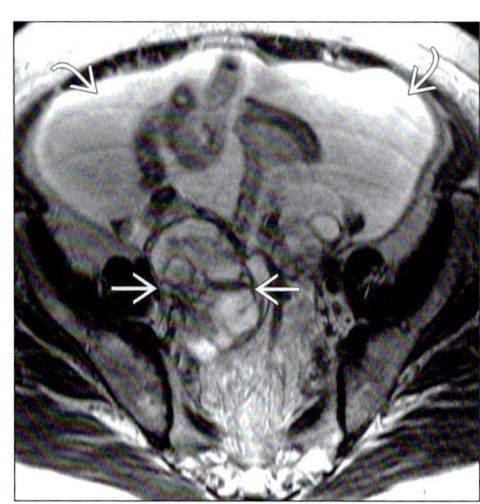

Typical

(Left) Sagittal T2WI MR shows an ovarian cancer seen as a complex mass with cystic ⇨ and solid ⇨ components. Layering hemorrhage ⇨ is seen in one of the cystic components. Ascites ⇨ is also noted. (Right) Axial CECT shows a large ovarian cancer with enhancing solid ⇨ and non-enhancing cystic ⇨ components. Note enhancing septations ⇨ in the cystic component of the mass.

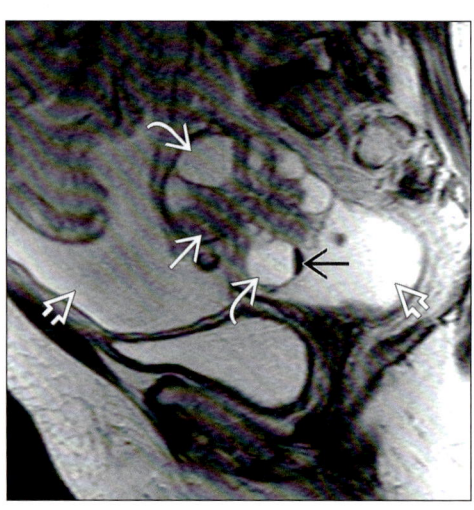
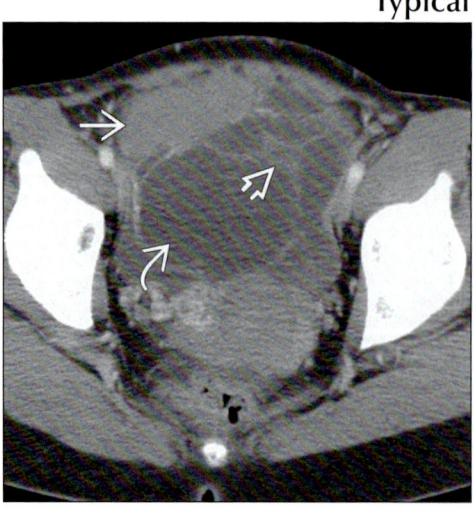

OVARIAN CANCER, CHARACTERIZATION & STAGING

Typical

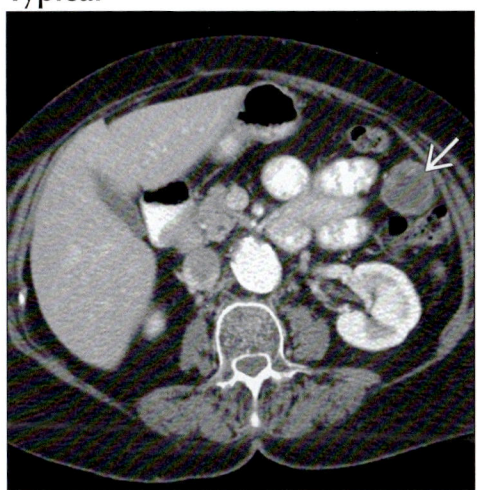
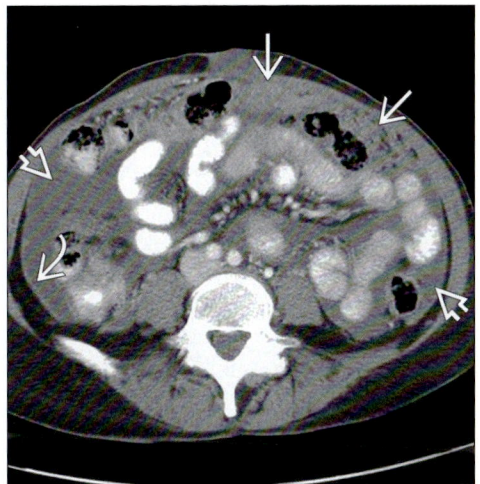

(**Left**) Axial CECT shows a peritoneal implant ➔ in the left upper quadrant in a patient with ovarian cancer. (**Right**) Axial CECT shows omental caking ➔, peritoneal thickening ➔ and ascites ➔ in a patient with ovarian cancer.

Typical

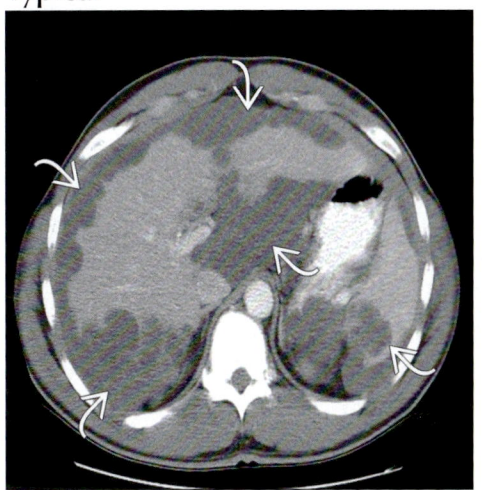
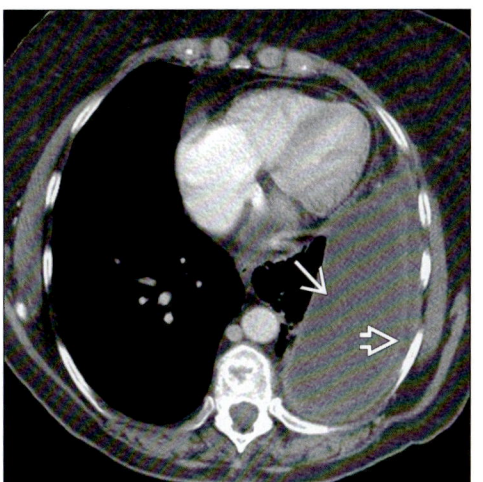

(**Left**) Axial CECT shows multiple cystic implants ➔ scalloping the surfaces of the liver and the spleen in a patient with ovarian cancer. (**Right**) Axial CECT shows a large, loculated malignant pleural effusion ➔ on the left. Note the thickening in the pleura ➔ due to pleural metastasis.

Typical

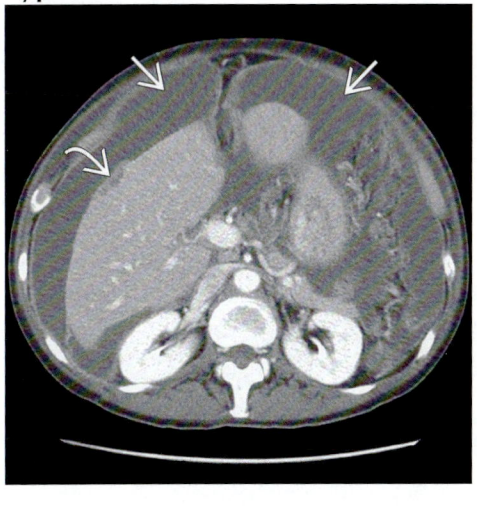
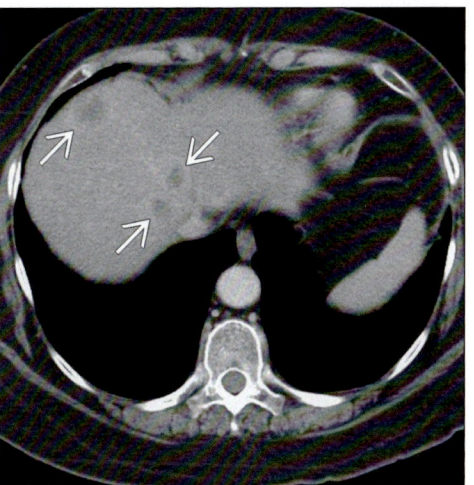

(**Left**) Axial CECT shows a liver surface implant ➔ and massive ascites ➔ in a patient with ovarian cancer. Note that liver surface implants are through peritoneal dissemination. (**Right**) Axial CECT shows multiple intrahepatic metastases ➔ in another patient with ovarian cancer. Note that intrahepatic metastases are through hematogenous dissemination.

OVARIAN CANCER, RECURRENT; RESECTABLE

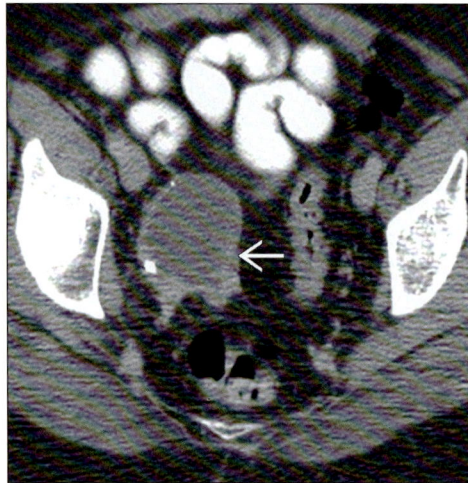

Axial CECT shows recurrent ovarian cancer seen as a mixed cystic and solid mass ➡ in the right pelvis. No pelvic side-wall invasion is seen.

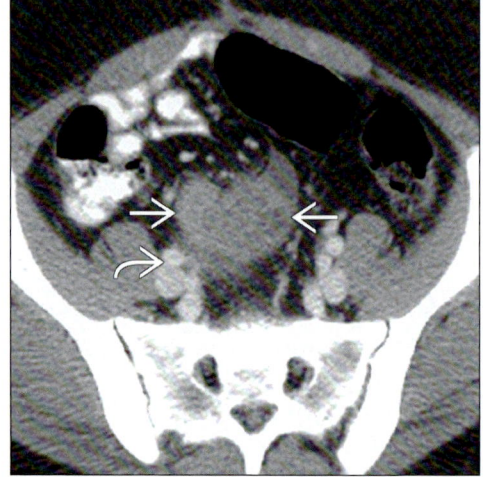

Axial CECT shows recurrent ovarian cancer seen as a solid mass ➡ in the pelvis. Note that the mass does not invade the adjacent external iliac vessels ➡.

TERMINOLOGY

Definitions
- Recurrent ovarian cancer amenable to optimal secondary cytoreduction
- **Recurrence is defined as disease relapse following**
  - Complete response to first line therapy
  - Negative second look operation
  - Disease-free interval greater than 6 months

IMAGING FINDINGS

General Features
- Best diagnostic clue
  - Recurrent mass without pelvic side wall or major vascular encasement/invasion
    - Pelvic sidewall invasion is ruled out if fat plane separating tumor from pelvic sidewall is > 3 mm
  - No evidence of disseminated disease
- Location
  - Most recurrences are in pelvis and abdomen
    - Vaginal cuff
    - Pelvic side wall
    - Peritoneum, mesentery
    - Liver, spleen
- Size: Varies from small nodules to large masses
- Morphology
  - Tumor recurrence may demonstrate different patterns
    - Well-defined nodules or lobulated masses
    - Thickening or infiltration in mesentery and along peritoneal surfaces

Radiographic Findings
- Radiography: Chest radiography may demonstrate pleural effusions due to pleural or lung metastases which indicate disseminated disease
- IVP
  - IVP may show hydroureteronephrosis with delayed nephrogram due to obstruction by recurrent mass
    - Obstruction may be due to invasion or just compression of ureter by recurrent mass
    - Tumor is unresectable if hydroureteronephrosis is due to invasion of ureter

Ultrasonographic Findings
- Grayscale Ultrasound

DDx: Recurrent Ovarian Cancer

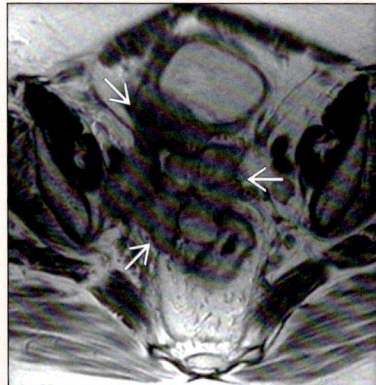

Unresectable: Pelvic Wall Invasion

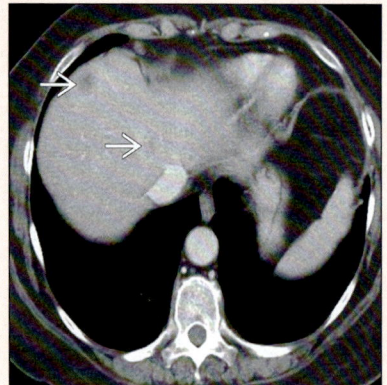

Unresectable: Liver Metastases

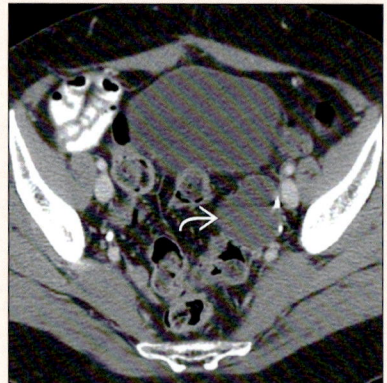

Lymphocele

OVARIAN CANCER, RECURRENT; RESECTABLE

Key Facts

Terminology
- Recurrent ovarian cancer amenable to optimal secondary cytoreduction
- **Recurrence is defined as disease relapse following**
- Complete response to first line therapy
- Negative second look operation
- Disease-free interval greater than 6 months

Clinical Issues
- Prognosis is better in patients with resectable recurrences than those with unresectable recurrences

Diagnostic Checklist
- **Imaging studies are used when**
- Tumor markers are elevated
- New clinical symptoms are present
- Imaging can assist in prediction of resectability
- Imaging findings aid the surgeon in surgical planning to optimize cytoreduction
- **Recurrent disease may present as**
- Well-defined nodules or lobulated masses
- Thickening or infiltration in the mesentery and along peritoneal surfaces
- Capsular implants indenting hepatic and splenic surfaces
- Intraparenchymal hepatic or splenic metastases, lung nodules
- **Indicators of tumor resectability in secondary cytoreduction are**
- No pelvic sidewall invasion (> 3 mm fat plane separating tumor from the pelvic sidewall)
- No bulky upper abdominal disease
- No hydronephrosis

- US is limited in assessment of extent of recurrent ovarian cancer and its resectability
- It may show large recurrences in pelvis and abdomen as solid or mixed solid and cystic masses
- US can also show or secondary signs of recurrence such as hydronephrosis, ascites, etc.

CT Findings
- CTA: Can be used to assess vascular invasion
- CECT: Heterogeneous attenuation solid or mixed solid and cystic masses

MR Findings
- T1WI: Intermediate signal intensity masses
- T2WI: Heterogeneous intensity solid or mixed solid and cystic masses
- T1 C+: Heterogeneous enhancement
- MRA: May be used to assess vascular invasion

Fluoroscopic Findings
- Small or large bowel obstruction can be seen due to
  - Invasion or compression by recurrent tumor
  - Peritoneal adhesions which may be due to peritoneal carcinomatosis or previous surgery

Nuclear Medicine Findings
- PET
  - FDG PET demonstrates radiotracer uptake at the site of recurrent tumor
  - However, FDG PET is insensitive to small-volume tumor implants
  - PET/CT facilitates to determine the exact anatomic location of recurrent masses

Imaging Recommendations
- Best imaging tool
  - CT is the most commonly used modality for detection of recurrent tumor
  - CT is very useful in determination of resectability and extent of tumor, and related complications (hydronephrosis, bowel obstruction, etc.)
    - Multidetector scanners and use of intravenous contrast facilitate detection of small-volume implants
  - MR is superior to CT in the assessment of local extent of disease due to its better soft tissue resolution
    - MR is best modality to assess pelvic sidewall invasion
    - Less than 3 mm fat plane between the mass and the pelvic side wall indicates non-resectability
    - MR can also accurately demonstrate adjacent organ and vascular invasion
  - FDG PET is accurate and useful when conventional studies are inconclusive or negative and tumor markers are rising
    - FDG PET can accurately show multiple foci of disseminated disease in abdomen and pelvis

DIFFERENTIAL DIAGNOSIS

Unresectable Recurrent Ovarian Cancer
- Recurrent mass with pelvic side wall, major vascular invasion or disseminated disease

Post-Operative Lymphocele
- Pelvic or retroperitoneal lymphoceles occur after radical pelvic lymphadenectomy
- They are entirely cystic and thin walled
- When infected they may have thickened walls
- But unlike recurrent tumor they do not have nodular solid components

PATHOLOGY

General Features
- General path comments: Pathologic findings are similar to the original type of ovarian cancer

CLINICAL ISSUES

Presentation
- Most common signs/symptoms
  - Pelvic mass

OVARIAN CANCER, RECURRENT; RESECTABLE

- Pelvic pain
- Pelvic pressure
- Abdominal distension due to recurrent masses and/or ascites
- Nausea, vomiting
- Other signs/symptoms
  - Change in bladder and bowel habits
  - Bowel obstruction
  - Hydronephrosis
- Clinical Profile
  - Serum tumor markers (CA-125) are used for follow-up
  - Tumor markers are elevated in most but not all patients with recurrent disease

Natural History & Prognosis
- Prognosis is better in patients with resectable recurrences than those with unresectable recurrences

Treatment
- Surgery with an attempt at complete resection, pelvic exenteration in cases of bladder and bowel invasion
- Surgical outcome and patient survival after secondary cytoreduction depends on tumor bulk and extent
  - In patients chosen for secondary cytoreduction, bulk of tumor is usually present in pelvis
  - Size of pelvic tumor does not affect surgical outcome, extent to pelvic sidewall does
  - Invasion of bladder and large bowel does not preclude secondary cytoreduction but requires more extensive surgery
- Second look surgery is no longer routine
- Adjuvant chemotherapy and radiation

DIAGNOSTIC CHECKLIST

Consider
- **Imaging studies are used when**
  - Tumor markers are elevated
  - New clinical symptoms are present
- Imaging can assist in prediction of resectability
  - Secondary cytoreduction is only justified if resection is possible with no residual tumor
- Imaging findings aid the surgeon in surgical planning to optimize cytoreduction

Image Interpretation Pearls
- **Recurrent disease may present as**
  - Well-defined nodules or lobulated masses
  - Thickening or infiltration in the mesentery and along peritoneal surfaces
  - Capsular implants indenting hepatic and splenic surfaces
  - Intraparenchymal hepatic or splenic metastases, lung nodules
- **Indicators of tumor resectability in secondary cytoreduction are**
  - No pelvic sidewall invasion (> 3 mm fat plane separating tumor from the pelvic sidewall)
  - No bulky upper abdominal disease
    - No parenchymal hepatic or splenic metastases
    - No bulky tumor implants in gastrohepatic and gastrosplenic ligaments, intersegmental fissure of liver, gallbladder fossa, mesenteric root
    - No suprarenal lymphadenopathy
  - No hydronephrosis

SELECTED REFERENCES
1. Chi DS et al: Guidelines and selection criteria for secondary cytoreductive surgery in patients with recurrent, platinum-sensitive epithelial ovarian carcinoma. Cancer. 106(9):1933-9, 2006
2. Simcock B et al: The impact of PET/CT in the management of recurrent ovarian cancer. Gynecol Oncol. 2006
3. Qayyum A et al: Role of CT and MR imaging in predicting optimal cytoreduction of newly diagnosed primary epithelial ovarian cancer. Gynecol Oncol. 96(2):301-6, 2005
4. Bristow RE et al: Clinically occult recurrent ovarian cancer: patient selection for secondary cytoreductive surgery using combined PET/CT. Gynecol Oncol. 90(3):519-28, 2003
5. Coakley FV et al: Peritoneal metastases: detection with spiral CT in patients with ovarian cancer. Radiology. 223(2):495-9, 2002
6. Salom E et al: Management of recurrent ovarian cancer: evidence-based decisions. Curr Opin Oncol. 14(5):519-27, 2002
7. Tay EH et al: Secondary cytoreductive surgery for recurrent epithelial ovarian cancer. Obstet Gynecol. 99(6):1008-13, 2002
8. Munkarah A et al: Secondary cytoreductive surgery for localized intra-abdominal recurrences in epithelial ovarian cancer. Gynecol Oncol. 81(2):237-41, 2001
9. Nakamoto Y et al: Clinical value of positron emission tomography with FDG for recurrent ovarian cancer. AJR Am J Roentgenol. 176(6):1449-54, 2001
10. Scarabelli C et al: Secondary cytoreductive surgery for patients with recurrent epithelial ovarian carcinoma. Gynecol Oncol. 83(3):504-12, 2001
11. Bristow RE et al: A model for predicting surgical outcome in patients with advanced ovarian carcinoma using computed tomography. Cancer. 89(7):1532-40, 2000
12. Eisenkop SM et al: The role of secondary cytoreductive surgery in the treatment of patients with recurrent epithelial ovarian carcinoma. Cancer. 88(1):144-53, 2000
13. Zang RY et al: Effect of cytoreductive surgery on survival of patients with recurrent epithelial ovarian cancer. J Surg Oncol. 75(1):24-30, 2000
14. Cormio G et al: Surgical treatment of recurrent ovarian cancer: report of 21 cases and a review of the literature. Eur J Obstet Gynecol Reprod Biol. 86(2):185-8, 1999

OVARIAN CANCER, RECURRENT; RESECTABLE

IMAGE GALLERY

Typical

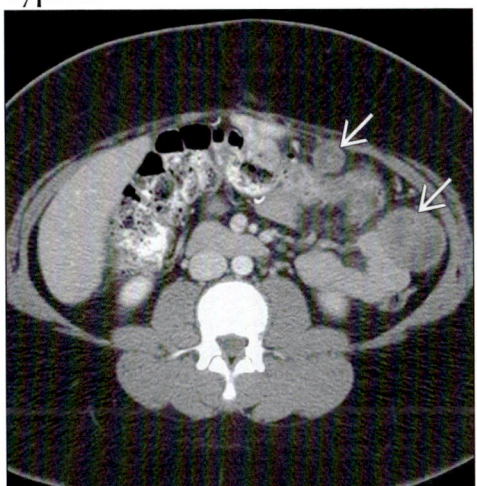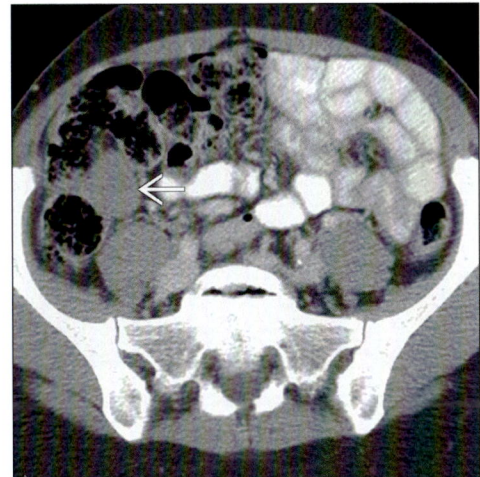

(Left) Axial CECT shows two peritoneal implants ➡ in a patient with recurrent ovarian cancer. No bowel invasion is seen. *(Right)* Axial CECT shows a solitary mass ➡ abutting the cecum in a patient with recurrent ovarian cancer. Note that the mass does not cause bowel obstruction.

Typical

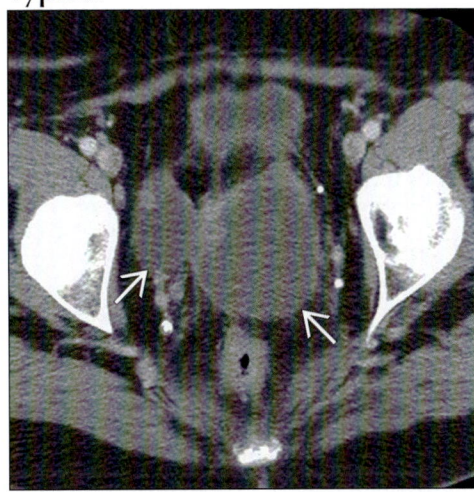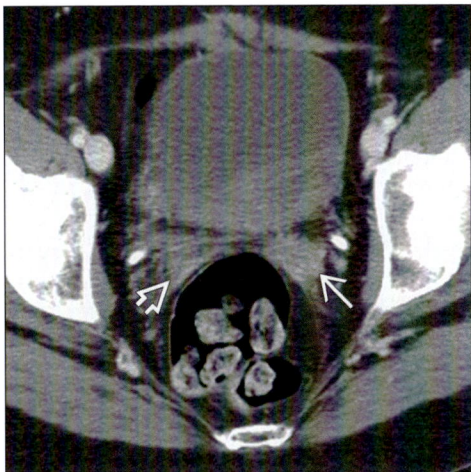

(Left) Axial CECT shows two large cystic masses ➡ in the pelvis in a patient with recurrent ovarian cancer. Note that the masses do not invade the pelvic side-wall. *(Right)* Axial CECT shows recurrent ovarian cancer seen as nodular soft tissue thickening ➡ in the left vaginal cuff. Note the normal appearance of the right vaginal cuff ➡.

Typical

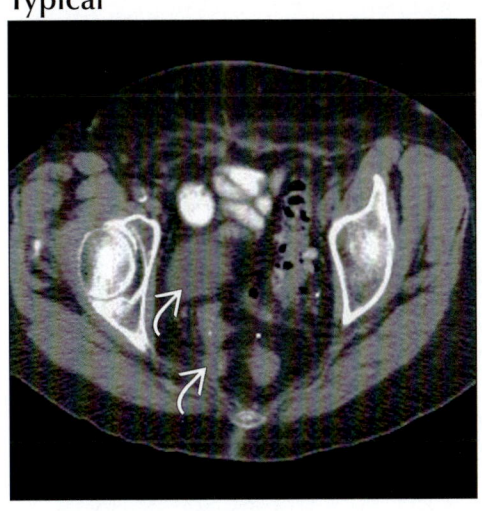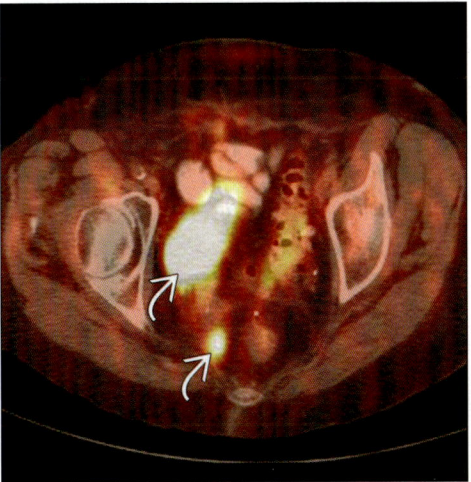

(Left) Axial NECT shows masses ➡ in the right pelvis in a patient with recurrent ovarian cancer. Note that there is no pelvic side-wall invasion. *(Right)* Axial fused PET/CT shows intense uptake ➡ in the recurrent masses.

OVARIAN CANCER, RECURRENT; UNRESECTABLE

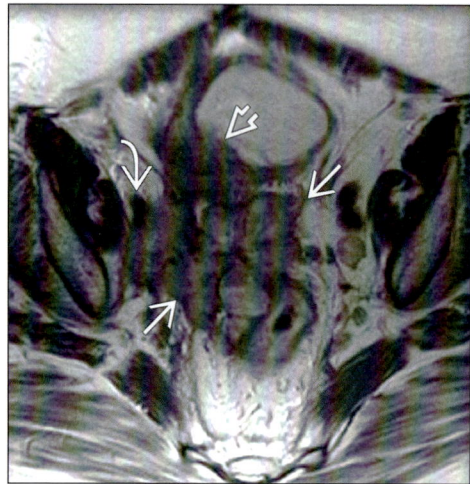

Axial T2WI MR shows recurrent ovarian cancer ➔ in the pelvis. Note that the mass invades the bladder ➔, encases the right external iliac vessels ➔ and abuts the right pelvic side wall.

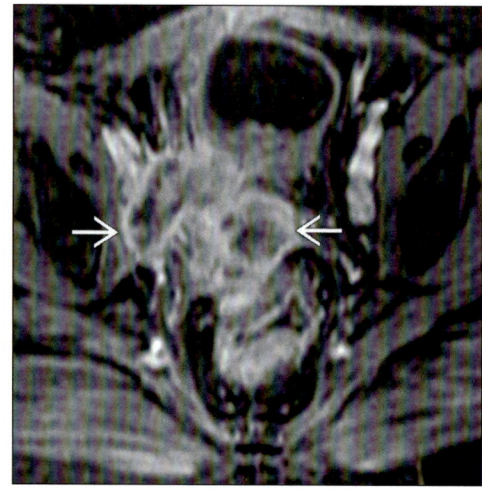

Axial T1 C+ FS MR shows that the recurrent ovarian cancer ➔ enhances heterogeneously.

TERMINOLOGY

Definitions
- Recurrent ovarian cancer (ROC) precluding optimal secondary cytoreduction
- **Recurrence defined as disease relapse following**
  - Complete response to first line therapy
  - Negative second look operation
  - Disease-free interval greater than 6 months

IMAGING FINDINGS

General Features
- Best diagnostic clue
  - Recurrent mass or masses in pelvis inseparable from pelvic sidewall
  - Disseminated tumor implants within mesentery and upper abdomen
- Location
  - Most recurrences in pelvis and abdomen
    - Vaginal cuff
    - Pelvic side wall
    - Peritoneum, mesentery
    - Liver, spleen
- Size: Varies from small nodules to large masses
- Morphology
  - Tumor recurrence may demonstrate different patterns
    - Well-defined nodules or lobulated masses
    - Thickening or infiltration in mesentery and along peritoneal surfaces

Radiographic Findings
- Radiography: Chest radiography may demonstrate pleural effusions due to pleural or lung metastases which indicate disseminated disease
- IVP
  - May show hydroureteronephrosis with delayed nephrogram due to obstruction by recurrent mass
    - Obstruction may be due to invasion or just compression of ureter by the recurrent mass
    - Mass is unresectable if hydronephrosis due to invasion of ureter

Ultrasonographic Findings
- Grayscale Ultrasound
  - US limited in assessment of extent of recurrent ovarian cancer and its resectability

DDx: Recurrent Ovarian Cancer

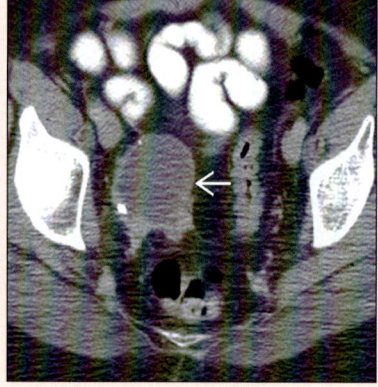

Resectable ROC

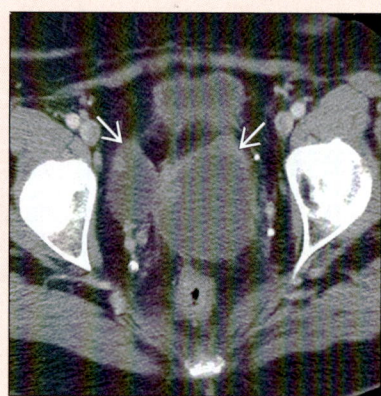

Resectable ROC

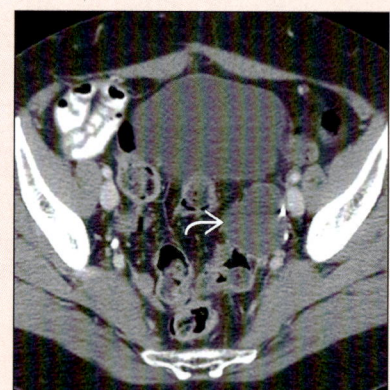

Lymphocele

OVARIAN CANCER, RECURRENT; UNRESECTABLE

Key Facts

Terminology
- Recurrent ovarian cancer (ROC) precluding optimal secondary cytoreduction
- **Recurrence defined as disease relapse following**
- Complete response to first line therapy
- Negative second look operation
- Disease-free interval greater than 6 months

Diagnostic Checklist
- **Imaging studies are used when**
- Tumor markers are elevated
- New clinical symptoms are present
- Imaging can assist in prediction of resectability to spare patients from unnecessary surgery
- **Recurrent disease may present as**
- Well-defined nodules or lobulated masses

- Thickening or infiltration in mesentery and along peritoneal surfaces
- Capsular implants indenting hepatic and splenic surfaces
- Intraparenchymal hepatic or splenic metastases, lung nodules
- **Indicators of tumor non-resectability in secondary cytoreduction**
- Pelvic sidewall invasion (< 3 mm fat plane separating tumor from pelvic sidewall)
- Bulky upper abdominal disease: Parenchymal hepatic or splenic metastases, tumor implants in gastrohepatic and gastrosplenic ligaments, intersegmental fissure of liver, gallbladder fossa, mesenteric root, and suprarenal lymphadenopathy
- Hydronephrosis

- May show large recurrences in pelvis and abdomen as solid or mixed solid and cystic masses
- US can also show or secondary signs of recurrence such as hydronephrosis, ascites, etc.

CT Findings
- CTA: Can be used to assess vascular invasion
- CECT: Heterogeneous attenuation solid or mixed solid and cystic masses

MR Findings
- T1WI: Intermediate signal intensity masses
- T2WI: Heterogeneous intensity solid or mixed solid and cystic masses
- T1 C+: Heterogeneous enhancement
- MRA: Can be used to assess vascular invasion

Fluoroscopic Findings
- Small or large bowel obstruction can be seen due to
  - Invasion or compression by recurrent tumor
  - Peritoneal adhesions which may be due to peritoneal carcinomatosis or previous surgery

Nuclear Medicine Findings
- PET
  - FDG PET demonstrates radiotracer uptake at site of recurrent tumor
  - FDG PET insensitive to small-volume tumor implants
  - PET/CT facilitates to determine exact anatomic location of recurrent masses

Imaging Recommendations
- Best imaging tool
  - CT is most commonly used modality for detection of recurrent tumor
  - CT is very useful in determination of resectability of recurrent tumor, extent of tumor in upper abdomen, and related complications (hydronephrosis, bowel obstruction, etc.)
    - Multidetector scanners and use of intravenous contrast facilitate detection of small-volume implants
  - MR is superior to CT in assessment of local extent of disease due to its better soft tissue resolution
    - MR is best modality to assess pelvic sidewall invasion
    - Less than 3 mm fat plane between mass and pelvic side wall indicates non-resectability
    - MR can also accurately demonstrate adjacent organ and vascular invasion
  - FDG PET is accurate and useful when conventional studies are inconclusive or negative and tumor markers are rising
    - FDG PET can accurately show multiple foci of disseminated disease in abdomen and pelvis

DIFFERENTIAL DIAGNOSIS

Resectable Ovarian Cancer
- Recurrent ovarian cancer without pelvic side-wall, major vascular invasion or disseminated disease

Post-Operative Lymphocele
- Pelvic or retroperitoneal lymphoceles occur after radical pelvic lymphadenectomy
- They are entirely cystic and thin walled
- When infected they may have thickened walls
- But unlike recurrent tumor they do not have nodular solid components

PATHOLOGY

General Features
- General path comments: Pathologic findings are similar to original type of ovarian cancer

CLINICAL ISSUES

Presentation
- Most common signs/symptoms
  - Pelvic mass
  - Pelvic pain

OVARIAN CANCER, RECURRENT; UNRESECTABLE

- Pelvic pressure
- Abdominal distension due to recurrent masses and/or ascites
- Nausea, vomiting
- Other signs/symptoms
  - Change in bladder or bowel habits
  - Bowel obstruction
  - Hydronephrosis
- Clinical Profile
  - Serum tumor markers (CA-125) are used for follow-up
  - Tumor markers are elevated in most but not all patients with recurrent disease

Natural History & Prognosis
- Prognosis worse in patients with unresectable recurrences than those with resectable recurrences

Treatment
- Recurrent ovarian cancer continues to be a therapeutic dilemma; no consensus for optimal treatment strategies
- Various therapeutic options have been proposed including
  - Chemotherapy for widespread abdominal disease
  - Pelvic irradiation for isolated unresectable disease in pelvis
  - Palliative surgery or interventions for bowel obstruction and hydronephrosis

DIAGNOSTIC CHECKLIST

Consider
- **Imaging studies are used when**
  - Tumor markers are elevated
  - New clinical symptoms are present
- Imaging can assist in prediction of resectability to spare patients from unnecessary surgery
  - Secondary cytoreduction only justified if resection is possible with no residual tumor
  - Imaging diagnosis of unresectable disease may obviate a second look laparotomy

Image Interpretation Pearls
- **Recurrent disease may present as**
  - Well-defined nodules or lobulated masses
  - Thickening or infiltration in mesentery and along peritoneal surfaces
  - Capsular implants indenting hepatic and splenic surfaces
  - Intraparenchymal hepatic or splenic metastases, lung nodules
- **Indicators of tumor non-resectability in secondary cytoreduction**
  - Pelvic sidewall invasion (< 3 mm fat plane separating tumor from pelvic sidewall)
  - Bulky upper abdominal disease: Parenchymal hepatic or splenic metastases, tumor implants in gastrohepatic and gastrosplenic ligaments, intersegmental fissure of liver, gallbladder fossa, mesenteric root, and suprarenal lymphadenopathy
  - Hydronephrosis

SELECTED REFERENCES

1. Chi DS et al: Guidelines and selection criteria for secondary cytoreductive surgery in patients with recurrent, platinum-sensitive epithelial ovarian carcinoma. Cancer. 106(9):1933-9, 2006
2. Murakami M et al: Whole-body positron emission tomography and tumor marker CA125 for detection of recurrence in epithelial ovarian cancer. Int J Gynecol Cancer. 16 Suppl 1:99-107, 2006
3. Simcock B et al: The impact of PET/CT in the management of recurrent ovarian cancer. Gynecol Oncol. 2006
4. Qayyum A et al: Role of CT and MR imaging in predicting optimal cytoreduction of newly diagnosed primary epithelial ovarian cancer. Gynecol Oncol. 96(2):301-6, 2005
5. Leitao MM Jr et al: Tertiary cytoreduction in patients with recurrent ovarian carcinoma. Gynecol Oncol. 95(1):181-8, 2004
6. Munkarah AR et al: Critical evaluation of secondary cytoreduction in recurrent ovarian cancer. Gynecol Oncol. 95(2):273-80, 2004
7. Ricke J et al: Prospective evaluation of contrast-enhanced MRI in the depiction of peritoneal spread in primary or recurrent ovarian cancer. Eur Radiol. 13(5):943-9, 2003
8. Togashi K. Related Articles et al: Ovarian cancer: the clinical role of US, CT, and MRI. Eur Radiol. 13 Suppl 4:L87-104, 2003
9. Coakley FV et al: Peritoneal metastases: detection with spiral CT in patients with ovarian cancer. Radiology. 223(2):495-9, 2002
10. Tay EH et al: Secondary cytoreductive surgery for recurrent epithelial ovarian cancer. Obstet Gynecol. 99(6):1008-13, 2002
11. Torizuka T et al: Ovarian cancer recurrence: role of whole-body positron emission tomography using 2-[fluorine-18]-fluoro-2-deoxy- D-glucose. Eur J Nucl Med Mol Imaging. 29(6):797-803, 2002
12. Munkarah A et al: Secondary cytoreductive surgery for localized intra-abdominal recurrences in epithelial ovarian cancer. Gynecol Oncol. 81(2):237-41, 2001
13. Eisenkop SM et al: The role of secondary cytoreductive surgery in the treatment of patients with recurrent epithelial ovarian carcinoma. Cancer. 88(1):144-53, 2000
14. Gadducci A et al: Complete salvage surgical cytoreduction improves further survival of patients with late recurrent ovarian cancer. Gynecol Oncol. 79(3):344-9, 2000
15. Zang RY et al: Effect of cytoreductive surgery on survival of patients with recurrent epithelial ovarian cancer. J Surg Oncol. 75(1):24-30, 2000
16. Low RN et al: Treated ovarian cancer: comparison of MR imaging with serum CA-125 level and physical examination--a longitudinal study. Radiology. 211(2):519-28, 1999

OVARIAN CANCER, RECURRENT; UNRESECTABLE

IMAGE GALLERY

Typical

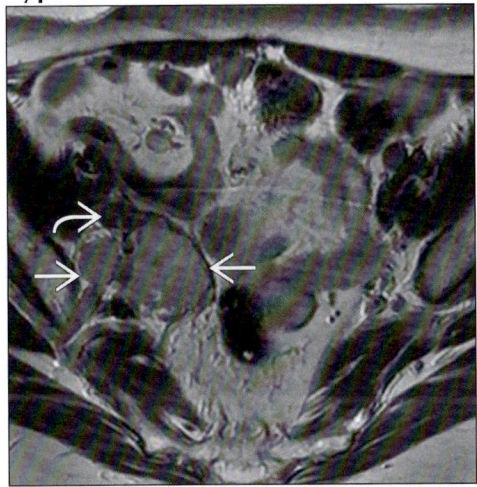
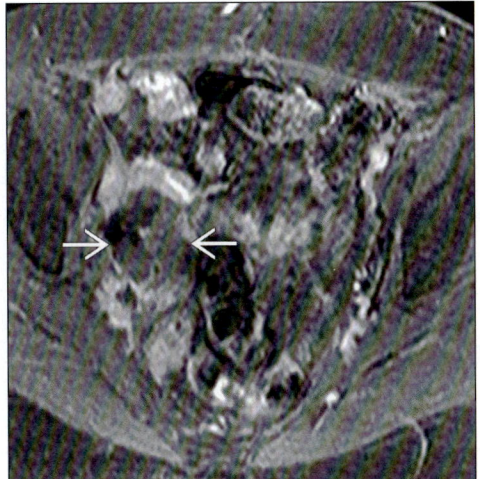

(Left) Axial T2WI MR shows recurrent ovarian cancer ➡ that is inseparable from the right external iliac vessels ➡. *(Right)* Axial T1 C+ FS MR shows that the mass ➡ enhances heterogeneously.

Typical

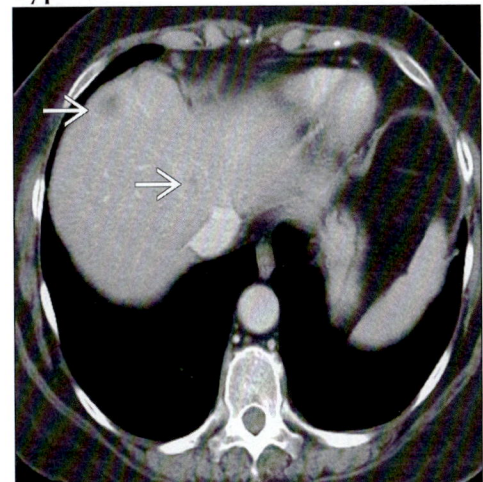
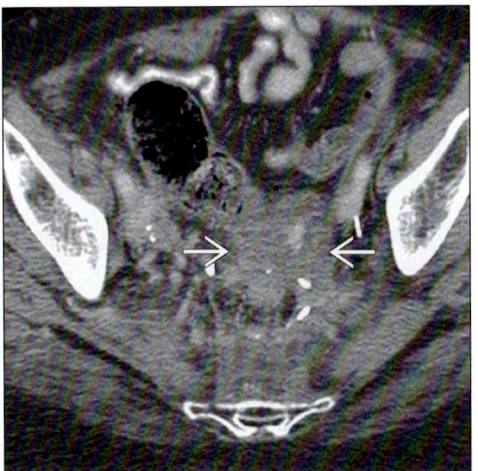

(Left) Axial CECT shows liver metastases ➡ in a patient with recurrent ovarian cancer. *(Right)* Axial CECT shows an infiltrative recurrent ovarian cancer ➡ in the left pelvis.

Typical

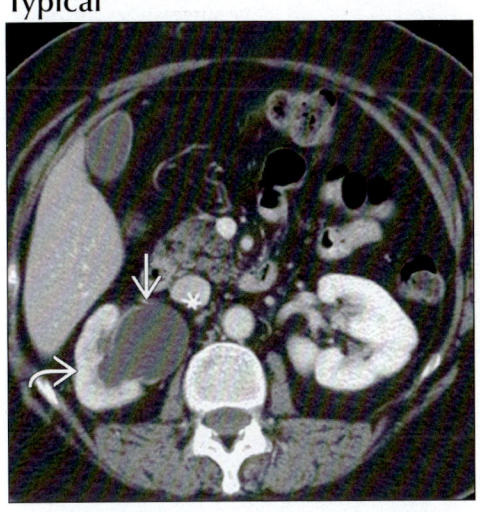
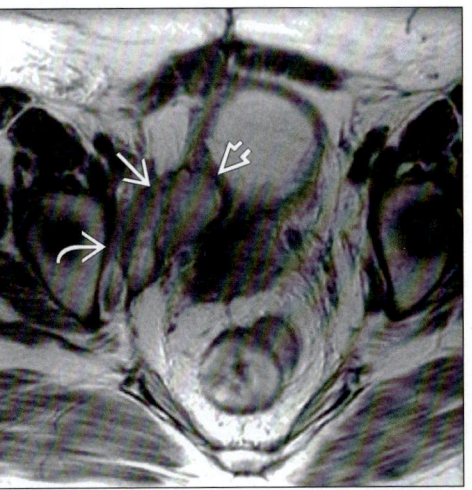

(Left) Axial CECT shows right hydronephrosis ➡ and delayed nephrogram ➡ due to invasion of right ureter in a patient with recurrent ovarian cancer in the pelvis. *(Right)* Axial T2WI MR shows recurrent ovarian cancer ➡ in the right pelvis. Note that the mass invades the urinary bladder ➡ and extends to the right pelvic side wall ➡.

CHORIOCARCINOMA, OVARY

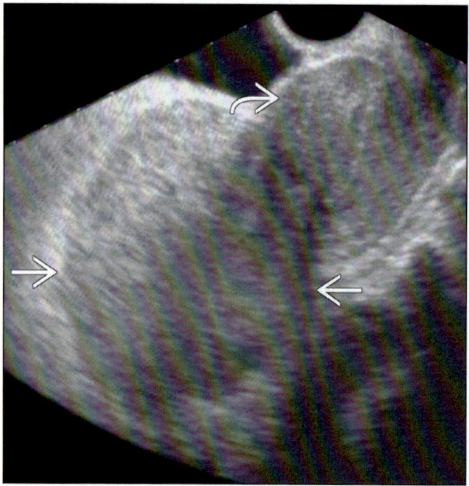

Longitudinal transvaginal ultrasound shows a heterogeneous solid adnexal lesion ➔ situated anterosuperior to the uterus ➔.

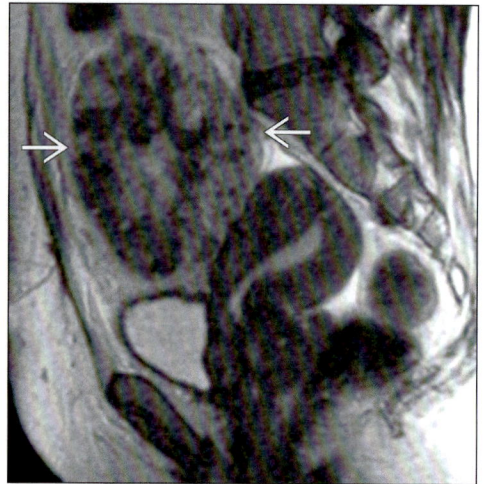

Sagittal T2WI MR shows a solid adnexal mass ➔ of mixed SI. Pathology: Pure non-gestational ovarian choriocarcinoma.

TERMINOLOGY

Abbreviations and Synonyms
- Primary choriocarcinoma of the ovary

Definitions
- Malignant tumor of ovary with trophoblastic differentiation
- Pure ovarian choriocarcinoma (germ cell tumor) is rare, in most cases the tumor is admixed with other malignant germ cell tumors (MGCT)
  - "Non gestational choriocarcinoma" is a malignant germ cell tumor showing partial or occasionally complete trophoblastic differentiation
  - Ovarian choriocarcinoma can occasionally represent a metastasis from primary gestational choriocarcinoma in the uterus
  - Rarely a gestational choriocarcinoma may arise from an ovarian pregnancy

IMAGING FINDINGS

General Features
- Best diagnostic clue: Typically unilateral, hypervascular adnexal mass with central hemorrhage and necrosis
- Location: Unilateral
- Size: Usually large mass
- Morphology: Solid mass with areas of necrosis and hemorrhage

Ultrasonographic Findings
- Grayscale Ultrasound
  - Predominantly solid adnexal mass
  - Anechoic cystic areas represent necrosis and hemorrhage
  - Intrauterine and ectopic pregnancy should be ruled out in cases of non-gestational ovarian choriocarcinoma
- Color Doppler: Marked blood flow within the solid components
- Power Doppler: Solid components demonstrate marked blood flow with low resistance

DDx: Adnexal Masses

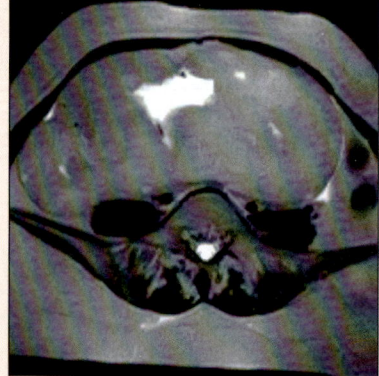

Dysgerminoma

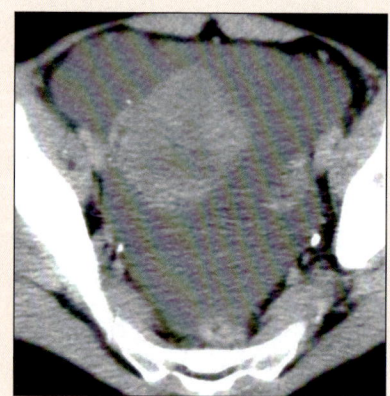

Yolk Sac Tumor

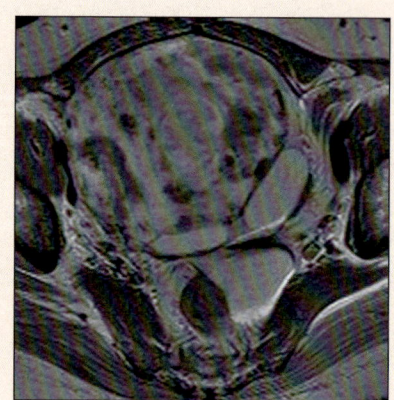

Sclerosing Stromal Tumor

CHORIOCARCINOMA, OVARY

Key Facts

Terminology
- Malignant tumor of ovary with trophoblastic differentiation
- Pure ovarian choriocarcinoma (germ cell tumor) is rare, in most cases the tumor is admixed with other malignant germ cell tumors (MGCT)
- Ovarian choriocarcinoma can occasionally represent a metastasis from primary gestational choriocarcinoma in the uterus
- Rarely a gestational choriocarcinoma may arise from an ovarian pregnancy

Imaging Findings
- Best diagnostic clue: Typically unilateral, hypervascular adnexal mass with central hemorrhage and necrosis
- Intrauterine and ectopic pregnancy should be ruled out in cases of non-gestational ovarian choriocarcinoma

Top Differential Diagnoses
- Gestational Ovarian Choriocarcinoma
- Other Malignant Germ Cell Tumors
- Sclerosing Stromal Tumor

Clinical Issues
- Signs and symptoms relating to pelvic mass
- Amenorrhea
- Other signs/symptoms: Elevated serum beta hCG

Diagnostic Checklist
- Vascular adnexal mass containing multiple cystic cavities in the solid portion and central necrosis/hemorrhage

CT Findings
- NECT
  - Large complex pelvic mass
  - Central low attenuation areas represent necrosis
  - Hemorrhage can appear as low as high attenuation
- CECT
  - Avid contrast medium enhancement is seen in the peripheral solid component of the mass
  - Enlarged irregular arterial vessels may be seen at the periphery of the mass during the arterial phase
  - Peritoneal thickening and/or peritoneal implants may be present
  - Ascites may be present occasionally
  - Distant metastases (lung, liver, brain) may be present at diagnosis

MR Findings
- T1WI
  - Pelvic mass of predominantly low SI
  - High SI areas are suggestive of hemorrhage
- T2WI
  - Solid pelvic mass of mixed SI
    - Low SI solid component
    - High SI cystic areas within the peripheral solid component
    - High SI central area representing necrosis/hemorrhage
  - Invasion of the adjacent organs (e.g. uterus) and pelvic side wall invasion may be seen at presentation
  - Liver metastases may be present at diagnosis
- T1 C+ FS
  - Avid gadolinium uptake in the peripheral solid portion of the mass
  - Peritoneal thickening and/or peritoneal implants, if present, are best appreciated on delayed (5-10 min) images

Imaging Recommendations
- Best imaging tool
  - US for initial diagnosis and to rule out intra/extrauterine pregnancy
  - CECT/MR for lesion characterization and evaluation of local extent of the tumor
  - CT for evaluation of distant metastases (lung, liver, brain)
- Protocol advice: MR: Sagittal, axial and coronal T2WI; axial T1WI; axial and coronal T1WI C+ FS

DIFFERENTIAL DIAGNOSIS

Gestational Ovarian Choriocarcinoma
- Evidence of intra/extrauterine trophoblastic disease, ovarian theca luteum cyst, or corpus luteum cyst
- Recent intra/extrauterine pregnancy
- Very high levels of beta hCG
- Differentiation is very difficult in the majority of cases and non-gestational type can be accurately diagnosed only in the pre-pubertal period

Other Malignant Germ Cell Tumors
- Dysgerminoma
  - Typically, a large solid mass containing multiple fibrovascular septae
  - May contain calcifications
- Yolk sac tumor
  - Elevated α-fetoprotein levels
  - Prominent intra-tumoral vessels and peripheral strong enhancement are characteristic

Sclerosing Stromal Tumor
- Normal β-hCG levels
- Characteristic appearances in MR with low SI nodules set against high SI stroma and the presence of a thin peripheral rim of low SI on T2WI
- Typical appearances on dynamic contrast-enhanced MR
  - Early striking peripheral enhancement with centripetal progression
  - Prolonged enhancement of central portion of the lesion

Tubo-Ovarian Abscess
- Normal β-hCG levels

CHORIOCARCINOMA, OVARY

- Preserved, peripherally placed ovarian follicles within edematous stroma

Massive Ovarian Edema
- Normal β-hCG levels
- Raised inflammatory markers, fever, vaginal discharge
- Tubular cystic adnexal lesions with rim-enhancement

PATHOLOGY

General Features
- Epidemiology: Pure ovarian choriocarcinomas account for < 1% of ovarian tumors
- Associated abnormalities
  - Intra/extrauterine pregnancy in the case of gestational type
  - Other MGCT's in the case of non-gestational type
  - Mucinous cystadenoma

Gross Pathologic & Surgical Features
- Large, unilateral, solid, white mass showing focal necrosis and hemorrhage

Microscopic Features
- Intimate admixture of cytotrophoblast and syncytiotrophoblast
- Cytotrophoblast
  - Medium-sized cells with clear or pink cytoplasm and a single nucleus with a prominent nucleolus
  - Positive for cytokeratin immunohistochemistry
  - Do not produce beta hCG
- Syncytiotrophoblast
  - Giant cells composed of abundant pink/vacuolated cytoplasm with multiple nuclei
  - Positive for cytokeratin, beta hCG immunohistochemistry
  - Produce beta hCG
- May have extensive hemorrhage and necrosis

CLINICAL ISSUES

Presentation
- Most common signs/symptoms
  - Signs and symptoms relating to pelvic mass
  - Amenorrhea
  - Isosexual pseudoprecocity in prepubertal girls
  - Bleeding from metastatic deposits
  - Signs suggestive of ectopic pregnancy
- Other signs/symptoms: Elevated serum beta hCG

Demographics
- Age
  - Non-gestational type occurs in prepubertal girls and postmenopausal women
  - Gestational type occurs during the reproductive years
- Gender: Female

Natural History & Prognosis
- Non-gestational choriocarcinoma is a highly malignant neoplasm showing invasion of pelvic structures and spread into the peritoneal cavity
- Non-gestational choriocarcinoma metastasizes via lymphatics and blood stream
- Non-gestational type has a worse prognosis than a gestational type
- Brain metastases occur in 10-20% of patients and are the leading cause of death; almost all patient with CNS involvement have lung metastases

Treatment
- Hysterectomy and bilateral oophorectomy
- Adjuvant chemotherapy

DIAGNOSTIC CHECKLIST

Consider
- Primary non-gestational ovarian choriocarcinoma in the differential diagnosis of a hypervascular ovarian tumor in the absence of uterine or extrauterine pregnancy

Image Interpretation Pearls
- Vascular adnexal mass containing multiple cystic cavities in the solid portion and central necrosis/hemorrhage

SELECTED REFERENCES

1. Allen SD et al: Radiology of gestational trophoblastic neoplasia. Clin Radiol. 61(4):301-13, 2006
2. Bazot M et al: Imaging of pure primary ovarian choriocarcinoma. AJR Am J Roentgenol. 182(6):1603-4, 2004
3. Ozaki Y et al: Choriocarcinoma of the ovary associated with mucinous cystadenoma. Radiat Med. 19(1):55-9, 2001
4. Simsek T et al: Primary pure choriocarcinoma of the ovary in reproductive ages: a case report. Eur J Gynaecol Oncol. 19(3):284-6, 1998
5. Sashi R et al: Infantile choriocarcinoma: a case report with MRI, angiography and bone scintigraphy. Pediatr Radiol. 26(12):869-70, 1996
6. Brammer HM 3rd et al: From the archives of the AFIP. Malignant germ cell tumors of the ovary: radiologic-pathologic correlation. Radiographics. 10(4):715-24, 1990
7. Grover V et al: Primary pure choriocarcinoma of the ovary. Gynecol Obstet Invest. 30(1):61-3, 1990
8. Axe SR et al: Choriocarcinoma of the ovary. Obstet Gynecol. 66(1):111-4, 1985
9. Jacobs AJ et al: Pure choriocarcinoma of the ovary. Obstet Gynecol Surv. 37(10):603-9, 1982

CHORIOCARCINOMA, OVARY

IMAGE GALLERY

Typical

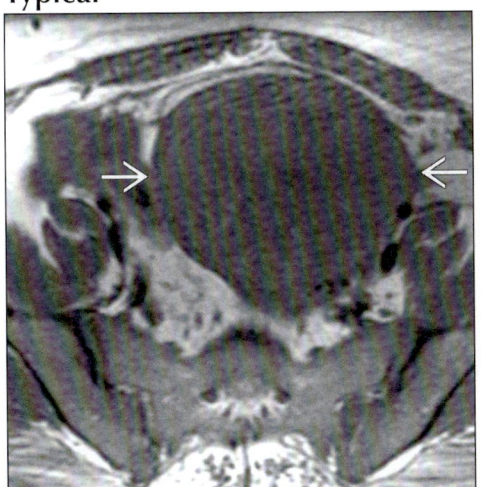
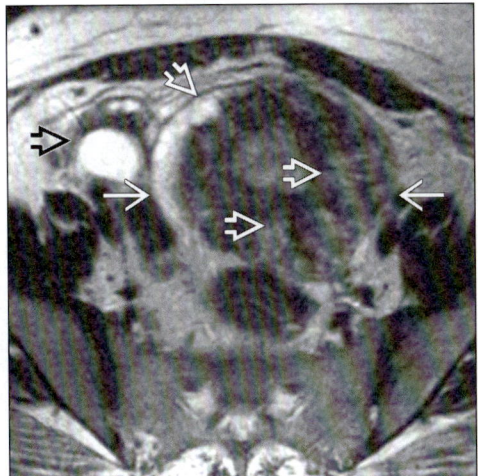

(Left) Axial T1WI MR shows a well-defined, low signal intensity left adnexal mass ➡. *(Right)* Axial T2WI MR in the same patient as previous image shows a left adnexal mass ➡ of mixed SI. Note presence of high SI areas ➡ within the peripheral solid component representing areas of necrosis and hemorrhage. A normal right ovary ➡ is also noted.

Typical

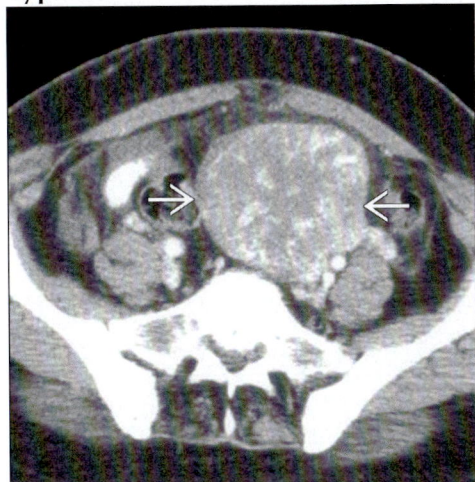
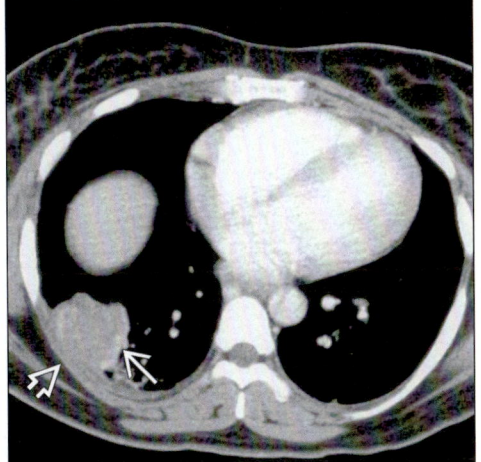

(Left) Axial CECT shows a solid left adnexal mass ➡ with avid peripheral enhancement. *(Right)* Axial CECT in the same patient as previous image shows a necrotic lung metastases ➡ in the right lower lobe. Note the peripheral rim-enhancement ➡. Pathology: Pure non-gestational ovarian choriocarcinoma.

Typical

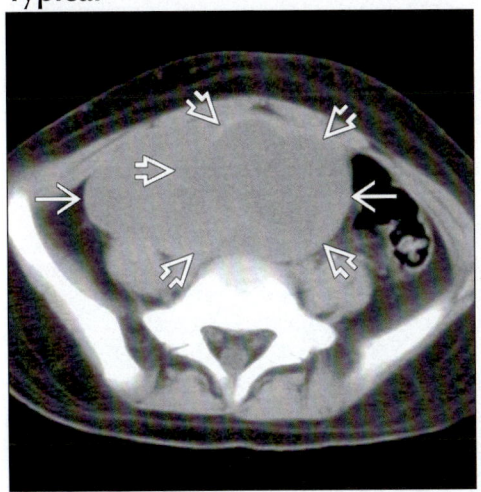
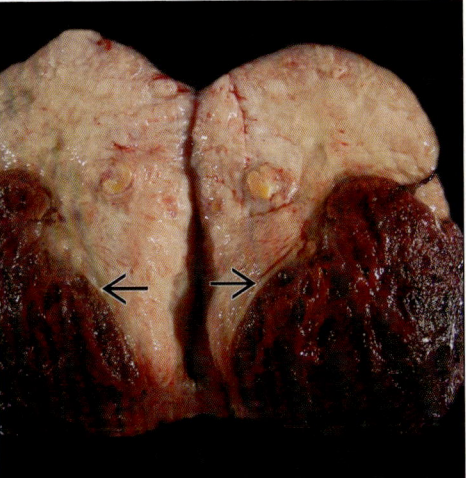

(Left) Axial CECT shows a large pelvic mass ➡ of mixed attenuation. Note the presence of a large low attenuation area ➡ indicative of necrosis/hemorrhage. *(Right)* Gross pathology in the same patient as previous image shows a solid mass with a large area of necrosis and hemorrhage ➡. Pathology: Pure non-gestational ovarian choriocarcinoma.

STRUMA OVARII

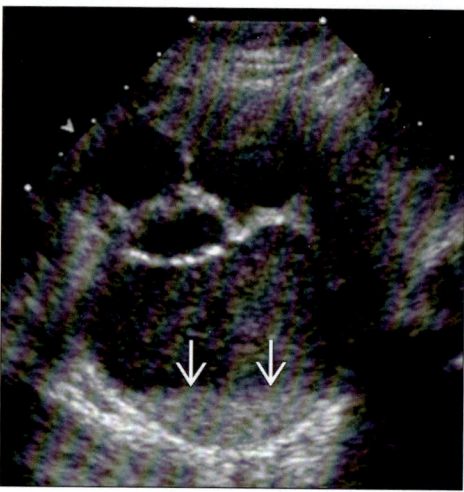

Transverse transabdominal ultrasound shows a complex cystic adnexal mass with internal septations and fat-fluid level ➡.

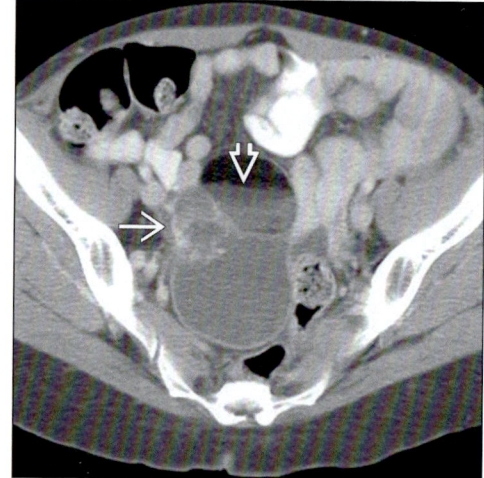

Axial CECT shows a complex cystic mass containing fat-fluid level ➡ and an avidly enhancing nodular soft tissue component ➡.

TERMINOLOGY

Abbreviations and Synonyms
- Monodermal ovarian teratoma
- Monodermal germ cell tumor

Definitions
- Monodermal teratomas are defined as teratomas composed predominantly or solely of a single tissue type
  o Struma ovarii, carcinoid and neural tumors belong to this group, with struma ovarii being the most common among them
- Struma ovarii is a monodermal teratoma in which thyroid tissue is exclusively present or constitutes > 50% of the tumor or is functionally active
  o Generally benign but can very occasionally be malignant

IMAGING FINDINGS

General Features
- Best diagnostic clue: Avidly enhancing soft tissue component due to vascular thyroid tissue within a teratoma-looking mass
- Location
  o Usually unilateral tumor
  o Right-sided in up to 65% of cases
- Size: Mean diameter 5 cm, range 3-9 cm
- Morphology: Multicystic or partially cystic/partially solid mass

Ultrasonographic Findings
- Cystic mass containing fat and an echogenic central solid component, resembling mature cystic teratoma
  o Low resistance blood flow is detected in highly vascular central echogenic portion on color/Doppler imaging
- Multicystic septated mass without solid component that can mimic benign cystic ovarian neoplasm

DDx: Ovarian Masses

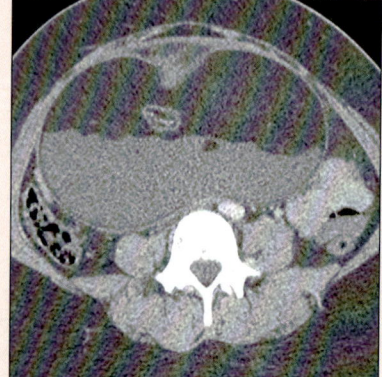

Mature Teratoma

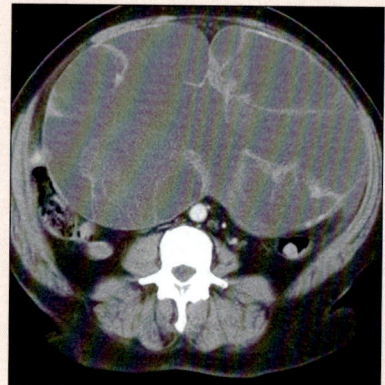

Mucinous Cystadenoma

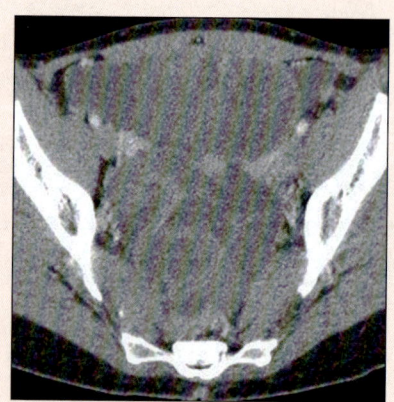

Mucinous Cystadenocarcinoma

STRUMA OVARII

Key Facts

Terminology
- Struma ovarii is a monodermal teratoma in which thyroid tissue is exclusively present or constitutes > 50% of the tumor or is functionally active
- Generally benign but can very occasionally be malignant

Imaging Findings
- Best diagnostic clue: Avidly enhancing soft tissue component due to vascular thyroid tissue within a teratoma-looking mass

Top Differential Diagnoses
- Mature Cystic Teratoma
- Mucinous Cystadenoma
- Mucinous Cystadenocarcinoma
- Thyroid Cancer Metastases to Ovary

Pathology
- Resembles normal thyroid with variably sized follicles containing colloid

Diagnostic Checklist
- Check thyroid function test in patient with teratoma-appearing ovarian mass which shows considerable enhancement of solid component on CT and MR and presence of low resistance flow on US
- Look for central solid component enhancement within teratoma since thyroid tissue is highly vascular
- Multicystic variant is radiographically indistinguishable from mucinous cystadenoma

CT Findings
- Cystic mass with fat-fluid level and brightly enhancing central soft tissue nodule
  - Calcifications may be present within the solid nodule
- Encapsulated multiloculated cystic mass with different density within the locules

MR Findings
- Cystic mass with solid component
  - Fatty components demonstrate drop in signal intensity with fat saturation technique
  - Calcifications within the solid component are more difficult to detect than on CT
  - Strong gadolinium enhancement of the solid component is characteristic
- Multiloculated mass with different SI among the cystic locules ("stained glass appearance") on T2WI caused by various concentrations of fluid
  - Often contents of some locules show prominent low signal intensity on both T1WI & T2WI caused by thyroid colloid within the cystic spaces

Nuclear Medicine Findings
- Iodine-123 uptake in mass

Imaging Recommendations
- Best imaging tool: MR
- Protocol advice: Gadolinium administration is essential

DIFFERENTIAL DIAGNOSIS

Mature Cystic Teratoma
- Fat containing mass with peripheral blood flow and avascular central mass (floating Rokitansky nodule on fat-fluid interface)

Mucinous Cystadenoma
- Multicystic ovarian mass with thin septations forming multiple locules
- Locules have different densities on CT or different signal intensities on MR reflecting various concentration of mucin

Mucinous Cystadenocarcinoma
- Malignant ovarian neoplasm that differs from benign counterpart by the presence of heterogeneous solid component
- Peritoneal and serosal implants are usually present at the time of presentation

Thyroid Cancer Metastases to Ovary
- Exceedingly rare
- Widespread metastatic disease should be documented to consider secondary thyroid neoplasm of the ovary

PATHOLOGY

General Features
- Epidemiology: Accounts for < 5% of mature teratomas
- Associated abnormalities
  - 50-60% are associated with a mature teratoma
  - Small percentage are associated with carcinoid tumors (strumal carcinoid) or mucinous cystadenomas of the same ovary
  - If associated with hyperthyroidism are generally > 6 cm in diameter

Gross Pathologic & Surgical Features
- Partially cystic and solid loculated mass filled with gelatinous material
- Usually seen as circumscribed nodules in wall of a mature teratoma
- Cut surface is soft or firm, red-brown tissue, may have areas of hemorrhage or necrosis

Microscopic Features
- Resembles normal thyroid with variably sized follicles containing colloid
- Can also show range of pathological changes such as colloid goiter, hyperplasia, rarely papillary thyroid carcinoma

STRUMA OVARII

- Immunohistochemistry is positive for thyroglobulin and chromogranin

CLINICAL ISSUES

Presentation
- Most common signs/symptoms
  - Incidental findings
  - Abdominal pain and other clinical symptoms related to ovarian torsion (nausea, vomiting, peritoneal irritation, etc.)
- Other signs/symptoms
  - One third have ascites (not associated with malignancy), which can be accompanied by Meigs syndrome (hydrothorax)
  - 5-15% have associated hyperthyroidism
  - Occasionally tumor marker CA-125 can be elevated

Demographics
- Age: Reproductive years, peak in fifth decade

Natural History & Prognosis
- 95% cases are benign with very good prognosis
- < 5% of struma ovarii cases are malignant, most commonly follicular carcinoma, papillary carcinoma or mixed pattern, similar to the types of thyroid carcinoma
- Even malignant struma ovarii rarely metastasizes, first by peritoneal implantation, subsequently by hematogenous spread to bone, liver, brain and lungs
- Metastatic spread from a thyroid carcinoma to ovary is exceedingly rare and should not be considered unless there is a history of primary thyroid carcinoma

Treatment
- Struma ovarii is treated by oophorectomy
- Pelvic clearance, thyroidectomy and radioactive Iodine is recommended for malignant tumors
  - Post-treatment follow-up is accomplished by serial serum thyroglobulin levels

DIAGNOSTIC CHECKLIST

Consider
- Check thyroid function test in patient with teratoma-appearing ovarian mass which shows considerable enhancement of solid component on CT and MR and presence of low resistance flow on US

Image Interpretation Pearls
- Look for central solid component enhancement within teratoma since thyroid tissue is highly vascular
- Multicystic variant is radiographically indistinguishable from mucinous cystadenoma

SELECTED REFERENCES

1. McDougall IR: Metastatic struma ovarii: the burden of truth. Clin Nucl Med. 31(6):321-4, 2006
2. Cherng SC et al: Malignant struma ovarii with peritoneal implants and pelvic structures and liver metastases demonstrated by I-131 SPECT and low-dose CT. Clin Nucl Med. 30(12):797-8, 2005
3. Garcia A et al: Malignant struma ovarii mimic clear cell carcinoma. Arch Gynecol Obstet. 271(3):251-5, 2005
4. Ciccarelli A et al: Thyrotoxic adenoma followed by atypical hyperthyroidism due to struma ovarii: clinical and genetic studies. Eur J Endocrinol. 150(4):431-7, 2004
5. Utsunomiya D et al: Struma ovarii coexisting with mucinous cystadenoma detected by radioactive iodine. Clin Nucl Med. 28(9):725-7, 2003
6. Van de Moortele K et al: Struma ovarii: US and CT findings. JBR-BTR. 86(4):209-10, 2003
7. Huh JJ et al: Struma ovarii associated with pseudo-Meigs' syndrome and elevated serum CA 125. Gynecol Oncol. 86(2):231-4, 2002
8. Robboy SJ et al: Pathology of the Female Genital Tract. 1st ed, Lon, Harcourt. 672-4, 2002
9. Outwater EK et al: Ovarian teratomas: tumor types and imaging characteristics. Radiographics. 21(2):475-90, 2001
10. Emoto M et al: Transvaginal color Doppler ultrasonic characterization of benign and malignant ovarian cystic teratomas and comparison with serum squamous cell carcinoma antigen. Cancer. 88(10):2298-304, 2000
11. Kim JC et al: MR findings of struma ovarii. Clin Imaging. 24(1):28-33, 2000
12. Matsuki M et al: Struma ovarii: MRI findings. Br J Radiol. 73(865):87-90, 2000
13. Okada S et al: Cystic struma ovarii: imaging findings. J Comput Assist Tomogr. 24(3):413-5, 2000
14. Zalel Y et al: Sonographic and clinical characteristics of struma ovarii. J Ultrasound Med. 19(12):857-61, 2000
15. Joja I et al: I-123 uptake in nonfunctional struma ovarii. Clin Nucl Med. 23(1):10-2, 1998
16. Joja I et al: Struma ovarii: appearance on MR images. Abdom Imaging. 23(6):652-6, 1998
17. Dohke M et al: Struma ovarii: MR findings. J Comput Assist Tomogr. 21(2):265-7, 1997
18. Yamashita Y et al: Struma ovarii: MR appearances. Abdom Imaging. 22(1):100-2, 1997
19. Zalel Y et al: Doppler flow characteristics of dermoid cysts: unique appearance of struma ovarii. J Ultrasound Med. 16(5):355-8, 1997
20. Brenner W et al: Radiotherapy with iodine-131 in recurrent malignant struma ovarii. Eur J Nucl Med. 23(1):91-4, 1996
21. Matsumoto F et al: Struma ovarii: CT and MR findings. J Comput Assist Tomogr. 14(2):310-2, 1990

STRUMA OVARII

IMAGE GALLERY

Typical

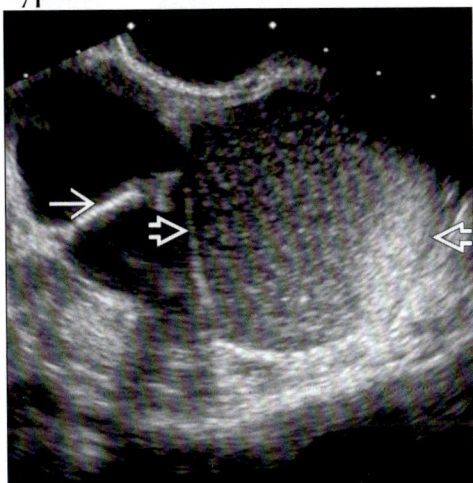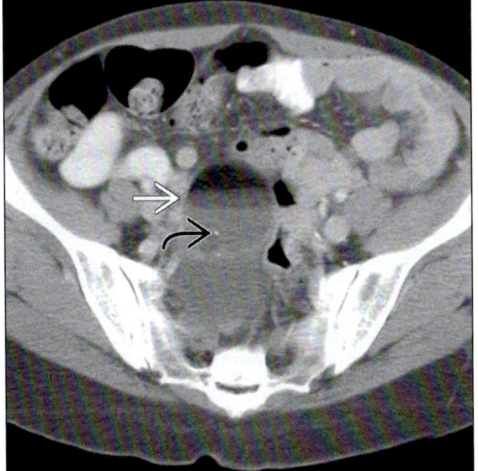

(Left) Longitudinal transvaginal ultrasound in a 53 year old patient shows a complex cystic mass with septations ➡. The largest portion of the mass is cystic with through transmission & low level internal echo ➡, suggesting the presence of colloid material. *(Right)* Axial CECT shows a complex cystic pelvic mass with fat-fluid level ➡ & punctate calcification ➡. The cystic component has higher attenuation than simple fluid, suggestive of proteinaceous/colloid material.

Typical

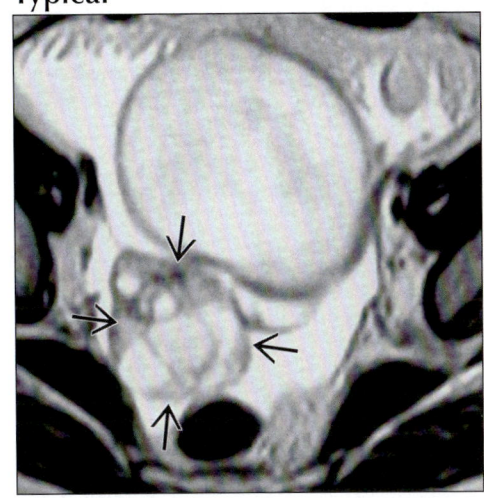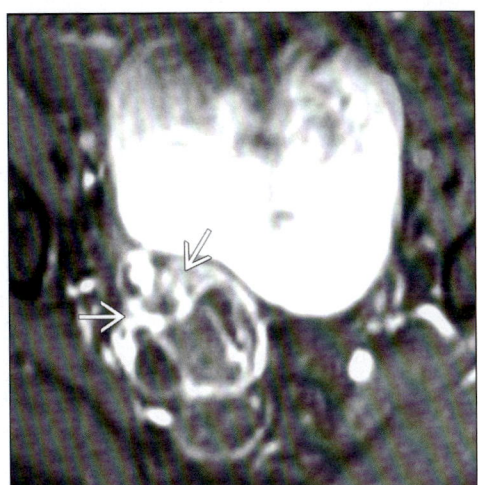

(Left) Axial T2WI MR in a 58 year old patient shows a complex cystic mass ➡ originating from the right ovary. *(Right)* Axial T1 C+ FS MR in the same patient as previous image shows avid enhancement of the solid components ➡ of the mass after administration of IV gadolinium. Pathology: Struma ovarii.

Variant

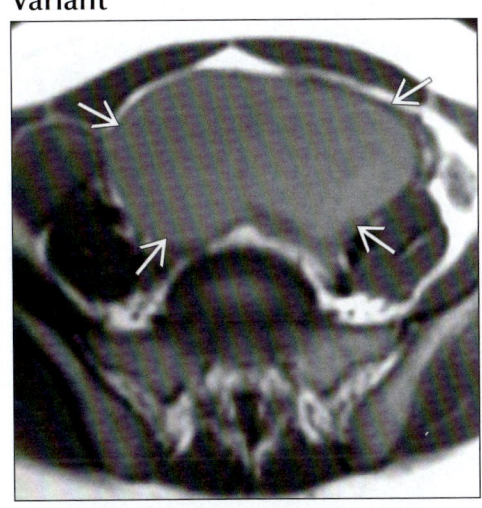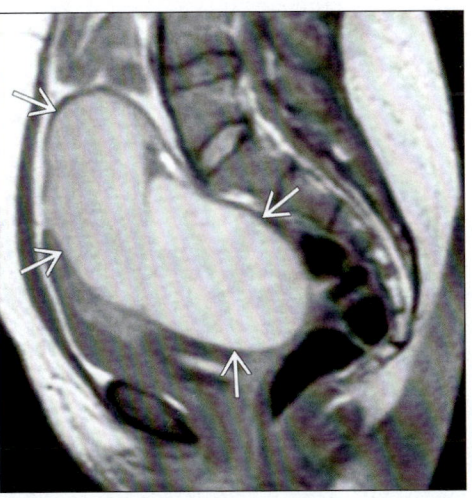

(Left) Axial T1WI MR shows a large multiloculated cystic mass ➡ of intermediate signal intensity suggestive of presence of proteinaceous/colloid fluid. *(Right)* Sagittal T2WI MR in the same patient as previous image confirms the presence of a large multiloculated cystic mass ➡ within the pelvis. Pathology: Mature teratoma containing mainly thyroid tissue.

CARCINOID, OVARY

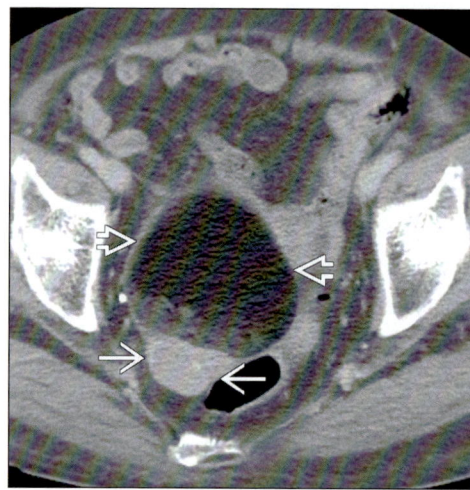
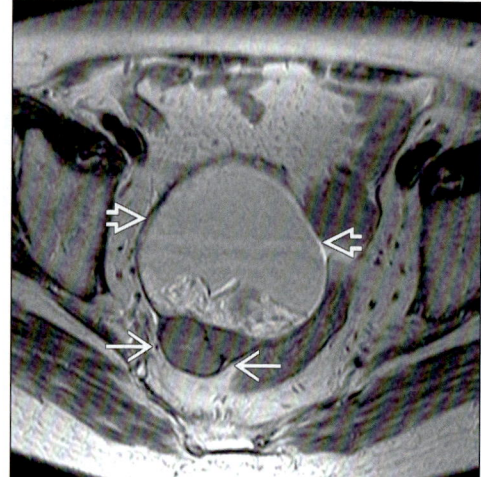

Axial CECT shows a central pelvic mass which contains a low attenuation component ⇨ consistent with fat and an enhancing solid nodule ➔ arising from the posterior wall.

Axial T2WI MR confirms the presence of an intermediate SI nodule ➔ in the posterior wall of a mature cystic teratoma ⇨. Pathology: Ovarian carcinoid.

TERMINOLOGY

Abbreviations and Synonyms
- Monodermal ovarian teratoma
- Monodermal germ cell tumor

Definitions
- Monodermal teratomas are defined as teratomas composed predominantly or solely of a single tissue type
  - Struma ovarii, carcinoid and neural tumors belong to this group
  - Ovarian carcinoid is generally a benign tumor, but very occasionally can be malignant

IMAGING FINDINGS

General Features
- Best diagnostic clue: Enhancing solid nodule in the wall of a mature cystic teratoma or an enhancing solid mass
- Location: Unilateral
- Size: Up to a maximum diameter of 10 cm
- Morphology: Solid ovarian tumor or solid nodule in the wall of a mature cystic teratoma (60-80%)
- When presenting as a solid mass, imaging features are usually indistinguishable from solid malignancies, although necrosis is less common in carcinoid tumors

Ultrasonographic Findings
- Grayscale Ultrasound
  - Solid nodule in the wall of a cystic mass which contains fat
  - Solid mass which may contain areas of necrosis
- Color Doppler: Blood flow is present in the solid mass or solid component

CT Findings
- Solid enhancing nodule in the wall of a mature cystic teratoma
  - Fat is present if associated with a mature cystic teratoma
- Solid enhancing mass
  - Necrosis is rare
  - Calcification may be present

MR Findings
- T1WI

DDx: Ovarian Masses

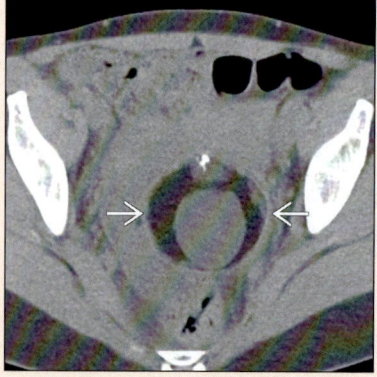
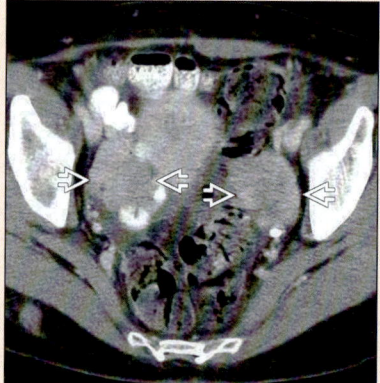
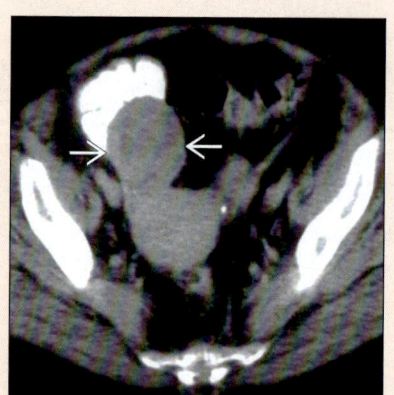

Mature Cystic Teratoma

Metastatic Carcinoid

Granulosa Cell Tumor

CARCINOID, OVARY

Key Facts

Terminology
- Monodermal ovarian teratoma

Imaging Findings
- Best diagnostic clue: Enhancing solid nodule in the wall of a mature cystic teratoma or an enhancing solid mass
- When presenting as a solid mass, imaging features are usually indistinguishable from solid malignancies, although necrosis is less common in carcinoid tumors
- Best imaging tool: MR
- Protocol advice: Fat-suppression sequences and gadolinium administration are essential

Top Differential Diagnoses
- Mature Cystic Teratoma
- Other Monodermal Teratomas
- Metastatic Carcinoid Tumor
- Granulosa Cell Tumor
- Krukenberg Tumor

Pathology
- Epidemiology: Primary carcinoid tumors constitute < 0.1% of all ovarian tumors and < 5% of ovarian teratomas
- 60-80% are components of a mature cystic teratoma
- Appear as firm yellow-tan colored nodule in the wall of a mature cystic teratoma or mucinous tumor

Diagnostic Checklist
- Mature cystic teratoma or mucinous tumors may be present in the contralateral ovary
- The majority of ovarian carcinoids appear as a solid component of a mature cystic teratoma

---

- Low signal intensity soft tissue nodule in the wall of a high signal intensity fat-containing lesion if associated with a mature cystic teratoma
- Low signal intensity solid mass
  - Mucinous types show intermediate signal intensity
- T1WI FS: Fatty component, if present, demonstrates suppressed signal intensity
- T2WI
  - Intermediate signal intensity soft tissue nodule in the wall of a high signal intensity fat-containing lesion if associated with a mature cystic teratoma
  - Intermediate signal intensity solid mass which may contain areas of high signal intensity suggestive of necrosis
    - Mucinous carcinoid can show higher signal intensity than other solid ovarian tumors because they contain high signal intensity mucin
    - Differentiation from other solid malignant ovarian tumors may be difficult
- T1 C+: Variable enhancement of the solid mass or solid component

Imaging Recommendations
- Best imaging tool: MR
- Protocol advice: Fat-suppression sequences and gadolinium administration are essential

DIFFERENTIAL DIAGNOSIS

Mature Cystic Teratoma
- Fat-containing mass with peripheral blood flow and avascular central solid portion (floating Rokitansky nodule on fat-fluid interface)

Other Monodermal Teratomas
- Struma ovarii, neural tumors
  - Soft tissue component of struma ovarii contains thyroid tissue and will avidly enhance

Metastatic Carcinoid Tumor
- Usually bilateral solid masses
- Extra ovarian metastases may be present

Granulosa Cell Tumor
- Usually solid in nature
- Can be difficult to distinguish on imaging and immunohistochemistry is required

Krukenberg Tumor
- Evidence of primary GI tumor is usually present
- Usually bilateral ovarian masses
- Occasionally can be difficult to distinguish on imaging and immunohistochemistry is required

Ovarian Carcinoma
- Mixed cystic and solid ovarian masses with peritoneal implants and ascites

PATHOLOGY

General Features
- Epidemiology: Primary carcinoid tumors constitute < 0.1% of all ovarian tumors and < 5% of ovarian teratomas
- Associated abnormalities: 15% have a mature cystic teratoma or mucinous tumor in the contralateral ovary

Gross Pathologic & Surgical Features
- 60-80% are components of a mature cystic teratoma
- Appear as firm yellow-tan colored nodule in the wall of a mature cystic teratoma or mucinous tumor
- May have cystic spaces

Microscopic Features
- Tumor cells are uniform in appearance with abundant pink cytoplasm and central round nuclei containing finely granular chromatin
- Carcinoids can be classified according to their microscopic patterns
  - Insular carcinoids (account for 50% of carcinoid tumors): Tumor cells arranged in round or angular islands with peripheral nuclear palisading
  - Trabecular carcinoids (33%): Cells are arranged in long wavy ribbons or cords

CARCINOID, OVARY

- ○ Strumal carcinoids (16%): Admixture of carcinoid and thyroid elements
- ○ Mucinous carcinoids (1%): Acini containing mucin, surrounded by columnar or cuboidal cells, may show extracellular mucin & signet ring cell forms
  - Differential for mucinous carcinoma includes a Krukenberg tumor (immunohistochemistry is helpful)
- Carcinoids demonstrate positive immunohistochemistry for neuroendocrine markers e.g., synaptophysin, NSE, CD56, chromogranin
- No histological features can reliably predict a malignant course for these tumors, however the following features have been noted in malignant cases
  - ○ Prominent mitotic activity (> 3 per high power field), conspicuous nucleoli, necrosis and a paucity of acini
- Metastatic carcinoids must be excluded: These are usually insular in type, almost always bilateral, multinodular & extraovarian metastases may be evident
- Granulosa cell tumors can be distinguished by their nuclear grooves and they are negative for neuroendocrine immunohistochemical markers

CLINICAL ISSUES

Presentation
- Most common signs/symptoms
  - ○ Most present with symptoms relating to an enlarging ovarian mass
  - ○ Can be an incidental finding
- Other signs/symptoms
  - ○ A small percentage present with symptoms of estrogen or androgen excess (abnormal uterine bleeding or virilization)
  - ○ Carcinoid syndrome has been rarely reported

Demographics
- Age: Most occur in postmenopausal women

Natural History & Prognosis
- Although ovarian carcinoids have a malignant potential, they usually show benign behavior clinically

Treatment
- Total abdominal hysterectomy, bilateral oophorectomy and omentectomy

DIAGNOSTIC CHECKLIST

Consider
- Mature cystic teratoma or mucinous tumors may be present in the contralateral ovary

Image Interpretation Pearls
- The majority of ovarian carcinoids appear as a solid component of a mature cystic teratoma

SELECTED REFERENCES

1. Diaz-Montes TP et al: Primary insular carcinoid of the ovary. Gynecol Oncol. 101(1):175-8, 2006
2. Netea-Maier RT et al: Virilization due to ovarian androgen hypersecretion in a patient with ectopic adrenocorticotrophic hormone secretion caused by a carcinoid tumour: case report. Hum Reprod. 21(10):2601-5, 2006
3. Kopf B et al: Locally advanced ovarian carcinoid. J Exp Clin Cancer Res. 24(2):313-6, 2005
4. McCluggage WG et al: Immunohistochemistry as a diagnostic aid in the evaluation of ovarian tumors. Semin Diagn Pathol. 22(1):3-32, 2005
5. Young RH: Sex cord-stromal tumors of the ovary and testis: their similarities and differences with consideration of selected problems. Mod Pathol. 18 Suppl 2:S81-98, 2005
6. Athavale RD et al: Primary carcinoid tumours of the ovary. J Obstet Gynaecol. 24(1):99-101, 2004
7. Chaowalit N et al: Carcinoid heart disease associated with primary ovarian carcinoid tumor. Am J Cardiol. 93(10):1314-5, 2004
8. van Luijk IF et al: Intraoperative detection of carcinoid tumor of the ovary by gamma probe. Clin Nucl Med. 29(6):343-5, 2004
9. Kuscu E et al: Primary carcinoid tumor of the ovary: a case report. Eur J Gynaecol Oncol. 24(6):574-6, 2003
10. Robboy SJ et al: Pathology of the Female Genital Tract. 1st ed, Lon, Harcourt. 674-7, 2002
11. Baker PM et al: Ovarian mucinous carcinoids including some with a carcinomatous component: a report of 17 cases. Am J Surg Pathol. 25(5):557-68, 2001
12. Doga M et al: Ectopic secretion of growth hormone-releasing hormone (GHRH) in neuroendocrine tumors: relevant clinical aspects. Ann Oncol. 12 Suppl 2:S89-94, 2001
13. Outwater EK et al: Ovarian teratomas: tumor types and imaging characteristics. Radiographics. 21(2):475-90, 2001
14. Kaltsas GA et al: How common are polycystic ovaries and the polycystic ovarian syndrome in women with Cushing's syndrome? Clin Endocrinol (Oxf). 53(4):493-500, 2000
15. Khadilkar UN et al: Ovarian strumal carcinoid--report of a case that matastasized. Indian J Pathol Microbiol. 43(4):459-61, 2000
16. Sabatini T et al: Primary carcinoid tumor of the ovary: report of an unusual case. Tumori. 86(1):91-4, 2000
17. Soga J et al: Carcinoids of the ovary: an analysis of 329 reported cases. J Exp Clin Cancer Res. 19(3):271-80, 2000
18. Kuhlman JE et al: Krukenberg tumors: CT features and growth characteristics. South Med J. 82(10):1215-9, 1989

CARCINOID, OVARY

IMAGE GALLERY

Typical

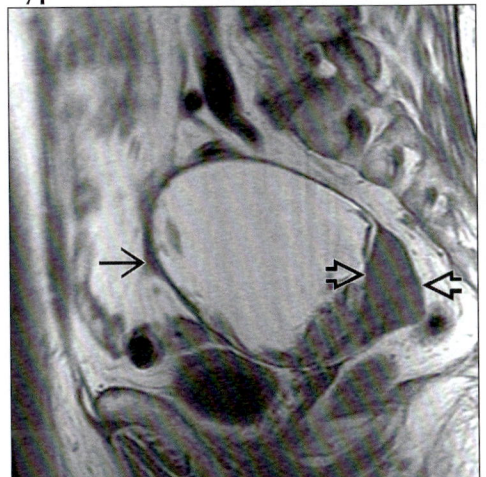
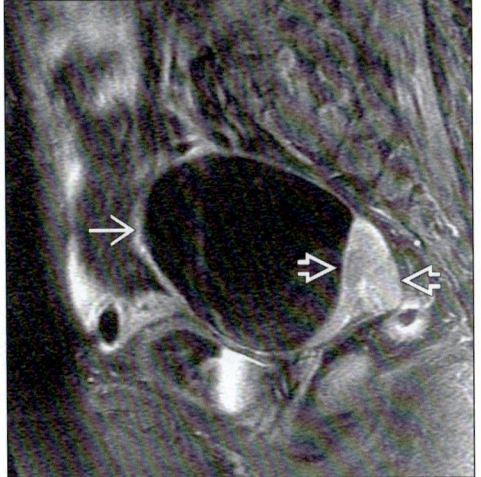

(Left) Sagittal T1WI MR shows a pelvic mass of mainly very high SI ➡ suggestive of fat. Note the presence of a low SI nodule arising from the posterior wall of the mass ➡. *(Right)* Sagittal T1 C+ FS MR in the same patient as previous image shows the presence of a pelvic mass. The drop in the SI of the large anterior component ➡ following fat-suppression confirms the presence of fat. Note moderate enhancement of the solid component ➡.

Typical

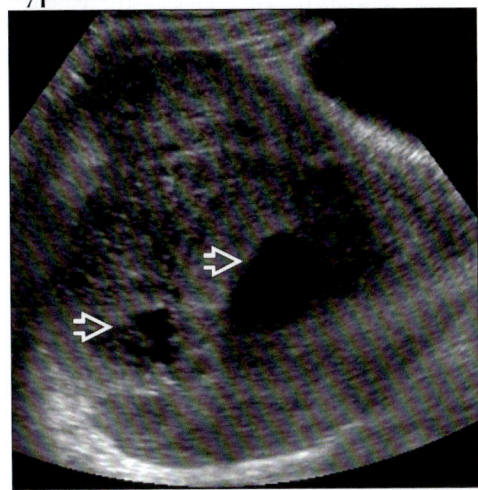
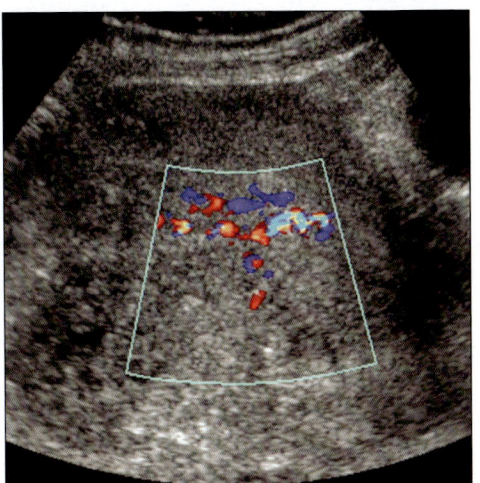

(Left) Longitudinal transabdominal ultrasound shows a solid heterogeneous mass arising from the right adnexa. Note the presence of anechoic areas ➡ suggestive of intratumoral necrosis. *(Right)* Longitudinal transabdominal ultrasound in the same patient as previous image shows presence of blood flow within the solid mass arising from the right ovary. Pathology: Ovarian carcinoid

Typical

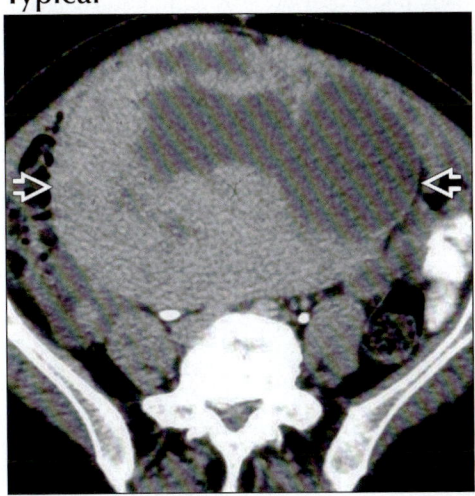
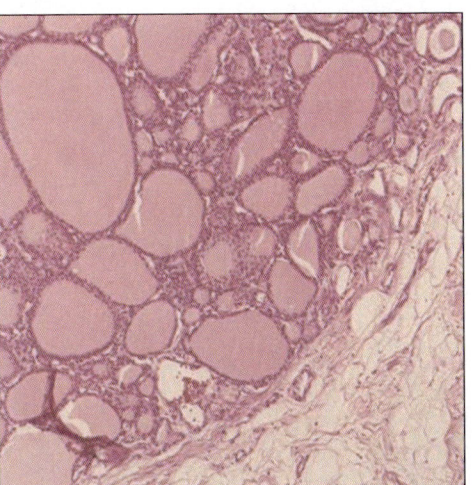

(Left) Axial CECT shows a large heterogeneous solid pelvic mass ➡ which contains multiple areas of necrosis. *(Right)* Micropathology in the same patient as previous image shows an admixture of carcinoid and thyroid elements. Pathology: Strumal carcinoid. (Courtesy of T. Cunha, MD).

UNDIFFERENTIATED CARCINOMA, OVARY

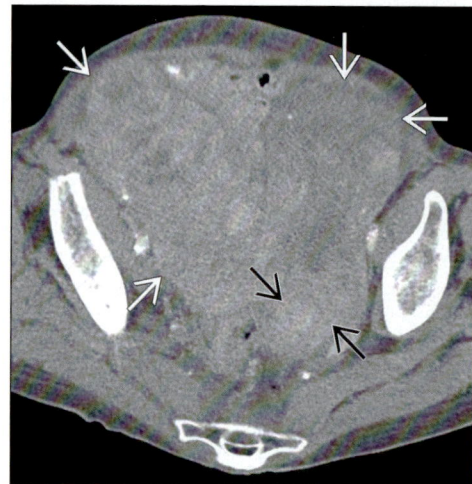

Axial CECT shows solid mass ➡ in the right hemipelvis extending to the pelvic sidewall and displacing the uterus ➡ to the left.

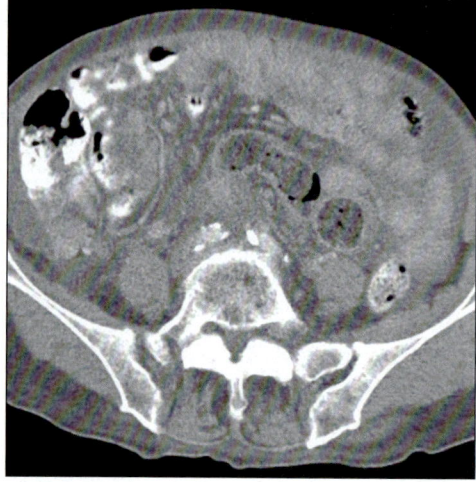

Axial CECT in the same patient as previous shows soft tissue nodules along the peritoneal surfaces with marbling of the mesentery and lymphadenopathy. Ascites with enhancing peritoneal reflections is present.

TERMINOLOGY

Definitions
- Diagnosed when solid areas of epithelial cells are predominant in the tumor
- Inclusion tumors with minimal differentiation such as mucin vacuoles, endometrial-like glands or psammoma bodies
- Cellular differentiation is not sufficient for the tumor to be categorized into one of the other categories

IMAGING FINDINGS

Ultrasonographic Findings
- Complex cystic mass with solid component
- May see papillary projections within cyst
- Increasing number & thickness of septations more associated with malignancy
- Fluid portion may be anechoic or with low level echoes
- Color Doppler US of ovarian mass can help identify vascularized tissue and differentiate solid tumor from nonvascularized structures
- Waveform analysis may distinguish benign from malignant masses
  - Malignant tumor vessels are morphologically abnormal
  - Malignant tumor vessels lack smooth muscle in their walls and demonstrate an irregular course
  - Arteriovenous shunt formation is commonly present
  - Generally with low impedance with high diastolic flow and low systolic-diastolic variation

CT Findings
- Walls and septa more than 3 mm thick
- Partially cystic-partially solid
- Disease may be confined to ovary or may see direct extension to adjacent structures
- Signs of direct spread
  - Localized distortion of the uterine contour
  - Irregular interface between the tumor and the myometrium
  - Loss of a tissue plane between the solid component of the tumor and the wall of the sigmoid colon or the bladder
  - Encasement of the sigmoid colon by the tumor or direct tumor extension to the sigmoid colon

DDx: Undifferentiated Carcinoma, Ovary

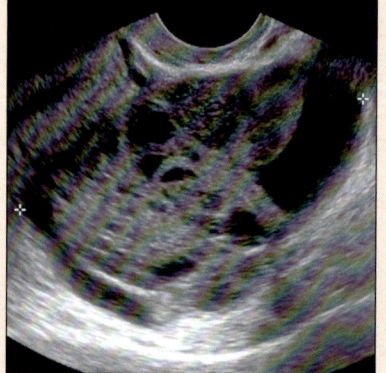

Granulosa Cell Tumor

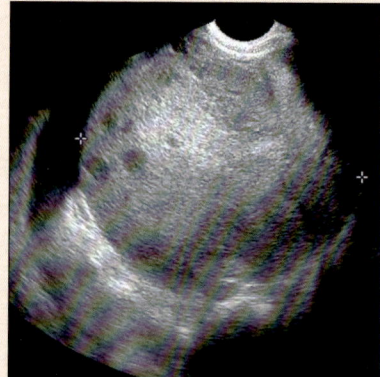

Krukenberg Tumor

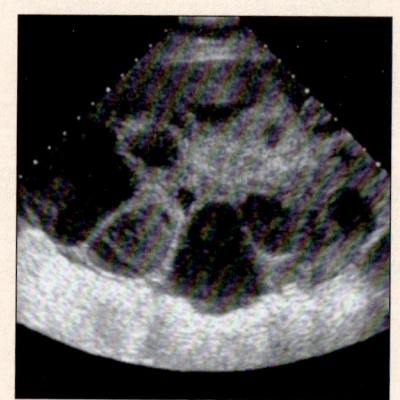

Ovarian Hyperstimulation

UNDIFFERENTIATED CARCINOMA, OVARY

Key Facts

Terminology
- Diagnosed when solid areas of epithelial cells are predominant in the tumor
- Inclusion tumors with minimal differentiation such as mucin vacuoles, endometrial-like glands or psammoma bodies

Imaging Findings
- Walls and septa more than 3 mm thick
- Partially cystic-partially solid
- Disease may be confined to ovary or may see direct extension to adjacent structures
- Best imaging tool: CT provides information for preop planning & determination of surgical resectability, demonstrates tumor response to therapy, & allows detection of persistent or recurrent disease

Top Differential Diagnoses
- Transitional Cell Carcinoma of the Ovary/Malignant Brenner Tumor
- Solid Tumors of Ovary
- Ovarian Hyperstimulation
- Metastases to the Ovary

Pathology
- Reported frequency varies due to lack of strict histologic criteria

Clinical Issues
- Most common signs/symptoms: Often silent, showing no obvious signs or symptoms until late in its course
- Most are stage III or IV at diagnosis (91%) with poor outcome

---

- Distance between the tumor and the pelvic side wall of less than 3 mm
- Iliac vessels surrounded or displaced by tumor

MR Findings
- Findings that suggest malignant behavior:
  - Pelvic organ or side wall invasion
  - Peritoneal, omental or mesenteric involvement
  - Ascites
  - Lymphadenopathy
- Cystic components are hyperintense on T2 weighted images and variable signal intensity on T1 weighted images
- Solid component with intermediate to high signal intensity on T2 weighted images
- Gadolinium-based contrast-enhancement of the solid component is helpful in making diagnosis
- Papillary projections best seen on contrast-enhanced images
- May present as lobulated solid mass

Imaging Recommendations
- Best imaging tool: CT provides information for preop planning & determination of surgical resectability, demonstrates tumor response to therapy, & allows detection of persistent or recurrent disease

DIFFERENTIAL DIAGNOSIS

Transitional Cell Carcinoma of the Ovary/Malignant Brenner Tumor
- Frequently confused pathologically
- Better response to chemotherapy than other types
- Multilocular cystic mass with large solid component

Solid Tumors of Ovary
- Include granulosa cell tumors, dysgerminomas, and fibrothecomas

Ovarian Hyperstimulation
- Enlarged ovaries with multiple thick-walled cysts simulating thick septations within a large ovarian cystic mass
- Associated with ascites which can be mistaken for sign of malignancy

Metastases to the Ovary
- Arise mainly from four sites: Gastrointestinal tract (stomach, biliary tract, pancreas, colon), breast, lymphatic tissue, pelvic structures
- Krukenberg tumors, more than other histologic types may have a predominantly solid appearance
- Spread to ovary is hematogenous and via lymphatics
- Often bilateral

PATHOLOGY

General Features
- Epidemiology
  - Reported frequency varies due to lack of strict histologic criteria
  - 4% of all ovarian carcinomas
  - 6-8% of ovarian epithelial tumors
  - Pure undifferentiated carcinoma is rare; most are mixed with areas of serous, glandular or transitional cell differentiation
  - All are malignant
- Associated abnormalities
  - Ovarian carcinomas in this category behave more aggressively than other tumors with a more differentiated histology
  - Often confused with transitional cell carcinoma of the ovary
  - Poor correlation between gross pathologic appearance and histologic type or aggressiveness of tumor

Gross Pathologic & Surgical Features
- Three types
  - Classical

UNDIFFERENTIATED CARCINOMA, OVARY

- Small cell carcinoma of hypercalcemic type
- Small cell carcinoma of pulmonary type

Microscopic Features
- Carcinoma with a predominantly solid epithelial histology area without Müllerian differentiation
- Diffuse solid areas lack a specific pattern
- Distinguished from TCC by the presence of thick, undulating papillae with smooth luminal borders in contrast to the pseudopapillae secondary to tumor cell necrosis in undifferentiated carcinoma
- Microspaces are more frequent in TCC
- Tumor cells in TCC have moderate cytoplasm

CLINICAL ISSUES

Presentation
- Most common signs/symptoms: Often silent, showing no obvious signs or symptoms until late in its course
- Other signs/symptoms: 2/3 of patients have tumors that have spread beyond the pelvis at the time of diagnosis

Natural History & Prognosis
- All are malignant
- Highly aggressive tumor
- Poorest outcome of any of the epithelial neoplasms & are often quite extensive at the time of presentation
- Most are stage III or IV at diagnosis (91%) with poor outcome
- Staging
  - I: Tumor limited to the ovaries
  - IA: Tumor limited to one ovary, no ascites
  - IB: Tumor limited to both ovaries; no ascites
  - Ic: Tumor stage IA or IB with ascites
  - II: Tumor involving one or both ovaries with pelvic extension
  - IIA: Extension or metastases to the uterus or fallopian tubes, no ascites
  - IIB: Extension to other pelvic tissues, no ascites
  - IIC: Tumor stage IIA or IIB with ascites
  - III: Tumor involving one or both ovaries with peritoneal implants outside the pelvis or positive retroperitoneal or inguinal nodes
  - IIIa: Tumor grossly limited to the true pelvis with histologically confirmed microscopic seeding of abdominal peritoneal surfaces
  - IIIB: Small implants (< or = 2 cm in diameter) of abdominal peritoneal surfaces
  - IIIC: Large abdominal implants (> 2 cm in diameter) or positive retroperitoneal or inguinal nodes
  - IV: Tumor involving one or both ovaries with distant metastases or parenchymal liver metastases
- Most common sites of direct involvement by spread
  - Anterior and posterior cul-de-sac
  - Sigmoid colon
  - Omentum
  - Small intestine
  - Pelvic wall peritoneum
  - Uterus
  - Fallopian tubes
  - Broad ligament
- May also spread by hematogenous dissemination and lymphatic invasion

Treatment
- At initial exploration, surgicopathologic staging and debulking of tumor
- Total abdominal hysterectomy, bilateral salpingo-oophorectomy and omentectomy with aspiration of ascites or peritoneal lavage for cytologic examination
- Random peritoneal biopsies including paracolic gutters and undersurface of hemidiaphragms
- Sampling of pelvic and paraaortic lymph nodes
- For patients with advanced ovarian cancer, surgical debulking followed by chemotherapy
- Volume of residual disease after cytoreduction surgery is directly correlated with survival
- May undergo second look surgery after induction chemotherapy to detect residual disease
- Others consider non-invasive imaging instead of second surgery more appropriate

DIAGNOSTIC CHECKLIST

Image Interpretation Pearls
- Consider the diagnosis when there is a large predominantly solid tumor with direct extension to adjacent structures
- Cannot easily determine site of origin due to large size and extension

SELECTED REFERENCES

1. Imaoka I et al: Developing an MR imaging strategy for diagnosis of ovarian masses. Radiographics. 26(5):1431-48, 2006
2. Prat J: Ovarian carcinomas, including secondary tumors: diagnostically challenging areas. Mod Pathol. 18 Suppl 2:S99-111, 2005
3. Georgescu CV et al: Value of immunohistochemistry in confirming undifferentiated ovarian carcinomas. Rom J Morphol Embryol. 45:133-42, 1999-2004
4. McCluggage WG: Ovarian neoplasms composed of small round cells: a review. Adv Anat Pathol. 11(6):288-96, 2004
5. Brown DL et al: Primary versus secondary ovarian malignancy: imaging findings of adnexal masses in the Radiology Diagnostic Oncology Group Study. Radiology. 219(1):213-8, 2001
6. Jeong YY et al: Imaging evaluation of ovarian masses. Radiographics. 20(5):1445-70, 2000
7. Kawamoto S et al: CT of epithelial ovarian tumors. Radiographics. 19 Spec No:S85-102; quiz S263-4, 1999
8. Kurtz AB et al: Diagnosis and staging of ovarian cancer: comparative values of Doppler and conventional US, CT, and MR imaging correlated with surgery and histopathologic analysis--report of the Radiology Diagnostic Oncology Group. Radiology. 212(1):19-27, 1999
9. Forstner R et al: Imaging of ovarian cancer. J Magn Reson Imaging. 5(5):606-13, 1995
10. Kuwashima Y et al: Cytopathological features of undifferentiated carcinoma of the ovary. Diagn Cytopathol. 12(3):254-8, 1995
11. Wagner BJ et al: From the archives of the AFIP. Ovarian epithelial neoplasms: radiologic-pathologic correlation. Radiographics. 14(6):1351-74; quiz 1375-6, 1994

UNDIFFERENTIATED CARCINOMA, OVARY

IMAGE GALLERY

Typical

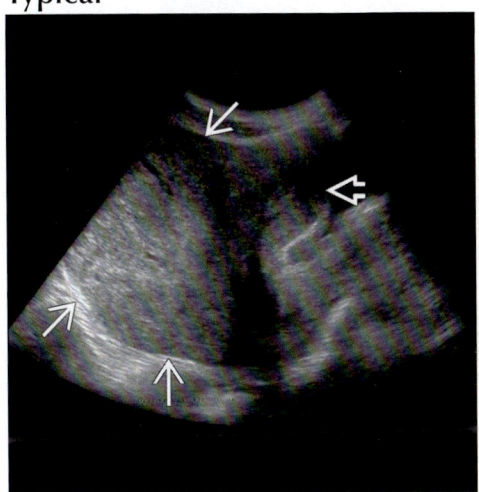
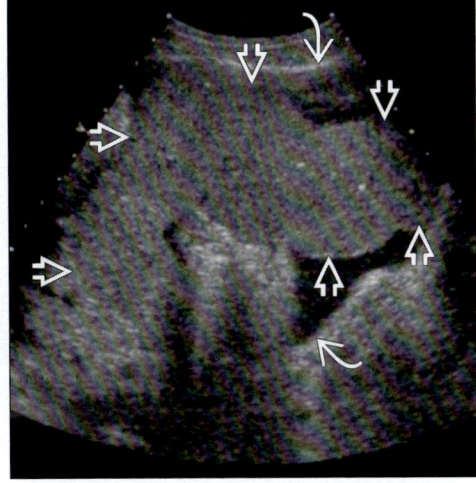

(Left) Sagittal transabdominal ultrasound shows large predominantly solid mass ➡ posterosuperior to the uterus ➡ and extending from the adnexa. *(Right)* Transverse transabdominal ultrasound in the same patient shows solid mass extending from the pelvis to encase bowel loops ➡. Note ascites ➡.

Typical

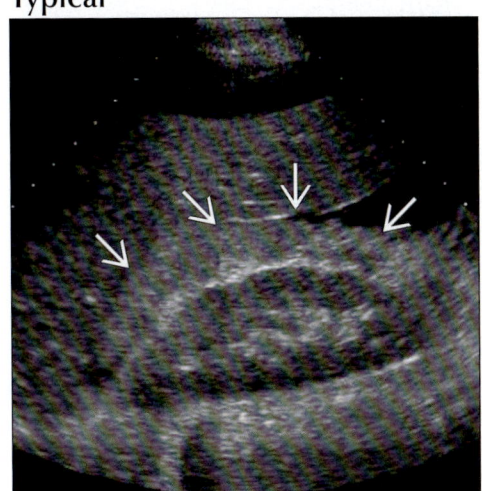
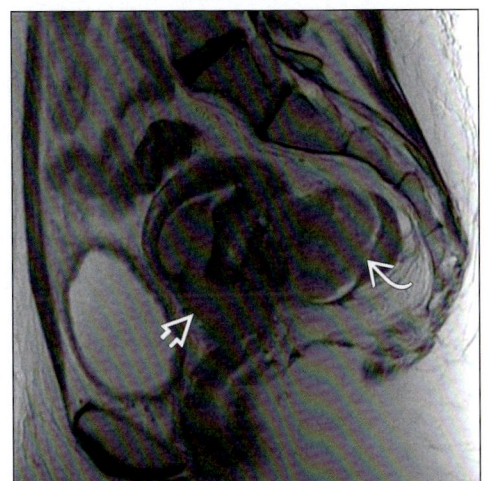

(Left) Longitudinal transabdominal ultrasound in the same patient as previous image shows an echogenic mass ➡ caking the hepatorenal fossa compatible with peritoneal spread of disease. Ascites is present. *(Right)* Sagittal T2WI MR shows a large adnexal mass ➡ that has metastasized to the cervix and extends to the lower uterine segment ➡.

Typical

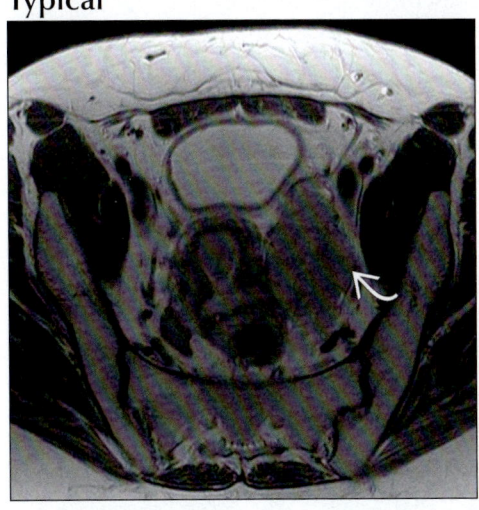
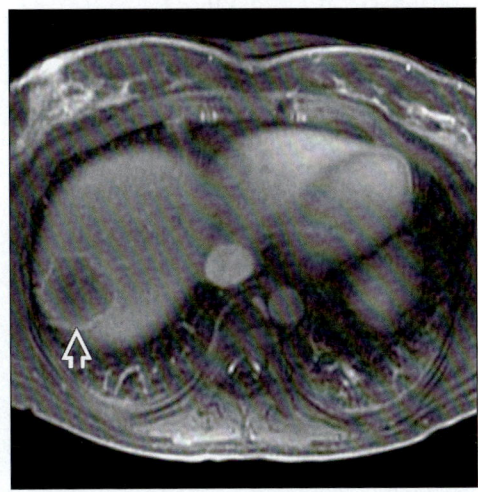

(Left) Axial T2WI MR in the same patient as previous image shows the left adnexal mass ➡ with uterine and cervical involvement. *(Right)* Axial T1 C+ FS MR in the same patient as previous image, shows a liver capsular deposit ➡.

EMBRYONAL CARCINOMA, OVARY

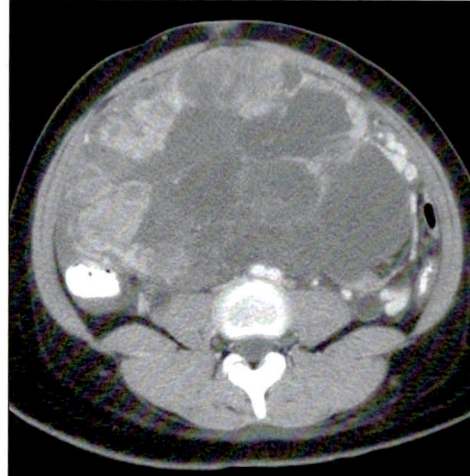

Axial CECT shows a large complex mass with multiple low-attenuation areas representing extensive necrosis and hemorrhage.

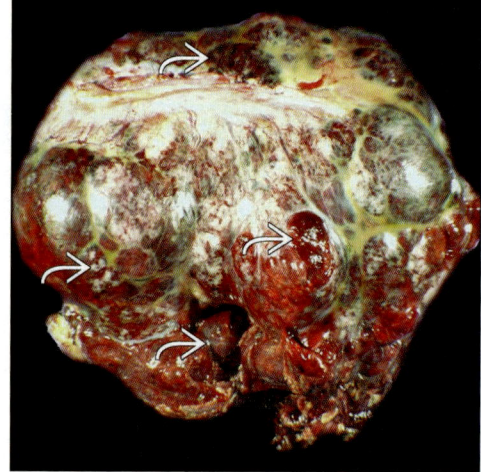

Gross pathology in the same patient shows a large mass with extensive necrosis/hemorrhage ➡. Pathology: MGCT composed predominantly of embryonal carcinoma (some yolk sac tumor also present).

TERMINOLOGY

Definitions
- Malignant germ cell tumor (MGCT) of the ovary

IMAGING FINDINGS

General Features
- Best diagnostic clue: Predominantly solid tumor containing areas of extensive necrosis and hemorrhage
- Location: Usually unilateral
- Size: Usually very large mass
- Morphology: Large, solid mass with extensive necrosis and hemorrhage

Ultrasonographic Findings
- Grayscale Ultrasound
  ○ TAS is mandatory as embryonal carcinomas are usually very large and may be missed on TVS alone
  ○ Predominantly solid adnexal mass
  ○ Anechoic cystic areas represent necrosis and hemorrhage
  ○ Ascites and peritoneal implants may be present
- Color Doppler: Marked blood flow within the solid components

CT Findings
- NECT
  ○ Large complex pelvic mass
  ○ Low attenuation areas represent extensive necrosis
  ○ High or low attenuation areas may also represent hemorrhage
- CECT
  ○ Solid component shows avid enhancement
  ○ Ascites and peritoneal implants may be present
  ○ Enlarged retroperitoneal lymph nodes may be seen
  ○ Distant spread (e.g., lung and liver metastases) may be present at diagnosis

MR Findings
- T1WI
  ○ Low SI large pelvic mass that may contain areas of high SI representing hemorrhage
  ○ Enlarged retroperitoneal lymph nodes
- T2WI
  ○ Large mass of predominantly high SI due to extensive necrosis
  ○ Ascites

DDx: Adnexal Masses

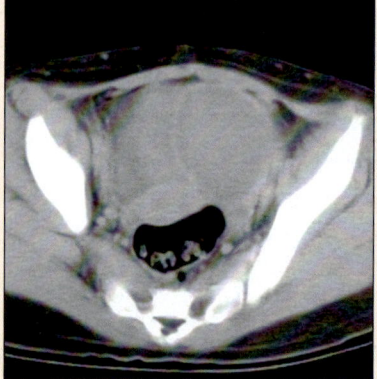

Choriocarcinoma

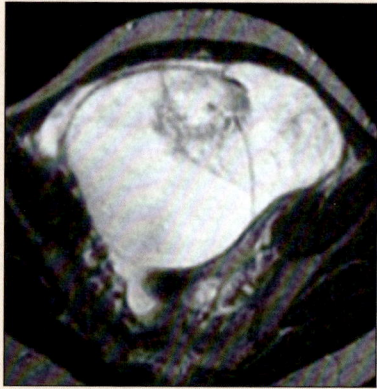

Immature Teratoma

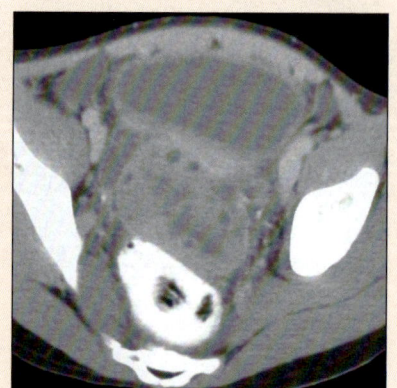

Ovarian Torsion

EMBRYONAL CARCINOMA, OVARY

Key Facts

Terminology
- Malignant germ cell tumor (MGCT) of the ovary

Imaging Findings
- Best diagnostic clue: Predominantly solid tumor containing areas of extensive necrosis and hemorrhage
- Ascites and peritoneal implants may be present
- Enlarged retroperitoneal lymph nodes may be seen
- Distant spread (e.g., lung and liver metastases) may be present at diagnosis
- Large mass of predominantly high SI due to extensive necrosis

Top Differential Diagnoses
- Other Malignant Germ Cell Tumors
- Mature/Immature Teratoma
- Ovarian Torsion

Pathology
- Epidemiology: Pure ovarian embryonal carcinomas are extremely rare; usually found as a component of a mixed GCT
- Embryonal carcinoma cells stain for alpha fetoprotein immunohistochemistry in 85% of cases

Clinical Issues
- Abdominal or pelvic mass
- Serum β-hCG levels are usually elevated

Diagnostic Checklist
- Malignant germ cell tumor of the ovary should be considered when a large, predominantly solid ovarian tumor is discovered in a girl or young woman

---

  - Peritoneal implants or simply peritoneal thickening
- T1 C+ FS
  - Avid enhancement of solid portions of tumor
  - Peritoneal thickening and/or implants, if present, are best appreciated on delayed gadolinium-enhanced images

Imaging Recommendations
- Best imaging tool
  - US for initial diagnosis
  - CT/MR for lesion characterization and evaluation of local extent of the tumor
  - CT for evaluation of hematogenous metastases (e.g., lung, liver)
- Protocol advice: MR: Sagittal, axial and coronal T2WI; axial T1WI, axial and coronal T1 C+ FS

DIFFERENTIAL DIAGNOSIS

Other Malignant Germ Cell Tumors
- Embryonal carcinoma may coexist with any type of malignant germ cell tumor (choriocarcinoma, yolk sac tumor, disgerminoma)
- Can be very difficult to distinguish on imaging alone

Mature/Immature Teratoma
- Embryonal carcinoma may coexist with both mature and immature teratoma therefore
  - The presence of well-defined cystic spaces or calcifications does not exclude a coexisting germ cell tumor
  - A coexisting germ cell tumor should be suspected when a significant solid component is present

Ovarian Torsion
- Typical clinical presentation with acute pelvic pain
- Smaller size of mass
- Multiple small peripheral follicles displaced due to edematous stroma
- Twisted vascular pedicle

Sex-Cord Stromal Tumors
- Granulosa cell and Sertoli-Leydig tumors may occur as predominantly solid tumor in young females but have distinct associated endocrine effects

Solid Ovarian Tumors
- Fibroma and fibrothecoma usually occur in older age group
- Typical low SI on T2WI

Ovarian Epithelial Neoplasms
- Predominantly cystic lesions that occur in middle-age or older women
- Extensive peritoneal disease and ascites is usually present at diagnosis
- Hematogenous metastases are rare

Endometriosis
- Frequently bilateral
- High SI cystic lesions on both T1WI and T1 FS images

Tubo-Ovarian Abscess
- Typical clinical presentation with severe pelvic pain and raised inflammatory markers
- Bilateral tubular cystic lesions with rim enhancement

PATHOLOGY

General Features
- Epidemiology: Pure ovarian embryonal carcinomas are extremely rare; usually found as a component of a mixed GCT
- Associated abnormalities
  - Other GCT's
  - Mature or immature teratoma

Gross Pathologic & Surgical Features
- Unilateral, large, solid, soft, yellow/grey masses with hemorrhage and necrosis

EMBRYONAL CARCINOMA, OVARY

Microscopic Features
- Solid sheets of large cells with vesicular nuclei and prominent nucleoli
- Mitoses are frequent
- Multinucleated syncytiotrophoblast cells producing beta β-hCG are common
- Embryonal carcinoma cells stain for alpha fetoprotein immunohistochemistry in 85% of cases
- Hyaline droplets are seen within and between cells
- Necrosis and hemorrhage are common
- Vascular invasion is seen

CLINICAL ISSUES

Presentation
- Most common signs/symptoms
  - Abdominal or pelvic mass
  - Two-thirds have have hormonal manifestations
    - Precocious pseudopuberty
    - Uterine bleeding
- Other signs/symptoms
  - Serum β-hCG levels are usually elevated
  - Serum AFP levels are occasionally elevated

Demographics
- Age
  - Most present in second or third decades
  - Median age is 15 years
- Gender
  - Female
    - Embryonal carcinoma of the ovary is much less common than that of the testis, but they are identical pathologically

Natural History & Prognosis
- Highly malignant neoplasm, locally aggressive
- Spread widely within the peritoneal cavity
- Metastasis to lungs, liver and retroperitoneal lymph nodes

Treatment
- Surgical removal of tumor with or without the ovary +/- adnexa
- Adjuvant chemotherapy and/or radiotherapy

DIAGNOSTIC CHECKLIST

Consider
- Malignant germ cell tumor of the ovary should be considered when a large, predominantly solid ovarian tumor is discovered in a girl or young woman

Image Interpretation Pearls
- Predominantly solid tumor with extensive necrosis and hemorrhage

SELECTED REFERENCES

1. De Backer A et al: Ovarian germ cell tumors in children: a clinical study of 66 patients. Pediatr Blood Cancer. 46(4):459-64, 2006
2. Baker PM et al: Immunohistochemistry as a tool in the differential diagnosis of ovarian tumors: an update. Int J Gynecol Pathol. 24(1):39-55, 2005
3. Ulbright TM: Germ cell tumors of the gonads: a selective review emphasizing problems in differential diagnosis, newly appreciated, and controversial issues. Mod Pathol. 18 Suppl 2:S61-79, 2005
4. Ulbright TM: Gonadal teratomas: a review and speculation. Adv Anat Pathol. 11(1):10-23, 2004
5. Nishida T et al: Ovarian mixed germ cell tumor comprising polyembryoma and choriocarcinoma. Eur J Obstet Gynecol Reprod Biol. 78(1):95-7, 1998
6. Borghi A et al: [An ovarian mass in childhood: a case report] Pediatr Med Chir. 15(4):413-5, 1993
7. Brammer HM 3rd et al: From the archives of the AFIP. Malignant germ cell tumors of the ovary: radiologic-pathologic correlation. Radiographics. 10(4):715-24, 1990
8. Kawai M et al: Alpha-fetoprotein in malignant germ cell tumors of the ovary. Gynecol Oncol. 39(2):160-6, 1990
9. Ueda G et al: Embryonal carcinoma of the ovary: a six-year survival. Int J Gynaecol Obstet. 31(3):287-92, 1990

EMBRYONAL CARCINOMA, OVARY

IMAGE GALLERY

Typical

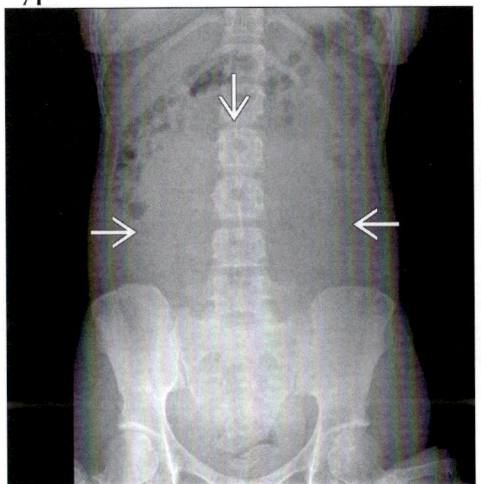
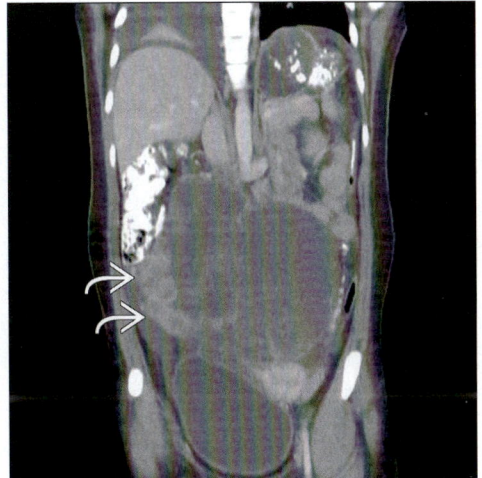

(Left) Radiograph shows a large soft tissue mass ➡ which is displacing the large bowel in a young girl. (Right) Coronal CECT in the same patient as on previous image shows a large abdomino-pelvic mass containing large areas of low-attenuation representing extensive necrosis/hemorrhage. Note avid enhancement of the solid components ➡.

Typical

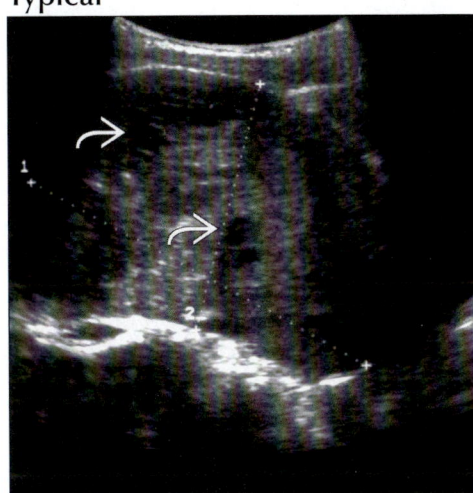
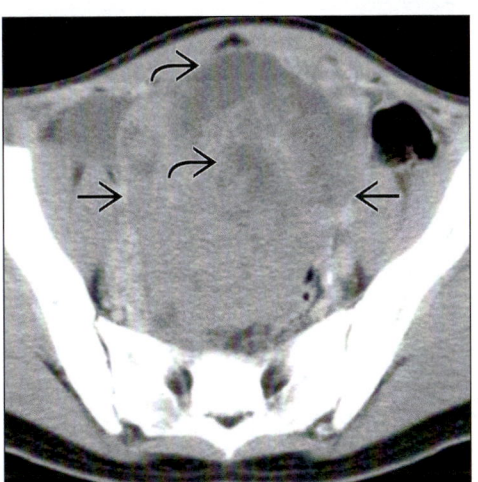

(Left) Transverse transabdominal ultrasound shows a large, predominantly solid adnexal mass (calipers) in a 14 year old girl. Note multiple anechoic areas ➡ representing necrosis/hemorrhage. (Right) Axial CECT in the same patient as previous image confirms the presence of a predominantly solid mass ➡ containing low-attenuation areas ➡ indicative of necrosis/hemorrhage. Note avid enhancement of the solid part of the mass.

Typical

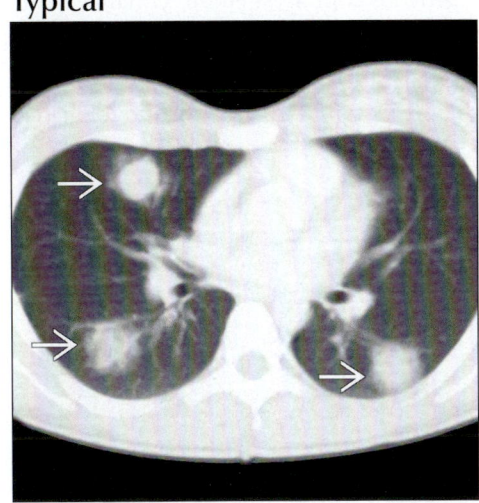
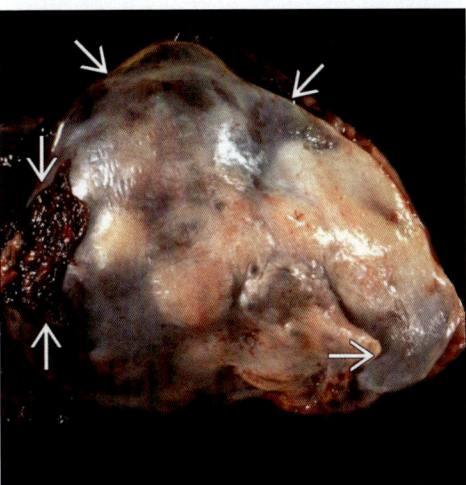

(Left) Axial CECT in the same patient as previous image shows multiple lung metastases ➡. (Right) Gross pathology in the same patient as previous image shows a large predominantly solid tumor with extensive areas of hemorrhage ➡. Pathology: MGCT composed of predominantly embryonal carcinoma.

MIXED MULLERIAN TUMOR, OVARY

Axial CECT shows a large heterogeneous pelvic mass ➡. Areas of low attenuation represent extensive necrosis. Note avid enhancement of the solid components.

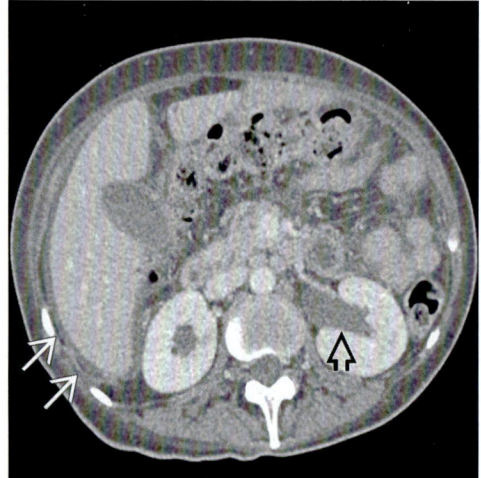

Axial CECT in the same patient as previous image shows left hydronephrosis ➡ caused by the large pelvic mass. Small amount of ascites ➡ is also seen around the liver. Pathology: MMMT of the ovary.

TERMINOLOGY

Abbreviations and Synonyms
- Malignant mixed mesodermal tumor (MMMT), carcinosarcoma

Definitions
- Malignant neoplasms composed of malignant epithelial (carcinoma) and malignant mesenchymal (sarcoma) elements
- MMMT are included in the endometrioid type of epithelial ovarian tumors

IMAGING FINDINGS

General Features
- Best diagnostic clue: Large mixed cystic and solid or multiseptated adnexal masses with invasion of the adjacent organs, ascites and peritoneal implants
- Location: Usually bilateral
- Size: Usually very large at presentation (> 10 cm)
- Morphology: Large, well-capsulated multinodular or multicystic tumors

Ultrasonographic Findings
- Grayscale Ultrasound
  - Large complex cystic and solid or multicystic adnexal masses
  - Relatively large peritoneal implants can be seen
  - Large amount of ascites is usually present
  - Technique of choice for guiding omental/peritoneal biopsy
- Color Doppler: Increased vascularity within the solid components or thick septa
- Power Doppler/Pulsed Doppler: Blood flow of low resistance within the solid component

CT Findings
- NECT
  - Large bilateral mixed solid and cystic adnexal masses
  - Multiseptated thick-walled cystic masses
- CECT
  - Avid, homogeneous contrast medium enhancement of the solid components
  - Strong contrast medium enhancement of the wall and internal septa of multicystic lesions
  - Loss of fat plane, marginal irregularity and lobulated contour of the uterus suggest direct invasion

DDx: Adnexal Masses

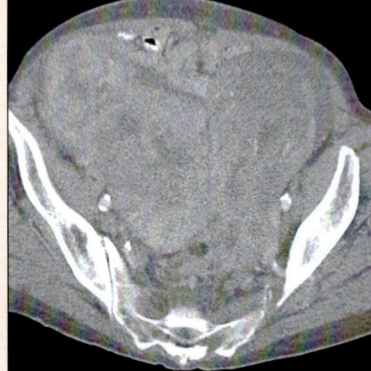

Undifferentiated Ovarian Carcinoma

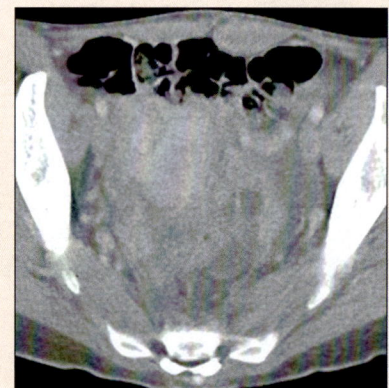

Krukenberg Tumor

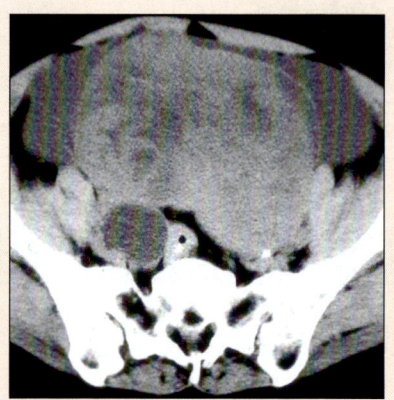

Metastases to the Ovary

MIXED MULLERIAN TUMOR, OVARY

Key Facts

Terminology
- Malignant mixed mesodermal tumor (MMMT), carcinosarcoma
- Malignant neoplasms composed of malignant epithelial (carcinoma) and malignant mesenchymal (sarcoma) elements

Imaging Findings
- Best diagnostic clue: Large mixed cystic and solid or multiseptated adnexal masses with invasion of the adjacent organs, ascites and peritoneal implants
- Avid, homogeneous contrast medium enhancement of the solid components
- Strong contrast medium enhancement of the wall and internal septa of multicystic lesions
- Loss of fat plane, marginal irregularity and lobulated contour of the uterus suggest direct invasion
- Focal wall thickening of bladder and sigmoid colon suggest invasion
- Enhancing solid or cystic peritoneal and omental implants of varying size are often present at diagnosis
- Large amount of ascites is usually present at diagnosis
- Best imaging tool: Contrast enhanced CT
- Prolonged oral contrast medium is essential for optimal bowel opacification to differentiate serosal implants from unopacified bowel loops
- Multiplanar reformatted images are very useful in evaluation of adjacent organ invasion and to distinguish liver capsular implants from intraparenchymal metastases

Top Differential Diagnoses
- Other Epithelial Ovarian Malignancies
- Krukenberg Tumor

- o Focal wall thickening of bladder and sigmoid colon suggest invasion
- o Presence of hydronephrosis indicate pelvic side wall invasion
- o Peritoneal thickening
- o Enhancing solid or cystic peritoneal and omental implants of varying size are often present at diagnosis
- o Enlarged retroperitoneal lymph nodes may be seen at presentation
- o Large amount of ascites is usually present at diagnosis
- o May present with small bowel obstruction
- o Hematogenous metastases (liver, lung, bone)
- It is useful for guiding biopsy for tissue diagnosis

MR Findings
- T1WI
  - o Large, bilateral adnexal masses of low SI
  - o Areas of intermediate SI represent proteinaceous fluid within the cystic components
  - o Areas of high SI indicate presence of hemorrhage
- T2WI
  - o Large, complex adnexal masses of predominantly high SI
  - o Invasion of adjacent organs such as uterus, bladder and rectum can be better appreciated on MR compared to CT
  - o Hydronephrosis indicating pelvic side wall invasion may be seen at presentation
  - o Peritoneal implants and ascites are usually present at diagnosis
- T1 C+ FS
  - o Avid enhancement of solid components or walls and internal septa of cystic lesions
  - o Enhancing implants along the peritoneal surface and peritoneal reflections, best appreciated on delayed images

Nuclear Medicine Findings
- PET/CT
  - o May be useful to evaluate the extent of disease especially if follow-up surgery is being considered
  - o It is of limited value in detection of small peritoneal implants as normal bowel uptake may obscure small lesions

Imaging Recommendations
- Best imaging tool: Contrast enhanced CT
- Protocol advice
  - o Intravenous contrast medium is mandatory
  - o Prolonged oral contrast medium is essential for optimal bowel opacification to differentiate serosal implants from unopacified bowel loops
  - o Scrolling through the images improves the ability to reliably detect subtle peritoneal implants
  - o Multiplanar reformatted images are very useful in evaluation of adjacent organ invasion and to distinguish liver capsular implants from intraparenchymal metastases

DIFFERENTIAL DIAGNOSIS

Other Epithelial Ovarian Malignancies
- MMMT's are more aggressive and larger than other epithelial ovarian tumors, however, imaging findings are not specific

Krukenberg Tumor
- Known primary tumor from the gastrointestinal tract
- Predominantly solid masses; large amount of ascites is rare

Ovarian Metastases
- Most ovarian metastases are predominantly solid
- Clinical presentation often due to primary tumor

PATHOLOGY

General Features
- General path comments: Large, well-capsulated multinodular or multicystic tumors
- Genetics: No genetic predisposition
- Etiology: Previous pelvic radiotherapy

MIXED MULLERIAN TUMOR, OVARY

- Epidemiology: Represent < 1% of all ovarian malignancies
- Associated abnormalities: Association with low parity has been described

Gross Pathologic & Surgical Features
- Hemorrhage and necrosis are usually present

Microscopic Features
- High grade malignant epithelial (carcinoma) and malignant mesenchymal (sarcoma) elements
- Either carcinomatous or sarcomatous component may predominate
- Epithelial element is most commonly serous carcinoma
- Bizarre epithelial giant cells are common
- Heterologous stromal elements (tissues not native to site) such as chondrosarcoma or malignant osteoid may be seen

CLINICAL ISSUES

Presentation
- Most common signs/symptoms
  - Lower abdominal pain
  - Abdominal distension
- Other signs/symptoms: Symptoms related to adjacent organ invasion and metastases

Demographics
- Age: More common in postmenopausal women
- Gender: Female

Natural History & Prognosis
- Almost 70% of the patient present with stage III or IV disease
- Poor prognosis with median survival of 8-21 months
- Older age at presentation and suboptimal debulking are related to worst prognosis

Treatment
- Surgical cytoreduction combined with platinum-based chemotherapy

DIAGNOSTIC CHECKLIST

Image Interpretation Pearls
- Large, aggressive bilateral adnexal lesions with invasion of adjacent organs, ascites and peritoneal implants at time of diagnosis

SELECTED REFERENCES

1. Mok JE et al: Malignant mixed mullerian tumors of the ovary: experience with cytoreductive surgery and platinum-based combination chemotherapy. Int J Gynecol Cancer. 16(1):101-5, 2006
2. Rutledge TL et al: Carcinosarcoma of the ovary-a case series. Gynecol Oncol. 100(1):128-32, 2006
3. Barnholtz-Sloan JS et al: Survival of women diagnosed with malignant, mixed mullerian tumors of the ovary (OMMMT). Gynecol Oncol. 93(2):506-12, 2004
4. Brown E et al: Carcinosarcoma of the ovary: 19 years of prospective data from a single center. Cancer. 100(10):2148-53, 2004
5. Harris MA et al: Carcinosarcoma of the ovary. Br J Cancer. 88(5):654-7, 2003
6. Inthasorn P et al: Malignant mixed mullerian tumour of the ovary: prognostic factor and response of adjuvant platinum-based chemotherapy. Aust N Z J Obstet Gynaecol. 43(1):61-4, 2003
7. Duska LR et al: Paclitaxel and platinum chemotherapy for malignant mixed mullerian tumors of the ovary. Gynecol Oncol. 85(3):459-63, 2002
8. Cho SB et al: Malignant mixed mullerian tumor of the ovary: imaging findings. Eur Radiol. 11(7):1147-50, 2001
9. Melilli GA et al: Malignant mixed mullerian tumor of the ovary: report of four cases. Eur J Gynaecol Oncol. 22(1):67-9, 2001
10. Wei LH et al: Carcinosarcoma of ovary associated with previous radiotherapy. Int J Gynecol Cancer. 11(1):81-4, 2001
11. Ariyoshi K et al: Prognostic factors in ovarian carcinosarcoma: a clinicopathological and immunohistochemical analysis of 23 cases. Histopathology. 37(5):427-36, 2000
12. Sit AS et al: Chemotherapy for malignant mixed Mullerian tumors of the ovary. Gynecol Oncol. 79(2):196-200, 2000
13. Krishnan E et al: Malignant mixed mullerian tumours of gynaecological origin: chemosensitive but aggressive tumours. Clin Oncol (R Coll Radiol). 10(4):246-9, 1998
14. Chang J et al: Carcinosarcoma of the ovary: incidence, prognosis, treatment and survival of patients. Ann Oncol. 6(8):755-8, 1995
15. Muntz HG et al: Malignant mixed mullerian tumors of the ovary: experience with surgical cytoreduction and combination chemotherapy. Cancer. 76(7):1209-13, 1995
16. Boucher D et al: Morphologic prognostic factors of malignant mixed mullerian tumors of the ovary: a clinicopathologic study of 15 cases. Int J Gynecol Pathol. 13(1):22-8, 1994
17. Costa MJ et al: Utility of immunohistochemistry in distinguishing ovarian sertoli-stromal cell tumors from carcinosarcomas. Hum Pathol. 23(7):787-97, 1992
18. Ehrmann RL et al: Malignant mixed mullerian tumor of the ovary with prominent neuroectodermal differentiation (teratoid carcinosarcoma). Int J Gynecol Pathol. 9(3):272-82, 1990

MIXED MULLERIAN TUMOR, OVARY

IMAGE GALLERY

Typical

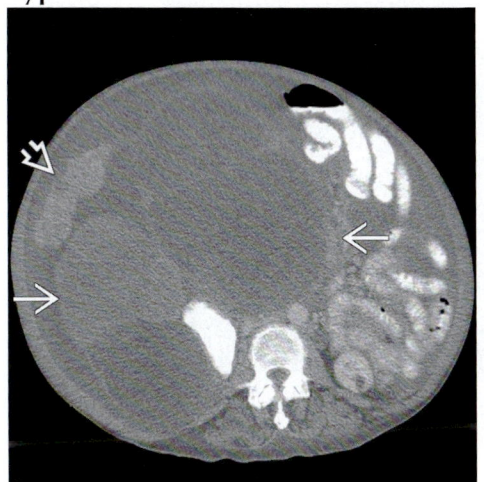
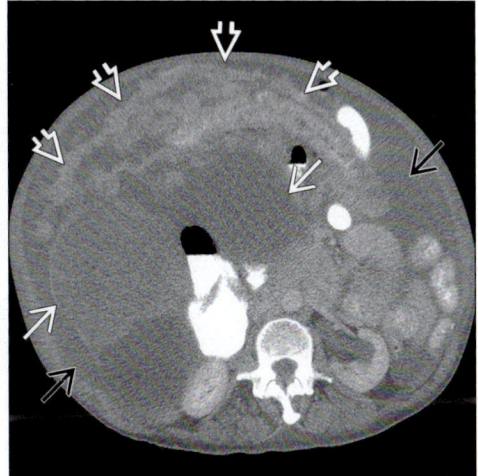

(Left) Axial CECT shows a very large multicystic mass ➡. Note presence of a peritoneal implant ➡ anterolateral to the mass. Moderate amount of ascites is also seen. *(Right)* Axial CECT in the same patient as previous image shows extension of the pelvic mass ➡ and associated extensive peritoneal implants ➡ anteriorly. Note also presence of ascites ➡.

Typical

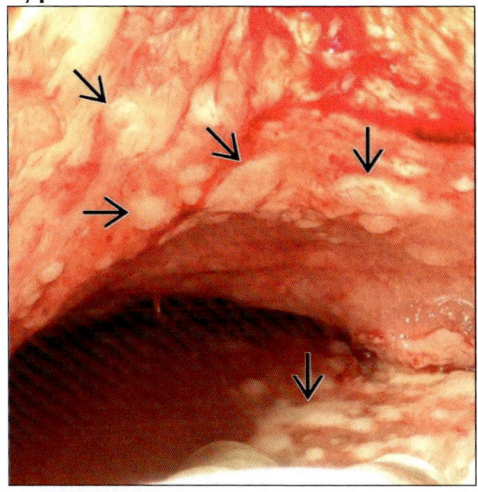
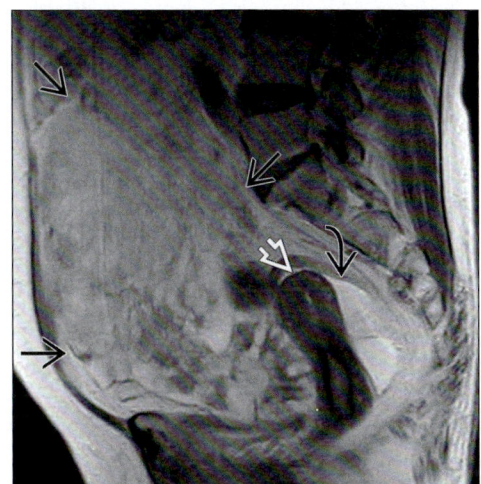

(Left) Intra-operative photograph in the same patient as previous image shows multiple peritoneal implants ➡. Pathology: MMMT of the ovary. *(Right)* Sagittal T2WI MR shows a large mass ➡ of high SI arising from the pelvis and extending into the abdominal cavity. The mass is displacing the uterus posteriorly ➡. Note presence of free fluid in the pouch of Douglas ➡.

Typical

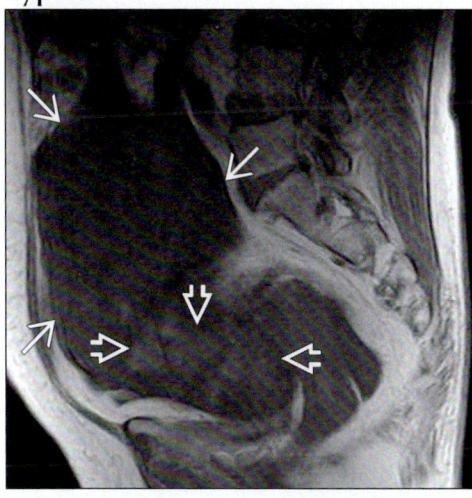
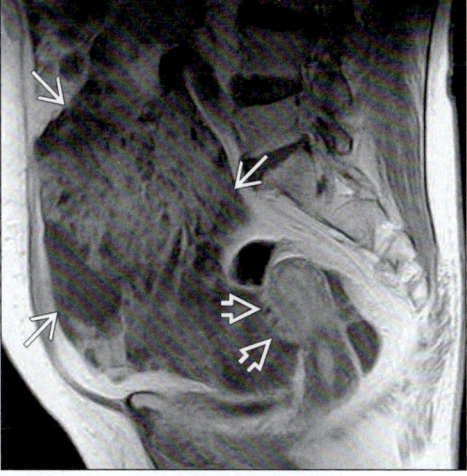

(Left) Sagittal T1WI MR in the same patient as previous image shows the large predominantly low SI pelvic mass ➡. Note the presence of high SI areas ➡ indicative of hemorrhage/necrosis. *(Right)* Sagittal T1 C+ MR in the same patient as previous image shows heterogeneous enhancement of the pelvic mass ➡. Note an irregular interface between the posterior aspect of the mass and the uterus ➡ suggesting direct invasion.

KRUKENBERG TUMOR

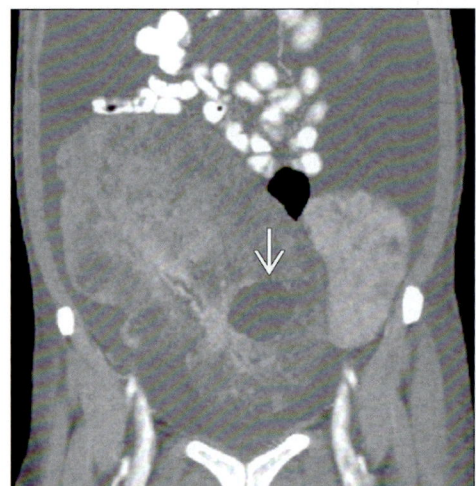

Coronal CECT in 36 year old patient shows massive ascites and large, bosselated, solid ovarian masses with an intratumoral cystic component ➔ in the larger mass.

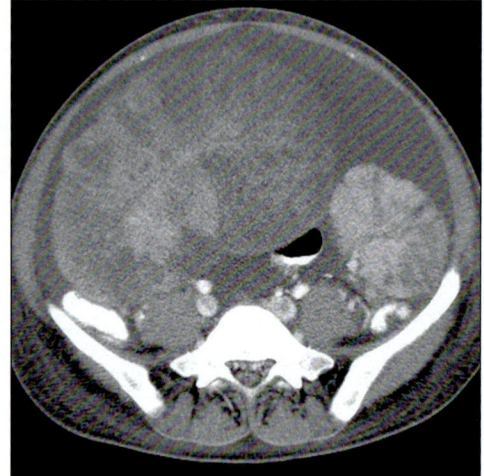

Axial CECT in same patient as previous image, shows enlarged ovaries which maintain oval shape and are replaced by predominantly solid masses from metastatic signet ring cell gastric adenocarcinoma.

TERMINOLOGY

Abbreviations and Synonyms
- Metastases to ovary from signet ring cell adenocarcinoma

Definitions
- Metastatic adenocarcinomas to ovary, most common from stomach → composed of mucin-filled signet ring cells and proliferation of ovarian stroma
  - Term should not be used with other types of ovarian metastases or primary bilateral tumors

IMAGING FINDINGS

General Features
- Best diagnostic clue: Bilateral, lobulated, predominantly solid ovarian masses
- Location: 80% bilateral, can be unilateral
- Size: Large, 2/3 are larger than 10 cm

Ultrasonographic Findings
- Grayscale Ultrasound
  - Bilateral, large lobulated ovarian masses
  - Predominantly solid, may be partially cystic
  - Ascites
- Color Doppler: Solid masses show rich vascularity

CT Findings
- Predominantly solid ovarian masses, can be partially cystic
- May detect peritoneal, omental or bowel implants
  - Easier to detect if there is free fluid
- May visualize gastric primary

MR Findings
- T1WI
  - Ovarian solid masses: Typical isointense signal, also heterogeneous or slightly hyperintense compared to myometrium
  - Peritoneal carcinomatosis: Nodules or peritoneal thickening of intermediate signal intensity in the cul de sac or parametrial regions
    - Omental and mesenteric lesions are hard to detect
  - 2/3 of patients present with ascites
- T2WI

DDx: Bilateral Ovarian Masses

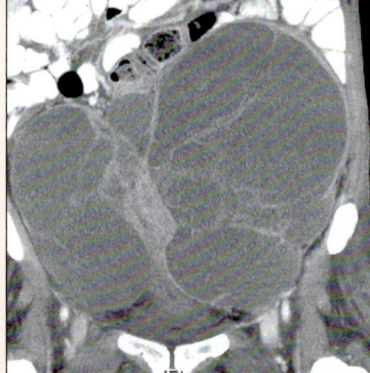

Primary Ovarian Tumors

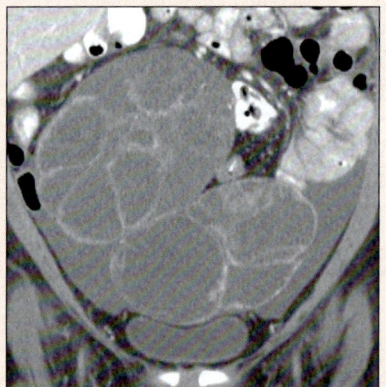

Ovarian Metastasis

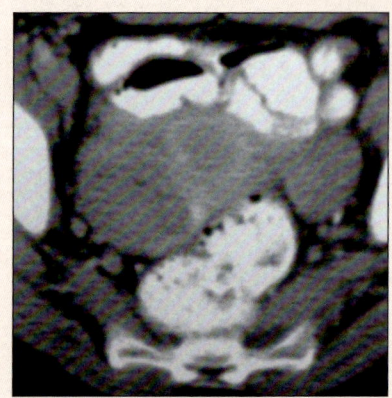

Lymphoma

KRUKENBERG TUMOR

Key Facts

Terminology
- Metastatic adenocarcinomas to ovary, most common from stomach → composed of mucin-filled signet ring cells and proliferation of ovarian stroma

Imaging Findings
- Best diagnostic clue: Bilateral, lobulated, predominantly solid ovarian masses
- Location: 80% bilateral, can be unilateral
- Solid, peripheral or diffuse hypointense components on T2WI are characteristic and related to dense stromal reaction or fibrosis
- Mucin produced by signet ring cells is usually hyperintense on T2WI
- Variable amounts of cystic components when solid masses increase in size

Top Differential Diagnoses
- Other Metastases to Ovaries

Pathology
- Gastric adenocarcinoma of signet ring cell type (infiltrative or diffuse gastric adenocarcinoma) is most common (and classic primary) → > 70% of cases
- Lymphatic metastasis → most likely pathway
- Ovarian metastasis may occur without involvement of other tissues

Clinical Issues
- Bad prognosis if primary tumor identified after metastasis to ovary and worse if primary tumor remains covert

---

- Solid, peripheral or diffuse hypointense components on T2WI are characteristic and related to dense stromal reaction or fibrosis
  - Ovaries retain oval shape
- Mucin produced by signet ring cells is usually hyperintense on T2WI
  - Solid components with free or intracellular mucin may appear relatively hyperintense
- Variable amounts of cystic components when solid masses increase in size
  - Common: Solid masses with intratumoral cysts
  - Less common: Predominantly cystic masses
  - Hyperintense or if hemorrhagic → hypointense rim
- T1 C+
  - Varying enhancement in solid components
  - Walls of intratumoral cysts may enhance

Imaging Recommendations
- Best imaging tool
  - Ultrasound for detection of ovarian involvement
  - CT for detection of primary

DIFFERENTIAL DIAGNOSIS

Other Metastases to Ovaries
- Patients with metastatic carcinomas tend to be older than patients with Krukenberg tumors
- Metastatic intestinal-type or mucinous carcinomas (large intestine, appendix, pancreas, biliary tract, stomach, cervix) or carcinoid tumors can be bilateral
- Multinodular growth pattern with surface implants and vascular space invasion
  - Predominantly cystic lesions with variable solid components

Lymphoma
- Bilateral, homogeneous solid masses, indistinguishable from other solid ovarian tumors

Primary Ovarian Tumors
- Primary ovarian tumors are usually unilateral
- Tend to be predominately cystic

Massive Ovarian Edema
- Diffuse hyperintense signal intensity on T2WI
- Typically unilateral

Polycystic Ovarian Syndrome
- Maintains ovarian contour
- Multiple, small peripheral cysts
- Not as large as Krukenberg tumors

PATHOLOGY

General Features
- Etiology
  - Signet ring cell adenocarcinomas of various organs metastasize more commonly to ovaries than other adenocarcinomas from same sites
    - Gastric adenocarcinoma of signet ring cell type (infiltrative or diffuse gastric adenocarcinoma) is most common (and classic primary) → > 70% of cases
    - Other primary sites: Carcinomas of breast, appendix, and colon
    - Rare causes of Krukenberg: Carcinoma of the gallbladder, biliary tract, pancreas, small intestine, rectum, ampulla of Vater, cervix, urinary bladder, urachus
  - Lymphatic metastasis → most likely pathway
  - Example of selective spread of cancers in the stomach-ovarian axis
    - Ovarian metastasis may occur without involvement of other tissues
    - Higher risk of metastasis with increased number of metastatic lymph nodes
    - Ascites is common and a bad prognostic sign
- Epidemiology
  - 1-2% of all ovarian tumors
  - Incidence higher if high prevalence of gastric carcinoma (17.8% in Japan)

KRUKENBERG TUMOR

- Incidence of metachronous Krukenberg tumors after curative surgery for gastric cancer → 6.7% at 3 years (median: 15 months)
- Associated abnormalities
  - History of prior carcinoma in 20-30% of cases
  - Primary carcinoma can be clinically occult (suspect pylorus or breast)

Gross Pathologic & Surgical Features
- Usually solid, one third of tumors have cysts
  - Ovary has round shape with fibrous, gelatinous or edematous sectioned surfaces
  - Capsular surface → smooth or bosselated contour
  - Fibrous adhesions or peritoneal deposits are rare
  - Marked proliferation of ovarian stroma may resemble fibrothecomas

Microscopic Features
- Multiple, ill-defined and coalescent nodules separated by normal stroma
  - Cellular in periphery
  - Edematous to gelatinous centrally
- Epithelial component: Mucin laden signet ring cells account for at least 10% of the neoplasm
  - Identification of intracytoplasmic mucin is essential for diagnosis
  - In classic Krukenberg tumors the signet ring cell lacks tubular formation
  - Tubular Krukenberg tumors and other unusual tubulo-glandular patterns are also described
- Mesenchymal component: Ovarian fibrous stroma → plump and spindle-shaped cells with minimal atypia
  - Stroma: Cellular to edematous, may form pseudocysts
  - Extracellular mucin can be associated with acellular stroma and give the appearance of feathery degeneration
  - Hypointense solid components seen on T2 weighted images correspond to areas of dense collagenous stroma
  - Desmoplastic reaction can be intense and obscure the signet ring pattern of the tumor

CLINICAL ISSUES

Presentation
- Most common signs/symptoms
  - Abdominal pain, distention, weight-loss
  - Vaginal bleeding (pre or postmenopausal)
  - Nonspecific gastrointestinal symptoms (nausea, vomiting, epigastric pain)
  - Endocrine manifestations: Virilization or hirsutism (with or without pregnancy)
  - Ascites in 50% of cases (malignant cells present), pleural effusions
  - Can be asymptomatic
- Other signs/symptoms
  - Massive intraperitoneal hemorrhage
  - Pre-operative serum CA 125 levels can be elevated

Demographics
- Age: Average: 45 years, more common premenopausal

Natural History & Prognosis
- Interval between diagnosis of primary carcinoma and discovery of ovarian metastasis: Less than 6 months
- Survival rates are low (14.7% at 2 years, mean survival is 7-14 months after diagnosis)
  - Bad prognosis if primary tumor identified after metastasis to ovary and worse if primary tumor remains covert
  - If the primary is occult, patients may not live long enough for the primary to become detectable
  - Limited extent of metastatic disease to the ovaries and complete gross resection are favorable prognostic factors for survival
  - Size of ovarian tumor is not good prognostic factor for survival
- If metastatic tumor is misinterpreted as primary tumor unnecessary major surgery or inappropriate chemotherapy or radiotherapy may occur

Treatment
- No optimal treatment strategy clearly established
  - Lower rate of resectability when primary tumor metastasizes to other sites
  - Surgery may be an option if ovarian lesion is the only metastatic lesion
- Chemotherapy and radiotherapy has no significant effect on prognosis
- No curative treatment
- Some consider prophylactic bilateral oophorectomy when resecting primary tumors → not well-studied

DIAGNOSTIC CHECKLIST

Consider
- High level of suspicion for metastasis to ovary if large or bilateral solid adnexal masses are found

Image Interpretation Pearls
- Search for primary site of malignancy

SELECTED REFERENCES
1. Al-Agha OM et al: An in-depth look at Krukenberg tumor: an overview. Arch Pathol Lab Med. 130(11):1725-30, 2006
2. Kiyokawa T et al: Krukenberg tumors of the ovary: a clinicopathologic analysis of 120 cases with emphasis on their variable pathologic manifestations. Am J Surg Pathol. 30(3):277-99, 2006
3. Valentin L et al: Ultrasound characteristics of different types of adnexal malignancies. Gynecol Oncol. 102(1):41-8, 2006
4. Ha HK et al: Krukenberg's tumor of the ovary: MR imaging features. AJR Am J Roentgenol. 164(6):1435-9, 1995

KRUKENBERG TUMOR

IMAGE GALLERY

Typical

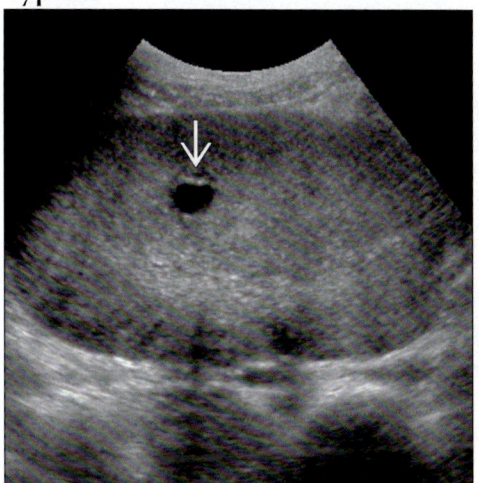
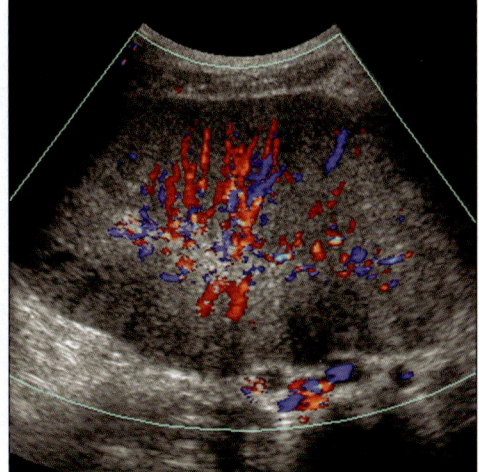

(Left) Sagittal transabdominal ultrasound shows solid ovarian mass with small intratumoral cyst ➡, peripheral hypoechogenicity and central hyperechogenicity in a patient with metastatic gastric adenocarcinoma. *(Right)* Sagittal color Doppler ultrasound in the same patient as previous image, shows enlarged ovary and increased vascularity.

Typical

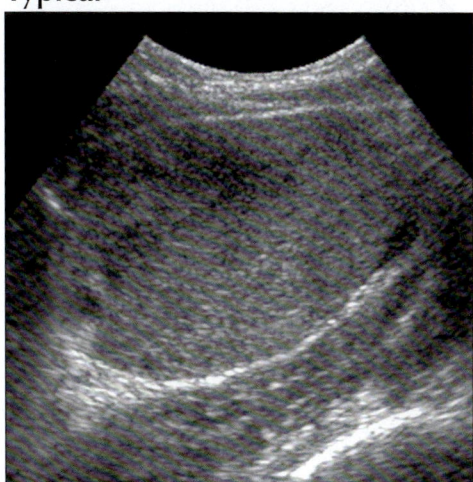
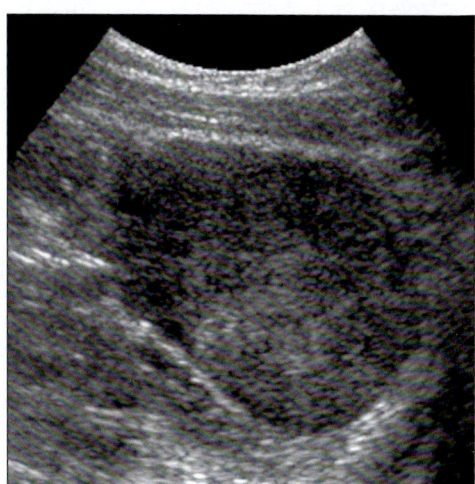

(Left) Sagittal ultrasound in a 39 year old patient who presented with severe left sided pain. The left ovary is enlarged and no flow was demonstrated on color Doppler. Krukenberg tumor with ovarian torsion was surgically confirmed. *(Right)* Sagittal ultrasound in the same patient as previous image, shows moderately enlarged right ovary with solid components.

Typical

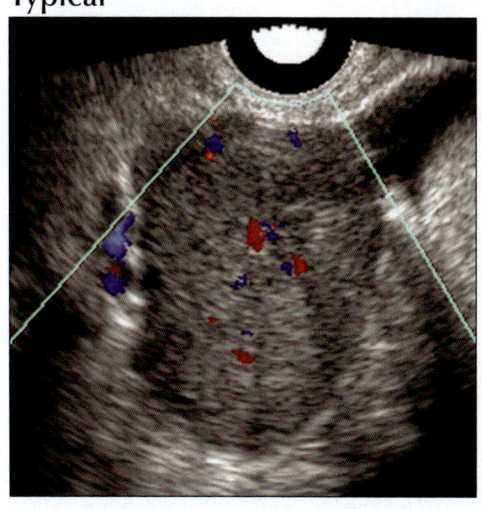
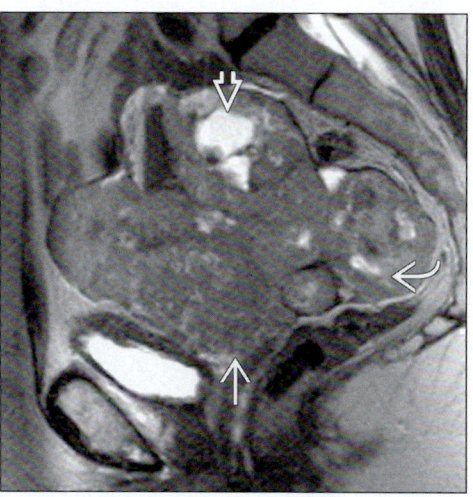

(Left) Color Doppler ultrasound of the right ovary in same patient, shows mildly increased vascularity. Patient had at the time of presentation an occult gastric adenocarcinoma. *(Right)* Sagittal T2WI MR shows multilobulated mass from Krukenberg tumor of gastrointestinal origin with predominantly solid components, some of which are relatively hypointense ➡. There are several hyperintense components from intratumoral cysts ➡ and mucin ➡.

INCLUSION CYST, OVARY

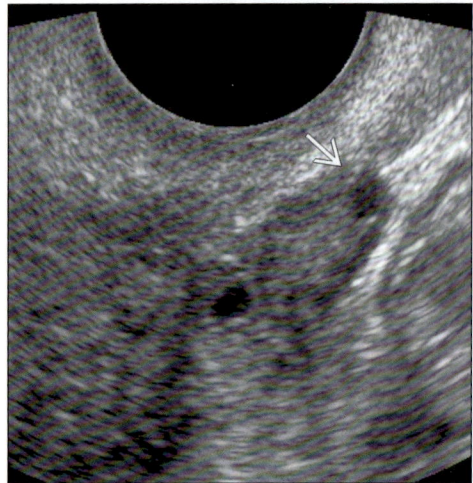

Sagittal oblique transvaginal ultrasound shows a 6 mm anechoic lesion ➔ in an ovary of a postmenopausal woman consistent with an inclusion cyst.

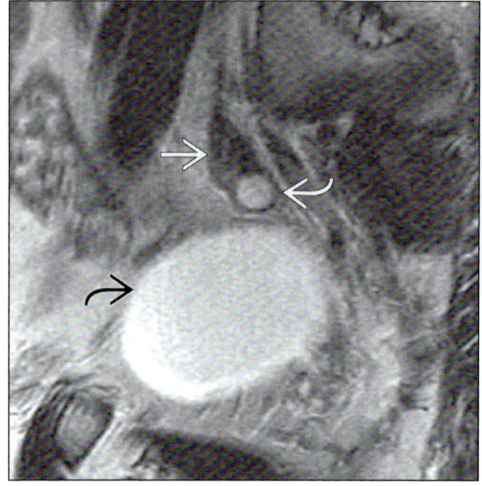

Sagittal T2WI MR shows a small hyperintense lesion in the right ovary ➔, presumed to be an ovarian inclusion cyst ➔. Also noted is a right para-ovarian cyst ➔.

TERMINOLOGY

Abbreviations and Synonyms
- Germinal inclusion cyst, epithelial inclusion cyst, cortical inclusion cyst

Definitions
- Invagination of ovarian cortical surface epithelium that has lost its connection with the surface

IMAGING FINDINGS

General Features
- Best diagnostic clue: Small caliber, simple, ovarian cyst in a postmenopausal woman
- Location
  - Superficial cortex of ovaries
    - Immediately beneath capsule or within 1-2 mm of the outer surface
- Size
  - Typically small, ranging from 1-13 mm
  - Rarely large cysts, up to 10 cm
- Morphology
  - Usually unilocular
    - Seldom multilocular
  - Thin, smooth wall
  - Fluid contents simple
  - Signs of complication: Wall irregularity and hemorrhage typically absent

Ultrasonographic Findings
- Grayscale Ultrasound
  - Sonographic features identical to ovarian follicles
  - Simple-appearing cyst < 16 mm
    - Anechoic thin-walled cyst
    - Posterior acoustic enhancement
    - Well-defined back wall
  - May manifest as punctate echogenic foci at periphery of ovaries
    - Associated psammoma bodies
- Color Doppler: No internal flow

CT Findings
- CECT
  - Hypodense round or oval-shaped lesion
  - Density of simple fluid (0-10 HU)
- CT can suggest presence of inclusion cyst, but is not diagnostic

DDx: Ovarian Cystic Lesions

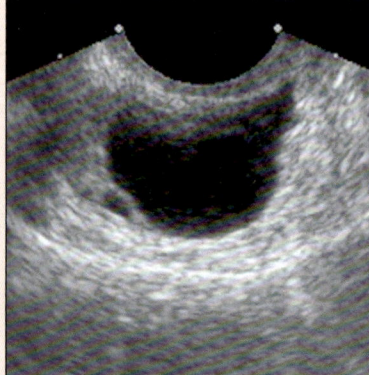

Follicular Cyst

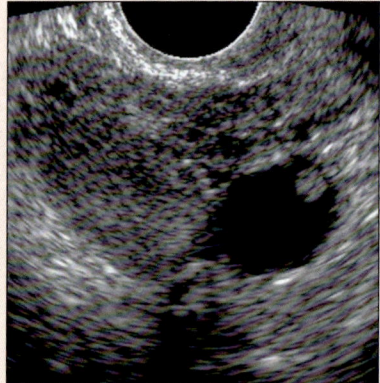

Mucinous Cystadenoma

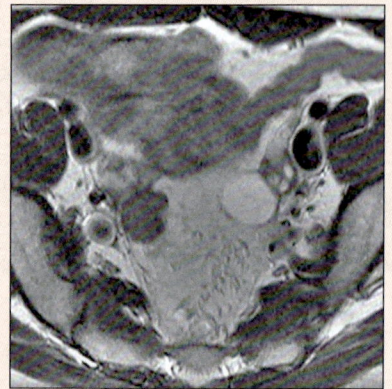

Paraovarian Cyst

INCLUSION CYST, OVARY

Key Facts

Terminology
- Invagination of ovarian cortical surface epithelium that has lost its connection with the surface

Imaging Findings
- Best diagnostic clue: Small caliber, simple, ovarian cyst in a postmenopausal woman
- Immediately beneath capsule or within 1-2 mm of the outer surface
- Typically small, ranging from 1-13 mm
- Usually unilocular
- May manifest as punctate echogenic foci at periphery of ovaries
- Transvaginal ultrasound (TVS) accurate for detection and characterization

Clinical Issues
- Either remain stable or involute
- Guidelines for management of simple unilocular postmenopausal cysts:
- Ovarian cysts < 16 mm may be left alone
- Ovarian cysts ≥ 16 mm and < 5 cm: Follow-up 4 months
- Ovarian cysts ≥ 5 cm are likely neoplastic, therefore managed surgically
- CA-125 should be obtained in cysts ≥ 16 mm; increased or rising levels warrant surgery

Diagnostic Checklist
- Consider epithelial inclusion cyst in a postmenopausal woman with a simple ovarian cyst < 16 mm

---

- Often not visualized on CT

MR Findings
- T1WI
  - Typical features of simple cyst
    - Low signal intensity (SI) lesion
    - SI lower than ovarian stroma
- T2WI
  - Typical features of simple cyst
    - High SI fluid contents
    - Thin wall, lower SI than ovarian stroma
- T1 C+
  - No enhancement of cyst contents
    - Cyst hypointense relative to surrounding ovarian cortex and stroma
  - Discrete enhancement of thin cyst wall

Imaging Recommendations
- Best imaging tool
  - Transvaginal ultrasound (TVS) accurate for detection and characterization
  - MR can be helpful as a problem solving modality
- Protocol advice: Adjust focal zones and gain on TVS to demonstrate simple nature of cyst

DIFFERENTIAL DIAGNOSIS

Ovarian Follicle
- Imaging appearance identical to inclusion cyst
- Not rare during menopause
  - Statistically inclusion cyst far more frequent than ovarian follicle at this age
- Most are atretic cystic follicles

Follicular Cyst
- Imaging appearance identical to inclusion cyst
- More common during reproductive age and early menopause
- More likely to exhibit signs of complication (hemorrhage, wall irregularity)
- Will spontaneously regress over time

Ovarian Epithelial Neoplasm
- Usually larger lesion
- Uni- to multilocular
- Septations, papillary projections, mural nodules
- Progression on follow-up imaging

Paraovarian/Paratubal Cyst
- Thin-walled, oblong adnexal cyst
- Ovary identified as separate structure
- Multilocular or unilocular

PATHOLOGY

General Features
- General path comments
  - Pathophysiology
    - After ovulation, surface epithelium is believed to cover the resultant defect as part of a reparative process
    - Invagination of surface epithelium is a frequent occurrence
    - Entrapment of surface mesothelial cells within stroma is responsible for inclusion cysts
  - Ovulation most common theory, although some evidence suggests inclusion cysts are not only caused by ovulation
    - Can increase in number after menopause
    - In some studies, more numerous in multiparous than nulliparous women
    - Can be seen in patients with polycystic ovary syndrome (PCOS)
  - Other theories
    - Entrapment of surface mesothelial cells by adhesions
    - Simple surface infolding
- Etiology: Sequela of ovulation
- Epidemiology
  - Very common, especially in postmenopausal women
  - May be found in women of all ages
- Associated abnormalities

INCLUSION CYST, OVARY

- Believed to be the site of origin of most common epithelial tumors of the ovary
- Patients with unilateral ovarian carcinoma have increased number of surface epithelial inclusion cysts in contralateral ovary

Gross Pathologic & Surgical Features
- Clear cyst on superficial cortex of ovary

Microscopic Features
- Cyst surrounded by ovarian stroma
- Lined by single layer of columnar epithelium, ciliated or non ciliated serous cuboidal epithelium, or flat epithelium
- Psammomatous calcifications may be seen within lumen of epithelial inclusion cysts
- By definition, an inclusion cyst measuring ≥ 1 cm is named a benign serous cystadenoma

CLINICAL ISSUES

Presentation
- Most common signs/symptoms: Asymptomatic

Demographics
- Age
  - Most common in postmenopausal women
  - May affect women of all ages: Fetuses, infants as well as adolescents

Natural History & Prognosis
- Either remain stable or involute
- May be site of ovarian carcinoma origin, although so prevalent that cannot be considered a pre-malignant lesion
  - As such their presence has no significance in identifying patients at increased risk of malignancy
  - Local environmental and hormonal influence may initiate phenotypic changes to Müllerian epithelium metaplasia and towards a neoplastic process

Treatment
- None for epithelial inclusion cysts
- Guidelines for management of simple unilocular postmenopausal cysts:
  - Ovarian cysts < 16 mm may be left alone
  - Ovarian cysts ≥ 16 mm and < 5 cm: Follow-up 4 months
  - Ovarian cysts ≥ 5 cm are likely neoplastic, therefore managed surgically
  - CA-125 should be obtained in cysts ≥ 16 mm; increased or rising levels warrant surgery

DIAGNOSTIC CHECKLIST

Consider
- Consider epithelial inclusion cyst in a postmenopausal woman with a simple ovarian cyst < 16 mm

Image Interpretation Pearls
- Small, simple ovarian cyst mimicking a follicle

SELECTED REFERENCES

1. Dikensoy E et al: Serum CA-125 is a good predictor of benign disease in patients with postmenopausal ovarian cysts. Eur J Gynaecol Oncol. 28(1):45-7, 2007
2. McDonald JM et al: The incidental postmenopausal adnexal mass. Clin Obstet Gynecol. 49(3):506-16, 2006
3. Heller DS et al: Are germinal inclusion cysts markers of ovulation? Gynecol Oncol. 96(2):496-9, 2005
4. Feeley KM et al: Precursor lesions of ovarian epithelial malignancy. Histopathology. 38(2):87-95, 2001
5. Kupfer MC et al: Transvaginal sonographic evaluation of multiple peripherally distributed echogenic foci of the ovary: prevalence and histologic correlation. AJR Am J Roentgenol. 171(2):483-6, 1998
6. Brandt KR et al: Focal calcifications in otherwise ultrasonographically normal ovaries. Radiology. 198(2):415-7, 1996
7. Outwater EK et al: Normal adnexa uteri specimens: anatomic basis of MR imaging features. Radiology. 201(3):751-5, 1996
8. Atri M et al: Endovaginal sonographic appearance of benign ovarian masses. Radiographics. 14(4):747-60; discussion 761-2, 1994
9. Mittal KR et al: Contralateral ovary in unilateral ovarian carcinoma: a search for preneoplastic lesions. Int J Gynecol Pathol. 12(1):59-63, 1993

INCLUSION CYST, OVARY

IMAGE GALLERY

Typical

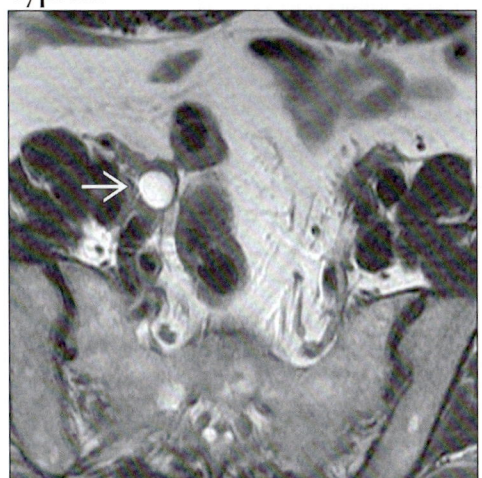
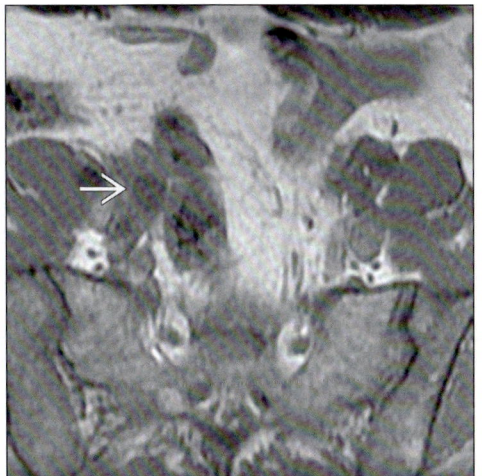

(Left) Axial T2WI MR shows a 12 mm hyperintense right ovarian cyst ➡ in a postmenopausal woman. The cyst is unilocular, homogeneous and thin-walled. The ovary is small in keeping with the patient's postmenopausal state. *(Right)* Axial T1WI MR in the same patient as previous image, shows that the right ovarian cyst is of low signal intensity ➡.

Typical

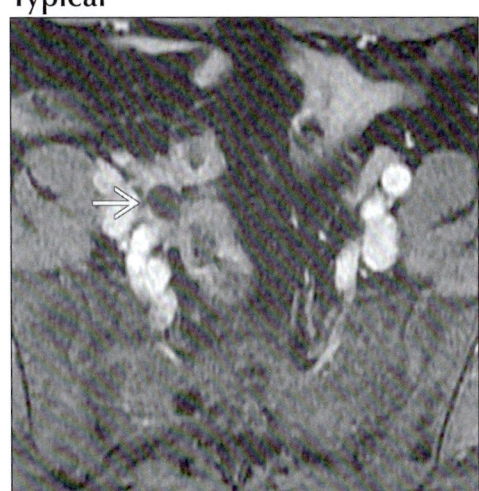
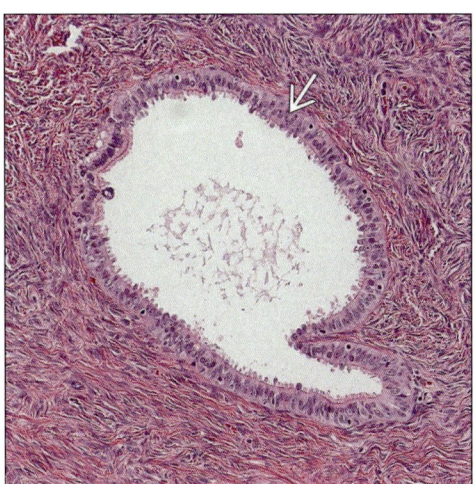

(Left) Axial T1 C+ FS MR in the same patient as previous image, shows no enhancement of the right ovarian cyst ➡. The surrounding ovarian stroma demonstrates normal enhancement. *(Right)* Micropathology of an ovarian cyst at high power shows that the cyst is lined by ciliated cuboidal serous epithelium ➡ without atypia, consistent with an epithelial inclusion cyst. (Courtesy V. Dubé, MD).

Typical

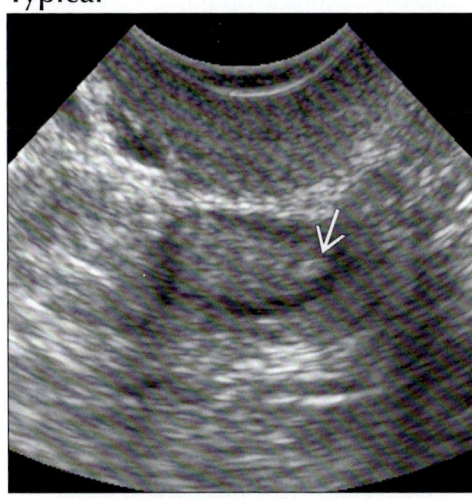
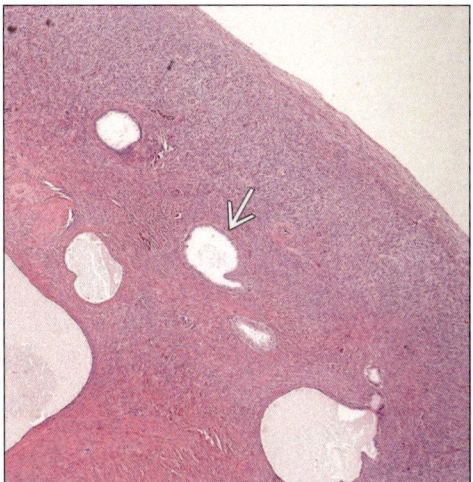

(Left) Sagittal transvaginal ultrasound shows a hyperechoic focus ➡ at the periphery of the left ovary in a postmenopausal woman in keeping with psammomatous calcification in an inclusion cyst. *(Right)* Micropathology in the same patient as previous image, shows the presence of several small inclusion cysts ➡ located in the superficial cortex of the ovary. (Courtesy V. Dubé, MD).

OVARIAN HYPERSTIMULATION SYNDROME

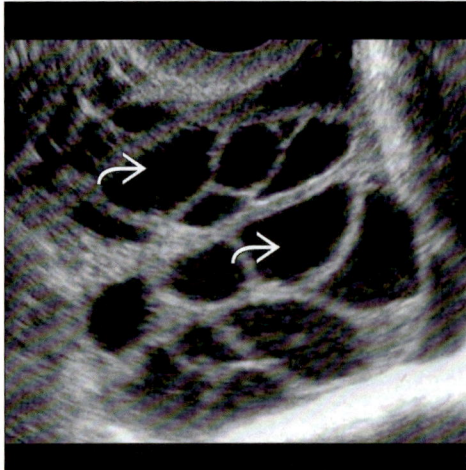

Transverse ultrasound shows an enlarged ovary containing grossly distended follicles ➔ in a patient admitted with abdominal swelling and pain while undergoing ovarian stimulation.

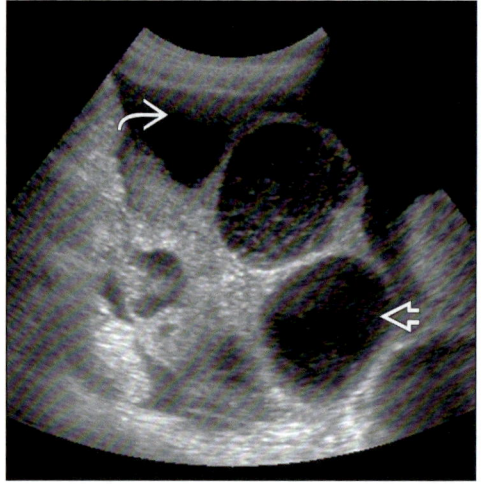

Transverse ultrasound shows peripherally placed enlarged anechoic luteal cysts ➔ in an ovary consistent with OHSS. Note the presence of ascites ➔.

TERMINOLOGY

Abbreviations and Synonyms
- Ovarian hyperstimulation syndrome (OHSS)

Definitions
- Rare complication of ovarian stimulation
  - Iatrogenic
  - Spontaneous, extremely rare

IMAGING FINDINGS

General Features
- Best diagnostic clue
  - Ovarian enlargement
    - Bilateral
    - Symmetrical
- Location: Adnexal
- Size: Ovarian enlargement ≥ 5 cm
- Morphology
  - Swelling of both ovaries
    - Multiple cystic changes
    - Variable sizes

Ultrasonographic Findings
- Grayscale Ultrasound
  - Abdominal and transvaginal US
  - Bilateral ovarian enlargement
  - Multiple peripheral cysts of variable size
  - Most cysts are anechoic
    - Some cysts may be complex due to hemorrhage
  - Centrally placed echogenic stromal tissue
  - Ascites
  - Pleural effusions
- Color Doppler
  - Grayscale Doppler US
    - Measures ovarian stromal blood flow
    - ↑ Ovarian stromal Doppler signal in moderate and severe OHSS
- Other imaging
  - Chest radiograph
    - Large bilateral pleural effusions
    - Effusions - isolated thoracic finding

CT Findings
- Ovarian enlargement with multiple low attenuation cysts

DDx: Multiple Cystic Adnexal Masses

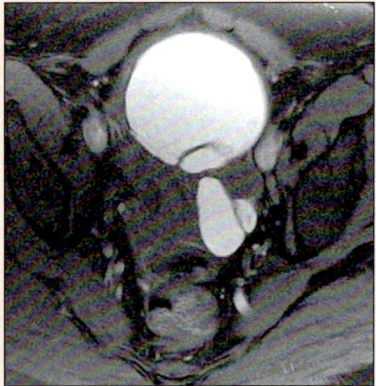

Endometriomas

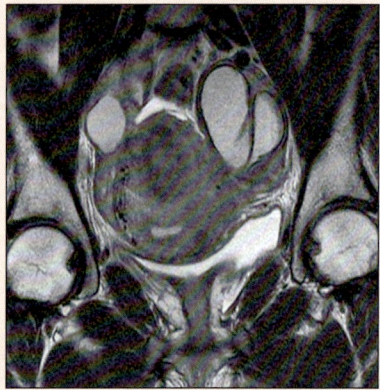

Bilateral Hydrosalpinx

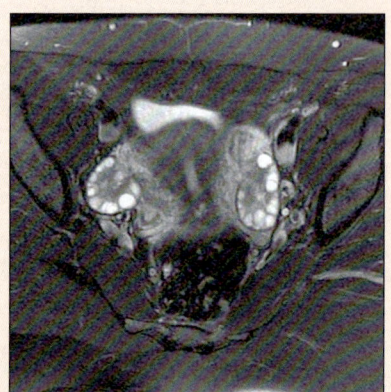

Polycystic Ovarian Syndrome

OVARIAN HYPERSTIMULATION SYNDROME

Key Facts

Terminology
- Rare complication of ovarian stimulation
- Iatrogenic
- Spontaneous, extremely rare

Imaging Findings
- T1WI
- Bilateral symmetrical low signal intensity (SI) rounded ovarian masses
- High SI seen within some loculi
- T1WI C+
- Bilateral symmetrical low SI rounded ovarian masses
- Classic "spoke wheel" appearance secondary to
- Secondary to enhancement of cyst walls and centrally located stromal tissue
- T2WI
- Bilateral homogeneous high SI of the cysts
- Intermediate to low SI of the centrally located stromal tissue (seen as high SI on T1WI)
- High SI ascites
- Abdominal and transvaginal US
- Bilateral ovarian enlargement
- Multiple peripheral cysts of variable size
- Most cysts are anechoic
- ↑ Ovarian stromal Doppler signal in moderate and severe OHSS

Top Differential Diagnoses
- Endometrioma
- Bilateral hydrosalpinx
- Polycystic ovarian syndrome
- Massive ovarian edema
- Ovarian cystic neoplasms

- Cysts may measure fluid density if simple or higher attenuation if complicated
- Ascites

MR Findings
- T1WI
  - Bilateral symmetrical low signal intensity (SI) rounded ovarian masses
  - High SI seen within some loculi
  - "Wheel spoke" appearance described
    - Enlarged follicles peripherally located
    - Stromal ovarian tissue located centrally
    - Also seen on CT
- T1WI C+
  - Bilateral symmetrical low SI rounded ovarian masses
  - Classic "spoke wheel" appearance secondary to
    - Secondary to enhancement of cyst walls and centrally located stromal tissue
- T2WI
  - Bilateral homogeneous high SI of the cysts
  - Intermediate to low SI of the centrally located stromal tissue (seen as high SI on T1WI)
  - High SI ascites

Imaging Recommendations
- Best imaging tool
  - US demonstrates ovarian enlargement best
  - MR is useful in differentiating ovarian swelling vs. tumor
- Protocol advice
  - Assessment with TV US and Doppler studies
  - Use MR if in doubt of nature of ovarian masses to characterize further

DIFFERENTIAL DIAGNOSIS

Non-Neoplastic
- Endometrioma
- Bilateral hydrosalpinx
- Polycystic ovarian syndrome
- Massive ovarian edema
- Degenerative uterine leiomyoma

Neoplastic
- Ovarian cystic neoplasms
  - Serous
  - Mucinous
  - Mature cystic teratoma
  - Fibrothecoma
  - Brenner tumor

PATHOLOGY

Gross Pathologic & Surgical Features
- Bilateral enlargement of the ovaries
- Mean diameter of 7.3 cm
- Multiple thin walled cysts
- Occasionally
  - Hemorrhage into the cysts
- Rarely
  - Torsion or rupture with intraabdominal bleeding

Microscopic Features
- Multiple large follicle cysts lined by
  - Hyperplastic, enlarged, luteinized granulosa cells
- Hyperplastic, luteinized theca cells lie underneath
- One or more corpora lutea
- Ovarian stroma
  - Typically markedly congested and edematous

CLINICAL ISSUES

Presentation
- Mild
  - Grade I
    - Ovarian enlargement
    - Abdominal distention
    - Low abdominal pain/adnexal discomfort
  - Grade II
    - Distention with nausea ± vomiting
  - Mild form common
- Moderate
  - Grade III

OVARIAN HYPERSTIMULATION SYNDROME

- Grade II and ultrasonic evidence of ascites
- Severe
  - Grade IV
    - Clinically apparent ascites with gross ovarian enlargement
    - ± Pleural effusions
    - Dyspnea
    - Chest pain
  - Grade V; additional changes
    - Reduced blood volume
    - Hemoconcentration
    - Clotting disorders
    - Abnormal renal function
  - Severe form
    - Rare
    - Life threatening
    - Accompanied by pleural effusions/chest symptoms
- Other signs/symptoms
  - Localized or generalized edema
- Complications
  - Gross ovarian enlargement → torsion
  - Distended luteal cysts → rupture

Demographics
- Age: Reproductive age
- Gender: Exclusively females

Natural History & Prognosis
- Usually self limiting
  - Occasionally life-threatening
- Patients undergoing fertility treatment
  - Complication of ovulation induction
  - Luteal phase of menstrual cycle
  - With the use of gonadotrophins
  - Rarely seen with Clomiphene
- Manifestations may persist after miscarriage/induced abortion
- Very rare in spontaneous pregnancy
- Women at risk
  - Ovaries demonstrating "necklace sign" on US
    - Multiple peripherally placed cysts
  - Young age (≤ 35 years) of lean habitus
  - Polycystic ovarian syndrome (PCOS)

Treatment
- Preventative
  - Monitoring during treatment
    - Sonographic, size and number of follicles, presence of ascites
    - Hormonal
- Conservative
  - Bed rest
  - Avoidance of further hormonal treatment
  - IV fluids ± albumin
  - Supportive treatment for
    - Renal failure
    - Coagulation abnormalities
    - Hypovolemia
    - Ascites and pleural effusions
- Usually spontaneous resolution

DIAGNOSTIC CHECKLIST

Consider
- In patients undergoing controlled ovarian hyperstimulation, especially
  - In high risk patients
    - Young age, PCOS, "necklace sign"
  - In symptomatic patients
    - Abdominal swelling and pain, dyspnea

Image Interpretation Pearls
- Bilateral symmetrically grossly enlarged ovaries with multiple cysts
  - Best seen on US
- Classic spoke wheel appearance on MR

SELECTED REFERENCES

1. Cepni I et al: Spontaneous ovarian hyperstimulation syndrome presenting with acute abdomen. J Postgrad Med. 52(2):154-5, 2006
2. Tamai K et al: MR features of physiologic and benign conditions of the ovary. Eur Radiol. 2006
3. Fox H et al: Hains and Taylor Obstetrical and Gynaecological pathology. 5th Ed, Edin, Churchill Livingstone. 675-7, 2003
4. Imaoka I et al: MR imaging of disorders associated with female infertility: use in diagnosis, treatment, and management. Radiographics. 23(6):1401-21, 2003
5. Bennett GL et al: Gynecologic causes of acute pelvic pain: spectrum of CT findings. Radiographics. 22(4):785-801, 2002
6. Delvigne A et al: Epidemiology and prevention of ovarian hyperstimulation syndrome (OHSS): a review. Hum Reprod Update. 8(6):559-77, 2002
7. McNeary M et al: Radiographic findings in ovarian hyperstimulation syndrome. J Thorac Imaging. 17(3):230-2, 2002
8. Jung BG et al: Severe spontaneous ovarian hyperstimulation syndrome with MR findings. J Comput Assist Tomogr. 25(2):215-7, 2001
9. Pinkas H et al: Doppler parameters of uterine and ovarian stromal blood flow in women with polycystic ovary syndrome and normally ovulating women undergoing controlled ovarian stimulation. Ultrasound Obstet Gynecol. 12(3):197-200, 1998
10. Kim IY et al: Ovarian hyperstimulation syndrome. US and CT appearances. Clin Imaging. 21(4):284-6, 1997
11. Levine CD et al: Benign extraovarian mimics of ovarian cancer. Distinction with imaging studies. Clin Imaging. 21(5):350-8, 1997
12. Man A et al: Pleural effusion as a presenting symptom of ovarian hyperstimulation syndrome. Eur Respir J. 10(10):2425-6, 1997
13. Levin MF et al: Thoracic manifestations of ovarian hyperstimulation syndrome. Can Assoc Radiol J. 46(1):23-6, 1995
14. Outwater EK et al: Imaging of the ovary and adnexa: clinical issues and applications of MR imaging. Radiology. 194(1):1-18, 1995
15. Takahashi K et al: Transvaginal ultrasonographic morphology in polycystic ovarian syndrome. Gynecol Obstet Invest. 39(3):201-6, 1995
16. Rankin RN et al: Ultrasound in the ovarian hyperstimulation syndrome. J Clin Ultrasound. 9(9):473-6, 1981

OVARIAN HYPERSTIMULATION SYNDROME

IMAGE GALLERY

Typical

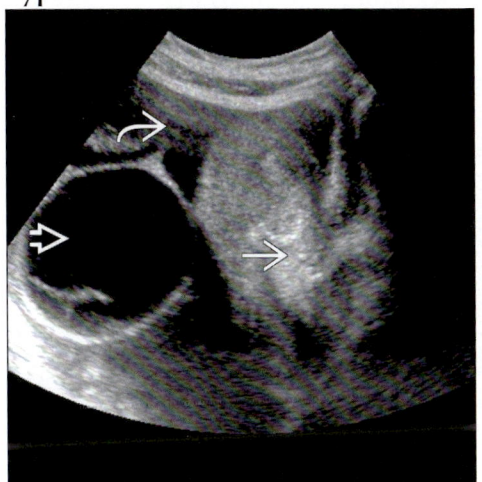
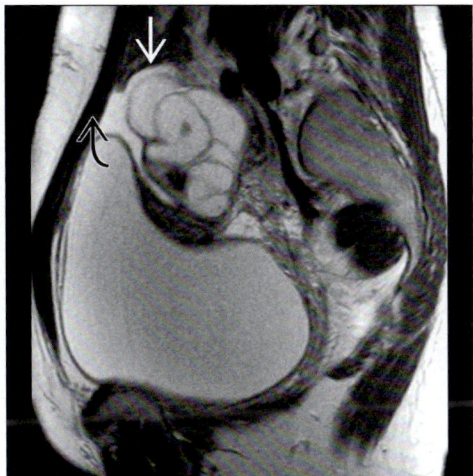

(Left) Longitudinal ultrasound shows enlarged ovarian follicles ⮕ and ascites ➔. Note the thickened endometrium ➔ consistent with ovulation induction therapy. *(Right)* Sagittal T2WI MR shows the grossly distended high SI ovarian follicles ⮕ in a patient undergoing ovarian stimulation. Note also the high SI ascites ➔.

Typical

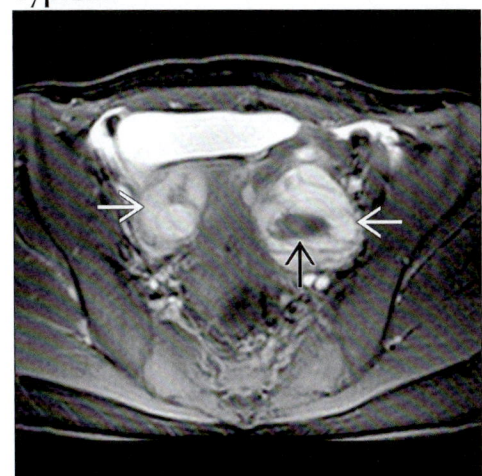
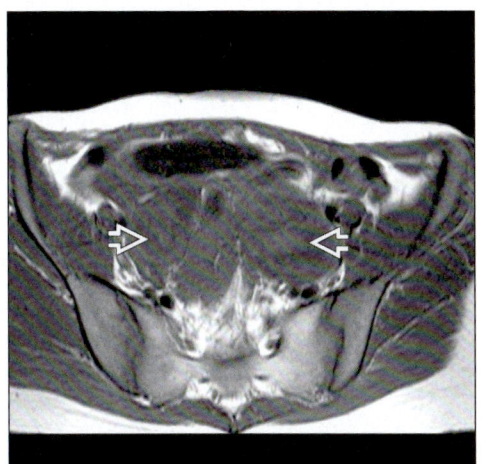

(Left) Axial T2WI FS MR shows bilateral symmetrical high SI ovarian swellings ⮕, typical of OHSS. The low SI ovarian stroma is seen centrally ➔. *(Right)* Axial T1WI MR shows bilateral symmetrical low SI ovarian swellings ⮕ in the same patient.

Typical

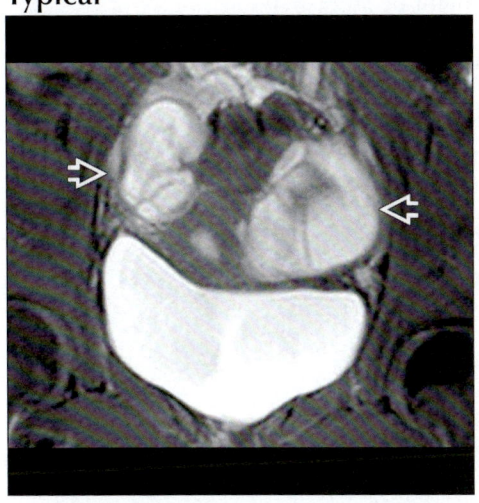
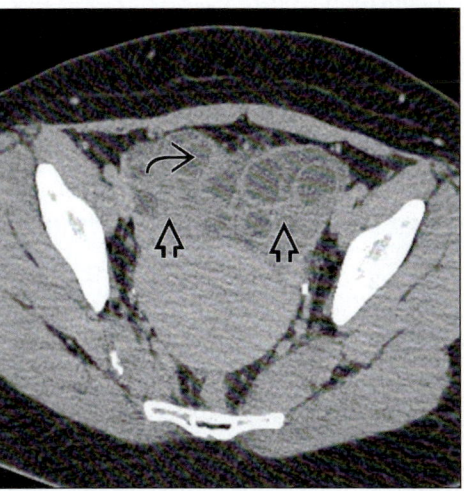

(Left) Axial T2WI FS MR shows bilateral high SI ovarian enlargement ⮕ in a patient undergoing ovarian stimulation. *(Right)* Axial CECT shows bilateral symmetrical ovarian enlargement ⮕. Note the low density distended follicles ➔.

PARAOVARIAN CYST

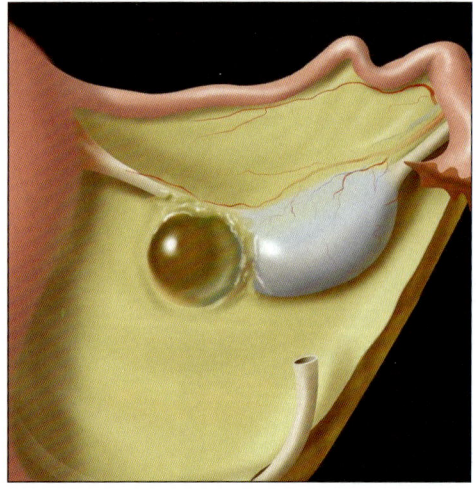

Graphic shows small paraovarian cyst adjacent to the medial aspect of the ovary.

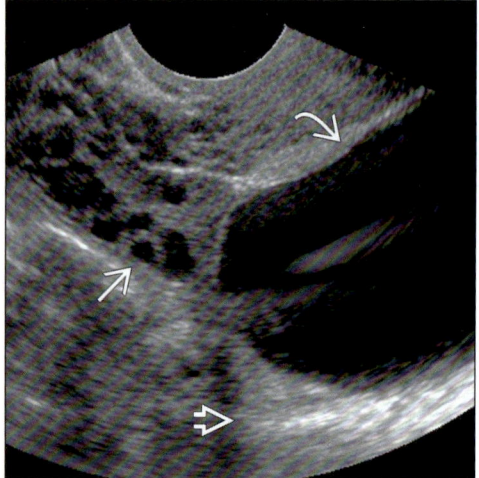

Sagittal transvaginal ultrasound shows paraovarian cyst ➡ adjacent to the ovary ➡. During dynamic exam the cyst moved separate from the ovary. Note increased through transmission ➡.

TERMINOLOGY

Abbreviations and Synonyms
- Paratubal cyst, broad ligament cyst

Definitions
- Cysts arising in broad ligament, more commonly in mesosalpinx between ovary and fallopian tube

IMAGING FINDINGS

General Features
- Best diagnostic clue: Cyst adjacent to but not originating from ipsilateral ovary
- Location
  o Anterior or posterior to the round ligament
  o Parovarium (mesosalpinx between ovary and fallopian tube)
- Size: Variable, up to 20 cm in diameter has been reported
- Morphology: Single or multicystic, unilateral or bilateral

Ultrasonographic Findings
- Grayscale Ultrasound
  o Majority are round or oval, anechoic or hypoechoic unilocular cysts with thin outer wall (< 3 mm) and smooth margins
    ▪ Minority of cases can be multilocular with variable number of thin and smooth septations dividing the cyst
    ▪ Can be bilateral and multiple
  o Normal ovary recognized adjacent but separate to cyst in 76% of cases with transabdominal and 92% of cases with transvaginal ultrasound
    ▪ Cyst not surrounded by follicular structures and does not arise from the ovary
    ▪ Dynamic evaluation with transvaginal ultrasound can show movement of cyst relative to other structures
    ▪ Ovarian contour is maintained despite displacement by large cysts
  o Up to 1/3 have papillary projections growing from cyst wall (usually small 2-8 mm in height)
- Color Doppler: Flow may be difficult to demonstrate within small papillary projections

DDx: Paraovarian Cyst

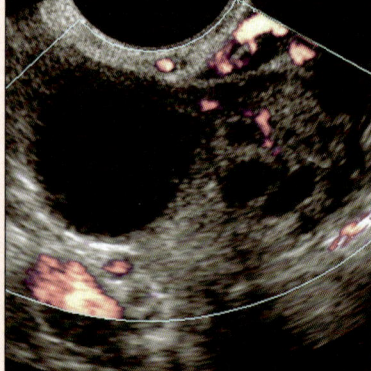

Exophytic Ovarian Cyst

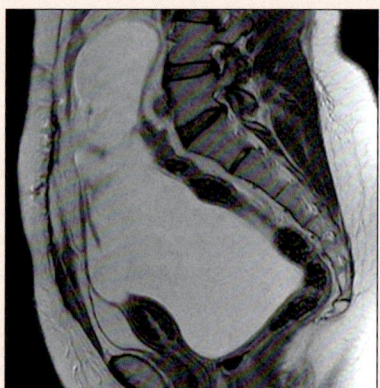

Peritoneal Inclusion Cyst

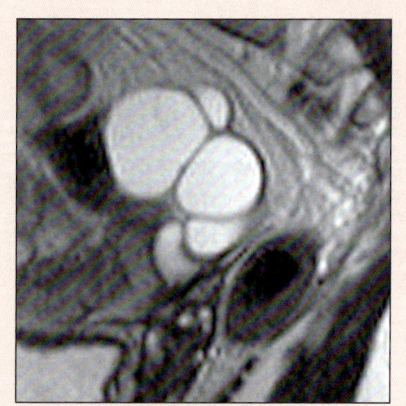

Hydrosalpinx

PARAOVARIAN CYST

Key Facts

Terminology
- Cysts arising in broad ligament, more commonly in mesosalpinx between ovary and fallopian tube

Imaging Findings
- T1WI: Low signal intensity related to muscle
- T2WI: Homogeneous, high signal intensity
- Majority are round or oval, anechoic or hypoechoic unilocular cysts with thin outer wall (< 3 mm) and smooth margins

Top Differential Diagnoses
- Eccentric, Functional Ovarian Cysts
- Peritoneal Inclusion Cysts (Peritoneal Pseudocysts)
- Hydrosalpinx

Pathology
- Not associated with history of pelvic surgery, pelvic inflammatory disease or trauma
- Epidemiology: 5-20% of adnexal masses in pathologic series

Clinical Issues
- If papillary projections are seen, surgery is indicated since benign or malignant tumors can arise within the cyst

Diagnostic Checklist
- Cyst adjacent to ipsilateral ovary
- Dynamic transvaginal exam may separate cyst from ovary and clarify diagnosis

CT Findings
- Fluid density, well-circumscribed adnexal cyst with no enhancement

MR Findings
- T1WI
  - T1WI: Low signal intensity related to muscle
    - If hemorrhagic may show moderate to high signal intensity
- T2WI
  - T2WI: Homogeneous, high signal intensity
    - Heterogeneous if hemorrhagic or torsed
    - Multiloculated with septations or single cavity
  - Ovary usually recognized adjacent but separate to cyst
    - Normal ovary may have follicles and low to intermediate signal
    - If cyst abuts ovary the contours of the cyst and ovary are not modified
    - The adnexa may be distorted with compression, displacement or stretching
    - In minority of cases paraovarian cysts may show a beak sign with ovarian stroma → confused with ovarian cysts
  - May have associated ascites
- T1 C+: No enhancement

Imaging Recommendations
- Best imaging tool: Transvaginal or transabdominal ultrasound
- Protocol advice: MR imaging may offer better delineation of lesion if large and causing adnexal distortion

DIFFERENTIAL DIAGNOSIS

Eccentric, Functional Ovarian Cysts
- Remaining "crescentic-shaped" ovarian tissue can be demonstrated along margin of cyst
- On follow-up exam they change size

Peritoneal Inclusion Cysts (Peritoneal Pseudocysts)
- Often large, multilocular, irregular cystic masses with poorly-defined walls (formed by adjacent organs)
  - Septations can be multiple and oscillate with dynamic technique
- Caused by accumulation of ovarian fluid that is contained by peritoneal adhesions
  - Ovary is inside or within the wall of the peritoneal inclusion cyst, but cyst does not distort the ovarian parenchyma
- Associated with pelvic adhesions due to pelvic surgery, pelvic inflammatory disease or endometriosis
  - Risk of recurrence after surgical resection is high (30-50%)

Hydrosalpinx
- Tubular elongated configuration, distinct wall, small hyperechoic mural nodules on cross section (beads on string)
- Shape of the ovary can be distorted by the hydrosalpinx from mass effect
- Hydrosalpinx with ovoid configuration may be indistinguishable from paraovarian cyst

Ovarian Serous Cystadenoma
- May be confused with multicystic paraovarian cyst
- They can be unilocular

Endometrioma
- Multifocal
- Low signal intensity on T2WI

Lymphocele
- History of radical lymphadenectomy for gynecologic malignancy or renal transplant
- Low attenuation cystic lesion which can have thick wall, septations and can become infected
- Wall consists of fibrotic tissue with no lining of epithelial cells

PARAOVARIAN CYST

Bowel Loops
- Look for peristalsis, change is size and tubular configuration

PATHOLOGY

General Features
- Etiology
  - Origin can be from pelvic mesothelium (68%), paramesonephric remnants (30%) or mesonephric remnants (2%)
  - Not associated with history of pelvic surgery, pelvic inflammatory disease or trauma
- Epidemiology: 5-20% of adnexal masses in pathologic series

Gross Pathologic & Surgical Features
- Cysts arise from mesosalpinx (the part of the broad ligament between the ovary and the fallopian tube)
- Ipsilateral ovary maintains normal configuration
- Tube may be stretched over smooth cyst wall

Microscopic Features
- Paraovarian cysts are lined by flat epithelium
- Paratubal cysts are lined by columnar epithelium containing ciliated and secretory cells
  - Papillary projections into the cyst simulating the normal fallopian tube can be seen
- No mural nodules or wall thickening

CLINICAL ISSUES

Presentation
- Most common signs/symptoms
  - Asymptomatic most commonly
  - Lower abdominal pain if torsion, hemorrhage or rupture has occurred
  - Abdominal fullness and increasing abdominal girth if large size
  - Menstrual irregularities rare
- Other signs/symptoms: Acute pain may be secondary to torsion or hemorrhage

Demographics
- Age: Wide range including pre and postmenopausal women, most commonly identified in third and fourth decades

Natural History & Prognosis
- If small they are usually asymptomatic and may not be detected by imaging
- If large they may become symptomatic when complicated by hemorrhage, torsion and rupture
- Reported incidence of malignancy is 2%
  - Reported cases of cystadenofibroma, cystadenoma, serous papillary borderline tumor, serous cystadenocarcinoma and mucinous cystadenocarcinoma arising within cyst

Treatment
- If paraovarian cyst is simple, asymptomatic and smaller than 5 cm surgery can be avoided
- If papillary projections are seen, surgery is indicated since benign or malignant tumors can arise within the cyst
- Surgical or laparoscopic removal can be performed if cyst is large and symptomatic due to rare complications like torsion, hemorrhage or rupture
- Ultrasound-guided aspiration of large cysts followed by laparoscopic removal has been described

DIAGNOSTIC CHECKLIST

Consider
- Adnexal cysts are frequently misinterpreted as ovarian in origin when they are paraovarian or paratubal

Image Interpretation Pearls
- Cyst adjacent to ipsilateral ovary
- Dynamic transvaginal exam may separate cyst from ovary and clarify diagnosis

SELECTED REFERENCES

1. Savelli L et al: Paraovarian/paratubal cysts: comparison of transvaginal sonographic and pathological findings to establish diagnostic criteria. Ultrasound Obstet Gynecol. 28(3):330-4, 2006
2. Kishimoto K et al: Paraovarian cyst: MR imaging features. Abdom Imaging. 27(6):685-9, 2002
3. Kim JS et al: Peritoneal inclusion cysts and their relationship to the ovaries: evaluation with sonography. Radiology. 204(2):481-4, 1997
4. Barloon TJ et al: Paraovarian and paratubal cysts: preoperative diagnosis using transabdominal and transvaginal sonography. J Clin Ultrasound. 24(3):117-22, 1996
5. Kim JS et al: Sonographic diagnosis of paraovarian cysts: value of detecting a separate ipsilateral ovary. AJR Am J Roentgenol. 164(6):1441-4, 1995

PARAOVARIAN CYST

IMAGE GALLERY

Typical

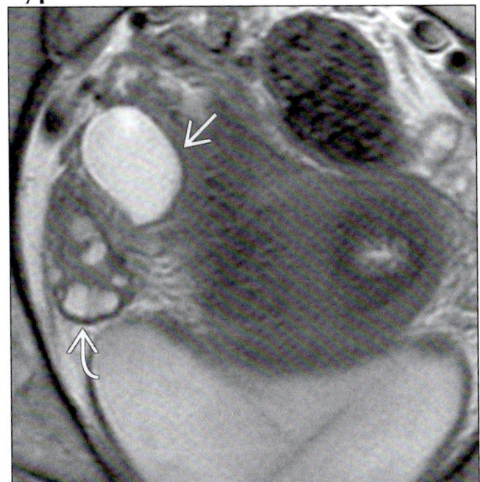 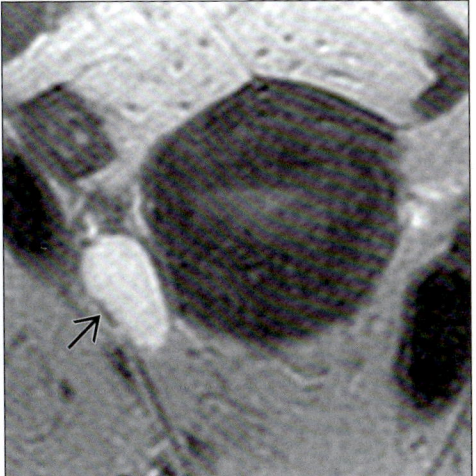

(Left) Coronal T2WI MR shows right adnexal cyst ➔ adjacent but separate from the right ovary ➔ and consistent with paraovarian cyst. *(Right)* Coronal T2WI MR shows a small right paraovarian cyst ➔ arising from the broad ligament, between the uterus and the right ovary (not shown).

Typical

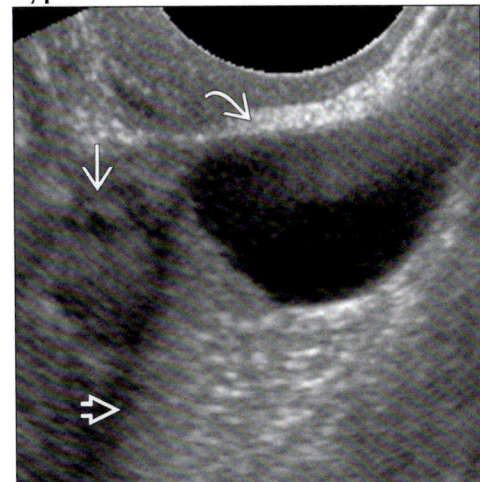 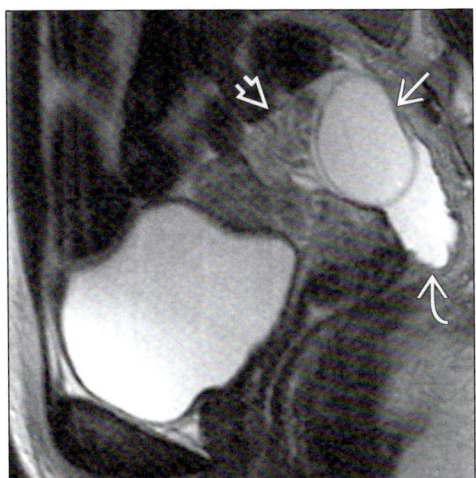

(Left) Transvaginal ultrasound shows small cyst ➔ with increased through transmission ➔, separate from the ovary ➔, consistent with a paraovarian cyst. *(Right)* Sagittal T2WI MR shows a cyst ➔ adjacent to the fallopian tube ➔ with surrounding free fluid ➔. The paratubal cyst served as a lead point and caused torsion of the fallopian tube.

Typical

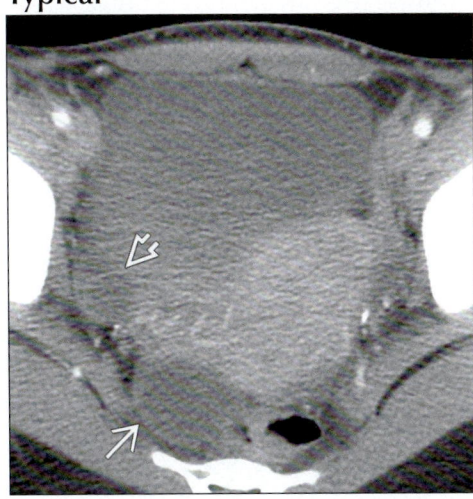 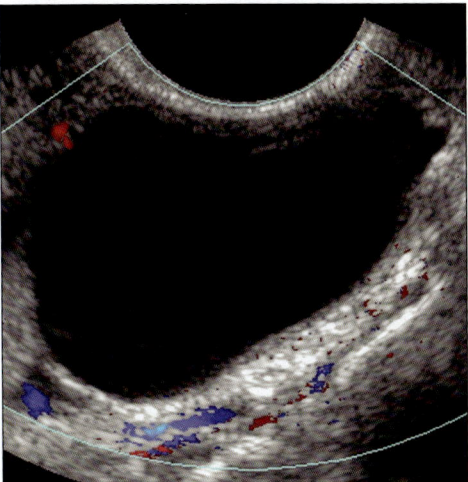

(Left) Axial CECT shows right hypodense, well-circumscribed round lesion ➔ in the right pelvis. The right ovary ➔ contains a small follicle. *(Right)* Sagittal color Doppler ultrasound transvaginal ultrasound on same patient as previous image shows large thin-walled cyst in the right pelvis with small amount of debris and no internal flow.

ENDOMETRIOMA

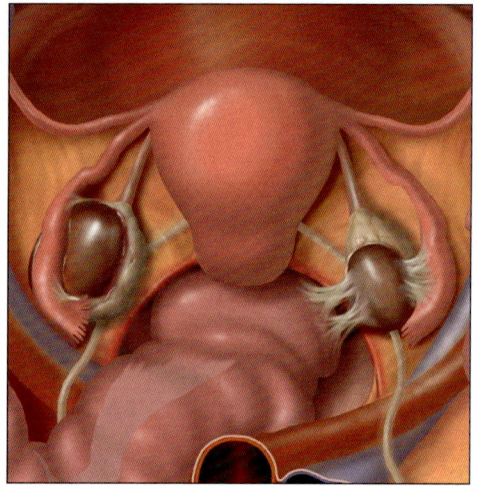

Graphic shows bilateral hemorrhagic ovarian cysts and adhesions between the left ovary, fallopian tube, and rectum.

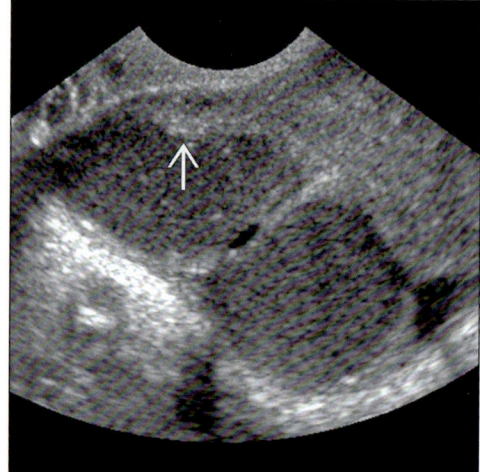

Axial transvaginal ultrasound shows two thick-walled ovarian cysts containing uniform low-level echoes. Note a solid-appearing nodule in one of the cysts ➡. The nodule demonstrated no vascularity on color Doppler.

TERMINOLOGY

Abbreviations and Synonyms
- Endometriotic cyst, chocolate cyst

Definitions
- Presence of endometrial epithelium & stroma outside of endometrium & myometrium

IMAGING FINDINGS

General Features
- Best diagnostic clue
  - "Chocolate cyst" with diffuse homogeneous low-level internal echoes
  - Multiple ovarian masses hyperintense on T1WI FS
  - Solitary ovarian mass hyperintense on T1WI FS, & hypointense on T2WI (shading)
- Location: Ovary
- Size: Less than 15 cm
- Morphology
  - May be solitary or multiple
    - Bilateral ovarian involvement in 30-50%
  - Complex cystic ovarian mass(es)
    - Contents most often homogeneous
    - May contain fluid-fluid levels
    - Typically thick-walled
    - Mural linear or punctate calcifications
  - Shape often not completely round, angulated margins
- Complicating malignancy in 0.3-0.8%
  - Most common tumor types: Endometrioid, clear cell, or carcinosarcoma
- Associated findings
  - Pelvic endometrial plaque
  - Pelvic adhesions

Ultrasonographic Findings
- Grayscale Ultrasound
  - Thick-walled ovarian cyst(s) with uniform low-level echoes: "Chocolate cyst"
    - May contain fluid-fluid level
    - Echogenic intracystic nodules representing adherent blood clot ± slight attenuation
    - Cyst contents may appear "solid", look for enhanced through transmission
    - Mural linear or punctate calcification

DDx: Endometrioma

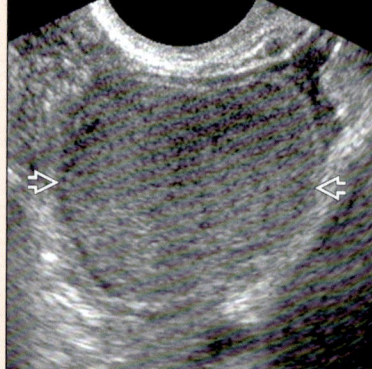

Functional Hemorrhagic Cyst

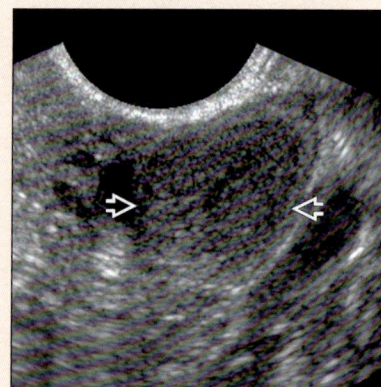

Fibrothecoma

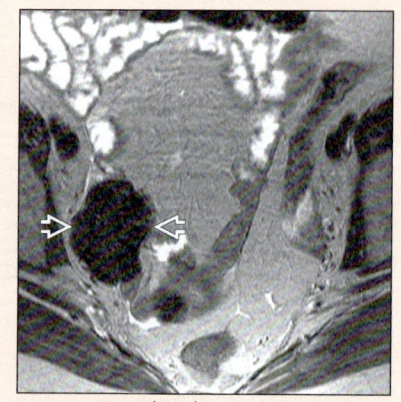

Fibrothecoma

ENDOMETRIOMA

Key Facts

Terminology
- Presence of endometrial epithelium & stroma outside of endometrium & myometrium

Imaging Findings
- "Chocolate cyst" with diffuse homogeneous low-level internal echoes
- Multiple ovarian masses hyperintense on T1WI FS
- Solitary ovarian mass hyperintense on T1W1 FS, & hypointense on T2WI (shading)
- Contents most often homogeneous
- Typically thick-walled
- Shape often not completely round, angulated margins
- Apply a low pulse repetition frequency (PRF) to detect flow in a neoplastic nodule & differentiate it from adherent blood clot
- T1WI must be acquired without & with fat-suppression
- Use subtraction images to diagnose an enhancing nodule within a high SI cyst

Top Differential Diagnoses
- Hemorrhagic Functional Cyst
- Dermoid
- Cystic Ovarian Neoplasm
- Fibrothecoma

Clinical Issues
- Increasing size with menses may occur
- 0.3-0.8% rate of malignancy, usually in endometriomas > 15 cm
- Pain responds to both GnRh-a & laser surgery, but infertility responds only to laser surgery

---

  - Ovaries adherent to adjacent structures
    - Ovaries remain fixed when pressure applied with transvaginal probe
- Color Doppler
  - Hypovascular wall
    - Less commonly, wall may show increased vascularity
  - Intracystic nodules show no flow on Doppler
  - Vascular mass within endometrioma suggests a complicating malignancy

CT Findings
- Nonenhancing hypoattenuating ovarian mass(es)
- No role in the diagnosis of endometrioma

MR Findings
- T1WI
  - Solitary hyperintense ovarian mass
  - Multiple hyperintense ovarian masses
  - Homogeneous appearance
- T1WI FS
  - Improved detection & characterization
  - Solitary ovarian mass with persistent high SI on fat-suppression (FS)
    - Nonspecific, most commonly a hemorrhagic ovarian cyst
    - Allows differentiation from dermoid cyst
  - Solitary ovarian mass with persistent high SI on FS, & markedly low SI on T2WI
    - Highly specific for endometrioma: 90-98%
    - Sensitivity: 68-82%
  - Multiple ovarian masses with persistent high SI on FS
    - Multiplicity increases specificity for diagnosing endometriomas
    - Neoplastic & functional cysts more commonly solitary
- T2WI
  - Range of low SI (shading) of ovarian mass
    - Markedly hypointense cyst content indicates hemoconcentration
  - May show intermediate to high SI
  - Low SI, thick, fibrous capsule composed of hemosiderin-laden macrophages
- T1 C+ FS
  - Variable degrees of mural enhancement but generally hypovascular
  - Enhancing mass within endometrioma suggests a complicating malignancy
- Additional findings
  - Low SI spiculated adhesive bands on T1WI & T2WI
  - Peritoneal plaque: Low signal T2WI ± high signal foci
  - Tethered bowel loops
  - Obliteration of cul-de-sac & organ interfaces

Imaging Recommendations
- Best imaging tool
  - Transvaginal ultrasound (TVS) for initial evaluation
  - MR imaging for indeterminate masses on TVS
- Protocol advice
  - Transvaginal ultrasound
    - Apply a low pulse repetition frequency (PRF) to detect flow in a neoplastic nodule & differentiate it from adherent blood clot
  - MR imaging
    - T1WI must be acquired without & with fat-suppression
    - Use subtraction images to diagnose an enhancing nodule within a high SI cyst

DIFFERENTIAL DIAGNOSIS

Hemorrhagic Functional Cyst
- Solitary
- More complex & heterogeneous content on TVS
  - Fine linear strands ("fish-net")
  - Retracting clot
- Shading on MR not typical
- Hypervascular wall

Dermoid
- Highly echogenic attenuating component on TVS
- Fat content on MR

ENDOMETRIOMA

○ High SI area(s) on T1WI become hypointense after fat-suppression

Cystic Ovarian Neoplasm
- Serous: Cyst content more commonly simple, enhancing mural nodules/septations
- Mucinous: Cyst content can overlap with endometrioma, typically multilocular with enhancing septations
- Enhancing solid component(s)
- Ascites & peritoneal seeding if malignant

Fibrothecoma
- Solid ovarian mass
  ○ Typically shows delayed enhancement
- Low to intermediate SI on T1WI

Ovarian Abscess
- History indicates infection
- Significant mural vascularity
- Evidence of adnexal fat stranding

PATHOLOGY

General Features
- Genetics: More common in some families
- Etiology
  ○ Seeding to ectopic locations through fallopian tubes or surgery
  ○ Metaplasia into endometrium at ectopic sites
- Epidemiology: Higher socioeconomic group
- Associated abnormalities
  ○ Extra-ovarian endometriosis
    ▪ Endometriotic plaque
    ▪ Fibrous adhesions
  ○ Adenomyosis
  ○ Complicating malignancy: Endometrioid, clear cell, or carcinosarcoma

Gross Pathologic & Surgical Features
- Surrounded by a fibrotic wall
- Content: Semifluid & chocolate colored

Microscopic Features
- Ectopic endometrial glands & stroma

CLINICAL ISSUES

Presentation
- Most common signs/symptoms
  ○ Dysmenorrhea, pain, dyspareunia, irregular bleeding, infertility
  ○ Symptoms may be cyclical
  ○ Unrelated to disease severity
- Other signs/symptoms
  ○ Large percentage asymptomatic
  ○ Ruptured endometrioma resulting in acute abdomen

Demographics
- Age
  ○ 80% premenopausal (25-40 years of age)
  ○ 10% adolescent
  ○ 5% postmenopausal

Natural History & Prognosis
- Self limited in most patients
- Increasing size with menses may occur
- Generally improve with pregnancy & menopause
- 0.3-0.8% rate of malignancy, usually in endometriomas > 15 cm
- Decidualized tissue may develop during pregnancy resulting in solid components that mimic malignancy

Treatment
- Gonadotropin releasing hormone agonist (GnRH-a)
- Laparoscopic surgery
- Pain responds to both GnRh-a & laser surgery, but infertility responds only to laser surgery

DIAGNOSTIC CHECKLIST

Consider
- Surgery for larger lesions
- Surgery for cyst with enhancing mural nodule(s) or solid component

Image Interpretation Pearls
- Bilateral cystic masses with low-level echoes on TVS
- Multiple ovarian masses hyperintense on T1WI FS
- Solitary ovarian mass hyperintense on T1W1 FS, & hypointense on T2WI (shading)
- Associated pelvic endometrial plaque

SELECTED REFERENCES

1. Kinkel K et al: Diagnosis of endometriosis with imaging: a review. Eur Radiol. 16(2):285-98, 2006
2. Lee SI: Radiological reasoning: imaging characterization of bilateral adnexal masses. AJR Am J Roentgenol. 187(3 Suppl):S460-6, 2006
3. Fruscella E et al: Sonographic features of decidualized ovarian endometriosis suspicious for malignancy. Ultrasound Obstet Gynecol. 24(5):578-80, 2004
4. Wu TT et al: Magnetic resonance imaging of ovarian cancer arising in endometriomas. J Comput Assist Tomogr. 28(6):836-8, 2004
5. Sala EJ et al: Magnetic resonance imaging of benign adnexal disease. Top Magn Reson Imaging. 14(4):305-27, 2003
6. Modesitt SC et al: Ovarian and extraovarian endometriosis-associated cancer. Obstet Gynecol. 100(4):788-95, 2002
7. Alcazar JL: Transvaginal colour Doppler in patients with ovarian endometriomas and pelvic pain. Hum Reprod. 16(12):2672-5, 2001
8. Guerriero S et al: Tumor markers and transvaginal ultrasonography in the diagnosis of endometrioma. Obstet Gynecol. 88(3):403-7, 1996
9. Atri M et al: Endovaginal sonographic appearance of benign ovarian masses. Radiographics. 14(4):747-60; discussion 761-2, 1994
10. Occhipinti KA et al: The ovary. Computed tomography and magnetic resonance imaging. Radiol Clin North Am. 31(5):1115-32, 1993
11. Outwater E et al: Characterization of hemorrhagic adnexal lesions with MR imaging: blinded reader study. Radiology. 186(2):489-94, 1993
12. Zawin M et al: Endometriosis: appearance and detection at MR imaging. Radiology. 171(3):693-6, 1989

ENDOMETRIOMA

IMAGE GALLERY

Typical

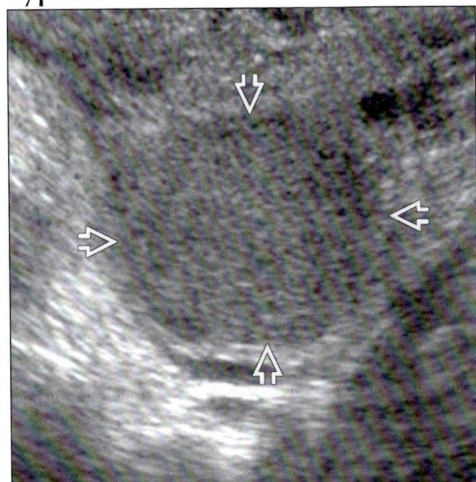
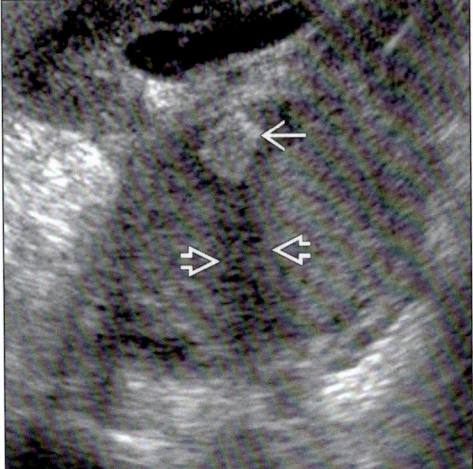

(Left) Axial transvaginal ultrasound shows a mass ➡ in the right ovary with uniform low-level echoes and posterior acoustic enhancement. *(Right)* Axial transvaginal ultrasound in the same patient as previous image, shows an echogenic nodule ➡ with sound attenuation ➡ within the complex cystic mass. The absence of flow on color Doppler favors an adherent blood clot.

Typical

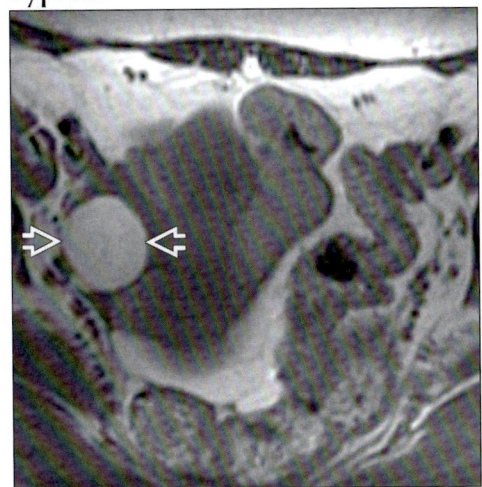
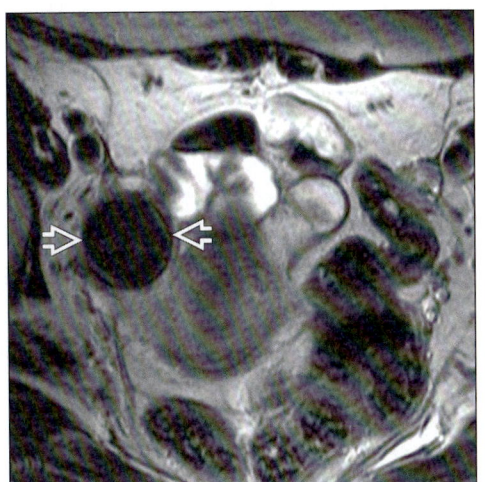

(Left) Axial T1WI MR in the same patient as previous image shows the mass ➡ to be hyperintense. There was persistent high SI on the fat-suppressed images (not shown). *(Right)* Axial T2WI MR on the same patient as previous image, shows the mass ➡ to be markedly hypointense (equivalent to skeletal muscle) indicating chronicity and hemoconcentration. The combination of findings is highly specific for an endometrioma.

Variant

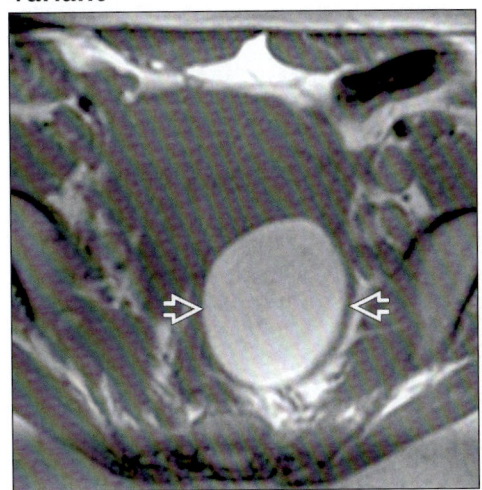
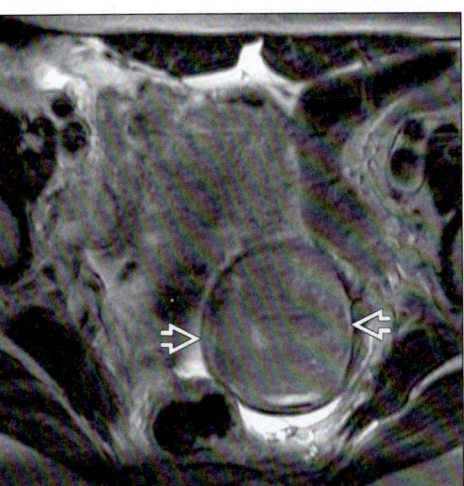

(Left) Axial T1WI MR shows a hyperintense left adnexal mass ➡ that remained bright on the T1WI FS (not shown). *(Right)* Axial T2WI MR on the same patient as previous image, shows the mass ➡ to be hypointense and somewhat heterogeneous, indicating hemorrhage of different stages.

ENDOMETRIOSIS

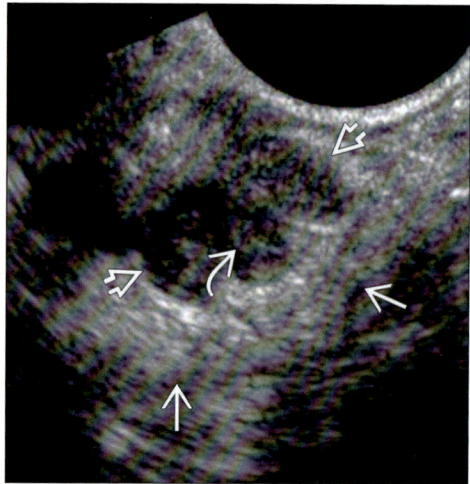

Sagittal transvaginal ultrasound shows a hypoechoic plaque ➡ on the anterior wall of the sigmoid colon ➡. Note pleating of the submucosa ➡.

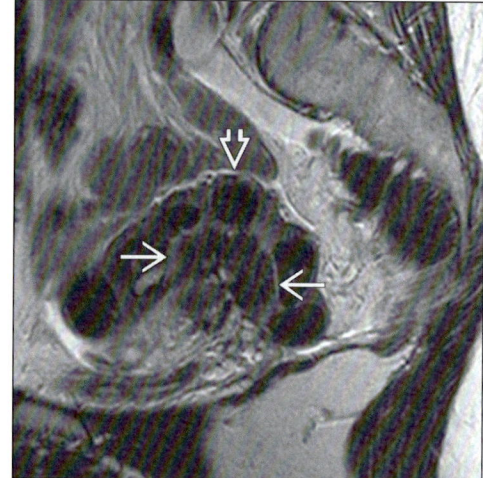

Sagittal T2WI MR in the same patient as previous image shows a hypointense plaque ➡ with foci of increased signal intensity (SI) on the anterior wall of the sigmoid colon ➡.

TERMINOLOGY

Definitions
- Presence of endometrial glands and stroma outside of endometrium and myometrium

IMAGING FINDINGS

General Features
- Best diagnostic clue
  - Endometrioma: Complex ovarian cyst
  - Plaque: Solid mass bridging cul-de-sac from dorsal surface of lower uterine segment to anterior surface of rectosigmoid
  - Adhesions
- Location
  - Ovary most common location
  - Peritoneal sites (in decreasing order of frequency): Uterine ligaments, cul-de-sac, pelvic peritoneum reflected over the uterus, fallopian tubes, rectosigmoid, laparotomy scars, and bladder
  - Rare extraperitoneal sites include lungs and central nervous system
- Size: Most plaques < 5 mm, plaques > 10 mm visible with imaging
- Morphology
  - Endometrioma: Thick-walled, complex cyst with debris ("chocolate cyst")
    - May be solitary or multiple
  - Complicated hydrosalpinx/hematosalpinx
  - Plaque-like structure ± hemorrhagic foci on peritoneal surface
    - Hourglass appearance of plaque between uterus and rectosigmoid
  - Oval-shaped mass on the surface of other structures
  - Tethering, adhesions and obliteration of organ interfaces

Radiographic Findings
- IVP: Bladder wall mass, rarely ureter

Ultrasonographic Findings
- Grayscale Ultrasound
  - Endometrioma
    - "Chocolate cyst" with diffuse, homogeneous, low-level internal echoes
    - Punctate calcifications in wall

DDx: Endometriosis

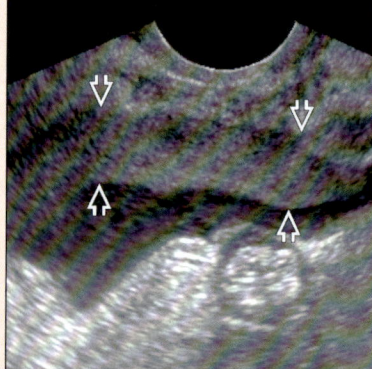

Peritoneal Tumor Implants

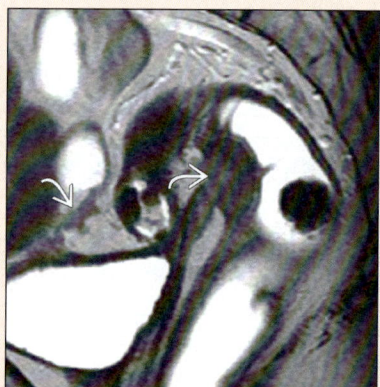

Peritoneal Tumor Implants

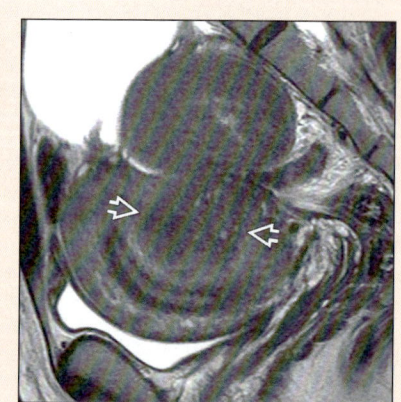

Adenomyoma

ENDOMETRIOSIS

Key Facts

Terminology
- Presence of endometrial glands and stroma outside of endometrium and myometrium

Imaging Findings
- Endometrioma: Thick-walled, complex cyst with debris ("chocolate cyst")
- Plaque-like structure ± hemorrhagic foci on peritoneal surface
- Hourglass appearance of plaque between uterus and rectosigmoid
- Tethering, adhesions and obliteration of organ interfaces
- Subserosal or myometrial endometriosis

Pathology
- Bilateral ovarian involvement in 30-50%

Clinical Issues
- Dysmenorrhea, pain, dyspareunia, irregular bleeding
- Large percentage asymptomatic
- Other signs/symptoms: Infertility 30-40%
- Symptoms may be cyclical and estrogen dependent
- 0.3-0.8% rate of malignancy in association with large (> 15 cm) ovarian endometriomas
- Rare endometrioid adenocarcinoma transformation of peritoneal endometriosis

Diagnostic Checklist
- Close examination of rectouterine space in all patients with unexplained pelvic pain, infertility or an ovarian mass suggestive of endometrioma
- Look for dark endometriotic plaque against the bright bowel submucosa

---

- Areas of clot may simulate solid mass but will not demonstrate internal flow
  - Peritoneal plaque
    - Hypoechoic flat, rounded, or oval-shaped
    - When anechoic can mimic fluid in posterior cul-de-sac
    - Pleating of submucosal layer of bowel
    - Tethering and kinking of bowel wall
  - "Kissing ovaries" due to adhesions causing proximity of ovaries to uterus
- Color Doppler
  - Generally hypovascular
  - May be moderately vascular and show vascularity perpendicular to long axis of plaque

CT Findings
- No role in the evaluation of endometriosis
- Nonspecific complex adnexal mass or peritoneal plaque

MR Findings
- T1WI
  - Endometrioma: High signal intensity (SI) cyst content
    - Maintains high SI on T1WI with fat suppression
  - Endometriotic plaque: Intermediate SI ± high SI foci
- T2WI
  - Endometrioma: Variable, low SI cyst content ("shading") is characteristic
  - Hypointense plaque ± high SI foci
    - SI of plaque often as low as skeletal muscle or air
- T1 C+ FS: Generally hypovascular, enhancement is usually delayed
- Common locations of endometriotic plaque seen on MR
  - Ventral aspect of rectosigmoid junction
  - Uterine surface extending into myometrium
    - Subserosal or myometrial endometriosis
    - Typically involves outer 10% of myometrium
    - Discontinuous with junctional zone
  - Junction of lower uterine segment and cervix dorsally ("torus uterinus")
  - Surface of ovary and adjacent ligaments

- Additional MR findings
  - Low SI spiculated bands on T1WI and T2WI
  - Angulated tethered bowel/ovaries on T1WI and T2WI
  - Obliteration of organ interfaces
  - Mixed SI masses on T1WI and T2WI in the bladder wall, bowel wall, abdominal wall with variable enhancement
    - Hypointense component on T2WI and hyperintense foci on T1WI allow differentiation from other masses

Imaging Recommendations
- Best imaging tool
  - Transvaginal ultrasound (TVS) for initial evaluation
    - MR for indeterminate masses on TVS
  - Neither TVS or MR sufficiently sensitive to screen for endometriotic plaque
    - MR more specific than TVS as a problem solving modality to differentiate from peritoneal seeding
- Protocol advice
  - Sensitivity of MR for detecting bright foci optimized
    - Images acquired during menstrual phase
    - Addition of fat-suppressed (FS) sequences
    - Volumetric acquisition (T1WI FS), thin sections and high resolution imaging parameters
  - Posterior cul de sac plaques can be assessed on transrectal sonography
  - Dynamic TVS scanning differentiates fixed endometrial plaque from pliable fluid in posterior cul de sac

DIFFERENTIAL DIAGNOSIS

Peritoneal Tumor Implants
- High signal intensity on T2WI, isointense on T1WI
- Ascites ± peritoneal enhancement without adhesions

Desmoid Tumor
- No hemorrhagic component
- Low SI on T2WI
- Delayed enhancement

ENDOMETRIOSIS

Post-Operative or Post-Infection Scar
- No hemorrhagic component
- Low SI on T2WI
- Delayed enhancement

Adenomyosis/Adenomyoma
- Morphology indistinguishable from subserosal endometriosis
- Adenomyosis typically continuous with junctional zone
- Acute angles with uterine serosal surface

PATHOLOGY

General Features
- General path comments
  - 80% of lesions show cyclic changes
  - Histologic evidence of recent or remote hemorrhage
- Genetics: More common in some families
- Etiology
  - "Metastasis" of endometrial tissue or cells to ectopic locations through fallopian tubes or at time of surgery
  - Metaplasia into endometrial tissue at ectopic peritoneal sites
- Epidemiology: Positive association with higher socioeconomic group and negative with gravidity
- Associated abnormalities
  - Adenomyosis of uterus
  - Obstructive uterine anomalies

Gross Pathologic & Surgical Features
- Superficial powder-burn or gunshot lesions on the ovaries, serosal surfaces and peritoneum
- Common: Black or blue-black plaques or puckered lesions
- Nodules or small cysts containing old hemorrhage surrounded by a variable extent of fibrosis
- Less common: White, yellow, red, and brown plaques
- Bilateral ovarian involvement in 30-50%

Microscopic Features
- Ectopic endometrial glands and stroma

CLINICAL ISSUES

Presentation
- Most common signs/symptoms
  - Dysmenorrhea, pain, dyspareunia, irregular bleeding
  - Large percentage asymptomatic
- Other signs/symptoms: Infertility 30-40%
- Clinical Profile
  - Symptoms may be cyclical and estrogen dependent
  - Different staging systems are used for patients with infertility and those with pain
    - Minimal: Isolated implants and no significant adhesions
    - Mild: Superficial implants less than 5 cm in aggregate, scattered on the peritoneum and ovaries
    - Moderate: Multiple implants, ± peritubal and periovarian adhesions
    - Severe: Multiple superficial and deep implants, including large endometriomas, filmy and dense adhesions

Demographics
- Age
  - 80% premenopausal (25-40 years of age)
  - 10% adolescent
  - 5% postmenopausal
- Ethnicity: Most common in Asian, followed by Caucasian and least common in black population

Natural History & Prognosis
- Self-limited in most patients
- Generally improve with pregnancy/menopause
- Size may increase with menses
- Malignant degeneration
  - 0.3-0.8% rate of malignancy in association with large (> 15 cm) ovarian endometriomas
    - Endometrioid, clear-cell type, or carcinosarcoma
  - Rare endometrioid adenocarcinoma transformation of peritoneal endometriosis

Treatment
- Laparoscopic laser surgery for infertility or pain
- Gonadotropin-releasing hormone agonist (GnRH-a) for pain

DIAGNOSTIC CHECKLIST

Consider
- Close examination of rectouterine space in all patients with unexplained pelvic pain, infertility or an ovarian mass suggestive of endometrioma

Image Interpretation Pearls
- Look for dark endometriotic plaque against the bright bowel submucosa
- Enhancement on MR and flow on color Doppler differentiates plaque from complex cul-de-sac fluid

SELECTED REFERENCES

1. Bazot M et al: Sonography and MR imaging for the assessment of deep pelvic endometriosis. J Minim Invasive Gynecol. 12(2):178-85; quiz 177, 186, 2005
2. Ghezzi F et al: "Kissing ovaries": a sonographic sign of moderate to severe endometriosis. Fertil Steril. 83(1):143-7, 2005
3. Kuligowska E et al: Pelvic pain: overlooked and underdiagnosed gynecologic conditions. Radiographics. 25(1):3-20, 2005
4. Okaro E et al: Diagnostic and therapeutic capabilities of ultrasound in the management of pelvic pain. Curr Opin Obstet Gynecol. 17(6):611-7, 2005
5. Bazot M et al: Deep pelvic endometriosis: MR imaging for diagnosis and prediction of extension of disease. Radiology. 232(2):379-89, 2004
6. Puglielli E et al: Rectal endometriosis: MRI study with rectal coil. Eur Radiol. 14(12):2362-3, 2004

ENDOMETRIOSIS

IMAGE GALLERY

Typical

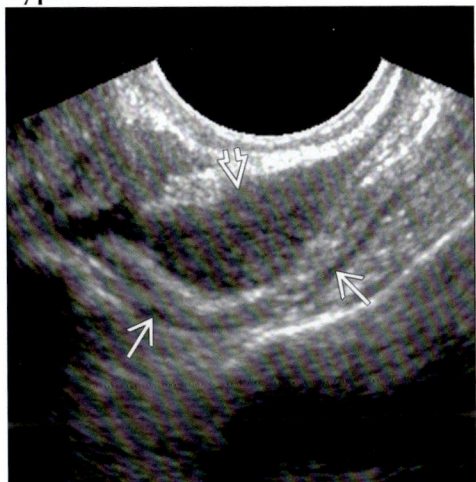
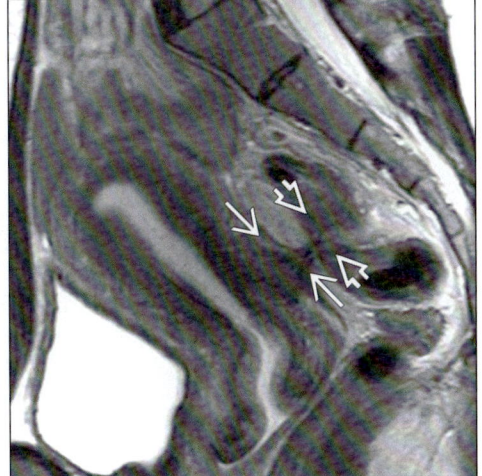

(Left) Sagittal transvaginal ultrasound shows a hypoechoic plaque ➡ on the anterior wall of the rectosigmoid colon ➡. This imaging appearance is nonspecific. *(Right)* Sagittal T2WI MR in the same patient as previous image, shows the plaque extending from the posterior aspect of the lower uterine segment ➡ to the anterior wall of the rectosigmoid colon ➡. The low SI is consistent with an endometriotic plaque.

Typical

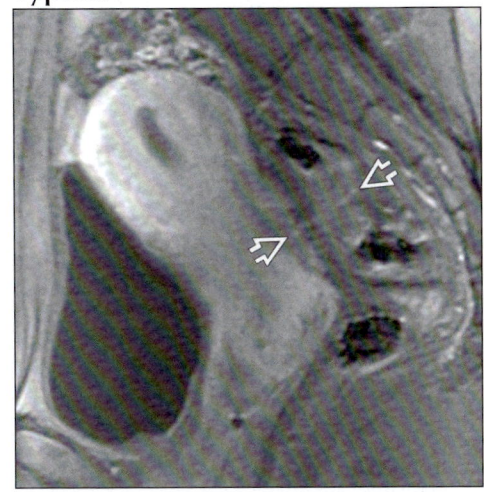
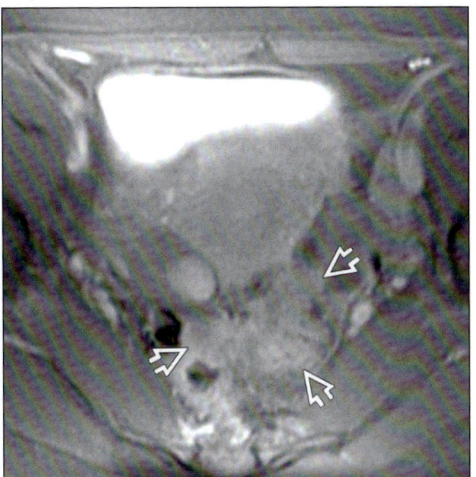

(Left) Sagittal T1 C+ FS MR in the same patient as previous image shows the enhancing plaque ➡ extending from the lower uterine segment to the rectosigmoid colon. *(Right)* Axial T1 C+ FS MR in the same patient as previous image, shows the enhancing plaque ➡ between the uterus and the rectosigmoid colon.

Typical

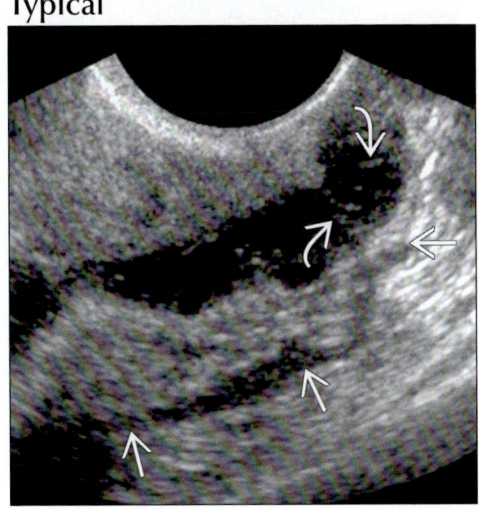
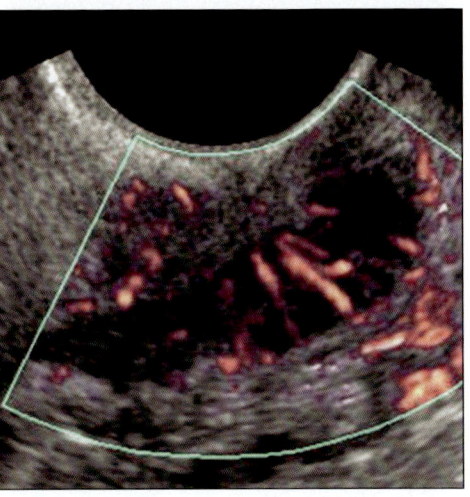

(Left) Sagittal transvaginal ultrasound shows a hypoechoic plaque with perpendicular tethering of the submucosa ➡ on the anterior wall of the rectosigmoid colon ➡. *(Right)* Sagittal color Doppler ultrasound of the same patient as previous image, shows increased vascularity of the plaque.

ENDOMETRIOSIS

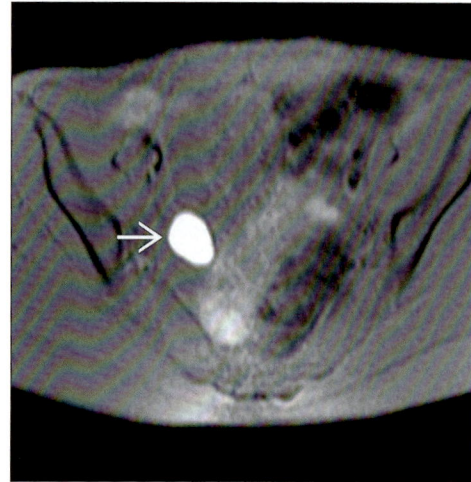
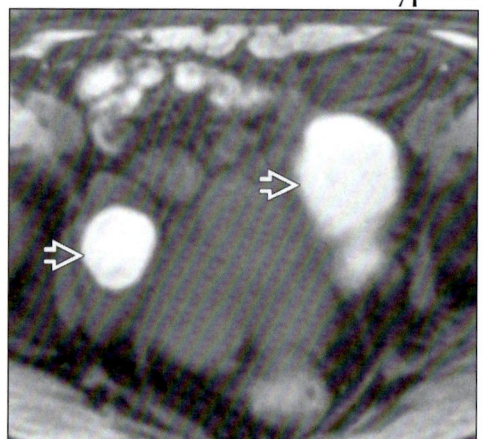

(Left) Axial T1WI FS MR shows a hyperintense right ovarian lesion ➡ proven to be an endometrioma at follow-up. Note the homogeneous signal intensity. (Right) Axial T1WI FS MR shows a typical case of bilateral ovarian endometriomas ➡ with high signal intensity and angulated margins. The specificity of MR increases in the setting of multiple hyperintense lesions.

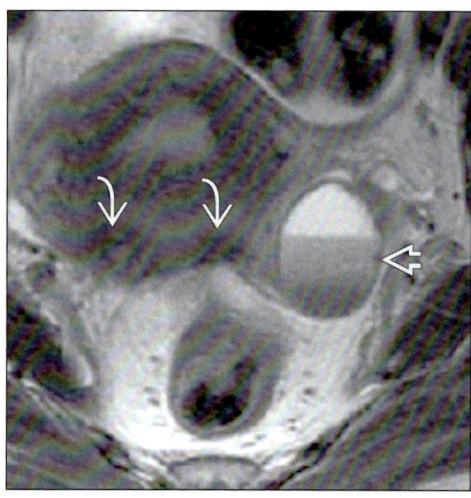
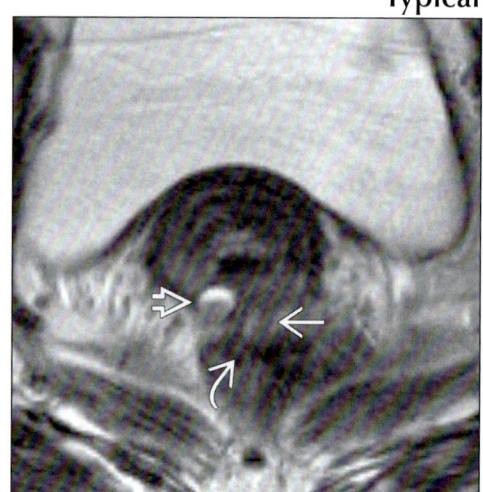

(Left) Axial T2WI MR shows layering of blood products ➡ within an ovarian endometrioma. The ovary is tethered to the uterus and there is subserosal endometriosis ➡ dorsally. (Right) Axial T2WI MR shows an endometrial implant ➡ posterior to the cervix. The sensitivity of small, hyperintense implants on T2WI is increased with fat-suppression. However, non fat-suppressed sequences are important for detecting low SI adhesions ➡ and plaque ➡.

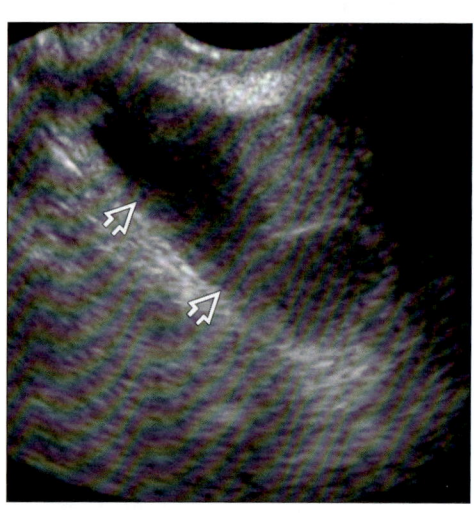
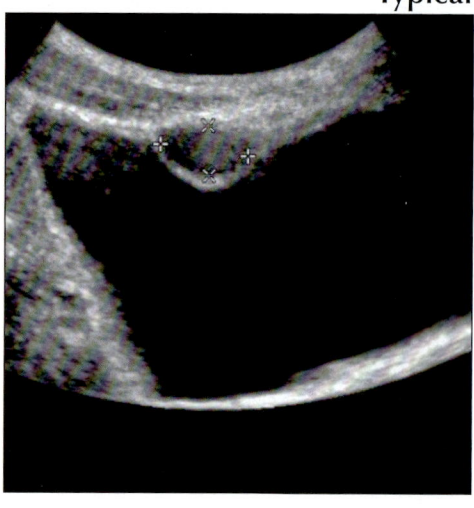

(Left) Oblique transvaginal ultrasound shows a distended fallopian tube ➡ filled with hemorrhagic debris in a patient with endometriosis. (Right) Sagittal transabdominal ultrasound shows a hypoechoic mass (calipers) impinging on the anterior bladder wall.

ENDOMETRIOSIS

Typical

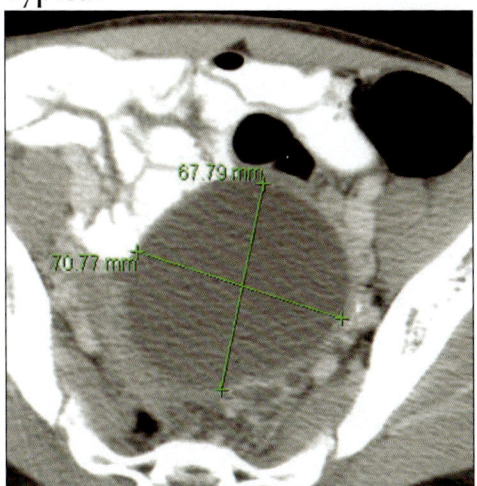
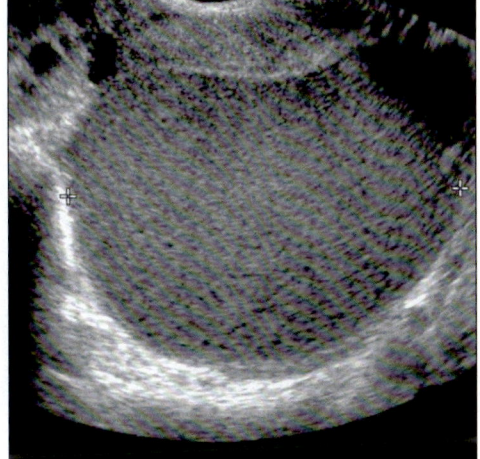

(Left) Axial CECT shows a non-specific, hypoattenuating, complex cystic pelvic mass *(calipers)* in a patient with endometriosis. *(Right)* Transverse transvaginal ultrasound in the same patient as the previous image, shows the classic appearance of a "chocolate cyst" *(calipers)* with diffuse homogeneous low-level internal echoes.

Variant

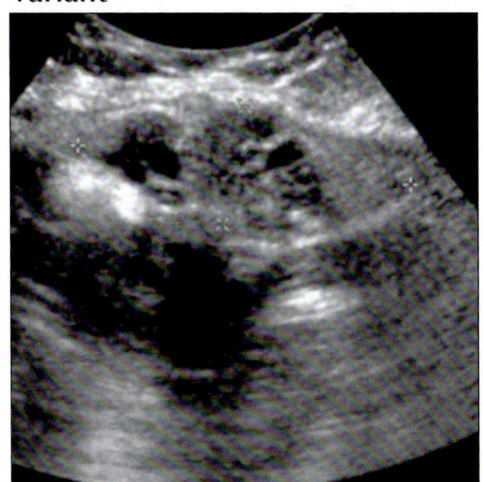
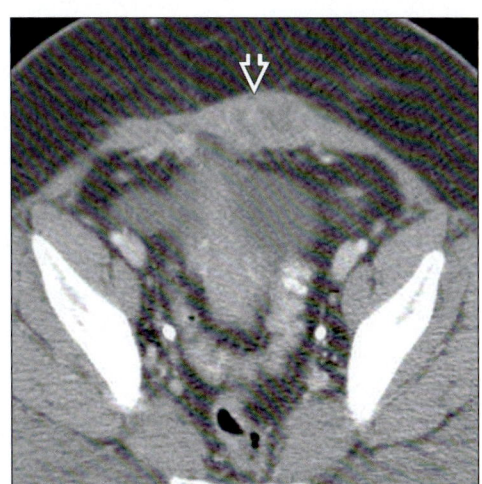

(Left) Transverse transabdominal ultrasound shows a heterogeneous mass *(calipers)* in the region of the rectus muscle. *(Right)* Axial CECT in the same patient as the previous image, shows the mass ➡ to enhance slightly. This was proven to be endometriosis in a prior laparotomy scar.

Variant

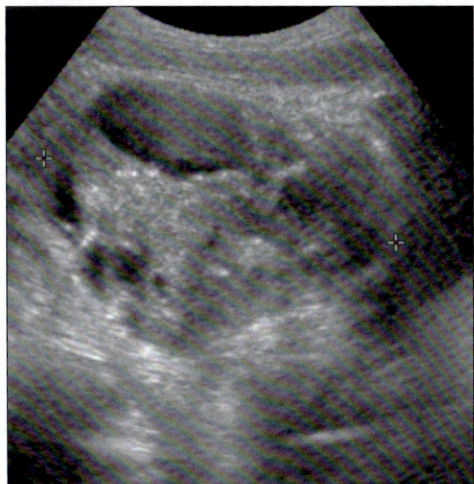
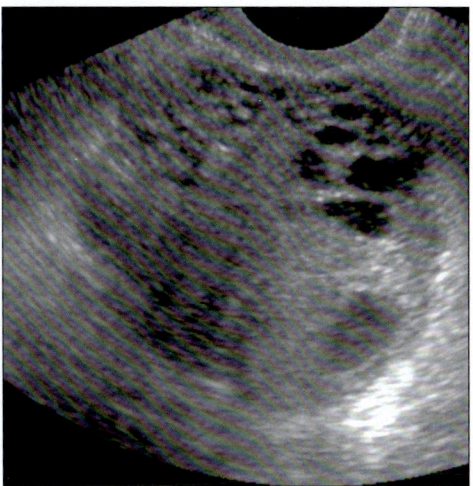

(Left) Transverse transabdominal ultrasound shows a heterogeneous cystic and solid mass *(calipers)* in a 27 year old woman with severe endometriosis. The solid portions represent fibrosis and adhesions. No malignancy was present. *(Right)* Sagittal transvaginal ultrasound shows a complex cystic pelvic mass with multiple septations in a patient with dense adhesions and endometriosis.

ADNEXAL TORSION

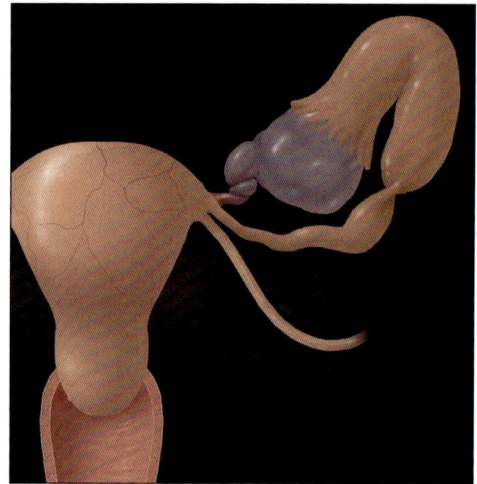

Graphic of tubal torsion associated with a dilated distal end of the left fallopian tube and ovarian enlargement on the ipsilateral side.

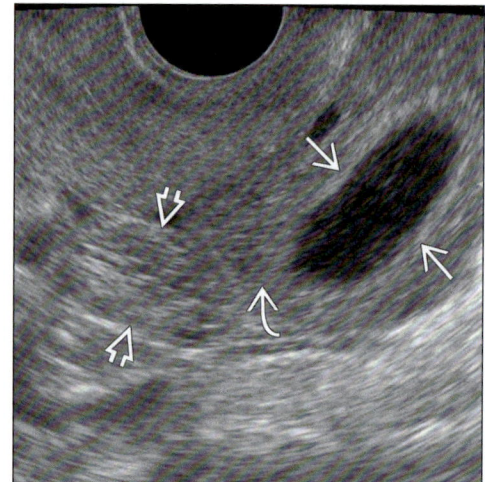

Transverse transvaginal ultrasound of the left adnexa shows a cystic lesion within the ovary ➡. The ovarian stroma is edematous ⤴ and there is thickening of the left fallopian tube ➡.

TERMINOLOGY

Abbreviations and Synonyms
- Fallopian tube (FT) torsion
- Ovarian torsion

Definitions
- Rotation of ovary, fallopian tube or both on its vascular pedicle

IMAGING FINDINGS

General Features
- Best diagnostic clue
  - Thickened fallopian tube with "twisted vascular pedicle" sign
  - Enlarged edematous ovary
    - In presence of ovarian mass, residual ovarian volume disproportionately prominent due to stromal edema
  - Uterine deviation towards torsed ovary
- Location
  - Ovary, fallopian tube or both
  - Torsed adnexa often located anteriorly in midline between abdominal wall and urinary bladder, cranial to fundus of uterus
    - May be misplaced to contralateral side or midline posteriorly
- Size
  - Variable
  - Ovary can become very large because of massive edema with subacute torsion
- Morphology
  - Imaging findings depend on degree and duration of torsion
  - Enlarged ovary ± hemorrhagic adnexal mass
    - Multiple follicles with debris due to hemorrhage
    - Follicles displaced peripherally due to edematous stroma and/or mass
    - Concentric or eccentric thickening of ovarian cyst wall
  - Thickened fallopian tube ± dilatation
    - Twisted vascular pedicle consisting of broad ligament, fallopian tube, and ovarian vessels
  - Adjacent fat stranding (correlates with necrosis)
  - Pelvic fluid may or may not be hemorrhagic
  - Calcified mass in chronic undiagnosed torsion

DDx: Enlarged Adnexa

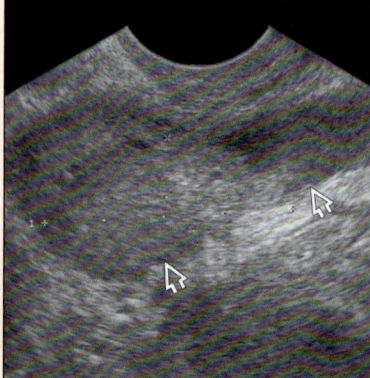
Pyosalpinx

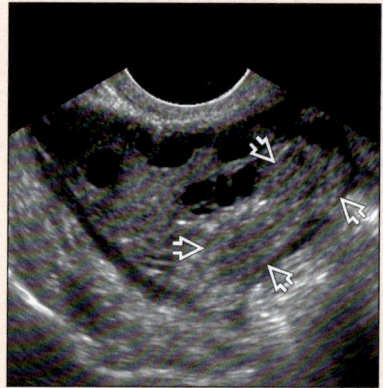
Hematosalpinx

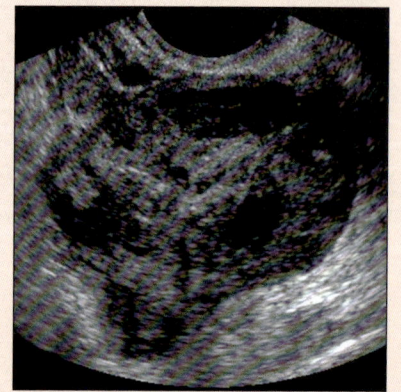
Ruptured Functional Cyst

ADNEXAL TORSION

Key Facts

Terminology
- Rotation of ovary, fallopian tube or both on its vascular pedicle

Imaging Findings
- Thickened fallopian tube with "twisted vascular pedicle" sign
- Enlarged edematous ovary
- Uterine deviation towards torsed ovary
- Adjacent fat stranding (correlates with necrosis)
- Pelvic fluid may or may not be hemorrhagic
- Beaked structure: Twisted fallopian tube
- Whirlpool sign: Coiled, twisted pedicle
- Early: No venous flow
- Late: High resistance arterial flow
- Spontaneously detorsed: Low resistance arterial flow

Pathology
- In adults, 50-80% accompanied by a nonneoplastic cyst or benign ovarian tumor
- In infants and children, most commonly no underlying mass
- Results in sequential venous, lymphatic, and arterial obstruction
- Vascular torsed adnexa likely viable
- Nonvascular torsed adnexa likely infarcted

Diagnostic Checklist
- In the appropriate clinical setting consider torsion even in the presence of normal flow
- Assess for abrupt change of vascularity on color Doppler in the vicinity of an enlarged ovary/adnexa from present to absent

Ultrasonographic Findings
- Grayscale Ultrasound
  - Most common finding: Enlarged, echogenic, edematous, ovarian stroma
  - Multiple follicles containing debris due to hemorrhage
  - Follicles displaced peripherally due to echogenic edematous stroma and/or mass
  - Twisted vascular pedicle (broad ligament, fallopian tube, and ovarian vessels)
    - Target sign: Round hyperechoic structure with multiple hypoechoic concentric rings
    - Beaked structure: Twisted fallopian tube
    - Heterogeneous tubular structure: Edematous fallopian tube
    - Whirlpool sign: Coiled, twisted pedicle
- Pulsed Doppler
  - Normal arterial and venous waveforms may be present in acute torsion
    - Presence of venous waveform is associated with ovarian viability
  - Early: No venous flow
  - Late: High resistance arterial flow
  - Spontaneously detorsed: Low resistance arterial flow
- Color Doppler
  - Normal adnexal flow
    - Early or incomplete torsion
    - Dual blood supply from ovarian and uterine artery
  - Diminished adnexal flow
  - No adnexal flow: Lack of vascularity on Doppler more common with nonviable ovary
  - Abrupt change of vascularity in vicinity of enlarged ovary/adnexa from present to absent
  - Whirlpool sign: Coiled twisted vessels

CT Findings
- NECT
  - Hemorrhagic FT/vascular pedicle > 50 HU
  - Hemorrhagic ovarian cyst > 50 HU
  - Nonspecific adnexal mass
- CECT
  - Adnexal mass with variable enhancement
  - Twisted ovarian vascular pedicle

MR Findings
- T1WI
  - Hyperintense fallopian tube/vascular pedicle due to hemorrhage
  - Hyperintense hemorrhagic cyst content/wall if present
- T2WI
  - Enlarged edematous stroma compared to contralateral side
    - Ovarian stroma hyperintense due to edema
    - Follicles displaced peripherally
  - Thickened fallopian tube
- T1 C+ FS
  - Ovary/adnexal mass with variable enhancement
  - Thickening of ovarian cyst wall, concentric or eccentric
    - Hemorrhage into cyst wall
    - Pseudothickening due to FT draped over cyst wall
  - Thickened fallopian tube
  - Twisted ovarian vascular pedicle

Imaging Recommendations
- Best imaging tool
  - Transvaginal US with Doppler initial imaging modality
  - CT/MR provide better overview of torsed pedicle and abnormal location of adnexa
- Protocol advice: Optimizing pulse repetition frequency (PRF) improves flow detection

DIFFERENTIAL DIAGNOSIS

Ruptured Functional Cyst
- Collapsing hemorrhagic cyst in a normal-sized ovary
- Clotted blood in pelvis

Pelvic Inflammatory Disease (PID)
- Uniformly thickened fallopian tubes ± pyosalpinx
- Enlarged ovaries ± tubo-ovarian abscess
- Pelvic fat inflammation more prominent

ADNEXAL TORSION

Ectopic Pregnancy
- Positive pregnancy test
- Extra-ovarian adnexal mass
- No inflammation of fat

Hematosalpinx
- Retrograde passage of blood into fallopian tube
- Positive pregnancy test if patient is bleeding with intra-uterine pregnancy
- History of vaginal bleeding
- No inflammation of fat

PATHOLOGY

General Features
- General path comments
  - Ovarian torsion, tubal torsion, most commonly both
    - Isolated torsed fallopian tube can occur
  - Torsed ovary may or may not show vascularity
  - Swollen hemorrhagic ± infarcted adnexa
  - Calcified mass in chronic cases
- Etiology
  - In adults, 50-80% accompanied by a nonneoplastic cyst or benign ovarian tumor
    - Most commonly dermoid and paraovarian cysts
  - In infants and children, most commonly no underlying mass
    - Hypermobility due to long mesosalpinx
  - Results in sequential venous, lymphatic, and arterial obstruction
- Epidemiology
  - Most common in first three decades
  - Increased incidence during pregnancy
  - Constitutes 3% of all gynecologic emergencies
- Associated abnormalities: Underlying ovarian mass in adults

Gross Pathologic & Surgical Features
- Swollen, hemorrhagic, and in some cases infarcted tubo-ovarian mass twisted on its pedicle
  - Twist ranges from 180 to 720 degrees

Microscopic Features
- Stromal edema & hemorrhage, vascular dilatation & congestion ± infarction

Staging, Grading or Classification Criteria
- Vascular torsed adnexa likely viable
- Nonvascular torsed adnexa likely infarcted

CLINICAL ISSUES

Presentation
- Most common signs/symptoms
  - Acute pelvic pain
  - Vomiting a helpful sign
- Other signs/symptoms: Adnexal mass
- Clinical Profile: Sudden onset of pain associated with vomiting

Demographics
- Age: Infants, children, pre and postmenopausal women

Natural History & Prognosis
- Spontaneous detorsion common
- Can recur especially in infants and children
- Early diagnosis prevents irreversible damage
- Autoamputation in rare asymptomatic patients

Treatment
- Laparoscopic surgical untwisting in non-infarcted adnexa
- Laparoscopic salpingo-oophorectomy in infarcted adnexa

DIAGNOSTIC CHECKLIST

Consider
- In the appropriate clinical setting consider torsion even in the presence of normal flow
- Assess for abrupt change of vascularity on color Doppler in the vicinity of an enlarged ovary/adnexa from present to absent

Image Interpretation Pearls
- Enlarged ovary or residual ovarian tissue disproportional to size of ovarian mass
- Twisted pedicle/thickened fallopian tube
- Twisted vascular pedicle in adnexa

SELECTED REFERENCES

1. Hiller N et al: CT features of adnexal torsion. AJR Am J Roentgenol. 189(1):124-9, 2007
2. Ghossain MA et al: Adnexal torsion: magnetic resonance findings in the viable adnexa with emphasis on stromal ovarian appearance. J Magn Reson Imaging. 20(3):451-62, 2004
3. Varras M et al: Uterine adnexal torsion: pathologic and gray-scale ultrasonographic findings. Clin Exp Obstet Gynecol. 31(1):34-8, 2004
4. Vijayaraghavan SB: Sonographic whirlpool sign in ovarian torsion. J Ultrasound Med. 23(12):1643-9; quiz 1650-1, 2004
5. Hurh PJ et al: Ultrasound of a torsed ovary: characteristic gray-scale appearance despite normal arterial and venous flow on Doppler. Pediatr Radiol. 32(8):586-8, 2002
6. Rha SE et al: CT and MR imaging features of adnexal torsion. Radiographics. 22(2):283-94, 2002
7. Albayram F et al: Ovarian and adnexal torsion: spectrum of sonographic findings with pathologic correlation. J Ultrasound Med. 20(10):1083-9, 2001
8. Bau A et al: Acute female pelvic pain: ultrasound evaluation. Semin Ultrasound CT MR. 21(1):78-93, 2000
9. Lee EJ et al: Diagnosis of ovarian torsion with color Doppler sonography: depiction of twisted vascular pedicle. J Ultrasound Med. 17(2):83-9, 1998
10. Richard HM 3rd et al: Torsion of the fallopian tube: progression of sonographic features. J Clin Ultrasound. 26(7):374-6, 1998
11. Baumgartel PB et al: Color Doppler sonography of tubal torsion. Ultrasound Obstet Gynecol. 7(5):367-70, 1996

ADNEXAL TORSION

IMAGE GALLERY

Typical

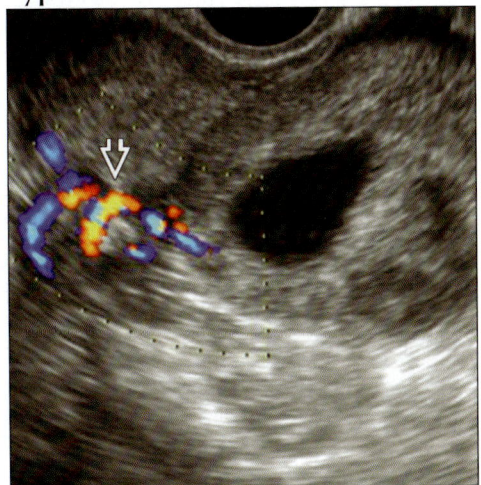
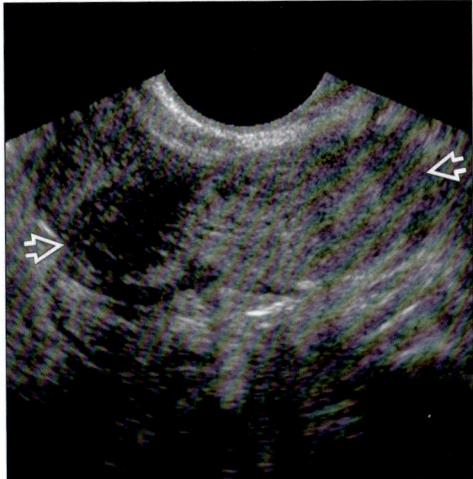

(Left) Transverse color Doppler ultrasound of the same patient as previous image shows the twisted vascular pedicle ➡ ("whirlpool" sign) at the level of the left fallopian tube. *(Right)* Oblique transvaginal ultrasound shows a thickened proximal fallopian tube ➡.

Typical

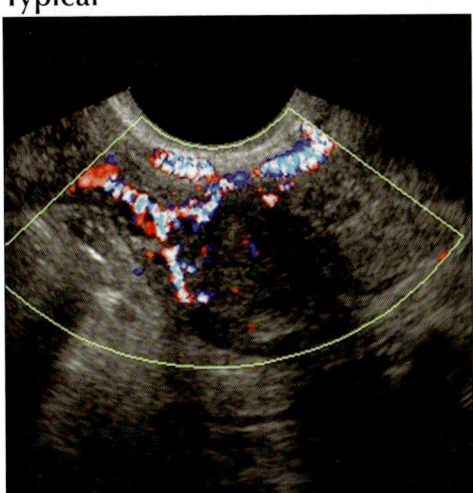
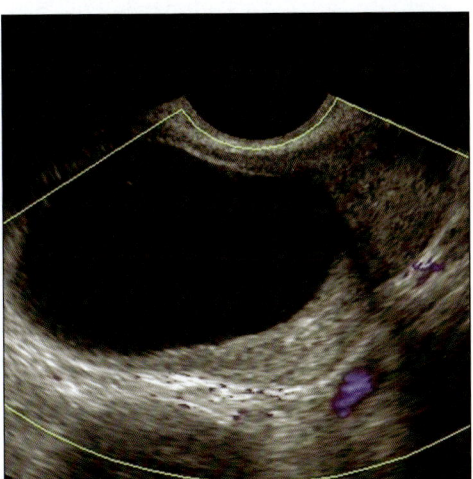

(Left) Oblique color Doppler ultrasound in the same patient as previous image shows vascularity of the thickened proximal fallopian tube. *(Right)* Axial color Doppler ultrasound in the same patient as previous image, shows lack of vascularity of the distended distal end of the fallopian tube.

Typical

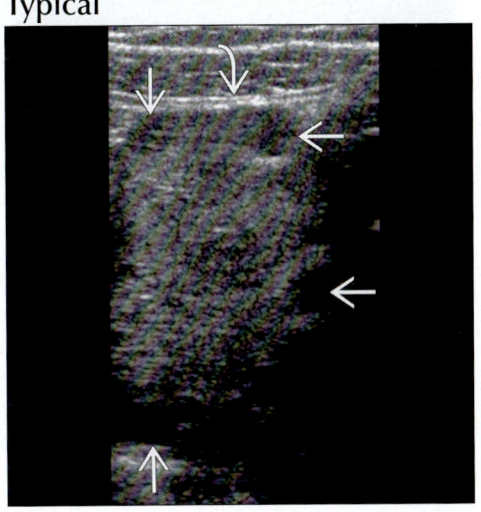
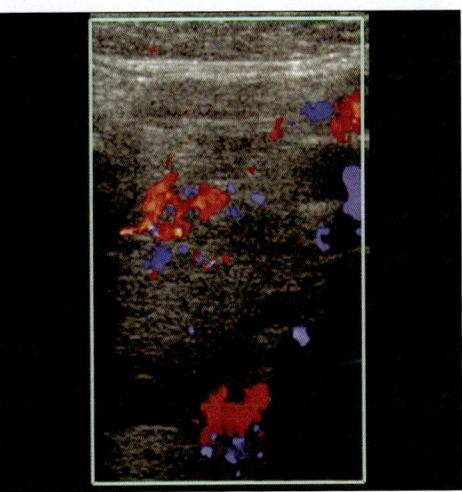

(Left) Sagittal high-resolution transabdominal ultrasound shows an enlarged ovary containing multiple small peripheral follicles ➡. The ovary is located immediately beneath the anterior abdominal wall ➡. *(Right)* Sagittal color Doppler ultrasound in the same patient as previous image, shows preservation of vascularity because of the dual blood supply to the ovary.

ADNEXAL TORSION

(Left) Axial oblique high-resolution transabdominal ultrasound in a pregnant woman shows enlargement of the right ovary ➡ with multiple, peripherally displaced follicles due to stromal edema. (Right) Axial oblique color Doppler ultrasound in the same patient as previous image, shows the "whirlpool" sign ➡ of ovarian torsion representing the coiled, twisted vessels.

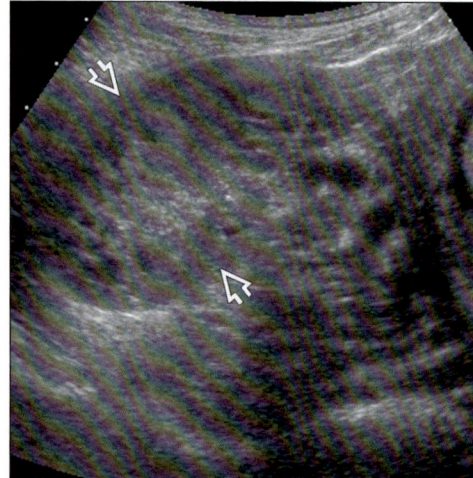
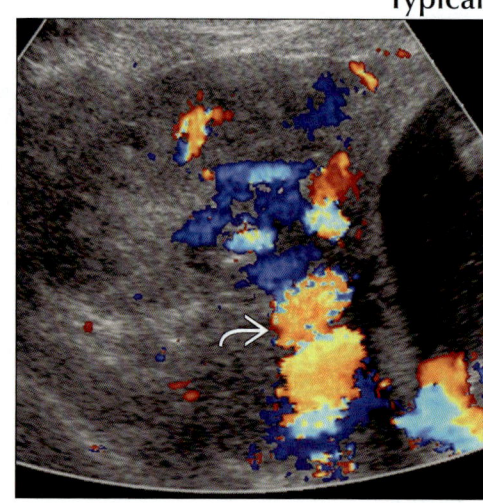

Typical

(Left) Axial transabdominal ultrasound shows a complex cystic mass (calipers) in the right lower quadrant in a patient with intermittent right lower abdominal pain. The thick rind of tissue ➡ at the periphery is avascular (not shown). (Right) Axial T2WI MR in the same patient as previous image, shows the large complex ovarian cyst with blood clot adherent to the wall ➡. There is a hematosalpinx ➡ with beaking ➡ due to torsion of the ovarian cyst and fallopian tube on its pedicle.

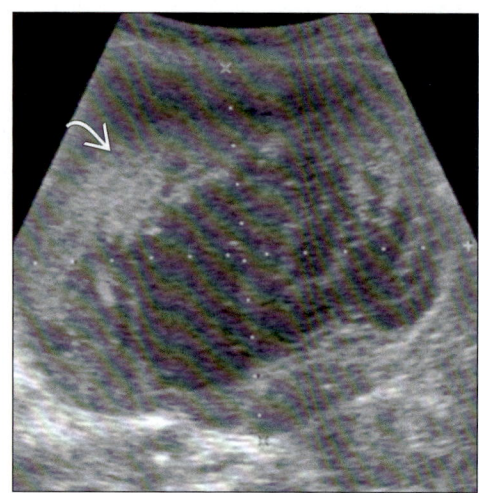
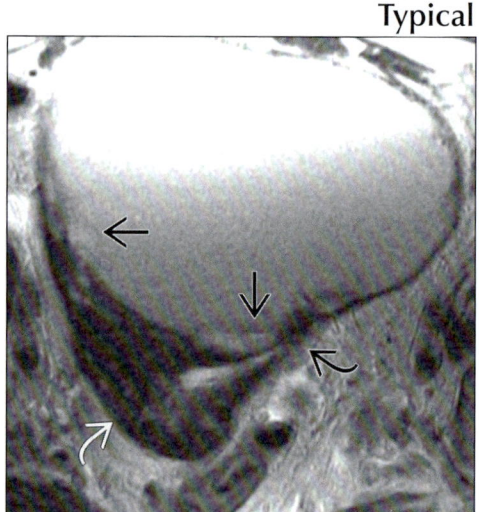

Typical

(Left) Axial T1WI FS MR (same patient as previous) shows the hyperintense contents of the cyst and adherent blood clot ➡ due to intra-cyst hemorrhage. (Right) Axial CECT shows a left ovarian dermoid cyst ➡ situated in the left lower quadrant immediately beneath the anterior abdominal wall. The residual rim of ovarian tissue ➡ is prominent and hypovascular. There is fat stranding posteriorly ➡.

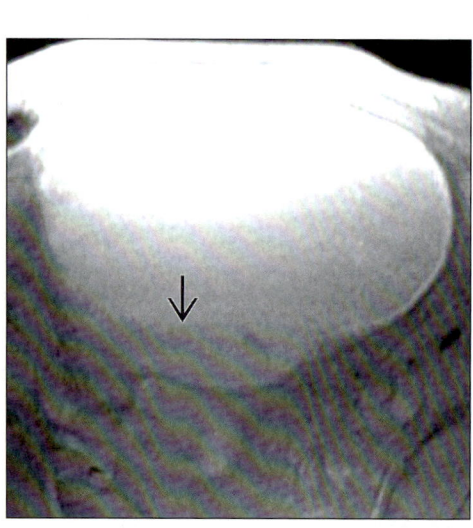
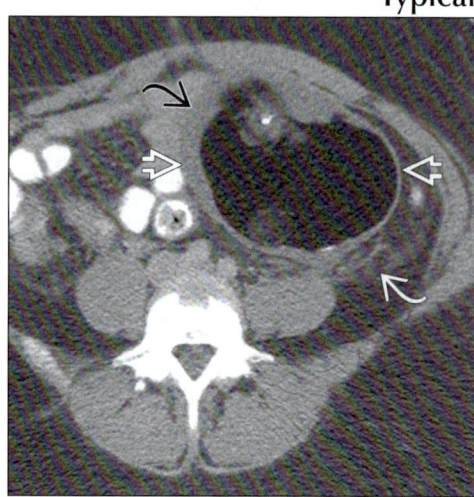

Typical

ADNEXAL TORSION

Typical

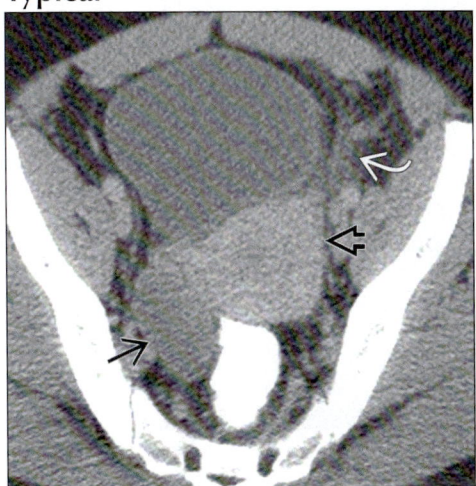
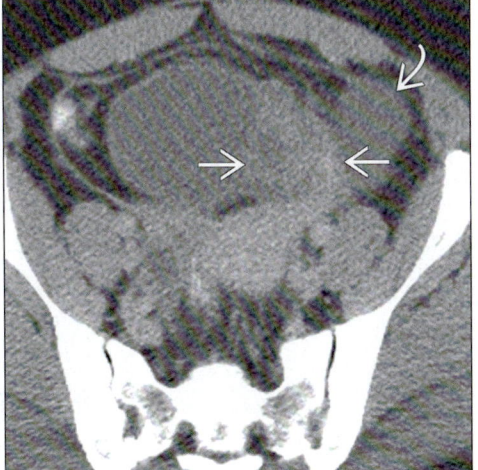

(Left) Axial CECT (same patient as previous) at the level of the uterus shows uterine deviation ⇨ towards the left ovary. Note the fat stranding ➔ in the left adnexa. A functional right ovarian cyst is present ➔. (Right) Axial CECT (same patient as previous), at a more cranial level, shows an intermediate density region ➔ in left adnexa proven to be a thickened fallopian tube due to a left tubo-ovarian torsion. Pocket of free fluid ➔ is present in left lower quadrant.

Typical

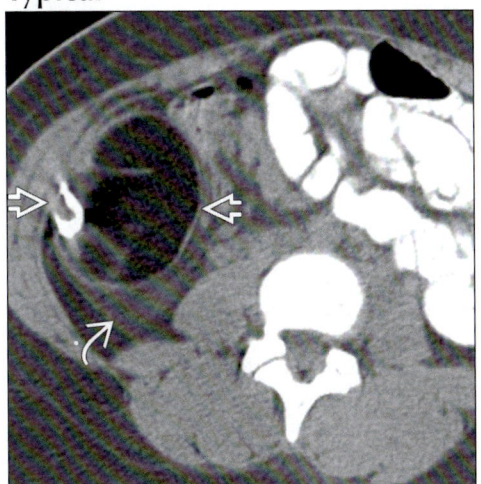
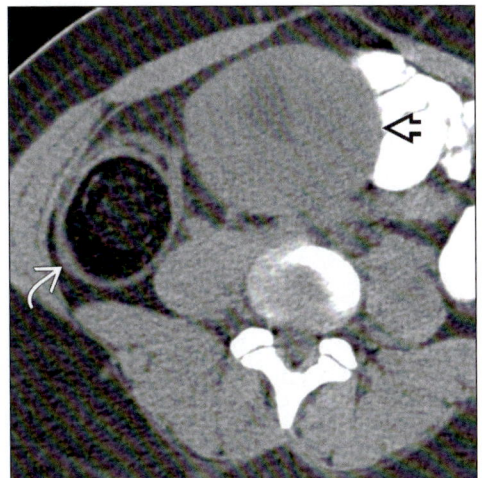

(Left) Axial NECT shows a mass ➔ containing fat and calcification consistent with a right ovarian dermoid, situated beneath the anterior abdominal wall in the right lower quadrant. There is fat stranding ➔ posteriorly. (Right) Axial NECT in the same patient as previous image, shows uterine deviation ⇨ towards the torsed right ovary. There is asymmetric thickening ➔ of the dermoid cyst wall.

Typical

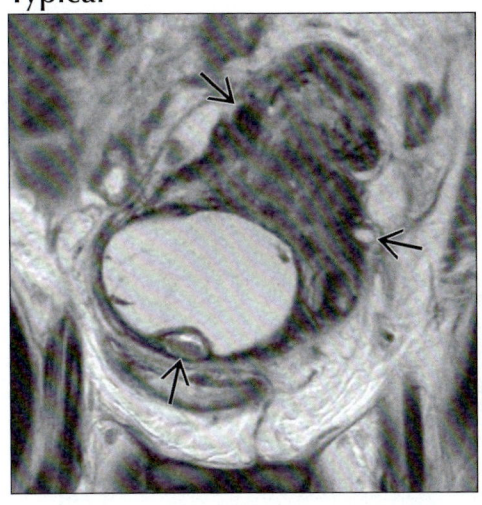
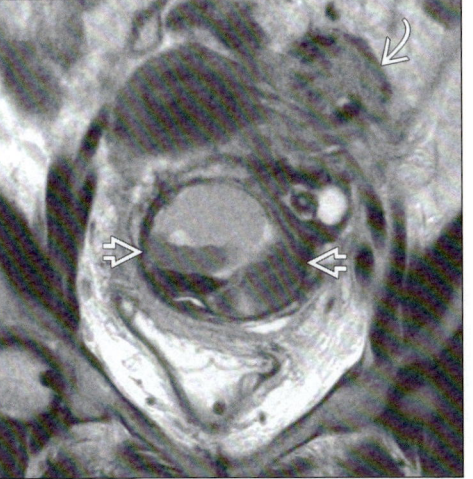

(Left) Coronal T2WI MR shows enlargement of the right ovary with stromal edema and peripherally displaced follicles ➔ containing hemorrhage. A functional cyst is present containing debris. (Courtesy J. Spencer, MD). (Right) Coronal T2WI MR acquired more posteriorly in the same patient as previous image, shows hemorrhage into the functional cyst ⇨. The fallopian tube ➔ is enlarged and edematous. (Courtesy J. Spencer, MD).

MASSIVE OVARIAN EDEMA

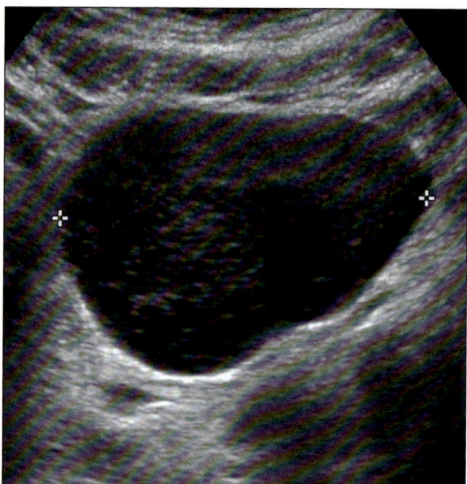

Transverse transabdominal ultrasound shows a 14 cm ovary (calipers). The stroma appears edematous.

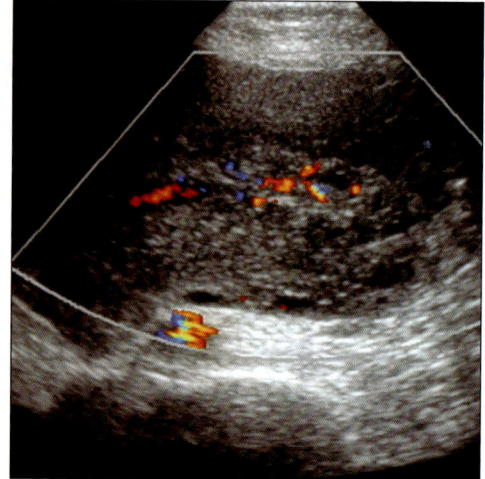

Transverse color Doppler ultrasound shows color flow centrally in a case of massive ovarian edema.

TERMINOLOGY

Definitions
- Partial or intermittent torsion leading to venous and lymphatic obstruction with subsequent ovarian enlargement

IMAGING FINDINGS

General Features
- Best diagnostic clue: Enlarged ovary with edematous appearance and peripheral follicles
- Location
  - Right: 75%
    - Predisposition of the right ovary may be due to elevated right ovarian vein pressure relative to the left reducing the tolerance of the right ovary to partial torsion
  - Bilateral: 15%
- Size: 5-35 cm, mean 11 cm
- Morphology
  - Ovoid shape
  - Massively enlarged ovary
  - Edematous appearance

Imaging Recommendations
- Best imaging tool
  - Ultrasound
    - Enlarged ovary
    - Well defined capsule
    - Focal tenderness while scanning
    - Doppler typically shows flow
    - Venous waveforms may be difficult to obtain
  - MR
    - Maintain ovarian configuration
    - High signal in ovarian stroma on T2WI
    - Signal intensity on T2WI increases with heavier T2 weighting
    - Low signal in ovarian stroma on T1WI
    - May show enhancement centrally
    - Central enhancement is stronger than enhancement in the remainder of ovary
    - Distinguish from tumor by presence of peripheral follicles
- Protocol advice: Presence of blood flow does not exclude this diagnosis

DDx: Massive Ovarian Edema

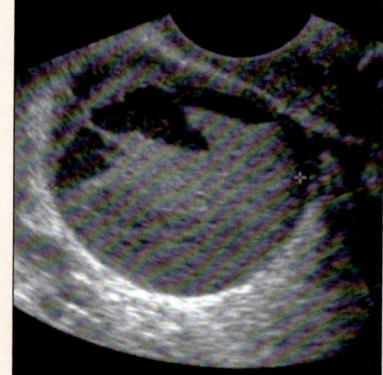

Hemorrhagic Cyst

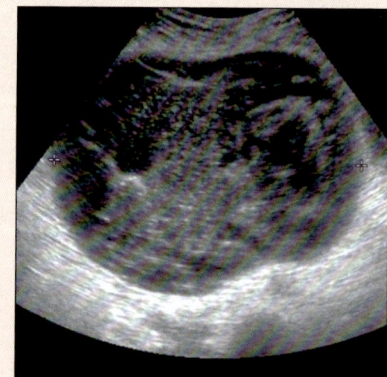

Necrotic Ovary

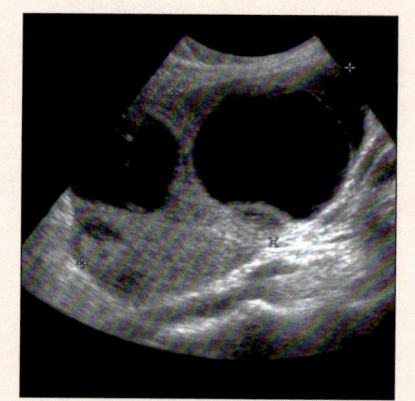

Hyperstimulated Ovary

MASSIVE OVARIAN EDEMA

Key Facts

Terminology
- Partial or intermittent torsion leading to venous and lymphatic obstruction with subsequent ovarian enlargement

Imaging Findings
- Best diagnostic clue: Enlarged ovary with edematous appearance and peripheral follicles
- Right: 75%
- Size: 5-35 cm, mean 11 cm
- Ovoid shape
- Protocol advice: Presence of blood flow does not exclude this diagnosis

Pathology
- Idiopathic theory attributes massive ovarian edema to recurrent partial torsion of the meso-ovarium
- Secondary theory attributes massive ovarian edema to underlying processes such as stromal hyperplasia or hyperthecosis
- Pre-existing ovarian lesion may be present with reported cases of cystadenoma, polycystic ovaries, fibrothecoma, and metastatic disease

Clinical Issues
- Long history of intermittent pain
- Typically in young women less than 33 years of age
- Conservative management with de-torsion and frozen section to exclude tumor; current treatment of choice
- May cause precocious puberty

DIFFERENTIAL DIAGNOSIS

Ovarian Torsion
- Enlarged ovary
- Ipsilateral pain
- Lack of flow in some cases, however flow may be present in cases of incomplete or partial torsion

Solid Ovarian Neoplasm
- Solid lesion
- Lack of peripheral follicles

Hemorrhagic Cyst
- Lack of internal flow
- Retractile clot

Ovarian Fibromatosis
- Edema may be present but is focal, not diffuse

Edematous Fibroma
- Lacks follicles within the ovarian stroma

Ovarian Myxoma
- Lacks follicles within the ovarian stroma

PATHOLOGY

General Features
- Etiology
  - Partial or intermittent torsion
  - Idiopathic theory attributes massive ovarian edema to recurrent partial torsion of the meso-ovarium
    - Obstruction to the venous and lymphatic return
    - Evidence of torsion is found only in half of the cases
  - Secondary theory attributes massive ovarian edema to underlying processes such as stromal hyperplasia or hyperthecosis
    - Facilitate torsion of an already abnormally enlarged ovary
  - Pre-existing ovarian lesion may be present with reported cases of cystadenoma, polycystic ovaries, fibrothecoma, and metastatic disease
- Associated abnormalities: Ovarian edema

Gross Pathologic & Surgical Features
- Unlike regular torsion, typically not associated with infarction or necrosis since this involves the venous and lymphatic flow rather than the arterial flow
- Ovary remains viable

Microscopic Features
- Diffuse edema centrally
- Capsule with dense collagen tissue spared from edema process
- Lymphedema leads to proliferation of the stromal cells and in some to conversion to lutein cells
- Follicles surrounded by edematous stroma

CLINICAL ISSUES

Presentation
- Most common signs/symptoms
  - Pain lateralized to side of torsion
  - Long history of intermittent pain
- Other signs/symptoms
  - Pelvic mass
  - At times will present as an incidental finding at laparotomy
  - Luteinization and stromal hyperplasia result in an increase in ovarian androgen and oestrogen production
    - Can lead to virilization and pubertal signs
    - May present as precocious puberty, reported in case as young as 6 months of age
    - May present with menstrual irregularities in patients after menarche

Demographics
- Age
  - Typically in young women less than 33 years of age
  - Mean age 21

MASSIVE OVARIAN EDEMA

- Gender: Female

Natural History & Prognosis
- Frequently surgically removed even though benign due to overlap in appearance with solid ovarian lesion
- Conservative management with de-torsion and frozen section to exclude tumor; current treatment of choice
- May cause precocious puberty
  - Precocious puberty can be reversed after surgical detorsion

Treatment
- Check histology on frozen section to exclude malignancy
- Wedge resection to debulk the ovary
- Detorsion (torsion occurs in half of cases)
- Bilateral gonadopexy to prevent both ipsilateral recurrence and contralateral occurrence

DIAGNOSTIC CHECKLIST

Consider
- Consider massive ovarian edema when an enlarged edematous appearing ovary is seen in a young woman
- Intra-operative biopsy is diagnostic and can lead to ovary sparing surgery

Image Interpretation Pearls
- An enlarged edematous appearing ovary with peripheral follicles should suggest this diagnosis
- Presence of blood flow does not exclude the diagnosis of massive ovarian edema

SELECTED REFERENCES
1. Cepni I et al: Massive edema of the ovary diagnosed with laparoscopic biopsy and frozen section. J Postgrad Med 51:336-337, 2005
2. Geist RR et al: Massive edema of the ovary: a case report and review of the pertinent literature. J Pediatr Adolesc Gynecol. 18(4):281-4, 2005
3. Natarajan A et al: Precocious puberty secondary to massive ovarian oedema in a 6-month-old girl. Eur J Endocrinol. 150(2):119-23, 2004
4. Bazot M et al. Massive ovarian edema revealing gastric carcinoma: a case report. Gynecol Oncol. 91: 648-50, 2003
5. Kocak M et al: Laparoscopic conservation of the ovaries in cases with massive ovarian oedema. Gynecol Obstet Invest 53:129-32, 2002
6. Guvenal T et al: Unilateral massive ovarian edema in a woman with polycystic ovaries. Eur J Obstet Gynecol Reprod Biol 99: 129-30, 2001
7. Dolgin SE et al: Maximizing ovarian salvage when treating idiopathic adnexal torsion J Pediatr Surg 35:624-626, 2000
8. Sakaki M et al. Ovarian fibrothecoma with massive edema. J Med Invest 47: 148-51, 2000
9. Umesaki N et al: Successful preoperative diagnosis of massive ovarian edema aided by comparative imaging study using magnetic resonance and ultrasound. Eur J Obstet Gynecol Reprod Biol 89:97-9, 2000
10. Roberts CL et al: Bilateral massive ovarian edema: a case report. Ultrasound Obstet Gynecol. 11(1):65-7, 1998
11. Hameed A et al. Ovarian mucinous cystadenoma associated with mural leiomyomatous nodule and massive ovarian edema. Gynecol Oncol 67: 226-9, 1997
12. Kramer LA et al. Massive edema of the ovary: high-resolution MR findings using a phased-array pelvic coil. J Magn Reson Imaging 75:758-60, 1997
13. Hall BP et al: Massive ovarian edema: ultrasound and MR characteristics. J Comput Assist Tomogr. 17(3):477-9, 1993
14. Hubbell GP et al: Conservative management of bilateral massive edema of the ovary. A case report. J Reprod Med.38: 61-4, 1993
15. Sageshima M et al: Massive ovarian edema associated with polycystic ovary. Acta Pathol Jpn 40: 73-8, 1990
16. Thorp JM Jr et al: Ovarian suspension in massive ovarian edema. Obstet Gynecol 76:912-4, 1990

MASSIVE OVARIAN EDEMA

IMAGE GALLERY

Typical

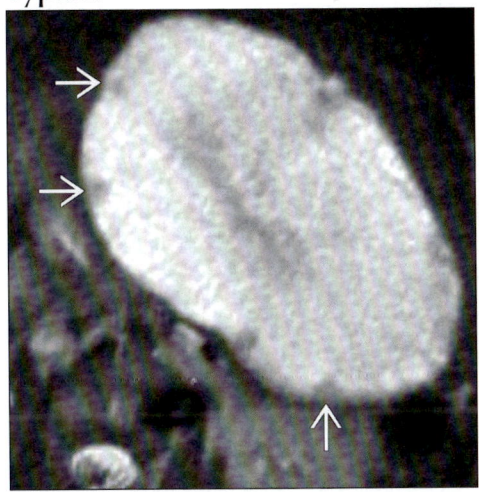
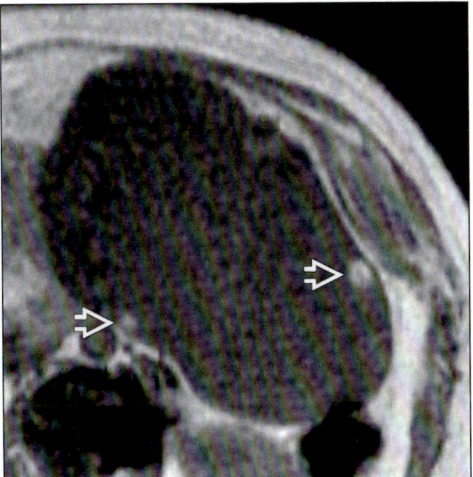

(Left) Axial T2WI MR shows enlarged edematous ovary with peripheral hemorrhagic follicles ➡. *(Right)* Transverse T1WI MR (same patient as previous image) shows low signal intensity in enlarged ovary with well-defined capsule and peripheral hemorrhagic follicles ➡.

Typical

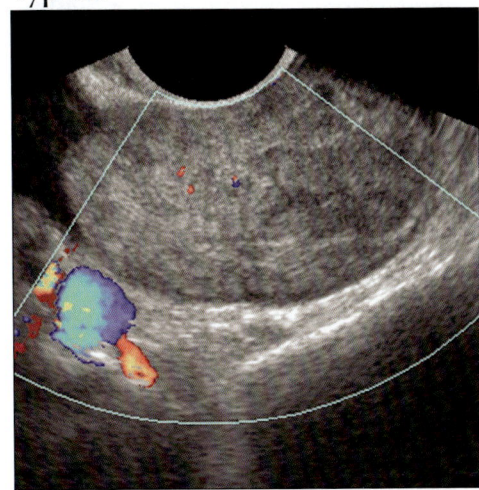
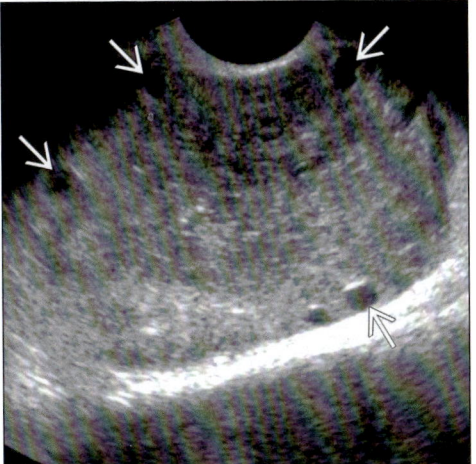

(Left) Axial oblique color Doppler ultrasound shows a small amount of blood in a solid appearing enlarged ovary. *(Right)* Oblique transvaginal ultrasound of the right ovary shows ovarian enlargement with multiple small, peripheral cysts ➡. Massive ovarian edema may be mistaken for a solid ovarian neoplasm. It is important to recognize this pattern and suggest the diagnosis preoperatively so more conservative surgery can be performed.

Variant

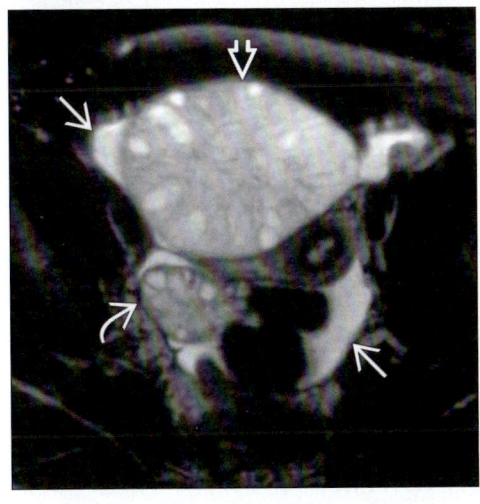
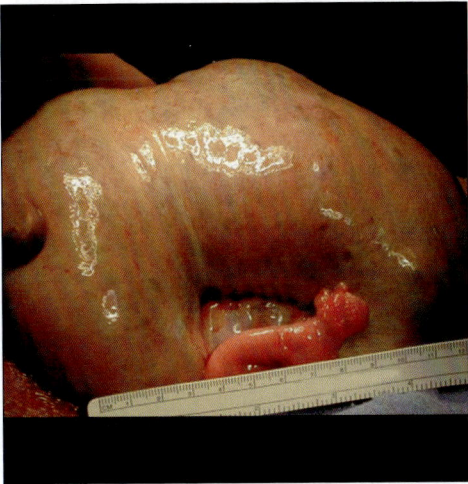

(Left) Axial T2WI FS MR of massive edema of the left ovary ➡. Note the high signal central stroma and small peripheral cysts. Free fluid ➡ is also present. The right ovary is normal ➡. *(Right)* Intra-operative photograph shows the massively enlarged ovary corresponding to the appearance seen on MR.

POLYCYSTIC OVARY SYNDROME

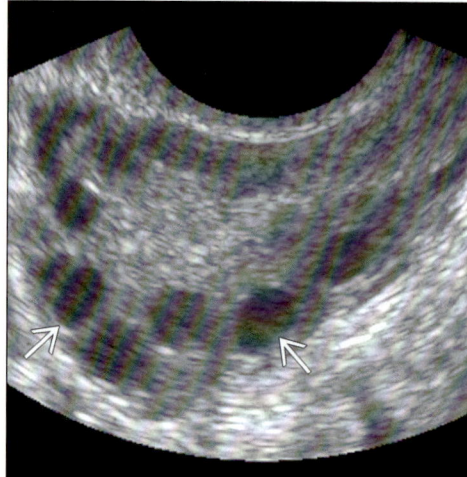

Axial transvaginal ultrasound in a patient with hirsutism & amenorrhea shows enlargement of the ovaries (right ovary shown) with multiple, small, peripheral follicles ➡ of uniform size. Ovarian stroma is prominent.

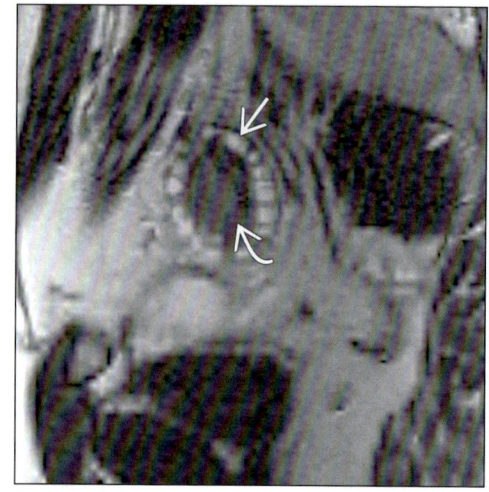

Sagittal T2WI MR shows a polycystic ovary in the setting of polycystic ovary syndrome (PCOS). Numerous peripheral follicles ➡ of similar size are noted around a central hypointense stroma ➡.

TERMINOLOGY

Abbreviations and Synonyms
- Stein-Leventhal syndrome, polycystic ovary syndrome (PCOS)

Definitions
- Association of hyperandrogenism and chronic anovulation without specific underlying adrenal or pituitary gland disease

IMAGING FINDINGS

General Features
- Best diagnostic clue
  - Enlarged ovaries with multiple small follicles arrayed around a prominent central stroma
    - "String-of-pearls" appearance
- Location: Usually bilateral and symmetric, may be unilateral
- Revised 2003 Rotterdam consensus imaging criteria
  - Ovarian volume ≥ 10 cm³
    - Ellipsoid volume formula: 0.52 x length x width x thickness
  - ≥ 12 follicles per ovary, ranging in size from 2-9 mm
  - No dominant follicle ≥ 10 mm or corpus luteum cyst
  - One ovary fitting these criteria sufficient for diagnosis
  - Peripheral follicular distribution and increased stromal echogenicity not included in the Rotterdam criteria
- Additional imaging findings
  - Ovaries more spherical in shape: Sphericity index (ovarian width to ovarian length ratio) ≥ 0.7
  - Follicles often show a peripheral distribution
  - Diffuse endometrial thickening due to prolonged proliferative phase or endometrial hyperplasia (30-40% of patients)

Ultrasonographic Findings
- Typical sonographic findings present in 60-90% of patients with one or more symptoms of PCOS
  - Multiple small anechoic cysts of similar size
    - Wall irregularity, increased echogenicity typically absent

DDx: Polycystic Ovaries

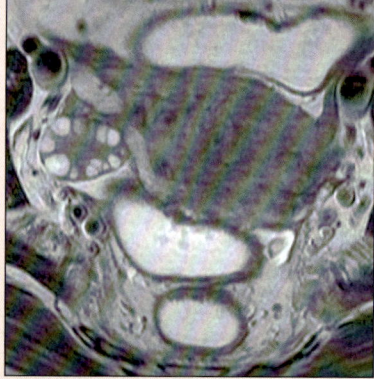
Multifollicular Ovary

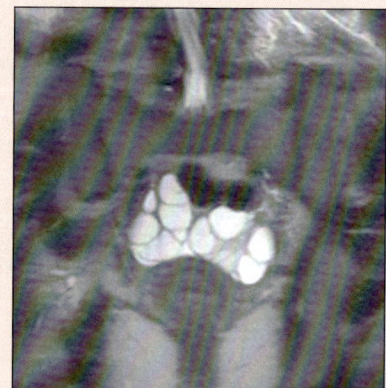
Theca Lutein Cysts

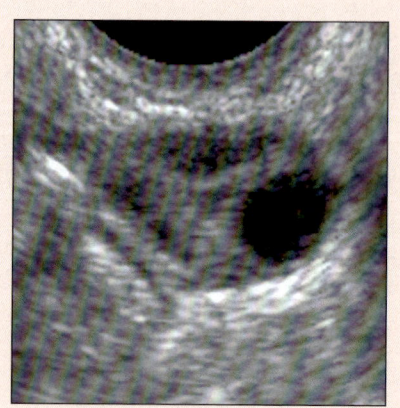
Normal Ovary

POLYCYSTIC OVARY SYNDROME

Key Facts

Terminology
- Stein-Leventhal syndrome, polycystic ovary syndrome (PCOS)
- Association of hyperandrogenism and chronic anovulation without specific underlying adrenal or pituitary gland disease

Imaging Findings
- Enlarged ovaries with multiple small follicles arrayed around a prominent central stroma
- "String-of-pearls" appearance
- Ovarian volume ≥ 10 cm^3
- ≥ 12 follicles per ovary, ranging in size from 2-9 mm
- No dominant follicle ≥ 10 mm or corpus luteum cyst
- One ovary fitting these criteria sufficient for diagnosis
- Regularly menstruating women: Scan during early follicular phase (day 3-5)
- Oligo/amenorrheic women: Scan randomly or 3-5 days after progestin-induced withdrawal bleeding

Top Differential Diagnoses
- Normal Ovaries
- Multifollicular Ovaries

Diagnostic Checklist
- Consider diagnosis of PCOS when 2 of 3 Rotterdam consensus criteria present:
- Clinical or biochemical evidence of hyperandrogenism
- Chronic anovulation
- Polycystic ovaries on imaging
- After exclusion of other etiologies (congenital adrenal hyperplasia, androgen-secreting tumor, Cushing syndrome)

- Increased ovarian stromal volume and echogenicity
  - Increased stromal echogenicity not included in Rotterdam criteria, may be artefactual due to peripheral location of follicles
  - Diffuse endometrial thickening due to hyperplasia
- 3D Ultrasound
  - Although diagnostic criteria elaborated with 2D ultrasound, 3D ultrasound seems promising in facilitating measurement of total ovarian and stromal volume, echogenicity, and blood flow
- Pulsed Doppler: Ovarian stroma
  - Decreased resistive and pulsatility index
  - Increased peak systolic velocity
- Color Doppler: Intra-ovarian stromal blood flow higher in PCOS

CT Findings
- CECT: May show enlarged ovaries with hypodense peripheral follicles and enhancing central stroma
- No role in primary diagnostic evaluation

MR Findings
- T1WI
  - Ovarian stroma isointense to myometrium
  - Follicles: Low to intermediate signal intensity
- T2WI
  - Thickened low signal intensity ovarian cortex
  - Central ovarian tissue increased in volume
    - Low to intermediate signal intensity
    - Reflects increased cellularity of medullary stroma
  - Follicles: High signal intensity with low signal intensity rim
    - Aside from size, number and location, follicles have same appearance as developing follicles in normal ovaries
    - Hemorrhage, wall irregularity typically absent
- T1 C+
  - Enhancement of highly vascularized stroma
    - Faster, greater enhancement and washout on time intensity curves
  - Follicles: Rim-enhancement

Imaging Recommendations
- Best imaging tool
  - TVS is the imaging modality of choice
  - MR useful when TVS cannot be performed or is technically suboptimal
- Protocol advice
  - Revised 2003 Rotterdam consensus imaging criteria
    - Regularly menstruating women: Scan during early follicular phase (day 3-5)
    - Oligo/amenorrheic women: Scan randomly or 3-5 days after progestin-induced withdrawal bleeding

DIFFERENTIAL DIAGNOSIS

Normal Ovaries
- Normal ovaries with multiple functional cysts
- Functional cysts typically vary in size and appearance
  - Presence of maturing follicles/corpus luteum cyst
  - May show features reflecting previous hemorrhage
- Normal volume of central ovarian stroma

Polycystic Ovaries
- Imaging criteria same as those for PCOS
- Clinical and biochemical evidence of PCOS absent

Multifollicular Ovaries
- Incomplete pulsatile gonadotropin (GnRH) stimulation of ovarian follicular development
  - Associated with hyperprolactinemia, hypothalamic anovulation, weight-related amenorrhea
  - Normal level of luteinizing hormone (LH) and testosterone
  - Reduced levels of follicle stimulating hormone (FSH)
- Occurs in mid to late normal puberty
- Imaging features
  - Normal or slightly enlarged ovary
  - Fewer follicles than PCOS: 6-10 per ovary (4-10 mm in diameter)
  - Normal amount of ovarian stroma
  - Distribution of cysts throughout ovary without stromal hypertrophy

POLYCYSTIC OVARY SYNDROME

- Return to normal following weight gain or treatment with pulsatile GnRH, while PCOS retain their appearance throughout reproductive life

Pelvic Congestion Syndrome
- Prominent ovaries, from polycystic pattern to clusters of 4-6 cysts
- Enlarged uterus, thickened endometrium
- Possible causes: Ovarian dysfunction, uterine veins engorgement, increased sensitivity or exposure to estrogens

PATHOLOGY

General Features
- Genetics: Genetic susceptibility, although inheritance pattern not precisely defined
- Epidemiology
  - One of the most common human endocrinopathies
    - 80-90% of women with oligomenorrhea have PCOS
    - Clinical symptoms of PCOS: 5-15% of reproductive age women
    - Sonographic findings of PCOS: 20% of ovulating women
- Associated abnormalities
  - Insulin resistance (type 2 diabetes)
  - Hypertension, altered lipid profile
  - Possible increased risk of cardiovascular disease later in life
  - Increased risk of endometrial cancer due to chronic anovulation with unopposed estrogen stimulation of endometrium (exact incidence unknown)
- Pathogenesis
  - Hypersecretion of LH, low level of FSH: Produce follicles that stay in suspended development
  - Stimulation of ovarian stroma by elevated LH causes excess androgen secretion, later converted into estrogens
  - Acyclical estrogen production coupled with progesterone deficiency contributes to
    - Unopposed estrogen effect on endometrium
    - Hypersecretion of LH, followed by depression of FSH; completing cycle

Gross Pathologic & Surgical Features
- Enlarged ovaries with thickened cortical tunica
- Abundance of primordial follicles typically located in outer cortex

Microscopic Features
- Fibrotic thickening of tunica albuginea
- Multiple cystic follicles, atretic follicles and/or degenerating granulosa cells
  - Hypertrophy and luteinization of inner theca cell layer

CLINICAL ISSUES

Presentation
- Most common signs/symptoms
  - Abnormal menstrual cycle: Amenorrhea/oligomenorrhea
  - Hyperandrogenism: Hirsutism, acne, male-pattern alopecia
  - Obesity, infertility
  - 20-30% of women with polycystic ovaries do ovulate, but 90% of these on closer examination will have at least one clinical or biochemical feature characteristic of PCOS
  - Raised serum concentrations of LH, testosterone and androstenedione
- Clinical Profile
  - Heterogeneous disorder with broad spectrum of clinical manifestations
  - Classic Stein-Leventhal syndrome (amenorrhea, hirsutism, sterility and obesity) is one extreme form in spectrum of PCOS

Demographics
- Age: Reproductive age female, although biochemical and ultrasound abnormalities may persist after menopause

Treatment
- Medical therapy directed at restoring ovulation and treating hirsutism
- Surgical management: Laparoscopic diathermy or laser "drilling"

DIAGNOSTIC CHECKLIST

Consider
- Consider diagnosis of PCOS when 2 of 3 Rotterdam consensus criteria present:
  - Clinical or biochemical evidence of hyperandrogenism
  - Chronic anovulation
  - Polycystic ovaries on imaging
  - After exclusion of other etiologies (congenital adrenal hyperplasia, androgen-secreting tumor, Cushing syndrome)

Image Interpretation Pearls
- Multiple, peripheral follicles, uniform in size, arrayed around large central stroma

SELECTED REFERENCES

1. Chang RJ: A practical approach to the diagnosis of polycystic ovary syndrome. Am J Obstet Gynecol. 191(3):713-7, 2004
2. Erdem CZ et al: Polycystic ovary syndrome: dynamic contrast-enhanced ovary MR imaging. Eur J Radiol. 51(1):48-53, 2004
3. Phy J et al: Transvaginal ultrasound detection of multifollicular ovaries in non-hirsute ovulatory women. Ultrasound Obstet Gynecol. 23(2):183-7, 2004
4. The Rotterdam ESHRE/ASRM-Sponsored PCOS consensus workshop group: Revised 2003 consensus on diagnostic criteria and long-term health risks related to polycystic ovary syndrome (PCOS). Hum Reprod. 19(1):41-7, 2004
5. Balen AH et al: Ultrasound assessment of the polycystic ovary: international consensus definitions. Hum Reprod Update. 9(6):505-14, 2003

POLYCYSTIC OVARY SYNDROME

IMAGE GALLERY

Typical

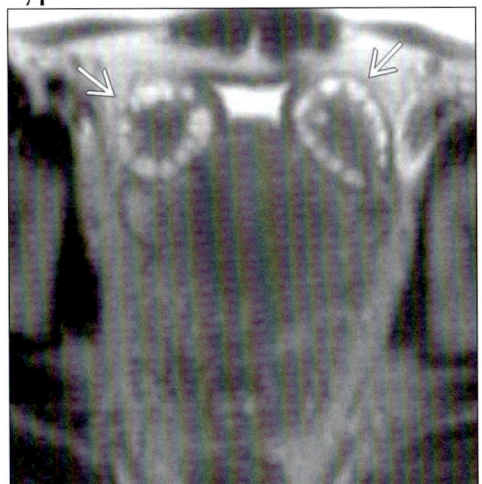
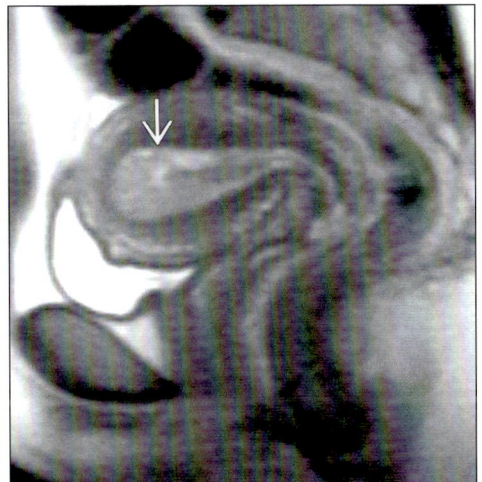

(Left) Axial T2WI MR shows polycystic ovaries ➡. There are multiple peripherally located hyperintense follicles and an enlarged intermediate signal intensity central stroma. *(Right)* Sagittal T2WI MR in the same patient as previous image, shows a thickened hypointense endometrial complex ➡. It proved to be endometrial hyperplasia with superficially invasive endometrial carcinoma.

Typical

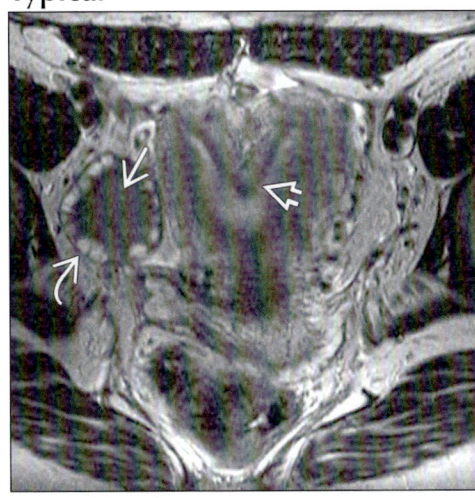
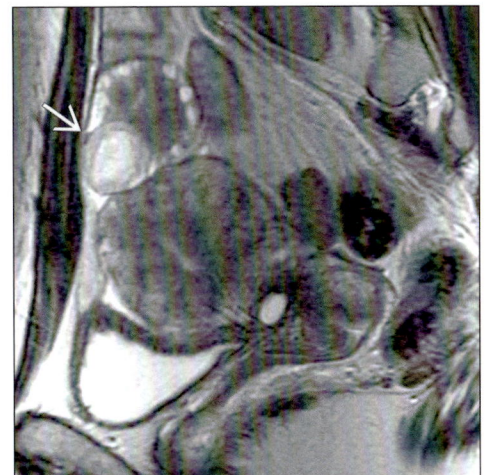

(Left) Axial T2WI MR of the right ovary in a patient with PCOS shows a prominent hypointense stroma ➡ surrounded by numerous peripheral follicles ➡. Incidental note is made of a septate uterus ➡. *(Right)* Sagittal T2WI MR in the same patient as previous image, shows a corpus luteum cyst ➡ arising from the left ovary, in keeping with recent ovulation (occurs in 20-30% of patients with PCOS). The underlying ovary has a polycystic appearance.

Typical

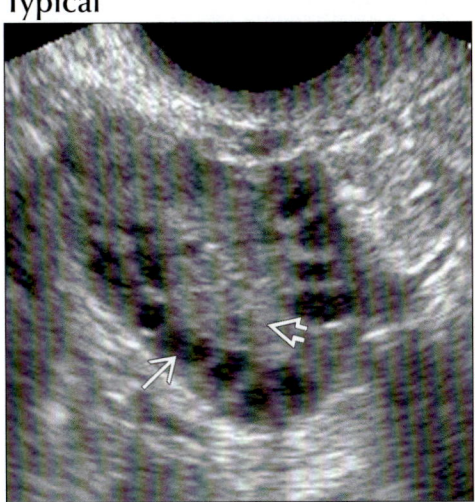
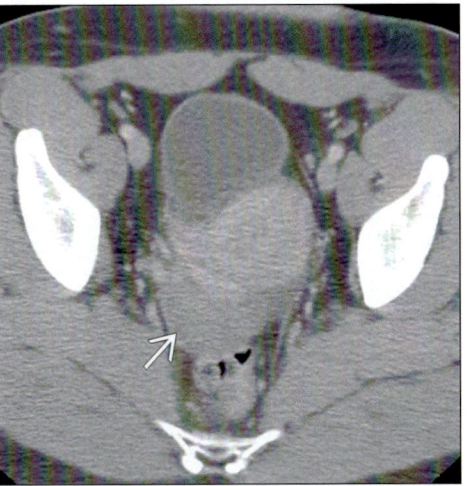

(Left) Sagittal transvaginal ultrasound shows a polycystic ovary in a patient with PCOS. Multiple, peripheral follicles ➡ are arranged as a "string-of-pearls" around a central echogenic stroma ➡. *(Right)* Axial CECT shows multiple peripheral hypodense follicles ➡ in the right ovary in a woman with amenorrhea and hirsutism.

FIBROMATOSIS, OVARY

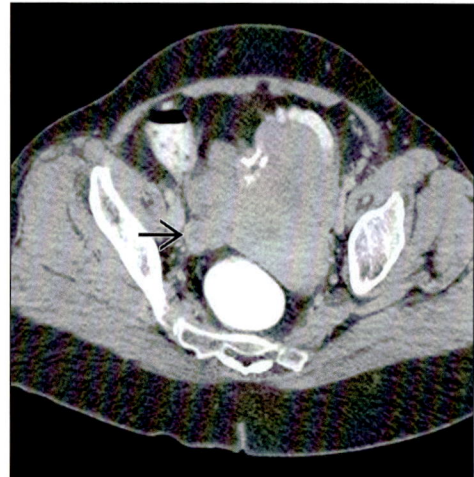

Axial CECT shows homogeneous soft tissue ➡ in expected location of the right ovary.

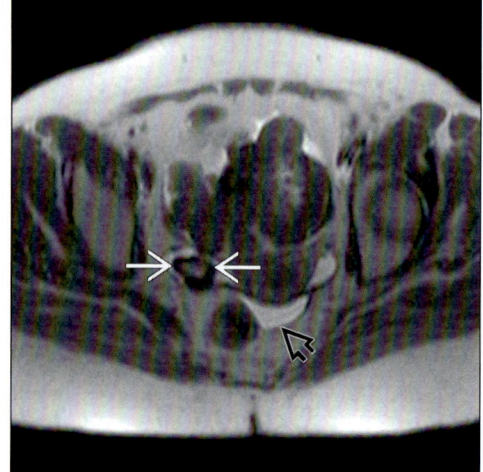

Axial T2WI MR in the same patient shows homogeneous low signal ➡ throughout the right ovarian cortex with sparing of the central ovarian stroma. A small amount of free fluid ⊳ is present.

TERMINOLOGY

Abbreviations and Synonyms
- Ovarian fibromatosis, stromal hyperplasia

Definitions
- Nonneoplastic proliferation of fibroblasts surrounding follicles

IMAGING FINDINGS

General Features
- Morphology: Lobulated

Ultrasonographic Findings
- Grayscale Ultrasound: Enlarged, bilateral, solid, lobulated ovarian masses

CT Findings
- Homogeneous, lobulated ovarian masses

MR Findings
- T1WI: Lobulated hypointense ovarian mass
- T2WI: Hypointense mass with few follicles interspersed
- T1 C+: No significant enhancement during parenchymal phase, mild enhancement on delayed imaging

Imaging Recommendations
- Best imaging tool: MR: Superior spatial resolution and multiplanar capabilities

DIFFERENTIAL DIAGNOSIS

Ovarian Fibroma
- Homogeneous ovarian masses without envelopment of normal follicles
- Typically low signal intensity on T2 weighted images

Ovarian Fibrothecoma
- May have mixed low and intermediate T2 signal

Polycystic Ovarian Syndrome
- Enlarged ovaries with peripherally arranged cysts

DDx: Ovarian Fibromatosis

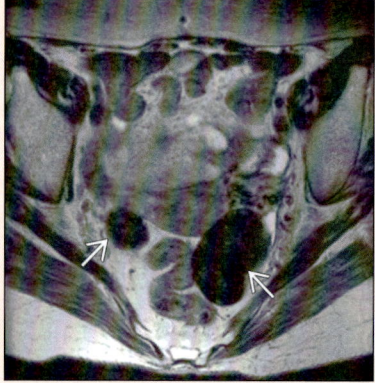

Fibromas

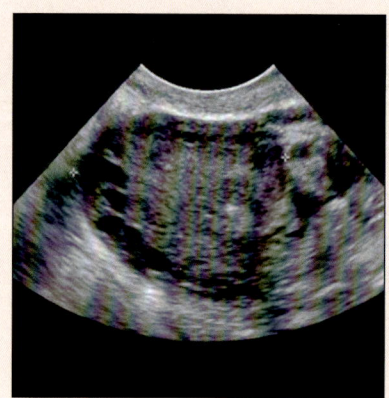

Polycystic Ovarian Disease

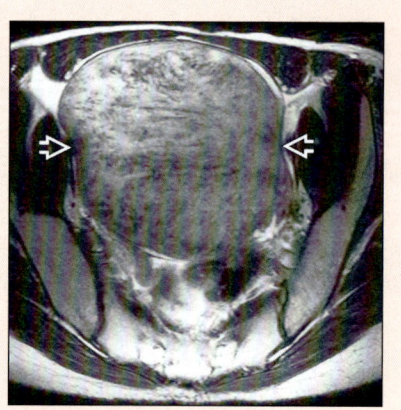

Fibrothecoma

FIBROMATOSIS, OVARY

Key Facts

Terminology
- Nonneoplastic proliferation of fibroblasts surrounding follicles

Imaging Findings
- T2WI: Hypointense mass with few follicles interspersed

Top Differential Diagnoses
- Ovarian Fibroma

- Ovarian Fibrothecoma
- Polycystic Ovarian Syndrome

Clinical Issues
- Most common signs/symptoms: Hyperandrogenism caused by the fibromatosis results in amenorrhea, menorrhagia, metrorrhagia, hirsutism, virilization
- Surgical excision: Wedge resection preferred to preserve ovarian function

PATHOLOGY

General Features
- Associated abnormalities: Omental fibrosis and idiopathic sclerosing peritonitis

Gross Pathologic & Surgical Features
- Firm, lobulated, yellow-white mass

Microscopic Features
- Proliferation of fibroblasts with bland nuclei
- Spindle cells encircle but do not destroy the normal follicles

CLINICAL ISSUES

Presentation
- Most common signs/symptoms: Hyperandrogenism caused by the fibromatosis results in amenorrhea, menorrhagia, metrorrhagia, hirsutism, virilization

Demographics
- Age: Premenopausal, younger patient population than that of fibromas or fibrothecomas

Treatment
- Surgical excision: Wedge resection preferred to preserve ovarian function

DIAGNOSTIC CHECKLIST

Image Interpretation Pearls
- Fibrous tumor-like tissue with sparing of normal ovarian structures

SELECTED REFERENCES

1. Onderoglu LS et al: Bilateral ovarian fibromatosis presenting with ascites and hirsutism. Gynecol Oncol. 94(1):223-5, 2004
2. Bazot M et al: Imaging of ovarian fibromatosis. AJR Am J Roentgenol. 180(5):1288-90, 2003
3. Frigerio L et al: Idiopathic sclerosing peritonitis associated with florid mesothelial hyperplasia, ovarian fibromatosis, and endometriosis: a new disorder of abdominal mass. Am J Obstet Gynecol. 176(3):721-2, 1997
4. Nielsen GP et al: Fibromatosis of soft tissue type involving the female genital tract: a report of two cases. Int J Gynecol Pathol. 16(4):383-6, 1997
5. Troiano RN et al: Fibroma and fibrothecoma of the ovary: MR imaging findings. Radiology. 204(3):795-8, 1997
6. Fukunishi H et al: Ovarian fibromatosis with minor sex cord elements. Arch Gynecol Obstet. 258(4):207-11, 1996
7. Scurry J et al: Ovarian fibromatosis, ascites and omental fibrosis. Histopathology. 28(1):81-4, 1996
8. Young RH et al: Fibromatosis and massive edema of the ovary, possibly related entities: a report of 14 cases of fibromatosis and 11 cases of massive edema. Int J Gynecol Pathol. 3(2):153-78, 1984

IMAGE GALLERY

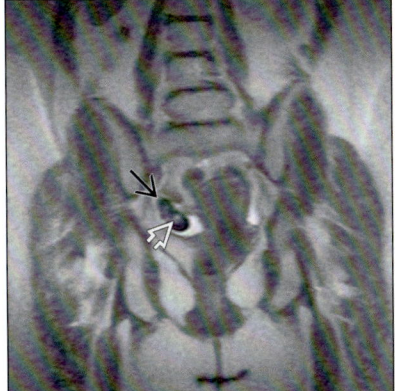 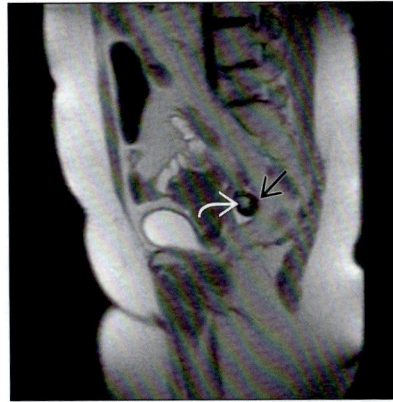 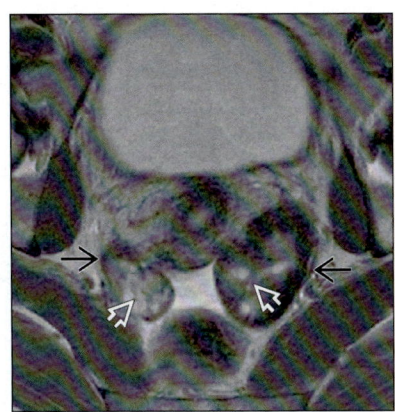

(Left) Coronal T2WI MR in the same patient shows dark signal of the entire ovarian cortex ➡ representing fibrous tissue, enveloping central follicles ▶. *(Center)* Sagittal T2WI MR in the same patient shows low signal intensity fibrous tissue ➡ surrounding a normal follicle ▶. *(Right)* Axial oblique T2WI MR shows bilateral ovarian enlargement with homogeneous low signal intensity peripherally ➡ and normal bright fluid-filled follicles centrally ▶.

HEMORRHAGIC CYSTS, OVARY

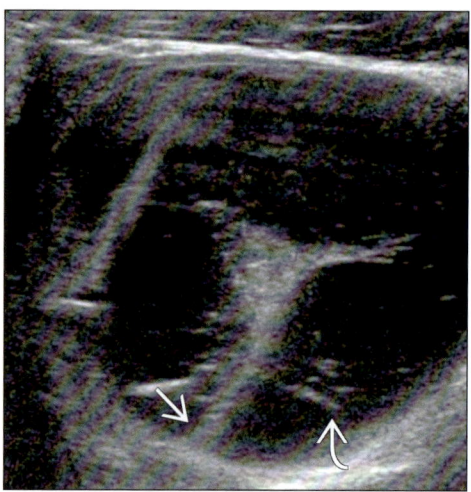

Axial transabdominal ultrasound of a hemorrhagic cyst shows echogenic component adjacent to the wall consistent with retracting clot. Note angular margins ➡ and surrounding fibrin strands ➡.

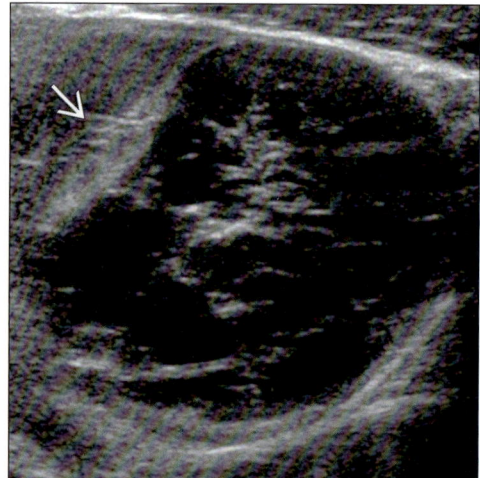

Axial transabdominal ultrasound of same hemorrhagic cyst shows linear, interdigitating echoes consistent with fibrin strands. Surrounding normal ovarian tissue ➡ is seen.

TERMINOLOGY

Abbreviations and Synonyms
- Hemorrhagic ovarian cyst, hemorrhagic corpus luteum cyst, ovarian functional hemorrhagic cysts

Definitions
- Acute hemorrhage in a follicular or corpus luteal cyst

IMAGING FINDINGS

General Features
- Best diagnostic clue: Presence of fibrin strands and a retracting clot within a cystic ovarian lesion
- Location: Intraovarian or exophytic ovarian cysts
- Size: Ranges from 2.5 cm to 10 cm in diameter
- Morphology: Round or ovoid, collapsed cyst → crenated

Ultrasonographic Findings
- Grayscale Ultrasound
  ○ Cystic features (well-defined wall, increased through transmission)
  ▪ Smooth, thick or thin wall
  ▪ Diffuse echogenic pattern ± small anechoic areas
  ▪ Fluid-debris or fluid-fluid levels
  ▪ Hemorrhagic cyst may be tender to direct pressure using transvaginal probe
  ○ Retracting clot (clumped echoes, concave or sharp angular shaped borders in the margin of lesion)
  ▪ Acute hemorrhage → more echogenic than ovarian parenchyma
  ▪ Remainder of mass → anechoic (contains serum)
  ○ Fibrin strands (innumerable reticular or linear echoes with a fishnet or lace-like appearance)
  ○ Fluid may be seen in Douglas pouch; if hemorrhagic may be complex
- Color Doppler
  ○ No flow in retracting clot or fibrin strands
  ▪ Motion in a clot may cause artifactual flow → confirm with pulsed Doppler
  ○ Ring of flow typically present in wall of corpus luteum

CT Findings
- NECT
  ○ Heterogeneous ovarian mass

DDx: Ovary: Hemorrhagic Cysts

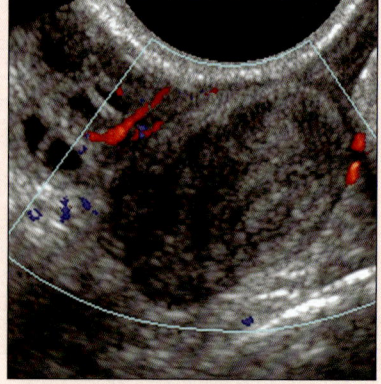

Ectopic Pregnancy

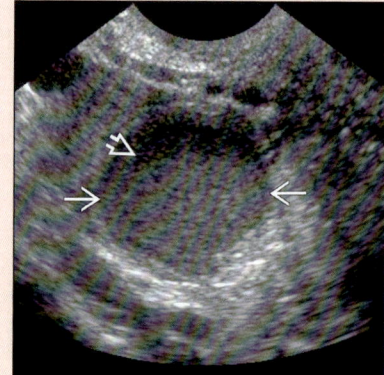

Endometrioma

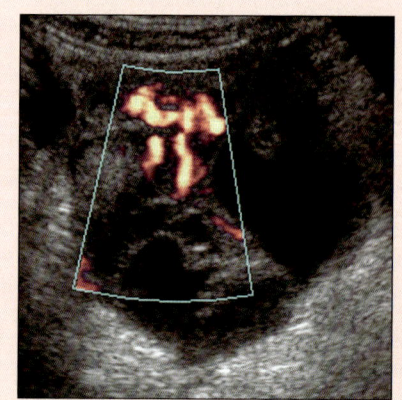

Ovarian Neoplasm

HEMORRHAGIC CYSTS, OVARY

Key Facts

Terminology
- Acute hemorrhage in a follicular or corpus luteal cyst

Imaging Findings
- Cystic features (well-defined wall, increased through transmission)
- Hemorrhagic cyst may be tender to direct pressure using transvaginal probe
- Retracting clot (clumped echoes, concave or sharp angular shaped borders in the margin of lesion)
- Fibrin strands (innumerable reticular or linear echoes with a fishnet or lace-like appearance)
- Fluid may be seen in Douglas pouch; if hemorrhagic may be complex
- No flow in retracting clot or fibrin strands
- Follow-up ultrasound → not necessary if appearance is typical and size is small (less than 3 cm)
- Short interval follow-up in 6 weeks to confirm diagnosis → safe alternative in appropriate cases
- Follow-up recommended for cysts larger than 3 cm or if not classic in appearance
- If mass persists diagnosis is usually endometrioma

Clinical Issues
- Negative pregnancy test crucial to distinguish from ruptured ectopic pregnancy
- Women of reproductive age

Diagnostic Checklist
- 90% of hemorrhagic ovarian cysts will exhibit either fibrin strands, retracting clot or both
- When free fluid with debris (blood) seen in pelvis, check up to assess for massive hemoperitoneum

---

- Hounsfield units in cystic component should be higher than water (> 10)
- CECT: Cyst wall may enhance

MR Findings
- T1WI
  - Majority (64%) → hypointense due to early age of hemorrhage and preexisting fluid
  - 36% → intermediate/high intensity in at least a portion of the cyst
  - Hemoperitoneum → hyperintense relative to urine
- T2WI
  - Majority → partially hyperintense, mostly heterogeneous
    - Up to 18% → homogeneously hyperintense (not distinguishable from nonhemorrhagic cysts)
    - Infrequently → layering or "hematocrit effect" (dependent hypointense and hyperintense nondependent components)
  - Cyst wall may be thick but usually smooth and hypointense
- T1 C+
  - Avid enhancement of outer wall
  - No enhancement of internal nodules if present

Nuclear Medicine Findings
- PET
  - Changes in the ovary associated with ovulation → can produce increased FDG uptake
    - Pitfall for staging cancers

Imaging Recommendations
- Best imaging tool: Transvaginal ultrasound
- Protocol advice
  - Follow-up ultrasound → not necessary if appearance is typical and size is small (less than 3 cm)
  - Short interval follow-up in 6 weeks to confirm diagnosis → safe alternative in appropriate cases
    - Follow-up recommended for cysts larger than 3 cm or if not classic in appearance
    - If mass persists diagnosis is usually endometrioma
    - More than 2 years postmenopause and not on hormonal treatment → surgery indicated

- Most hemorrhagic ovarian cysts are nonneoplastic
- Hemorrhage in a neoplasm is most common in benign, but cystic ovarian cancer can also bleed

DIFFERENTIAL DIAGNOSIS

Endometrioma
- Classic appearance → diffuse homogeneous low level echoes and hyperechoic wall foci
- May have fibrin strands (if there has been recent hemorrhage), retracting clot usually not seen
- Increased through transmission and internal septations
- On T1WI: High signal → chronic, repetitive hemorrhage
- Clinical history: Chronic cyclic pain or infertility
- Will persist on follow-up ultrasound

Tubo-Ovarian Abscess
- Fever, leucocytosis and pelvic pain
- There may be multiple complex fluid collections with ill-definition of ovarian margins

Ectopic Pregnancy
- Positive pregnancy test and no intrauterine pregnancy
- Pain and palpable adnexal mass
- May have adnexal ring sign
- Typically arise from the tube, not the ovary; real time scanning with gentle palpation may help distinction

Dermoid Cyst
- Echogenic mass or nodule; no flow within nodule or around lesion
- Fibrin strands → resemble bright echoes from hair
  - No change in appearance in short term follow-up
- Poor through transmission
- Fluid-debris levels

Degenerating Leiomyoma
- Exophytic, necrotic fibroid extending to adnexa can mimic a hemorrhagic cyst
- Connected to uterus and separate to ovary

HEMORRHAGIC CYSTS, OVARY

Hydrosalpinx
- Tubular morphology and mucosal pattern
- Fluid may be simple or complex

Cystadenoma/Cystadenocarcinoma
- Tumor nodule will show flow on color Doppler
- Mucinous tumor → low level echoes and septations
- Ruptured hemorrhagic cyst surrounded by hematoma may appear as a complex adnexal or solid mass
- If cyst does not change or resolve on follow-up exam surgical removal should be considered

Ovarian Torsion
- Heterogeneous, hypoechoic or solid with peripheral cysts
- May be predisposed by ovarian mass
- Focal tenderness while scanning ovary
- Absent or diminished flow
- Torsion due to hemorrhagic cyst is rare

Paraovarian Cysts
- Usually anechoic, may be hemorrhagic
- Extraovarian in location

PATHOLOGY

General Features
- Etiology
  - Follicular cysts develop when the follicles fail to regress or ovulate
    - Contain simple fluid or small amount of blood
  - Corpus luteum cysts forms on release of an oocyte in mid menstrual cycle
    - Cysts with hemorrhage are typically visualized at end of luteal phase or during pregnancy
    - May or may not be symptomatic
    - Contain variable amounts of blood products
    - Rarely complicated with massive ovarian bleeding
- Epidemiology: Women of menstrual age

Gross Pathologic & Surgical Features
- Macroscopically corpora lutea are bright yellow masses (recent corpus luteum) or white masses (degenerating corpus luteum) with a small cystic center
- Cystic and hemorrhagic appearance is common

Microscopic Features
- Histologic hallmark of recent corpus luteum is prominent luteinization of granulosa cell layers
  - Plump granulosa cells are arranged in cerebriform convoluted mass, with internal folds that contain small luteinized theca cells
  - Granulosa cells → produce progesterone, theca cells → produce estrogen
  - With the onset of menstruation granulosa and theca cells undergo apoptosis and loose their distinct architecture
- Degenerated corpus luteum: ↓ Size within two cycles
  - Luteal cells are reduced to small rounded nuclei with scant cytoplasm
- Corpus luteum of pregnancy: Persistence of the corpus luteum that accompanies conception
  - Most prominent in the first 8 weeks, later regresses
  - Characterized by enlargement of the granulosa lutein cells and presence of cytoplasmic vacuoles and hyaline droplets

CLINICAL ISSUES

Presentation
- Most common signs/symptoms
  - Abrupt onset of pelvic or lower quadrant pain
  - Negative pregnancy test crucial to distinguish from ruptured ectopic pregnancy
  - May be asymptomatic
- Other signs/symptoms
  - Palpable mass
  - 25% of patients → recurrent or prior ovarian cysts

Demographics
- Age
  - Women of reproductive age
  - Rarely occur in postmenopausal women receiving hormonal treatment but need to be followed carefully in this age group
  - Infrequent in childhood and adolescence
- Gender: Female

Natural History & Prognosis
- Hemorrhagic cysts change rapidly in appearance due to changing appearance of blood clot
- Most cases resolve by 2 menstrual cycles, one third of cases resolve by two weeks

Treatment
- Nonsurgical unless patient's condition is hemodynamically unstable from massive bleeding
  - After conservative treatment patient usually followed with ultrasound

DIAGNOSTIC CHECKLIST

Image Interpretation Pearls
- 90% of hemorrhagic ovarian cysts will exhibit either fibrin strands, retracting clot or both
- When free fluid with debris (blood) seen in pelvis, check up to assess for massive hemoperitoneum

SELECTED REFERENCES

1. Kanso HN et al: Variable MR findings in ovarian functional hemorrhagic cysts. J Magn Reson Imaging. 24(2):356-61, 2006
2. Patel MD et al: The likelihood ratio of sonographic findings for the diagnosis of hemorrhagic ovarian cysts. J Ultrasound Med. 24(5):607-14; quiz 615, 2005
3. Swire MN et al: Various sonographic appearances of the hemorrhagic corpus luteum cyst. Ultrasound Q. 20(2):45-58, 2004
4. Jain KA. Related Articles et al: Sonographic spectrum of hemorrhagic ovarian cysts. J Ultrasound Med. 21(8):879-86, 2002

HEMORRHAGIC CYSTS, OVARY

IMAGE GALLERY

Typical

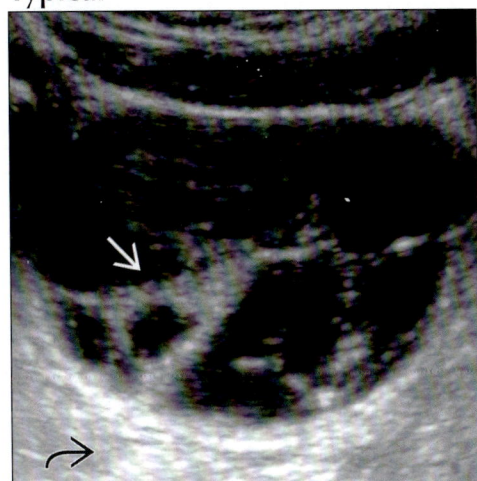
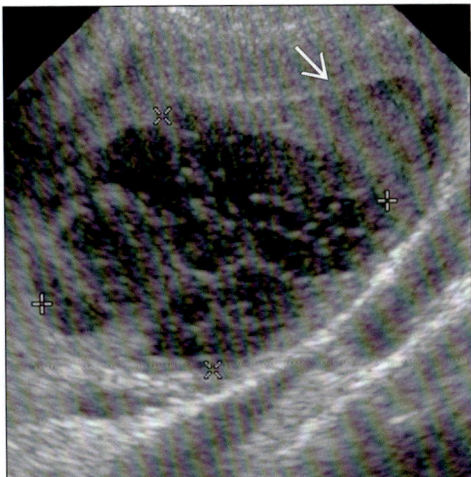

(Left) Axial transabdominal ultrasound shows cyst with retracting clot ➡ adjacent to wall, linear borders, and apparent septations. Note increased through transmission ➡. *(Right)* Longitudinal transvaginal ultrasound shows hemorrhagic cyst (calipers) with fine interdigitating strands. Normal ovarian tissue ➡ is visualized superiorly.

Typical

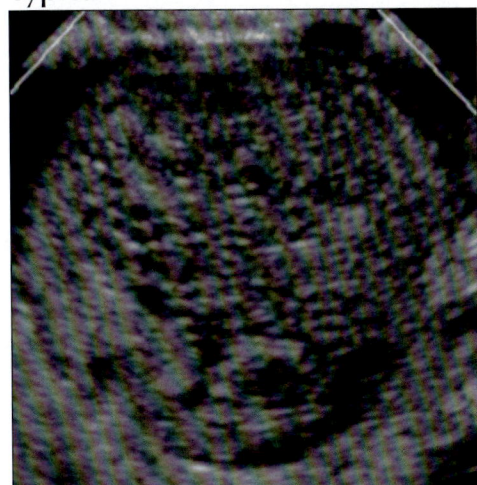
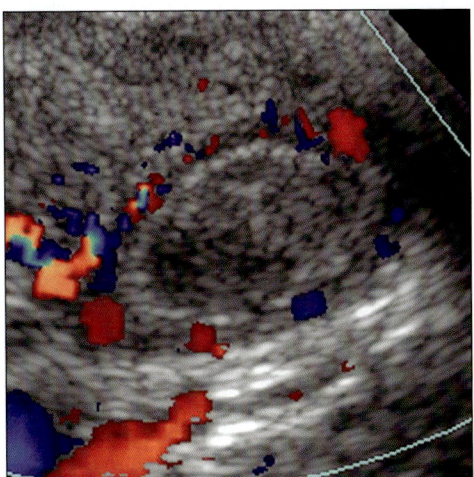

(Left) Transverse transvaginal ultrasound shows slightly heterogeneous cyst with multiple low level echoes. *(Right)* Transvaginal ultrasound shows small hemorrhagic ovarian cyst with increased echogenicity peripherally, which was originally mistaken for a dermoid. The cyst resolved on follow-up exam.

Typical

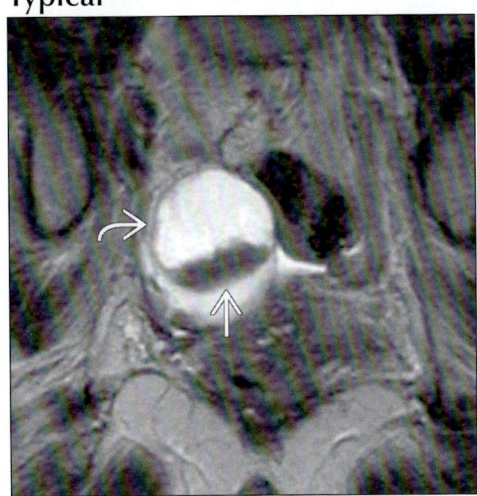
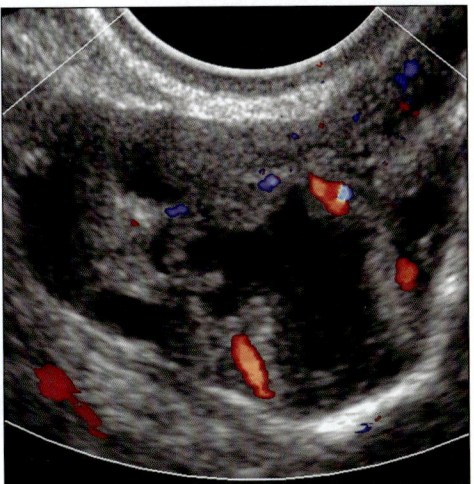

(Left) Coronal T2WI MR shows ovarian cyst with low signal intensity components ➡ consistent with blood products and hyperintense fluid component ➡. *(Right)* Sagittal color Doppler ultrasound shows ovary with resolving corpus luteum with wall with crenated appearance and subtle echogenic debris in the dependent portion of the cyst. There is increased flow in the wall.

HEMORRHAGIC CYSTS, OVARY

Typical

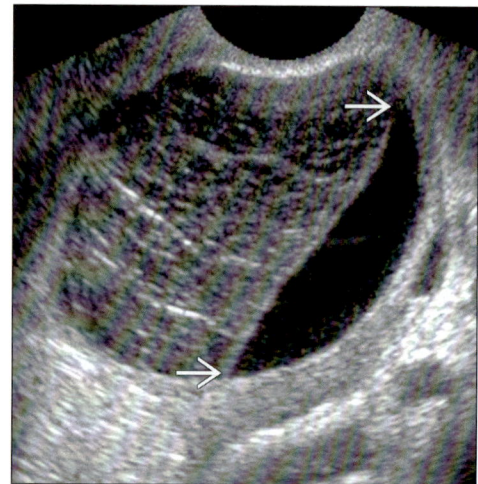 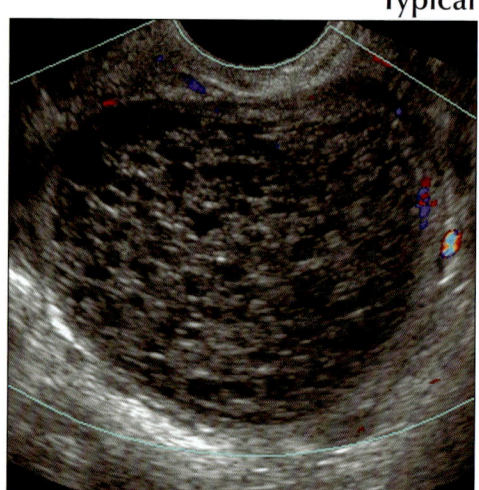

(Left) Sagittal transvaginal ultrasound shows cyst with retractile clot. Note the acute angles ➡ of the clot with the cyst wall. *(Right)* Transverse color Doppler ultrasound shows cyst with heterogeneous internal echoes and a small amount of flow in the wall of the cyst.

Variant

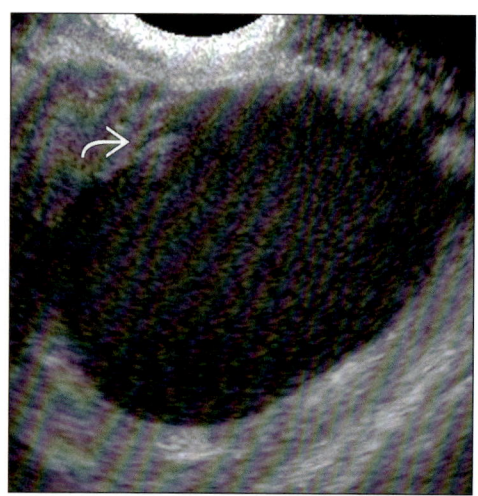 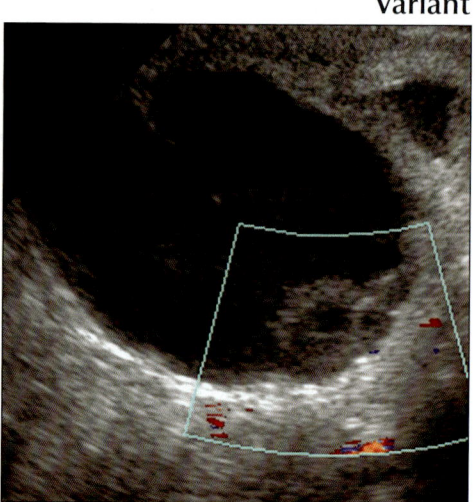

(Left) Transverse transvaginal ultrasound shows cyst with diffuse low level internal echoes and a nodular component ➡. This appearance is worrisome for endometrioma or tumor, but the cyst resolved on follow-up. *(Right)* Sagittal color Doppler ultrasound shows no flow in a solid-appearing component. This is consistent with retractile clot, but follow-up is needed to ensure resolution.

Typical

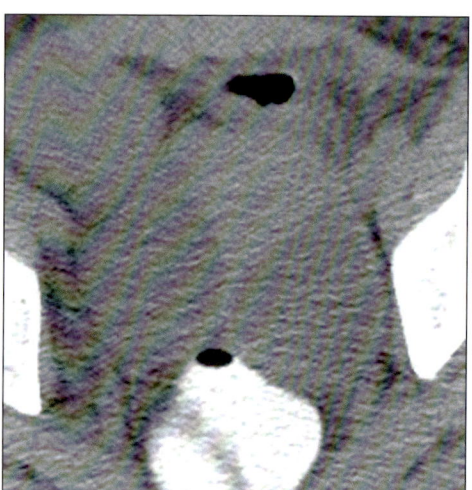 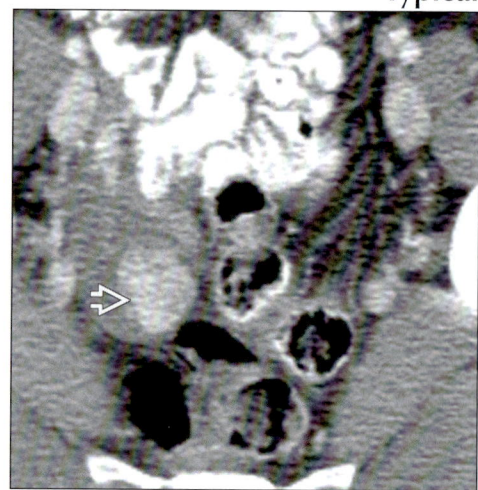

(Left) Axial NECT shows bilateral adnexal cysts with slightly heterogeneous internal echoes. *(Right)* Axial CECT shows high attenuation cyst ➡.

HEMORRHAGIC CYSTS, OVARY

Typical

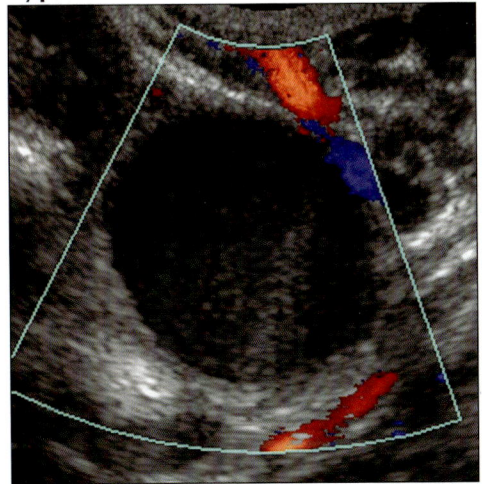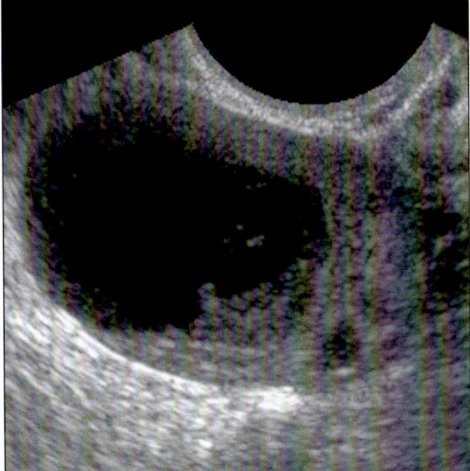

(Left) Sagittal color Doppler ultrasound shows complex cyst with hematocrit level in a postmenopausal woman on tamoxifen. This cyst resolved on follow-up. (Right) Sagittal transvaginal ultrasound shows cyst with dependent debris.

Typical

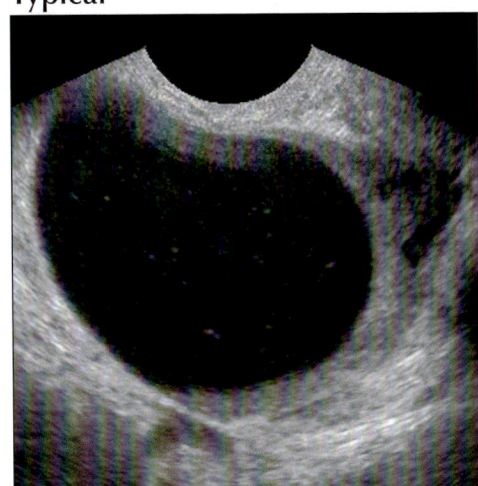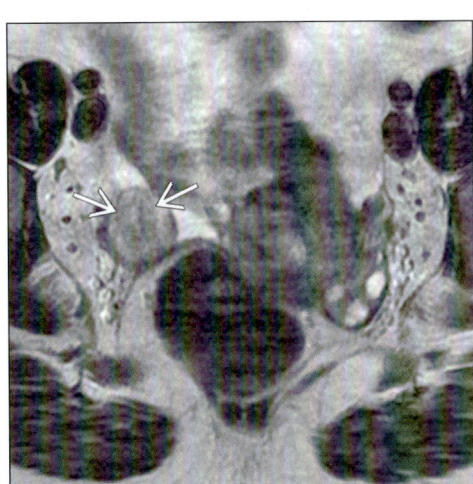

(Left) Sagittal transvaginal ultrasound shows cyst with scattered floating internal echoes. (Right) Axial T2WI MR shows heterogeneous cyst with slightly low signal intensity wall ➔.

Typical

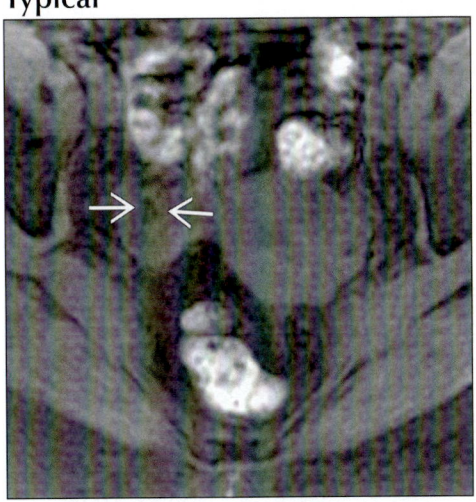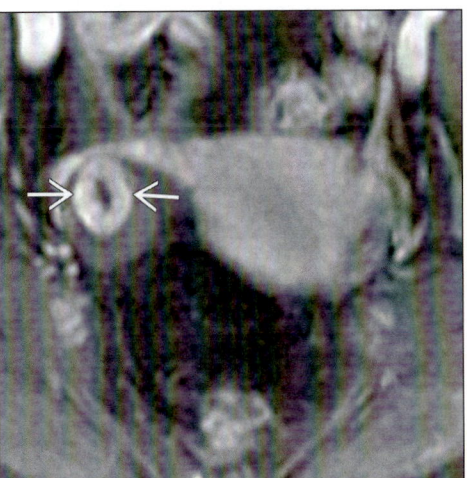

(Left) Axial T1WI MR shows heterogeneous cyst ➔. (Right) Axial T1 C+ MR in same case as previous image shows intense peripheral enhancement ➔ post gadolinium.

MEIGS SYNDROME

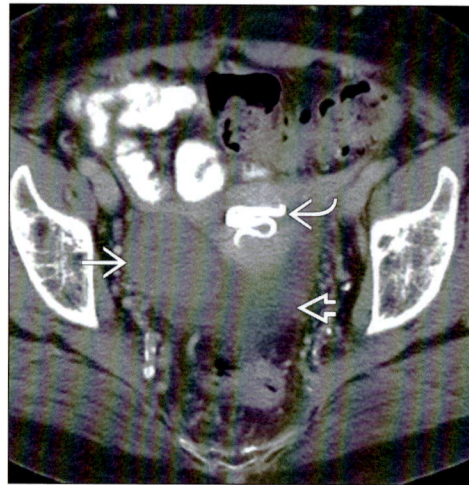

Axial CECT shows solid, homogeneous low-attenuation right ovarian mass ➡ and small amount of pelvic ascites ➡. Intrauterine contraceptive device ➡ is present in the endometrial cavity.

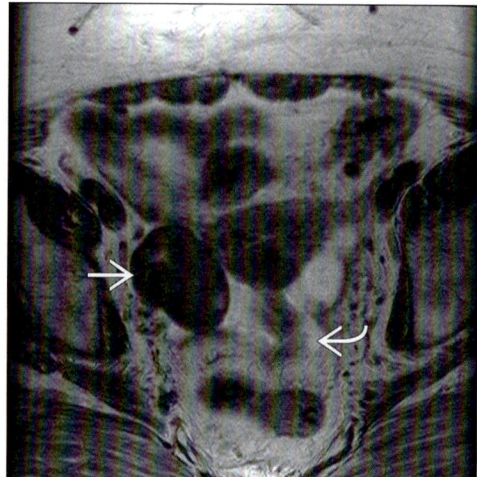

Axial T2WI MR shows a well-defined low signal intensity right ovarian mass consistent with fibroma ➡ and small amount of pelvic ascites ➡.

TERMINOLOGY

Abbreviations and Synonyms
- Demons-Meigs syndrome

Definitions
- Presence of ascites and pleural effusion that disappear after removal of a benign ovarian tumor
  - Over 80% of tumors associated with Meigs syndrome are fibromas
  - Most of the remainder are thecomas and granulosa cell tumors and rarely Brenner tumors
- Pseudo-Meigs syndrome: Phenomenon of ascites and hydrothorax that disappear after removal of any other type of histologically benign ovarian or uterine tumor

IMAGING FINDINGS

General Features
- Best diagnostic clue: Well-defined, lobulated, solid adnexal mass with ascites and pleural effusion in the absence of findings indicating malignancy
- Location: One or both ovaries may be involved
- Size: Medium to large size masses
- Morphology: Well-defined, solid, homogeneous masses

Radiographic Findings
- Radiography: Chest radiography confirms pleural effusion

Ultrasonographic Findings
- Grayscale Ultrasound
  - Well-defined masses with homogeneous echogenicity
  - Ascites is easily seen with ultrasound

CT Findings
- NECT
  - Homogeneous, well-defined adnexal mass
  - Ascites and pleural effusion can be easily detected
- CECT
  - Well-defined, homogeneous, solid adnexal mass
  - Usually diffuse enhancement
  - Central low-attenuation areas of hemorrhage or necrosis can be present

DDx: Ovarian Masses

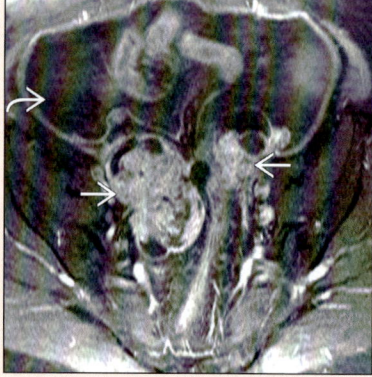
Ovarian Cancer & Malignant Ascites

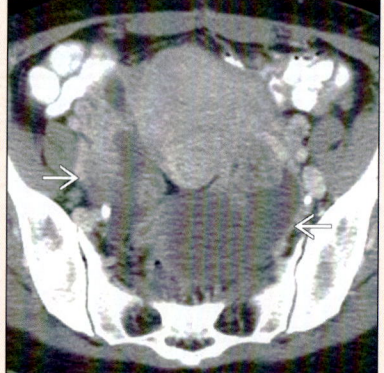
Ovarian Metastasis

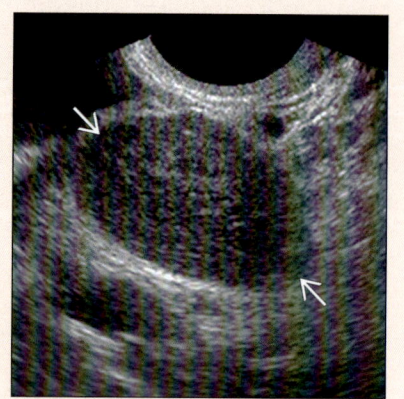
Ovarian Lymphoma

MEIGS SYNDROME

Key Facts

Terminology
- Presence of ascites and pleural effusion that disappear after removal of a benign ovarian tumor
- Over 80% of tumors associated with Meigs syndrome are fibromas
- Most of the remainder are thecomas and granulosa cell tumors and rarely Brenner tumors
- Pseudo-Meigs syndrome: Phenomenon of ascites and hydrothorax that disappear after removal of any other type of histologically benign ovarian or uterine tumor

Imaging Findings
- Best diagnostic clue: Well-defined, lobulated, solid adnexal mass with ascites and pleural effusion in the absence of findings indicating malignancy

Top Differential Diagnoses
- Pedunculated Uterine Leiomyoma
- Ovarian Cancer with Malignant Ascites
- Ovarian Lymphoma
- Ovarian Metastasis

Diagnostic Checklist
- Importance of Meigs syndrome is that the presence of ascites and pleural effusion does not necessarily indicate that a pelvic mass is malignant
- However, Meigs syndrome is a diagnosis of exclusion and the initial workup should be done to rule out malignancy
- Findings suggestive of malignant ascites (e.g., peritoneal nodules and thickening) should be carefully scrutinized to rule out malignancy on imaging studies

---

  - Ascites and pleural effusion are not associated with enhancing peritoneal or pleural nodules and/or thickening

MR Findings
- T1WI
  - Medium to low signal intensity adnexal mass
  - Ascites is of low signal intensity
- T2WI
  - Homogeneous, well-defined, low signal intensity adnexal mass
  - Necrotic component in large tumors may be of high signal intensity
  - Ascites is of high signal intensity
- T1 C+
  - Usually homogeneous enhancement
  - Central low-attenuation areas of hemorrhage or necrosis can be present
  - Ascites is not associated with enhancing peritoneal nodules and/or thickening

Imaging Recommendations
- Best imaging tool
  - US, CT or MR can be used to detect and characterize an adnexal mass
  - MR is superior to US and CT in tumor characterization due to its better soft tissue resolution
  - Ovarian fibromas have characteristic low-signal intensity on T2WI

DIFFERENTIAL DIAGNOSIS

Pedunculated Uterine Leiomyoma
- Similar signal intensity characteristics on MR
- Identification of normal ovaries suggests uterine origin
- Demonstration of connecting vessels between pedunculated leiomyoma and uterus is helpful in determining the origin of the mass

Ovarian Cancer with Malignant Ascites
- Ovarian cancers are usually mixed cystic masses
- Peritoneal implants and lymphadenopathy suggest malignancy

Ovarian Lymphoma
- Typically solid ovarian masses
- Extensive lymphadenopathy suggest lymphoma
- Ascites is not common

Ovarian Metastasis
- Most ovarian metastases are solid or a mixture of solid and cystic tumors
- Ascites and pleural effusions can be seen
- Clinical presentation is often due to primary disease

PATHOLOGY

General Features
- Etiology
  - Ascites
    - Irritation of the peritoneal surfaces by a hard, solid ovarian tumor
    - Secretion of fluid from the tumor
    - Pressure of mass on surrounding lymphatics and vessels
    - Hormonal stimulation or release of mediators by tumor, leading to increased capillary permeability
  - Pleural effusion
    - Passage of ascitic fluid through diaphragm via lymphatics or congenital defects which are more common on the right side
- Epidemiology
  - Ovarian fibroma is found in 2-5% of surgically removed ovarian tumors
  - Meigs syndrome is observed in about 1%

Gross Pathologic & Surgical Features
- Fibromas are chalky-white, edematous, hard masses
- They may contain cystic degeneration

Microscopic Features
- Spindle cells producing collagen and arranged in intersecting bundles

MEIGS SYNDROME

- Fan-shaped plaques of hyalinized collagen are common
- Varying degrees of intercellular edema may give myxoid appearance

CLINICAL ISSUES

Presentation
- Most common signs/symptoms
  - Abdominal distention due to large pelvic mass and/or ascites
  - Shortness of breath
  - Cough
  - Menstrual irregularity
- Other signs/symptoms
  - Fatigue
  - Cachexia as a result of protein loss
- Clinical Profile
  - Ascites is usually a transudate; however, on occasion it can be serosanguineous or frankly bloody
  - Pleural effusion is right-sided in 2/3, left-sided in 1/9 and bilateral in 1/4 of cases
  - CA-125 may be elevated and complicates differentiation from malignant tumors
  - Degree of elevation of CA-125 does not correlate with malignancy

Demographics
- Age
  - 3rd-7th decade
  - Meigs syndrome in prepubertal girls has been reported

Natural History & Prognosis
- Very good; recurrence is extremely rare
- Ascites and pleural effusion resolve dramatically within a few weeks to months after removal of the pelvic mass
- Serum CA-125 level also returns to normal after surgery

Treatment
- Surgery
  - Unilateral salpingo-oophorectomy in women of reproductive age
  - Bilateral salpingo-oophorectomy with total hysterectomy or unilateral salpingo-oophorectomy in postmenopausal women
  - Wedge resection of ovary or unilateral salpingo-oophorectomy in prepubertal girls
- Symptomatic relief of ascites and pleural effusion by means of therapeutic paracentesis and thoracentesis

DIAGNOSTIC CHECKLIST

Consider
- Importance of Meigs syndrome is that the presence of ascites and pleural effusion does not necessarily indicate that a pelvic mass is malignant
- However, Meigs syndrome is a diagnosis of exclusion and the initial workup should be done to rule out malignancy

- An elevated serum CA-125 level does not always indicate malignancy

Image Interpretation Pearls
- Findings suggestive of malignant ascites (e.g., peritoneal nodules and thickening) should be carefully scrutinized to rule out malignancy on imaging studies
- Ovarian fibromas have characteristic low signal intensity on T2WI

SELECTED REFERENCES

1. Moran-Mendoza A et al: Elevated CA125 level associated with Meigs' syndrome: case report and review of the literature. Int J Gynecol Cancer. 16 Suppl 1:315-8, 2006
2. Gucer F et al: Ovarian dysgerminoma associated with Pseudo-Meigs' syndrome and functioning ovarian stroma: a case report. Gynecol Oncol. 97(2):681-4, 2005
3. Kurai M et al: Leiomyoma of the ovary presenting with Meigs' syndrome. J Obstet Gynaecol Res. 31(3):257-62, 2005
4. Loizzi V et al: Pseudo-Meigs syndrome and elevated CA125 associated with struma ovarii. Gynecol Oncol. 97(1):282-4, 2005
5. Schmitt R et al: Pseudo-pseudo Meigs' syndrome. Lancet. 366(9497):1672, 2005
6. Bildirici K et al: Sclerosing stromal tumor of the ovary associated with Meigs' syndrome: a case report. Eur J Gynaecol Oncol. 25(4):528-9, 2004
7. Nemeth AJ et al: Meigs syndrome revisited. J Thorac Imaging. 18(2):100-3, 2003
8. Kebapci M et al: Pedunculated uterine leiomyoma associated with pseudo-Meigs' syndrome and elevated CA-125 level: CT features. Eur Radiol. 12 Suppl 3:S127-9, 2002
9. Buttin BM et al: Meigs' syndrome with an elevated CA 125 from benign Brenner tumors. Obstet Gynecol. 98(5 Pt 2):980-2, 2001
10. Chan CY et al: A large abdominal mass in a young girl. Br J Radiol. 73(872):913-4, 2000
11. Abad A et al: Meigs' syndrome with elevated CA125: case report and review of the literature. Eur J Obstet Gynecol Reprod Biol. 82(1):97-9, 1999
12. Giannacopoulos K et al: Pseudo-Meigs' syndrome caused by paraovarian fibroma. Eur J Gynaecol Oncol. 19(4):389-90, 1998
13. Outwater EK et al: Ovarian fibromas and cystadenofibromas: MRI features of the fibrous component. J Magn Reson Imaging. 7(3):465-71, 1997
14. Troiano RN et al: Fibroma and fibrothecoma of the ovary: MR imaging findings. Radiology. 204(3):795-8, 1997
15. Timmerman D et al: Meigs' syndrome with elevated serum CA 125 levels: two case reports and review of the literature. Gynecol Oncol. 59(3):405-8, 1995
16. Bierman SM et al: Meigs syndrome and ovarian fibroma: CT findings. J Comput Assist Tomogr. 14(5):833-4, 1990

MEIGS SYNDROME

IMAGE GALLERY

Typical

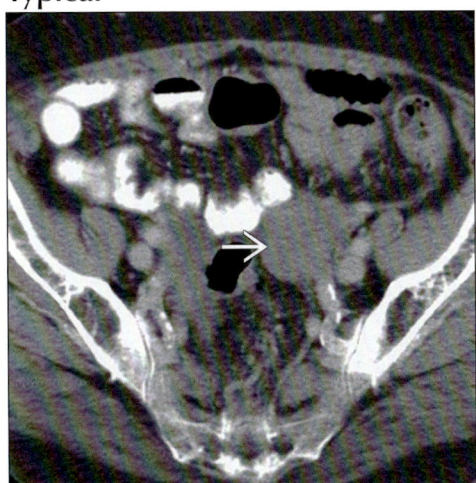
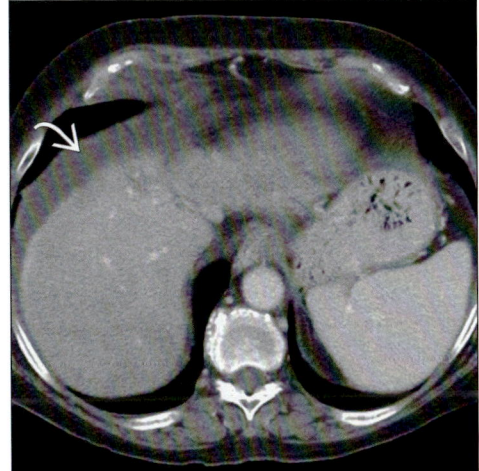

(Left) Axial CECT shows a fibroma seen as a homogeneous, low density mass ➡ in the left ovary. *(Right)* Axial CECT shows ascites ➡ in the abdomen.

Typical

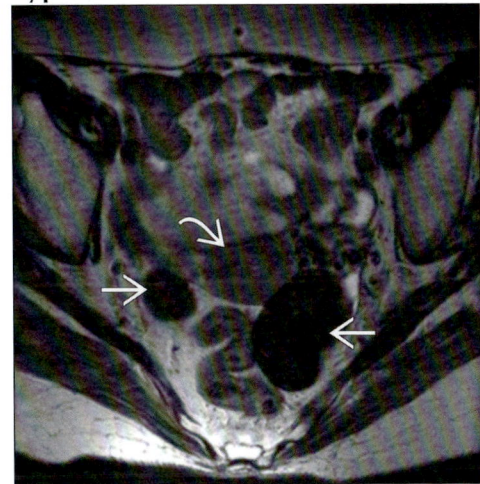
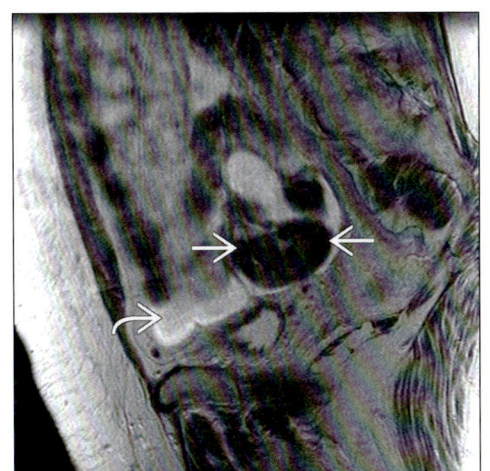

(Left) Axial T2WI MR shows bilateral ovarian fibromas ➡ with homogeneous low signal intensity. Uterus ➡ is also seen. *(Right)* Sagittal T2WI MR shows low signal intensity ovarian fibroma ➡ and pelvic ascites ➡.

Typical

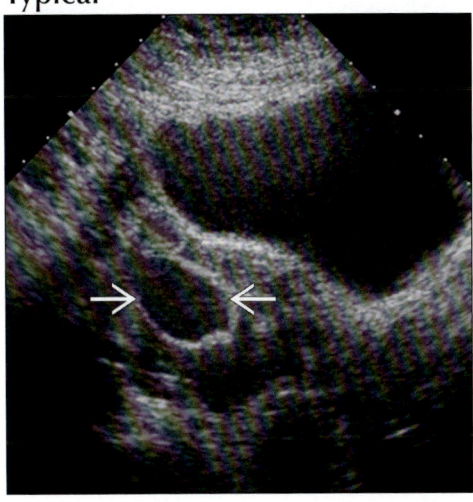
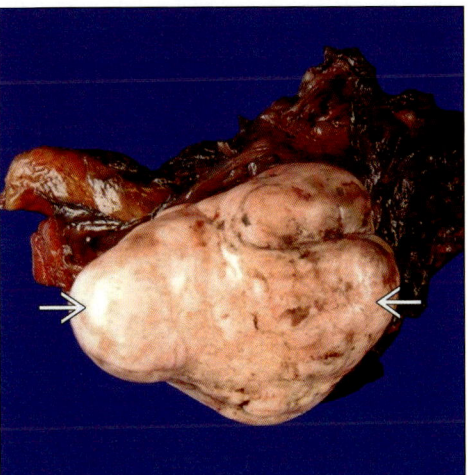

(Left) Sagittal oblique transabdominal ultrasound shows an ovarian fibroma ➡ with well-defined margins and homogeneous echogenicity. *(Right)* Gross pathology shows an ovarian fibroma ➡ seen as a well-defined, solid, white mass.

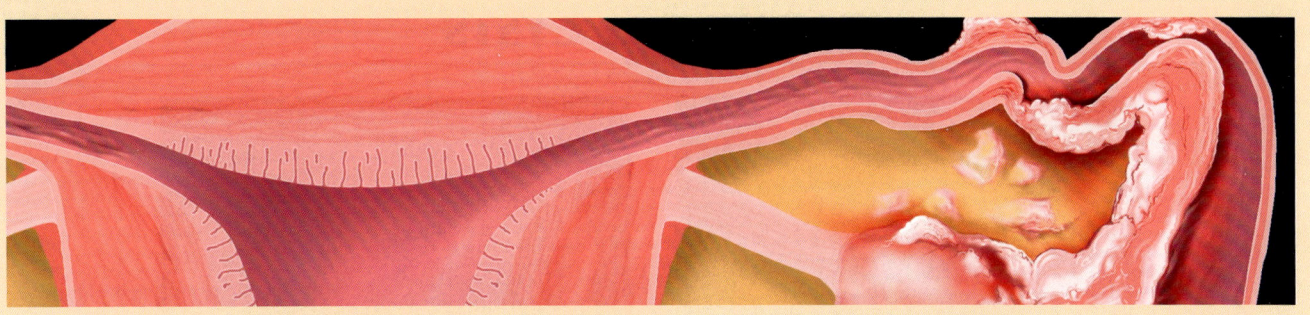

SECTION 8: Fallopian Tubes

Congenital
Paratubal Cysts   8-2

Inflammation/Infection
Hydrosalpinx   8-6
Salpingitis   8-10
Genital Tuberculosis   8-14
Actinomycosis   8-18
Salpingitis Isthmica Nodosa   8-22
Tubo-Ovarian Abscess   8-26

Neoplasm, Benign
Leiomyoma, Fallopian Tube   8-32

Neoplasm, Malignant
Tubal Carcinoma, Characterization   8-36
Tubal Carcinoma, Staging/Prognosis   8-42
Metastases, Tubal   8-48

Miscellaneous
Hematosalpinx   8-50

PARATUBAL CYSTS

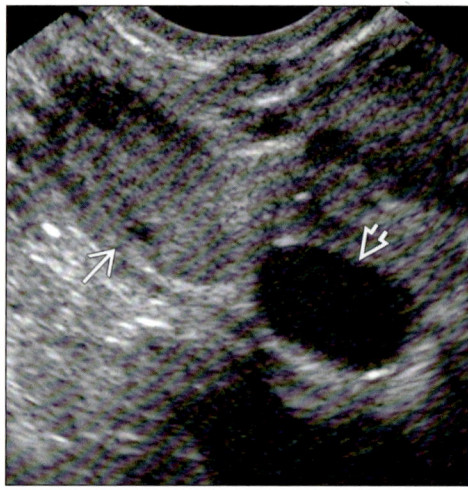

Coronal transvaginal ultrasound right ovary ➡ separate from anechoic paratubal cyst ➡.

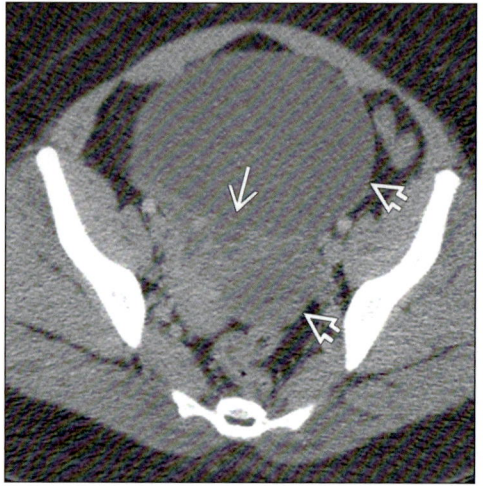

Axial NECT shows large multilocular mass ➡ in patient presenting with acute pelvic pain from torsed left paratubal cyst. Note solid component representing ovary ➡.

TERMINOLOGY

Abbreviations and Synonyms
- Paraovarian cyst, hydatid cyst, cyst of Morgagni, extraovarian cyst

Definitions
- Simple cyst lined by ciliated epithelium separate from, but near the ipsilateral ovary
  - Do not arise from ovary
  - Typically develop in broad ligament
  - May also arise from
    - Fallopian tube
    - Mesosalpinx
    - Peritoneum
    - Ovarian surface
  - Almost always benign
    - Rare incidence of malignancy (serous neoplasm)
    - 2-3% if cystic mass > 5 cm
    - Incidence much lower if cystic mass < 5 cm
  - Account for 10-20% of adnexal masses

IMAGING FINDINGS

General Features
- Best diagnostic clue
  - Simple unilocular cyst separate from nearby ovary
    - Anechoic
    - Inapparent thin wall
    - Variable in size, mean size 8 cm
    - Rare multilocular cysts
- Location: Variable, can be anywhere in relation to the ipsilateral ovary
- Size
  - Can vary greatly in size
    - Reports of up to 18 cm
- Morphology
  - Unilateral
    - Rare bilateral cysts
  - Ipsilateral ovary retains its ovoid shape
  - Unilocular
    - Septated or multiloculated cysts are uncommon

Ultrasonographic Findings
- Color Doppler: No color flow
- Transvaginal ultrasound (TVS) findings

DDx: Paratubal Cyst

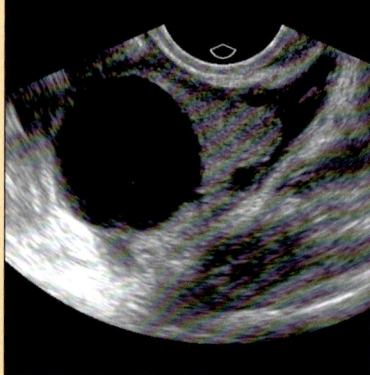
Ovarian Cyst

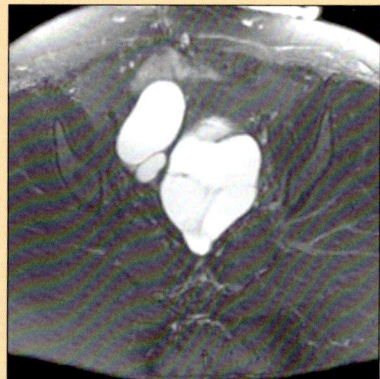
Lymphocele

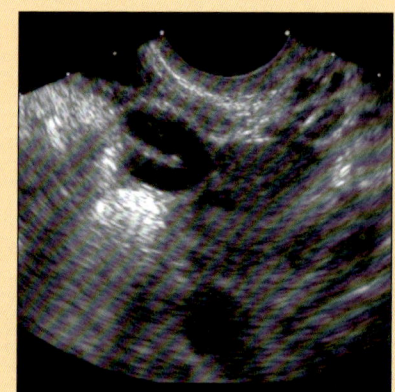
Hydrosalpinx

PARATUBAL CYSTS

Key Facts

Terminology
- Paraovarian cyst, hydatid cyst, cyst of Morgagni, extraovarian cyst
- Simple cyst lined by ciliated epithelium separate from, but near the ipsilateral ovary
- Typically develop in broad ligament
- Almost always benign
- Account for 10-20% of adnexal masses

Imaging Findings
- Simple unilocular cyst separate from nearby ovary
- Anechoic
- Inapparent thin wall
- Variable in size, mean size 8 cm
- Ipsilateral ovary retains its ovoid shape
- NECT: Not readily distinguished from other adnexal cysts on CT scans
- CECT: No contrast-enhancement

Top Differential Diagnoses
- Ovarian Cysts
- Peritoneal Inclusion Cysts
- Lymphocele
- Hydrosalpinx
- Ectopic Tubal Pregnancy

Pathology
- Paratubal cysts may arise from a number of epithelial origins
- Hydatid cyst of Morgagni is most common

Clinical Issues
- Usually asymptomatic unless complicated by hemorrhage, torsion, or rupture
- If symptomatic, may be removed laparoscopically

- Cyst contents are anechoic or may show low-level echoes or debris
- Not commonly septated
- Show no vegetations or solid components
- Thin wall
- Through transmission
- Ovary retains intact ovoid shape
- Ovary sometimes can be separated from cyst with gentle pressure on transvaginal transducer

CT Findings
- NECT: Not readily distinguished from other adnexal cysts on CT scans
- CECT: No contrast-enhancement

MR Findings
- T1WI
  - Cyst shows low signal intensity
    - High signal intensity suggests hemorrhage into cyst and/or torsion
- T2WI
  - Cyst shows very high signal intensity
    - Heterogeneity in the cyst fluid suggests hemorrhage due to torsion
- T1 C+: Cyst does not enhance

Imaging Recommendations
- Best imaging tool: TVS
- Protocol advice
  - Ovary can sometimes be separated from paraovarian cyst by gentle pressure on transvaginal transducer
  - If paraovarian cyst diagnosed on TVS, further follow-up is probably unnecessary because malignancy is rare
  - Value of ultrasound-guided fine needle aspiration of paraovarian cysts is not clear

DIFFERENTIAL DIAGNOSIS

Ovarian Cysts
- Ovarian cysts of all histologic types may resemble paraovarian cysts
- Ovarian cysts cause crescentic shape of ovary instead of intact ovoid appearance

Peritoneal Inclusion Cysts
- Also called peritoneal pseudocysts, entrapped ovarian cysts
- Requires presence of hormonally active ovary producing fluid and peritoneal adhesions
  - Fluid entrapped by adhesions
- Associated with a history of prior surgery, trauma, endometriosis, pelvic inflammatory disease
- Always include the ovary as part of the lesion either within cyst or within cyst wall

Lymphocele
- Results from expansions of lymphatic channels in pelvic sidewall
- Associated with prior surgery on the lymphatic chains, most commonly lymphadenectomy
- Located in pelvic sidewall rather than in adnexal region
- Non-mobile

Hydrosalpinx
- Usually able to clearly define a tubular configuration
- Often contains folds
- Ovary is usually outside of hydrosalpinx

Ectopic Tubal Pregnancy
- Clinical setting of positive pregnancy test
- Not anechoic
- May see complex free fluid

Pedunculated Subserosal Leiomyomas
- Cystic degeneration may mimic adnexal cyst
- Not anechoic

Fallopian Tube Neoplasms
- Solid elements are present

PARATUBAL CYSTS

PATHOLOGY

General Features
- General path comments
  - Represent 10-20% of all adnexal masses
  - Paratubal cysts may arise from a number of epithelial origins
    - Mesonephric (Wolffian) structures
    - Paramesonephric (Müllerian) structures
    - Mesothelial inclusions
    - Hydatid cyst of Morgagni related to fallopian fimbria
  - Hydatid cyst of Morgagni is most common
  - Commonly range in size from 2-10 mm
- Etiology
  - Believed to arise from embryological remnants
  - Rare in children or adolescents
  - Derived from mesonephric (Wolffian), paramesonephric (Müllerian) structures, or from mesothelial inclusions
  - Peak incidence 3rd-4th decades
  - Classically believed to be hormone insensitive inclusion cysts, however growth reported in pregnant patients
- Associated abnormalities
  - Complications include
    - Hemorrhage
    - Rupture
    - Torsion

Gross Pathologic & Surgical Features
- Simple unilocular cyst filled with clear serous fluid
- May cause torsion because arise on a thin pedicle attached to fallopian tube, broad ligament, or ovary
- Lining of cyst is smooth

Microscopic Features
- Paratubal cysts contain clear serous fluid
- Lined by ciliated and non-ciliated cells
- Atrophy and compression may lead to flattening of epithelium causing nonspecific appearance
- Uncommon benign and malignant neoplasms reported with paratubal cysts include
  - Papillary serous cystadenoma
    - May be associated with Von Hippel Lindau disease
  - Endometrioid cystadenocarcinoma
  - Serous cystadenocarcinoma
  - Mucinous cystadenocarcinoma

CLINICAL ISSUES

Presentation
- Most common signs/symptoms
  - Usually asymptomatic unless complicated by hemorrhage, torsion, or rupture
    - Sever acute pain if complicated by above
  - Larger cysts may cause pelvic pain due to bulk effects
- Other signs/symptoms
  - Postulated as a cause of infertility
    - Cyst interferes with egg transfer from adjacent ovary

Natural History & Prognosis
- Benign

Treatment
- No treatment necessary for vast majority
- If symptomatic, may be removed laparoscopically

DIAGNOSTIC CHECKLIST

Image Interpretation Pearls
- Paratubal cyst if cyst is adjacent to ovary and ovary retains ovoid shape

SELECTED REFERENCES

1. Letourneur B et al: [Management of a giant paraovarian cyst] Gynecol Obstet Fertil. 34(3):239-41, 2006
2. Pansky M et al: Adnexal torsion involving hydatids of Morgagni: a rare cause of acute abdominal pain in adolescents. Obstet Gynecol. 108(1):100-2, 2006
3. Puig F et al: Serous cystadenoma of borderline malignancy arising in a parovarian paramesonephric cyst. Eur J Gynaecol Oncol. 27(4):417-8, 2006
4. Quinlan D: Paratubal cyst. J Obstet Gynaecol Can. 28(4):275-6, 2006
5. Breitowicz B et al: Torsion of bilateral paramesonephric cysts in young girls. Acta Obstet Gynecol Scand. 84(2):199-200, 2005
6. Dietrich JE et al: Uteroovarian ligament torsion of the due to a paratubal cyst. J Pediatr Adolesc Gynecol. 18(2):125-7, 2005
7. Low SC et al: Paratubal cyst complicated by tubo-ovarian torsion: computed tomography features. Australas Radiol. 49(2):136-9, 2005
8. Salamon C et al: Borderline endometrioid tumor arising in a paratubal cyst: a case report. Gynecol Oncol. 97(1):263-5, 2005
9. Fujii T et al: Parovarian cystadenoma: sonographic features associated with magnetic resonance and histopathologic findings. J Clin Ultrasound. 32(3):149-53, 2004
10. Macarthu M et al: Laparoscopy in the diagnosis and management of a complicated paraovarian cyst. Surg Endosc. 17(10):1676-7, 2003
11. Kishimoto K et al: Paraovarian cyst: MR imaging features. Abdom Imaging. 27(6):685-9, 2002
12. Korbin CD et al: Paraovarian cystadenomas and cystadenofibromas: sonographic characteristics in 14 cases. Radiology. 208(2):459-62, 1998
13. Kim JS et al: Peritoneal inclusion cysts and their relationship to the ovaries: evaluation with sonography. Radiology. 204(2):481-4, 1997
14. Barloon TJ et al: Paraovarian and paratubal cysts: preoperative diagnosis using transabdominal and transvaginal sonography. J Clin Ultrasound. 24(3):117-22, 1996
15. Kim JS et al: Sonographic diagnosis of paraovarian cysts: value of detecting a separate ipsilateral ovary. AJR Am J Roentgenol. 164(6):1441-4, 1995
16. Athey PA et al: Sonographic features of parovarian cysts. AJR Am J Roentgenol. 144(1):83-6, 1985
17. Samaha M et al: Paratubal cysts: frequency, histogenesis, and associated clinical features. Obstet Gynecol. 65(5):691-4, 1985
18. Alpern MB et al: Sonographic features of parovarian cysts and their complications. AJR Am J Roentgenol. 143(1):157-60, 1984

PARATUBAL CYSTS

IMAGE GALLERY

Typical

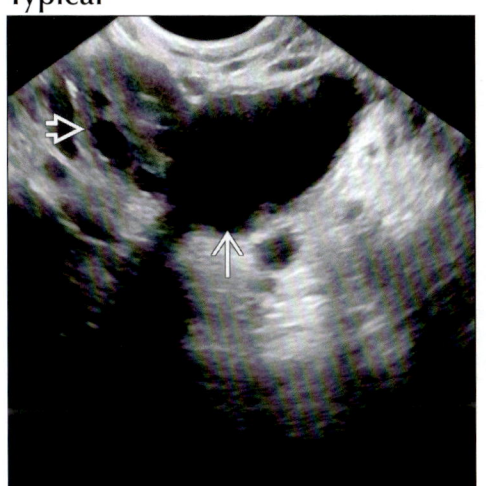
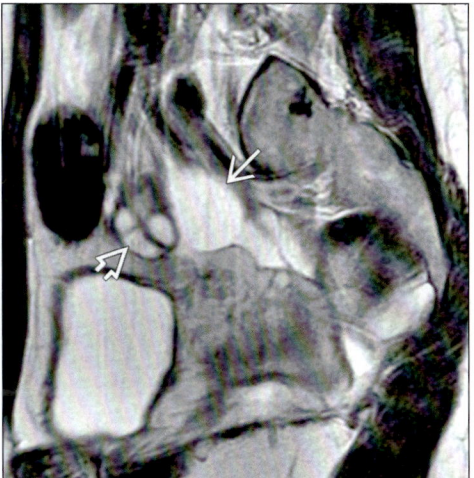

(Left) Sagittal transvaginal ultrasound shows paratubal cyst ➡ adjacent to the left ovary ➡. *(Right)* Sagittal T2WI MR shows unilocular paraovarian cyst ➡ dorsal to ovary ➡.

Variant

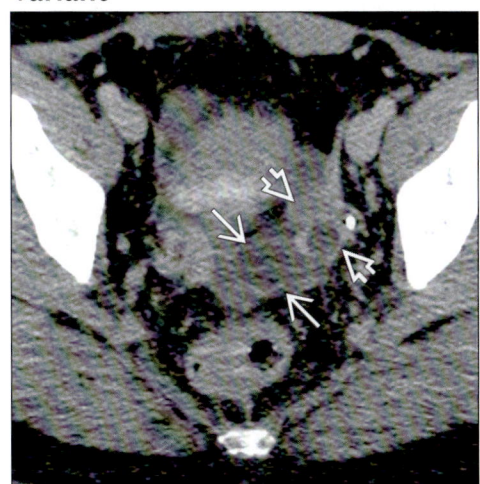
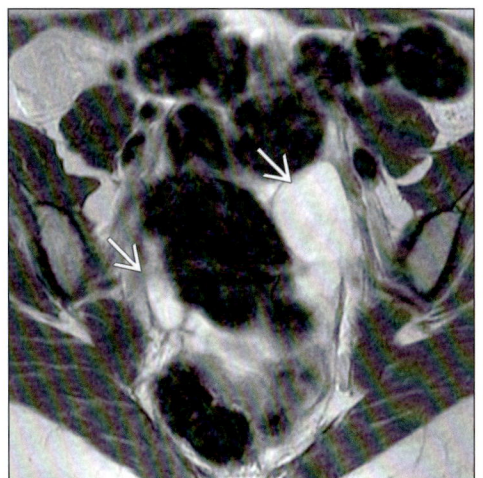

(Left) Axial CECT shows multiloculated paratubal cyst ➡ medial to ovary ➡. *(Right)* Axial T2WI MR shows bilateral paratubal cysts ➡ left greater than right containing bright signal intensity fluid.

Variant

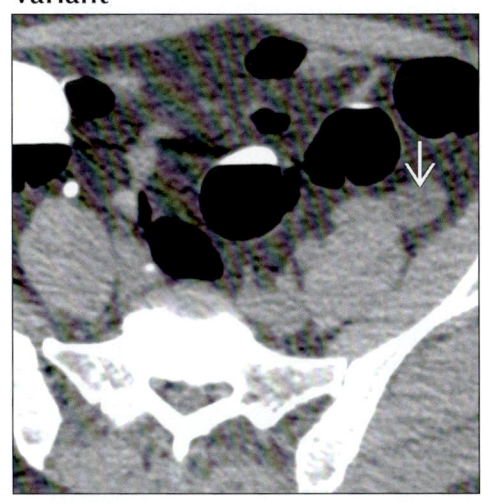
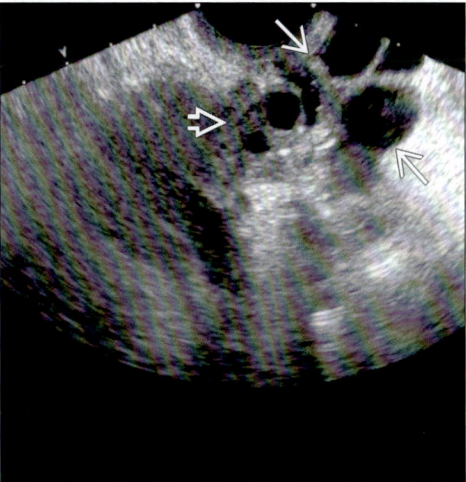

(Left) Axial CECT shows subtle septation ➡ in paratubal cyst. *(Right)* Sagittal transvaginal ultrasound shows a multiloculated paratubal cyst ➡ adjacent to ovary ➡.

HYDROSALPINX

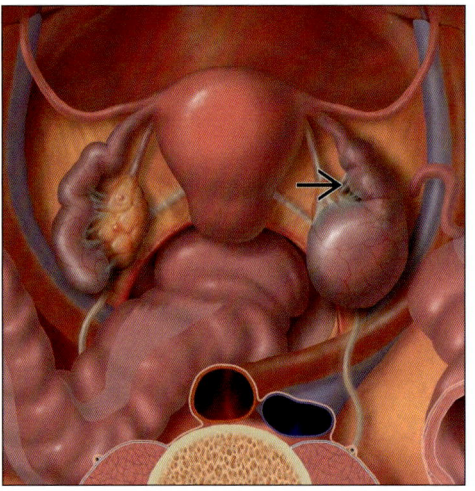

Coronal graphic of the female pelvis. The left fallopian tube ➔ is asymmetrically dilated when compared with the right.

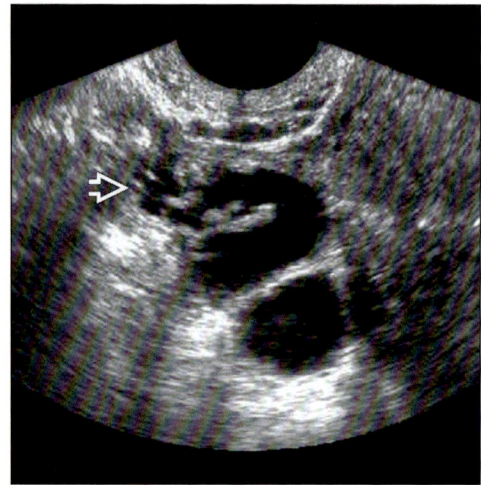

Coronal transvaginal ultrasound demonstrates a tortuous structure containing anechoic fluid consistent with hydropsalpinx. Notice the fimbriated portion ➔.

TERMINOLOGY

Definitions
- Dilated, fluid-filled fallopian tube
- Distinguished from hematosalpinx and pyosalpinx by its contents

IMAGING FINDINGS

General Features
- Best diagnostic clue: Dilated adnexal tubular structure separate from and leading to ovary with incomplete septations

Radiographic Findings
- Hysterosalpingogram (HSG) findings
  - Dilated fallopian tube(s)

Ultrasonographic Findings
- Grayscale Ultrasound: On transabdominal ultrasound may have a very nonspecific appearance and often indistinguishable from other pelvic fluid collections and complex cystic masses

- Transvaginal ultrasound (TVS) findings
  - Dilated tubular structure with folded configuration
  - May be anechoic or contain low-level echoes
  - Walls of the structure are typically well-defined and echogenic
  - "Cogwheel" sign: Sonolucent cogwheel-shaped structure visible in cross section of affected tube; the cogs consist of short linear echoes protruding into the lumen
  - "Beads-on-a-string" sign: Hyperechoic mural nodules, measuring 2-3 mm, seen on the cross section of a fluid-filled distended structure representing flattened and fibrotic endosalpingeal folds secondary to progressive fluid accumulation and distention of a blocked tube (57% of chronic cases)
  - Incomplete septae correlate with folds or kinks in dilated tube
  - Longitudinal folds may be present if not effaced
  - Thickening of tube wall > 5 mm in 3% of chronic cases
  - Should demonstrate extraovarian origin/relationship

DDx: Hydrosalpinx

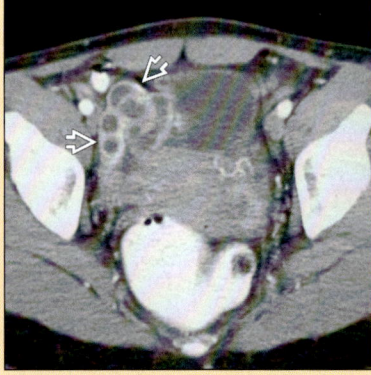
Pyosalpinx

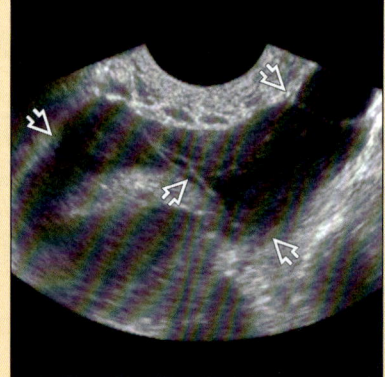
Peritoneal Inclusion Cysts

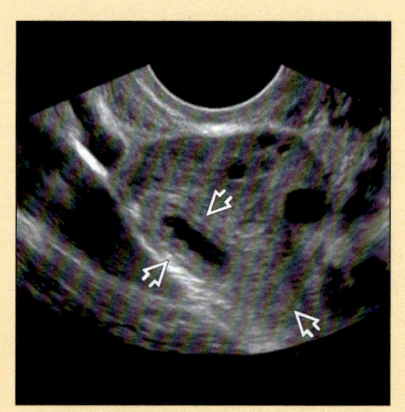
Acute Appendicitis

HYDROSALPINX

Key Facts

Terminology
- Dilated, fluid-filled fallopian tube
- Distinguished from hematosalpinx and pyosalpinx by its contents

Imaging Findings
- Best diagnostic clue: Dilated adnexal tubular structure separate from and leading to ovary with incomplete septations
- **Transvaginal ultrasound (TVS) findings**
- Dilated tubular structure with folded configuration
- May be anechoic or contain low-level echoes
- "Cogwheel" sign: Sonolucent cogwheel-shaped structure visible in cross section of affected tube; the cogs consist of short linear echoes protruding into the lumen
- "Beads-on-a-string" sign: Hyperechoic mural nodules, measuring 2-3 mm, seen on the cross section of a fluid-filled distended structure representing flattened and fibrotic endosalpingeal folds secondary to progressive fluid accumulation and distention of a blocked tube (57% of chronic cases)

Top Differential Diagnoses
- Peritoneal Inclusion Cysts
- Cystic Ovarian Neoplasm
- Paraovarian Cysts
- Appendicitis
- Distended Pelvic Veins

Clinical Issues
- Usually asymptomatic

- Presence of substantial adhesions may result in atypical appearances and even simulate ovarian neoplasm
- Can distinguish from dilated bowel loops by the absence of peristalsis

CT Findings
- Serpentine structures with internal fluid attenuation
- Enhancing walls
- Separate from ovaries
- Separate from bowel by absence of intraluminal enteric contrast

MR Findings
- T1WI
  - Signal intensity (SI) depends on tube contents
    - Simple fluid: Low SI
    - Proteinaceous fluid: Intermediate to high SI
  - High SI of the tubal fluid is significantly correlated with endometriosis in the pelvis and tubes
- T2WI
  - Fluid-filled tubular structure with relatively thin walls
  - Folded configuration: Sausage-, C-, S-shaped cystic masses
  - Thin, longitudinally oriented folds along the interior of the tube represent incompletely effaced mucosal or submucosal plicae
  - Lower SI contents have been reported in acute salpingitis
- T1 C+: Intense enhancement more suggestive of inflammation & active pelvic inflammatory disease
- Best seen in coronal views

Imaging Recommendations
- Distinguishing dilated fallopian tubes from other adnexal masses is important in the differentiation of benign from malignant adnexal disease
- Hysterosalpingography is considered the mainstay of evaluation of tubal patency, whereas laparoscopy is preferred for assessment of the peritubal environment
- MR imaging can aid in noninvasive assessment of tubal dilatation and peritubal disease

DIFFERENTIAL DIAGNOSIS

Peritoneal Inclusion Cysts
- Trapping by peritoneal adhesions of fluid that is normally produced by active ovaries
- Similar causative factors to that of hydrosalpinx
- Ovary is characteristically surrounded by septations and fluid
- In hydrosalpinx, the ovary is not surrounded by a cystic lesion (dilated tube) but rather adjacent to and separate from it
- Does not present with echogenic walls
- Adhesions may extend across the entire width of a fluid collection unlike the incomplete septations in hydrosalpinx

Cystic Ovarian Neoplasm
- Can be confused with tumor with small internal papillations and septae
  - Tumor papillary formations are usually dissimilar in size along a wall that may show variable thickness
- No tubular structures

Tubo-Ovarian Abscess/Pelvic Inflammatory Disease
- Patient symptomatic
- Usually with intense enhancement
- Contents of tube more complex
- Fallopian tube walls tend to be much thicker with surrounding inflammatory change
- Patient tender during transvaginal examination of this area

Paraovarian Cysts
- Usually round or ovoid
- Separate from ovary
- Absence of longitudinal folds
- Thin-walled

Appendicitis
- Blind-ending tubular structure contiguous with cecum and separate from adnexa
- Distinct bowel wall layers

HYDROSALPINX

Distended Pelvic Veins
- Also have a tubular appearance when imaged along their long axis
- Blood flow within produces multiple low level moving echoes on real time sonography
- Color Doppler may establish the diagnosis if flow is detected
- When flow is too slow, spectral Doppler can be performed to confirm venous flow

PATHOLOGY

General Features
- General path comments: Characterized by obliteration of the fimbriated end and dilatation of the fallopian tube, usually ampullary & infundibular portions
- Etiology
  - Caused by adhesions around the fimbriated portion of tube
  - Usually a result of chlamydial or gonococcal infection
  - 8% of patients with PID or endometriosis
  - Can be seen as a complication of anything that causes salpingitis or peritubal inflammation
  - Common component of tuboovarian abscess, endometrioma and neoplasm

Gross Pathologic & Surgical Features
- Dilatation of usually the ampullary and infundibular portions of the tube
- Tube usually contains clear serous fluid
- Most of the epithelial lining is flattened and cuboidal
- Occasional plica with intact columnar epithelium may persist
- When thin-walled, tube grossly distended with straw colored fluid which makes it appear translucent
- If chronic, thick-walled with fibrous wall, small lumen and contains little fluid

CLINICAL ISSUES

Presentation
- Usually asymptomatic
- Seen in the setting of obstruction, prior pelvic inflammatory disease, endometriosis
- Detected incidentally or in setting of infertility workup
- Its presence bilaterally is diagnostic of tubal infertility
- More complicated forms (hematosalpinx/pyosalpinx) detected in setting of infection

Natural History & Prognosis
- Depends on severity of associated conditions

Treatment
- Surgical: Lysis of adhesions, fimbrioplasty (freeing up fimbria) or tuboplasty (creating new fimbria)
- Radiologic catheter recanalization for proximal tubal obstruction (similar to angioplasty)

DIAGNOSTIC CHECKLIST

Image Interpretation Pearls
- Extraovarian tubular structure with incomplete septations

SELECTED REFERENCES
1. Patel MD et al: Likelihood ratio of sonographic findings in discriminating hydrosalpinx from other adnexal masses. AJR Am J Roentgenol. 186(4):1033-8, 2006
2. Imaoka I et al: MR imaging of disorders associated with female infertility: use in diagnosis, treatment, and management. Radiographics. 23(6):1401-21, 2003
3. Bennett GL et al: Gynecologic causes of acute pelvic pain: spectrum of CT findings. Radiographics. 22(4):785-801, 2002
4. Sam JW et al: Spectrum of CT findings in acute pyogenic pelvic inflammatory disease. Radiographics. 22(6):1327-34, 2002
5. Dohke M et al: Comprehensive MR imaging of acute gynecologic diseases. Radiographics. 20(6):1551-66, 2000
6. Guerriero S et al: Transvaginal ultrasonography associated with colour Doppler energy in the diagnosis of hydrosalpinx. Hum Reprod. 15(7):1568-72, 2000
7. Jain KA: Imaging of peritoneal inclusion cysts. AJR Am J Roentgenol. 174(6):1559-63, 2000
8. Thurmond AS: Sonographic imaging in infertility. In: Callen PW, ed. Ultrasonography in obstetrics and gynecology. 4th ed. Philadelphia, Pa: Saunders. 897-911, 2000
9. Outwater EK et al: Dilated fallopian tubes: MR imaging characteristics. Radiology. 208(2):463-9, 1998
10. Kim JS et al: Peritoneal inclusion cysts and their relationship to the ovaries: evaluation with sonography. Radiology. 204(2):481-4, 1997
11. Timor-Tritsch IE et al: Transvaginal sonographic markers of tubal inflammatory disease. Ultrasound Obstet Gynecol. 22:20, 1995
12. Atri M et al: Accuracy of endovaginal sonography for the detection of fallopian tube blockage. J Ultrasound Med. 13(6):429-34, 1994
13. Atri M et al: Endovaginal sonographic appearance of benign ovarian masses. Radiographics. 14(4):747-60; discussion 761-2, 1994
14. Cacciatore B et al: Transvaginal sonographic findings in ambulatory patients with suspected pelvic inflammatory disease. Obstet Gynecol. 80(6):912-6, 1992
15. Terry J et al: Sonographic demonstration of salpingitis. Potential confusion with appendicitis. J Ultrasound Med. 8(1):39-41, 1989
16. Tessler FN et al: Endovaginal sonographic diagnosis of dilated fallopian tubes. AJR Am J Roentgenol. 153(3):523-5, 1989

HYDROSALPINX

IMAGE GALLERY

Typical

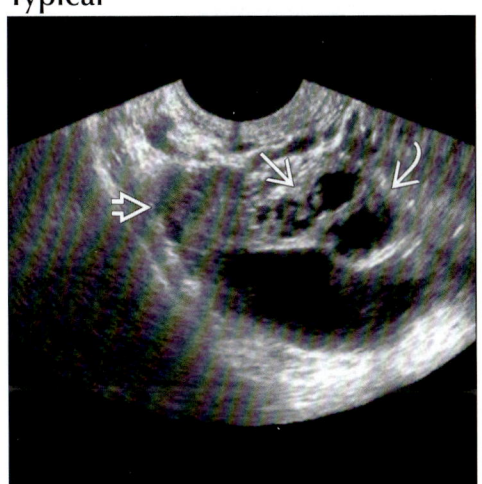
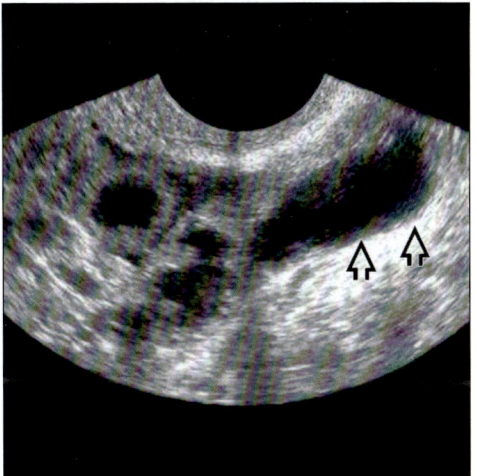

(Left) Coronal transvaginal ultrasound shows a cluster of cystic structures ⇒ adjacent to the ovary ⇒. Echogenic nodules ⇒ line the walls of the structures. (Right) Sagittal transvaginal ultrasound of the same patient as previous image shows that the cystic structures elongate into a tubular structure ⇒ in a different plane consistent with hydrosalpinx.

Typical

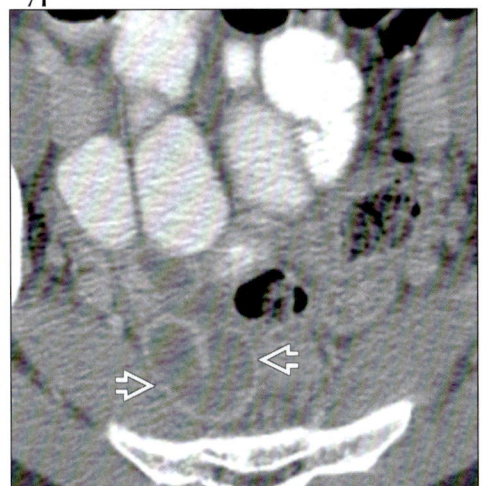
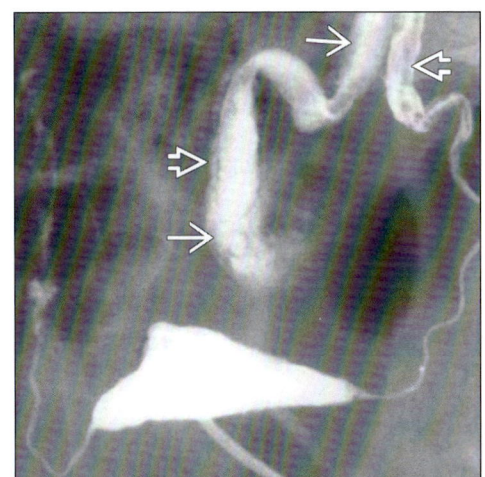

(Left) Coronal CECT shows bowel-like enhancing tubular structure in folded configuration ⇒. This structure did not fill with enteric contrast. (Right) Oblique hysterosalpingogram shows dilated left fallopian tube ⇒. Note the thin longitudinally oriented folds ⇒.

Typical

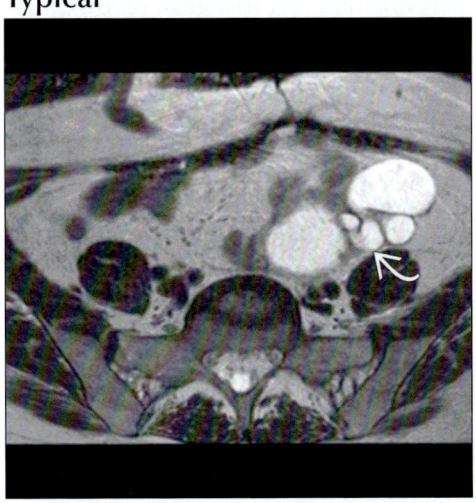
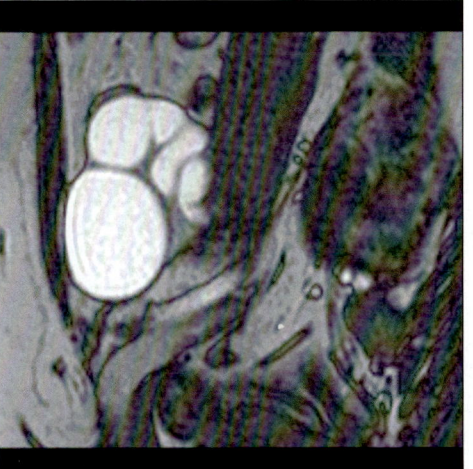

(Left) Axial T2WI MR shows a cluster of high signal intensity "cysts" ⇒. (Courtesy D. Mitchell, MD). (Right) Sagittal T2WI MR in the same patient as previous image, in an orthogonal plane, shows the "cysts" are actually connected in a tubular configuration consistent with hydrosalpinx. (Courtesy D. Mitchell, MD).

SALPINGITIS

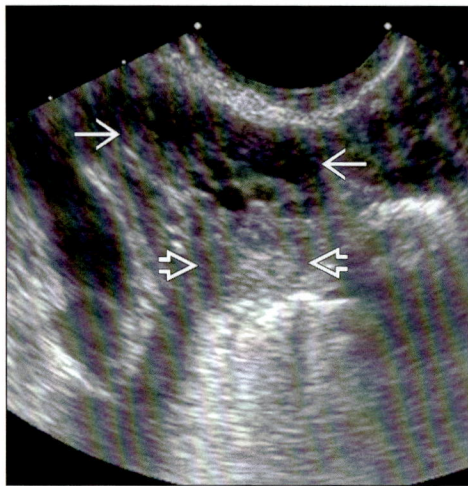

Axial transvaginal ultrasound shows a thickened fallopian tube ⇨ adjacent to the right ovary ➡ mimicking an enlarged ovary.

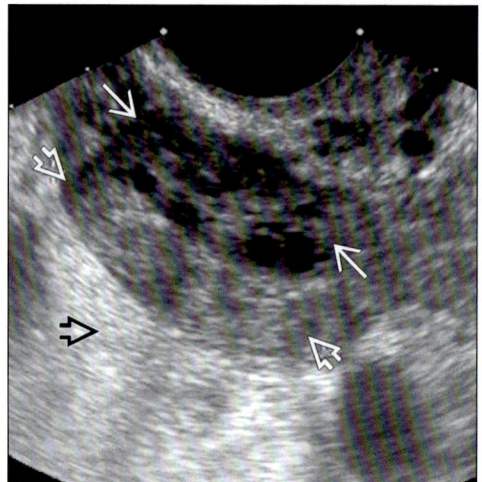

Sagittal transvaginal ultrasound of the same patient as previous image, shows the elongated fallopian tube ⇨ adjacent to the right ovary ➡. Note the increased echogenicity of the surrounding inflamed fat ⇨.

TERMINOLOGY

Definitions
- Inflammation of fallopian tubes (FT)
- Acute salpingitis is a purulent inflammatory process usually secondary to passage of bacteria from uterine cavity into fallopian tubes
- Chronic salpingitis may result from residual changes in tubes after acute salpingitis resolves

IMAGING FINDINGS

General Features
- Best diagnostic clue
  - Thick-walled fallopian tube ± fluid distention (pyosalpinx)
  - Enlarged edematous ovaries
  - Inflammatory changes in pelvic fat and other pelvic structures
- Location: Typically bilateral
- Early or mild salpingitis
  - Enhancement and thickening of FT ± hydrosalpinx
  - Mild pelvic edema
  - Haziness/stranding of pelvic fat with obscuration of fascial planes
  - Enhancing peritoneum
- Advanced salpingitis
  - Pyosalpinx
    - Greater degree of wall thickening and enhancement
    - Filled with complex fluid, fluid-debris level

Ultrasonographic Findings
- Transvaginal ultrasound (TVS)
  - Salpingitis can present as a pear-shaped or ovoid collection either anechoic or containing low-level echoes
    - When surrounded by fluid, a thickened edematous hyperemic tube can be visualized, even without intraluminal fluid
  - Wall of the collection has incomplete hyperechoic septae
    - These septae originate as a triangular protrusion from one of the walls, but do not reach the opposite wall

DDx: Thickened Fallopian Tube

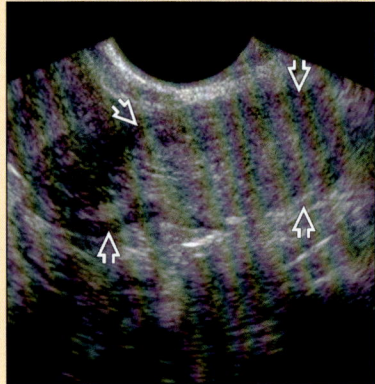

Fallopian Tube Torsion

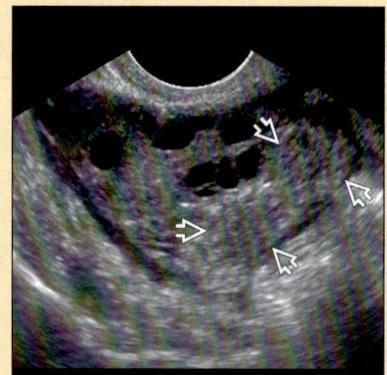

Hematosalpinx

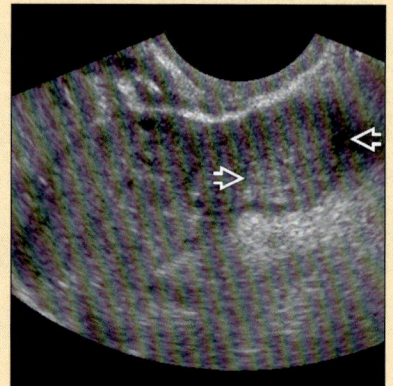

Ectopic Pregnancy

SALPINGITIS

Key Facts

Terminology
- Acute salpingitis is a purulent inflammatory process usually secondary to passage of bacteria from uterine cavity into fallopian tubes
- Chronic salpingitis may result from residual changes in tubes after acute salpingitis resolves

Imaging Findings
- Thick-walled fallopian tube ± fluid distention (pyosalpinx)
- Enlarged edematous ovaries
- Inflammatory changes in pelvic fat and other pelvic structures
- Location: Typically bilateral

Top Differential Diagnoses
- Ectopic Pregnancy
- Adnexal Torsion
- Hemorrhagic Ovarian Cyst

Pathology
- Most commonly infectious cause: Neisseria gonorrhoeae or Chlamydia trachomatis
- Three-fold increased risk of PID with use of an intra-uterine contraceptive device (IUCD)

Clinical Issues
- Fever
- Abdominal and pelvic pain
- Gonococcal salpingitis has typical onset of pain a few days after menses

Diagnostic Checklist
- Patient very tender on TVS examination

- Beads-on-a-string (chronic disease) due to degenerated and flattened endosalpingeal fold remnants
- Cogwheel sign (acute disease)
- Chronic salpingitis can have a thin or thick wall
- Pulsed Doppler
  - Low resistance flow
- Color Doppler
  - Increased vascularity of fallopian tube or wall of pyosalpinx
  - Increased vascularity of peritubal/pelvic fat

CT Findings
- CECT
  - May be normal in very mild cases
  - Dilated enhancing fallopian tubes
  - Prominent adnexa with enlarged heterogeneous enhancement of ovaries
  - Fat stranding with enhancing bands
  - Abscess, and fluid in advanced cases

MR Findings
- T1WI
  - Fluid contents: Hypointense to intermediate signal intensity
  - Abscess wall: 1-3 mm hyperintense inner rim (granulation tissue)
- T2WI: Fluid contents: Intermediate to high signal intensity
- T1 C+ FS
  - Enhancing thickened/dilated fallopian tubes
  - Enlarged heterogeneous enhancing ovaries with tiny nonenhancing foci corresponding to microabscesses
  - Pelvic, or in more severe cases, abdominal peritoneal enhancement, enhancing bands in the peritoneal fat

Imaging Recommendations
- Best imaging tool
  - TVS: Initial evaluation and follow-up; ultrasound guidance for transvaginal or transabdominal (TA) drainage of abscess or pyosalpinx
  - CT: Complicated PID, cause of pain/fever uncertain at TVS, guidance for TA or transgluteal drainage
  - MR: Differentiate an abnormal FT from a multicystic ovarian mass
- Protocol advice: On MR, add fat-suppression to T2WI and T1 C+ images to better appreciate inflammatory changes

DIFFERENTIAL DIAGNOSIS

Ectopic Pregnancy
- Positive serum β-hCG
- Generally rounded or oval-shaped, extraovarian, solid adnexal mass
- No inflammation of fat
- Unilateral

Adnexal Torsion
- Twisted pedicle sign
- Normal to diminished vascularity of adnexa
- More significant enlargement of ovary
- High signal intensity on T1WI and T2WI
- Less inflammation of pelvic fat
- Unilateral

Hemorrhagic Ovarian Cyst
- High signal on T1WI
- Little or no pelvic fat inflammation
- No thickening of fallopian tube
- Unilateral disease

Blood Filled Fallopian Tube
- Patient has vaginal bleeding
- Avascular blood filled fallopian tube
- No pelvic fat inflammation
- Particulate free intraperitoneal fluid

PATHOLOGY

General Features
- General path comments
  - Salpingitis is most commonly due to a bacterial infection

SALPINGITIS

- Granulomatous, fungal and parasitic infections can also be seen
- Etiology
  - 30-40% polymicrobial
  - Most commonly infectious cause: Neisseria gonorrhoeae or Chlamydia trachomatis
  - Three-fold increased risk of PID with use of an intra-uterine contraceptive device (IUCD)
    - Actinomycosis is the infecting organism when associated with prolonged use of IUCD

Gross Pathologic & Surgical Features
- Thickened inflamed fallopian tubes covered by fibrinous exudates and pus exuding from the fimbriated end

Microscopic Features
- Purulent inflammatory process results in cell lysis and sloughing, vascular engorgement and edema of all tubal layers
- Fibrinous exudates on the serosal surface in severe cases

CLINICAL ISSUES

Presentation
- Most common signs/symptoms
  - Fever
  - Abdominal and pelvic pain
    - Due to cell necrosis, distension of tube(s) and focal peritonitis
- Other signs/symptoms
  - Gonococcal salpingitis has typical onset of pain a few days after menses
    - Because gonococcus gains access to tubes most easily during menstruation

Demographics
- Age: Sexually active women

Natural History & Prognosis
- Salpingitis can lead to infertility and ectopic pregnancies if not diagnosed and treated in early stages
- Hydrosalpinx is one of complications of salpingitis

Treatment
- IUCD removed if present
- Antibiotic therapy
- Image-guided or surgical drainage of pelvic abscess
- Transvaginal, transrectal or laparoscopic tuboplasty in patients with infertility and confirmed tube blockage

DIAGNOSTIC CHECKLIST

Consider
- Thickened FT as a cause of apparent "ovarian enlargement" in the appropriate clinical setting
  - FT may be closely related/adherent to the ovary and as such mistaken for ovary

Image Interpretation Pearls
- Patient very tender on TVS examination

- Thickened/distended fallopian tube
- Inflamed adnexal fat

SELECTED REFERENCES

1. Horrow MM: Ultrasound of pelvic inflammatory disease. Ultrasound Q. 20(4):171-9, 2004
2. Nishie A et al: Fitz-Hugh-Curtis syndrome. Radiologic manifestation. J Comput Assist Tomogr. 27(5):786-91, 2003
3. Nishino M et al: Magnetic resonance imaging findings in gynecologic emergencies. J Comput Assist Tomogr. 27(4):564-70, 2003
4. Varras M et al: Tubo-ovarian abscesses: spectrum of sonographic findings with surgical and pathological correlations. Clin Exp Obstet Gynecol. 30(2-3):117-21, 2003
5. Bennett GL et al: Gynecologic causes of acute pelvic pain: spectrum of CT findings. Radiographics. 22(4):785-801, 2002
6. Sam JW et al: Spectrum of CT findings in acute pyogenic pelvic inflammatory disease. Radiographics. 22(6):1327-34, 2002
7. Ueda H et al: Adnexal masses caused by pelvic inflammatory disease: MR appearance. Magn Reson Med Sci. 1(4):207-15, 2002
8. Bau A et al: Acute female pelvic pain: ultrasound evaluation. Semin Ultrasound CT MR. 21(1):78-93, 2000
9. Nelson AL et al: Transrectal ultrasonographically guided drainage of gynecologic pelvic abscesses. Am J Obstet Gynecol. 182(6):1382-8, 2000
10. Corsi PJ et al: Transvaginal ultrasound-guided aspiration of pelvic abscesses. Infect Dis Obstet Gynecol. 7(5):216-21, 1999
11. Hawnaur JM et al: Magnetic resonance imaging of actinomycosis presenting as pelvic malignancy. Br J Radiol. 72(862):1006-11, 1999
12. McCormack WM: Pelvic inflammatory disease. N Engl J Med. 330(2):115-9, 1994

SALPINGITIS

IMAGE GALLERY

Typical

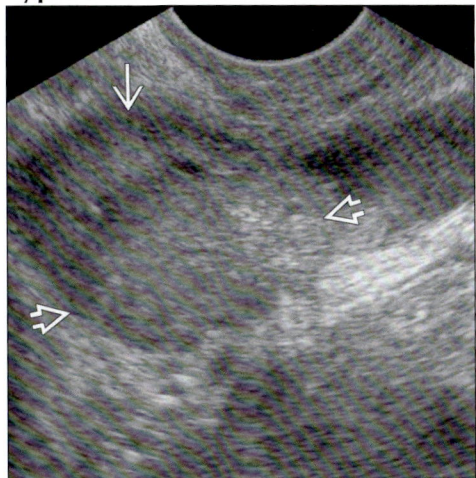
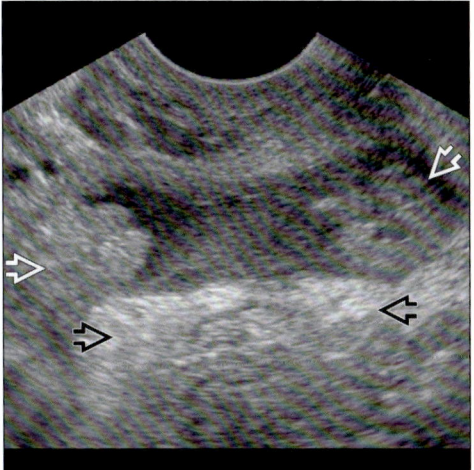

(Left) Sagittal transvaginal ultrasound shows a distended fallopian tube ➔ adjacent to the right ovary ➔. *(Right)* Sagittal transvaginal ultrasound of the same patient as previous image, shows the distended fallopian tube ➔ containing pus of different echogenicity. Note the increased echotexture of the adjacent inflamed fat ➔.

Typical

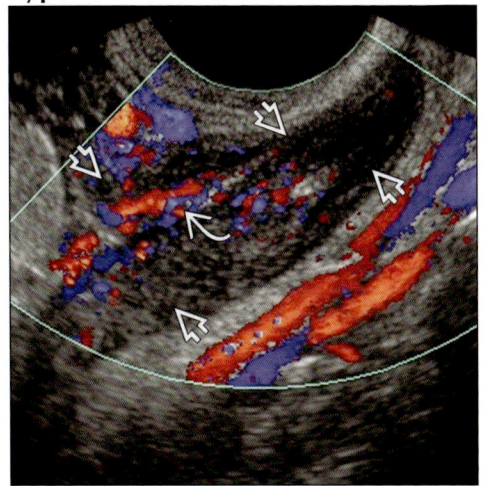
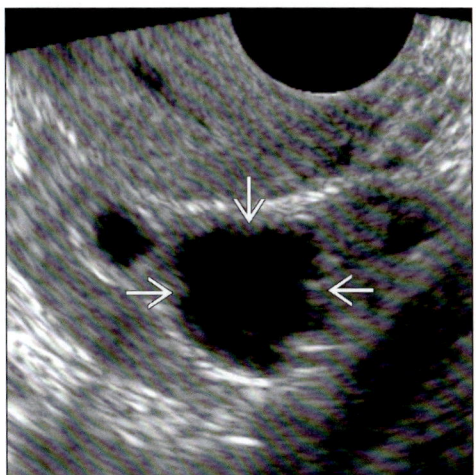

(Left) Axial color Doppler ultrasound shows increased vascularity ➔ of the thickened fallopian tube ➔. *(Right)* Transvaginal ultrasound shows beads-on-a-string appearance due to degenerated and flattened endosalpingeal fold remnants ➔ in a patient with chronic salpingitis.

Typical

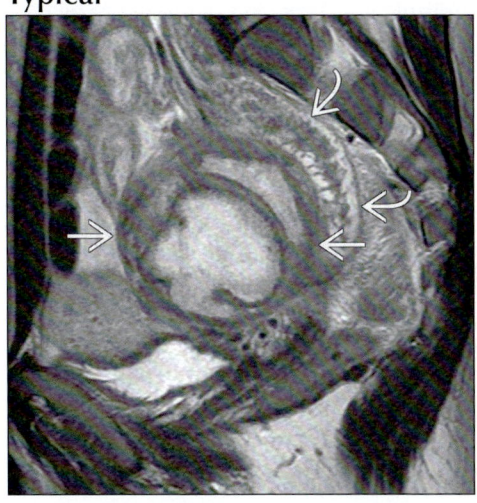
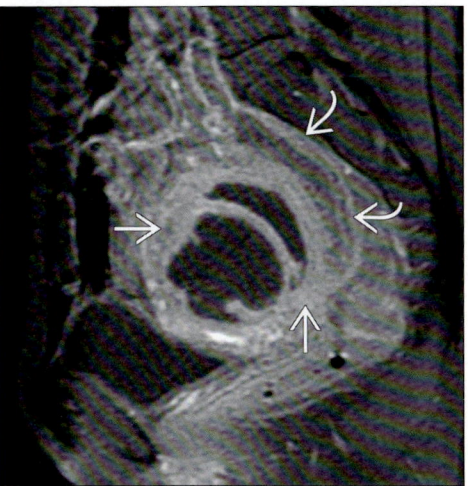

(Left) Sagittal T2WI MR shows a multiloculated cystic mass ➔ compressing a thick-walled inflamed sigmoid colon ➔. This represents a tubo-ovarian abscess encompassing a folded pyosalpinx. *(Right)* Sagittal T1 C+ FS MR shows significant enhancement of the non-cystic components ➔ of the mass seen on the left. Note enhancement of the rectosigmoid wall ➔ and pelvic fat.

GENITAL TUBERCULOSIS

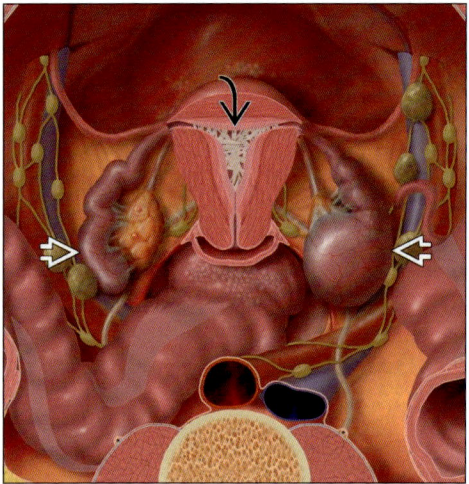

Frontal graphic shows evidence of genital TB with bilateral hydrosalpinges, peritubal adhesions and endometrial synechiae. Enlarged lymph nodes are also present.

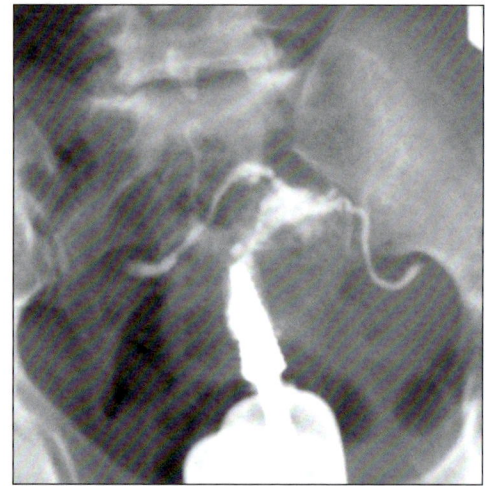

Frontal hysterosalpingogram shows a featureless appearance of the fallopian tubes without peritoneal spillage. The endometrial cavity is irregular consistent with multiple synechiae. (Courtesy A. Lotfy, MD).

TERMINOLOGY

Abbreviations and Synonyms
- Female genital tuberculosis (TB), TB pelvic inflammatory disease (TB PID), TB salpingitis

Definitions
- Involvement of female genital tract by Mycobacterium Tuberculosis

IMAGING FINDINGS

General Features
- Best diagnostic clue
  - Klein diagnostic criteria
    - Calcified nodes or small, irregular calcifications in adnexal area
    - Obstruction of FT in zone of transition between isthmus and ampulla
    - Multiple FT constrictions (beading)
    - Endometrial adhesion ± deformity or obliteration of endometrial cavity
- Location
  - Involvement typically bilateral
  - FT most common (95%), endometrium (60-70%), peritoneum (50%), ovary (15%), cervix (5%)
- Tubo-ovarian abscesses: Bilateral complex cystic and solid adnexal masses ± calcification
  - May extend through peritoneum into extraperitoneal compartment
- Endometritis (60%)
  - Diffuse endometrial thickening
  - Fluid within endometrial cavity
  - Synechiae
- Peritonitis (50%)
  - "Wet-type" with ascites most common (90%)
    - Large amounts of free or loculated fluid
    - Transudate early on, becomes complex later
  - "Dry or plastic type" peritonitis least frequent (10%)
- "Omental cake" or nodular infiltration of omentum
- Mesenteric mass with "stellate appearance"
- Lymphadenopathy: More common with abdominal TB
  - Typically multiple and large, 2-3 cm in diameter
- Bowel wall thickening, strictures and fistula formation

Radiographic Findings
- Radiography

DDx: Genital Tuberculosis

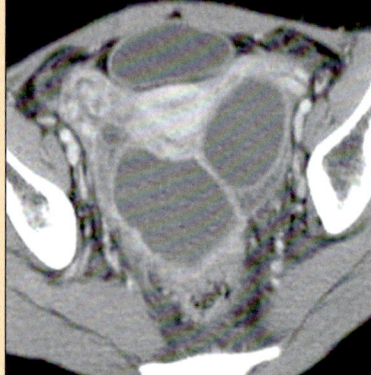

Acute Pelvic Inflammatory Disease

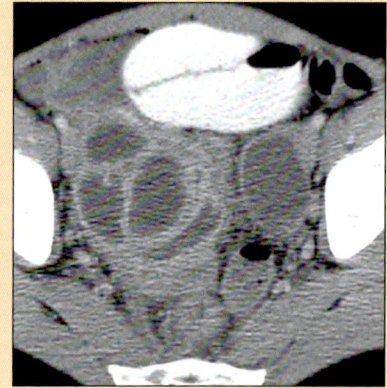

Actinomycosis

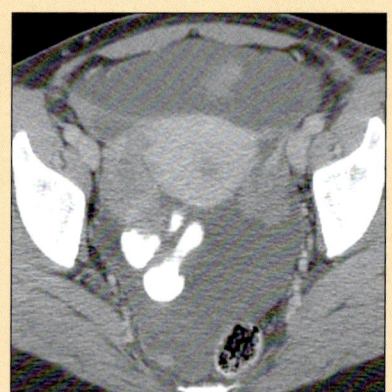

Ovarian Carcinoma

GENITAL TUBERCULOSIS

Key Facts

Terminology
- Involvement of female genital tract by Mycobacterium Tuberculosis

Imaging Findings
- Calcified nodes or small, irregular calcifications in adnexal area
- Multiple FT constrictions (beading)
- Tubo-ovarian abscesses: Bilateral complex cystic and solid adnexal masses ± calcification
- May extend through peritoneum into extraperitoneal compartment
- Fluid within endometrial cavity
- Peritonitis (50%)
- "Omental cake" or nodular infiltration of omentum
- Lymphadenopathy common
- HSG best modality for evaluating FT patency and morphology

Top Differential Diagnoses
- PID/Actinomycosis
- Ovarian Carcinoma

Clinical Issues
- Most common signs/symptoms: Infertility
- CA-125 may be significantly elevated due to peritoneal inflammation

Diagnostic Checklist
- Consider TB in the setting of bilateral complex cystic adnexal masses with obliteration of pelvic fat planes, lymphadenopathy and peritoneal disease

---

- Healed or active pulmonary TB on chest radiograph
  - Normal chest radiograph in up to 75% of cases
- Hysterosalpingography (HSG)
  - Tubal obstructive findings most common, mainly at isthmus and ampulla
    - Flask-shaped dilation with obstruction at fimbriae
  - Non-obstructive tubal changes
    - "Tufted" appearance of ampulla due to surrounding diverticular cavities
    - Multiple FT constrictions: "Beaded" appearance
    - Featureless "rigid pipe stem" appearance
  - Peritubal adhesions
    - Convoluted or corkscrew FT, loculated spillage of contrast material
  - Endometrial tuberculosis
    - Irregular and stellate synechiae with well-demarcated borders
    - "Pseudounicornuate" uterus due to obliteration of cavity on one side

Ultrasonographic Findings
- Grayscale Ultrasound
  - Dilated FT with thickened wall, containing simple or echogenic fluid
  - Mixed echogenicity solid or complex cystic adnexal masses
  - Endometrial thickening ± fluid (anechoic to echogenic)
    - Synechiae: Echogenic bands traversing cavity
  - Peritoneal/omental/mesenteric disease
    - Hypoechoic nodules/masses
  - Lymphadenopathy typically hypoechoic, with echogenic centers due to caseation necrosis

CT Findings
- NECT: Superior for demonstrating calcification of FTs, ovaries, and periadnexal nodes
- CECT
  - Dilated FT with simple or dense fluid (25-45 HU)
    - Tubal wall thickened showing marked enhancement
  - Mixed density solid/complex cystic adnexal masses
  - Characteristic high-density (20-45 HU) ascites
    - Multiloculated collections in cul-de-sac
  - Thickening and nodularity of the peritoneal surfaces, mesentery, omentum, bowel wall
    - Nodular peritoneal enhancement
    - "Omental cake" or nodular infiltration
    - "Stellate appearance" of mesenteric mass due to fixing of bowel and mesentery
  - Lymphadenopathy common
    - Typical: Peripheral rim-enhancement of enlarged nodes with hypodense centers
    - Less common: Homogeneous, low-density nodes
  - Inflammatory changes including thickening of ligaments and obliteration of fat planes

MR Findings
- T1WI
  - Multiloculated cystic adnexal masses
    - Irregularly thickened walls/septa of intermediate to high signal intensity (SI)
  - Hydrosalpinx of variable SI: Intermediate to high
- T2WI
  - Multiloculated cystic adnexal masses
    - Irregularly thickened walls/septa of low SI
    - Fluid contents variable: Intermediate to high SI
  - Predominantly solid adnexal masses
    - Mottled high SI (caseation) on background of low SI (dense fibrosis)
  - Diffusely thickened, iso- to hypointense endometrium
    - Pyometra: Intermediate to high SI
    - Synechiae: Low SI bands traversing cavity
  - Intermediate SI of plaque-like or nodular peritoneal deposits
  - Majority of enlarged nodes demonstrating high SI due to liquefactive necrosis/caseation
    - Obliteration of perinodal fat with high SI due to capsular disruption
    - Central nodal hypointensity due to paramagnetic free radicals of active phagocytic cells
- T1 C+
  - Marked enhancement of walls/septa of adnexal masses with inner wall serration/nodularity
  - Avidly enhancing, thickened endometrium ± fluid

GENITAL TUBERCULOSIS

- Peripheral lymph node enhancement most common
  - Highly vascular perinodal inflammatory response
  - Homogeneous, heterogeneous or no nodal enhancement less common

Imaging Recommendations
- Best imaging tool
  - HSG best modality for evaluating FT patency and morphology
  - CT optimal for showing peritoneal, omental, mesenteric and nodal disease
  - Transvaginal ultrasound and MR best for characterizing adnexal masses

DIFFERENTIAL DIAGNOSIS

PID/Actinomycosis
- No significant lymphadenopathy, peritoneal involvement or calcification
- History of long-standing IUD use in patients with pelvic actinomycosis

Ovarian Carcinoma
- Tubal pathology not a predominant feature
- Coarse calcification typically absent
- Inflammatory changes not present

PATHOLOGY

General Features
- Etiology: Hematogenous spread from primary TB site
- Epidemiology
  - 5-15% of patients with pulmonary TB
  - Frequent and important cause of chronic PID and infertility in developing countries
  - Rare disease in developed countries, incidence on the rise

Gross Pathologic & Surgical Features
- Miliary tubercles on the serosal surface
- Rarely Fitz-Hugh-Curtis syndrome (perihepatitis with violin-string adhesions)

Microscopic Features
- Tubercle formation in tubal wall and mucosa
  - Granulomas composed of epithelioid histiocytes with or without langhan giant cells
- Caseation in advanced cases, followed by fibrosis in later stages

CLINICAL ISSUES

Presentation
- Most common signs/symptoms: Infertility
- Other signs/symptoms
  - Pelvic pain, fever, dysmenorrhea, dyspareunia
  - Abnormal bleeding most common symptom in postmenopausal women
  - Up to 11% of patients asymptomatic
- Clinical Profile
  - Laboratory findings: Leukocytosis, positive Tuberculin test, elevated ESR
  - CA-125 may be significantly elevated due to peritoneal inflammation

Demographics
- Age
  - Most common between 26-35 years in developing countries
  - Most patients older than 40 years in developed countries

Natural History & Prognosis
- Poor rate of successful pregnancy after treatment
  - 28.6% success rate with in vitro fertilization
- Increased risk of ectopic pregnancy

Treatment
- Excellent response to multi-drug regimen
- Surgery for fistulae and large tubo-ovarian abscesses
- Total abdominal hysterectomy and bilateral salpingo-oophorectomy
  - Indicated with persistent disease

DIAGNOSTIC CHECKLIST

Consider
- Consider TB in the setting of bilateral complex cystic adnexal masses with obliteration of pelvic fat planes, lymphadenopathy and peritoneal disease

Image Interpretation Pearls
- Beading of FT ± calcification

SELECTED REFERENCES

1. Kitajima K et al: Magnetic resonance imaging findings of tuberculous endometritis: a report of 2 cases. J Comput Assist Tomogr. 30(1):62-4, 2006
2. De Backer A et al: Female genital tract tuberculosis with peritoneal involvement: CT and MR imaging features. European Journal of Radiology Extra. 53(2):71-5, 2005
3. De Backer AI et al: Abdominal tuberculous lymphadenopathy: MRI features. Eur Radiol. 15(10):2104-9, 2005
4. Hassoun A et al: Female genital tuberculosis: uncommon presentation of tuberculosis in the United States. Am J Med. 118(11):1295-6, 2005
5. Matos MJ et al: Genitourinary tuberculosis. Eur J Radiol. 55(2):181-7, 2005
6. Chavhan GB et al: Female genital tuberculosis: hysterosalpingographic appearances. Br J Radiol. 77(914):164-9, 2004
7. Kim SH et al: Unusual causes of tubo-ovarian abscess: CT and MR imaging findings. Radiographics. 24(6):1575-89, 2004
8. Vanhoenacker FM et al: Imaging of gastrointestinal and abdominal tuberculosis. Eur Radiol. 14 Suppl 3:E103-15, 2004
9. Sharma JB et al: Fitz-Hugh-Curtis syndrome as a result of genital tuberculosis: a report of three cases. Acta Obstet Gynecol Scand. 82(3):295-7, 2003
10. Palmer V: The imaging of tuberculosis with epidemiological, pathological and clinical correlation. Springer-Verlag, Berlin, Germany. 67-83, 2002

GENITAL TUBERCULOSIS

IMAGE GALLERY

Typical

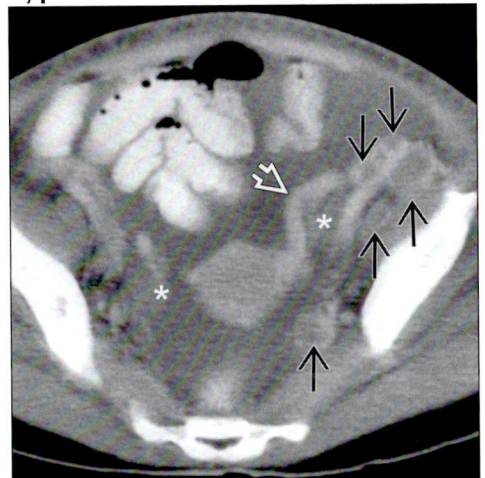
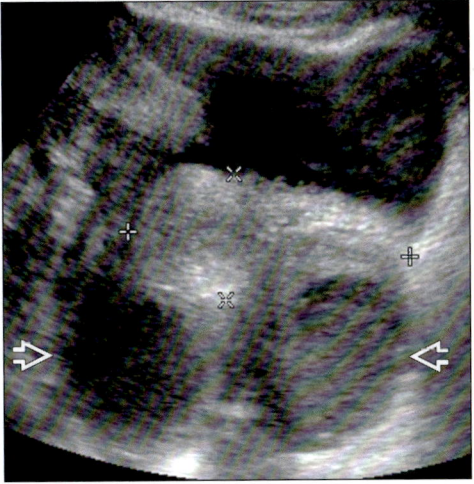

(Left) Axial CECT shows an enhancing thick-walled fallopian tube ➡ without fluid distention. The ovaries (*) are normal. Multiple rim-enhancing, left internal and external iliac lymph nodes ➡ are identified. There is a moderate amount of ascites. *(Right)* Sagittal transabdominal ultrasound shows bilateral complex cystic masses ➡ consistent with tubo-ovarian abscesses (TOAs) situated behind the uterus. The uterus (calipers) has a normal appearance.

Typical

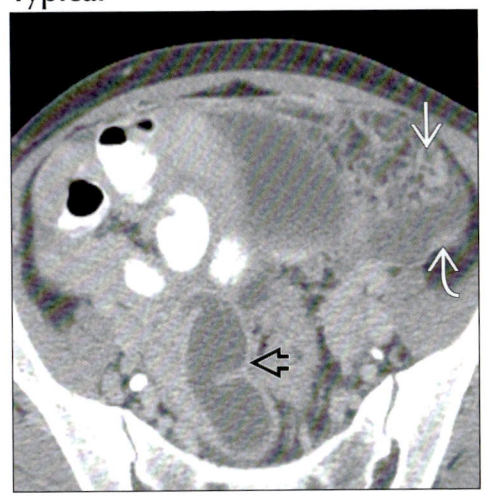
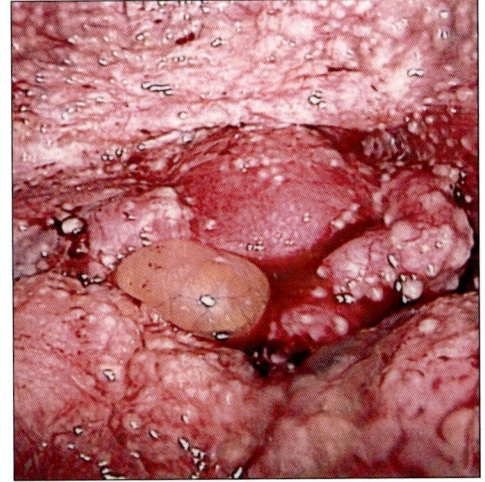

(Left) Axial CECT in the same patient as previous image, shows a thick-walled pyosalpinx ➡ with nodular infiltration of the omentum ➡ and dense ascites. There is nodular peritoneal enhancement ➡. Note the obliteration of the fat planes, particularly, in the right hemipelvis. *(Right)* Intra-operative photograph in the same patient as previous image, shows miliary deposits on the peritoneal surface proven to be tuberculosis.

Typical

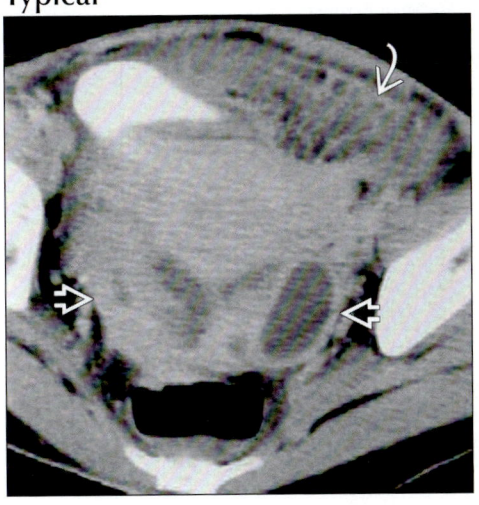
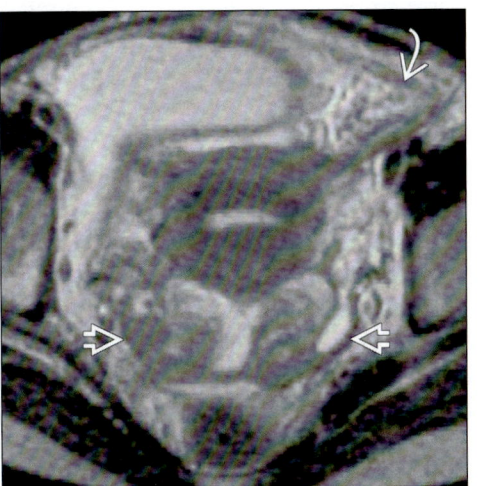

(Left) Axial CECT shows bilateral complex solid and cystic adnexal masses ➡. There is extensive infiltration of the omentum ➡. Note the diffuse obliteration of the pelvic fat planes. *(Right)* Axial T2WI MR in the same patient as previous image, shows bilateral complex adnexal masses ➡ with the solid components primarily of low signal intensity (SI). The mottled high SI foci represent caseation. The infiltration of the omentum ➡ is again seen.

ACTINOMYCOSIS

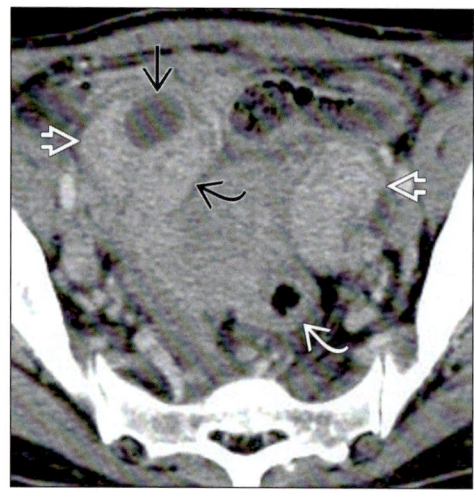

Axial CECT shows enlarged ovaries ➡, a hypodense right ovarian lesion ➡, and thickening of the right fallopian tube ➡. The wall of the sigmoid colon ➡ is thickened and there is obliteration of the fat planes.

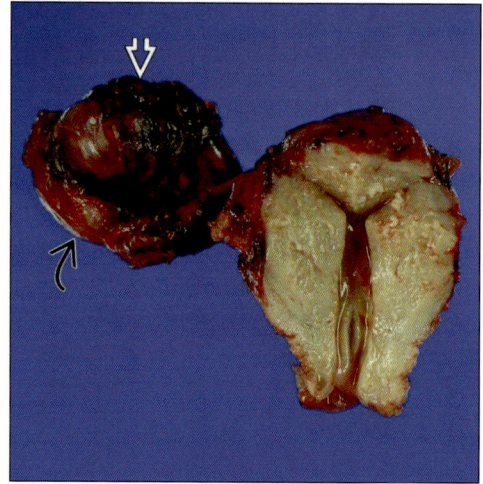

Gross pathology in the same patient as left shows the thickened fallopian tube ➡ draped around an enlarged ovary ➡ containing an abscess. This patient went to surgery for presumed ovarian malignancy.

TERMINOLOGY

Definitions
- Gram-positive anaerobic infection caused by actinomycetes, usually A. israelii

IMAGING FINDINGS

General Features
- Best diagnostic clue
  ○ Infiltrative adnexal mass mimicking a malignant process
    ▪ Associated inflammatory features and discordant lack of lymphadenopathy/ascites (given disease extent) allow differentiation from pelvic malignancy
  ○ Intrauterine device (IUD) visible within endometrial cavity
- Location: Most commonly unilateral
- Morphology
  ○ Ill-defined solid adnexal mass
    ▪ Chronic oophoritis ± thickened fallopian tube
  ▪ Pelvic phlegmon (pseudotumoral inflammatory tissue)
  ○ Ill-defined, thick-walled, complex cystic mass
    ▪ Tubo-ovarian and/or pelvic abscess, pyosalpinx
  ○ IUD in situ ± uterine enlargement
  ○ Obliteration of tissue planes with extension to contiguous structures irrespective of anatomic barriers
  ○ Mild reactive lymphadenopathy in 25%
- Additional findings
  ○ Hydroureteronephrosis, bladder wall thickening
  ○ Concentric or eccentric thickening of sigmoid colon wall with preservation of mucosa
    ▪ Extrinsic tethering of sigmoid colon mimicking endometriosis
    ▪ "Diverticulitis-like" picture with extraluminal mass, serrated margins, fold thickening and nodularity
  ○ Anorectal fistulae and sinus tract formation mimicking Crohn disease

Ultrasonographic Findings
- Grayscale Ultrasound
  ○ IUD present ± uterine enlargement

DDx: Pelvic Actinomycosis

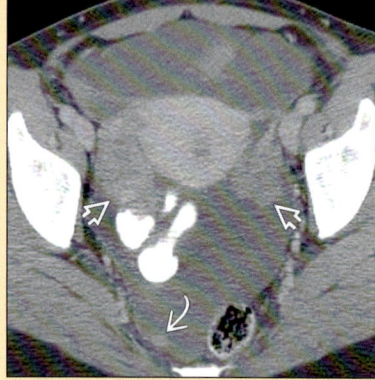
Ovarian Carcinoma

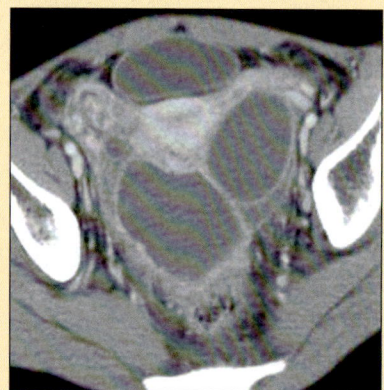
Acute Pelvic Inflammatory Disease

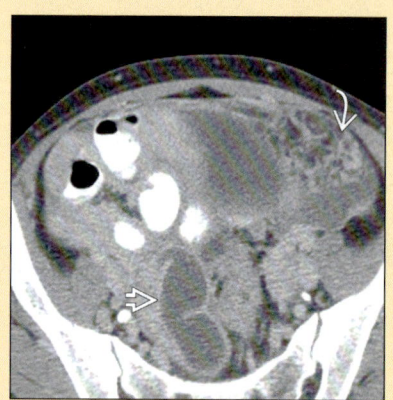
Genital Tuberculosis

ACTINOMYCOSIS

Key Facts

Terminology
- Gram-positive anaerobic infection caused by actinomycetes, usually A. israelii

Imaging Findings
- Ill-defined solid adnexal mass
- Ill-defined, thick-walled, complex cystic mass
- IUD in situ ± uterine enlargement
- Obliteration of tissue planes with extension to contiguous structures irrespective of anatomic barriers
- Multiple tiny intraovarian hypointensities with ring-like enhancement consistent with intraovarian microabscesses: "Salt and pepper" appearance of ovaries

Top Differential Diagnoses
- Ovarian Malignancy
- Acute Pelvic Inflammatory Disease (PID)
- Tuberculous PID
- Pelvic Abscess from Other Cause

Clinical Issues
- CA-125 typically normal or only mildly elevated
- Long-term (up to 1 year) high-dose penicillin ± percutaneous or surgical drainage

Diagnostic Checklist
- Consider actinomycosis in the differential diagnosis of an infiltrative adnexal mass with inflammatory features and a history of long-term IUD use

---

- Oophoritis ± pelvic phlegmon
  - Ill-defined solid adnexal mass typically hypoechoic, occasionally isoechoic
- Tubo-ovarian and/or pelvic abscess
  - Thick-walled cystic mass with anechoic/hypoechoic contents
- Pyosalpinx
  - Thick-walled tubular structure with anechoic/hypoechoic contents
- Hyperechoic pelvic fat consistent with inflammation
- Thick-walled sigmoid colon
- Color Doppler
  - Patchy increased vascularity on color/power Doppler imaging
  - Wall of tubo-ovarian abscess shows increased flow on color/power Doppler imaging

CT Findings
- CECT
  - Nonspecific adnexal enlargement
    - Predominantly solid pelvic mass with focal hypodense areas
    - Marked inhomogeneous enhancement of solid components in 80%
    - Thick-walled cystic masses with wall enhancement
  - Enhancement of pelvic fat, obliteration of tissue planes
  - No significant free fluid in pelvis, absence of peritoneal implants
  - Mildly enlarged reactive lymph nodes may be present
  - Diffuse bowel wall and ureteral thickening

MR Findings
- T1WI
  - Adnexal mass/pseudotumoral inflammatory tissue: Low to intermediate signal intensity (SI)
  - Abscess/pyosalpinx: Low to intermediate SI
- T2WI
  - Adnexal mass/pseudotumoral inflammatory tissue: Low to intermediate SI (atypical for malignancy)
  - Abscess/pyosalpinx: Intermediate to high SI fluid contents
  - Inflammatory changes of pelvic fat
  - No significant free fluid in pelvis
  - Mild reactive lymph nodes may be present
- T1 C+
  - Marked heterogeneous enhancement of adnexal mass/pseudotumoral inflammatory tissue
    - Multiple tiny intraovarian hypointensities with ring-like enhancement consistent with intraovarian microabscesses: "Salt and pepper" appearance of ovaries
  - Pyosalpinx/abscesses show enhancement of thickened wall
  - Enhancement of pelvic fat, obliteration of tissue planes
  - Marked enhancement of affected pelvic organs/structures (bowel, bladder, ureter)

Imaging Recommendations
- Best imaging tool
  - Transvaginal ultrasound (TVS) first line modality to assess overall morphology of pelvic organs
  - CT for better depiction of disease extent, associated pelvic inflammatory changes, sinus tracts/fistulae
  - MR best modality to confirm invasive nature of disease, delineate extent, demonstrate inflammatory component and intraovarian microabscesses
- Protocol advice
  - Contrast administration improves diagnostic accuracy of CT and MR imaging
  - Core needle biopsy/aspiration can be performed under TVS or CT guidance

DIFFERENTIAL DIAGNOSIS

Ovarian Malignancy
- Pelvic inflammatory changes absent
- Ascites and lymphadenopathy present in advanced disease
- Higher SI of ovarian mass on T2WI, absence of "salt and pepper" appearance on T1 C+

ACTINOMYCOSIS

Acute Pelvic Inflammatory Disease (PID)
- Inflammatory changes more acute and edematous
- Greater preservation of tissue planes

Tuberculous PID
- Lymphadenopathy ± calcification
- Peritoneal involvement

Pelvic Abscess from Other Cause
- Diverticulitis, Crohn disease: Complex cystic lesion
- Paraovarian structures are less likely to be involved
- Presence of gas more common

PATHOLOGY

General Features
- General path comments
  - Chronic, suppurative, granulomatous disease
  - Colonies macroscopically described as "sulfur granules"
  - Characterized by extensive fibrosis with multiple abscesses and sinus tract formation
- Etiology
  - Saprophytic genus Actinomycetales, mainly A. israelii
  - Fastidious, slow-growing, anaerobic, Gram-positive, filamentous bacterium
  - Saprophytic organism, part of normal oral, intestinal and female genital flora
- Epidemiology
  - As high as 27% vaginal carriage in women not using an IUD
  - Increasing incidence in the past two decades
- Pathogenesis
  - Colonization of vagina secondary to anal contamination and urogenital contact
  - Local breakdown of tissue/mucosal barrier (as in IUD use) necessary for infection
    - Unable to cross intact mucous membranes due to low virulence
  - Once established, infection spreads irrespective of anatomic barriers due to organism's proteolytic enzymes
  - Eradication of colonization by removal of IUD or replacement by copper device

Gross Pathologic & Surgical Features
- Actinomycotic "sulfur granules" presenting as yellow material in fistulous discharge
- Infiltrated, indurated pelvis at laparotomy mimicking malignancy

Microscopic Features
- Identification of actinomycotic "sulfur granules"
- Clumps of actinomycetes on Pap smear: "Gupta bodies"
- Diagnosis by direct immunofluorescence or anaerobic culture

CLINICAL ISSUES

Presentation
- Most common signs/symptoms: Abdominal pain, weight loss, vaginal discharge and fever
- Other signs/symptoms: Pelvic mass without signs/symptoms of inflammation, even in the presence of established infection
- Clinical Profile: IUD in place for more than 3 years, average 8 years
- Laboratory findings
  - Anemia, leukocytosis, elevated ESR
  - CA-125 typically normal or only mildly elevated

Demographics
- Age: Most common in 4th decade

Natural History & Prognosis
- Diagnosis frequently not considered pre-operatively
  - Leading to unnecessary total abdominal hysterectomy (TAH) and bilateral salpingo-oophorectomy (BSO) for presumed ovarian cancer
- Surgery for undiagnosed cases complicated by multiple draining fistulae with "sulfur granule" discharge

Treatment
- Removal of IUD
- Long-term (up to 1 year) high-dose penicillin ± percutaneous or surgical drainage
- Secondary surgery for residual abscesses, sinuses or strictures

DIAGNOSTIC CHECKLIST

Consider
- Consider actinomycosis in the differential diagnosis of an infiltrative adnexal mass with inflammatory features and a history of long-term IUD use

Image Interpretation Pearls
- Classical presentation with tubo-ovarian abscess formation
- "Salt and pepper" ovaries due to ring-enhancing hypointense microabscesses

SELECTED REFERENCES

1. Baird AS: Pelvic actinomycosis: still a cause for concern. J Fam Plann Reprod Health Care. 31(1):73-4, 2005
2. Kim SH et al: Unusual causes of tubo-ovarian abscess: CT and MR imaging findings. Radiographics. 24(6):1575-89, 2004
3. Alfuhaid T et al: Pelvic actinomycosis associated with intrauterine device use. Can Assoc Radiol J. 54:160-2, 2003
4. Lee I et al: Abdominopelvic actinomycosis involving the gastrointestinal tract: CT features. Radiology. 220:76-80, 2001
5. Hawnaur JM et al: Magnetic resonance imaging of actinomycosis presenting as pelvic malignancy. Br J Radiol. 72(862):1006-11, 1999
6. Müller-Holzner E: IUD-associated pelvic actinomycosis: a report of five cases. Int J Gynecol Pathol. 14:70-4, 1995

ACTINOMYCOSIS

IMAGE GALLERY

Typical

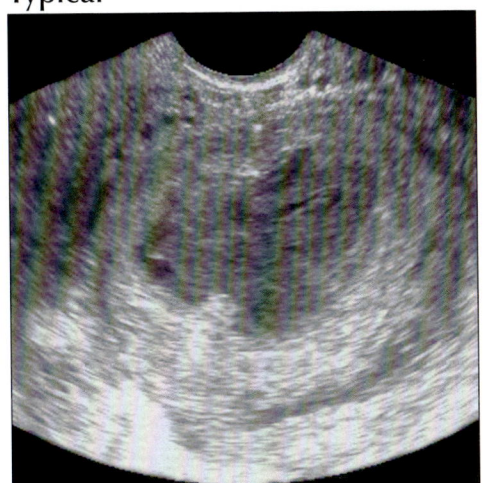
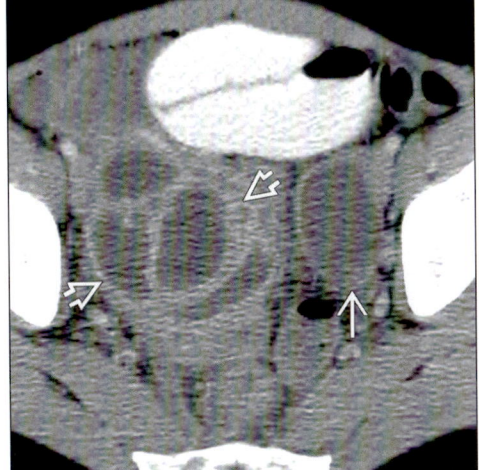

(Left) Sagittal oblique transvaginal ultrasound shows a complex thick-walled right adnexal mass with hypoechoic contents. (Right) Axial CECT in the same patient as left shows a complex, thick-walled right adnexal mass ➡ consistent with a tubo-ovarian abscess. The pelvic fat shows inflammatory changes and there is obliteration of the fat planes. Incidentally there is a hemorrhagic left ovarian cyst ➡.

Typical

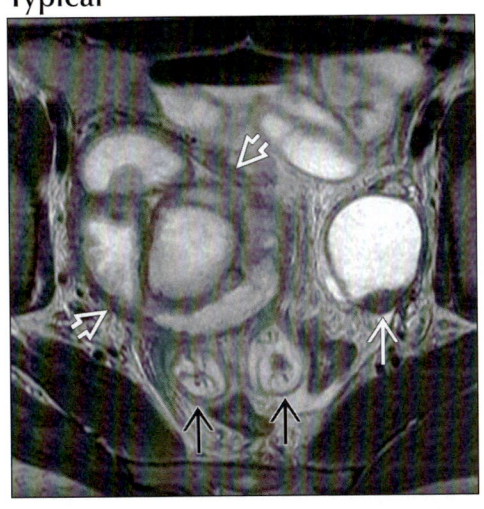
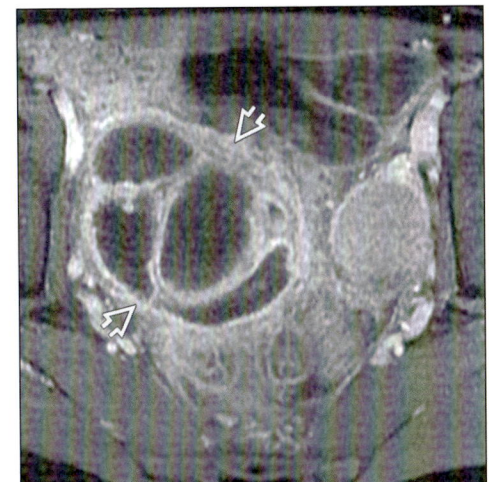

(Left) Axial T2WI MR in the same patient as previous image shows the right tubo-ovarian abscess ➡. The extensive stranding of the pelvic fat is better appreciated on the MR exam. There is thickening of pelvic small bowel loops ➡. Debris can be seen in the dependent portion of the hemorrhagic left ovarian cyst ➡. (Right) Axial T1 C+ FS MR in same patient as left shows the right tubo-ovarian abscess ➡ & extensive fat stranding with obliteration of pelvic fat planes.

Typical

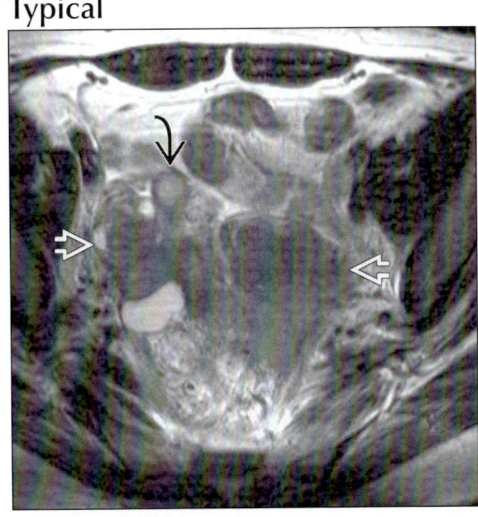
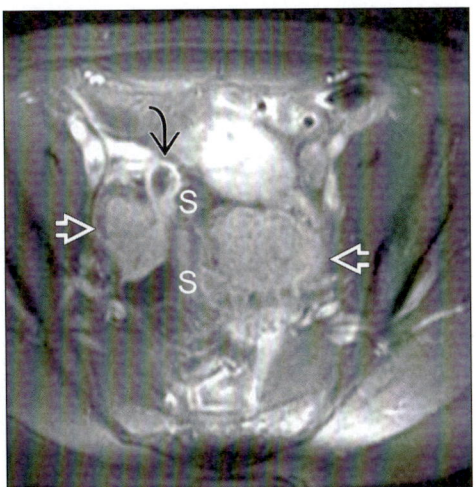

(Left) Axial T2WI MR shows bilateral low signal-intensity (SI) ovarian masses ➡. There is a right-sided pyosalpinx ➡ with intermediate SI fluid contents. Note the inflamed pelvic fat. (Right) Axial T1 C+ FS MR in the same patient as left shows the "salt and pepper" appearance of both ovarian masses ➡ consistent with intraovarian microabscesses. There is a thick-walled right pyosalpinx ➡. Note the secondary involvement of the sigmoid colon (S).

SALPINGITIS ISTHMICA NODOSA

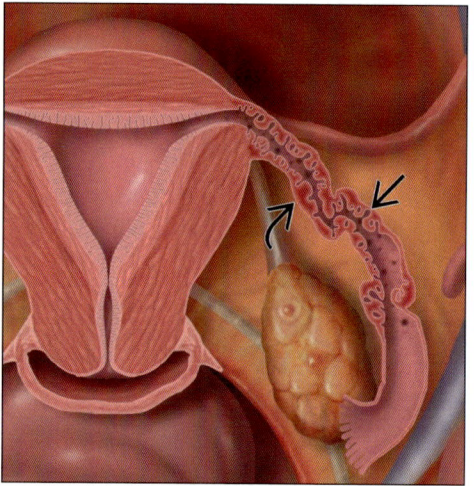

Coronal graphic shows multiple diverticula ➔ involving the intramural and isthmic portions of the fallopian tube with areas of nodular hyperplasia of the surrounding muscle ➔.

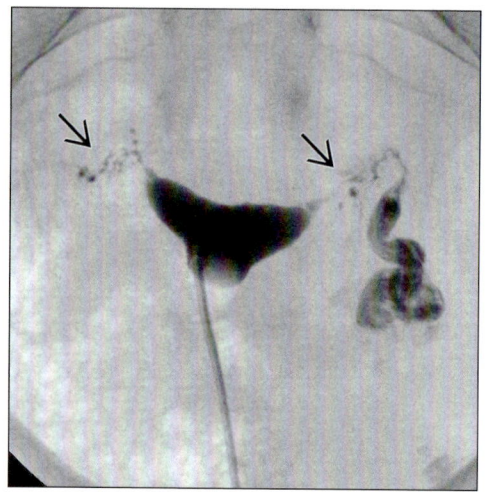

Frontal view from hysterosalpingogram shows bilateral multiple diverticula ➔ in the isthmic portions of the fallopian tubes. Free spillage is seen on the left. (Courtesy A. Thurmond, MD).

TERMINOLOGY

Abbreviations and Synonyms
- Salpingitis isthmica nodosa (SIN)
- Tubal diverticulosis
- Tubal adenomyosis

Definitions
- Small outpouchings or diverticula from the isthmic portion of the fallopian tube

IMAGING FINDINGS

General Features
- Best diagnostic clue: Small diverticula in the proximal two thirds of the fallopian tube
- Location
  - Bilateral in 60-80% of cases
  - Tubes may be asymmetrically affected
- Size: Typically outpouchings are 2 mm in diameter and clustered over tubal length of 1-2 cm

Ultrasonographic Findings
- Cystic changes usually not demonstrated
- Sonohysterosalpingogram does not show anatomy of the tube as well as hysterosalpingogram (HSG)

MR Findings
- Tiny or large cystic spaces in wall of fallopian tube
- Small nodules of hypertrophic muscle
- May be associated with hydrosalpinx

Fluoroscopic Findings
- Hysterosalpingogram → classic appearance: Multiple small diverticula extending from the lumen of the fallopian tube into the wall
  - Larger nodular areas from larger diverticula can be seen
  - Extraluminal channels are frequently seen in the more severe cases
  - Tubal lumen may appear narrowed and irregular in severe cases
  - Decreased free spillage as lesions increase in severity or extent
  - Often associated with proximal obstruction or ampullary dilatation

DDx: Fallopian Tube Abnormalities

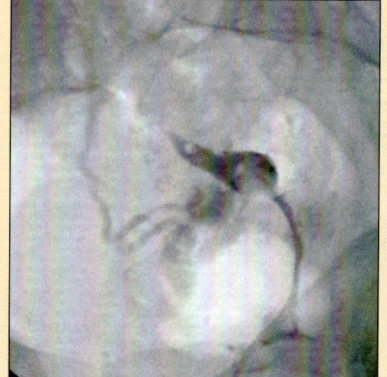
Venous Intravasation

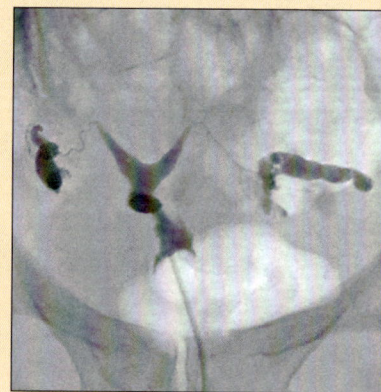
Hydrosalpinx

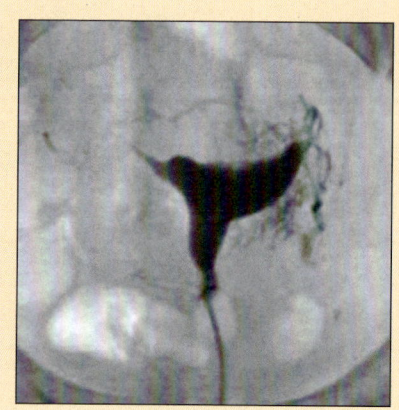
Lymphatic Intravasation

SALPINGITIS ISTHMICA NODOSA

Key Facts

Terminology
- Small outpouchings or diverticula from the isthmic portion of the fallopian tube

Imaging Findings
- Bilateral in 60-80% of cases
- Hysterosalpingogram → classic appearance: Multiple small diverticula extending from the lumen of the fallopian tube into the wall
- Decreased free spillage as lesions increase in severity or extent

Top Differential Diagnoses
- Salpingitis
- Tuberculosis

Pathology
- Prevalence in healthy, fertile women → 0.6-11%
- SIN is a common cause of proximal tubal disease → 23-60% in histologically documented cases
- Nodules composed of hypertrophic myosalpinx and glandular spaces lines by tubal epithelium

Clinical Issues
- Infertility (38%)
- Ectopic pregnancy (9%; they also have greater risk of recurrent ectopic pregnancy or infertility)

Diagnostic Checklist
- Fallopian tube catheterization has increased ability to diagnose SIN → ability to fill isthmic diverticula beyond proximally occluded tube

---

- More commonly seen in the isthmus and intramural segments, less often in the ampullary segment
- SIN is found in 50% of patients on post recanalization HSG

Imaging Recommendations
- Best imaging tool: Hysterosalpingogram best demonstrates the small outpouchings
- Protocol advice: Magnified spot films are useful

DIFFERENTIAL DIAGNOSIS

Salpingitis
- Chronic salpingitis histologically presents as fibrous adhesions of plica forming follicle-like architecture and often accompanied by hydrosalpinx
- Tissue between the epithelial cysts consists of fibrosis rather than smooth muscle

Tuberculosis
- Isthmic diverticulosis identical to SIN can be seen
- Associated tubal narrowing and contraction of the ampulla
- May have calcified pelvic lymph nodes, tubes or ovaries

Tubal Endometriosis
- Pathology shows presence of endometrial glands and stroma
- Occlusive SIN may be associated with endometriosis

Adenomyosis
- Cysts in cornual regions can mimic tubal outpouchings

PATHOLOGY

General Features
- Etiology: Unknown, associated with pelvic inflammatory disease
- Epidemiology
  - Prevalence in healthy, fertile women → 0.6-11%
  - More common in setting of ectopic pregnancy and infertility
  - SIN is a common cause of proximal tubal disease → 23-60% in histologically documented cases
- Associated abnormalities
  - Most patients have history of pelvic infection
  - Perihepatic adhesions or adnexal adhesions frequently coexist

Gross Pathologic & Surgical Features
- Discrete nodular swelling in the more proximal portion of the tube
  - Superficial adhesions can be observed on laparoscopy
  - Nodular tissue firm to touch
  - Nodules composed of hypertrophic myosalpinx and glandular spaces lines by tubal epithelium
  - Isthmic portion of the tube has a thick muscular wall and luminal dilatation is very rare
- Involves isthmic portion in 72% of cases and isthmic portion and ampulla in 28% of cases

Microscopic Features
- Swelling consists of multiple discrete lumina encased in smooth muscle
  - Concentrically arranged lumina in the wall of the fallopian tube, analogous to adenomyosis of the uterus
- Salpingitis isthmica nodosa may coexist with chronic salpingitis → unclear relationship between the two
  - Central tubal lumen is narrowed in most cases
  - Slight inflammatory response found with lymphocytes and fibrosis
  - Antibodies to Chlamydia have been associated

CLINICAL ISSUES

Presentation
- Most common signs/symptoms
  - Infertility (38%)
  - Ectopic pregnancy (9%; they also have greater risk of recurrent ectopic pregnancy or infertility)

SALPINGITIS ISTHMICA NODOSA

- Other signs/symptoms: May have prior history of PID

Demographics
- Age: Develops during reproductive years, mean age of diagnosis 30

Natural History & Prognosis
- Patients are at risk for recurrent ectopic pregnancy
  - Incidence of SIN associated with ectopic tubal pregnancies → range 2.8-57%
  - Incidence of SIN in pathologic specimens from isthmic tubal ectopic pregnancy → 46-57%

Treatment
- Microsurgical approaches are successful in patients with infertility or ectopic pregnancy
  - Microsurgical resection and tubocornual anastomosis of nonocclusive SIN decreases the time to conceive an intrauterine pregnancy
    - Postsurgical studies have described intrauterine pregnancy rates of 46-56%
  - Also may reduce risk for ectopic pregnancy
    - Postsurgical ectopic rate of 11%
- Fluoroscopic transcervical fallopian tube recanalization is an option in women with SIN and favored by some authors since it is not invasive
  - Incidence of post treatment intrauterine pregnancy is 23-30%
  - Incidence of post treatment ectopic pregnancy is 4.5-10%
- Management of isthmic ectopic pregnancy associated with SIN depends on patient's desire for future fertility
  - Post-operative HSG is recommended with an abnormal contralateral tube or when SIN is noted in the resected tubal segment
- Management is controversial if found in fertile women, since process can be progressive and may affect fertility
- In cases of occlusive SIN associated with endometriosis, patency of fallopian tubes has been reported after treatment with GnRH agonist

DIAGNOSTIC CHECKLIST

Consider
- Fallopian tube catheterization has increased ability to diagnose SIN → ability to fill isthmic diverticula beyond proximally occluded tube

Image Interpretation Pearls
- Radiographic diagnosis of SIN may be pressure dependent

SELECTED REFERENCES

1. Eng CW et al: Hysterosalpingography: current applications. Singapore Med J. 48(4):368-73; quiz 374, 2007
2. Simpson WL Jr et al: Hysterosalpingography: a reemerging study. Radiographics. 26(2):419-31, 2006
3. Almeida OD Jr: Microlaparoscopy and a GnRH agonist: a combined minimally invasive approach for the diagnosis and treatment of occlusive salpingitis isthmica nodosa associated with endometriosis. JSLS. 9(4):431-3, 2005
4. Awartani K et al: Microsurgical resection of nonocclusive salpingitis isthmica nodosa is beneficial. Fertil Steril. 79(5):1199-203, 2003
5. Houston JG et al: Salpingitis isthmica nodosa: technical success and outcome of fluoroscopic transcervical fallopian tube recanalization. Cardiovasc Intervent Radiol. 21(1):31-5, 1998
6. Lang EK et al: Recanalization of obstructed fallopian tube by selective salpingography and transvaginal bougie dilatation: outcome and cost analysis. Fertil Steril. 66(2):210-5, 1996
7. Thurmond AS et al: Salpingitis isthmica nodosa: results of transcervical fluoroscopic catheter recanalization. Fertil Steril. 63(4):715-22, 1995
8. Gurgan T et al: Salpingoscopic findings in women with occlusive and nonocclusive salpingitis isthmica nodosa. Fertil Steril. 61(3):461-3, 1994
9. Hovsepian DM et al: Fallopian tube recanalization in an unrestricted patient population. Radiology. 190(1):137-40, 1994
10. Kutluay L et al: Tubal histopathology in ectopic pregnancies. Eur J Obstet Gynecol Reprod Biol. 57(2):91-4, 1994
11. Jenkins CS et al: Salpingitis isthmica nodosa: a review of the literature, discussion of clinical significance, and consideration of patient management. Fertil Steril. 60(4):599-607, 1993
12. Gomel V et al: Infertility surgery: microsurgery. Curr Opin Obstet Gynecol. 4(3):390-9, 1992
13. Saracoglu FO et al: Salpingitis isthmica nodosa in infertility and ectopic pregnancy. Gynecol Obstet Invest. 34(4):202-5, 1992
14. Letterie GS et al: Histology of proximal tubal obstruction in cases of unsuccessful tubal canalization. Fertil Steril. 56(5):831-5, 1991
15. Skibsted L et al: Salpingitis isthmica nodosa in female infertility and tubal diseases. Hum Reprod. 6(6):828-31, 1991
16. Yoder IC et al: Hysterosalpingography in the 1990s. AJR Am J Roentgenol. 157(4):675-83, 1991
17. Stock RJ: Histopathology of fallopian tubes with recurrent tubal pregnancy. Obstet Gynecol. 75(1):9-14, 1990
18. Green LK et al: Histopathologic findings in ectopic tubal pregnancy. Int J Gynecol Pathol. 8(3):255-62, 1989
19. McComb PF et al: Salpingitis isthmica nodosa: evidence it is a progressive disease. Fertil Steril. 51(3):542-5, 1989
20. Creasy JL et al: Salpingitis isthmica nodosa: radiologic and clinical correlates. Radiology. 154(3):597-600, 1985

SALPINGITIS ISTHMICA NODOSA

IMAGE GALLERY

Typical

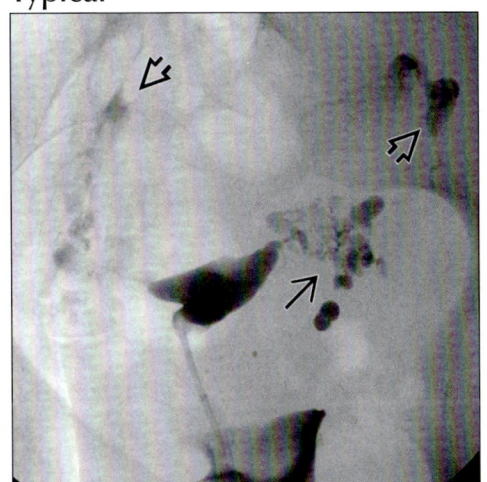
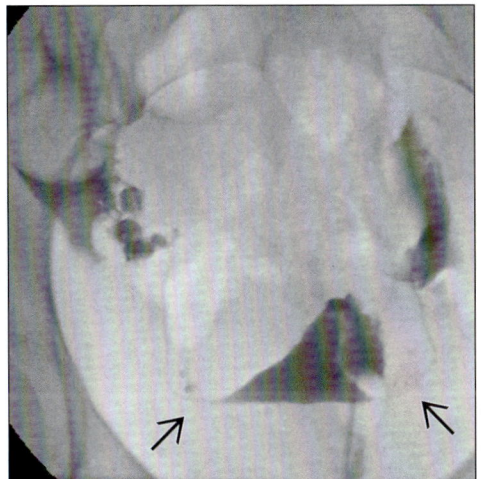

(Left) Prone oblique image from a hysterosalpingogram shows prominent diverticula in the proximal portions of the fallopian tube ➡. Free spillage was demonstrated bilaterally ➡. (Courtesy A. Thurmond, MD). *(Right)* Hysterosalpingogram shows tiny diverticula arising from the isthmic portion of both fallopian tubes ➡ in a patient with a prior history of ruptured appendicitis and primary infertility.

Typical

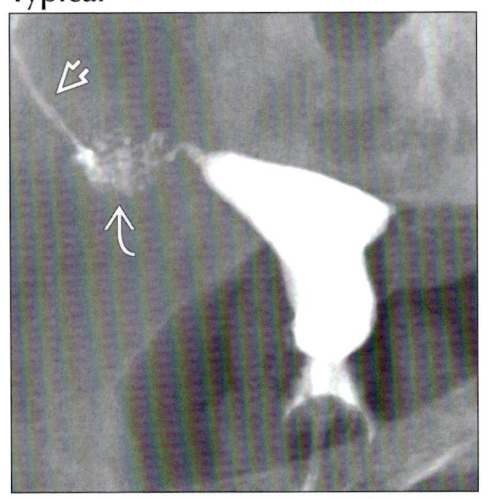
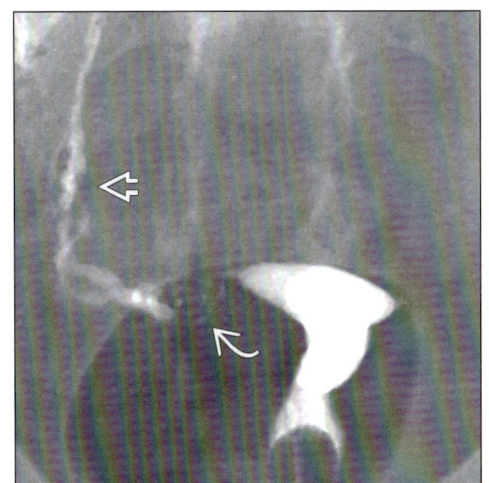

(Left) Anteroposterior view from a hysterosalpingogram shows multiple tiny diverticula ➡ in the isthmus of the right fallopian tube associated with tubal obstruction and lymphatic extravasation ➡. *(Right)* Anteroposterior more delayed view from hysterosalpingogram in same patient as previous image shows prominent venous extravasation ➡ in a patient with salpingitis isthmica nodosa ➡ and proximal tubal obstruction.

Typical

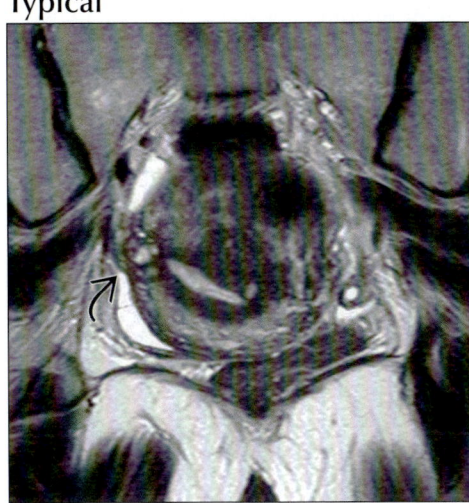
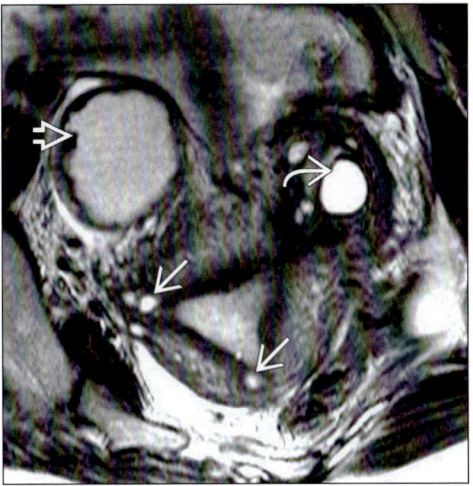

(Left) Coronal T2WI MR shows multiple small diverticula ➡ in the interstitial portion of the fallopian tubes, best seen on the right. (Courtesy A. Thurmond, MD). *(Right)* Axial T2WI MR shows bilateral cystic spaces in the proximal portions of both fallopian tubes surrounded by hypertrophic muscle ➡. Note Nabothian cyst ➡ and corpus luteum ➡. (Courtesy A. Thurmond, MD).

TUBO-OVARIAN ABSCESS

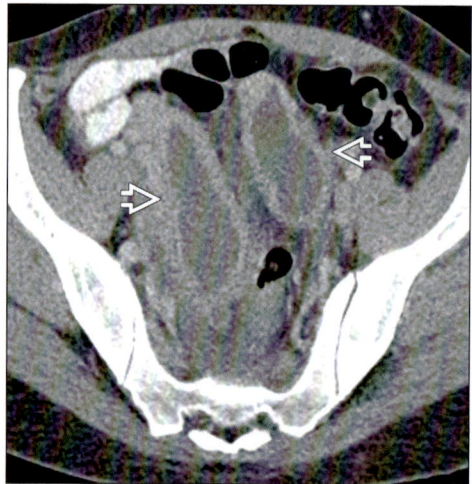

Axial CECT shows bilateral thick-walled tubular cystic masses ➲ with enhancing walls corresponding to bilateral TOAs.

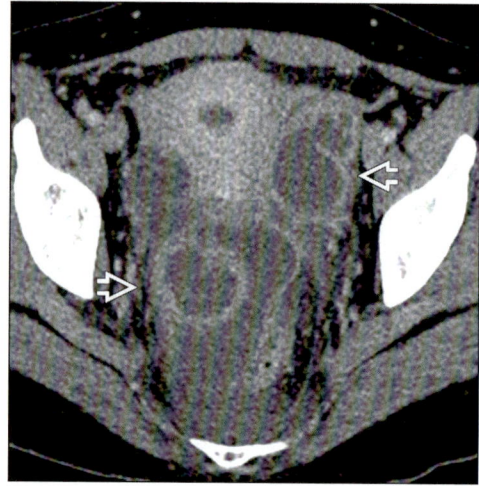

Axial CECT shows another example of bilateral TOAs ➲ appearing as thick-walled enhancing cystic lesions.

TERMINOLOGY

Abbreviations and Synonyms
- TOA/acute pyogenic pelvic inflammatory disease (PID)

Definitions
- Infection of upper female genital tract including endometrium, fallopian tubes (FT), and ovaries

IMAGING FINDINGS

General Features
- Best diagnostic clue
  - Thick-walled fallopian tube
  - ± Fluid distention (pyosalpinx), enlarged edematous ovaries, TOA/pelvic abscess, with inflammatory changes in pelvic fat and other pelvic structures, and free intrapelvic fluid
- Location: Within the pelvis
- Size: Variable; can be greater than 10 cm in size
- Early PID
  - Mild pelvic edema
    - Haziness/stranding of pelvic fat with obscuration of fascial planes
  - Mild salpingitis: Enhancement and thickening of FT ± hydrosalpinx
  - Mild oophoritis: Enlarged and heterogeneously enhancing ovaries ± polycystic-like appearance of ovaries
  - Abnormal endometrial/endocervical enhancement with fluid in cavity
  - Enhanced peritoneum
- Advanced PID
  - Pyosalpinx
    - Greater degree of wall thickening and enhancement
    - Filled with complex fluid, fluid-debris level
  - Tubo-ovarian or pelvic abscess
    - Complex fluid collection ± internal septa
    - Thick-walled with ill-defined outer borders
    - Inner borders may be irregular
    - Presence of air uncommon
  - Involvement of adjacent structures
    - Small or large bowel ileus/obstruction
    - Thickening of small/large bowel wall or bladder wall

DDx: Pelvic Cystic Lesions

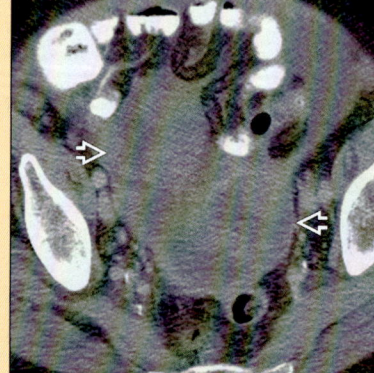

Bilateral Ovarian Carcinoma

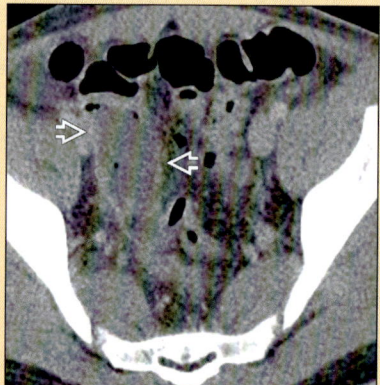

Appendicular Abscess

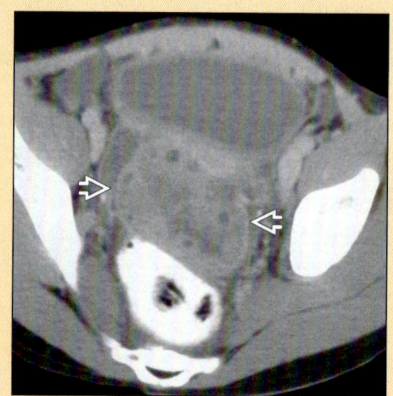

Ovarian Torsion

TUBO-OVARIAN ABSCESS

Key Facts

Terminology
- TOA/acute pyogenic pelvic inflammatory disease (PID)
- Infection of upper female genital tract including endometrium, fallopian tubes (FT), and ovaries

Imaging Findings
- Thick-walled fallopian tube
- ± Fluid distention (pyosalpinx), enlarged edematous ovaries, TOA/pelvic abscess, with inflammatory changes in pelvic fat and other pelvic structures, and free intrapelvic fluid
- TVS and CT used for image-guided drainage of abscess

Top Differential Diagnoses
- Ovarian Neoplasm
- Adnexal Torsion
- Hemorrhagic Ovarian Cyst/Endometriosis
- Pelvic Abscess from Another Cause

Pathology
- Most commonly Neisseria gonorrhoeae or Chlamydia trachomatis
- 30-40% polymicrobial
- Risk factors for pelvic inflammatory disease i.e., multiple sexual partners, intrauterine contraceptive device (IUCD), lower socioeconomic class

Clinical Issues
- Most common signs/symptoms: Fever, abdominal or pelvic pain
- Can lead to infertility and ectopic pregnancies if not diagnosed and treated in early stages

---

- Ureteropelvicaliectasis (functional or mechanical obstruction)
- Fitz-Hugh and Curtis syndrome (inflammation of right upper quadrant peritoneal surfaces, thick gallbladder wall, heterogeneous enhancement of liver)

Ultrasonographic Findings
- Transvaginal ultrasound (TVS) findings
  - Early PID
    - May be normal
    - Increased echogenicity of pelvic fat
    - Thickening of FT ± distention with simple fluid
    - Enlarged ovaries with indistinct margins and multiple cysts
  - Advanced PID
    - Pyosalpinx: Cogwheel sign/incomplete septa; increased thickening of FT wall (> 5 mm); increased echogenicity of FT wall
    - Tubo-ovarian or pelvic abscess: Multilocular/unilocular, complex, thick-walled, cystic adnexal mass
  - Accuracy: Variable, highest in patients with advanced PID
    - Sensitivity 30-85%; specificity 80-100%

CT Findings
- CECT
  - Early PID
    - Abnormal enhancement of cervix and endometrium with endometrial fluid in keeping with cervicitis and endometritis
    - Engorged, abnormally enhancing ovaries in keeping with oophoritis
    - Enhancing, thickened FT in keeping with salpingitis
    - Stranding of pelvic fat
  - Advanced PID
    - Pyosalpinx; appears as enhancing dilated fallopian tubes filled with complex fluid
    - TOA appearing as unilateral or bilateral uni/multilocular thick walled adnexal masses of fluid density with wall enhancement; may see internal gas bubbles
    - +/- Associated thickening and anterior displacement of mesosalpinges
    - +/- Associated thickening of uterosacral ligaments
    - +/- Hydronephrosis or hydroureter due to serosal involvement of ureters
    - +/- Serosal thickening of rectosigmoid colon
    - +/- Para-aortic lymphadenopathy

MR Findings
- T1WI
  - Advanced PID
    - Pyosalpinx; tortuous, dilated, fluid-filled fallopian tube; contents are of low signal intensity
    - TOA; ill-defined adnexal mass with thick irregular walls containing fluid of low signal intensity
    - Abscess wall: 1-3 mm hyperintense inner rim (granulation tissue)
- T2WI
  - Early PID
    - Free fluid of high signal intensity, enlarged ovaries with a polycystic appearance
  - Advanced PID
    - Pyosalpinx; tortuous dilated fluid-filled fallopian tube; contents are of intermediate to high signal intensity
    - TOA; ill-defined adnexal mass with thick irregular walls containing fluid of intermediate to high signal intensity
    - Abscess wall: Low to intermediate signal intensity
- T1 C+
  - Advanced PID
    - Marked enhancement of pyosalpinx or abscess wall (corresponding to inner rim of granulation tissue)
  - Accuracy: Limited data available
    - Sensitivity: 95%; specificity: 90%

Imaging Recommendations
- Best imaging tool

TUBO-OVARIAN ABSCESS

- o TVS/CT/MR all helpful in the diagnosis
- o TVS and CT used for image-guided drainage of abscess
- Protocol advice
  - o US
    - Initial evaluation and follow-up; guidance for transvaginal or transabdominal drainage of abscess or pyosalpinx
  - o CT
    - Complicated PID, and cause of pain/fever uncertain at TVS; guidance for transabdominal or transgluteal drainage of abscess
  - o MR
    - Differentiate between a multicystic mass and an abnormal FT

DIFFERENTIAL DIAGNOSIS

Ovarian Neoplasm
- Mixed cystic solid lesion
- Large amount of free fluid
- No stranding of fat
- +/- Peritoneal deposits

Adnexal Torsion
- Twisted pedicle sign
- Normal to diminished vascularity of adnexa
- High signal intensity on T1WI and T2WI, with layering on T2WI

Hemorrhagic Ovarian Cyst/Endometriosis
- High signal on T1WI
- Little or no pelvic fat stranding

Pelvic Abscess from Another Cause
- E.g., diverticulitis, Crohn; complex cystic lesion
- Parovarian structures are less likely to be involved
- Unilateral rather than bilateral
- Presence of gas more common than for TOA

PATHOLOGY

General Features
- General path comments
  - o Most commonly Neisseria gonorrhoeae or Chlamydia trachomatis
  - o 30-40% polymicrobial
  - o Rare causes: Actinomycosis, TB, xanthogranulomatous inflammation
- Etiology
  - o Results from untreated or unrecognized ascending vaginal or cervical infection that progresses to endometritis, salpingitis, then tubo-ovarian abscess
  - o Postmenopausal tubo-ovarian abscesses may be associated with concomitant gynecological malignancy in up to 50% of cases
- Epidemiology
  - o Premenopausal females
  - o Risk factors for pelvic inflammatory disease i.e., multiple sexual partners, intrauterine contraceptive device (IUCD), lower socioeconomic class

CLINICAL ISSUES

Presentation
- Most common signs/symptoms: Fever, abdominal or pelvic pain
- Other signs/symptoms
  - o Vaginal discharge, cervical/adnexal tenderness
  - o May be asymptomatic
- Clinical Profile: Prior history of pelvic inflammatory disease

Demographics
- Age: Premenopausal
- Gender: Females

Natural History & Prognosis
- Can lead to infertility and ectopic pregnancies if not diagnosed and treated in early stages

Treatment
- IUCD removed if present
- Antibiotic therapy ± image-guided or surgical drainage of pelvic abscess

DIAGNOSTIC CHECKLIST

Consider
- Diagnosis of TOA in a sexually active female presenting with pyrexia, abdominal/pelvic pain and enhancing complex cystic adnexal masses on CECT or MR

Image Interpretation Pearls
- Unilocular/multilocular adnexal cystic masses with wall enhancement

SELECTED REFERENCES

1. Harisinghani MG et al: Transgluteal approach for percutaneous drainage of deep pelvic abscesses: 154 cases. Radiology. 228(3):701-5, 2003
2. Sam JW et al: Spectrum of CT findings in acute pyogenic pelvic inflammatory disease. Radiographics. 22:1327-34, 2002
3. Bau A et al: Acute female pelvic pain: ultrasound evaluation. Seminars in Ultrasound, CT, and MR. 21:78-93, 2000
4. Tukeva TA et al: MR imaging in pelvic inflammatory disease: comparison with laparoscopy and US. Radiology. 210(1):209-16, 1999
5. Ha HK et al: MR imaging of tubo-ovarian abscess. Acta Radiol. 36(5):510-4, 1995
6. McCormack WM: Pelvic inflammatory disease. NEJM. 330:115-9, 1994
7. Wilbur AC et al: CT findings in tuboovarian abscess. AJR Am J Roentgenol. 158(3):575-9, 1992
8. Lande IM et al: Adnexal and cul-de-sac abnormalities: transvaginal sonography. Radiology. 166(2):325-32, 1988

TUBO-OVARIAN ABSCESS

IMAGE GALLERY

Typical

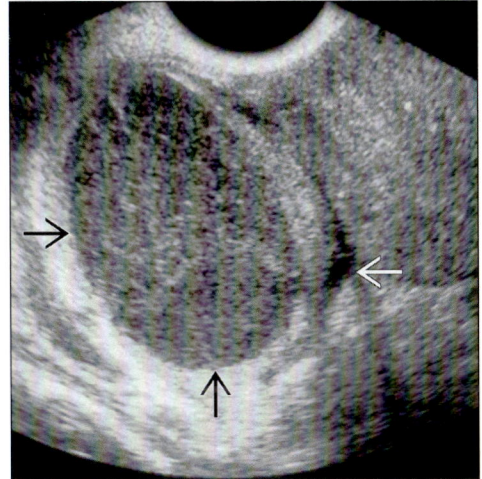
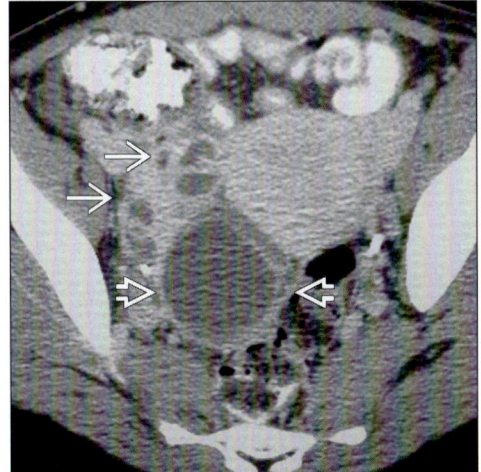

(Left) Longitudinal transvaginal ultrasound shows a typical case of right TOA in a young patient presenting with acute pelvic pain and raised inflammatory markers. Note the large heterogeneous cyst ➡ in the right adnexa. A trace of free fluid ➡ is also present. *(Right)* Axial CECT in the same patient as previous image shows a thick-wall adnexal cystic lesion ➡ with rim-enhancement. Note the presence of dilated right fallopian tube ➡ with thickened walls.

Typical

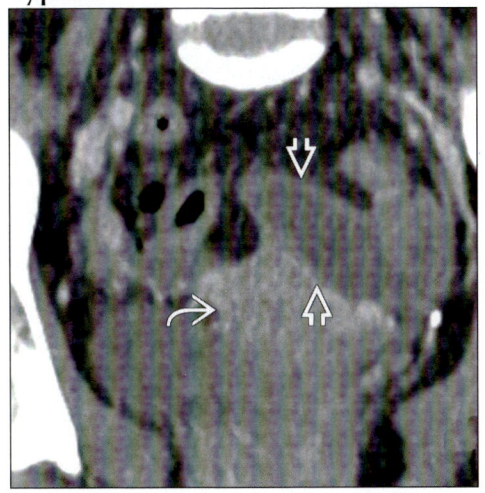
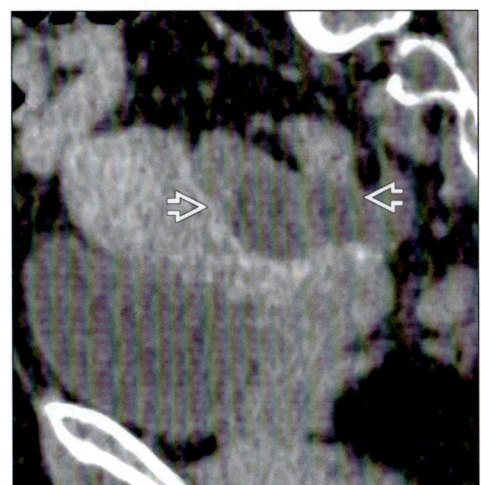

(Left) Coronal CECT shows a left TOA as enhancing tubular cystic structure ➡ located superior and to the left of the uterus ➡. *(Right)* Sagittal CECT in the same patient as previous image confirms the presence of the left TOA ➡ as an enhancing tubular cystic structure located posterior to the uterus. Note the presence of high attenuation material within the dilated fallopian tube.

Typical

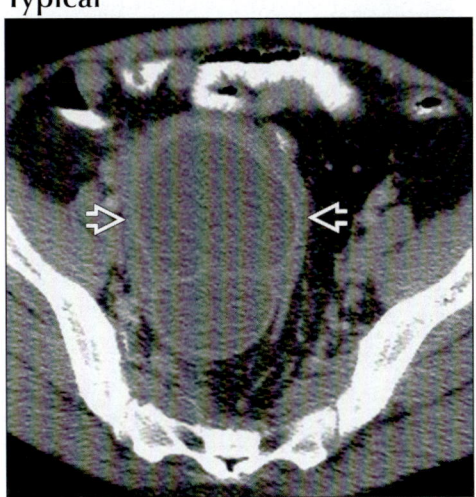
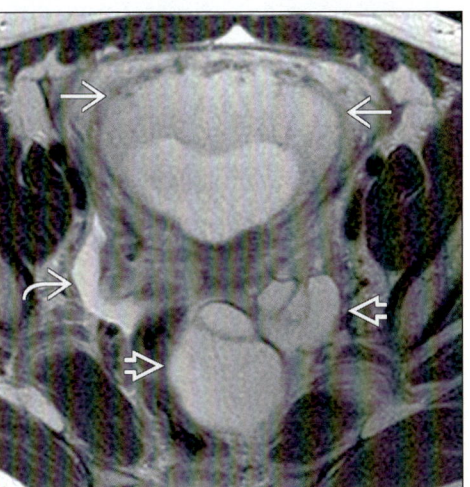

(Left) Axial CECT shows a right TOA ➡ appearing as a thick-walled enhancing adnexal cystic lesion displacing the sigmoid colon to the left of the midline. *(Right)* Axial T2WI MR shows a dilated left fallopian tube of high signal intensity ➡ in a pregnant patient presenting with vaginal discharge, abdominal pain and fever. Note the presence of free fluid ➡ posterior to the pregnant uterus ➡. Overall appearances are those of a left salpingitis.

TUBO-OVARIAN ABSCESS

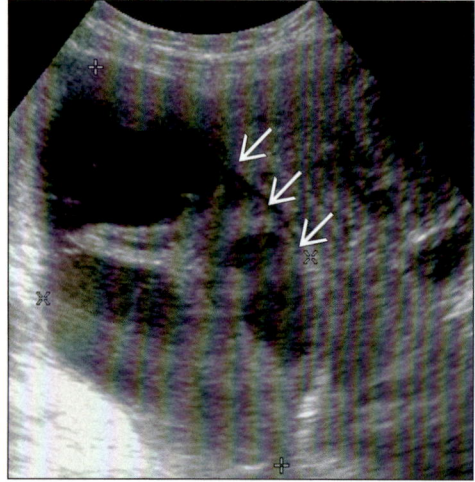
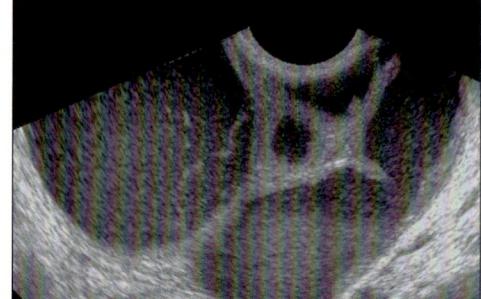

(Left) Transverse transabdominal ultrasound shows a large heterogeneous multiseptated cystic mass (calipers) to the right of the uterus ➡. Note how the margins between the cystic mass and the uterus are ill-defined. (Right) Transverse transvaginal ultrasound shows a dilated tube folded on itself with thick walls and heterogeneous internal contents.

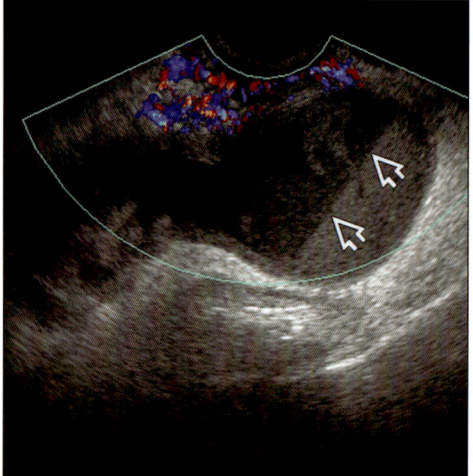
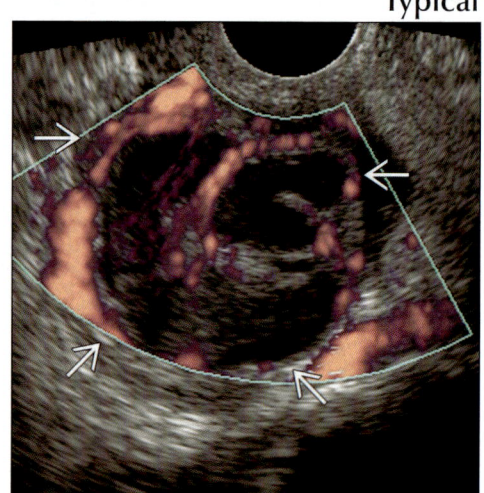

(Left) Transverse color Doppler ultrasound shows a dilated thick-walled tube with fluid-fluid layer ➡ due to dependent debris in the tube. Note the hyperemia around the tube. (Right) Transverse transvaginal ultrasound shows a heterogeneous hyperemic multiseptated cystic mass ➡.

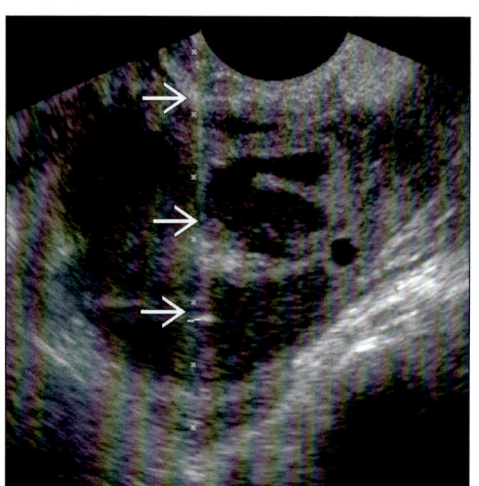
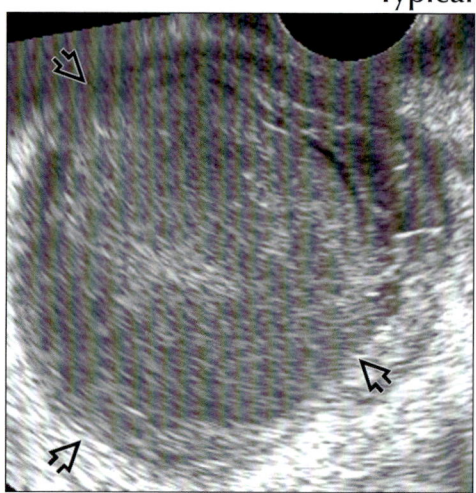

(Left) Longitudinal transvaginal ultrasound shows a needle guide and needle ➡ during transvaginal aspiration of TOA. (Right) Longitudinal transvaginal ultrasound shows an enlarged heterogeneous cyst ➡ in the right adnexa.

TUBO-OVARIAN ABSCESS

Typical

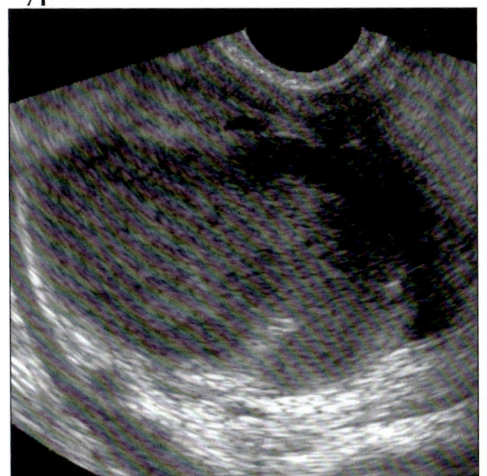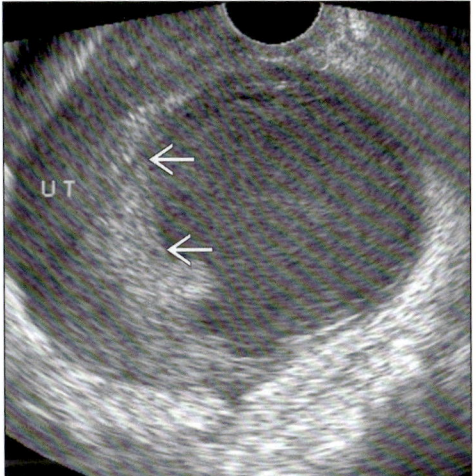

(Left) Transverse transvaginal ultrasound shows a dilated thick-walled tube filled with debris. *(Right)* Transverse transvaginal ultrasound shows a heterogeneous fluid collection adjacent to the uterus (UT). Note how the margins ➡ of the uterus and the cyst wall are indistinct.

Typical

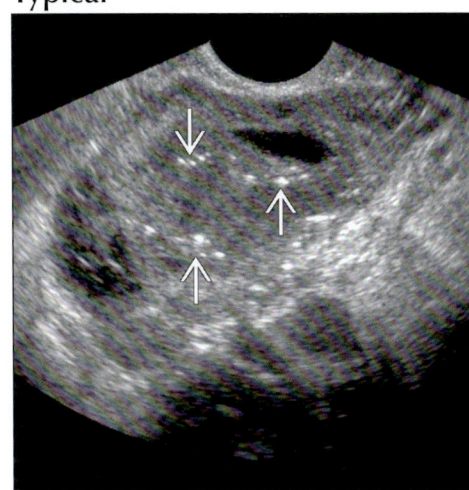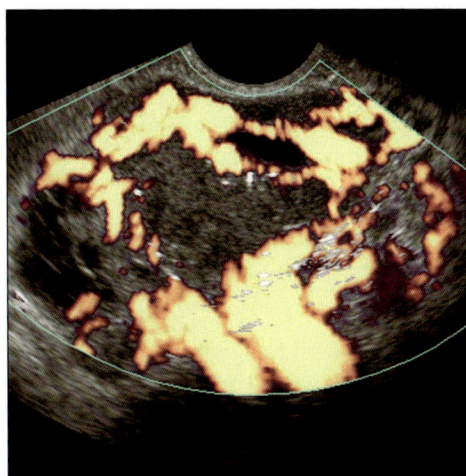

(Left) Transverse transvaginal ultrasound in patient with TOA after egg retrieval. Note the punctate echogenicities ➡ in the heterogeneous mass due to gas bubbles. *(Right)* Transverse power Doppler ultrasound in same patient as on left shows the marked hyperemia associated with the process.

Typical

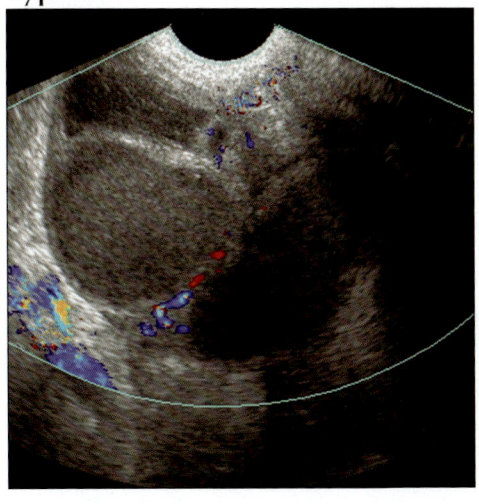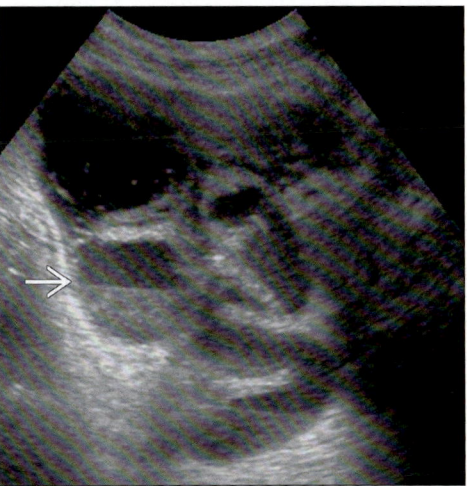

(Left) Transverse color Doppler ultrasound shows a multiseptated mass with heterogeneous fluid contents and mild hyperemia of walls of the tube. *(Right)* Sagittal oblique transabdominal ultrasound shows a heterogeneous multiloculated fluid collection. Some of the fluid collection is in the tube with fluid-fluid layers ➡ due to layering debris.

LEIOMYOMA, FALLOPIAN TUBE

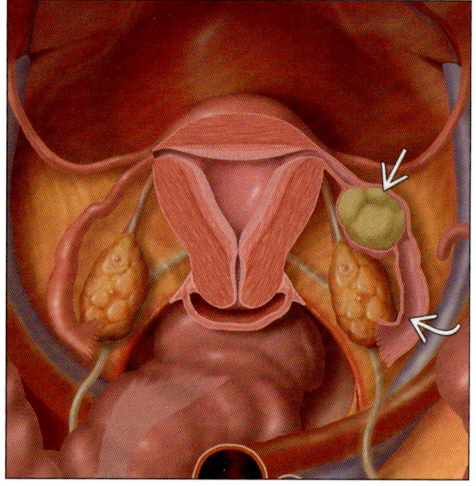

Coronal graphic shows a left fallopian tube leiomyoma arising from the muscular wall and distending the tubal lumen.

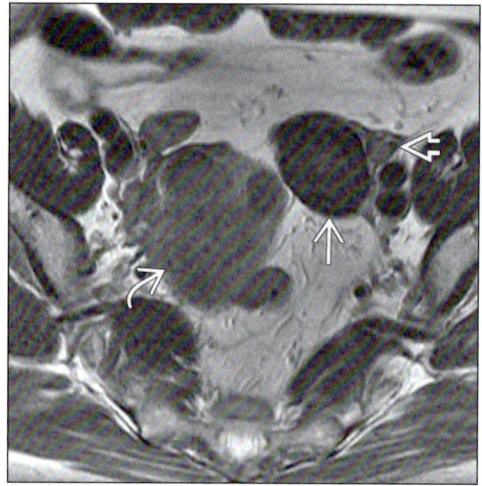

Axial T2WI MR shows a hypointense mass located between the uterus and left ovary.

TERMINOLOGY

Definitions
- Benign smooth muscle tumor arising from muscular layer of fallopian tube (FT)

IMAGING FINDINGS

General Features
- Best diagnostic clue: Solid adnexal mass with imaging characteristics of uterine leiomyoma, situated between uterus and ovary
- Location
  o Ampullary-isthmic junction
  o Unilateral
    ▪ Reported to involve left side more commonly
- Size: Typically small, < 3 cm
- Morphology
  o Solid adnexal mass separate from uterus and ovary
    ▪ Absent "claw" sign with uterus/ovary
    ▪ Absent "bridging vessel" sign with myometrium
  o Usually solitary
  o Most commonly homogeneous
  o Pedunculated or broad-based

Ultrasonographic Findings
- Grayscale Ultrasound
  o Hypoechoic solid mass distinct from uterus and ovary
    ▪ Moves separately from uterus/ovary on transvaginal ultrasound (TVS)
  o Poor sound transmission
  o Although most often homogeneous, may be of mixed echogenicity: Hypo- and hyperechoic
- Pulsed Doppler: Low impedance flow

CT Findings
- NECT: Mass isodense to uterus
- CECT: Variable degree of enhancement

MR Findings
- T1WI
  o Intermediate signal intensity (SI) mass, isointense to myometrium
  o May be hyperintense if associated with hemorrhagic degeneration
- T2WI
  o Hypointense to myometrium

DDx: Adnexal Masses

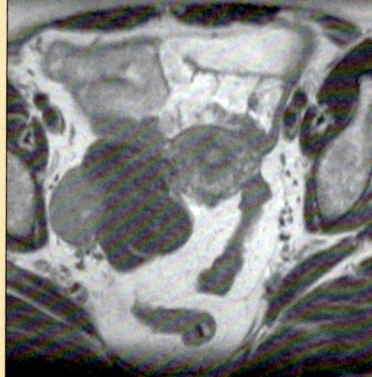
Broad Ligament Leiomyoma

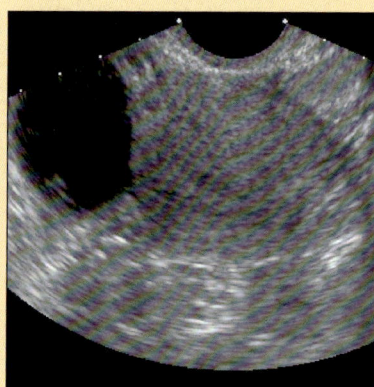
Ovarian Fibroma

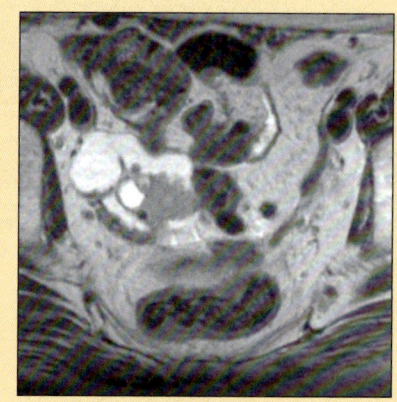
Fallopian Tube Carcinoma

LEIOMYOMA, FALLOPIAN TUBE

Key Facts

Terminology
- Benign smooth muscle tumor arising from muscular layer of fallopian tube (FT)

Imaging Findings
- Best diagnostic clue: Solid adnexal mass with imaging characteristics of uterine leiomyoma, situated between uterus and ovary
- Size: Typically small, < 3 cm
- Absent "claw" sign with uterus/ovary
- Absent "bridging vessel" sign with myometrium
- Most commonly homogeneous
- Hypervascular rim surrounds a portion or entire circumference of the mass
- Moves separately from uterus/ovary on transvaginal ultrasound (TVS)
- Best imaging tool: TVS and MR are the modalities of choice for detection and characterization

Top Differential Diagnoses
- Subserosal/Broad Ligament Leiomyoma
- Ovarian Leiomyoma/Fibroma
- Tubal Adenocarcinoma
- Other Mesodermal Tubal Tumors
- Mature Teratoma of Fallopian Tube

Diagnostic Checklist
- Consider fallopian tube leiomyoma in the setting of a small solid adnexal mass distinct from the uterus and ovary
- Solid adnexal mass with imaging characteristics of uterine leiomyoma
- "Rim" sign on MR helps suggest tubal origin

- ○ May show foci of hyperintensity when cystic degeneration present
  - Less common than in uterine leiomyomas, since FT leiomyomas typically smaller
- ○ Separate uterus/ovary identified
- ○ Tubal origin may be seen in some cases
  - Intermediate to low SI rim surrounds a portion or entire circumference of the mass
- T1 C+ FS
  - ○ Variable enhancement
    - Hypo- to isovascular with myometrium
  - ○ Tubal origin may be seen in some cases
    - Hypervascular rim surrounds a portion or entire circumference of the mass

Imaging Recommendations
- Best imaging tool: TVS and MR are the modalities of choice for detection and characterization
- Protocol advice
  - ○ MR: Phased array body coil
  - ○ High-resolution FSE T2WI
    - Slice thickness ≤ 4 mm
    - Transverse, sagittal and coronal images help demonstrate absence of connection to uterus/ovary
  - ○ T1 C+ FS best sequence to demonstrate tubal wall surrounding mass as a complete or incomplete hypervascular rim

DIFFERENTIAL DIAGNOSIS

Subserosal/Broad Ligament Leiomyoma
- Imaging appearance mimics FT leiomyoma
- Often larger and multiple
- Vascular pedicle connecting mass to uterus
  - ○ "Bridging vessel" sign

Ovarian Leiomyoma/Fibroma
- Imaging appearance mimics FT leiomyoma
- Mass draped by ovarian tissue
- No cleavage plane with ovary

Tubal Adenocarcinoma
- Malignant tumors of FT more frequently encountered than benign
- Heterogeneous solid adnexal mass
- Often manifests as a complex hydrosalpinx with enhancing mural nodules/papillary projections

Other Mesodermal Tubal Tumors
- Fibroma, lipoma, hemangioma, mesothelioma, lymphangioma, fibroadenoma, papilloma, mucosal polyp, adenomatoid tumor

Mature Teratoma of Fallopian Tube
- Same imaging appearance as ovarian dermoid
- Mixed cystic/solid mass
- Fat content, calcifications

PATHOLOGY

General Features
- General path comments
  - ○ Very low growth potential
    - Clinically significant late in life
    - Fail to undergo malignant transformation
  - ○ Derive from müllerian ducts as do uterine leiomyomas
    - Unlike uterine leiomyomas do not arise on a background of muscularis propria hypertrophy
  - ○ Possible explanation for low prevalence of FT leiomyomas compared to uterine leiomyomas
    - Myometrium demonstrates marked morphologic and functional changes during menstrual cycle and pregnancy due to hormonal responsiveness
    - Tubal musculature fails to exhibit significant changes even during pregnancy
- Epidemiology: Rare entity, less common than uterine leiomyomas
- Associated abnormalities
  - ○ Uterine leiomyomas
  - ○ Complications
    - Excessive growth

LEIOMYOMA, FALLOPIAN TUBE

- Torsion
- Degenerative or purulent changes
- Ectopic pregnancy

Gross Pathologic & Surgical Features
- Fusiform swelling of tubal wall with dome-like projection in compressed lumen
- Pedunculated mass
- Ovoid, smooth, firm mass

Microscopic Features
- Elongated smooth muscle elements arranged in interweaving, intersecting bundles and fascicles
- Positivity for alpha smooth muscle actin on immunohistochemistry
- Continuity with tubal muscularis layer

CLINICAL ISSUES

Presentation
- Most common signs/symptoms: Asymptomatic
- Other signs/symptoms
  - Vague pelvic discomfort
  - Abdominal pain 2° to obstruction of tubal lumen
  - Acute abdomen when FT leiomyoma complicated by: Torsion, ectopic pregnancy, degeneration
  - Palpable adnexal mass

Demographics
- Age: Pre and postmenopausal women

Natural History & Prognosis
- Usually asymptomatic and incidentally found at autopsy or unrelated surgical procedure
- No report of malignant transformation

Treatment
- Tubal sparing surgery when possible
- Salpingectomy when diagnosis uncertain or in complicated cases
- Confirmation of tubal patency after tumor resection

DIAGNOSTIC CHECKLIST

Consider
- Consider fallopian tube leiomyoma in the setting of a small solid adnexal mass distinct from the uterus and ovary

Image Interpretation Pearls
- Solid adnexal mass with imaging characteristics of uterine leiomyoma
  - Distinct from uterus and ovary
  - "Rim" sign on MR helps suggest tubal origin

SELECTED REFERENCES

1. Yang CC et al: Primary leiomyoma of the fallopian tube: preoperative ultrasound findings. J Chin Med Assoc. 70(2):80-3, 2007
2. Berzal-Cantalejo F et al: Solitary fibrous tumor arising in the fallopian tube. Gynecol Oncol. 96(3):880-2, 2005
3. Wen KC et al: Primary fallopian tube leiomyoma managed by laparoscopy. J Minim Invasive Gynecol. 12(3):193, 2005
4. Misao R et al: Leiomyoma of the fallopian tube. Gynecol Obstet Invest. 49(4):279-80, 2000
5. Mroueh J et al: Tubal pregnancy associated with ampullary tubal leiomyoma. Obstet Gynecol. 81(5 (Pt 2)):880-2, 1993
6. Schust D et al: Leiomyomas of the fallopian tube. A case report. J Reprod Med. 38(9):741-2, 1993
7. Escoffery CT et al: Leiomyoma of the fallopian tube: an unusual cause of abdominal pain. Int J Gynaecol Obstet. 38(2):128-9, 1992
8. Moore OA et al: Leiomyoma of the fallopian tube: a cause of tubal pregnancy. Am J Obstet Gynecol. 134(1):101-2, 1979
9. Crissman JD et al: Leiomyoma of uterine tube: report of a case. Am J Obstet Gynecol. 126(8):1046, 1976
10. Honore LH et al: Leiomyoma of the Fallopian tube. A case report and review of the literature. Arch Gynakol. 221(1):47-50, 1976

LEIOMYOMA, FALLOPIAN TUBE

IMAGE GALLERY

Typical

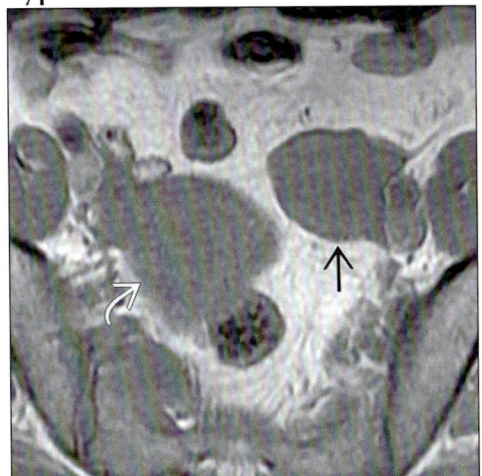 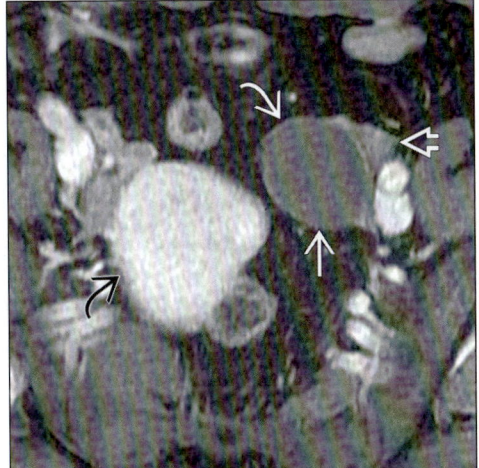

(Left) Axial T1WI MR in the same patient as previous image shows the mass ➡ to be isointense to the myometrium ➡. *(Right)* Axial T1 C+ FS MR in the same patient as previous, shows the mass ➡ to be hypovascular relative to the myometrium ➡ and adjacent ovary ➡. Note the hypervascular rim ➡ surrounding a portion of the mass, a clue to the tubal origin of this leiomyoma.

Typical

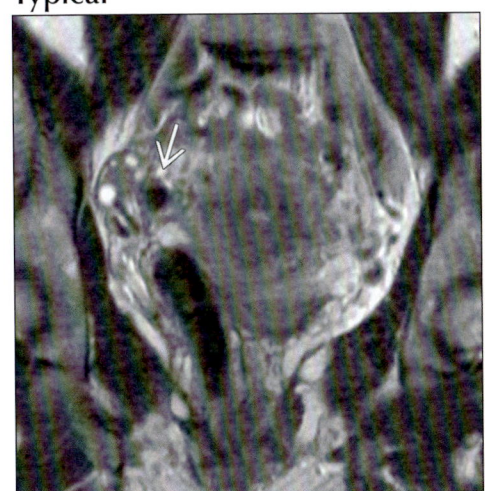 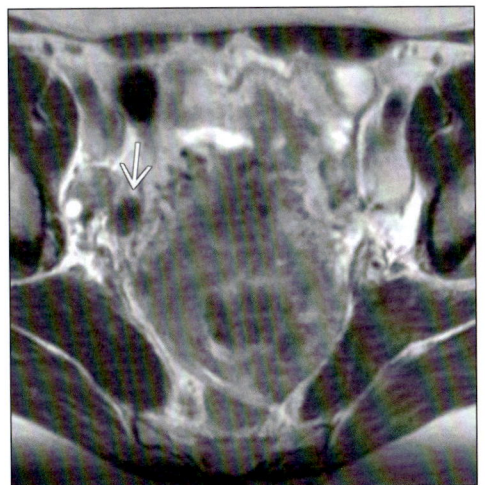

(Left) Coronal T2WI MR shows a small, round, hypointense lesion ➡ situated between the uterus and right ovary. No connection to either the uterus or ovary is seen. *(Right)* Axial T2WI MR in the same patient as previous image, shows the hypointense mass ➡ consistent with a small fallopian tube leiomyoma.

Typical

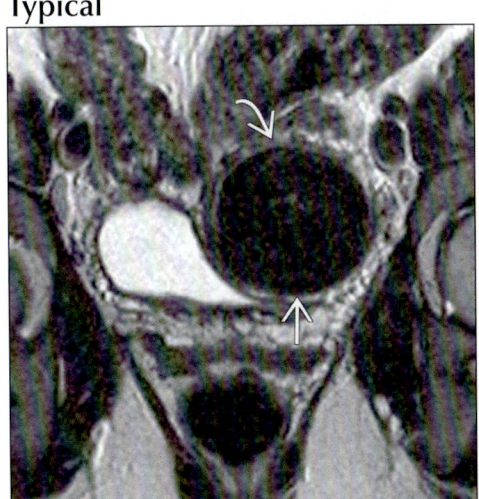 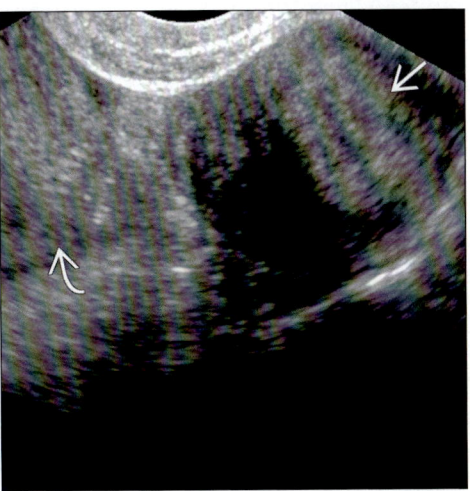

(Left) Coronal T2WI MR in a patient with a previous hysterectomy shows a round, hypointense adnexal mass ➡ that is distinct from the left ovary (not shown) and proved to be a fallopian tube leiomyoma. Note the incomplete rim ➡ of intermediate signal intensity surrounding the mass. *(Right)* Oblique transvaginal ultrasound shows a hypoechoic attenuating lesion ➡ in the left adnexa that is completely separate from the uterus ➡ and ovary (not shown).

TUBAL CARCINOMA, CHARACTERIZATION

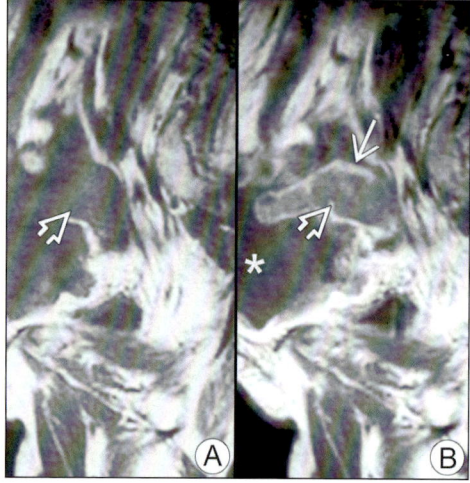

Sagittal T1WI MR (A) and T1 C+ MR (B) show tubular adnexal mass ➡. Note enhancing fallopian tube wall ➡ around mass on (B). Ascites (*).

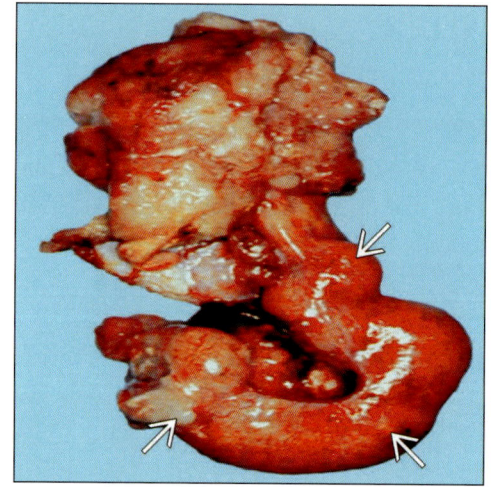

Gross pathology shows expanded fallopian tube with intraluminal tumoral growth ➡.

TERMINOLOGY

Abbreviations and Synonyms
- Fallopian tube carcinoma

Definitions
- Primary malignant neoplasm of fallopian tube

IMAGING FINDINGS

General Features
- Best diagnostic clue
  - Solid or partly solid and cystic adnexal mass which expands fallopian tube lumen
  - Hydrosalpinx is seen when fallopian tube lumen is obstructed
  - Other associated findings include intrauterine fluid and peritumoral ascites
- Location: Usually unilateral but both fallopian tubes can be involved
- Morphology
  - Tubal carcinoma can show nodular, papillary, infiltrative, or diffuse growth patterns
  - Fallopian tube may remain intact or it may show swelling and sausage-like expansion

Ultrasonographic Findings
- Grayscale Ultrasound
  - Solid or partly solid and cystic adnexal mass with variable echotexture
  - Associated hydrosalpinx is seen as anechoic or hypoechoic tubular structure
- Color Doppler: Solid components of tubal carcinoma demonstrate low-resistance vascular flow
- Power Doppler: Tumor vascularity in the solid components of tubal carcinoma is augmented with power Doppler
- 3D: Useful in better visualization of tubal wall irregularities such as papillary projections and pseudosepta.

CT Findings
- CECT
  - Heterogeneously enhancing, solid or partly solid and cystic adnexal mass
  - Tubular configuration of mass and associated hydrosalpinx can be seen

DDx: Adnexal Masses

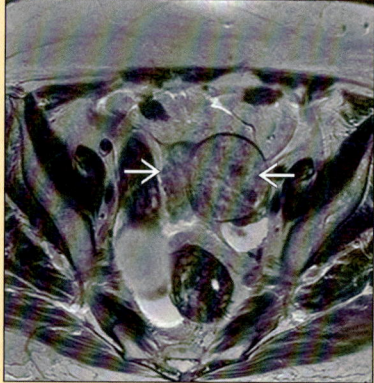

Ovarian Cancer

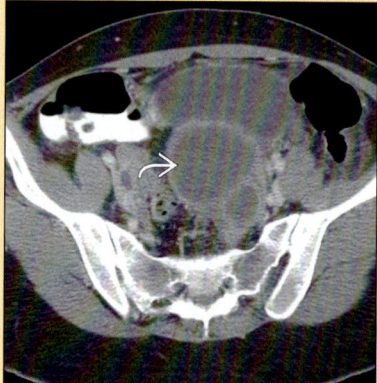

Tubo-Ovarian Abscess

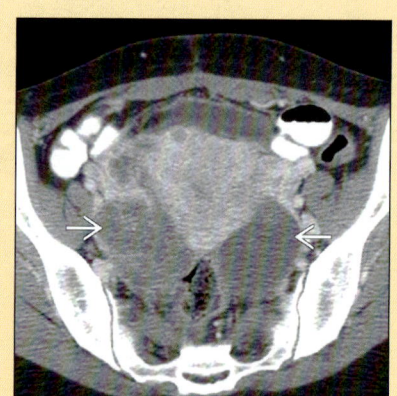

Metastases to Fallopian Tubes

TUBAL CARCINOMA, CHARACTERIZATION

Key Facts

Terminology
- Primary malignant neoplasm of fallopian tube

Imaging Findings
- Solid or partly solid and cystic adnexal mass which expands fallopian tube lumen
- Hydrosalpinx is seen when fallopian tube lumen is obstructed
- Other associated findings include intrauterine fluid and peritumoral ascites
- Location: Usually unilateral but both fallopian tubes can be involved
- Tubal carcinoma can show nodular, papillary, infiltrative, or diffuse growth patterns
- Fallopian tube may remain intact or it may show swelling and sausage-like expansion

Pathology
- Most common histologic type of primary adenocarcinoma of fallopian tube is papillary serous carcinoma, which is histologically identical to ovarian serous adenocarcinoma
- Tubal carcinoma spreads in a similar fashion as ovarian cancer
- Lymphatic spread is more common in tubal carcinoma compared to ovarian carcinoma

Diagnostic Checklist
- On imaging, it may be difficult to differentiate tubal carcinoma from other ovarian masses
- Enhancing fallopian tube wall around mass and tubular shape of mass are helpful in diagnosis

---

  ○ Enhancing thickened tubal walls can be seen around mass

MR Findings
- T1WI: Intermediate signal intensity adnexal mass
- T2WI
  ○ Heterogeneous, intermediate to high signal intensity mass
  ○ Associated hydrosalpinx is seen as high signal intensity tubular structure
- T1 C+
  ○ Solid elements of the mass and papillary projections show heterogeneous enhancement
  ○ Enhancing thickened tubal walls can be seen around the mass

Nuclear Medicine Findings
- PET: Useful in detecting metastases and recurrences

Imaging Recommendations
- Best imaging tool
  ○ Initial imaging method is usually US in patients with suspected adnexal mass
  ○ MR can be used as a problem solving tool for initial diagnosis of tubal carcinoma
  ○ CT and MR can be used for staging purposes

DIFFERENTIAL DIAGNOSIS

Ovarian Cancer
- It may be difficult to differentiate tubal carcinoma from ovarian cancer on imaging studies
- Enhancing wall around mass, tubular configuration of mass and intact ovaries suggest diagnosis of tubal carcinoma

Benign Hydrosalpinx, Pyosalpinx or Hematosalpinx
- Absence of obstructing mass is helpful in differentiation between benign hydrosalpinx and malignant hydrosalpinx

Tubo-Ovarian Abscess
- Unilocular/multilocular adnexal cystic masses with wall enhancement
- Clinical findings of fever, pelvic pain with complex adnexal mass on imaging in a sexually active female is characteristic for tubo-ovarian abscess

Metastasis to Fallopian Tube
- Metastasis to fallopian tube is more common than primary tubal carcinoma
- Ovarian, uterine, breast and gastrointestinal cancers most commonly metastasize to fallopian tube
- Imaging findings of metastatic and primary fallopian cancer are similar

PATHOLOGY

General Features
- General path comments
  ○ Most common histologic type of primary adenocarcinoma of fallopian tube is papillary serous carcinoma, which is histologically identical to ovarian serous adenocarcinoma
  ○ These tumors tend to produce large amounts of serous fluid
  ○ Tubal carcinoma spreads in a similar fashion as ovarian cancer
    ▪ Peritoneal dissemination
    ▪ Contiguous invasion
    ▪ Transluminal migration
    ▪ Hematogenous dissemination
  ○ Lymphatic spread is more common in tubal carcinoma compared to ovarian carcinoma
- Epidemiology
  ○ Primary tubal carcinoma is a very rare tumor
  ○ It accounts for approximately 0.14-1.8% of female genital tract malignancies
  ○ Bilateral involvement can occur in 7% of early stages and in 30% of late stages
  ○ There is predilection for nulliparous women (25-30% of cases occur in nulliparous women)

TUBAL CARCINOMA, CHARACTERIZATION

Gross Pathologic & Surgical Features
- Swollen and expanded fallopian tube with intraluminal papillary or solid tumoral growth

Microscopic Features
- Serous tumors may show papillary patterns, cords or sheets of pleomorphic cells

Staging, Grading or Classification Criteria
- Similar to FIGO staging of ovarian cancer

CLINICAL ISSUES

Presentation
- Most common signs/symptoms
  - Typical triad of symptoms are seen only in a small number of cases
    - Intermittent profuse serosanguineous vaginal discharge
    - Colicky pain relieved by discharge
    - Abdominal or pelvic mass
  - **Hydrops tubae profluens** is a pathognomonic feature of tubal carcinoma but is rarely seen
    - Intermittent discharge of clear or bloody fluid, either spontaneous or caused by pressure, followed by shrinkage of adnexal mass
- Clinical Profile: CA-125 is a useful tumor marker for diagnosis, assessment of response to treatment, and detection of recurrence

Demographics
- Age
  - Tubal carcinoma most frequently occurs between the fourth and sixth decades of life
    - Median age: 55 years; range: 17-88 years

Natural History & Prognosis
- Most important prognostic factor is stage of disease
- 5 year survival rate is 80% in early stages and 20% in advanced disease

Treatment
- Surgery is primary method of treatment
  - Surgery consists of total abdominal hysterectomy, bilateral salpingo-oophorectomy, omentectomy, tumor debulking and lymph node dissection
- Chemotherapy is useful for advanced and recurrent disease
- Role of radiotherapy is limited due to availability of effective chemotherapy

DIAGNOSTIC CHECKLIST

Consider
- Diagnosis of tubal carcinoma is rarely made pre-operatively
- Tubal carcinoma is similar to ovarian cancer in staging, treatment and prognosis

Image Interpretation Pearls
- Prognosis of tubal carcinoma is related to stage of disease

- Therefore, familiarity with imaging findings of tubal carcinoma is important for establishing an early diagnosis
- On imaging, it may be difficult to differentiate tubal carcinoma from other ovarian masses
- Enhancing fallopian tube wall around mass and tubular shape of mass are helpful in diagnosis
- Detection of solid components and papillary projections is augmented by administration of contrast
- Other associated findings include peritumoral ascites, intrauterine fluid and hydrosalpinx

SELECTED REFERENCES

1. Hosokawa C et al: Bilateral primary fallopian tube carcinoma: findings on sequential MRI. AJR Am J Roentgenol. 186(4):1046-50, 2006
2. Pectasides D et al: Fallopian tube carcinoma: a review. Oncologist. 11(8):902-12, 2006
3. Ajithkumar TV et al: Primary fallopian tube carcinoma. Obstet Gynecol Surv. 60(4):247-52, 2005
4. Haratz-Rubinstein N et al: Sonographic diagnosis of Fallopian tube carcinoma. Ultrasound Obstet Gynecol. 24(1):86-8, 2004
5. Patlas M et al: Sonographic diagnosis of primary malignant tumors of the fallopian tube. Ultrasound Q. 20(2):59-64, 2004
6. Varras M et al: Primary fallopian tube adenocarcinoma: preoperative diagnosis, treatment and follow-up. Eur J Gynaecol Oncol. 25(5):640-6, 2004
7. Mikami M et al: Preoperative diagnosis of fallopian tube cancer by imaging. Abdom Imaging. 28(5):743-7, 2003
8. Szklaruk J et al: MR imaging of common and uncommon large pelvic masses. Radiographics. 23(2):403-24, 2003
9. Makhija S et al: Positron emission tomography/computed tomography imaging for the detection of recurrent ovarian and fallopian tube carcinoma: a retrospective review. Gynecol Oncol. 85(1):53-8, 2002
10. Patel PV et al: PET-CT localizes previously undetectable metastatic lesions in recurrent fallopian tube carcinoma. Gynecol Oncol. 87(3):323-6, 2002
11. Kurjak A et al: Preoperative diagnosis of the primary fallopian tube carcinoma by three-dimensional static and power Doppler sonography. Ultrasound Obstet Gynecol. 15(3):246-51, 2000
12. Schneider C et al: Primary carcinoma of the fallopian tube. A report of 19 cases with literature review. Eur J Gynaecol Oncol. 21(6):578-82, 2000
13. Slanetz PJ et al: Imaging of fallopian tube tumors. AJR Am J Roentgenol. 169(5):1321-4, 1997

TUBAL CARCINOMA, CHARACTERIZATION

IMAGE GALLERY

Typical

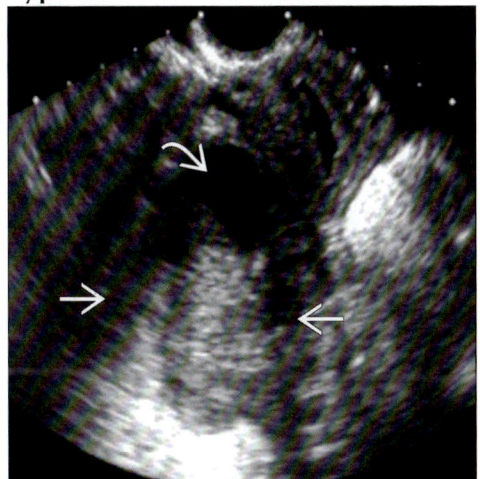
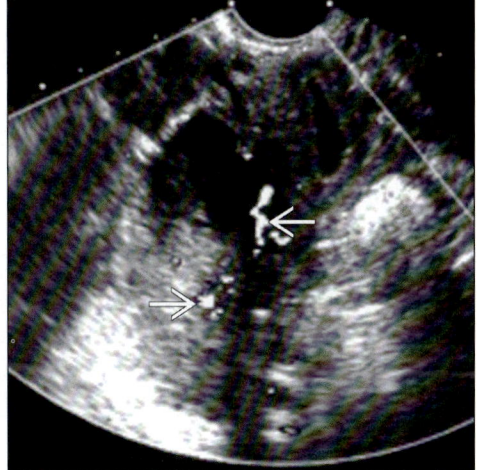

(Left) Coronal oblique transvaginal ultrasound shows tubal carcinoma seen as a solid ➡ and cystic ➡ mass in the right adnexal region. *(Right)* Coronal oblique black and white image from color Doppler examination shows vascularity ➡ in the solid components of the tubal carcinoma.

Typical

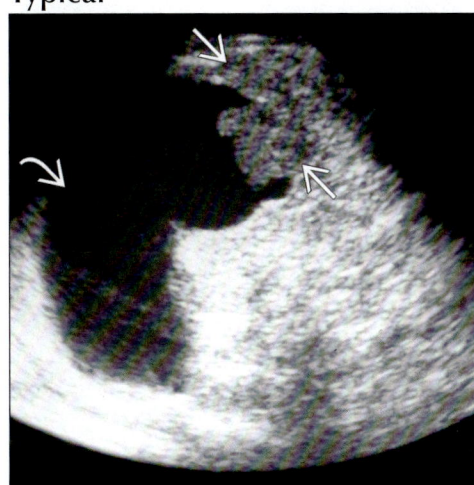
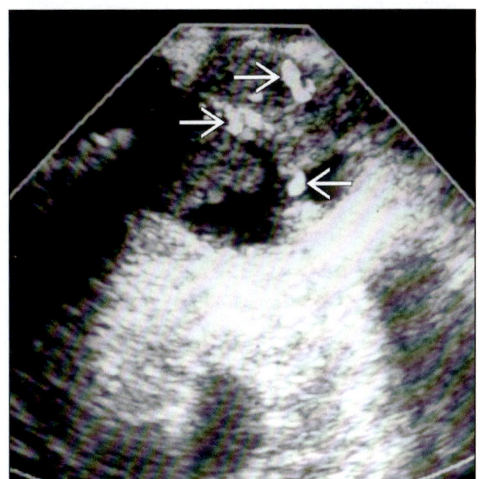

(Left) Axial oblique transabdominal ultrasound shows tubal carcinoma ➡ expanding the fallopian tube with associated hydrosalpinx ➡. *(Right)* Axial oblique black and white image from color Doppler examination shows vascularity ➡ in tubal carcinoma in the same patient.

Typical

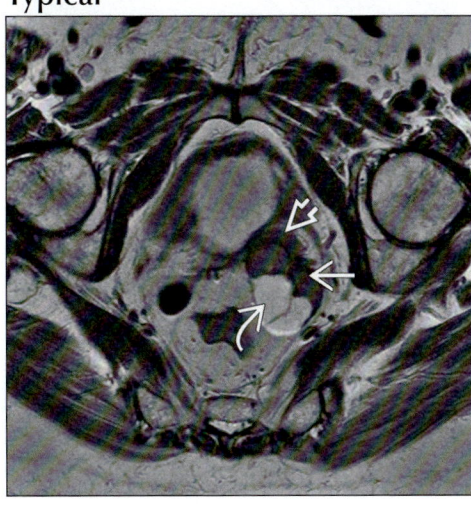
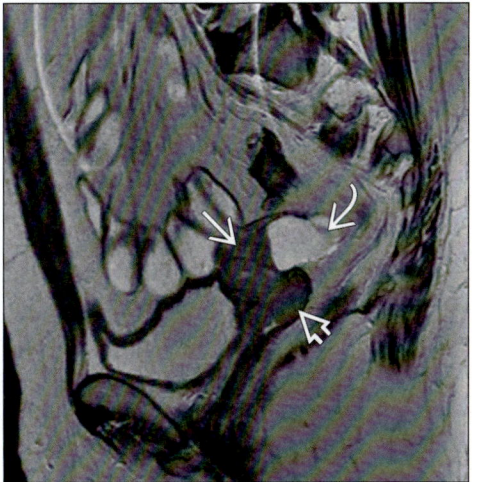

(Left) Axial oblique T2WI MR shows tubal carcinoma seen as a solid mass ➡ with associated hydrosalpinx ➡. Note that the mass invades the vaginal cuff ➡. *(Right)* Sagittal T2WI MR shows tubal carcinoma ➡ and associated hydrosalpinx ➡. Invasion to vaginal cuff ➡ is better visualized on this image.

TUBAL CARCINOMA, CHARACTERIZATION

(Left) Axial CECT shows tubal carcinoma seen as a solid enhancing mass ➡ with associated hydrosalpinx ➡ and ascites ➡. *(Right)* Axial CECT shows tubal carcinoma seen as a heterogeneously enhancing solid mass ➡, expanding the fallopian tube. Ascites ➡ is also seen.

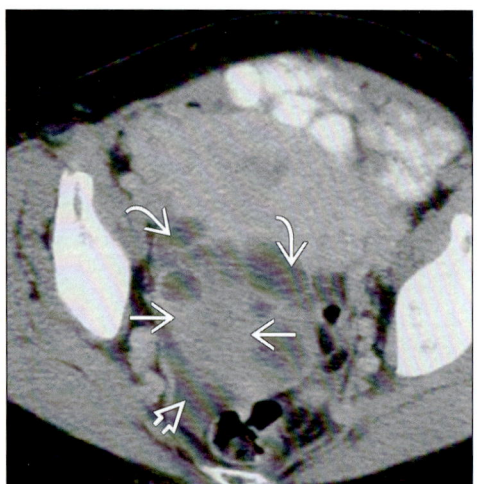
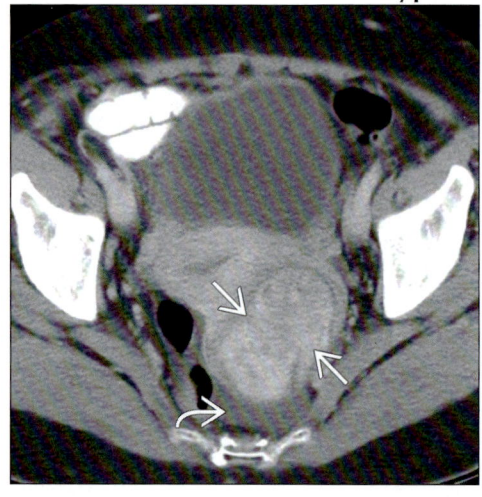

Typical

(Left) Axial CECT shows tubal carcinoma seen as an enhancing mass ➡ with tubular configuration in the right adnexal region. *(Right)* Axial CECT shows tubal carcinoma ➡ and associated dilated tube ➡ in the same patient as previous image.

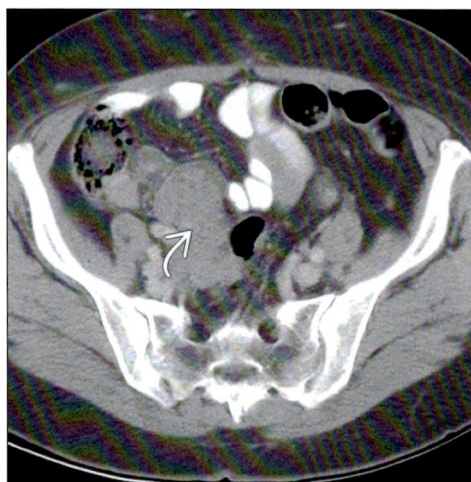
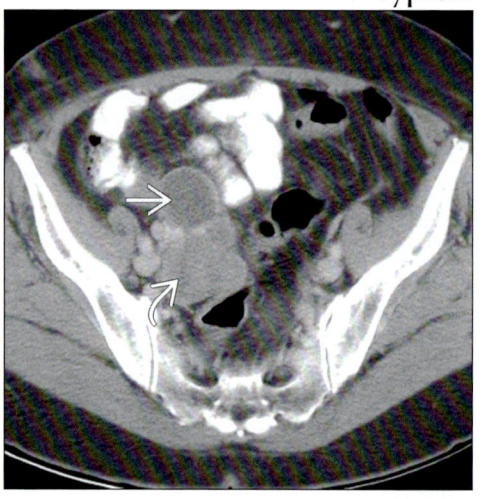

Typical

(Left) Axial CECT shows tubal carcinoma ➡ and associated hydrosalpinx ➡. *(Right)* Axial CECT shows tubal carcinoma ➡ and hydrosalpinx ➡. Note that the mass invades the rectosigmoid ➡.

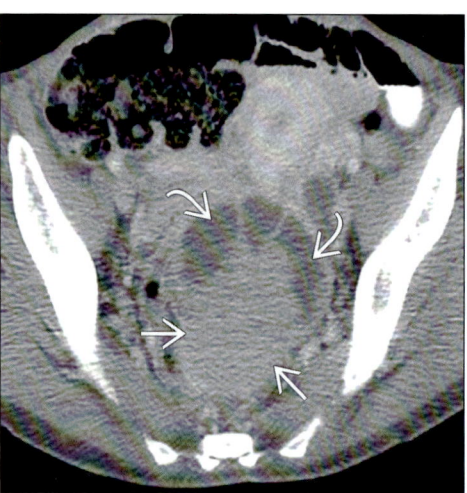
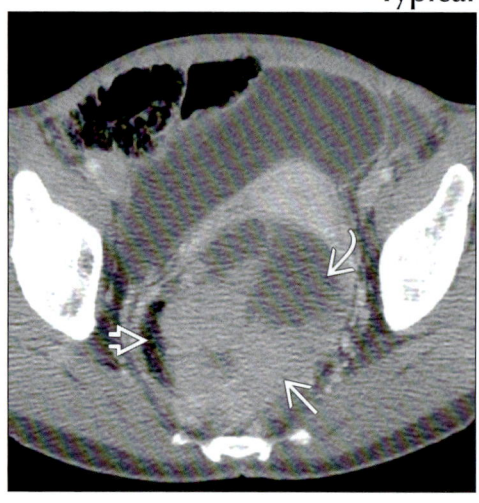

Typical

TUBAL CARCINOMA, CHARACTERIZATION

Typical

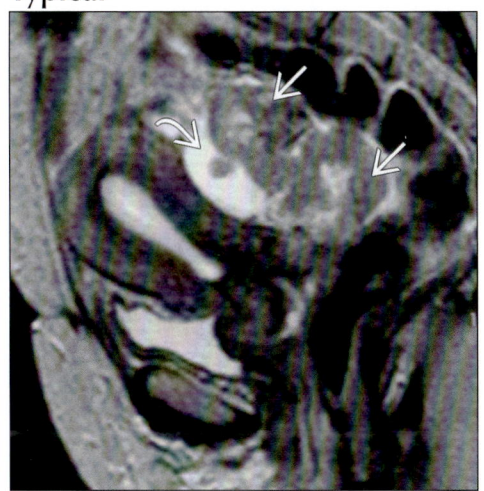 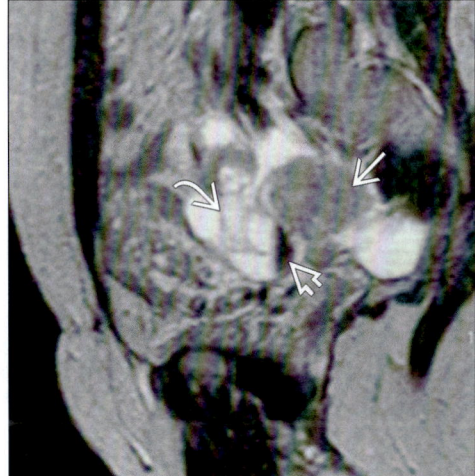

(Left) Sagittal T2WI MR shows tubal carcinoma seen as a heterogeneous mass ➡ with associated hydrosalpinx ➡. *(Right)* Sagittal T2WI MR shows tubal carcinoma ➡ and dilated fallopian tube ➡. Note the layering, low-signal intensity blood ➡ in the dependent portion of the fallopian tube.

Typical

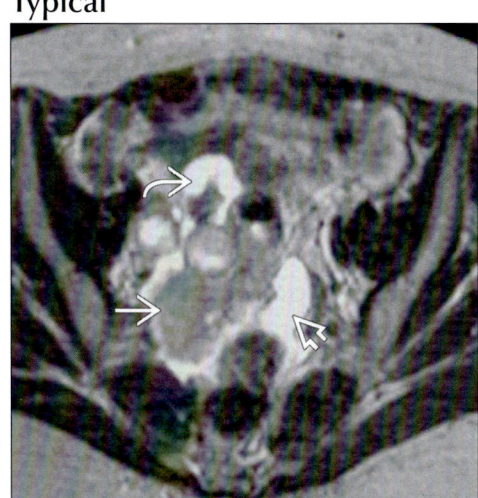 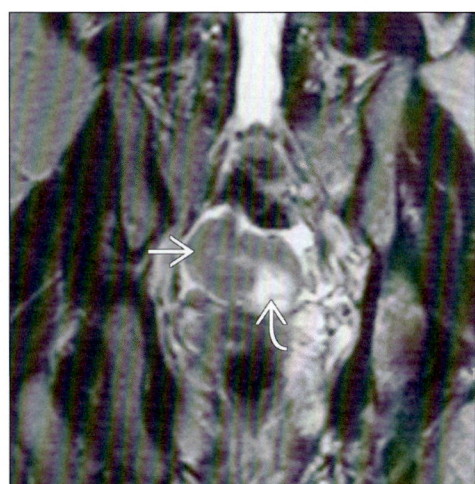

(Left) Axial T2WI MR shows tubal carcinoma ➡ with associated dilated fallopian tube ➡ and ascites ➡. *(Right)* Coronal T2WI MR shows tubal carcinoma seen as a heterogeneous mass with solid ➡ and cystic ➡ components.

Typical

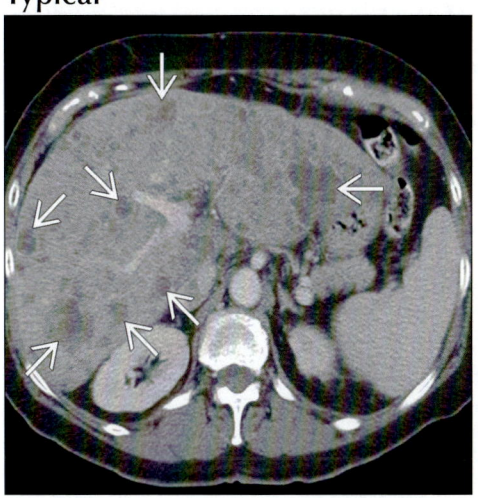 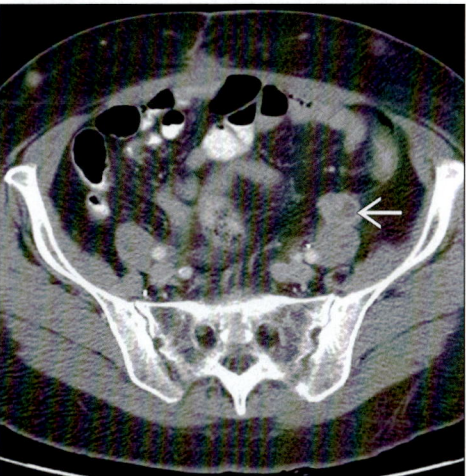

(Left) Axial CECT shows multiple liver metastases ➡ in a patient with tubal carcinoma. *(Right)* Axial CECT shows a tumor implant ➡, anterior to left psoas muscle, in a patient with metastatic tubal carcinoma.

TUBAL CARCINOMA, STAGING/PROGNOSIS

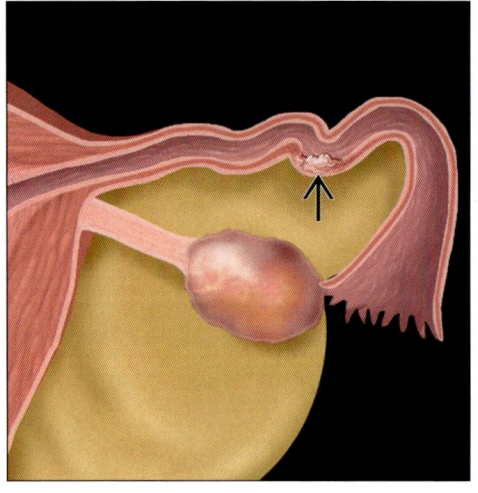

Coronal graphic shows growth limited to one tube ➔ with no penetration to serosal surfaces or ascites. Compatible with stage IA.

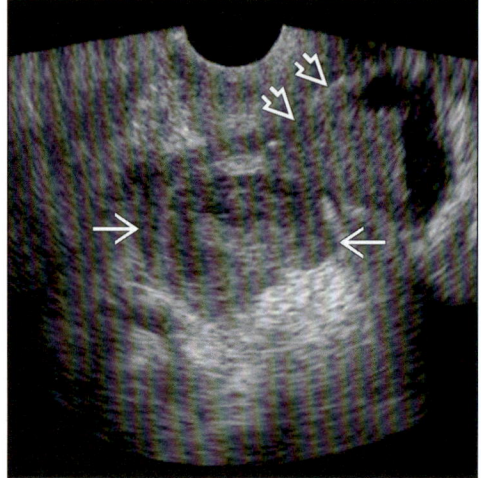

Coronal transvaginal ultrasound shows hypoechoic material filling the tube ➔. Compatible with stage I fallopian tube tumor. The tube and mass are separate from ovary ➔.

TERMINOLOGY

Abbreviations and Synonyms
- Fallopian tubal carcinoma

Definitions
- Cancer of fallopian tube origin
- Rarest female gynecologic malignancy with similarities to ovarian epithelial carcinoma

IMAGING FINDINGS

General Features
- Ultrasonography (US), MR or CT can be useful in confirming the finding of a pelvic mass or ascites but are not diagnostic for tubal carcinoma per se
- With both CT & MR imaging, the lesion can appear relatively small, solid & lobulated when not associated with hydrosalpinx
  - On CT the attenuation is usually equal to other soft tissue masses & enhances less than myometrium
  - On T1WI tumor is usually hypointense
  - On T2WI tumor is most often homogeneously hyperintense
  - Associated findings include peritumoral ascites, intrauterine fluid collection & hydrosalpinx

DIFFERENTIAL DIAGNOSIS

Lesions Arising from Ovary or Uterus
- With extension or involvement of fallopian tube
- When large, may not be able to decide origin

Tubo-Ovarian Abscess
- Dilated fallopian tube containing pus & inseparable from complex solid and cystic lesion involving adjacent ovary
- Simulates mass

Hydrosalpinx
- Benign, simple fluid-filled fallopian tube
- May be an associated finding with tubal cancer

DDx: Tubal Carcinoma

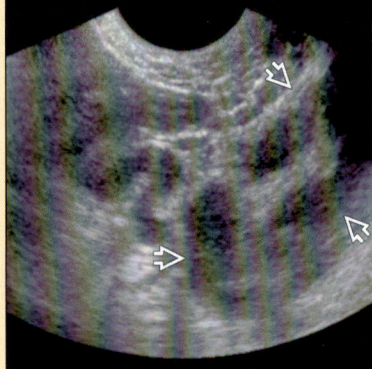
Hydrosalpinx

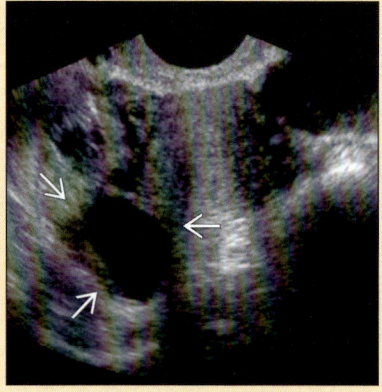
Tubo-Ovarian Abscess

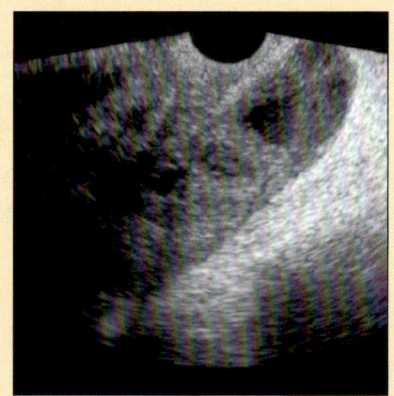
Tumor of Ovarian Origin

TUBAL CARCINOMA, STAGING/PROGNOSIS

Key Facts

Imaging Findings
- Ultrasonography (US), MR or CT can be useful in confirming the finding of a pelvic mass or ascites but are not diagnostic for tubal carcinoma per se

Top Differential Diagnoses
- Lesions Arising from Ovary or Uterus
- Tubo-Ovarian Abscess
- Hydrosalpinx

Pathology
- If the tube & ovary are both involved with tumor, the bulk of the tumor should be in the tube
- Most common histology is adenocarcinoma with papillary features and serous type (more than 90%)
- Stage I: Growth is limited to the fallopian tube
- Stage II: Growth involving one or both fallopian tubes with pelvic extension
- Stage III: Tumor involves one or both fallopian tubes with peritoneal implants outside of the pelvis and/or positive retroperitoneal or inguinal lymph nodes; superficial liver metastasis; tumor limited to the pelvis but with histologically proven malignant extension to the small bowel or omentum
- Stage IIIC: Abdominal implants more than 2 cm in diameter and/or positive retroperitoneal or inguinal nodes
- Stage IV: Growth involving one or both tubes with distant metastases; if pleural effusion is present there must be positive cytology to be stage IV; parenchymal liver metastases equals stage IV

PATHOLOGY

General Features
- Epidemiology: True incidence is probably underestimated because advanced cases may be incorrectly diagnosed clinically & histologically as primary ovarian carcinoma

Gross Pathologic & Surgical Features
- May see gross, diffuse intra-abdominal spread of disease at surgery similar to ovarian epithelial cancer
- Original pathologic criteria for diagnosing carcinoma primary to the fallopian tube was established by Hu et al in 1950
- Hu's criteria was then modified in 1978 by Sedlis
  - Tumor must arise from the endosalpinx
  - Histologic pattern is of mucosal tubal epithelium
  - Transition from benign to malignant epithelium must be present
  - Endometrium & ovaries are either normal or the tumor in these organs is smaller than the tumor in the tube
  - If the tube & ovary are both involved with tumor, the bulk of the tumor should be in the tube
  - Tubal mucosa should be involved & should show a papillary pattern
  - If tubal wall is completely involved, the transition between benign & malignant tubal epithelium should be demonstrable

Microscopic Features
- Most resemble serous carcinoma of the ovary
- Most common histology is adenocarcinoma with papillary features and serous type (more than 90%)

Staging, Grading or Classification Criteria
- Staging is based on laparotomy & resection of tubal masses as well as hysterectomy with biopsies of all suspicious sites including omentum, mesentery, liver diaphragm & pelvic & paraaortic lymph nodes
- Staging (FIGO nomenclature)
  - Stage 0: Carcinoma in situ (limited to tubal mucosa)
  - Stage I: Growth is limited to the fallopian tube
  - Stage IA: Growth is limited to one tube with extension into the submucosa and/or muscularis but not penetrating the serosal surface; no ascites
  - Stage IB: Growth is limited to both tubes with extension to submucosa and/or muscularis but not penetrating the serosal surface; no ascites
  - Stage IC: Tumor either stage IA or IB but with extension through or onto the tubal serosa or with ascites present containing malignant cells or with positive peritoneal washing
  - Stage II: Growth involving one or both fallopian tubes with pelvic extension
  - Stage IIA: Extension or metastasis to the uterus and/or ovaries
  - Stage IIB: Extension to other pelvic tissues
  - Stage IIC: Tumor either stage IIA or IIB but with extension through or onto the tubal serosa, or with ascites present containing malignant cells or with positive peritoneal washing
  - Stage III: Tumor involves one or both fallopian tubes with peritoneal implants outside of the pelvis and/or positive retroperitoneal or inguinal lymph nodes; superficial liver metastasis; tumor limited to the pelvis but with histologically proven malignant extension to the small bowel or omentum
  - Stage IIIA: Tumor is grossly limited to true pelvis with negative nodes and with histologically confirmed microscopic seeding of the abdominal peritoneal surface
  - Stage IIIB: Tumor involving one or both tubes with histologically confirmed implants of abdominal peritoneal surfaces, not exceeding 2 cm in diameter; lymph nodes are negative
  - Stage IIIC: Abdominal implants more than 2 cm in diameter and/or positive retroperitoneal or inguinal nodes
  - Stage IV: Growth involving one or both tubes with distant metastases; if pleural effusion is present there must be positive cytology to be stage IV; parenchymal liver metastases equals stage IV
- Surface involvement of the liver occurs in stage II as do inguinal nodal metastases

TUBAL CARCINOMA, STAGING/PROGNOSIS

- In stage III, classification of the tumor is based on the findings at the time of entry into the abdominal cavity, not on the residual at the end of debulking
- At surgery, 20-25% are stage I, 20-25% are stage II and 40-50% with disease beyond the pelvis

CLINICAL ISSUES

Presentation
- Most common signs/symptoms
  - Triad of **hydrops tubae profluens** is pathognomonic of tubal cancer
    - Profuse vaginal discharge
    - Colicky abdominal pain (± relief with vaginal discharge)
    - Abdominal pelvic mass
  - Other rare presenting symptoms: Respiratory insufficiency, urinary urgency, inguinal node & umbilical metastases, bowel movement dysfunction, ureteral obstruction, back pain, abnormal neurologic findings (subacute cerebellar degeneration), & exfoliative dermatitis
  - Diagnosis is rarely made before surgery because of nonspecific presentation & findings

Natural History & Prognosis
- Compared to ovarian cancer, fallopian tube cancer
  - Presents earlier
  - Has a worse prognosis stage for stage
  - Has similar pattern of relapse
- Prognostic factors
  - Size of residual tumor at the termination of surgery, nodal status & type of treatment post-operatively
  - Presence of ascites & histologic grade
- Early stage of disease & absence of residual tumor at the end of the initial surgical procedure are considered strongest predictors of survival
- Prognosis of early stage disease is proportional to the involvement of the tubal wall
- Presence of residual tumor nodules over 2 cm after debulking surgery is an adverse prognostic factor
- Survival has been correlated with nodal status; 76 months when nodes negative & 33 months when nodes positive
- Time to first recurrence: Within first 2 years after diagnosis
- Mortality from recurrence is high
- Patterns of spread
  - Spreads first by exfoliation of the clonogenic cells into the lumen of the fallopian tube, expanding & distending it
  - Direct extension from tube to adjacent uterus & ovaries
  - May migrate into & throughout intraperitoneal cavity
  - Fimbriated end may be obliterated preventing peritoneal spread
  - Other patterns include lymphatic & less likely vascular routes
- Survival rates at 5 years
  - Stage I 60-80%
  - Stage II & above 29%

Treatment
- Treated with the same surgical & chemotherapeutic approach as ovarian carcinoma because the two diseases often have analogous histologic & biologic features
- Correct staging prior to & optimal debulking at surgery is considered single most important factor predicting survival

DIAGNOSTIC CHECKLIST

Image Interpretation Pearls
- Three-dimensional Doppler sonography can allow a more accurate pre-operative diagnosis because it allows a precise depiction of tubal wall irregularities such as papillary protrusions & pseudosepta & depiction of vascular abnormalities
- MR is superior to CT & US in depicting local tumor infiltration of bladder, pelvic fat, vagina, pelvic sidewall and bowel

SELECTED REFERENCES

1. Benoit MF et al: A 10-year review of primary fallopian tube cancer at a community hospital: a high association of synchronous and metachronous cancers. Int J Gynecol Cancer. 16(1):29-35, 2006
2. Paulsen T et al: Improved short-term survival for advanced ovarian, tubal, and peritoneal cancer patients operated at teaching hospitals. Int J Gynecol Cancer. 16 Suppl 1:11-7, 2006
3. Singhal P et al: Primary fallopian tube carcinoma: a retrospective clinicopathologic study. Eur J Gynaecol Oncol. 27(1):16-8, 2006
4. Acikalin MF et al: Mixed serous and endometrioid carcinoma of the fallopian tube: a case report with literature review. Eur J Gynaecol Oncol. 26(3):342-4, 2005
5. Ajithkumar TV et al: Primary fallopian tube carcinoma. Obstet Gynecol Surv. 60(4):247-52, 2005
6. Clayton NL et al: Primary fallopian tube carcinoma - the experience of a UK cancer centre and a review of the literature. J Obstet Gynaecol. 25(7):694-702, 2005
7. Liapis A et al: Primary fallopian tube cancer--a ten year review. Clinicopathological study of 12 cases. Eur J Gynaecol Oncol. 25(4):522-4, 2004
8. Takeshima N et al: Treatment of fallopian tube cancer. Review of the literature. Arch Gynecol Obstet. 264(1):13-9, 2000
9. Alvarado-Cabrero I et al: Carcinoma of the fallopian tube: a clinicopathological study of 105 cases with observations on staging and prognostic factors. Gynecol Oncol. 72(3):367-79, 1999
10. Nikrui N et al: Fallopian tube carcinoma. Surg Oncol Clin N Am. 7(2):363-73, 1998
11. Rosen A et al: Primary carcinoma of the fallopian tube--a retrospective analysis of 115 patients. Austrian Cooperative Study Group for Fallopian Tube Carcinoma. Br J Cancer. 68(3):605-9, 1993
12. Meyer JS et al: Ultrasound presentation of primary carcinoma of the fallopian tube. J Clin Ultrasound. 15(2):132-4, 1987

TUBAL CARCINOMA, STAGING/PROGNOSIS

IMAGE GALLERY

Typical

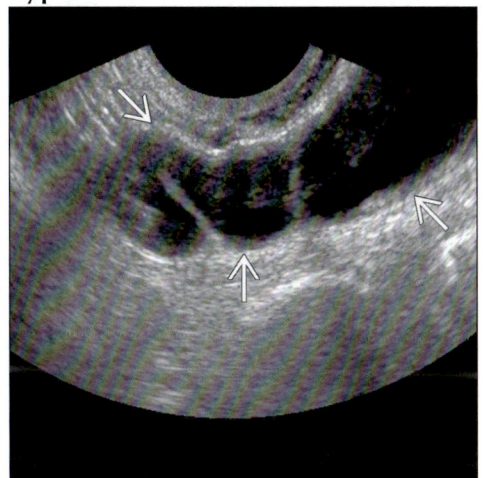
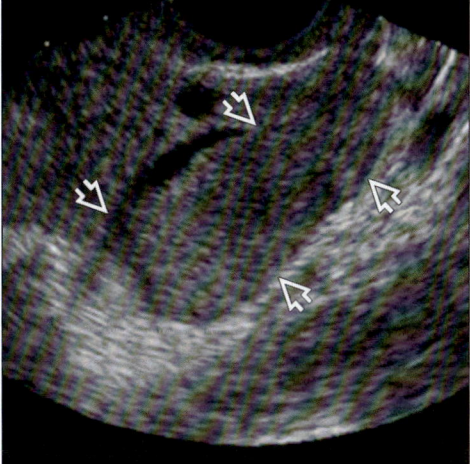

(Left) Sagittal transvaginal ultrasound shows hydrosalpinx ➡ without visible obstructing mass. The contralateral fallopian tube was not dilated. This was stage I at surgery. *(Right)* Coronal transvaginal ultrasound shows a tubular mass ➡ distending and conforming to the fallopian tube, one of the described appearances of stage I fallopian tube cancer.

Typical

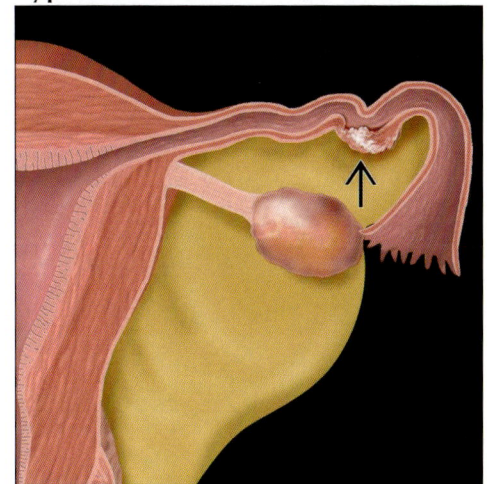
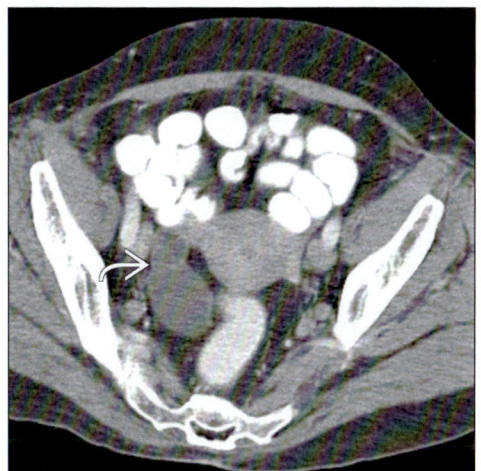

(Left) Graphic shows extension to the serosal surface ➡ compatible with stage IC. *(Right)* Axial CECT shows unilateral dilatation of right fallopian tube ➡.

Typical

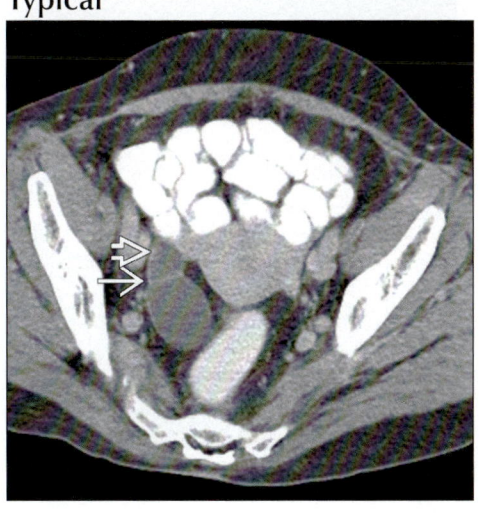
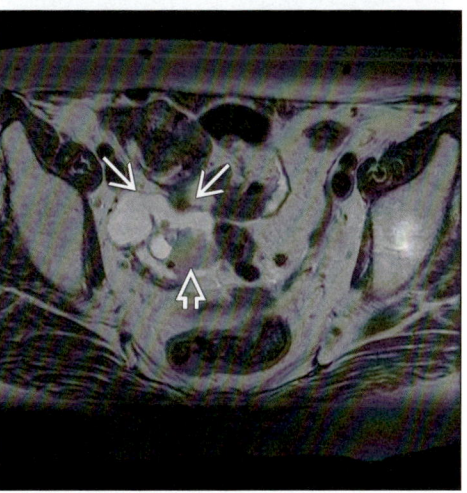

(Left) Axial CECT (delayed phase) in the same patient as previous image, shows a unilateral hydrosalpinx ➡ with a subtle mass ➡. The patient presented with watery discharge and pelvic pain and had stage IC disease. *(Right)* Axial T2WI MR shows a distended fallopian tube ➡ with an associated soft tissue mass ➡ in a patient with hydrops tubae profluens.

TUBAL CARCINOMA, STAGING/PROGNOSIS

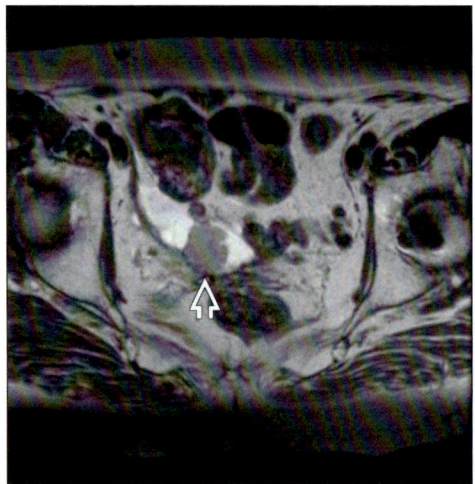
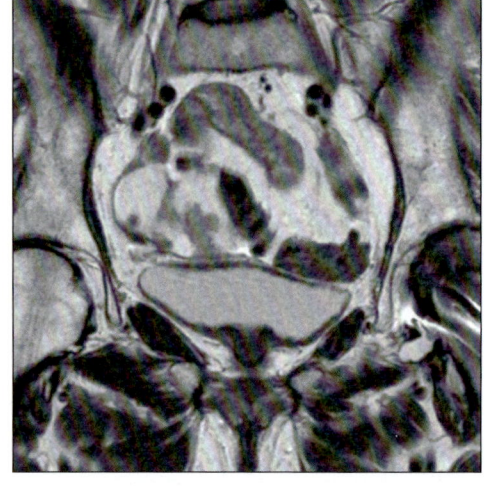

Typical

(Left) Axial T2WI MR in the same patient as previous image, more inferiorly shows the obstructing fallopian tube tumor ➡. *(Right)* Coronal T2WI MR in the same patient as previous image, shows tumor nodules within the hydrosalpinx.

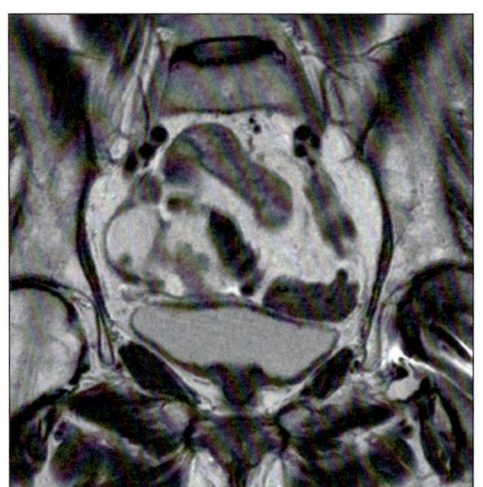

Typical

(Left) Coronal T2WI MR in the same patient as previous image, shows the combination of tumor and distended fallopian tube. *(Right)* Coronal T2WI MR in the same patient as previous image, shows tumor expanding and obstructing ➡ the fallopian tube. At surgery this was a stage IIB mixed endometrioid and papillary serous tubal carcinoma.

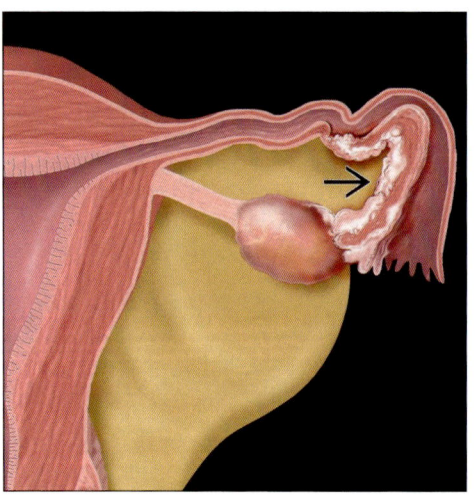
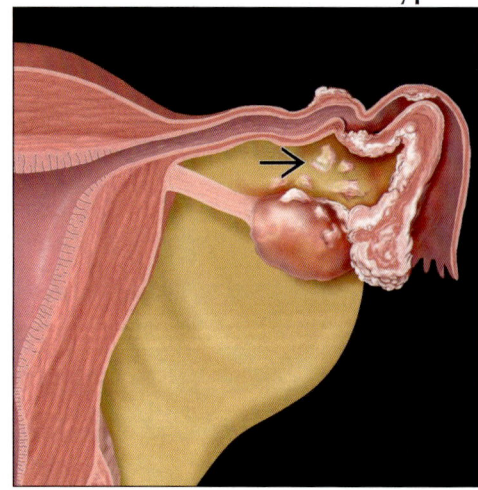

Typical

(Left) Graphic shows extension of tumor to ovary and growth on tubal serosa ➡ which meets criteria for stage IIC. *(Right)* Graphic shows implants onto peritoneal surfaces ➡ not exceeding 2 cm in diameter. If the lymph nodes are negative, this is stage IIIB.

TUBAL CARCINOMA, STAGING/PROGNOSIS

Typical

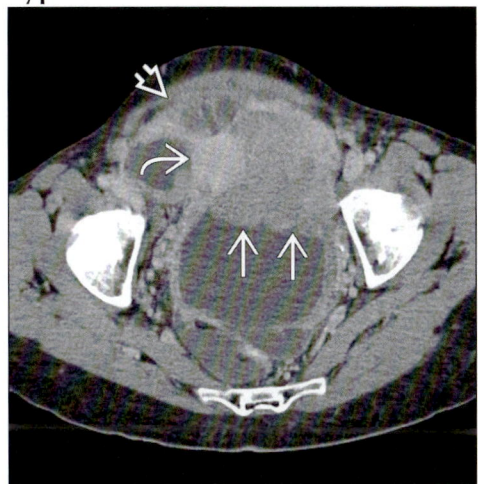
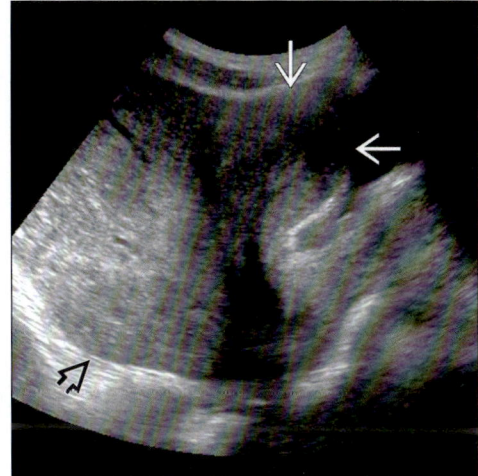

(Left) Axial CECT shows soft tissue mass ➡ inseparable from the uterus ➡ on the left, ascites and peritoneal nodularity ➡ compatible with stage IIIB. *(Right)* Sagittal transabdominal ultrasound shows large solid appearing mass ➡ superior to the uterus ➡.

Typical

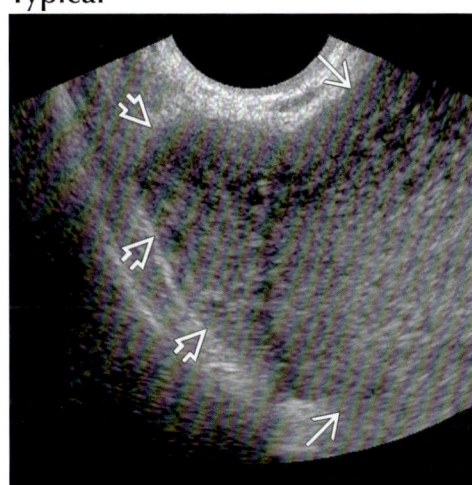
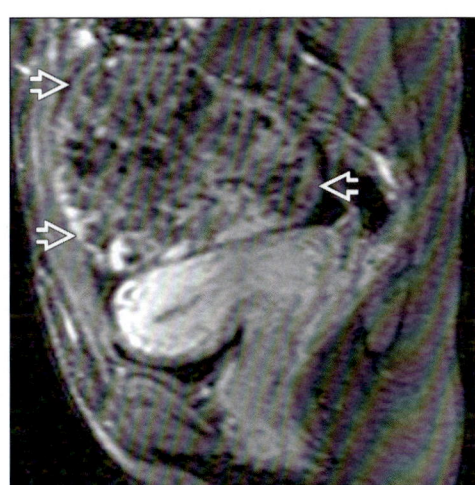

(Left) Coronal transabdominal ultrasound in the same patient as previous image, shows the same mass ➡ adjacent to but separate from the right ovary ➡. *(Right)* in the same patient as previous image, shows the mass ➡ superior to the uterus. Both solid and cystic components are present.

Typical

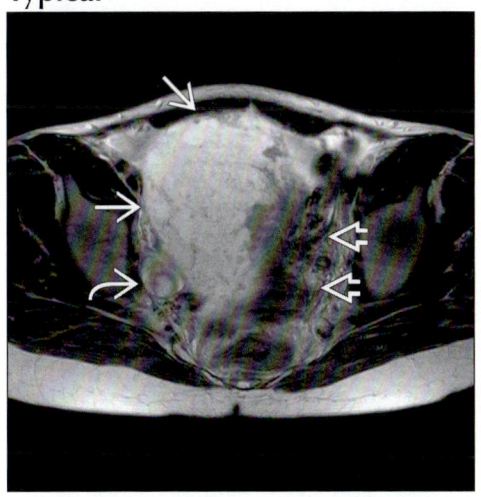
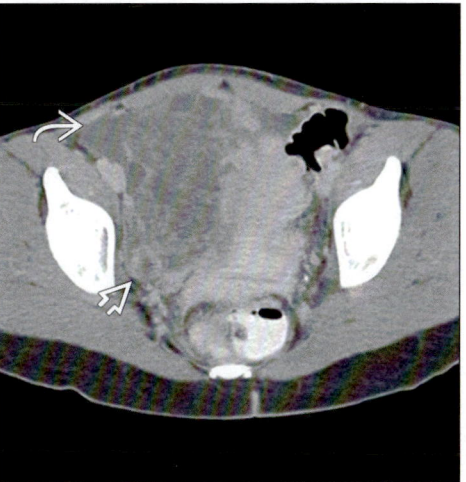

(Left) Axial T2WI MR in the same patient as previous image, shows the mass ➡ abutting, displacing and invading the uterus ➡. The right ovary is separate ➡. *(Right)* Axial CECT in the same patient as previous image. The ovary ➡ is adjacent to, but separate from the complex mass. Ascites is also present ➡. The patient had stage IIIB disease.

METASTASES, TUBAL

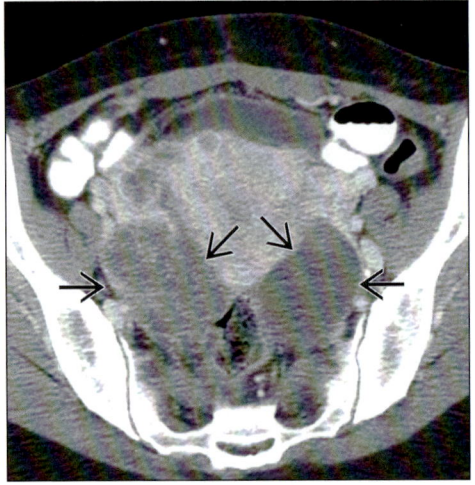

Axial CECT shows complex cystic lesions ➔ in both adnexa.

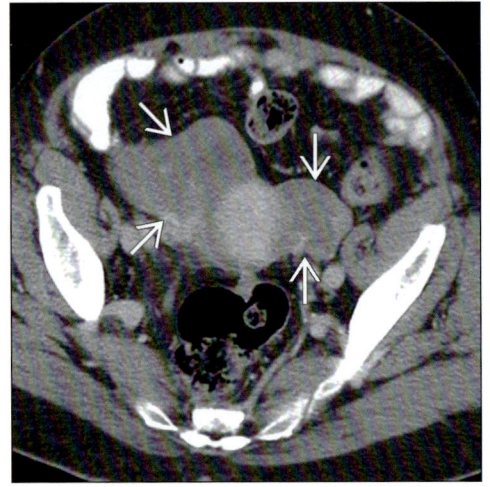

Axial CECT shows bilateral adnexal low attenuation soft tissue masses ➔.

TERMINOLOGY

Definitions
- Neoplastic spread to the fallopian tubes
  - Most commonly seen in patients with primary ovarian cancer

IMAGING FINDINGS

General Features
- Location: Adnexa
- Size: Variable
- Morphology: Commonly mixed cystic and solid

Ultrasonographic Findings
- Cystic or echogenic adnexal masses

CT Findings
- CECT
  - Variable appearance
  - Solid or cystic adnexal masses
  - Enhancement is typical

MR Findings
- As in CT, variable appearance but usually enhancing adnexal masses

DIFFERENTIAL DIAGNOSIS

Primary Fallopian Tube Carcinoma
- Adenocarcinoma and transitional cell carcinoma

Endometriosis
- Cystic and hemorrhagic lesions scattered throughout the pelvis

Tubo-Ovarian Abscess
- Cystic lesions in pelvis caused by pelvic inflammatory disease

Ectopic Pregnancy
- May see sac-like structure with yolk sac or even fetal pole in the fallopian tube

Epithelial Polyp
- Usually seen in women with history of tubal sterilization

DDx: Tubal Metastases

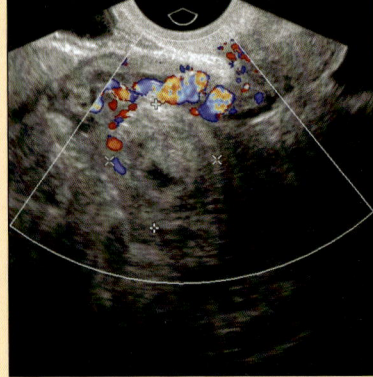

Ectopic Pregnancy

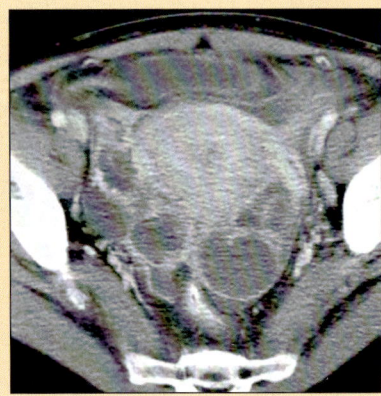

Tubo-Ovarian Abscesses

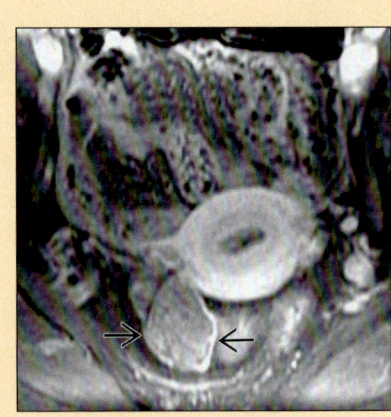

Fallopian Tube Carcinoma

METASTASES, TUBAL

Key Facts

Terminology
- Neoplastic spread to the fallopian tubes
- Most commonly seen in patients with primary ovarian cancer

Imaging Findings
- Solid or cystic adnexal masses
- Enhancement is typical

Pathology
- Microscopic features will reflect the primary malignancy

Clinical Issues
- Most common signs/symptoms: Abdominal pain, pelvic mass, vaginal bleeding
- Other signs/symptoms: May be asymptomatic
- Age: Any age, but usually older women who are at higher risk for malignancy

Teratoma of the Fallopian Tube
- Extremely rare, majority are cystic

Hydatidiform Mole of the Fallopian Tube
- Elevated β-hCG levels should raise suspicion of this lesion

PATHOLOGY

General Features
- Primary cancers that metastasize to fallopian tubes include ovarian, vaginal & vulvar cancer
  - Ovarian cancer
    - Stage IIA is defined as extension or metastases to the tubes or uterus
  - Vaginal cancer: Mesonephric adenocarcinoma
  - Endometrial cancer: Serous adenocarcinoma
    - Method of spread to peritoneum is via transtubal route

Microscopic Features
- Microscopic features will reflect the primary malignancy

CLINICAL ISSUES

Presentation
- Most common signs/symptoms: Abdominal pain, pelvic mass, vaginal bleeding
- Other signs/symptoms: May be asymptomatic

Demographics
- Age: Any age, but usually older women who are at higher risk for malignancy

Treatment
- Total hysterectomy, bilateral salpingo-oophorectomy, omentectomy, lymphadenectomy, and tumor debulking
- Chemotherapy with or without radiotherapy

SELECTED REFERENCES
1. Ersahin C et al: Mesonephric adenocarcinoma of the vagina with a 3-year follow-up. Gynecol Oncol. 99:757-60, 2005
2. Heatley MK: Brief communication polyp of the fallopian tube. Pathology. 33, 538-9, 2001
3. Kurtz AB et al: Diagnosis and staging of ovarian cancer: comparative values of Doppler and conventional US, CT, and MR imaging correlated with surgery and histopathologic analysis--report of the Radiology Diagnostic Oncology Group. Radiology. 212:19-27, 1999
4. Forstner R et al: Imaging of ovarian cancer. JMRI. 5:606-13, 1995
5. Baginski L et al: Immature (malignant) teratoma of the fallopian tube. Am J Obstet Gynecol. 160:671-2, 1989
6. Horn T et al: Benign cystic teratoma of the fallopian tube. Arch Pathol Lab Med. 48:107, 1983
7. Govender NS et al: Metastatic tubal mole and coexisting intrauterine pregnancy. Obstetrics and Gynecology. 49:67-9s, 1977

IMAGE GALLERY

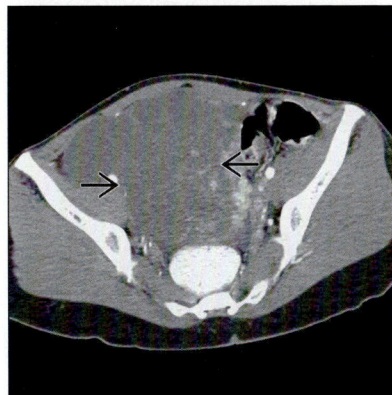 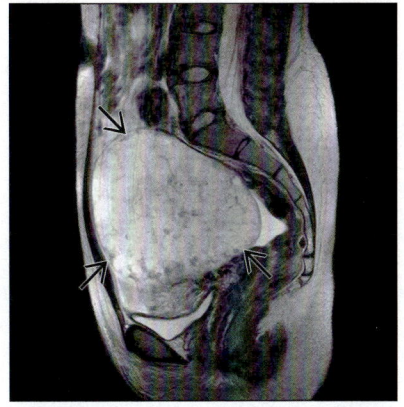 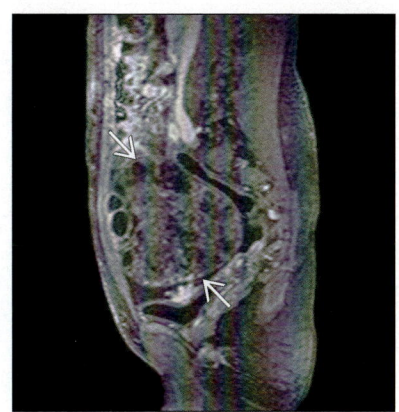

(Left) Axial CECT shows a large complex cystic mass ➔ in the right pelvis. Pathology revealed this to be a large tubal metastasis from gastric adenocarcinoma. *(Center)* Sagittal T2WI MR in the same patient shows a massive multiseptated cystic pelvic mass ➔. *(Right)* Sagittal T1 C+ FS MR of this same mass ➔ shows heterogeneous enhancement within the mass which contains both septation between cystic elements and a more confluent soft tissue component.

HEMATOSALPINX

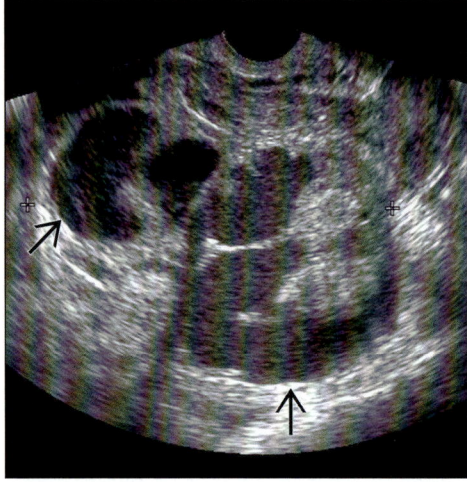

Sagittal oblique transvaginal ultrasound shows a distended fallopian tube with low level echoes ➡, blood, in a patient with a ruptured ectopic pregnancy.

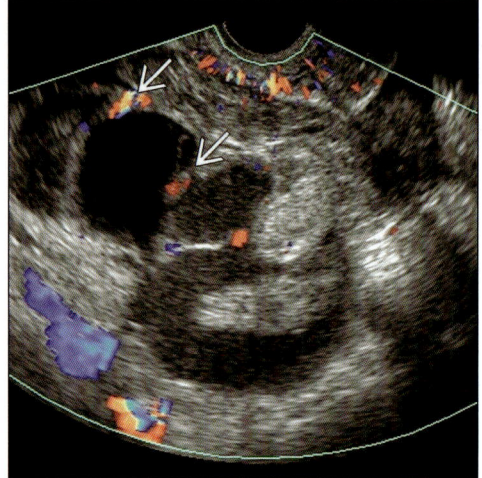

Sagittal oblique color Doppler ultrasound in the same patient shows flow to the wall of the tube ➡. There is no flow to the blood within the hematosalpinx.

TERMINOLOGY

Definitions
- Blood-filled fallopian tube
- Often associated with a tubal ectopic pregnancy (EP), though many other etiologies

IMAGING FINDINGS

General Features
- Best diagnostic clue
  - Distended fallopian tube containing blood-like material ± associated mass
    - Folded appearance of tube may mimic a complex cystic adnexal mass
  - If tubal EP: Extra-ovarian solid adnexal mass with or without cystic components
- Location
  - Extra-ovarian adnexal
  - Hematosalpinx is associated with 95% of EP
    - 75-80% in ampullary end
    - 10-15% in isthmus
    - 5% in fimbrial end of tube
- Size: Few mm to multiple cm
- Morphology: Tubular shape

Ultrasonographic Findings
- Pulsed Doppler
  - High resistive index (RI) in the wall of a blood-filled fallopian tube
  - Low RI when associated with a fallopian tube mass
  - RI of hematosalpinx in EP ranges from very high (> 0.7) to very low (< 0.4)
- Color Doppler
  - No color flow if isolated hematosalpinx without associated mass or EP
  - Vascularity of hematosalpinx in EP on US ranges from avascular to extremely vascular
  - Increased vascularity in the solid component when associated with a fallopian tube mass
- Transvaginal ultrasound (TVS) features
  - Distended fallopian tube containing particulate material ± fallopian tube mass
  - Free intra-peritoneal fluid containing particles suggesting blood
  - Etiology of hematosalpinx may be identified

DDx: Extra-Ovarian Complex Adnexal Mass

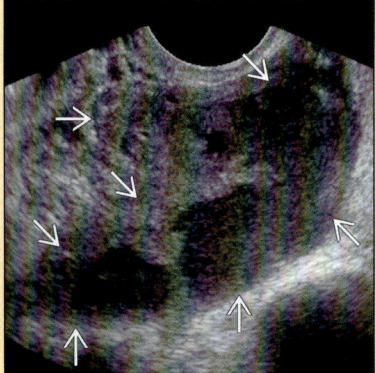

Pyosalpinx

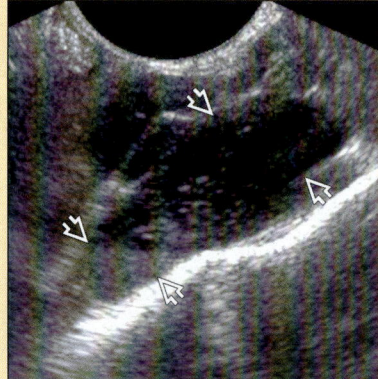

Tarlov Cyst

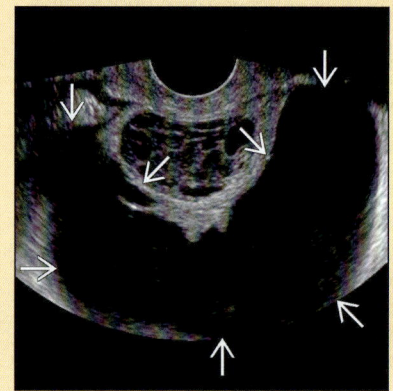

Peritoneal Inclusion Cyst

HEMATOSALPINX

Key Facts

Terminology
- Blood-filled fallopian tube
- Often associated with a tubal ectopic pregnancy (EP), though many other etiologies

Imaging Findings
- Distended fallopian tube containing blood-like material ± associated mass
- TVS is primary imaging examination to evaluate hematosalpinx
- Scanning in multiple planes will allow "elongation" of tube and aid diagnosis

Top Differential Diagnoses
- Pyosalpinx
- Tarlov Cyst
- Peritoneal Inclusion Cyst

Pathology
- **Predisposing factors**
- EP or history of EP
- Pelvic inflammatory disease (PID)
- Endometriosis
- Tuboplasty
- Intrauterine device (IUD)
- Tubal ligation
- Müllerian duct anomalies
- Assisted reproductive technique
- Cervical stenosis
- Fallopian tube mass

Clinical Issues
- Most common signs/symptoms: If associated with an EP: Pain, vaginal bleeding, ± adnexal mass

---

- EP: Extra-ovarian solid adnexal mass with or without cystic elements associated with positive pregnancy test: Sensitivity of hematosalpinx is 90-95% & specificity of hematosalpinx is 92-99% in appropriate clinical setting
  - Müllerian duct anomaly: Unicornuate uterus etc.
  - Endometrioma
  - Other adnexal mass: Fallopian tube cancer, metastases to fallopian tube etc.

MR Findings
- T1WI: High signal intensity tubular structure due to blood-filled fallopian tube
- T2WI
  - Variable SI tubular structure due to blood-filled fallopian tube
    - Low SI if associated with different stages of blood products similar to endometriomas
    - High SI if met hemoglobin
  - Mixed signal intensity extra-ovarian adnexal mass ± cystic component
  - Free intra-peritoneal fluid and/or blood
- T1 C+ FS
  - Distended fallopian tube + an enhancing mass when associated with fallopian tube mass
  - Fallopian tube wall enhancement

Imaging Recommendations
- Best imaging tool
  - TVS is primary imaging examination to evaluate hematosalpinx
  - MR can supplement TVS for assessment of endometriosis or fallopian tube cancer
- Protocol advice
  - Scanning in multiple planes will allow "elongation" of tube and aid diagnosis
  - Once hematosalpinx identified, try to find etiology
  - Always start without color Doppler in the case of EP
    - Flash artifact may obscure small hematosalpinx in EP
  - Color Doppler increases specificity of TVS in EP

DIFFERENTIAL DIAGNOSIS

Pyosalpinx
- Distended fallopian tube containing particulate material and hypervascular wall
- Enlarged ovary
- Inflamed pelvic fat

Tarlov Cyst
- Vascular appearance overlaps EP-associated hematosalpinx but resistive index > 0.3

Peritoneal Inclusion Cyst
- Complex cystic mass with entrapped or eccentrically-located ovary

PATHOLOGY

General Features
- General path comments: Pathology is a function of etiology with hematosalpinx being the common imaging manifestation
- Etiology
  - Causes are multifactorial
    - Retrograde passage of blood from endometrial canal into tube
    - Mass associated with tube
  - **Predisposing factors**
    - EP or history of EP
    - Pelvic inflammatory disease (PID)
    - Endometriosis
    - Tuboplasty
    - Intrauterine device (IUD)
    - Tubal ligation
    - Müllerian duct anomalies
    - Assisted reproductive technique
    - Cervical stenosis
    - Fallopian tube mass
- Epidemiology: Incidence is 1% in general population increasing to 10% when previous history of EP
- Associated abnormalities: Chronic pelvic inflammatory disease in EP

HEMATOSALPINX

Gross Pathologic & Surgical Features
- Distended blood-filled fallopian tube

Microscopic Features
- Depend on etiology, for example
  - Chorionic villi seen in blood-filled and dilated tubal lumen in EP
  - Trophoblast behaves as in placenta increta penetrating deep into muscularis layer
  - Cancer foci in the wall of the tube when associated with fallopian tube cancer

CLINICAL ISSUES

Presentation
- Most common signs/symptoms: If associated with an EP: Pain, vaginal bleeding, ± adnexal mass
- Other signs/symptoms: If ruptured EP: Hemorrhagic shock
- Clinical Profile: Varies with etiology

Demographics
- Age: Child bearing age; peak: 35-44 years of age in EP, premenopausal in endometriosis, postmenopausal in FT cancer

Natural History & Prognosis
- Natural history & prognosis of hematosalpinx reflects etiology, for example
  - In ectopic pregnancy
    - Spontaneous resolution due to spontaneous expulsion from fimbrial end or involution of conceptus
    - Continuous growth and rupture if untreated
    - Chronic EP presenting as hemorrhagic inflammatory adnexal mass, often with negative serum β-hCG test
    - Favorable with early diagnosis and treatment
  - In endometriosis
    - Some may resolve with conservative therapy
    - More advanced cases may require laparoscopy and/or laparotomy

Treatment
- Varies with etiology of hematosalpinx, for example
- In ectopic pregnancy
  - Expectant management with dropping serum β-hCG level indicating trophoblast regression
  - Intramuscular methotrexate (MTX)
  - Intrathecal injection of MTX/KCL in the interstitial EP
  - Surgery
  - Imaging can impact management by determining size, vascularity & lack of rupture of EP
- In fallopian tube cancer
  - TAH BSO
- In endometriosis
  - ± Surgery depending on size or symptoms
- In Müllerian duct anomaly
  - ± Surgery depending on type and severity of symptoms
- In infection
  - Conservative therapy initially, may need surgery in cases refractive to medical therapy

DIAGNOSTIC CHECKLIST

Consider
- Majority of hematosalpinx related to EP are within 2 cm of ovaries
- Hematosalpinx in patients with EP, endometriosis or any condition that leads to retrograde menses

Image Interpretation Pearls
- Folded appearance of tube in hematosalpinx may mimic a complex cystic adnexal mass

SELECTED REFERENCES

1. Krasevic M et al: Serous borderline tumor of the fallopian tube presented as hematosalpinx: a case report. BMC Cancer. 5:129, 2005
2. Lin SK et al: Hematosalpinx: an unusual complication after medical abortion with oral mifepristone and misoprostol. Ultrasound Obstet Gynecol. 25(4):416-7, 2005
3. Datta S et al: Tubal endometriosis mimicking an ectopic pregnancy. J Obstet Gynaecol. 24(7):838-9, 2004
4. Elson J et al: Expectant management of tubal ectopic pregnancy: prediction of successful outcome using decision tree analysis. Ultrasound Obstet Gynecol. 23(6):552-6, 2004
5. Stein MW et al: Sonographic comparison of the tubal ring of ectopic pregnancy with the corpus luteum. J Ultrasound Med. 23(1):57-62, 2004
6. Atri M: Ectopic pregnancy versus corpus luteum cyst revisited: best Doppler predictors. J Ultrasound Med. 22(11):1181-4, 2003
7. Mikami M et al: Preoperative diagnosis of fallopian tube cancer by imaging. Abdom Imaging. 28(5):743-7, 2003
8. Oyelese Y et al: Sonography and magnetic resonance imaging in the diagnosis of cervico-isthmic pregnancy. J Ultrasound Med. 22(9):981-3, 2003
9. Atri M et al: Expectant management of ectopic pregnancy: clinical and ultrasonographic predictors. AJR. 176:123-7, 2001
10. Bakos O et al: Imperforate hymen and ruptured hematosalpinx: a case report with a review of the literature. J Adolesc Health. 24(3):226-8, 1999
11. Fujimoto VY et al: Late-onset hematometra and hematosalpinx in a woman with a noncommunicating uterine horn. A case report. J Reprod Med. 43(5):465-7, 1998
12. Tanaka YO et al: Uterus didelphys associated with obstructed hemivagina and ipsilateral renal agenesis: MR findings in seven cases. Abdom Imaging. 23(4):437-41, 1998
13. Yamamoto K et al: Tubal endometriosis diagnosed within one month after menarche: a case report. Tohoku J Exp Med. 181(3):385-7, 1997
14. Atri M et al: Role of endovaginal sonography in the diagnosis and management of ectopic pregnancy. Radiographics. 16:755-74, 1996
15. Nyberg DA et al: MR imaging of hemorrhagic adnexal masses. J Comput Assist Tomogr. 11(4):664-9, 1987
16. Subramanyam BR et al: Hematosalpinx in tubal pregnancy: sonographic-pathologic correlation. AJR Am J Roentgenol. 141(2):361-5, 1983
17. Pent D et al: The natural history of an hematosalpinx. Obstet Gynecol. 47(1):2S-4S, 1976

HEMATOSALPINX

IMAGE GALLERY

Typical

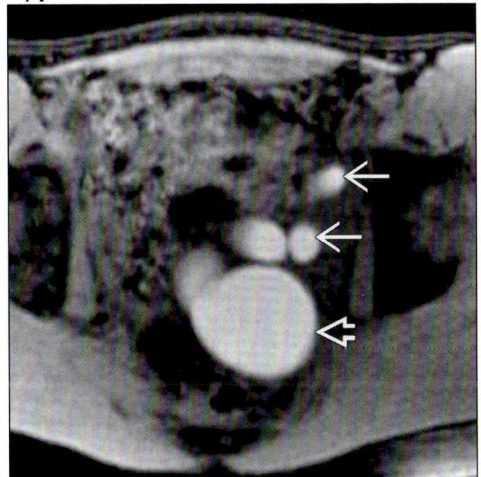
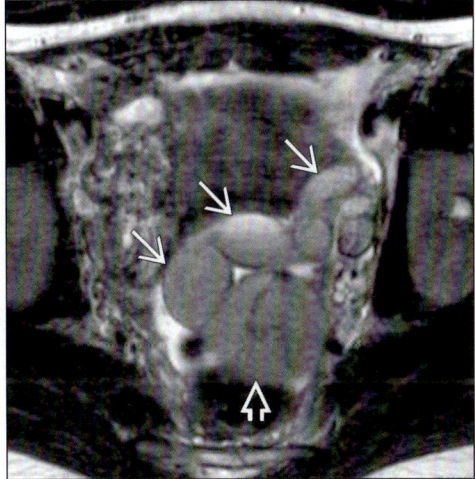

(Left) Axial T1WI FS MR shows a serpiginous blood-filled tubular structure ➡, hematosalpinx, which terminates at an endometrioma ➡. *(Right)* Axial T2WI MR in the same patient as previous image shows the hematosalpinx ➡ and endometrioma ➡ have lower SI than simple fluid. The patient had a unicornuate uterus with a non communicating cavitary rudimentary horn.

Typical

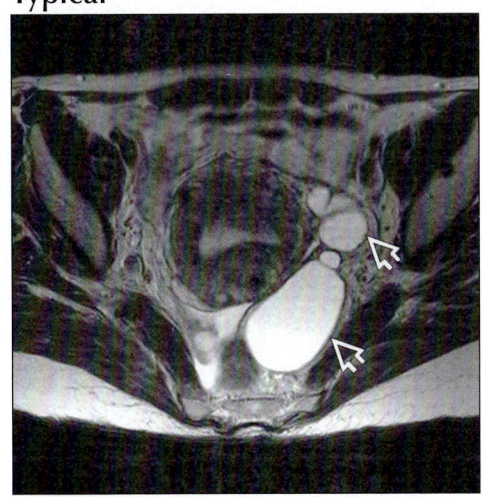
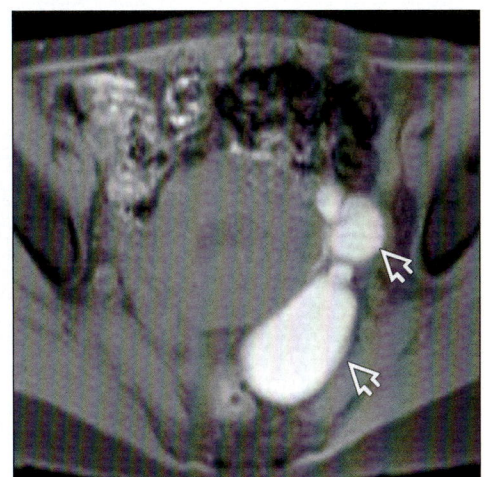

(Left) Axial T2WI MR shows a complex "cystic" left adnexal mass ➡. *(Right)* Axial T1WI FS MR in the same patient as previous image shows the mass is high signal ➡ consistent with blood products and the possibility of endometriomas was raised.

Typical

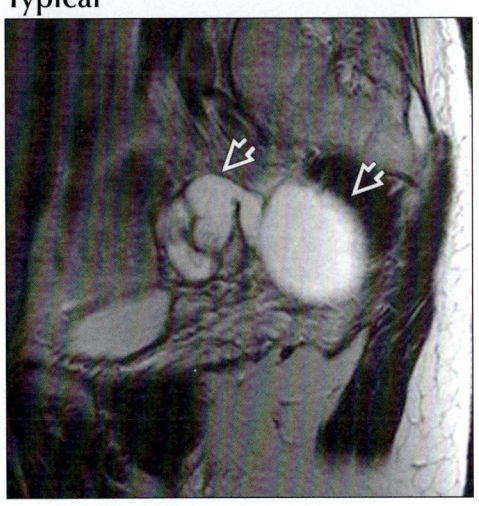
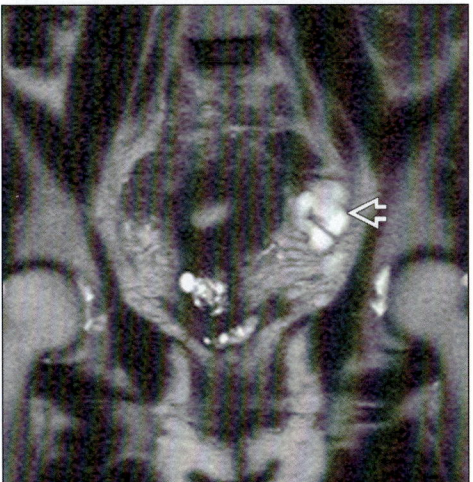

(Left) Sagittal T2WI MR in the same patient as previous image shows the left adnexal "cystic" mass is a contiguous tubular structure ➡, the fallopian tube. The diagnosis of hematosalpinx can be made with confidence. *(Right)* Coronal T2WI MR in the same patient as previous image shows the serpiginous nature of the hematosalpinx ➡. Imaging in multiple planes helps differentiate a complex cyst from a dilated fallopian tube.

HEMATOSALPINX

Typical

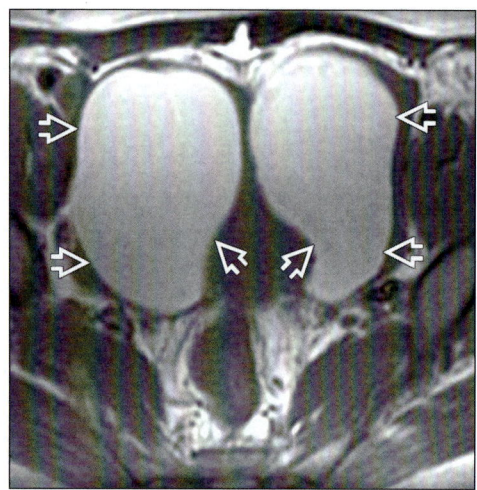 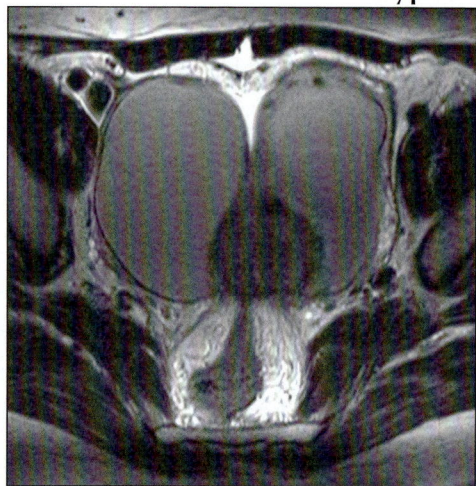

(Left) Axial T1WI MR shows bilateral elongated cystic structures ➡ with high signal content in a patient with endometriosis consistent with hydrosalpinges. (Right) Axial T2WI MR in the same patient as previous image, shows low signal (shading) associated with blood products in the fallopian tubes.

Typical

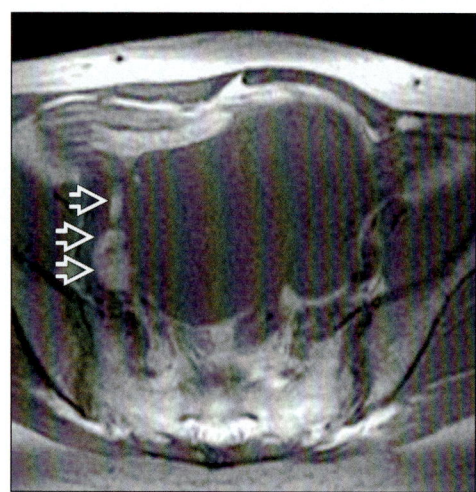 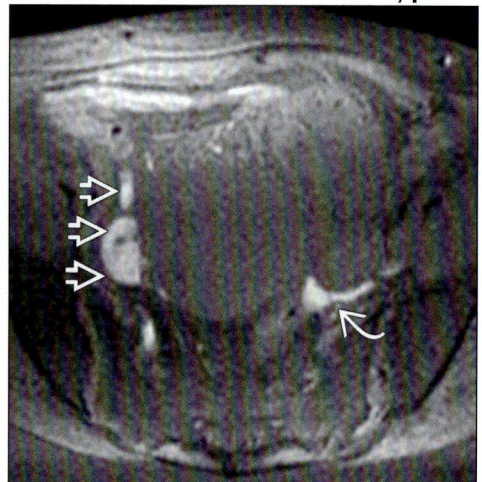

(Left) Axial T1WI MR shows ovoid high signal intensity in the right adnexa ➡. (Right) Axial T1WI FS MR in the same patient as previous image shows the ovoid masses retain their high signal intensity consistent with blood products ➡. Note a small amount of blood in the pelvis ➡.

Typical

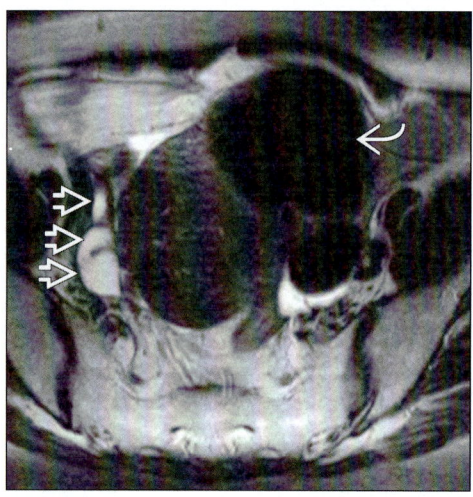 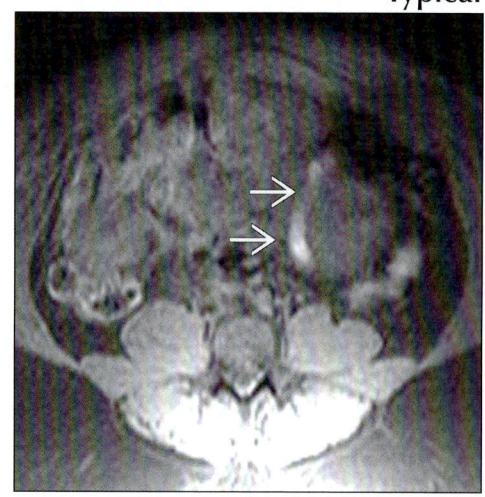

(Left) Axial T2WI MR in the same patient as previous image shows the right tubular adnexal mass ➡. Note the masses are contiguous. The uterus is myomatous ➡. (Right) Axial T1WI FS MR shows a blood-filled, distended, left fallopian tube ➡ in a patient with endometriosis.

HEMATOSALPINX

Typical

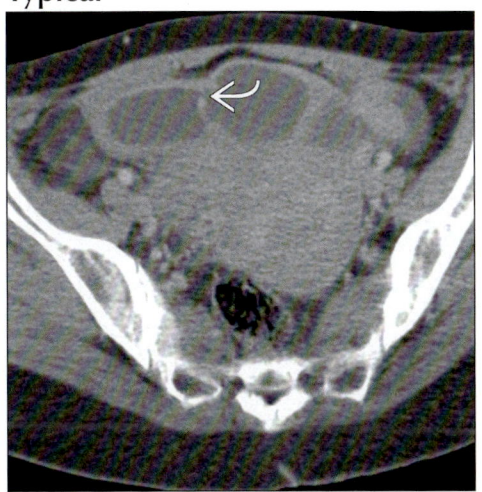
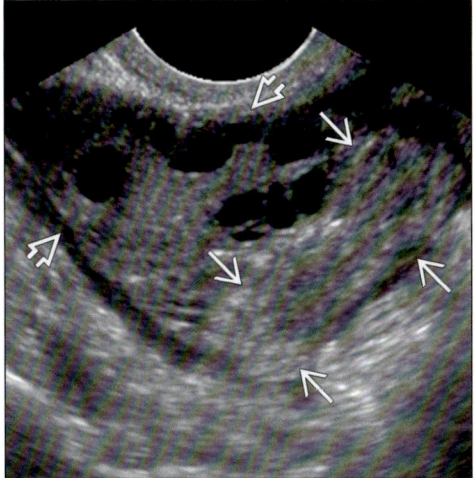

(Left) Axial CECT shows a markedly dilated blood-filled fallopian tube. Note the connection between the different "locules" ➔. At surgery the fallopian tube was torsed. *(Right)* Transverse transvaginal ultrasound shows an elongated structure ➔ lying adjacent to the ovary ➔ in a patient with vaginal bleeding due to retrograde passage of blood.

Typical

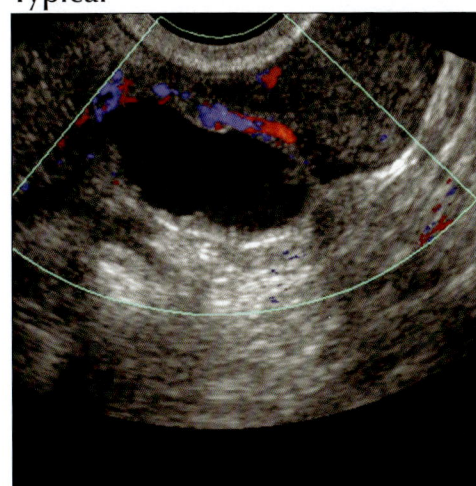
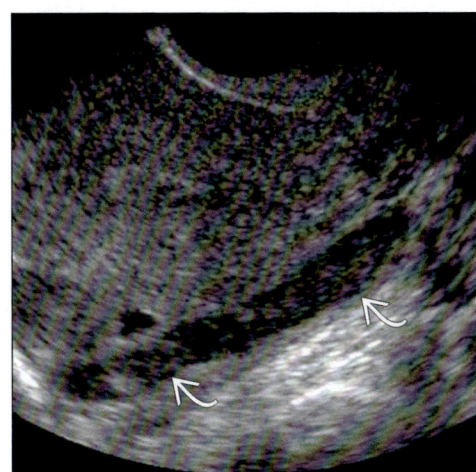

(Left) Sagittal oblique color Doppler ultrasound shows an oblong structure with low level echoes in a patient with cervical stenosis and retrograde menses. *(Right)* Sagittal transabdominal ultrasound shows a tubular structure filled with low level echoes ➔, blood, in a patient with endometriosis.

Typical

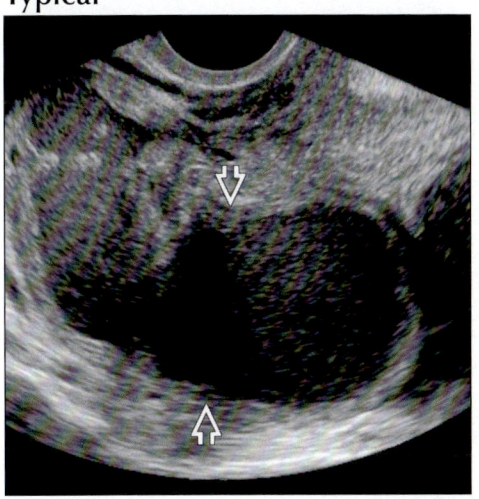
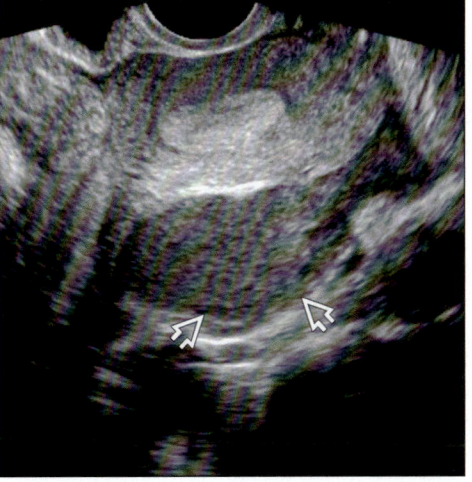

(Left) Sagittal oblique transvaginal ultrasound shows an oblong tubular structure with low level echoes ➔ associated with a hematosalpinx. In a patient with endometriosis. *(Right)* Axial transvaginal ultrasound in the same patient as previous image shows an endometrioma ➔ with typical low level echoes. Retrograde menses likely accounts for both the hematosalpinx and endometrioma.

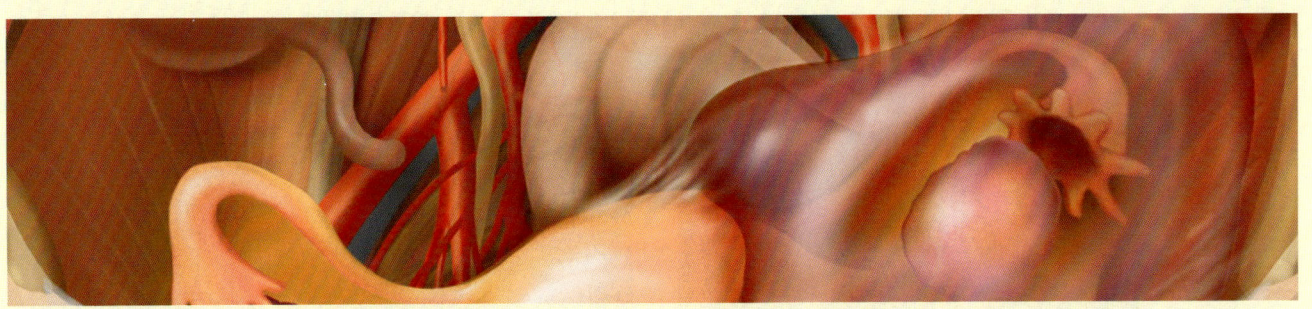

SECTION 9: Peritoneum

Pseudolesions

Peritoneal Inclusion Cysts   9-2

Neoplasm, Malignant

Pseudomyxoma Peritonei   9-6
Peritoneal Mesothelioma   9-8
Peritoneal Metastases   9-12

PERITONEAL INCLUSION CYSTS

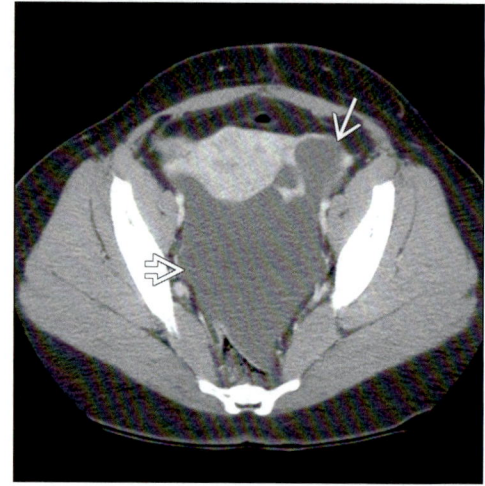

Frontal graphic shows peritoneal inclusion cyst ➡ conforming to pelvic structures. Peritoneal adhesions ➡ are also seen.

Axial CECT demonstrates cystic pelvic mass ➡ with neither wall enhancement nor any solid nodular component. Note displaced left ovary ➡ contains follicles.

TERMINOLOGY

Abbreviations and Synonyms
- Benign cystic mesothelioma
- Peritoneal pseudocyst
- Inflammatory cysts of the pelvic peritoneum

Definitions
- Benign cystic pelvic masses secondary to nonneoplastic reactive mesothelial proliferation
- Occur almost exclusively in premenopausal females who have active ovaries and pelvic adhesions with impaired absorption of peritoneal fluid

IMAGING FINDINGS

General Features
- Best diagnostic clue
  ○ Cystic mass with centrally located ovary entrapped by thick irregular adhesions (spider web appearance)
  ○ Cystic mass with eccentrically-located ovary
  ○ Peritoneal inclusion cysts can also be seen as oblong cystic lesions adjacent to the uterus
- Location: They are most commonly located in the pelvis; around the ovaries
- Size: Ranges from a few millimeters to large cystic masses
- Morphology: Frequently conformed to peritoneal cavity

Ultrasonographic Findings
- Grayscale Ultrasound
  ○ Anechoic cystic mass with through transmission adherent to normal or distorted ovary
  ○ Sometimes cystic loculations can contain echogenic fluid
- Color Doppler: Low-resistance flow can be detected within the septations due to vessels running in the mesothelial tissue

CT Findings
- NECT
  ○ Unilateral or bilateral fluid-density cystic masses
  ○ Density of fluid may be higher than simple fluid in cases with hemorrhage
- CECT
  ○ Unilateral or bilateral cystic masses without enhancing solid components

DDx: Pelvic Cystic Masses

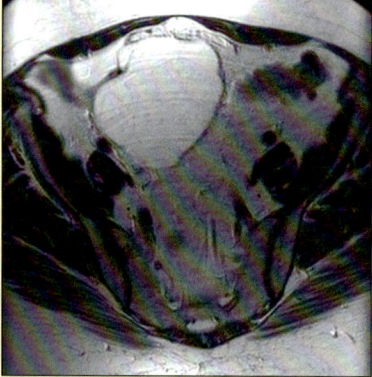
Paraovarian Cyst

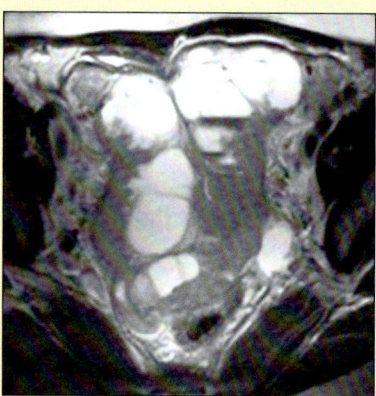
Ovarian Cancer

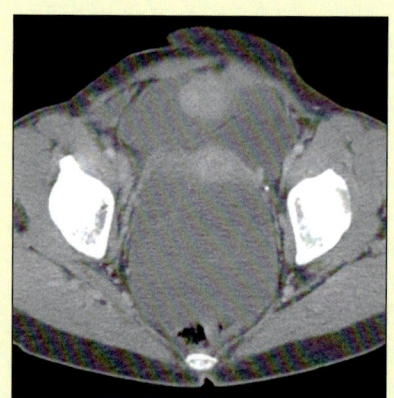
Loculated Ascites

PERITONEAL INCLUSION CYSTS

Key Facts

Terminology
- Benign cystic pelvic masses secondary to nonneoplastic reactive mesothelial proliferation
- Occur almost exclusively in premenopausal females who have active ovaries and pelvic adhesions with impaired absorption of peritoneal fluid

Imaging Findings
- Cystic mass with centrally located ovary entrapped by thick irregular adhesions (spider web appearance)
- Cystic mass with eccentrically-located ovary
- Peritoneal inclusion cysts can also be seen as oblong cystic lesions adjacent to the uterus

Top Differential Diagnoses
- Paraovarian Cyst
- Hydrosalpinx
- Pyosalpinx
- Ovarian Cancer
- Loculated Ascites

Pathology
- Peritoneal inclusion cysts are secondary to nonneoplastic reactive mesothelial proliferation
- Peritoneal inclusion cysts occur in cases where an active ovary and peritoneal adhesions are present

Diagnostic Checklist
- Diagnosis of peritoneal inclusion cysts should be considered in patients with typical clinical setting
- Imaging diagnosis depends on the presence of normal ovary with surrounding loculated fluid conforming to pelvis

---

  - Ovary adjacent to or within peritoneal inclusion cyst enhances and should not be confused with a solid nodule

MR Findings
- T1WI
  - Cystic masses with low signal intensity
    - Occasionally old blood in the peritoneal inclusion cysts cause high signal intensity
- T2WI
  - Cystic masses with high signal intensity
    - Occasionally old blood in the peritoneal inclusion cysts causes low signal intensity
  - Ovary adjacent to or within peritoneal inclusion cyst can easily be recognized on T2WI
- T1 C+
  - No enhancing solid components
    - Ovary adjacent to or within peritoneal inclusion cyst enhances and should not be confused with a solid nodule

Imaging Recommendations
- Best imaging tool
  - US is most commonly used modality to detect and characterize
  - MR may be used in problematic cases
  - US and CT can be used for imaging-guided aspiration

DIFFERENTIAL DIAGNOSIS

Paraovarian Cyst
- Paraovarian cysts are seen as single or multiple cystic pelvic masses within broad ligament
- They are often seen as cystic lesions separate from a normal ipsilateral ovary

Hydrosalpinx
- Oblong peritoneal inclusion cyst may mimic hydrosalpinx
- Folded, tubular appearance of the fallopian tube is typical in case of hydrosalpinx

Pyosalpinx
- Occasionally peritoneal inclusion cysts may contain echogenic fluid mimicking pyosalpinx
- Patients are often symptomatic and have fever in case of pyosalpinx

Ovarian Cancer
- Complex unilateral or bilateral mixed solid and cystic masses without identifiable ovaries
- In advanced ovarian cancer cases, ascites and peritoneal carcinomatosis are seen

Loculated Ascites
- Focal accumulation of fluid within most dependent portions of peritoneal cavity secondary to inflammatory or malignant adhesions
- Presence of thick peritoneal enhancement is a characteristic feature

PATHOLOGY

General Features
- General path comments
  - Peritoneal inclusion cysts are secondary to nonneoplastic reactive mesothelial proliferation
  - Peritoneal inclusion cysts occur in cases where an active ovary and peritoneal adhesions are present
    - Peritoneal fluid is predominantly formed by the ovary
    - This is supported by the fact that high concentration of ovarian steroid hormones is seen in peritoneal fluid
    - Peritoneal fluid absorption decreases when the peritoneum is infected or adhesions are present
- Etiology
  - Non-neoplastic reactive mesothelial proliferation causing
    - Decreased absorption of ovarian fluid by peritoneum
    - Gradual accumulation of locules of fluid between peritoneal layers and/or adhesions

PERITONEAL INCLUSION CYSTS

Gross Pathologic & Surgical Features
- Loculated cystic masses filled with clear or yellow serous fluid

Microscopic Features
- Locules are lined by one or several layers of flat and cuboidal mesothelial cells
- Occasionally, cuboid cells can undergo squamous metaplasia

CLINICAL ISSUES

Presentation
- Most common signs/symptoms
  - Pelvic pain
  - Pelvic mass or swelling
  - Pelvic discomfort
- Other signs/symptoms
  - Asymptomatic cases are not rare
  - Peritoneal inclusion cysts may be incidentally detected on US performed for other reasons
- Clinical Profile
  - Premenopausal females with functioning ovaries and history of any of the following
    - Pelvic surgery
    - Pelvic trauma
    - Endometriosis
    - Pelvic inflammatory disease

Demographics
- Age: Postmenarche to premenopause

Natural History & Prognosis
- Peritoneal inclusion cysts have no malignant potential despite the occasional occurrence of metaplasia
- Peritoneal inclusion cysts tend to grow slowly
- Risk of recurrence is 30-50% following surgery

Treatment
- Oral contraceptives to decrease ovarian fluid production by suppressing ovulation
- US- or CT-guided fluid aspiration
- Sclerotherapy following catheter insertion
- Pain control
- Surgical resection of adhesions

DIAGNOSTIC CHECKLIST

Consider
- Diagnosis of peritoneal inclusion cysts should be considered in patients with typical clinical setting
- Imaging findings suggesting a peritoneal inclusion cyst is helpful in treatment planning by selection of conservative treatment

Image Interpretation Pearls
- Imaging diagnosis depends on the presence of normal ovary with surrounding loculated fluid conforming to pelvis
- Peritoneal inclusion cysts are adherent to the surface of the ovary but do not involve the ovarian parenchyma
- Peritoneal fluid accumulation within adhesions may appear as a complex multicystic adnexal mass on imaging
- Extensive adhesions, thick septations and complex fluid content of a paraovarian cyst may mimic a malignant ovarian neoplasm
- In such cases, identification of normal ovaries helps in correct diagnosis

SELECTED REFERENCES

1. Durak E et al: Multilocular peritoneal inclusion cyst. Surgery. 137(5):580, 2005
2. Guerriero S et al: Role of transvaginal sonography in the diagnosis of peritoneal inclusion cysts. J Ultrasound Med. 23(9):1193-200, 2004
3. Savelli L et al: Transvaginal sonographic appearance of peritoneal pseudocysts. Ultrasound Obstet Gynecol. 23(3):284-8, 2004
4. Toprak U et al: Sonographic, CT, and MRI findings of endometrial stromal sarcoma located in the myometrium and associated with peritoneal inclusion cyst. AJR Am J Roentgenol. 182(6):1531-3, 2004
5. Adolph AJ et al: Benign multicystic mesothelioma: a case report. J Obstet Gynaecol Can. 24(3):246-7, 2002
6. Jeong JY et al: Sclerotherapy of peritoneal inclusion cysts: preliminary results in seven patients. Korean J Radiol. 2(3):164-70, 2001
7. Omeroglu A et al: Multilocular peritoneal inclusion cyst (benign cystic mesothelioma). Arch Pathol Lab Med. 125(8):1123-4, 2001
8. Brustmann H: Multilocular peritoneal inclusion cyst with extensive xanthogranulomatous stromal changes: a differential diagnosis of cystic pelvic tumors in women. Ann Diagn Pathol. 4(5):308-10, 2000
9. Jain KA: Imaging of peritoneal inclusion cysts. AJR Am J Roentgenol. 174(6):1559-63, 2000
10. Nozawa S et al: Gonadotropin-releasing hormone analogue therapy for peritoneal inclusion cysts after gynecological surgery. J Obstet Gynaecol Res. 26(6):389-93, 2000
11. Kim JS et al: Peritoneal inclusion cysts and their relationship to the ovaries: evaluation with sonography. Radiology. 204(2):481-4, 1997
12. Hoffer FA et al: Peritoneal inclusion cysts: ovarian fluid in peritoneal adhesions. Radiology. 169(1):189-91, 1988
13. McFadden DE et al: Peritoneal inclusion cysts with mural mesothelial proliferation. A clinicopathological analysis of six cases. Am J Surg Pathol. 10(12):844-54, 1986

PERITONEAL INCLUSION CYSTS

IMAGE GALLERY

Typical

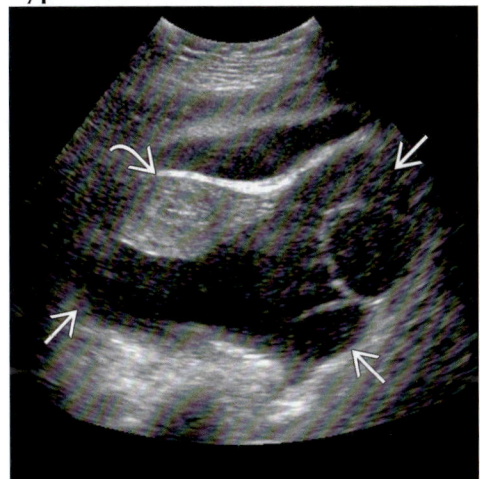
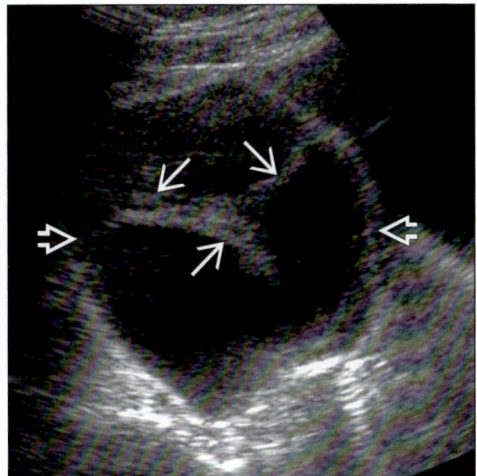

(Left) Axial transabdominal ultrasound shows a large peritoneal inclusion cyst ➔ in the pelvis. Uterus ➔ is also seen. *(Right)* Axial transabdominal ultrasound shows thick septations ➔ that mimic malignancy in a peritoneal inclusion cyst ➔.

Typical

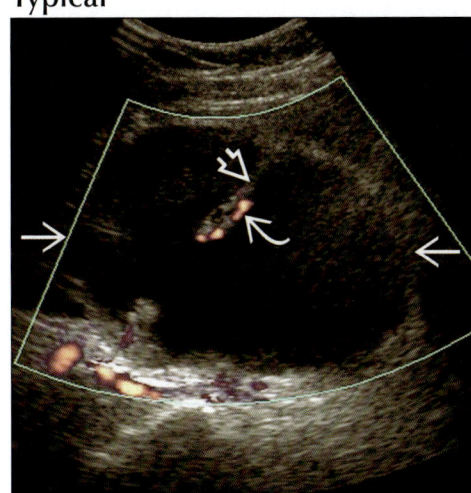
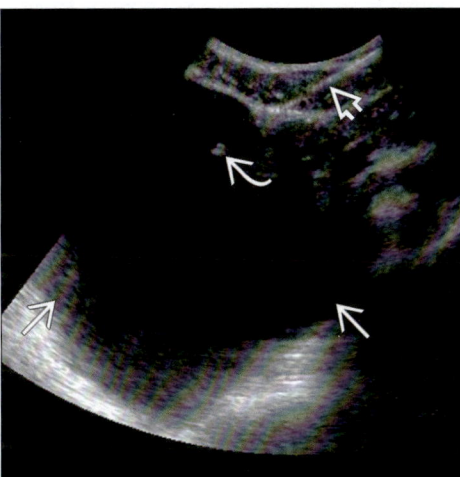

(Left) Axial oblique power Doppler ultrasound shows a peritoneal inclusion cyst ➔ with a septation ➔. Note the vascular flow ➔ in the septation. *(Right)* Axial transabdominal ultrasound shows US-guided drainage of a peritoneal inclusion cyst ➔. Note the needle ➔ with its tip ➔ in the cyst.

Typical

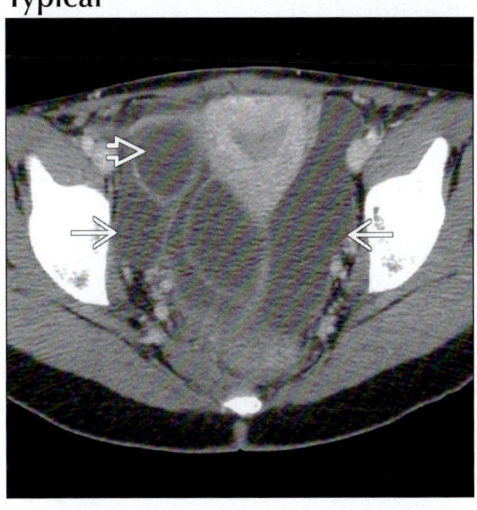
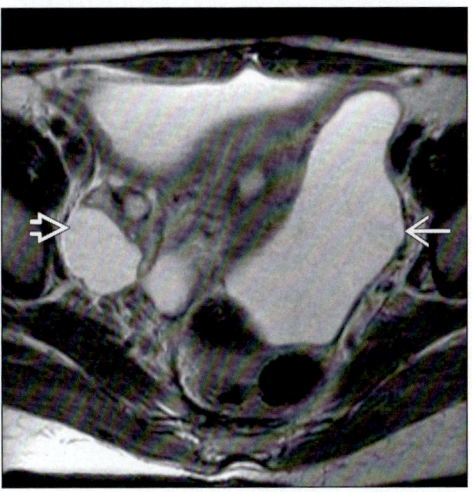

(Left) Axial CECT shows multiloculated peritoneal inclusion cyst ➔ in the pelvis. An ovarian cyst is seen on the right ➔. *(Right)* Axial T2WI MR shows an oblong peritoneal inclusion cyst ➔ in the pelvis on the left. Note there is a cyst in the right ovary ➔.

PSEUDOMYXOMA PERITONEI

Coronal T2WI MR demonstrates numerous high signal intensity masses ➡ in peritoneal cavity. Note that masses cause scalloping on liver surface.

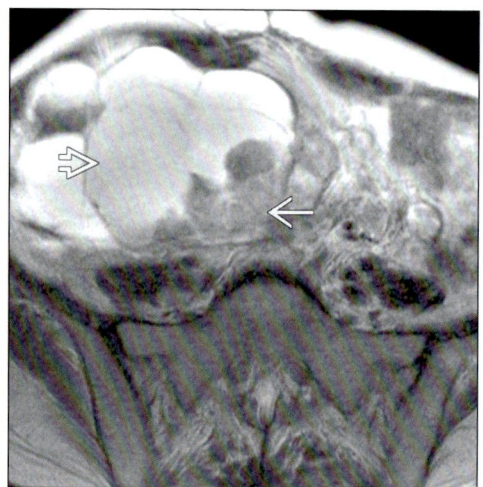

Axial T2WI MR demonstrates right ovarian mucinous adenocarcinoma (M). Note that the mass has cystic ➡ and solid components ➡.

TERMINOLOGY

Definitions
- Massive gelatinous accumulations often arranged in locular fashion in peritoneal cavity

IMAGING FINDINGS

General Features
- Best diagnostic clue: Loculated collections of mucinous fluid in peritoneal cavity, scalloping liver and splenic surfaces and displacing bowel loops
- Location: Initially seeds at sites of relative stasis and as large-volume disease develops, it fills the remaining spaces in peritoneal cavity

Ultrasonographic Findings
- Grayscale Ultrasound: Echogenic ascites reflecting the mucinous nature of fluid

CT Findings
- CECT
  - Low attenuation loculated collections
  - Areas of high attenuation, septa and calcification can be seen

MR Findings
- T1WI: Low signal intensity locules
- T2WI: High signal intensity locules

DIFFERENTIAL DIAGNOSIS

Ascites
- Ascites do not cause scalloping of liver and splenic surfaces
- In uncomplicated ascites bowel loops are mobile and free-floating

Peritoneal Carcinomatosis
- Ascites and peritoneal thickening and/or soft tissue nodules

Peritoneal Inclusion Cysts
- Benign cystic masses in the pelvis

DDx: Mimics of Pseudomyxoma Peritonei

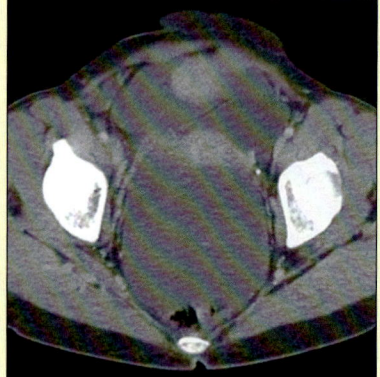

Loculated Ascites

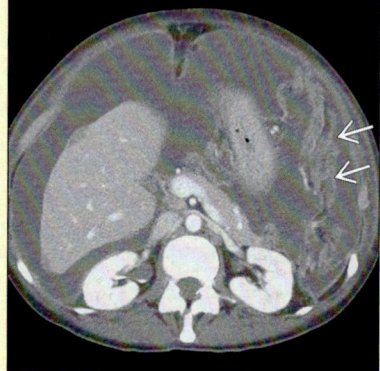

Peritoneal Carcinomatosis

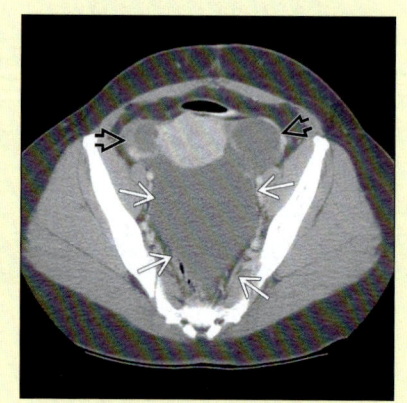

Peritoneal Inclusion Cysts

PSEUDOMYXOMA PERITONEI

Key Facts

Terminology
- Massive gelatinous accumulations often arranged in locular fashion in peritoneal cavity

Imaging Findings
- Best diagnostic clue: Loculated collections of mucinous fluid in peritoneal cavity, scalloping liver and splenic surfaces and displacing bowel loops

Pathology
- Most commonly associated with benign, borderline, or malignant mucinous tumors of ovary or appendix
- On rare occasions can be seen in tumors of colon, stomach, uterus, pancreas, common bile duct, urachal duct, or omphalomesenteric duct
- Synchronous ovarian and appendiceal tumors are present in 90% of patients

PATHOLOGY

General Features
- General path comments
  - Pseudomyxoma peritonei results from peritoneal implants of columnar epithelium associated with progressive accumulation of mucinous ascites
  - Most commonly associated with benign, borderline, or malignant mucinous tumors of ovary or appendix
    - On rare occasions can be seen in tumors of colon, stomach, uterus, pancreas, common bile duct, urachal duct, or omphalomesenteric duct
    - Synchronous ovarian and appendiceal tumors are present in 90% of patients
  - Extraperitoneal spread can be seen on rare occasions

Gross Pathologic & Surgical Features
- Peritoneal cavity is filled with large amounts of gelatinous material with mucinous globules

Microscopic Features
- Strips of single layer of mature cells filled with mucin
- Individual epithelial cells can be found floating within gelatinous material

CLINICAL ISSUES

Presentation
- Most common signs/symptoms: Abdominal distention, pain and weight loss
- Other signs/symptoms: Bowel obstruction in advanced cases

Natural History & Prognosis
- Recurrences are common
- Patients with adenocarcinoma of the ovary or appendix have a worse prognosis than those with a benign neoplasm
- Overall 5 year survival is 40-50%

Treatment
- Surgical debulking is main treatment option
- Role of intraperitoneal chemotherapy, radiotherapy or application of mucolytic therapy remains uncertain

DIAGNOSTIC CHECKLIST

Image Interpretation Pearls
- Scalloping of liver and splenic surfaces and displacement of bowel loops due to pressure effects suggest pseudomyxoma peritonei

SELECTED REFERENCES
1. Hanbidge AE et al: US of the peritoneum. Radiographics. 23(3):663-84; discussion 684-5, 2003
2. Sulkin TV et al: CT in pseudomyxoma peritonei: a review of 17 cases. Clin Radiol. 57(7):608-13, 2002
3. Buy JN et al: Magnetic resonance imaging of pseudomyxoma peritonei. Eur J Radiol. 9(2):115-8, 1989

IMAGE GALLERY

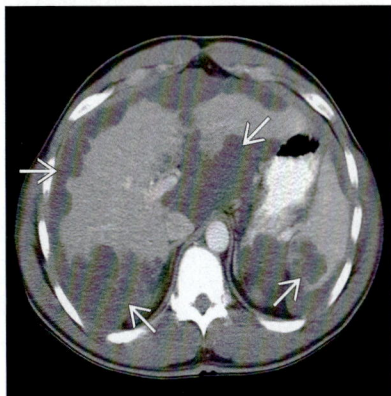 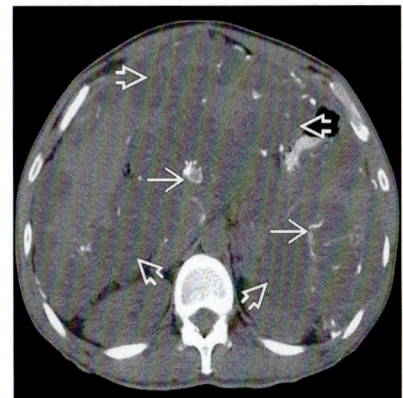 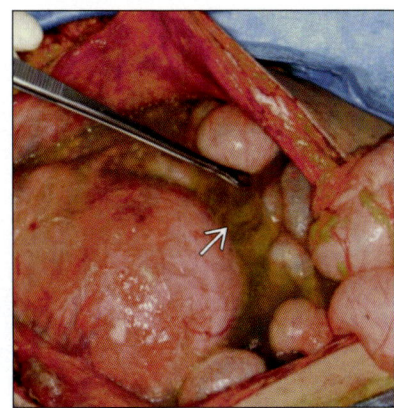

(Left) Axial CECT shows multiple cystic masses ➡ scalloping the surfaces of liver and spleen. *(Center)* Axial NECT shows multiple cystic masses ➡ with calcifications ➡. *(Right)* Intra-operative photograph shows gelatinous material ➡ filling the abdominal cavity in a patient with pseudomyxoma peritonei.

PERITONEAL MESOTHELIOMA

Axial CECT shows peritoneal mesothelioma ➡ seen as an infiltrative soft tissue mass. The normal uterus and ovaries are effaced.

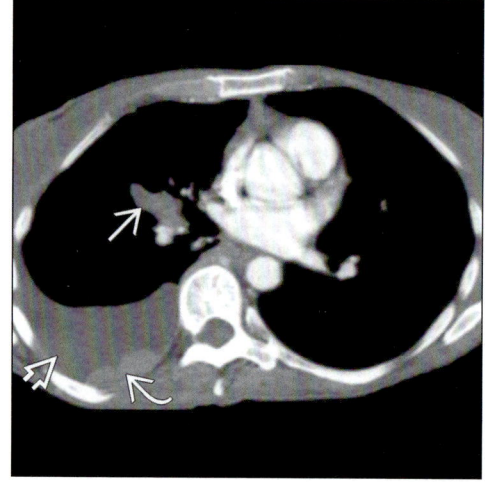

Axial CECT in the same patient shows a right pleural effusion ➡, a bilobed pleural mass ➡ and a pulmonary mass ➡.

TERMINOLOGY

Abbreviations and Synonyms
- Malignant peritoneal mesothelioma (MPM)

Definitions
- Rare, rapidly fatal mesothelial neoplasm

IMAGING FINDINGS

General Features
- Best diagnostic clue
  - Soft tissue mass within mesentery, omentum or peritoneum
    - Scant ascites in relation to amount of soft tissue mass
    - Lymphadenopathy rare
    - No known primary tumor (ovary, stomach, colon)
- Location: May affect thorax, abdomen and/or pelvis
- Size: Variable
- Morphology
  - Spreads along serosal surfaces
    - Liver and colon most commonly affected
  - Direct invasion of hollow and solid viscera
    - Liver is most common viscera invaded
  - Less commonly, infiltrating mass or multiple small nodules
    - Nodule becomes more confluent with time

Radiographic Findings
- Radiography
  - Chest X-ray: May see pleural involvement
    - Pleural mass (+/- calcification) and/or effusion
- IVP: May see displacement and/or encasement of ureters

CT Findings
- CECT
  - Enhancing soft tissue mass within mesentery, omentum or peritoneum and/or small nodules and/or infiltrating mass
  - Small amount of ascites in relation to tumor
  - Lack of bulky lymphadenopathy
  - Direct invasion of solid and hollow viscera
    - Liver is most solid viscera invaded
  - Serosal involvement
    - Liver
    - Colon

DDx: Peritoneal Mesothelioma

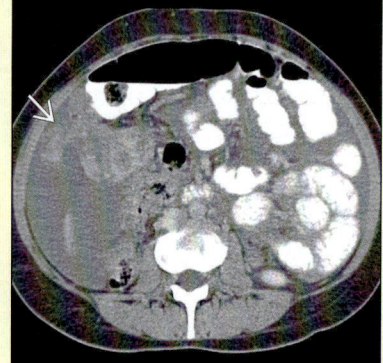

Peritoneal Carcinomatosis

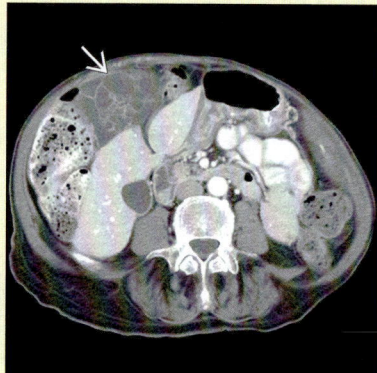

Cystic Mesothelioma

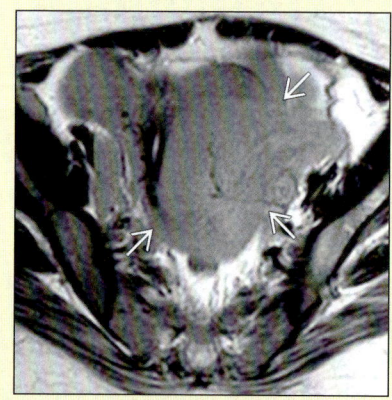

Lymphoma

PERITONEAL MESOTHELIOMA

Key Facts

Terminology
- Rare, rapidly fatal mesothelial neoplasm

Imaging Findings
- Location: May affect thorax, abdomen and/or pelvis
- Enhancing soft tissue mass within mesentery, omentum or peritoneum and/or small nodules and/or infiltrating mass
- Small amount of ascites in relation to tumor
- Lack of bulky lymphadenopathy
- Direct invasion of solid and hollow viscera
- Serosal involvement
- CT classification schema
- Class I: No small bowel or mesenteric abnormality
- Class II: Tumor involvement of small bowel or its mesentery; the mesentery appears stellate or pleated
- Class III: Increased solid tumor involvement of the small bowel and its mesentery; mesentery appears distorted and thickened
- Best imaging tool: CECT is modality of choice

Top Differential Diagnoses
- Peritoneal Carcinomatosis
- Cystic Mesothelioma
- Metastatic Peritoneal Lymphomatosis
- Pseudomyxoma Peritonei

Pathology
- Arises from peritoneal mesothelial cells
- Asbestos exposure has been implicated in pathogenesis

Clinical Issues
- Three clinical types: "Dry-painful," "wet," "mixed"

- Pleural disease
  - Enhancing solid masses
  - Asbestos-related plaques (with or without calcification)
  - Effusion
- CT classification schema
  - Class I: No small bowel or mesenteric abnormality
  - Class II: Tumor involvement of small bowel or its mesentery; the mesentery appears stellate or pleated
  - Class III: Increased solid tumor involvement of the small bowel and its mesentery; mesentery appears distorted and thickened

MR Findings
- T1WI: Low to intermediate signal intensity
- T2WI: Intermediate to high signal intensity
- T1 C+: Solid elements enhance

Fluoroscopic Findings
- Barium enema: May see displacement and/or encasement of bowel

Imaging Recommendations
- Best imaging tool: CECT is modality of choice

DIFFERENTIAL DIAGNOSIS

Peritoneal Carcinomatosis
- Ovary, colon, or gastric primary cancer
- Moderate or marked ascites & lymphadenopathy
- May develop dystrophic calcification
- Pleural metastases are rare

Cystic Mesothelioma
- Benign neoplasm derived from peritoneal mesothelium
- Rare, but female predilection
- Recurs in 25-50% of cases
- Involvement of the pelvis is characteristic
  - Peritoneum-based multilocular cystic mass or multiple unilocular thin-walled cysts
  - No mass effect, invasion, nor prominent soft tissue

Metastatic Peritoneal Lymphomatosis
- Non-Hodgkin lymphoma predominates
- Ascites, omental infiltration, peritoneal & pelvic involvement
- Bulky lymphadenopathy
- Soft masses; pushes & envelops adjacent organs

Pseudomyxoma Peritonei
- Mucinous ascites
  - Associated with ruptured mucocele, cystadenoma, or low grade carcinoma arising from the appendix, colon or ovary
- Mucinous deposits insinuate themselves throughout peritoneal cavity, but do not invade adjacent viscera
- Pleural metastases are rare

Well-Differentiated Papillary Mesothelioma
- Female predominance
- Indolent, considered benign
  - Negative immunostain for calretinin
- May have psammoma body calcifications

Peritoneal Leiomyomatosis
- Benign, non-destructive smooth muscle nodules in women
  - May occur in conjunction with uterine leiomyomas
  - Others postulate multicentric leiomyomatous growths
- May "metastasize" to lung parenchyma, pleural involvement is rare

Tuberculosis Peritonitis
- Irregular soft tissue densities in the omentum
- Low attenuation intraabdominal masses, lymphadenopathy & ascites
- Visceral invasion is rare

PATHOLOGY

General Features
- General path comments
  - Arises from peritoneal mesothelial cells

PERITONEAL MESOTHELIOMA

- Rarely arises from pericardium or tunica vaginalis
- Approximately 30% arise solely from peritoneum
- Asbestos exposure has been implicated in pathogenesis
  - About 1/2 of patients report asbestos exposure
- Etiology
  - Asbestos exposure
    - Primarily crocidolite variety
- Epidemiology
  - Overall prevalence in US is 1-2 cases per million
    - Annual US incidence: 300-400 cases
  - Constitute 12-20% of all mesotheliomas
  - Most cases in 5th & 6th decades

Gross Pathologic & Surgical Features
- Solid and lobular

Microscopic Features
- Epithelioid histological pattern predominates
  - Sarcomatoid histological pattern is rare
- Marked cytologic diversity of tumor cells
  - Tumor cells form tubulopapillary & solid arrangements
- Need to distinguish MPM from adenocarcinoma
  - Diagnostic accuracy increases with sample size & use of immunohistochemistry
    - Positive immunostain for calretinin, cytokeratin 5/6 & mesothelin
    - Negative BerEp4, CEA & LeuM1

Staging, Grading or Classification Criteria
- Histopathological staging according to nuclear size and estimated 3 year survival
  - I: 10-20 um and 100%, respectively
  - II: 21-30 um and 87%, respectively
  - III: 31-40 um and 27%, respectively
  - IV: > 40 um and 0%, respectively

CLINICAL ISSUES

Presentation
- Three clinical types: "Dry-painful," "wet," "mixed"
  - "Dry-painful" form most common: Localized pain related to a dominant tumor mass with little or no ascites
  - "Wet non-painful" form: Ascites and abdominal distention
  - "Mixed": A combination of "dry" and "wet" types

Demographics
- Age: Most cases occur in 5th & 6th decades
- Gender: Male predominance

Natural History & Prognosis
- Rapidly fatal
- Poor: 5-12 months in most series
  - Median survival of 50-60 months with aggressive treatment
- Improved prognosis following cytoreduction and perioperative intraperitoneal chemotherapy for histopathological class I patients
  - Mesotheliomas with small nuclear size (< 20 um)

Treatment
- Important diagnosis as treatment differs from ovarian cancer
- Resection
- Debulking if tumors are found late in their course
- Management of involved organs depends largely on specific organ
- Intra-operative intraperitoneal chemotherapy with cisplatin & doxorubicin
- Early post-operative intraoperative paclitaxel
- Perioperative treatment
  - Adjuvant intraoperative paclitaxel & second look cytoreduction

DIAGNOSTIC CHECKLIST

Consider
- MPM when an extensive and infiltrative mass is seen, especially if
  - Associated pleural disease
  - Scant ascites
  - Absent bulky lymphadenopathy

Image Interpretation Pearls
- Soft tissue mass within mesentery, omentum or peritoneum in case of no known primary malignancy of other organs

SELECTED REFERENCES

1. Yan TD et al: Prognostic Indicators for Patients Undergoing Cytoreductive Surgery and Perioperative Intraperitoneal Chemotherapy for Diffuse Malignant Peritoneal Mesothelioma(dagger). Ann Surg Oncol. 14(1):41-9, 2007
2. Pickhardt PJ et al: Primary neoplasms of peritoneal and sub-peritoneal origin: CT findings. Radiographics. 25(4):983-95, 2005
3. Yan TD et al: Abdominal computed tomography scans in the selection of patients with malignant peritoneal mesothelioma for comprehensive treatment with cytoreductive surgery and perioperative intraperitoneal chemotherapy. Cancer. 103(4):839-49, 2005
4. Yan TD et al: Computed tomographic characterization of malignant peritoneal mesothelioma. Tumori. 91(5):394-400, 2005
5. Chung DJ et al: Deciduoid peritoneal mesothelioma: CT findings with pathologic correlation. Abdom Imaging. 28(5):614-6, 2003
6. Kebapci M et al: CT findings and serum ca 125 levels in malignant peritoneal mesothelioma: report of 11 new cases and review of the literature. Eur Radiol. 13(12):2620-6, 2003
7. Sethna K et al: Peritoneal cystic mesothelioma: a case series. Tumori. 89(1):31-5, 2003
8. Busch JM et al: Malignant peritoneal mesothelioma. Radiographics. 22:1511-5, 2002
9. Puvaneswary M et al: Peritoneal mesothelioma: CT and MRI findings. Australas Radiol. 46(1):91-6, 2002
10. Sugarbaker PH et al: Diagnosis and treatment of peritoneal mesothelioma: The Washington Cancer Institute experience. Semin Oncol. 29:51-61, 2002
11. Loggie BW: Malignant peritoneal mesothelioma. Curr Treat Options Oncol. 2(5):395-9, 2001

PERITONEAL MESOTHELIOMA

IMAGE GALLERY

Typical

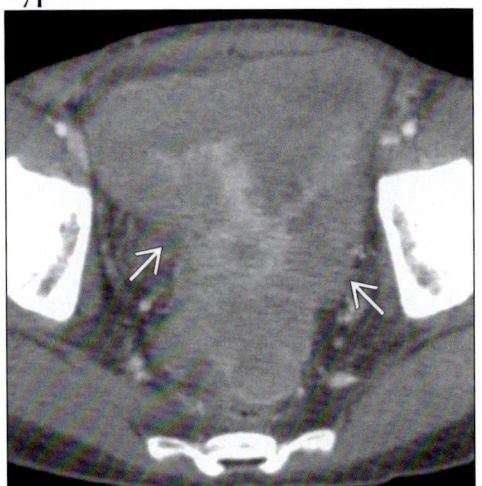
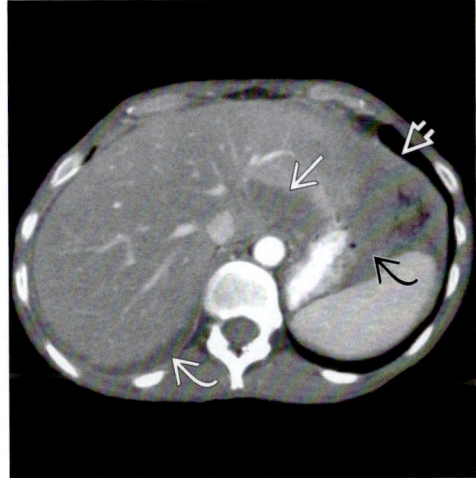

(Left) Axial CECT in the same person shows the destructive mass ➡ encasing the pelvic viscera. Lymphadenopathy and massive ascites are absent. *(Right)* Axial CECT in the same person shows scant ascites ➡ and soft tissue occupying the gastrosplenic ligament ➡, gastrohepatic ligament ➡ and the omentum ➡.

Typical

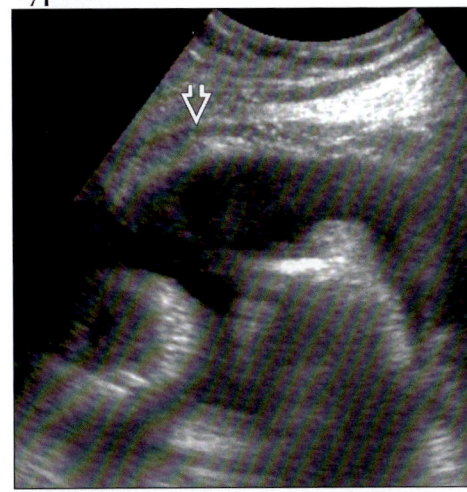
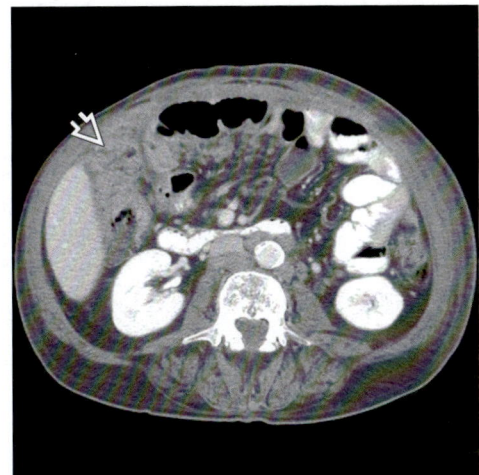

(Left) Axial oblique transabdominal ultrasound shows ascites and peritoneal thickening ➡ in a patient with the "mixed" type of disease. *(Right)* Axial CECT in the same patient shows peritoneal ➡ and serosal soft tissue masses.

Typical

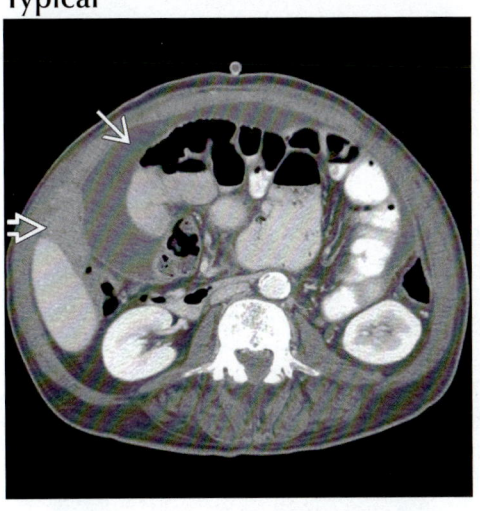
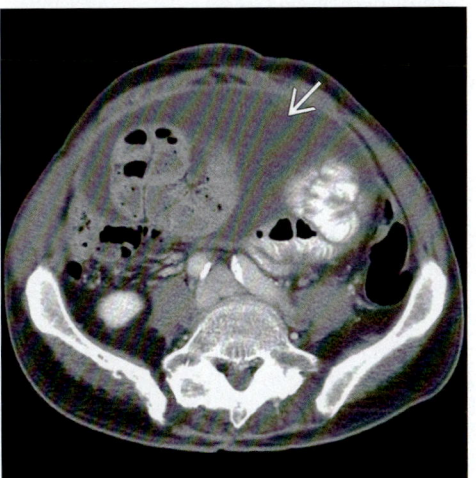

(Left) Axial CECT in the same patient shows both "wet" (ascites ➡) and "dry" (solid ➡) elements within the abdomen in a case of "mixed" disease. *(Right)* Axial CECT in the same patient shows ascites ➡ extending into the false pelvis.

PERITONEAL METASTASES

Axial CECT shows peritoneal implants along the right lobe of the liver, falciform ligament, and left upper quadrant lateral to the descending colon. Also note the presence of a liver capsular implant.

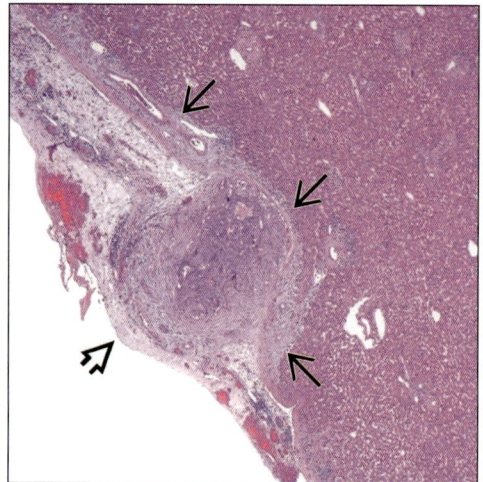

Micropathology in the same patient shows a liver capsular implant indenting the normal liver parenchyma. Pathology: Stage 3 serous papillary carcinoma of the ovary.

TERMINOLOGY

Abbreviations and Synonyms
- Peritoneal implants, peritoneal carcinomatosis

Definitions
- Metastatic tumor deposits throughout the peritoneal cavity

IMAGING FINDINGS

General Features
- Best diagnostic clue: Peritoneal thickening or multiple peritoneal masses in typical locations frequently associated with ascites
- Location
  o Malignant cells follow normal clockwise peritoneal fluid flow facilitated by bowel peristalsis and implant in dependent portion of peritoneal cavity
    - Anterior and posterior cul-de-sac
    - Paracolic gutters
    - Sigmoid colon at the site of sigmoid turn
    - Ileocecal junction
    - Omentum
    - Subphrenic space
    - Peritoneal reflections around the liver (falciform ligament and fissure of ligamentum teres)
    - Splenic hilum
- Size: Varies from microscopic nodular thickening and sand-paper appearance of the peritoneal surface to large implants
- Morphology: Solid or cystic lesions, solid lesions may demonstrate necrosis

Ultrasonographic Findings
- Grayscale Ultrasound
  o Hyperechoic, isoechoic or hypoechoic lesions
  o Relatively large tumor implants can be depicted with ultrasound
  o Small peritoneal implants in patients with little or no ascites can be difficult to visualize
- Color Doppler: Increased vascularity of peritoneal implants
- TV US
  o Particularly useful in detecting implants in the Pouch of Douglas and characterizing adnexal masses

DDx: Peritoneal Lesions

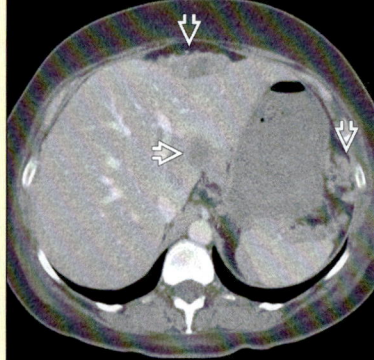

Primary Peritoneal Cancer

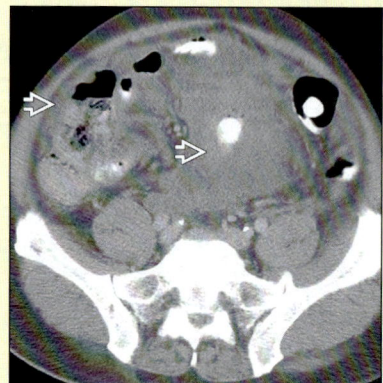

Lymphoma

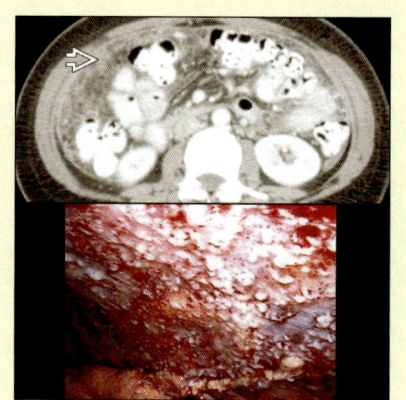

Tuberculosis

PERITONEAL METASTASES

Key Facts

Imaging Findings
- Best diagnostic clue: Peritoneal thickening or multiple peritoneal masses in typical locations frequently associated with ascites
- Malignant cells follow normal clockwise peritoneal fluid flow facilitated by bowel peristalsis and implant in dependent portion of peritoneal cavity

Top Differential Diagnoses
- Primary Papillary Serous Carcinoma of Peritoneum
- Lymphoma
- Extrapulmonary Tuberculosis
- Peritoneal Mesothelioma

Pathology
- Any tumor can potentially metastasize to the peritoneal cavity

- Most common malignant neoplasms are metastatic adenocarcinoma and lymphoma
- Immunohistochemistry may help to determine the site of the primary tumor

Diagnostic Checklist
- PET/CT for equivocal cases when tumor markers (serum CA-125, CEA, etc.) are elevated but conventional CECT or MR shows no evidence of disease
- Both ovarian and colon cancer can present with ascites, adnexal masses and typical location tumor deposits throughout the peritoneal cavity
- Peritoneal thickening or multiple peritoneal masses which tend to form in peritoneal reflections, associated with ascites

---

- Technique of choice for guiding omental/peritoneal biopsy

CT Findings
- Peritoneal thickening or enhancing solid or cystic peritoneal deposits of varying sizes
- Frequently outlined by ascites which facilitates their detection
- Calcifications may be present
- Small bowel obstruction may be present
- Primary tumor such as ovary, colon etc. may be visualized
- It is crucial to distinguish liver capsular implants from parenchymal metastases in ovarian cancer
  - Liver capsular implants represent operable disease (stage 3)
  - Liver parenchymal metastases represent inoperable disease (stage 4)
- It is useful for guiding biopsy for tissue diagnosis

MR Findings
- Peritoneal thickening or enhancing masses along the peritoneal surface and peritoneal reflections
- Better appreciated on delayed gadolinium enhanced fat suppressed T1WI
- Single shot breath-hold gradient echo technique allows elimination of motion artifact from respirations, bowel peristalsis and cardiac activity

Nuclear Medicine Findings
- PET/CT
  - May be useful to define disease extent, particularly when follow-up surgery is being considered
  - It is of limited value in small implants which may be obscured by normal FDG uptake in the bowel

Imaging Recommendations
- Best imaging tool: Contrast-enhanced CT
- Protocol advice
  - Intravenous contrast administration is necessary
  - Adequate amount of oral contrast is essential for bowel opacification to prevent misinterpretation of tumor implants vs. unopacified bowel loops
  - Scrolling through images improves the ability to reliably detect subtle peritoneal implants and distinguish them from normal bowel
  - Two-dimensional multiplanar reformatted images are very useful to distinguish liver capsular implants from intraparenchymal liver metastases

DIFFERENTIAL DIAGNOSIS

Primary Papillary Serous Carcinoma of Peritoneum
- Very rare
- Absence of an ovarian mass is critical for excluding metastatic papillary serous ovarian carcinoma, as identical appearance on imaging and histology

Lymphoma
- Frequently affects bowel at the same time, usually small bowel
- Omental caking is indistinguishable from other forms of peritoneal carcinomatosis and ascites can be present

Extrapulmonary Tuberculosis
- More common in endemic areas
- Absence of ovarian mass is crucial
- Usually sand-like tiny peritoneal plaques
- Enlarged, usually necrotic abdomino-pelvic lymph nodes may be present

Peritoneal Mesothelioma
- Related to asbestos exposure
- Pleural involvement is common
- Small amount of ascites, disproportional to amount of peritoneal thickening/masses

Other Primary Neoplasms of Peritoneal and Subperitoneal Origin
- Desmoplastic tumors, gastrointestinal stromal tumor, liposarcoma, malignant fibrous histiocytoma, leiomyosarcoma, angiosarcoma, etc.

PERITONEAL METASTASES

PATHOLOGY

General Features
- Genetics: No genetic predisposition
- Etiology
  o Any tumor can potentially metastasize to the peritoneal cavity
  o Most common malignant neoplasms are metastatic adenocarcinoma and lymphoma
    ▪ Among carcinomas, the most frequent primaries are colon, ovarian, uterine, gastric, pancreatic, bile ducts and breast carcinoma
    ▪ Hepatocellular carcinoma, renal cell carcinoma and urothelial neoplasms have been reported as rare origin of peritoneal carcinomatosis
  o Gliomatosis peritonei is a rare condition consisting of peritoneal implants composed of mature glial tissue
    ▪ Can be associated with a solid ovarian teratoma
    ▪ Tears in the ovarian capsule of a mature teratoma has lead to belief that this entity occurs due to gliomatous tissue leaking into the peritoneal cavity
    ▪ May occasionally be seen in patients with a ventriculo-peritoneal shunt for hydrocephalus
    ▪ Good prognosis, although recurrences can occur
- Associated abnormalities: Ascites and bowel obstruction

Microscopic Features
- Serosal or capsular invasion of visceral peritoneum can occur
- Immunohistochemistry may help to determine the site of the primary tumor
  o More common sources of metastases are from female genital tract (ovary, uterus & cervix)
    ▪ Immunohistochemical stains are positive for cytokeratin 7 (CK7 +ve) and negative for cytokeratin 20 (CK20 -ve)
  o Gastro-intestinal tract
    ▪ Gastric: CK 7 +ve, CK20 +ve or -ve
    ▪ Colorectal: CK 7 -ve, CK 20 +ve
    ▪ Pancreatico-biliary: CK 7 +ve, CK20 +ve or -ve, Ca19-9 +ve
  o Breast: CK 7+ve, CK20 -ve, estrogen receptor +ve or -ve
  o Lung: CK7+ve, CK 20 -ve, TTF 1 +ve
  o Prostate: Prostate specific antigen (PSA) +ve

CLINICAL ISSUES

Presentation
- Most common signs/symptoms: Abdominal pain and distension, increased abdominal girth, early satiety, nausea and vomiting
- Other signs/symptoms: Weight loss, bowel obstruction, malnutrition, and cachexia

Natural History & Prognosis
- Dismal prognosis, most patients die after developing multilevel bowel obstruction due to widespread peritoneal implants and adhesions
- Elevated CA-125 values are associated with poor outcome

Treatment
- Surgery to remove the bulk of the tumor, followed by systemic chemotherapy and occasionally by radiation for local residual or recurrent disease
- Intraperitoneal chemotherapy

DIAGNOSTIC CHECKLIST

Consider
- PET/CT for equivocal cases when tumor markers (serum CA-125, CEA, etc.) are elevated but conventional CECT or MR shows no evidence of disease
- Both ovarian and colon cancer can present with ascites, adnexal masses and typical location tumor deposits throughout the peritoneal cavity

Image Interpretation Pearls
- Peritoneal thickening or multiple peritoneal masses which tend to form in peritoneal reflections, associated with ascites

SELECTED REFERENCES

1. Barnetson RJ et al: Immunohistochemical analysis of peritoneal mesothelioma and primary and secondary serous carcinoma of the peritoneum: antibodies to estrogen and progesterone receptors are useful. Am J Clin Pathol. 125(1):67-76, 2006
2. Blake MA et al: Pearls and pitfalls in interpretation of abdominal and pelvic PET-CT. Radiographics. 26(5):1335-53, 2006
3. Spencer JA et al: Image guided biopsy in the management of cancer of the ovary. Cancer Imaging. 6:144-7, 2006
4. Testa AC et al: Ultrasound and color power Doppler in the detection of metastatic omentum: a prospective study. Ultrasound Obstet Gynecol. 27(1):65-70, 2006
5. Pickhardt PJ et al: Primary neoplasms of peritoneal and sub-peritoneal origin: CT findings. Radiographics. 25(4):983-95, 2005
6. Qayyum A et al: Role of CT and MR imaging in predicting optimal cytoreduction of newly diagnosed primary epithelial ovarian cancer. Gynecol Oncol. 96(2):301-6, 2005
7. Savelli L et al: Transvaginal sonographic features of peritoneal carcinomatosis. Ultrasound Obstet Gynecol. 26(5):552-7, 2005
8. Ricke J et al: Prospective evaluation of contrast-enhanced MRI in the depiction of peritoneal spread in primary or recurrent ovarian cancer. Eur Radiol. 13(5):943-9, 2003
9. Coakley FV et al: Peritoneal metastases: detection with spiral CT in patients with ovarian cancer. Radiology. 223(2):495-9, 2002
10. Tempany CM et al: Staging of advanced ovarian cancer: comparison of imaging modalities--report from the Radiological Diagnostic Oncology Group. Radiology. 215(3):761-7, 2000
11. Hamrick-Turner JE et al: Neoplastic and inflammatory processes of the peritoneum, omentum, and mesentery: diagnosis with CT. Radiographics. 12(6):1051-68, 1992

PERITONEAL METASTASES

IMAGE GALLERY

Typical

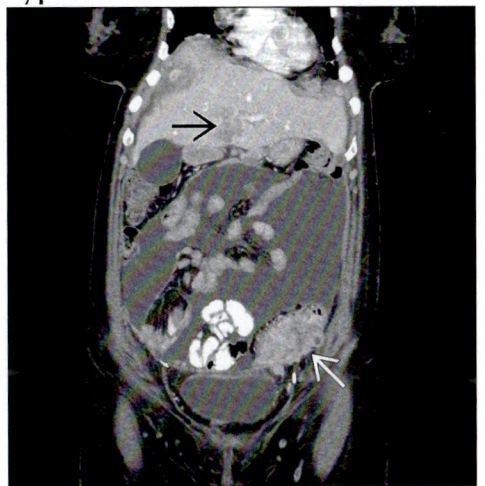
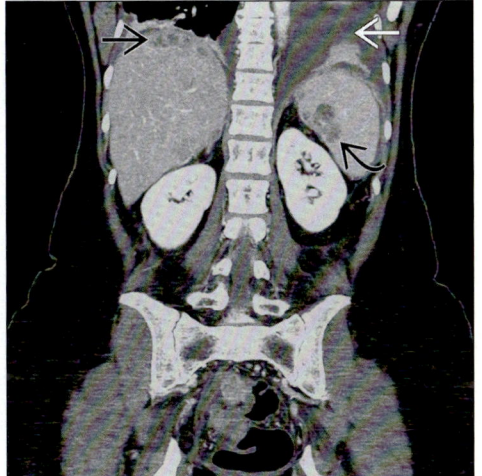

(Left) Coronal CECT shows peritoneal implants in the porta hepatis ➔ and serosal implants along the sigmoid colon ➔. *(Right)* Coronal CECT of the same patient shows peritoneal implants on the liver capsule ➔ and in the splenic hilum ➔. Note the presence of left pleural effusion ➔ in this patient with stage 4 ovarian cancer (malignant pleural effusion on cytology).

Typical

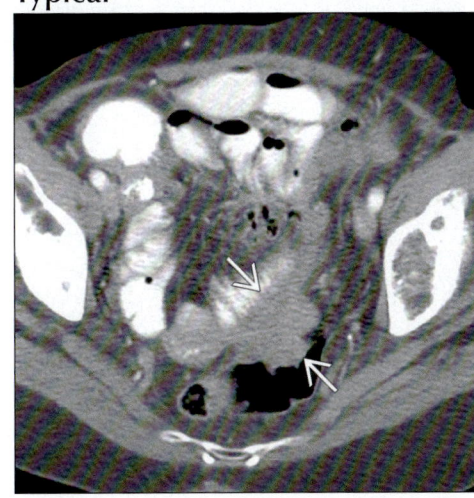
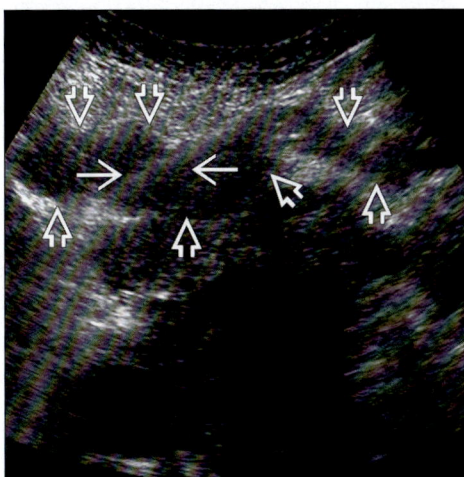

(Left) Axial CECT shows peritoneal metastases in cul-de-sac ➔ in a patient with stage 3 ovarian cancer. *(Right)* Axial ultrasound guided biopsy image shows a hypoechoic omental cake ➔ in a patient with ovarian cancer. Note the needle track ➔ through the lesion confirming the accurate position of the needle within the lesion.

Variant

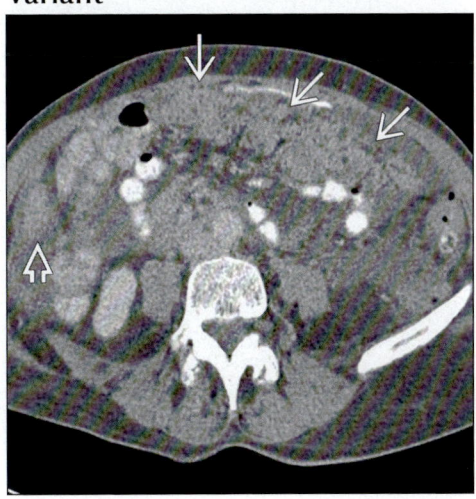
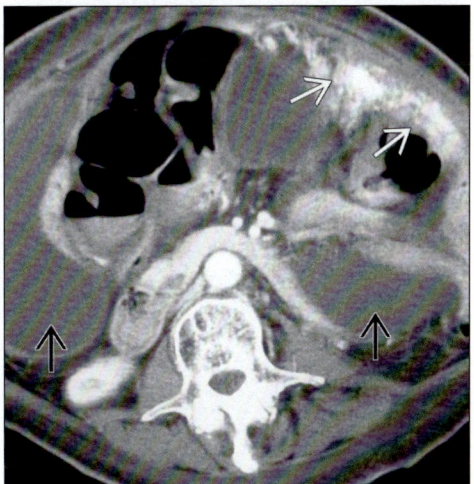

(Left) Axial CECT shows the presence of omental metastases ➔ and a peritoneal implant ➔ in the right paracolic gutter in a patient with stage 3 ovarian cancer. *(Right)* Axial CECT shows calcified omental metastases ➔ in a patient with ovarian cancer. Large amount of ascites ➔ is also present.

PERITONEAL METASTASES

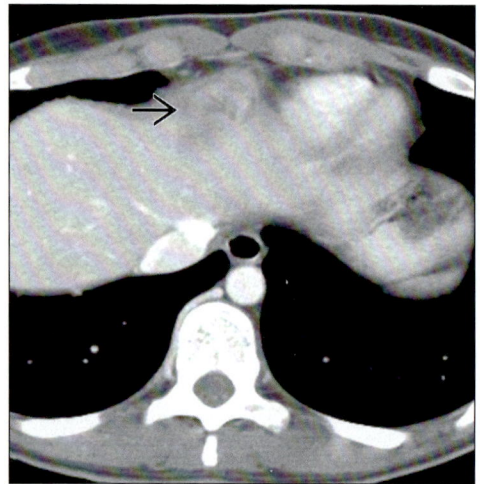 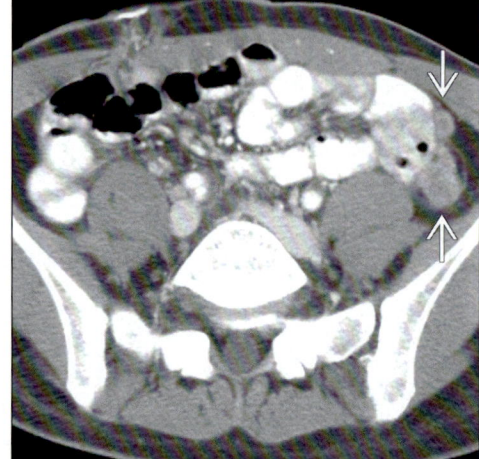

(Left) Axial CECT shows a peritoneal implant on the surface of the dome of the liver ➡ in a patient with metastatic colon cancer. *(Right)* Axial CECT in the same patient shows peritoneal implants ➡ in left paracolic gutter.

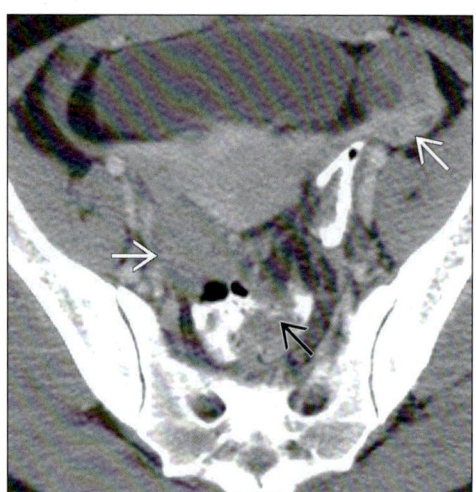 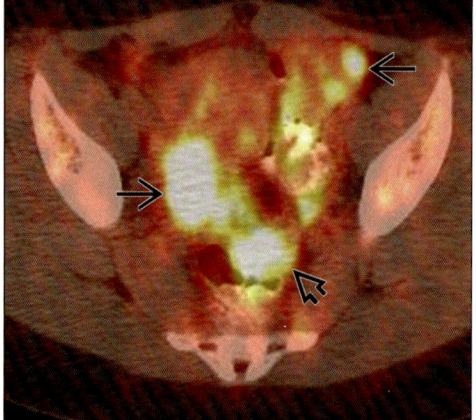

(Left) Axial CECT shows bilateral ovarian metastases ➡ in a patient with colon cancer. Also note presence of a serosal deposit in the sigmoid colon ➡. *(Right)* Axial fused PET/CT in the same patient shows increased radiotracer uptake in both ovaries ➡ and on the surface of the sigmoid colon ➡ confirming presence of metastases suspected on the CECT image.

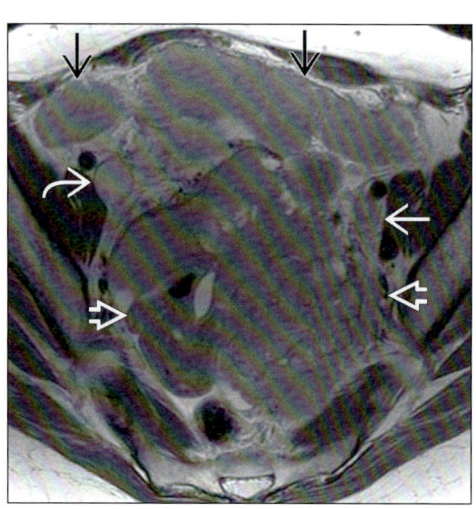 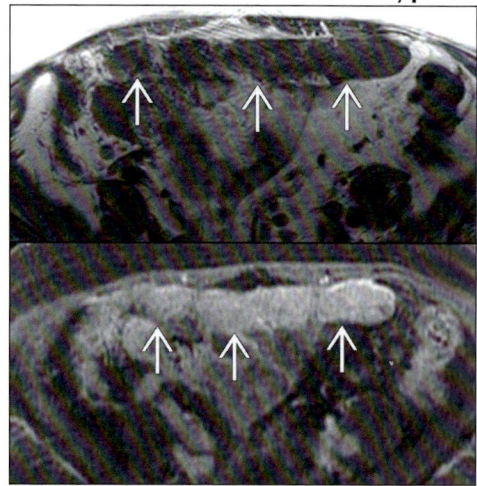

(Left) Axial T2WI MR shows omental metastases ➡ and bilateral ovarian masses ➡ in a patient with ovarian cancer. Also note presence of an enlarged left external iliac lymph node ➡ and thrombus within the right external iliac vein ➡. *(Right)* Axial T1WI and axial T1 C+ FS MR (delayed images at 5 minutes) show omental metastases which demonstrate prominent enhancement ➡ in a patient with stage 3 ovarian cancer.

PERITONEAL METASTASES

Variant

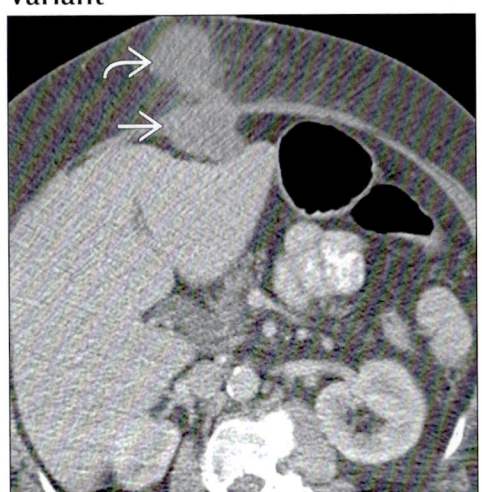 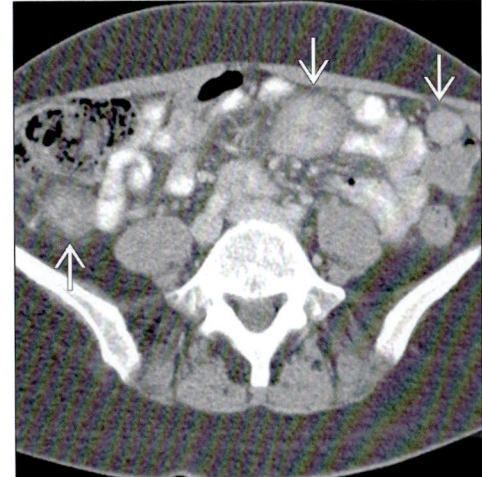

(Left) Axial CECT shows a peritoneal implant indenting the left lobe liver surface ➡ and extending into the subcutaneous fat ➡ in a patient with papillary serous carcinoma of the endometrium. *(Right)* Axial CECT shows multiple peritoneal metastases ➡ in a patient with endometrial stromal sarcoma of the uterus.

Variant

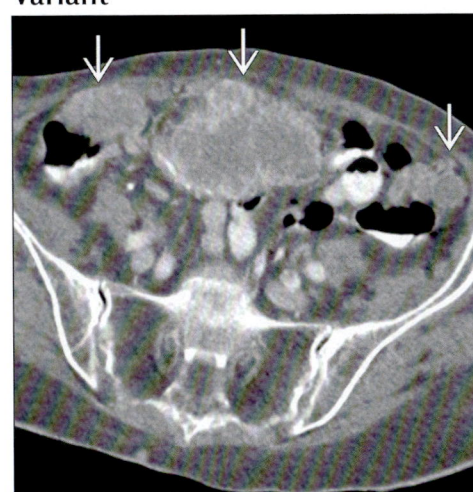 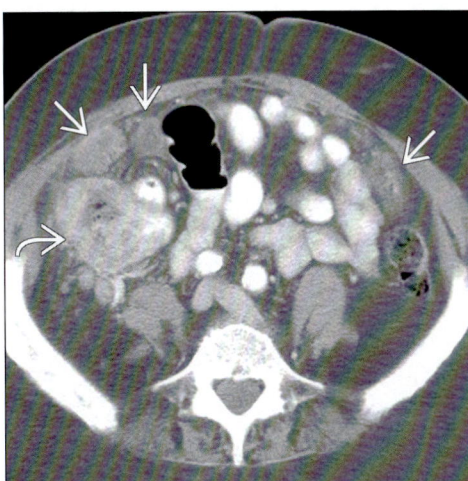

(Left) Axial CECT shows multiple necrotic peritoneal metastases ➡ in a patient with metastatic adenocarcinoma of the tail of the pancreas. *(Right)* Axial CECT shows multiple peritoneal metastases ➡ in a patient with metastatic invasive ductal carcinoma of the breast. Also note the presence of the serosal implants in the caecum ➡.

Variant

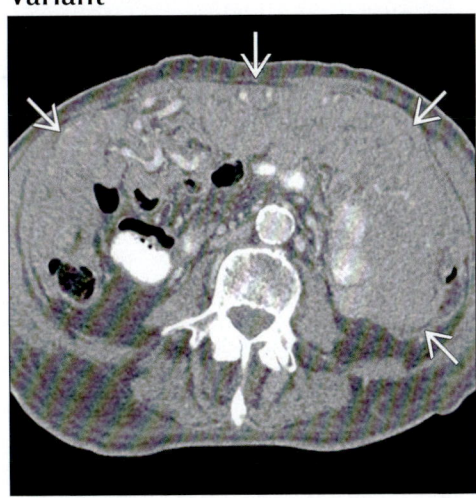 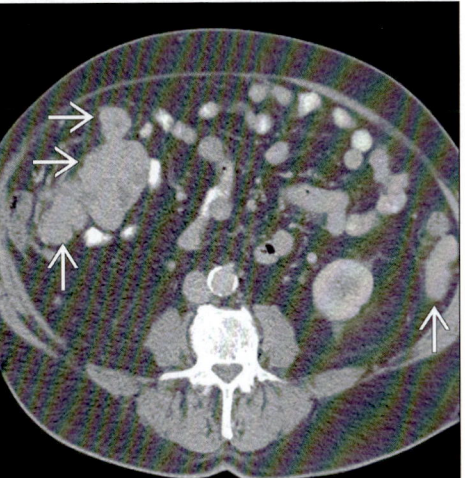

(Left) Axial CECT shows extensive omental metastases ➡ in a patient with metastatic melanoma. *(Right)* Axial CECT shows multiple peritoneal metastases ➡ in a liver transplant patient with recurrent hepatocellular carcinoma.

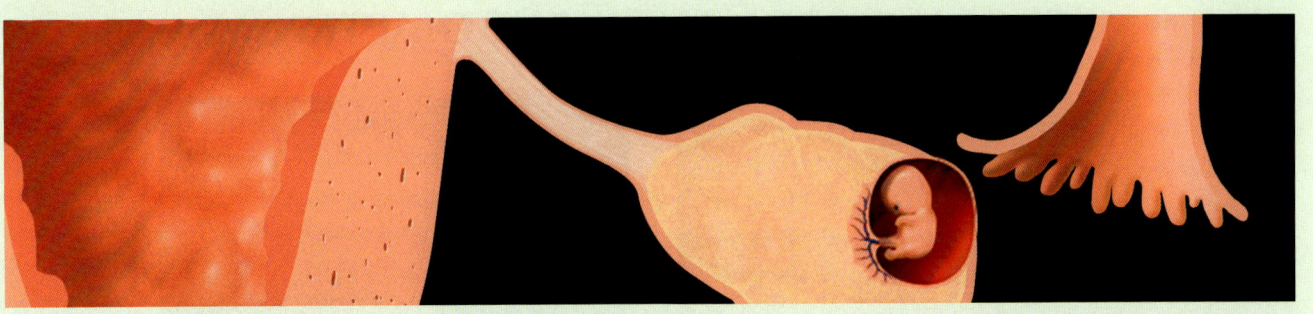

SECTION 10: Ectopic Pregnancy

Ectopic Pregnancy, Endometrium	10-2
Ectopic Pregnancy, Tubal	10-4
Ectopic Pregnancy, Interstitial	10-10
Ectopic Pregnancy, Cervical	10-16
Ectopic Pregnancy, Ovarian	10-20
Ectopic Pregnancy, Heterotopic	10-22
Ectopic Pregnancy, Abdominal	10-26
Ectopic Pregnancy, Rupture	10-28

ECTOPIC PREGNANCY, ENDOMETRIUM

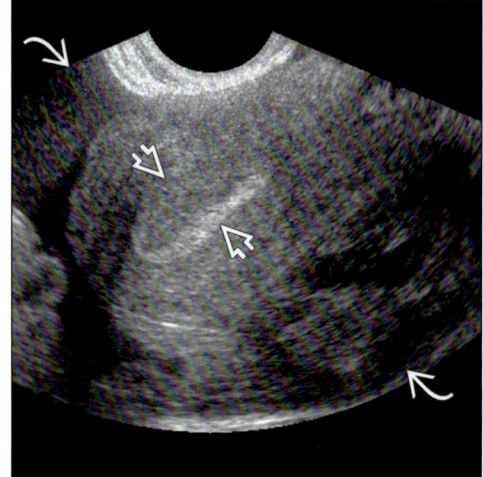

Sagittal transabdominal ultrasound shows heterogeneous debris ⇨ in endometrium in patient with ectopic pregnancy.

Sagittal transvaginal ultrasound shows thickened slightly heterogeneous appearance to endometrium ⇨ in patient with ruptured ectopic pregnancy. Note blood clot around uterus ➡.

TERMINOLOGY

Definitions
- Pseudosac: Collection of blood products/debris centrally located in endometrial cavity
- Decidual cysts: Tiny cysts in endometrium without surrounding echogenic rim
- Decidual reaction in the endometrium gives a thickened echogenic appearance

IMAGING FINDINGS

General Features
- Best diagnostic clue
  - Differentiate pseudosac and decidual cysts from gestational sac by location in endometrial cavity
    - Pseudosac is centrally located and does not have an echogenic rim around it
    - Decidual cysts at periphery of the endometrium and do not have echogenic rims
- Location
  - Pseudosac centrally located
  - Decidual cysts at periphery of endometrium

- Morphology
  - Pseudosac may have anechoic fluid, fluid with debris, solid appearing clot
  - Decidual reaction in the endometrium gives a thickened echogenic appearance

Imaging Recommendations
- Best imaging tool: Transvaginal ultrasound
- Protocol advice
  - Assess for appearance of fluid in endometrial cavity
  - Look for changing appearance of endometrial fluid to suggest pseudosac

DIFFERENTIAL DIAGNOSIS

Intradecidual Sac Sign
- Sac eccentrically located in endometrial cavity but abuts the endometrial cavity
- Echogenic rim around sac
- Round appearance
- Present at 4.5 menstrual weeks

DDx: Endometrial Findings in Ectopic Pregnancy

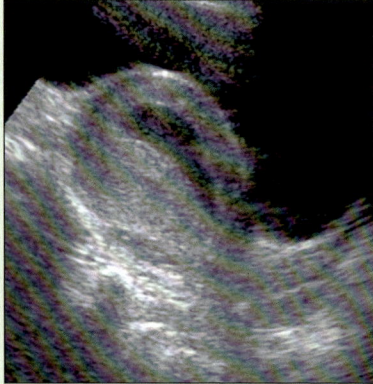
Empty Gestational Sac

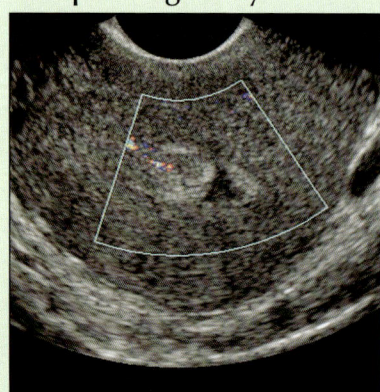
Retained Products of Conception

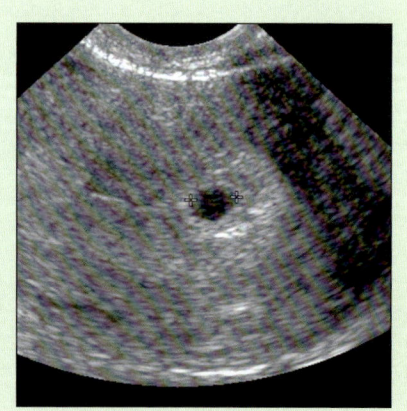
Intradecidual Sac Sign

ECTOPIC PREGNANCY, ENDOMETRIUM

Key Facts

Imaging Findings
- Differentiate pseudosac and decidual cysts from gestational sac by location in endometrial cavity
- Pseudosac is centrally located and does not have an echogenic rim around it
- Decidual cysts at periphery of the endometrium and do not have echogenic rims

Pathology
- Pseudosac and decidual cysts will not show chorionic villi

Diagnostic Checklist
- Consider ectopic pregnancy when fluid seen centrally in endometrial cavity and no definite intrauterine gestational sac visualized

Double Decidual Sac Sign
- Inner rim of chronic villi surrounded by a thin crescent of fluid in the endometrial cavity, surrounded by the outer echogenic rim of the decidua vera

Intrauterine Gestational Sac with Yolk Sac
- 100% specific for intrauterine pregnancy
- Normal intrauterine gestational sacs grow 0.8 mm per day thus will increase in size on follow-up

Miscarriage
- Human chorionic gonadotropin (hCG) reverts to normal over time
- May visualize echogenic rim around sac or embryonic parts in sac

PATHOLOGY

Microscopic Features
- Pseudosac and decidual cysts will not show chorionic villi

CLINICAL ISSUES

Presentation
- Most common signs/symptoms: Pain, bleeding in first trimester

Demographics
- Age: Reproductive age
- Gender: F

Natural History & Prognosis
- Typically associated with tubal ectopic pregnancy

Treatment
- Laparoscopy if clinically unstable
- Methotrexate if meet selection/exclusion
- Watchful waiting if clinically stable and meet section/exclusion criteria

DIAGNOSTIC CHECKLIST

Consider
- Consider ectopic pregnancy when fluid seen centrally in endometrial cavity and no definite intrauterine gestational sac visualized

SELECTED REFERENCES

1. Chiang G et al: The intradecidual sign: is it reliable for diagnosis of early intrauterine pregnancy? AJR Am J Roentgenol. 183(3):725-31, 2004
2. Nyberg DA et al: Endovaginal sonographic evaluation of ectopic pregnancy: a prospective study. AJR Am J Roentgenol. 149(6):1181-6, 1987
3. Yeh HC et al: Intradecidual sign: a US criterion of early intrauterine pregnancy. Radiology. 161(2):463-7, 1986
4. Bradley WG et al: The double sac sign of early intrauterine pregnancy: use in exclusion of ectopic pregnancy. Radiology. 143(1):223-6, 1982

IMAGE GALLERY

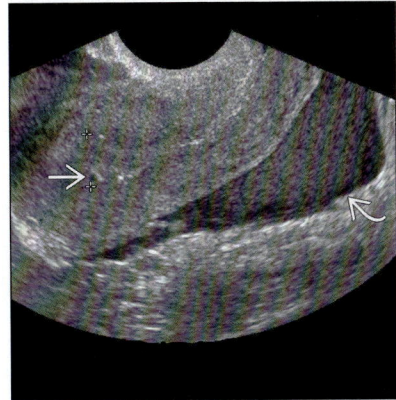
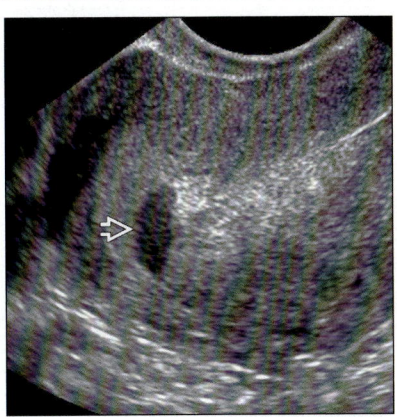
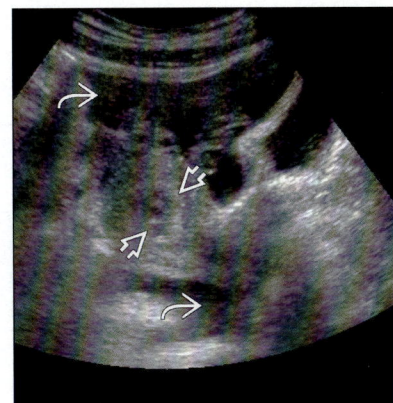

(Left) Sagittal transvaginal ultrasound shows tiny decidual cyst ➡ in endometrium in patient with ectopic pregnancy. Note blood in cul-de-sac ➡. (Center) Sagittal transvaginal ultrasound shows pseudosac ➡ of blood in endometrial cavity. (Right) Sagittal transabdominal ultrasound shows heterogeneous material ➡ in endometrial cavity in patient with ruptured ectopic pregnancy. Note blood products ➡ around uterus.

ECTOPIC PREGNANCY, TUBAL

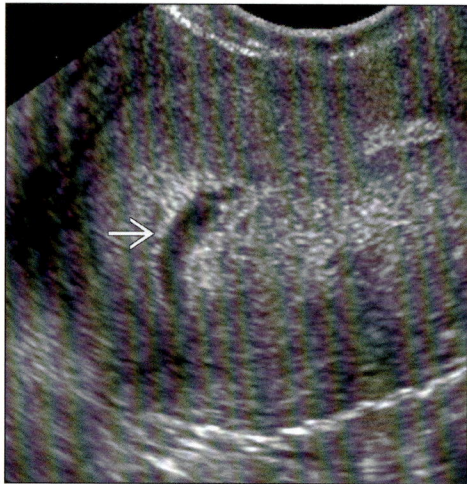

Sagittal transvaginal ultrasound shows fluid in endometrial cavity ➡ but no intrauterine gestational sac.

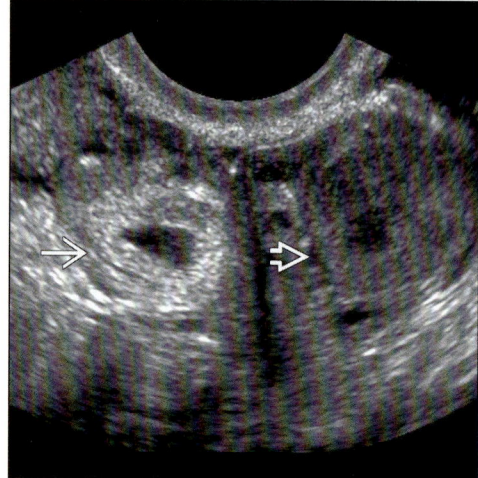

Axial oblique transvaginal ultrasound shows echogenic ring-like mass ➡ adjacent to ovary with corpus luteum cyst ➡.

TERMINOLOGY

Abbreviations and Synonyms
- Ectopic pregnancy, tubal ectopic pregnancy

Definitions
- Pregnancy located within the fallopian tube

IMAGING FINDINGS

General Features
- Best diagnostic clue
  - Typical presentation is at 5-6 weeks after last menstrual period
  - Echogenic mass adjacent to ovary with embryonic pole with cardiac activity
- Location
  - In the fallopian tube, seen sonographically as adjacent to the ovary
  - Moves separately from ovary at real time scanning
- Size
  - 2-5 cm
  - May be larger if there is a large amount of clot
  - May be larger at gestational ages greater than 6 weeks
- Morphology
  - Echogenic ring-like mass
  - Gestational sac with yolk sac
  - Gestational sac with yolk sac and embryonic pole
  - Amorphous mass due to blood clot

Ultrasonographic Findings
- Endometrium
  - No intrauterine pregnancy
  - Pseudosac
    - Fluid centrally located in endometrial cavity
    - May change in appearance over time
  - Decidual cysts
    - Located away from endometrial cavity
    - Do not have echogenic rim around them
- Tube
  - Amorphous mass may be due to blood clot
    - Ectopic pregnancy is the most common cause of hematosalpinx
  - Ring-like mass separate from ovary
    - May have yolk sac

DDx: Mimics of Tubal Ectopic Pregnancy

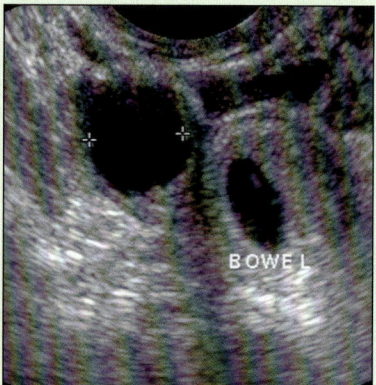

Bowel Next to Ovary

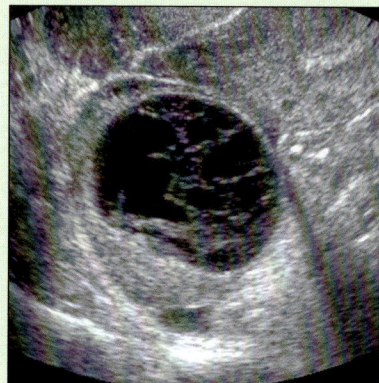

Hemorrhagic Cyst

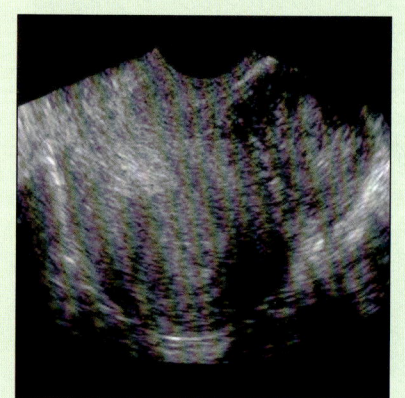

Exophytic Leiomyoma

ECTOPIC PREGNANCY, TUBAL

Key Facts

Imaging Findings
- Typical presentation is at 5-6 weeks after last menstrual period
- In the fallopian tube, seen sonographically as adjacent to the ovary
- Moves separately from ovary at real time scanning
- No intrauterine pregnancy
- Pseudosac
- Fluid centrally located in endometrial cavity
- Ring-like mass separate from ovary
- Fluid with debris suggests hemorrhage
- Large amount of fluid will be seen in upper abdomen, if rupture has occurred
- Ring of color around an adnexal mass may be due to either hemorrhagic cyst or ectopic
- Color can be helpful to locate an ectopic hidden in bowel gas

Top Differential Diagnoses
- If diagnosis is unclear, a follow-up sonogram and hCG will be helpful

Pathology
- High risk in patients with tubal disease, prior ectopic pregnancy, infertility treatment, use of intrauterine device
- 90% of ectopic pregnancies are located in the fallopian tubes

Clinical Issues
- May resolve spontaneously
- May rupture and bleed leading to life-threatening hemoperitoneum

---

    - May have embryonic pole with or without cardiac activity
- Free fluid
  - Fluid with debris suggests hemorrhage
  - Large amount of fluid will be seen in upper abdomen, if rupture has occurred
  - Fluid with debris in a pregnant patient has a 90% positive predictive value for ectopic pregnancy
- Color Doppler
  - Ring of color around an adnexal mass may be due to either hemorrhagic cyst or ectopic
  - Color can be helpful to locate an ectopic hidden in bowel gas

CT Findings
- Fluid with high Hounsfield units (due to blood) in pelvis
- Heterogeneous adnexal mass separate from ovary

MR Findings
- Fluid with signal characteristics of blood in the pelvis
- Heterogeneous adnexal mass separate from ovary

Imaging Recommendations
- Best imaging tool: Ultrasound
- Protocol advice
  - Begin with a full bladder
    - Assess for pregnancies located in or around the uterus
    - Assess for masses out of the plane of the vaginal probe
  - Endovaginal scan
    - Scan uterus to check for intrauterine pregnancy
    - Scan adnexa to check for mass separate from ovary
    - Ovarian mass is more likely to be corpus luteum than ectopic pregnancy
    - If no extra ovarian adnexal mass is visualized, scan with color to find ectopic hidden between bowel loops
    - Ectopic pregnancy may not be on same side as corpus luteum
    - Check cul-de-sac for free fluid
    - Check by kidneys for hemoperitoneum

DIFFERENTIAL DIAGNOSIS

Intrauterine Pregnancy with Hemorrhagic Corpus Luteum Cyst
- Intrauterine pregnancy diagnosed with intradecidual sign, double decidual sac sign, yolk sac, or embryo
- Adnexal cyst will be in ovary, not adjacent to ovary
- Cyst wall will be less echogenic than wall of ectopic pregnancy
- Anechoic cyst is unlikely to be ectopic pregnancy
- If diagnosis is unclear, a follow-up sonogram and hCG will be helpful

Heterotopic Pregnancy
- Combined intra- and extrauterine pregnancy
- Pregnancies are typically of similar gestational age

No Pregnancy Visualized with Positive Pregnancy Test
- Early intrauterine pregnancy, too early to visualize
  - β-hCG should rise normally (doubling time of 2 days)
- Miscarriage
  - β-hCG should not rise normally or should decrease
  - Retrograde flow of blood into tube can mimic ectopic pregnancy
- Ectopic pregnancy, too early to visualize
  - β-hCG should not rise normally or should decrease
  - 21% of ectopic pregnancies have β-hCG that rises similar to intrauterine pregnancy

Exophytic Leiomyoma
- Broad base of attachment to uterus
- Similar echogenicity to other leiomyomas

Tubo-Ovarian Abscess
- Cervical motion tenderness
- Elevated white blood cell count

ECTOPIC PREGNANCY, TUBAL

Tubal Cyst
- Thin-walled anechoic cyst
- Separate from ovary

PATHOLOGY

General Features
- Etiology: Pregnancy implants in tube instead of in uterus
- Epidemiology
  - High risk in patients with tubal disease, prior ectopic pregnancy, infertility treatment, use of intrauterine device
  - 1:150 pregnancies

Gross Pathologic & Surgical Features
- 90% of ectopic pregnancies are located in the fallopian tubes
- Fertilized ovum undergoes its usual development
- Implantation site develops decidual changes
- Intratubal hemorrhage can occur without tubal rupture

Microscopic Features
- Endometrial biopsy may show decidual changes
- Endometrial biopsy will not show chorionic villi (unless heterotopic pregnancy)
- Tubal pregnancy will show chorionic villi

CLINICAL ISSUES

Presentation
- Most common signs/symptoms
  - Early pregnancy
  - Pain
  - Bleeding
  - Adnexal mass
  - Triad of pain, bleeding, and adnexal mass present in 45% of patients with ectopic pregnancy

Demographics
- Age: Reproductive age
- Gender: Female

Natural History & Prognosis
- May resolve spontaneously
  - Reliable and clinically stable patients with small ectopic pregnancies can be watched
- After treatment with methotrexate, may enlarge and cause pain
- May rupture and bleed leading to life-threatening hemoperitoneum

Treatment
- Watchful waiting in stable patients
- Methotrexate in reliable patients with ectopic pregnancy less than 5 cm and no cardiac activity
- Laparoscopy

DIAGNOSTIC CHECKLIST

Consider
- Hemorrhagic cyst masquerading as ectopic pregnancy

Image Interpretation Pearls
- Check that mass is in tube not in ovary
- Check that echogenicity of mass is greater than that of corpus luteum cyst

SELECTED REFERENCES

1. Dialani V et al: Ectopic pregnancy: a review. Ultrasound Q. 20(3):105-17, 2004
2. Stein MW et al: Sonographic comparison of the tubal ring of ectopic pregnancy with the corpus luteum. J Ultrasound Med. 23(1):57-62, 2004
3. Ferrero S et al: Seventy-five ectopic pregnancies. Medical and surgical management. Minerva Ginecol. 54(6):471-82, 2002
4. Frates MC et al: Comparison of tubal ring and corpus luteum echogenicities: a useful differentiating characteristic. J Ultrasound Med. 20(1):27-31; quiz 33, 2001
5. Aboud E: A five-year review of ectopic pregnancy. Clin Exp Obstet Gynecol. 24(3):127-9, 1997
6. Atri M et al: Role of endovaginal sonography in the diagnosis and management of ectopic pregnancy. Radiographics. 16(4):755-74; discussion 775, 1996
7. Buster JE et al: Ectopic pregnancy: new advances in diagnosis and treatment. Curr Opin Obstet Gynecol. 7(3):168-76, 1995
8. Mol BW et al: Contraception and the risk of ectopic pregnancy: a meta-analysis. Contraception. 52(6):337-41, 1995
9. Brown DL et al: Transvaginal sonography for diagnosing ectopic pregnancy: positivity criteria and performance characteristics. J Ultrasound Med. 13(4):259-66, 1994
10. Frates MC et al: Tubal rupture in patients with ectopic pregnancy: diagnosis with transvaginal US. Radiology. 191(3):769-72, 1994
11. Atri M et al: Accuracy of transvaginal ultrasonography for detection of hematosalpinx in ectopic pregnancy. J Clin Ultrasound. 20(4):255-61, 1992
12. Jurkovic D et al: Transvaginal color Doppler study of blood flow in ectopic pregnancies. Fertil Steril. 57(1):68-73, 1992
13. Rottem S et al: Classification of tubal gestations by transvaginal sonography. Ultrasound Obstet Gynecol. 1(3):197-201, 1991
14. Fleischer AC et al: Ectopic pregnancy: features at transvaginal sonography. Radiology. 174(2):375-8, 1990
15. Herman A et al: The role of tubal pathology and other parameters in ectopic pregnancies occurring in in vitro fertilization and embryo transfer. Fertil Steril. 54(5):864-8, 1990
16. Kivikoski AI et al: Transabdominal and transvaginal ultrasonography in the diagnosis of ectopic pregnancy: a comparative study. Am J Obstet Gynecol. 163(1 Pt 1):123-8, 1990
17. Fernandez H et al: Spontaneous resolution of ectopic pregnancy. Obstet Gynecol. 71(2):171-4, 1988
18. Sauer MV et al: Nonsurgical management of unruptured ectopic pregnancy: an extended clinical trial. Fertil Steril. 48(5):752-5, 1987
19. Breen JL: A 21 year survey of 654 ectopic pregnancies. Am J Obstet Gynecol. 106(7):1004-19, 1970

ECTOPIC PREGNANCY, TUBAL

IMAGE GALLERY

Typical

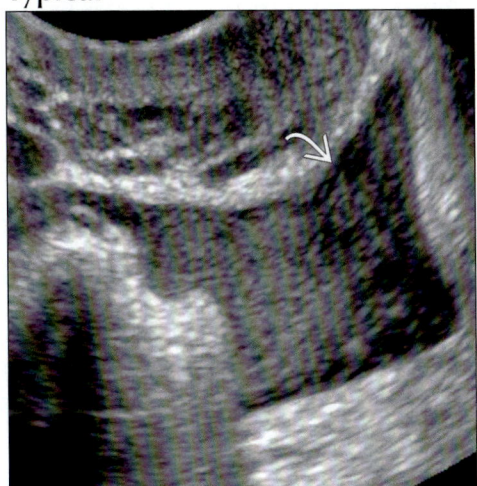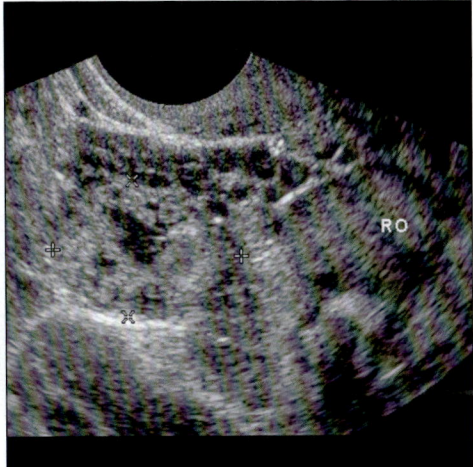

(Left) Sagittal transvaginal ultrasound shows fluid with debris in cul-de-sac ➔. *(Right)* Axial oblique transvaginal ultrasound shows ring-like mass (calipers) adjacent to the right ovary (RO).

Typical

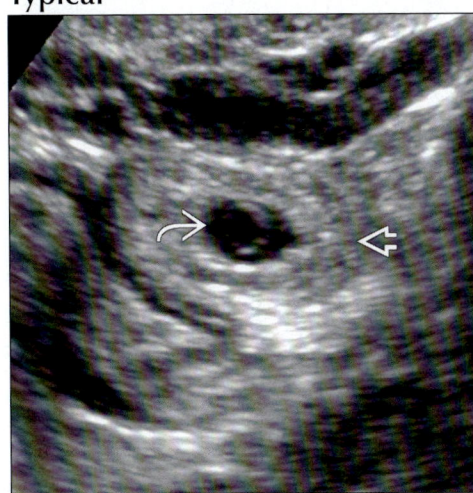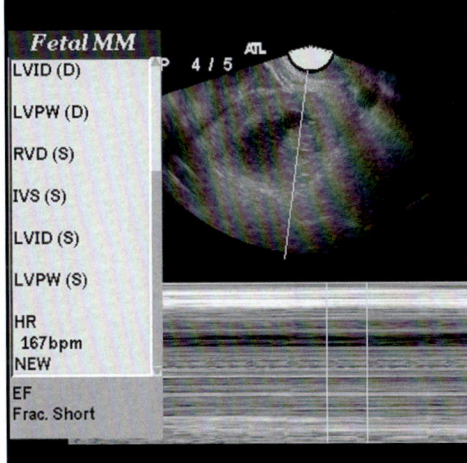

(Left) Axial transvaginal ultrasound shows echogenic ring-like mass ➔ with yolk sac ➔. *(Right)* Oblique transvaginal ultrasound shows M-mode of cardiac activity in a live ectopic.

Typical

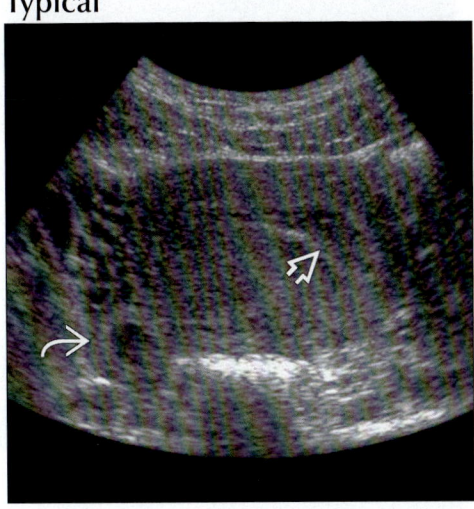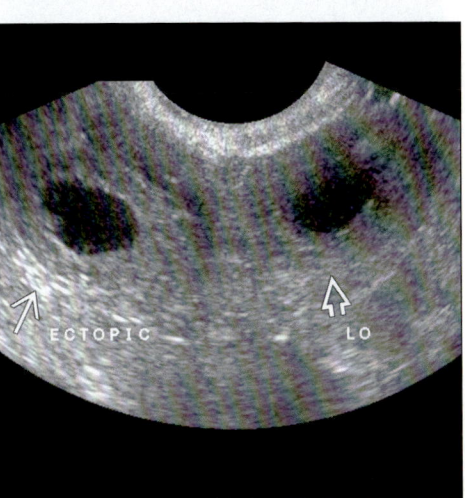

(Left) Transverse transabdominal ultrasound shows a pseudosac ➔ and a ring-like adnexal mass posterior to the uterus ➔. *(Right)* Axial oblique transvaginal ultrasound shows an ectopic pregnancy ➔ located medial to the left ovary ➔.

ECTOPIC PREGNANCY, TUBAL

(Left) Transverse transabdominal ultrasound shows a left sided ectopic pregnancy ➔, with free fluid ➔. Note the empty uterus (UT) and normal appearing right ovary (RTO). *(Right)* Transverse transvaginal ultrasound shows an echogenic round mass ➔ inferomedial to the right ovary ➔.

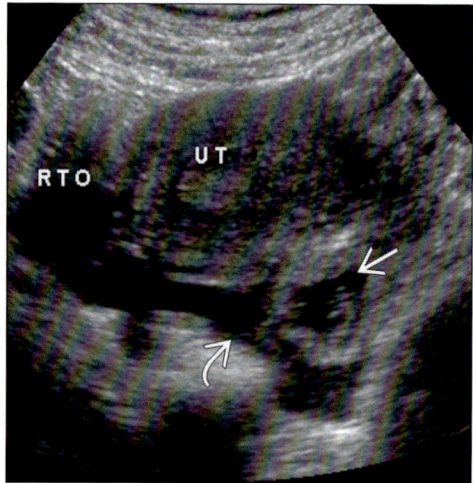
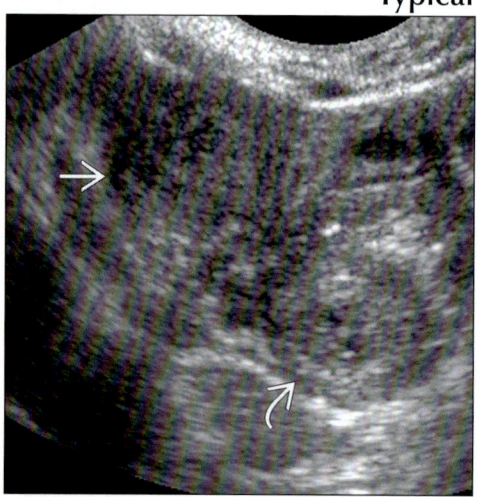

(Left) Transverse transabdominal ultrasound shows an ectopic pregnancy ➔ inferomedial to the left ovary (LT O). Note that the uterus (UT) is empty. *(Right)* Sagittal transabdominal ultrasound shows a gestational sac ➔ posterior to the uterus ➔.

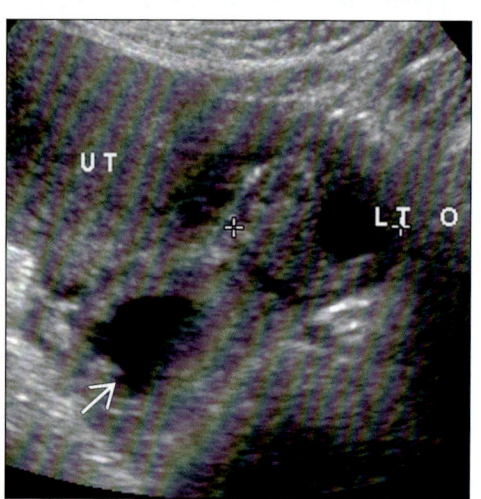
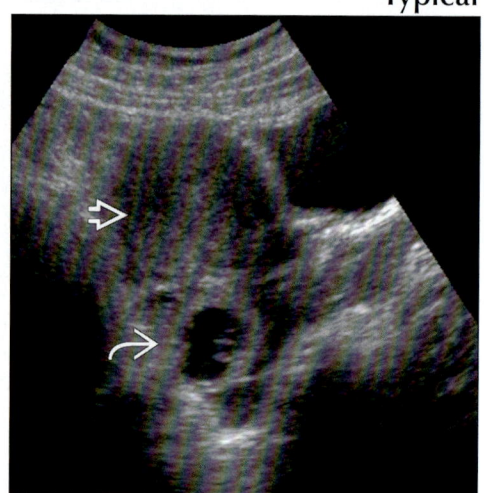

(Left) Axial oblique transvaginal ultrasound shows an ill-defined oblong hypoechoic mass ➔ consistent with hematosalpinx. *(Right)* Transverse transvaginal ultrasound shows a slightly echogenic round mass (calipers). At real-time imaging this was separate from the right ovary and consistent with an ectopic pregnancy.

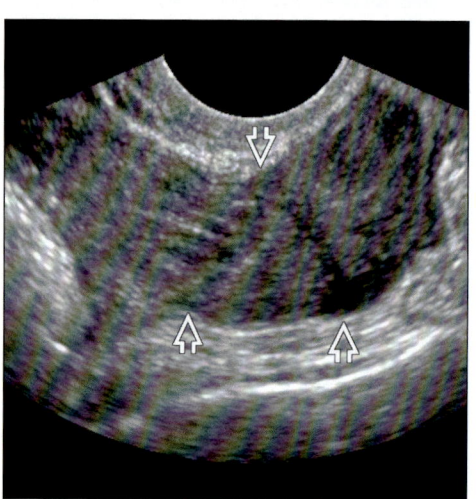
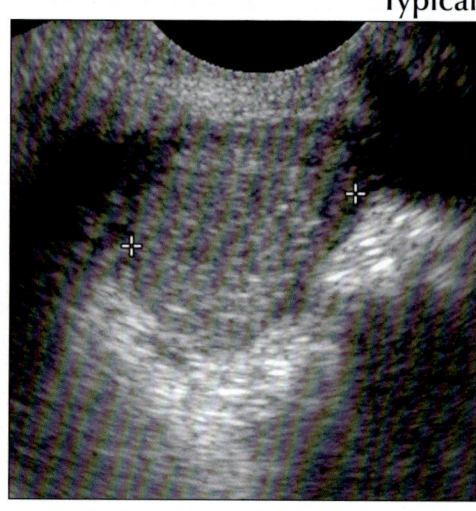

ECTOPIC PREGNANCY, TUBAL

Typical

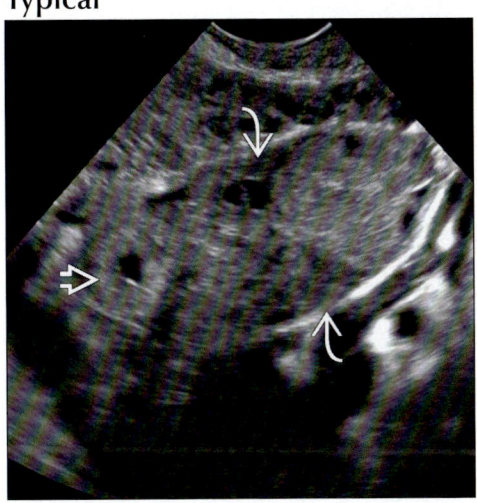
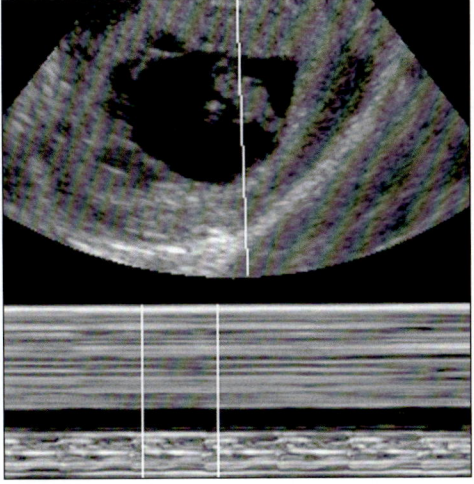

(Left) Sagittal oblique transvaginal ultrasound shows an echogenic ring-like mass ➡ inferomedial to the left ovary ➡. *(Right)* Axial oblique M-mode shows cardiac activity in an ectopic pregnancy.

Typical

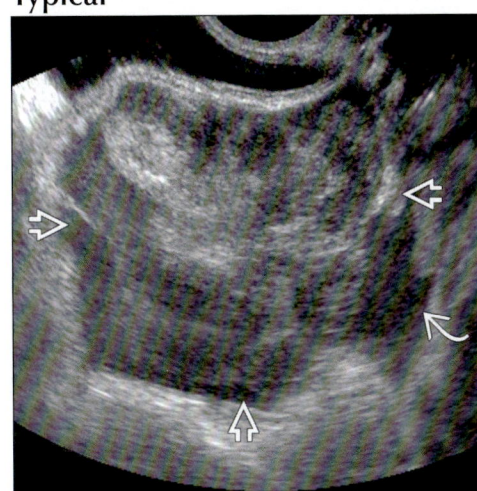
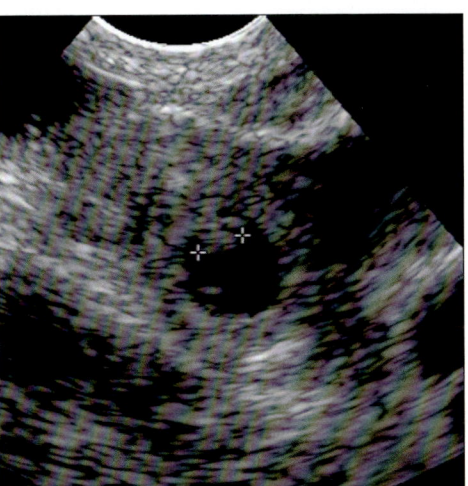

(Left) Sagittal oblique transvaginal ultrasound shows a heterogeneous mass in the right adnexa consistent with blood clot ➡. Note that there is adjacent free fluid ➡ in this patient with a ruptured ectopic pregnancy. *(Right)* Transverse transvaginal ultrasound shows a ring-like mass with an embryo (calipers). Other images documented a yolk sac and cardiac activity in a live ectopic pregnancy.

Typical

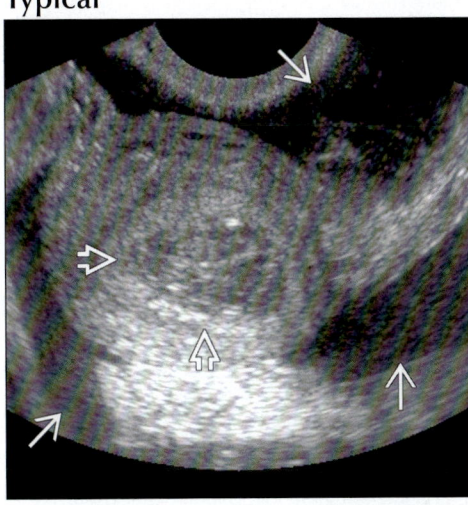
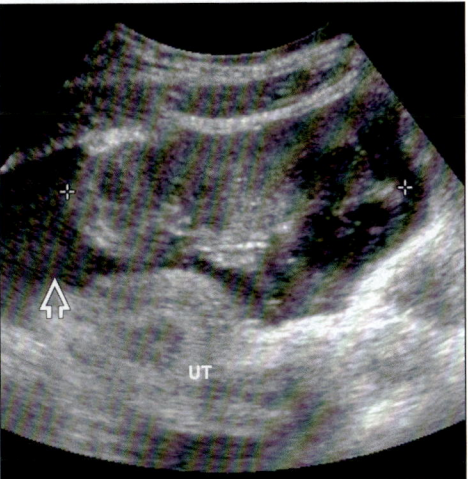

(Left) Transverse transvaginal ultrasound shows a uterus with debris in the endometrial cavity ➡ but no gestational sac. A moderate amount of surrounding free fluid ➡ suggests rupture of ectopic or cyst. *(Right)* Transverse transabdominal ultrasound shows a blood clot (calipers) and free fluid ➡ with no gestational sac in the uterus (UT) in a patient with ruptured ectopic pregnancy.

ECTOPIC PREGNANCY, INTERSTITIAL

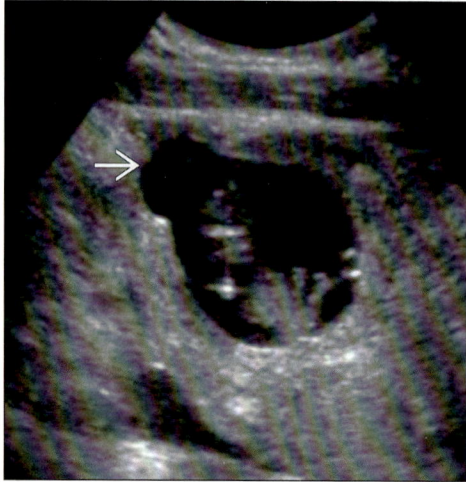

Sagittal oblique transabdominal ultrasound shows 11 week fetus with gestational sac bulging ➡ beyond the confines of the uterus.

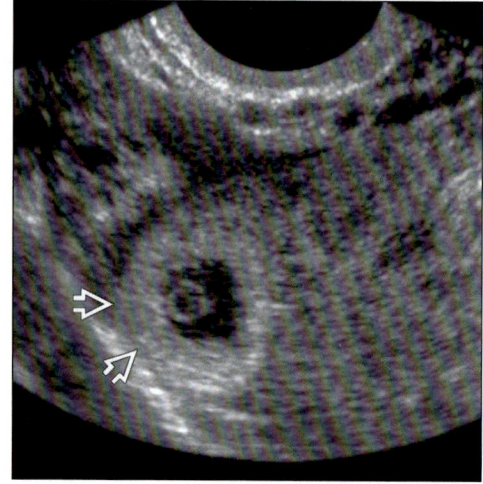

Coronal oblique transvaginal ultrasound shows gestational sac with yolk sac without surrounding myometrium ➡ peripherally.

TERMINOLOGY

Abbreviations and Synonyms
- Cornual ectopic, interstitial ectopic

Definitions
- Interstitial ectopics are in interstitial portion of tube as it enters uterus
- Isthmic ectopics are in portion of tube adjacent to myometrium
- Cornual ectopics are in cornu of bicornuate uterus

IMAGING FINDINGS

General Features
- Best diagnostic clue: Pregnancy located high in uterus without surrounding myometrium
- Location: Interstitial portion of tube as it enters uterus
- Size
  ○ Typically presents at 8-10 weeks of gestation
  ○ May present earlier with rupture
- Morphology
  ○ Gestational sac with less than 5 mm of surrounding myometrium
  ○ May rupture into pelvis with surrounding hematoma

Ultrasonographic Findings
- Gestational sac high in uterus
  ○ May have yolk sac, embryonic pole, cardiac activity
  ○ Very vascular due to blood supply from ovarian and uterine arteries
- Eccentric location of gestational sac (40% sensitivity, 62% specificity)
- Sac does not communicate with endometrial cavity
- Less than 5 mm of myometrium around sac (40% sensitivity, 74% specificity)
- May see bulge in uterine contour
- Lack of double decidual sac sign
- Interstitial line sign
  ○ Echogenic line extends up to middle of gestational sac or mass
  ○ 80% sensitivity, 99% specificity

CT Findings
- Exophytic mass off fundal portion of uterus
- Blood products will be of high attenuation

DDx: Interstitial Ectopic Pregnancy Mimics

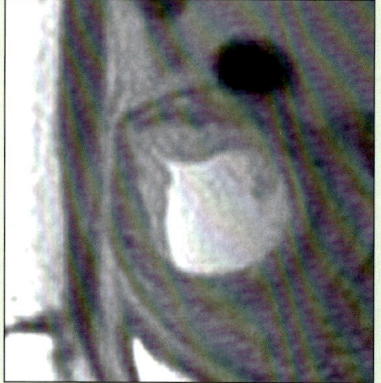

Scar Pregnancy

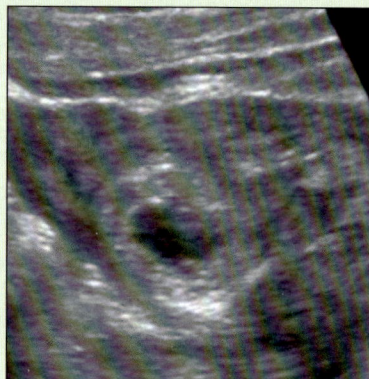

Tubal Ectopic Pregnancy

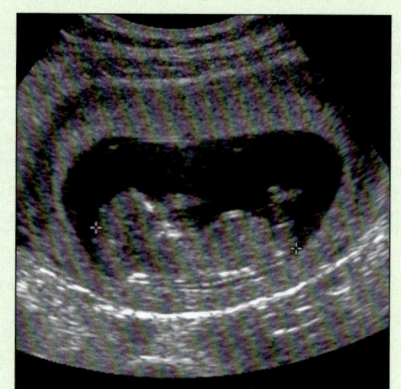

Normal Intrauterine Pregnancy

ECTOPIC PREGNANCY, INTERSTITIAL

Key Facts

Terminology
- Interstitial ectopics are in interstitial portion of tube as it enters uterus
- Isthmic ectopics are in portion of tube adjacent to myometrium
- Cornual ectopics are in cornu of bicornuate uterus

Imaging Findings
- Best diagnostic clue: Pregnancy located high in uterus without surrounding myometrium
- Typically presents at 8-10 weeks of gestation
- May rupture into pelvis with surrounding hematoma
- Very vascular due to blood supply from ovarian and uterine arteries
- Eccentric location of gestational sac (40% sensitivity, 62% specificity)
- Sac does not communicate with endometrial cavity
- Less than 5 mm of myometrium around sac (40% sensitivity, 74% specificity)
- May see bulge in uterine contour
- Best imaging tool: Ultrasound
- Scan transabdominally and transvaginally to get best view of entire gestational sac

Pathology
- 2-3% of all ectopic pregnancies
- Mortality rate of 2-2.5% much higher than for tubal ectopics

Clinical Issues
- Rupture later than tubal ectopics since myometrium more distensible than tube
- Increased vascularity of interstitial ectopics can lead to hemorrhage and death

MR Findings
- Gestational sac off fundal portion of uterus
- Blood products will be of varying signal intensity depending on age

Imaging Recommendations
- Best imaging tool: Ultrasound
- Protocol advice
  - Scan transabdominally and transvaginally to get best view of entire gestational sac
  - Carefully assess endometrial cavity to ensure that gestational sac entirely located within endometrium
  - Document yolk sac, embryonic pole, crown rump length, cardiac activity
  - Interstitial line sign seen when echogenic line of endometrium extends to midportion of interstitial ectopic
  - Follow-up sonography helpful in cases when unclear whether there is sufficient myometrium around sac located high in uterus and patient is stable
  - Always check for free fluid on pregnancy sonograms
    - If free fluid with debris present, suggests either ruptured cyst or ruptured ectopic pregnancy
    - Check up by kidneys to see if large hemoperitoneum present

DIFFERENTIAL DIAGNOSIS

Normal Intrauterine Pregnancy
- Will have at least 5 mm of surrounding myometrium
- May have double decidual sac sign
- If unsure of diagnosis and patient stable, bring patient back in few days

Pregnancy in Atrophic Horn of Uterus with Duplication Anomaly
- Two separate uterine horns will be visualized
- Measure endometrium around sac
- Cesarean section may be needed for delivery

Tubal Ectopic Pregnancy
- Will be separate from uterus
- Typical appearance of tubal ectopic
  - Ring-like mass adjacent to ovary
  - May have yolk sac or embryonic pole

PATHOLOGY

General Features
- Etiology: Implantation within tubal segment that penetrates uterine wall
- Epidemiology
  - 1:2,500-5,000 live births
  - 2-3% of all ectopic pregnancies
  - Predisposing factors
    - Ipsilateral salpingectomy
    - Previous ectopic pregnancy
    - In vitro fertilization
  - Mortality rate of 2-2.5% much higher than for tubal ectopics

Gross Pathologic & Surgical Features
- Bulge in external contour of uterus
- Uterine rupture common
- Hemoperitoneum

Microscopic Features
- Dilatation and curettage will not show chorionic villi
- Surgical specimen will show chorionic villi

CLINICAL ISSUES

Presentation
- Most common signs/symptoms
  - Rupture
    - Rupture later than tubal ectopics since myometrium more distensible than tube
    - Increased vascularity of interstitial ectopics can lead to hemorrhage and death
- Other signs/symptoms

ECTOPIC PREGNANCY, INTERSTITIAL

- Can rupture and lead to abdominal pregnancy
  - In rare instances there can be surviving fetus
- Can occur as heterotopic pregnancy
  - Local injection or local resection of interstitial pregnancy can be utilized to treat ectopic pregnancy without loss of coexistent intrauterine pregnancy

Demographics
- Age: Reproductive age
- Gender: Female

Natural History & Prognosis
- Tend to present later than tubal ectopic pregnancies since myometrium more expansile than fallopian tube
- Present with pain lateralized to side of ectopic
- When rupture occurs can present with hypotension from hemorrhage
- Only rare cases of live-born pregnancies have been reported, typically after uterine rupture has occurred
- May result in maternal death

Treatment
- Surgery
  - Laparoscopic removal of ectopic or cornual resection
  - Laparotomy with hysterectomy or cornual resection (no longer preferred treatment in most cases)
- Methotrexate intramuscular
- Sonographic guidance of direct injection of ectopic pregnancy
  - Local methotrexate injection
  - Local potassium chloride injection
  - May use either transabdominal or transvaginal guidance, depending on location of ectopic
  - Excellent method for treatment of heterotopic pregnancy, since co-existent intrauterine pregnancy can survive after direct injection of interstitial pregnancy
- Expectant management

DIAGNOSTIC CHECKLIST

Consider
- Normal intrauterine pregnancy can be located high in uterus and mimic an interstitial ectopic
- If attention not paid to myometrium surrounding an interstitial pregnancy, diagnosis can be missed
  - Delay in diagnosis of interstitial ectopic pregnancy can lead to life-threatening hemorrhage

Image Interpretation Pearls
- Always check myometrium around any presumed intrauterine pregnancy
- Look for free fluid in all pregnancies, if present, check up by kidneys for hemoperitoneum

SELECTED REFERENCES

1. Brewer H et al: Asymptomatic uterine rupture of a cornual pregnancy in the third trimester: a case report. J Reprod Med. 50(9):715-8, 2005
2. Dilbaz S et al: Treating cornual pregnancy with a single methotrexate injection: a report of 3 cases. J Reprod Med. 50(2):141-4, 2005
3. Dialani V et al: Ectopic pregnancy: a review. Ultrasound Q. 20(3):105-17, 2004
4. Doubilet PM et al: Sonographically guided minimally invasive treatment of unusual ectopic pregnancies. J Ultrasound Med. 23(3):359-70, 2004
5. Jermy K et al: The conservative management of interstitial pregnancy. BJOG. 111(11):1283-8, 2004
6. Tulandi T et al: Interstitial pregnancy: results generated from the Society of Reproductive Surgeons Registry. Obstet Gynecol. 103(1):47-50, 2004
7. Chan LY et al: Pitfalls in diagnosis of interstitial pregnancy. Acta Obstet Gynecol Scand. 82(9):867-70, 2003
8. Chan LY et al: Successful treatment of ruptured interstitial pregnancy with laparoscopic surgery. A report of 2 cases. J Reprod Med. 48(7):569-71, 2003
9. Bouyer J et al: Sites of ectopic pregnancy: a 10 year population-based study of 1800 cases. Hum Reprod. 17(12):3224-30, 2002
10. Ghazeeri GS et al: Live birth after treatment of a heterotopic cornual pregnancy with fetal intrathoracic KCl. A case report. J Reprod Med. 47(12):1038-40, 2002
11. Haimov-Kochman R et al: Conservative management of two ectopic pregnancies implanted in previous uterine scars. Ultrasound Obstet Gynecol. 19(6):616-9, 2002
12. Sills ES et al: Uncomplicated pregnancy and normal singleton delivery after surgical excision of heterotopic (cornual) pregnancy following in vitro fertilization/embryo transfer. Arch Gynecol Obstet. 266(3):181-4, 2002
13. Idama TO et al: Survival of cornual (interstitial) pregnancy. Eur J Obstet Gynecol Reprod Biol. 84(1):103-5, 1999
14. Grobman WA et al: Conservative laparoscopic management of a large cornual ectopic pregnancy. Hum Reprod. 13(7):2002-4, 1998
15. Bassil S et al: A magnetic resonance imaging approach for the diagnosis of a triplet cornual pregnancy. Fertil Steril. 64(5):1029-31, 1995
16. Chen GD et al: Diagnosis of interstitial pregnancy with sonography. J Clin Ultrasound. 22(7):439-42, 1994
17. Ackerman TE et al: Interstitial line: sonographic finding in interstitial (cornual) ectopic pregnancy. Radiology. 189(1):83-7, 1993
18. Timor-Tritsch IE et al: Sonographic evolution of cornual pregnancies treated without surgery. Obstet Gynecol. 79(6):1044-9, 1992
19. Fernandez H et al: The place of methotrexate in the management of interstitial pregnancy. Hum Reprod. 6(2):302-6, 1991
20. Jafri SZ et al: Sonographic detection of interstitial pregnancy. J Clin Ultrasound. 15(4):253-7, 1987

ECTOPIC PREGNANCY, INTERSTITIAL

IMAGE GALLERY

Typical

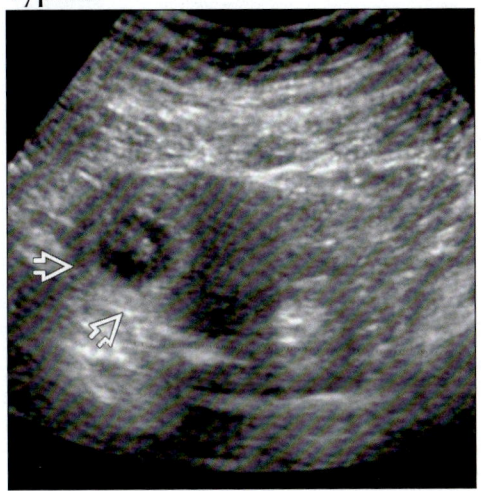
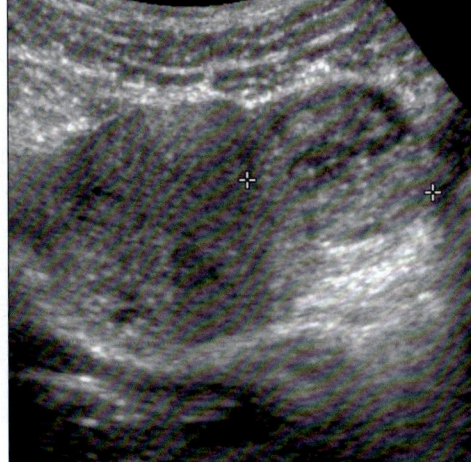

(Left) Coronal oblique transabdominal ultrasound shows gestational sac located high in the uterus without myometrium ➡ laterally. *(Right)* Axial oblique transabdominal ultrasound shows gestational sac (calipers) exophytic from the uterus. It is difficult to tell if this is an interstitial or isthmic ectopic pregnancy.

Typical

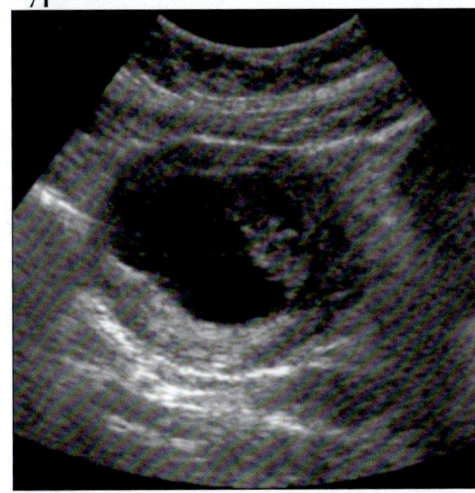
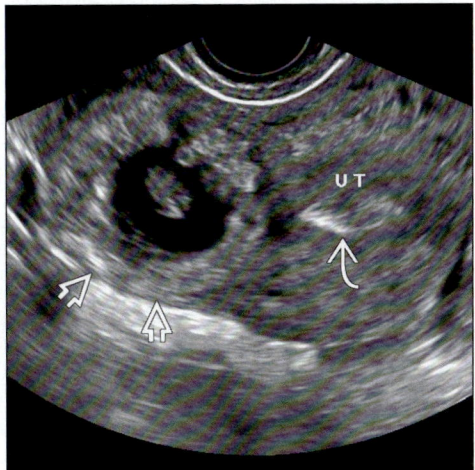

(Left) Axial transabdominal ultrasound shows gestational sac. In this plane, the connection to the uterus is not apparent. Note lack of surrounding myometrium. *(Right)* Coronal oblique transvaginal ultrasound shows ectopic pregnancy in interstitial region. Note lack of surrounding myometrium ➡. Note endometrium ➡ in uterus (UT) separate from gestational sac.

Typical

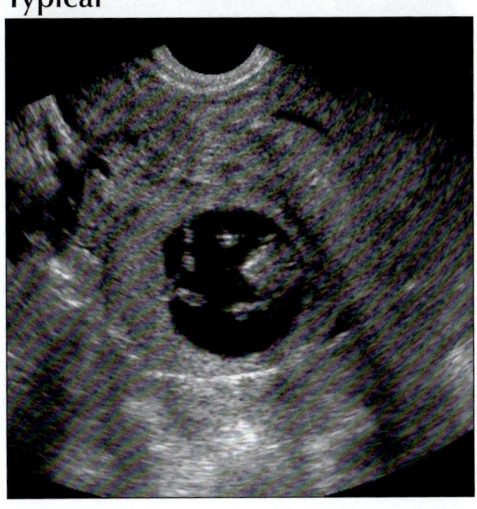
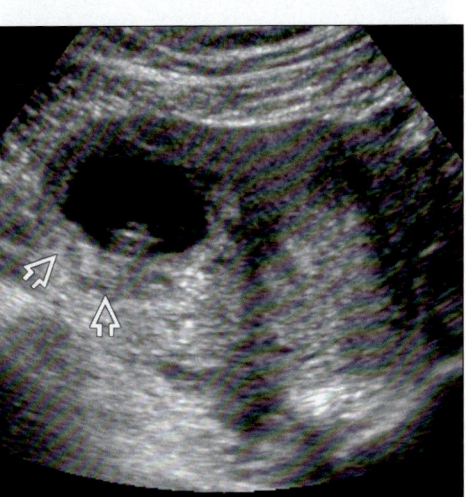

(Left) Sagittal oblique transvaginal ultrasound shows gestational sac protruding from the uterus. Note lack of surrounding myometrium. *(Right)* Axial oblique transabdominal ultrasound shows gestational sac in left interstitial region. Note lack of surrounding myometrium ➡.

ECTOPIC PREGNANCY, INTERSTITIAL

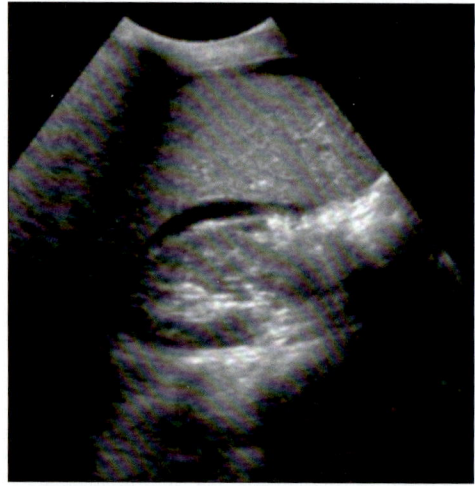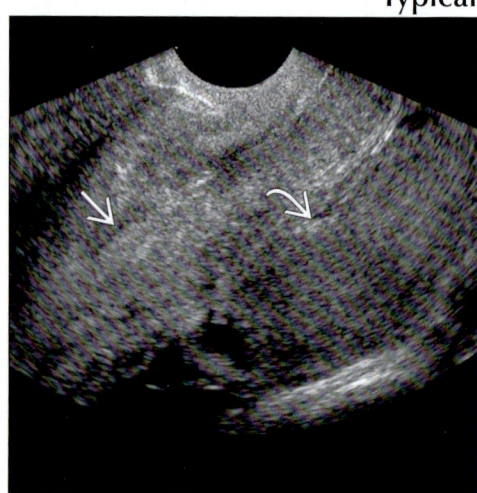

(Left) Sagittal transabdominal ultrasound shows blood by liver and kidney in patient with hemoperitoneum from ruptured interstitial ectopic pregnancy. *(Right)* Sagittal transvaginal ultrasound on same patient as previous image shows an empty endometrial cavity ➡ and blood clot ➡ in the cul-de-sac.

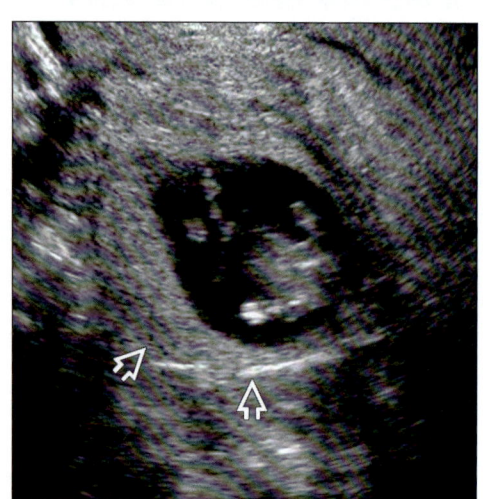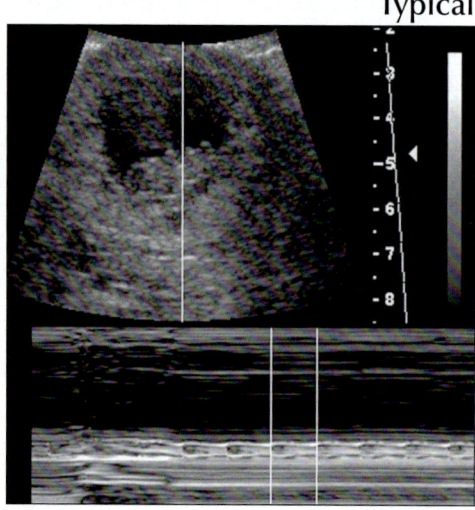

(Left) Sagittal oblique transvaginal ultrasound shows ectopic pregnancy in interstitial region. Note lack of surrounding myometrium ➡. *(Right)* Axial transabdominal ultrasound M-mode in same patient as previous image shows embryonic cardiac activity.

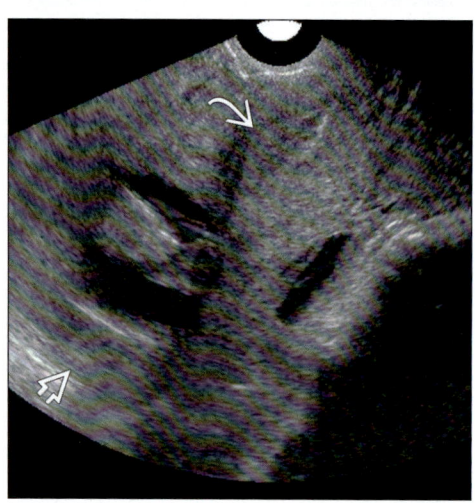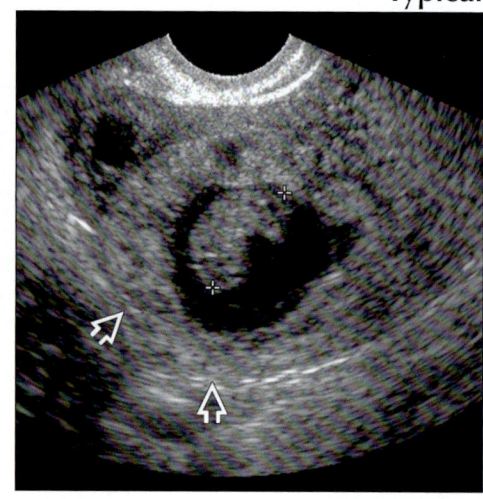

(Left) Sagittal transvaginal ultrasound shows ectopic pregnancy in interstitial region. Note lack of surrounding myometrium ➡. Also note how endometrium ➡ appears separate from gestational sac. *(Right)* Sagittal oblique transvaginal ultrasound shows ectopic pregnancy in interstitial region. Note lack of surrounding myometrium ➡. Calipers indicate embryonic crown rump length.

ECTOPIC PREGNANCY, INTERSTITIAL

Typical

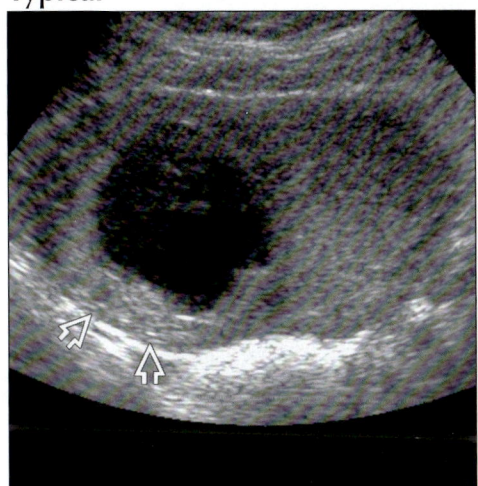
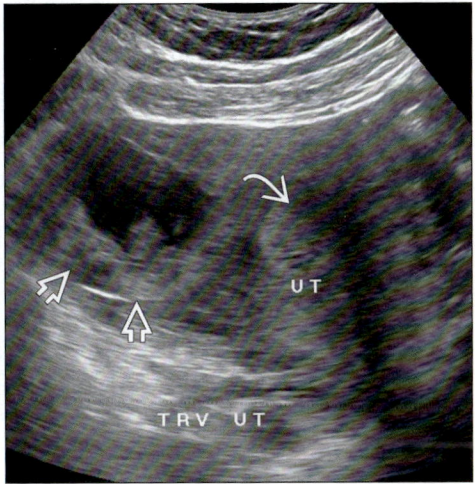

(Left) Transverse transabdominal ultrasound shows right sided interstitial ectopic pregnancy. Note lack of myometrium posteriorly ➡. *(Right)* Transverse transabdominal ultrasound shows ectopic pregnancy in interstitial region. Note lack of surrounding myometrium ➡. Note endometrium ➡ separate from sac in uterus (UT).

Typical

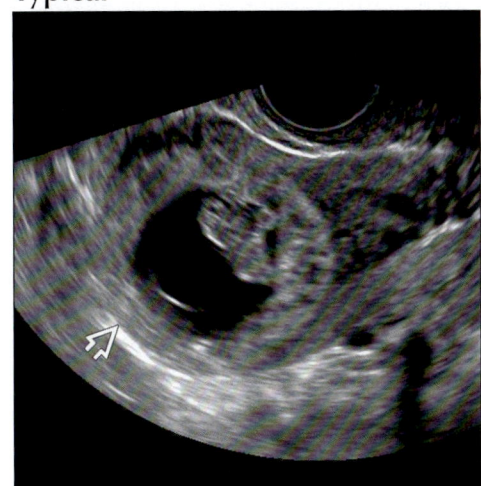
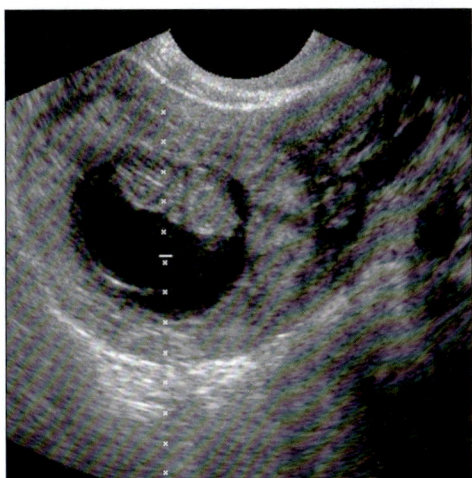

(Left) Sagittal oblique transvaginal ultrasound shows ectopic pregnancy in interstitial region. Note lack of surrounding myometrium ➡. *(Right)* Sagittal oblique transvaginal ultrasound in same patient as previous image shows needle guide for percutaneous injection of potassium chloride to treat interstitial ectopic pregnancy.

Other

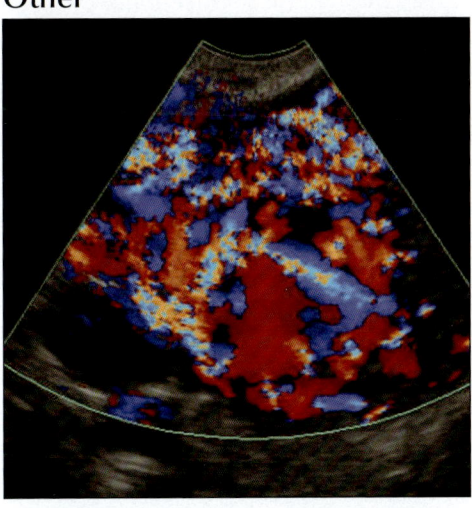
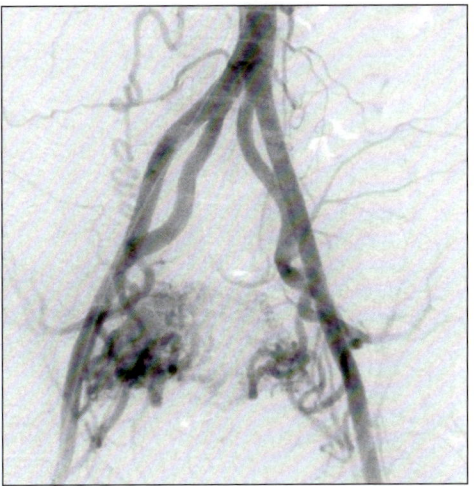

(Left) Sagittal oblique color Doppler ultrasound shows tangle of vessels in patient after dilatation and evacuation of interstitial ectopic pregnancy. *(Right)* Anteroposterior angiogram in same patient as previous image shows tangle of vessels in patient after dilatation and evacuation of interstitial ectopic.

ECTOPIC PREGNANCY, CERVICAL

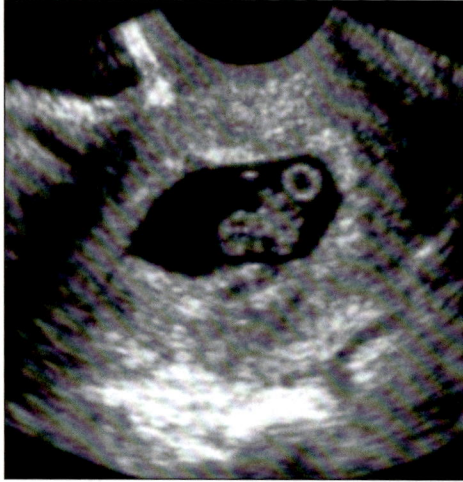

Sagittal transvaginal ultrasound shows gestational sac with embryo and yolk sac in cervix. Real-time scanning (not shown) showed cardiac activity.

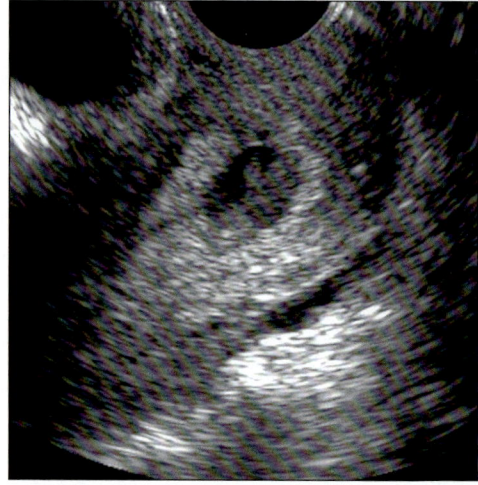

Sagittal transvaginal ultrasound shows gestational sac in cervix. Real-time scanning (not shown) demonstrated cardiac activity.

TERMINOLOGY

Abbreviations and Synonyms
- Cervical ectopic

Definitions
- Pregnancy located in the cervix

IMAGING FINDINGS

General Features
- Best diagnostic clue: Embryo with cardiac activity seen in sac in the cervix
- Location: Cervix
- Size: 5-8 weeks gestational age
- Morphology: Gestational sac with yolk sac and embryonic pole in the cervix

Ultrasonographic Findings
- Gestational sac in the cervix, typically eccentrically located
- Endocervical canal distended by gestational sac
  ○ Gestational sac round or oval
  ○ Yolk sac may be present
  ○ Embryonic pole may be present
  ○ Doppler demonstrates flow to gestational sac
  ○ Cardiac activity virtually pathognomonic
    ▪ Cardiac activity indicates live cervical pregnancy
    ▪ Rare care report of abortion in progress with cardiac activity in cervix
  ○ When gestational sac is large it may "balloon" out of cervix into lower uterine segment giving "hourglass" appearance
- Lack of gestational sac in endometrial cavity (unless heterotopic intrauterine and cervical pregnancies)
- Endometrial cavity may have pseudosac
- Normal appearance of the adnexa

CT Findings
- Gestational sac in cervix
- Endometrial cavity may appear normal or have blood/debris

MR Findings
- Gestational sac in cervix
- Endometrial cavity may appear normal or have blood/debris

DDx: Cervical Pregnancy Mimics

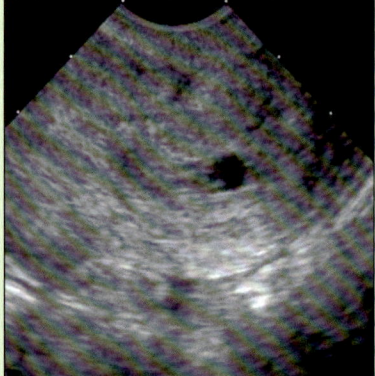
Abortion in Progress

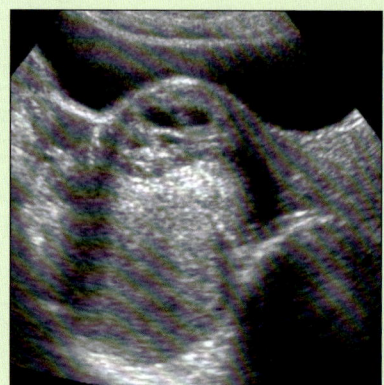
C-Section Scar Pregnancy

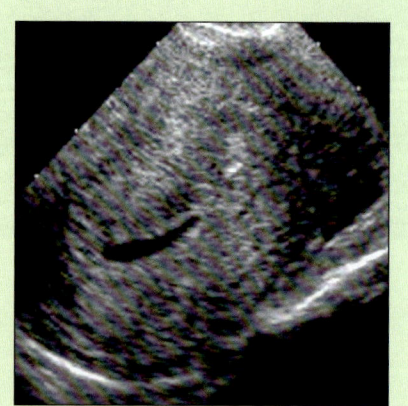
Intrauterine Pregnancy

ECTOPIC PREGNANCY, CERVICAL

Key Facts

Terminology
- Pregnancy located in the cervix

Imaging Findings
- Best diagnostic clue: Embryo with cardiac activity seen in sac in the cervix
- Size: 5-8 weeks gestational age
- Embryonic pole may be present
- Cardiac activity indicates live cervical pregnancy
- Best imaging tool: Transvaginal ultrasound

Pathology
- Epidemiology: Less than 1% of all ectopic pregnancies
- Close attachment of placenta to the cervix

Clinical Issues
- Bleeding in early pregnancy: With or without pain
- Soft cervix that is disproportionately enlarged compared with the uterus
- Profuse hemorrhage on manipulation of the cervix
- Other signs/symptoms: Clinical diagnosis is suspected when dilation and curettage for presumed incomplete abortion results in unexpected hemorrhage
- If dilatation and curettage is performed, due to high vascularity of the cervix, this can lead to life-threatening hemorrhage
- Transvaginal guided injection is current procedure of choice

Imaging Recommendations
- Best imaging tool: Transvaginal ultrasound
- Protocol advice
  - Scan entire uterus to ensure that there is no pregnancy in endometrial cavity
  - Scan cervix to ensure that gestational sac is in cervix
  - Use M-mode to demonstrate cardiac activity in embryo
  - If it is too early to demonstrate cardiac activity (less than 6 weeks gestational age), color Doppler can show flow to the sac in the cervix

DIFFERENTIAL DIAGNOSIS

Pregnancy in a Cesarian Section Scar
- Endocervical canal not dilated
- Lack of cervical tissue/myometrium between gestational sac and serosa

Abortion in Progress
- In the endocervical canal
- Oblong appearance
- Crenated shape
- Typically without a heart beat
- Change in position over time
- Endometrial cavity may show blood and products of conception
- "Sliding sign" present
  - Gentle pressure on the cervix with vaginal probe leads to motion of gestational sac

Low Position of Intrauterine Pregnancy
- Located above the cervix
- Will not have "hourglass" appearance
- Has poor prognosis, but may result in live birth
- Needs follow-up to assess for viability

PATHOLOGY

General Features
- Etiology
  - Risk factors include
    - Prior dilation and curettage
    - Intrauterine device (IUD) use (decreases overall pregnancy rate, but if patient gets pregnant, location is more likely to be ectopic compared to general population)
    - Pelvic inflammatory disease
    - In vitro fertilization
- Epidemiology: Less than 1% of all ectopic pregnancies

Gross Pathologic & Surgical Features
- Close attachment of placenta to the cervix
- Cervical glands present opposite the implantation site
- Placental location below uterine vessel insertion or below anterior and posterior reflections of the visceral peritoneum of the uterus

Microscopic Features
- Dilatation and curettage will show chorionic villi

CLINICAL ISSUES

Presentation
- Most common signs/symptoms
  - Bleeding in early pregnancy: With or without pain
  - Physical examination
    - Soft cervix that is disproportionately enlarged compared with the uterus
    - Partially open external os
    - Profuse hemorrhage on manipulation of the cervix
    - Blue/purple cervical lesion
- Other signs/symptoms: Clinical diagnosis is suspected when dilation and curettage for presumed incomplete abortion results in unexpected hemorrhage

Demographics
- Age: Reproductive age

ECTOPIC PREGNANCY, CERVICAL

- Gender: Female

Natural History & Prognosis
- May spontaneous resolve
- Due to high risk of life-threatening hemorrhage is typically treated either medically or surgically (or both)
- If dilatation and curettage is performed, due to high vascularity of the cervix, this can lead to life-threatening hemorrhage
  - Interventional radiology embolization of uterine arteries can be life saving in cases of hemorrhage
- Future fertility has been documented in patients treated with uterine artery embolization for cervical ectopic

Treatment
- Stable patient
  - Medical therapy
    - Systemic methotrexate
  - Transvaginal guided injection is current procedure of choice
    - Intra-amniotic potassium chloride
    - Intra-amniotic methotrexate
    - Intracervical vasopressin
  - Close follow-up of patients treated medically is needed due to potential for life-threatening hemorrhage
    - Serial sonograms to assess for size of gestational sac and any vascularity
    - Serial hCG to document falling values
  - Some centers perform dilatation and curettage 1 week after medical therapy
- Unstable patient
  - Selective embolotherapy
  - Cervical artery ligation
  - Intracervical balloon tamponade
  - Hysterectomy previously was commonly performed, but now reserved for uncontrollable bleeding or patients who do not desire future fertility

DIAGNOSTIC CHECKLIST

Consider
- Abortion in progress when no cardiac activity and oblong appearance of centrally located sac
- Cervical ectopic when cardiac activity present in cervical sac

Image Interpretation Pearls
- Consider cervical ectopic when gestational sac is located in cervix
- Unchanging appearance over time and cardiac activity in the embryo are pathognomonic

SELECTED REFERENCES
1. Kirk E et al: The conservative management of cervical ectopic pregnancies. Ultrasound Obstet Gynecol. 27(4):430-7, 2006
2. Einarsson JI et al: Delayed spontaneous expulsion of a cervical ectopic pregnancy: a case report. J Minim Invasive Gynecol. 12(2):165-7, 2005
3. Mesogitis S et al: Management of early viable cervical pregnancy. BJOG. 112(4):409-411,2005
4. Trambert JJ et al: Uterine artery embolization in the management of vaginal bleeding from cervical pregnancy: a case series. J Reprod Med. 50(11):844-50, 2005
5. Dialani V et al: Ectopic pregnancy: a review. Ultrasound Q. 20(3):105-17, 2004
6. Doubilet PM et al: Sonographically guided minimally invasive treatment of unusual ectopic pregnancies. J Ultrasound Med. 23(3):359-70, 2004
7. Hwang JL et al: Successful treatment of a cervical pregnancy by intracervical vasopressin. BJOG. 111(4):387-8, 2004
8. Kumar S et al: Heterotopic cervical and intrauterine pregnancy in a spontaneous cycle. Eur J Obstet Gynecol Reprod Biol. 112(2):217-20, 2004
9. Celik C et al: Methotrexate for cervical pregnancy. A case report. J Reprod Med. 48(2):130-2, 2003
10. Loureiro T et al: Non-viable cervico-isthmic pregnancy: the importance of an accurate sonographic diagnosis to preserve fertility. Fetal Diagn Ther. 18(5):289-91, 2003
11. Sherer DM et al: Viable cervical pregnancy managed with systemic Methotrexate, uterine artery embolization, and local tamponade with inflated Foley catheter balloon. Am J Perinatol. 20(5):263-7, 2003
12. Suzumori N et al: Conservative treatment by angiographic artery embolization of an 11-week cervical pregnancy after a period of heavy bleeding. Fertil Steril. 80(3):617-9, 2003
13. Bouyer J et al: Sites of ectopic pregnancy: a 10 year population-based study of 1800 cases. Hum Reprod. 17(12):3224-30, 2002
14. Chew S et al: Medical management of cervical pregnancy--a report of two cases. Singapore Med J. 42(11):537-9, 2001
15. Ushakov FB et al: Cervical pregnancy: past and future. Obstet Gynecol Surv. 52(1):45-59,1997
16. Jurkovic D et al: Diagnosis and treatment of early cervical pregnancy: a review and a report of two cases treated conservatively. Ultrasound Obstet Gynecol. 8(6):373-80, 1996
17. Monteagudo A et al: Successful transvaginal ultrasound-guided puncture and injection of a cervical pregnancy in a patient with simultaneous intrauterine pregnancy and a history of a previous cervical pregnancy. Ultrasound Obstet Gynecol. 8(6):381-6, 1996
18. Pattinson HA et al: Cervical pregnancy following in vitro fertilization: evacuation after uterine artery embolization with subsequent successful intrauterine pregnancy. Aust N Z J Obstet Gynaecol. 34(4): 492-3, 1994
19. Meyerovitz MF et al: Preoperative uterine artery embolization in cervical pregnancy. J Vasc Interv Radiol. 2(1):95-7, 1991
20. Parente JT et al: Cervical pregnancy analysis: a review and report of five cases. Obstet Gynecol. 62(1):79-82, 1983

ECTOPIC PREGNANCY, CERVICAL

IMAGE GALLERY

Typical

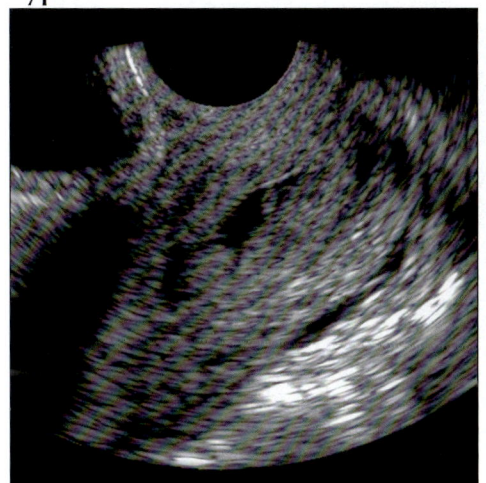
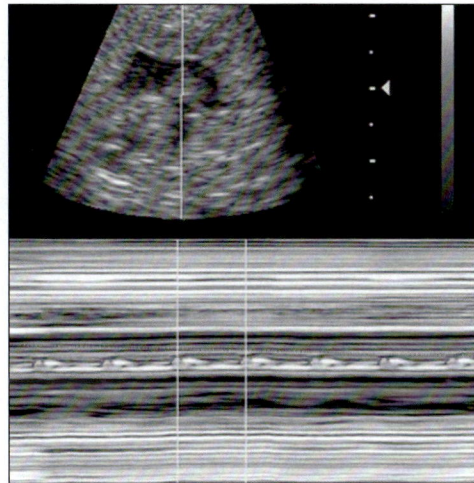

(Left) Sagittal transvaginal ultrasound shows gestational sac in cervix. *(Right)* Sagittal oblique transvaginal ultrasound in same patient as left image shows M-mode documenting cardiac activity.

Typical

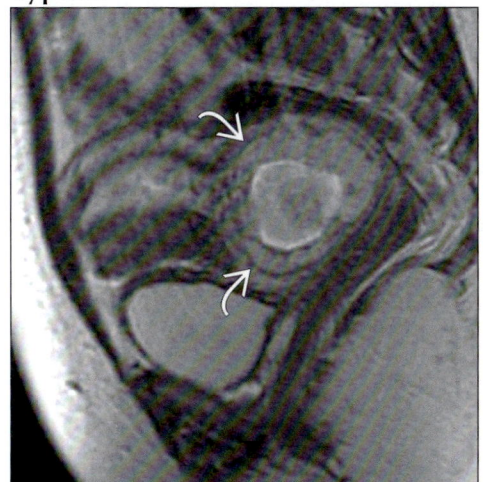
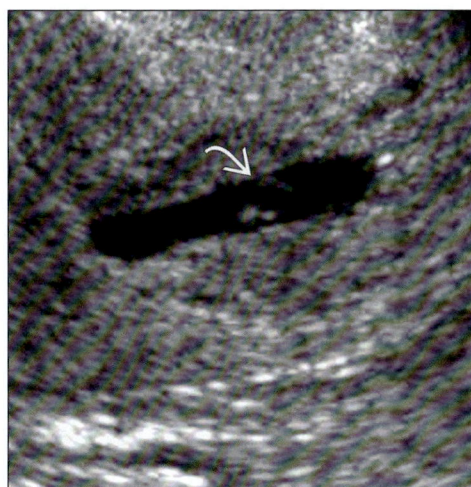

(Left) Sagittal T2WI MR shows gestational sac ➤ expanding the endocervical canal with empty uterus. *(Right)* Sagittal transvaginal ultrasound shows oblong gestational sac with yolk sac ➤ in cervix. M-mode (not shown) documented cardiac activity.

Typical

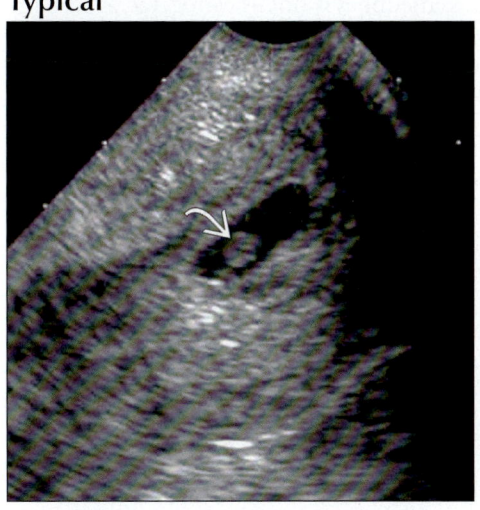
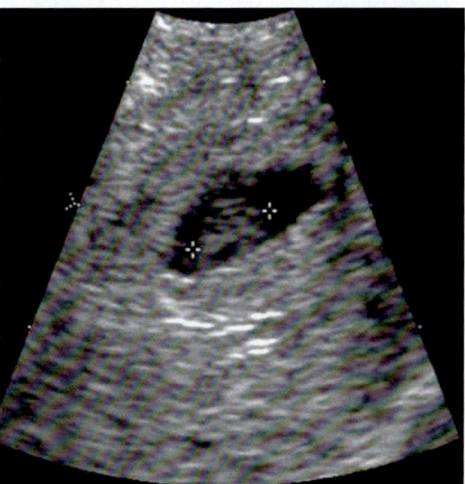

(Left) Sagittal transvaginal ultrasound shows gestational sac with yolk sac ➤ in cervix. *(Right)* Sagittal oblique transvaginal ultrasound in same case as on left shows embryonic pole (calipers) in the gestational sac.

ECTOPIC PREGNANCY, OVARIAN

Transverse transabdominal ultrasound of the left adnexa shows an ectopic pregnancy (calipers) outside of uterus.

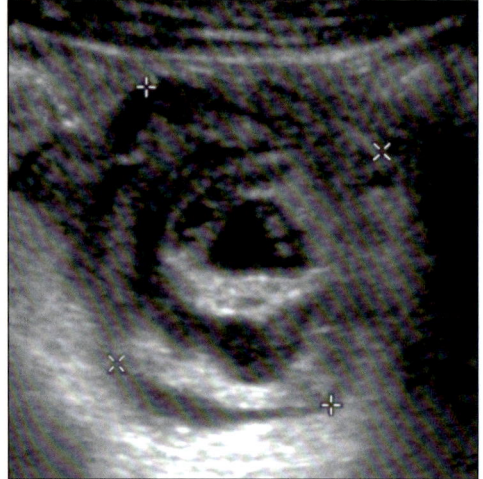

Transverse transabdominal ultrasound shows ectopic pregnancy surrounded by blood clot (calipers).

TERMINOLOGY

Definitions
- Ectopic pregnancy arising from ovary

IMAGING FINDINGS

General Features
- Best diagnostic clue: Gestational sac with live embryo inseparable from ovarian tissue
- Location: Ovary
- Size: Typically at least 5 weeks gestational age

Ultrasonographic Findings
- Appearance overlaps with that of tubal ectopic pregnancy and may be indistinguishable if tubal pregnancy near ovary
  - Echogenic ring
    - Echogenicity of ring greater than that of adjacent ovary
    - Ring with yolk sac with or without embryonic pole
    - Live embryo inseparable from ovarian tissue is diagnostic
- Uterine cavity either empty or with heterogeneous debris
- Free fluid with debris (blood) in cul-de-sac

Imaging Recommendations
- Best imaging tool: Transvaginal ultrasound
- Protocol advice
  - Transabdominal sonography to assess uterine contents and free fluid
  - Transvaginal sonography to assess ovaries and adnexa
  - M-mode to document cardiac activity

DIFFERENTIAL DIAGNOSIS

Hemorrhagic Corpus Luteum Cyst
- Ring of corpus luteum cyst not as echogenic as ring of ectopic pregnancy
- Blood clot may have heterogeneous appearance, at times mimicking yolk sac or embryo

DDx: Ovarian Ectopic Pregnancy Mimics

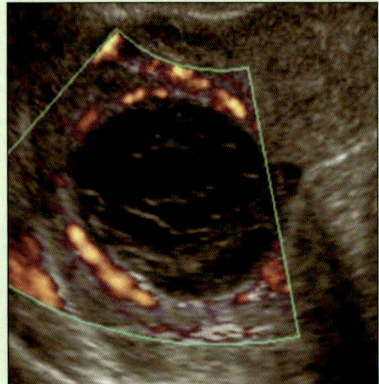
Hemorrhagic Cyst

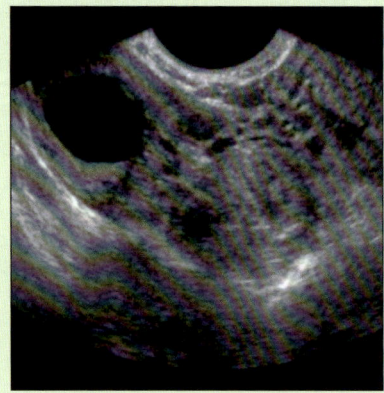
Tubal Ectopic Pregnancy

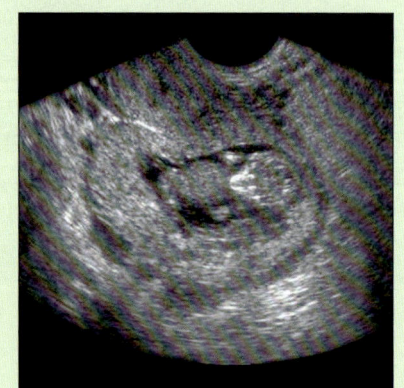
Abdominal Ectopic Pregnancy

ECTOPIC PREGNANCY, OVARIAN

Key Facts

Terminology
- Ectopic pregnancy arising from ovary

Imaging Findings
- Appearance overlaps with that of tubal ectopic pregnancy and may be indistinguishable if tubal pregnancy near ovary
- Echogenicity of ring greater than that of adjacent ovary

Top Differential Diagnoses
- Ring of corpus luteum cyst not as echogenic as ring of ectopic pregnancy

Clinical Issues
- Expectant management if patient stable, low human chorionic gonadotropin (hCG), no embryonic cardiac activity, small gestational sac
- Laparoscopy if clinically unstable or cardiac activity present

Tubal Ectopic Pregnancy
- Ring of ectopic pregnancy will move separately from ovary
- Located between ovary and uterus

Abdominal Pregnancy
- Pregnancy located in abdomen, not attached to ovary or tube
- Blood supply from adjacent organs or mesentery

PATHOLOGY

General Features
- Etiology: 0.5% of ectopic pregnancy
- Epidemiology
  - Same risk factors as tubal ectopic pregnancy
  - Incidence may be increased with in vitro fertilization patients and those using IUDs

CLINICAL ISSUES

Presentation
- Most common signs/symptoms: Pain and bleeding in early pregnancy

Demographics
- Age: Reproductive age
- Gender: Female

Natural History & Prognosis
- May resolve spontaneously

Treatment
- Expectant management if patient stable, low human chorionic gonadotropin (hCG), no embryonic cardiac activity, small gestational sac
- Methotrexate if no contraindications
- Laparoscopy if clinically unstable or cardiac activity present
  - Oophorectomy, ovarian wedge resection, or ovarian cystectomy

SELECTED REFERENCES

1. Comstock, C et al: The Ultrasonographic Appearance of Ovarian Ectopic Pregnancies. Obstet Gynecol. 105:42-45, 2005
2. Melilli GA et al: Combined intrauterine and ovarian pregnancy after in vitro fertilization and embryo transfer: a case report. Clin Exp Obstet Gynecol. 28:100-1, 2001
3. Marcus SF et al: Primary ovarian pregnancy after in vitro fertilization and embryo transfer: report of seven cases. Fertil Steril. 60:167-9, 1993
4. Sandvei R et al: History and findings in ectopic pregnancies in women with and without an IUD. Contracept Deliv Syst. 1:131-8, 1980

IMAGE GALLERY

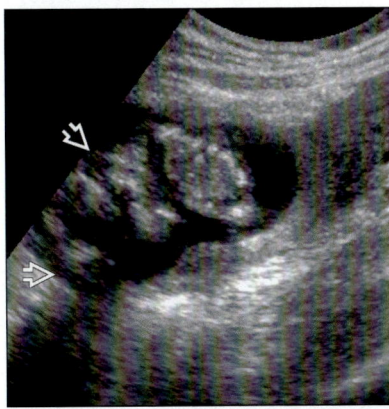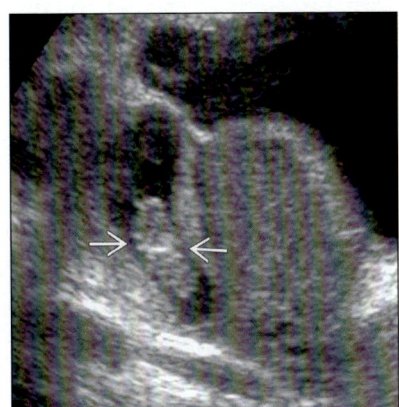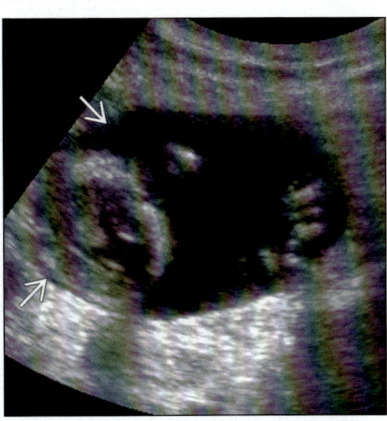

(Left) Sagittal oblique transabdominal ultrasound shows ectopic pregnancy in right ovary, outside of uterus. Note lack of myometrium ➡ around gestational sac. *(Center)* Sagittal transabdominal ultrasound shows ectopic pregnancy ➡ posterior to uterus. *(Right)* Axial oblique transabdominal ultrasound shows heterotopic pregnancy located in ovary. Note lack of surrounding myometrium ➡.

ECTOPIC PREGNANCY, HETEROTOPIC

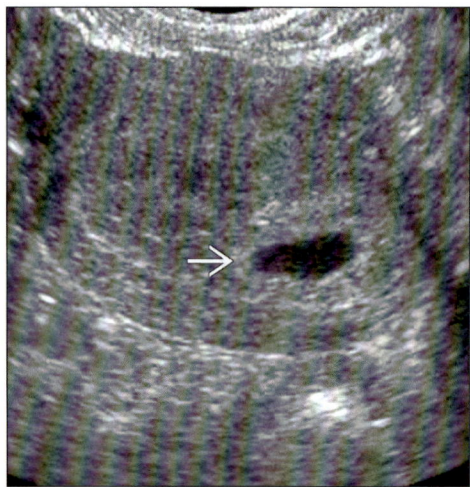

Coronal oblique ultrasound shows an intrauterine pregnancy ➡.

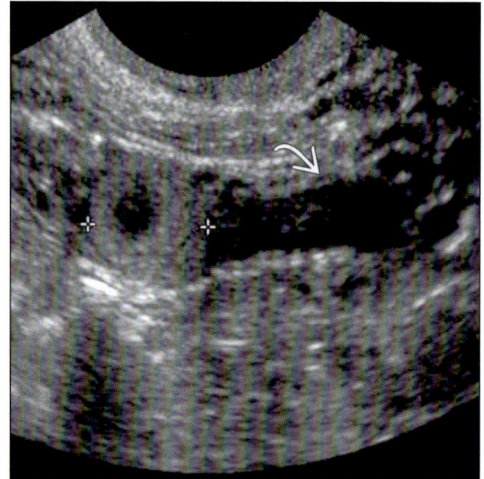

Sagittal transvaginal ultrasound in same patient as previous image shows a ring-like mass (calipers) with some adjacent fluid ➡. This was seen at real-time to be separate from the ovary.

TERMINOLOGY

Abbreviations and Synonyms
- Combined intra- and extrauterine pregnancies
- Intrauterine pregnancy (IUP) and ectopic pregnancy

Definitions
- Concurrent IUP and ectopic pregnancies

IMAGING FINDINGS

General Features
- Best diagnostic clue: Combination of live pregnancy inside uterus and outside uterus
- Location
  - Intrauterine and extrauterine
  - Extrauterine pregnancy can be in any ectopic location
  - Tubal pregnancy will have an appearance similar to tubal ectopic pregnancy
    - May have a ring-like mass separate from the ovary
    - May have a yolk sac
    - May have an embryonic pole with or without cardiac activity
  - Abdominal pregnancy will be out of uterus separate from ovary
    - May appear to be in a duplicate uterine horn
    - Careful search for surrounding myometrium will be the clue to the diagnosis
  - Ovarian pregnancy is rare
    - The ectopic pregnancy arises from ovary
    - It will appear similar to an abdominal ectopic pregnancy but will not move separately from ovary
  - Cesarean section scar will show a pregnancy in the lower uterine segment anteriorly
    - To distinguish this from a twin pregnancy low in uterus, note lack of myometrium anteriorly near bladder
  - Cervical pregnancy will be located in cervix with blood flow to gestational sac
  - Isthmic pregnancy will be located high in uterus without a complete rim of surrounding myometrium
- Size: Depends on gestational age and if hematosalpinx is present

DDx: Heterotopic Pregnancy Mimics

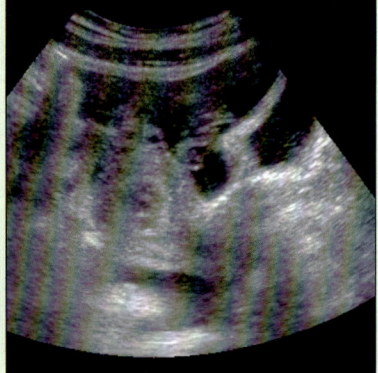

Ruptured Ectopic Pregnancy

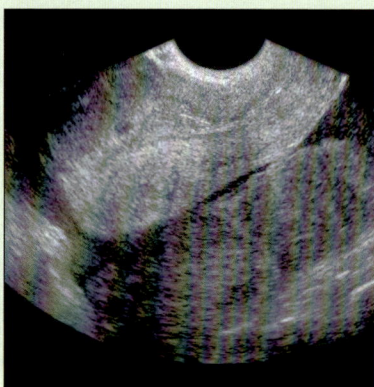

Ruptured Hemorrhagic Cyst and IUP

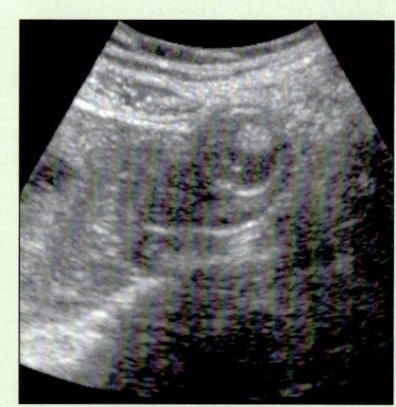

Dermoid in Pregnant Patient

ECTOPIC PREGNANCY, HETEROTOPIC

Key Facts

Imaging Findings
- Best diagnostic clue: Combination of live pregnancy inside uterus and outside uterus
- Extrauterine pregnancy can be in any ectopic location
- Classic appearance of intrauterine pregnancy with a pregnancy of similar age in an ectopic location
- Adnexal mass with yolk sac, embryonic pole, embryonic/fetal cardiac activity are definitive signs of ectopic pregnancy
- Can also occur in isthmic, cervical, abdominal and ovarian locations
- If pregnancy is advanced, ectopic pregnancy may mimic twin pregnancy in duplicated uterus
- Evaluate adnexa in all early pregnancies, especially in patients who have undergone in vitro fertilization (IVF)

Clinical Issues
- If not treated, heterotopic pregnancies can rupture, leading to life-threatening hemorrhage
- Heterotopic pregnancies can be operated upon without loss of the intrauterine pregnancy

Diagnostic Checklist
- Transabdominal and transvaginal sonography may both be needed to adequately assess for combined intra- and extrauterine pregnancies
- MR is helpful in assessing vascularity of the heterotopic pregnancy and planning surgical management

---

- Morphology
  - Adnexal mass separate from ovary
    - Ectopic mass with yolk sac, embryonic pole, embryonic cardiac activity are definitive signs

Ultrasonographic Findings
- Classic appearance of intrauterine pregnancy with a pregnancy of similar age in an ectopic location
  - Adnexal mass with yolk sac, embryonic pole, embryonic/fetal cardiac activity are definitive signs of ectopic pregnancy
  - Can also occur in isthmic, cervical, abdominal and ovarian locations
  - If pregnancy is advanced, ectopic pregnancy may mimic twin pregnancy in duplicated uterus
    - Ectopic pregnancy will not have normal myometrium surrounding the gestational sac

CT Findings
- CT should not be performed since most patients are known to be pregnant
  - If performed (i.e., rule out appendicitis), then a combined intrauterine pregnancy and ectopic mass will be visualized
- Free fluid with high Hounsfield units suggests blood

MR Findings
- Combined intrauterine pregnancy and ectopic mass
- Fluid with heterogeneous high signal on T1WI and heterogeneous intermediate signal on T2WI due to hemoperitoneum
- Helpful in determining exact location of heterotopic pregnancy
- Helpful in demonstrating vascular supply for surgical planning

Imaging Recommendations
- Best imaging tool
  - Ultrasound
  - MR may be needed for surgical planning in the second and third trimesters
- Protocol advice
  - Evaluate adnexa in all early pregnancies, especially in patients who have undergone in vitro fertilization (IVF)
  - Presence of an intrauterine gestational sac should not negate need for careful evaluation of adnexa and follow-up sonography in symptomatic patients
  - Hyper-stimulated ovaries make visualization of an ectopic pregnancy difficult
  - Transabdominal scanning may demonstrate a heterotopic that cannot be visualized transvaginally

DIFFERENTIAL DIAGNOSIS

Intrauterine Pregnancy with Hemorrhagic Corpus Luteum Cyst
- Hemorrhagic corpus luteum cyst can masquerade as an ectopic pregnancy
- Look for ovary separate from a tubal pregnancy
- Intrauterine pregnancy with hemoperitoneum
- Free fluid in the cul-de-sac can be due to ruptured cyst or ruptured ectopic pregnancy

Ruptured Ectopic Pregnancy
- Pseudosac may mimic an intrauterine pregnancy
- Note changing appearance of material within intrauterine cavity

Intrauterine Pregnancy with Ovarian Tumor
- Ovarian mass with characteristics of tumor, not pregnancy
- Dermoid is most common ovarian tumor found in pregnancy

PATHOLOGY

General Features
- Etiology: Twin pregnancy, with one implanted in the uterus and one in an ectopic location
- Epidemiology
  - Occurs in 1-2% of IVF patients
  - Occurs 1:7,000 spontaneous pregnancies

ECTOPIC PREGNANCY, HETEROTOPIC

- o Incidence is increasing due to ovulation induction, IVF, embryo transfer, previous pelvic surgery, and history of previous ectopic pregnancy managed conservatively and by salpingostomy

Gross Pathologic & Surgical Features
- Findings in the adnexa will be similar to any adnexal ectopic pregnancy
- Chorionic villi will be present

CLINICAL ISSUES

Presentation
- Most common signs/symptoms
  - o Pain localized to the side of the heterotopic
  - o If ruptured, hemodynamic instability may result

Demographics
- Age: Patients of menstrual age
- Gender: Female

Natural History & Prognosis
- Some ectopic pregnancies associated with intrauterine pregnancies resolve spontaneously
- If not treated, heterotopic pregnancies can rupture, leading to life-threatening hemorrhage
- Heterotopic pregnancies can be operated upon without loss of the intrauterine pregnancy
- When diagnosed at late gestational age, live deliveries of both gestations can occur

Treatment
- Surgery
- Percutaneous potassium chloride injection into the heterotopic
- Percutaneous hyperosmolar glucose into the heterotopic
- If diagnosed late in pregnancy, and patient is stable, the intrauterine pregnancy can be delivered vaginally and the ectopic pregnancy can be delivered by laparotomy

DIAGNOSTIC CHECKLIST

Consider
- Transabdominal and transvaginal sonography may both be needed to adequately assess for combined intra- and extrauterine pregnancies
- MR is helpful in assessing vascularity of the heterotopic pregnancy and planning surgical management

Image Interpretation Pearls
- Always evaluate the adnexa in pregnant patients

SELECTED REFERENCES

1. Amagada JO et al: Spontaneous heterotopic pregnancy remains a diagnostic enigma. J Obstet Gynaecol. 25(1):72-3, 2005
2. Korkontzelos I et al: Ruptured heterotopic pregnancy with successful obstetrical outcome: a case report and review of the literature. Clin Exp Obstet Gynecol. 32(3):203-6, 2005
3. Rabbani I et al: Heterotopic pregnancy is not rare. A case report and literature review. J Obstet Gynaecol. 25(2):204-5, 2005
4. Sohail S: Hemorrhagic corpus luteum mimicking heterotopic pregnancy. J Coll Physicians Surg Pak. 15(3):180-1, 2005
5. Tan PL et al: Incidental heterotopic pregnancy demonstrated on magnetic resonance imaging. Australas Radiol. 49(1):75-8, 2005
6. Umezurike CC et al: Heterotopic pregnancy with spontaneous vaginal delivery at 36 weeks and laparotomy at term--a case report. Afr J Reprod Health. 9(1):162-5, 2005
7. Breyer MJ et al: Heterotopic gestation: another possibility for the emergency bedside ultrasonographer to consider. J Emerg Med. 26(1):81-4, 2004
8. Cheng PJ et al: Heterotopic pregnancy in a natural conception cycle presenting as hematometra. Obstet Gynecol. 104(5 Pt 2):1195-8, 2004
9. Chiang G et al: Imaging of adnexal masses in pregnancy. J Ultrasound Med. 23(6):805-19, 2004
10. Chin HY et al: Heterotopic pregnancy after in vitro fertilization-embryo transfer. Int J Gynaecol Obstet. 86(3):411-6, 2004
11. Doubilet PM et al: Sonographically guided minimally invasive treatment of unusual ectopic pregnancies. J Ultrasound Med. 23(3):359-70, 2004
12. Fernandez H et al: Ectopic pregnancies after infertility treatment: modern diagnosis and therapeutic strategy. Hum Reprod Update. 10(6):503-13, 2004
13. Kumar S et al: Heterotopic cervical and intrauterine pregnancy in a spontaneous cycle. Eur J Obstet Gynecol Reprod Biol. 112(2):217-20, 2004
14. Shaya A: Heterotopic twin delivery of live infants. Trop Doct. 34(3):190-1, 2004
15. Strelec M et al: Heterotopic triplet pregnancy with laparoscopic resection of the ruptured tube at 10 weeks of gestation. Eur J Obstet Gynecol Reprod Biol. 117(1):117-8, 2004
16. Yazicioglu HF et al: An unusual case of heterotopic twin pregnancy managed successfully with selective feticide. Ultrasound Obstet Gynecol. 23(6):626-7, 2004
17. Hoopmann M et al: Heterotopic triplet pregnancy with bilateral tubal and intrauterine pregnancy after IVF. Reprod Biomed Online. 6(3):345-8, 2003
18. Porpora MG et al: Heterotopic cervical pregnancy: a case report. Acta Obstet Gynecol Scand. 82(11):1058-9, 2003
19. Ludwig M et al: Heterotopic pregnancy in a spontaneous cycle: do not forget about it! Eur J Obstet Gynecol Reprod Biol. 87(1):91-3, 1999
20. Maaita ME et al: Advanced heterotopic pregnancy. J Obstet Gynaecol. 19(6):677-8, 1999

ECTOPIC PREGNANCY, HETEROTOPIC

IMAGE GALLERY

Typical

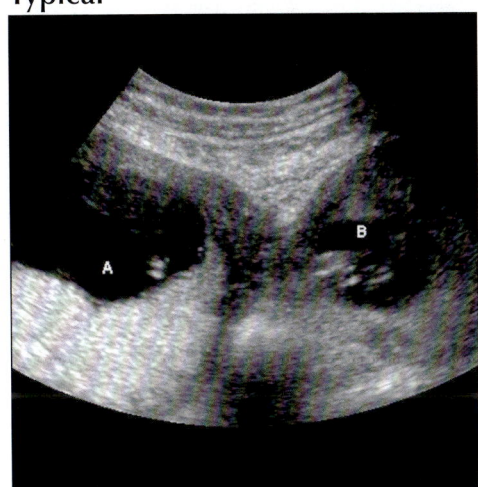 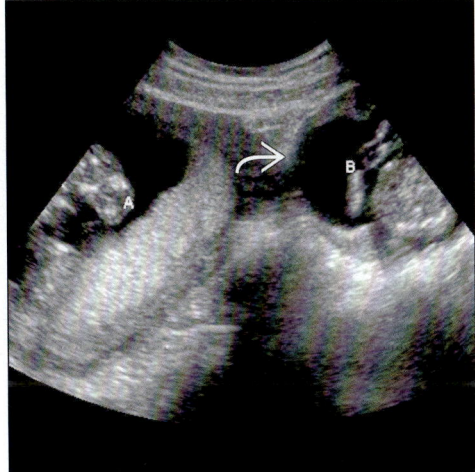

(Left) Transverse transabdominal ultrasound shows 2 gestational sacs. "A" is located in the uterus with normal surrounding myometrium. "B" is heterotopic. *(Right)* Transverse transabdominal ultrasound shows same patient as previous image. Note the lack of myometrium around the sac of "B" ➔.

Typical

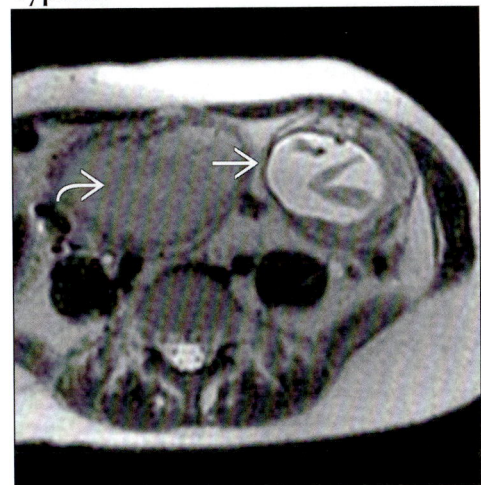 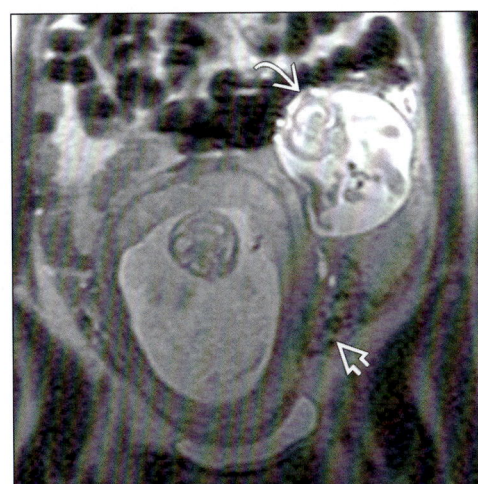

(Left) Transverse T2WI MR shows same case as above, with placenta of the intrauterine pregnancy ➔ and gestational sac of the heterotopic ➔. *(Right)* Coronal T2WI MR shows same as previous image with intrauterine pregnancy and ectopic pregnancy. Note the lack of myometrium around the ectopic gestational sac ➔. Note vascularity ➔.

Typical

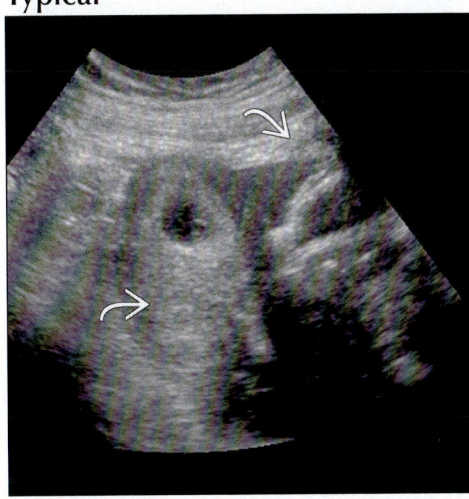 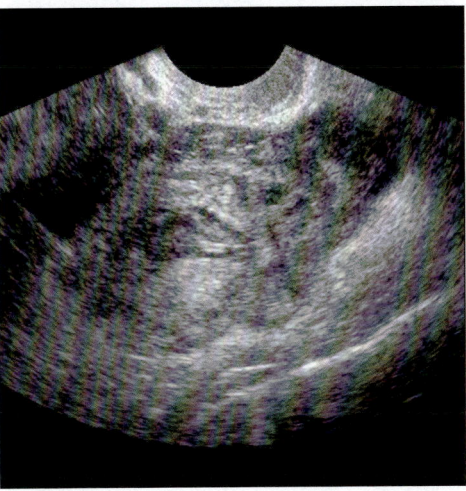

(Left) Sagittal transabdominal ultrasound shows intrauterine pregnancy with surrounding blood products ➔. *(Right)* Sagittal transvaginal ultrasound shows same patient as previous image with heterogeneous mass that was separate from ovary, consistent with ruptured heterotopic pregnancy.

ECTOPIC PREGNANCY, ABDOMINAL

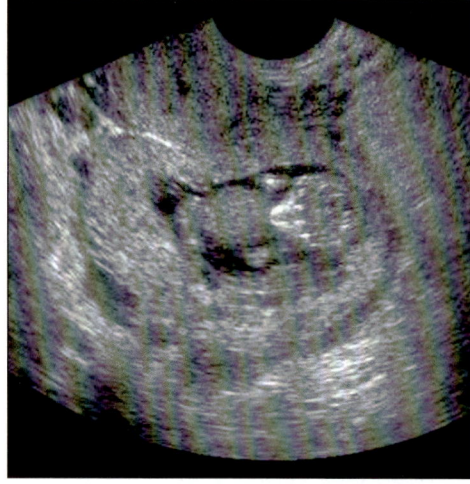

Sagittal transvaginal ultrasound shows pregnancy in cul-de-sac.

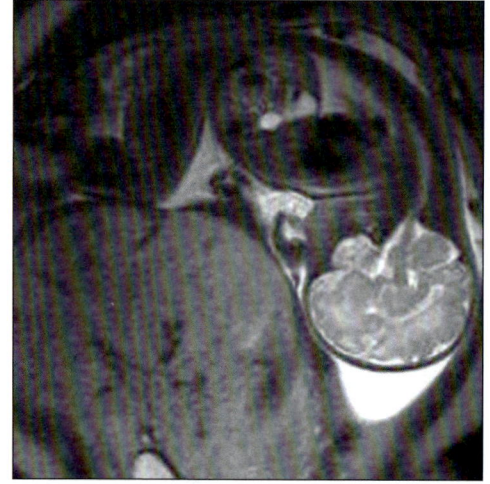

Coronal T2WI MR shows abdominal pregnancy. (Courtesy S. Ulrich, MD).

TERMINOLOGY

Abbreviations and Synonyms
- Abdominal pregnancy, peritoneal pregnancy

Definitions
- Pregnancy outside of uterus with blood supply from within the peritoneal cavity

IMAGING FINDINGS

General Features
- Best diagnostic clue: Pregnancy outside of the uterus

Imaging Recommendations
- Best imaging tool
  - Ultrasound for screening for location of ectopic pregnancy
  - MR for pre-operative planning in cases of advanced gestational age
- Protocol advice: If surgery is indicated, then use of gadolinium is reasonable to determine site of placental attachment

DIFFERENTIAL DIAGNOSIS

Tubal Ectopic Pregnancy
- Located in fallopian tube with characteristic appearance

Ovarian Ectopic Pregnancy
- May not be possible to distinguish from abdominal ectopic pregnancy

Interstitial Ectopic Pregnancy
- Less than 5 mm of endometrium around entire sac
- Lateral location of gestational sac

Pregnancy in Horn of Bicornuate Uterus
- See myometrium around entire gestational sac

PATHOLOGY

General Features
- Etiology
  - Primary abdominal pregnancy originates in abdomen (rare)

DDx: Abdominal Ectopic Pregnancy Mimics

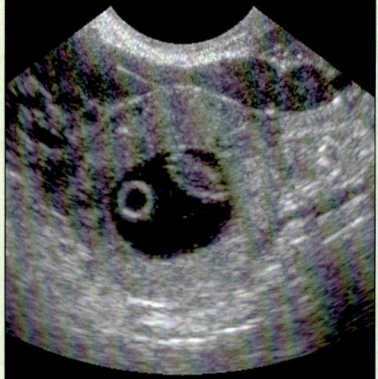

Tubal Ectopic

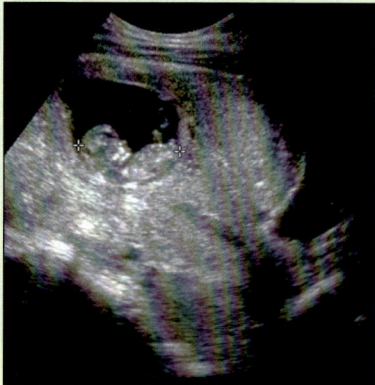

Interstitial Ectopic

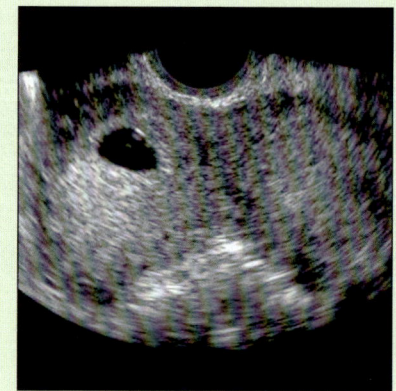

Gestational Sac in Bicornuate Uterus

ECTOPIC PREGNANCY, ABDOMINAL

Key Facts

Terminology
- Pregnancy outside of uterus with blood supply from within the peritoneal cavity

Pathology
- Primary abdominal pregnancy originates in abdomen (rare)
- Secondary abdominal pregnancy originates in tube or uterus with subsequent rupture
- 1% of all ectopic pregnancy

- Risk factors: Infertility, endometriosis, in vitro fertilization, prior ectopic pregnancy, tubal reconstructive surgery

Clinical Issues
- Mortality rate of abdominal pregnancy is 7 times higher than that of tubal ectopic pregnancy
- Placenta frequently left in situ, patient treated medically to aid in placental regression with later removal of the placenta

---

  - Secondary abdominal pregnancy originates in tube or uterus with subsequent rupture
- Epidemiology
  - 1% of all ectopic pregnancy
  - Risk factors: Infertility, endometriosis, in vitro fertilization, prior ectopic pregnancy, tubal reconstructive surgery
- Associated abnormalities: If secondary abdominal pregnancy there may be evidence of uterine or tubal rupture

CLINICAL ISSUES

Presentation
- Most common signs/symptoms: Lower abdominal pain, bleeding

Demographics
- Age: Reproductive age
- Gender: Female

Natural History & Prognosis
- Mortality rate of abdominal pregnancy is 7 times higher than that of tubal ectopic pregnancy
  - Maternal mortality: 0.5-18%
  - Perinatal mortality: 40-95%
- MR is helpful in demonstrating location and adherence of placenta which directly affects decision whether to remove or leave placenta in situ

Treatment
- Laparoscopy if early and no hemoperitoneum
- Laparotomy if late and hemoperitoneum
- If diagnosed late in gestation, a viable neonate may be delivered by laparotomy
- Placental attachment to mesentery can limit ability to remove entire placenta
  - Placenta frequently left in situ, patient treated medically to aid in placental regression with later removal of the placenta

DIAGNOSTIC CHECKLIST

Consider
- Abdominal pregnancy when gestational sac is seen outside of uterus in second or third trimester

SELECTED REFERENCES

1. Lockhat F, et al: The value of magnetic resonance imaging in the diagnosis and management of extra-uterine abdominal pregnancy. Clin Radiol. 61:264-9, 2006
2. Atrash H et al: Abdominal pregnancy in the United States: frequency and maternal mortality. Obstet Gynecol. 69:333-7, 1987

IMAGE GALLERY

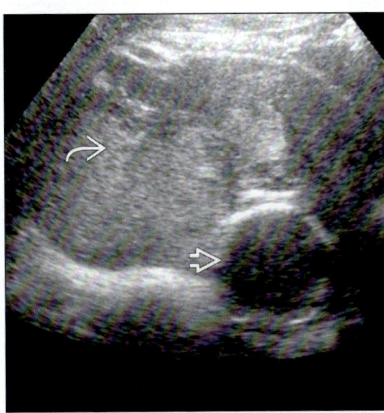 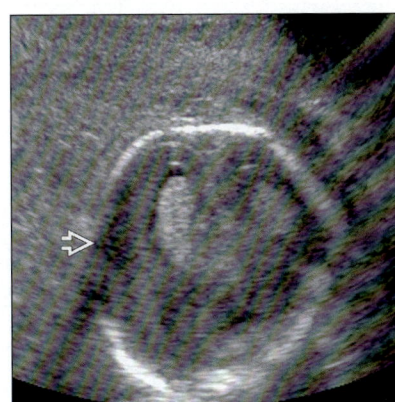 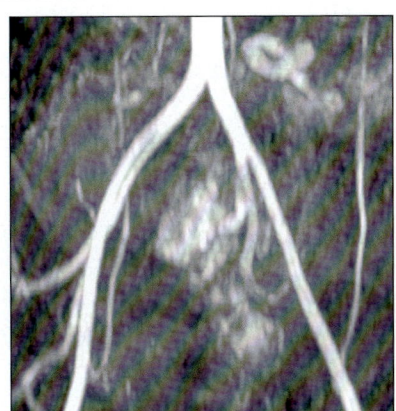

(Left) Sagittal transabdominal ultrasound shows fetal head ➡ in cul-de-sac. Note empty endometrial cavity ➡. (Center) Sagittal transvaginal ultrasound in same patient as previous image shows fetal head ➡ in cul-de-sac. (Right) Coronal T1 C+ MR in same patient as previous image shows blood supply to abdominal ectopic.

ECTOPIC PREGNANCY, RUPTURE

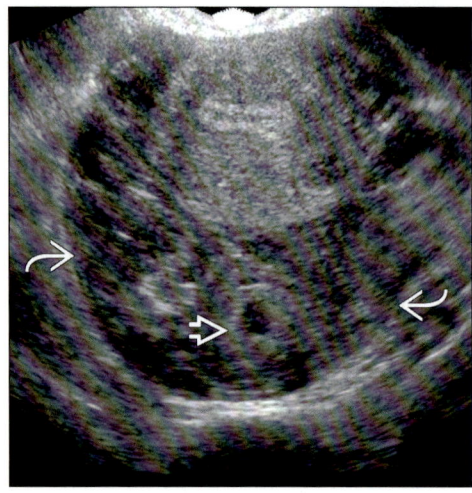

Transverse transvaginal ultrasound shows tubal ring ➡ surrounded by clot ➡.

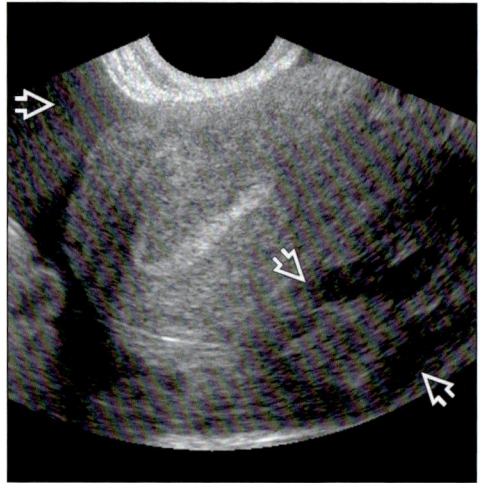

Sagittal transvaginal ultrasound shows heterogeneous material consistent with blood ➡ surrounding the uterus.

TERMINOLOGY

Definitions
- Pregnancy located outside of the endometrial cavity that has ruptured

IMAGING FINDINGS

General Features
- Best diagnostic clue: Large amount of hemoperitoneum in pregnant patient
- Location
  - Most commonly in fallopian tubes
  - Ectopic pregnancy in ovary, abdomen, rudimentary horn can all rupture
- Size: Large masses are more likely to have ruptured, but there is overlap in size of ruptured and non-ruptured ectopic pregnancies
- Morphology
  - Tubal ring
  - Tubal ring with yolk sac and/or embryonic pole
  - Ill-defined mass
  - Hemoperitoneum

Ultrasonographic Findings
- Findings of ectopic pregnancy
  - Pseudosac in uterus
    - Fluid centrally located in endometrial cavity
    - May change in appearance over time
  - Decidual cysts
    - Located away from endometrial cavity
    - Do not have echogenic rim around them (as would be seen in intradecidual sign)
  - Mass separate from ovary in fallopian tube
    - Amorphous mass may be due to blood clot
    - Ectopic pregnancy is the most common cause of hematosalpinx
    - Ring-like mass separate from ovary represents ectopic pregnancy
    - Extra-ovarian mass may have yolk sac or embryonic pole
  - Color flow may or may not be present around the ectopic pregnancy
    - Ring of color around an adnexal mass may be due to either hemorrhagic cyst or ectopic
    - Color can be helpful to locate an ectopic hidden in bowel gas

DDx: Ruptured Ectopic Pregnancy Mimics

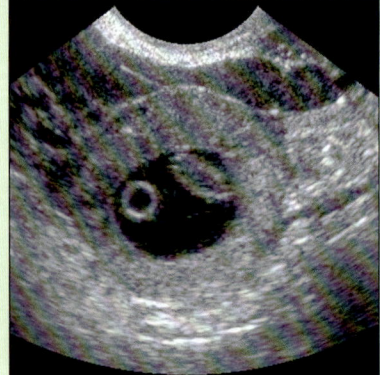

Unruptured Ectopic

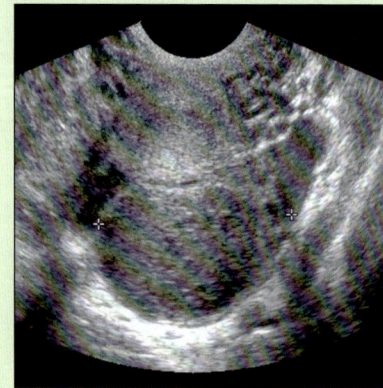

Hemorrhagic Cyst

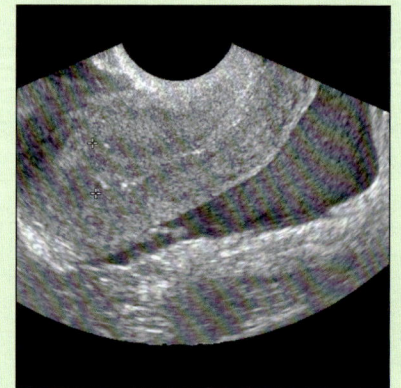

Blood in Cul-de-Sac

ECTOPIC PREGNANCY, RUPTURE

Key Facts

Imaging Findings
- Hematoma may obscure the ectopic pregnancy
- Blood may collect in the fallopian tube giving the appearance of an elongated, enlarged heterogeneous tube
- Mass greater than 3.5 cm is more likely to be ruptured, but rupture can occur in small mass as well
- Image up by kidneys to assess for large amount of hemoperitoneum

Top Differential Diagnoses
- Corpus luteum located in ovary whereas ectopic pregnancy more likely to be in tube
- Hemoperitoneum can be life-threatening

Clinical Issues
- Pain and bleeding in first trimester
- Increased pain after treatment with methotrexate
- Hemodynamic instability is a highly specific sign of rupture
- Heart rate and blood pressure are insensitive for prediction of rupture
- Ruptured ectopic pregnancy is the leading cause of maternal death
- Due to hemodynamic instability, this can be a surgical emergency

Diagnostic Checklist
- Suspect ruptured ectopic pregnancy when a large amount of hemoperitoneum is present
- In a pregnant patient without visualized intrauterine or extrauterine pregnancy and a moderate amount of hemoperitoneum, the diagnosis of ruptured ectopic pregnancy should be considered

---

  - Hematoma may obscure the ectopic pregnancy
  - Blood may collect in the fallopian tube giving the appearance of an elongated, enlarged heterogeneous tube
  - Free fluid
    - Fluid with debris suggests hemorrhage
    - Large amount of fluid may be seen in upper abdomen
- Mass greater than 3.5 cm is more likely to be ruptured, but rupture can occur in small mass as well

CT Findings
- NECT
  - High-attenuation fluid surrounding adnexal mass
  - Heterogeneous adnexal mass separate from ovary

MR Findings
- T1WI: Fluid with high signal due to blood products surrounding adnexal mass
- T2WI: Heterogeneous signal intensity fluid surrounding adnexal mass that is separate from ovary

Imaging Recommendations
- Best imaging tool: Ultrasound
- Protocol advice
  - Image up by kidneys to assess for large amount of hemoperitoneum
  - Transabdominal scan to assess for ectopic located high in the pelvis
    - If a large amount of free fluid is seen, exam may need to be curtailed if patient is hemodynamically unstable
  - Transvaginal scan to best assess the fallopian tubes and ovaries
    - Scan uterus to check for intrauterine pregnancy
    - Scan adnexal to check for mass separate from ovary
    - Ovarian mass is more likely to be corpus luteum than ectopic pregnancy
    - If no extra-ovarian adnexal mass is visualized, scan with color to find ectopic hidden between bowel loops
    - Ectopic pregnancy may not be on same side as corpus luteum

DIFFERENTIAL DIAGNOSIS

Unruptured Ectopic Pregnancy
- May be indistinguishable from ruptured ectopic pregnancy
- Tend to be smaller in size with less hemoperitoneum

Ruptured Hemorrhagic Corpus Luteum Cyst
- Corpus luteum located in ovary whereas ectopic pregnancy more likely to be in tube
- Hemoperitoneum can be life-threatening

Ovarian Torsion
- Enlarged ovary with or without mass
- Patient acutely tender on the side of the torsion
- Arterial and venous flow may be present due to the dual blood supply of the ovary

Blood in Cul-de-Sac
- Small amount of blood in the cul-de-sac can be seen in patients with normal intrauterine pregnancy

Tubo-Ovarian Abscess
- Cervical motion tenderness
- Elevated white blood cell count

PATHOLOGY

General Features
- Etiology: Pregnancy implants in tube (or other location) instead of in uterus
- Epidemiology
  - Ectopic pregnancy risk is increased in patients with tubal disease, prior ectopic pregnancy, infertility treatment, use of intrauterine device
  - Serum beta-hCG by itself cannot predict whether a tubal ectopic pregnancy is likely to be ruptured
  - There is no safe lower limit in hCG titer below which ruptured ectopic is not seen

ECTOPIC PREGNANCY, RUPTURE

- hCG values prior to ectopic diagnosis that increase at least 66% over 48 hours and rising hCG values after treatment with methotrexate are independent predictors of tubal rupture
- Heterotopic pregnancies can rupture

Gross Pathologic & Surgical Features
- 90% of ectopic pregnancies are located in the fallopian tubes
- Swelling of tube at site of pregnancy with evidence of rupture and hemorrhage, associated hemoperitoneum
- Fluid with debris has a 90% sensitivity for prediction of ectopic pregnancy in pregnant patient without intrauterine pregnancy

Microscopic Features
- Disrupted, dilated tube wall with admixed blood clot, chorionic villi and trophoblast

CLINICAL ISSUES

Presentation
- Most common signs/symptoms
  - Pain and bleeding in first trimester
  - Increased pain after treatment with methotrexate
- Other signs/symptoms
  - Hemodynamic instability is a highly specific sign of rupture
  - Heart rate and blood pressure are insensitive for prediction of rupture

Demographics
- Age: Reproductive age

Natural History & Prognosis
- Ruptured ectopic pregnancy is the leading cause of maternal death
- Due to hemodynamic instability, this can be a surgical emergency

Treatment
- Laparoscopy in centers with experience
- Laparotomy

DIAGNOSTIC CHECKLIST

Consider
- Suspect ruptured ectopic pregnancy when a large amount of hemoperitoneum is present

Image Interpretation Pearls
- In a pregnant patient without visualized intrauterine or extrauterine pregnancy and a moderate amount of hemoperitoneum, the diagnosis of ruptured ectopic pregnancy should be considered
- If a large amount of hemoperitoneum is visualized and no ectopic pregnancy is seen, this could be either a ruptured ectopic pregnancy or ruptured corpus luteum cyst, both of which will require surgery if the patient is hemodynamically unstable

SELECTED REFERENCES
1. Latchaw G et al: Risk factors associated with the rupture of tubal ectopic pregnancy. Gynecol Obstet Invest. 60(3):177-80, 2005
2. Dialani V et al: Ectopic pregnancy: a review. Ultrasound Q. 20(3):105-17, 2004
3. Dudley PS et al: Characterizing ectopic pregnancies that rupture despite treatment with methotrexate. Fertil Steril. 82(5):1374-8, 2004
4. Stein MW et al: Sonographic comparison of the tubal ring of ectopic pregnancy with the corpus luteum. J Ultrasound Med. 23(1):57-62, 2004
5. Ferrero S et al: Seventy-five ectopic pregnancies. Medical and surgical management. Minerva Ginecol. 54(6):471-82, 2002
6. Frates MC et al: Comparison of tubal ring and corpus luteum echogenicities: a useful differentiating characteristic. J Ultrasound Med. 20(1):27-31; quiz 33, 2001
7. Aboud E: A five-year review of ectopic pregnancy. Clin Exp Obstet Gynecol. 24(3):127-9, 1997
8. Atri M et al: Role of endovaginal sonography in the diagnosis and management of ectopic pregnancy. Radiographics. 16(4):755-74; discussion 775, 1996
9. Buster JE et al: Ectopic pregnancy: new advances in diagnosis and treatment. Curr Opin Obstet Gynecol. 7(3):168-76, 1995
10. Mol BW et al: Contraception and the risk of ectopic pregnancy: a meta-analysis. Contraception. 52(6):337-41, 1995
11. Brown DL et al: Transvaginal sonography for diagnosing ectopic pregnancy: positivity criteria and performance characteristics. J Ultrasound Med. 13(4):259-66, 1994
12. Frates MC et al: Tubal rupture in patients with ectopic pregnancy: diagnosis with transvaginal US. Radiology. 191(3):769-72, 1994
13. Atri M et al: Accuracy of transvaginal ultrasonography for detection of hematosalpinx in ectopic pregnancy. J Clin Ultrasound. 20(4):255-61, 1992
14. Jurkovic D et al: Transvaginal color Doppler study of blood flow in ectopic pregnancies. Fertil Steril. 57(1):68-73, 1992
15. Rottem S et al: Classification of tubal gestations by transvaginal sonography. Ultrasound Obstet Gynecol. 1(3):197-201, 1991
16. Fleischer AC et al: Ectopic pregnancy: features at transvaginal sonography. Radiology. 174(2):375-8, 1990
17. Herman A et al: The role of tubal pathology and other parameters in ectopic pregnancies occurring in in vitro fertilization and embryo transfer. Fertil Steril. 54(5):864-8, 1990
18. Kivikoski AI et al: Transabdominal and transvaginal ultrasonography in the diagnosis of ectopic pregnancy: a comparative study. Am J Obstet Gynecol. 163(1 Pt 1):123-8, 1990
19. Breen JL: A 21 year survey of 654 ectopic pregnancies. Am J Obstet Gynecol. 106(7):1004-19, 1970

ECTOPIC PREGNANCY, RUPTURE

IMAGE GALLERY

Typical

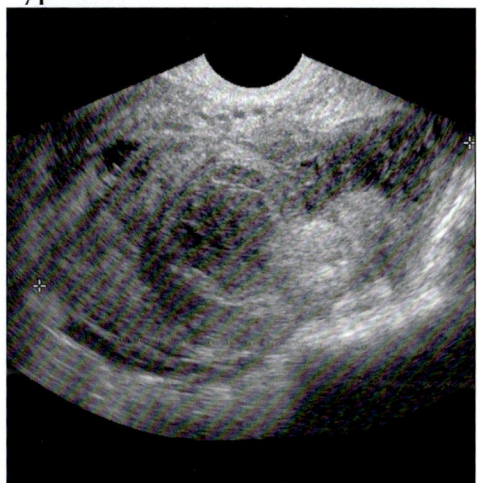
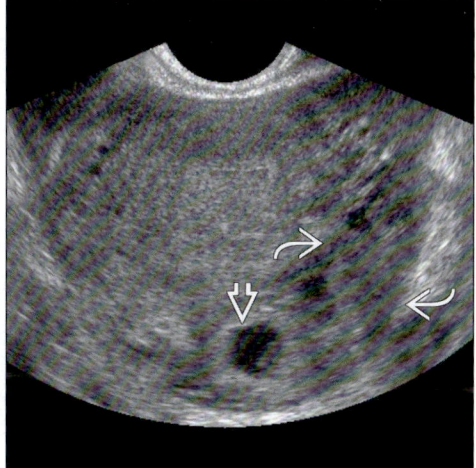

(Left) Sagittal transvaginal ultrasound shows heterogeneous material *(calipers)* consistent with blood in the adnexal region. *(Right)* Transverse transvaginal ultrasound shows ectopic sac ➡ surrounded by blood clot ➡ in a patient with ruptured ectopic pregnancy after treatment with methotrexate.

Typical

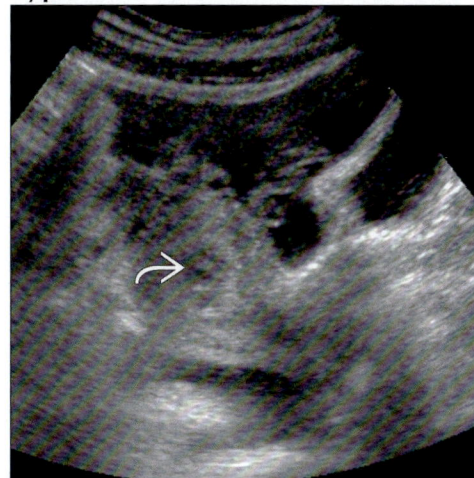
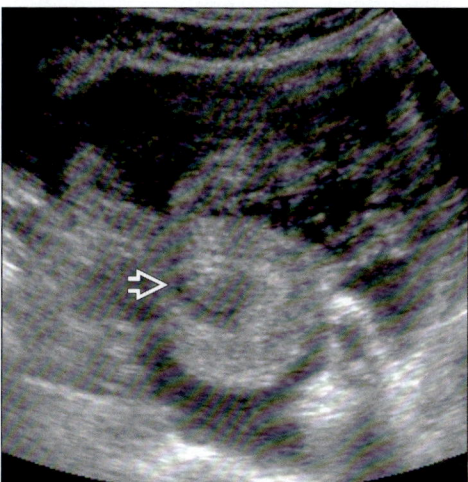

(Left) Sagittal transabdominal ultrasound shows blood surrounding the uterus. Note the pseudosac ➡ within the endometrial cavity. *(Right)* Transverse transabdominal ultrasound shows blood surrounding the uterus. Note the pseudosac ➡ within the endometrial cavity.

Typical

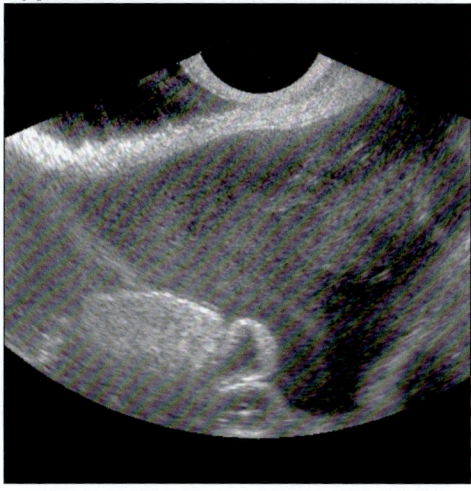
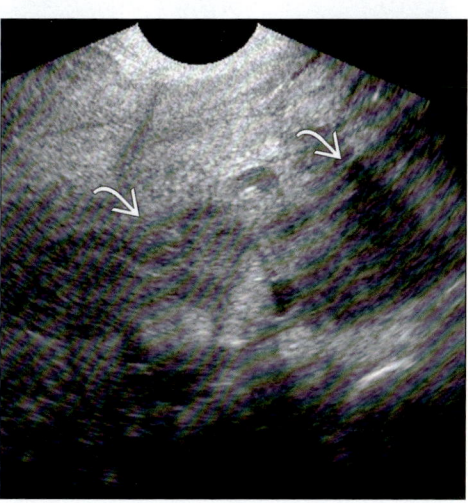

(Left) Sagittal oblique transvaginal ultrasound shows fluid with debris in the pelvis, consistent with blood in a patient with ruptured ectopic pregnancy. *(Right)* Sagittal transvaginal ultrasound shows heterogeneous material ➡ behind the uterus, consistent with blood clot.

ECTOPIC PREGNANCY, RUPTURE

Typical

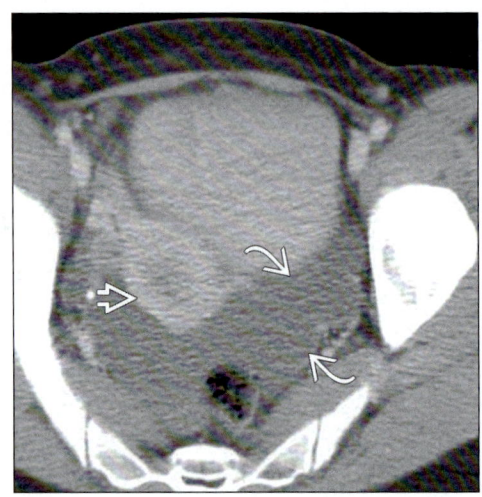 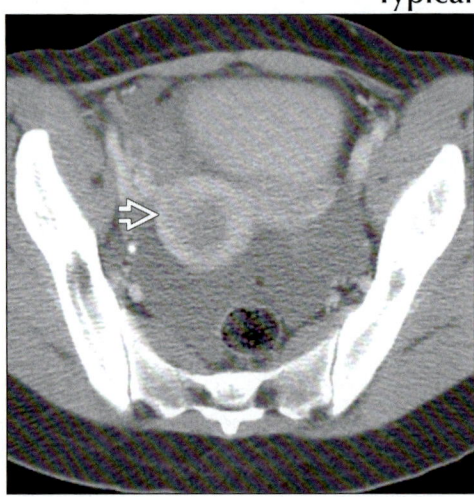

(Left) Transverse CECT shows tubal ring ➡ in a patient with free fluid/blood clot ➡ posterior to the uterus and tubal ring. *(Right)* Transverse CECT (same patient as previous image) shows tubal ring ➡ with surrounding fluid. The fluid had high Hounsfield units consistent with blood.

Typical

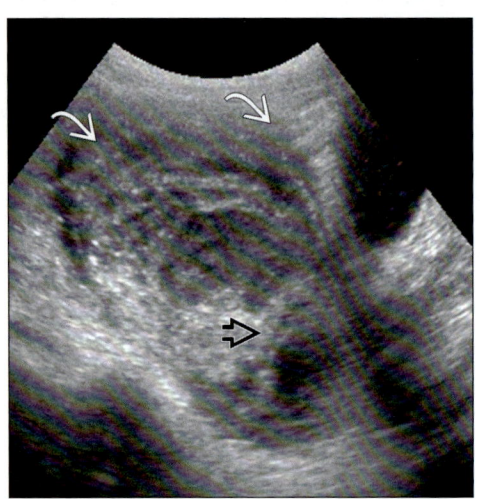 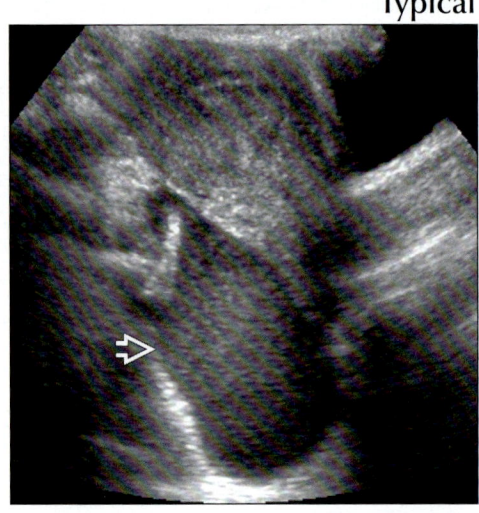

(Left) Sagittal transabdominal ultrasound shows heterogeneous material ➡ in the pelvis consistent with blood clot. The ectopic is located posteriorly ➡. *(Right)* Sagittal transabdominal ultrasound shows a large amount of blood ➡ posterior to the uterus.

Typical

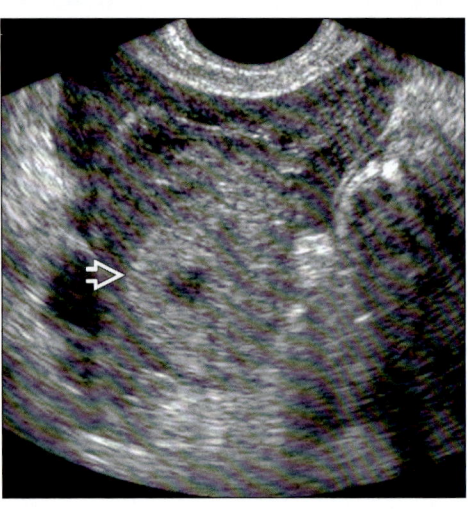 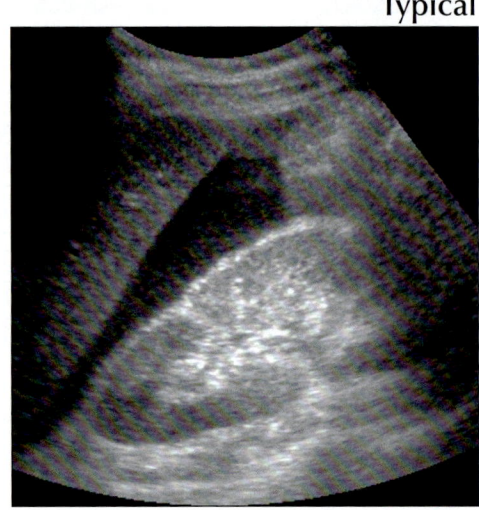

(Left) Transverse transvaginal ultrasound shows blood and debris surrounding a tubal ring ➡. *(Right)* Sagittal transabdominal ultrasound shows hemoperitoneum in the right flank.

ECTOPIC PREGNANCY, RUPTURE

Typical

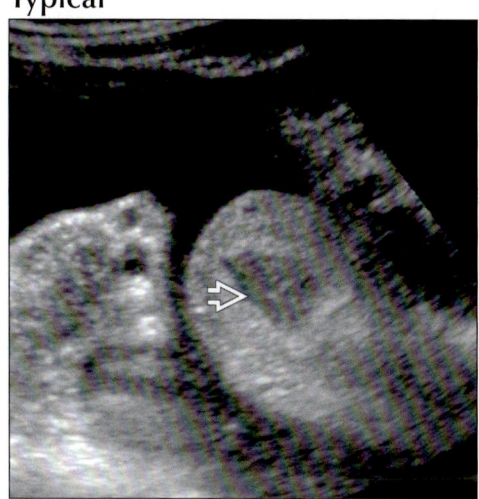
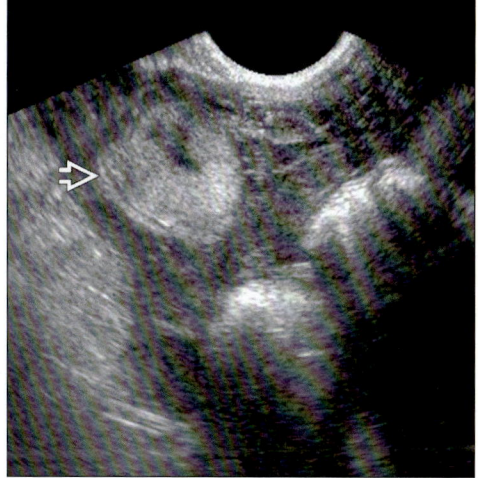

(Left) Transverse transabdominal ultrasound shows a large amount of fluid around the uterus. Note the pseudosac ➤ in the uterus. *(Right)* Sagittal oblique transvaginal ultrasound shows echogenic ring-like mass ➤ surrounded by blood.

Typical

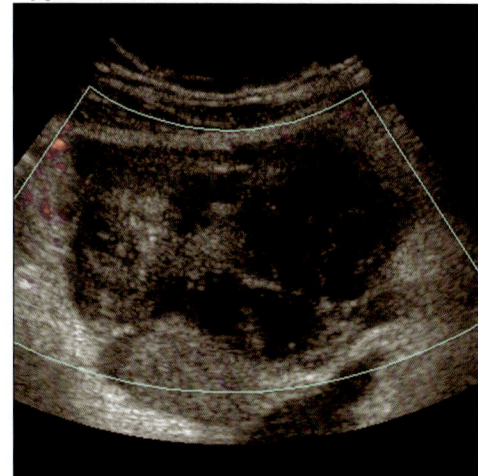
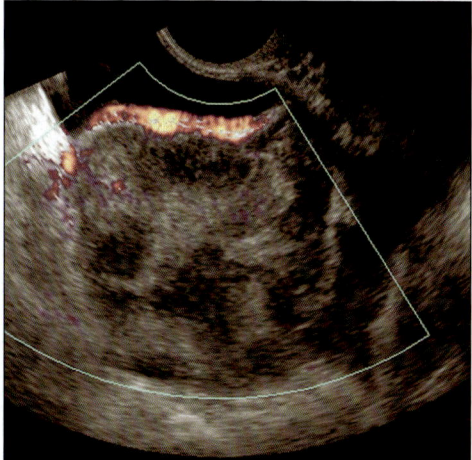

(Left) Transverse power Doppler ultrasound in pelvis of pregnant patient shows a large amount of blood clot in a patient with a ruptured ectopic pregnancy. Note the lack of vascularity in the clot. *(Right)* Sagittal power Doppler ultrasound transvaginal ultrasound in same patient as previous, shows a heterogeneous mass. At real time this was seen separate from the ovary.

Typical

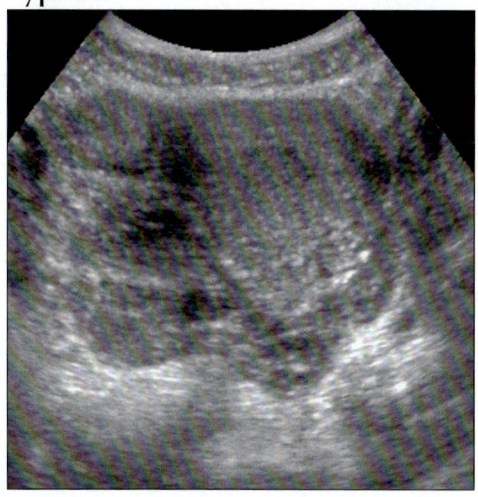
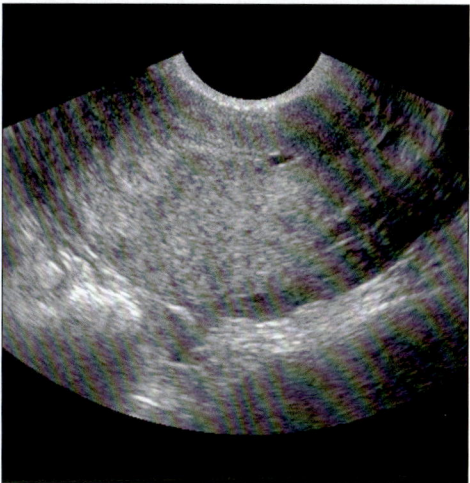

(Left) Transverse transabdominal ultrasound shows blood surrounding the uterus. Note how the uterine contour is indistinct due to the surrounding debris. *(Right)* Sagittal transvaginal ultrasound in same patient as previous image. Note the indistinct margins of the uterus secondary to the surrounding clot.

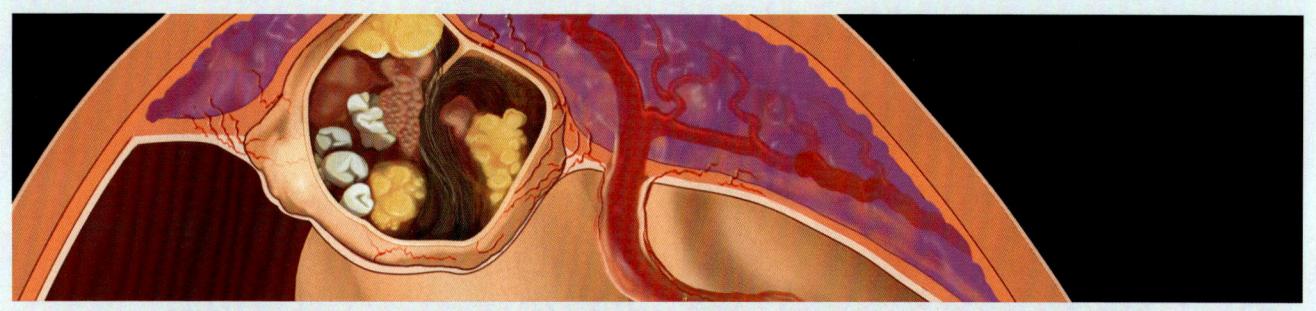

SECTION 11: Placenta

Neoplasm, Benign

Teratoma, Placenta	11-2
Hydatiform Mole, Complete Mole	11-4
Hydatiform Mole, Partial Mole	11-10

Neoplasm, Malignant

Invasive Mole	11-16
Placental Site Trophoblastic Tumor	11-20

Miscellaneous

Hematoma, Placenta	11-24
Chorioangioma, Placenta	11-30

TERATOMA, PLACENTA

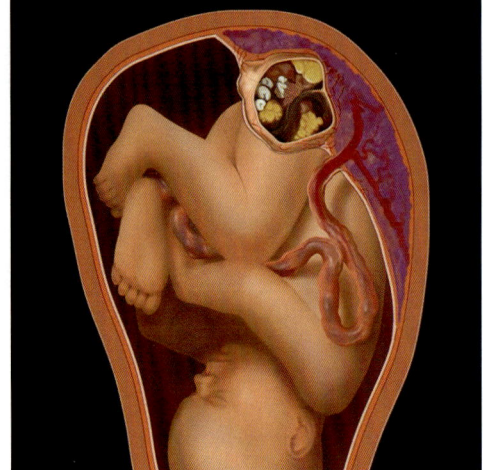

Graphic shows internal contents of a benign placental teratoma on cross-section. Mature components such as hair, teeth, muscle, bones and fat may be recognized macroscopically.

Sagittal graphic shows a placental teratoma situated between the amnion and the chorion and bulging on the fetal side of the placenta. The blood supply is through placental arteries and not the umbilical vessels.

TERMINOLOGY

Definitions
- Benign tumor of the placenta
- Very rare, less than 20 reported cases

IMAGING FINDINGS

General Features
- Best diagnostic clue
  - Smooth round or oval tumors with heterogeneous contents
  - Usual appearance of a benign teratoma
- Location
  - Lies between the amnion and the chorion
  - Usually on the fetal surface of placenta
  - Rarely in membranes
- Size: 2.5-7.5 cm in diameter
- Morphology
  - Smooth round or oval tumors
  - May contain hair, teeth, bone etc.

Ultrasonographic Findings
- Presence of tissues of varied echogenicity such as calcification, fat, and fluid
- Absence of organized skeletal structures
- Absence of an umbilical cord
- Less vascular than the placenta on color Doppler imaging

Imaging Recommendations
- Best imaging tool: Prenatal US with color Doppler

DIFFERENTIAL DIAGNOSIS

Chorioangioma
- No calcifications
- Vascular: May cause hydrops

Twin Reversed Arterial Perfusion
- Twin gestation with an acardiac twin
- Has a separate umbilical cord (may be poorly developed or rudimentary)
- Has axial organization with development of a central skeleton

DDx: Placental Teratoma

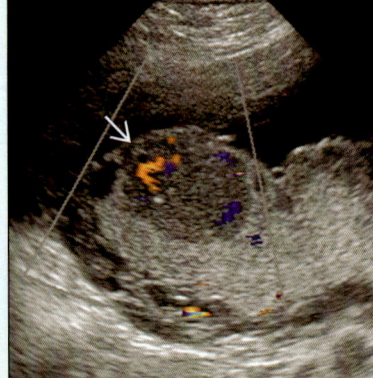
Chorioangioma

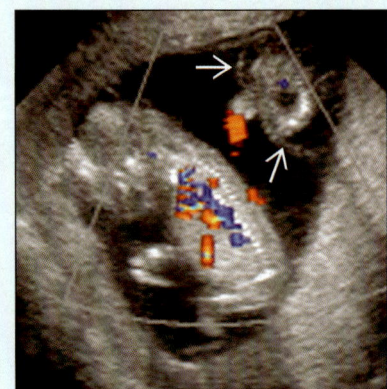
TRAP Twin

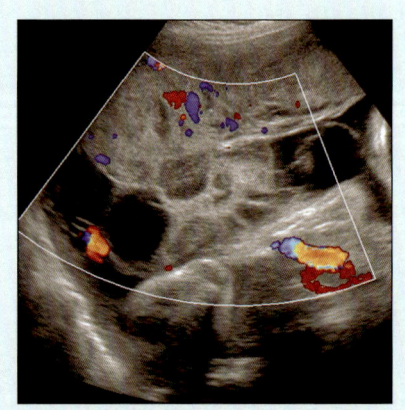
Placental Hematoma

TERATOMA, PLACENTA

Key Facts

Terminology
- Benign tumor of the placenta

Imaging Findings
- Smooth round or oval tumors with heterogeneous contents
- Presence of tissues of varied echogenicity such as calcification, fat, and fluid

Top Differential Diagnoses
- Chorioangioma

Pathology
- Absence of segmental organization of the skeletal structures
- Arterial supply most commonly from a placental arterial branch, not the umbilical cord

Placental Hematoma
- No internal blood flow on Doppler US

PATHOLOGY

General Features
- Etiology: Aberrant migration of embryonic germ cells

Gross Pathologic & Surgical Features
- Smooth round exterior
- Brownish contents which may contain fat, calcifications, teeth, hair and more

Microscopic Features
- Mixture of different tissues derived from all three germ cell layers: Skin with dermal appendages, ganglion-like cells, and nervous structures, gut structures, osteocartilaginous and smooth and striated muscle
- Absence of segmental organization of the skeletal structures
- Fully matured with no evidence of malignancy
- Arterial supply most commonly from a placental arterial branch, not the umbilical cord

CLINICAL ISSUES

Presentation
- Most common signs/symptoms
  - Incidental finding
  - No clear clinical significance

DIAGNOSTIC CHECKLIST

Consider
- Round or oval solid mass of the placenta bulging on the fetal side with heterogeneous sonographic appearance

Image Interpretation Pearls
- Presence of calcification, fat and fluid
- No connection to the umbilical cord

SELECTED REFERENCES

1. Ahmed N et al: Sonographic diagnosis of placental teratoma. J Clin Ultrasound. 32(2):98-101, 2004
2. Elagoz S et al: Placental teratoma. A case report. Eur J Obstet Gynecol Reprod Biol. 80(2):263-5, 1998
3. Wang L et al: Placental teratoma. A case report and review of the literature. Pathol Res Pract. 191(12):1267-70; discussion 1270, 1995
4. Williams VL et al: Placental teratoma: prenatal ultrasonographic diagnosis. J Ultrasound Med. 13(7):587-9, 1994
5. Block D et al: Placental teratoma. Int J Gynaecol Obstet. 34(4):377-80, 1991
6. Nickell KA et al: Placental teratoma: a case report. Pediatr Pathol. 7(5-6):645-50, 1987
7. Fox H et al: Pathology of the placenta. In: major problems in pathology. Volume 7. Philadelphia: WB Saunders. 355-6, 1978

IMAGE GALLERY

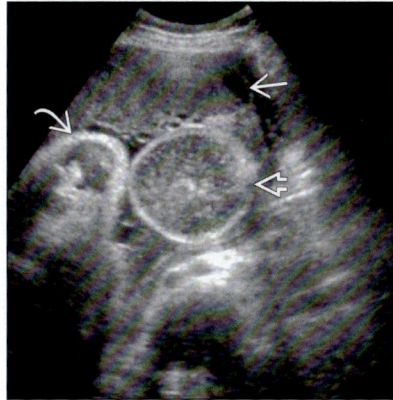 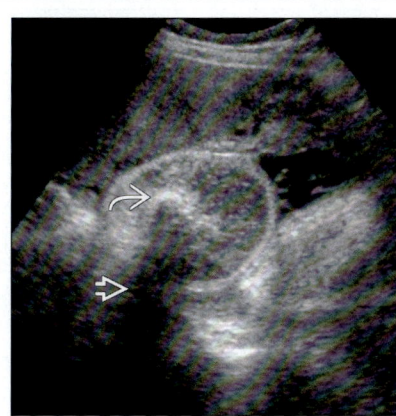 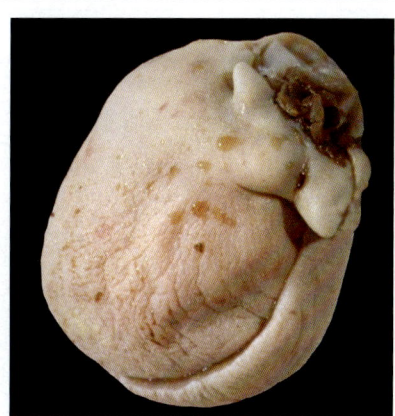

(Left) Axial ultrasound shows a round, well-defined mass ➡ on the fetal surface of the placenta ➡. Fetal extremities ➡ are also seen. *(Center)* Ultrasound focused on the mass shows it contains calcifications ➡, which are causing posterior shadowing ➡. *(Right)* Gross pathology of the resected mass shows it is skin covered. It was located between the membranes of the placenta and was separate from the umbilical cord. Histologically it contained fat, cartilage, teeth, bone and respiratory tissue.

HYDATIFORM MOLE, COMPLETE MOLE

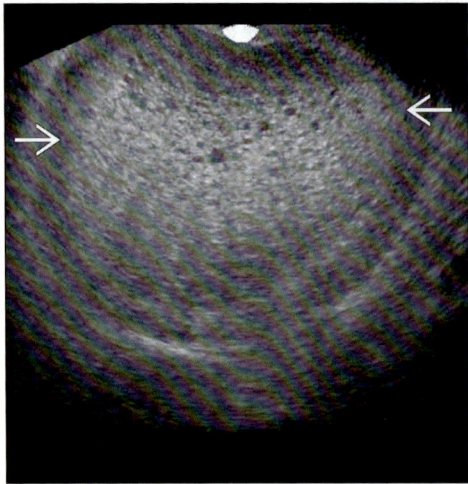

Sagittal transvaginal ultrasound with cystic & solid areas ➡ within the uterine cavity. Normal myometrium can be easily defined. Note the "snowstorm" appearance relating to multiple interfaces produced by tiny cysts.

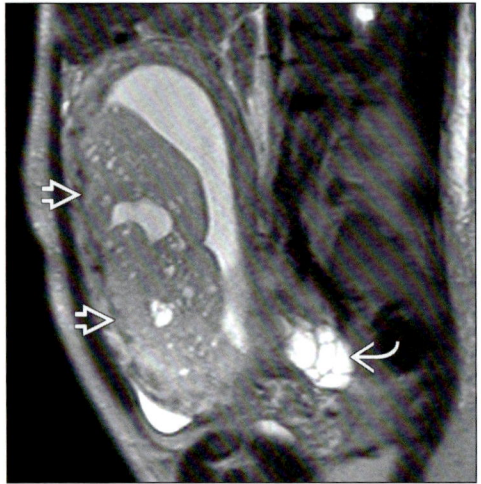

Sagittal T2WI MR shows enlarged, thickened placenta ➡ with innumerable tiny cystic structures. Note the enlarged ovary with theca lutein cysts ➡.

TERMINOLOGY

Abbreviations and Synonyms
- Hydatidiform mole
- Classic mole
- Benign form of gestational trophoblastic disease (GTD)

Definitions
- Abnormal proliferation of pregnancy-associated trophoblastic tissue with malignant potential

IMAGING FINDINGS

General Features
- Best diagnostic clue: Thickened endometrial cavity with multiple cystic spaces in pregnancy

Ultrasonographic Findings
- Color Doppler
  - Tend to be very vascular with very high velocity blood flow
  - High impedance flow in myometrium
  - When low impedance flow (RI < 0.4) is detected, invasive pathology is suspected
  - High diastolic flow is result of decreased vessel tone
- Transvaginal ultrasound (TVS) findings
  - Best imaging clue: "Bunch of grapes"
    - Hydropic villi & trophoblastic tissue
    - Uterine cavity filled with multiple sonolucent areas of varying size & shape
    - Vesicles 1-30 mm in diameter & seem to increase in size with gestational age
  - More uniform appearance with relatively smaller villi seen in earlier gestation
  - Doppler ultrasound: High velocities & low resistance to flow in uterine arterial circulation
  - First trimester moles may have a sonographic appearance simulating that of an incomplete abortion
  - Ovaries
    - Theca lutein cysts secondary to very high beta human chorionic gonadotropin (β-HCG) levels in up to 50% of cases
    - "Soap-bubble" or "spoke wheel" appearance
    - Enlarged

DDx: Pregnancy Related Pathologies

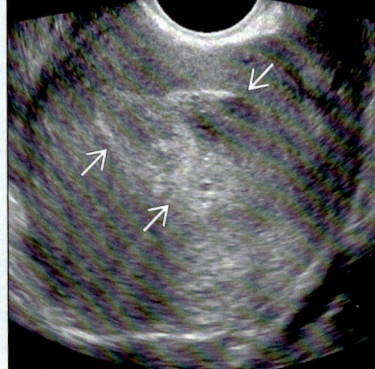
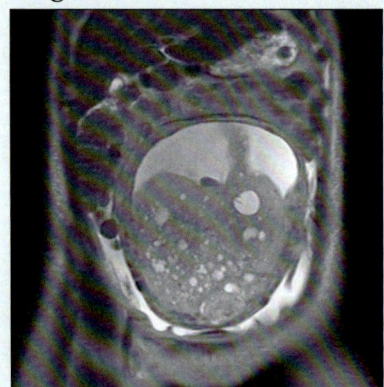
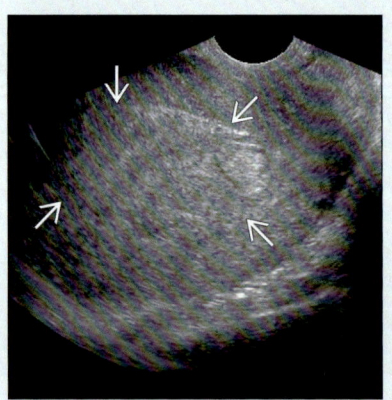

Spontaneous Abortion | Partial Mole | Retained Products of Conception

HYDATIFORM MOLE, COMPLETE MOLE

Key Facts

Terminology
- Hydatidiform mole
- Benign form of gestational trophoblastic disease (GTD)
- Abnormal proliferation of pregnancy-associated trophoblastic tissue with malignant potential

Imaging Findings
- Best imaging clue: "Bunch of grapes"
- Uterine cavity filled with multiple sonolucent areas of varying size & shape
- Theca lutein cysts secondary to very high beta human chorionic gonadotropin (β-HCG) levels in up to 50% of cases
- Best imaging tool: Ultrasonography has replaced all other means in early screening & is examination of choice for initial diagnosis

Top Differential Diagnoses
- Hydropic Placental Degeneration
- Retained Products of Conception
- Incomplete Abortion
- Invasive Mole & Choriocarcinoma

Pathology
- No fetal tissue present

Clinical Issues
- Vaginal bleeding late in first trimester, during 2nd trimester
- Hyperemesis gravidarum
- Patients with complete mole present with vaginal bleeding, uterine enlargement greater than expected for gestational age, & abnormally high level of serum β-HCG (> 100,000)

CT Findings
- Variable
- Normal-sized uterus with areas of low attenuation
- Enlarged heterogeneous uterus with central areas of low attenuation
- Hypoattenuating foci surrounded by markedly-enhancing areas in myometrium

MR Findings
- T2WI: Numerous cystic spaces may be present in the mass
- T1 C+: Characteristic numerous cystic areas are clearly seen in the mass
- T2WI
- Heterogeneous mass of high signal intensity that distends endometrial cavity
- May see numerous cystic spaces within mass
- Usually extremely hypervascular with signal voids representing dilated vessels prominent within mass, adjacent myometrium and parametrium

Imaging Recommendations
- Best imaging tool: Ultrasonography has replaced all other means in early screening & is examination of choice for initial diagnosis
- CT & MR used for extrauterine extension

DIFFERENTIAL DIAGNOSIS

Hydropic Placental Degeneration
- Chorionic villi are engorged
- Trophoblastic proliferation absent

Uterine Dysgerminoma
- Most frequent malignant germ cell tumor in women
- Heterogeneous uterine mass with multiple echolucent spaces
- HCG not elevated

Retained Products of Conception
- Also occurs in reproductive-aged women with irregular vaginal bleeding & elevated β-HCG titer
- Differentiate from GTD by correlating with clinical presentation, pattern of β-HCG progression & US appearance
- Unlike GTD, not centered in myometrium, no placental venous lakes

Incomplete Abortion
- Widening of the endometrial canal due to the presence of blood products
- May see fetal parts

Invasive Mole & Choriocarcinoma
- Diagnosis usually made on the basis of consistent or rising gonadotropin levels in the absence or following evacuation of a pregnancy
- Patients may present with persistent bleeding
- Otherwise, US findings are indistinguishable from those of a complete mole (unless see myometrial invasion)

PATHOLOGY

General Features
- General path comments
  - No fetal tissue present
  - Rarely coexist with a normal pregnancy
    - When it does, it is thought to be due to molar transformation of one twin placenta
- Genetics
  - 90% of complete moles result of dispermic fertilization of an empty ovum usually 46,XX
  - XY has been reported
  - In both XX & XY molar chromosomes have been shown to be entirely of paternal origin
- Epidemiology
  - Most common form of gestational trophoblastic disease
  - Occurs in 1 of every 1,000-2,000 pregnancies
  - Incidence estimated as high as 1 in 41 miscarriages
  - Can occur in a pregnant woman of any age but more common in those in their teens or between 40-50 years old

HYDATIFORM MOLE, COMPLETE MOLE

- ○ Women who have had a previous molar gestation are at increased risk to develop a similar subsequent lesion
- ○ Risk increases with the number of spontaneous abortions
- ○ North American and European countries with low or intermediate rates of risk
- ○ Asian and Latin American nations with high rates of disease
- Associated abnormalities: Ovarian theca lutein cysts in 25-60% of cases, resulting from overstimulation of lutein elements by large amounts of β-HCG produced by proliferating trophoblast

Gross Pathologic & Surgical Features
- Occupy uterine cavity & rarely present in fallopian tubes or ovaries
- Chorionic villi are converted into a mass of clear vesicles that resemble a cluster of grapes

Microscopic Features
- Characterized by diffuse hydropic villi, atypical trophoblastic proliferation, paucity of recognizable vessels
- Hydropic villous swelling with prominent acellular spaces
- Noninvasive process

CLINICAL ISSUES

Presentation
- Most common signs/symptoms
  - ○ Vaginal bleeding late in first trimester, during 2nd trimester
  - ○ Hyperemesis gravidarum
- Other signs/symptoms
  - ○ In early stages of development, cannot distinguish clinically from a normal pregnancy
  - ○ Uterus large for dates
  - ○ May present with pregnancy-induced hypertension
  - ○ Hyperthyroidism may occur because of the thyroid stimulating properties of β-HCG
  - ○ Anemia may occur as a result of plasma volume expansion
- Clinical Profile
  - ○ Patients with complete mole present with vaginal bleeding, uterine enlargement greater than expected for gestational age, & abnormally high level of serum β-HCG (> 100,000)
  - ○ HCG levels in both blood and urine greatly exceed that of a normal pregnancy at the same stage; serial determinations indicate rapidly mounting level
  - ○ Presence & course of disease can be monitored with quantitative levels of β-HCG
  - ○ Present with dyspnea, neurologic symptoms & abdominal pain a few weeks or months after last pregnancy

Natural History & Prognosis
- After uterine evacuation, a persistent trophoblastic tumor may develop
- May take 2-4 months for the theca lutein cysts to regress after molar evacuation
- Majority of moles, however, remain benign & present no further difficulty
  - ○ 20% of complete moles are followed by the malignant sequelae of invasive mole or choriocarcinoma

Treatment
- Suction curettage followed by metastatic disease work-up
- Hysterectomy advocated by gynecologists in patients over 35 years old who are not interested in preserving fertility
- After evacuation, β-HCG level should be monitored weekly until it is undetectable followed by monthly monitoring for 6-24 months
- In women with persistent disease or chemotherapy resistant disease, angiography useful in work-up of myometrial invasion and surgical management
- Pregnancy should be postponed to avoid confusing the clinical picture while monitoring β-HCG levels

DIAGNOSTIC CHECKLIST

Consider
- Once the diagnosis is made, patient should be evaluated for metastatic disease & molar pregnancy terminated

Image Interpretation Pearls
- Classic sonographic appearance of solid collection of echoes with numerous anechoic spaces

SELECTED REFERENCES

1. Bertel C et al: Sonographic diagnosis of gestational trophoblastic disease and comparison with retained products of conception. J Ultrasound Med. 25:985-93, 2006
2. Zhou Q et al: Sonographic and Doppler imaging in the diagnosis and treatment of gestational trophoblastic disease. A 12-year experience. J Ultrasound Med. 24:15-24, 2005
3. Leyendecker JR et al: MR imaging of maternal diseases of the abdomen and pelvis during pregnancy and the immediate postpartum period. Radiographics. 24:1301-16, 2004
4. Williams P et al: US of abnormal uterine bleeding. Radiographics. 23:703-18, 2003
5. Jung SE et al: MR imaging of maternal diseases in pregnancy. AJR. 177:1293-300, 2001
6. Green CL et al: Gestational trophoblastic disease: a spectrum of radiologic diagnosis. Radiographics. 16:1371-84, 1996
7. Wagner BJ et al: Gestational trophoblastic disease: radiologic-pathologic Correlation. Radiographics. 16:131-48, 1996

HYDATIFORM MOLE, COMPLETE MOLE

IMAGE GALLERY

Typical

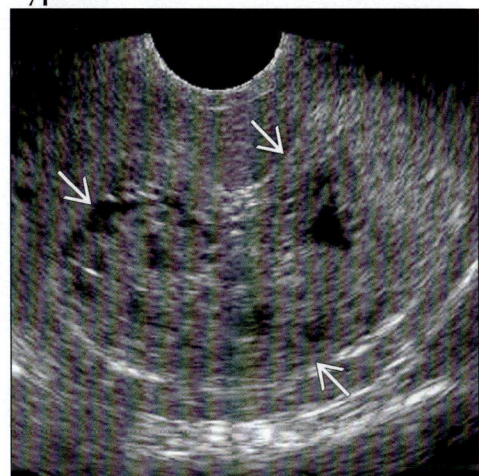
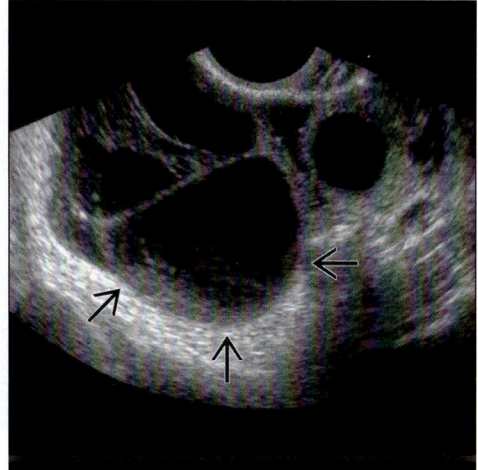

(Left) Sagittal transvaginal ultrasound shows multiple cystic structures ➡ filling the gestational sac. *(Right)* Coronal transvaginal ultrasound shows an enlarged ovary in the same patient with replacement of parenchyma with multiple multilocular cysts ➡ giving the ovary a "soap-bubble" appearance.

Typical

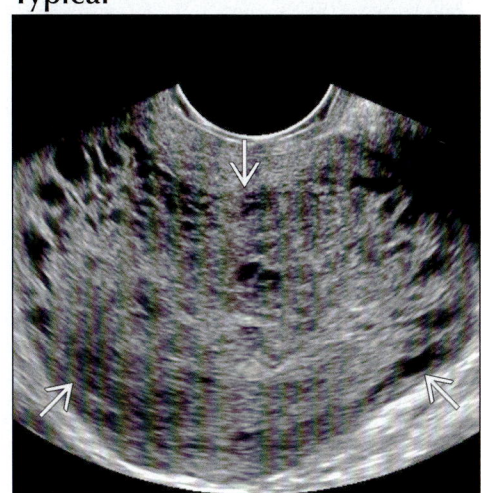
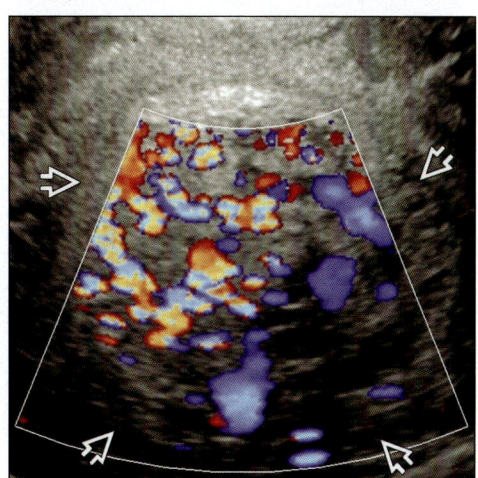

(Left) Transverse transvaginal ultrasound shows multiple cystic structures ("cluster of grapes") ➡ filling the uterine cavity and absence of fetal parts. *(Right)* Coronal color Doppler ultrasound of the same patient shows the lesion ➡ to be very vascular.

Typical

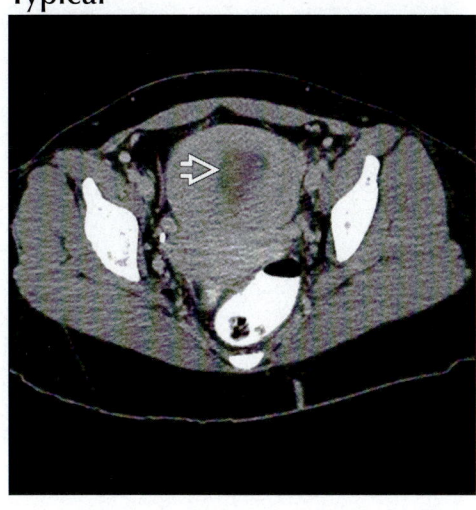
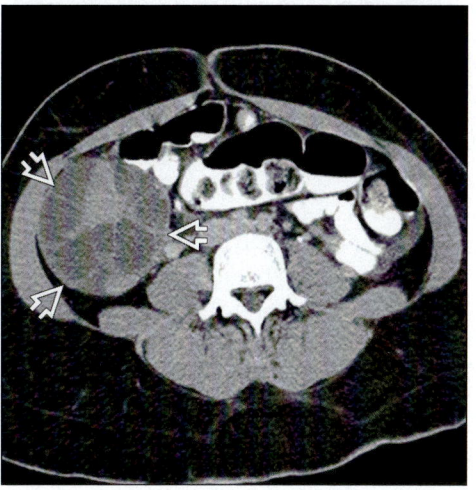

(Left) Axial CECT shows normal sized uterus with cystic components ➡ in uterine cavity. *(Right)* Axial CECT in the same patient shows right ovary with multiple thick-walled theca lutein cysts in the "spoke wheel" pattern ➡.

HYDATIFORM MOLE, COMPLETE MOLE

(Left) Sagittal transvaginal ultrasound in a 53 year old woman with 3 months of amenorrhea shows heterogeneous material in the endometrial cavity. This was an unexpected pregnancy that was a complete mole. (Right) Sagittal color Doppler ultrasound in same patient as on left shows a paucity of blood flow to the endometrial contents.

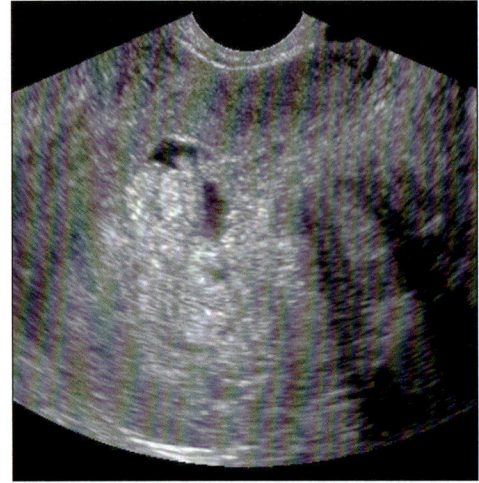

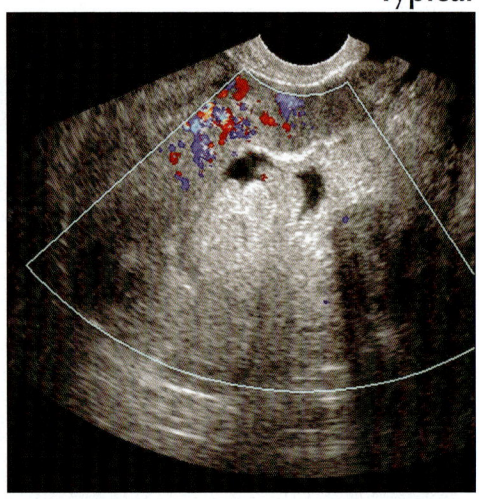
Typical

(Left) Sagittal transabdominal ultrasound shows distension of the endometrial cavity ➡ with multiple cystic spaces and an ovary with multiple theca lutein cysts ➡. (Right) Sagittal transvaginal ultrasound in same patient as left shows the multiple thin walled cysts in the ovary. Some of the cysts have some hemorrhagic debris within them.

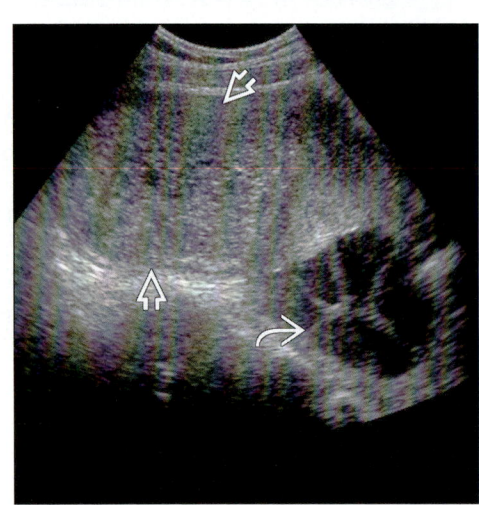

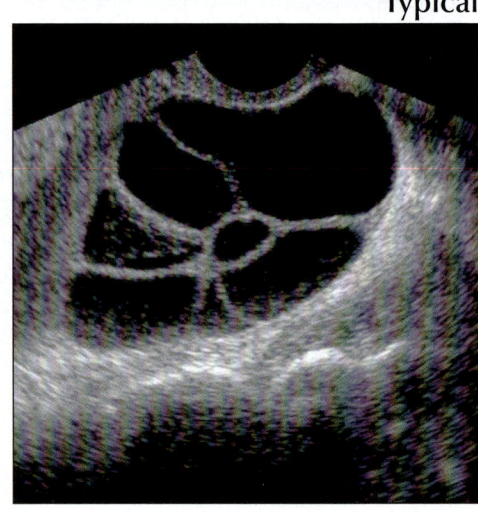
Typical

(Left) Sagittal transabdominal ultrasound shows an endometrial cavity with irregularly thickened endometrium and some fluid. This appearance of a molar pregnancy could be mistaken for a miscarriage. (Right) Transverse transvaginal ultrasound in same patient as on left shows the irregularity of the material within the endometrial cavity. Histology was a complete molar pregnancy.

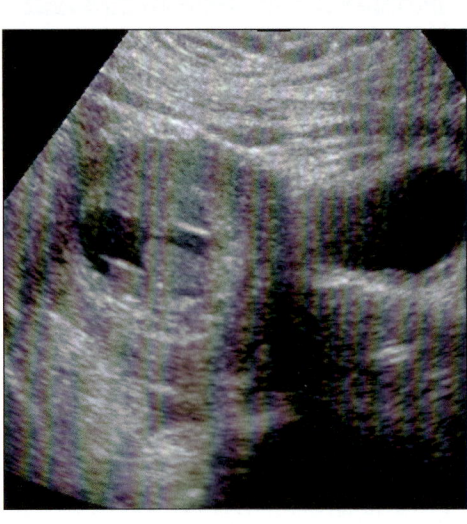

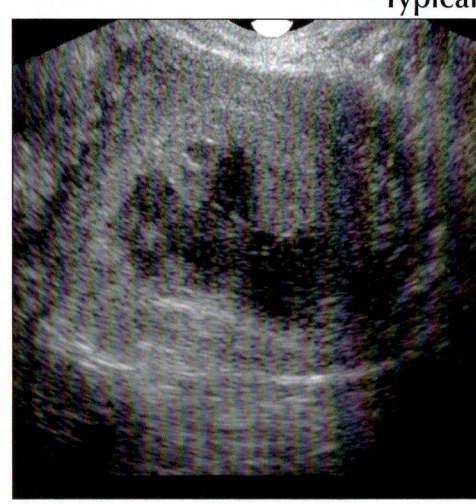
Typical

HYDATIFORM MOLE, COMPLETE MOLE

Typical

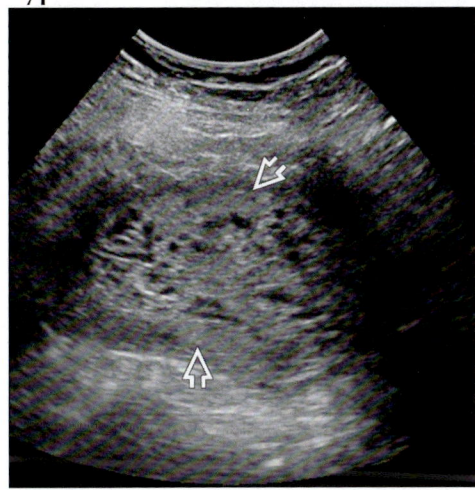
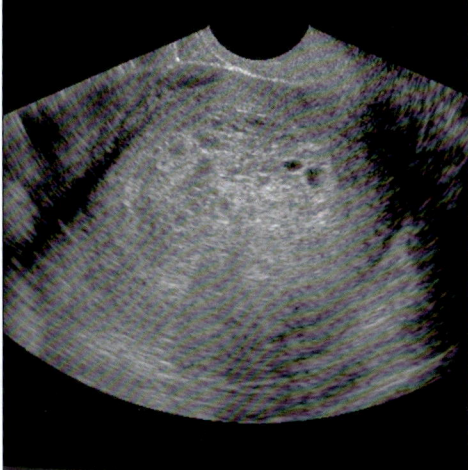

(Left) Transverse transabdominal ultrasound shows an enlarged uterus with thickened endometrium ➤ with multiple cystic spaces. *(Right)* Sagittal transvaginal ultrasound shows a distended endometrial cavity with multiple cystic spaces in a 40 year old with complete hydatidiform mole.

Typical

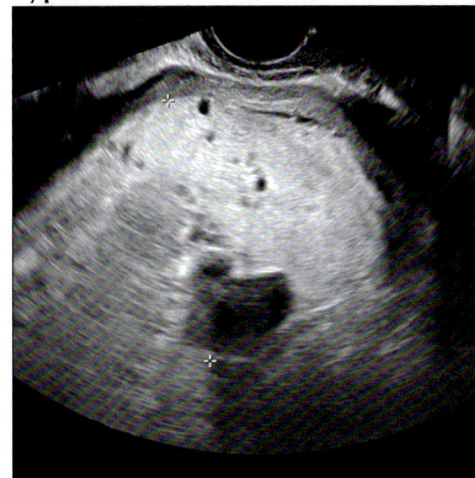
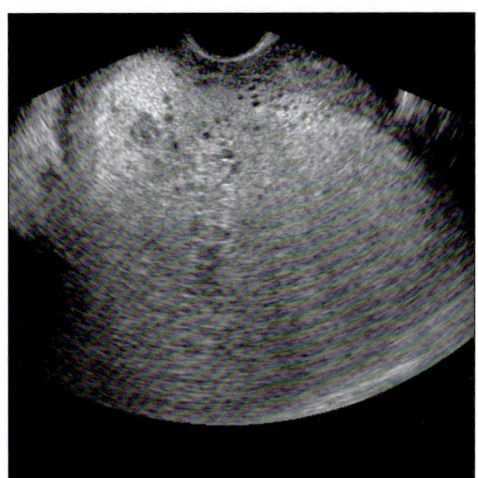

(Left) Sagittal transvaginal ultrasound shows a thickened endometrial cavity (calipers) with cystic spaces in patient with molar pregnancy. *(Right)* Sagittal transvaginal ultrasound shows a dramatically thickened endometrial cavity. The margins of the myometrium are ill-defined. Histology was complete molar pregnancy.

Typical

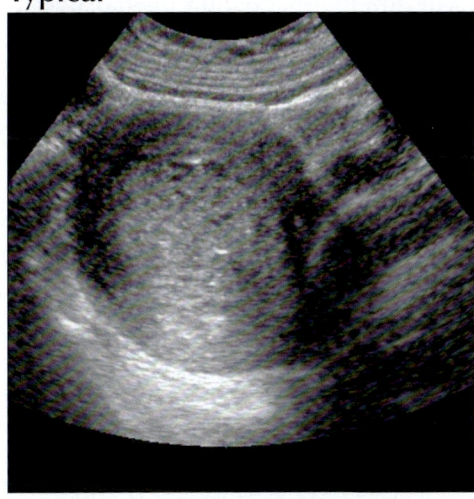
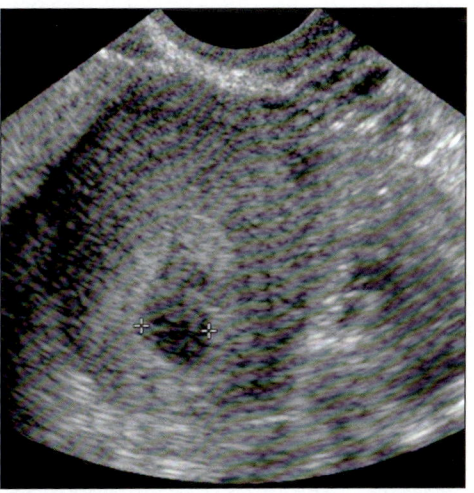

(Left) Sagittal transabdominal ultrasound shows a thickened endometrial cavity in a woman with a molar pregnancy. *(Right)* Sagittal transvaginal ultrasound shows a fluid collection (calipers) in the endometrial cavity with some debris. This could be a pseudosac or an abnormal early pregnancy. Histology was complete mole.

HYDATIFORM MOLE, PARTIAL MOLE

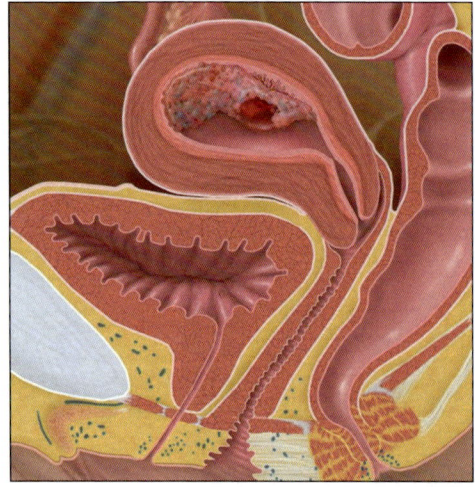

Sagittal graphic shows cystic placenta in partial hydatidiform mole.

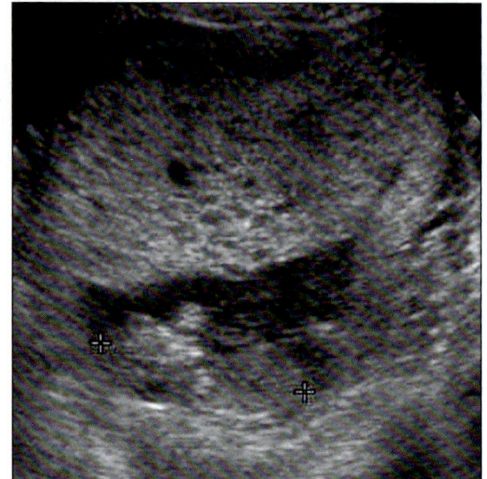

Transverse transabdominal ultrasound at 13 weeks shows a small fetus (calipers) and a large cystic placenta.

TERMINOLOGY

Abbreviations and Synonyms
- Gestational trophoblastic disease

Definitions
- Usually paternally derived triploid conceptions → embryonal development associated with trophoblastic hyperplasia and focal hydropic chorionic villi

IMAGING FINDINGS

General Features
- Best diagnostic clue: Intrauterine gestation with focal placental thickening and cystic changes

Ultrasonographic Findings
- Grayscale Ultrasound
  ○ Thickened placenta with focal cystic changes or increased echogenicity
    ▪ In first trimester placental changes are limited
  ○ Abnormal gestational sac
    ▪ Ratio of transverse to anteroposterior dimension of gestational sac greater than 1.5
    ▪ May present as empty sac (mean diameter ≥ 20 mm or no change in size after 1-2 weeks)
    ▪ May present as delayed miscarriage (embryonic pole ≥ 6 mm with no cardiac activity)
  ○ If fetal tissue present → 80% growth restricted
    ▪ ± Fetal cardiac activity
    ▪ Multiple anomalies (hand and cardiac abnormalities, cerebral ventriculomegaly, micrognathia)
    ▪ Fetal nuchal translucency at 10-14 weeks → above 95th percentile in 59% of cases
  ○ Amniotic fluid may be reduced
  ○ Theca lutein cysts are uncommon
- Color Doppler
  ○ Tissue typically hypervascular
    ▪ High velocity, low impedance flow (high diastolic flow) during first and early second trimester → mean arterial resistive indices of 0.56
    ▪ Mean arterial resistive indices for: Normal pregnancy → 0.66, complete mole → 0.55, invasive mole → 0.28, choriocarcinoma → 0.25

DDx: Placental Disorders

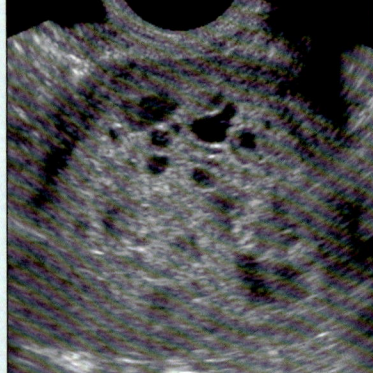
Complete Mole

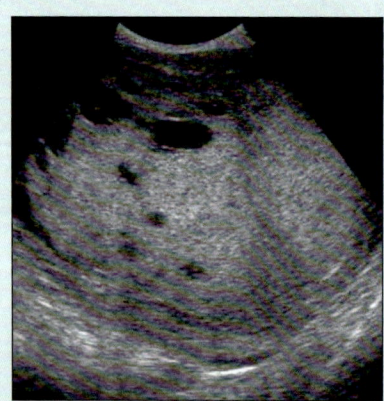
Beckwith Wiedemann Syndrome

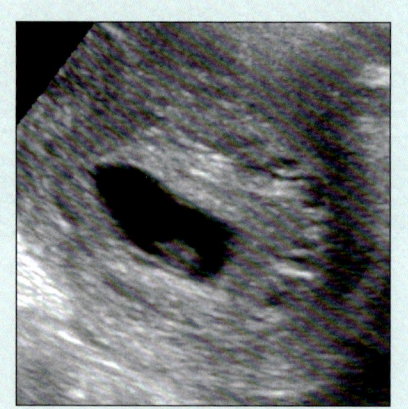
Hydropic Abortion

HYDATIFORM MOLE, PARTIAL MOLE

Key Facts

Terminology
- Usually paternally derived triploid conceptions → embryonal development associated with trophoblastic hyperplasia and focal hydropic chorionic villi

Imaging Findings
- Best diagnostic clue: Intrauterine gestation with focal placental thickening and cystic changes
- Ratio of transverse to anteroposterior dimension of gestational sac greater than 1.5
- May present as empty sac (mean diameter ≥ 20 mm or no change in size after 1-2 weeks)
- May present as delayed miscarriage (embryonic pole ≥ 6 mm with no cardiac activity)
- If fetal tissue present → 80% growth restricted
- Multiple anomalies (hand and cardiac abnormalities, cerebral ventriculomegaly, micrognathia)
- Detection rates improve after 14 weeks, most frequently diagnosed between 15-20 weeks

Top Differential Diagnoses
- Incomplete or Missed Miscarriage
- Complete Hydatidiform Mole
- Placental Mesenchymal Dysplasia
- Twin Pregnancy Complicated by a Co-Existing Molar Pregnancy

Clinical Issues
- Vaginal bleeding (usually late first trimester)
- Risk of progression to persistent gestational trophoblastic disease → 2-4%

Imaging Recommendations
- Best imaging tool
  - Overall detection rates for ultrasound: 18-49% of partial moles → majority diagnosed as miscarriage
    - Sensitivity 20% and positive predictive value 22%
    - Detection rates improve after 14 weeks, most frequently diagnosed between 15-20 weeks
    - False positive rates 20% (hydropic miscarriages)
- Protocol advice: Combined testing of ultrasound and serum hCG improves diagnostic accuracy

DIFFERENTIAL DIAGNOSIS

Incomplete or Missed Miscarriage
- Hydropic degeneration of placenta characterized by edematous villi with attenuated trophoblastic lining
  - Prolonged retention in utero (missed miscarriages)
  - Focal hydropic changes can be found in aneuploidy

Complete Hydatidiform Mole
- No fetal tissue present
- Villi show hydropic change and central cistern formation, both often mild at early gestations
  - Diffuse, circumferential trophoblastic hyperplasia
- Ploidy analysis and p 57 immunohistochemistry will distinguish from partial mole in difficult cases

Placental Mesenchymal Dysplasia
- Characterized by placentomegaly and cystic placenta
  - Histologically distinguished from partial mole because of absence of trophoblastic proliferation
  - Associated with normal fetus, growth restriction or features of overgrowth (Beckwith Wiedemann syndrome)
    - Beckwith-Wiedemann syndrome: Rare, congenital overgrowth syndrome → caused by mutation in chromosome 11p15.5 region
    - Placenta → marked umbilical edema, large villi with central cavitation
    - Fetus has omphalocele, mild microcephaly, ear lobe creases, macrosomia, macroglossia, visceromegaly, increased incidence of childhood tumors

Twin Pregnancy Complicated by a Co-Existing Molar Pregnancy
- Rare for both to coexist, also reported with triplets
- Pregnancy may progress to delivery but high risk of complications → important to distinguish early
  - 25% chance of a live birth
  - 35% → develop persistent trophoblastic disease
  - 20% of cases develop early onset of preeclampsia
- Mole does not grow proportionally with normal placenta → at 17-20 weeks it may partially cover normal placenta (difficult to distinguish from partial mole)
- Most cases → normal placenta separate from the mole

PATHOLOGY

General Features
- Genetics
  - Partial moles have a triploid karyotype in which two of the three chromosomal complements are derived from the father → diandric monogynic (70% → 69, XXY; 27% → 69, XXX; 3% → 69 XYY)
    - 75% of cases → normal ovum (one set of haploid maternal chromosomes) fertilized by two spermatozoa (two sets of haploid paternal chromosomes)
    - 25% of cases → non-disjunction in meiosis I or meiosis II of spermatogenesis results in extra set of paternal chromosomes in one sperm (diandric) which fertilizes a haploid (monogynic) ovum
  - Not all triploid gestations present as partial moles → 10% occur due to non-disjunction in meiosis I or meiosis II of oogenesis (digynic) and one haploid set of paternal chromosomes (monoandric)

HYDATIFORM MOLE, PARTIAL MOLE

- If two of the three chromosomal complements are derived from mother → triploidy will present with intrauterine growth retardation, normal placenta
  - Rare reported cases of non-triploid partial moles (likely misdiagnosed early complete moles)
- Epidemiology
  - Occurs in 1 of 700 conceptions
  - Incidence is 2-3 times higher than complete mole

Gross Pathologic & Surgical Features
- Variable gross appearance, depends on gestational age, mimics spontaneous abortion
  - Focal hydropic change develops in second trimester, vesicles are few or absent macroscopically
  - Placental tissue → not as bulky as complete mole
  - Fetal parts, membranes and cord frequently found

Microscopic Features
- Two populations of villi → normal and hydropic (mild and focal involvement)
  - Some villi are large and cavitated, others have scalloped borders with trophoblastic inclusions
  - Focal areas of trophoblastic hyperplasia, mild atypia
- Stromal vessels → contain nucleated fetal red blood cells
- Fetal tissue with multiple malformations → marked growth retardation, prominent forehead, micrognathia, microphthalmia, hypogonadism, ambiguous genitalia, hand or toe syndactyly
  - Absence of fetal tissue does not exclude diagnosis
- Accuracy of histologic diagnosis enhanced by flow cytometry or image analysis → ploidy analysis of DNA
- Positive stain for p57 and PHLDA2 (complete moles have no immunoreactivity)

CLINICAL ISSUES

Presentation
- Most common signs/symptoms
  - Most present as missed or incomplete miscarriages
    - Vaginal bleeding (usually late first trimester)
- Other signs/symptoms
  - Theca lutein cysts, hyperthyroidism, hyperemesis rarely seen
  - Preeclampsia in 2.5%
  - Small or appropriate uterine size (96% of cases)
  - Levels of hCG typically in low to normal range
    - 6% → excessive levels over 100,000 mIU/mL

Demographics
- Age: Women of all reproductive ages
- Ethnicity
  - Maternal Asian race is major risk factor
    - Incidence in Southeast Asia is 7 to 10 times higher than in Europe or North America
    - Poor individuals show 10 fold greater increased risk than wealthy individuals

Natural History & Prognosis
- Clinical diagnosis in 90% of cases → incomplete or missed miscarriage (correct diagnosis on histology)
- Majority of partial moles miscarry before 10-12 weeks
  - Less often associated with placental molar changes in first trimester than in second or third trimester
- Risk of progression to persistent gestational trophoblastic disease → 2-4%
  - Lungs are most common site of metastasis
- Risk of second molar pregnancy is 1.7%

Treatment
- Evacuation of uterine contents by suction curettage followed by sharp curettage (confirms removal)
- If no desire for future fertility, hysterectomy eliminates risk of local invasion but does not prevent metastasis
- Managed as low-risk disease; followed to exclude persistent mole
  - Beta hCG levels are monitored serially → every week until < 5 mIU/mL for 3 weeks, then every month for 6 months, then every year for 1-3 years
  - Normalize on average after 2 months
  - Persistent mole suspected if levels persist or increase
  - If serum hCG levels spontaneously decline and become undetectable → virtually no risk of developing gestational trophoblastic neoplasia → shorter period of hCG followup may be reasonable
- Contraception for 6-12 months

DIAGNOSTIC CHECKLIST

Consider
- Partial molar pregnancies examined in first trimester may not have developed the degree of hydropic villus change detectable by ultrasound or histology
- Majority of partial molar cases present as missed miscarriage → histological criteria should provides final diagnosis
- Few small anechoic spaces can be present in the placenta without clinical significance

Image Interpretation Pearls
- Consider partial mole if cystic changes in placenta are associated with empty sac, missed miscarriage, severe intrauterine growth restriction or multiple congenital anomalies

SELECTED REFERENCES
1. Garner EI et al: Gestational trophoblastic disease. Clin Obstet Gynecol. 50(1):112-22, 2007
2. Kirk E et al: The accuracy of first trimester ultrasound in the diagnosis of hydatidiform mole. Ultrasound Obstet Gynecol. 29(1):70-5, 2007
3. Parveen Z et al: Placental mesenchymal dysplasia. Arch Pathol Lab Med. 131(1):131-7, 2007
4. Fowler DJ et al: Routine pre-evacuation ultrasound diagnosis of hydatidiform mole: experience of more than 1000 cases from a regional referral center. Ultrasound Obstet Gynecol. 27(1):56-60, 2006
5. Johns J et al: A prospective study of ultrasound screening for molar pregnancies in missed miscarriages. Ultrasound Obstet Gynecol. 25(5):493-7, 2005
6. Jauniaux E: Partial moles: from postnatal to prenatal diagnosis. Placenta. 20(5-6):379-88, 1999

HYDATIFORM MOLE, PARTIAL MOLE

IMAGE GALLERY

Typical

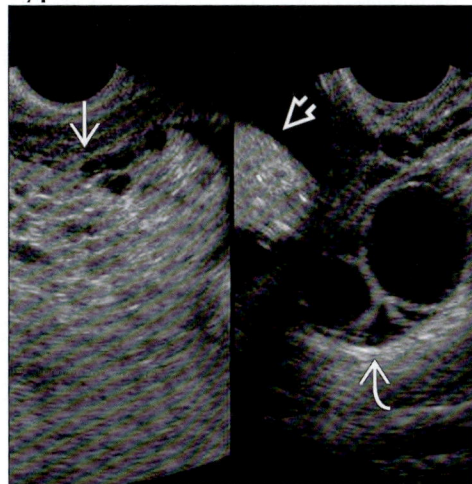
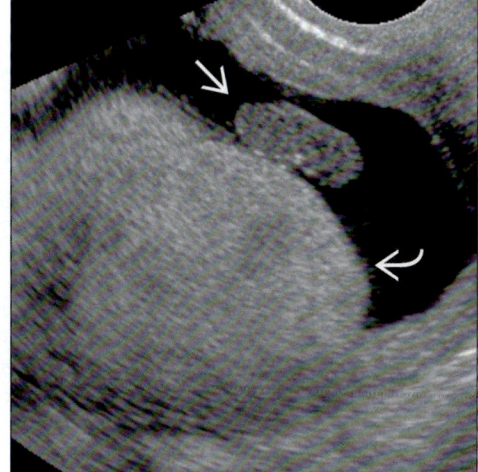

(Left) Transvaginal ultrasound shows cystic placental changes ➡ with areas of increased echogenicity ➡ and multicystic ovary ➡. *(Right)* Transvaginal ultrasound shows thickened ➡ echogenic placenta and a live intrauterine gestation ➡ with size less than dates (ultrasound size of 8 weeks 5 days, age by dates: 14 weeks 6 days).

Typical

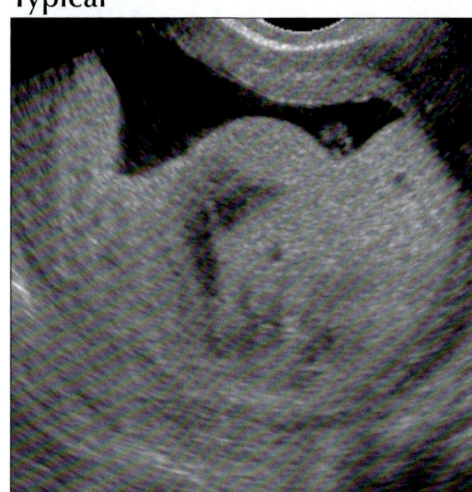
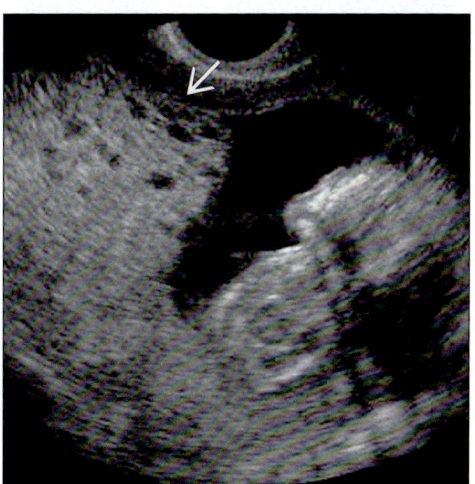

(Left) Transvaginal ultrasound shows thickened placenta with cystic changes. The histologic diagnosis was partial mole. *(Right)* Transvaginal ultrasound in a partial mole shows a live intrauterine gestation with cystic changes of the placenta ➡.

Typical

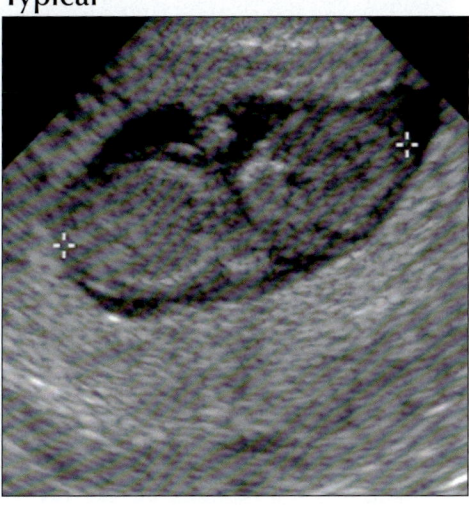
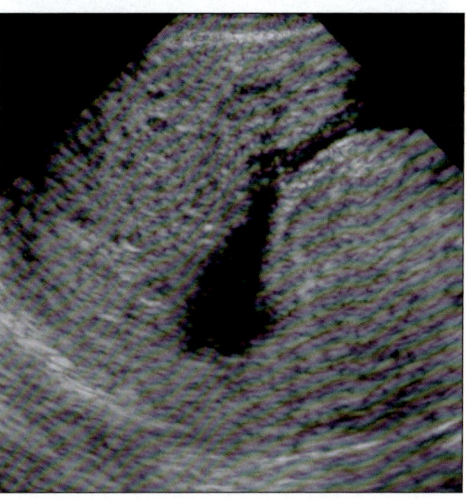

(Left) Transvaginal ultrasound shows an intrauterine gestation (calipers) with no heart rate, low amniotic fluid and a crown rump length that corresponds to 10 weeks and 5 days, two weeks less than dates. *(Right)* Transvaginal ultrasound in the same patient as previous image, shows thickening of the placenta associated with cystic changes. The histologic diagnosis was partial mole.

HYDATIFORM MOLE, PARTIAL MOLE

(Left) Transverse transabdominal ultrasound in an Asian patient with a 15 week pregnancy by dates, demonstrates a partial mole with an empty sac and a thickened and cystic placenta. *(Right)* Transabdominal ultrasound of a histologically proven partial mole shows a live embryo with early IUGR, ventriculomegaly ➡, low amniotic fluid and no obvious placental abnormalities.

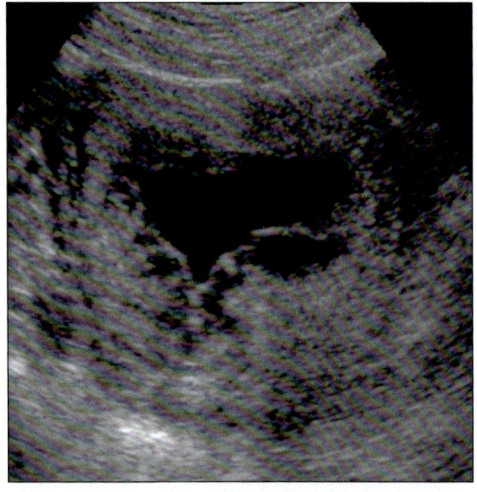
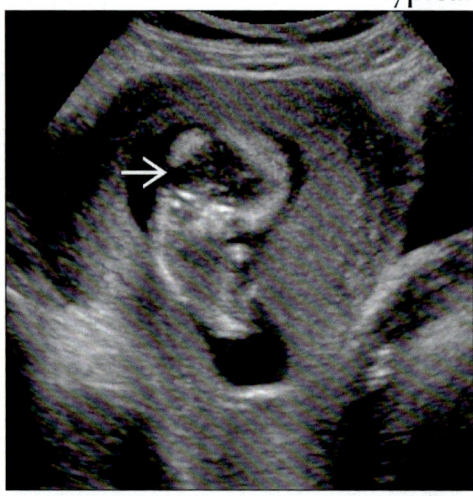

(Left) Axial transvaginal ultrasound in the same fetus as previous image shows ventriculomegaly (calipers). *(Right)* Sagittal transabdominal ultrasound shows growth restricted fetus with oligohydramnios. Histology showed a partial mole.

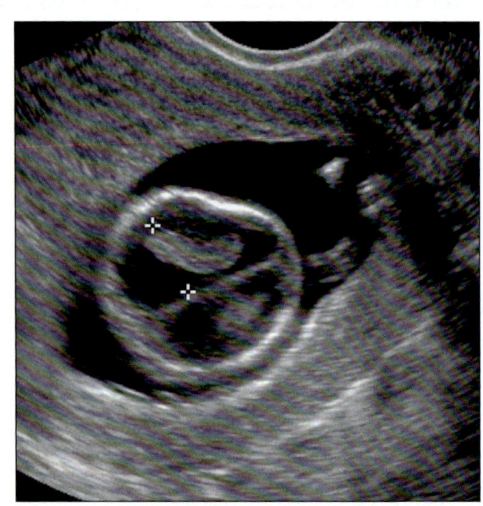
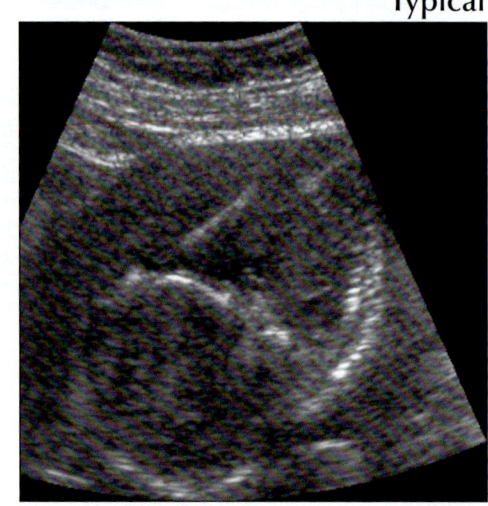

(Left) Sagittal transvaginal ultrasound shows early pregnancy at 8 weeks, one week less than dates with no other anomalies. *(Right)* Sagittal transvaginal ultrasound shows thick cystic placenta and embryonic pole ➡ in a patient with partial mole.

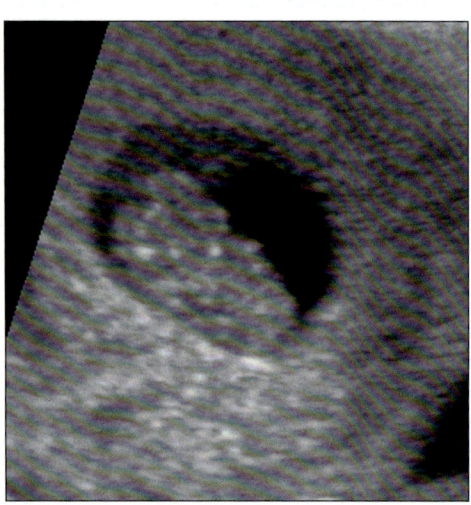
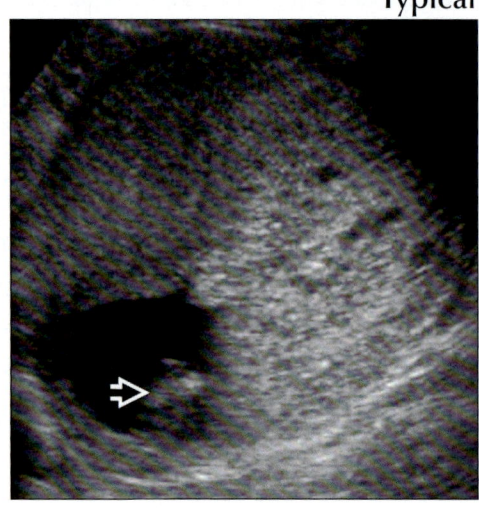

HYDATIFORM MOLE, PARTIAL MOLE

Typical

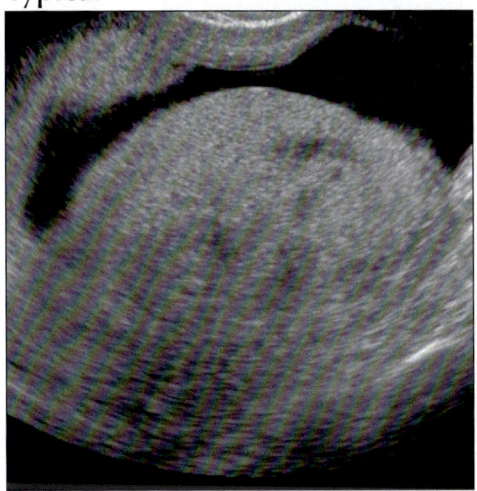 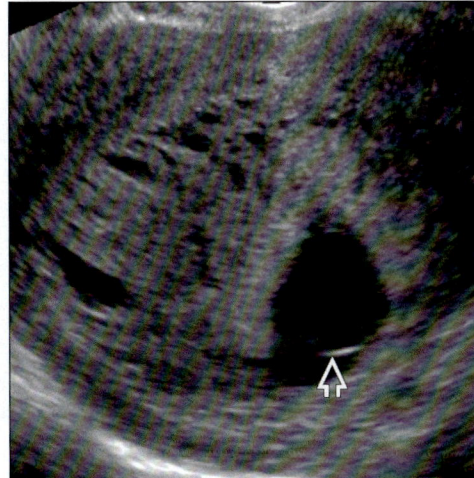

(Left) Lateral transvaginal ultrasound shows thick cystic placenta in patient with partial mole. *(Right)* Sagittal transvaginal ultrasound shows cystic placenta and empty amnion ➲ in a patient with partial mole.

Typical

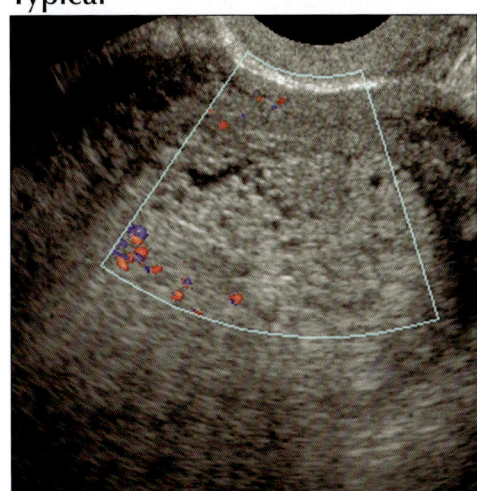 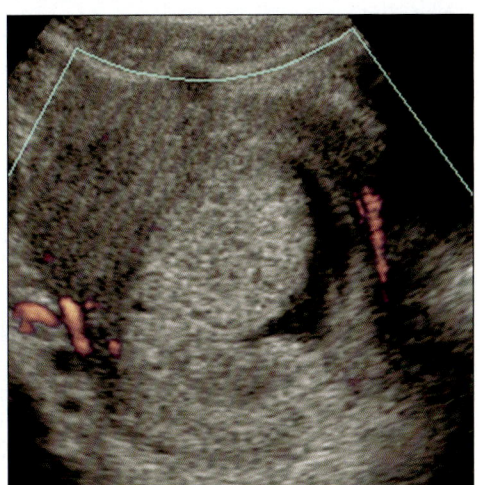

(Left) Axial color Doppler ultrasound shows cystic placenta with paucity of vascularity. B-hCG was 160,000 mIU/mL. *(Right)* Sagittal power Doppler ultrasound at 12 weeks gestation shows thickened placenta with small cysts. Histology was partial mole.

Typical

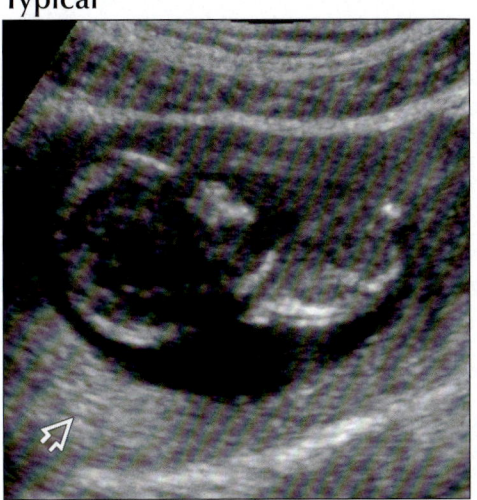 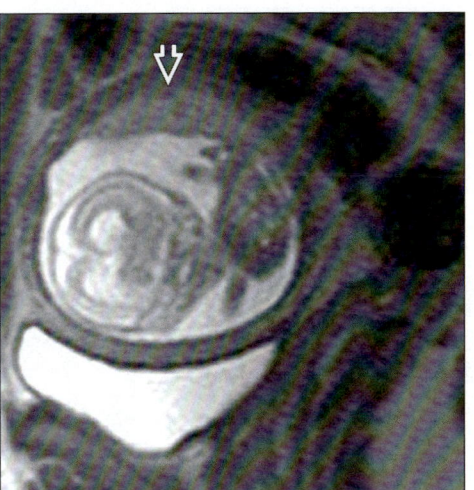

(Left) Axial transabdominal ultrasound shows growth restricted fetus. Note the small chest size with respect to the fetal head. The placenta is small ➲. *(Right)* Sagittal T2WI MR in same fetus as previous image, shows growth restricted fetus with ventriculomegaly and small placenta ➲.

INVASIVE MOLE

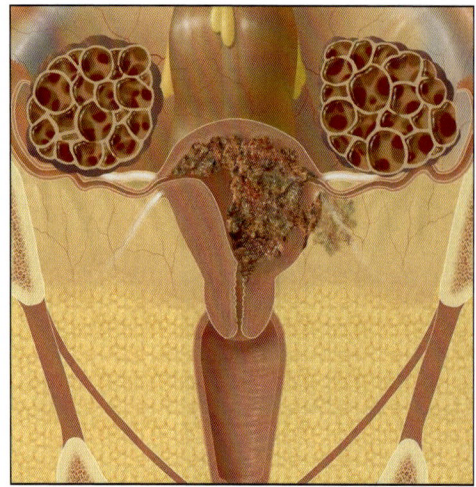

Coronal graphic shows an invasive mole characterized by villi that invade the underlying myometrium, traverse the serosa and extend into the left broad ligament. Note the bilateral theca lutein cysts.

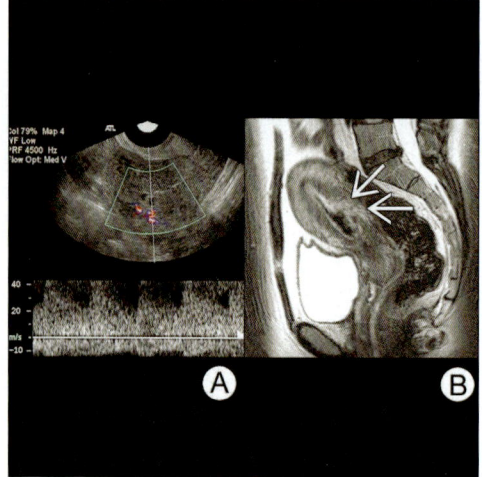

(A) Duplex TVS shows a vascular echogenic mass with myometrial lucencies & high velocity, low resistance flow. (B) Sagittal T2WI shows abnormal signal extending from endometrium into myometrium ➡.

TERMINOLOGY

Abbreviations and Synonyms
- Invasive gestational trophoblastic disease or neoplasia
- Invasive GTD or invasive GTN
- Persistent gestational trophoplastic neoplasia
- Chorioadenoma destruens

Definitions
- Severe trophoblastic overgrowth & penetration by trophoblastic elements, including whole villi, deep into myometrium
  - There may be penetration into peritoneum, parametrium or vagina
  - While locally invasive, rarely metastasize to distant sites (unlike choriocarcinoma)

IMAGING FINDINGS

General Features
- Best diagnostic clue
  - Highly vascular tumor
  - Endometrial solid mass punctuated by cystic spaces (4-5 mm) with associated invasion of adjacent myometrium, parametrium & other pelvic structures
  - Focal areas of abnormality within myometrium
- Location: Uterine

Radiographic Findings
- Radiography: Soft tissue density representing enlarged uterus

Ultrasonographic Findings
- Color Doppler
  - Increased velocities
  - Low resistance: Low resistive indices (RI) ranging from 0.2 to 0.45
- Power Doppler: Increased vascularity
- Transvaginal ultrasound (TVS) findings
  - Heterogeneous, echogenic mass punctuated by anechoic lucencies within the endometrial cavity & extending into underlying myometrium
  - Alternatively, focal nodules of increased echogenicity within myometrium
  - Rarely image extension outside of uterus
  - May see theca lutein cysts

DDx: Invasive Mole

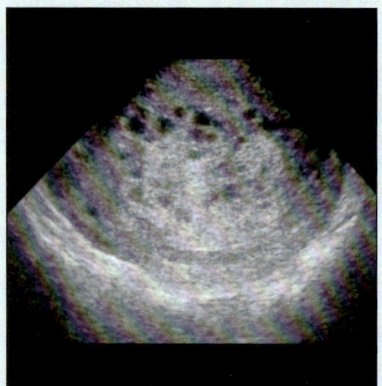

Choriocarcinoma

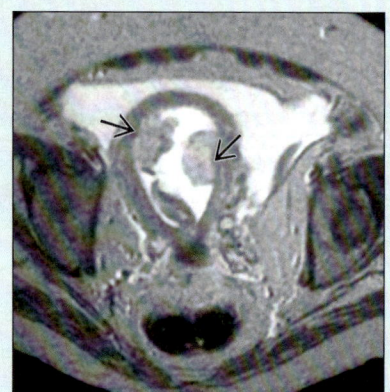

Endometrial Cancer

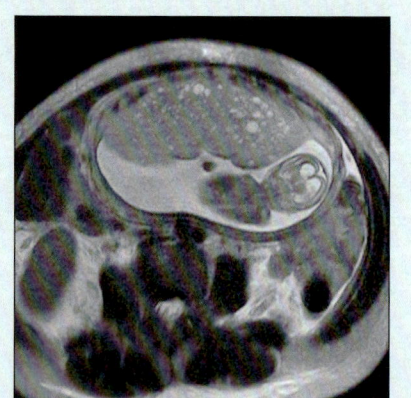

Partial Mole

INVASIVE MOLE

Key Facts

Terminology
- Invasive gestational trophoblastic disease or neoplasia
- Severe trophoblastic overgrowth & penetration by trophoblastic elements, including whole villi, deep into myometrium
- There may be penetration into peritoneum, parametrium or vagina

Imaging Findings
- Highly vascular tumor
- Endometrial solid mass punctuated by cystic spaces (4-5 mm) with associated invasion of adjacent myometrium, parametrium & other pelvic structures
- Focal areas of abnormality within myometrium
- Ill-defined, heterogeneous markedly enhancing lesion with low-attenuation nonenhancing foci (hydropic villi) that involves the endometrium & myometrium & may extend beyond uterus
- Theca lutein cysts may be present

Top Differential Diagnoses
- Choriocarcinoma
- Complete Mole
- Abnormal cystic placenta with abnormal fetus
- Endometrial Cancer
- Placental Site Trophoblastic Tumor

Clinical Issues
- May present with heavy vaginal bleeding
- Diagnosis is important for management: Chemotherapy is often curative

CT Findings
- CECT
  - Ill-defined, heterogeneous markedly enhancing lesion with low-attenuation nonenhancing foci (hydropic villi) that involves the endometrium & myometrium & may extend beyond uterus
  - Marked focal enhancement within myometrium with low-attenuation nonenhancing foci that may extend beyond uterus
  - May see enlarged, enhancing pelvic vessels
  - Theca lutein cysts may be present

MR Findings
- T1WI
  - Foci of high signal intensity (SI): Hemorrhage
  - Serpiginous signal voids: Dilated vessels
- T2WI
  - Heterogeneous, irregular, high SI mass invading & expanding myometrium
  - Indistinct boundary between tumor & myometrium
  - Complete or partial loss of zonal anatomy
    - Disruption of junctional zone
  - Prominent serpiginous signal voids of enlarged blood vessels
  - Parametrial involvement characterized by abnormal high SI beyond confines of the uterus
- T1 C+: Marked enhancement of tumor mass & associated blood vessels
- Enlarged uterus
- Ovarian theca lutein cysts may be present
- Decrease in uterine volume & tumor size, return of zonal anatomy & regression of hypervascularity parallels decrease in HCG with treatment
  - HCG levels may still be elevated even when MR returns to normal

Angiographic Findings
- Conventional: Abnormal vessels originating from internal iliac arteries

Imaging Recommendations
- Transvaginal ultrasound for initial evaluation
- MR for further evaluation to include myometrial invasion
- CT or MR for distant metastases
- HCG levels remain arbiter of management decisions

DIFFERENTIAL DIAGNOSIS

Choriocarcinoma
- May be indistinguishable from invasive mole on imaging
- HCG levels are usually higher than with invasive mole
- Discrete central invasive uterine mass with hemorrhage & necrosis
- Distant metastases (usually to lung) aid diagnosis
- No hydropic villi in choriocarcinoma (vs. invasive mole)

Complete Mole
- Hyperechoic mass with numerous cystic space filling uterine cavity

Partial Mole
- Abnormal cystic placenta with abnormal fetus

Endometrial Cancer
- Usually postmenopausal women who present with bleeding
- No temporal association with gravid state
- Not as vascular as invasive mole

Placental Site Trophoblastic Tumor
- Rare tumor that develops in women who have recently been pregnant
- May occur at any site in uterus & may be indistinguishable from mole

PATHOLOGY

General Features
- General path comments: Hydropic villi invade the myometrium, blood vessels & beyond
- Genetics: Errant fertilization

INVASIVE MOLE

- Etiology
  - Majority arise from hydatidiform mole (50%)
  - Can arise from abortion (25%)
  - May even arise following apparent normal or ectopic pregnancy (25%)
- Epidemiology: 6-10x more frequent than choriocarcinoma

Gross Pathologic & Surgical Features
- Erosive, hemorrhagic lesion extending from uterine cavity into myometrium forming a ragged irregular mass
- Invasion can range from superficial penetration to extension through wall, with perforation into adjacent structures
- Molar vesicles are often grossly apparent

Microscopic Features
- Excessive trophoblastic overgrowth with extensive penetration by hydropic villi & trophoblastic elements deep into myometrium & beyond
- Trophoblastic atypia is common (slightly proliferative to extreme atypia)

CLINICAL ISSUES

Presentation
- Most common signs/symptoms
  - May present with heavy vaginal bleeding
    - Usually after evacuation of molar pregnancy
- Other signs/symptoms: Fever and signs of sepsis can evolve if uterine rupture occurs
- Diagnosis is suggested on basis of consistent or rising human chorionic gonadotropin (HCG) levels in absence of, or following evacuation of a pregnancy
- Diagnosis is important for management: Chemotherapy is often curative
- Heavy vaginal bleeding, usually after evacuation of a molar pregnancy

Demographics
- Age: Reproductive age women

Natural History & Prognosis
- Tumor locally invades pelvis; may regress spontaneously
  - Vector of spread: Local invasion into myometrium, peritoneum, parametrium, vagina, broad ligament & vulva
- Rarely metastasize
- Excellent following therapy: Cure rate of > 95%
- If untreated, highly fatal
- Degree of myometrial invasion is prognostic factor
- Resistive indices measured on Doppler have shown to prognosticate response to chemotherapy
  - Higher RIs associated with better response to fewer courses of single chemotherapeutic agent
  - Lower RIs associated with poorer response and increased need for combined chemotherapy
- Lower pre-treatment β-hCG have less need for multiple courses of chemotherapy

Treatment
- Chemotherapy is mainstay of therapy
- Hysterectomy in select cases

DIAGNOSTIC CHECKLIST

Consider
- Invasive mole in a reproductive age woman with a hypervascular endometrial & myometrial mass with elevated β-hCG in the absence of a current pregnancy

Image Interpretation Pearls
- Vascular endometrial mass showing extension into the myometrium
- Possible thecal lutein cysts

SELECTED REFERENCES

1. Allen SD et al: Radiology of gestational trophoblastic neoplasia. Clin Radiol. 61(4):301-13, 2006
2. Taskin S et al: Invasive mole in a postmenopausal woman. Int J Gynaecol Obstet. 93(2):156-7, 2006
3. Jain KA: Gestational trophoblastic disease: pictorial review. Ultrasound Q. 21(4):245-53, 2005
4. Zhou Q et al: Sonographic and Doppler imaging in the diagnosis and treatment of gestational trophoblastic disease: a 12-year experience. J Ultrasound Med. 24(1):15-24, 2005
5. Leyendecker JR et al: MR imaging of maternal diseases of the abdomen and pelvis during pregnancy and the immediate postpartum period. Radiographics. 24(5):1301-16, 2004
6. Oguz S et al: Doppler study of myometrium in invasive gestational trophoblastic disease. Int J Gynecol Cancer. 14(5):972-9, 2004
7. Tsukihara S et al: Ultrasound-guided local injection of methotrexate to treat an invasive hydatidiform mole. J Obstet Gynaecol Res. 30(3):202-4, 2004
8. Altieri A et al: Epidemiology and aetiology of gestational trophoblastic diseases. Lancet Oncol. 4(11):670-8, 2003
9. Cheung AN: Pathology of gestational trophoblastic diseases. Best Pract Res Clin Obstet Gynaecol. 17(6):849-68, 2003
10. Köhorn EI et al: Nonmetastatic gestational trophoblastic neoplasia. Role of ultrasonography and magnetic resonance imaging. J Reprod Med. 43(1):14-20, 1998
11. Green CL et al: Gestational trophoblastic disease: a spectrum of radiologic diagnosis. Radiographics. 16(6):1371-84, 1996
12. Preidler KW et al: Magnetic resonance imaging in patients with gestational trophoblastic disease. Invest Radiol. 31(8):492-6, 1996
13. Wagner BJ et al: From the archives of the AFIP. Gestational trophoblastic disease: radiologic-pathologic correlation. Radiographics. 16(1):131-48, 1996
14. Ha HK et al: Gestational trophoblastic tumors of the uterus: MR imaging--pathologic correlation. Gynecol Oncol. 57(3):340-50, 1995
15. Kaczmarek JC et al: Intrapartum uterine rupture in a primiparous patient previously treated for invasive mole. Obstet Gynecol. 83(5 Pt 2):842-4, 1994
16. Cunningham FG et al: Diseases and abnormalities of the placenta. In: Licht J, ed. Williams's obstetrics. 19th ed. Norwalk, Conn: Appleton & Lange. 748-59, 1993

INVASIVE MOLE

IMAGE GALLERY

Typical

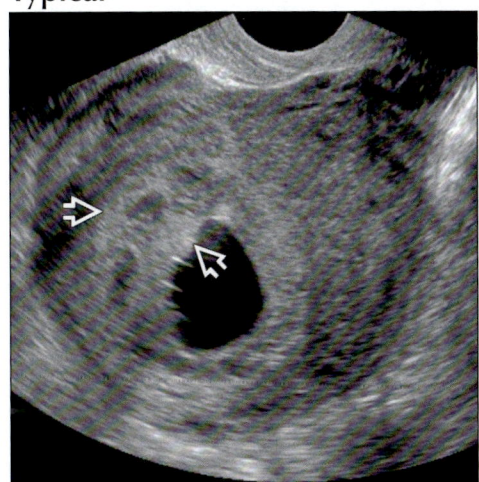
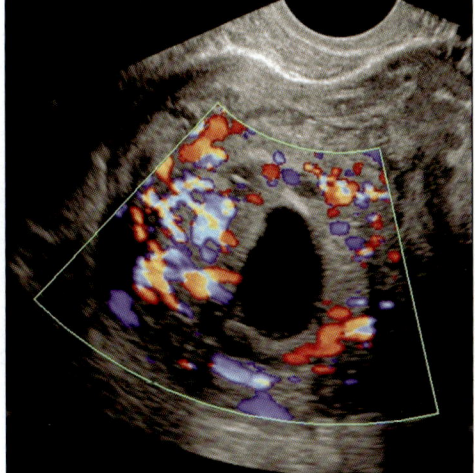

(Left) Sagittal transvaginal ultrasound shows heterogeneous echogenic soft tissue ➡ within the endometrium, extending into the myometrium. *(Right)* Sagittal transvaginal ultrasound in the same patient as previous image, shows marked vascularity of the abnormal soft tissue.

Typical

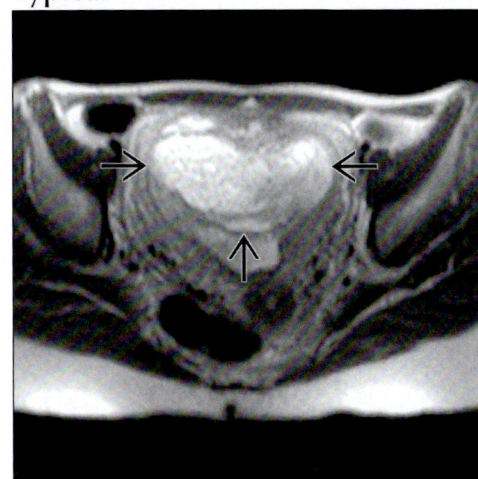
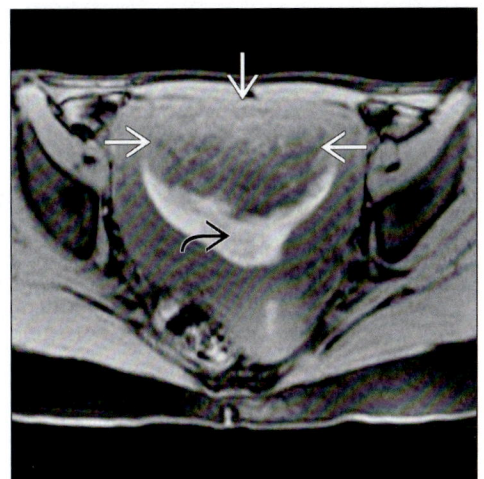

(Left) Axial T2WI MR shows a large T2 hyperintense mass ➡ involving the anterior uterine endometrium and myometrium. *(Right)* Axial T1WI FS MR in the same patient as previous image, shows a somewhat heterogeneous T1 hypointense mass ➡ within the anterior uterus. Blood products distend the endometrial cavity posteriorly ➡.

Typical

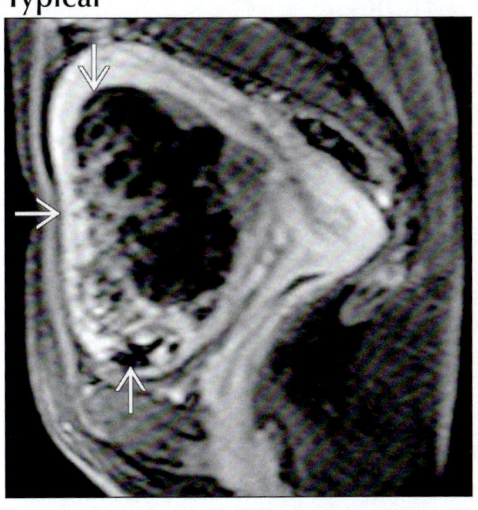
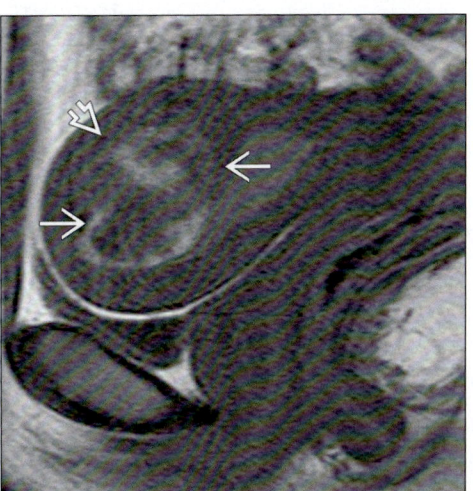

(Left) Sagittal T1 C+ FS MR shows a largely necrotic, heterogeneously enhancing mass ➡ that involves both the endometrium and myometrium. *(Right)* Sagittal T2WI MR shows a distended endometrial cavity containing heterogeneous soft tissue ➡ invading the myometrium superiorly ➡.

PLACENTAL SITE TROPHOBLASTIC TUMOR

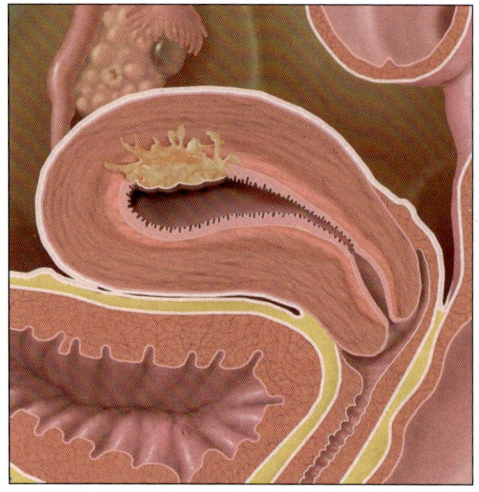

Graphic shows irregular mass within the endometrial cavity which demonstrates infiltration into the myometrium. This is typical of placental site trophoblastic tumor.

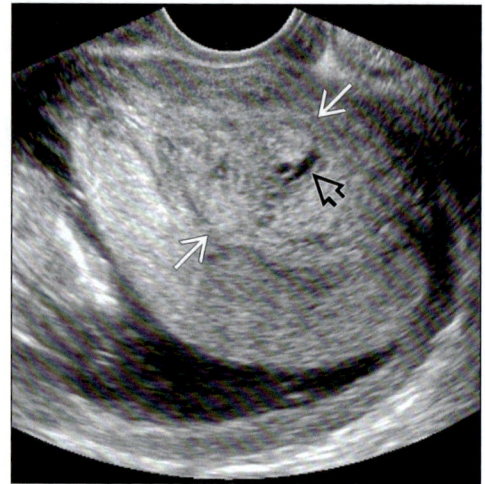

Sagittal transvaginal ultrasound shows a large heterogeneous mass ➡ expanding the endometrial cavity. Small cystic spaces are seen centrally ▷.

TERMINOLOGY

Abbreviations and Synonyms
- Placental site trophoblastic tumor (PSTT)

Definitions
- Rare gestational trophoblastic neoplasm (GTN) with malignant potential

IMAGING FINDINGS

General Features
- Location: Uterine wall
- Size: Variable
- Morphology
  - Imaging findings are nonspecific
  - May predominantly invade myometrium or extend into endometrial cavity

Ultrasonographic Findings
- Grayscale Ultrasound
  - Enlarged uterus
  - Multiple, small, rounded, fluid-filled structures within uterine wall
- Color Doppler: May be hypervascular
- Power Doppler: Vascularity extending into the myometrium may help demonstrate invasive nature of the tumor

CT Findings
- CECT
  - Strong enhancement of mass
  - Dilatation of gonadal vessels
- Enlarged uterus
- Mass can contain both solid & cystic elements

MR Findings
- T1WI: Isointense to normal myometrium
- T2WI: May be hypointense or hyperintense to normal myometrium
- T1 C+ FS: Marked enhancement

Angiographic Findings
- Conventional: Hypervascular blush with enlarged uterine & ovarian arteries

DDx: Placental Site Trophoblastic Tumor

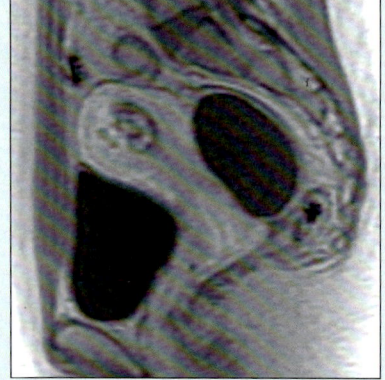

Choriocarcinoma

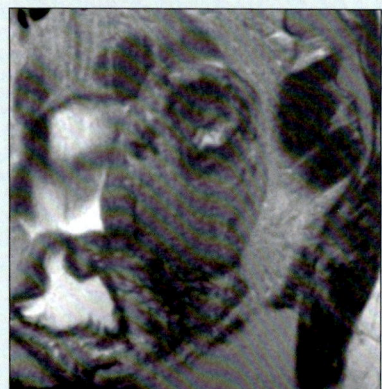

Retained Products of Conception

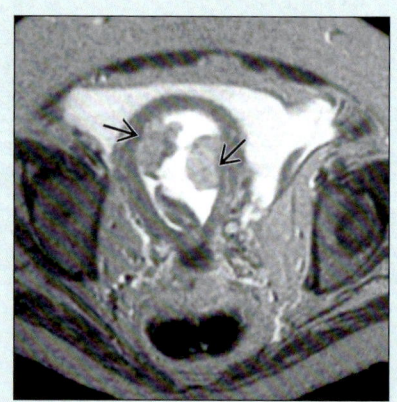

Endometrial Cancer

PLACENTAL SITE TROPHOBLASTIC TUMOR

Key Facts

Imaging Findings
- Imaging findings are nonspecific
- May predominantly invade myometrium or extend into endometrial cavity

Top Differential Diagnoses
- Hydatiform Mole
- Choriocarcinoma
- Invasive Mole
- Endometrial Carcinoma
- Retained Products of Conception
- Endometrial Hyperplasia/Polyp
- Adenomyosis

Pathology
- Etiology: Can occur after normal pregnancy, abortion, miscarriage or molar pregnancy

- Epidemiology: Rarest form of GTN
- β-human chorionic gonadotropin (HCG) levels are either normal or mildly elevated

Clinical Issues
- Most common signs/symptoms: Irregular vaginal bleeding
- 10-15% are malignant
- Lungs most common site of metastasis
- Treated with abdominal hysterectomy with bilateral salpingo-oophorectomy
- Treated with adjuvant chemotherapy

Diagnostic Checklist
- Consider PSTT in patients with amorphous uterine wall lesions, particularly with history of recent pregnancy

Imaging Recommendations
- Best imaging tool: MR because of superior soft tissue detail & multiplanar capabilities

DIFFERENTIAL DIAGNOSIS

Hydatiform Mole
- May be complete or partial depending on coexistence of fetus
- Uterine mass with numerous cystic spaces

Choriocarcinoma
- Much higher levels of hCG than those seen in PSTT
- Heterogeneous appearance due to hemorrhage & necrosis

Invasive Mole
- Ill-defined mass extending into myometrium
- May be indistinguishable from PSTT

Endometrial Carcinoma
- Primarily disease of postmenopausal women

Retained Products of Conception
- Heterogeneous, vascular material within endometrial cavity

Endometrial Hyperplasia/Polyp
- Hyperplasia
  - Proliferation of endometrial glands of irregular shape & size
  - Typically presents as diffuse endometrial thickening
- Polyp
  - Pedunculated or sessile focal lesion arising from the endometrium without myometrial invasion

Adenomyosis
- Thickening of junctional zone of myometrium
- Myometrial cysts

PATHOLOGY

General Features
- Etiology: Can occur after normal pregnancy, abortion, miscarriage or molar pregnancy
- Epidemiology: Rarest form of GTN
- Associated abnormalities
  - β-human chorionic gonadotropin (HCG) levels are either normal or mildly elevated
    - HCG levels do not correlate with degree of tumor burden or malignant behavior
    - Limited HCG production is result of minimal syncytiotrophoblast proliferation (as compared with choriocarcinoma)

Microscopic Features
- Monomorphic population of implantation-like intermediate trophoblastic cells
  - In contrast, other forms of gestational trophoblastic disease demonstrate mixture of cell types
    - For example, choriocarcinoma composed of cytotrophoblasts and syncytiotrophoblasts
- Invasion between myometrial muscle fibers
- Avillous
- Immunohistochemistry demonstrates keratin & human placental lactogen
- Intermediate trophoblastic cells produce human placental lactogen
- Extensive necrosis is not common

Staging, Grading or Classification Criteria
- Two types
  - Hypervascular type
  - Hypovascular type

CLINICAL ISSUES

Presentation
- Most common signs/symptoms: Irregular vaginal bleeding
- Other signs/symptoms
  - Amenorrhea

PLACENTAL SITE TROPHOBLASTIC TUMOR

- Abdominal pain
- Galactorrhea
- Virilization
- Nephrotic syndrome
- Polycythemia

Demographics
- Age
  - Women of reproductive age
  - Few reported cases of PSTT in postmenopausal women

Natural History & Prognosis
- Unpredictable course
- 10-15% are malignant
- Poor prognostic factors
  - Metastases
  - Antecedent pregnancy interval longer than 4 years
  - Older than 40 years of age
- Lungs most common site of metastasis

Treatment
- Treated with abdominal hysterectomy with bilateral salpingo-oophorectomy
  - Ovaries can be preserved if not involved
- Treated with adjuvant chemotherapy
  - Etoposide
  - Methotrexate
  - Actinomycin-etoposide
  - Vincristine
- Radiation therapy
  - Palliative only

DIAGNOSTIC CHECKLIST

Consider
- Consider PSTT in patients with amorphous uterine wall lesions, particularly with history of recent pregnancy

Image Interpretation Pearls
- Radiographic appearance is nonspecific & can resemble that of choriocarcinoma or invasive mole

SELECTED REFERENCES

1. Allen SD et al: Radiology of gestational trophoblastic neoplasia. Clin Radiol. 61(4):301-13, 2006
2. Hassadia A et al: Placental site trophoblastic tumour: clinical features and management. Gynecol Oncol. 99(3):603-7, 2005
3. Takeuchi M et al: Pathologies of the uterine endometrial cavity: usual and unusual manifestations and pitfalls on magnetic resonance imaging. Eur Radiol. 15(11):2244-55, 2005
4. Zhou Q et al: Sonographic and Doppler imaging in the diagnosis and treatment of gestational trophoblastic disease: a 12-year experience. J Ultrasound Med. 24(1):15-24, 2005
5. Bonazzi C et al: Placental site trophoblastic tumor: an overview. J Reprod Med. 49(8):585-8, 2004
6. Nigam S et al: Placental site trophoblastic tumor in a postmenopausal female--a case report. Gynecol Oncol. 93(2):550-3, 2004
7. Oguz S et al: Doppler study of myometrium in invasive gestational trophoblastic disease. Int J Gynecol Cancer. 14(5):972-9, 2004
8. Altieri A et al: Epidemiology and aetiology of gestational trophoblastic diseases. Lancet Oncol. 4(11):670-8, 2003
9. Davis PC et al: Sonohysterographic findings of endometrial and subendometrial conditions. Radiographics. 22(4):803-16, 2002
10. Papadopoulos AJ et al: Twenty-five years' clinical experience with placental site trophoblastic tumors. J Reprod Med. 47(6):460-4, 2002
11. Feltmate CM et al: Placental site trophoblastic tumor: a 17-year experience at the New England Trophoblastic Disease Center. Gynecol Oncol. 82(3):415-9, 2001
12. Sumi Y et al: Placental site trophoblastic tumor: imaging findings. Radiat Med. 17(6):427-30, 1999
13. Green CL et al: Gestational trophoblastic disease: a spectrum of radiologic diagnosis. Radiographics. 16(6):1371-84, 1996
14. Schneider D et al: Placental-site trophoblastic tumor following metastatic gestational trophoblastic neoplasia. Gynecol Oncol. 63(2):267-9, 1996
15. Wagner BJ et al: From the archives of the AFIP. Gestational trophoblastic disease: radiologic-pathologic correlation. Radiographics. 16(1):131-48, 1996
16. Rutgers JL et al: Placental site trophoblastic tumour: clinicopathologic study of 64 cases. Mod Pathol. 8:96A, 1995
17. Abulafia O et al: Unusual endovaginal ultrasonography and magnetic resonance imaging of placental site trophoblastic tumor. Am J Obstet Gynecol. 170(3):750-2, 1994
18. Mangili G et al: Transvaginal ultrasonography in persistent trophoblastic tumor. Am J Obstet Gynecol. 169(5):1218-23, 1993
19. Bagshawe KD: Choriocarcinoma. A model for tumour markers. Acta Oncol. 31(1):99-106, 1992
20. Brewer CA et al: Erythrocytosis associated with a placental-site trophoblastic tumor. Obstet Gynecol. 79(5 (Pt 2)):846-9, 1992
21. Fisher RA et al: Genetic evidence that placental site trophoblastic tumours can originate from a hydatidiform mole or a normal conceptus. Br J Cancer. 65(3):355-8, 1992
22. Caspi B et al: Invasive mole and placental site trophoblastic tumor. Two entities of gestational trophoblastic disease with a common ultrasonographic appearance. J Ultrasound Med. 10(9):517-9, 1991
23. Finkler NJ: Placental site trophoblastic tumor. Diagnosis, clinical behavior and treatment. J Reprod Med. 36(1):27-30, 1991
24. Heintz AP et al: Placental-site trophoblastic tumor: diagnosis, treatment, and biological behavior. Int J Gynecol Pathol. 4(1):75-82, 1985
25. Nagelberg SB et al: Clinical and laboratory investigation of a virilized woman with placental-site trophoblastic tumor. Obstet Gynecol. 65(4):527-34, 1985

PLACENTAL SITE TROPHOBLASTIC TUMOR

IMAGE GALLERY

Typical

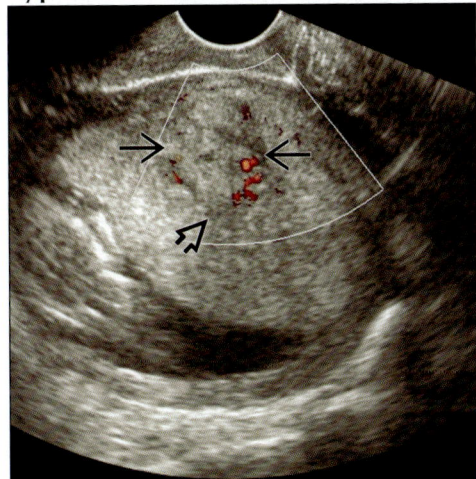
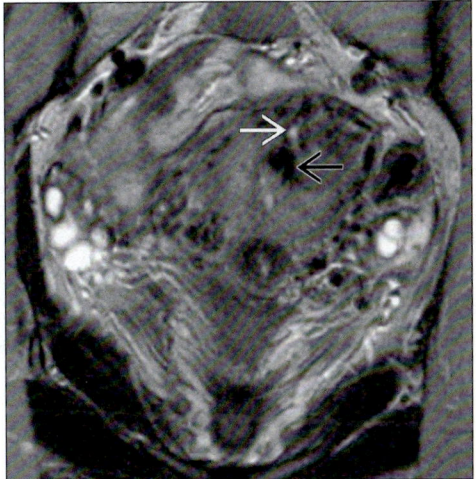

(Left) Axial oblique power Doppler ultrasound in the same patient as previous image, shows the infiltrative, heterogeneous vascular mass ➔ within the endometrial cavity. There is ill-defined extension of this mass into the myometrium ➔. *(Right)* Coronal T2WI MR shows marked heterogeneity of the uterine body with loss of the normal zonal anatomy. Both T2 bright ➔ and low T2 ➔ signal intensity areas are noted within the uterus.

Typical

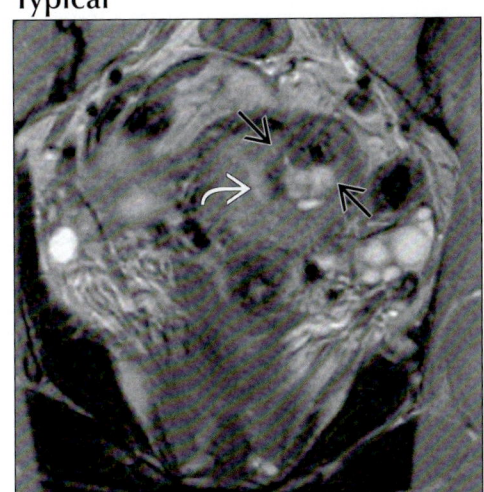
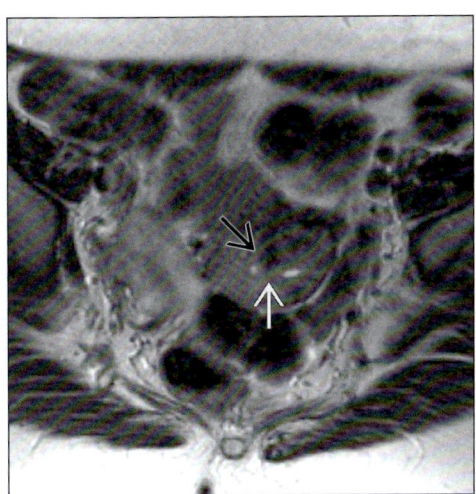

(Left) Coronal T2WI MR in the same patient as previous image, shows a mixed signal intensity mass within the left uterine fundus/body ➔. The endometrium ➔ is indistinct, involved by tumor. *(Right)* Axial T2WI MR in the same patient as previous image, shows a predominantly low T2 signal intensity mass extending from the endometrium ➔ into the fundus ➔.

Typical

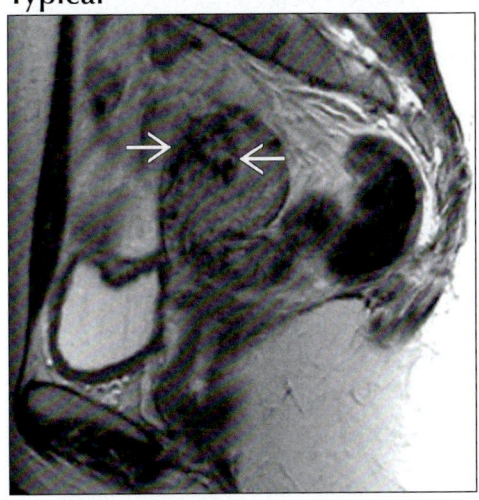
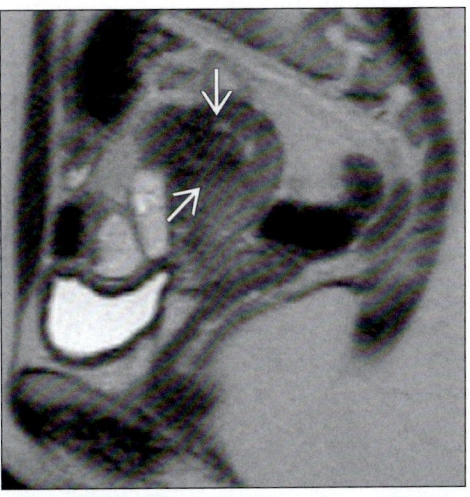

(Left) Sagittal T2WI MR in the same patient as previous image, shows obliteration of the normal endometrial cavity by a predominantly low T2 signal mass ➔ that infiltrates into the anterior myometrium. *(Right)* Sagittal T2WI MR in the same patient as previous image, shows a mixed solid/cystic ill-defined mass ➔ within the uterus.

HEMATOMA, PLACENTA

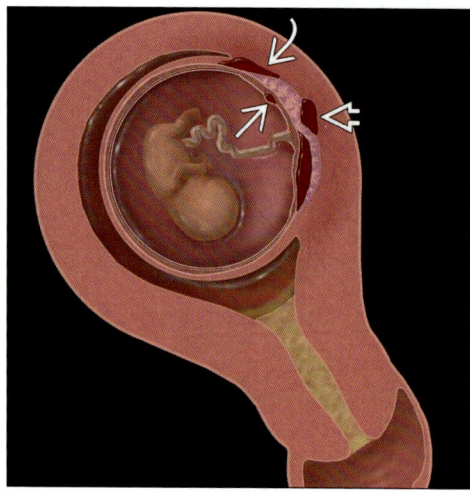

Graphic shows subtypes of placenta hematoma, the most common is marginal subchorionic ➔, less frequently seen are retroplacental ➔, and preplacental hematoma (including subamniotic ➔).

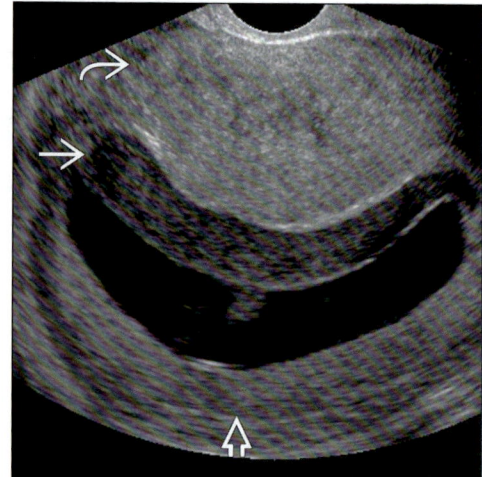

Transvaginal ultrasound in a 13 week gestation shows large marginal subchorionic hematoma ➔. The placenta is posterior ➔, and there is an anterior contraction ➔.

TERMINOLOGY

Abbreviations and Synonyms
- Intrauterine, perigestational, subchorionic, subamniotic, preplacental or retroplacental hematoma; Breus mole, massive subchorionic thrombohematoma

Definitions
- Collection adjacent to gestational sac which results from hemorrhage at decidual-placental interface

IMAGING FINDINGS

General Features
- Location
  - Subchorionic hematoma occurs between chorion and uterine wall, external to chorion laeve
  - Retroplacental hematoma occurs behind the placenta, external to chorion frondosum
  - Subamniotic hematoma occurs under the amniotic layer covering the fetal chorionic plate
  - Massive subchorionic hematoma occurs in fetal chorionic plate
- Size
  - Size of hematoma is compared to size of gestational sac → small (< 20%), medium (20-50%), large (> 50%)
  - Others estimate volume: Small → < 1 mL, medium → between 1-10 mL and large → > 10 mL

Ultrasonographic Findings
- Grayscale Ultrasound
  - Subchorionic (marginal) hematoma
    - Crescent-shaped collection
    - Between chorion and uterine wall, commonly slightly elevates edge of placenta
    - May be in site remote from margin of placenta, dissects around endometrial cavity
    - May compress and distort gestational sac
    - Isoechoic or echogenic when acute
    - As hematoma evolves → becomes hypoechoic to anechoic (cystic), ± fluid-fluid levels, ↓ size
  - Retroplacental hematoma
    - Collection behind placenta → separates placenta from myometrium

DDx: Placental Collection or Mass

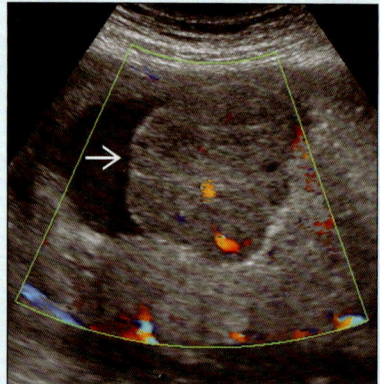
Chorioangioma

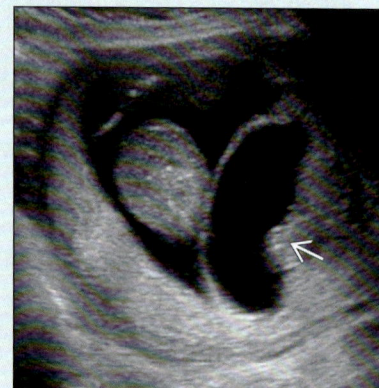
Vanishing Twin

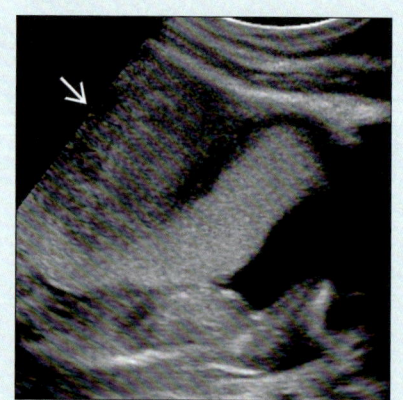
Uterine Contraction

HEMATOMA, PLACENTA

Key Facts

Imaging Findings
- Subchorionic hematoma occurs between chorion and uterine wall, external to chorion laeve
- Retroplacental hematoma occurs behind the placenta, external to chorion frondosum
- Subamniotic hematoma occurs under the amniotic layer covering the fetal chorionic plate
- Massive subchorionic hematoma occurs in fetal chorionic plate
- Size of hematoma is compared to size of gestational sac → small (< 20%), medium (20-50%), large (> 50%)
- Between chorion and uterine wall, commonly slightly elevates edge of placenta
- May be in site remote from margin of placenta, dissects around endometrial cavity
- May compress and distort gestational sac
- Collection behind placenta → separates placenta from myometrium
- Preplacental hematoma → includes subamniotic and massive subchorionic hematoma
- Oval-shaped cystic mass overlying fetal plate of placenta → covered by thin membrane
- Multiple anechoic spaces elevating fetal chorionic plate → projects focally into amniotic cavity
- No blood flow or feeding vessels within hematoma
- Cord insertion seen close to preplacental hematoma

Pathology
- Subchorionic → tears of marginal veins
- Retroplacental → hemorrhage from spiral arteries
- Subamniotic hematomas → excessive traction on umbilical cord (usually at delivery)

- Acute hematoma → echogenic and isoechoic to placenta or thickening posterior to placenta
- If large and involves 30-40% of maternal placental surface → hypoxia to fetus is likely
- Follow-up for growth restriction or in-utero demise
- Preplacental hematoma → includes subamniotic and massive subchorionic hematoma
- Subamniotic hematoma
  - Oval-shaped cystic mass overlying fetal plate of placenta → covered by thin membrane
  - Recent hematoma is echogenic and may mimic subchorionic hematoma
  - Follow-up → predominantly cystic with retracting clot and fibrin strands
  - Cord vessels seen close to hematoma
- Massive subchorionic or preplacental hematoma
  - Multiple anechoic spaces elevating fetal chorionic plate → projects focally into amniotic cavity
  - Mass extends from anterior placental surface
- Color Doppler
  - No blood flow or feeding vessels within hematoma
    - Flow in periphery delineates isoechoic hematoma
  - Cord insertion seen close to preplacental hematoma
  - Umbilical artery Doppler evaluation → exclude signs of vascular compromise in fetus (third trimester)

MR Findings
- Hematoma signal depends on age of blood products; typically low signal on T2WI and high signal on T1WI

Imaging Recommendations
- Best imaging tool: Transvaginal ultrasound ± Doppler

DIFFERENTIAL DIAGNOSIS

Chorioamniotic Separation
- Normal before 14 weeks, should fuse by 16 weeks
  - Associated with aneuploidy (Trisomy 21)
- No history of vaginal bleeding
- Fluid is less complex than subchorionic hematoma
  - Placenta edge not lifted

Twin Pregnancy with Empty Sac
- During early pregnancy → intact gestational sac with adjacent anechoic area (distinguish on real time)
- Empty sac tends to disappear before week 12
- Elevated levels maternal serum alfa fetoprotein ± vaginal bleeding

Chorioangioma
- Most common tumor of placenta (hamartoma)
  - Seen in 1% of examined placentas, clinically significant lesions are rare (1 in 9,000 deliveries)
- Solid mass protruding from fetal surface of placenta
  - Well-delineated, isoechoic or hypoechoic mass, may have thin septations and calcification
  - Color Doppler demonstrates feeding vessels from fetal circulation and blood flow within the mass
  - Follow-up scans → increasing size of mass
- If large (≥ 5 cm) may be associated with polyhydramnios, premature delivery, fetal anemia, hydrops, growth restriction, fetal congestive heart failure, maternal coagulopathy and toxemia

Placental Lakes
- Multicystic areas, ± at least 1 cm, surrounded by normal echogenic placenta
- Normal finding seen in 17% of second trimester scans, may be found in up to 67% of placentas
- Slow blood flow on real-time scanning
- Occasionally large spaces seen in association with elevated maternal serum alpha fetoprotein, fetal growth restriction and premature delivery
- More prevalent with increasing placental thickness

Uterine Contraction or Retroplacental Leiomyoma
- May mimic a heterogeneous hematoma

Cord Cyst
- Round, anechoic, nonvascular mass attached to cord
- Prevalence is 3% in the first trimester, 20% associated with fetal chromosomal or structural defects
- Usually small (may be > 5 cm)

HEMATOMA, PLACENTA

Placental Cysts (Cytotrophoblastic Cysts)
- Within the placenta or under the fetal plate
- Contain gelatinous material rather than blood
- Not associated with poor perinatal outcome

Circumvallate Placenta
- Mass limited to marginal zone of placenta, no change throughout pregnancy
- Abnormal implantation → transition of membranous to villous chorion at a distance from placental edge
- Associated with premature rupture of membranes

PATHOLOGY

General Features
- Etiology
  - Unknown
    - Reported with autoimmune and immunologic diseases, thrombolysis or anticoagulation
    - Subchorionic → tears of marginal veins
    - Retroplacental → hemorrhage from spiral arteries
    - Subamniotic hematomas → excessive traction on umbilical cord (usually at delivery)
- Epidemiology
  - Incidence of intrauterine hematoma associated with vaginal bleeding → 4-39% (different patient populations, study design, range of gestational ages)
  - Incidence of intrauterine hematoma in first trimester of single intrauterine pregnancy → 3.1% in general obstetric population → 1.3% in low risk
  - Subamniotic hematomas are rare, the majority reported in the third trimester or at delivery

Gross Pathologic & Surgical Features
- Subchorionic hematoma: Bleeding of maternal origin pooling beneath chorionic membrane and uterine wall
- Subamniotic hematoma: Bleeding of fetal origin → rupture of chorionic vessels near cord insertion
  - Cyst contains thrombotic mass arising from amniotic membrane → attaches to fetal surface
- Massive subchorionic thrombohematoma (Breus mole) → rare but serious condition; large amount of maternal blood collects and dissects fetal plate from villous chorion
  - Thrombus is found in trophoblast-lined intervillous space and hematoma dissects beyond confines of this space and between layers of chorionic plate
  - Involvement of much of placental surface area with blood clot measuring at least 1 cm in thickness
  - Frequently associated with fetal demise, intrauterine growth restriction or onset of premature labor

Microscopic Features
- Intervillous, subamniotic or subchorionic thrombosis with fibrin deposition

CLINICAL ISSUES

Presentation
- Most common signs/symptoms
  - Symptoms of threatened abortion (vaginal bleeding ± cramping), spontaneous abortion
  - Asymptomatic (29% of patients)
- Other signs/symptoms: Elevated maternal serum alpha fetoprotein from direct placental injury

Natural History & Prognosis
- Vaginal bleeding in first trimester → 14% have intrauterine hematoma
  - 20% likelihood of miscarriage if diagnosis of intrauterine hematoma made before 9 weeks
  - Spontaneous abortion is affected by hematoma size → 18.8% with large, 9.2% with moderate and 7.7% with small hematoma
  - Very large hematomas → adverse outcome in 46%
  - Size of the hematoma → not a reliable estimation of severity since some blood is lost through cervix
- 70% of subchorionic hematomas spontaneously resolve by end of second trimester, some persist until end of pregnancy and may cause problems → chorioamnionitis, abortion and premature labor
- Intrauterine hematoma → ↑ rate premature delivery (16% in general obstetric population; 32% in high risk)
  - Higher risk for preeclampsia, abruption, adherent placentation, growth restriction, perinatal mortality
- Subamniotic hematomas → most found after birth from excessive traction on umbilical cord at delivery, rarely reported in utero (from 18-34 weeks)

Treatment
- Large hematomas are followed to assess fetal growth velocity, amniotic fluid volume and compromise of the fetal-placental circulation (Doppler studies)

DIAGNOSTIC CHECKLIST

Consider
- Follow-up since there is ↑ maternal and fetal morbidity

Image Interpretation Pearls
- False negative exams occur despite bleeding if all of the blood leaves the uterus through the cervix
- Blood can appear isoechoic to placenta, and thus be difficult to detect sonographically

SELECTED REFERENCES
1. Leite J et al: Prognosis of very large first-trimester hematomas. J Ultrasound Med. 25(11):1441-5, 2006
2. Maso G et al: First-trimester intrauterine hematoma and outcome of pregnancy. Obstet Gynecol. 105(2):339-44, 2005
3. Johns J et al: Obstetric outcome after threatened miscarriage with and without a hematoma on ultrasound. Obstet Gynecol. 102(3):483-7, 2003
4. Deans A et al: Prenatal diagnosis and outcome of subamniotic hematomas. Ultrasound Obstet Gynecol. 11(5):319-23, 1998
5. Bennett GL et al: Subchorionic hemorrhage in first-trimester pregnancies: prediction of pregnancy outcome with sonography. Radiology. 200(3):803-6, 1996

HEMATOMA, PLACENTA

IMAGE GALLERY

Typical

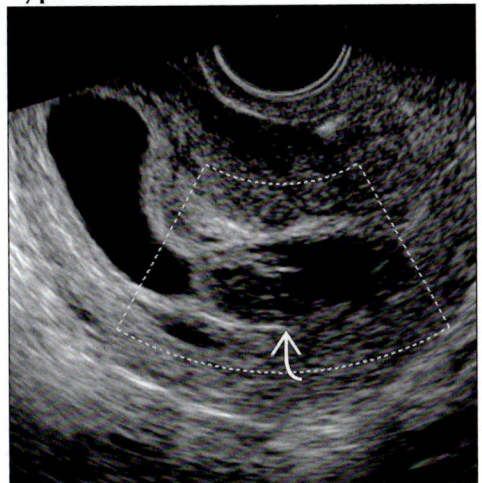
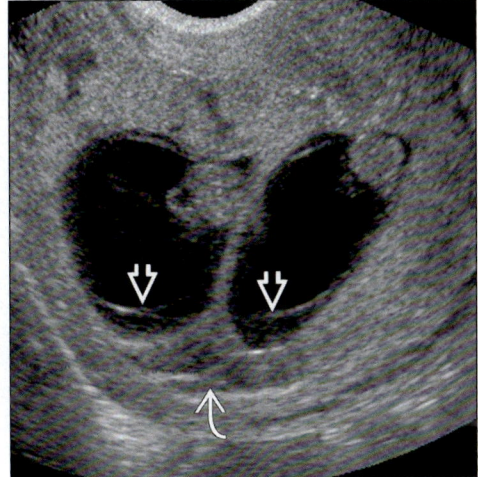

(Left) Transvaginal color Doppler ultrasound in an 8 week gestation shows a marginal subchorionic hematoma that resembles a second gestational sac ➙. *(Right)* Transvaginal ultrasound shows dichorionic diamniotic twin gestation with normal chorioamniotic separation ➙. There is a small marginal subchorionic hematoma ➙.

Typical

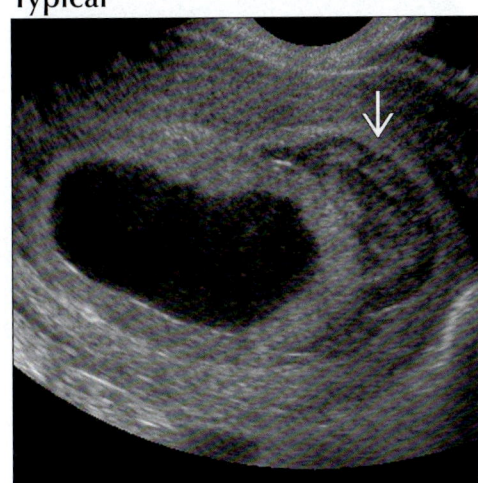
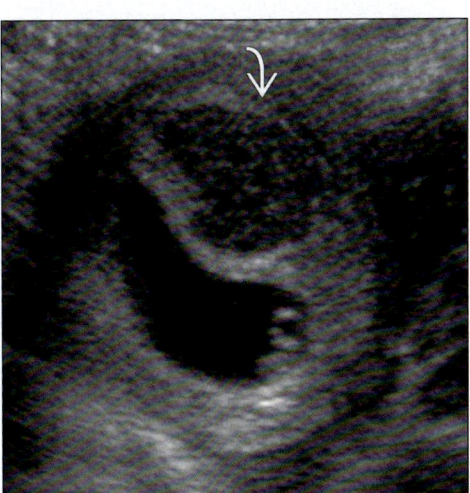

(Left) Transvaginal ultrasound in a 7 week gestation shows a moderate subchorionic hematoma ➙ that resolved in the second trimester. *(Right)* Transvaginal ultrasound in a 7 week gestation shows a moderate subchorionic marginal hematoma ➙ that slightly deforms the gestational sac.

Typical

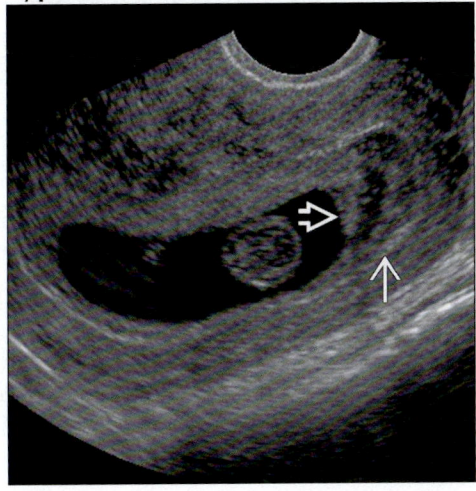
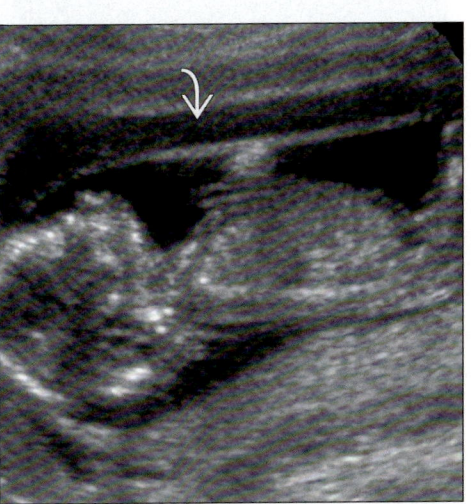

(Left) Transvaginal ultrasound in a 10 week gestation shows a small marginal subchorionic hematoma ➙ that slightly elevates the margin of the placenta ➙. *(Right)* Transabdominal ultrasound of same patient as previous image with continued vaginal bleeding at 14 weeks gestation, shows enlarging marginal subchorionic hematoma ➙ that has dissected anteriorly.

HEMATOMA, PLACENTA

(Left) Transvaginal ultrasound at 9 weeks gestation in a patient with bleeding shows a large, marginal, subchorionic hematoma ➡ which lifts the border of the anterior placenta ➡. *(Right)* Transvaginal ultrasound at 7 weeks gestation shows a large subchorionic hematoma ➡ with distortion of the gestational sac.

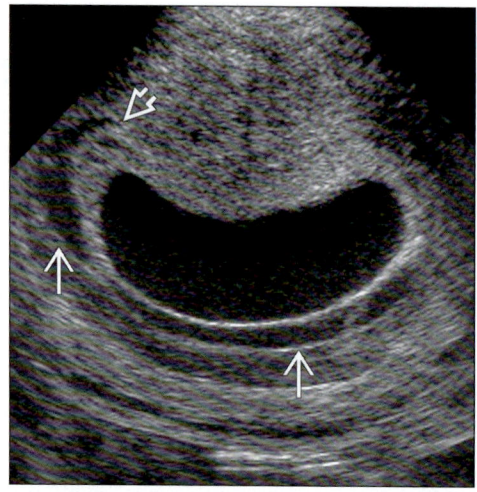

(Left) Transabdominal ultrasound at 13 weeks gestation shows marginal subchorionic ➡ and retroplacental ➡ hematoma. Note maternal bladder ➡ and myometrial contraction ➡. *(Right)* Color Doppler ultrasound at 13 weeks gestation shows a marginal subchorionic ➡ and retroplacental ➡ hematoma. Note the umbilical cord ➡ and maternal bladder ➡.

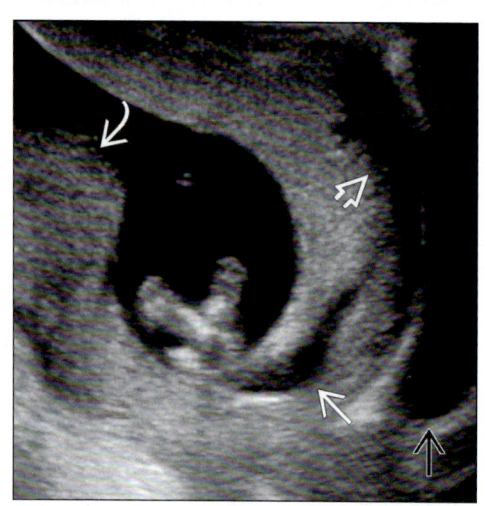 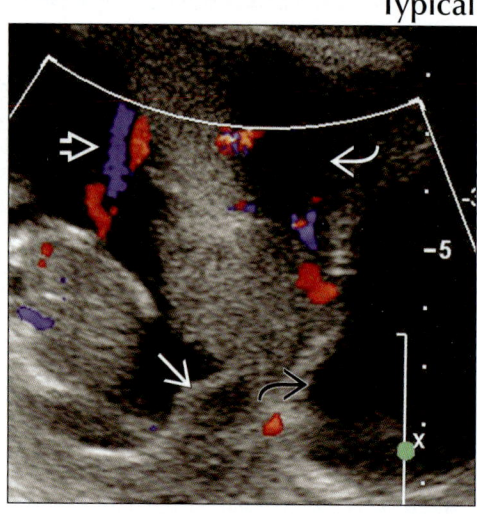

(Left) Coronal T2WI MR shows twin pregnancy with low signal between the membranes ➡ due to blood products. *(Right)* Axial T1WI MR in the same case as previous image, shows heterogeneous high signal ➡ material consistent with blood products.

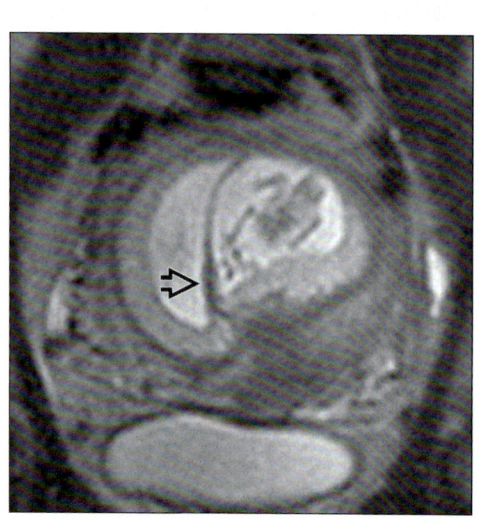 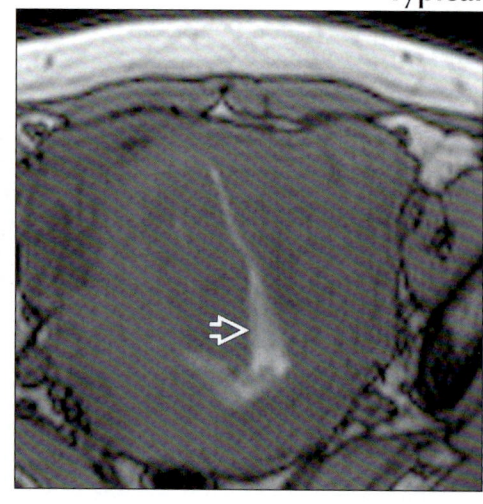

HEMATOMA, PLACENTA

Typical

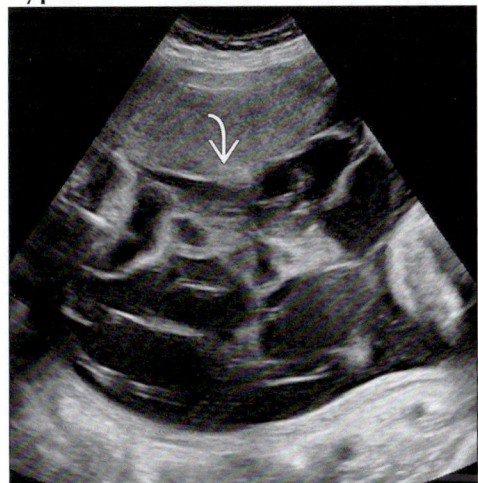 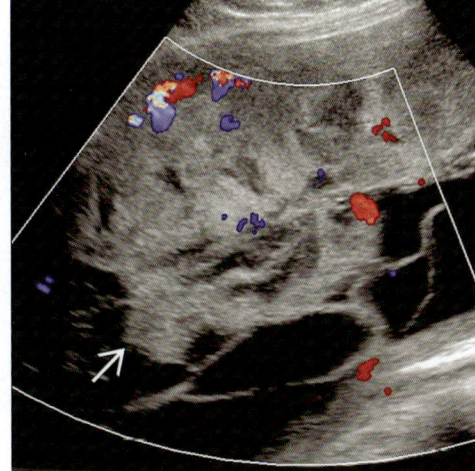

(Left) Transabdominal ultrasound shows heterogeneous collection originating in the fetal chorionic plate ➡ in a patient with preeclampsia and massive subchorionic hemorrhage. The patient had premature onset of labor. *(Right)* Color Doppler ultrasound in the same patient as previous image, shows heterogeneous organizing collection ➡ projecting into the amniotic cavity. There is flow in the normal placenta.

Typical

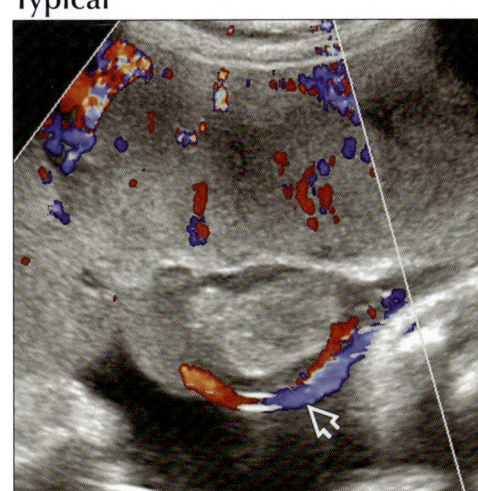 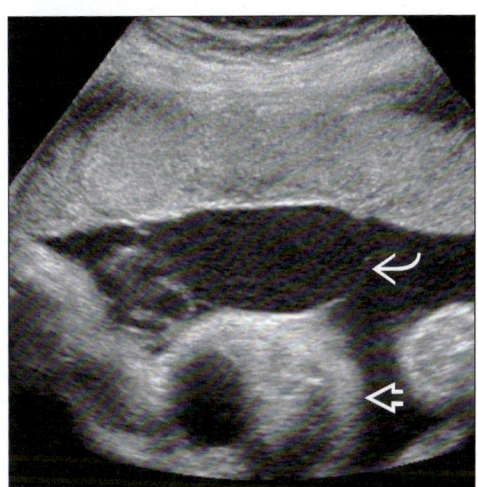

(Left) Transabdominal ultrasound color Doppler sonogram shows heterogeneous clot with adjacent umbilical cord ➡. *(Right)* Transabdominal ultrasound at 29 weeks gestation shows a preplacental homogeneous hypoechoic collection which is surrounded by a thin membrane ➡ and abuts the fetus ➡.

Typical

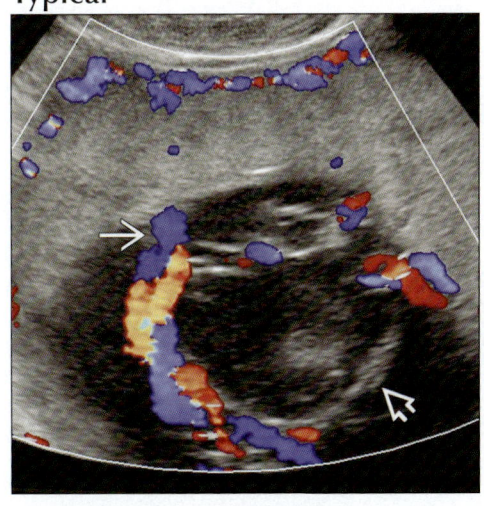 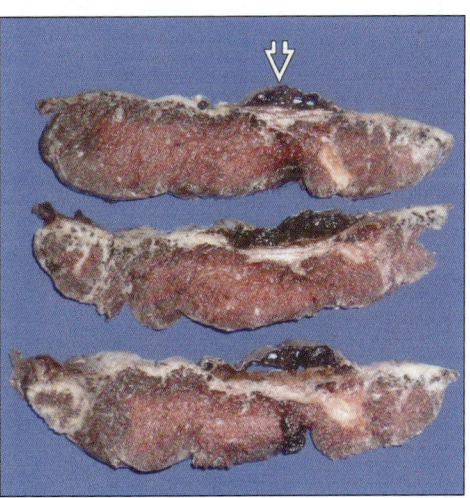

(Left) Color Doppler ultrasound in the same patient as previous image, one week later shows a hypoechoic collection ➡ in close proximity to the cord insertion ➡. *(Right)* Gross pathology in same patient as previous image, shows the hematoma ➡.

CHORIOANGIOMA, PLACENTA

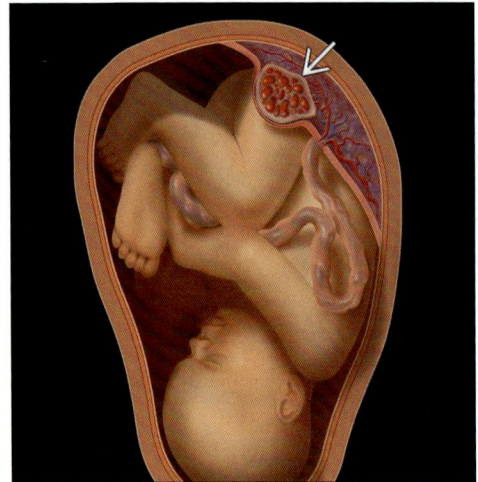

Sagittal graphic shows a placental chorioangioma ➡, typically bulging on the fetal aspect of the placenta. The blood-filled sinusoids are responsible for the red-purple appearance of the mass.

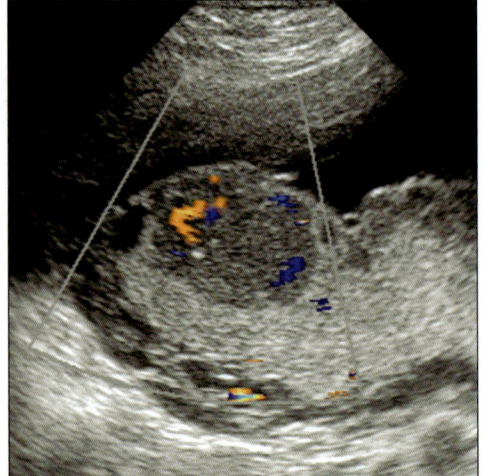

Color Doppler ultrasound shows a placental mass with internal blood flow. Chorioangiomas may have substantial arteriovenous shunting and are a potential cause of fetal hydrops.

TERMINOLOGY

Abbreviations and Synonyms
- Chorangioma
- Placental hemangioma

Definitions
- Most common placental tumor
- Benign vascular tumor of the placenta

IMAGING FINDINGS

General Features
- Best diagnostic clue: Vascular mass-like lesion in placenta
- Location
  ○ More common on fetal surface
  ○ Subchorionic lesions
  ○ Entirely intraplacental
- Size
  ○ Ranges from a few millimeters in diameter to 10 centimeters
  ○ Largest reported placental chorioangioma weighed 780 grams
  ○ Usually not clinically significant when smaller than 4-5 centimeters
  ○ May grow rapidly
- Morphology
  ○ When large and externally visible, usually have a red-purple encapsulated outer appearance
  ○ When opened, contain large sinusoids filled with blood

Ultrasonographic Findings
- Solid intraplacental mass
- Hypoechoic to isoechoic to normal placenta
- Bulging protuberance on fetal surface of placenta
- Usually solitary but may be multiple
- Shows vascularity throughout mass on color Doppler US
  ○ Vascularity may help differentiate it from other placental masses
  ○ Amount of flow in mass is quite variable
  ○ Greater arterial flow increases risk of developing fetal hydrops

DDx: Placental Chorioangioma

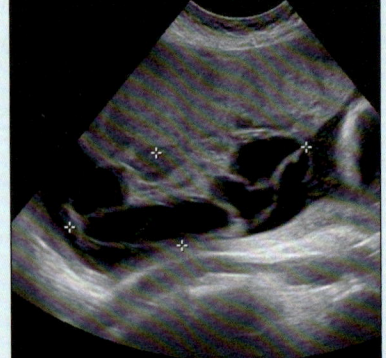
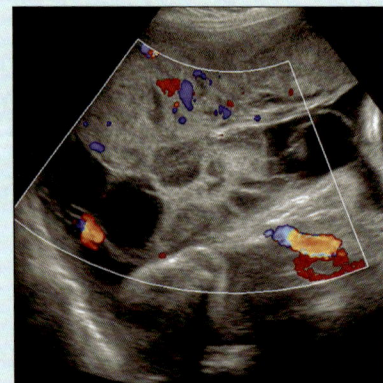
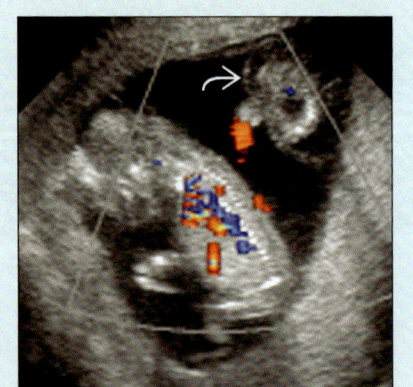

Placental Hematoma | Placental Hematoma | TRAP Twin

CHORIOANGIOMA, PLACENTA

Key Facts

Terminology
- Most common placental tumor

Imaging Findings
- Best diagnostic clue: Vascular mass-like lesion in placenta
- Usually not clinically significant when smaller than 4-5 centimeters
- Solid intraplacental mass
- Shows vascularity throughout mass on color Doppler US
- Vascularity may help differentiate it from other placental masses
- Amount of flow in mass is quite variable
- Greater arterial flow increases risk of developing fetal hydrops

Pathology
- Incidence about 1% of placentas
- Large, clinically important chorioangiomas present in about 1:8,000-1:9,000 pregnancies

Clinical Issues
- Polyhydramnios (16-33%), more common with larger tumors
- Predisposition for premature onset of labor, more common with polyhydramnios
- Complications in the newborn include cardiomegaly (high output state), generalized edema
- Chorioangiomas of the skin and other organs more frequent than in the general population
- Elevated maternal alpha-fetoprotein with no elevation of amniotic alpha-fetoprotein

MR Findings
- T1WI
  - Isointense to normal placenta
  - May have areas of heterogeneously increased signal intensity
- T2WI
  - Increased signal intensity
  - May be heterogeneous with low signal rim from hemorrhage

Imaging Recommendations
- Best imaging tool: Antenatal US with color Doppler imaging

DIFFERENTIAL DIAGNOSIS

Placental Hemorrhage
- Well-circumscribed solid or solid and cystic mass
- Will not show marked vascularization on color Doppler US

Placental Teratoma
- Heterogeneous content on US
  - Fat, calcifications, soft tissue
- No internal blood flow on color Doppler US
- Lies between the amnion and the chorion

Partial Mole (Triploidy)
- Multicystic lesion on US
- Intervillous lesion
- Fetus is abnormal
  - Multiple anomalies
  - Severe growth restriction
- Clinically, uterine size usually small for date

Maternal Placental Metastasis
- Very rare!
- Most commonly a solid mass
- Malignant melanoma is most common origin
- Usually in the intervillous space
- Fetal neuroblastoma also reported to metastasize to placenta

Twin Reversed Arterial Perfusion (TRAP, Fetus Acardius Amorphus)
- Twin gestation with an acardiac twin
- Mass with separate umbilical cord and development of a central skeleton

PATHOLOGY

General Features
- Etiology
  - Hamartomas or benign neoplasm of unknown etiology
  - Malformations of primitive angioblastic tissue of the early placenta
- Epidemiology
  - Incidence about 1% of placentas
  - Large, clinically important chorioangiomas present in about 1:8,000-1:9,000 pregnancies
- Associated abnormalities
  - Usually associated to shunting of blood by a large chorioangioma
  - Fetal abnormalities may include
    - Cardiomegaly
    - Anemia
    - Thrombocytopenia

Gross Pathologic & Surgical Features
- Lesion is entirely intraplacental
- Usually single but may be multiple
- Rarely a placenta may be diffusely infiltrated by hemangiomatous tissue
- Round, oval or reniform
  - May be deeply grooved by fibrous tissue
- Smooth firm encapsulated mass

Microscopic Features
- Three pathological types (often various transitions between types in a single tumor)
  - Angiomatous type
    - Numerous blood vessels set in a loose fibrous stroma

CHORIOANGIOMA, PLACENTA

- Vessels are usually the size of capillaries, rarely they may be dilated with a cavernous appearance
  - Cellular type
    - Primarily a loose cellular mesenchymal tumor containing only a few not well-formed blood vessels
  - Degenerate type
    - Tumor showing myxoid changes, hyalinization, necrosis and calcification
    - Rarely fat may be present
- Mitotic figures may be seen
- No capsular invasion
- No evidence of malignant behavior

CLINICAL ISSUES

Presentation
- Most common signs/symptoms
  - During pregnancy
    - Polyhydramnios (16-33%), more common with larger tumors
    - Association with pre-eclampsia
    - Antepartum bleeding may be caused by a retroplacental chorioangioma
    - Predisposition for premature onset of labor, more common with polyhydramnios
  - During labor
    - Usually normal labor
    - Rarely, tumor may remain in the uterus after placental expulsion, leading to postpartum hemorrhage
    - If very large, may obstruct vaginal delivery
  - Complications to the fetus or neonate
    - Minimal increase in perinatal mortality may be seen with very large or multiple tumors
    - Hydrops fetalis and fetal anemia with or without thrombocytopenia
    - May be related to low birth weight
    - Complications in the newborn include cardiomegaly (high output state), generalized edema
    - Chorioangiomas of the skin and other organs more frequent than in the general population
- Other signs/symptoms
  - Elevated maternal alpha-fetoprotein with no elevation of amniotic alpha-fetoprotein
  - If large, may cause shunting of blood and fetal heart failure

Natural History & Prognosis
- May enlarge rapidly
- Polyhydramnios/hydrops may decrease on follow-up if chorioangioma thromboses

Treatment
- Close monitoring and follow-up
- Consider laser ablation when very large

DIAGNOSTIC CHECKLIST

Consider
- Vascular mass in the placenta with or without polyhydramnios

Image Interpretation Pearls
- Most common tumor of the placenta
- Subchorionic solid vascular mass on US
- Only large chorioangiomas are clinically significant
- Large chorioangiomas associated with polyhydramnios, fetal cardiomegaly and hydrops fetalis

SELECTED REFERENCES

1. Hata T et al: Three-dimensional sonographic features of placental abnormalities. Gynecol Obstet Invest. 57(2):61-5, 2004
2. Sepulveda W et al: Perinatal outcome after prenatal diagnosis of placental chorioangioma. Obstet Gynecol. 102(5 Pt 1):1028-33, 2003
3. Blaustein's Pathology of the Female Genital Tract. 5th ed. Robert J. Kurman ed. New York, SpringerVerlag. 1171-3, 2002
4. Kawamotoa S et al: Chorioangioma: antenatal diagnosis with fast MR imaging. Magn Reson Imaging. 18(7):911-4, 2000
5. Prapas N et al: Color Doppler imaging of placental masses: differential diagnosis and fetal outcome. Ultrasound Obstet Gynecol. 16(6):559-63, 2000
6. Sepulveda W et al: Placental chorioangioma. Ultrasound Obstet Gynecol. 16(6):597-8, 2000
7. Harris RD et al: Sonography of the placenta with emphasis on pathological correlation. Semin Ultrasound CT MR. 17(1):66-89, 1996
8. Mann L et al: Placental haemangioma. Case report. Br J Obstet Gynaecol. 90(10):983-6, 1983
9. Fox H. Pathology of the placenta. In: Benninger JL, series editor. Major problems in pathology. Vol 7. Philadelphia, WB Saunders. 343, 1978

CHORIOANGIOMA, PLACENTA

IMAGE GALLERY

Typical

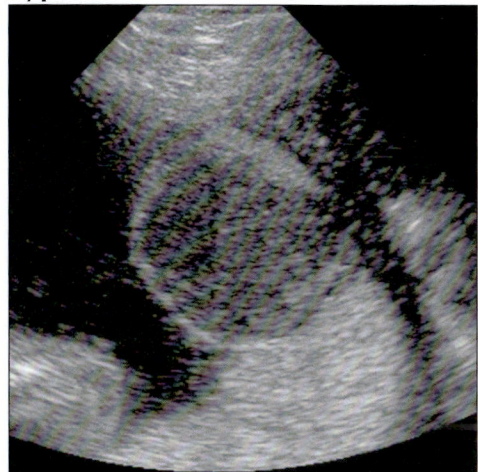
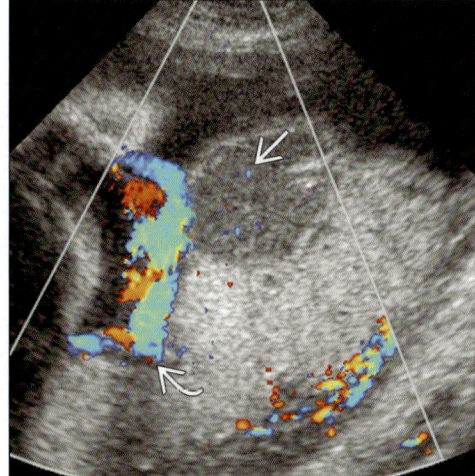

(Left) Ultrasound of the placenta in the second trimester shows a well-defined, hypoechoic mass. *(Right)* Color Doppler ultrasound shows mild vascularity ➡ within the mass (➡ placental cord insertion). Always interrogate placental masses with Doppler to evaluate for flow.

Typical

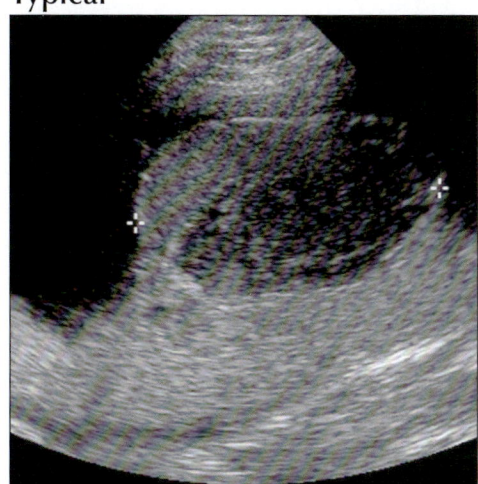
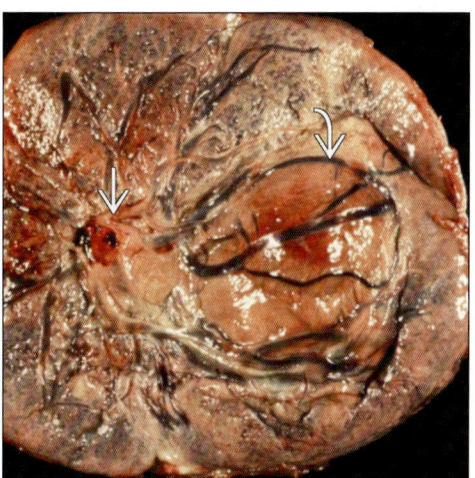

(Left) Ultrasound in the third trimester (same patient as previous image) shows an increase in the size of the mass (calipers). Despite this increase in size, it had no adverse effect on the fetus. *(Right)* Gross pathology of the placenta shows the chorangioma ➡ bulging the fetal surface, near the placental cord insertion site ➡. This is a very typical appearance.

Typical

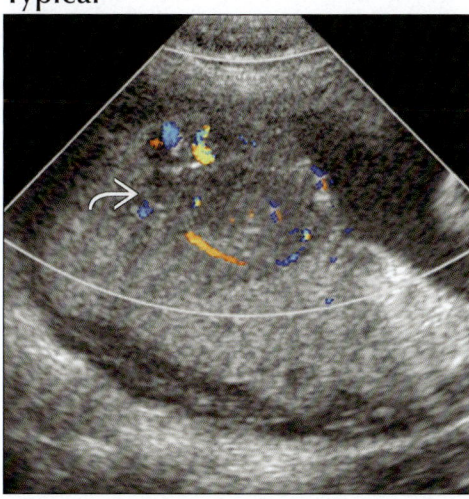
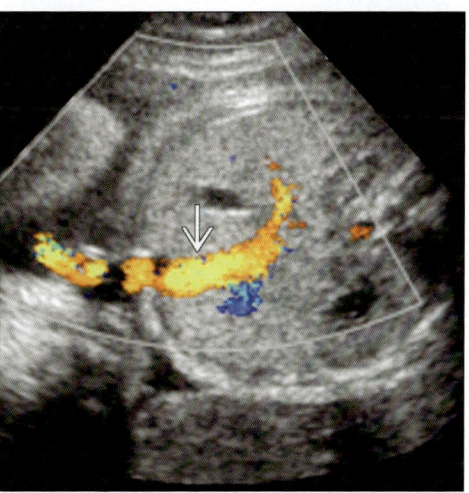

(Left) Color Doppler ultrasound shows a moderately vascular placental mass ➡, which was detected during a routine fetal screening. *(Right)* Transverse color Doppler ultrasound through the fetal abdomen shows an enlarged umbilical vein ➡. In addition, the fetus had mild cardiomegaly but never developed hydrops.

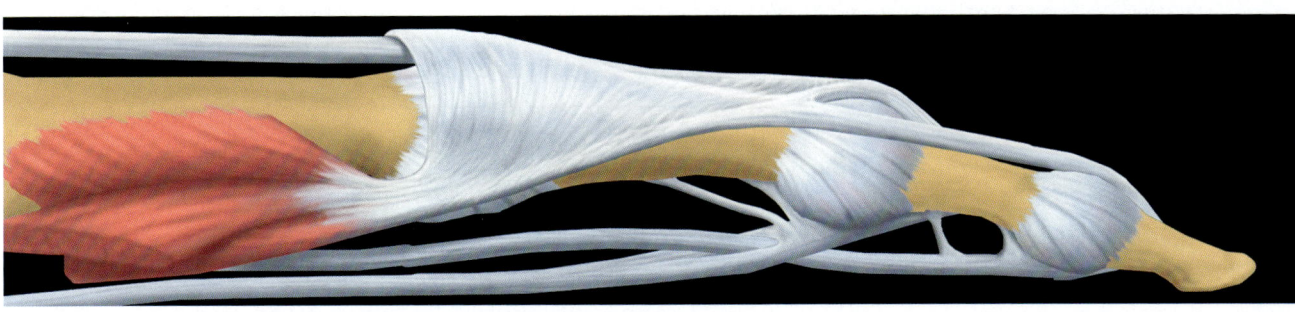

INDEX

A

Abortion
    failed, vs. uterine rupture, 2:229
    hydropic, vs. partial hydatiform mole, **11:10i**, 11:11
    incomplete
        complete hydatiform mole vs., **11:4i**, 11:5
        partial hydatiform mole vs., 11:11
    missed
        partial hydatiform mole vs., 11:11
        retained products of conception vs., **2:232i**, 2:233
    spontaneous
        cervical ectopic pregnancy vs., **10:16i**, 10:17
        endometrial ectopic pregnancy vs., 10:3
        tubal ectopic pregnancy vs., 10:5

Abscess
    appendicular
        tubo-ovarian abscess vs., **8:26i**, 8:28
        yolk sac tumor vs., **7:88i**, 7:89
    bladder flap hematoma vs., 1:49
    ovarian. *See also* Tubo-ovarian abscess
        corpus luteal cyst vs., 7:13
        endometrioma vs., 7:168
        follicular cyst vs., 7:9
    pelvic
        actinomycosis vs., 8:20
        tubo-ovarian abscess vs., 8:28
    periurethral, 6:23

Actinomycosis, 8:18–20, **8:21i**
    differential diagnosis, **8:18i**, 8:19–20
    genital tuberculosis vs., **8:14i**, 8:16

Adenocarcinoma
    Bartholin gland, vs. Bartholin cysts, 4:59
    cervical, 3:26–28, **3:29i**
        cervical glandular hyperplasia vs., **3:64i**, 3:65
        differential diagnosis, **3:26i**, 3:27
        endometrioid cervical, 3:48–50, **3:51i**
            differential diagnosis, **3:48i**, 3:49

Adenofibroma, 7:32–33, **7:32i**

Adenoma malignum, 3:38–39
    cervical cancer vs., **3:14i**, 3:15
        stage IB-IIA., **3:20i**, 3:21
        stage IIB-IVB, 3:23
    cervical glandular hyperplasia vs., **3:64i**
    differential diagnosis, **3:38i**, 3:39
    nabothian cysts vs., **3:60i**, 3:61

Adenomyoma, 2:198–200, **2:201i**
    adenomyosis vs., 2:193
    degenerated leiomyoma vs., **2:110i**, 2:111
    differential diagnosis, **2:198i**, 2:199–200
    endometriosis vs., **7:170i**, 7:172
    submucosal leiomyoma vs., **2:92i**, 2:93
    uterine peristalsis vs., **2:22i**, 2:23

Adenomyosis, 2:192–194, **2:195i–197i**
    adenomyoma vs., 2:199
    adenosarcoma vs., **2:166i**, 2:167
    age-related changes vs., **2:12i**, 2:14
    benign metastasizing leiomyoma vs., **2:118i**, 2:119
    cystic, 2:202–204, **2:205i**
        differential diagnosis, **2:202i**, 2:203
        unicornuate uterus vs., **2:34i**, 2:35–36
    degenerated leiomyoma vs., **2:110i**, 2:111
    differential diagnosis, **2:192i**, 2:193–194
    early stage endometrial cancer vs., **2:144i**, 2:146
    endometrial atrophy vs., **2:18i**, 2:19
    endometrial stromal sarcoma vs., **2:162i**, 2:163
    endometriosis vs., 7:172
    failed uterine artery embolization for, **2:218i**, 2:219
    intramural leiomyoma vs., **2:98i**, 2:99
    leiomyosarcoma vs., 2:177
    malignant mixed mesodermal tumor vs., 2:173
    nabothian cysts vs., 3:61
    placental site trophoblastic tumor vs., 11:21
    submucosal leiomyoma vs., **2:92i**, 2:93
    uterine peristalsis vs., **2:22i**, 2:23

Adenomyositis, 8:23

Adenosarcoma, 2:166–168, **2:169i–171i**
    differential diagnosis, **2:166i**, 2:167
    endocervical polyp vs., 3:7
    endometrial stromal sarcoma vs., **2:162i**, 2:163–164

Adnexal mass, cystic
    degenerated leiomyoma vs., **2:110i**, 2:111
    nabothian cysts vs., 3:61

Adnexal torsion, 7:176–178, **7:179i–181i**
    differential diagnosis, **7:176i**, 7:177–178
    embryonal carcinoma vs., **7:142i**, 7:143
    hemorrhagic cyst vs., 7:194
    massive ovarian edema vs., 7:183
    ovarian vein thrombosis vs., 1:41
    ruptured ectopic pregnancy vs., 10:29
    salpingitis vs., **8:10i**, 8:11

INDEX

tubo-ovarian abscess vs., **8:26i**, 8:28
Air in vagina, **4:62i**, 4:64
Ambiguous genitalia, 4:18–20, **4:21i**. *See also* MRKH (Mayer-Rokitansky-Kuster-Hauser) syndrome; Pseudohermaphrodite
    differential diagnosis, **4:18i**, 4:20
    gonadal dysgenesis vs., 4:23
    hermaphrodite vs. androgen insensitivity syndrome, **4:14i**, 4:15
Anal cancer
    enterocele/rectocele vs., **1:64i**, 1:66
    mucinous, **1:56i**, 1:57
Anatomic imaging issues
    ovary, 7:2–3, **7:5i–7i**
    pelvis
        computed tomography, 1:11, **1:13i–15i**
        magnetic resonance imaging, 1:17–18, **1:19i–21i**
        PET/CT technique, 1:22–24, **1:25i–27i**
        ultrasound, 1:2–4, **1:5i**
    urethra, 6:2, **6:5i**
    uterus, 2:2–3, **2:5i–7i**
    vagina, 4:2–2
    vulva, 5:2
Androgen insensitivity syndrome, 4:14–16, **4:17i**
    differential diagnosis, **4:14i**, 4:15
    gonadal dysgenesis vs., **4:22i**, 4:23
    MRKH syndrome vs., **4:4i**, 4:5
    uterine hypoplasia/agenesis vs., **2:30i**, 2:31
Angiolipoma, 1:37
Angiomatosis, 1:37
Angiomyofibroblastoma, **5:16i**, 5:17
Angiomyxoma, aggressive, 5:16–18, **5:19i**
    differential diagnosis, **5:16i**, 5:17
    leiomyosarcoma vs., **5:10i**
Appendicitis
    hydrosalpinx vs., **8:6i**, 8:7
    ovarian vein thrombosis vs., **1:40i**, 1:41
Appendicular abscess
    tubo-ovarian abscess vs., **8:26i**, 8:28
    yolk sac tumor vs., **7:88i**, 7:89
Arcuate artery calcifications, **2:242i**, 2:243
Arcuate uterus, 2:58–59
    bicornuate uterus vs., 2:48
    DES-exposed uterus vs., 2:61
    differential diagnosis, **2:58i**, 2:59
    septate uterus vs., **2:52i**, 2:53
Arteriovenous malformation
    pelvic congestion syndrome vs., **1:52i**, 1:53
    uterine, 2:206–208, **2:206i, 2:209i–211i**
Ascites, loculated
    peritoneal inclusion cyst vs., **9:2i**, 9:3
    pseudomyxoma peritonei vs., **9:6i**
Asherman syndrome, 2:68–70, **2:71i–73i**
    DES-exposed uterus vs., **2:60i**, 2:61
    differential diagnosis, **2:68i**, 2:69

B

Bartholin cysts, 4:58–60, **4:61i**
    Bartholin gland cancer vs., **4:54i**
    bartholinitis vs., **4:30i**, 4:31
    differential diagnosis, **4:58i**, 4:59
    Gartner duct cysts vs., **4:26i**, 4:27
    Merkel cell tumor vs., **5:22i**, 5:23
    urethral diverticulum vs., **6:18i**, 6:19
    urethral prolapse vs., **6:22i**, 6:23
    vaginal carcinoma vs., 4:41
    vulvar carcinoma vs., **5:4i**, 5:5
    vulvar hemangioma vs., **5:24i**, 5:25
Bartholin gland cancer, 4:54–55
    Bartholin cysts vs., 4:59
    bartholinitis vs., **4:30i**
    differential diagnosis, **4:54i**
Bartholin glands, anatomy, 5:2
Bartholinitis, 4:30–31
    aggressive angiomyxoma vs., **5:16i**, 5:17
    differential diagnosis, **4:30i**, 4:31
    vulvar carcinoma vs., 5:5
    vulvar leiomyosarcoma vs., **5:10i**
Bicornuate uterus, 2:46–48, **2:49i–51i**
    arcuate uterus vs., 2:59
    complex duplication anomalies vs., **2:64i**, 2:65
    didelphys uterus vs., **2:40i**, 2:41
    differential diagnosis, **2:46i**, 2:47–48
    ectopic pregnancy
        abdominal ectopic pregnancy vs., **10:26i**
        interstitial ectopic pregnancy vs., 10:11
    septate uterus vs., **2:52i**, 2:53
    unicornuate uterus vs., **2:34i**, 2:35
Bladder
    non-distended, vs. bladder flap hematoma, **1:48i**, 1:49
    overdistention vs. cervical incompetence, **3:68i**, 3:69
Blood clots
    endocervical polyp vs., **3:6i**, 3:7
    endometrial
        Asherman syndrome vs., 2:69
        synechiae vs., **2:74i**, 2:75
    intrauterine, vs. endometritis, 2:79
    retained products of conception vs., **2:232i**, 2:233
    vaginal, vs. foreign body, 4:64
Bowel
    dermoid vs., **7:22i**, 7:23
    loops vs. paraovarian cyst, 7:164
    next to ovary, vs. tubal pregnancy, **10:4i**
Brenner tumor, 7:60–62, **7:63i**
    cystadenofibroma vs., **7:44i**, 7:45
    differential diagnosis, **7:60i**, 7:61
    fibrothecoma vs., **7:28i**, 7:29
    ovarian hyperstimulation syndrome vs., 7:159

INDEX

undifferentiated ovarian carcinoma vs., 7:139
Broad ligament
   cyst. *See* Paraovarian cyst
   fibroma vs. fibrothecoma, **7:28i**
   hematoma vs. ovarian vein thrombosis, 1:41
   leiomyoma
      fallopian tube leiomyoma vs., **8:32i**, 8:33
      subserosal leiomyoma vs., **2:104i**, 2:105

C

Cancer. *See specific sites and histologic types*
Carcinoid, ovarian, 7:134–136, **7:137i**
   differential diagnosis, **7:134i**, 7:135
Carcinoma
   Bartholin gland, vs. bartholinitis, **4:30i**
   cervical. *See* Cervical carcinoma
   endometrial. *See* Endometrial carcinoma
   fallopian tube. *See* Tubal carcinoma
   Müllerian, vs. parasitic leiomyoma, 2:115
   ovarian. *See* Ovarian carcinoma
   peritoneal
      primary vs. metastases, **9:12i**, 9:13
      pseudomyxoma peritonei vs., **9:6i**
   renal cell, vs. intravenous leiomyomatosis, **2:86i**, 2:87
   urethral. *See* Urethral carcinoma
   vaginal. *See* Vaginal carcinoma
   vulvar. *See* Vulvar carcinoma
Carcinomatosis, peritoneal
   disseminated peritoneal leiomyomatosis vs., **2:90i**
   mesothelioma vs., **9:8i**, 9:9
Cardiac thrombosis, right heart, **2:86i**, 2:87
Cervical adenocarcinoma, 3:26–28, **3:29i**
   cervical glandular hyperplasia vs., **3:64i**, 3:65
   differential diagnosis, **3:26i**, 3:27
Cervical cancer
   adenoma malignum vs., **3:38i**
   characterization, 3:14–16, **3:17i–19i**
      differential diagnosis, **3:14i**, 3:15
   endocervical polyp vs., **3:6i**, 3:7
   leiomyoma vs., **3:10i**, 3:11
   lymphoma vs., **3:40i**, 3:41
   metastasis. *See* Cervical metastasis
   recurrence, 3:34–36, **3:37i**
      differential diagnosis, **3:34i**, 3:35
      post trachelectomy appearances vs., **3:72i**, 3:73
   stage IB-IIA, 3:20–21
      differential diagnosis, **3:20i**, 3:21
      stage IIB-IVB vs., **3:22i**, 3:23
   stage IIB-IVB, 3:22–24, **3:25i**
      differential diagnosis, **3:22i**, 3:23
   vaginal carcinoma vs., 4:41

Cervical carcinoma
   cervical metastasis vs., **3:56i**, 3:57
   endocervical polyp vs., **3:6i**, 3:7
   late stage endometrial cancer vs., **2:150i**, 2:152
   leiomyosarcoma vs., **4:48i**, 4:49
   recurrence vs. post-radiation cervix, **3:76i**, 3:77
   sarcoma vs., **3:44i**, 3:45
   small cell, 3:30–32, **3:30i**, **3:33i**
   vaginal leiomyoma vs., **4:38i**, 4:39
Cervical glandular hyperplasia, 3:64–66, **3:67i**
   adenoma malignum vs., 3:38
   cervical adenocarcinoma vs., **3:26i**, 3:27
   differential diagnosis, **3:64i**, 3:65
Cervical incompetence, 3:68–70, **3:71i**
   differential diagnosis, **3:68i**, 3:69
Cervical leiomyoma, 3:10–12, **3:13i**
   cervical stenosis vs., 3:3
   differential diagnosis, **3:10i**, 3:11
   endocervical polyp vs., **3:6i**, 3:7
   lymphoma vs., **3:40i**, 3:41
Cervical lymphoma, 3:40–42, **3:43i**
   adenoma malignum vs., **3:38i**, 3:39
   cervical cancer vs., **3:14i**, 3:15
      stage IB-IIA, **3:20i**, 3:21
      stage IIB-IVB, 3:23
   differential diagnosis, **3:40i**, 3:41
   endometrioid cervical adenocarcinoma vs., 3:49
   melanoma vs., **3:52i**, 3:53
   metastasis vs., **3:56i**, 3:57
   sarcoma vs., **3:44i**, 3:45
   small cell carcinoma vs., **3:30i**, 3:31
Cervical metastasis, 3:56–58, **3:59i**
   cervical cancer vs., 3:15, 3:21
   differential diagnosis, **3:56i**, 3:57
   endometrioid cervical adenocarcinoma vs., **3:48i**, 3:49
   lymphoma vs., 3:41
   sarcoma vs., **3:44i**, 3:45
   small cell carcinoma vs., **3:30i**, 3:31
Cervical polyp. *See* Endocervical polyp
Cervical sarcoma, 3:44–46, **3:47i**
   differential diagnosis, **3:44i**, 3:45
   endometrioid cervical adenocarcinoma vs., 3:49
   melanoma vs., 3:53
   metastasis vs., **3:56i**, 3:57
Cervical stenosis, 3:2–4, **3:5i**
   cervical glandular hyperplasia vs., 3:65
   differential diagnosis, **3:2i**, 3:3
   endometritis vs., **2:78i**, 2:79
   retained products of conception vs., **2:232i**, 2:233
Cervix uteri, 3:2–3:79
   adenocarcinoma, 3:26–28, **3:29i**
      endometrioid cervical, 3:48–50, **3:51i**
   adenoma malignum, 3:38–39

INDEX

cervical cancer
    characterization, 3:14–16, **3:17i–19i**
    metastasis, 3:56–58, **3:59i**
    recurrence, 3:34–36, **3:37i**
    stage IB-IIA, 3:20–21
    stage IIB-IVB, 3:22–24, **3:25i**
cervical glandular hyperplasia, 3:64–66, **3:67i**
cervical incompetence, 3:68–70, **3:71i**
cervical stenosis, 3:2–4, **3:5i**
endocervical polyp, 3:6–8, **3:9i**
leiomyoma, 3:10–12, **3:13i**
lymphoma, 3:40–42, **3:43i**
melanoma, 3:52–54, **3:55i**
nabothian cysts, 3:60–62, **3:63i**
normal effacement vs. cervical incompetence, 3:69
post-radiation cervix, 3:76–78, **3:79i**
post trachelectomy appearances, 3:72–74, **3:75i**
sarcoma, 3:44–46, **3:47i**
small cell carcinoma, 3:30–32, **3:33i**
Cesarian section
    normal incision vs. uterine rupture, 2:229
    normal postoperative changes, 2:26–28, **2:29i**
        bladder flap hematoma vs., **1:48i**, 1:49
        cervical ectopic pregnancy vs., **10:16i**, 10:17
        differential diagnosis, **2:26i**, 2:27
        interstitial ectopic pregnancy vs., **10:10i**
Chordoma
    sacral, vs. extraperitoneal sarcoma, **1:32i**, 1:33
    sacrococcygeal, vs. sacral teratoma, **1:28i**, 1:29
Chorioamnionitis, 3:69
Chorioamniotic separation, 11:25
Chorioangioma, placental, 11:30–32, **11:33i**
    differential diagnosis, **11:30i**, 11:31
    hematoma vs., **11:24i**, 11:25
    teratoma vs., **11:2i**
Choriocarcinoma
    ovarian, 7:126–128, **7:129i**
        differential diagnosis, **7:126i**, 7:127–128
        embryonal carcinoma vs., **7:142i**, 7:143
        gestational, 7:127
        yolk sac tumor vs., 7:89
    uterine, 2:184–186, **2:187i**
        arteriovenous malformation vs., **2:206i**, 2:207
        complete hydatiform mole vs., 11:5
        differential diagnosis, **2:184i**, 2:185
        invasive mole vs., **11:16i**, 11:17
        placental site trophoblastic tumor vs., **11:20i**, 11:21
Circumvallate placenta, 11:26
Clear cell carcinoma
    ovarian, 7:96–98, **7:99i**
        differential diagnosis, **7:96i**, 7:97
        endometrioid carcinoma vs., 7:75
    vaginal, vs. yolk sac tumor, 4:53
Clitoris, anatomy, 5:2
Colitis, ulcerative, **1:68i**, 1:69
Collagen injection, periurethral
    Bartholin cysts vs., **4:58i**, 4:59
    Gartner duct cysts vs., 4:27
    urethral metastasis vs., **6:14i**, 6:15
Complex duplication anomalies of uterus, 2:64–66, **2:67i**
    bicornuate uterus vs., 2:47
    differential diagnosis, **2:64i**, 2:65
    uterus didelphys vs., **2:40i**, 2:41
Computed tomography (CT), pelvic
    combined PET/CT technique, 1:22–24, **1:25i–27i**
    technique and anatomy, 1:10–12, **1:13i–15i**
Condyloma acuminatum, 6:23
Corpus luteal cyst, 7:12–14, **7:15i**
    differential diagnosis, **7:12i**, 7:13
    hemorrhagic
        heterotopic pregnancy vs., **10:22i**, 10:23
        ovarian ectopic pregnancy vs., **10:20i**
        ruptured ectopic pregnancy vs., **10:28i**, 10:29
        tubal ectopic pregnancy vs., **10:4i**, 10:5
    mucinous cystadenoma vs., 7:55
    serous cystadenoma vs., **7:48i**, 7:49
Crohn disease
    actinomycosis vs., 8:20
    parasitic leiomyoma vs., 2:115
    tubo-ovarian abscess vs., 8:28
Cryptorchidism, 4:20
Cul-de-sac
    fluid vs. bladder flap hematoma, **1:48i**, 1:49
    ruptured ectopic pregnancy vs. blood in, **10:28i**, 10:29
Cyst of Müllerian origin, 4:27
Cystadenocarcinoma
    cystadenofibroma vs., **7:44i**, 7:45
    hemorrhagic cyst vs., **7:192i**, 7:194
    mucinous, 7:64–66, **7:67i–69i**
        clear cell carcinoma vs., **7:96i**, 7:97
        cystadenoma vs., **7:54i**, 7:55
        differential diagnosis, **7:64i**, 7:65
        dysgerminoma vs., 7:85
        endometrioid carcinoma vs., **7:74i**, 7:75
        granulosa cell tumor vs., 7:35
        serous cystadenocarcinoma vs., **7:70i**, 7:71
        struma ovarii vs., **7:130i**, 7:131
    ovarian hyperstimulation syndrome vs., 7:159
    parasitic leiomyoma vs., 2:115
    serous, 7:70–72, **7:73i**
        clear cell carcinoma vs., **7:96i**, 7:97
        cystadenoma vs., **7:48i**, 7:49
        differential diagnosis, **7:70i**, 7:71
        dysgerminoma vs., **7:84i**, 7:85
        endometrioid carcinoma vs., **7:74i**, 7:75

INDEX

granulosa cell tumor vs., 7:35
mucinous cystadenocarcinoma vs., **7:64i**, 7:65
theca lutein cyst vs., **7:16i**
Cystadenofibroma, 7:44–46, **7:47i**
differential diagnosis, **7:44i**, 7:45
Cystadenoma
mucinous, 7:54–56, **7:57i–59i**
clear cell carcinoma vs., 7:97
cystadenocarcinoma vs., **7:64i**, 7:65
differential diagnosis, **7:54i**, 7:55
endometrioid carcinoma vs., 7:75
granulosa cell tumor vs., 7:35
inclusion cyst vs., **7:154i**, 7:155
luteoma of pregnancy vs., **7:20i**
serous cystadenocarcinoma vs., 7:71
serous cystadenoma vs., 7:49–50
struma ovarii vs., **7:130i**, 7:131
ovarian hyperstimulation syndrome vs., 7:159
parasitic leiomyoma vs., 2:115
serous, 7:48–50, **7:51i–53i**
clear cell carcinoma vs., 7:97
cystadenocarcinoma vs., **7:70i**, 7:71
differential diagnosis, **7:48i**, 7:49–50
endometrioid carcinoma vs., 7:75
granulosa cell tumor vs., 7:35
mucinous cystadenoma vs., 7:55
paraovarian cyst vs., 7:163
Cystic adenomyosis, 2:202–204, **2:205i**
differential diagnosis, **2:202i**, 2:203
unicornuate uterus vs., **2:34i**, 2:35–36
Cystitis, 1:57
Cystocele, 1:60–62, **1:63i**
differential diagnosis, **1:60i**, 1:61–62
urethral diverticulum vs., **6:18i**, 6:19
Cytotrophoblastic cysts, 11:26

D

Dermoid cyst, 7:22–24, **7:25i–27i**
Brenner tumor vs., **7:60i**, 7:61
carcinoid vs., **7:134i**, 7:135
differential diagnosis, **7:22i**, 7:23
embryonal carcinoma vs., 7:143
endometrioma vs., 7:167
fibrothecoma vs., 7:29
follicular cyst vs., **7:8i**, 7:9
hemorrhagic cyst vs., 7:193
heterotopic pregnancy vs., **10:22i**, 10:23
immature teratoma vs., **7:100i**, 7:101
lipomatous uterine tumor vs., **2:124i**, 2:125
mucinous cystadenoma vs., 7:55
ovarian cancer vs., 7:113
ovarian hyperstimulation syndrome vs., 7:159
parasitic leiomyoma vs., **2:114i**
sacral teratoma vs., 1:29

serous cystadenoma vs., **7:48i**, 7:50
struma ovarii vs., **7:130i**, 7:131
yolk sac tumor vs., **7:88i**, 7:89
DES-exposed uterus, 2:60–62, **2:63i**
differential diagnosis, **2:60i**, 2:61
MRKH syndrome vs., 4:5
uterine hypoplasia/agenesis vs., 2:32
Desmoid tumor, 7:171
Diethystilbestrol (DES) exposure. *See* DES-exposed uterus
Diverticulitis
actinomycosis vs., 8:20
post-radiation pelvis vs., 1:72
tubo-ovarian abscess vs., 8:28
Diverticulum, urethral, 6:18–6:20, **6:21i**
carcinoma vs., **6:10i**, 6:11
differential diagnosis, **6:18i**, 6:19
leiomyoma vs., **6:6i**
metastasis vs., **6:14i**, 6:15
prolapse vs., 6:23
schwannoma vs., **6:8i**, 6:9
Double decidual sac sign, 10:3
Duplication cyst
enterocele/rectocele vs., **1:64i**
sacral teratoma vs., 1:29
Dysgerminoma
ovarian, 7:84–86, **7:87i**
choriocarcinoma vs., **7:126i**, 7:127
differential diagnosis, **7:84i**, 7:85
embryonal carcinoma vs., 7:143
lymphoma vs., 7:93
undifferentiated ovarian carcinoma vs., 7:139
yolk sac tumor vs., 7:89
uterine, vs. complete hydatiform mole, 11:5

E

Ectopic pregnancy, 10:2–33
abdominal, 10:26–27
differential diagnosis, **10:26i**
ovarian pregnancy vs., **10:20i**, 10:21
adnexal torsion vs., 7:178
cervical, 10:16–18, **10:19i**
cervical glandular hyperplasia vs., 3:65
differential diagnosis, **10:16i**, 10:17
endometrial, 10:2–3, **10:2i**
hemorrhagic cyst vs., **7:192i**, 7:193
heterotopic, 10:22–24, **10:25i**
interstitial, 10:10–12, **10:13i–15i**
abdominal ectopic pregnancy vs., **10:26i**
differential diagnosis, **10:10i**, 10:11
ovarian, 10:20–21
abdominal pregnancy vs., 10:26
differential diagnosis, **10:20i**, 10:21
parasitic leiomyoma vs., 2:115

INDEX

ruptured, 10:28–30, **10:31i–33i**
    differential diagnosis, **10:28i**, 10:29
    heterotopic pregnancy vs., **10:22i**, 10:23
  tubal, 10:4–6, **10:7i–9i**. *See also* Tubal ectopic pregnancy
Edema, bullous, **2:150i**, 2:152
Embryology
  ovary, 7:4
  uterus, 2:4
  vagina, 4:3
Embryonal carcinoma, 7:142–144, **7:145i**
  differential diagnosis, **7:142i**, 7:143
  yolk sac tumor vs., 7:89
Endocervical polyp, 3:6–8, **3:9i**
  adenocarcinoma vs., **3:26i**, 3:27
  cervical cancer vs., **3:14i**, 3:15
    stage IB-IIA, **3:20i**, 3:21
    stage IIB-IVB, **3:22i**, 3:23
  differential diagnosis, **3:6i**, 3:7
  late stage endometrial cancer vs., **2:150i**, 2:152
  leiomyoma vs., **3:10i**, 3:11
  lymphoma vs., **3:40i**, 3:41
Endocervicitis, papillary, 3:65
Endometrial atrophy, 2:18–20, **2:21i**
  differential diagnosis, **2:18i**, 2:19
Endometrial calcifications, **2:78i**, 2:79
Endometrial cancer. *See also specific cancer names and histologic types*
  adenomyosis vs., 2:194
  adenosarcoma vs., **2:166i**, 2:167
  age-related changes vs., **2:12i**, 2:14
  characterization, 2:140–142, **2:140i**, **2:143i**
  early stage, 2:144–146, **2:144i**, **2:147i–149i**
  hyperplasia vs., **2:134i**, 2:135
  invasive mole vs., **11:16i**, 11:17
  late stage, 2:150–152, **2:153i–155i**
    differential diagnosis, **2:150i**, 2:151–152
    endometrioid cervical adenocarcinoma vs., **3:48i**, 3:49
  leiomyosarcoma vs., **2:176i**, 2:177
  polyps vs., **2:128i**, 2:129
  recurrence, 2:156–158, **2:156i**, **2:159i–161i**
  submucosal leiomyoma vs., 2:93
  synechiae vs., 2:75
  tamoxifen-induced cancer vs., **2:238i**, 2:240
Endometrial carcinoma
  adenosarcoma vs., **2:166i**, 2:167
  age-related changes vs., **2:12i**, 2:14
  choriocarcinoma vs., **2:184i**, 2:185
  endometrial stromal sarcoma vs., **2:162i**, 2:163–164
  hyperplasia vs., **2:134i**, 2:135
  lymphoma vs., **2:180i**, 2:181
  malignant mixed mesodermal tumor vs., **2:172i**, 2:173
  placental site trophoblastic tumor vs., **11:20i**, 11:21
  polyps vs., **2:128i**, 2:129
  submucosal leiomyoma vs., 2:93
  uterine artery embolization complications vs., **2:222i**, 2:223–224
  uterine metastases vs., **2:188i**, 2:189
Endometrial hyperplasia, 2:134–136, **2:137i–139i**
  age-related changes vs., 2:14
  differential diagnosis, **2:134i**, 2:135
  early stage endometrial cancer vs., **2:144i**, 2:146
  endometrial cancer vs., 2:141
  focal, vs. polyps, **2:128i**, 2:129
  placental site trophoblastic tumor vs., 11:21
  synechiae vs., 2:75
Endometrial polyps, 2:128–130, **2:131i–133i**
  adenomatous, vs. adenosarcoma, **2:166i**, 2:167
  adenomyoma vs., 2:200
  age-related changes vs., **2:12i**, 2:14
  Asherman syndrome vs., **2:68i**, 2:69
  cystic, vs. endometrial atrophy, **2:18i**, 2:19
  differential diagnosis, **2:128i**, 2:129
  early stage endometrial cancer vs., **2:144i**, 2:146
  endocervical polyp vs., 3:7
  endometrial cancer vs., 2:141
  endometrial synechiae vs., **2:74i**, 2:75
  hyperplasia vs., **2:134i**, 2:135
  placental site trophoblastic tumor vs., 11:21
  submucosal leiomyoma vs., **2:92i**, 2:93
  tamoxifen-induced polyps vs., **2:238i**, 2:240
  uterine artery embolization complications vs., **2:222i**, 2:223
Endometrial stromal nodule, benign, 2:163
Endometrial stromal sarcoma, 2:162–164, **2:165i**
  adenomyosis vs., **2:192i**, 2:194
  characterization, **2:140i**, 2:141
  differential diagnosis, **2:162i**, 2:163–164
  endocervical polyp vs., 3:7
  leiomyosarcoma vs., **2:176i**, 2:177
  lymphoma vs., 2:181
  malignant mixed mesodermal tumor vs., **2:172**i, 2:173
Endometrial synechiae, 2:74–76, **2:77i**
  Asherman syndrome vs., **2:68i**, 2:69
  differential diagnosis, **2:74i**, 2:75
Endometrioid carcinoma, ovarian, 7:74–76, **7:77i–79i**
  adenofibroma vs., **7:32i**
  differential diagnosis, **7:74i**, 7:75
Endometrioid cervical adenocarcinoma, 3:48–50, **3:51i**
  differential diagnosis, **3:48i**, 3:49
Endometrioma, 7:166–168, **7:169i**
  clear cell carcinoma vs., **7:96i**, 7:97
  corpus luteal cyst vs., 7:13
  cystadenofibroma vs., 7:45

INDEX

dermoid vs., **7:22i**, 7:23
differential diagnosis, **7:166i**, 7:167–168
endometrioid carcinoma vs., **7:74i**, 7:75
follicular cyst vs., **7:8i**, 7:9
hemorrhagic cyst vs., **7:192i**, 7:193
mucinous cystadenoma vs., 7:55
ovarian hyperstimulation syndrome vs., **7:158i**, 7:159
paraovarian cyst vs., 7:163
serous cystadenoma vs., 7:49
spinal meningeal cyst vs., **1:44i**, 1:45
Endometriosis, 7:170–172, **7:173i–175i**
    cervical, vs. glandular hyperplasia, 3:65
    differential diagnosis, **7:170i**, 7:171–172
    disseminated peritoneal leiomyomatosis vs., **2:90i**
    embryonal carcinoma vs., 7:143
    failed uterine artery embolization for, **2:218i**, 2:219
    mucinous cystadenoma vs., **7:54i**
    ovarian cancer vs., 7:113
    parasitic leiomyoma vs., 2:115
    subserosal, **2:198i**, 2:200
    tubal, 8:23
    tubal metastases vs., 8:48
    vulvar, vs. hemangioma, 5:25
Endometritis, 2:78–80, **2:81i**
    cervical stenosis vs., **3:2i**, 3:3
    differential diagnosis, **2:78i**, 2:79
    endometrial hyperplasia vs., 2:135
    pyomyoma vs., 2:83
    retained products of conception vs., 2:233
    tuberculous, vs. synechiae., 2:75
    uterine rupture vs., **2:228i**, 2:229
Endometrium
    nondistention of cavity vs. synechiae., 2:75
    normal lining vs. intrauterine device, **2:242i**, 2:243
    premenstrual, 2:146
    secretory, vs. hyperplasia, **2:134i**, 2:135
Enterocele, 1:64–66, **1:67i**
    differential diagnosis, **1:64i**, 1:65–1:66
Epidermal inclusion cyst, 4:31
Epidermoid cyst, 1:29
Epithelial polyp, 8:48
Epithelial tumor
    ovarian, vs. theca lutein cyst, 7:17
    surface
        corpus luteal cyst vs., 7:13
        follicular cyst vs., 7:9

F

Fallopian tubes, 8:2–8:55. *See also* Tubal ectopic pregnancy
    actinomycosis, 8:18–20, **8:21i**
    cysts, vs. ectopic pregnancy, 10:6
    genital tuberculosis, 8:14–16, **8:17i**
    hematosalpinx, 8:50–52, **8:53i–55i**
    hydrosalpinx, 8:6–8, **8:9i**
    leiomyoma, 8:32–34, **8:35i**
    metastases, 8:48–49
    paratubal cysts, 8:2–4, **8:5i**
    salpingitis, 8:10–12, **8:13i**
    salpingitis isthmica nodosa, 8:22–24, **8:25i**
    torsion. *See* Adnexal torsion
    tubal carcinoma
        characterization, 8:36–38, **8:39i–41i**
        staging and prognosis, 8:42–44, **8:45i–47i**
    tubo-ovarian abscess, 8:26–28, **8:29i–31i**
Fibroids. *See* Leiomyoma
Fibrolipomatosis. *See* Lipomatosis, pelvic
Fibroma
    broad ligament, vs. fibrothecoma, **7:28i**
    edematous, vs. massive ovarian edema, 7:183
    ovarian
        adenofibroma vs., **7:32i**
        Brenner tumor vs., 7:61
        cystadenofibroma vs., **7:44i**, 7:45
        embryonal carcinoma vs., 7:143
        fallopian tube leiomyoma vs., **8:32i**, 8:33
        fibromatosis vs., **7:190i**
        lymphoma vs., **7:92i**, 7:93
        parasitic leiomyoma vs., **2:114i**, 2:115
        sclerosing stromal tumor vs., **7:40i**, 7:41
        serous cystadenoma vs., 7:50
        Sertoli-Leydig cell tumor vs., 7:81
    with focal degeneration, **7:34i**, 7:35
Fibromatosis, ovarian, 7:190–191
    differential diagnosis, **7:190i**
    massive ovarian edema vs., 7:183
Fibrothecoma, ovarian, 7:28–30, **7:31i**
    Brenner tumor vs., 7:61
    cystadenofibroma vs., **7:44i**, 7:45
    differential diagnosis, **7:28i**, 7:29
    embryonal carcinoma vs., 7:143
    endometrioma vs., **7:166i**, 7:168
    fibromatosis vs., **7:190i**
    granulosa cell tumor vs., **7:34i**, 7:35
    lymphoma vs., 7:93
    ovarian hyperstimulation syndrome vs., 7:159
    Sertoli-Leydig cell tumor vs., **7:80i**, 7:81
    undifferentiated ovarian carcinoma vs., 7:139
Fistula
    urethral, vs. carcinoma, **6:10i**, 6:11
    vaginal, 4:32–34, **4:35i–37i**
        differential diagnosis, **4:32i**
        foreign body vs., **4:62i**, 4:64
Follicular cyst, 7:8–10, **7:11i**
    differential diagnosis, **7:8i**, 7:9
    inclusion cyst vs., **7:154i**, 7:155
    mucinous cystadenoma vs., 7:55
    serous cystadenoma vs., **7:48i**, 7:49

INDEX

Foreign bodies, vaginal, 4:62–64, **4:65i**
    differential diagnosis, **4:62i**, 4:64

G

Gartner duct cysts, 4:26–28, **4:29i**
    Bartholin cysts vs., **4:58i**, 4:59
    Bartholin gland cancer vs., **4:54i**
    bartholinitis vs., 4:31
    cervical glandular hyperplasia vs., 3:65
    cystic adenomyosis vs., **2:202i**, 2:203
    differential diagnosis, **4:26i**, 4:27
    nabothian cysts vs., **3:60i**, 3:61
    urethral diverticulum vs., 6:19
Gas, intrauterine
    endometritis vs., 2:79
    retained products of conception vs., 2:233
Genitalia, ambiguous. *See* Ambiguous genitalia
Germ cell tumor, 7:13
Gestational sac, empty
    endometrial ectopic pregnancy vs., **10:2i**, 10:3
    in twin pregnancy, vs. placental hematoma, **11:24i**, 11:25
Gestational trophoblastic disease. *See* Choriocarcinoma, uterine; Hydatiform mole
Gonadal dysgenesis, 4:22–24, **4:25i**
    androgen insensitivity syndrome vs., 4:15
    differential diagnosis, **4:22i**, 4:23
    MRKH syndrome vs., 4:5
    uterine hypoplasia/agenesis vs., 2:31
Granuloma, post-surgical, **2:156i**, 2:157
Granulosa cell tumor, 7:34–36, **7:37i–39i**
    carcinoid vs., **7:134i**, 7:135
    corpus luteal cyst vs., **7:12i**, 7:13
    differential diagnosis, **7:34i**, 7:35
    embryonal carcinoma vs., 7:143
    lymphoma vs., 7:93
    Sertoli-Leydig cell tumor vs., **7:80i**, 7:81
    theca lutein cyst vs., 7:17
    undifferentiated ovarian carcinoma vs., **7:138i**, 7:139

H

Hemangioendothelioma, 1:37
Hemangioma
    pelvic, 1:36–38, **1:39i**
        differential diagnosis, **1:36i**, 1:37
    urethral, vs. metastasis, 6:15
    uterine, vs. arteriovenous malformation, 2:208
    vulvar, 5:24–25
        differential diagnosis, **5:24i**, 5:25
        lymphoma vs., **5:20i**, 5:21
        urethral prolapse vs., 6:23
Hemangiopericytoma
    aggressive angiomyxoma vs., **5:16i**, 5:17
    extraperitoneal sarcoma vs., **1:32i**, 1:33
    pelvic hemangioma vs., **1:36i**, 1:37
Hematoma
    bladder flap, 1:48–50, **1:51i**
        differential diagnosis, **1:48i**, 1:49
        uterine rupture vs., **2:228i**, 2:229
    broad ligament, vs. ovarian vein thrombosis, 1:41
    placental, 11:24–26, **11:27i–29i**
        chorioangioma vs., **11:30i**, 11:31
        differential diagnosis, **11:24i**, 11:25–26
        teratoma vs., **11:2i**, 11:3
    subfascial vs. bladder flap, 1:49
    urethral prolapse vs., 6:23
Hematometra
    cystic adenomyosis vs., **2:202i**, 2:203
    endometrial polyps vs., **2:128i**, 2:129
Hematosalpinx, 8:50–52, **8:53i–55i**
    adnexal torsion vs., **7:176i**, 7:178
    differential diagnosis, **8:50i**, 8:51
    salpingitis vs., **8:10i**, 8:11
    tubal carcinoma vs., 8:37
Hemorrhage, placental, 11:31
Hemorrhagic cysts, 7:192–194, **7:195i–197i**
    adnexal torsion vs., **7:176i**, 7:177
    dermoid vs., **7:22i**, 7:23
    differential diagnosis, **7:192i**, 7:193–194
    functional, vs. endometrioma, **7:166i**, 7:167
    granulosa cell tumor vs., **7:34i**, 7:35
    luteoma of pregnancy vs., **7:20i**
    massive ovarian edema vs., **7:182i**, 7:183
    ovarian cancer vs., 7:113
    salpingitis vs., 8:11
    tubo-ovarian abscess vs., 8:28
Hermaphrodite, **4:14i**, 4:15
Heterotopic pregnancy, 10:22–24, **10:25i**
    differential diagnosis, **10:22i**, 10:23
    tubal ectopic pregnancy vs., 10:5
Histiocytoma, malignant fibrous, 2:115
Hydatiform mole
    complete mole, 11:4–6, **11:7i–9i**
        differential diagnosis, **11:4i**, 11:5
        invasive mole vs., 11:17
        partial mole vs., **11:10i**, 11:11
    fallopian tube, vs. tubal metastases, 8:49
    invasive, 11:16–18, **11:19i**
        complete mole vs., 11:5
        differential diagnosis, **11:16i**, 11:17
        placental site trophoblastic tumor vs., 11:21
    partial mole, 11:10–12, **11:13i–15i**
        chorioangioma vs., 11:31
        complete mole vs., **11:4i**, 11:5
        differential diagnosis, **11:10i**, 11:11
        invasive mole vs., **11:16i**, 11:17
    placental site trophoblastic tumor vs., 11:21

INDEX

Hydrometrocolpos, **4:50i**, 4:51
Hydrosalpinx, 8:6–8, **8:9i**
   differential diagnosis, **8:6i**, 8:7–8
      hemorrhagic cyst vs., 7:194
      ovarian hyperstimulation syndrome vs., **7:158i**, 7:159
      ovarian vein thrombosis vs., **1:40i**, 1:41
      paraovarian cyst vs., **7:162i**, 7:163
      paratubal cysts vs., **8:2i**, 8:3
      pelvic congestion syndrome vs., **1:52i**, 1:53
      peritoneal inclusion cyst vs., 9:3
      salpingitis isthmica nodosa vs., **8:22i**
      spinal meningeal cyst vs., **1:44i**, 1:45
      tubal carcinoma vs., 8:37, **8:42i**
Hymen. *See* Imperforate hymen
Hypogonadism, hypogonadotropic, **4:22i**, 4:23
Hysterectomy
   MRKH syndrome vs., **4:4i**, 4:6
   uterine hypoplasia/agenesis vs., **2:30i**, 2:32
Hysterosalpingography, 1:6–8, **1:9i**
   problems and complications, 1:8
   procedure, 1:7–8

I

Imaging issues. *See* Anatomic imaging issues; Pathologic imaging issues
Imperforate hymen, 4:10–11
   differential diagnosis, **4:10i**, 4:11
   Gartner duct cysts vs., 4:27
   urethral prolapse vs., 6:23
   vaginal atresia vs., **4:8i**, 4:9
   vaginal septae vs., **4:12i**, 4:13
Inclusion cysts
   epidermal, 4:31
   ovarian, 7:154–156, **7:157i**
      differential diagnosis, **7:154i**, 7:155
   peritoneal. *See* Peritoneal inclusion cysts
   squamous, vs. Bartholin cyst, 4:59
   urethral diverticulum vs., 6:19
Inferior vena cava, 1:41
Intraductal sac sign, **10:2i**
Intrauterine device evaluation, 2:242–244, **2:245i–247i**
   differential diagnosis, **2:242i**, 2:243
Introitus, anatomy, 5:2
Intussusception, rectal
   enterocele/rectocele vs., 1:65
   pelvic floor descent vs., 1:57
Invasive mole. *See* Hydatiform mole, invasive

K

Kallmann syndrome, **4:22i**, 4:23
Krukenberg tumor, 7:150–152, **7:153i**
   Brenner tumor vs., **7:60i**, 7:61
   carcinoid vs., 7:135
   differential diagnosis, **7:150i**, 7:151
   mixed Mullerian tumor vs., **7:146i**, 7:147
   sclerosing stromal tumor vs., **7:40i**, 7:41
   undifferentiated ovarian carcinoma vs., **7:138i**, 7:139

L

Labia
   adhesions, 4:11
   anatomy, 5:2
Leiomyoma
   adenomyoma vs., **2:198i**, 2:199
   adenomyosis vs., **2:192i**, 2:193
   air in, vs. uterine rupture, **2:228i**, 2:229
   autoinfarction, **2:212i**, 2:213
   benign metastasizing, 2:118–120, **2:121i**
      differential diagnosis, **2:118i**, 2:119
      disseminated peritoneal leiomyomatosis vs., 2:90
   broad ligament
      fallopian tube leiomyoma vs., **8:32i**, 8:33
      subserosal leiomyoma vs., **2:104i**, 2:105
   cervical. *See* Cervical leiomyoma
   degenerated, 2:110–112, **2:113i**
      cystic adenomyosis vs., **2:202i**, 2:203
      differential diagnosis, **2:110i**, 2:111
      endometrial stromal sarcoma vs., 2:163
      hemorrhagic, unicornuate uterus vs., 2:35
      hemorrhagic cyst vs., 7:193
      lipomatous uterine tumor vs., **2:124i**, 2:125
      ovarian hyperstimulation syndrome vs., 7:159
      pyomyoma vs., **2:82i**, 2:83
   exophytic, vs. tubal ectopic pregnancy, **10:4i**, 10:5
   fallopian tube, 8:32–34, **8:35i**
      differential diagnosis, **8:32i**, 8:33
      paratubal cyst vs., 8:3
   intramural, 2:98–100, **2:101i–103i**
      differential diagnosis, **2:98i**, 2:99
      uterine peristalsis vs., **2:22i**
   leiomyosarcoma vs., 2:177
   luteoma of pregnancy vs., **7:20i**
   malignant mixed mesodermal tumor vs., 2:173
   parasitic, 2:114–116, **2:117i**
      differential diagnosis, **2:114i**, 2:115
      subserosal leiomyoma vs., **2:104i**, 2:105
   prolapsing, **1:56i**
   retroplacental, vs. placental hematoma, 11:25
   submucosal, 2:92–94, **2:95i–97i**
      arcuate uterus vs., **2:58i**, 2:59
      Asherman syndrome vs., 2:69
      cervical stenosis vs., 3:3
      differential diagnosis, **2:92i**, 2:93–2:94

INDEX

endometrial cancer vs., 2:141
endometrial polyps vs., 2:129
tamoxifen-induced, **2:238i**, 2:239
uterine artery embolization complications vs., **2:222i**, 2:223
uterine peristalsis vs., **2:22i**, 2:23
vaginocele/cystocele vs., **1:60i**
subserosal, 2:104–106, **2:107i–109i**
Brenner tumor vs., 7:61
differential diagnosis, **2:104i**, 2:105
fallopian tube leiomyoma vs., **8:32i**, 8:33
unicornuate uterus vs., **2:34i**, 2:35–36
urethral. *See* Urethral leiomyoma
uterine. *See* Uterine leiomyoma
vaginal. *See* Vaginal leiomyoma
with hemorrhagic infarction, vs. pyomyoma, 2:83
Leiomyomatosis
benign metastasizing, 2:87
diffuse uterine, 2:122–123
differential diagnosis, **2:122i**, 2:123
intravenous leiomyomatosis vs., 2:87
disseminated peritoneal, 2:90–91
benign metastasizing leiomyoma vs., 2:119
differential diagnosis, **2:90i**, 2:91
diffuse uterine leiomyomatosis vs., 2:122
intravenous leiomyomatosis vs., 2:87
intravenous, 2:86–88, **2:89i**
differential diagnosis, **2:86i**, 2:87
diffuse uterine leiomyomatosis vs., **2:122i**, 2:123
disseminated peritoneal leiomyomatosis vs., 2:91
endometrial stromal sarcoma, 2:164
peritoneal, 9:9
Leiomyosarcoma
failed uterine artery embolization for, **2:218i**, 2:219
uterine. *See* Uterine leiomyosarcoma
uterine artery embolization imaging for, **2:212i**, 2:213
vaginal, 4:48–49
differential diagnosis, **4:48i**, 4:49
leiomyoma vs., **4:38i**
vulvar, 5:10–11, **5:10i**
Lipoleiomyoma
ovarian, vs. lipomatous uterine tumor, 2:125
pedunculated, vs. dermoid, 7:23
Lipoma, 2:125
Lipomatosis, pelvic, 1:68–69, **1:68i**
Lipomatous uterine tumors, 2:124–126, **2:127i**
differential diagnosis, **2:124i**, 2:125–126
Liposarcoma
hemangioma vs., **1:36i**, 1:37
pelvic, vs. lipomatous uterine tumor, **2:124i**, 2:126

Luteoma of pregnancy, 7:20–21
differential diagnosis, **7:20i**
theca lutein cyst vs., **7:16i**, 7:17
Lymphadenopathy
necrotic, vs. ovarian vein thrombosis, 1:41
parasitic leiomyoma vs., 2:115
pelvic congestion syndrome vs., **1:52i**, 1:53
Lymphangioleiomyomatosis, **2:118i**, 2:119
Lymphatic intravasation, **8:22i**
Lymphocele
cervical cancer recurrence vs., **3:34i**, 3:35
endometrial cancer recurrence vs., 2:157
paraovarian cyst vs., 7:163
paratubal cysts vs., **8:2i**, 8:3
pelvic, vs. endometrial cancer recurrence, **2:156i**, 2:157
postoperative
recurrent resectable ovarian cancer vs., **7:118i**, 7:119
recurrent unresectable ovarian cancer vs., **7:122i**, 7:123
Lymphoma
cervical. *See* Cervical lymphoma
extraperitoneal sarcoma vs., 1:33
ovarian. *See* Ovarian lymphoma
peritoneal
mesothelioma vs., **9:8i**, 9:9
metastasis vs., **9:12i**, 9:13
uterine, 2:180–182, **2:183i**
differential diagnosis, **2:180i**, 2:181
metastases vs., 2:189
vaginal, 4:46–47
carcinoma vs., **4:40i**, 4:41
differential diagnosis, **4:46i**, 4:47
metastases vs., **4:56i**
vulvar, 5:20–21
differential diagnosis, **5:20i**, 5:21
urethral prolapse vs., **6:22i**, 6:23

M

Magnetic resonance imaging (MRI)
pelvis, technique and anatomy, 1:16–18, **1:19i–21i**
Malignant mixed mesodermal tumor, 2:172–174, **2:175i**
adenosarcoma vs., 2:167
characterization of, **2:140i**, 2:141
differential diagnosis, **2:172i**, 2:173
leiomyosarcoma vs., **2:176i**
lipomatous uterine tumor vs., 2:125
Malignant teratoma. *See* Teratoma, immature (malignant)
Mature teratoma. *See* Dermoid cyst

INDEX

Mayer-Rokitansky-Kuster-Hauser (MRKH) syndrome. *See* MRKH (Mayer-Rokitansky-Kuster-Hauser) syndrome
Meigs syndrome, 7:198–200, **7:201i**
    differential diagnosis, **7:198i**, 7:199
Melanocytic nevus, 5:13
Melanoma
    cervical, 3:52–54, **3:55i**
        differential diagnosis, **3:52i**, 3:53
        metastasis vs., 3:57
    vaginal, **4:40i**, 4:41
    vulvar. *See* Vulvar melanoma
Meningeal cysts, spinal, 1:44–46, **1:47i**
    differential diagnosis, **1:44i**, 1:45
Menstrual cycle, imaging issues, 2:2
Merkel cell tumor, 5:22–23
    carcinoma vs., **5:4i**, 5:5
    differential diagnosis, **5:22i**, 5:23
    melanoma vs., **5:12i**, 5:13
Mesenchymal dysplasia, **11:10i**, 11:11
Mesodermal tumor, malignant mixed. *See* Malignant mixed mesodermal tumor
Mesothelioma
    cystic vs. peritoneal, **9:8i**, 9:9
    papillary vs. peritoneal, 9:9
    peritoneal, 9:8–10, **9:11i**
        differential diagnosis, **9:8i**, 9:9
        metastasis vs., 9:13
Metastases
    bone, vs. post-radiation pelvis, 1:72
    carcinoid, **7:134i**, 7:135
    cervical. *See* Cervical metastasis
    cervical cancer stage IIB-IVB vs., **3:22i**, 3:23
    fallopian tube, 8:48–49
        differential diagnosis, **8:48i**, 8:49
        tubal carcinoma vs., **8:36i**, 8:37
    leiomyosarcoma, vs. benign metastasizing leiomyoma., **2:118i**, 2:119
    malignant melanoma., **3:52i**, 3:53
    maternal placental, vs. chorioangioma, 11:31
    ovarian. *See* Ovarian metastases
    peritoneal, 9:12–14, **9:15i–17i**
        differential diagnosis, **9:12i**, 9:13
        disseminated peritoneal leiomyomatosis vs., **2:90i**
        lymphomatosis vs. mesothelioma, 9:9
    thyroid, vs. struma ovarii, 7:131
    urethral, 6:14–6:16, **6:17i**
        differential diagnosis, **6:14i**, 6:15
    uterine, 2:188–190, **2:191i**
        adenomyosis vs., 2:194
        differential diagnosis, **2:188i**, 2:189
        granulosa cell tumor vs., 7:35
    vaginal, 4:56–57
        carcinoma vs., **4:40i**, 4:41
        differential diagnosis, **4:56i**, 4:57
        lymphoma vs., **4:46i**
    vulvar, vs. melanoma, **5:12i**, 5:13
Miscarriage. *See* Abortion
Mixed Mullerian tumor
    ovarian, 7:146–148, **7:149i**
        differential diagnosis, **7:146i**, 7:147
        uterine lymphoma vs., 2:181
        uterine metastases vs., **2:188i**, 2:189
Molar pregnancy. *See also* Hydatiform mole
    choriocarcinoma vs., **2:184i**, 2:185
    co-existing with twin pregnancy, 11:11
    retained products of conception vs., 2:233
MRKH (Mayer-Rokitansky-Kuster-Hauser) syndrome, 4:4–6, **4:7i**
    ambiguous genitalia vs., **4:18i**, 4:20
    androgen insensitivity syndrome vs., **4:14i**, 4:15
    differential diagnosis, **4:4i**, 4:5–6
    post-operative pelvis vs., **1:74i**, 1:76
Mucocele, 7:55
Müllerian duct anomalies
    Class I. *See* Uterine hypoplasia/agenesis
    Class II. *See* Unicornuate uterus
    Class III. *See* Uterus didelphys
    Class IV. *See* Bicornuate uterus
    Class V. *See* Septate uterus
    Class VI. *See* Arcuate uterus
    Class VII. *See* DES-exposed uterus
Myelomeningocele, **1:28i**, 1:29
Myoma, uterine, **7:34i**, 7:35
Myomectomy scar, **2:26i**, 2:27
Myometrial contraction
    adenomyoma vs., **2:198i**, 2:199
    adenomyosis vs., **2:192i**, 2:193
    cervical incompetence vs., **3:68i**, 3:69
    placental hematoma vs., **11:24i**, 11:25
    submucosal leiomyoma vs., **2:92i**, 2:94
    uterine peristalsis vs., **2:22i**, 2:23
Myometrial cyst, **2:26i**, 2:27
Myometrial hypertrophy, diffuse, 2:193
Myxoma
    extraperitoneal sarcoma vs., 1:33
    massive ovarian edema vs., 7:183

N

Nabothian cysts, 3:60–62, **3:63i**
    adenoma malignum vs., **3:38i**
    Bartholin cysts vs., 4:59
    cervical adenocarcinoma vs., 3:27
    cervical cancer vs., 3:15
    cervical glandular hyperplasia vs., **3:64i**, 3:65
    differential diagnosis, **3:60i**, 3:61
    Gartner duct cysts vs., **4:26i**, 4:27
Neural tumors, 7:135
Neurofibroma
    extraperitoneal sarcoma vs., 1:33

INDEX

pelvic hemangioma vs., **1:36i**, 1:37
vulvar hemangioma vs., **5:24i**
Nevus, melanocytic, 5:13

O

Ovarian abscess. *See also* Tubo-ovarian abscess
    corpus luteal cyst vs., 7:13
    endometrioma vs., 7:168
    follicular cyst vs., 7:9
Ovarian cancer. *See also* Ovarian metastases; *specific cancer names and histologic types*
    bilateral, vs. metastases, **7:106i**, 7:107
    borderline, vs. serous cystadenoma, 7:49
    Brenner tumor vs., **7:60i**, 7:61
    characterization and staging, 7:112–114, **7:112i, 7:115i–117i**
    cystic
        endometrioma vs., 7:168
        hydrosalpinx vs., 8:7
        ovarian hyperstimulation syndrome vs., 7:159
        spinal meningeal cyst vs., **1:44i**, 1:45
    epithelial
        embryonal carcinoma vs., 7:143
        inclusion cyst vs., 7:155
    hemorrhagic cyst vs., **7:192i**, 7:194
    heterotopic pregnancy vs., **10:22i**, 10:23
    immature teratoma vs., **7:100i**, 7:101
    luteoma of pregnancy vs., **7:20i**
    mucinous, vs. follicular cyst, **7:8i**, 7:9
    peritoneal inclusion cyst vs., **9:2i**, 9:3
    primary
        Krukenberg tumor vs., **7:150i**, 7:151
        metastases vs., 7:107
    recurrent
        resectable, 7:118–120, **7:118i, 7:121i**
        unresectable, 7:122–124, **7:122i, 7:125i**
    subserosal leiomyoma vs., **2:104i**, 2:105
    tubal carcinoma vs., **8:36i**, 8:37, **8:42i**
    tubo-ovarian abscess vs., **8:26i**, 8:28
Ovarian carcinoma
    actinomycosis vs., **8:18i**, 8:19
    carcinoid vs., 7:135
    clear cell, 7:96–98, **7:99i**
        differential diagnosis, **7:96i**, 7:97
        endometrioid carcinoma vs., 7:75
    embryonal, 7:142–144, **7:145i**
        differential diagnosis, **7:142i**, 7:143
        yolk sac tumor vs., 7:89
    genital tuberculosis vs., **8:14i**, 8:16
    immature teratoma vs., **7:100i**, 7:101
    lymphoma vs., **7:92i**, 7:93
    recurrent unresectable, 7:122–124, **7:125i**
    sclerosing stromal tumor vs., **7:40i**, 7:41
    solid tumors vs. massive ovarian edema, 7:183
    transitional cell. *See* Brenner tumor
    tubo-ovarian abscess vs., **8:26i**, 8:28
    undifferentiated, 7:138–140, **7:141i**
        differential diagnosis, **7:138i**, 7:139
        mixed Mullerian tumor vs., **7:146i**
    with malignant ascites, **7:198i**, 7:199
    yolk sac tumor vs., 7:89
Ovarian cysts
    exophytic, vs. paraovarian cyst, **7:162i**, 7:163–164
    functional
        mucinous cystadenoma vs., 7:55
        serous cystadenoma vs., **7:48i**, 7:49
    paratubal cysts vs., **8:2i**, 8:3
Ovarian edema, massive, 7:182–184, **7:185i**
    choriocarcinoma vs., 7:128
    differential diagnosis, **7:182i**, 7:183
    Krukenberg tumor vs., 7:151
    ovarian hyperstimulation syndrome vs., 7:159
    sclerosing stromal tumor vs., 7:41
Ovarian hyperstimulation syndrome, 7:158–160, **7:161i**
    differential diagnosis, **7:158i**, 7:159
    massive ovarian edema vs., **7:182i**, 7:183
    undifferentiated ovarian carcinoma vs., **7:138i**, 7:139
Ovarian lymphoma, 7:92–94, **7:95i**
    differential diagnosis, **7:92i**, 7:93
    Krukenberg tumor vs., **7:150i**, 7:151
    Meigs syndrome vs., **7:198i**, 7:199
    metastases vs., **7:106i**, 7:107
    primary cancer vs., **7:112i**, 7:113
Ovarian metastases, 7:106–108, **7:109i–111i**. *See also* Krukenberg tumor
    adenofibroma vs., 7:32
    clear cell carcinoma vs., 7:97
    cystadenofibroma vs., **7:44i**, 7:45
    differential diagnosis, **7:106i**, 7:107
    dysgerminoma vs., **7:84i**, 7:85
    Krukenberg tumor vs., **7:150i**, 7:151
    lymphoma vs., **7:92i**, 7:93
    Meigs syndrome vs., **7:198i**, 7:199
    mixed Mullerian tumor vs., **7:146i**, 7:147
    mucinous cystadenocarcinoma vs., **7:64i**, 7:65
    primary cancer vs., **7:112i**, 7:113
    sclerosing stromal tumor vs., 7:41
    serous cystadenocarcinoma vs., **7:70i**, 7:71
    undifferentiated ovarian carcinoma vs., 7:139
Ovarian torsion. *See* Adnexal torsion
Ovarian vein thrombosis, 1:40–42, **1:43i**
    differential diagnosis, **1:40i**, 1:41
    intravenous leiomyomatosis vs., **2:86i**, 2:87
Ovary, 7:2–7:201
    adenofibroma, 7:32–33
    adnexal torsion, 7:176–178, **7:179i–181i**
    anatomy and imaging issues, 7:2–4, **7:5i–7i**

INDEX

Brenner tumor, 7:60–62, **7:63i**
carcinoid, 7:134–136, **7:137i**
carcinoma, undifferentiated, 7:138–140, **7:141i**
choriocarcinoma, 7:126–128, **7:129i**
clear cell carcinoma, 7:96–98, **7:99i**
corpus luteal cyst, 7:12–14, **7:15i**
cystadenocarcinoma
    mucinous, 7:64–66, **7:67i–69i**
    serous, 7:70–72, **7:73i**
cystadenofibroma, 7:44–46, **7:47i**
cystadenoma
    mucinous, 7:54–56, **7:57i–59i**
    serous, 7:48–50, **7:51i–53i**
dermoid (mature teratoma), 7:22–24, **7:25i–27i**
dysgerminoma, 7:84–86, **7:87i**
edema, massive, 7:182–184, **7:185i**
embryonal carcinoma, 7:142–144, **7:145i**
endometrioma, 7:166–168, **7:169i**
endometriosis, 7:170–172, **7:173i–175i**
endometroid carcinoma, 7:74–76, **7:77i–79i**
fibromatosis, 7:190–191
fibrothecoma, 7:28–30, **7:31i**
follicle vs. inclusion cyst, 7:155
follicular cyst, 7:8–10, **7:11i**
granulosa cell tumor, 7:34–36, **7:37i–39i**
hemorrhagic cysts, 7:192–194, **7:195i–197i**
inclusion cyst, 7:154–156, **7:157i**
Krukenberg tumor, 7:150–152, **7:153i**
luteoma of pregnancy, 7:20–21
lymphoma, 7:92–94, **7:95i**
Meigs syndrome, 7:198–200, **7:201i**
metastases, 7:106–108, **7:109i–111i**
mixed Mullerian tumor, 7:146–148, **7:149i**
multifollicular, vs. polycystic ovary syndrome, **7:186i**, 7:187
necrotic, vs. massive ovarian edema, **7:182i**, 7:183
normal, vs. polycystic ovary syndrome, **7:186i**, 7:187
ovarian hyperstimulation syndrome, 7:158–160, **7:161i**
paraovarian cyst, 7:162–164, **7:165i**
polycystic, vs. polycystic ovary syndrome, 7:187
polycystic ovary syndrome, 7:186–188, **7:189i**
sclerosing stromal tumor, 7:40–42, **7:43i**
Sertoli-Leydig cell tumor, 7:80–82, **7:83i**
struma ovarii, 7:130–132, **7:133i**
teratoma, immature, 7:100–102, **7:103i–106i**
theca lutein cysts, 7:16–18, **7:19i**
yolk sac tumor, 7:88–90, **7:91i**

P

Paget disease, vs. vulvar melanoma, 5:13
Papilloma, vulvar, 6:23
Paraovarian cyst, 7:162–164, **7:165i**
    differential diagnosis, **7:162i**, 7:163–164
    hemorrhagic cyst vs., 7:194
    hydrosalpinx vs., 8:7
    inclusion cyst vs., **7:154i**, 7:155
    peritoneal inclusion cyst vs., **9:2i**, 9:3
    spinal meningeal cyst vs., 1:45
Paratubal cysts, 8:2–4, **8:5i**
    differential diagnosis, **8:2i**, 8:3
    serous cystadenoma vs., 7:49
    spinal meningeal cyst vs., 1:45
Pathologic imaging issues
    ovary, 7:4, **7:5i–7i**
    urethra, 6:2–4, **6:5i**
    uterus, 2:3–4. **2:5i–7i**
    vulva, 5:2–3
Pelvic abscess
    actinomycosis vs., 8:20
    tubo-ovarian abscess vs., 8:28
Pelvic congestion syndrome, 1:52–54, **1:55i**
    differential diagnosis, **1:52i**, 1:53
    polycystic ovary syndrome vs., 7:188
    uterine arteriovenous malformation vs., **2:206i**, 2:208
Pelvic floor descent, 1:56–58, **1:59i**
    differential diagnosis, **1:56i**, 1:57
Pelvic inflammatory disease
    actinomycosis vs., **8:18i**, 8:20
    adnexal torsion vs., 7:177
    genital tuberculosis vs., **8:14i**, 8:16
    hydrosalpinx vs., 8:7
Pelvic veins, 8:8
Pelvis, 1:2–1:77
    bladder flap hematoma, 1:48–50, **1:51i**
    enterocele/rectocele, 1:64–66, **1:67i**
    extraperitoneal sarcoma, 1:32–34, **1:35i**
    hemangioma, 1:36–38, **1:39i**
    lipomatosis, 1:68–69
    normal variant vs. lipomatosis, 1:69
    ovarian vein thrombosis, 1:40–42, **1:43i**
    pelvic congestion syndrome, 1:52–54, **1:55i**
    pelvic floor descent, 1:56–58, **1:59i**
    post-operative, 1:74–76, **1:77i**
    post-radiation, 1:70–72, **1:73i**
    radiologic procedures
        CT technique and anatomy, 1:10–12, **1:13i–15i**
        hysterosalpingography, 1:6–8, **1:9i**
        MRI technique and anatomy, 1:16–18, **1:19i–21i**
        PET/CT technique and issues, 1:22–24, **1:25i–27i**
        ultrasound technique and anatomy, 1:2–4, **1:5i**
    sacral teratoma, 1:28–30, **1:31i**
    spinal meningeal cysts, 1:44–46, **1:47i**
    vaginocele/cystocele, 1:60–62, **1:63i**

INDEX

Perineal trauma, 6:23
Peristalsis, uterine, 2:22–24, **2:25i**
    differential diagnosis, **2:22i**, 2:23
Peritoneal inclusion cysts, 9:2–4, **9:5i**
    differential diagnosis, **9:2i**, 9:3
    hematosalpinx vs., **8:50i**, 8:51
    hydrosalpinx vs., **8:6i**, 8:7
    mucinous cystadenoma vs., 7:55
    paraovarian cyst vs., **7:162i**, 7:163
    paratubal cysts vs., 8:3
    pseudomyxoma peritonei vs., **9:6i**
    spinal meningeal cyst vs., **1:44i**, 1:45
Peritoneal tumors. *See also* Metastases, peritoneal
    implants vs. endometriosis, **7:170i**, 7:171
    primary vs. metastases, **9:12i**, 9:13
    pseudomyxoma peritonei vs., **9:6i**
Peritoneum, 9:2–17
    inclusion cyst, 9:2–4, **9:5i**
    mesothelioma, 9:8–10, **9:11i**
    metastases, 9:12–14, **9:15i–17i**
    pseudomyxoma peritonei, 9:6–7
Periurethral abscess, 6:23
Placenta, 11:2–33
    abruption
        cervical incompetence vs., 3:69
        uterine rupture vs., 2:229
    chorioangioma, 11:30–32, **11:33i**
    cysts vs. hematoma, 11:26
    hematoma, 11:24–26, **11:27i–29i**
    hydatiform mole
        complete mole, 11:4–6, **11:7i–9i**
        partial mole, 11:10–12, **11:13i–15i**
    hydropic degeneration, 11:5
    invasive mole, 11:16–18, **11:19i**
    mesenchymal dysplasia, **11:10i**, 11:11
    placental site trophoblastic tumor, 11:20–22, **11:23i**
    teratoma, 11:2–3
Placental site trophoblastic tumor, 11:20–22, **11:23i**
    differential diagnosis, **11:20i**, 11:21
    invasive mole vs., 11:17
Polycystic ovary syndrome, 7:186–188, **7:189i**
    differential diagnosis, **7:186i**, 7:187–188
    fibromatosis vs., **7:190i**
    Krukenberg tumor vs., 7:151
    ovarian hyperstimulation syndrome vs., **7:158i**, 7:159
    theca lutein cyst vs., **7:16i**, 7:17
Polyps
    cervical. *See* Endocervical polyp
    urethral
        carcinoma vs., 6:11
        metastasis vs., 6:15
    uterine. *See* Endometrial polyps
    vulvar, vs. urethral prolapse, 6:23
Positron emission tomography (PET)
    pelvis, combined PET/CT technique, 1:22–24, **1:25i–27i**
Post-operative changes, 3:35. *See also* Cesarian section
    cervical
        cervical cancer recurrence vs., **3:34i**, 3:35
            post-conization defect vs. nabothian cysts, 3:61
            post-radiation cervix vs., **3:76i**, 3:77
            post trachelectomy appearances, 3:72–74, **3:75i**
            differential diagnosis, **3:72i**, 3:73
    granuloma, vs. endometrial cancer recurrence, **2:156i**, 2:157
    lymphocele
        recurrent resectable ovarian cancer vs., **7:118i**, 7:119
        recurrent unresectable ovarian cancer vs., **7:122i**, 7:123
    pelvis, 1:74–76, **1:77i**
        differential diagnosis, 1:74–76, **1:77i**
        normal post-operative C-section changes, 2:26–28, **2:29i**
    scars vs. endometriosis, 7:172
Postpartum uterus, normal, 2:233
Post-radiation changes
    cervix, 3:76–78, **3:79i**
        cervical cancer recurrence vs., **3:34i**, 3:35
        differential diagnosis, **3:76i**, 3:77
        post trachelectomy appearances vs., **3:72i**, 3:73
    pelvis, 1:70–72, **1:73i**
        differential diagnosis, **1:70i**, 1:72
        endometrial cancer recurrence vs., 2:157
    vagina
        lymphoma vs., **4:46i**, 4:47
        metastases vs., **4:56i**, 4:57
Pregnancy. *See also* Ectopic pregnancy
    early intrauterine, vs. tubal pregnancy, 10:5
    failed termination vs. uterine rupture, 2:229
    molar. *See* Molar pregnancy
    normal
        cervical ectopic pregnancy vs., **10:16i**, 10:17
        interstitial ectopic pregnancy vs., **10:10i**, 10:11
Proctitis, 1:69
Prostate cancer, **1:68i**, 1:69
Pseudocysts, peritoneal. *See* Peritoneal inclusion cysts
Pseudodilatation/funneling, cervical, 3:69
Pseudohermaphrodite
    androgen insensitivity syndrome vs., 4:15
    MRKH syndrome vs., **4:4i**, 4:5
    uterine hypoplasia/agenesis vs., **2:30i**, 2:31
Pseudomyxoma peritonei, 9:6–7
    differential diagnosis, **9:6i**

INDEX

mesothelioma vs., 9:9
Pyomyoma, 2:82–84, **2:85i**
   differential diagnosis, **2:82i**, 2:83
Pyomyomata, **2:228i**, 2:229
Pyosalpinx
   adnexal torsion vs., **7:176i**
   hematosalpinx vs., **8:50i**, 8:51
   hydrosalpinx vs., **8:6i**
   ovarian vein thrombosis vs., **1:40i**, 1:41
   peritoneal inclusion cyst vs., 9:3
   tubal carcinoma vs., 8:37

R

Radiation necrosis, **3:72i**, 3:73. *See also* Post-radiation changes
Radiologic procedures
   computed tomography, 1:10–12, **1:13i–15i**
   cystourethrography, voiding, 6:3
   hysterosalpingography, 1:6–8, **1:9i**
   MRI technique and anatomy, 1:16–18, **1:19i–21i**
   PET/CT technique and issues, 1:22–24, **1:25i–27i**
   sonohysterography, 2:8–10, **2:11i**
   ultrasound technique and anatomy, 1:2–4, **1:5i**
   urethrography, double-balloon, 5:2–3
Rectal cancer
   enterocele/rectocele vs., **1:64i**, 1:66
   mucinous, vs. pelvic floor descent, **1:56i**, 1:57
Rectocele, 1:64–66, **1:67i**
   differential diagnosis, **1:64i**, 1:65–1:66
Retained products of conception, 2:232–234, **2:235i–237i**
   choriocarcinoma vs., **2:184i**, 2:185
   complete hydatiform mole vs., **11:4i**, 11:5
   differential diagnosis, **2:232i**, 2:233
   endometrial ectopic pregnancy vs., **10:2i**
   endometritis vs., **2:78i**, 2:79
   intrauterine device vs., **2:242i**, 2:243
   placental site trophoblastic tumor vs., **11:20i**, 11:21
   uterine arteriovenous malformation vs., **2:206i**, 2:207
Retroperitoneal neoplasms, 1:69
Rhabdomyosarcoma
   bladder, **4:50i**, 4:51
   embryonal, 4:50–51
      differential diagnosis, **4:50i**, 4:51
      yolk sac tumor vs., **4:52i**, 4:53
   sacral teratoma vs., **1:28i**, 1:29
   vaginal, vs. leiomyoma, **4:38i**, 4:39
Rhabdosarcoma, 2:181

S

Sacral teratoma, 1:28–30, **1:31i**
   differential diagnosis, **1:28i**, 1:29

Salpingitis, 8:10–12, **8:13i**
   differential diagnosis, **8:10i**, 8:11
   parasitic leiomyoma vs., 2:115
   salpingitis isthmica nodosa vs., 8:23
Salpingitis isthmica nodosa, 8:22–24, **8:25i**
   differential diagnosis, **8:22i**, 8:23
Sarcoidosis, 2:115
Sarcoma
   cervical. *See* Cervical sarcoma
   extraperitoneal, 1:32–34, **1:35i**
      differential diagnosis, **1:32i**, 1:33
   ovarian, vs. lymphoma, 7:93
   pelvic, vs. sacral teratoma, **1:28i**, 1:29
   soft tissue, vs. hemangioma, **1:36i**, 1:37
   uterine. *See* Uterine sarcoma
Sarcoma botryoides
   endocervical polyp vs., 3:7
   vaginal yolk sac tumor vs., **4:52i**
Schwannoma
   extraperitoneal sarcoma vs., **1:32i**, 1:33
   urethral, 6:8–6:9
      differential diagnosis, **6:8i**, 6:9
      leiomyoma vs., **6:6i**, 6:7
Septate uterus, 2:52–54, **2:55i–57i**
   arcuate uterus vs., **2:58i**, 2:59
   bicornuate uterus vs., **2:46i**, 2:47
   complex duplication anomalies vs., **2:64i**, 2:65
   DES-exposed uterus vs., **2:60i**, 2:61
   differential diagnosis, **2:52i**, 2:53
Sertoli-Leydig cell tumor, 7:80–82, **7:83i**
   corpus luteal cyst vs., **7:12i**, 7:13
   differential diagnosis, **7:80i**, 7:81
   embryonal carcinoma vs., 7:143
   lymphoma vs., 7:93
Sexual abuse, 6:23
Skene gland cyst
   Bartholin cysts vs., 4:59
   Gartner duct cysts vs., 4:27
   urethral prolapse vs., **6:22i**, 6:23
Small cell carcinoma, cervical, 3:30–32, **3:33i**
   differential diagnosis, **3:30i**, 3:31
Sonohysterography, 2:8–10, **2:11i**
Squamous cell carcinoma, cervical
   adenocarcinoma vs., **3:26i**, 3:27
   endometrioid cervical adenocarcinoma vs., **3:48i**, 3:49
   melanoma vs., **3:52i**, 3:53
   nabothian cysts vs., **3:60i**, 3:61
Squamous inclusion cyst, 4:59
Stromal tumor
   ovarian, vs. parasitic leiomyoma, **2:114i**, 2:115
   sclerosing, 7:40–42, **7:43i**
      choriocarcinoma vs., **7:126i**, 7:127
      cystadenofibroma vs., 7:45
      differential diagnosis, **7:40i**, 7:41
      Sertoli-Leydig cell tumor vs., **7:80i**, 7:81
   sex-cord

INDEX

corpus luteal cyst vs., 7:13
dysgerminoma vs., 7:85
embryonal carcinoma vs., 7:143
Struma ovarii, 7:130–132, **7:133i**
    carcinoid vs., 7:135
    differential diagnosis, 7:130i, 7:131

T

Tamoxifen-induced uterine changes, 2:238–240, **2:242i**
    differential diagnosis, 2:238i, 2:239–240
Tarlov cyst, **8:50i**, 8:51
Teratoma
    fallopian tube
        leiomyoma vs., 8:33
        tubal metastases vs., 8:49
    immature (malignant), 7:100–102, **7:103i–106i**
        differential diagnosis, **7:100i**, 7:101
        dysgerminoma vs., **7:84i**, 7:85
        embryonal carcinoma vs., **7:142i**, 7:143
    mature ovarian. *See* Dermoid cyst
    parasitic leiomyoma vs., 2:115
    placental, 11:2–3
        chorioangioma vs., 11:31
        differential diagnosis, **11:2i**, 11:3
Testicular feminization. *See* Androgen insensitivity syndrome
Theca lutein cysts, 7:16–18, **7:19i**
    differential diagnosis, **7:16i**, 7:17
    polycystic ovary syndrome vs., **7:186i**, 7:187
Thecoma, 7:81
Trachelectomy, postoperative appearances, 3:72–74, **3:75i**
    differential diagnosis, **3:72i**, 3:73
    post-radiation cervix vs., **3:76i**, 3:77
Transitional cell carcinoma of ovary. *See* Brenner tumor
TRAP (twin reversed arterial perfusion)
    chorioangioma vs., **11:30i**, 11:31
    placental teratoma vs., **11:2i**
Tubal carcinoma
    characterization, 8:36–38, **8:39i–41i**
        differential diagnosis, **8:36i**, 8:37
    leiomyoma vs., **8:32i**, 8:33
    paratubal cyst vs., 8:3
    staging and prognosis, 8:42–44, **8:42i, 8:45i–47i**
    tubal metastases vs., **8:48i**
Tubal cyst, vs. ectopic pregnancy, 10:6
Tubal ectopic pregnancy, 10:4–6, **10:7i–9i**
    abdominal ectopic pregnancy vs., **10:26i**
    differential diagnosis, **10:4i**, 10:5–6
    interstitial pregnancy vs., **10:10i**, 10:11
    ovarian pregnancy vs., **10:20i**, 10:21
    paratubal cyst vs., 8:3
    salpingitis vs., **8:10i**, 8:11

tubal metastases vs., **8:48i**
Tuberculosis
    extrapulmonary, vs. peritoneal metastasis, **9:12i**, 9:13
    genital, 8:14–16, **8:17i**
        actinomycosis vs., **8:18i**, 8:20
        differential diagnosis, **8:14i**, 8:16
        salpingitis isthmica nodosa vs., 8:23
    peritonitis vs. mesothelioma, 9:9
Tubo-ovarian abscess, 8:26–28, **8:29i–31i**
    choriocarcinoma vs., 7:127
    degenerated leiomyoma vs., 2:111
    differential diagnosis, **8:26i**, 8:28
    embryonal carcinoma vs., 7:143
    hemorrhagic cyst vs., 7:193
    hydrosalpinx vs., 8:7
    immature teratoma vs., **7:100i**, 7:101
    mucinous cystadenoma vs., **7:54i**, 7:55
    ovarian cancer vs., **7:112i**, 7:113
    ruptured ectopic pregnancy vs., 10:29
    tubal carcinoma vs., **8:36i**, 8:37, **8:42i**
    tubal ectopic pregnancy vs., 10:5
    tubal metastases vs., **8:48i**
    yolk sac tumor vs., **7:88i**, 7:89
Tumor recurrence
    post-radiation pelvis vs., **1:70i**, 1:72
    in vaginal vault, **1:74i**, 1:76
Twin pregnancy
    with co-existing molar pregnancy, 11:11
    with empty sac, vs. placental hematoma, **11:24i**, 11:25
Twin reversed arterial perfusion (TRAP)
    chorioangioma vs., **11:30i**, 11:31
    placental teratoma vs., **11:2i**

U

Ulcerative colitis, **1:68i**, 1:69
Ultrasound, pelvic
    problems with, 1:4
    technique and anatomy, 1:2–4, **1:5i**
Umbilical cord cyst, 11:25
Unicornuate uterus, 2:34–36, **2:37i–39i**
    bicornuate uterus vs., **2:46i**, 2:47
    didelphys vs., **2:40i**, 2:41
    differential diagnosis, **2:34i**, 2:35–36
    septate uterus vs., 2:53
Urachus, 2:229
Ureter, dilated, **1:40i**, 1:41
Urethra, 6:2–6:25
    anatomy and imaging issues, 6:2–6:4, **6:5i**
    carbuncle vs. Bartholin cyst, 4:59
    carcinoma, 6:10–6:12, **6:13i**
    diverticulum, 6:18–6:20, **6:21i**
    duplication vs. diverticulum, 6:19
    leiomyoma, 6:6–6:7

INDEX

metastasis, 6:14–6:16, **6:17i**
prolapse, 6:22–6:24, **6:25i**
schwannoma, 6:8–6:9
Urethral carcinoma, 6:10–6:12, **6:13i**
   differential diagnosis, **6:10i**, 6:11
   diverticulum vs., **6:18i**, 6:19
   leiomyoma vs., **6:6i**
   metastasis vs., **6:14i**, 6:15
   prolapse vs., 6:23
   schwannoma vs., **6:8i**, 6:9
Urethral diverticulum
   Bartholin cysts vs., **4:58i**, 4:59
   Gartner duct cysts vs., **4:26i**, 4:27
   vaginocele/cystocele vs., **1:60i**
Urethral leiomyoma, 6:6–6:7
   carcinoma vs., 6:11
   differential diagnosis, **6:6i**, 6:7
   metastasis vs., 6:15
   schwannoma vs., **6:8i**
Urethral prolapse, 6:22–6:24, **6:25i**
   differential diagnosis, **6:22i**, 6:23
Urethritis, atrophic
   pelvic floor descent vs., 1:57
   vaginocele/cystocele vs., 1:61
Urethrocele, prolapsed, 4:59
Urethrography, double-balloon, 5:2–3
Uterine agenesis. *See* Uterine hypoplasia/agenesis
Uterine artery embolization
   complications, 2:222–224, **2:225i–227i**
      differential diagnosis, **2:222i**, 2:223–224
      failed, 2:218–220, **2:221i**
         differential diagnosis, **2:218i**, 2:219
         UAE imaging for, **2:212i**, 2:214
      imaging, 2:212–214, **2:215i–217i**
         differential diagnosis, **2:212i**, 2:213–214
      normal uterus following, vs. pyomyoma., **2:82i**, 2:83
Uterine cancer. *See also* Endometrial cancer; Metastases, uterine; *specific histologic type*
   lipomatous tumors, 2:124–126, **2:127i**
      differential diagnosis, **2:124i**, 2:125–126
   lower segment, vs. cervical stenosis, 3:2i, 3:3
   malignant, vs. intramural leiomyoma, **2:98i**, 2:99
   tubal carcinoma vs., 8:42
Uterine hypoplasia/agenesis, 2:30–32, **2:33i**
   ambiguous genitalia vs., **4:18i**, 4:20
   DES-exposed uterus vs., 2:61
   differential diagnosis, **2:30i**, 2:31–32
   post-operative pelvis vs., **1:74i**, 1:76
Uterine leiomyoma
   adenofibroma vs., **7:32i**, 7:33
   endocervical polyp vs., 3:7
   fibrothecoma vs., **7:28i**, 7:29
   lymphoma vs., **2:180i**, 2:181
   Meigs syndrome vs., 7:199

metastases vs., 2:189
multiple, vs. diffuse leiomyomatosis, **2:122i**
obscured endometrium vs. endometrial atrophy., **2:18i**, 2:19
pedunculated
   cervical leiomyoma vs., 3:11
   disseminated peritoneal leiomyomatosis vs., 2:91
   unicornuate uterus vs., 2:35
Uterine leiomyosarcoma, 2:176–178, **2:179i**
   benign metastasizing leiomyoma vs., **2:118i**, 2:119
   characterization of, **2:140i**, 2:141
   degenerated leiomyoma vs., **2:110i**, 2:111
   differential diagnosis, **2:176i**, 2:177
   diffuse uterine leiomyomatosis vs., **2:122i**, 2:123
   disseminated peritoneal leiomyomatosis vs., **2:90i**
   intramural leiomyoma vs., **2:98i**, 2:99
   intravenous leiomyomatosis vs., **2:86i**, 2:87
   lymphoma vs., **2:180i**, 2:181
   malignant mixed mesodermal tumor vs., **2:172i**, 2:173
   metastases vs., **2:188i**, 2:189
   parasitic leiomyoma vs., 2:115
   pyomyoma vs., **2:82i**, 2:83
Uterine peristalsis, 2:22–24, **2:25i**
   adenomyosis vs., **2:192i**, 2:193
   differential diagnosis, **2:22i**, 2:23
Uterine rupture, 2:228–230, **2:231i**
   differential diagnosis, **2:228i**, 2:229
Uterine sarcoma. *See also* Endometrial stromal sarcoma
   adenosarcoma vs., 2:167
   diffuse uterine leiomyomatosis vs., **2:122i**, 2:123
   early stage endometrial cancer vs., 2:146
   endometrial cancer vs., **2:140i**, 2:141
   endometrial stromal sarcoma vs., 2:163
   intramural leiomyoma vs., **2:98i**, 2:99
   late stage endometrial cancer vs., **2:150i**, 2:151
   leiomyosarcoma vs., 2:177
Uterocele, prolapsed, 6:23
Uterus, 2:2–2:247. *See also* Cervix uteri
   adenomyoma, 2:198–200, **2:201i**
   adenomyosis, 2:192–194, **2:195i–197i**
      cystic, 2:202–204, **2:205i**
   adenosarcoma, 2:166–168, **2:169i–171i**
   age-related changes, **2:12i**, 2:14
   age-related physiologic alterations, 2:12–14, **2:15i–17i**
   anatomy and imaging issues, 2:2–4, **2:5i–7i**
   anteflexion, **2:26i**, 2:27
   arcuate, 2:58–59
   arteriovenous malformation, 2:206–208, **2:209i–211i**
   Asherman syndrome, 2:68–70, **2:71i–73i**

INDEX

bicornuate, 2:46–48, **2:49i–51i**
choriocarcinoma, 2:184–186, **2:187i**
complex duplication anomalies, 2:64–66, **2:67i**
congenital anomalies
    cervical stenosis vs., **3:2i**, 3:3
contraction. *See* Myometrial contraction
cysts vs. cystic adenomyosis, **2:202i**, 2:203
dehiscence vs. bladder flap hematoma, 1:49
DES-exposed, 2:60–62, **2:63i**
didelphys, 2:40–42, **2:43i–45i**
diffuse leiomyomatosis, 2:122–123
endometrial atrophy, 2:18–20, **2:21i**
endometrial cancer
    characterization, 2:140–142, **2:143i**
    early stage, 2:144–146, **2:147i–149i**
    late stage, 2:150–152, **2:153i–155i**
    recurrence, 2:156–158, **2:159i–161i**
endometrial hyperplasia, 2:134–136,
    2:137i–139i
endometrial polyps, 2:128–130, **2:131i–133i**
endometrial stromal sarcoma, 2:162–164, **2:165i**
endometrial synechiae, 2:74–76, **2:77i**
endometritis, 2:78–80, **2:81i**
hypoplasia/agenesis, 2:30–32, **2:33i**
intrauterine device evaluation, 2:242–244,
    2:245i–247i
leiomyoma
    benign metastasizing, 2:118–120, **2:121i**
    degeneration, 2:110–112, **2:113i**
    intramural, 2:98–100, **2:101i–103i**
    parasitic, 2:114–116, **2:117i**
    submucosal, 2:92–94, **2:95i–97i**
    subserosal, 2:104–106, **2:107i–109i**
leiomyomatosis
    disseminated peritoneal, 2:90–91
    intravenous, 2:86–88, **2:89i**
leiomyosarcoma, 2:176–178, **2:179i**
lipomatous uterine tumors, 2:124–126, **2:127i**
lymphoma, 2:180–182, **2:183i**
malignant mixed mesodermal tumor, 2:172–174,
    2:175i
metastases, 2:188–190, **2:191i**
normal post c-section changes, 2:26–28, **2:29i**
partial septum vs. endometrial synechiae., **2:74i**,
    2:75
peristalsis, 2:22–24, **2:25i**
pyomyoma, 2:82–84, **2:85i**
retained products of conception, 2:232–234,
    2:235i–237i
rupture, 2:228–230, **2:231i**
septate, 2:52–54, **2:55i–57i**
sonohysterography, 2:8–10, **2:11i**
tamoxifen-induced changes, 2:238–240, **2:242i**
unicornuate, 2:34–36, **2:37i–39i**
uterine artery embolization
    complications, 2:222–224, **2:225i–227i**
    failed, 2:218–220, **2:221i**
    imaging techniques, 2:212–214, **2:215i–217i**
Uterus didelphys, 2:40–42, **2:43i–45i**
    bicornuate uterus vs., **2:46i**, 2:47
    complex duplication anomalies vs., **2:64i**, 2:65
    differential diagnosis, **2:40i**, 2:41
    septate uterus vs., **2:52i**, 2:53
    unicornuate uterus vs., 2:35
    with obstructed hemivagina, 4:27

V

Vagina, 4:2–4:65
    ambiguous genitalia, 4:18–20, **4:21i**
    anatomy and imaging issues, 4:2–3
    androgen insensitivity syndrome, 4:14–16, **4:17i**
    atresia, 4:8–9
    Bartholin cysts, 4:58–60, **4:61i**
    Bartholin gland cancer, 4:54–55
    bartholinitis, 4:30–31
    carcinoma, 4:40–42, **4:43i–45i**
    fistula, 4:32–34, **4:35i–37i**
    foreign bodies, 4:62–64, **4:65i**
    Gartner duct cysts, 4:26–28, **4:29i**
    gonadal dysgenesis, 4:22–24, **4:25i**
    imperforate hymen, 4:10–11
    leiomyoma, 4:38–39
    leiomyosarcoma, 4:48–49
    lymphoma, 4:46–47
    metastasis, 4:56–57
    MRKH syndrome, 4:4–6, **4:7i**
    rhabdomyosarcoma, embryonal, 4:50–51
    septae, 4:12–13
    yolk sac tumor, 4:52–53
Vaginal agenesis
    androgen insensitivity syndrome vs., **4:14i**, 4:15
    with uterine hypoplasia
        imperforate hymen vs., 4:11
        vaginal atresia vs., 4:9
        vaginal septae vs., 4:13
Vaginal atresia, 4:8–9
    differential diagnosis, **4:8i**, 4:9
    imperforate hymen vs., **4:10i**, 4:11
    vaginal septae vs., **4:12i**, 4:13
Vaginal carcinoma, 4:40–42, **4:43i–45i**
    clear cell, vs. yolk sac tumor, 4:53
    differential diagnosis, **4:40i**, 4:41
    foreign body vs., **4:62i**, 4:64
    leiomyosarcoma vs., **4:48i**, 4:49
    lymphoma vs., **4:46i**
    metastases vs., **4:56i**
    recurrence in vaginal vault, **1:74i**, 1:76
    urethral carcinoma vs., **6:10i**, 6:11
    urethral prolapse vs., 6:23
Vaginal fistula, 4:32–34, **4:35i–37i**
    differential diagnosis, **4:32i**

INDEX

foreign body vs., **4:62i**, 4:64
Vaginal leiomyoma, 4:38–39
    differential diagnosis, **4:38i**, 4:39
    Gartner duct cysts vs., 4:27
    leiomyosarcoma vs., **4:48i**, 4:49
    vaginocele/cystocele vs., **1:60i**, 1:62
Vaginal septae, 4:12–13
    differential diagnosis, **4:12i**, 4:13
    imperforate hymen vs., **4:10i**, 4:11
    vaginal atresia vs., **4:8i**, 4:9
Vaginitis
    atrophic, vaginocele/cystocele vs., 1:61
    atrophic, vs. pelvic floor descent., 1:57
    vaginal carcinoma vs., 4:41
Vaginitis emphysematosa, **4:62i**, 4:64
Vaginocele, 1:60–62, **1:63i**
    differential diagnosis, **1:60i**, 1:61–62
Vena cava, inferior, 1:41
Venous intravasation, **8:22i**
Vestibular bulbs, anatomy, 5:2
Voiding cystourethrography, 6:3
Vulva, 5:2–5:25
    anatomy and imaging issues, 5:2–3
    angiomyxoma, aggressive, 5:16–18, **5:19i**
    carcinoma, 5:4–6, **5:7i–9i**
    hemangioma, 5:24–25
    leiomyosarcoma, 5:10–11
    lymphoma, 5:20–21
    melanoma, 5:12–14, **5:15i**
    Merkel cell tumor, 5:22–23
Vulvar carcinoma, 5:4–6, **5:7i–9i**
    aggressive angiomyxoma vs., **5:16i**, 5:17
    Bartholin gland cancer vs., **4:54i**
    bartholinitis vs., **4:30i**, 4:31
    differential diagnosis, **5:4i**, 5:5
    hemangioma vs., **5:24i**
    leiomyosarcoma vs., **5:10i**
    lymphoma vs., **5:20i**, 5:21
    melanoma vs., **5:12i**, 5:13
    Merkel cell tumor vs., **5:22i**
Vulvar melanoma, 5:12–14, **5:15i**
    carcinoma vs., **5:4i**, 5:5
    differential diagnosis, **5:12i**, 5:13
    lymphoma vs., **5:20i**, 5:21
    Merkel cell tumor vs., **5:22i**

differential diagnosis, **7:88i**, 7:89
embryonal carcinoma vs., 7:143
vaginal, 4:52–53
    differential diagnosis, **4:52i**, 4:53
    embryonal rhabdomyosarcoma vs., **4:50i**, 4:51

W

Wilms tumor, extrarenal, 1:29

Y

Yolk sac tumor
    ovarian, 7:88–90, **7:91i**
        choriocarcinoma vs., **7:126i**, 7:127